MW00846339

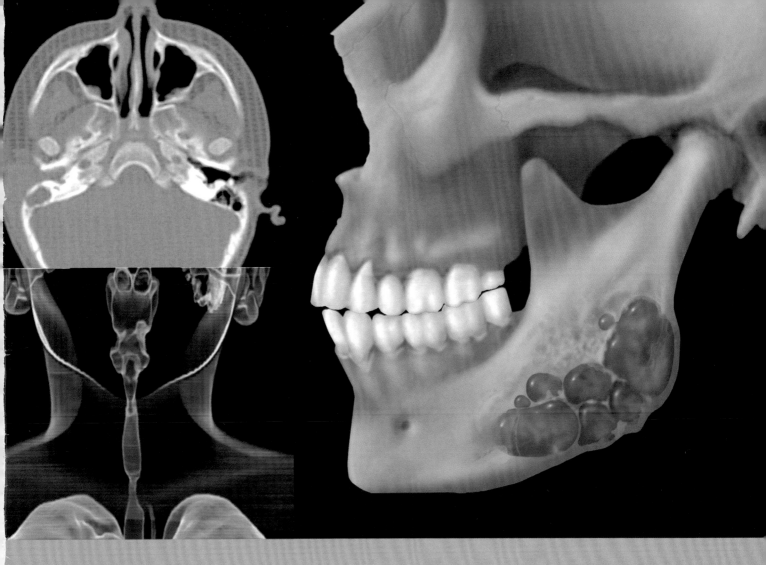

Diagnostic Imaging

Head and Neck

THIRD EDITION

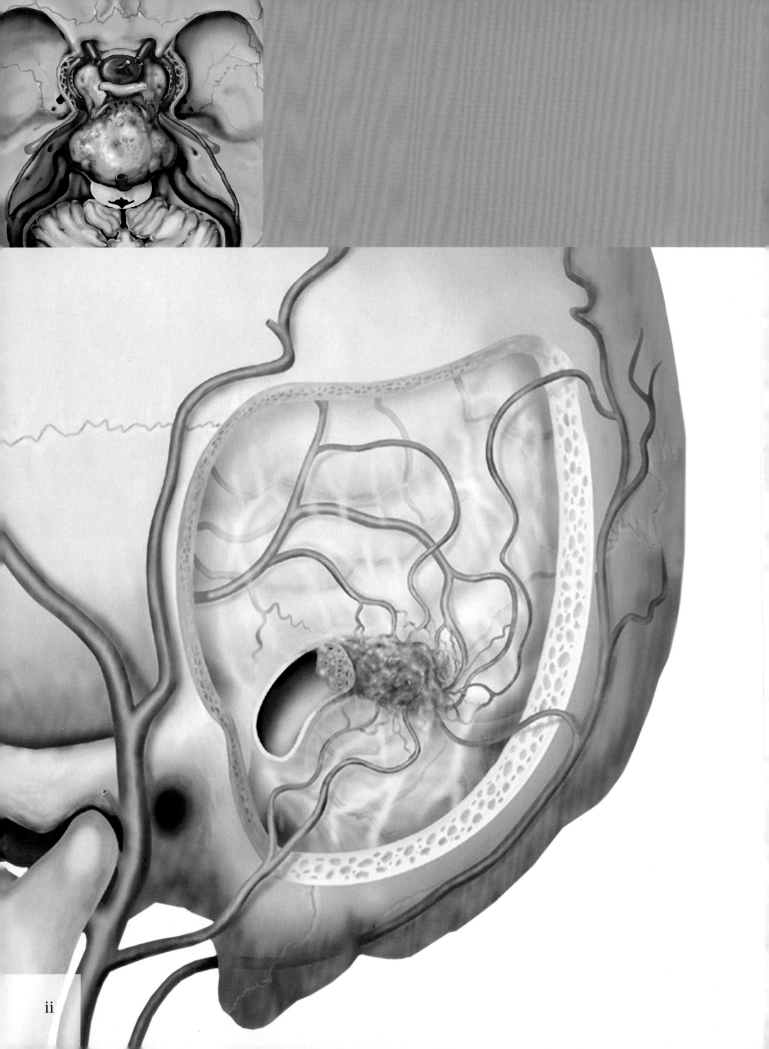

Diagnostic Imaging

Head and Neck

THIRD EDITION

Bernadette L. Koch, MD

Associate Director of Radiology
Cincinnati Children's Hospital Medical Center
Professor of Clinical Radiology and Pediatrics
University of Cincinnati College of Medicine
Cincinnati, Ohio

Bronwyn E. Hamilton, MD

Professor of Radiology
Director of Head & Neck Radiology
Oregon Health & Science University
Portland, Oregon

Patricia A. Hudgins, MD, FACR

Professor of Radiology and Otolaryngology
Director of Head & Neck Radiology
Department of Radiology and Imaging Sciences
Emory University School of Medicine
Atlanta, Georgia

H. Ric Harnsberger, MD

R.C. Willey Chair in Neuroradiology
Professor of Radiology and Otolaryngology
University of Utah School of Medicine
Salt Lake City, Utah

ELSEVIER

1600 John F. Kennedy Blvd.
Ste 1800
Philadelphia, PA 19103-2899

DIAGNOSTIC IMAGING: HEAD AND NECK, THIRD EDITION　　　　　　　　　　　　ISBN: 978-0-323-44301-2

Copyright © 2017 by Elsevier. All rights reserved.

No part of this publication may be reproduced or transmitted in any form or by any means, electronic or mechanical, including photocopying, recording, or any information storage and retrieval system, without permission in writing from the publisher. Details on how to seek permission, further information about the Publisher's permissions policies and our arrangements with organizations such as the Copyright Clearance Center and the Copyright Licensing Agency, can be found at our website: www.elsevier.com/permissions.

This book and the individual contributions contained in it are protected under copyright by the Publisher (other than as may be noted herein).

Notices

Knowledge and best practice in this field are constantly changing. As new research and experience broaden our understanding, changes in research methods, professional practices, or medical treatment may become necessary.

Practitioners and researchers must always rely on their own experience and knowledge in evaluating and using any information, methods, compounds, or experiments described herein. In using such information or methods they should be mindful of their own safety and the safety of others, including parties for whom they have a professional responsibility.

With respect to any drug or pharmaceutical products identified, readers are advised to check the most current information provided (i) on procedures featured or (ii) by the manufacturer of each product to be administered, to verify the recommended dose or formula, the method and duration of administration, and contraindications. It is the responsibility of practitioners, relying on their own experience and knowledge of their patients, to make diagnoses, to determine dosages and the best treatment for each individual patient, and to take all appropriate safety precautions.

To the fullest extent of the law, neither the Publisher nor the authors, contributors, or editors, assume any liability for any injury and/or damage to persons or property as a matter of products liability, negligence or otherwise, or from any use or operation of any methods, products, instructions, or ideas contained in the material herein.

Publisher Cataloging-in-Publication Data

Names: Koch, Bernadette L. | Hamilton, Bronwyn E. | Hudgins, Patricia A. | Harnsberger, H. Ric.
Title: Diagnostic imaging. Head & neck / [edited by] Bernadette L. Koch, Bronwyn E. Hamilton,
　　Patricia A. Hudgins, and H. Ric Harnsberger.
Other titles: Head & neck. | Head and neck.
Description: Third edition. | Salt Lake City, UT : Elsevier, Inc., [2016] | Includes
　　bibliographical references and index.
Identifiers: ISBN 978-0-323-44301-2
Subjects: LCSH: Head--Imaging--Handbooks, manuals, etc. | Neck--Imaging--Handbooks, manuals, etc. |
　　MESH: Head--pathology--Atlases. | Neck--pathology--Atlases. | Diagnostic Imaging--Atlases. |
　　Head--radiography--Atlases. | Neck--radiography--Atlases.
Classification: LCC RC936.D515 2016 | NLM WE 39 | DDC 617.5'10754--dc23

International Standard Book Number: 978-0-323-44301-2

Cover Designer: Tom M. Olson, BA
Cover Art: Richard Coombs, MS

Printed in Canada by Friesens, Altona, Manitoba, Canada

Last digit is the print number: 9　8　7　6　5　4　3　2　1

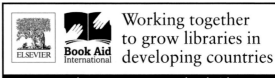

Working together to grow libraries in developing countries

www.elsevier.com • www.bookaid.org

Dedications

To the most important things in life: My husband, Peter; children, Jay and Katherine; my mother (a.k.a. "Granny"); and siblings for their unconditional love, support, understanding, and encouragement.

BLK

Gary & Rhiannon: Thank you for being my light & inspiration.
Mum, Dad, & Mark: Thank you for all your love and for always being there.
Doug: I feel your spirit in the open spaces we shared. Rest in peace.

BEH

I dedicate my portion of this book, with sincerity and admiration, to all the residents, fellows, and students who have kept me honest, asked me the hard questions, and kept me climbing on that steep portion of the learning curve. Thank you for keeping my spirit young and my inquisitive nature active. And I dedicate this to all the patients who hopefully will benefit from these hard-working radiologists-in-training who have mastered Head and Neck Imaging.

PAH

Thank you to my wife, Janet, for anchoring our lives in what matters. You and our family (Dave, Dan, Dylan, Danielle, and Roen) are my reason for being and the loves of my life. To Doris and Hutch, thank you for giving me more than enough love to get me through.

HRH

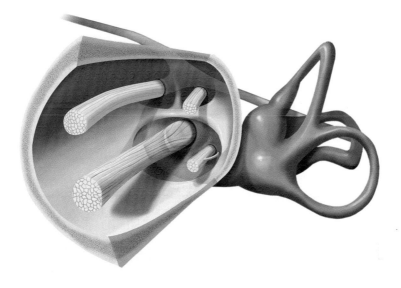

Contributing Authors

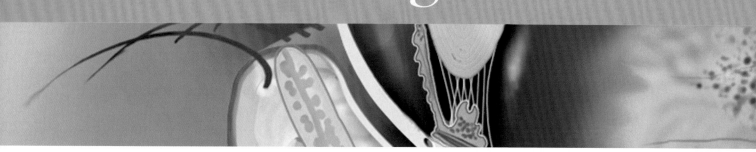

Nicholas A. Koontz, MD
Director of Fellowship Programs
Assistant Professor of Radiology
Department of Radiology and Imaging Sciences
Indiana University School of Medicine
Indianapolis, Indiana

Caroline D. Robson, MBChB
Operations Vice Chair, Radiology
Chief, Neuroradiology & Head and Neck Imaging
Boston Children's Hospital
Associate Professor of Radiology
Harvard Medical School
Boston, Massachusetts

Luke N. Ledbetter, MD
Assistant Professor of Radiology
Division of Neuroradiology
University of Kansas Medical Center
Kansas City, Kansas

H. Christian Davidson, MD
Professor of Radiology
University of Utah School of Medicine
Salt Lake City, Utah

C. Douglas Phillips, MD, FACR
Professor of Radiology
Director of Head and Neck Imaging
Weill Cornell Medical College
NewYork-Presbyterian Hospital
New York, New York

Daniel E. Meltzer, MD
Associate Clinical Professor of Radiology
Icahn School of Medicine at Mount Sinai
New York, New York

Troy A. Hutchins, MD
Assistant Professor of Radiology
University of Utah School of Medicine
Salt Lake City, Utah

Kristine M. Mosier, DMD, PhD
Associate Professor of Radiology
Chief, Head and Neck Radiology
Indiana University School of Medicine
Department of Radiology & Imaging Sciences
Indianapolis, Indiana

Philip R. Chapman, MD
Section Chief, Neuroradiology
Associate Professor
University of Alabama Birmingham
Birmingham, Alabama

Hilda E. Stambuk, MD
Attending Radiologist
Clinical Head of Head and Neck Imaging
Memorial Sloan-Kettering Cancer Center
Professor of Clinical Radiology
Weill Medical College of Cornell University
New York, New York

Karen L. Salzman, MD
Professor of Radiology
Chief of Neuroradiology
Leslie W. Davis Endowed Chair in Neuroradiology
University of Utah School of Medicine
Salt Lake City, Utah

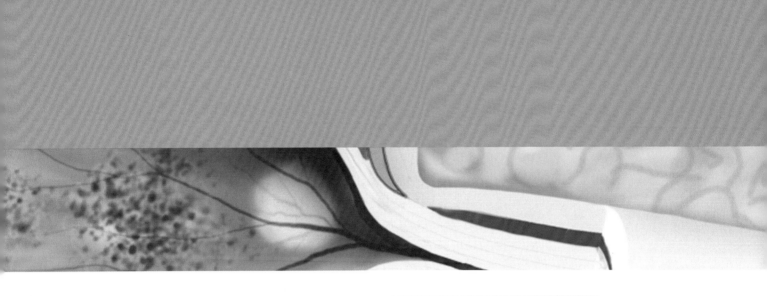

Richard H. Wiggins, III, MD, CIIP, FSIIM
Director of Head and Neck Imaging
Director of Imaging Informatics
Professor, Departments of Radiology,
Otolaryngology, Head and Neck Surgery, and
BioMedical Informatics
University of Utah Health Sciences Center
Salt Lake City, Utah

Yoshimi Anzai, MD, MPH
Professor of Radiology
Associate Chief Medical Quality Officer
University of Utah
Salt Lake City, Utah

Blair A. Winegar, MD
Assistant Professor of Medical Imaging
Division of Neuroradiology
University of Arizona College of Medicine
Banner - University Medical Center
Tucson, Arizona

Additional Contributors

Anne G. Osborn, MD, FACR
Barton F. Branstetter, IV, MD, FACR
A. Carlson Merrow, Jr., MD
Chang Yueh Ho, MD

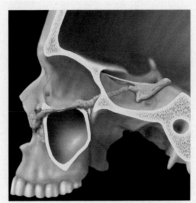

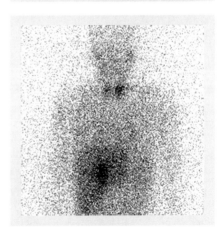

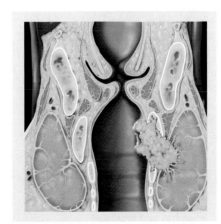

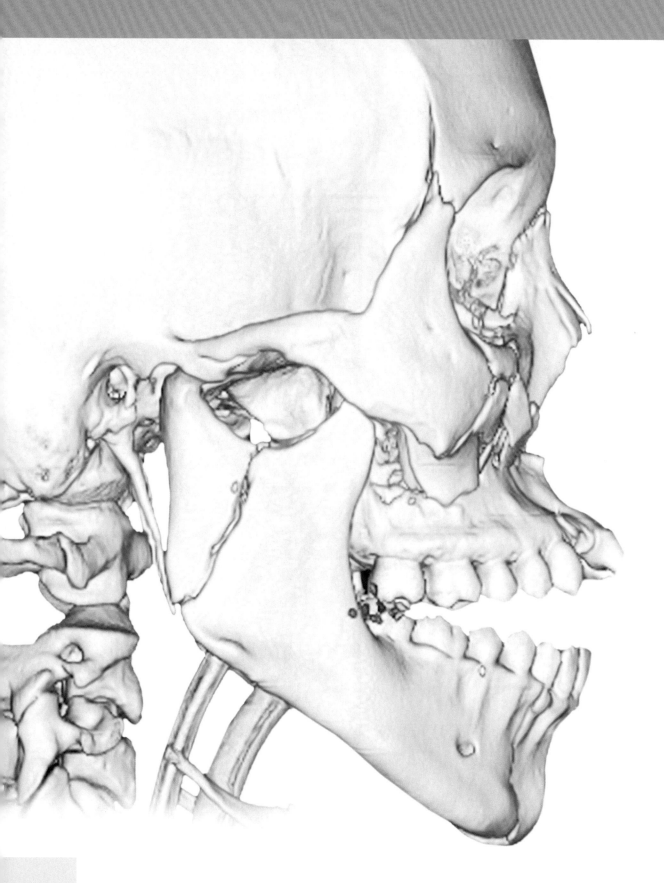

Preface

This stunning third edition of *Diagnostic Imaging: Head and Neck* represents the most comprehensive single volume textbook in the field of head and neck imaging today. It appears six years after the second edition and is full of new imaging information as a result. There are also many new and exciting features. The layout has been improved but still maintains the basic organization of presenting the same information in the same easy-to-find place—every time, in every chapter. We've added 75 new diagnoses, 250 new gallery images, and 35 new signature color graphics. The references in all diagnoses have been updated to within a few weeks of publication.

What else makes the third edition different? We have updated the 23 prose introductions at the front of each of the book's sections. The goal of these introductions is to tie together the imaging techniques and indications, embryology, area imaging anatomy, imaging issues, and clinical implications. An anatomy-based differential diagnosis for each overview chapter is also presented. Another key update is seen in the diagnosis chapter gallery images where updated, higher resolution images have replaced older, lower resolution images from previous editions. The 2,200 images in the eBook galleries (645 of them new) give a rich additional perspective for each diagnosis chapter.

On a global content level, the third edition of *Diagnostic Imaging: Head and Neck* now contains the updated Squamous Cell Carcinoma section that follows the same primary site organization (pharynx, oral cavity, and larynx) of the American Joint Committee on Cancer. Why was this added and updated? Because diagnosis, staging, and treatment of head and neck cancer is going through changes we never anticipated. New virus-related cancers have been discovered, and with developments in surgical, radiation, and chemotherapy treatments, accurate staging is even more critical. Who better to stage a cancer than the radiologist! A second, fully updated portion of the book is seen in the 29-chapter Pediatric Lesions and Syndromic Diseases sections.

In the simplest terms, our reason for writing this book was to contribute to the process of demystifying head and neck imaging. We want *Diagnostic Imaging: Head and Neck*, Third Edition to be your favorite head and neck imaging text—used, worn, dog-eared, and loved. Thanks for making the books in the Diagnostic Imaging series the bestsellers they are. We hope you enjoy this fully updated sequel!

The Third Edition Lead Editorial Team

Bernadette, Bronwyn, Pat, & Ric

a.k.a. Drs. Koch, Hamilton, Hudgins, & Harnsberger

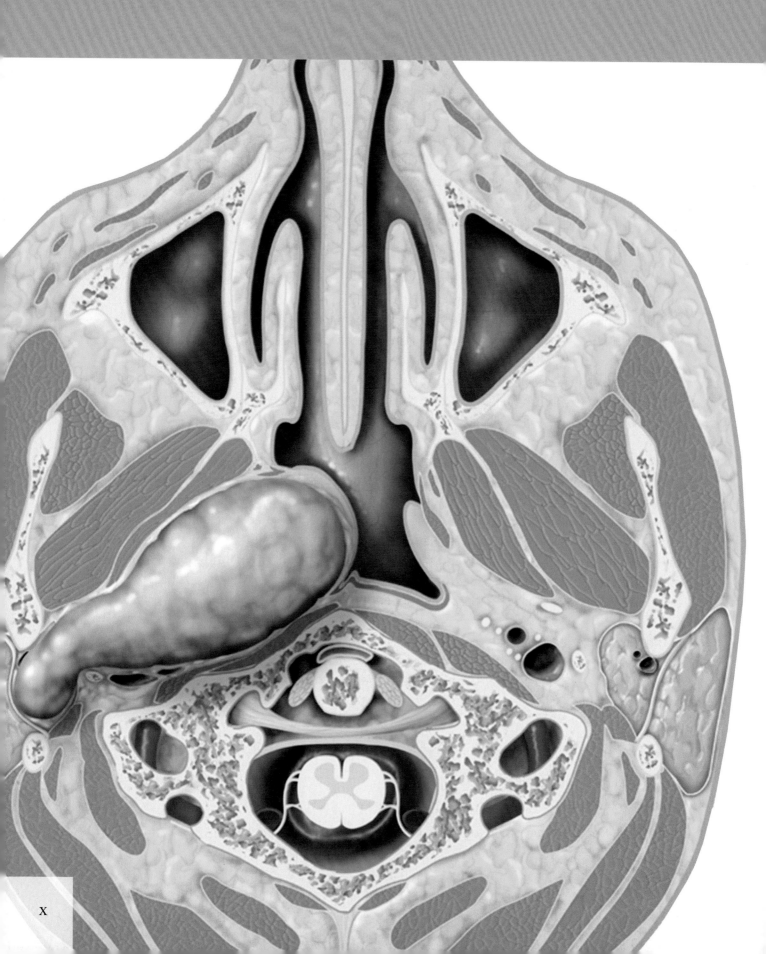

Acknowledgments

Text Editors

Arthur G. Gelsinger, MA
Terry W. Ferrell, MS
Lisa A. Gervais, BS
Karen E. Concannon, MA, PhD
Matt W. Hoecherl, BS
Megg Morin, BA

Image Editors

Jeffrey J. Marmorstone, BS
Lisa A. M. Steadman, BS

Illustrations

Richard Coombs, MS
Lane R. Bennion, MS
Laura C. Sesto, MA

Art Direction and Design

Tom M. Olson, BA
Laura C. Sesto, MA

Lead Editor

Nina I. Bennett, BA

Production Coordinators

Angela M. G. Terry, BA
Rebecca L. Hutchinson, BA
Emily Fassett, BA

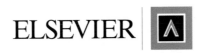

Sections

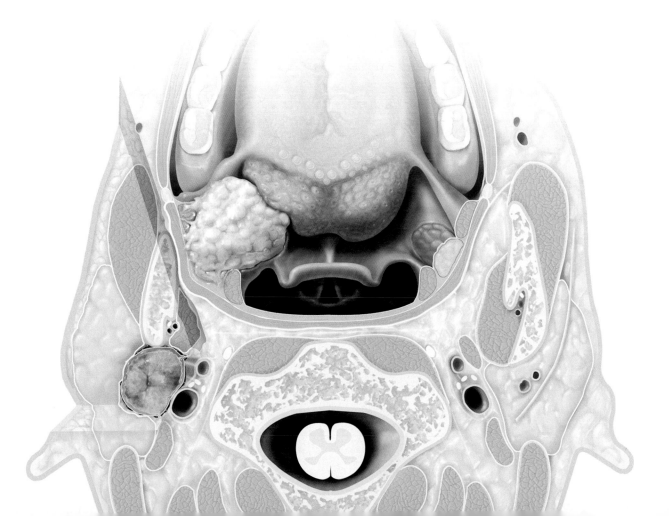

TABLE OF CONTENTS

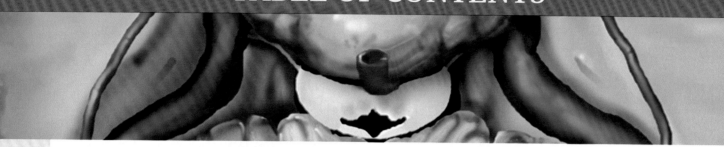

TABLE OF CONTENTS

TABLE OF CONTENTS

TABLE OF CONTENTS

TABLE OF CONTENTS

TABLE OF CONTENTS

TABLE OF CONTENTS

TABLE OF CONTENTS

TABLE OF CONTENTS

TABLE OF CONTENTS

TABLE OF CONTENTS

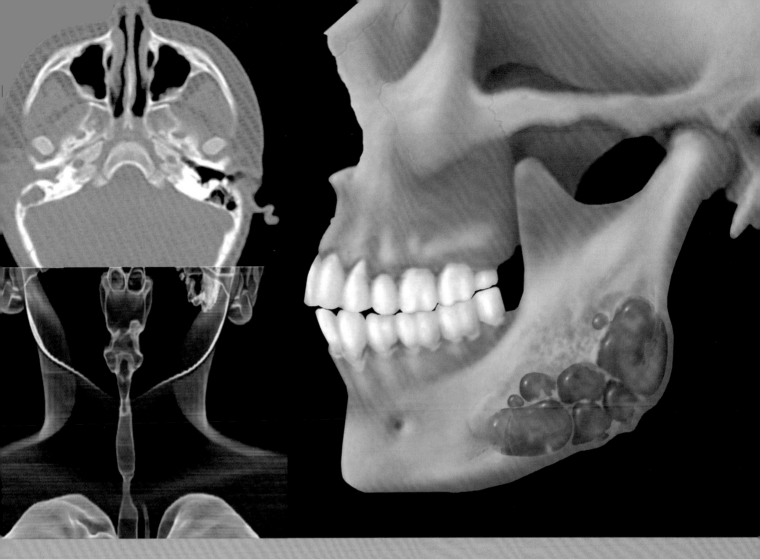

Diagnostic Imaging

Head and Neck

THIRD EDITION

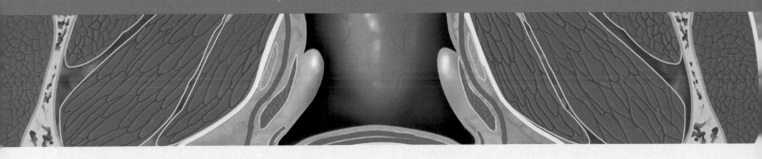

SECTION 1
Introduction and Overview of Suprahyoid and Infrahyoid Neck

Imaging Approaches & Indications

Neither CT nor MR is a perfect modality in imaging the extracranial H&N. MR is most useful in the suprahyoid neck (SHN) because it is less affected by oral cavity dental amalgam artifact. Because the SHN tissue is less affected by motion compared with the infrahyoid neck (IHN), MR image quality is not degraded by movement seen in the IHN. Axial and coronal T1 fat-saturated enhanced MR is superior to CECT in defining soft tissue extent of tumor, perineural tumor spread, and dural/intracranial spread. When MR is combined with bone CT of the facial bones and skull base, precise preoperative lesion mapping results.

CECT is the modality of choice when IHN and mediastinum are imaged. Swallowing, coughing, and breathing makes this area a "moving target" for the imager. MR image quality is often degraded as a result. Multislice CT with multiplanar reformations now permits exquisite images of the IHN unaffected by movement.

High-resolution ultrasound also has a role. Superficial lesions, thyroid disease, and nodal evaluation with biopsy are best done by skilled ultrasonographers.

Many indications exist for imaging the extracranial H&N. Exploratory imaging, tumor staging, and abscess search comprise three common reasons imaging is ordered in this area. Exploratory imaging, an imaging search for any lesion that may be causing the patient's symptoms, is best completed with CECT from skull base to the clavicles.

Squamous cell carcinoma (SCCa) staging is best started with CECT, as both the primary tumor and nodes must be imaged, requiring imaging from the skull base to clavicles. MR imaging times and susceptibility to motion artifact make it a less desirable exam in this setting. Instead, MR is best used when specific delineation of exact tumor extent, perineural tumor, or intracranial invasion is needed.

When the type and cause of H&N infection are sought, CECT is the best exam. CECT can readily differentiate cellulitis, phlegmon, and abscess. CT can also identify salivary gland ductal calculi, teeth infection, mandible osteomyelitis, and intratonsillar abscess as causes of infection.

Imaging Anatomy

In discussing the extracranial H&N soft tissues, a few definitions are needed. The **SHN** is defined as deep facial spaces **above the hyoid bone**, including parapharyngeal space (PPS), pharyngeal mucosal space (PMS), masticator space (MS), parotid space (PS), carotid space (CS), retropharyngeal space (RPS), danger space (DS), and perivertebral (PVS) space. The **IHN** soft tissue spaces are predominantly **below the hyoid bone**, with some continuing inferiorly into the mediastinum or superiorly into the SHN, including the visceral space (VS), posterior cervical space (PCS), CS, RPS, and PVS.

Important **SHN** space **anatomic relationships** include their interactions with the skull base, oral cavity, and infrahyoid neck. When one thinks about the SHN spaces and their relationships with the skull base, perhaps the most important consideration is to examine each space alone to see what critical structures (cranial nerves, arteries, veins) are at the point of contact between the space and the skull base. Space

by space, the **skull base interactions** above and IHN extension below are apparent.

- **PPS** has bland triangular skull base abutment without critical foramen involved; it empties inferiorly into submandibular space (SMS)
- **PMS** touches posterior basisphenoid and anterior basiocciput, including **foramen lacerum**; PMS includes nasopharyngeal, oropharyngeal, and hypopharyngeal mucosal surfaces
- **MS** superior skull base interaction includes zygomatic arch, condylar fossa, skull base including **foramen ovale (CNV3)**, and **foramen spinosum** (middle meningeal artery); MS ends at inferior surface of body of mandible
- **PS** abuts floor of external auditory canal, mastoid tip including **stylomastoid foramen (CNVII)**; parotid tail extends inferiorly into posterior SMS
- **CS** meets **jugular foramen (CNIX-XI)** floor, hypoglossal canal (CNXII), and petrous internal carotid artery canal; CS can be followed inferiorly to aortic arch
- **RPS** contacts skull base along lower clivus without involvement of critical structures; it continues inferiorly to empty into DS at T3 level
- **PVS** touches low clivus, encircles occipital condyles and foramen magnum; PVS continues inferiorly to level into thorax

In addition to skull base interactions, the relationships of the SHN spaces to the fat-filled PPSs are key to analyzing SHN masses. The PPSs are a pair of fat-filled spaces in the lateral SHN surrounded by the PMS, MS, PS, CS, and RPS. When a mass enlarges in one of these spaces, it displaces the PPS fat. Larger masses define their space of origin based on this displacement pattern.

- Medial PMS mass displaces PPS laterally
- The more anterior MS mass displaces PPS posteriorly
- Lateral PS mass displaces PPS medially
- Posterolateral CS mass displaces styloid process and PPS anteriorly
- The more posteromedial lateral RPS nodal mass displaces PPS anterolaterally

The **IHN** space **anatomic relationships** are defined by their superior and inferior projections. The VS has **no** SHN component, instead projecting only inferiorly into the superior mediastinum. The PCS extends superiorly to the mastoid tip and ends inferiorly at the clavicle. It is predominantly an IHN space, however. The CS begins at the floor of jugular foramen and carotid canal and extends inferiorly to the aortic arch. The RPS begins at the ventral clivus superiorly and traverses SHN-IHN to T3 level. The DS is immediately posterior to the RPS but continues beyond T3 level into mediastinum. For imaging purposes, RPS and DS can be considered a single entity. The PVS can be defined from skull base above to clavicle below. The PVS is divided by fascial slip into prevertebral and paraspinal components.

Nobody likes to study the **deep cervical fasciae (DCF)** of the neck. However, it is these fasciae that define the very spaces we use to subdivide neck diseases and construct space-specific DDx lists. It is imperative that a clear understanding of these fasciae be grasped by any imager involved in evaluating this area.

Many nomenclatures have been used to describe the neck fascia. The following is a practical distillate meant to simplify this challenging subject. There are three main DCF in the neck.

Common Tumors in Spaces of Neck

Pharyngeal mucosal space	Warthin tumor	Posterior cervical space
Pharyngeal SCCa	**Carotid space**	Pharyngeal SCCa nodal metastasis
Tonsillar NHL	Glomus vagale paraganglioma	NHL nodal disease
Masticator space	Carotid body paraganglioma	Differentiated thyroid carcinoma nodes
Sarcoma	Schwannoma of CNIX-XII	**Visceral space**
Perineural CNV3 SCCa	**Retropharyngeal space**	Differentiated thyroid carcinoma
Parotid space	SCCa nodal metastasis	Anaplastic thyroid carcinoma
Mucoepidermoid carcinoma	NHL nodal disease	Thyroid NHL
Adenoid cystic carcinoma	**Perivertebral space**	Cervical esophageal carcinoma
Malignant nodal metastases	Vertebral body systemic metastasis	Parathyroid adenoma
Benign mixed tumor	Brachial plexus schwannoma	

SCCa = squamous cell carcinoma; NHL = non-Hodgkin lymphoma.

The same names are used in the SHN and IHN. The superficial layer (**SL-DCF**), the middle layer (**ML-DCF**), and deep layer of DCF (**DL-DCF**) are the three important fascia in the neck.

In the SHN, the **SL-DCF** circumscribes **MS** and **PS** and contributes to the carotid sheath. In the IHN, it "invests" neck by surrounding the infrahyoid strap, sternocleidomastoid, and trapezius muscles. It also contributes to the carotid sheath of the CS in the IHN.

The **ML-DCF** in the SHN defines the deep margin of the PMS. It contributes to carotid sheath in both the SHN and IHN. In the IHN, it also circumscribes the VS.

In both the SHN and IHN, the **DL-DCF** surrounds **PVS**. A slip of DL-DCF dives medially to the transverse process, dividing PVS into prevertebral and paraspinal components. Another slip of DL-DCF, the alar fascia, provides the lateral wall to RPS and DS, as well as the posterior wall to RPS, separating RPS from DS. DL-DCF contributes to carotid sheath, like the SL and ML-DCF.

The internal structures of the spaces of the neck are for the most part responsible for the diseases there. Let us begin by defining the **critical contents of the SHN spaces**:

- **PPS** contains fat with rare minor salivary glands
- **PMS** contains mucosa, lymphatic ring, and minor salivary glands; in nasopharyngeal mucosal space, opening of eustachian tube, torus tubarius, adenoids, superior constrictor, and levator palatini muscles can be seen; oropharyngeal mucosal space contains anterior and posterior tonsillar pillars, palatine, and lingual tonsils
- **MS** includes posterior mandibular body and ramus, TMJ, CNV3, masseter, medial and lateral pterygoid and temporalis muscles, and pterygoid venous plexus
- **PS** houses parotid, extracranial CNVII, nodes, retromandibular vein, and external carotid artery
- **CS** contains the CNIX-XII, internal jugular vein, and internal carotid artery
- **RPS** has fat and medial and lateral RPS nodes inside
- Prevertebral **PVS** contains vertebral body, veins and arteries, and prevertebral muscles (longus colli and capitis); in paraspinal PVS resides the posterior elements of vertebra and paraspinal muscles

The **critical contents** of **IHN spaces** are defined next:

- **VS** contains thyroid and parathyroid glands, trachea, esophagus, recurrent laryngeal nerves, and pretracheal and paratracheal nodes
- **PCS** has fat, CNXI, and level V nodes inside
- **CS** houses common carotid artery, internal jugular vein, and CNX
- **IHN RPS** has **no** nodes and contains only fat
- Prevertebral **PVS** has brachial plexus and phrenic nerve, vertebral body, veins, arteries, and prevertebral and scalene muscles within; paraspinal PVS contains only posterior vertebra elements and paraspinal muscles

Approaches to Imaging Issues in SHN & IHN

It's crucial that the imager has a method of analysis when a mass is found in the neck. In the SHN, mass evaluation methodology begins with defining mass **space of origin** (PMS, MS, PS, CS, lateral RPS). When small, this is simple, as the mass is seen within the confines of one space. In larger masses, ask, "How does the mass displace the PPS?" Next, utilize a **space-specific DDx** list. Match the imaging findings to the diagnoses within this list to narrow your differential.

With IHN masses, a similar evaluation methodology can be employed. First, determine what space the mass originates in (VS, CS, PCS). Then, review space-specific DDx list. Match radiologic findings of your case to this DDx list. In all neck masses, knowing the clinical findings can be very helpful.

Lesions of posterior midline spaces (RPS and PVS) of the neck need different image evaluation. When a lesion is defined here, first ask, "How does mass displace prevertebral muscles (PVM)?" In the case of an **RPS mass**, PVMs are flattened posteriorly or invaded from anterior to posterior. Contrast this imaging appearance to that of the **PVS mass** in which the PVMs are lifted anteriorly or invaded from posterior to anterior. Since most PVS lesions arise from vertebral body, vertebral body destruction and epidural disease will be linked. The DL-DCF "forces" PVS disease into the epidural space.

Selected References

1. Harnsberger HR et al: Differential diagnosis of head and neck lesions based on their space of origin. 1. The suprahyoid part of the neck. AJR Am J Roentgenol. 157(1):147-54, 1991
2. Smoker WR et al: Differential diagnosis of head and neck lesions based on their space of origin. 2. The infrahyoid portion of the neck. AJR Am J Roentgenol. 157(1):155-9, 1991

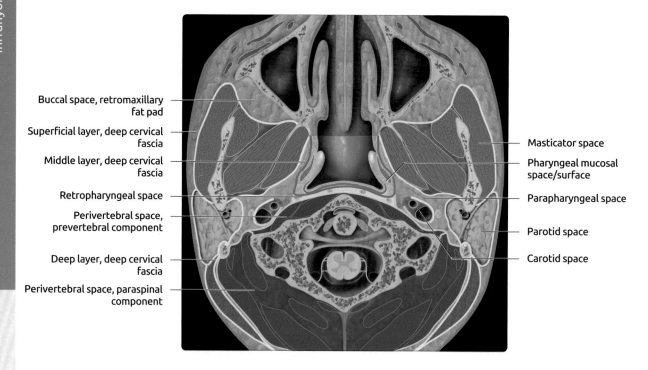

Buccal space, retromaxillary fat pad

Superficial layer, deep cervical fascia

Middle layer, deep cervical fascia

Retropharyngeal space

Perivertebral space, prevertebral component

Deep layer, deep cervical fascia

Perivertebral space, paraspinal component

Masticator space

Pharyngeal mucosal space/surface

Parapharyngeal space

Parotid space

Carotid space

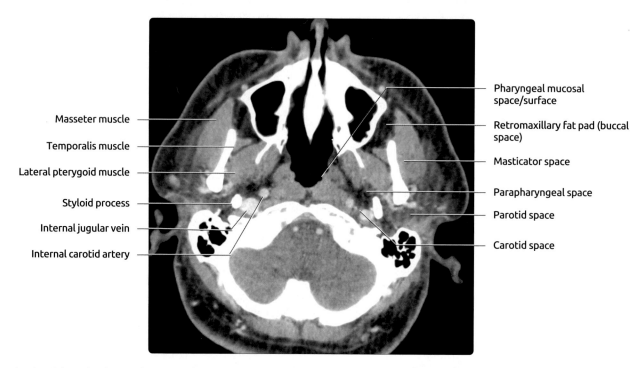

Masseter muscle

Temporalis muscle

Lateral pterygoid muscle

Styloid process

Internal jugular vein

Internal carotid artery

Pharyngeal mucosal space/surface

Retromaxillary fat pad (buccal space)

Masticator space

Parapharyngeal space

Parotid space

Carotid space

(Top) *Axial graphic depicts the spaces of the suprahyoid neck. Surrounding the paired fat-filled parapharyngeal spaces (PPS) are the 4 critical paired spaces of this region, the pharyngeal mucosal (PMS), masticator (MS), parotid (PS), and carotid spaces (CS). Retropharyngeal (RPS) and perivertebral spaces (PVS) are the midline nonpaired spaces. A PMS mass pushes the PPS laterally, an MS mass pushes the PPS posteriorly, a PS mass pushes the PPS medially, and a CS mass pushes the PPS anteriorly. Lateral RPS mass pushes PPS anteriorly without lifting styloid process. The superficial (yellow line), middle (pink line), & deep (turquoise line) layers of deep cervical fascia outline the spaces.* **(Bottom)** *Axial CECT at the level of the nasopharyngeal suprahyoid neck shows the 4 key spaces surrounding the PPS: The PMS, MS, PS, and CS. Notice the retropharyngeal fat stripe is not seen in the high nasopharynx between the prevertebral muscles and the pharyngeal mucosal surface.*

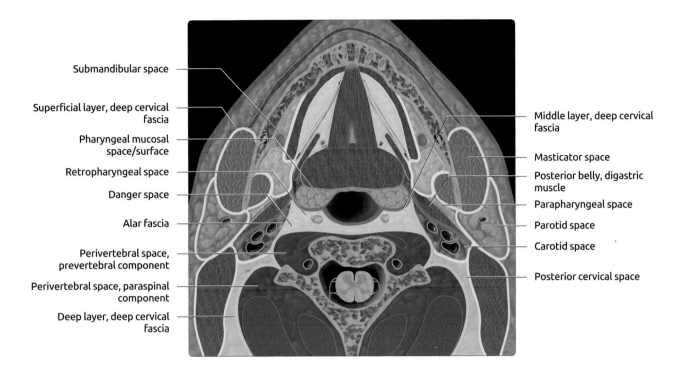

Submandibular space

Superficial layer, deep cervical fascia

Pharyngeal mucosal space/surface

Retropharyngeal space

Danger space

Alar fascia

Perivertebral space, prevertebral component

Perivertebral space, paraspinal component

Deep layer, deep cervical fascia

Middle layer, deep cervical fascia

Masticator space

Posterior belly, digastric muscle

Parapharyngeal space

Parotid space

Carotid space

Posterior cervical space

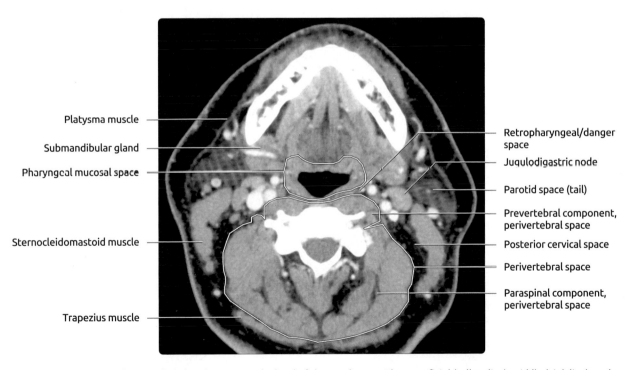

Platysma muscle

Submandibular gland

Pharyngeal mucosal space

Sternocleidomastoid muscle

Trapezius muscle

Retropharyngeal/danger space

Juqulodigastric node

Parotid space (tail)

Prevertebral component, perivertebral space

Posterior cervical space

Perivertebral space

Paraspinal component, perivertebral space

(Top) *Axial graphic shows the suprahyoid neck spaces at the level of the oropharynx. The superficial (yellow line), middle (pink line), and deep (turquoise line) layers of deep cervical fascia outline the suprahyoid neck spaces. Notice the lateral borders of the RPS & danger spaces are called the alar fascia, which represents a slip of the deep layer of deep cervical fascia. The CS has a tricolored fascial representation for the carotid sheath. This is because all 3 layers of deep cervical fascia contribute to the carotid sheath. **(Bottom)** In this image, through the low oropharynx, the PMS and the PVS have been outlined. The space between them is the RPS. The alar fascia that makes up the lateral borders of the RPS is not shown.*

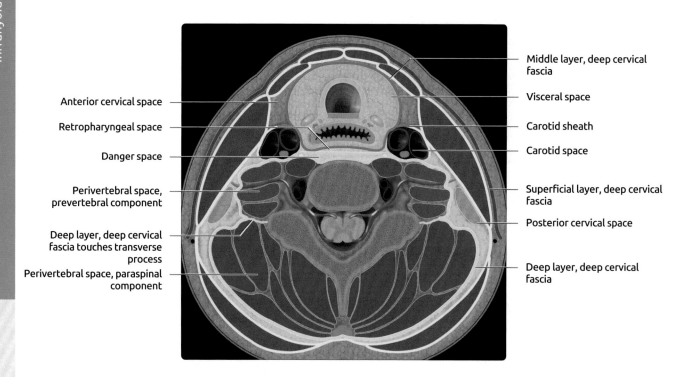

Middle layer, deep cervical fascia

Visceral space

Carotid sheath

Carotid space

Superficial layer, deep cervical fascia

Posterior cervical space

Deep layer, deep cervical fascia

Anterior cervical space

Retropharyngeal space

Danger space

Perivertebral space, prevertebral component

Deep layer, deep cervical fascia touches transverse process

Perivertebral space, paraspinal component

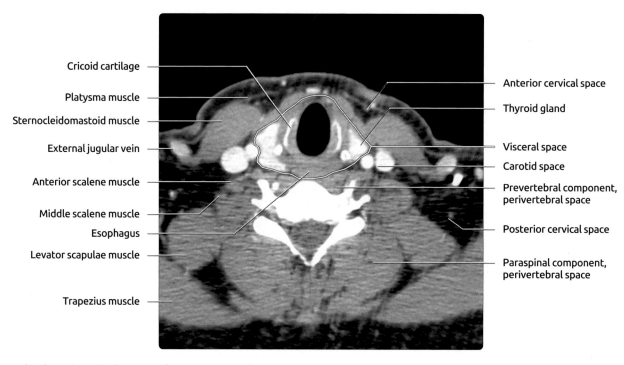

Cricoid cartilage

Platysma muscle

Sternocleidomastoid muscle

External jugular vein

Anterior scalene muscle

Middle scalene muscle

Esophagus

Levator scapulae muscle

Trapezius muscle

Anterior cervical space

Thyroid gland

Visceral space

Carotid space

Prevertebral component, perivertebral space

Posterior cervical space

Paraspinal component, perivertebral space

(Top) *Axial graphic depicts the fascia and spaces of the infrahyoid neck. The 3 layers of deep cervical fascia are present in the suprahyoid and infrahyoid neck. The carotid sheath is made up of all 3 layers of deep cervical fascia (tricolor line around CS). Notice the deep layer (turquoise line) completely circles the PVS, diving in laterally to divide it into prevertebral and paraspinal components. The middle layer (pink line) circumscribes the visceral space, while the superficial layer (yellow line) "invests" the neck deep tissues.*
(Bottom) *In this axial CECT, the middle layer of deep cervical fascia is drawn to delineate the margins of the visceral space. The visceral space contains the high-density thyroid gland, the upper cervical esophagus, and the cricoid cartilage. The CS are lateral to the visceral space, while the RPS and PVS are posterior.*

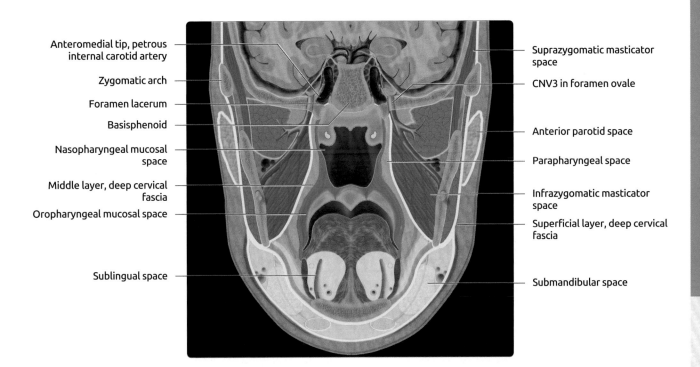

Anteromedial tip, petrous internal carotid artery

Zygomatic arch

Foramen lacerum

Basisphenoid

Nasopharyngeal mucosal space

Middle layer, deep cervical fascia

Oropharyngeal mucosal space

Sublingual space

Suprazygomatic masticator space

CNV3 in foramen ovale

Anterior parotid space

Parapharyngeal space

Infrazygomatic masticator space

Superficial layer, deep cervical fascia

Submandibular space

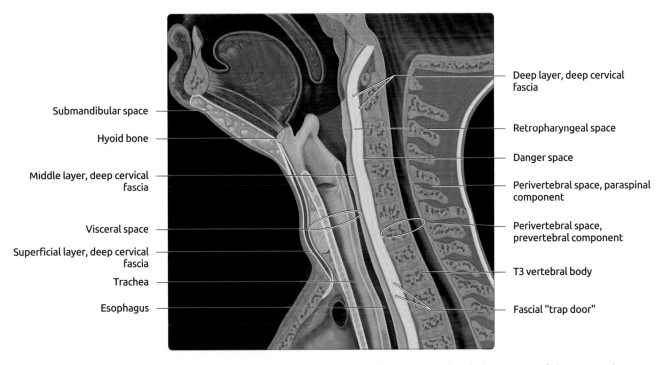

Submandibular space

Hyoid bone

Middle layer, deep cervical fascia

Visceral space

Superficial layer, deep cervical fascia

Trachea

Esophagus

Deep layer, deep cervical fascia

Retropharyngeal space

Danger space

Perivertebral space, paraspinal component

Perivertebral space, prevertebral component

T3 vertebral body

Fascial "trap door"

(Top) *Coronal graphic shows suprahyoid neck spaces as they interact with the skull base. The MS has the largest area of abutment with the skull base, including CNV3. The PMS abuts the basisphenoid and foramen lacerum. The foramen lacerum is the cartilage-covered floor of the anteromedial petrous internal carotid artery (ICA) canal.* **(Bottom)** *Sagittal graphic depicts longitudinal spatial relationships of the infrahyoid neck. Anteriorly, the visceral space is seen surrounded by middle layer of deep cervical fascia (pink line). Just anterior to the vertebral column, the RPS and danger space run inferiorly toward the mediastinum. Notice the fascial "trap door" found at the approximate level of T3 vertebral body that serves as a conduit from the RPS to the danger space. RPS infection or tumor may access the mediastinum via this route of spread.*

SECTION 2
Parapharyngeal Space

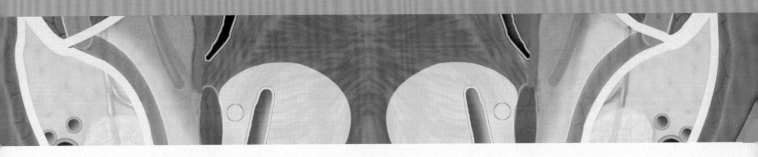

Summary Thoughts: Parapharyngeal Space

The four key spaces of the suprahyoid neck surround the parapharyngeal space (PPS), which is the central fat-filled lateral suprahyoid neck (SHN) space. When large lesions of the SHN become hard to localize to a space of origin, the direction of the PPS displacement may be used in combination with the space where most of the tumor is located to make a definite determination as to where the lesion originated. Once a space of origin is assigned, the space-specific differential diagnosis can be applied to narrow the diagnostic possibilities.

Imaging Anatomy

The parapharyngeal spaces are paired central, fat-filled spaces in the lateral suprahyoid neck around which most of the important spaces are located. These surrounding important spaces are the pharyngeal mucosal space (PMS), masticator space (MS), parotid space (PS), carotid space (CS), and the lateral retropharyngeal space (RPS). The PPS contents are limited; therefore, few lesions actually occur in this space. Diseases (tumor and infection) of PPS usually arise in adjacent spaces (PMS, MS, PS, CS), spreading secondarily into PPS.

The importance of the fat-filled PPS is its conspicuity on CT and MR. Even when large lesions are present in the SHN, it is still usually possible to find the PPS. Identifying the direction of displacement of the PPS by a mass lesion from a surrounding space can be a **key finding** in determining its **space of origin**. The PPS displacement direction defines the space of the primary lesion.

- PMS mass lesion pushes PPS laterally
- MS mass lesion pushes PPS posteriorly
- PS mass lesion pushes PPS medially
- CS mass lesion pushes PPS anteriorly
- Lateral retropharyngeal space mass (nodal) pushes PPS anterolaterally

The PPS is a crescent-shaped, fat-filled space in craniocaudal dimension extending from the skull base superiorly to the superior cornu of hyoid bone inferiorly. As paired fatty tubes separating other SHN spaces from one another, the PPS functions as an elevator shaft through which infection and tumor from these adjacent spaces may travel from the skull base to the hyoid bone.

The PPS has multiple important **anatomic relationships** with surrounding spaces. As there is no fascia separating the inferior PPS from the submandibular space (SMS), open communication between the PPS and posterior SMS exists. Superiorly PPS interacts with the skull base in bland triangular area on the inferior surface of the petrous apex. No exiting skull base foramina are found in this area of attachment. In the axial plane the PMS is medial, the MS anterior, the PS lateral, the CS posterior, and the lateral RPS posteromedial to the parapharyngeal space.

PPS **internal structures** are few. There is no mucosa, muscle, bone, nodes, or major salivary gland tissue within the PPS boundaries. The PPS principal content is **fat**. **Minor salivary glands** can be found there but are ectopic and rare. Although most of the **pterygoid venous plexus** is in the deep portion of the masticator space, a part of the plexus spills into the PPS.

The **fascia** surrounding the PPS is complex. Different layers of the deep cervical fascia combine to circumscribe the PPS. The medial fascial margin of PPS is made up of the middle layer of the deep cervical fascia as it curves around the lateral margin of PMS. The lateral fascial margin of the PPS is comprised of

the medial slip of the superficial layer of deep cervical fascia along the deep border of the MS and PS. The posterior fascial margin of the PPS is formed by the deep layer of the deep cervical fascia on the anterolateral margin of the retropharyngeal space and the anterior part of the carotid sheath (made up of components of all three layers of deep cervical fascia).

Clinical Implications

Since the PPS empties inferiorly into the SMS, PPS infection or malignancy spread inferiorly from the upper SHN to present as angle of mandible mass.

Approaches to Imaging Issues of Parapharyngeal Space

When you discover a lesion in the PPS on CT or MR, answer the following question first: "Is this lesion really primary to the PPS?" This question needs to be answered because there are so few things that occur initially in the PPS. In fact, the vast majority of lesions of the PPS arise in adjacent spaces and spread from there into the PPS. To conclude that a lesion is primary to the PPS, it must be completely surrounded by PPS fat. In most cases where a lesion is thought to be primary to the PPS, careful observation will find a connection to one of the surrounding spaces.

Lesions that are primary to the PPS itself include atypical 2nd branchial cleft cyst, benign mixed tumor, and lipoma. All are rare. Far more common lesions can be seen spreading into the PPS, such as intratonsillar abscess becoming peritonsillar and squamous cell carcinoma of the nasopharynx and oropharyngeal palatine tonsil. When a large, parotid deep lobe benign mixed tumor pedunculates into the PPS, it may at first glance appear to be primary to the PPS. Careful inspection will reveal a connection to the deep lobe of the parotid in the vast majority of cases.

Differential Diagnosis

DDx of parapharyngeal space lesion includes:
- Congenital: Atypical 2nd branchial cleft cyst, lymphatic malformation, venous malformation
- Inflammatory: Large diving ranula spreading from submandibular space into PPS
- Infection: Spreading from PMS, MS, PS or RPS; most commonly peritonsillar abscess from palatine tonsil (PMS) involves parapharyngeal space
- Benign tumor: Lipoma, benign mixed tumor (from minor salivary gland rest in parapharyngeal space)
- Malignant tumor: Spreading from PMS, MS, PS or RPS into PPS; most commonly squamous cell carcinoma spreading from naso- or oropharynx (PMS) into parapharyngeal space

Selected References

1. Mendelsohn AH et al: Parapharyngeal space pleomorphic adenoma: a 30-year review. Laryngoscope. 119(11):2170-4, 2009
2. Piccin O et al: Branchial cyst of the parapharyngeal space: report of a case and surgical approach considerations. Oral Maxillofac Surg. 12(4):215-7, 2008
3. Stambuk HE et al: Imaging of the parapharyngeal space. Otolaryngol Clin North Am. 41(1):77-101, vi, 2008
4. Monobe H et al: Peritonsillar abscess with parapharyngeal and retropharyngeal involvement: incidence and intraoral approach. Acta Otolaryngol Suppl. (559):91-4, 2007

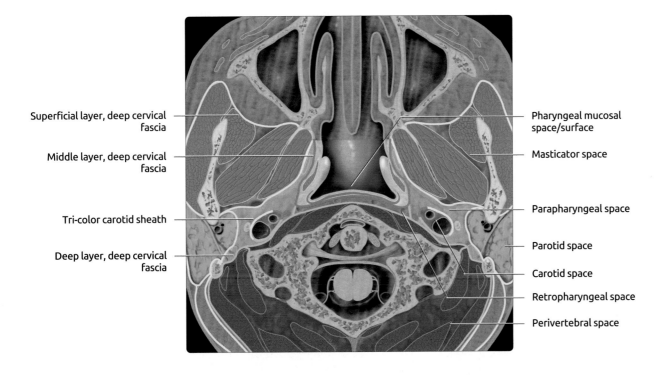

Superficial layer, deep cervical fascia

Middle layer, deep cervical fascia

Tri-color carotid sheath

Deep layer, deep cervical fascia

Pharyngeal mucosal space/surface

Masticator space

Parapharyngeal space

Parotid space

Carotid space

Retropharyngeal space

Perivertebral space

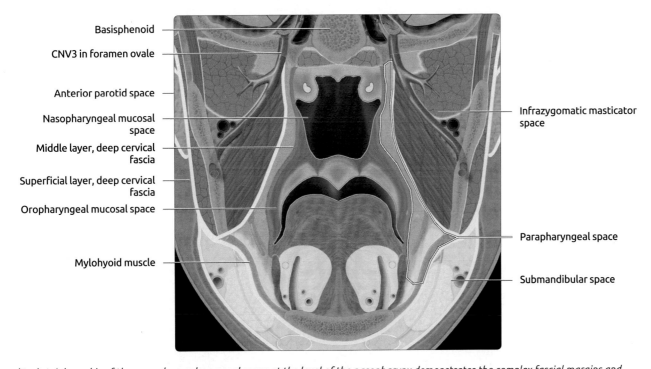

Basisphenoid

CNV3 in foramen ovale

Anterior parotid space

Nasopharyngeal mucosal space

Middle layer, deep cervical fascia

Superficial layer, deep cervical fascia

Oropharyngeal mucosal space

Mylohyoid muscle

Infrazygomatic masticator space

Parapharyngeal space

Submandibular space

(Top) *Axial graphic of the normal parapharyngeal space at the level of the nasopharynx demonstrates the complex fascial margins and the fat-only contents. Mass lesions originating in the surrounding pharyngeal mucosal, masticator, parotid, and carotid spaces can extend into the parapharyngeal space. The resulting displacement pattern of the parapharyngeal space may be helpful in defining the space of origin of a mass in the suprahyoid neck.* **(Bottom)** *Coronal graphic shows suprahyoid neck spaces as they interact with the skull base superiorly and submandibular space inferiorly. The parapharyngeal space interacts with no critical structures as it abuts the skull base. Inferiorly it empties into the posterior submandibular space along the posterior margin of the mylohyoid muscle. As a consequence of this anatomic arrangement, it is possible for an infection or a malignant tumor that breaks into the parapharyngeal space to present inferiorly as an angle of mandible mass.*

Parapharyngeal Space Benign Mixed Tumor

TERMINOLOGY

- Synonyms: Pleomorphic adenoma, parapharyngeal space (PPS)
- Surgeons often describe lesions as parapharyngeal whether arising in PPS, parotid deep lobe, PMS, or pterygoid muscles

IMAGING

- Rounded, well-defined lesion within PPS fat
  - Distinct from parotid deep lobe
- Well-defined, rounded lesion when small
- More lobulated when larger
- Marked T2 hyperintensity similar to CSF

TOP DIFFERENTIAL DIAGNOSES

- Benign mixed tumor, parotid deep lobe
- Neurogenic tumor, PPS
- Pterygoid venous plexus asymmetry
- 2nd branchial cleft cyst

PATHOLOGY

- Benign tumor arising in aberrant salivary gland rests
- Solid but often heterogeneous with hemorrhage, cystic degeneration, or necrosis
- Occasional ossific or calcific degeneration

CLINICAL ISSUES

- Most asymptomatic, or minimally so, because of deep location and slow growth
- Small lesion usually incidental imaging finding
- Larger lesion may be found at dental/oral exam

DIAGNOSTIC CHECKLIST

- Primary parapharyngeal space lesions are uncommon
- MR: T2 signal similar to CSF, but solidly enhances
- Look for fat plane to distinguish from parotid deep lobe benign mixed tumor

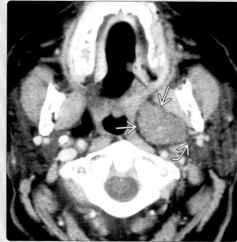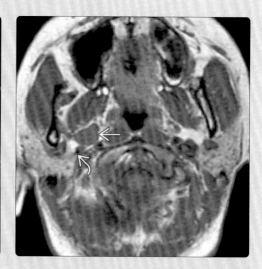

(Left) Axial CECT demonstrates a well-defined, slightly lobulated mass ➡ within the left parapharyngeal space. The mass is completely surrounded by fat separating it from pharyngeal mucosal space medially, parotid deep lobe laterally ➡, and carotid space posteriorly. (Right) Axial T1WI MR reveals a well-defined mass within the right deep face ➡, completely surrounded by parapharyngeal fat. Note the mass is distinct from medial aspect of the right parotid deep lobe ➡.

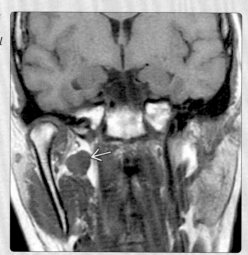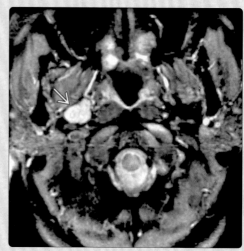

(Left) Coronal T1WI MR shows a well-defined mass ➡ to be surrounded by parapharyngeal fat. The mass is too small to have mass effect on adjacent tissues and was incidentally found on brain MR. (Right) Axial T2WI FS MR shows homogeneous hyperintensity of a slightly lobulated mass ➡. Hyperintensity similar to CSF is typically seen with benign mixed tumors, although postcontrast images confirm it to be a solid mass.

TERMINOLOGY

Abbreviations

- Benign mixed tumor, parapharyngeal space (BMT-PPS)

Synonyms

- Pleomorphic adenoma, PPS

Definitions

- Benign tumor arising from aberrant minor salivary gland rests in parapharyngeal space
- Surgeons often describe lesions as parapharyngeal whether arising in PPS, parotid deep lobe, pharyngeal mucosal, or masticator space

IMAGING

General Features

- Best diagnostic clue
  - Rounded, well-defined lesion within PPS fat
    - Distinct from parotid deep lobe
- Location
  - Within parapharyngeal fat of deep face
- Size
  - Variable: 1-8 cm
  - Large lesion often indistinguishable from parotid deep lobe tumor
- Morphology
  - Well-defined, rounded lesion when small
  - More lobulated with increasing size

Imaging Recommendations

- Best imaging tool
  - Readily detected on CT or MR
  - MR allows better characterization & improved delineation from adjacent structures
    - Parotid deep lobe, internal carotid artery
- Protocol advice
  - T1 MR best to delineate parotid deep lobe

CT Findings

- CECT
  - Heterogeneous, well-defined mass within PPS fat
  - Occasional focal ossification or calcification

MR Findings

- T1WI
  - Well-circumscribed rounded lesion within PPS fat
- T2WI FS
  - Marked hyperintensity similar to CSF
- T1WI C+ FS
  - Heterogeneous enhancement especially when large

DIFFERENTIAL DIAGNOSIS

Benign Mixed Tumor, Parotid Deep Lobe

- Identical appearance but **within** parotid deep lobe

Pterygoid Venous Plexus Asymmetry

- Tubular enhancing structures in PPS or medial masticator space

Neurogenic Tumor, PPS

- Well-defined, oval mass
- Intermediate T2, homogeneous CE if small

2nd Branchial Cleft Cyst

- Type IV branchial cleft cyst lies within PPS
- Cystic mass abutting lateral pharyngeal wall

PATHOLOGY

General Features

- Etiology
  - Benign tumor arising in aberrant salivary gland rests

Gross Pathologic & Surgical Features

- Solid but often heterogeneous with hemorrhage, cystic degeneration, or necrosis
- Occasional ossific or calcific degeneration

Microscopic Features

- As name implies, morphologically diverse
  - Epithelial and myoepithelial cells, mesenchymal or stromal elements

CLINICAL ISSUES

Presentation

- Most common signs/symptoms
  - Most asymptomatic because of deep location and slow growth
    - Small lesion usually incidental imaging finding
    - Large lesion may be found at dental/oral exam
  - Large mass often has minimal symptoms
    - Painless oral swelling or dysphagia

Demographics

- Age
  - Adults; peak in 5th decade
- Gender
  - Slight female predominance

Natural History & Prognosis

- Slow growing; may be asymptomatic even when large
- Uncommonly degenerates to malignant mixed tumor (carcinoma ex pleomorphic adenoma)

Treatment

- Resection for definitive pathological diagnosis or if large and symptomatic
- Operative tumor cell spillage may result in recurrence

DIAGNOSTIC CHECKLIST

Image Interpretation Pearls

- Primary PPS lesions are uncommon
  - Should be entirely surrounded by fat
- Look for fat at posterolateral margin to distinguish BMT of PPS from parotid deep lobe lesion

SELECTED REFERENCES

1. Pelaz AC et al: Simultaneous pleomorphic adenomas of the hard palate and parapharyngeal space. J Craniofac Surg. 20(4):1298-9, 2009
2. Zhi K et al: Management of parapharyngeal-space tumors. J Oral Maxillofac Surg. 67(6):1239-44, 2009

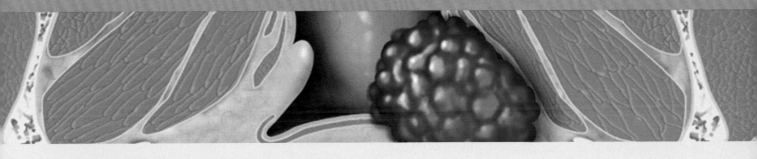

Summary Thoughts: Pharyngeal Mucosal Space

The pharyngeal mucosal space (PMS) is a key suprahyoid neck (SHN) space that represents the pharyngeal mucosal surface. The PMS has on its nonairway surface the **middle layer of deep cervical fascia**. Important pharyngeal mucosal space contents include the mucosal surface of the pharynx, pharyngeal lymphatic ring (adenoidal, palatine, and lingual tonsils), and submucosal minor salivary glands.

An enlarging PMS mass of the palatine tonsil or nasopharyngeal lateral pharyngeal recess displaces the parapharyngeal space fat laterally. Disruption of the mucosal and submucosal landmarks also occurs in PMS masses.

Important pharyngeal mucosal space malignancies include squamous cell carcinoma (SCCa) arising from the mucosal surface, non-Hodgkin lymphoma (NHL) from the pharyngeal lymphatic ring, and minor salivary gland carcinoma from the normal submucosal minor salivary glands. Of these, SCCa is by far the most frequent and the most important. Staging of SCCa primary and nodal disease is one of the most common reasons for imaging studies in the head and neck.

The pharyngeal mucosal space is not a true space as it is not enclosed on all sides by fascia. It is an imaging construct to overcome the problems encountered in describing a lesion of the pharynx as nasopharyngeal, oropharyngeal, and hypopharyngeal. These terms, although universally applied to lesions of the pharyngeal surface, do not address the deep tissue component of an invasive PMS mass. Describing a lesion as primary to the PMS with extension into the adjacent suprahyoid neck spaces clearly delineates lesion extent in a radiologic report.

Imaging Techniques & Indications

Both CECT and enhanced MR can be used to image the pharyngeal mucosal space. If tonsillar or peritonsillar abscess is the major clinical concern, CECT of the soft tissues with bone CT of the mandible is a better choice. When pharyngeal squamous cell carcinoma tumor staging is requested, enhanced fat-saturated multiplanar MR is the better exam. MR is usually less affected by dental amalgam artifact than CT and visualizes perineural and perivascular tumor spread more readily. In larger tumors of the oropharynx and nasopharynx already imaged with MR, the addition of noncontrast bone CT provides information regarding bone invasion that may be difficult to derive from MR imaging.

Imaging Anatomy

The **anatomic relationships** of the pharyngeal mucosal space and surrounding deep tissue anatomy are extremely important because both PMS malignancy and infection readily spread into these adjacent areas. Directly posterior to the PMS is the retropharyngeal space (RPS). The parapharyngeal space (PPS) is lateral to the PMS.

Superiorly, the **pharyngeal mucosal space** abuts the **skull base** along the roof and posterosuperior portion of the nasopharynx. This broad abutment with the skull base includes the posterior basisphenoid (sphenoid sinus floor) and the anterior basiocciput (anterior clival margin). The **foramen lacerum** (cartilaginous floor of the anteromedial petrous ICA canal) is a key area of abutment of the PMS with the skull base. Nasopharyngeal carcinoma accesses the intracranial compartment via the **perivascular spread** along the ICA beginning at the foramen lacerum.

The PMS extends from the roof of the nasopharynx above to the hypopharynx below as a continuous mucosal sheet. This mucosal space/surface is subdivided into **nasopharyngeal**, **oropharyngeal**, and **hypopharyngeal** components.

The PMS is a space with fascia on each deep margin but no superficial fascia. With no fascia on the surface of the PMS, it is not a true fascia-enclosed space. In fact it represents a conceptual construct to complete the spatial map of the suprahyoid neck. The term pharyngeal mucosal surface functions just as well as pharyngeal mucosal space.

The **middle layer of deep cervical fascia** (ML-DCF) defines the deep margin of the PMS. Just below the skull base, the ML-DCF encircles the lateral and posterior margins of the pharyngobasilar fascia (tough aponeurosis connecting the superior constrictor muscle to the skull base). In the more inferior nasopharynx and oropharynx, the ML-DCF resides on the deep margin of the superior and middle constrictor muscles.

Important **PMS internal structures** include the mucosa, lymphatic ring (of Waldeyer), and minor salivary glands. The pharyngeal lymphatic ring is divided into three components: The nasopharyngeal **adenoids** and the oropharyngeal **palatine** (faucial) and **lingual tonsils** (base of tongue). The lymphatic tissue normally declines in volume with age. Minor salivary glands are found in the submucosa throughout the oral cavity, pharynx, larynx, and trachea. Their highest concentration is found in the oral cavity and at the hard-soft palate junction.

The nasopharyngeal mucosal space also contains the superior constrictor muscle and the **pharyngobasilar fascia**. Along the posterosuperior margin of the pharyngobasilar fascia, there is a notch referred to as the **sinus of Morgagni**. The levator palatini muscle and the distal eustachian tube (torus tubarius) project into the PMS through this notch. Nasopharyngeal carcinoma may escape the PMS through this notch.

Approaches to Imaging Issues of Pharyngeal Mucosal Space

The answer to the question, "**What imaging findings define a pharyngeal mucosal space mass**?" depends on the area of the PMS where the mass originates. The most common PMS mass arises in the lateral pharyngeal recess of the nasopharynx or in the palatine tonsil of the oropharynx. As such, it is medial to the PPS, displacing the PPS fat laterally as it enlarges. A PMS mass of the lingual tonsil projects into the posterior sublingual space of the tongue as it enlarges. The rare posterior nasopharyngeal or oropharyngeal wall mass pushes posteriorly into the RPS as it grows. No matter where in the PMS a mass grows, disruption of the mucosal and submucosal architecture occurs. In addition, the growing airway side of the mass projects out into the adjacent PMS airway.

Traditionally, the pharynx is divided into the nasopharynx, oropharynx, and hypopharynx as a method to describe where on the this continuous sheet of mucosa a SCCa is found. This **surface of the pharynx** is referred to here as the **pharyngeal mucosal space**. To unify these two terminologies, it is possible to refer to the nasopharyngeal, oropharyngeal, or hypopharyngeal mucosal space. It is not helpful to merely refer to a tumor as either of the oropharynx or found in the oropharyngeal mucosal space. The radiologist must also describe what other deep facial spaces are involved by a PMS

Differential Diagnosis of Pharyngeal Mucosal Space

Pseudolesions	Malignant tumor
Asymmetric lateral pharyngeal recess	Nasopharyngeal carcinoma
Fluid in lateral pharyngeal recess	Oropharyngeal squamous cell carcinoma
Asymmetric tonsillar tissue	Palatine tonsil SCCa
Inflammatory lesions	Lingual tonsil SCCa
Mucosal inflammation (pharyngitis, post radiation)	Non-Hodgkin lymphoma
Tonsillar lymphoid hyperplasia	Minor salivary gland carcinoma
Retention cyst	Rhabdomyosarcoma
Postinflammatory dystrophic calcifications	Extraosseous chordoma
Tonsillar inflammation	**Miscellaneous**
Infectious lesions	Tornwaldt cyst
Tonsillar/peritonsillar abscess	Patulous lateral pharyngeal recess + palate atrophy
Benign tumor	In proximal vagal neuropathy
Benign mixed tumor, minor salivary gland	

tumor. This requires bringing the other deep facial spaces affected into the radiologic report, including the PPS, MS, parotid space (PS), CS, RPS, and perivertebral space (PVS).

When the PMS lesion is identified on CT or MR imaging, there are a limited number of common diseases to consider. If the patient is imaged to evaluate for possible infection, three lesions may be identified. **Tonsillar lymphoid hyperplasia** is commonly found in children and young adults, resulting from multiple bouts of tonsillar inflammation. **Tonsillar inflammation** is suggested when enhancing, enlarged tonsil(s) possess "stripes." **Tonsillar abscess** is diagnosed when focal rim-enhancing pus collections are seen. If the abscess has ruptured from the tonsil into the adjacent PPS, RPS, or masticator space (MS), the term **peritonsillar abscess** may be used.

If the PMS lesion lacks a clinical infectious context but has invasive imaging features, a limited group of **malignant tumors** must be considered. Squamous cell carcinoma is by far the most common malignancy of the PMS with non-Hodgkin lymphoma (NHL), next in frequency followed by minor salivary gland carcinoma. These neoplasms arise from the normal structures found within the PMS.

- Mucosa → **squamous cell carcinoma**
- Pharyngeal lymphatic ring → **NHL**
- Minor salivary glands → **minor salivary gland carcinoma**
- Notochordal remnant → extraosseous chordoma
- Constrictor and levator palatini muscles → rhabdomyosarcoma

The most common **interpretation pitfall** associated with the PMS occurs when the radiologist overcalls large adenoidal tonsillar tissue as tumor. Recurrent tonsillar inflammation in the young may lead to disturbingly prominent, often asymmetric tonsillar hyperplasia on CT or MR imaging. If the prominent lymphatic tissue in the PMS has no invasive deep margins, demonstrates inflammatory septa, and is found in a patient under 20 years of age, lymphoid hyperplasia is the most likely explanation.

A second common interpretation pitfall occurs when the lateral pharyngeal recess is asymmetric either because of retained secretions, retention cysts, or unevenly distributed adenoidal tissue. Suggesting nasopharyngeal carcinoma

(NPCa) in this setting creates great patient and physician consternation. Suggesting normal asymmetry and recommending clinical inspection usually suffice to clear the nasopharynx of significant pathology.

Clinical Implications

Remember that the referring clinician can usually directly visualize a lesion of the PMS. Lesions of the lateral pharyngeal recess of the nasopharynx may be the exception to this rule. In the case of SCCa, the appearance of the mucosal lesion is often diagnostic. Knowing what the physical examination of the pharynx shows at the time of rendering your radiologic report allows for a richly detailed and highly relevant interpretation.

If the requisition requests a staging CT or MR of a **SCCa of the PMS**, the report should comment on both the **primary tumor (T) and nodal (N) stage**. The 2010 AJCC staging manual defining the T and N stages of each of the subsites of the pharynx is an important reference for the radiologist doing this type of work. Familiarity with the routes of spread of SCCa of the PMS by primary site and subsite also permit directed radiologic reports to be rendered.

NPCa, because of its proximity to the skull base, spreads early into the intracranial compartment. The middle layer of deep cervical fascia and the pharyngobasilar fascia direct NPCa superiorly where it will invade directly into the upper clivus, floor of the sphenoid sinuses, and the foramen lacerum. When the tumor invades through the foramen lacerum, it accesses the anteromedial internal carotid artery. **Perivascular spread** takes it into the cavernous sinus from there. The proximity of the nasopharyngeal CS to lateral pharyngeal recess NPCa makes early invasion of the internal carotid artery and cranial nerves IX-XII likely.

Selected References

1. Gamss C et al: Imaging evaluation of the suprahyoid neck. Radiol Clin North Am. 53(1):133-44, 2015
2. Parker GD et al: The pharyngeal mucosal space. Semin Ultrasound CT MR. 11(6):460-75, 1990

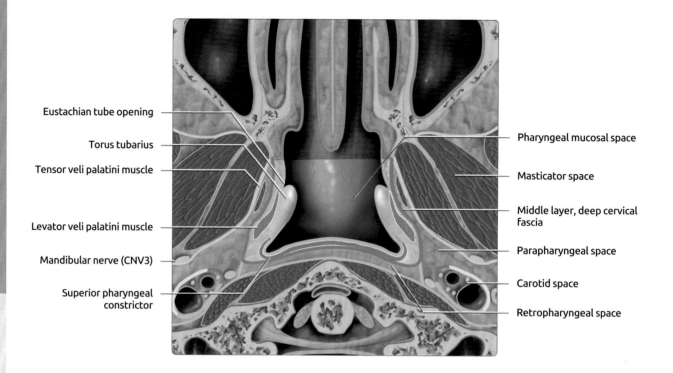

Eustachian tube opening

Torus tubarius

Tensor veli palatini muscle

Levator veli palatini muscle

Mandibular nerve (CNV3)

Superior pharyngeal constrictor

Pharyngeal mucosal space

Masticator space

Middle layer, deep cervical fascia

Parapharyngeal space

Carotid space

Retropharyngeal space

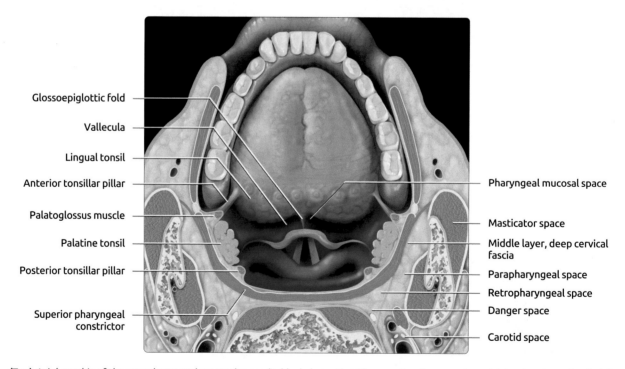

Glossoepiglottic fold

Vallecula

Lingual tonsil

Anterior tonsillar pillar

Palatoglossus muscle

Palatine tonsil

Posterior tonsillar pillar

Superior pharyngeal constrictor

Pharyngeal mucosal space

Masticator space

Middle layer, deep cervical fascia

Parapharyngeal space

Retropharyngeal space

Danger space

Carotid space

(Top) *Axial graphic of the nasopharyngeal mucosal space (in blue) shows that the superior pharyngeal constrictor, levator veli palatini muscles, and the cartilaginous eustachian tube ending (torus tubarius) are within the space. The levator veli palatini and eustachian tube access the pharyngeal mucosal space via the sinus of Morgagni in the upper margin of the pharyngobasilar fascia. The middle layer of deep cervical fascia provides a deep margin to the space. The retropharyngeal space is behind and the parapharyngeal space is lateral to the pharyngeal mucosal space.* **(Bottom)** *Axial graphic of the oropharyngeal mucosal space (in blue) viewed from above reveals that the superior pharyngeal constrictor and the tonsillar pillars along with the palatine and lingual tonsils are all occupants of this space. The middle layer of deep cervical fascia provides a deep margin to the space. The retropharyngeal space is behind and the parapharyngeal space is lateral to the pharyngeal mucosal space.*

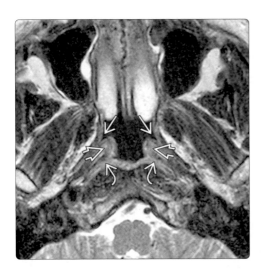

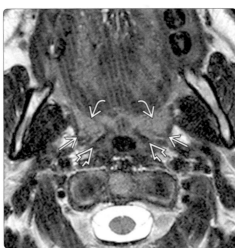

(Left) Axial T2WI MR shows the pharyngeal mucosal space at the level of the nasopharynx. Notice the opening to the eustachian tube ➡ and torus tubarius ➡. The lateral pharyngeal recess is collapsed ➡ with the 2 mucosal surfaces touching each other. (Right) Axial T2WI MR through the midoropharynx reveals the palatine tonsil ➡ as the main occupant of the PMS. The superior constrictor muscle ➡ and the palatopharyngeus muscles ➡ are visible.

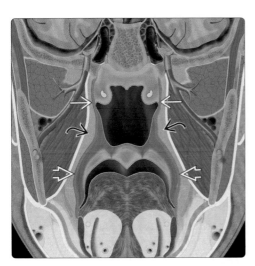

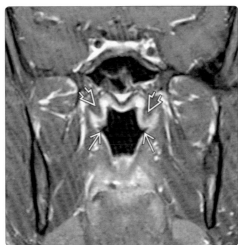

(Left) Coronal graphic shows nasopharyngeal and oropharyngeal mucosal space. Note the middle layer of deep cervical fascia defining the lateral margin of the nasopharyngeal PMS ➡ and the oropharyngeal PMS ➡. The parapharyngeal spaces are paired fatty spaces ➡ lateral to the pharyngeal mucosal space. (Right) Coronal C+ FS T1WI MR reveals the normal enhancing sheet of mucosa. Notice the torus tubarius (cartilaginous eustachian tube) ➡ & lateral pharyngeal recesses ➡.

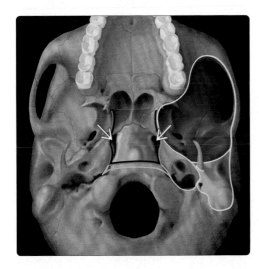

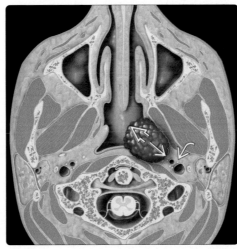

(Left) Skull base graphic viewed from below highlights area of PMS abutment (blue). Note posterior basisphenoid & clival basiocciput both are involved. Foramen lacerum ➡ are both within abutment area. (Right) Axial graphic through the nasopharynx depicts a generic PMS mass. The lesion projects into the nasopharyngeal airway ➡ as well as pushes from medial to lateral on the adjacent parapharyngeal space ➡. Notice the close proximity of the nasopharyngeal carotid space ➡ with CNIX-XII.

Tornwaldt Cyst

TERMINOLOGY

- Tornwaldt cyst (TC) definition
  - Benign developmental midline cyst in pharyngeal mucosal space (PMS) covered by mucosa anteriorly & bounded by longus muscles posteriorly

IMAGING

- Ovoid, cystic mass in midline nasopharyngeal mucosal space
- MR findings
  - T1: Intermediate to high signal depending on cyst fluid protein concentration
  - T2: Homogeneously high signal with no deep extension into surrounding structures
    - Low signal if contains highly proteinaceous fluid
  - T1 C+: May have minimal enhancement of cyst wall

TOP DIFFERENTIAL DIAGNOSES

- Adenoidal hyperplasia

- PMS retention cyst
- PMS benign mixed tumor
- Nasopharyngeal carcinoma

PATHOLOGY

- TC represents **notochordal remnant** where embryologic notochord & endoderm of primitive pharynx come into contact

CLINICAL ISSUES

- Usually asymptomatic and incidental
  - Seen on **5%** of routine brain MR
- Most common lesion of nasopharyngeal mucosal space occurring in 4% at autopsy
- Rarely, chronically infected large cyst (> 2 cm) causes periodic halitosis and unpleasant taste in mouth

DIAGNOSTIC CHECKLIST

- If invasion into prevertebral muscles, think nasopharyngeal carcinoma

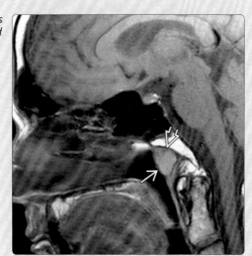
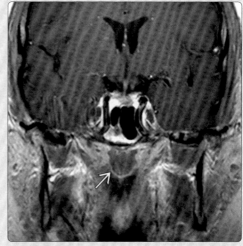

(Left) Sagittal T1WI MR shows a patient with a medium-sized Tornwaldt cyst ➡. The cyst is slightly hyperintense presumably due to increased protein content. Subtle internal septation ➡ is present. (Right) Coronal enhanced fat-saturated MR through the pituitary gland in the same patient reveals the nonenhancing Tornwaldt cyst ➡ within the otherwise enhancing nasopharyngeal mucosal space.

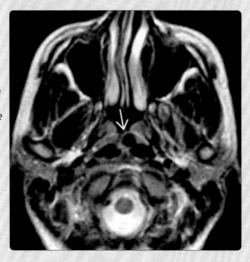
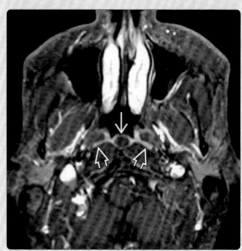

(Left) Axial T2WI MR reveals a Tornwaldt cyst ➡ in the midline nasopharyngeal mucosal space that is hypointense due to proteinaceous contents. Tornwaldt cysts are often high signal when water content is higher. Note the discrete plane between cyst and deep muscles indicating its mucosal surface location. (Right) Axial T1WI C+ fat-saturated MR demonstrates a classic small nonenhancing Tornwaldt cyst ➡. The mucosal surface enhances ➡ and is seen as a thin white line.

TERMINOLOGY

Abbreviations
- Tornwaldt cyst (TC)

Synonyms
- Nasopharyngeal bursa, Thornwaldt cyst

Definitions
- Benign developmental nasopharyngeal (NP) midline cyst covered by mucosa anteriorly & bounded by longus muscles posteriorly

IMAGING

General Features
- Best diagnostic clue
  - Midline, well-circumscribed pharyngeal mucosal space (PMS) cyst on posterior nasopharyngeal wall between prevertebral muscles
- Size
  - TC ranges from a few mm to 2-3 cm in diameter
- Morphology
  - Round or ovoid cyst

CT Findings
- NECT
  - Midline low-density cyst on posterior NP wall
- CECT
  - Rim of cyst may enhance only; TC remains low density

MR Findings
- T1WI
  - TC intermediate to high signal depending on cyst fluid protein concentration
- T2WI
  - Homogeneously high intensity NP cyst **without** deep extension into surrounding structures
  - Lower T2 signal possible with high protein content
- T1WI C+
  - May have minimal enhancement of cyst wall

DIFFERENTIAL DIAGNOSIS

Adenoidal Hyperplasia
- T2 high signal, diffuse soft tissue filling nasopharyngeal PMS

PMS Retention Cyst
- Often multiple, lateral pharyngeal recess lesions hyperintense on T2

PMS Benign Mixed Tumor
- Rare, well-circumscribed submucosal enhancing mass

Nasopharyngeal Carcinoma
- Invasive nasopharyngeal mucosal space mass
- T2 intermediate signal
- T1 C+ diffuse enhancement except in necrotic portions

PATHOLOGY

General Features
- Embryology
  - TC is **notochordal remnant** where embryologic notochord & endoderm of primitive pharynx come into contact
  - If adhesion occurs at point of contact, small midline diverticulum lined by pharyngeal mucosa is formed as notochord ascends into clivus

Gross Pathologic & Surgical Features
- Smooth, translucent cyst if uninfected
- Thick-walled if prior infection
- Rarely associated with median basal canal

Microscopic Features
- Cyst lining: Respiratory epithelium, little or no lymphoid tissue is seen in cyst wall
- Cyst fluid: Usually with high protein concentration

CLINICAL ISSUES

Presentation
- Most common signs/symptoms
  - Rarely symptomatic
- Tornwaldt syndrome (rare)
  - Chronically infected large cyst (> 2 cm)
  - Causes periodic halitosis, unpleasant taste

Demographics
- Age
  - Most common in young adults
- Epidemiology
  - Most common lesion of nasopharyngeal mucosal space, occurring in 4% at autopsy
  - Seen on ~ **5%** of routine brain MR

Natural History & Prognosis
- Incidental finding on MR with no clinical significance

Treatment
- Asymptomatic cysts require no treatment
- Chronically infected, painful lesions treated with endoscopic marsupialization

DIAGNOSTIC CHECKLIST

Consider
- TC if **high signal** intensity **midline** NP cyst on T2 MR

Image Interpretation Pearls
- TC on routine brain MR is of **no** clinical significance

Reporting Tips
- If invasion into prevertebral muscles, think nasopharyngeal carcinoma

SELECTED REFERENCES

1. Jyotirmay H et al: Recent trends in the management of Thornwaldts cyst: a case report. J Clin Diagn Res. 8(8):KD03-4, 2014

TERMINOLOGY

- Retention cyst (RC) of pharyngeal mucosal space (PMS)
- Synonyms: Postinflammatory cyst, tonsillar cyst
- RC: Benign, asymptomatic PMS cyst

IMAGING

- RC of PMS in nasopharynx or oropharynx
  - Usually < 1 cm
  - Smooth, well circumscribed, round or ovoid
  - **Pear-shaped** when in **lateral pharyngeal recess nasopharynx**
  - Discrete plane between cyst and underlying constrictor muscles
- Simple cyst in PMS on CT or MR
  - T1 MR: May be hyperintense if proteinaceous
  - T2 MR: Homogeneously hyperintense mucosal cyst
  - CT or MR: No significant enhancement in wall

TOP DIFFERENTIAL DIAGNOSES

- Thyroglossal duct cyst at foramen cecum
- Tornwaldt cyst
- PMS benign mixed tumor
- Vallecular cyst

CLINICAL ISSUES

- Incidental PMS lesion usually found on lowest images of routine brain MR
- Common **incidental lesion** found on brain or C-spine MR imaging
- Cyst in lateral pharyngeal recess may rarely obstruct eustachian tube with middle ear-mastoid fluid

DIAGNOSTIC CHECKLIST

- Important to recognize PMS RC as benign "leave alone" lesion

(Left) Sagittal T1WI MR shows characteristic smooth retention cyst ➡ at the posterior nasopharyngeal wall. This lesion mimics a Tornwaldt cyst, but axial images showed the cyst was paramedian. (Right) Axial T1WI MR in the same patient shows the characteristic pear-shaped retention cyst ➡ in the lateral pharyngeal recess. Note the high signal within the cyst, suggesting that cyst contents are either hemorrhagic or proteinaceous.

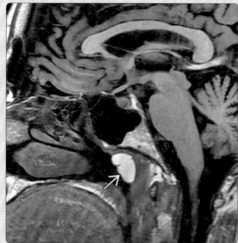
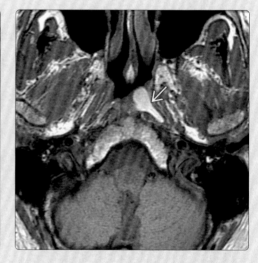

(Left) Axial T2WI MR shows bilateral nasopharyngeal retention cysts ➡, larger on the right. Note that the small left retention cyst is septated. The right mastoid is partially opacified. (Right) Axial CECT at base of tongue in an adult reveals a right vallecular retention cyst ➡. The left vallecula is partially filled with enhancing lingual tonsillar tissue ➦. A foramen cecum thyroglossal duct cyst would be more midline and not fill the vallecula. This lesion is different from the congenital vallecular cyst of the newborn.

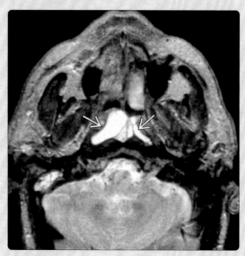
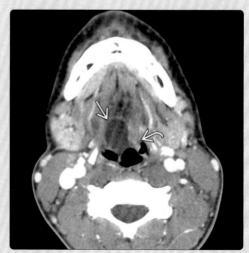

Retention Cyst of Pharyngeal Mucosal Space

TERMINOLOGY

Abbreviations
- Retention cyst (RC) of pharyngeal mucosal space (PMS)

Synonyms
- Postinflammatory cyst, tonsillar cyst

Definitions
- RC: Benign, asymptomatic PMS cyst

IMAGING

General Features
- Best diagnostic clue
  - Simple cyst in PMS on CT or MR
- Location
  - Usually on posterior wall of PMS in nasopharynx or oropharynx
  - Lateral nasopharyngeal recess common but can occur anywhere on PMS surface
- Size
  - Usually < 1 cm
  - Occasionally very large, > 1 cm
- Morphology
  - Smooth, well circumscribed, round or ovoid
    - **Pear-shaped** when in **lateral recess of nasopharynx**
  - Usually unilocular but occasionally multiple or septated

CT Findings
- NECT
  - Low-density PMS cyst with no deep extension
- CECT
  - No significant enhancement in cyst wall

MR Findings
- T1WI
  - Difficult to detect when fluid-filled & isointense to muscle
  - Often slightly hyperintense to muscle due to proteinaceous contents
- T2WI
  - Homogeneously hyperintense, superficial mucosal cyst
  - Discrete plane between cyst and underlying constrictor muscles when on posterior wall
- T1WI C+
  - No significant enhancement in wall

Imaging Recommendations
- Best imaging tool
  - T2 MR of PMS best displays RC
- Protocol advice
  - T2 axial & coronal MR images make RC diagnosis straightforward

DIFFERENTIAL DIAGNOSIS

Thyroglossal Duct Cyst, Foramen Cecum
- Benign embryologic remnant cyst of thyroglossal duct occurring at foramen cecum

Tornwaldt Cyst
- Benign embryologic notochordal remnant at midline of posterior nasopharyngeal wall

Benign Mixed Tumor, PMS
- Solid, homogeneously enhancing PMS lesion

Vallecular Cyst
- May be congenital in newborn
- In adult usually postinflammatory

PATHOLOGY

General Features
- Etiology: Postinflammatory in origin

Gross Pathologic & Surgical Features
- Soft discrete cyst lying on mucosal surface of nasopharynx or oropharynx

Microscopic Features
- Epithelial-lined cyst filled with serous fluid
- Rare cyst contains old blood products or proteinaceous fluid

CLINICAL ISSUES

Presentation
- Most common signs/symptoms
  - **Incidental PMS lesion** usually found on lowest images of routine brain MR
  - Cyst in lateral pharyngeal recess may obstruct eustachian tube with middle ear-mastoid fluid
  - Rare large cyst may present with dysphagia

Demographics
- Age
  - Usually found in adults
- Epidemiology
  - Common incidental lesion found on brain or cervical spine MR imaging

Natural History & Prognosis
- Incidental finding with no progression to symptoms

Treatment
- Rarely, large symptomatic cysts may be surgically excised

DIAGNOSTIC CHECKLIST

Consider
- If cyst in midline nasopharynx: Tornwaldt cyst, not retention cyst

Image Interpretation Pearls
- Important to recognize PMS RC as it is benign "leave alone" lesion

SELECTED REFERENCES
1. Matsumoto Y et al: Intra-adenoid cyst: a case report with an immunohistochemical study and review of literature. Clin Med Insights Case Rep. 8:41-5, 2015
2. Woodfield CA et al: Pharyngeal retention cysts: radiographic findings in seven patients. AJR Am J Roentgenol. 184(3):793-6, 2005
3. Yousem DM et al: Oral cavity and pharynx. Radiol Clin North Am. 36(5):967-81, vii, 1998

KEY FACTS

TERMINOLOGY

- Synonyms
  - Tonsillitis/tonsillopharyngitis
  - Tonsillar/peritonsillar phlegmon
  - Tonsillar/peritonsillar cellulitis
- Definition: Acute, nonsuppurative tonsillar inflammation

IMAGING

- Bilateral > unilateral tonsillar enlargement with variable attenuation/intensity/enhancement
- CECT to distinguish acute tonsillitis from tonsillar/peritonsillar (TA/PTA)
  - Well-formed capsule and homogeneous internal hypodensity in TA/PTA
- **Striated pattern** of internal enhancement (tiger stripe sign) relatively specific for **nonsuppurative tonsillitis**
- Reactive adenopathy common

TOP DIFFERENTIAL DIAGNOSES

- Tonsillar/peritonsillar abscess
- Tonsillar hyperplasia (hypertrophy)
- Palatine tonsil squamous cell carcinoma
- Pharyngeal mucosal space non-Hodgkin lymphoma

PATHOLOGY

- Most commonly secondary to respiratory virus
- 30-40% bacterial: Group A β-hemolytic streptococci most common

CLINICAL ISSUES

- Children and young adults
  - > 6 million office visits/year by children (< 15 years)

DIAGNOSTIC CHECKLIST

- Striated pattern of internal enhancement, absence of well-defined capsule help rule out TA/PTA

(Left) Axial CECT in a child with fever and sore throat shows the typical striated ➡ appearance of the bilaterally enlarged tonsils, consistent with nonsuppurative tonsillitis. (Right) Axial CECT in a child with a fever and sore throat shows that both palatine tonsils ➡ are enlarged and are "kissing" in the midline. There is also a well-defined, low-attenuation focus within the left tonsil ➡, which did not yield pus at aspiration, consistent with phlegmon.

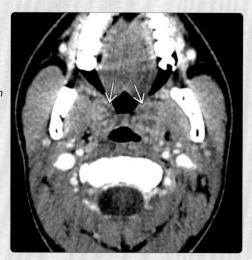
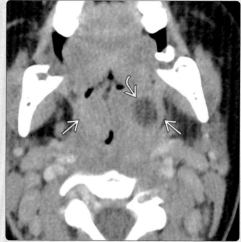

(Left) Coronal CECT demonstrates diffuse, bilateral enlargement of the palatine tonsils, both with small areas of heterogeneity ➡, consistent with edema, without frank abscess. (Right) Axial T1WI C+ FS MR shows bilateral tonsillar enlargement and pronounced enhancement ➡. Small internal areas of low signal ➡ are compatible with submucosal edema/exudate.

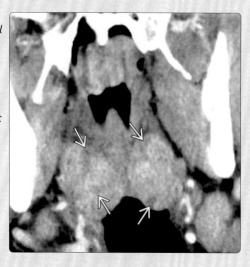
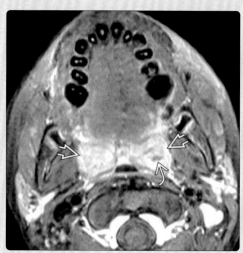

TERMINOLOGY

Synonyms
- Tonsillitis/tonsillopharyngitis
  - Tonsillar/peritonsillar phlegmon
  - Tonsillar/peritonsillar cellulitis

Definitions
- Acute, **nonsuppurative** tonsillar inflammation

IMAGING

General Features
- Best diagnostic clue
  - Bilateral tonsillar enlargement with variable attenuation/enhancement
    - Distinguish from tonsillar/peritonsillar abscess (TA/PTA), which demonstrates well-formed capsule and homogeneous internal fluid attenuation
    - **Striated pattern** of internal enhancement (tiger stripe sign) relatively specific for nonsuppurative tonsillitis
- Location
  - Lateral oropharyngeal wall
    - May be associated with enlargement of adenoids/lingual tonsils
- Size
  - Bilateral > unilateral tonsillar enlargement

Imaging Recommendations
- Best imaging tool
  - CECT to distinguish acute tonsillitis from TA/PTA
  - Intraoral ultrasound may be used to define abscess collection, though evaluation of deep extent of disease is limited

DIFFERENTIAL DIAGNOSIS

Tonsillar/Peritonsillar Abscess
- Well-defined capsule and central hypodensity

Tonsillar Hyperplasia (Hypertrophy)
- Lacks pronounced enhancement & acute symptomatology

Palatine Tonsil Squamous Cell Carcinoma
- Older age group
- Subacute, noninfectious presentation

Pharyngeal Mucosal Space Non-Hodgkin Lymphoma
- Homogeneous enhancement, subacute presentation

PATHOLOGY

General Features
- Etiology
  - Most commonly secondary to respiratory virus
    - Adenovirus, influenza virus, parainfluenza virus, rhinovirus, respiratory syncytial virus
  - 30-40% bacterial: Group A β-hemolytic streptococci most common
    - Occasional *Neisseria, Arcanobacterium, Mycoplasma, Chlamydia*

CLINICAL ISSUES

Presentation
- Most common signs/symptoms
  - Signs: Tonsillar swelling, redness, exudate
    - Typically bilateral; unilateral tonsillar deviation more commonly associated with TA/PTA
  - Symptoms: Fever, sore throat
    - Stridor, odynophagia, dysphagia, trismus indicate severe inflammation and airway compromise

Demographics
- Age
  - Children and young adults
- Epidemiology
  - One of most common infections encountered by pediatricians and family physicians
    - > 6 million office visits/year by children (< 15 years)
    - Additional 1.8 million visits by adolescents and young adults aged 15-24 years

Natural History & Prognosis
- Types of tonsillar disease: Acute tonsillitis, recurrent acute tonsillitis
  - Chronic: Chronic tonsillitis, tonsillar hyperplasia (hypertrophy)
- Nonsuppurative complications: Scarlet fever, rheumatic fever, poststreptococcal glomerulonephritis
- Suppurative complications: Tonsillar/peritonsillar (parapharyngeal, retropharyngeal) cellulitis ± abscess
  - Rarely Lemierre (septic internal jugular venous thrombophlebitis & metastatic abscesses), descending mediastinitis

Treatment
- Antibiotics
  - Given preponderance of viral etiology, some advocate observation
- Tonsillectomy may be performed in cases of recurrent acute or chronic tonsillitis

DIAGNOSTIC CHECKLIST

Image Interpretation Pearls
- **Striated pattern** of internal enhancement highly suggestive of **acute tonsillitis**
  - TA/PTA distinguished by well-defined rim and homogeneous internal hypodensity

SELECTED REFERENCES

1. Ulualp SO et al: Management of intratonsillar abscess in children. Pediatr Int. 55(4):455-60, 2013
2. Janjanin S et al: Acute lingual tonsillitis: an overlooked cause of severe sore throat in adults who have had a palatine tonsillectomy? Med J Aust. 191(1):44, 2009
3. Islam A et al: Cervical necrotising fasciitis and descending mediastinitis secondary to unilateral tonsillitis: a case report. J Med Case Reports. 2:368, 2008
4. Pinto A et al: Infections of the neck leading to descending necrotizing mediastinitis: Role of multi-detector row computed tomography. Eur J Radiol. 65(3):389-94, 2008
5. Van Howe RS et al: Diagnosis and management of pharyngitis in a pediatric population based on cost-effectiveness and projected health outcomes. Pediatrics. 117(3):609-19, 2006
6. Bell Z et al: Mediastinitis: a life-threatening complication of acute tonsillitis. J Laryngol Otol. 119(9):743-5, 2005

TERMINOLOGY

- Definitions
  - Tonsillar abscess (TA): Palatine tonsil suppurates, with abscess forming within tonsil
  - Peritonsillar abscess (PTA): TA spreads to adjacent parapharyngeal ± masticator ± submandibular spaces

IMAGING

- CECT
  - TA: Swollen tonsil with central low-density & peripheral enhancing rim
  - PTA: Focal low-density pus in adjacent PPS ± MS ± SMS
  - Reactive bulky bilateral cervical adenopathy common
  - Important to differentiate tonsillar inflammation from TA
    - Tonsillar abscess may be treated with incision & drainage
  - CECT recommended when TA or PTA suspected
    - Especially if trismus present

TOP DIFFERENTIAL DIAGNOSES

- Tonsillar hyperplasia (hypertrophy)
  - Chronic; palatine, ± adenoid, ± lingual tonsil enlargement
  - Tonsils do not significantly enhance or show low-density center (TA)
- Tonsillar inflammation (tonsillitis)
  - Acute; unilateral or bilateral palatine tonsil enlargement with enhancement but without low-density center (TA)
- Tonsillar retention cyst
  - Chronic; incidental CECT finding
  - Focal tonsillar fluid without tonsillar enhancement or enhancing rim
- Retropharyngeal space (RPS) abscess
  - Acute; suppurative RPS node ruptures into RPS
- Palatine tonsil SCCa
  - Chronic; invasive tonsil mass with local invasion

DIAGNOSTIC CHECKLIST

- Carefully differentiate tonsillar edema from TA or PTA

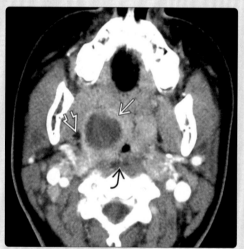
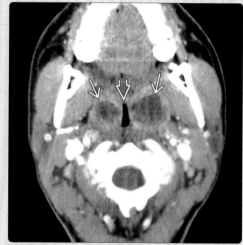

(Left) Axial CECT shows a large, low-density tonsillar abscess ➡. No extension through the capsule into PPS ⇗ is present. The left tonsil is prominent and enhancing, but no abscess is seen. Note sympathetic effusion in the retropharyngeal space ➡. (Right) Axial CECT reveals bilateral tonsillar abscesses ➡, the left larger than the right. Note the mass effect on both PPS but no extension of inflammatory process into the surrounding spaces. The airway is narrowed with a slit-like appearance ➡.

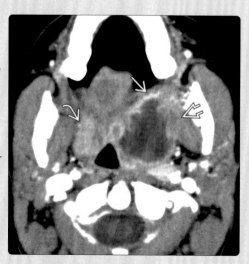
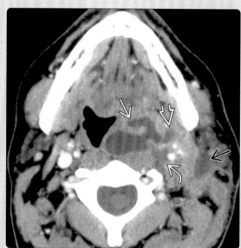

(Left) Axial CECT demonstrates left tonsillar and peritonsillar abscess with extension through the capsule into the posterior buccal space ➡ and medial pterygoid muscle ➡ of the masticator space. Note enhancement in the inflamed right tonsil ➡ without abscess formation. (Right) Axial CECT reveals a complicated large left tonsillar abscess ➡. Infection has ruptured posteriorly into the carotid space ➡, anterolaterally into the upper submandibular space ➡, and laterally into the inferior parotid space ➡.

TERMINOLOGY

Abbreviations
- Tonsillar abscess (TA), peritonsillar abscess (PTA)

Synonyms
- Intratonsillar abscess

Definitions
- Tonsillar abscess: Abscess within palatine tonsil
- Peritonsillar abscess: TA spreads to adjacent spaces

IMAGING

General Features
- Best diagnostic clue
  - TA: Fluid within large tonsil + peripheral enhancement

CT Findings
- CECT
  - TA: Large palatine tonsil(s) with central low-density & peripheral enhancing rim
    - Differentiating tonsillar edema from discrete abscess may be difficult on CECT
    - Important to differentiate tonsillar inflammation from TA as treatment may differ
    - Inflammatory stranding in adjacent spaces
  - PTA: TA extends into adjacent spaces
    - Parapharyngeal (PPS), masticator (MS), submandibular (SMS) spaces
  - Reactive bulky bilateral cervical adenopathy common in both adolescents & adults

MR Findings
- T2WI
  - Hyperintense, edematous tonsil with edema in surrounding spaces
- T1WI C+
  - Peripheral rim enhancement around abscess
  - Diffuse tonsillar enhancement when inflammation present without discrete TA

Ultrasonographic Findings
- Hypoechoic foci within tonsil suggests abscess

Imaging Recommendations
- Best imaging tool
  - CECT better than MR; faster in sick patient

DIFFERENTIAL DIAGNOSIS

Tonsillar Hyperplasia (Hypertrophy)
- Clinical: Chronic, recurrent tonsillitis
  - May be incidental imaging finding
- Imaging: Large, bilateral adenoidal, ± palatine ± lingual tonsils
  - Tonsils enhance less than in tonsillar inflammation

Tonsillar Inflammation (Tonsillitis)
- Clinical: Acute bilateral tonsillar nonsuppurative inflammation, sore throat, fever
- Imaging: Bilateral > unilateral tonsillar enlargement
  - Enlarged, enhancing tonsil(s)
  - Tonsillar striations suggests nonsuppurative tonsillitis

Tonsillar Retention Cyst
- Clinical: Asymptomatic; incidental imaging finding
- Imaging: Discrete, focal tonsillar fluid without surrounding enhancement or edema

Retropharyngeal Space Abscess
- Clinical: Bulging posterior pharyngeal wall in septic child
- Imaging: Retropharyngeal space abscess fluid with enhancing rim + tonsillar inflammation

Palatine Tonsil Squamous Cell Carcinoma
- Clinical: Adult with unilateral tonsillar mass with mucosal ulcer
- Imaging: Mildly enhancing, poorly circumscribed tonsillar mass with local invasion

PATHOLOGY

General Features
- Etiology
  - Acute exudative tonsillitis undergoes internal cavitation & suppuration, creating TA
  - TA rupture into PPS, MS, or SMS creates PTA

Microscopic Features
- Abscess commonly **polymicrobial**
  - Diverse aerobic & anaerobic flora common
  - Group A β-hemolytic streptococci often dominant bug

CLINICAL ISSUES

Presentation
- Most common signs/symptoms
  - Fever, sore throat, dysphagia, & tender cervical nodes
  - Other signs/symptoms
    - Trismus & uvular deviation common, even with uncomplicated tonsillitis
    - Imaging recommended if severe trismus to exclude PTA & determine local extension of pus

Demographics
- Age
  - Usually occurs in child or young adult

Treatment
- Tonsillar phlegmon or cellulitis treated with antibiotics & clinical observation
- TA now initially treated with IV antibiotics alone if **no** PTA or airway compromise
- TA or PTA with airway compromise treated with incision & drainage & IV antibiotics

SELECTED REFERENCES

1. Ulualp SO et al: Management of intratonsillar abscess in children. Pediatr Int. 55(4):455-60, 2013
2. Klug TE et al: Significant pathogens in peritonsillar abscesses. Eur J Clin Microbiol Infect Dis. 30(5):619-27, 2011
3. Windfuhr J: Malignant neoplasia at different ages presenting as peritonsillar abscess. Otolaryngol Head Neck Surg. 126(2):197-8, 2002
4. Schraff S et al: Peritonsillar abscess in children: a 10-year review of diagnosis and management. Int J Pediatr Otorhinolaryngol. 57(3):213-8, 2001
5. Buckley AR et al: Diagnosis of peritonsillar abscess: value of intraoral sonography. AJR Am J Roentgenol. 162(4):961-4, 1994

TERMINOLOGY

- Benign mixed tumor (BMT) of minor salivary gland (MSG)
- Synonym: Pleomorphic adenoma

IMAGING

- Palate > > oropharyngeal mucosal space (lingual or faucial tonsil) > nasopharyngeal mucosal space
- Size: Variable, but usually > 2 cm
- Shape: Oval to round, well-circumscribed mass without invasive margins
- CECT findings
  - Variable enhancing, well-circumscribed **palatal or pharyngeal mucosal space (PMS) mass**
- MR findings
  - **T2** signal variable but usually **hyperintense** to muscle
  - **T1 C+ enhancement** pattern variable but most commonly **homogeneous** enhancement

TOP DIFFERENTIAL DIAGNOSES

- PMS retention cyst
- Nasopalatine duct (incisive canal) cyst
- PMS squamous cell carcinoma
- PMS non-Hodgkin lymphoma
- PMS minor salivary gland malignancy
- Thyroglossal duct cyst in foramen cecum

CLINICAL ISSUES

- Submucosal mass of palate or pharyngeal surface

DIAGNOSTIC CHECKLIST

- BMT-MSG if mucosal space lesion is submucosal with no deep extension
- T2 MR in multiple planes often best imaging modality for BMT visualization

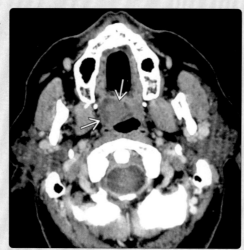
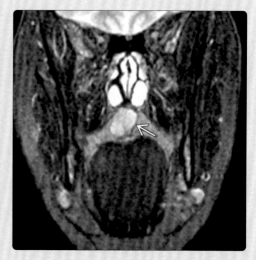

(Left) *Axial CECT demonstrates low-density soft palate benign mixed tumor (BMT) ➔ with smooth margins. Without adequate clinical history, lesion would be easily overlooked. Lack of enhancement makes squamous cell carcinoma unlikely.* (Right) *Coronal T2WI FS MR reveals BMT of midportion of hard palate ➔ as a smooth, oval mass elevating floor of nasal cavity. Note low SI rim. Mass enhanced with contrast, excluding palatal or incisive cyst.*

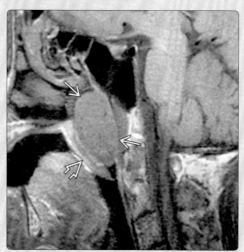
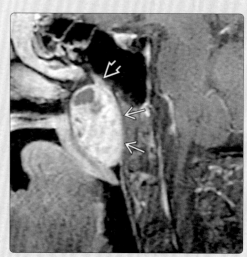

(Left) *Sagittal T1WI MR shows an oval, smooth BMT ➔ arising from nasopharyngeal mucosa with mass effect on soft palate ➔.* (Right) *Sagittal T1WI C+ FS MR in the same patient displays robust but heterogeneous enhancement of the mass. Note lack of deep invasion into longus capitis muscle ➔ or floor of sphenoid sinus ➔, characteristic of benign lesion. Lesion is entirely submucosal without ulceration, unlike squamous cell carcinoma.*

TERMINOLOGY

Abbreviations

- Benign mixed tumor (BMT) of minor salivary gland (MSG)
- Pleomorphic adenoma of oral mucosal (OMS) or pharyngeal mucosal space (PMS)

Synonyms

- Pleomorphic adenoma (PA)

Definitions

- Benign, heterogeneous tumor of MSG origin with epithelial, myoepithelial, and stromal components

IMAGING

General Features

- Best diagnostic clue
  - Solitary, sharply marginated, submucosal mass often pedunculated when large
- Location
  - Submucosal, anywhere in upper aerodigestive tract
- Size
  - Variable, but usually > 2 cm
- Morphology
  - Oval to round, well-circumscribed, mobile mass

CT Findings

- CECT
  - Variable enhancing, well-circumscribed **palatal or PMS mass**
  - If tumor is adjacent to bone (e.g., hard palate), benign-appearing remodeling on bone CT

MR Findings

- T2WI
  - Signal variable but usually **hyperintense** with respect to muscle
    - Dark rim often present
  - Well circumscribed but may be lobulated with **no deep invasion**
- DWI
  - ADC values increased compared to malignant salivary neoplasms
- T1WI C+
  - Variable enhancement but most commonly homogeneous

Imaging Recommendations

- Protocol advice
  - T2 MR best sequence as BMT in PMS often isodense on CECT

DIFFERENTIAL DIAGNOSIS

PMS Retention Cyst

- Postinflammatory PMS cyst without enhancement

Thyroglossal Duct Cyst at Foramen Cecum

- Midline base of tongue cyst

Nasopalatine Duct (Incisive Canal) Cyst

- Sharply marginated hard palate fissural cyst of incisive canal

PMS Squamous Cell Carcinoma

- Poorly circumscribed mass in pharyngeal mucosal space with deep invasion
  - Usually only slightly hyperintense on T2 MR

PMS Non-Hodgkin Lymphoma

- Diffuse adenoidal prominence or asymmetric faucial or lingual tonsil mass

PMS Minor Salivary Gland Malignancy

- Poorly circumscribed PMS mass
- Aggressive bone changes when malignancy develops in MSG of hard palate

PATHOLOGY

General Features

- Etiology
  - Benign tumor arising spontaneously from MSG that normally line all surfaces of upper aerodigestive tract

Gross Pathologic & Surgical Features

- Exophytic, 1-4 cm in size, smooth mass projecting into pharyngeal airway

Microscopic Features

- Interspersed epithelial, myoepithelial, and stromal cellular components must be identified to diagnose BMT-MSG
- Malignancy may develop in 2-10% of BMT
  - Carcinoma ex pleomorphic adenoma most common malignancy

CLINICAL ISSUES

Presentation

- Most common signs/symptoms
  - Painless submucosal mass of palate or pharyngeal surface

Demographics

- Age
  - Most common at presentation: 30-60 years
- Gender
  - M:F = 1:2

Natural History & Prognosis

- Slow-growing, painless, benign tumor
- Excellent prognosis after complete resection

Treatment

- Complete surgical resection of mass

DIAGNOSTIC CHECKLIST

Consider

- BMT-MSG if mucosal space lesion is submucosal with no mucosal ulceration or deep extension

Image Interpretation Pearls

- T2 MR in multiple planes often best imaging modality

SELECTED REFERENCES

1. Zaghi S et al: MRI criteria for the diagnosis of pleomorphic adenoma: a validation study. Am J Otolaryngol. 35(6):713-8, 2014

Minor Salivary Gland Malignancy of Pharyngeal Mucosal Space

TERMINOLOGY

- Minor salivary gland malignancy (MSGM) of pharyngeal mucosal space (PMS)
- Rare, aggressive tumors arising from MSG in PMS
- Most common pathology: Adenoid cystic carcinoma (ACCa) > mucoepidermoid carcinoma (MECa) > adenocarcinoma (ADCa)

IMAGING

- Locations: Oral cavity (**hard palate**) > > oropharynx (**soft palate**, base of tongue) > > nasal cavity/sinus
- Enhancing, infiltrating mass centered in PMS
- Hard palate, skull base, mandible invasion common
- MR: Submucosal mass usually **high T2 signal intensity**
  - T1 helpful to detect mandible or maxilla invasion, perineural tumor
  - T1 C+ FS helps define perineural spread

TOP DIFFERENTIAL DIAGNOSES

- PMS benign mixed tumor
- PMS squamous cell carcinoma
  - Nasopharyngeal carcinoma
  - Palatine tonsil SCCa
  - Lingual tonsil SCCa
- PMS non-Hodgkin lymphoma

CLINICAL ISSUES

- Painful submucosal pharyngeal surface mass
- ACCa often presents with pain & V2, V3 neuropathy
- Metastatic adenopathy at presentation rare unless high-grade histology
- Preoperative image-guided biopsy usually needed if mass not palpable

DIAGNOSTIC CHECKLIST

- Consider MSGM if T2-hyperintense PMS lesion has bone invasion or perineural spread

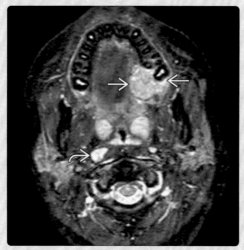
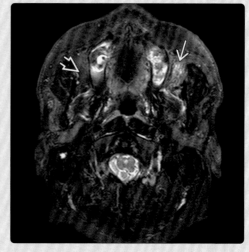

(**Left**) *Axial T2WI FS MR shows a high signal intensity mass ➡, mucoepidermoid carcinoma, at left maxillary alveolar ridge and lateral hard palate. The patient is young, so retropharyngeal node ➡ could be reactive.* (**Right**) *Axial T2WI FS MR shows a relatively hyperintense, small mucoepidermoid carcinoma ➡ filling left buccal fat pad. Note normal buccal fat pad on the right ➡. Poorly defined margins of the mass suggest a malignant histology; however, the imaging features are otherwise nonspecific.*

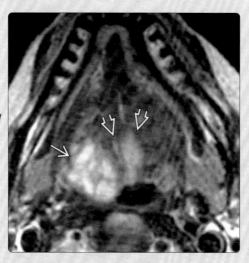
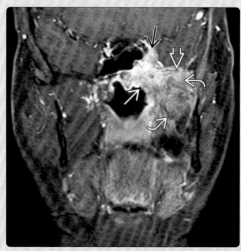

(**Left**) *Axial T2WI MR shows a high signal intensity lobulated adenoid cystic carcinoma ➡ involving the base of tongue and floor of mouth. Note extension into genioglossus muscles ➡ bilaterally.* (**Right**) *Coronal T1WI C+ FS MR shows an aggressive mucoepidermoid carcinoma ➡ of nasopharyngeal PMS. Note extension into deep masticator space with pterygoid muscle invasion ➡ and destruction of floor of middle cranial fossa ➡. Cavernous sinus involvement ➡ likely resulted from direct extension of tumor.*

TERMINOLOGY

Abbreviations

- Minor salivary gland malignancy (MSGM) of pharyngeal mucosal space (PMS)

Definitions

- Rare, aggressive tumors arising from MSG in PMS
- Most common pathology: Adenoid cystic carcinoma (ACCa) > mucoepidermoid carcinoma (MECa) > adenocarcinoma (ADCa)

IMAGING

General Features

- Best diagnostic clue
  - Enhancing, infiltrating PMS mass often with deep extension into adjacent structures
- Location
  - Oral cavity (**hard palate, floor of mouth**) > oropharynx (**soft palate**, base of tongue) > buccal mucosa & nasal cavity/paranasal sinus

CT Findings

- CECT
  - Enhancing, infiltrating mass on pharyngeal surface
  - Hard palate, skull base, mandible invasion common

MR Findings

- T1WI
  - PMS lesion usually isointense to muscle
  - T1 helpful to detect mandible or maxilla invasion, perineural tumor
- T2WI
  - PMS mass hyperintense when low grade
  - ↓ T2 signal mass (more cellular) generally has worse prognosis than high-signal mass (less cellular)
- T1WI C+
  - Enhancing mass with infiltrating margins
  - Fat saturation helps define **perineural spread**
    - Hard/soft palate MSGM → palatine nerve → CNV2

Nuclear Medicine Findings

- PET
  - Tumors usually are FDG avid

Imaging Recommendations

- Protocol advice
  - Recommend T1, T2, & T1 C+ MR with fat saturation in all planes
  - Perineural spread common
    - Image entire CNV2, CNV3 distributions

DIFFERENTIAL DIAGNOSIS

PMS Benign Mixed Tumor

- Well-circumscribed, submucosal, ↑ ↑ T2 mass

PMS Squamous Cell Carcinoma

- Poorly circumscribed PMS lesion malignant adenopathy
- Sites to consider
  - Nasopharyngeal, palatine tonsil, lingual tonsil carcinoma

PMS Non-Hodgkin Lymphoma

- Adenoidal, tonsillar, or lingual lymphoid tissue mass usually ↓ ↓ on T2 MR
  - Large, nonnecrotic nodes present 50% of time

PATHOLOGY

Staging, Grading, & Classification

- Staged according to anatomic site of origin: Nasopharynx, oral cavity, oropharynx, sinuses

Microscopic Features

- ACCa: Unencapsulated neoplasm of small, darkly staining epithelial cells with cribriform appearance
- MECa: Admixture of epidermoid, mucus-secreting, intermediate & squamous cells
- ADCa: Encapsulated neoplasm composed of cells of glandular origin

CLINICAL ISSUES

Presentation

- Most common signs/symptoms
  - Submucosal, painful pharyngeal surface mass
  - More invasive lesions, especially ACCa, present with pain & CNV2 & CNV3 neuropathy
- Other signs/symptoms
  - Metastatic adenopathy at presentation most common for higher grade malignancies

Demographics

- Age
  - Range: 35-80 yr
- Epidemiology
  - Rare, compared to major salivary gland malignancy (1/10 as common)

Natural History & Prognosis

- Begin as slow-growing tumors that tend to recur late
- 5-yr survival: 80%
- 20-yr survival: 20%

Treatment

- Preoperative image-guided biopsy usually needed if mass not palpable
- Wide surgical removal is treatment of choice
  - Transoral robotic surgery reserved for T1 or T2 tumors
- Neck dissection controversial, but often done for higher grade MSGM

DIAGNOSTIC CHECKLIST

Reporting Tips

- Carefully assess surrounding hard palate, skull base, mandible for bony invasion
- **Perineural spread** impacts prognosis & treatment

SELECTED REFERENCES

1. Kato H et al: CT and MR imaging findings of palatal tumors. Eur J Radiol. 83(3):e137-46, 2014
2. Villanueva NL et al: Transoral robotic surgery for the management of oropharyngeal minor salivary gland tumors. Head Neck. 36(1):28-33, 2014
3. Singh Nanda KD et al: Fine-needle aspiration cytology: a reliable tool in the diagnosis of salivary gland lesions. J Oral Pathol Med. 41(1):106-12, 2012

TERMINOLOGY

- Non-Hodgkin lymphoma (NHL) of pharyngeal mucosal space (PMS)
- Multiple subtypes, usually B- or T-cell categories
- 3 subsites of Waldeyer lymphatic ring
  - Nasopharyngeal adenoids
  - Palatine tonsils
  - Lingual tonsil

IMAGING

- CECT: Minimally enhancing bulky mass filling PMS airway, often without deep extension
  - Associated NHL nodal disease present 50% of time
- T2WI MR: Varies in signal intensity depending on cellularity
- DWI MR: Restricted because of high cellularity

TOP DIFFERENTIAL DIAGNOSES

- Tonsillar lymphoid hyperplasia
- PMS benign mixed tumor
- Nasopharyngeal carcinoma
- Palatine tonsil SCCa
- Lingual tonsil SCCa
- Inflammatory pseudotumor/IgG4 disease
- PMS minor salivary gland malignancy

PATHOLOGY

- When in H&N, commonly involves Waldeyer ring

CLINICAL ISSUES

- Increased incidence in patients with AIDS, Sjögren syndrome, Hashimoto thyroiditis, IgG4 disease, some autoimmune conditions

DIAGNOSTIC CHECKLIST

- Consider NHL of PMS when imaging shows bulky mass of adenoids, tonsils, or base of tongue
- Note local or deep extension & associated adenopathy for staging & treatment planning

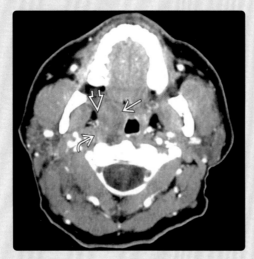
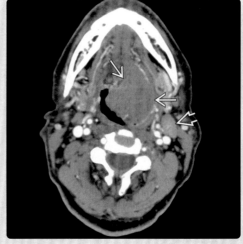

(Left) CECT shows a large, low-density mass ⟹ in right tonsil. Smooth interface between parapharyngeal fat ⟹ implies no extension through lateral capsule, but note fullness in right prevertebral muscles ⟹, suggesting mass has invaded through posterior tonsillar capsule. (Right) Large, exophytic, minimally enhancing NHL ⟹ arises in left lingual lymphoid tissue, with near-complete airway obstruction. Note level IIA node ⟹ with no central necrosis, a common finding in nodal lymphoma.

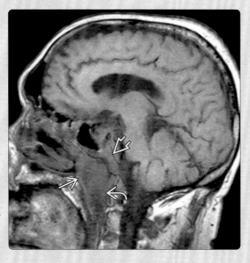
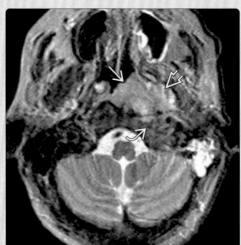

(Left) Sagittal T1WI MR shows a bulky nasopharyngeal mass ⟹ extending to oropharyngeal level ⟹. Abnormal signal intensity in clivus ⟹ implies central skull base invasion. (Right) Axial T2WI FS MR in the same patient reveals mass ⟹ is relatively low signal intensity, with invasion of prevertebral muscles ⟹ & parapharyngeal space ⟹. Note mastoid opacification from tumor invasion of eustachian tube orifice. Nasopharyngeal carcinoma could exactly mimic this imaging appearance.

TERMINOLOGY

Abbreviations

- Non-Hodgkin lymphoma (NHL) of pharyngeal mucosal space (PMS)

Synonyms

- Multiple subtypes, usually B- or T-cell categories
  o B-cell types: Burkitt, diffuse large, follicular, immunoblastic large cell, mantle cell, chronic lymphocytic lymphoma (CLL), mucosa-associated lymphoid tissue (MALT)
  o T-cell types: Anaplastic large cell, precursor T-lymphoblastic, mycosis fungoides

Definitions

- 3 subsites of Waldeyer lymphatic ring: Adenoids, palatine tonsils, lingual tonsil

IMAGING

General Features

- Best diagnostic clue
  o Large PMS mass with associated cervical adenopathy > 50% of time
  o Imaging findings **may be identical to squamous cell carcinoma** (SCCa) of PMS
- Location
  o Most common sites of NHL of PMS
    – Palatine tonsil > nasopharyngeal adenoids > lingual tonsil
    – More than one site often involved
  o Nonnodal, extralymphatic NHL of sinus, orbit, parotid, larynx, or thyroid can rarely occur
- Size
  o Large, usually > 4 cm, at presentation
- Morphology
  o Poorly defined, diffusely infiltrative mass most common (mimics SCCa)
  o Unilateral, asymmetric, smooth mass in tonsil less common (mimics benign mixed tumor)

CT Findings

- CECT
  o Minimally enhancing bulky mass filling PMS airway
    – Often without deep extension into surrounding spaces
  o Associated NHL nodal disease present 50% of time
    – **Nodes** usually **large**, > 2 cm & nonnecrotic
    – Nodes may be centrally necrotic in high-grade NHL
      □ Especially AIDS-related NHL

MR Findings

- T1WI
  o Large PMS mass isointense to muscle
- T2WI
  o Varies in signal intensity (SI), depending on cellularity, but usually homogeneously intermediate SI
    – Highly cellular lesions generally less hyperintense on T2WI
  o Invasion into surrounding structures, including skull base, PPS, and prevertebral muscles, is common

- DWI
  o Restricted diffusion especially for FDG-avid lymphoma types
- T1WI C+
  o Enhancing palatine, lingual, or adenoidal tonsillar mass
  o No internal enhancing septa present, as compared with benign lymphoid hyperplasia or tonsillar infection

Nuclear Medicine Findings

- PET
  o NHL FDG avid
  o MALT type lymphomas less FDG avid
  o PET/CT used to stage disease & for surveillance of posttreatment imaging
    – PET/CT limited sensitivity for lower grade NHL

Imaging Recommendations

- Best imaging tool
  o PET/CT best staging & surveillance modality
  o CECT recommended as part of PET/CT imaging
- Protocol advice
  o Imaging (CT or MR) should cover entire extracranial H&N from sellar floor above to clavicles below
    – Coverage should include PMS primary site as well as potential cervical adenopathy

DIFFERENTIAL DIAGNOSIS

Tonsillar Lymphoid Hyperplasia

- Patients < 20 years old (NHL usually > 40 years old)
- Symmetric enlargement of adenoidal & tonsillar tissue

Nasopharyngeal Carcinoma

- Poorly circumscribed nasopharyngeal PMS mass
  o Often mimics NHL on imaging alone
- Associated malignant, often necrotic, adenopathy

Palatine Tonsil SCCa

- Invasive palatine tonsil mass
  o Often mimics NHL on imaging alone

Lingual Tonsil SCCa

- Invasive lingual tonsil mass
  o Often mimics NHL on imaging alone

PMS Minor Salivary Gland Malignancy

- May be indistinguishable from H&N SCCa
- Associated nodal metastases are rare

PMS Benign Mixed Tumor

- Well-circumscribed, noninvasive PMS mass

Inflammatory Pseudotumor/IgG4 Disease

- Poorly defined autoimmune disease can present as PMS mass
- Spectrum that includes Sjögren syndrome, thyroiditis, autoimmune disease

PATHOLOGY

General Features

- Etiology
  o Primary malignancy of lymphatic system
  o PMS NHL usually of B-cell origin

- Genetics
  - Cytogenetics of NHL complicated & related to subtype of lymphoma
- Associated abnormalities
  - Sjögren syndrome & Hashimoto thyroiditis associated with MALT, B-cell type, NHL
    - Currently being redefined as IgG4 disease
  - Posttransplant lymphoproliferative disorders (PTLDs) associated with NHL from iatrogenic immunosuppression used for transplant patients
    - Spectrum of diseases from prominent lymphoid hyperplasia to malignant NHL

Staging, Grading, & Classification

- 2 prognostic groups: Indolent & aggressive
- NHL clinical staging (I-IV) Ann Arbor staging system
  - Stage I or IE
    - Single lymphatic site: Waldeyer lymphatic ring
    - IE: Single extralymphatic site + no nodal disease
  - Stage II or IIE
    - ≥ 2 nodal regions on same side of diaphragm
    - IIE: Single extralymphatic site and > 1 nodal region on same side of diaphragm
  - Stage III, IIIE, IIIS
    - ≥ 2 nodal regions on both sides of diaphragm
    - IIIE: Extralymphatic extension with adjacent lymph node involvement
    - IIIS: Splenic involvement
  - Stage IV: Diffuse or disseminated involvement of ≥ 1 extralymphatic organ(s) ± lymph node involvement

Gross Pathologic & Surgical Features

- Soft, bulky PMS lesion, may be submucosal or ulcerative

Microscopic Features

- Any of NHL patterns & cell types can be seen
- Most common histologic pattern is diffuse with immunoblastic or large cell (B cell) cytologic features & markers
  - Immunochemistry differentiates nasopharyngeal carcinoma (NPC) from NHL
    - Leukocyte common antigen (LCA) vs. cytokeratin
    - NHL, immunoblastic or large cell type: LCA positive, cytokeratin negative
    - NPC, undifferentiated: LCA negative, cytokeratin positive

CLINICAL ISSUES

Presentation

- Most common signs/symptoms
  - Presenting signs similar to SCCa
    - Nasopharyngeal adenoidal NHL: Nasal obstruction, serous otitis media
    - Palatine or lingual tonsil NHL: Sore throat, otalgia, tonsillar mass
  - Other signs/symptoms
    - B symptoms: Systemic complaints such as fever, sweats, weight loss
    - Children with large PMS NHL may present with airway compromise
- Clinical profile

- Most common presentation: Adult with PMS mass & neck mass
- Increased incidence in patients with AIDS, Sjögren syndrome, Hashimoto thyroiditis, and other autoimmune conditions

Demographics

- Age
  - Adult more common than pediatric; > 50 years
- Gender
  - M:F = 1.5:1
- Epidemiology
  - NHL 5x as common as Hodgkin disease in H&N
  - 35% of extranodal NHL in H&N occurs in PMS
  - PMS is most common extranodal site in H&N
    - Palatine tonsil involved (50%)
    - Nasopharyngeal adenoids involved (35%)
    - Lingual tonsil involved (15%)
  - 50% of PMS NHL have malignant lymph nodes at presentation

Natural History & Prognosis

- Prognosis determined by both stage & aggressive vs. indolent types
  - High histopathologic grade & recurrent disseminated disease have poorest prognosis
  - AIDS-related NHL generally has poorer prognosis
- 2/3 of patients have remission after initial therapy
  - Of these, 2/3 are cured & have no further relapse
- 75% of those who relapse after achieving remission die of NHL

Treatment

- Based on clinical stage and aggressive vs. indolent subtypes at presentation
- Treatment regimens range from "watch and wait" for indolent types especially in elderly, to combined chemoradiotherapy
- Complete remission & cure rates improved with development of combined chemotherapy options
- **Overall survival rate** for H&N PMS NHL is **60%**

DIAGNOSTIC CHECKLIST

Consider

- NHL of PMS when imaging shows bulky mass of adenoidal, tonsillar, or base of tongue (lingual tonsil)

Image Interpretation Pearls

- Local or deep extension important to recognize & map for staging & radiotherapy
- Associated cervical adenopathy common
  - Must scan entire neck

Reporting Tips

- Describe primary PMS lesion & adenopathy as both affect accurate staging

SELECTED REFERENCES

1. Heacock L et al: PET/MRI for the evaluation of patients with lymphoma: initial observations. AJR Am J Roentgenol. 204(4):842-8, 2015
2. Aiken AH et al: Imaging Hodgkin and non-Hodgkin lymphoma in the head and neck. Radiol Clin North Am. 46(2):363-78, ix-x, 2008

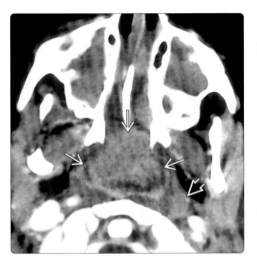

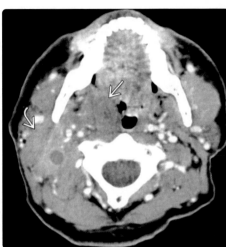

(Left) *Axial CECT in a child with AIDS shows heterogeneous enhancement in bulky adenoidal NHL* ⮕. *Note large left retropharyngeal lymph node* ⮕ *and near occlusion of nasopharyngeal airway. Benign secretions fill bilateral maxillary sinuses and nasal cavity.* (Right) *Axial CECT shows multifocal NHL with involvement in right tonsil* ⮕ *and level II matted nodal mass* ⮕ *with extranodal extension. Cervical adenopathy is present more than 50% of time with NHL of PMS.*

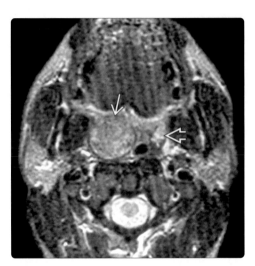

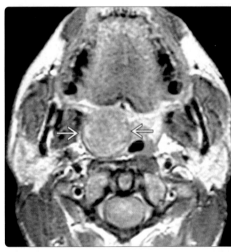

(Left) *Axial T2WI FS MR shows a well-circumscribed right tonsillar NHL* ⮕. *Small left tonsil* ⮕ *is normal for adult, as lymphoid tissue involutes with age. Squamous cell carcinoma of tonsil or benign mixed tumor could have identical appearance, and only biopsy would confirm NHL.* (Right) *Axial T1WI C+ MR in the same patient reveals homogeneous enhancement in tonsillar NHL* ⮕. *Tonsillar infection should have striated enhancement pattern; intratonsillar abscess would be centrally necrotic.*

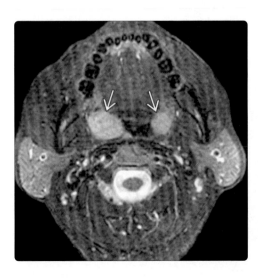

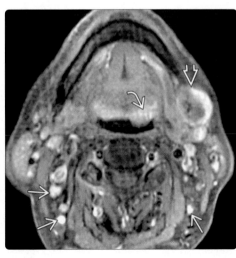

(Left) *Axial T2WI FS MR demonstrates multifocal NHL in both palatine tonsils* ⮕. *Well-circumscribed appearance suggests that tumor remains within tonsillar capsules.* (Right) *Axial T1WI C+ FS MR in the same patient shows additional sites of NHL in left base of tongue lymphoid tissue* ⮕ *and large necrotic left IB node* ⮕. *Multiple small cervical nodes* ⮕ *are present, and only a metabolic study such as PET/CT could determine involvement by NHL.*

SECTION 4
Masticator Space

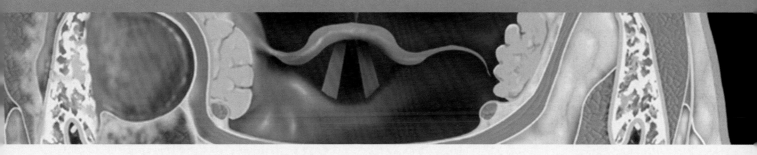

Summary Thoughts: Masticator Space

The three most frequently encountered abnormalities in the masticator space (MS) are infection, infection, and infection. Odontogenic infection should always cross the radiologist's mind first when evaluating abnormalities in this space.

When evaluating tumors of the MS, the presence of **perineural CNV3 tumor spread (PNT)** is of critical importance, because it is easily overlooked but can have a dramatic effect on treatment and prognosis.

The MS includes the posterior body and ramus of the mandible, the four muscles of mastication (masseter, temporalis, medial pterygoid, lateral pterygoid), and the mandibular branch of the trigeminal nerve (CNV3). It has greater extension in the craniocaudal dimension than commonly recognized, as it reaches from the bottom of the mandible nearly to the vertex of the skull.

The MS is divided at the level of the zygomatic arch into the suprazygomatic MS (**temporal fossa**) and the infrazygomatic MS (**infratemporal fossa**).

Imaging Techniques & Indications

Because **odontogenic infection** is by far the **most likely pathology** to affect the MS, CECT is the preferred imaging modality. The tooth of origin can be best identified with bone CT. This is important because the infection will recur until the offending tooth is treated. To be sure that a worrisome tooth is the true site of origin, look for mandibular cortical erosions that communicate between the apical tooth abscess and the soft tissue MS abscess. Contrast is needed to determine how far the infection has spread into soft tissues. Contrast also helps differentiate cellulitis and phlegmon from surgically drainable abscess.

Any cross-sectional imaging exam should cover the entire length of CNV3 in the MS, in the jaw, and up to the skull base to assess for PNT. Ideally, imaging should include the lateral pons, Meckel cave, foramen ovale, the mandibular foramen (where the inferior alveolar nerve enters the mandible), the entire inferior alveolar canal, and the mental foramen.

Imaging Anatomy

The masticator space is the largest suprahyoid neck space. In the superior direction its suprazygomatic component extends along the parietal skull almost to the vertex, enclosing the temporalis muscle. There is a broad abutment of the MS to the skull base. Within this area of contact with the skull base is the foramen ovale (CNV3) and the foramen spinosum (middle meningeal artery). Inferiorly, the MS terminates at the inferior margin of the posterior body of the mandible.

MS regional anatomic relationships are important as both tumor and infection of the MS tend to spread into adjacent spaces. The buccal space is found anteriorly, including retromaxillary fat pad. The parotid space is posterolateral, while the parapharyngeal space is posteromedial to the MS. The relationship between the MS & PPS is important because the PPS fat will be displaced posteromedially by an enlarging MS mass. Medial to the MS is the pharyngeal mucosal space. The subcutaneous fat of the cheek is seen lateral to the MS.

The **superficial layer** of the **deep cervical fascia** divides around the the inferior margin of the mandible. This split fascia encases the mandible and the muscles of mastication. The medial slip of the fascia runs along the deep surface of the pterygoid muscles to insert on the undersurface of the skull base just **medial** to **foramen ovale**. The medial slip is also known as the medial pterygoid fascia. The lateral slip covers the superficial surface of the masseter muscle and attaches to the zygomatic arch, where the masseter muscle originates. This lateral fascia continues over the temporalis muscle to the top of the suprazygomatic MS. There is no fascia separating the suprazygomatic and infrazygomatic portions of the MS. In fact, there are no horizontal fascia anywhere in the MS, facilitating craniocaudal spread of disease.

Most of the MS is filled by the **four muscles of mastication**. The masseter muscle originates at the zygomatic arch and inserts on the inferior mandibular body. The temporalis muscle takes its origin from a semicircular area of bone splayed across parietal skull. Inferiorly, the temporalis inserts on the coronoid process of mandible. The medial pterygoid arises from the medial pterygoid plate and inserts on the lingual surface of mandibular angle and ramus. The lateral pterygoid muscle originates from the lateral pterygoid plate and greater wing of sphenoid and inserts on the pterygoid fovea under the mandibular condyle. The lateral pterygoid is unique among the muscles of mastication because it serves to open the jaw instead of close it.

The mandibular division of the trigeminal nerve (**CNV3**) emerges into the MS from the middle cranial fossa via the **foramen ovale**. CNV3 gives off a masticator branch (motor innervation to the muscles of mastication), a mylohyoid branch (motor innervation to the mylohyoid and anterior digastric muscles), and an auriculotemporal branch (sensory innervation to the skin overlying the parotid gland). The nerve continues as the inferior alveolar nerve, entering the mandible via the **mandibular foramen** on the lingual surface of the mandibular ramus.

The remaining contents of the MS are the inferior alveolar artery and veins (which accompany the inferior alveolar nerve into the mandibular foramen), the **pterygoid venous plexus** (which lies amongst the fibers of the pterygoid muscles), and the ramus and posterior body of the mandible. The posterior teeth are considered part of the oral cavity, not the MS. Remember the TMJ is within the superior aspect of the infrazygomatic MS. Tumefactive TMJ lesions must be considered in the differential diagnosis of MS mass.

Approaches to Imaging Issues of Masticator Space

The answer to the question, "What imaging findings define an MS mass?" depends on what part of the MS is primarily involved. If the lesion is in the infrazygomatic MS, the muscles of mastication, ramus, and posterior body of the mandible are involved. If a larger mass is present, the parapharyngeal fat is displaced posteromedially. If the lesion begins in the suprazygomatic MS, it is within or immediately adjacent to the temporalis muscle in the temporal fossa.

The MS is one of the suprahyoid neck spaces that is connected to the intracranial compartment via a major cranial nerve branch, CNV3. As a result, all MS masses should be assessed for possible **perineural tumor spread (PNT)** along CNV3 into the middle cranial fossa. Squamous cell carcinoma from the chin skin, alveolar ridge, and retromolar trigone may demonstrate PNT spreading through foramen ovale into Meckel cave and beyond. Alternatively, a parotid space malignancy may travel along the **auriculotemporal nerve** to

Differential Diagnosis of Masticator Space

Pseudolesions	Malignant tumor, primary
Asymmetric pterygoid venous plexus	Chondrosarcoma
Asymmetric accessory parotid lobe	Osteosarcoma
Motor denervation CNV3 (acute or chronic)	Synovial sarcoma
Benign masticator muscle hypertrophy	Rhabdomyosarcoma
Infectious	Malignant schwannoma
Odontogenic abscess	Non-Hodgkin lymphoma (primary H&N)
Inflammatory	**Malignant tumor, metastatic**
Postradiation scarring	SCCa from retromolar trigone (direct invasion)
Vascular	SCCa from oral cavity (perineural spread along V3)
Benign tumor	SCCa from nasopharynx (direct spread)
Nodular fasciitis	Systemic hematogenous metastasis
Schwannoma (CNV3)	Non-Hodgkin lymphoma (systemic)
Neurofibroma	Non-Hodgkin lymphoma (direct invasion from jaw primary)
Venous or venolymphatic malformation	Intracranial tumor spread (glioblastoma, meningioma)
Infantile hemangioma	

CNV3, then through foramen ovale to the intracranial compartment.

When CNV3 is injured, the muscles that undergo denervation are the muscles of mastication, the tensor tympani and palatini, anterior belly of the digastric, and the mylohyoid. Remember that in acute-subacute denervation, the muscles often swell and enhance, whereas in more chronic denervation, the muscles lose volume and fatty infiltrate.

There are at least four **pseudolesions** that can mimic pathology in the masticator space. The most challenging of these is the **pterygoid venous plexus**. This structure has a wide range of size in normal individuals. It lies within and around the pterygoid muscles in the medial MS. Asymmetric pterygoid venous plexus can mimic an infiltrative mass or PNT involving the pterygoid muscles.

A second pseudolesion of note is **denervation of the muscles of mastication**. In the acute phase of denervation, the affected muscles may be mistaken for tumor infiltration as they enlarge and enhance. The sparing of the muscle ligaments is an important clue to the true diagnosis. In late denervation, muscular atrophy can be mistaken for a tumor (due to asymmetric normal muscle bulk) on the contralateral side.

Similarly, **benign masticator muscle hypertrophy** is a third potential pseudolesion. This can mimic a mass lesion due to asymmetric enlargement of the muscles of mastication; however, normal muscle attenuation and signal, lack of enhancement, and preserved internal architecture (with normal striated appearance typical of muscle tissue) helps distinguish this pseudolesion from pathology.

Finally, **prominent or asymmetric accessory lobe of the parotid gland** can mimic a mass on clinical examination, especially when asymmetrically enlarged on one side. The accessory lobe typically has the same density or signal and enhancement pattern as the remainder of the parotid gland on CT or MR imaging.

Clinical Implications

A common clinical presentation of a masticator space mass is **trismus**. Trismus is defined as an inability to open the mouth due to masticator muscle spasm or fibrosis. Patients with trismus are notoriously difficult to examine clinically. Imaging plays an even more important role in the assessment of these patients.

The most frequent primary neoplasm of the masticator space is **sarcoma**, either from the mandible or soft tissues. However, extension of **oral cavity SCCa** from the **mandibular alveolar ridge** is far more common than primary masticator space malignancy, so evidence of a mucosal origin should always be sought.

The presence of PNT is critical to the prognosis and care of cancer patients. PNT may require additional surgery, chemotherapy, &/or radiation therapy. If PNT reaches the intracranial compartment, the tumor may be rendered unresectable. Remember that enhanced, fat-saturated MR is far more sensitive than CT for PNT. As a result, MR should be recommended in patients who are at risk for PNT. One final caveat regarding PNT: Only a high degree of suspicion during image analysis will allow the radiologist to make the diagnosis of subtle PNT.

Tumefactive TMJ lesions must also be considered whenever there is a mass found in the peri-TMJ portion of the masticator space. Pigmented villonodular synovitis, calcium pyrophosphate dihydrate deposition disease, and synovial chondromatosis are the principal TMJ lesions that must be added to the list of tumor-like lesions in the masticator space.

Selected References

1. Faye N et al: The masticator space: from anatomy to pathology. J Neuroradiol. 36(3):121-30, 2009
2. Schuknecht B et al: Masticator space abscess derived from odontogenic infection: imaging manifestation and pathways of extension depicted by CT and MR in 30 patients. Eur Radiol. 18(9):1972-9, 2008
3. Wei Y et al: Masticator space: CT and MRI of secondary tumor spread. AJR Am J Roentgenol. 189(2):488-97, 2007
4. Curtin HD: Separation of the masticator space from the parapharyngeal space. Radiology. 163(1):195-204, 1987

Masticator Space Overview

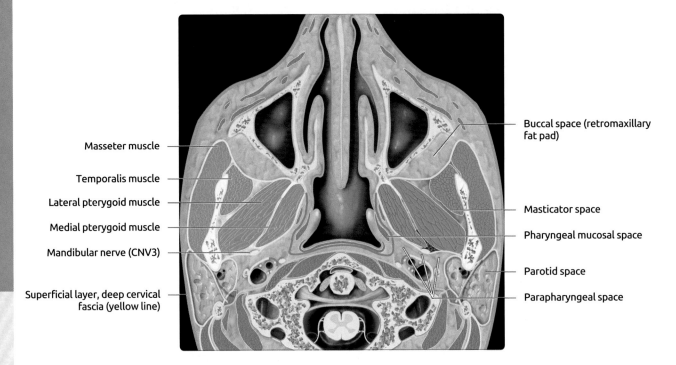

Masseter muscle

Temporalis muscle

Lateral pterygoid muscle

Medial pterygoid muscle

Mandibular nerve (CNV3)

Superficial layer, deep cervical fascia (yellow line)

Buccal space (retromaxillary fat pad)

Masticator space

Pharyngeal mucosal space

Parotid space

Parapharyngeal space

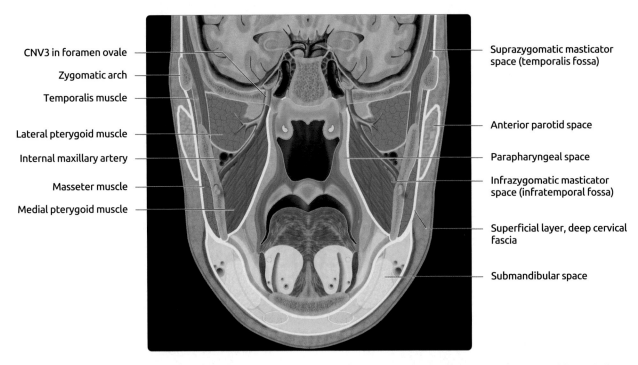

CNV3 in foramen ovale

Zygomatic arch

Temporalis muscle

Lateral pterygoid muscle

Internal maxillary artery

Masseter muscle

Medial pterygoid muscle

Suprazygomatic masticator space (temporalis fossa)

Anterior parotid space

Parapharyngeal space

Infrazygomatic masticator space (infratemporal fossa)

Superficial layer, deep cervical fascia

Submandibular space

(Top) *Axial graphic shows the masticator space (MS) enclosed by the superficial layer (investing layer) of the deep cervical fascia (yellow line). The muscles of mastication from medial to lateral are the medial and lateral pterygoid, temporalis, and masseter muscles. Note the mandibular nerve (CNV3 main trunk) lies just posterior to the medial pterygoid muscle inside the superficial layer of deep cervical fascia. The buccal space is anterior, while the parapharyngeal and parotid space are posterior to the MS. The pharyngeal mucosal space is medial.* (Bottom) *Coronal graphic of the MS shows the suprazygomatic & infrazygomatic components. Note the medial slip of the superficial layer of the deep cervical fascia attaching to the skull base just medial to the foramen ovale, while the lateral slip continues over the zygomatic arch and up the parietal bone.*

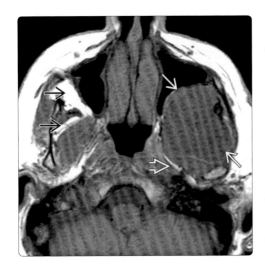
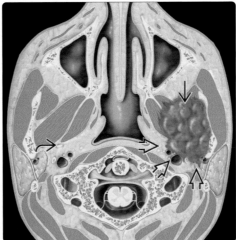

(Left) *Axial T1WI MR shows a large MS mass* ➡️. *Parapharyngeal fat* ➡️ *is displaced posteromedially. The muscles of mastication are invaded, and surrounding fat planes are replaced by tumor. Note preserved fat planes in the contralateral MS* ➡️ *for comparison.* (Right) *Axial graphic shows a generic MS mass* ➡️ *invading the surrounding parapharyngeal space* ➡️ *from anterior to posterior. The mandibular nerve is engulfed by the tumor. Note normal contralateral mandibular nerve* ➡️ *for comparison.*

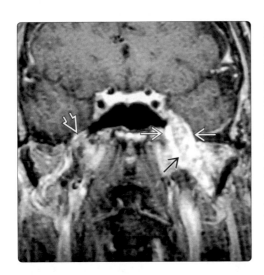
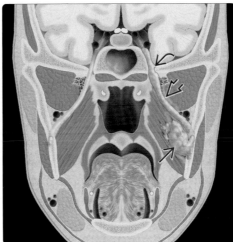

(Left) *Coronal T1WI C+ FS MR shows perineural tumor* ➡️ *along CNV3, widening foramen ovale* ➡️ *as it extends intracranially. Compare the perineural tumor to the opposite normal size of the contralateral foramen* ➡️, *where normal perineural enhancement can be seen.* (Right) *Coronal graphic of the suprahyoid neck demonstrates a generic malignant tumor of the MS* ➡️ *spreading in a perineural fashion along CNV3* ➡️. *Notice the tumor traversing the foramen ovale* ➡️ *into the intracranial compartment.*

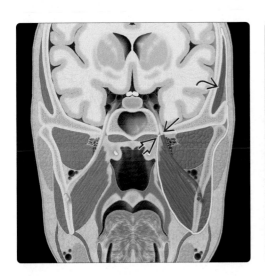
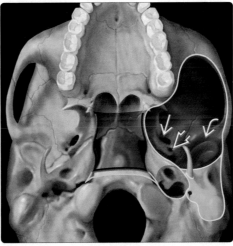

(Left) *Coronal graphic shows craniocaudal extent of MS. CNV3 passes through foramen ovale* ➡️ *near the medial attachment of superficial layer of the deep cervical fascia* ➡️. *Note more superior suprazygomatic MS* ➡️. (Right) *Axial skull base graphic depicts the large area of abutment of the MS (purple). The yellow line around the outer MS margin represents the superficial layer of deep cervical fascia. Note the foramen ovale* ➡️ *& spinosum* ➡️ *and TMJ* ➡️ *within the MS abutment.*

Pterygoid Venous Plexus Asymmetry

TERMINOLOGY

- PVP asymmetry: Unilateral prominence of deep facial venous network draining cavernous sinus
- Usually incidental finding at time of brain or neck imaging

IMAGING

- Tubular enhancing structures in medial masticator space (MS) & parapharyngeal space
- Postcontrast imaging shows identical enhancement to other neck veins
- Relevant imaging anatomy
  - Cavernous sinus drains to PVP through foramina ovale, spinosum, & lacerum
  - PVP also connects with ophthalmic veins through inferior orbital fissure & anterior facial vein via deep facial branch
  - Receives tributaries from pterygopalatine maxillary artery
  - PVP drainage 1: Maxillary vein → retromandibular vein → internal jugular vein (IJV)
  - PVP drainage 2: Posterior & common facial veins → IJV
- Flow signal is often seen in left > right PVP on 3T MRA images in normal patients
  - This may reflect flow reversal and should not be considered indicative of occult DAVF

TOP DIFFERENTIAL DIAGNOSES

- Prominent internal maxillary arterial branches
- Venous vascular malformation
- Perineural V3 tumor, pterygopalatine fossa
- Carotid cavernous fistula

DIAGNOSTIC CHECKLIST

- Consider ipsilateral CCF if there are referable symptoms
- Differentiate PVP asymmetry from CNV3 PNT

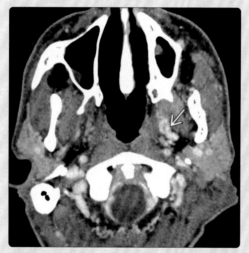 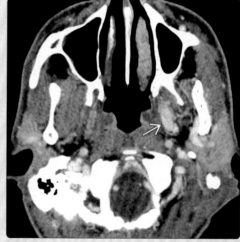

(Left) Axial CECT shows curvilinear enhancement in the medial masticator and parapharyngeal spaces ➡ representing incidental enlarged asymmetric left PVT. Note enhancement is similar density compared to other veins. (Right) Axial CECT at a level just above the previous image shows more mass-like appearance of incidental asymmetric enlarged pterygoid venous plexus ➡. Although this might raise concern for perineural tumor spread, the enhancement does not parallel the expected course of CNV3.

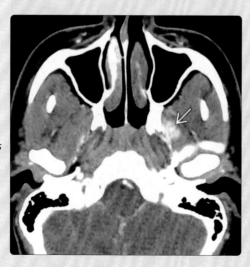 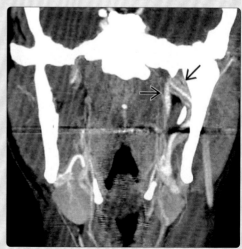

(Left) Axial CECT shows mass-like enhancement in the medial masticator space ➡ representing incidental asymmetric enlargement of the left pterygoid venous plexus. (Right) Coronal CECT reconstructed from the previous axial image better demonstrates the linear converging vascular structures ➡ representing incidental asymmetric enlargement of the left pterygoid venous plexus.

Pterygoid Venous Plexus Asymmetry

TERMINOLOGY

Abbreviations

- Pterygoid venous plexus (PVP) asymmetry

Synonyms

- Pterygoid plexus

Definitions

- Unilateral prominence of deep facial venous network draining cavernous sinus
  - Usually incidental finding at time of brain or neck imaging
    - May be secondary to carotid cavernous fistula (CCF)

IMAGING

General Features

- Best diagnostic clue
  - Tubular enhancing structures in medial masticator space (MS) & parapharyngeal space
- Location
  - PVP is medial to pterygoid muscle of MS & in parapharyngeal spaces (PPS)
- Size
  - Several mm width, runs anteromedially several centimeters
- Morphology
  - Serpiginous structures in deep MS, anterior PPS
- Relevant imaging anatomy
  - Cavernous sinus drains to PVP through foramen ovale, spinosum, & lacerum
  - PVP also connects with ophthalmic veins through inferior orbital fissure & anterior facial vein via deep facial branch
    - Receives tributaries from pterygopalatine maxillary artery
  - PVP drainage
    - Maxillary vein → retromandibular vein → internal jugular vein (IJV)
    - Posterior and common facial veins → IJV

CT Findings

- NECT
  - Poorly seen without contrast
- CECT
  - Asymmetric curvilinear enhancement in MS & PPS
- CTA
  - Thin-slice CTA/CTV may best clarify with venous phase
    - Enhancement identical or similar to other veins

MR Findings

- T1WI
  - Serpiginous flow voids in medial MS & anterior PPS
- T2WI
  - Serpiginous flow voids in medial MS & anterior PPS
- T1WI C+
  - Uniform enhancement of PVP (similar to other veins)
  - Looks like small area of worms
- MRA
  - Flow signal is often seen in left > right PVP on 3T MRA images in normal patients
    - This may reflect flow reversal and should not be considered indicative of occult DAVF

Angiographic Findings

- AP projection best demonstrates drainage of cavernous sinus through skull base to PVP

Imaging Recommendations

- Best imaging tool
  - Either CT or MR may detect this anomaly
- Protocol advice
  - Postcontrast imaging shows identical enhancement to other neck veins
  - Dynamic phase CTA or CTV may best confirm

DIFFERENTIAL DIAGNOSIS

Prominent Internal Maxillary Arterial Branches

- Arise from internal maxillary artery of external carotid artery

Venous Vascular Malformation

- Transspatial lobulated or cystic masses with high T2 signal intensity
- Venous component may have phleboliths

Perineural V3 Tumor, Pterygopalatine Fossa

- Search for perineural tumor (PNT) may yield conspicuous PVP asymmetry
  - Must sort out PNT from PVP asymmetry
  - Linear anatomical nerve course in PNT helps distinguish from serpiginous veins in PVP

Carotid Cavernous Fistula

- Enlarged ipsilateral superior ophthalmic vein, cavernous sinus, & inferior petrosal sinus

CLINICAL ISSUES

Presentation

- Most common signs/symptoms
  - Asymptomatic, incidental CT or MR finding
  - May be produced by a carotid cavernous fistula, symptoms are then of high- or low-flow carotid cavernous fistula

Demographics

- Epidemiology
  - Reasonably frequent finding on brain or neck imaging

Natural History & Prognosis

- If incidental finding, then of no clinical concern
- If related to CCF, requires interventional treatment

DIAGNOSTIC CHECKLIST

Consider

- Differentiate PVP asymmetry from CNV3 PNT
- Consider ipsilateral CCF if there are referable symptoms

SELECTED REFERENCES

1. Kim E et al: MRI and MR angiography findings to differentiate jugular venous reflux from cavernous dural arteriovenous fistula. AJR Am J Roentgenol. 202(4):839-46, 2014

IMAGING

- Smooth, diffuse enlargement of masticator muscles
  - Masseter, temporalis, medial, and lateral pterygoids
  - Masseter muscle most obviously affected
  - Masticator muscles enhance normally
- 50% bilateral, usually asymmetric
- CT: Enlarged, normal-density masticator muscles
  - Cortical thickening affecting mandible & zygomatic arch
- MR: Enlarged, normal-intensity masticator muscles

TOP DIFFERENTIAL DIAGNOSES

- Masticator space (MS) pseudolesion
- MS abscess
- MS sarcoma
- MS squamous cell carcinoma (SCCa)
  - SCCa enters MS directly (from retromolar trigone, palatine tonsil)
  - Skin of chin or mandibular alveolar ridge SCCa enters MS via perineural CNV3 route

PATHOLOGY

- **Bruxism** (nocturnal teeth grinding)
- Habitual gum chewing
- TMJ dysfunction
- Anabolic steroids ± unilateral chewing

CLINICAL ISSUES

- Nontender lateral facial mass that enlarges with jaw clenching
  - Masseter muscle most obvious clinical finding
- Slowly progressive masticator muscle enlargement
- Treatment
  - Surgery only for cosmetic reasons
  - Botulinum toxin A injection
  - Treat TMJ dysfunction

DIAGNOSTIC CHECKLIST

- Enlarged muscle(s) should be isodense (CT) or isointense (MR) to normal skeletal muscle

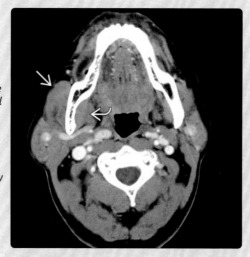
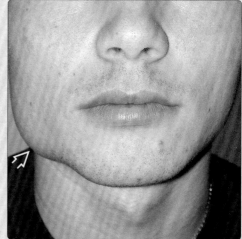

(Left) *Axial CECT demonstrates incidental asymmetric enlargement of the right masseter ➡ and medial pterygoid ➡ muscle. Enhancement and density of these muscles are equal to the opposite side.* (Right) *A clinical photograph demonstrates the clinical appearance of a patient with unilateral benign masticator muscle hypertrophy. Note the broad, smooth cheek bulge secondary to the enlarged masseter muscle ➡.*

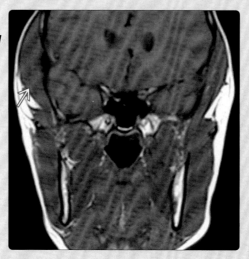
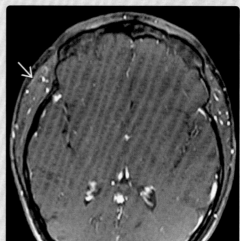

(Left) *Coronal T1 MR shows asymmetric enlargement of the right temporalis muscle ➡ in a young teenager complaining of the cosmetic deformity when wearing her hair pulled back in a ponytail. Although masseter hypertrophy is more common, any muscle can be involved.* (Right) *Axial T1 C+ FS MR shows normal muscle signal intensity in the enlarged right temporalis without enhancement ➡ in the same patient.*

TERMINOLOGY

Abbreviations
- Benign masticator muscle hypertrophy (BMMH)

Synonyms
- Benign masseteric hypertrophy

Definitions
- BMMH: Benign enlargement of muscles of mastication (temporalis, masseter, medial, & lateral pterygoids)

IMAGING

General Features
- Best diagnostic clue
  o Smooth, diffuse enlargement of masticator muscles
- Location
  o Masticator space (MS); masseter muscle most obviously affected
  o 50% bilateral, usually asymmetric

Radiographic Findings
- Radiography
  o May have flaring of mandibular angle with exostosis at masseteric insertion

CT Findings
- NECT
  o Enlarged, normal-density masticator muscles
- CECT
  o Enlarged masticator muscles enhance normally
- Bone CT
  o Cortical thickening of mandible & zygomatic arch

MR Findings
- T1WI
  o Enlarged, normal-intensity masticator muscles
  o Decreased marrow signal in areas of cortical thickening (mandible, zygomatic arch)
- T2WI
  o Enlarged, normal-intensity masticator muscles
- T1WI C+
  o Enlarged masticator muscles enhance normally

Ultrasonographic Findings
- Enlarged masseter muscle with normal echogenicity

Nuclear Medicine Findings
- May have intense FDG uptake on PET

Other Modality Findings
- Sialography: Parotid duct displaced by large masseter

Imaging Recommendations
- Best imaging tool
  o CECT or T1 C+ MR excellent in evaluating MS lesions
- Protocol advice
  o Bone & soft tissue algorithms on CECT data

DIFFERENTIAL DIAGNOSIS

MS Pseudolesion
- Contralateral small masticator muscles make normal MS appear hypertrophic

MS Abscess
- Rim-enhancing fluid in MS ± mandibular osteomyelitis

MS Sarcoma
- Primary malignancy of MS

MS Squamous Cell Carcinoma, Direct Invasion or Perineural Tumor (V3)
- Enters MS directly (retromolar trigone, faucial tonsil)
- Enters MS via perineural V3 from chin skin squamous cell carcinoma (SCCa) or SCCa (mandibular alveolar ridge)

PATHOLOGY

General Features
- Etiology
  o **Bruxism** (nocturnal teeth grinding), gum chewing, TMJ dysfunction
  o Anabolic steroids ± unilateral chewing

Microscopic Features
- Normal skeletal muscle
- Process may involve hyperplasia (↑ number of fibers) rather than true hypertrophy

CLINICAL ISSUES

Presentation
- Most common signs/symptoms
  o Nontender lateral facial mass that enlarges with jaw clenching

Demographics
- Age
  o BMMH usually begins in adolescence
- Gender
  o M:F = 2:1

Natural History & Prognosis
- Slowly progressive masticator muscle enlargement

Treatment
- Surgery only for cosmetic reasons
- Botulinum toxin A injection
- Treat TMJ dysfunction

DIAGNOSTIC CHECKLIST

Image Interpretation Pearls
- Enlarged muscle(s) should be isodense (CT) or isointense (MR) to normal skeletal muscle

SELECTED REFERENCES
1. Andreadis D et al: Bilateral masseter and internal pterygoid muscle hypertrophy: a diagnostic challenge. Med Princ Pract. 23(3):286-8, 2014
2. Connor SE et al: Masticator space masses and pseudomasses. Clin Radiol. 59(3):237-45, 2004
3. Palacios E et al: Benign asymmetric hypertrophy of the masticator muscles. Ear Nose Throat J. 79(12):915, 2000

CNV3 Motor Denervation

TERMINOLOGY

- Abbreviations: Trigeminal nerve (CNV)
- Mandibular nerve: 3rd division of CNV (CNV3) only division with motor function
- CNV3 denervation atrophy: Alteration in appearance of muscle groups from loss of innervation
  - **Acute** (< 1 month): Muscles slightly enlarged with edema; enhancement seen
  - **Subacute** (≤ 12-20 months): Fatty replacement and atrophy begins
  - **Chronic** (> 12-20 months): Fatty atrophic muscles with significant volume loss

IMAGING

- Involved muscles: Masticator space (muscles of mastication), nasopharynx (tensor veli palatini), and anterior belly digastric and mylohyoid muscles
- **Acute**: Increased T2 signal intensity with edema of muscles and abnormal contrast enhancement

- **Subacute**: T2 prolongation and abnormal contrast enhancement (diminishing) with early fatty replacement
- **Chronic**: Fatty infiltration of muscles with volume loss of muscles of mastication
- MR imaging tips
  - Fat saturation/STIR makes ↑ T2 signal more evident
  - Fat saturation on T1 C+ ↑ enhancement visibility

PATHOLOGY

- Malignant or benign tumors involving CNV3
- Surgical trauma 2nd most frequent cause

DIAGNOSTIC CHECKLIST

- 1st determine that CNV3 denervation present by analyzing muscles involved
- 2nd determine cause of CNV3 denervation
- Review history for obvious episodes of trauma or surgery
- If none, malignant tumor must be excluded
  - Search for CNV3 perineural tumor

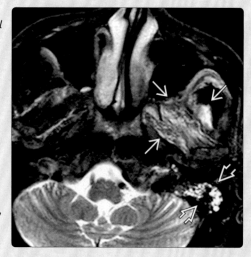
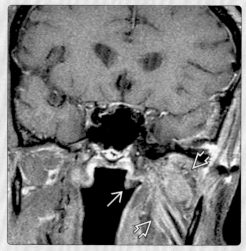

(Left) Axial T2WI FS MR demonstrates increased signal in the pterygoid muscles and deep portion of temporalis muscle ➡. Mastoid opacification ➡ indicates eustachian tube obstruction due to tensor veli palatini dysfunction. This patient had meningioma in Meckel cave (not shown). (Right) Coronal T1WI C+ FS MR in the same patient shows mild pterygoid muscle enhancement ➡ as well as small size of left torus tubarius ➡, consistent with subacute denervation atrophy of CNV3.

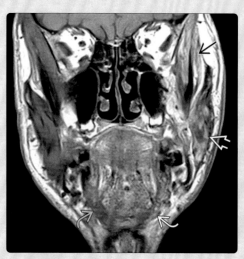
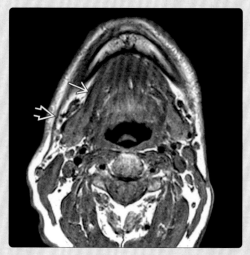

(Left) Coronal T1WI MR reveals chronic fatty atrophy of left temporalis ➡ and masseter ➡ muscle indicating chronic CNV3 injury. Left mylohyoid muscle ➡ is also small with fatty infiltration compared to the normal right ➡. (Right) Axial T1WI MR in the same patient demonstrates the normal right mylohyoid muscle ➡ and platysma muscle ➡. Absence/marked atrophy on the left indicates that both CNV3 (mylohyoid) and CNVII (platysma) are chronically injured.

TERMINOLOGY

Abbreviations

- Trigeminal nerve (CNV)
  - Mandibular nerve: 3rd division (CNV3) of CNV (only division with motor function)

Synonyms

- Denervation atrophy

Definitions

- CNV3 motor denervation: Alteration in appearance of muscle groups from loss of innervation by CNV3
- Denervation pattern identified
  - **Acute** (< 1 month): Muscles slightly enlarged with edema; enhancement seen
  - **Subacute** (≤ 12-20 months): Fatty replacement and atrophy begins
  - **Chronic** (> 12-20 months): Fatty atrophic muscles with significant volume loss

IMAGING

General Features

- Best diagnostic clue
  - Acute: Increased T2 signal intensity with edema of muscles and abnormal contrast enhancement
  - Subacute: T2 prolongation and abnormal contrast enhancement with early fatty replacement
  - Chronic: Fatty infiltration of muscles with volume loss
- Location
  - Most frequently unilateral process
  - **Masticator space** (muscles of mastication), tensor veli palatini in nasopharynx and anterior belly digastric and mylohyoid muscles
  - Ipsilateral parotid atrophy can accompany chronic CNV3 denervation; proposed theories on etiology
    - Involvement of auriculotemporal nerve
    - Disuse atrophy from decreased ipsilateral mastication and decreased salivary flow
- Size
  - Acute: Muscles slightly enlarged
  - Subacute: Muscles may be normal size
  - Chronic: Muscles atrophic
- Morphology
  - Initially muscle edema; later fatty replacement and atrophy
- CNV3 motor innervation
  - Muscles of mastication
    - Medial and lateral pterygoid, masseter, and temporalis muscles
  - Tensor muscles
    - Tensor veli palatini and tensor tympani muscles
  - Mylohyoid and anterior belly digastric muscles

CT Findings

- CECT
  - Acute and subacute CNV3 denervation atrophy
    - Altered density and enhancement may be difficult to identify (MR more sensitive)
  - Chronic CNV3 denervation atrophy
    - Fatty atrophic change readily evident

MR Findings

- T1WI
  - Acute: Reduced muscle signal intensity from edema
  - Subacute: Increased signal intensity starts with fatty replacement
  - Chronic: Increased signal intensity with fatty atrophy
- T2WI
  - Acute: Increased T2 signal intensity of muscles (edema)
  - Subacute: Increased T2 signal intensity (early fat)
  - Chronic: Volume loss and fatty infiltration
- T1WI C+
  - **Acute**: Muscle **enhancement**
  - Subacute: Muscle enhancement more subtle
  - Chronic: No contrast enhancement

Imaging Recommendations

- Best imaging tool
  - MR best characterizes changes of muscles
    - Most sensitive to altered contrast enhancement
  - CT readily identifies chronic fatty atrophic changes
    - Relatively insensitive to earlier changes
- Protocol advice
  - Fat saturation/STIR makes T2 ↑ signal more evident
    - Fat saturation on T1 C+ makes enhancement more evident
  - Contrast distinguishes acute and subacute from chronic

DIFFERENTIAL DIAGNOSIS

Masticator Space Perineural Tumor, CNV3

- Clinical: Usually from SCCa of chin skin, mandible alveolar ridge, deep palatine tonsil
- CT/MR: Thickened, enhancing CNV3
  - If nerve injury present, perineural tumor and CNV3 motor atrophy may coexist

Masticator Muscle Hypertrophy

- Clinical: TMJ dysfunction or bruxism (nocturnal teeth grinding)
- CT/MR: Normal side appears too small compared to hypertrophic muscles
  - Masseter most frequently enlarged of masticator muscles
  - Mylohyoid, anterior belly digastric not affected
  - Normal muscle signal intensity and no abnormal contrast enhancement

Masticator Space Abscess

- Clinical: Presents with pain, fever, and elevated WBC
- CT/MR: Will not involve all muscle groups
  - Look particularly at temporalis, mylohyoid, and digastric muscles
  - Look for dental source of infection

Masticator Space Sarcoma

- Clinical: History of new or treated deep facial malignancy
- CT/MR: Will not involve all muscle groups

PATHOLOGY

General Features

- Etiology

- o Malignant or benign tumors involving mandibular division CNV
- o Surgical trauma 2nd most frequent cause
- o Hemifacial atrophy can rarely occur from unilateral bulbar poliomyelitis infection
- o Infarcts involving pontine trigeminal nucleus may rarely cause isolated trigeminal motor neuropathy and denervation
- Associated abnormalities
  - o Other cranial nerves may also be affected
    - – CNVII, X, XI, ± XII (depending on size/location of offending lesion)
- 2 denervation patterns are recognized
  - o Injury to CNV3 **proximal to** masticator nerve ramification (occurs just after CNV3 emerges from foramen ovale)
    - – All muscles innervated by CNV3 undergo stages of atrophy
      - □ Medial and lateral pterygoid, masseter, temporalis
      - □ Tensor veli palatini and tensor tympani
      - □ Mylohyoid and anterior belly digastric
  - o **Distal to** mandibular nerve ramification
    - – Mylohyoid and anterior belly digastric muscles alone undergo stages of atrophy
    - – Muscles of mastication spared
  - o May be helpful in identifying site of injury
    - – If only mylohyoid and anterior belly of digastric muscle involved, lesion is between skull base and mandibular foramen
    - – If all CNV3 innervated muscles involved, lesion is between root exit zone of lateral pons and foramen ovale

Gross Pathologic & Surgical Features

- Loss of muscle bulk and tone with fatty change

Microscopic Features

- Denervated muscle shows relatively increased tissue water
- Atrophy of muscle fibers develops in subacute to chronic phases with fatty infiltration
- Denervated, atrophic muscle shows greater concentration of capillaries for muscle volume

CLINICAL ISSUES

Presentation

- Most common signs/symptoms
  - o Difficulty chewing
  - o In chronic atrophy, facial asymmetry from masseter muscle volume loss visible
  - o Denervation difficult to detect clinically
    - – Paralysis, loss of tone and reflexes, fasciculations
  - o MR STIR signal intensity changes precede electromyography (EMG) changes
- Other signs/symptoms
  - o Serous otitis media from eustachian tube dysfunction with tensor veli palatini denervation

Demographics

- Age: Adults due to ↑ H&N tumors + surgery vs. children
- Epidemiology: CNV most frequent of cranial nerves to show motor denervation

Natural History & Prognosis

- With peripheral neuropathies, acute and subacute changes may resolve spontaneously or with nerve grafting
  - o Not so with cranial neuropathies
  - o Cranial nerve grafting does not significantly reverse CNV3 atrophy
- Acute denervation signal intensity and contrast enhancement pattern expected to progress to chronic pattern with time

Treatment

- No effective treatment

DIAGNOSTIC CHECKLIST

Consider

- If CNV3 atrophy is discovered without known cause, search for causal lesion must be completed

Image Interpretation Pearls

- 1st determine that CNV3 denervation is present by analyzing muscles involved
  - o Look at all muscles innervated by CNV3
    - – Muscles of mastication
    - – Mylohyoid, anterior belly digastric muscles
    - – Tensor veli palatini dysfunction → small torus tubarius and ipsilateral middle ear/mastoid fluid
    - – Tensor tympani dysfunction not apparent by imaging
- Next determine cause of CNV3 denervation
  - o Review history for obvious episodes of trauma or surgery
    - – If none, malignant tumor must be excluded
      - □ Check for perineural CNV3 malignancy
      - □ Check for masticator space malignancy
      - □ Follow course of CNV from lateral pons to mandibular foramen
- Finally look for MR evidence of other CN dysfunction (especially CNVII, X-XII)

SELECTED REFERENCES

1. Kim DH et al: Pure motor trigeminal neuropathy in a woman with tegmental pontine infarction. J Clin Neurosci. 20(12):1792-4, 2013
2. Chong V: Imaging the cranial nerves in cancer. Cancer Imaging. 4 Spec No A:S1-5, 2004
3. Kato K et al: Motor denervation of tumors of the head and neck: changes in MR appearance. Magn Reson Med Sci. 1(3):157-64, 2002
4. Fischbein NJ et al: MR imaging in two cases of subacute denervation change in the muscles of facial expression. AJNR Am J Neuroradiol. 22(5):880-4, 2001
5. Russo CP et al: MR appearance of trigeminal and hypoglossal motor denervation. AJNR Am J Neuroradiol. 18(7):1375-83, 1997
6. Davis SB et al: Masticator muscle enhancement in subacute denervation atrophy. AJNR Am J Neuroradiol. 16(6):1292-4, 1995
7. Petersilge CA et al: Denervation hypertrophy of muscle: MR features. J Comput Assist Tomogr. 19(4): 596-600, 1995
8. Fleckenstein JL et al: Denervated human skeletal muscle: MR imaging evaluation. Radiology. 187(1):213-8, 1993
9. Uetani M et al: Denervated skeletal muscle: MR imaging. Work in progress. Radiology. 189(2): 511-5, 1993
10. Schellhas KP: MR imaging of muscles of mastication. AJR Am J Roentgenol. 153(4):847-55, 1989
11. Polak JF et al: Magnetic resonance imaging of skeletal muscle. Prolongation of T1 and T2 subsequent to denervation. Invest Radiol. 23(5): 365-9, 1988
12. Shabas D et al: Magnetic resonance imaging examination of denervated muscle. Comput Radiol. 11(1): 9-13, 1987
13. Harnsberger HR et al: Major motor atrophic patterns in the face and neck: CT evaluation. Radiology. 155(3):665-70, 1985

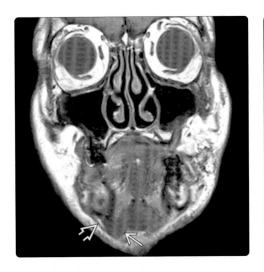

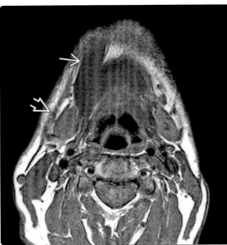

(Left) *Coronal T1WI MR reveals normal right anterior belly of digastric muscle ➡ and platysma muscle ➡. The left-sided mylohyoid and platysma are poorly seen as a result of chronic CNV3 and CNVII injury, respectively.* (Right) *Axial T1WI MR in the same patient shows a normal right anterior belly of digastric muscle ➡ and normal platysma muscle ➡. Both muscles on the left have undergone fatty atrophy and are not visible. Skull base malignant tumor was found affecting the foramen ovale and geniculate fossa.*

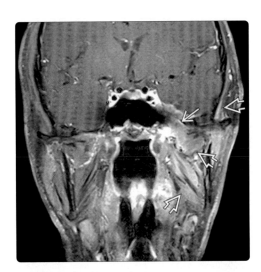

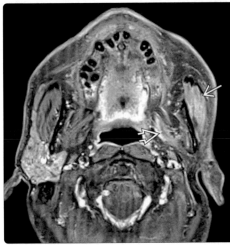

(Left) *Coronal T1WI FS enhanced MR reveals adenoid cystic carcinoma spreading intracranially through the foramen ovale ➡. Subacute masticator muscle denervation ➡ causes muscle enhancement.* (Right) *Axial T1WI FS MR in the same patient demonstrates masseter ➡ and lateral pterygoid ➡ muscle enhancement typical of subacute denervation. Muscles are beginning to lose volume, indicating that they are in the late subacute phase of denervation.*

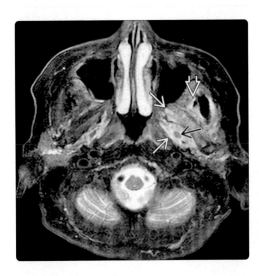

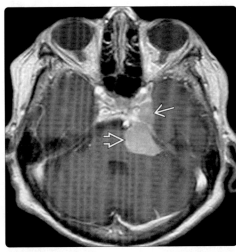

(Left) *Axial T2WI FS MR demonstrates T2 hyperintensity and swelling in pterygoid ➡ and temporalis ➡ muscles, indicating acute to subacute denervation atrophy. The mandibular nerve ➡ is visible here as a lower signal intensity structure within the masticator space.* (Right) *Axial T1WI C+ MR in the same patient shows cavernous sinus ➡ and prepontine cistern ➡ meningioma, which is the cause of the denervation changes. Imaging findings of CNV schwannoma would appear similar.*

Masticator Space Abscess

TERMINOLOGY

- Abscess in masticator space (MS) from molar tooth infection or following dental procedure

IMAGING

- **CECT** preferred imaging modality in suspected infection
- **Focal fluid density** within muscles of mastication with thick **enhancing rim** = MS abscess
  - Adjacent muscles are swollen, enhancing without associated fluid = myositis
- Bone CT findings
  - Tooth radiolucency or extraction socket ± gas
  - Osteomyelitis: Periosteal elevation ± cortical erosion
- Soft tissue and bone algorithm CECT is best imaging approach in acutely infected patients with trismus

TOP DIFFERENTIAL DIAGNOSES

- Cellulitis-phlegmon of MS
- Mandibular osteonecrosis
- Masticator muscle atrophy
- TMJ degenerative disease
- Masticator muscle hypertrophy
- Sarcoma of MS

CLINICAL ISSUES

- Principal symptom: Trismus
- Initial presentation may be confused clinically with TMJ disease (i.e., TMJ pain and trismus)
- Early MS abscess treated with involved molar extraction + aggressive IV antibiotics
- Late abscess treatment: Surgical drainage + IV antibiotics

DIAGNOSTIC CHECKLIST

- Questions for radiologist to answer in MS abscess
  - What is potential source (offending tooth)?
  - Is mandibular osteomyelitis present?
  - Is MS only space with abscess?
  - Is suprazygomatic MS involved?

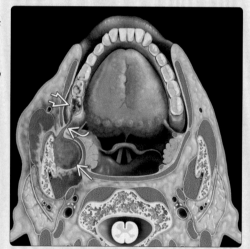
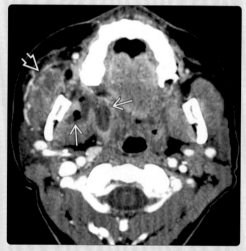

(Left) *Axial graphic depicts masticator space (MS) abscess ➡ arising from infected posterior mandibular molar tooth ➡. Notice the fistula tract ➡ leading from tooth to abscess.* (Right) *Axial CECT in a 31 year old presenting with facial swelling, pain, and trismus demonstrates right medial MS abscess containing gas ➡. There is inflammatory change in the lateral MS with edema and enlargement of the masseter muscle ➡.*

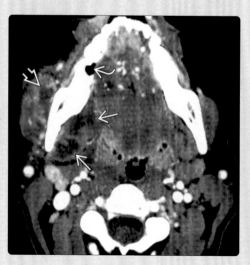
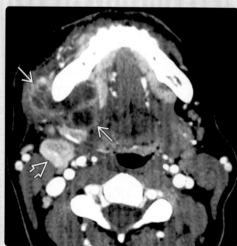

(Left) *Axial CECT in the same patient shows further inferior extent of the medial MS abscess ➡ as well as lateral MS abscess ➡. Dental caries involving posterior molar tooth is the origin of this patient's infection ➡.* (Right) *Axial CECT in the same patient reveals inferior extension of abscess into the right submandibular space ➡. There is reactive level II lymphadenopathy present ➡.*

TERMINOLOGY

Definitions

- Masticator space (MS) abscess: Abscess within MS usually arises from molar tooth (odontogenic) infection or following dental procedure

IMAGING

General Features

- Best diagnostic clue
  - CECT: **Fluid with enhancing wall** within MS ± posterior mandibular osteomyelitis
- Location
  - Lower MS adjacent to posterior body and ramus of mandible
- Size
  - Early abscess: Often small (1 cm) fluid collection adjacent to mandible
  - Late, severe MS abscess: May be many centimeters, filling entire MS and beyond
- Morphology
  - Ovoid to round
  - If breaks into adjacent deep facial spaces, may be lobulated and irregular

CT Findings

- CECT
  - MS mass lesion with compression of parapharyngeal space from anterolateral to posteromedial
  - Focal fluid density within muscles of mastication with thick enhancing rim = **MS abscess**
    - Adjacent muscles are swollen, enhancing without associated fluid = **myositis**
    - Adjacent fatty planes are "dirty" = **cellulitis**
  - **Linear markings** in subcutaneous fat and thickening of skin when associated help differentiate infection from malignant tumor
- Bone CT
  - Typically 2nd or 3rd molar tooth infection ± findings of posterior body and ramus mandible osteomyelitis
    - **Mandibular osteomyelitis**: Cortical destruction with periosteal elevation
    - **Signs of molar tooth infection or suggesting dental source**
      - □ Empty socket (from extraction) ± gas
      - □ Radiolucency ± gas involving tooth itself (caries) ± periodontal lucency surrounding molar tooth root
      - □ Fistula = radiolucent line leading from tooth area through bone into adjacent soft tissue
- CTA
  - If abscess extends to parapharyngeal or retropharyngeal spaces, proximal internal carotid artery (ICA) may show **spasm**

MR Findings

- T1WI
  - Low-signal fluid adjacent to mandible
- T2WI
  - Focal high-signal fluid collections = MS abscess
- DWI
  - High signal (low ADC) characteristic of abscess

- T1WI C+
  - Focal low-signal area surrounded by enhancing wall defines MS abscess
  - Sinus tract from mandible may be visible
- MRA
  - If MS abscess has spread to involve either parapharyngeal or retropharyngeal spaces, ICA spasm may be seen
    - More common in children, usually self-limited

Nuclear Medicine Findings

- Bone scan
  - Can be used to follow mandibular osteomyelitis response to antibiotic therapy

Dental X-Ray or Panorex

- Moth-eaten posterior mandibular body in vicinity of decaying molar tooth with associated root abscess

Imaging Recommendations

- Best imaging tool
  - **CECT** preferred imaging modality in suspected infection
    - Better assessment of dentition, bones, and foci of gas
    - MR less specific for dental infection and osteomyelitis
- Protocol advice
  - CECT viewed in soft tissue and bone algorithm is best imaging approach in setting of acutely infected patient with trismus (limited jaw movement)
    - Rapid scan time, important for sick patient
    - Shows extent of soft tissue abscess cavity
    - Identifies offending tooth and extent of osteomyelitis if not obscured by dental amalgam artifact

DIFFERENTIAL DIAGNOSIS

Cellulitis-Phlegmon of MS

- Clinical: Painful, swollen MS; same as with MS abscess
- Imaging: Swollen MS with cellulitis, myositis ± fasciitis **without** focal rim-enhancing fluid

Mandibular Osteonecrosis

- Clinical: Usually associated with prior H&N radiation therapy or bisphosphonate use
  - **Radionecrosis** in setting of **prior H&N radiation**
    - Imaging: Permeative-destructive change of mandible bone ± soft tissue swelling
    - Rarely fluid with enhancing wall
      - □ May require needle aspiration to exclude infection
  - **Bisphosphonate-related osteonecrosis of jaws**
    - Bisphosphonates (IV or oral) are used to treat metabolic bone disorders, primary or metastatic bone tumors, and hypercalcemia of malignancy
    - Imaging: Osseous sclerosis on CT ranging from subtle thickening of lamina dura and alveolar crest to attenuated osteopetrosis-like sclerosis
      - □ May also be associated with infection

Masticator Muscle Atrophy

- Clinical: Mandibular branch of CNV injured
- Imaging: Muscle of mastication atrophy with normal side appearing enlarged

TMJ Degenerative Disease

- Clinical: TMJ pain and trismus
- Imaging: Degenerative findings in TMJ; no MS abscess seen

Masticator Muscle Hypertrophy

- Clinical: Asymmetric chewing, TMJ disease, or nocturnal grinding
- Imaging: Masticator muscles show unilateral enlargement
  - No focal rim-enhancing fluid or other cellulitis, myositis, or fasciitis

Sarcoma of MS

- Clinical: Rock-hard cheek mass ± CNV symptoms
- Imaging: Infiltrating MS mass with significant enhancement and minimal adjacent skin or soft tissue changes
  - Lacks cellulitis, myositis, or fasciitis to suggest infection

PATHOLOGY

General Features

- Etiology
  - Dental infection (molar) from caries ± periodontal disease or dental manipulation spreads via cortical dehiscence, rupturing pus into MS ± osteomyelitis of posterior body of mandible
- Anatomic considerations
  - Superficial layer, deep cervical fascia circumscribes MS tissues
  - MS contains muscles of mastication, posterior body, ramus and condyle of mandible, and CNV3 as it passes into mandibular foramen
  - 2nd and 3rd molar abut anterior surface of MS
  - Temporal fossa = suprazygomatic MS
  - Infratemporal fossa = nasopharyngeal MS + retromaxillary fat pad (high posterior buccal space)

Gross Pathologic & Surgical Features

- Irregular cystic lesion filled with green-white, thick fluid (pus) surrounded by thick wall made up of fibrous connective tissue
- Surrounding tissues are edematous

CLINICAL ISSUES

Presentation

- Most common signs/symptoms
  - Principal symptom: **Trismus**
  - Other signs/symptoms
    - Fever, high white blood cell count
    - Tender, swollen cheek
    - History of **bad dentition** or recent **dental manipulation** common
    - Physical exam: Tenderness and limited mouth opening makes examination difficult
    - CECT becomes critical part of physical exam when patient cannot open mouth
- Other signs/symptoms
  - Initial presentation may clinically mimic **TMJ disease** (i.e., TMJ pain and trismus)

Demographics

- Age
  - Increasing incidence with increasing age
  - Dental problems generally increase in older people
- Epidemiology
  - Common cause of MS lesion
  - In countries where antibiotics and dental care are readily available, MS involvement rare
  - When dental care and antibiotics are unavailable, MS abscess from dental decay is common

Natural History & Prognosis

- Previous oral antibiotic treatment has inadequately treated simmering MS infection
- After termination of oral antibiotic, clinical recrudescence occurs
- Adequate drainage of pus leads to rapid cure
- Potential source of deep neck infection or necrotizing fasciitis if untreated

Treatment

- Remove decayed molars 1st
- Aggressive intravenous antibiotics for early abscess
- Surgical drainage combined with intravenous antibiotics needed in most cases
- Mandibular osteomyelitis may require subperiosteal drain and prolonged intravenous antibiotics

DIAGNOSTIC CHECKLIST

Consider

- Questions for radiologist to answer in MS abscess
  - What is potential source (offending tooth)?
  - Is mandibular osteomyelitis present?
    - If so, requires more extensive surgical intervention and protracted antibiotic therapy
  - Is MS only space with abscess?
    - Surgeon needs 1 drain per space or break through adjacent fascia
  - Is suprazygomatic MS involved?
    - Infection tends to spread upward because superficial layer, deep cervical fascia is firmly attached to inferior margin of mandible below

Image Interpretation Pearls

- Differentiate cellulitis in MS from abscess
- If subtle fluid is seen, consider delayed CECT
  - Multidetector CT may finish data acquisition before contrast reaches abscess wall
  - If so, existing abscess may be missed

SELECTED REFERENCES

1. Kos M: Incidence and risk predictors for osteonecrosis of the jaw in cancer patients treated with intravenous bisphosphonates. Arch Med Sci. 11(2):319-24, 2015
2. Schuknecht B et al: Masticator space abscess derived from odontogenic infection: imaging manifestation and pathways of extension depicted by CT and MR in 30 patients. Eur Radiol. 18(9):1972-9, 2008
3. Jones KC et al: Chronic submasseteric abscess: anatomic, radiologic, and pathologic features. AJNR Am J Neuroradiol. 24(6):1159-63, 2003
4. Yonetsu K et al: Deep facial infections of odontogenic origin: CT assessment of pathways of space involvement. AJNR Am J Neuroradiol. 19(1):123-8, 1998
5. Kim HJ et al: Odontogenic versus nonodontogenic deep neck space infections: CT manifestations. J Comput Assist Tomogr. 21(2):202-8, 1997
6. Hardin CW et al: Infection and tumor of the masticator space: CT evaluation. Radiology. 157(2):413-7, 1985
7. Braun IF et al: Computed tomography of the buccomasseteric region: 2. Pathology. AJNR Am J Neuroradiol. 5(5):611-6, 1984

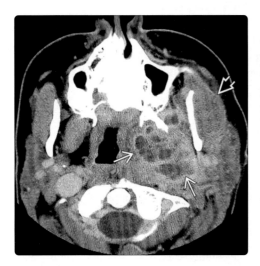
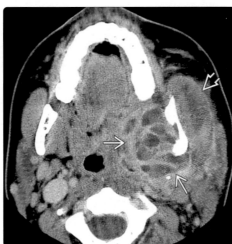

(Left) *Axial CECT demonstrates a large, multiloculated medial MS abscess involving the pterygoid musculature ➡. Note edema and swelling in the masseter muscle in the lateral MS ➡. The patient is a 21-year-old woman who underwent a left molar tooth extraction 9 months previously. Since then, she has complained of trismus and otalgia misdiagnosed as TMJ syndrome.* (Right) *Axial CECT in the same patient shows further inferior extent of medial MS abscess ➡ and masseter edema ➡.*

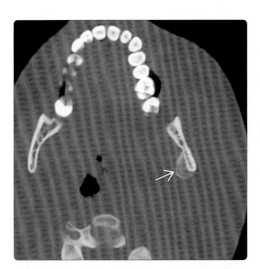
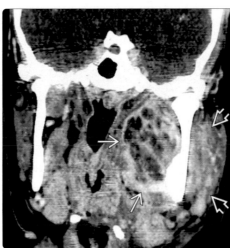

(Left) *Axial bone CT in the same patient reveals periosteal new bone formation indicative of mandibular osteomyelitis ➡.* (Right) *Coronal CECT in the same patient demonstrates medial MS multiloculated abscess ➡ and lateral MS masseter muscle edema and enlargement ➡.*

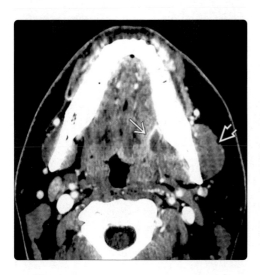
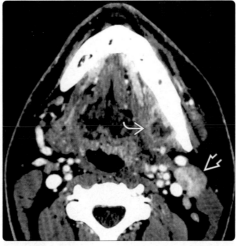

(Left) *Axial CECT in a 22 year old with infected molar tooth not responding to antibiotic treatment presenting with pain, swelling, and trismus demonstrates left medial MS abscess involving the inferior aspect of the medial pterygoid muscle ➡ with masseter muscle myositis ➡.* (Right) *Axial CECT in the same patient reveals inferior spread of abscess into the left submandibular space ➡. Level II reactive lymphadenopathy is also seen ➡.*

TERMINOLOGY

- CNV3 schwannoma: Encapsulated tumor of Schwann cell origin, which displaces rather than infiltrates fascicles of CNV3 in masticator space (MS)

IMAGING

- Well-circumscribed, smoothly marginated soft tissue mass along course of CNV3
- Bone CT findings
  - **Smooth enlargement of bony foramen** involved
  - Foramen ovale most commonly enlarged
  - Mandibular foramen, inferior alveolar nerve canal, or mental foramen enlargement occurs with distal CNV3 schwannoma
- Enhanced MR findings
  - Homogeneous or heterogeneous enhancement
  - **Intramural cysts** are characteristic of schwannoma
  - Masticator muscle atrophy possible

TOP DIFFERENTIAL DIAGNOSES

- **CNV3 neurofibroma**
- **Perineural tumor** CNV3 in MS
- CNV3 **malignant nerve sheath tumor**
- Keratocystic odontogenic tumor (odontogenic keratocyst)
- Ameloblastoma

CLINICAL ISSUES

- Treatment: Surgery, gamma knife, or observation

DIAGNOSTIC CHECKLIST

- Mass in MS without history of H&N SCCa or infection (MS abscess) should suggest sarcoma
  - Sarcoma may mimic CNV3 schwannoma if centered on CNV3
  - Rapid growth suggests malignancy
- **Well-circumscribed, fusiform, or ovoid mass following course of CNV3 suggests schwannoma**

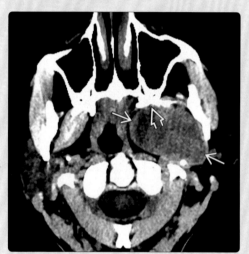
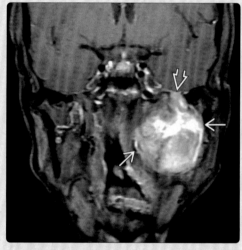

(Left) Axial NECT in a patient with CNV3 schwannoma shows a circumscribed, heterogeneous, solid mass in the left masticator space ➡ with remodeling of the pterygoid plates ➡ suggesting a slow-growing lesion. (Right) Coronal T1 C+ FS MR in the same patient demonstrates a heterogeneously enhancing masticator space schwannoma ➡ minimally projecting intracranially through an enlarged foramen ovale ➡.

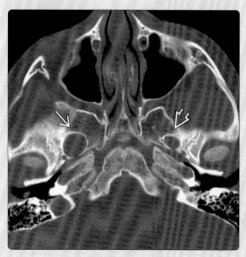
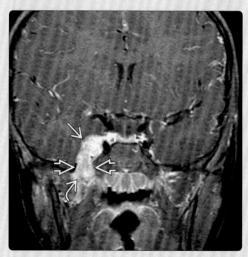

(Left) Axial bone CT in a patient with known neurofibromatosis type 2 reveals a large right foramen ovale ➡. Note the normal left foramen ovale ➡. This foraminal enlargement with preservation of its cortical margin is characteristic of benign nerve sheath tumors. (Right) Coronal T1 C+ FS MR in the same patient shows a tubular, enhancing CNV3 schwannoma coursing from the parasellar region ➡ through the enlarged foramen ovale ➡ into the nasopharyngeal masticator space ➡.

TERMINOLOGY

Abbreviations

- Masticator space (MS) CNV3 (mandibular branch, trigeminal nerve) schwannoma

Synonyms

- Neuroma, neurilemmoma, neurinoma

Definitions

- Encapsulated tumor of Schwann cell, which displaces rather than infiltrates fascicles of CNV3 in MS

IMAGING

General Features

- Best diagnostic clue
  - Well-circumscribed, smoothly marginated soft tissue mass along course of CNV3 branch of CNV
- Location
  - From Meckel cave to MS along CNV3
  - Rarely affects CNV3 branches (inferior alveolar or mental nerves)
- Morphology
  - Ovoid to fusiform/tubular

Radiographic Findings

- Radiography
  - Enlargement of inferior alveolar nerve canal or mental foramen on plain films, panorex, or bite-wing films

CT Findings

- CECT
  - Lesion enhances mildly to moderately
  - Homogeneous or heterogeneous enhancement
- Bone CT
  - **Smooth enlargement** of bony foramen involved
    - **Foramen ovale** most commonly enlarged

MR Findings

- T1WI
  - Isointense or hypointense to muscles of mastication
  - Variable signal if hemorrhage or cysts present
  - Masticator muscle denervation may be present
- T2WI
  - Variable, isointense to hyperintense
    - More cellular tumors, isointense to muscle
  - Myxoid or cystic changes: ↑ signal intensity
  - Hypointense foci (blood) common in larger tumors
- T1WI C+
  - Homogeneous or heterogeneous enhancement
    - **Intramural cysts** somewhat characteristic
  - Sometimes rim enhances, lesion appear mostly cystic

Imaging Recommendations

- Best imaging tool
  - T1WI C+ FS MR in axial & coronal plane

DIFFERENTIAL DIAGNOSIS

CNV3 Neurofibroma

- Neurofibromatosis type 1; rarely isolated

Perineural Tumor CNV3 in Masticator Space

- Typically known SCCa from chin skin, mandibular alveolar ridge, oral tongue, oropharynx

CNV3 Malignant Nerve Sheath Tumor

- Invasive mass centered on CNV3 within MS

Keratocystic Odontogenic Tumor

- Unilocular or multilocular cystic lesion of mandible
- Lesion envelops or incorporates crown & tooth root

Ameloblastoma

- Bubbly, multilocular, cystic-solid tumor, mandible or maxilla

PATHOLOGY

General Features

- Etiology
  - Unknown in sporadic cases
- Genetics
  - Associated with neurofibromatosis type 2 (NF2)
    - Mutation on chromosome 22

Microscopic Features

- Proliferating Schwann cells in collagenous matrix with fibrous capsule
- 2 Antoni tissue types (may coexist in single lesion)
  - Antoni A type: Compact, hypercellular
  - Antoni B type: Looser architecture; cystic changes
- Cystic degeneration (intramural cysts) common

CLINICAL ISSUES

Presentation

- Most common signs/symptoms
  - Most common asymptomatic neoplasm in deep facial soft tissues
    - Even large lesions may be asymptomatic
  - Other signs/symptoms
    - Atypical facial pain, ↓ chin sensation

Demographics

- Age
  - Predominantly 3rd-4th decade
    - Younger in patients with NF2
- Epidemiology
  - Peripheral CNV3 schwannomas account for 5% of all trigeminal schwannomas

Natural History & Prognosis

- Gradually enlarging masticator space mass

Treatment

- Options, risks, complications
  - Some cases may be managed conservatively (observed)
- Surgical resection (open & endoscopic techniques used)
- Gamma knife

SELECTED REFERENCES

1. Agarwal A: Intracranial trigeminal schwannoma. Neuroradiol J. 28(1):36-41, 2015
2. Majoie CB et al: Primary nerve-sheath tumours of the trigeminal nerve: clinical and MRI findings. Neuroradiology. 41(2):100-8, 1999

TERMINOLOGY

- Perineural tumor (PNT) of masticator space (MS) is malignant spread along CNV3 (mandibular branch of trigeminal nerve)

IMAGING

- PNT occurs along all or part of V3 from mental foramen to lateral pons root entry zone of CNV
  - Nerve enlarged; may reach 1 cm in diameter
  - CNV3 may be normal size in early PNT
- Bone CT findings
  - **Enlarged** mandibular **inferior alveolar canal, mandibular foramen, foramen ovale**
- MR findings
  - Coronal T1 C+ best shows CNV3 abnormal enhancing PNT
  - Fat saturation (FS) ↑ conspicuity of PNT
  - T1 MR without contrast and **without FS** useful for obliteration of fat pads below foramen ovale

- CECT less sensitive for PNT; MR recommended
- MR very sensitive but not specific for CNV3 PNT

TOP DIFFERENTIAL DIAGNOSES

- Normal pterygoid venous plexus asymmetry
- Normal vasa nervosa CNV3
- CNV3 schwannoma
- CNV3 neurofibroma
- Skull base meningioma

CLINICAL ISSUES

- **Often asymptomatic (40%)**
- Lower face paresthesias, numbness, MS denervation

DIAGNOSTIC CHECKLIST

- Primary malignancies that may yield CNV3 PNT
  - Skin cancers of chin & jaw (SCCa, BCC, melanoma)
  - Oral cavity or pharynx primaries (SCCa, ACC)
  - MS malignancy (sarcoma, non-Hodgkin lymphoma)
  - Parotid primary (spread via auriculotemporal nerve)

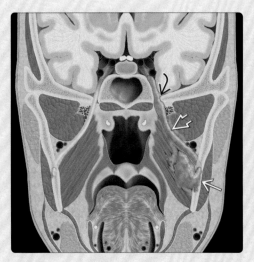
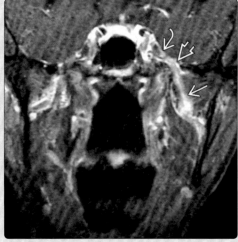

(Left) Coronal graphic depicts classic example of malignant masticator space tumor ➡ with perineural V3 spread ➡ through foramen ovale ⊡ into intracranial compartment. (Right) Patient presents with a history of treated buccal space adenoid cystic carcinoma. New chin numbness creates concern for perineural CNV3 recurrence. Coronal T1WI C+ MR reveals perineural tumor involving CNV3 in nasopharyngeal masticator space ➡, passing through foramen ovale ➡, & beginning to invade Meckel cave ➡.

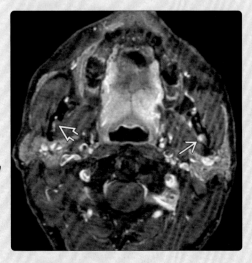
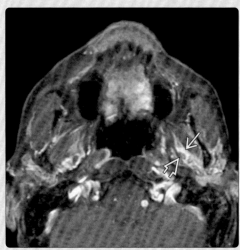

(Left) Axial T1WI C+ FS MR in the same patient demonstrates the perineural tumor at the mandibular foramen ➡. Notice the minimal enhancement in the contralateral mandibular foramen ➡. Clearly if the radiologist does not look for this specific finding, the observation of perineural tumor will not be made. (Right) Axial T1WI C+ FS MR in the same patient shows enhancing perineural tumor ➡ surrounding the CNV3 ➡ on its way to the foramen ovale.

TERMINOLOGY

Abbreviations

- Perineural tumor (PNT) of masticator space (MS) is malignant spread along CNV3 (mandibular branch of trigeminal nerve)

Synonyms

- PNT spread, PNT invasion
- Trigeminal ganglion = gasserian ganglion, semilunar ganglion

Definitions

- CNV3: 3rd division of trigeminal nerve (CNV)
- CNV3 PNT: Extension of malignancy along CNV3 allowing spread from MS though foramen ovale into Meckel cave (MC)
- MC: Small cistern for CNV
  - Contains trigeminal ganglion in anterior aspect of MC

IMAGING

General Features

- Best diagnostic clue
  - T1 C+ MR shows **enlarged enhancing CNV3**
- Location
  - PNT can occur along all or segments of CNV3 from mental foramen to root entry zone of CNV on lateral pons
    - **Inferior alveolar nerve**: In inferior alveolar canal from mental foramen to mandibular foramen
    - **Mandibular branch, CNV3**: Extends from mandibular foramen to foramen ovale in MS
    - **Foramen ovale**: Skull base foramen through which CNV3 passes
    - **MC**: Cistern inferior & lateral to cavernous sinus; contains trigeminal ganglion
    - **Preganglionic segment CNV**: Spans distance from MC to root entry zone on lateral pons
- Size
  - Nerve usually enlarged; may reach 1 cm in diameter
  - Nerve may be normal in size early
- Morphology
  - Linear, along expected course of CNV3

CT Findings

- CECT
  - CNV3 enhancement & enlargement
  - Abnormal enhancement of enlarged cavernous sinus & MC
- Bone CT
  - Enlarged inferior alveolar canal in mandible
  - Widened mandibular foramen
  - Foramen ovale enlargement

MR Findings

- T1WI
  - Infiltration of MS muscle & fat surrounding CNV3
  - Tissue within mandibular foramen; intermediate to low signal replacing marrow fat of mandibular ramus
  - Obliteration of fat pad below foramen ovale
  - Enlargement of CNV3

  - Early edema in MS muscles with chronic fatty atrophy
- T2WI
  - Enlarged MC with loss of normal fluid signal
  - ↑ signal of edematous nerve difficult & unreliable sign
- T1WI C+
  - Enlarged, enhancing extracranial CNV3
    - Inferior alveolar canal of mandible (inferior alveolar nerve)
    - Mandibular foramen to foramen ovale (mandibular nerve)
  - Enhancement of nerve in foramen ovale
    - Normal nerve: Low signal
    - Beware vasa nervosa (veins accompanying nerve)
    - Beware normal pterygoid venous plexus enhancement
  - Enlargement, enhancement of MC
  - Enhancing MS muscles (acute-subacute CNV3 denervation)

Nuclear Medicine Findings

- PET
  - Uptake along CNV3 often difficult to differentiate from brain & primary tumor
  - Combined PET/CT useful; not as good as MR

Imaging Recommendations

- Best imaging tool
  - CECT less sensitive for PNT; MR recommended
  - MR very sensitive but not specific for CNV3 PNT
    - Normal nerves asymmetrically enhance in 5% of patients
- Protocol advice
  - Coronal T1 C+ best shows CNV3 abnormal enhancing PNT
    - Good quality FS ↑ conspicuity of PNT
    - Beware FS susceptibility artifacts that obscure PNT
  - Coronal T1 MR without contrast and **without FS** useful for obliteration of fat pads below foramen ovale

DIFFERENTIAL DIAGNOSIS

Pterygoid Venous Plexus Asymmetry

- Normal venous plexus in & around pterygoid muscles in MS
- May extend to foramen ovale but does not enter
- Asymmetry common

CNV3 Schwannoma in Masticator Space

- Benign neoplasm of CNV3 nerve sheath
- Intermediate T1, heterogeneously bright T2
- Heterogeneous enhancement with intramural cysts possible
- When crossing foramen ovale, dumbbell-shaped on coronal images
- May arise anywhere along course of CNV

CNV3 Neurofibroma

- Uncommon site for neurofibroma
- When crossing foramen ovale, dumbbell-shaped on coronal images
- Uniform enhancement
- May follow branches of CNV3

Normal Skull Base Marrow Around Foramen Ovale

- Marrow fat in skull base around foramen ovale has inherent high T1 signal
- High T1 signal alongside foramen ovale
- Dark cortical bone separates marrow from nerve within foramen
- T1 FS clarifies fat vs. enhancement

Skull Base Meningioma

- Benign neoplasm of brain coverings
- Isodense to brain on T1 & T2 images
- Uniform, brisk enhancement
- May extend into foramen ovale & beyond

Vasa Nervosa CNV3

- Normal small veins accompanying CNV3 through foramen ovale
- Vague peripheral enhancement on T1 C+ MR
- Nerve itself remains dark on T1 C+ MR

Normal Fat Pad, CNV3

- Fat pads normally seen at exit points of cranial nerves
- High inherent T1 signal surrounding nerve
- Does not extend into foramen ovale
- T1 C+ FS MR or compare T1 C+ MR to T1 MR without contrast to clarifiy fat vs. enhancement

PATHOLOGY

General Features

- Etiology
  - "Path of least resistance" for tumors predisposed to PNT spread
  - Tumor expression of nerve growth factor or neural cell adhesion molecules may correlate with propensity to PNT spread
- Tumor may spread outside nerve sheath or involve support tissues within sheath (endoneurium, perineurium, epineurium)
- Any malignant tumor may undergo PNT spread

Gross Pathologic & Surgical Features

- Enlargement of nerve complex
- Encasement-replacement of CNV3

Microscopic Features

- Perineural spread = gross pathologic or radiographic diagnosis of tumor along nerve
- Perineural invasion = microscopic finding of tumor within nerve bundles

CLINICAL ISSUES

Presentation

- Most common signs/symptoms
  - **Often asymptomatic (40%)**
  - Paresthesias of lower face
  - Jaw pain or numbness
  - Masticator muscle denervation atrophy

Demographics

- Age

- 50-80 years (reflects demographics of common primary tumors)
- Gender
  - M > F, because squamous cell carcinoma (SCCa) more common in men
- Epidemiology
  - Tumors with greatest propensity for PNT spread
    - **Adenoid cystic carcinoma (ACC)**
    - **SCCa, pharynx or skin**
    - Desmoplastic melanoma, skin
    - Non-Hodgkin lymphoma
    - Mucoepidermoid carcinoma
    - Basal cell carcinoma (BCC)

Natural History & Prognosis

- PNT spread strongly affects patient prognosis
- **PNT is very poor prognostic sign**
  - ↑ local recurrence
  - ↑ distant metastases
  - ↑ meningeal carcinomatosis
  - ↓ survival
- Cranial nerve defects unlikely to resolve with therapy

Treatment

- Radiotherapy ± surgery and chemotherapy

DIAGNOSTIC CHECKLIST

Consider

- Primary malignancy sites of origin that may yield CNV3 PNT spread
  - **Skin of chin & jaw** (SCCa, melanoma, or BCC)
  - **Alveolar ridge, retromolar trigone** (deep tonsillar & nasopharyngeal SCCa)
  - MS malignancy (sarcoma, non-Hodgkin lymphoma)
  - Parotid malignancy (especially ACC)
    - May spread from CNVII along **auriculotemporal nerve** to CNV3
- Some CNV3 PNT patients have no known primary
  - Patients with remote skin cancer history may not recall or mention prior diagnosis

Image Interpretation Pearls

- Inspect CNV from mental foramen of mandible to root entry zone of lateral pons
  - Look for asymmetric CNV3 enlargement & enhancement
  - Axial & coronal **T1 C+ FS MR ↑** lesion conspicuity
    - Remove FS if susceptibility artifacts obscure PNT
- Do not confuse pterygoid venous plexus with PNT
  - Look for CNV3 nerve enhancement to distinguish
- Beware of "**skip lesions**"
  - Normal nerve between noncontiguous areas of PNT

SELECTED REFERENCES

1. Singh FM et al: Patterns of spread of head and neck adenoid cystic carcinoma. Clin Radiol. 70(6):644-53, 2015
2. Curtin HD: Detection of perineural spread: fat suppression versus no fat suppression. AJNR Am J Neuroradiol. 25(1):1-3, 2004
3. Ginsberg LE: MR imaging of perineural tumor spread. Magn Reson Imaging Clin N Am. 10(3):511-25, vi, 2002

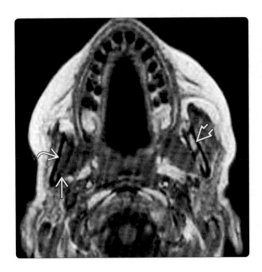

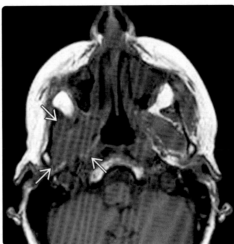

(Left) *Axial T1WI MR in a patient presenting with a history of previously treated nasopharyngeal squamous cell carcinoma shows replacement of the normal marrow fat in the right mandibular ramus ➡ & abnormal soft tissue at the level of mandibular foramen ➡ related to perineural tumor spread along CNV3. Note normal high-signal marrow fat in left mandibular ramus ➡.* (Right) *Axial T1WI MR in the same patient shows CNV3 perineural tumor spread with obliteration of normal fat planes in masticator space ➡.*

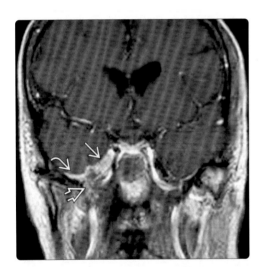

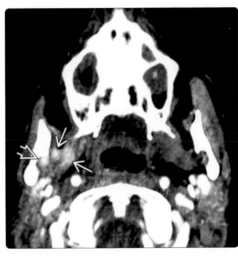

(Left) *Coronal T1WI C+ MR in the same patient demonstrates perineural tumor extending along CNV3 through the foramen ovale ➡ and into Meckel cave ➡. There is also spread of tumor laterally along the dura ➡ of the middle cranial fossa.* (Right) *Axial CECT in the same patient shows enhancing tumor in the right mandibular foramen ➡ as well as areas of abnormal enhancement along the mandibular branch of CNV3 in the masticator space ➡.*

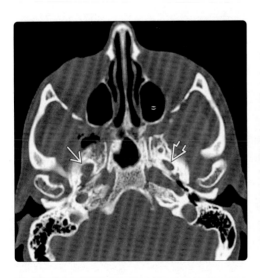

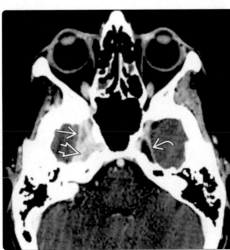

(Left) *Axial bone CT reveals an enlarged right foramen ovale ➡ compared to the normal left foramen ovale ➡. CNV3 perineural tumor is responsible for the foramen enlargement.* (Right) *Axial CECT shows that the perineural CNV3 tumor has extended through foramen ovale into Meckel cave ➡ and the middle cranial fossa ➡. Note the normal CSF density Meckel cave on the left ➡.*

Masticator Space Chondrosarcoma

TERMINOLOGY

- Chondrosarcoma (CSa), masticator space (MS)

IMAGING

- Enhancing soft tissue mass in MS in or adjacent to mandible with variable calcification (Ca^{++}) pattern
- Molar region and ramus most frequent in mandible
- May extend down from skull base or TMJ
- CT shows characteristic Ca^{++}, but MR better delineates extent of tumor
- Bone CT findings
  - **Radiolucent lesion ± areas of Ca^{++}**
  - Rings and crescents of calcium: Low-grade tumors
  - Amorphous or no Ca^{++}: High-grade tumors
  - When using CECT, view bone windows
- MR findings
  - Greater T1 C+ enhancement in high-grade CSa
  - T1 C+ heterogeneous, predominantly peripheral enhancement

- Invasion of bone best delineated on T1 without contrast
- High signal typical on T2
  - Extraosseous CSa tends to have intermediate signal
  - Flow voids may be present in extraosseous CSa

TOP DIFFERENTIAL DIAGNOSES

- MS infection
- TMJ synovial chondromatosis
- Odontoma
- Mandibular ossifying fibroma
- Mandibular fibrous dysplasia
- Mandibular osteosarcoma

DIAGNOSTIC CHECKLIST

- Infection far more common than sarcoma in MS
  - Consider infection 1st if no Ca^{++} present
- MS masses should be followed to resolution to ensure that they are not sarcomas

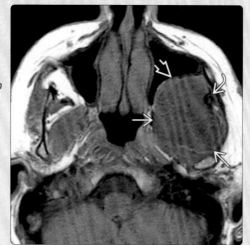
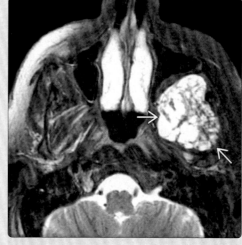

(Left) *Axial T1WI MR shows intermediate-signal mass ➜ distending the masticator space and causing anterior bowing of posterior wall of the left maxillary sinus ➡. A large focal calcification is seen as low signal intensity on all sequences ➡.* **(Right)** *Axial T2WI MR in the same patient shows the mass ➜ with characteristic pronounced T2 hyperintensity of chondroid tumors.*

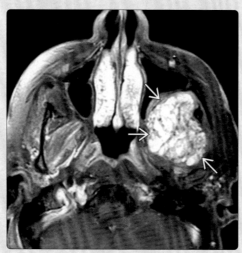
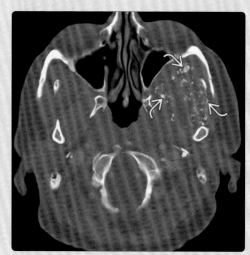

(Left) *Axial T1WI C+ MR in the same patient shows the tumor ➜ is generally heterogeneous with intense enhancement with gadolinium.* **(Right)** *Axial CECT in bone window in the same patient shows a large mass with intrinsic calcifications ➡, which are "fluffy," with rings and arcs. These are typical of chondroid calcifications. Chondrosarcoma with visible chondroid calcifications usually indicates low-grade tumor is present.*

Masticator Space Chondrosarcoma

TERMINOLOGY

Abbreviations

- Chondrosarcoma (CSa)

Definitions

- CSa-masticator space (MS): Malignant tumor of cartilage that originates in MS

IMAGING

General Features

- Best diagnostic clue
  - Enhancing soft tissue mass in MS in or adjacent to mandible with variable calcification (Ca^{++}) pattern
- Location
  - Adjacent to (inseparable from) bone of origin
  - Mandible, molar region, and ramus most frequent
  - May extend down from skull base or TMJ
  - Extraosseous CSa without bony involvement is uncommon (2%)
- Size
  - At presentation, most > 3 cm
- Morphology
  - Round with lobular margin
  - Soft tissue mass may be well circumscribed

Radiographic Findings

- Radiography
  - Symmetrically widened periodontal space on panoral radiographs

CT Findings

- CECT
  - Heterogeneous, predominantly peripheral enhancement
- Bone CT
  - Mass with ill-defined osseous borders and long zone of transition
  - Shows radiolucent lesion ± areas of **Ca^{++}**
    - Presence and degree of Ca^{++} depends on tumor grade
    - **Rings and crescents** of Ca^{++} most characteristic of **low-grade tumors**
    - **Amorphous Ca^{++}** or no Ca^{++} typical of **high-grade tumors**
  - Erosion of bone of origin and surrounding bones (e.g., skull base)
  - Widening of joint (when arising from TMJ)
  - Periosteal reaction usually mild, if present

MR Findings

- T1WI
  - Homogeneous intermediate signal
  - Cartilage matrix or Ca^{++} make signal heterogeneous
  - Invasion of bone best delineated on unenhanced T1WI
    - Replacement of marrow fat
- T2WI
  - **High signal** most typical on **T2**
    - Extraosseous CSa tends to have intermediate signal
    - Flow voids may be present in extraosseous CSa
  - Homogeneous or heterogeneous, depending on degree and type of Ca^{++}

- Marrow, soft tissue edema may be seen
- T1WI C+
  - Enhancement may be focal (often peripheral) or diffuse
  - Extent of enhancement depends on tumor grade
    - Greater T1 C+ MR enhancement in high-grade CSa

Imaging Recommendations

- Best imaging tool
  - CT shows characteristic Ca^{++}, but MR better delineates extent of tumor
- Protocol advice
  - When using CECT, view bone windows
    - Bone CT most likely to show characteristic Ca^{++}

DIFFERENTIAL DIAGNOSIS

Masticator Space Infection

- Most frequent cause of MS mass
- Usually of dental origin
- Noncalcifying CSa-MS may mimic MS infection on imaging

TMJ Synovial Chondromatosis

- TMJ filled with tiny loose bodies
- Multiple foci of free cartilage, variably calcified
- Grains of rice appearance
- Abnormalities usually confined to expanded synovial cavity but can erode skull base

Odontoma

- Compound variant: Small teeth identified within mass
- Complex variant: Amorphous Ca^{++} with areas of dense enamel

Mandibular Ossifying Fibroma

- Benign solitary jaw tumor
- Radiodense periphery surrounding fibrous center
- Characteristic stellate Ca^{++} pattern

Mandibular Fibrous Dysplasia

- Expanded bone with characteristic matrix
- Ground-glass and cystic patterns, usually in combination
- Expansile, rather than erosive like CSa-MS
- Confined to bone without soft tissue mass

Mandibular Osteosarcoma

- Most frequent MS sarcoma of bone
- Cumulus cloud pattern of new bone formation
- Sunburst pattern of periosteal reaction
- Osteosarcoma has poorer prognosis than CSa-MS

Mandibular Metastasis

- Ca^{++} seen in lung, prostate, breast, colon metastases
- Amorphous Ca^{++} of mucinous metastases may be confused with chondroid calcification
- Sites of metastasis include jaw, skull base, soft tissues

PATHOLOGY

General Features

- Etiology
  - CSa-MS mostly sporadic (75%)
  - Predisposing conditions
    - Osteochondroma

- – Enchondroma
- – Ollier disease
- – Maffucci syndrome
- – Paget disease
- – Fibrous dysplasia
- – Synovial chondromatosis
- – Radiation exposure
- – Thorotrast exposure
- CSa-MS may or may not occur at cartilaginous joints (TMJ)
  - TMJ CSa represents tumoral differentiation of pluripotent mesenchymal cells

Staging, Grading, & Classification

- Osseous vs. extraosseous
- Central (medullary) vs. peripheral (juxtacortical)
- Primary vs. secondary (secondary = associated with enchondroma or osteochondroma)
- Histological subtype
  - Conventional
  - Myxoid
  - Clear cell
  - Mesenchymal
  - Dedifferentiated
- Histologic grade
  - Grade I (well-differentiated): Ca++ and bone formation frequent
  - Grade II (moderately differentiated): Matrix more myxoid than chondroid
  - Grade III (poorly differentiated): No matrix, high mitotic rate (rare)

Gross Pathologic & Surgical Features

- Firm, nodular mass
- Tan-white to opalescent blue-gray
- Gross hemorrhage in high-grade tumors

Microscopic Features

- Matrix of lobular hyaline cartilage
- Multinucleated lacunes with variable nucleoli
- May be difficult to distinguish from chondroblastic osteosarcoma
- Low-grade neoplasms hard to distinguish from enchondroma

CLINICAL ISSUES

Presentation

- Most common signs/symptoms
  - Expanding, painless preauricular mass
    - – Rate of enlargement depends on tumor grade
    - – May be mistaken for parotid mass
  - Other signs/symptoms
    - – Headache
    - – Loose teeth
    - – CNV3 dysfunction
    - – CSa arising from TMJ often painful

Demographics

- Age
  - Any age
  - 30-45 years most common
- Epidemiology

- 2nd most common malignancy of bone (after osteosarcoma, excluding multiple myeloma)
- CSa = 15% of malignant bone tumors
- 5-10% of CSa occur in H&N
  - – Larynx, jaws, facial bones, skull base, TMJ affected
  - – Orbit more common location in children

Natural History & Prognosis

- Local recurrence problematic (50%)
  - Late recurrence (10-20 years) possible
- Metastases unusual (7%)
- 5-year overall survival: 68% (90% grade I; 50% combined grades II and III)
- Overall prognosis depends on tumor grade, size at presentation
  - Lower survival if systemic metastases present at presentation
- May dedifferentiate into osteosarcoma, malignant fibrous histiocytoma, or fibrosarcoma

Treatment

- Wide local excision
- Role of radiation, chemotherapy, cryosurgery, and immunotherapy are controversial and evolving

DIAGNOSTIC CHECKLIST

Consider

- Infection far more common than sarcoma in MS
  - If no calcifications, consider infection 1st
- If MS mass without clinical suggestion of infection, consider tumor as possibility
  - 1st consider perineural tumor on V3 from squamous cell carcinoma (SCCa) of chin skin, mandibular alveolar ridge, retromolar trigone
  - If no evidence for SCCa invasion of MS, then consider primary MS sarcoma

Image Interpretation Pearls

- MS masses should be followed to resolution to ensure that they are not sarcomas
- Unless characteristic calcifications seen, variable appearance of CSa makes precise diagnosis difficult
  - Suggestion of tumor is critical; exact pathology can be determined at surgery

SELECTED REFERENCES

1. Meltzer DE et al: Masticator space: imaging anatomy for diagnosis. Otolaryngol Clin North Am. 45(6):1233-51, 2012
2. Murphey MD et al. Imaging of primary chondrosarcoma: radiologic-pathologic correlation. RadioGraphics 23:1245-1278. 2003
3. Gorsky M et al: Craniofacial osseous and chondromatous sarcomas in British Columbia--a review of 34 cases. Oral Oncol. 36(1):27-31, 2000
4. Koch BB et al: National cancer database report on chondrosarcoma of the head and neck. Head Neck. 22(4):408-25, 2000
5. Saito K et al: Chondrosarcoma of the jaw and facial bones. Cancer. 76(9):1550-8, 1995
6. Ormiston IW et al: Chondrosarcoma of the mandible presenting as periodontal lesions: report of 2 cases. J Craniomaxillofac Surg. 22(4):231-5, 1994
7. Wanebo HJ et al: Head and neck sarcoma: report of the Head and Neck Sarcoma Registry. Society of Head and Neck Surgeons Committee on Research. Head Neck. 14(1):1-7, 1992
8. Garrington GE et al: Chondrosarcoma. II. Chondrosarcoma of the jaws: analysis of 37 cases. J Oral Pathol. 17(1):12-20, 1988

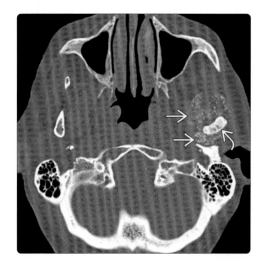

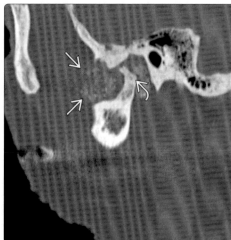

(Left) *Axial bone CT of typical chondrosarcoma through the left TMJ reveals irregular sclerotic appearance of mandibular condyle ➡ and multiple small, focal calcifications ➡ within and around the joint. Although this may be difficult to distinguish from synovial chondromatosis, both are treated surgically, and histology can confirm.* **(Right)** *Sagittal reformat in the same patient shows condylar deformity ➡ and also suggests that some of the calcifications ➡ reside within a soft tissue component outside the joint.*

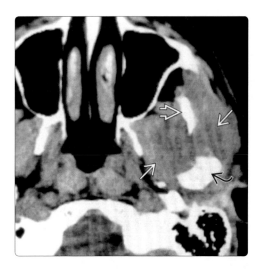

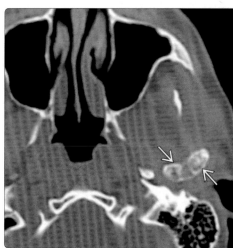

(Left) *CECT with soft tissue window, in a variant case of masticator space chondrosarcoma without calcifications, shows a low-density mass ➡ surrounding the ramus of the mandible, extending around the coronoid process ➡ and condyle ➡.* **(Right)** *Axial bone CT shows expansion of the condyle and neck of the mandible containing chondroid calcifications ➡. The absence of the characteristic calcifications of chondrosarcoma in the soft tissue component makes the diagnosis difficult in this case.*

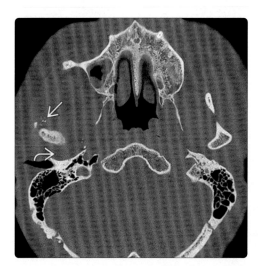

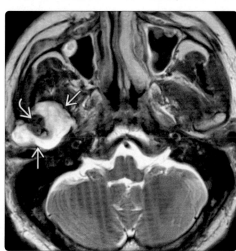

(Left) *Typical axial bone CT in a case of low-grade TMJ chondrosarcoma shows small, dystrophic calcifications or calcified matrix of this mass ➡ with extensive remodeling/destruction of glenoid fossa ➡.* **(Right)** *Axial T2WI MR in the same patient demonstrates that the lobulated mass ➡ is markedly hyperintense but with well-defined margins. Mass clearly surrounds condyle ➡.*

Masticator Space Sarcoma

TERMINOLOGY

- Sarcoma, masticator space (SA-MS): Malignant tumor of soft tissue origin (fat, muscle, nerve, joint, blood vessel, or deep skin tissues) in MS of suprahyoid neck

IMAGING

- Aggressive, poorly marginated MS mass with bone destruction and invasion of adjacent fascial planes/spaces
- Imaging recommendations: Thin-section bone CT and C+ MR
- Bone CT: Allows assessment of SA matrix ± bone destructive changes
  - **Bone production** or **calcification** can be present in any SA
  - **Invasive MS mass** with **bone destruction**
- MR: Evaluation of soft tissues, possible mandibular invasion
  - Perineural tumor spread along CNV3

TOP DIFFERENTIAL DIAGNOSES

- MS abscess
- Mandibular osteomyelitis
- Invasive SCCa
  - Palatine tonsil SCCa, retromolar trigone SCCa
- Mandible metastasis
- MS venous malformation
- Keratocystic odontogenic tumor
- Perineural tumor of CNV3 in MS

CLINICAL ISSUES

- Enlarging soft tissue mass over mandible with ↑ pain
- Mean age: 35 years old
- SA location, in addition to pathology and TNM stage, is important when planning treatment

DIAGNOSTIC CHECKLIST

- Absent known malignancy or infectious signs, MS mass should suggest diagnosis of SA

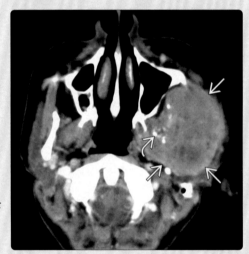
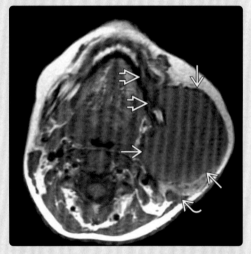

(Left) Axial CECT shows a large, heterogeneous, centrally necrotic mass ➡ with scattered coarse calcifications ➔ in the masticator space (MS). The lesion surrounds the mandible and engulfs the medial and lateral pterygoid muscles, the temporalis, and the masseter muscle. (Right) Axial T1WI MR in the same patient shows the mass ➡ to be slightly hyperintense relative to normal sternocleidomastoid muscle ➔. Loss of marrow fat within the mandible ➔ suggests tumor infiltration.

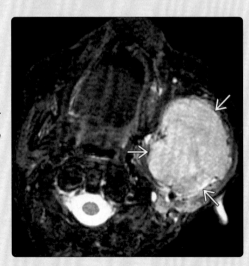
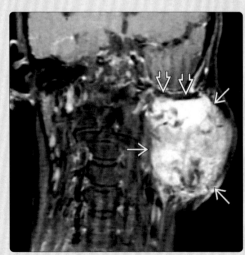

(Left) Axial T2WI MR in the same patient shows the mass ➡ is diffusely increased in signal. (Right) Coronal T1WI C+ FS MR in the same patient shows heterogeneous enhancement of the mass ➡, which abuts the skull base ➔. This patient had a history of prior irradiation, putting them at risk for radiation-induced sarcoma (SA). In this case, the lesion was an unusual tumor, an undifferentiated pleomorphic SA.

TERMINOLOGY

Synonyms

- Sarcoma, masticator space (SA-MS)
- Many types: Rhabdomyosarcoma, leiomyosarcoma, Ewing sarcoma, synovial sarcoma, liposarcoma, fibrosarcoma

Definitions

- SA-MS: Malignant tumor of soft tissue origin (fat, muscle, nerve, joint, blood vessel, or deep skin tissues) in MS of suprahyoid neck

IMAGING

General Features

- Best diagnostic clue
  o Aggressive, poorly marginated MS mass with bone destruction and invasion of adjacent fascial planes-spaces
- Location
  o MS; frequently extends outside of MS
- Size
  o Often **large** (> 4 cm) despite superficial MS location
- Morphology
  o Poorly marginated ± multilobulated

CT Findings

- CECT
  o Variable enhancement pattern
    – Typically heterogeneous
- Bone CT
  o **Invasive MS mass** with mandibular, zygomatic arch, or pterygoid plate **destruction**
    – Jaw osteosarcomas show soft tissue extension in most (86%)
  o **Bone production** or **calcification** can be present in any SA
    – Most commonly seen in osteosarcoma (72%), chondrosarcoma, synovial and Ewing SA
    – Periosteal reaction seen in 62% of jaw osteosarcoma

MR Findings

- T1WI
  o Iso- to hyperintense to normal muscle, often heterogeneous
  o Mandible involvement shows replacement of normal marrow signal
- T2WI
  o Heterogeneously hyperintense to muscle
- STIR
  o Heterogeneously hyperintense to muscle
- DWI
  o Quantitative ADC values may help distinguish between infection and SA
  o Suggested ADC value cutoff = 1.20 x 10-3 mm² s-1
    – Higher values suggest infection
    – Lower values suggest malignancy
- T1WI C+
  o Heterogeneous enhancement is typical

Nuclear Medicine Findings

- Bone scan

- Tc-99m can assist with evaluation
- PET
  o F-18 fluorodeoxyglucose (FDG) avid
  o Role in directing biopsy, predicting tumor grade, and assessing treatment response under investigation

Imaging Recommendations

- Best imaging tool
  o Thin-section bone CT combined with T1 C+ MR
    – MR for evaluation of soft tissues, possible mandibular invasion, and evaluation for **perineural tumor spread along CNV3**
    – Bone CT allows assessment of SA matrix ± bone destructive changes

DIFFERENTIAL DIAGNOSIS

Masticator Space Abscess

- Rim-enhancing MS fluid collection ± mandibular osteomyelitis

Mandibular Osteomyelitis

- Bony destruction without osteoid formation
- May see sequestrum formation

Invasive Squamous Cell Carcinoma

- Palatine tonsil squamous cell carcinoma (SCCa)
  o Palatine tonsil mass invades subjacent MS
- Retromolar trigone SCCa
  o Retromolar triangle mass invades MS

Mandible Metastasis

- Aggressive bony destructive changes
- Without periosteal reaction or tumoral calcification

Masticator Space Venous Malformation

- Multiloculated mass with possible flow voids and calcified phleboliths

Keratocystic Odontogenic Tumor (Odontogenic Keratocyst)

- Cystic mass arising from mandible with benign expansile changes

Perineural Tumor of CNV3 in Masticator Space

- Chin skin SCCa or SCCa primary of oral cavity or oropharynx
- Malignancy spreads along CNV3 into MS

PATHOLOGY

General Features

- Etiology
  o **Ionizing radiation** (most commonly from XRT to treat other tumors)
    – Accounts for < 5% of SAs
    – 10 years is average time between XRT and SA diagnosis
  o Family history
    – Gardner syndrome: Risk of desmoid tumors (low-grade fibrosarcoma) in abdomen
    – Li-Fraumeni syndrome: Increased risk of developing soft tissue SAs and bone SAs
    – Retinoblastoma (inherited form): Increased risk of developing bone or soft tissue SAs

- o Nodal injury
  - − Lymphangiosarcomas rarely found following surgical nodal dissection or in XRT fields
- Genetics
  - o DNA mutations common in soft tissue SA

Staging, Grading, & Classification

- Histologic grading system
  - o G1: Microscopically normal tissue (slow growing)
  - o G2: Microscopically similar to normal tissue (somewhat faster growing)
  - o G3: Microscopically only slightly similar to normal tissue (faster growing)
  - o G4: Microscopically abnormal (fastest growing)
- T-staging system
  - o T1: Tumor < 5 cm
  - o T2: Tumor > 5 cm
    - − a: Superficial tumor
    - − b: Deep tumor
- American Joint Committee on Cancer anatomic stages/prognostic groups
  - o Stage IA: G1-2, T1 (a or b), N0, M0
  - o Stage IB: G1-2, T2a, N0, M0
  - o Stage IIA: G1-2, T2b, N0, M0
  - o Stage IIB: G3-4, T1 (a or b), N0, M0
  - o Stage IIC: G3-4, T2a, N0, M0
  - o Stage III: G3-4, T2b, N0, M0
  - o Stage IVA: Any G, any T, N1, M0
  - o Stage IVB: Any G, any T, any N, M1

Gross Pathologic & Surgical Features

- Pathologic findings depend on SA type
- Heterogeneous mass with ossified (yellow-white, firm) and nonossified components (soft, tan, with foci of hemorrhage ± necrosis)
- Periosteal reaction: Lamellae of new bone at lesion periphery

Microscopic Features

- Low-grade lesions
  - o Few mitotic figures, little if any cellular atypia, and relatively noninfiltrative growth pattern
- High-grade lesions
  - o Marked cellular atypia, hyperchromatism, nuclear pleomorphism, and infiltrative growth pattern

CLINICAL ISSUES

Presentation

- Most common signs/symptoms
  - o Enlarging soft tissue mass over mandible with increasing pain
  - o Other signs/symptoms
    - − Cranial nerve deficits common if skull base involved

Demographics

- Age
  - o Mean: 35 years old
- Gender
  - o M:F = 2:1
- Epidemiology
  - o About 8,000 new cases per year in USA

Natural History & Prognosis

- Stage I = 5-year survival: 99%; recurrence: 20%
- Stage II = 5-year survival: 80%; recurrence: 35%
- Stage III = 5-year survival: 50%; recurrence: 65%
- Stage IVB = 5-year survival: 10%

Treatment

- SA location, in addition to pathology and TNM stage, is important when planning treatment
  - o Multimodality treatment usually recommended
- Stage I: Surgically removed; XRT may be added if inadequate margins
  - o XRT may be utilized primarily if tumor unresectable (i.e., encasing critical structures)
- Stage II: Surgical excision with 2-cm normal margin is goal
  - o Pre- or postoperative XRT common, chemotherapy less commonly given
- Stage III: Surgery and XRT commonly used with chemotherapy to reduce recurrences
- Stage IV: Surgery and XRT, with metastatic surgical excision
- Experimental treatments, such as interleukin-2 immunotherapy, are being researched
- Possible role for adjuvant chemotherapy in unusual cases
- Radiofrequency ablation has been used in recurrent rhabdomyosarcoma

DIAGNOSTIC CHECKLIST

Consider

- Absent known systemic malignancy or signs of infection, MS mass should suggest diagnosis of SA
- Mandibular destruction ± perineural tumor spread along CNV3 toward skull base both suggest SA diagnosis from imaging perspective

Image Interpretation Pearls

- CT or MR of MS mass suspected of being malignant
  - o Carefully evaluate inferior alveolar canal, mandibular foramen, foramen ovale, and remainder of CNV3 course for perineural tumor spread

SELECTED REFERENCES

1. Abdel Razek AA et al: Role of diffusion-weighted MRI in differentiation of masticator space malignancy from infection. Dentomaxillofac Radiol. 42(4):20120183, 2013
2. Wang S et al: Osteosarcoma of the jaws: demographic and CT imaging features. Dentomaxillofac Radiol. 41(1):37-42, 2012
3. Makimoto Y et al: Imaging findings of radiation-induced sarcoma of the head and neck. Br J Radiol. 80(958):790-7, 2007
4. Pandey M et al: Soft tissue sarcoma of the head and neck region in adults. Int J Oral Maxillofac Surg. 32(1):43-8, 2003
5. Potter BO et al: Sarcomas of the head and neck. Surg Oncol Clin N Am. 12(2):379-417, 2003
6. Folpe AL et al: (F-18) fluorodeoxyglucose positron emission tomography as a predictor of pathologic grade and other prognostic variables in bone and soft tissue sarcoma. Clin Cancer Res. 6(4):1279-87, 2000
7. Patel SG et al: Radiation induced sarcoma of the head and neck. Head Neck. 21(4):346-54, 1999
8. Som PM et al: A re-evaluation of imaging criteria to assess aggressive masticator space tumors. Head Neck. 19(4):335-41, 1997
9. Lyos AT et al: Soft tissue sarcoma of the head and neck in children and adolescents. Cancer. 77(1):193-200, 1996
10. Le Vay J et al: An assessment of prognostic factors in soft-tissue sarcoma of the head and neck. Arch Otolaryngol Head Neck Surg. 120(9):981-6, 1994
11. Wanebo HJ et al: Head and neck sarcoma: report of the Head and Neck Sarcoma Registry. Society of Head and Neck Surgeons Committee on Research. Head Neck. 14(1):1-7, 1992

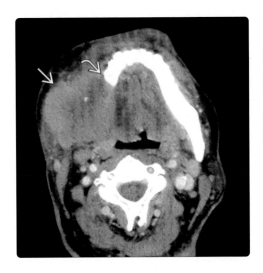

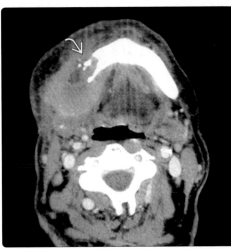

(Left) *Axial CECT shows an MS and mandible malignant fibrous histiocytoma. The lesion is seen as a solid, mildly enhancing right MS mass ➡️ with mandible destruction ➡️, including both the ramus and body. The MS is known as a deep facial location where SA arises.* (Right) *Axial CECT in the same patient again demonstrates a solid, mildly enhancing right MS mass with extensive mandible destruction ➡️.*

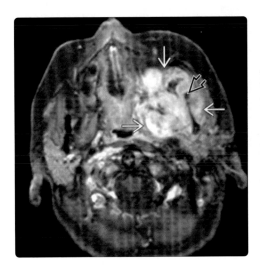

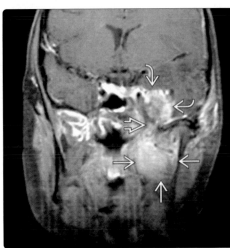

(Left) *Axial T1WI C+ FS MR shows a high-grade leiomyosarcoma of the MS. The tumor is a heterogeneously enhancing mass ➡️ involving the mandible ➡️. It is not possible to differentiate most SA-MS types with imaging unless osteo- or chondrosarcoma matrix is present.* (Right) *Coronal T1WI C+ FS MR in the same patient shows an enhancing mass ➡️ with intracranial spread through foramen ovale ➡️, which allows the tumor to involve the cavernous sinus ➡️.*

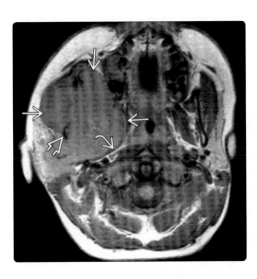

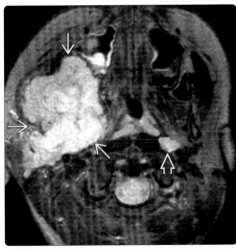

(Left) *Axial T1WI MR shows a Ewing SA arising in the MS. Notice the very large mass is hyperintense to muscle on T1WI ➡️. Mandible destruction is present with only a small fragment still visible ➡️. The parapharyngeal fat stripe ➡️ can be seen displaced medially.* (Right) *Axial T2WI FS MR in the same patient shows the tumor is markedly hyperintense but heterogeneous on T2WI ➡️. A prominent left retropharyngeal node ➡️ is incidentally noted.*

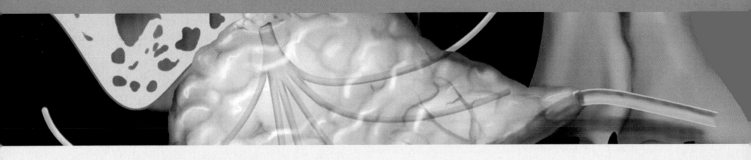

SECTION 5
Parotid Space

Summary Thoughts: Parotid Space

The parotid space (PS) lies in the lateral suprahyoid neck in the cheek anterior to the external auditory canal. The main content of the PS is the parotid gland, but many other critical structures, such as the facial nerve (CNVII), external carotid branches, and intraparotid lymph nodes, also lie within the boundaries of this space.

The PS is traditionally divided into **superficial and deep compartments**. The true dividing line between these compartments is the CNVII, but the nerve is not visible radiologically, so an imaginary line between the stylomastoid foramen and the lateral margin of the retromandibular vein serves as a radiologic surrogate.

The deep PS compartment lies anterior to the styloid process and lateral to the parapharyngeal fat. The deep compartment was previously called the **"prestyloid parapharyngeal space"** to emphasize these anatomic relationships. Recalling the older name may help when determining the site of origin of a parapharyngeal mass; a mass arising anterior to the styloid process, displacing the parapharyngeal fat medially, is parotid in origin.

In the setting of a PS mass, the key findings are benign vs. aggressive margins, unifocal vs. multifocal, and homogeneity vs. heterogeneity. Potential involvement of CNVII must be carefully sought.

The main goal of imaging a parotid mass is not to provide a precise diagnosis (since this is often difficult). Instead, the **main goal is to guide the next step in the work-up**. For example, would a fine-needle aspiration be useful? Does the patient need an oncologic excision with neck dissection?

Key findings in PS inflammation include calculi, ductal dilatation, and the number of glands affected.

Imaging Techniques

Either CECT or MR can be used to evaluate diseases of the PS. The choice is often based on regional preferences.

In the setting of suspected inflammatory disease, CT is preferred because it can identify small calculi. Unenhanced CT images through the parotid before CECT may allow identification of subtle intraparotid calcification that might be mistaken for enhancing vessels on CECT. Enhanced CT images through the entire neck from the skull base to clavicles follow. The patient's head should be positioned such that streak artifact from dental amalgam does not interfere with evaluation of the gland or the parotid duct (Stenson duct). Unfortunately, the punctum of the parotid duct lies alongside the second maxillary molar, so dental amalgam often interferes with evaluation of the punctum. Open-mouthed images can avoid this pitfall.

MR is preferred in the setting of CNVII paralysis because it can better identify **perineural spread**. MR also allows sialography, in which heavily T2-weighted images emphasize the ductal system in settings like Sjögren syndrome.

Catheter sialography, once a mainstay of parotid radiology, has now become rare because of competition from MR sialography and sialoendoscopy.

Imaging Anatomy

The parotid space is a suprahyoid neck space only. PS anatomic relationships include the medial parapharyngeal space (PPS), anterior masticator space (MS), and posteromedial carotid space. The tail of the parotid projects into the posterior submandibular space below. Superiorly, the PS abuts the undersurface of the external auditory canal and the mastoid tip.

The superficial layer of deep cervical fascia circumscribes the PS. This fascia surrounds the **superficial and deep lobes** of the parotid gland. The superficial lobe is about twice as large as the deep lobe. There is an inconstant third lobe, the **accessory lobe**, that lies superficial to the masseter muscle and occurs in 20% of patients.

The parotid duct emerges from the anterior PS and runs along the surface of masseter muscle. It then arches through the buccal space to pierce the buccinator muscle at the level of the maxillary second molar. The normal duct is small and often not appreciable on cross-sectional imaging.

CNVII runs through the center of the PS. Although not usually visible radiographically, its course may be approximated by an imaginary line from the stylomastoid foramen to lateral aspect of the retromandibular vein. CNVII divides within the parotid, with five major branches arrayed in a sagittal plane. Superior to inferior, they are **temporal, zygomatic, buccal, marginal, and cervical branches**.

The external carotid artery is the medial and smaller of the two vessels seen just posterior to the mandibular ramus in the PS. The lateral and larger of the two vessels is the retromandibular vein.

Because the parotid gland undergoes late encapsulation during development, mature **lymph nodes are present within the parenchyma of the gland**. This differentiates the parotid gland from the other salivary glands and results in a longer differential diagnosis for parotid masses (including metastases, lymphoma, BLEL-HIV, and Warthin tumors). The intraparotid lymph nodes serve as 1st-order drainage for malignancies in the scalp, the EAC, and the deep face. Each gland contains approximately 20 nodes.

The parotid glands undergo progressive fatty degeneration throughout life. In childhood, the glands display radiodensity similar to that of underlying masseter muscle on CT. With age, the glands progressively decrease in density due to normal fatty degeneration. Occasionally, one parotid gland will undergo premature fatty degeneration.

Clinical Implications

Eighty percent of parotid masses are **benign**. Unfortunately, most parotid masses cannot be diagnosed by imaging findings alone. As a result, until biopsy or resection is performed, the exact diagnosis remains in question. Some benign lesions (BMT in particular) need to be surgically removed because they might degenerate into malignancy, for cosmetic reasons, or to relieve mass effect on surrounding structures.

BMT accounts for the majority of parotid masses. Although benign, it can undergo malignant degeneration. Consequently, **all BMT should be surgically removed**. BMT also has a high rate of local recurrence, so superficial or total parotidectomy is needed to avoid tumor "spillage."

Because a specific diagnosis is usually not possible radiographically, the goal of imaging is to **determine the next step in the diagnostic process**.

- If discrete PS mass is seen, fine-needle aspiration or biopsy is most frequently employed; goal is not to

Parotid Space Overview

Congenital	Infectious-Inflammatory	Degenerative	Benign Tumor	Malignant Tumor, Primary	Neoplasm, Metastatic
Infantile hemangioma	Acute parotitis	Atrophy	Benign mixed tumor	Mucoepidermoid carcinoma	Skin cancer nodal metastasis
Venolymphatic malformation	Reactive adenopathy	Sialosis	Warthin tumor	Adenoid cystic carcinoma	NHL nodal metastasis
1st branchial cleft cyst	Chronic parotitis		Oncocytoma	Acinic cell carcinoma	Systemic nodal metastasis
	Benign lymphoepithelial lesions		Facial nerve schwannoma	Mammary analogue secretory carcinoma	
	Kimura disease		Lipoma	Adenocarcinoma	
	Kikuchi disease			Primary parotid non-Hodgkin lymphoma (NHL)	
				Salivary ductal carcinoma	
				Sebaceous carcinoma	

prevent surgery but to determine extent of surgery needed; malignancies often require wider excision ± neck dissection since surgical goal is to perform all procedures in single operative setting; palpable lesions can be needled without imaging guidance; sonographic guidance is most appropriate for superficial lobe lesions; CT guidance is most appropriate for deep lobe lesions

- If aggressive lesion present that clearly represents malignancy, resection and neck dissection may be performed even without definitive cytologic diagnosis; frozen section guidance is employed in such cases

Advanced imaging techniques, such as dynamic CT, dynamic MR, and quantitative ADC analysis, may increase diagnostic confidence in the probable diagnosis of a PS mass. However, they cannot provide a definitive diagnosis. As a result, the goal of imaging continues to be guidance of the next clinical step.

Facial nerve palsy in the setting of a PS mass suggests a malignant etiology. Imaging is aimed at determining if the deep PS lobe is affected, if perineural tumor (PNT) is present, and if malignant adenopathy exists. MR is recommended in this setting as it is particularly sensitive to the presence of PNT. In addition to PNT spread along the CNVII into the stylomastoid foramen, tumors may extend along the **auriculotemporal branch** of the trigeminal nerve. This PNT route runs through the parotid gland, around the posterior edge of the mandibular ramus, joining the main trunk of CNV3 in the masticator space below the foramen ovale.

Approaches to Imaging Issues of Parotid Space

The answer to the question, "What imaging findings define a PS mass?" is simple in a smaller intraparotid mass where the lesion is partially or completely surrounded by parotid tissue. It can be difficult to determine the space of origin for a larger, deep lobe PS mass, but in most cases **PPS fat** is **displaced medially** with the MS pterygoid muscles pushed anteriorly. The stylomandibular tunnel is also often widened by a deep lobe mass.

When developing a differential diagnosis for parotid masses, the most important consideration is **multiplicity**. Solitary lesions should be distinguished from unilateral multifocal lesions and from bilateral lesions.

- **Multiple bilateral lesions** suggest unique differential diagnosis, including Sjögren syndrome, BLEL-HIV, Warthin tumor, NHL, and systemic metastases; for multifocal unilateral lesions, primary parotid lymphoma and regional metastases should be more strongly considered; BMT is not consideration in multifocal parotid masses
- Solitary intraparotid lesion is most often BMT; although Warthin tumor may be multifocal, most are actually solitary

Parotid mass margins can be used to suggest if a lesion is benign or malignant. Ill-defined, aggressive margins suggest a malignant lesion is present. A well-circumscribed lesion is usually benign. However, a **well-defined parotid mass should not be assumed to be benign** since a low-grade malignancy may have an imaging appearance identical to that of BMT.

Although there are no truly specific imaging findings to distinguish parotid masses, some diagnoses have characteristic features that may be helpful.

- BMT at times will have hyperintense T2 signal (> CSF); when present, this finding strongly suggests BMT
- Warthin tumor may appear as well-defined, cystic, rim-enhancing mass; unfortunately, PS carcinoma (especially MECa) may have areas of cystic degeneration mimicking this appearance
- PNT spread is hallmark of malignancy; although adenoid cystic carcinoma is known for this tendency, lymphoma, MECa, and SCCa can spread this way

Always note the relationship of a PS mass to the CNVII plane. Designate the mass as superficial, deep, or in same plane as the intraparotid CNVII. Superficial lobe masses are removed by superficial parotidectomy, while deep lobe masses require total parotidectomy. Parotid tail masses must be identified as intraparotid or their excision may injure CNVII. Remember that the platysma and sternocleidomastoid muscles are the superficial and deep borders of the parotid tail, respectively.

Parotid Space Overview

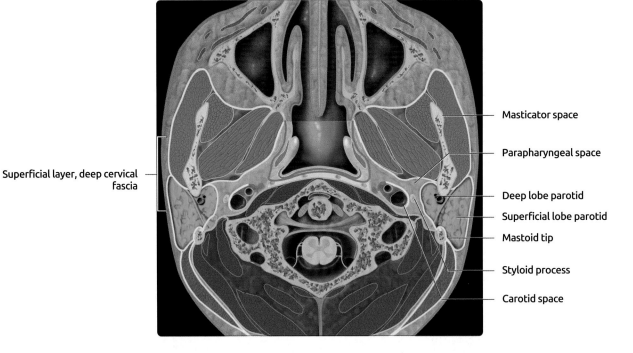

Superficial layer, deep cervical fascia

Masticator space

Parapharyngeal space

Deep lobe parotid

Superficial lobe parotid

Mastoid tip

Styloid process

Carotid space

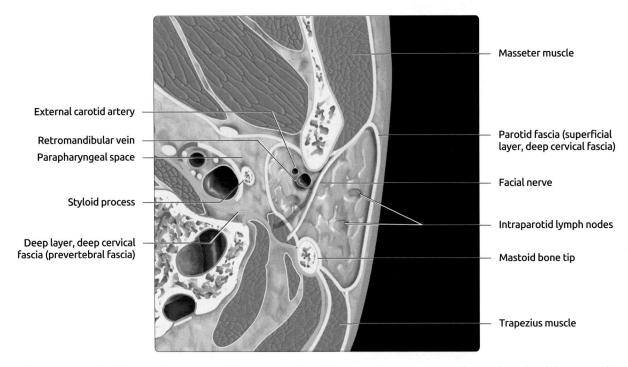

External carotid artery

Retromandibular vein

Parapharyngeal space

Styloid process

Deep layer, deep cervical fascia (prevertebral fascia)

Masseter muscle

Parotid fascia (superficial layer, deep cervical fascia)

Facial nerve

Intraparotid lymph nodes

Mastoid bone tip

Trapezius muscle

(Top) *Axial graphic of the suprahyoid neck soft tissues shows the relationships between the parotid space (green) and the surrounding spaces on the right. Notice the masticator space is anterior, while the parapharyngeal space is medial and the carotid space is posteromedial. On the left, the superficial layer of deep cervical fascia (yellow line) is seen to circumscribe both the masticator and parotid spaces.* **(Bottom)** *Axial graphic at the level of C1 vertebral body shows the contents of the parotid space. The intraparotid course of the facial nerve (not seen with imaging) extends from just medial to the mastoid tip to a position just lateral to the retromandibular vein. Within the superficial lobe (parotid superficial to the facial nerve), only parotid tissue and nodes are present. Within the deep lobe, notice the medial external carotid artery spand retromandibular vein. The parapharyngeal space fat lies just medial to the deep lobe of the gland.*

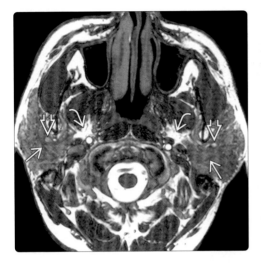 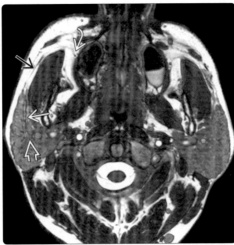

(Left) Axial T2WI high-resolution MR shows the intraparotid facial nerve ➡ dividing the parotid space into superficial and deep lobes. The retromandibular vein ➡ is visible just medial to the CNVII projected course. The parapharyngeal space fat ➡ is immediately medial to the deep lobe. (Right) Axial T2WI high-resolution MR reveals the intraparotid duct ➡ and radicals ➡. The duct is seen superficial to the masseter muscle ➡. It continues anteromedially to pierce the buccinator muscle ➡.

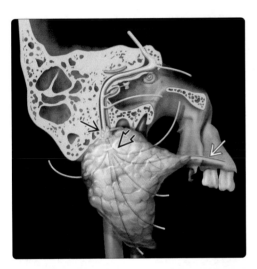 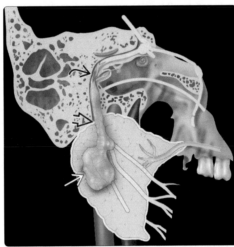

(Left) Sagittal graphic of the parotid shows the facial nerve exiting the temporal bone through the stylomastoid foramen ➡, then branching ➡ into its 5 components. The facial nerve plane defines the parotid superficial and deep lobes. Note also the parotid duct ➡. (Right) Sagittal graphic of a parotid malignancy ➡ shows perineural tumor spread following the intraparotid facial nerve through the stylomastoid foramen ➡ along the mastoid segment to the posterior genu area ➡.

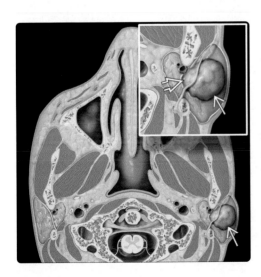 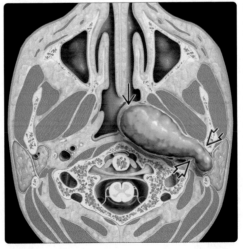

(Left) Axial graphic of intraparotid well-circumscribed tumor ➡ shows it is primarily in the superficial lobe but has a small component ➡ crossing the facial nerve plane. If tumor needle biopsy revealed BMT diagnosis, it still may be possible to remove it via superficial parotidectomy. (Right) Axial graphic of a deep lobe parotid mass shows medial displacement of the parapharyngeal space fat ➡. Note widening of the stylomandibular tunnel ➡. Total parotidectomy is necessary for removal.

Acute Parotitis

TERMINOLOGY

- Acute inflammation of parotid gland
  - Bacterial: Localized bacterial infection; ± abscess
  - Viral: Usually from systemic viral infection
  - Calculus-induced: Ductal obstruction by sialolith
  - Autoimmune: Acute episode of chronic disease

IMAGING

- Appearance: Enlargement of parotid gland with stranding of surrounding fat
  - Parotid retains normal configuration as it enlarges
- Bacterial parotitis
  - CECT shows enlarged, enhancing gland
  - Periparotid cellulitis/stranding common
  - Intra- or periparotid abscess may occur
- Parotitis with duct calculus
  - CECT shows large duct and intraluminal stone
- Viral parotitis
  - Clinical diagnosis; imaging rarely required

- Autoimmune parotitis
  - Diagnose with serum markers
  - Sialography for chronic complications
  - Usually involves entire gland, but can be focal

TOP DIFFERENTIAL DIAGNOSES

- Sjögren syndrome
- Benign lymphoepithelial lesions of HIV
- Parotid sialosis
- Infected 1st branchial cleft anomaly
- Parotid sarcoidosis

DIAGNOSTIC CHECKLIST

- Sialography for recurrent disease to assess complications
- Reimage parotid if residual mass after acute infection resolves to exclude underlying malignancy or abscess

(Left) *Axial CECT in a child demonstrates diffuse enlargement and asymmetric enhancement of the right parotid gland ➡. There is associated facial cellulitis ⇨ and myositis ➡ that is typical of acute bacterial parotitis.* (Right) *Axial CECT shows a low-density collection ➡ replacing the left parotid gland. There is substantial surrounding fat stranding, indicating infectious source. These findings suggest abscess complicating acute bacterial parotitis.*

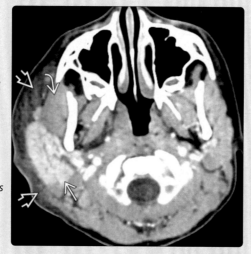
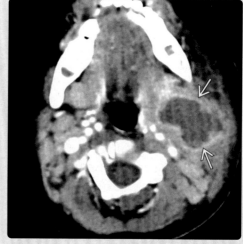

(Left) *Axial CECT shows a nonenhancing, irregular collection ➡ within the enlarged, asymmetrically enhancing right parotid gland ➡. Lack of rim enhancement suggests phlegmon rather than abscess; this resolved with IV antibiotics.* (Right) *Axial CECT demonstrates a peripherally enhancing abscess ➡ in the enlarged, asymmetrically enhancing left parotid gland ➡. Pus was drained at surgery.*

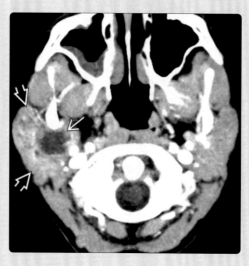
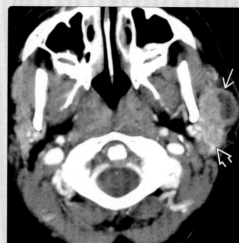

TERMINOLOGY

Synonyms

- Acute sialadenitis

Definitions

- Acute inflammation of parotid gland
  - Bacterial: Localized infection may become suppurative, with central abscess
  - Viral: Usually from systemic viral infection
  - Calculus-induced: Ductal obstruction by sialolith
  - Autoimmune: Acute episode of chronic disease

IMAGING

General Features

- Best diagnostic clue
  - Enlarged parotid(s) with surrounding fat stranding
- Location
  - Bacterial: Usually unilateral
  - Viral: 75% bilateral; submandibular and sublingual glands may also be involved
  - Calculus induced: Unilateral, with radiopaque stone in parotid duct
    - Most frequent locations for calculus: Hilum of gland, distal parotid duct
  - Autoimmune: Usually bilateral
- Morphology
  - Parotid retains normal configuration as it enlarges
  - Usually involves entire gland but can be focal

CT Findings

- NECT
  - Bacterial: Hyperdense enlarged parotid, ill-defined margins
  - Viral: Hyperdense enlarged parotids
  - Calculus-induced: Parotid duct calculus usually evident when sought
  - Autoimmune: Less involvement of surrounding fat
- CECT
  - Bacterial: Enlarged, diffusely enhancing parotid
    - Inflammatory stranding of surrounding fat
    - Ring enhancement of low-density abscesses (if present)
  - Viral: Enlarged parotids with mild enhancement
  - Calculus-induced: Parotid duct dilated with enhancing walls, otherwise like bacterial
  - Autoimmune: Less stranding of surrounding fat
    - May have ductal dilatation if longstanding disease

MR Findings

- T2WI
  - Diffuse high signal ± focal areas of high signal (microabscesses or dilated ducts)
- T1WI C+
  - Enlarged parotid gland with diffuse, moderate enhancement
  - Abscesses: Rim-enhancing fluid collections

Ultrasonographic Findings

- Enlarged, hypoechoic, heterogeneous gland
- Sensitive for detection of calculi
- Focal, hypoechoic collection suggests abscess formation
- US can be used to guide aspiration

Other Modality Findings

- Sialography contraindicated in acute suppurative parotitis
  - Useful in evaluating recurrent disease and complications when sialendoscopy not available

Imaging Recommendations

- Best imaging tool
  - Bacterial and calculus-induced infection: CECT best for detection of calculi or abscess
  - Viral parotitis is clinical diagnosis
    - Imaging rarely required
  - Autoimmune disease diagnosed with serum markers
    - Sialography for chronic complications
- Protocol advice
  - Optimize CT scan plane (parallel to upper fillings) so dental amalgam artifact does not obscure calculus in parotid duct
  - Additional NECT images optional
    - Calculus large enough to obstruct will be considerably more dense than contrast in vessels
    - Intraglandular stones better detected with NECT

DIFFERENTIAL DIAGNOSIS

Sjögren Syndrome

- Dry eyes and mouth; arthritis
- Cystic and solid intraparotid lesions

Benign Lymphoepithelial Lesions of HIV

- May be found prior to HIV seroconversion
- Bilateral heterogeneous glands, ± cystic and solid lesions
- Prominent Waldeyer ring and cervical nodes
- Affects parotid only, not other salivary glands

Parotid Sialosis

- Bilateral, prolonged, painless, soft parotid (and occasionally submandibular) gland enlargement
- Associated with alcoholism, endocrinopathies (especially diabetes mellitus), malnutrition (including anorexia nervosa, bulimia)

Infected 1st Branchial Cleft Anomaly

- 1st branchial cleft cyst in or adjacent to parotid gland
- Superinfection presents as parotid abscess
- Recurrent infections associated with upper respiratory illnesses

Parotid Sarcoidosis

- Rare manifestation of H&N sarcoidosis
- Nodal or parenchymal inflammatory changes

Parotid Malignancy

- Parotid adenoid cystic carcinoma
- Parotid mucoepidermoid carcinoma
  - CNVII dysfunction should raise suspicion of malignant neoplasm
  - Unilateral focal (low-grade) or ill-defined (high-grade) parotid mass
  - High-grade tumors associated with nodal metastases

PATHOLOGY

General Features

- Etiology
  - Bacterial: Usually due to ascending infection
    - May result from adjacent cellulitis
    - *Staphylococcus aureus* (50-90%) > *Streptococcus*, *Haemophilus*, *Escherichia coli*, anaerobes
    - Neonatal suppurative parotitis may be bilateral, due to bacteremia
      - □ More common in premature infants, males
  - Viral: Mumps paramyxovirus most common cause; so-called epidemic parotitis
    - Also influenza, parainfluenza, Coxsackie A & B, ECHO, lymphocytic choriomeningitis viruses
    - CMV, adenovirus reported with HIV infection
  - Juvenile recurrent parotitis = recurrent parotitis of childhood
    - Recurrent episodes mimic mumps
    - Usually begin by age 5 years; resolves by age 10-15
    - Patient often has unilateral symptoms but bilateral sialographic abnormalities
    - Sialographically mimics Sjögren syndrome
    - Etiology unknown
  - Other lesions that may have acute parotitis presentation
    - Sjögren syndrome
    - Mikulicz syndrome
    - Sicca syndrome, acute phase
- Bacterial and calculus induced usually unilateral
- Viral and autoimmune more frequently bilateral

CLINICAL ISSUES

Presentation

- Most common signs/symptoms
  - Bacterial: Sudden-onset parotid pain and swelling
  - Viral: Prodromal symptoms of headaches, malaise, myalgia followed by parotid pain, earache, trismus
  - Calculus induced: Recurrent episodes of swollen, painful gland, usually related to eating
  - Autoimmune: Recurrent episodes of tender gland swelling, accompanied by dry mouth
- Clinical profile
  - Bacterial: Acutely painful, enlarged parotid in debilitated patient or neonate
  - Predisposing factors
    - Dehydration, surgery, diuretics, or anticholinergics reducing salivary flow
    - Duct obstruction by calculus
    - Immunosuppression, poor oral hygiene, malnutrition
  - Viral: More frequently seen in children who have not received MMR vaccine

Demographics

- Age
  - Bacterial: > 50 years and neonates
  - Viral: Most < 15 years; peak age 5-9 years
    - Adults usually immune from childhood exposure or MMR vaccine

Natural History & Prognosis

- Bacterial parotitis mortality may reach 20%
  - Due to occurrence in debilitated elderly patients
- Responds well to early treatment, though number of complications recognized
  - Early complications
    - Abscess formation → rupture to deep neck spaces, external auditory canal (EAC), or TMJ
    - Thrombophlebitis of retromandibular or facial veins → internal jugular vein thrombosis
    - CNVII dysfunction rarely found; usually resolves
  - Long-term complications
    - Sialectasis (ductal dilation) with recurrent infections, reduced salivation, pain
- Viral parotitis self-limited; swelling lasts ≤ 2 weeks
  - Systemic mumps paramyxovirus has complications
    - Orchitis, meningoencephalitis, thyroiditis, sensorineural hearing loss, pancreatitis
- Autoimmune: Slowly progressive disease
  - May be complicated by non-Hodgkin lymphoma

Treatment

- Bacterial parotitis
  - Broad spectrum antibiotics, rehydration, good oral hygiene, sialogogues
  - Surgical drainage of abscesses
- Viral parotitis
  - Supportive treatment with rest, hydration
- Juvenile recurrent parotitis
  - Sialendoscopy ± corticosteroid application
- Calculus-induced parotitis
  - Extract smaller stones from duct (perorally)
  - Larger proximal stones may require surgical removal ± parotidectomy
- Autoimmune parotitis
  - Immunosuppressive medications (steroids)

DIAGNOSTIC CHECKLIST

Consider

- Sialography for recurrent disease to assess complications
- Reimage parotid if residual mass after resolution of acute infection to exclude underlying malignancy or abscess

Image Interpretation Pearls

- Carefully inspect entire parotid duct for calculi

SELECTED REFERENCES

1. Ramakrishna J et al: Sialendoscopy for the management of juvenile recurrent parotitis: A systematic review and meta-analysis. Laryngoscope. 125(6):1472-9, 2015
2. Roby BB et al: Treatment of juvenile recurrent parotitis of childhood: an analysis of effectiveness. JAMA Otolaryngol Head Neck Surg. 141(2):126-9, 2015
3. Francis CL et al: Pediatric sialadenitis. Otolaryngol Clin North Am. 47(5):763-78, 2014
4. Lampropoulos P et al: Acute suppurative parotitis: a dreadful complication in elderly surgical patients. Surg Infect (Larchmt). 13(4):266-9, 2012

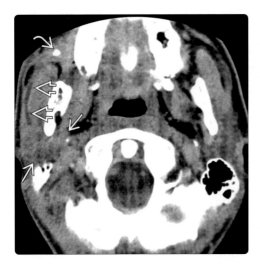

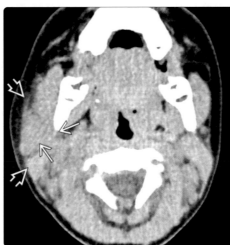

(Left) *Axial CECT in a teenage boy with calculus-induced parotitis shows typical enlargement and asymmetric enhancement of the right parotid gland ➡, enlargement of the parotid duct ➡, and distal intraluminal stone ➡.* (Right) *Axial NECT in a patient with recent blunt trauma demonstrates diffuse enlargement of the right parotid gland ➡ and edema in the overlying subcutaneous fat ➡.*

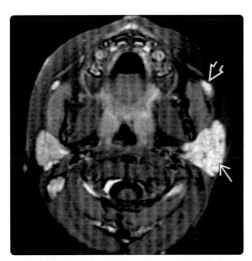

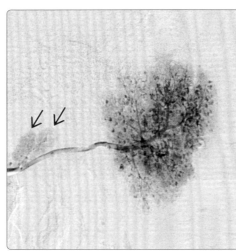

(Left) *Axial T1 C+ FS MR in a child with recurrent parotitis shows a enlarged, asymmetrically enhancing left parotid gland ➡, without significant cellulitis. Notice moderate enhancement in the ipsilateral accessory glandular tissue as well ➡.* (Right) *Lateral sialogram in the same child demonstrates multiple small puddles/collections of contrast throughout the left parotid gland and a few within the accessory parotid tissue ➡. Notice normal caliber of the ducts.*

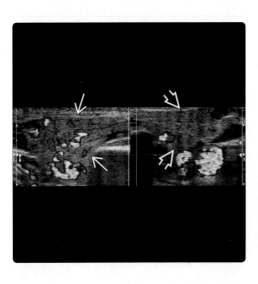

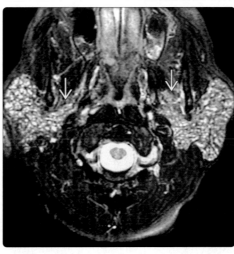

(Left) *Transverse color Doppler ultrasound of both parotid glands in a patient with right parotitis shows diffuse enlargement and increased vascularity of the right parotid gland ➡ compared to the left ➡.* (Right) *Axial T2 FS MR shows diffuse enlargement of both parotid glands with numerous foci of increased signal. This patient has an acute exacerbation of autoimmune sialadenitis. Note that the diffuse involvement includes the deep parotid lobes ➡.*

Parotid Sjögren Syndrome

TERMINOLOGY

- SjS: Chronic systemic **autoimmune exocrinopathy** that causes salivary & lacrimal gland tissue destruction
  - Primary SjS: Dry eyes & mouth; no collagen vascular disease (CVD)
  - Secondary SjS: Dry eyes & mouth with CVD, most commonly associated with **rheumatoid arthritis**

IMAGING

- Imaging appearance depends on stage of disease & presence or absence of lymphocyte aggregates within parotid
  - Earliest stage SjS: Parotids may appear normal
  - Intermediate stage SjS: Miliary pattern of **small cysts** diffusely throughout both parotids
  - Late stage SjS: Larger cystic (parenchymal destruction) & solid masses (lymphocyte aggregates) in both parotids
- Punctate diffuse **calcifications** in both parotids
- Conventional sialography
  - Alternating areas of ductal stenosis and dilatation (string of beads pattern)
  - Acinar spill into enlarged acini (apple tree pattern)
- MR sialography is replacing conventional sialography

TOP DIFFERENTIAL DIAGNOSES

- Chronic infectious or obstructive parotitis
- Benign lymphoepithelial lesions of HIV
- Warthin tumor
- Parotid NHL nodes

CLINICAL ISSUES

- Tender bilateral parotid gland swelling
- Striking **female** predominance (90-95%)
- Increased risk of malignancy in primary SjS
  - **Relative risk of NHL = 13.8**

DIAGNOSTIC CHECKLIST

- Dominant parotid mass ± cervical adenopathy worrisome for **lymphomatous transformation**

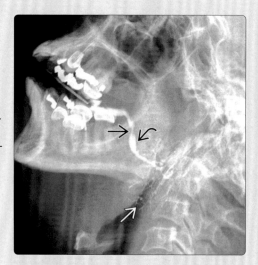
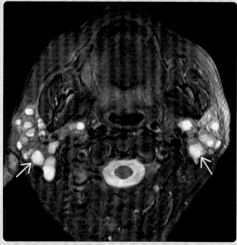

(Left) *Lateral parotid sialogram shows stenosis ➡ and dilation ➡ in Stensen duct (string of beads). Intraglandular branches are truncated, with cystic spaces (apple tree) ➡. Findings can be seen in any chronic sialadenitis but are classic for Sjögren syndrome.* (Right) *Axial T2WI FS MR shows high-signal masses ➡ within both parotid glands. These represent cystic dilatation of the intraglandular ducts in Sjögren syndrome but are indistinguishable from lymphoepithelial lesions in HIV.*

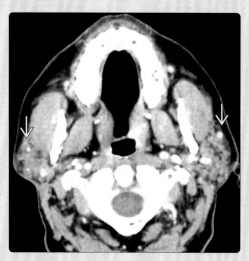
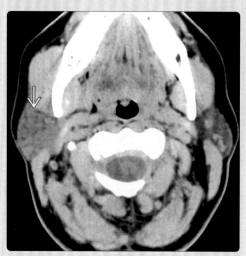

(Left) *Axial CECT shows multiple calcifications ➡ in parotid glands that have a multilobular configuration with fatty involution. Lobules of edematous glandular tissue with intervening fat and scattered calculi are characteristic of Sjögren syndrome.* (Right) *Axial NECT shows enlargement and increased density of the right parotid gland ➡, indicating inflammation. Although Sjögren syndrome affects both parotid glands, acute exacerbations may be unilateral.*

TERMINOLOGY

Abbreviations
- Sjögren syndrome (SjS)

Synonyms
- Sicca syndrome
- Sicca complex

Definitions
- SjS: Chronic systemic **autoimmune exocrinopathy** that causes salivary and lacrimal gland tissue destruction
  - Primary SjS: Dry eyes and mouth; no collagen vascular disease (CVD)
  - Secondary SjS: Dry eyes and mouth with CVD, most commonly associated with **rheumatoid arthritis**
- Mikulicz syndrome
  - Autoimmune exocrinopathy affecting salivary and lacrimal glands
  - Previously thought to be variant of primary SjS
  - Considered separate entity with abnormalities of IgG4
- Juvenile SjS
  - Predilection for male children until teen years
  - Usually resolves with puberty

IMAGING

General Features
- Best diagnostic clue
  - CT shows **bilateral enlarged parotids** with multiple **cystic** and **solid** intraparotid lesions ± smooth, round intraglandular calcifications
- Location
  - Bilateral salivary and lacrimal glands
- Size
  - Sub-mm to macrocysts or mixed solid-cystic masses > 2 cm
- Morphology
  - Diffuse bilateral parotid enlargement acute, atrophy late
  - Variant morphology: Dominant solid nodule mimics tumor
  - Premature fat deposition progresses over time
- Imaging appearance depends on stage of disease and presence or absence of lymphocyte aggregates within parotid
  - Early stage SjS: Parotids may appear normal
  - Intermediate stage SjS: Miliary pattern of **small cysts** diffusely throughout both parotids
  - Late stage SjS: Larger cystic (parenchymal destruction) & solid masses (lymphocyte aggregates) in both parotids
  - Any stage may have solid intraparotid masses that mimic tumor secondary to lymphocytic accumulation
  - Dominant parotid mass ± cervical adenopathy worrisome for **lymphomatous transformation**

CT Findings
- NECT
  - Symmetric parotid enlargement with increased CT density & heterogeneity
  - Punctate diffuse **calcifications** in both parotids
- CECT
  - Wide range of appearances based on SjS stage
    - Early, diffuse, sub-mm fluid density cystic lesions
    - Cysts mimic lymphoepithelial lesions of HIV ± solid nodules, which may mimic neoplasm
    - Chronic SjS shows atrophy and fatty change
  - Heterogeneous enhancement of solid components

MR Findings
- T1WI
  - Discrete collections of low signal intensity, reflecting watery saliva within dilated ducts and acini
- T2WI
  - Diffuse, bilateral, high T2, 1- to 2-mm foci (early stages, I & II)
  - Multiple high T2-signal foci > 2 mm (late stages, III & IV)
- T1WI C+
  - Heterogeneous, mild enhancement of nodular parenchyma & fibrosis with nonenhancing cystic changes
- MR sialography
  - Sensitive to diagnosis of SjS (approaching 95% sensitivity & specificity)
  - Stages severity of SjS
  - Display punctate, globular, cavitary, or destructive parotid distal ductal changes of SjS as focal high T2 signal
  - Replacing conventional sialography
  - Competes with sialoendoscopy

Ultrasonographic Findings
- Early stage miliary (≤ 1 mm punctate cystic changes) may be missed, but late stages readily apparent
- Increased vascularity on color Doppler

Nonvascular Interventions
- Conventional sialography
  - Reference standard for staging
  - Alternating areas of ductal stenosis and dilatation (string of beads pattern)
  - Acinar spill into enlarged acini (apple tree pattern)
  - Truncated intraglandular ductal branching pattern
- Sialoendoscopy
  - Accuracy of staging unknown
  - Not widely utilized

Imaging Recommendations
- Best imaging tool
  - MR with sialography
    - Allows cross-sectional analysis & staging

DIFFERENTIAL DIAGNOSIS

Chronic Infectious or Obstructive Parotitis
- Irregular dilatation and stenosis of ducts
- Lacks solid masses
- Multiple calculi may be present
  - Sialoliths are usually oblong, sharp, or pointed
  - Calcification in SjS is round, regular

Benign Lymphoepithelial Lesions of HIV
- Mixed cystic & solid lesions enlarging both parotids **may exactly mimic SjS**
- Tonsillar hyperplasia & cervical reactive adenopathy
- Lack glandular calcifications

Warthin Tumor

- 20% are multiple; may be unilateral or bilateral
- Tumors characteristically heterogeneous
- Mural nodules present if cystic

Parotid NHL Nodes

- Solid masses in parotid usually without cystic change
- Cervical adenopathy may or may not be present
- Chronic systemic NHL often already apparent

Parotid Metastatic Disease

- Primary malignancy & other metastatic deposits often concurrently present
- Skin cancers of scalp, face, external ear
- Unilateral or bilateral, single or multiple parotid masses with invasive margins

Parotid Sarcoidosis

- Rare manifestation of sarcoidosis
- Cervical & mediastinal lymph nodes
- Mixed cystic & solid masses enlarging both parotids with associated reactive-appearing cervical adenopathy

PATHOLOGY

General Features

- Etiology
  - Poorly understood immune-mediated disease
  - Viral infection, hormonal or epigenetic changes proposed as initiating events
- Periductal lymphocyte aggregates destroy salivary acini
- Autoimmune dysregulation leads to destruction of acinar cells & ductal epithelia of lacrimal & salivary glands
- Activated lymphocytes selectively injure lacrimal & salivary glands leading to tissue damage

Staging, Grading, & Classification

- Based on conventional or MR sialography
  - Stage I: Punctate contrast/high signal ≤ 1 mm
  - Stage II: Globular contrast/high signal 1-2 mm
  - Stage III: Cavitary contrast/high signal > 2 mm
  - Stage IV: Parotid gland parenchymal destruction
- Modest correlation with disease duration

Gross Pathologic & Surgical Features

- Enlarged parotid glands with multiple small to large cysts & lymphocyte aggregates

Microscopic Features

- Labial biopsy: CD4(+) T-cell lymphocytes
- Periductal lymphocyte & plasma cell infiltration & epimyoepithelial islands
  - Early stages: Lymphocyte-plasma cell infiltration obstructs intercalated ducts with enlarged distal ducts throughout parotids
  - Late stages: Activated lymphocytes destroy salivary tissue, leaving larger cysts & solid lymphocyte aggregates

CLINICAL ISSUES

Presentation

- Most common signs/symptoms
  - Tender, bilateral parotid gland swelling

- Other signs/symptoms
  - Dry eyes, mouth, and skin
  - **Secondary SjS associations: Rheumatoid arthritis** > > systemic lupus erythematosus > progressive systemic sclerosis
- Clinical profile
  - Patient complains of recurrent acute episodes of tender glandular swelling
  - Less common: Chronic glandular enlargement with superimposed acute attacks
  - Less common: Nontender parotid enlargement
- Laboratory
  - **Positive labial biopsy** or **autoantibody against Sjögren-associated A or B antigen** for definitive diagnosis
  - Rheumatoid factor positive in 95%
  - ANA positive in 80%
  - Positive Schirmer test (decreased tear production)

Demographics

- Age
  - 50-70 years old
- Gender
  - Striking **female** predominance (90-95%)
  - Most common in menopausal women
- Epidemiology
  - Incidence of SjS: ~ 0.5%
  - 2nd most common autoimmune disorder after rheumatoid arthritis
- Juvenile SjS
  - Males < 20 years old
  - High rate of recurrent parotitis
  - Most resolve spontaneously at puberty

Natural History & Prognosis

- Slowly progressive syndrome that evolves over years
- Increased risk of malignancy in primary SjS
  - **Relative risk of NHL = 13.8**

Treatment

- Symptomatic moisture-replacing therapy
- If systemic disease, immunotherapy may be used

DIAGNOSTIC CHECKLIST

Consider

- MR sialography to analyze both ducts and parenchyma

Image Interpretation Pearls

- Invasive margins, dominant solid mass, & cervical lymphadenopathy suggest malignant transformation

SELECTED REFERENCES

1. Liang Y et al: Primary Sjogren's syndrome and malignancy risk: a systematic review and meta-analysis. Ann Rheum Dis. 73(6):1151-6, 2014
2. Sun Z et al: Diagnostic accuracy of parotid CT for identifying Sjögren's syndrome. Eur J Radiol. 81(10):2702-9, 2012
3. Lee S et al: Mikulicz's disease: a new perspective and literature review. Eur J Ophthalmol. 16(2):199-203, 2006
4. Hamilton BE et al: Earring lesions of the parotid tail. AJNR Am J Neuroradiol. 24(9): 1757-64, 2003

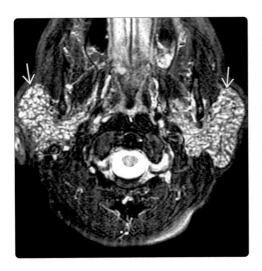
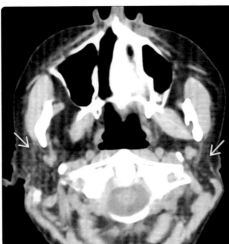

(Left) *Axial T2WI FS MR shows innumerable tiny cysts completely replacing both parotid glands ➡. The glands are markedly enlarged. This represents the acute phase of Sjögren syndrome.* (Right) *Axial NECT shows complete atrophy of both parotid glands ➡ with replacement of parenchyma by fat. This represents the chronic phase of Sjögren syndrome.*

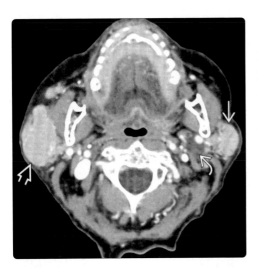
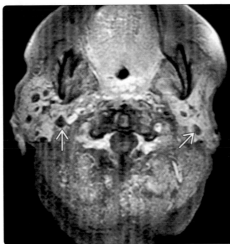

(Left) *Axial CECT shows dense, hyperenhancing parotid glands ➡ with cystic areas ➡. In the right parotid gland, there is a solid, uniformly enhancing mass ➡, representing lymphoma. Patients with Sjögren syndrome are at high risk for intraparotid lymphoma. Any solid glandular mass should be biopsied.* (Right) *Axial T1WI C+ FS MR shows numerous cystic lesions ➡ scattered throughout both parotid glands. Each lesion has a thin rim of enhancement, as expected in Sjögren syndrome.*

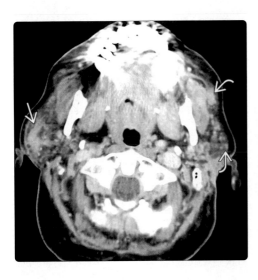
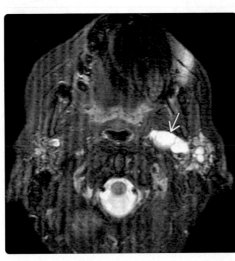

(Left) *Axial CECT shows diffuse fatty replacement of the parotid glands, with areas of scarring ➡ and lobular edema ➡. These findings are characteristic of late-stage Sjögren syndrome.* (Right) *Axial T2WI FS MR shows a septate cystic mass ➡ in the deep lobe of the parotid gland. This is a dilated duct from Sjögren syndrome, but it might be easily mistaken for a neoplasm.*

Benign Lymphoepithelial Lesions of HIV

TERMINOLOGY

- 3-tiered classification
  - Persistent generalized parotid lymphadenopathy: **Solid** intraparotid lesions
  - Benign lymphoepithelial lesions (BLEL): **Mixed** solid and cystic lesions
  - Benign lymphoepithelial (BLE) cysts: **Cystic** lesions

IMAGING

- Enhanced CT or MR: Multiple bilateral, well-circumscribed cystic and solid masses within enlarged parotid glands
  - BLE cyst wall may be nodular (lymphoid follicles)
- Look for other CECT findings associated with HIV
  - **Reactive cervical adenopathy**
  - **Tonsillar hypertrophy**

TOP DIFFERENTIAL DIAGNOSES

- 1st branchial cleft cyst
- Parotid Sjögren syndrome

- Warthin tumor
- Non-Hodgkin lymphoma in parotid nodes
- Metastatic disease to parotid nodes

CLINICAL ISSUES

- Bilateral painless enlargement of both parotid glands
  - BLEL may precede HIV seroconversion
  - **HIV testing** should be done on **any patient with BLEL**
- Historically, **5%** of HIV-positive patients develop BLEL
- BLEL seen less frequently now because HAART therapy treats this manifestation of HIV

DIAGNOSTIC CHECKLIST

- Nonnecrotic cervical adenopathy with tonsillar hypertrophy can be important clue to BLEL diagnosis with CECT
- When BLE cysts present as unilateral cystic intraparotid mass, may be mistaken for 1st branchial cleft cyst
- When BLEL presents as unilateral solid intraparotid mass, may be mistaken for parotid tumor

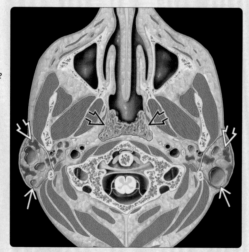
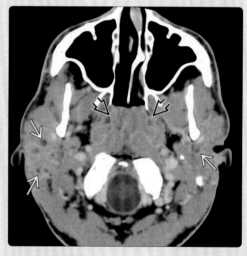

(Left) Classic findings of benign lymphoepithelial lesions (BLEL) as bilateral intraparotid cysts ⟹ are mixed with bilateral solid lymphoid aggregates ⟹. Note associated adenoidal hypertrophy ⟹ in the nasopharynx. Reactive adenopathy (not shown) is also a part of the imaging picture in LEL-HIV. (Right) Axial CECT shows microcysts ⟹ scattered throughout both hyperdense parotid glands in an HIV-positive patient, findings most consistent with BLE cysts. Note associated adenoidal hypertrophy ⟹.

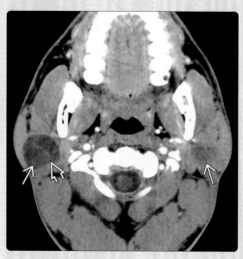
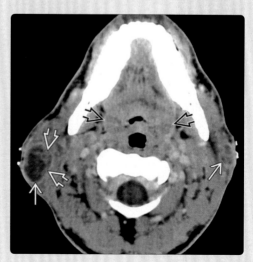

(Left) Axial CECT in an HIV-positive patient shows larger loculated cystic lesions ⟹ in both parotid glands. Septations can sometimes be seen within BLE cysts ⟹. (Right) Axial CECT in an HIV-positive patient shows bilateral cystic masses ⟹ with mural nodularity ⟹ (lymphoid follicles) in both parotid glands. BLEL can have both cystic and solid components. Note the associated tonsillar hypertrophy ⟹.

TERMINOLOGY

Abbreviations

- Benign lymphoepithelial lesions (BLEL)-HIV

Synonyms

- AIDS-related parotid cysts (ARPC)
  - Patient need only be HIV-positive to manifest BLEL
    - May not have full-blown AIDS with BLEL
    - Avoid ARPC synonym

Definitions

- Multifocal mixed **cystic** and **solid** intraparotid masses found in HIV-infected patients
- 3-tiered classification
  - Persistent generalized parotid gland lymphadenopathy: Solid lesions
  - Benign lymphoepithelial lesions: Mixed solid and cystic lesions
  - Benign lymphoepithelial cysts: Cystic lesions

IMAGING

General Features

- Best diagnostic clue
  - Multiple cystic and solid masses enlarging both parotid glands associated with **tonsillar hyperplasia** and **reactive cervical adenopathy**
- Location
  - Intraglandular
  - Rarely seen in submandibular or sublingual salivary glands
    - Only parotid has intrinsic lymphoid tissue
- Size
  - Variable: Typically several mm, up to 3.5 cm
- Morphology
  - Cysts are well circumscribed, rounded
  - Solid lymphoid aggregates may be poorly defined
  - **Bilateral** parotid enlargement
  - Often innumerable small masses

CT Findings

- NECT
  - Multiple bilateral, well-circumscribed cystic and solid masses within enlarged parotid glands
- CECT
  - Bilateral parotid **hyperdensity** and enlargement
  - Thin rim enhancement of **cystic** lesions with heterogeneous enhancement of **solid** lesions
  - Other CECT findings associated with HIV
    - **Reactive cervical adenopathy**
    - **Adenoidal, palatine, and lingual tonsillar hypertrophy**

MR Findings

- T1WI
  - Low signal intensity cystic lesions
  - Heterogeneous variable signal in solid lesions
    - Normal parotid fat provides good inherent contrast
- T2WI
  - Hyperintense, bilateral, well-circumscribed, round to ovoid intraparotid lesions
  - Hyperintense, bilateral cervical lymphadenopathy
  - Waldeyer lymphatic ring enlargement with high signal
- STIR
  - Improves lesion conspicuity
- T1WI C+
  - Thin rim enhancement in cystic lesions with variable heterogeneous enhancement of solid lesions
    - Cystic lesions solid mural nodules (enlarged lymph follicles)
  - Solid lesions may be less conspicuous on enhanced than unenhanced T1WI because of surrounding fat

Ultrasonographic Findings

- Spectrum of sonographic findings ranging from simple cysts to mixed masses with predominantly solid components
  - Cystic lesions not purely anechoic but contain internal network of thin septa supplied by vessel pedicles
    - 40% have mural nodules
  - Solid lesions may resemble parotid neoplasms

Imaging Recommendations

- Best imaging tool
  - Neck CECT shows signature findings of bilateral cystic to solid parotid masses, tonsillar hyperplasia, & cervical adenopathy

DIFFERENTIAL DIAGNOSIS

1st Branchial Cleft Cyst

- Clinical: Recurrent unilateral, inflammatory parotid mass
- Imaging: Unilateral, oval cystic intraparotid mass

Parotid Sjögren Syndrome

- Clinical: Older female patient with Sicca syndrome (dry eyes, mouth, and skin) and connective tissue disorder (rheumatoid arthritis); antinuclear antibodies
- Imaging: May be identical to benign lymphoepithelial (BLE) cysts

Parotid Sarcoidosis

- Clinical: Intraparotid sarcoid is very rare
- Imaging: Cervical and mediastinal lymph nodes
  - May be identical to BLEL

Warthin Tumor

- Clinical: Solitary or multifocal parotid masses
- Imaging
  - Solid or mixed cystic-solid parotid masses with nodular walls
  - 20% are multifocal but never innumerable
  - Lacks associated tonsillar hyperplasia and cervical adenopathy

Non-Hodgkin Lymphoma in Parotid Nodes

- Clinical: Chronic systemic non-Hodgkin lymphoma usually already apparent
- Imaging: Bilateral solid masses in parotid

Metastatic Disease to Parotid Nodes

- Clinical: Primary malignancy and other metastatic deposits already apparent
- Imaging: Unilateral, multifocal solid parotid masses

Parotid Space

PATHOLOGY

General Features

- Etiology
  - Lymphoepithelial lesion (LEL) formation occurs in glandular epithelium ± intraparotid nodes
  - Intraparotid LELs lined by benign epithelium with enlarged, irregularly shaped lymphoid follicles in wall
- Associated abnormalities
  - Cervical lymphadenopathy and nasopharyngeal lymphofollicular hyperplasia

Microscopic Features

- Thin, smooth-walled cysts measuring few mm to 3-4 cm
- Cyst aspirate: Fluid reveals foamy macrophages, lymphoid and epithelial cells, and **multinucleated giant cells**

Immunohistochemistry

- Lymphoid component includes reactivity for B-cell lineage and T-cell lineage markers
- Epithelial markers (e.g., cytokeratins, EMA, others) delineate squamous epithelial-lined cysts
- **HIV p24** core antigen immunoreactivity found in **germinal centers** and **multinucleated giant cells**
  - Multinucleated giant cells also S100 protein and p55 positive

CLINICAL ISSUES

Presentation

- Most common signs/symptoms
  - Bilateral painless parotid gland enlargement
- Other signs/symptoms
  - Cervical lymphadenopathy
  - Tonsillar swelling
- Clinical profile
  - BLEL may be 1st symptom of HIV infection
  - Bilateral parotid masses in HIV-positive patient
    - Initially seen in HIV-positive patients prior to AIDS onset
      - □ BLEL may precede HIV seroconversion
      - □ BLEL not considered precursor to AIDS
  - **HIV testing** should be done on **any patient with BLEL**

Demographics

- Age
  - Any age infected with HIV
  - Most commonly seen in men
- Epidemiology
  - Historically, **5%** of HIV-positive patients develop BLEL
  - BLEL seen less frequently since institution of combination antiviral therapy

Natural History & Prognosis

- If left untreated, grows into chronic, mumps-like state with significant bilateral parotid enlargement
- Patient prognosis dependent on other HIV- and AIDS-related diseases, not on BLEL
- Rarely may transform into B-cell lymphoma

Treatment

- HAART for HIV will completely or partially treat BLEL of parotid glands
- BLE cysts: Intralesional doxycycline or alcohol sclerotherapy if painful or if not antiviral candidate
- Surgical excision: **Not** recommended in AIDS patients

DIAGNOSTIC CHECKLIST

Consider

- Use CECT as 1st imaging modality if suspect LEL-HIV
- Image from skull base to clavicles to fully evaluate extent of parotid involvement and adenopathy

Image Interpretation Pearls

- Bilateral cystic and solid masses within enlarged parotids in HIV-positive patient should be considered BLEL until proven otherwise
- Nonnecrotic cervical adenopathy with tonsillar hypertrophy can be important clue to BLEL diagnosis
- When BLE cysts present as unilateral cystic intraparotid mass, may be mistaken for 1st branchial cleft cyst
- When BLEL presents as unilateral solid intraparotid mass, may be mistaken for parotid tumor

Reporting Tips

- BLE may be 1st sign of HIV infection
  - Call clinician with HIV testing recommendation in characteristic cases

SELECTED REFERENCES

1. Sujatha D et al: Parotid lymphoepithelial cysts in human immunodeficiency virus: a review. J Laryngol Otol. 127(11):1046-9, 2013
2. Kreisel FH et al: Cystic lymphoid hyperplasia of the parotid gland in HIV-positive and HIV-negative patients: quantitative immunopathology. Oral Surg Oral Med Oral Pathol Oral Radiol Endod. 109(4):567-74, 2010
3. Wu L et al: Lymphoepithelial cyst of the parotid gland: its possible histopathogenesis based on clinicopathologic analysis of 64 cases. Hum Pathol. 40(5):683-92, 2009
4. Marsot-Dupuch K et al: Head and neck lesions in the immunocompromised host. Eur Radiol. 14 Suppl 3:E155-67, 2004
5. Mandel L: Ultrasound findings in HIV-positive patients with parotid gland swellings. J Oral Maxillofac Surg. 59(3): 283-6, 2001
6. Uccini S et al: The benign cystic lymphoepithelial lesion of the parotid gland is a viral reservoir in HIV type 1-infected patients. AIDS Res Hum Retroviruses. 15(15): 1339-44, 1999
7. Chetty R: HIV-associated lymphoepithelial cysts and lesions: morphological and immunohistochemical study of the lymphoid cells. Histopathology. 33(3): 222-9, 1998
8. Craven DE et al: Response of lymphoepithelial parotid cysts to antiretroviral treatment in HIV-infected adults. Ann Intern Med. 128(6): 455-9, 1998
9. Kooper DP et al: Management of benign lymphoepithelial lesions of the parotid gland in human immunodeficiency virus-positive patients. Eur Arch Otorhinolaryngol. 255(8): 427-9, 1998
10. Maiorano E et al: Lymphoepithelial cysts of salivary glands: an immunohistochemical study of HIV-related and HIV-unrelated lesions. Hum Pathol. 29(3): 260-5, 1998
11. Martinoli C et al: Benign lymphoepithelial parotid lesions in HIV-positive patients: spectrum of findings at gray-scale and Doppler sonography. AJR Am J Roentgenol. 165(4): 975-9, 1995
12. Som PM et al: Nodal inclusion cysts of the parotid gland and parapharyngeal space: a discussion of lymphoepithelial, AIDS-related parotid, and branchial cysts, cystic Warthin's tumors, and cysts in Sjogren's syndrome. Laryngoscope. 105(10): 1122-8, 1995
13. Kirshenbaum KJ et al: Benign lymphoepithelial parotid tumors in AIDS patients: CT and MR findings in nine cases. AJNR Am J Neuroradiol. 12(2):271-4, 1991
14. Holliday RA et al: Benign lymphoepithelial parotid cysts and hyperplastic cervical adenopathy in AIDS-risk patients: a new CT appearance. Radiology. 168(2):439-41, 1988

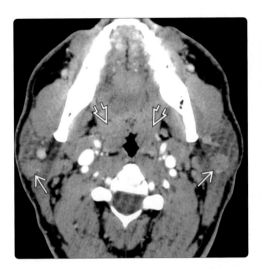

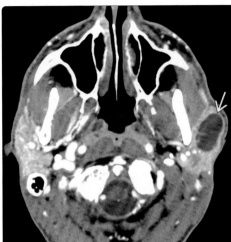

(Left) Axial CECT shows bilateral, well-defined, enhancing solid masses ➡ in both parotid glands. Although metastases and lymphoma may have a similar appearance, the presence of tonsillar hypertrophy ➡ should suggest the diagnosis of BLEL or persistent parotid gland lymphadenopathy from HIV. (Right) Axial CECT shows a solitary cystic, septated mass ➡ in the left parotid gland. BLEL are generally multiple but can present as a solitary mass. First branchial cleft cyst may be misdiagnosed in this setting.

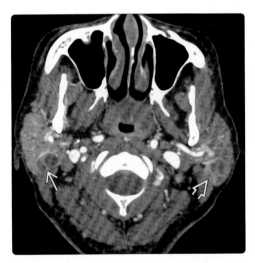

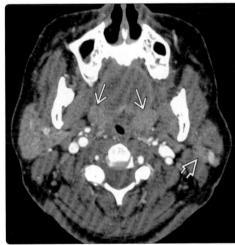

(Left) Axial CECT in a patient presenting with a left neck mass shows bilateral hyperdense parotids with a septated cystic lesion on the right ➡ and a mixed cystic-solid lesion on the left ➡. (Right) Axial CECT in the same patient reveals a left periparotid enlarged, solid node ➡, and palatine tonsillar hypertrophy ➡. Based on the CT findings, HIV testing was recommended, which revealed the patient to be HIV positive.

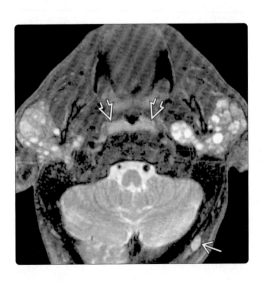

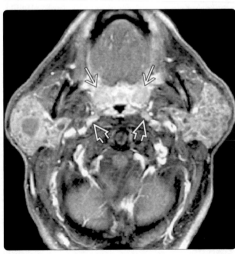

(Left) Axial STIR MR shows bilateral, intraparotid, hyperintense, cystic lymphoepithelial lesions of HIV. Notice both superficial and deep lobes are involved. Note the associated reactive occipital node ➡. Only minimal tonsillar hyperplasia is visible ➡. (Right) Axial T1WI C+ FS MR reveals bilateral cystic and solid intraparotid lesions of HIV. Palatine tonsils ➡ are hyperplastic and associated with reactive lateral retropharyngeal nodes ➡.

Parotid Benign Mixed Tumor

TERMINOLOGY

- Synonym: Pleomorphic adenoma

IMAGING

- Choice of imaging tool: CECT, MR, or US
  - CT or MR adequate to answer most imaging questions
    - MR best if specific signs (↑ T2 signal, ↑ ADC) present
  - Alternate approach leading with combination of US and FNAC
    - If US shows superficial lobe benign lesion and FNAC shows BMT cells, no further imaging needed
- CT findings
  - Smooth, homogeneously enhancing, ovoid mass
  - **Pear-shaped** when in deep lobe
- MR findings
  - ↑ T1 signal in hemorrhagic lesions
  - **Very high T2 signal specific for BMT**
  - ADC values higher than other parotid tumors
- US findings

- Well-demarcated, homogeneous, hypoechoic mass with posterior enhancement
- Larger BMT shows heterogeneous hypoechogenicity

TOP DIFFERENTIAL DIAGNOSES

- Warthin tumor
- Metastatic nodes in parotid
- Parotid adenoid cystic carcinoma
- Mucoepidermoid carcinoma
- Parotid non-Hodgkin lymphoma

CLINICAL ISSUES

- Painless, slow-growing cheek mass most common
- Multifocal primary BMT rare (< 1%)
- Rapid enlargement concerning for malignant degeneration

DIAGNOSTIC CHECKLIST

- Infiltrative margins, multicentricity, or hypointense T2 signal suggests malignancy
- Relationship of BMT to CNVII critical for surgical planning

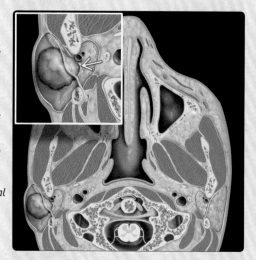
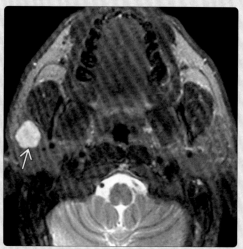

(Left) Axial graphic depicts a small, predominantly superficial lobe benign mixed tumor (BMT). Notice on insert the tongue of tumor that has insinuated itself between 2 facial nerve branches to involve the deep lobe ➡. (Right) Axial T2 FS MR reveals a sharply circumscribed, high-signal BMT ➡ in the superficial lobe of the parotid gland. This tumor at the very least abuts, if not crosses, the plane of the intraparotid facial nerve.

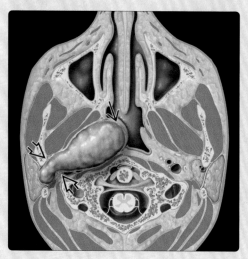
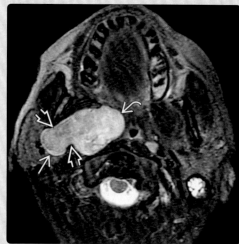

(Left) Axial graphic reveals a pear-shaped BMT of the deep lobe of the parotid gland. Despite the size of this tumor, the parapharyngeal fat can still be seen ➡ as it is pushed superomedially. Note widened stylomandibular notch ➡. (Right) Axial T2 FS MR shows a pear-shaped mass extending from the deep lobe of the parotid gland ➡, through the enlarged stylomandibular notch ➡, displacing the parapharyngeal fat and palatine tonsil medially ➡. Large, deep lobe parotid tumors are almost always benign mixed tumors.

TERMINOLOGY

Abbreviations
- Benign mixed tumor (BMT)

Synonyms
- Pleomorphic adenoma

Definitions
- Benign, histologically **heterogeneous** tumor of parotid
- Epithelial, myoepithelial, and stromal components

IMAGING

General Features
- Best diagnostic clue
  - Small BMT (< 2 cm): Sharply marginated, intraparotid ovoid mass with uniform enhancement
  - Large BMT (> 2 cm): Lobulated mass with heterogeneous enhancement
- Location
  - Parotid space; usually superficial lobe
- Size
  - Variable; may be > 10 cm if in deep lobe or neglected
- Morphology
  - Round or oval
  - Pear-shaped when arising in deep lobe and extending into stylomandibular tunnel

CT Findings
- CECT
  - **Small BMT**
    - Smooth, homogeneously enhancing, ovoid mass
  - **Large BMT**
    - Inhomogeneously enhancing, lobulated mass with areas of lower attenuation representing foci of degenerative necrosis and old hemorrhage
    - Dystrophic calcification may be present
      - □ Calcifications unusual in other parotid tumors
  - **Deep lobe BMT**
    - Variably enhancing **pear-shaped mass** displacing parapharyngeal space (PPS) fat medially
    - Widening of stylomandibular notch

MR Findings
- T1WI
  - Small BMT: Sharply marginated intraparotid mass with uniform hypointensity
  - Large BMT: Lobulated intraparotid mass with heterogeneous signal
    - Hyperintense signal can be seen if hemorrhagic
- T2WI
  - Small BMT: Well-circumscribed intraparotid mass with **uniform high signal**
  - Large BMT: **Lobulated** intraparotid mass with heterogeneous high signal
  - May show peripheral low signal intensity capsule
  - If **very high T2** signal present, **specific for BMT**
- STIR
  - Lesions more conspicuous than on standard T2
- DWI

- On average, BMT has **higher ADC value** than other benign lesions and cancers
  - DWI not yet accurate enough to avoid fine-needle aspiration cytology (FNAC)
- T1WI C+
  - Variable, mild to moderate enhancement
  - Dynamic contrast curve shows **quick uptake, then plateau** (contrast retention)
    - Not yet accurate enough to avoid FNAC

Ultrasonographic Findings
- Grayscale ultrasound
  - Well-demarcated, homogeneous, **hypoechoic** mass with **posterior enhancement**
    - Larger BMT shows heterogeneous hypoechogenicity
      - □ Secondary to hemorrhage and necrosis
  - Only visible when located in parotid superficial lobe
- Color Doppler
  - ↑ peripheral vessels, mainly venous: Often sparse

Nuclear Medicine Findings
- Cold on Tc-99m pertechnetate and PET/CT
  - Helps differentiate from Warthin tumor (hot) but not from malignancy (cold)

Imaging Recommendations
- Best imaging tool
  - Either CECT or MR adequate to answer most imaging questions
  - MR best when specific signs (high T2 signal, high ADC) are present
    - May be able to avoid neck dissection without performing FNAC and rely on surgical excisional biopsy as primary treatment
    - Advanced MR sequences (quantitative ADC, dynamic contrast) may become standard of care in future
  - Alternate approach leading with combination of US and FNAC
    - If US shows **superficial lobe benign lesion** and **FNAC shows BMT cells**, no further imaging needed
- Define facial nerve plane
  - CNVII plane projects from stylomastoid foramen, anteroinferiorly to lateral aspect of retromandibular vein, then anteriorly over surface of masseter muscle
  - CNVII plane represents imaging estimation of line dividing superficial and deep lobes of parotid gland
  - Relationship of BMT to facial nerve critical for surgical planning; comment in radiology report appropriate
    - e.g., "BMT is in superficial lobe of parotid or abuts facial nerve plane or is in deep lobe"
- Risk of malignant degeneration
  - Rapid enlargement concerning for **carcinoma ex pleomorphic adenoma**

DIFFERENTIAL DIAGNOSIS

Warthin Tumor
- Clinical: Adult male smoker
- Imaging: Inhomogeneous but well-circumscribed intraparotid mass
  - Multicentric (20%)

- o Warthin tumor does not calcify, but BMT may have calcification

Parotid Nodal Metastatic Disease

- Systemic nodal metastases
  - o Intraparotid nodes may be site of systemic nodal metastases
- Regional nodal drainage
  - o Clinical: Known primary periauricular skin malignancy
  - o Imaging: Single or multiple pathologic nodes seen

Primary Parotid Carcinoma

- Parotid adenoid cystic carcinoma (ACCa)
- Mucoepidermoid carcinoma (MECa)
  - o Clinical for either carcinoma: Gradual-onset facial nerve paresis
  - o Imaging for either carcinoma: Heterogeneous infiltrating mass with poorly defined margins
    - Low-grade malignancy may be well demarcated
    - Perineural tumor spread common for ACCa
    - Adjacent node common for MECa

Parotid Non-Hodgkin Lymphoma

- Clinical: Chronic systemic NHL may already be present
- Imaging: Solitary, multiple, or bilateral solid masses of parotid gland

PATHOLOGY

General Features

- Etiology
  - o Unknown; may arise from minor salivary gland rests
  - o Benign tumor arising from distal portions of parotid ductal system, including intercalated ducts and acini

Gross Pathologic & Surgical Features

- Lobulated heterogeneous mass with **fibrous capsule**
- Soft tan lobules representing epithelial component interspersed among lobulated firm, white, gritty chondromyxoid component

Microscopic Features

- Interspersed **epithelial, myoepithelial, and stromal cellular components** needed to diagnose BMT
- Sites of necrosis, hemorrhage, hyalinization, and calcification may be present

CLINICAL ISSUES

Presentation

- Most common signs/symptoms
  - o Painless cheek mass
  - o Location-dependent symptoms and signs
    - Superficial lobe or accessory parotid: Cheek mass
    - Parotid tail: Angle of mandible mass
    - Deep lobe: Enlarging mass pushes palatine tonsil into pharyngeal airway
  - o Facial nerve paralysis is rare and suggests malignancy

Demographics

- Age
  - o Most common > 40 years
  - o Range: 30-60 years

- Ethnicity
  - o Most common in Caucasians, rare in African Americans
- Epidemiology
  - o **Most common parotid space tumor (80%)**
  - o 80% of BMT arise in parotid glands
    - 8% in submandibular glands; 6.5% arise from minor salivary glands in pharyngeal mucosal space
  - o 80-90% of parotid BMTs involve superficial lobe
  - o Multifocal BMT rare (< 1%)
    - Multiple lesions not suggestive of primary BMT
    - May be seen in **recurrent BMT**

Natural History & Prognosis

- Slowly growing, painless, benign tumor
- Recurrent tumor typically from incomplete resection or cellular spillage at surgery
  - o Recurrent BMT **multifocal** (cluster of grapes)
- Malignant transformation reported up to 15% if left untreated
  - o Referred to as **carcinoma ex pleomorphic adenoma**
  - o Various histologies

Treatment

- Complete surgical resection of encapsulated mass within adequate margin of surrounding parotid gland tissue to avoid cellular spillage and seeding
- Recurrent tumor difficult to treat
  - o Radiation treatment of uncertain effectiveness

DIAGNOSTIC CHECKLIST

Consider

- **Large asymptomatic** masses arising from **deep lobe of parotid** almost always **BMT**

Image Interpretation Pearls

- Define facial nerve plane and identify deep parotid lobe component as this may be missed clinically
- Infiltrative margins, multicentricity, or hypointense T2 signal suggests malignancy
- Must distinguish deep lobe parotid BMT from true parapharyngeal BMT
  - o Look for fat plane between parotid tissue and BMT

SELECTED REFERENCES

1. Dong Y et al: Diagnostic value of CT perfusion imaging for parotid neoplasms. Dentomaxillofac Radiol. 43(1):20130237, 2014
2. Brennan PA et al: Is ultrasound alone sufficient for imaging superficial lobe benign parotid tumours before surgery? Br J Oral Maxillofac Surg. 50(4):333-7, 2012
3. Christe A et al: MR imaging of parotid tumors: typical lesion characteristics in MR imaging improve discrimination between benign and malignant disease. AJNR Am J Neuroradiol. 32(7):1202-7, 2011
4. Dumitriu D et al: Ultrasonographic and sonoelastographic features of pleomorphic adenomas of the salivary glands. Med Ultrason. 12(3):175-83, 2010
5. Habermann CR et al: Diffusion-weighted echo-planar MR imaging of primary parotid gland tumors: is a prediction of different histologic subtypes possible? AJNR Am J Neuroradiol. 30(3):591-6, 2009
6. Yabuuchi H et al: Parotid gland tumors: can addition of diffusion-weighted MR imaging to dynamic contrast-enhanced MR imaging improve diagnostic accuracy in characterization? Radiology. 249(3):909-16, 2008
7. Ikeda K et al: The usefulness of MR in establishing the diagnosis of parotid pleomorphic adenoma. AJNR Am J Neuroradiol. 17(3):555-9, 1996
8. Joe VQ et al: Tumors of the parotid gland: MR imaging characteristics of various histologic types. AJR Am J Roentgenol. 163(2):433-8, 1994

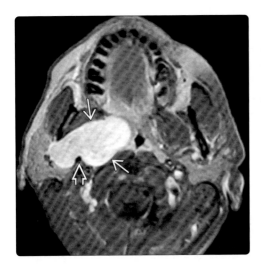

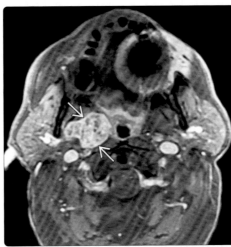

(Left) *Axial T1WI C+ FS MR shows a large, lobulated, homogeneously enhancing mass ➡ in the deep lobe of the parotid. The styloid process ➡ indents the posterior aspect of the mass, indicating that the mass is in the parotid space, suggesting BMT.* (Right) *Axial T1WI C+ FS MR shows a heterogeneously enhancing mass ➡ in the deep lobe of the parotid. BMTs enhance to variable degrees. Homogeneous, heterogeneous, and poorly enhancing tumors may be seen.*

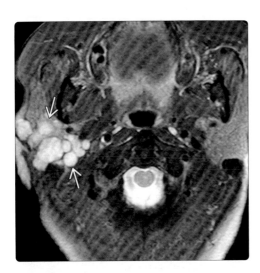

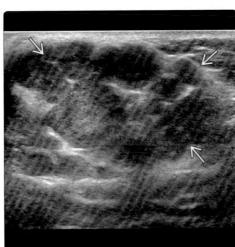

(Left) *Axial T2WI FS MR in a patient with previous removal of a right parotid BMT shows the typical cluster of grapes high-signal multifocal recurrent BMTs ➡ in the parotid bed. (From DI: Ultrasound.)* (Right) *Longitudinal grayscale US shows a cluster of solid, hypoechoic nodules at the postoperative site ➡ in a patient with previous surgery for BMT. Multifocal benign mixed tumors by themselves are rare (< 1%) but are often seen in recurrent BMT as in this case. (From DI: Ultrasound.)*

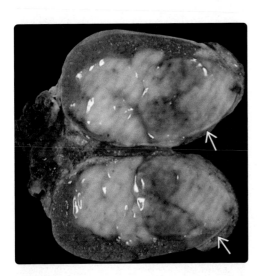

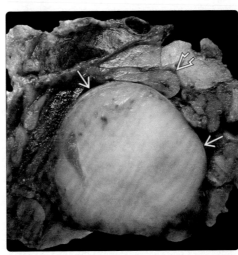

(Left) *Gross photograph shows a well-circumscribed, oval BMT. Bisection shows a tan-pink to white surface and a thin fibrous capsule ➡. This fibrous capsule must not be violated during surgical removal or multifocal recurrence may ensue. (From DP: Head & Neck.)* (Right) *Gross photograph shows a formalin-fixed BMT with a well-defined fibrous capsule ➡ surrounded by normal parotid gland ➡. This specimen illustrates why BMT in the parotid gland is so well circumscribed when imaged. (From DP: Head & Neck.)*

Warthin Tumor

TERMINOLOGY

- Benign tumor arising from salivary-lymphoid tissue in intraparotid & periparotid nodes
- Most common mass to arise in parotid tail superficial to angle of mandible

IMAGING

- Contrast-enhanced CT or MR provides adequate presurgical information
- **20% multifocal**
  - May be multiple lesions in 1 gland or bilateral lesions
  - May be synchronous or metachronous
- Sharply marginated **parotid tail** mass
- **Parenchymal heterogeneity** is characteristic
- Cystic component in 30% with thin, uniform walls & CT density of 10-20 HU
  - Difficult to differentiate from 1st branchial cleft cyst, infected lymph node, or other cystic mass
- Increased uptake of FDG
- Incidentally PET/CT finding
- Ultrasound highly suggestive
  - Well-defined hypoechoic mass or masses with multiple hypoechoic areas at lower pole of superficial parotid
  - Heterogeneous cystic & solid internal architecture
  - Multiseptated with debris

TOP DIFFERENTIAL DIAGNOSES

- Benign lymphoepithelial lesions-HIV
- Parotid benign mixed tumor
- Parotid adenoid cystic carcinoma
- Parotid mucoepidermoid carcinoma
- Parotid metastatic nodal disease
- Parotid non-Hodgkin lymphoma

CLINICAL ISSUES

- Angle of mandible (tail of parotid) mass in **smoker**
- **2nd** most frequent benign parotid tumor
  - BMT most common parotid tumor

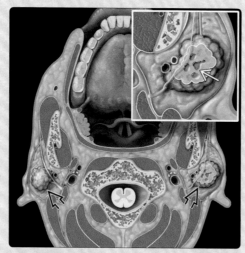
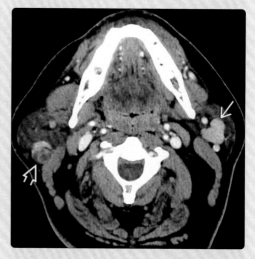

(Left) Axial graphic depicts bilateral, mixed solid/cystic, parotid tail Warthin tumors ➔. A larger left intraparotid tumor is cut in the insert to show characteristic parenchymal cystic changes ➔. (Right) Axial CECT shows bilateral parotid masses. The left-sided lesion ➔ is homogeneously enhancing. The right-sided lesion ➔ is heterogeneous. Twenty percent of Warthin tumors are multifocal.

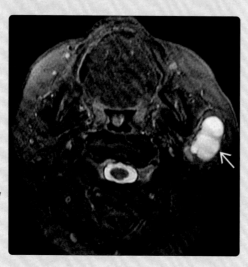
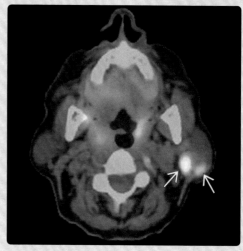

(Left) Axial T2WI FS MR shows a high-intensity mass ➔ with thin septations in the superficial lobe of the parotid gland. Thirty percent of Warthin tumors appear cystic on imaging. (Right) Axial PET/CT shows marked FDG uptake in 2 parotid masses ➔. Some benign glandular tumors, such as oncocytomas and Warthin tumors, are FDG avid, but multifocality suggests Warthin tumor. These lesions must be sampled to exclude metastatic disease.

TERMINOLOGY

Synonyms

- Papillary cystadenoma lymphomatosum, adenolymphoma, lymphomatous adenoma

Definitions

- Benign tumor with characteristic histopathologic appearance: Papillary structures, mature lymphocytic infiltrate, & cystic changes

IMAGING

General Features

- Best diagnostic clue
  o Sharply marginated parotid tail mass with heterogeneous parenchyma
- Location
  o Intraparotid > > periparotid > upper cervical nodes
  o Most common mass to arise in parotid tail superficial to angle of mandible
  o **20% multifocal**
    – Multiple lesions in 1 gland or bilateral lesions
    – May be synchronous or metachronous
- Size
  o Typically 2- to 4-cm diameter
  o Neglected lesions > 10-cm diameter
- Morphology
  o Round to ovoid, well-circumscribed, encapsulated mass or masses
  o **Parenchymal heterogeneity** is **characteristic**

CT Findings

- CECT
  o Solitary small, ovoid, smoothly marginated masses in posterior aspect of superficial lobe of parotid
  o No calcification
  o Cystic component in 30% with thin, uniform walls & CT density of 10-20 HU
    – Large cystic component, septa or multiple adjacent cystic lesions
      □ May be difficult to differentiate from 1st branchial cleft cyst, infected lymph node, or other cystic mass
    – **Mural nodule** more suggestive of Warthin tumor
  o Minimal enhancement of solid components
  o Dynamic CT behavior
    – Rapid enhancement with rapid washout

MR Findings

- T1WI
  o Low signal in both solid & cystic components
  o Cystic areas may show high signal secondary to proteinaceous debris ± hemorrhage
- T2WI
  o Intermediate to high T2 signal in solid component
  o High T2 signal in cystic foci
- STIR
  o Lesions more conspicuous, especially cystic component
- DWI
  o ADC values lower than benign mixed tumor (BMT), but similar to carcinoma
- T1WI C+

  o Minimal contrast enhancement of solid components
  o Dynamic contrast imaging: Rapid enhancement with rapid washout
    – Similar to some carcinomas

Nuclear Medicine Findings

- PET
  o Increased uptake of FDG
    – Benign parotid tumors (Warthin, oncocytoma) often incidentally seen on PET
- Technetium-99m
  o Increased uptake within mitochondrial-rich oncocytes of Warthin tumors
  o Delayed "washout" following sialogogue administration

Imaging Recommendations

- Best imaging tool
  o Contrast-enhanced CT or MR provides adequate presurgical information

DIFFERENTIAL DIAGNOSIS

Benign Lymphoepithelial Lesions-HIV

- When unilateral & singular, may strongly mimic Warthin tumor
- Tonsillar hyperplasia & cervical adenopathy help differentiate

Parotid Benign Mixed Tumor

- Well-circumscribed, homogeneous, intraparotid mass when small
- Larger lesions may be heterogeneous & mimic Warthin

Malignant Parotid Tumor

- Parotid adenoid cystic carcinoma
  o Low-grade tumor may be well demarcated & mimic Warthin tumor
  o High-grade tumor invasive appearance is distinctive
  o Perineural tumor spread common
- Parotid mucoepidermoid carcinoma
  o Low-grade tumor may be well demarcated & mimic Warthin tumor
  o High-grade tumor invasive appearance is distinctive
  o Adjacent malignant nodes common

Parotid Metastatic Nodal Disease

- Primary malignancy on or around skin of ear
- Single or multiple parotid masses with invasive margins
- Central necrosis may mimic cystic change of Warthin tumor

Parotid Non-Hodgkin Lymphoma

- Multiple solid, uniformly enhancing, intraparotid lesions
- Cervical adenopathy may help differentiate from Warthin tumor

PATHOLOGY

General Features

- Etiology
  o **Smoking-induced**, benign tumor arising from salivary-lymphoid tissue **in** intraparotid & periparotid nodes
  o Theorized heterotopic salivary gland parenchyma present in preexisting intra- or periparotid lymph nodes

o Reported association with **Epstein-Barr virus**
  – Patients with multifocal or bilateral lesions
- Associated abnormalities
  o Increased incidence in patients with autoimmune disorders
- Embryology
  o Parotid gland undergoes "**late encapsulation**," incorporating lymphoid tissue-nodes within superficial layer of deep cervical fascia
    – Warthin tumor arises within this lymphoid tissue

Gross Pathologic & Surgical Features

- Encapsulated, soft, ovoid mass with smooth, lobulated surface
- Tan tissue with cystic spaces that contain tenacious, mucoid, brown fluid or thin, yellow fluid with cholesterol crystals
  o Papillary projections can be seen within cystic areas

Microscopic Features

- Epithelial & lymphoid components dominate histopathologic picture
- Papillary projections are lined with double epithelial layer
  o Inner-luminal layer: Tall columnar cells with nuclei oriented toward lumen
  o Outer-basal layer: Cuboidal or polygonal cells with vesicular nuclei
- Inner lymphoid component of papillary projection is composed of mature lymphoid aggregates with germinal centers

CLINICAL ISSUES

Presentation

- Most common signs/symptoms
  o Angle of mandible (tail of parotid) mass
  o Painless
  o Multiple masses ~ 20%
- Other signs/symptoms
  o Facial nerve weakness very rare
    – Suggests malignancy
- Clinical profile
  o **90%** of patients with Warthin tumor **smoke**
  o Increased incidence with radiation exposure

Demographics

- Age
  o Mean age at presentation = 60 years
- Gender
  o Earlier reports have M:F = 3:1
  o More recent reports show more equal gender incidence (likely related to smoking patterns)
- Epidemiology
  o **2nd** most frequent benign parotid tumor (after benign mixed tumor)
  o 10% of all salivary gland epithelial tumors
  o 12% of benign parotid gland tumors
  o 20% multifocal: May be unilateral or bilateral, synchronous or metachronous
  o **5-10%** arise in **extraparotid** locations (periparotid & upper neck lymph nodes)

Natural History & Prognosis

- Slowly growing, benign tumor
- Malignant transformation (carcinoma or lymphoma) reported in < 1%
- "Recurrent" Warthin tumor may be from inadequate resection or metachronous 2nd lesion

Treatment

- Biopsy (or excision) needed for confirmation of benign nature
- Resection of mass within a collar of normal parotid tissue without injury to intraparotid facial nerve is treatment goal

DIAGNOSTIC CHECKLIST

Consider

- Consider CECT to help identify cystic areas within Warthin tumor to help differentiate from small BMT
- Enhanced T1 with fat saturation to determine intra- vs. periparotid tumor location & to define plane of facial nerve

Image Interpretation Pearls

- Be sure to carefully examine for multiplicity & bilaterality
- Well-circumscribed heterogeneous multiple or bilateral parotid masses in asymptomatic smoker should be considered Warthin tumor

SELECTED REFERENCES

1. Dell'Aversana Orabona G et al: Surgical management of benign tumors of the parotid gland: extracapsular dissection versus superficial parotidectomy--our experience in 232 cases. J Oral Maxillofac Surg. 71(2):410-3, 2013
2. Teymoortash A et al: Is Warthin's tumour of the parotid gland a lymph node disease? Histopathology. 59(1):143-5, 2011
3. Habermann CR et al: Diffusion-weighted echo-planar MR imaging of primary parotid gland tumors: is a prediction of different histologic subtypes possible? AJNR Am J Neuroradiol. 30(3):591-6, 2009
4. Yabuuchi H et al: Parotid gland tumors: can addition of diffusion-weighted MR imaging to dynamic contrast-enhanced MR imaging improve diagnostic accuracy in characterization? Radiology. 249(3):909-16, 2008
5. Hamilton BE et al: Earring lesions of the parotid tail. AJNR Am J Neuroradiol. 24(9):1757-64, 2003
6. Parwani AV et al: Diagnostic accuracy and pitfalls in fine-needle aspiration interpretation of Warthin tumor. Cancer. 99(3):166-71, 2003
7. Laane CJ et al: Role of Epstein-Barr virus and cytomegalovirus in the etiology of benign parotid tumors. Head Neck. 24(5):443-50, 2002
8. Lewis PD et al: Mitochondrial DNA mutations in the parotid gland of cigarette smokers and non-smokers. Mutat Res. 518(1):47-54, 2002
9. Maiorano E et al: Warthin's tumour: a study of 78 cases with emphasis on bilaterality, multifocality and association with other malignancies. Oral Oncol. 38(1):35-40, 2002
10. Raymond MR et al: Accuracy of fine-needle aspiration biopsy for Warthin's tumours. J Otolaryngol. 31(5):263-70, 2002
11. Webb AJ et al: Parotid Warthin's tumour Bristol Royal Infirmary (1985-1995): a study of histopathology in 33 cases. Oral Oncol. 38(2):163-71, 2002
12. Miyake H et al: Warthin's tumor of parotid gland on Tc-99m pertechnetate scintigraphy with lemon juice stimulation: Tc-99m uptake, size, and pathologic correlation. Eur Radiol. 11(12):2472-8, 2001
13. Joe VQ et al: Tumors of the parotid gland: MR imaging characteristics of various histologic types. AJR Am J Roentgenol. 163(2):433-8, 1994
14. Minami M et al: Warthin tumor of the parotid gland: MR-pathologic correlation. AJNR Am J Neuroradiol. 14(1):209-14, 1993

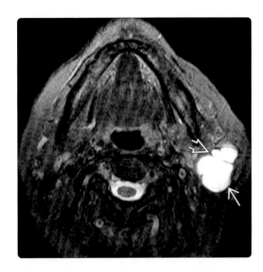

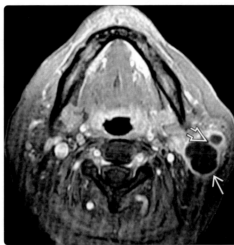

(Left) *Axial T2WI FS MR shows a high-intensity mass ➡ with septations ⮞ in the superficial lobe of the parotid gland. Cystic Warthin tumors can be confused with simple cysts.* (Right) *Axial T1WI C+ FS MR in the same patient reveals a septated ⮞ low-intensity mass ➡ with an enhancing rim. This enhancement can help to distinguish Warthin tumors from simple cysts but may be mistaken for parotid abscess. Note the lack of surrounding fat stranding, which argues against abscess.*

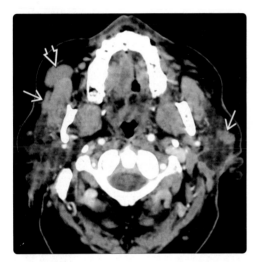

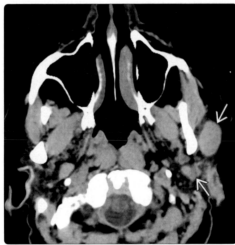

(Left) *Axial CECT shows multiple bilateral, ovoid, poorly enhancing Warthin tumors ➡ within the parotid glands. Note, in particular, the tumor involving the right accessory parotid lobe ⮞.* (Right) *Axial NECT shows multiple well-defined, ovoid Warthin tumors ➡ of varying size within the left parotid gland. Twenty percent of patients with Warthin tumor have multifocal disease, which may be multiple lesions in a single gland or bilateral lesions.*

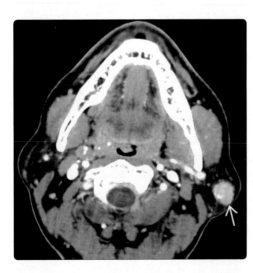

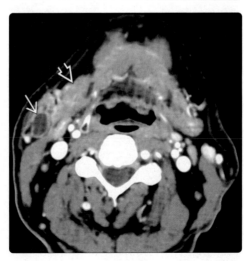

(Left) *Axial CECT shows a round, uniformly enhancing mass ➡ in the superficial lobe of the parotid gland. Smaller Warthin tumors may enhance homogeneously, but larger tumors are generally heterogeneous.* (Right) *Axial CECT shows a cystic mass ➡ lateral to the submandibular gland ⮞, near the parotid tail. Although most Warthin tumors arise within the parotid gland, some are found in periparotid lymph nodes.*

KEY FACTS

TERMINOLOGY

- Benign nerve sheath neoplasm from Schwann cells of intraparotid facial nerve (CNVII)

IMAGING

- Heterogeneously enhancing tumor with intramural cystic areas when large
  - Cystic areas may be small, multifocal, or large
- May extend toward or into stylomastoid foramen
- Similar appearance to schwannomas in other anatomic locations

TOP DIFFERENTIAL DIAGNOSES

- Parotid benign mixed tumor
- Warthin tumor
- Parotid metastatic nodal disease
- Parotid mucoepidermoid carcinoma
- Perineural tumor spread, CNVII

PATHOLOGY

- < 10% CNVII schwannoma = extratemporal (intraparotid), remaining = intratemporal or intracranial
- Type A: Exophytic off CNVII branch; no CNVII resection required
- Type B: Intrinsic to facial nerve branch; branch resection required
- Type C: Intrinsic to facial nerve trunk; resection and reconstruction required
- Type D: Encases main trunk and branches; resection and reconstruction required

CLINICAL ISSUES

- Presents like any parotid mass; difficult to differentiate clinically or radiographically
  - Facial nerve palsy uncommon
- Associated with neurofibromatosis type 2
- Treatment goal: Preserve facial nerve function
  - Controversial: Observation vs. surgery vs. radiation

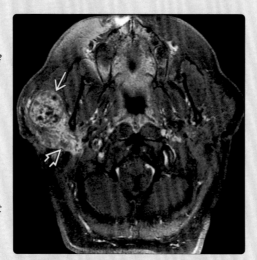
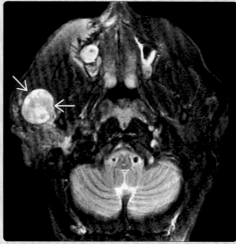

(Left) Axial T1WI C+ FS MR shows a rounded mass ➡ in the anterior aspect of the superficial parotid lobe. There are areas of heterogeneous enhancement with scattered cystic regions. Note the parotitis ⬆ that results from ductal obstruction by the schwannoma. (Right) Axial T2WI FS MR shows a round mass ➡ with heterogeneous high signal in the anterior aspect of the superficial parotid lobe. This lesion appearance would be difficult to distinguish from the far more common benign mixed tumor.

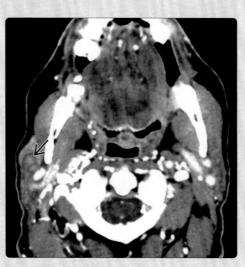
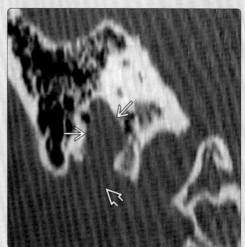

(Left) Axial CECT in a patient with neurofibromatosis type 2 shows a round, subcentimeter mass ➡ in the anterior aspect of the superficial parotid lobe. This schwannoma has heterogeneous enhancement but no cystic areas because of its small size. (Right) Coronal bone CT shows smooth expansion of the vertical segment of the facial canal ➡. The facial nerve schwannoma extends from the parotid gland ➡ up through the stylomastoid foramen.

Parotid Schwannoma

TERMINOLOGY

Synonyms

- Facial neuroma, intraparotid neurilemmoma

Definitions

- Benign nerve sheath neoplasm from Schwann cells of intraparotid facial nerve (CNVII)

IMAGING

General Features

- Best diagnostic clue
  - Heterogeneously enhancing + **intramural cysts**
- Location
  - Course of intraparotid CNVII ± stylomastoid foramen

Imaging Recommendations

- Best imaging tool
  - T1WI C+ FS MR best demonstrates cystic areas

CT Findings

- CECT
  - Well-defined, intraparotid, round or oval mass
  - Intramural cysts within larger (> 2 cm) lesions
  - Enlarged stylomastoid foramen in proximal lesions

MR Findings

- T1WI
  - Tumor isointense to muscle, well defined
- T2WI
  - Slightly hyperintense to brain, muscle
  - Larger lesions with high-intensity cysts
- T1WI C+ FS
  - Enhancing & cystic regions + peripheral enhancement

DIFFERENTIAL DIAGNOSIS

Parotid Benign Mixed Tumor

- Appears similar to schwannoma on CT & MR
  - Benign mixed tumor classically with bosselated margins

Warthin Tumor

- Cystic areas present as in schwannoma
- Can be multiple, bilateral, & favor parotid tail

Parotid Metastatic Nodal Disease

- Often multiple; have primary lesion (e.g., skin, lymphoma)

Parotid Mucoepidermoid Carcinoma

- Low-grade form of mucoepidermoid carcinoma
  - Well defined

Perineural Tumor Spread, CNVII

- Parotid or skin primary lesion

PATHOLOGY

General Features

- Etiology
  - Arises from differentiated neoplastic Schwann cells of CNVII nerve sheath
  - < 10% CNVII schwannoma = extratemporal (intraparotid), remaining = intratemporal or intracranial

Staging, Grading, & Classification

- Type A: Exophytic off CNVII branch; no CNVII resection required
- Type B: Intrinsic to CNVII branch; branch resection required
- Type C: Intrinsic to CNVII trunk; resection & reconstruction required
- Type D: Encases main CNVII trunk & branches; resection & reconstruction required

Gross Pathologic & Surgical Features

- Smooth, rubbery, yellow, encapsulated fusiform mass

Microscopic Features

- Same as schwannomas in other anatomic locations

CLINICAL ISSUES

Presentation

- Most common signs/symptoms
  - Painless, slowly enlarging cheek mass
- Other signs/symptoms
  - Presents like any parotid mass; difficult to differentiate clinically or radiographically
    - Rarely diagnosed preoperatively unless biopsied
  - CNVII palsy uncommon: ↑ risk if intratemporal extension
  - Associated with neurofibromatosis type 2

Demographics

- Age: Can affect any age group

Natural History & Prognosis

- Slow, continuous enlargement
- May eventually cause mass effect or cosmetic issues

Treatment

- Controversial: Observation vs. surgery vs. radiation
  - Goal: CNVII function preservation & facial cosmesis
  - Can dissect tumor off of nerve, but CNVII palsy may still result
  - Types C and D lesions at greater risk of postoperative CNVII palsy
  - Treatment depends on CNVII function & location of tumor
- Stereotactic radiosurgery may be used if CNVII intact

DIAGNOSTIC CHECKLIST

Consider

- Which branch of facial nerve involved
  - Main trunk most common
- Relationship of mass to stylomastoid foramen
  - Extent into mastoid segment of bony facial nerve canal

Image Interpretation Pearls

- Difficult to make radiographic diagnosis
  - Tissue sampling required but excisional biopsy risky
  - Image-guided biopsy (CT or US) very useful
    - Core needle biopsy required (FNA inadequate)

SELECTED REFERENCES

1. Zhang GZ et al: Clinical retrospective analysis of 9 cases of intraparotid facial nerve schwannoma. J Oral Maxillofac Surg. pii: S0278-2391(16)00165-8, 2016

Parotid Mucoepidermoid Carcinoma

KEY FACTS

TERMINOLOGY

- Malignant epithelial salivary gland neoplasm composed of mixture of both epidermoid & mucus-secreting cells arising from ductal epithelium

IMAGING

- Imaging appearance based on histologic grade
  - **Low-grade MECa**: Well-circumscribed, heterogeneous PS mass
  - **High-grade MECa**: Invasive, ill-defined PS mass with associated malignant nodes
- If lesion high grade, infiltrative, or near stylomastoid foramen, **perineural spread** along **CNVII** may occur
- High-grade MECa often has **nodal metastases**
- MR findings
  - **Low T2** areas characteristic but not pathognomonic
  - T1 C+ shows heterogeneous tumor enhancement
  - Enhanced images may "hide" lesion

- MR useful for extent of lesion and facial nerve **perineural spread**

TOP DIFFERENTIAL DIAGNOSES

- Parotid benign mixed tumor
- Warthin tumor
- Parotid adenoid cystic carcinoma
- Parotid non-Hodgkin lymphoma
- Parotid metastatic nodes

CLINICAL ISSUES

- MECa is most common primary parotid malignancy
- Recurrence & survival rates depend heavily on histologic grade
- Late local recurrence (after 5 years) possible

DIAGNOSTIC CHECKLIST

- Low-grade MECa may exactly mimic BMT
- High-grade MECa has invasive appearance

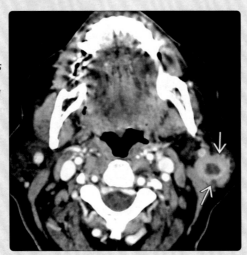
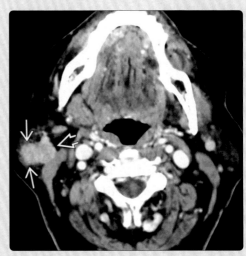

(Left) Axial CECT reveals a well-defined mass ➡ in the superficial lobe of the parotid gland. It has a thick rind of peripheral enhancement and is centrally cystic or necrotic. This is a characteristic imaging appearance for a low-grade mucoepidermoid carcinoma (MECa). (Right) Axial CECT shows a mass in the parotid gland with ill-defined lateral borders ➡ and well-defined medial borders ➡. The tumor enhances uniformly. Although nonspecific, this is the expected appearance of an intermediate-grade MECa.

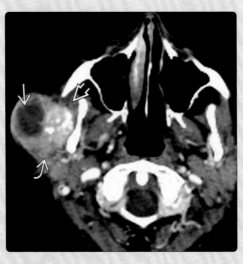
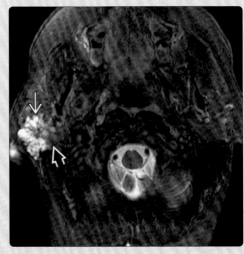

(Left) Axial CECT shows a large, heterogeneous mass with cystic areas ➡, heterogeneous enhancement, and ill-defined borders ➡. The masseter muscle is invaded ➡. This is a characteristic appearance of a high-grade MECa. (Right) Axial T2WI FS MR shows an irregular mass in the parotid with mixed T2 signal. Laterally, there are high-signal cystic areas ➡, but medially there is a low-signal region ➡. Low T2 signal within the solid components of the tumor is characteristic of MECa.

TERMINOLOGY

Abbreviations

- Mucoepidermoid carcinoma (MECa)

Definitions

- Malignant epithelial salivary gland neoplasm composed of variable mixture of both epidermoid & mucus-secreting cells arising from ductal epithelium

IMAGING

General Features

- Best diagnostic clue
  - Imaging appearance based on histologic grade
  - Low-grade MECa: Well-circumscribed, heterogeneous PS mass
  - High-grade MECa: **Invasive**, ill-defined PS mass with associated **malignant nodes**
- Location
  - Superficial lobe > > deep lobe parotid
- Size
  - Usually 1-4 cm at presentation
- Morphology
  - Low grade: Ovoid, well circumscribed
    - Cystic areas may be single & large or small & multifocal
  - High grade: Amorphous, infiltrating mass
- **Malignant adenopathy** often present
  - 1st order nodes = jugulodigastric nodes (level II)
  - Intrinsic parotid nodes & parotid tail nodes also involved

CT Findings

- CECT
  - Low-grade MECa
    - Enhancing heterogeneous mass with well-defined margins
    - Mucous deposits create cystic areas
    - Calcification may occur
  - High-grade MECa
    - Enhancing invasive mass with ill-defined margins
    - Intraparotid & cervical metastatic nodes

MR Findings

- T1WI
  - Low-grade MECa: Heterogeneous, well-defined mass with predominantly low signal
  - High-grade MECa: Solid, infiltrative mass with intermediate signal
- T2WI
  - Low-grade MECa: Heterogeneous signal
    - Areas of low signal are characteristic but not pathognomonic
    - Cystic areas have high signal
  - High-grade MECa: Intermediate signal infiltrating mass
- DWI
  - ADC value lower than benign mixed tumor (BMT) but similar to Warthin tumor
    - Not reliable enough to avoid biopsy
- T1WI C+
  - Heterogeneous enhancement
    - Cystic areas have no enhancement
  - If lesion high grade, infiltrative, or near stylomastoid foramen, perineural spread on CNVII may occur

Nuclear Medicine Findings

- No pertechnetate uptake (unlike Warthin tumor)

Imaging Recommendations

- Best imaging tool
  - MR useful for extent of lesion and perineural spread
  - No radiographic modality provides definitive diagnosis
- Protocol advice
  - T1 unenhanced images best delineate MECa because high-signal fat of normal parotid tissue provides natural contrast
  - Enhanced images may "hide" lesion even if fat saturation used
  - Long-term (at least 10 years) imaging follow-up recommended because of late recurrences

DIFFERENTIAL DIAGNOSIS

Parotid Benign Mixed Tumor

- Most common parotid mass
- Small: Well demarcated, solid, homogeneous, ovoid
- Large: Heterogeneous, lobulated
- Low-grade MECa may be confused with BMT

Warthin Tumor

- Multicentric (20%)
- CECT: 30% with cystic components
- T1WI C+ MR: Heterogeneous enhancement, well circumscribed
- Cystic areas of low-grade MECa appear similar to cystic areas of Warthin tumor

Parotid Adenoid Cystic Carcinoma

- 2nd most common parotid malignancy
- Homogeneous; may be well defined or poorly defined, depending on grade
- Prone to perineural spread

Parotid Non-Hodgkin Lymphoma

- Primary parotid lymphoma: Invasive parenchymal tumor indistinguishable from high-grade MECa or adenoid cystic carcinoma (ACCa)
- Primary nodal lymphoma: Multiple bilateral intraparotid masses

Parotid Metastatic Nodes

- Primary lesion usually on or around skin of ear (SCCa, melanoma)
- Multiple intraparotid masses, often with central necrosis

Parotid Ductal Carcinoma

- Salivary ductal carcinoma similar to high-grade MECa on CT and MR
- Low T2 signal, infiltrative mass characteristic of both histologies
- Cannot differentiate preoperatively

PATHOLOGY

General Features

- Etiology

- Exposure risk: Radiation
  - Latency: 7-32 years

Staging, Grading, & Classification

- TNM staging
  - T1: Tumor ≤ 2 cm without extraparenchymal extension
  - T2: Tumor 2-4 cm without extraparenchymal extension
  - T3: Tumor 4-6 cm with extraparenchymal extension
  - T4: Tumor > 6 cm or invades adjacent structures
    - Mandible, skull base, deep spaces of suprahyoid neck
- Histologic grading (low vs. intermediate vs. high) correlates best with prognosis

Gross Pathologic & Surgical Features

- Gray, tan-yellow, or pink

Microscopic Features

- Mixture of epidermoid & mucus-secreting cells, with some cells intermediate between
- Cellular atypia & pleomorphism
- Arises in glandular ductal epithelium

CLINICAL ISSUES

Presentation

- Most common signs/symptoms
  - Palpable parotid mass, usually rock-hard
  - Other signs/symptoms: Facial pain, otalgia, facial nerve paralysis
    - Other cranial nerve involvement (CNV3)
  - Clinical presentation depends on tumor grade
    - Low grade: Painless, mobile, slowly enlarging
    - High grade: Painful, immobile, rapidly enlarging

Demographics

- Age
  - Usually 35-65 years old
  - May be seen in pediatric population
- Epidemiology
  - **MECa** is **most common** primary parotid malignancy
  - MECa: 10% of all salivary gland tumors
  - MECa: 30% of all salivary gland malignancies
  - Majority (60%) occur in parotid
    - Also other salivary glands, any mucosal surface (esp. larynx), or within bone (mandible)

Natural History & Prognosis

- Recurrence & survival rates depend heavily on histologic grade
  - Low grade: 6% local recurrence; 90% 10-year survival rate
  - Intermediate grade: 20% local recurrence; 80% 10-year survival rate
  - High grade: 78% local recurrence; 27% 10-year survival rate
  - Distant mets common in high grade; uncommon in low/intermediate
- Poor prognostic signs
  - Male sex
  - Age > 40 years
  - Fixed tumor, invasion of surrounding structures
  - Higher TNM stage or histologic grade

- Cellular markers (p53, Ki-67)
- Late local recurrence (after 5 years) possible

Treatment

- Low-grade MECa
  - Wide local excision with preservation of facial nerve
  - Superficial parotidectomy if possible
  - Total parotidectomy may be necessary if tumor involves deep lobe
  - Postoperative radiotherapy
- High-grade MECa
  - Wide local excision; extended total parotidectomy
  - Facial nerve sacrifice often necessary
  - Neck dissection routine
  - Postoperative radiotherapy with large port

DIAGNOSTIC CHECKLIST

Consider

- In all parotid masses, check for **perineural spread** along **CNVII**
  - Replaced fat in stylomastoid foramen
  - Enhancement of vertical (mastoid) segment of CNVII
  - Extension along CNV3 (foramen ovale) if deep lobe parotid or **auriculotemporal nerve** involved
- Check for invasion of surrounding structures: Mandible, skull base, deep fascial spaces

Image Interpretation Pearls

- Low-grade MECa may exactly mimic BMT
- High-grade MECa has nonspecific invasive appearance
  - Remember to look for nodal metastases
  - Also check stylomastoid foramen & mastoid segment CNVII for perineural tumor spread
- General evaluation of parotid space masses
  - 1st decide whether lesion is **intraparotid** (BMT, Warthin, MECa, ACCa) or **extraparotid** (skin or different suprahyoid space)
  - If intraparotid, distinguish superficial vs. deep lobe
    - Divided by facial nerve plane, just lateral to retromandibular vein
  - Sharpness of margins helps distinguish benign from malignant lesions
    - Caveat: Benign tumors can incite sialadenitis, & low-grade malignancy may have sharp margins

SELECTED REFERENCES

1. Kashiwagi N et al: MRI findings of mucoepidermoid carcinoma of the parotid gland: correlation with pathological features. Br J Radiol. 85(1014):709-13, 2012
2. Singh Nanda KD et al: Fine-needle aspiration cytology: a reliable tool in the diagnosis of salivary gland lesions. J Oral Pathol Med. 41(1):106-12, 2012
3. Christe A et al: MR imaging of parotid tumors: typical lesion characteristics in MR imaging improve discrimination between benign and malignant disease. AJNR Am J Neuroradiol. 32(7):1202-7, 2011
4. Boukheris H et al: Incidence of carcinoma of the major salivary glands according to the WHO classification, 1992 to 2006: a population-based study in the United States. Cancer Epidemiol Biomarkers Prev. 18(11):2899-906, 2009
5. Pinkston JA et al: Incidence rates of salivary gland tumors: results from a population-based study. Otolaryngol Head Neck Surg. 120(6):834-40, 1999
6. Goode RK et al: Mucoepidermoid carcinoma of the major salivary glands: clinical and histopathologic analysis of 234 cases with evaluation of grading criteria. Cancer. 82(7):1217-24, 1998
7. Freling NJ et al: Malignant parotid tumors: clinical use of MR imaging and histologic correlation. Radiology. 185(3):691-6, 1992

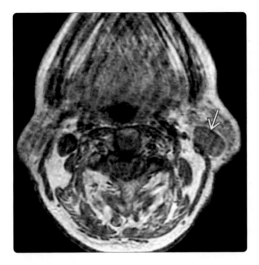
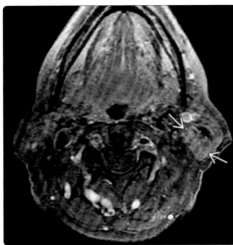

(Left) Axial T1WI MR shows a well-defined, ovoid mass ➡ of intermediate signal in the parotid tail. Note that this low-grade MECa is easily distinguished from the surrounding gland on this unenhanced image. (Right) Axial T1WI C+ FS MR in the same patient shows a well-defined, ovoid MECa ➡ that is almost indistinguishable from the surrounding parotid gland. The administration of contrast can sometimes obscure parotid masses if the enhancement matches the inherent fat signal in the gland.

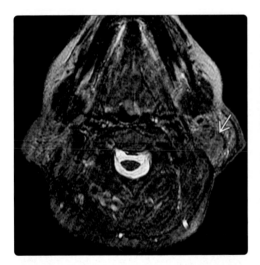
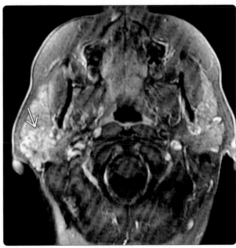

(Left) Axial T2WI FS MR in the same patient demonstrates a low-signal, well-defined, ovoid mass ➡ in the parotid gland. Low T2 signal is unusual and is most frequently a sign of MECa. (Right) Axial T1WI C+ FS MR shows a lobular, well-defined mass ➡ in the parotid gland with numerous smaller cystic spaces. The cystic areas in MECa can be either 1 large cyst or multiple smaller cysts.

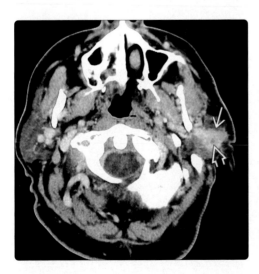
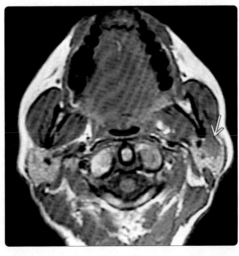

(Left) Axial CECT reveals an ill-defined, enhancing mass ➡ in the left parotid gland with a small, central cystic area ➡. This is a characteristic imaging appearance for intermediate-grade MECa. (Right) Axial T1WI MR shows a well-defined, intermediate-signal mass ➡ in the superficial lobe of the parotid gland. There are no features that specifically distinguish this mass as a low-grade MECa, which is why biopsy is needed in almost all parotid masses.

Parotid Adenoid Cystic Carcinoma

KEY FACTS

TERMINOLOGY

- Malignant salivary gland neoplasm arising in peripheral parotid ducts

IMAGING

- **Low-grade ACCa**: Well-circumscribed, homogeneously enhancing parotid mass
- **High-grade ACCa**: Infiltrative, homogeneously enhancing parotid mass
- MR findings
  - Moderate T2 signal intensity
  - High-grade ACCa: Lower in signal intensity
  - Look for **perineural tumor** CNVII or CNV3

TOP DIFFERENTIAL DIAGNOSES

- Parotid space benign mixed tumor
- Warthin tumor
- Parotid space mucoepidermoid carcinoma
- Intraparotid metastatic nodal disease

PATHOLOGY

- Tumor grading based on dominant histologic pattern
  - Tubular = grade 1
  - Cribriform = grade 2
  - Solid = grade 3

CLINICAL ISSUES

- Greatest propensity of all H&N tumors to spread via perineural pathway
- 33% present with pain & CNVII paralysis
- Treat with complete resection (parotidectomy)
- Postoperative radiotherapy for all but lowest grade
- Favorable short-term but poor long-term prognosis
- Metastatic spread to lungs & bones more frequent than lymph nodes
- Nodal metastasis very uncommon
- **Late local recurrence**, up to 20 years after diagnosis, is not uncommon

(Left) *Axial T1WI C+ FS MR shows an infiltrative, uniformly enhancing mass ➡ replacing the deep lobe of the parotid gland. Tumor extends into the mandibular foramen ⇨ along the inferior alveolar nerve. The perineural spread provides a clue that this is ACCa but is not a specific finding.* **(Right)** *Axial T2WI FS MR shows an ill-defined, intermediate-signal mass ➡ in the deep lobe of the parotid gland. Unlike MECa, this ACCa lacks cystic areas and low T2 signal.*

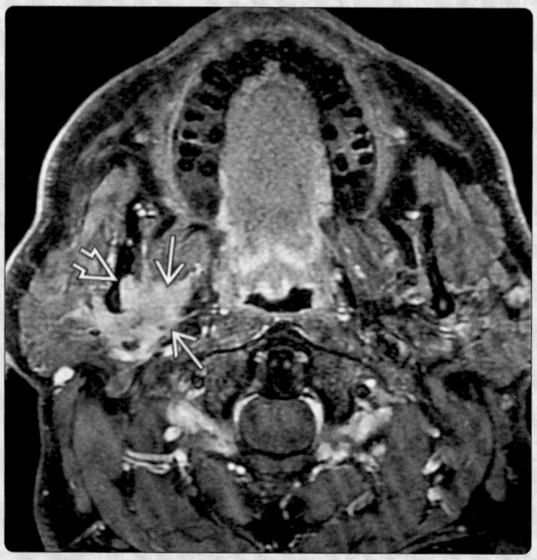

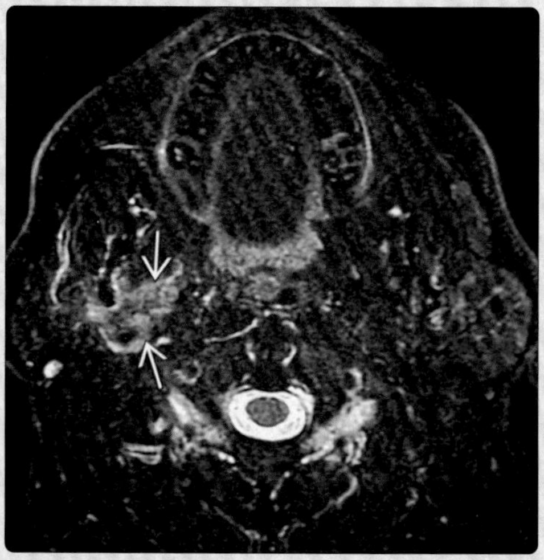

(Left) *Axial graphic depicts high-grade parotid adenoid cystic carcinoma spreading in perineural fashion along proximal facial nerve toward the stylomastoid foramen ➡ & via the auriculotemporal nerve ⇨ to the mandibular branch (CNV3) of the trigeminal nerve ⇨.* **(Right)** *Axial T1WI C+ FS MR shows marked thickening and enhancement of the auriculotemporal nerve ➡ from perineural spread of ACCa that originated in the superficial lobe of the parotid gland ⇨.*

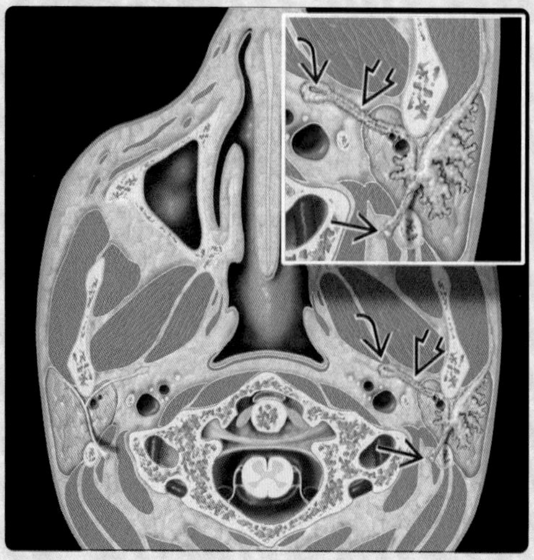

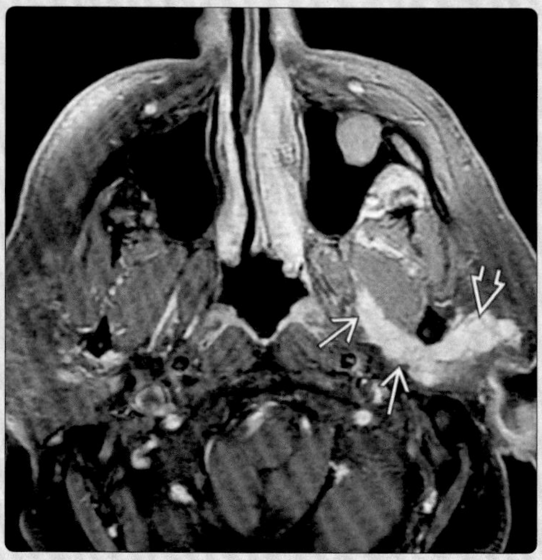

TERMINOLOGY

Abbreviations

- Adenoid cystic carcinoma (ACCa)

Definitions

- Malignant salivary gland neoplasm arising in peripheral parotid ducts
- **2nd most frequent** parotid malignancy (after mucoepidermoid carcinoma)

IMAGING

General Features

- Best diagnostic clue
  - **Low-grade ACCa**: Well-circumscribed, homogeneously enhancing parotid mass
  - **High-grade ACCa**: Infiltrative, homogeneously enhancing parotid mass
- Location
  - May involve superficial or deep lobe

CT Findings

- CECT
  - Homogeneously enhancing parotid space (PS) mass with well- (low-grade) or ill-defined (high-grade) margins

MR Findings

- T1WI
  - Low to intermediate signal intensity PS mass
- T2WI
  - Moderate signal intensity PS mass
  - High-grade tumors usually lower in signal intensity
- T1WI C+
  - Homogeneously enhancing PS mass
  - **Perineural tumor** spread on **mastoid CNVII**

DIFFERENTIAL DIAGNOSIS

Parotid Space Benign Mixed Tumor

- Well-defined, homogeneous, ovoid PS mass indistinguishable from low-grade ACCa

Warthin Tumor

- Well-defined PS mass, more heterogeneously enhancing

Parotid Space Mucoepidermoid Carcinoma

- Well-defined or infiltrative PS mass; depends on grade
- More likely cystic or with low T2 signal than ACCa

Intraparotid Metastatic Nodal Disease

- Primary lesion on skin of ear, forehead, or EAC
- Often central necrosis; may be multiple nodes

PATHOLOGY

Staging, Grading, & Classification

- Tumor grading based on dominant histologic pattern
  - Tubular = grade 1, cribriform = grade 2, solid = grade 3

Gross Pathologic & Surgical Features

- Pink-tan with mottled surface; rarely necrotic
- Infiltrative margins; no capsule

Microscopic Features

- 3 distinct histological patterns
  - Cribriform, tubular, and solid
  - Tumor may have 1, 2, or 3 of these

CLINICAL ISSUES

Presentation

- Most common signs/symptoms
  - Painful hard parotid mass; present months to years
  - 33% present with pain & CNVII paralysis

Demographics

- Age
  - Peak: 5th to 7th decades; rarely < 20 years
- Epidemiology
  - 7-18% of parotid tumors
  - Greatest propensity of all H&N tumors to spread via perineural pathway

Natural History & Prognosis

- **Late local recurrence**
  - ≤ 20 years after diagnosis
- Favorable short-term but poor long-term prognosis
- Metastatic spread to lungs & bones more frequent than lymph nodes
- Predictors of distant metastasis: Tumor > 3 cm, solid pattern, local recurrence, node disease

Treatment

- Surgical plan is wide resection with negative margins
- Postoperative radiotherapy for all but lowest grade

DIAGNOSTIC CHECKLIST

Consider

- Look carefully for **perineural tumor** with any parotid neoplasm but particularly ACCa
  - CNVII & CNV
  - **Auriculotemporal nerve** runs behind mandible
    - Alternate course for intracranial spread via CNV3
- Ill-defined margins suggest higher grade lesion

Image Interpretation Pearls

- Imaging findings often nonspecific & similar to other parotid tumors
- Imaging is for extent of mass and perineural tumor

SELECTED REFERENCES

1. Hirvonen K et al: Pattern of recurrent disease in major salivary gland adenocystic carcinoma. Virchows Arch. 467(1):19-25, 2015
2. Christe A et al: MR imaging of parotid tumors: typical lesion characteristics in MR imaging improve discrimination between benign and malignant disease. AJNR Am J Neuroradiol. 32(7):1202-7, 2011

Parotid Acinic Cell Carcinoma

TERMINOLOGY

- Slow-growing variant of adenocarcinoma arising in parotid glandular tissue
- 3rd most frequent primary parotid malignancy after mucoepidermoid and adenoid cystic carcinoma
- Rare in other salivary glands

IMAGING

- Generally indistinguishable from other low-grade parotid neoplasms
- CT: Well defined, usually homogeneously enhancing; may have cystic areas
- MR: Variable signal from cystic areas, necrosis, hemorrhage, but typically hyperintense on T2 and solid component enhances uniformly
- PET: Variable uptake; high-grade acinic cell carcinoma (AciCC) uncommon but has intense FDG uptake

TOP DIFFERENTIAL DIAGNOSES

- Parotid benign mixed tumor
- Parotid mucoepidermoid carcinoma
- Warthin tumor

PATHOLOGY

- Considered to be low-grade tumors

CLINICAL ISSUES

- Mean age 44 yr; younger than most parotid malignancies
- Favorable prognosis: 80% 10-yr survival
- Indolent course; recurrences and metastases may occur many years after treatment

DIAGNOSTIC CHECKLIST

- Important to describe location, extent, adenopathy
- Always look for CNVII perineural tumor

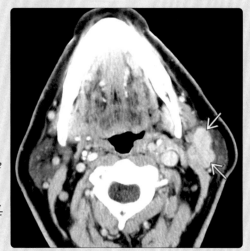
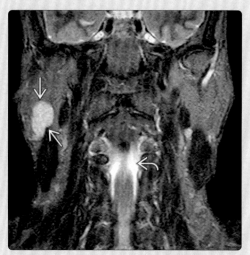

(Left) Axial CECT shows a lobulated, well-demarcated, homogeneous mass ➡ in the superficial lobe of the right parotid gland. There are no specific imaging features that would suggest AciCC over the more common benign mixed tumor. (Right) Coronal T2WI FS MR in a different patient shows a lobulated, well-defined mass ➡ with uniform high T2 signal in the tail of the right parotid gland. The solid component of AciCC is typically uniformly high signal, although not as intense as CSF ➡.

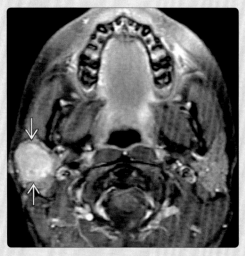
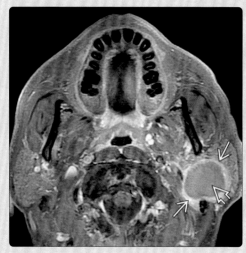

(Left) Axial T1WI C+ FS MR shows a uniformly enhancing mass ➡ expanding the superficial lobe of right parotid gland. Most AciCC are uniformly enhancing and have no imaging features to distinguish them from more common parotid neoplasms. (Right) Axial T1WI C+ FS MR in a different patient shows a large left superficial lobe mass with solidly enhancing periphery ➡ and a nonenhancing, cystic, necrotic core ➡. This AciCC showed no vascular or perineural invasion or abnormal mitoses; however, it was 90% necrotic.

Parotid Acinic Cell Carcinoma

TERMINOLOGY

Synonyms

- Acinic cell carcinoma (AciCC)
- Synonyms: Acinar cell carcinoma, acinous cell carcinoma

Definitions

- Slow-growing **variant of adenocarcinoma** arising in parotid glandular tissue
- **3rd most frequent** primary parotid malignancy after mucoepidermoid and adenoid cystic carcinoma

IMAGING

General Features

- Best diagnostic clue
  - Well-circumscribed, lobulated, homogeneously enhancing parotid mass
  - Cystic areas may be present
  - Usually **indistinguishable from other parotid neoplasms**
- Location
  - Most often superficial lobe parotid and parotid tail
  - Rare in other salivary glands
  - Can be multicentric, bilateral
- Size
  - Variable; generally 1-3 cm

CT Findings

- CECT
  - Well defined, usually homogeneously enhancing, but may have cystic areas
  - No calcification

MR Findings

- T1WI: **Variable signal from cystic areas, necrosis, hemorrhage**
- T2WI: High signal overall, but variable from cysts, necrosis, hemorrhage
- DWI: Low ADC values like other malignancies
- T1WI C+: Predominantly uniformly enhancing ± focal nonenhancing cyst

Nuclear Medicine Findings

- PET
  - Overall, AciCC has variable uptake
  - High grade (uncommon) has intense uptake

DIFFERENTIAL DIAGNOSIS

Parotid Benign Mixed Tumor

- Well defined, typically markedly T2 hyperintense
- Calcifications may be present

Parotid Mucoepidermoid Carcinoma

- Low-grade variant is well defined, uniform
- Most common parotid malignancy

Warthin Tumor

- Well-defined mass with central low density
- May be multiple, bilateral

PATHOLOGY

General Features

- Etiology
  - Associated with prior radiation, family history
- Epidemiology
  - **5-17% of parotid malignancies**

Gross Pathologic & Surgical Features

- Lobular, tan to red, well defined, solid or cystic, 1-3 cm

Microscopic Features

- Polygonal cells in sheets, uniform nuclei, vacuolated cells, locally infiltrative
  - ± microcysts, microhemorrhage, focal necrosis
- **Considered to be low-grade tumors**, although no uniform grading system
  - Poorer prognosis if perineural or vascular invasion, many or atypical mitoses, necrosis, or nodal metastasis

CLINICAL ISSUES

Presentation

- Most common signs/symptoms
  - Painless parotid mass for several years
- Other signs/symptoms
  - **Facial paresis rare**
  - May be exquisitely painful during FNA

Demographics

- Age
  - Median: 52 yr; mean: 44 yr
- Gender
  - F:M = 3:2

Natural History & Prognosis

- Favorable prognosis: 80% 10-yr survival
- **Generally indolent course**; recurrences and metastases may occur many years after treatment
  - 35% recur locally
  - Distant metastases occur in lungs, bone

Treatment

- Wide surgical excision ± radiation; chemoresistant

DIAGNOSTIC CHECKLIST

Consider

- Not usually possible to differentiate malignant parotid tumors prior to biopsy

Image Interpretation Pearls

- Important to describe location, extent, adenopathy; look for CNVII perineural tumor

SELECTED REFERENCES

1. Mamlouk MD et al: Paediatric parotid neoplasms: a 10 year retrospective imaging and pathology review of these rare tumours. Clin Radiol. 70(3):270-7, 2015
2. Suh SI et al: Acinic cell carcinoma of the head and neck: radiologic-pathologic correlation. J Comput Assist Tomogr. 29(1):121-6, 2005
3. Sakai O et al: Acinic cell Carcinoma of the parotid gland: CT and MRI. Neuroradiology. 38(7):675-9, 1996

Parotid Malignant Mixed Tumor

TERMINOLOGY

- Definition: Malignant tumor arising within preexisting BMT
- 2 types of malignant mixed tumor (MMT)
  - Carcinoma ex pleomorphic adenoma (most)
  - Carcinosarcoma (very rare)

IMAGING

- Early: Encapsulated mass, looks like BMT
- Late: Extensive aggressive parotid mass with invasion of surrounding structures
  - Encapsulated benign-appearing portion often present
- MR best for extent of lesion, invasion, & characterizing different tumor regions
  - Unenhanced T1 MR very useful due to inherent contrast from parotid gland fat
  - Native BMT has high T2 signal, but most carcinomas have lower T2 signal
  - Native BMT has high diffusivity, but carcinomas have low diffusivity

TOP DIFFERENTIAL DIAGNOSES

- Parotid benign mixed tumor
- Warthin tumor
- Parotid mucoepidermoid carcinoma
- Parotid adenoid cystic carcinoma

CLINICAL ISSUES

- Rapid enlargement of longstanding parotid mass is most suggestive history
- Other signs
  - Facial nerve weakness & pain
- Early MMT may be incidentally discovered on histologic examination of pleomorphic adenoma
- Prior radiation may increase risk
- 5-10% of BMT degrade into MMT
- All BMT should be surgically removed before they transform into MMT

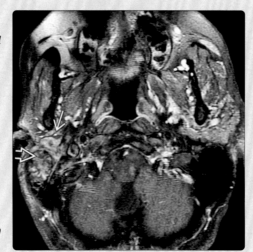
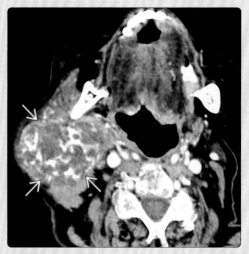

(Left) Axial T1WI C+ FS MR shows an aggressive mass ➡ at the stylomandibular tunnel with direct invasion of the mastoid bone ➡. This appearance is consistent with any aggressive parotid tumor, but histology revealed a myoepithelial carcinoma arising within a BMT. (Right) Axial CECT reveals a heterogeneously enhancing, irregularly calcified mass ➡ centered in the region of the parotid tail. Although BMT may calcify, these calcifications are from a chondrosarcoma that arose in a BMT.

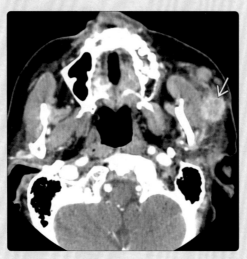
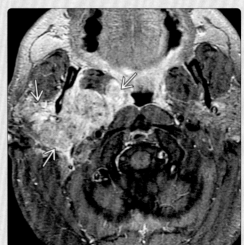

(Left) Axial CECT shows an ill-defined, invasive mass ➡ in the accessory lobe of the parotid, where the patient had sudden enlargement of a longstanding mass. This is salivary ductal carcinoma, the most common malignancy to arise from a BMT. (Right) Axial T1WI C+ FS MR shows an aggressive, heterogeneously enhancing mass ➡ replacing the parotid gland. Histologically, this malignancy showed areas of carcinoma & sarcoma, as well as residual BMT, which confirmed the diagnosis of true malignant mixed tumor (MMT).

Parotid Malignant Mixed Tumor

TERMINOLOGY

Abbreviations
- Malignant mixed tumor (MMT)

Synonyms
- Carcinoma ex pleomorphic adenoma

Definitions
- Malignant tumor arising within parotid benign mixed tumor (BMT)
- 2 types of MMT
  o **Carcinoma ex pleomorphic adenoma**
    – Common MMT type
    – Consists of single malignant cell type
  o **Carcinosarcoma** (true MMT)
    – Consists of multiple malignant cell types
    – Very rare (< 70 cases in literature)

IMAGING

General Features
- Best diagnostic clue
  o Early MMT: Not distinguishable from surrounding BMT
  o Late MMT: Aggressive parotid mass with extensive invasion of surrounding tissues
    – Tumor has characteristics of malignant cell type
    – Residual well-circumscribed BMT component often still visible

MR Findings
- T2WI
  o Native BMT has high T2 signal, often heterogeneous
  o Carcinomas (mucoepidermoid, salivary ductal) often have low T2 signal
- DWI
  o Native BMT has high diffusivity (↓ DWI signal)
  o Carcinomas have low diffusivity (↑ DWI signal)

Imaging Recommendations
- Best imaging tool
  o MR best for extent of lesion, invasion, & characterizing different tumor regions
- Protocol advice
  o Unenhanced T1 sequences very useful because of inherent contrast from parotid gland fat

DIFFERENTIAL DIAGNOSIS

Parotid Benign Mixed Tumor
- Sharp margins
- MR: T2 mostly hyperdense; T1 C+ heterogeneous

Warthin Tumor
- Typically at tail of parotid
- May be multiple, solid, or cystic
- MR: T2 bright if cystic or solid

Parotid Mucoepidermoid Carcinoma
- Well-defined or infiltrative parotid space (PS) mass
- MR: Lower T2 signal than ACCa; nodes common

Parotid Adenoid Cystic Carcinomafps
- Well-defined or infiltrative PS mass
- MR: Higher T2 signal than MECa; perineural tumor

PATHOLOGY

General Features
- Carcinoma ex pleomorphic adenoma: Malignant degeneration of 1 cell line in BMT
  o Most often salivary ductal carcinoma
  o Residual BMT needed to definitively diagnose carcinoma ex pleomorphic adenoma
- Parotid carcinosarcoma: Etiology controversial
  o Likely represents malignancy from pluripotent cell that differentiates in multiple directions while maintaining malignant potential
  o May represent collision tumor of multiple carcinomas ex pleomorphic adenoma
  o Carcinoma component of true MMT usually salivary gland carcinoma
    – Sarcoma component usually chondrosarcoma
    – Glandular and spindle cell components common

CLINICAL ISSUES

Presentation
- Most common signs/symptoms
  o Rapid enlargement of longstanding parotid mass
- Other signs/symptoms
  o Facial nerve weakness & pain
  o Early MMT may be incidentally discovered on histologic evaluation of pleomorphic adenoma

Demographics
- Prior radiation may increase risk
- 5-10% of BMT degrade into MMT
  o All BMTs should be surgically removed before they degrade

Natural History & Prognosis
- Carcinoma ex pleomorphic adenoma: Prognosis depends on histologic type, grade, & stage
- Carcinosarcoma: Aggressive tumor with poor prognosis
  o Mean survival: 3.6 yr, even with treatment

Treatment
- Trimodal therapy (surgery, chemotherapy, radiation)

DIAGNOSTIC CHECKLIST

Image Interpretation Pearls
- Sudden enlargement of longstanding parotid mass is suggestive history
- Look for CNVII and CNV perineural spread

SELECTED REFERENCES

1. Kashiwagi N et al: Carcinoma ex pleomorphic adenoma of the parotid gland. Acta Radiol. 53(3):303-6, 2012
2. Lüers JC et al: Carcinoma ex pleomorphic adenoma of the parotid gland. Study and implications for diagnostics and therapy. Acta Oncol. 48(1):132-6, 2009
3. Kato H et al: Carcinoma ex pleomorphic adenoma of the parotid gland: radiologic-pathologic correlation with MR imaging including diffusion-weighted imaging. AJNR Am J Neuroradiol. 29(5):865-7, 2008

Parotid Non-Hodgkin Lymphoma

TERMINOLOGY

- 3 forms of parotid involvement with non-Hodgkin lymphoma (NHL)
- **Nodal NHL**
  - **Primary nodal NHL**
  - **Systemic NHL** involving parotid nodes
- **Primary parenchymal NHL**, often mucosa-associated lymphoid tissue (MALT)

IMAGING

- Nodal NHL: Multiple well-defined, homogeneous parotid masses
- Primary parotid NHL: Infiltrative or focal solid mass, uncommonly cystic
- Often periparotid & upper cervical lymphadenopathy
- Ultrasound shows hypoechoic intraparotid mass(es)
- Color Doppler shows hypervascular mass(es)
- PET/CT typically markedly FDG avid
- MALT-type primary NHL variable; often less FDG avid

TOP DIFFERENTIAL DIAGNOSES

- Benign lymphoepithelial lesions-HIV
- Parotid Sjögren syndrome
- Warthin tumor
- Parotid nodal metastatic disease

CLINICAL ISSUES

- Overall 5-year survival = 72%
- Systemic NHL involves parotid in 1-8%
- Primary parotid NHL ~ 2-5% of parotid malignancies

DIAGNOSTIC CHECKLIST

- Beware: Isodense NHL may be "invisible" on CECT
- Parotid lesions best seen on T1 or T2 FS/STIR
- Heterogeneous parotids with new parotid mass
  - Suspect NHL complicating Sjögren disease
  - Sjögren may not be previously diagnosed

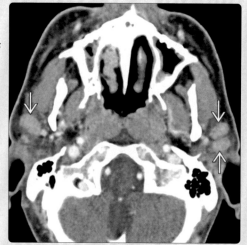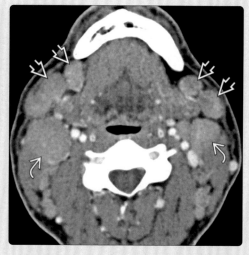

(Left) Axial CECT shows multiple bilateral, well-defined, homogeneously enhancing masses ➡. Nodules ≥ 1 cm in parotid gland deserve further evaluation as they may represent multiple Warthin tumors, multiple metastatic nodes, or multiple lymphoma nodes. Remaining neck should be evaluated for lymphadenopathy as 1st step. *(Right)* Axial CECT shows extensive lymphadenopathy in upper neck, including level I ➡ & II ➡ nodes. This case shows parotid node involvement with systemic lymphoma.

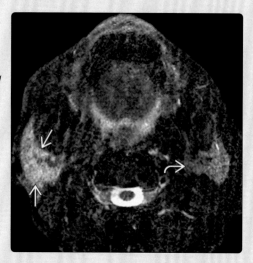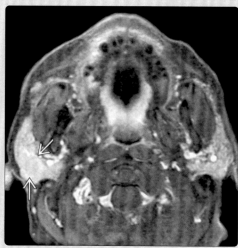

(Left) Axial T2WI FS MR in a patient presenting with fullness of right cheek demonstrates subtle enlargement and diffuse hyperintensity of right parotid gland ➡ as compared to left side ➡. Prior CECT study had no reported abnormality or calculi. *(Right)* Axial T1 C+ FS MR reveals diffuse enhancement of right parotid with more conspicuous ill-defined but homogeneous lesion ➡ in superficial lobe. Fine needle aspiration revealed mucosa-associated lymphoid tissue (MALT)-type primary parotid lymphoma.

TERMINOLOGY

Abbreviations
- Non-Hodgkin lymphoma (NHL)
- Mucosa-associated lymphoid tissue (MALT) lymphoma

Definitions
- 3 forms of parotid involvement with NHL
  - Nodal NHL
    - **Primary nodal NHL**
    - **Systemic NHL** involving parotid nodes
  - **Primary parenchymal lymphoma**
    - Most often MALT-type NHL

IMAGING

General Features
- Best diagnostic clue
  - Nodal NHL: Multiple homogeneous, well-defined parotid masses & upper cervical adenopathy
  - Parenchymal NHL: Infiltrative parotid mass
- Location
  - Parotid gland ± ipsilateral neck nodes
- Size
  - Nodal masses: 1-3 centimeters
  - Primary lymphoma may involve most of gland
- Morphology
  - Most often: Multiple round or ovoid well-circumscribed masses
    - Unilateral with primary or systemic NHL
    - Bilateral with systemic NHL
  - Primary parotid lymphoma: Diffusely infiltrating process
    - Occasionally bilateral parotid masses
    - May be solid and cystic mass

CT Findings
- CECT
  - Nodal NHL: Multiple well-defined intraparotid masses
    - Mild to moderate homogeneous enhancement
    - Necrosis, calcification, & hemorrhage rare
  - Primary parenchymal NHL: Invasive mass or solid/cystic mass
  - Periparotid & upper cervical lymphadenopathy often present

MR Findings
- T1WI
  - Homogeneous intermediate signal nodules or infiltrative mass; seen in hypointense parotid
- T2WI FS
  - FS or STIR makes parotid lesions more conspicuous
  - Homogeneous intermediate to low signal intensity nodules or solid/cystic mass
- T1WI C+
  - Mild to moderate homogeneous enhancement

Ultrasonographic Findings
- Grayscale ultrasound
  - Solitary or multiple uniform **hypoechoic** intraparotid masses
- Color Doppler
  - **Hypervascular** compared to adjacent parotid parenchyma

Nuclear Medicine Findings
- PET/CT
  - **Nodal NHL typically markedly FDG avid**
    - Multifocal nodular uptake in parotid ± neck nodes
    - Benign parotid lesions may also be FDG avid
  - **MALT lymphoma variable, often less FDG avid**
    - Role of PET controversial
- Ga-67 scintigraphy
  - Foci of ↑ activity within normal parotid uptake
  - Improved visualization with SPECT
  - Sialadenitis after chemotherapy or radiation therapy (XRT) may have identical appearance
- Tc-99m pertechnetate
  - Cold lesion(s) within normal uptake of parotid

Other Modality Findings
- MR sialography or conventional sialography
  - Smooth displacement of ducts around ovoid masses
  - Normal arborization pattern without dilatation of parotid ductal system
    - Unless in setting of Sjögren syndrome

Imaging Recommendations
- Best imaging tool
  - CECT to identify intraparotid lesions & allow evaluation of cervical lymphadenopathy for staging
    - Beware: Isodense lesions may be "invisible"
  - Intraparotid lesions more conspicuous on T1 or with T2 FS or STIR
- Protocol advice
  - Be sure to image from skull base to clavicles to aid in staging
  - PET/CT typically performed for complete staging

DIFFERENTIAL DIAGNOSIS

Benign Lymphoepithelial Lesions-HIV
- Mixed cystic & solid intraparotid lesions enlarge both parotid glands
- If AIDS patient has NHL, imaging may be complex

Parotid Sjögren Syndrome
- Older female patient with connective tissue disease, dry eyes, dry mouth
- Bilateral enlarged parotid glands, small or large cysts ± lymphoid aggregates
- Chronic: Atrophied, heterogeneous glands ± calcifications
- Sjögren syndrome has 40x incidence of NHL

Warthin Tumor
- Painless parotid mass in older male smoker
- Solid, cystic, or mixed
- 20% multiple, may be bilateral
- Lacks periparotid & cervical lymphadenopathy

Parotid Nodal Metastatic Disease
- Multiple unilateral or bilateral masses with invasive margins, often central necrosis
- Often other nodal metastases: Levels II & V
- Periparotid skin and scalp primaries most frequent

PATHOLOGY

General Features

- Etiology
  - Unknown; possibly multifactorial
    - Environmental, genetic, viral, prior radiation
  - Increased incidence with autoimmune disorders
    - **Primary Sjögren syndrome** has **13x** relative risk of NHL
    - Rheumatoid arthritis, systemic lupus
  - Increased incidence with **immunosuppression**

Staging, Grading, & Classification

- **Modified Ann Arbor staging system** is for clinical staging, treatment, and prognosis of NHL
  - Stage I: Single node region or lymphoid structure (e.g., spleen) or single extralymphatic site (IE)
  - Stage II: ≥ 2 node regions on same side of diaphragm (II) or contiguous extranodal organ/site + regional nodes ± other nodes on same side of diaphragm (IIE)
  - Stage III: Node regions on both sides of diaphragm (III), spleen (IIIS), extranodal (IIIE), both (IIISE)
  - Stage IV: Disseminated disease: ≥ 1 extranodal organ or tissue, ± nodes or isolated extralymphatic disease with distant nodes
- **World Health Organization** is for NHL histological classification (2008)
  - Based on immunophenotype & morphology
  - B-cell (≤ 85%), T-cell, & putative NK-cell neoplasms

Gross Pathologic & Surgical Features

- Well-circumscribed, encapsulated, soft fleshy masses

Microscopic Features

- Sheets of homogeneous lymphoid cells arranged in diffuse or follicular pattern
  - Subdivided into small-cleaved & large-cell variants
- Primary parotid lymphoma
  - Most often MALT-type NHL
  - Unilateral diffuse invasion of ductal & acinar tissue

CLINICAL ISSUES

Presentation

- Most common signs/symptoms
  - Slowly enlarging painless parotid mass ± cervical lymphadenopathy
- Other signs/symptoms
  - Systemic "B" symptoms: Fever, weight loss, night sweats
- Clinical profile
  - Middle-aged male patient with painless cheek mass

Demographics

- Age
  - Mean age at presentation = 55 years
- Gender
  - M:F = 1.5:1
- Ethnicity
  - Caucasian > > African American, Hispanic, or Asian
  - Rare T-cell lymphomas more common in young African American males
- Epidemiology

- Primary parotid NHL uncommon; 2-5% of parotid malignancies
- Systemic NHL involves parotid in 1-8%

Natural History & Prognosis

- Depends on histology, morphology, and stage
- **Overall 5-year survival = 72%**
  - High-grade disease: Rapidly progressive, aggressive
  - Low-grade lesions: Indolent, minimal treatment, and slow progression over years
    - Best prognosis: Small-cleaved cell & follicular forms
- Generally good prognosis with primary parotid NHL
  - Usually diagnosed early: Stage I or II
  - XRT ± chemotherapy

Treatment

- Tumor debulking of parotid mass may be performed for cosmetic purposes
- Chemotherapy & XRT remain mainstays of treatment

DIAGNOSTIC CHECKLIST

Consider

- CECT from skull base to clavicles for intraparotid lesions & to fully evaluate extent of cervical disease
- Beware: Isodense NHL may be "invisible" on CECT
- When using T2 MR, FS, or STIR make intraparotid lesions more conspicuous

Image Interpretation Pearls

- Carefully evaluate contralateral parotid glands, other salivary & lacrimal glands, and extent of cervical nodes
- PET/CT typically performed as work-up for systemic lymphoma
- In patient with new parotid mass, background heterogeneous parotids suggest NHL + Sjögren
  - **Sjögren may not be previously diagnosed**

SELECTED REFERENCES

1. Liang Y et al: Primary Sjogren's syndrome and malignancy risk: a systematic review and meta-analysis. Ann Rheum Dis. 73(6):1151-6, 2014
2. Cohen C et al: 18F-fluorodeoxyglucose positron emission tomography/computer tomography as an objective tool for assessing disease activity in Sjögren's syndrome. Autoimmun Rev. 12(11):1109-14, 2013
3. Feinstein AJ et al: Parotid gland lymphoma: prognostic analysis of 2140 patients. Laryngoscope. 123(5):1199-203, 2013
4. Zhu L et al: Non-Hodgkin lymphoma involving the parotid gland: CT and MR imaging findings. Dentomaxillofac Radiol. 42(9):20130046, 2013
5. Kato H et al: Mucosa-associated lymphoid tissue lymphoma of the salivary glands: MR imaging findings including diffusion-weighted imaging. Eur J Radiol. 81(4):e612-7, 2012
6. Aiken AH et al: Imaging Hodgkin and non-Hodgkin lymphoma in the head and neck. Radiol Clin North Am. 46(2):363-78, ix-x, 2008
7. Gasparotto D et al: Extrasalivary lymphoma development in Sjogren's syndrome: clonal evolution from parotid gland lymphoproliferation and role of local triggering. Arthritis Rheum. 48(11):3181-6, 2003
8. Hamilton BE et al: Earring lesions of the parotid tail. AJNR Am J Neuroradiol. 24(9):1757-64, 2003
9. Eichhorn KW et al: Malignant non-Hodgkin's lymphoma mimicking a benign parotid tumor: sonographic findings. J Clin Ultrasound. 30(1):42-4, 2002
10. Stein ME et al: Diagnosis and treatment of primary non-Hodgkin's lymphoma of the parotid gland: a retrospective study - Experience at the Northern Israel Oncology Center (1977-1999). J BUON. 7(3):229-33, 2002
11. Yencha MW: Primary parotid gland Hodgkin's lymphoma. Ann Otol Rhinol Laryngol. 111(4):338-42, 2002
12. Abbondanzo SL: Extranodal marginal-zone B-cell lymphoma of the salivary gland. Ann Diagn Pathol. 5(4):246-54, 2001

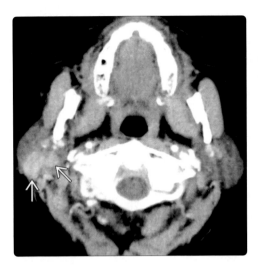

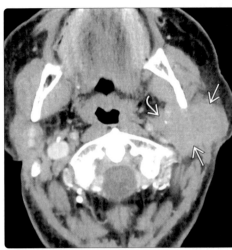

(Left) *Axial CECT shows multiple unilateral intraparotid masses ➡ with well-defined borders and uniform enhancement on right side. No evidence of disease was found elsewhere, so this patient was diagnosed with primary parotid nodal non-Hodgkin lymphoma.* **(Right)** *Axial CECT demonstrates primary MALT lymphoma of the parotid. Infiltrative mass involves superficial ➡ and deep ➡ lobes mimicking aggressive primary salivary gland malignancy. Lymphocytic lymphomas may have better defined margins.*

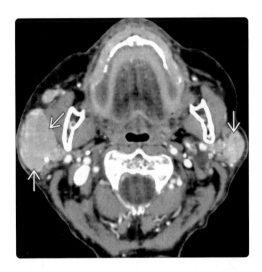

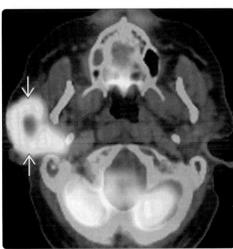

(Left) *Axial CECT shows bilateral, homogeneous enhancing parotid fullness ➡ found to be bilateral primary lymphoma in a patient with long-standing Sjögren. Primary Sjögren syndrome carries a 13x relative risk of lymphoma. This case is typical of MALT-type parotid lymphoma.* **(Right)** *Corresponding axial fused PET/CT shows marked FDG uptake ➡ that is typically found with lymphoma. Interestingly, for such homogeneous lesion on CT, lesion has little central uptake, suggesting necrosis.*

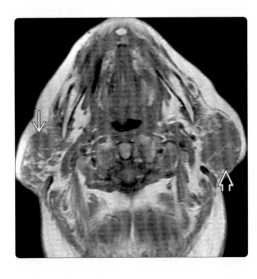

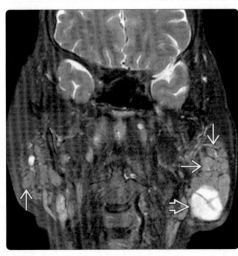

(Left) *Axial T1WI MR demonstrates markedly heterogeneous appearance of enlarged parotid glands. Patient reported 10-year history of Sjögren disease and now palpable left parotid mass ➡. Clinician felt additional mass on right ➡.* **(Right)** *Coronal T2WI FS MR reveals multiple intermediate-signal masses bilaterally ➡ and a solid and cystic lesion on the left side ➡. Aspiration of this and right parotid revealed MALT lymphoma in both. Patient was treated with radiation therapy.*

Metastatic Disease of Parotid Nodes

TERMINOLOGY

- Lymphangitic or hematogeneous tumor spread to intraglandular parotid lymph nodes
- Parotid and periparotid nodes = **1st-order nodal station for skin** squamous cell carcinoma (SCCa) and melanoma from scalp, auricle, and face ("forgotten nodal station")

IMAGING

- Nodes usually well defined but infiltrative if extranodal spread
- Nodes may be homogeneous or heterogeneous with central necrosis
- PET/CT most sensitive for identification of small nodes
- MR most sensitive for extranodal spread and perineural tumor spread on CNVII

TOP DIFFERENTIAL DIAGNOSES

- Benign lymphoepithelial lesions
- Parotid Sjögren disease

- Warthin tumor
- Parotid non-Hodgkin lymphoma

PATHOLOGY

- **Skin cancers** of face, external ear, and scalp account for 75% of primary tumors
- **Metastatic SCCa is 2nd most common parotid malignancy**
- Systemic metastases to parotid nodes rare

CLINICAL ISSUES

- Prognosis depends on presence of extracapsular spread (8% vs. 79% local recurrence)
- Metastatic SCCa involving parotid gland and neck nodes is aggressive form of SCCa with tendency for infiltrative growth pattern and multiple recurrences

DIAGNOSTIC CHECKLIST

- If asked to image parotid nodal metastases from skin cancer, also scan cervical nodes to clavicle

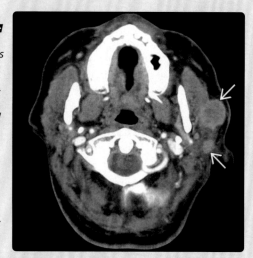
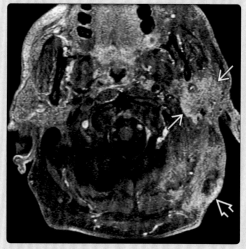

(Left) Axial CECT shows multiple enhancing masses ➡ of varying size within the left parotid gland. This patient has squamous cell carcinoma of the face, and these nodes represent 1st-order lymphatic drainage. (Right) Axial T1WI C+ FS MR shows an ill-defined mass ➡ replacing the left parotid gland. The primary tumor, postauricular squamous cell carcinoma, is partially visible ➡. The ill-defined margins of the intraparotid metastasis indicate extracapsular spread.

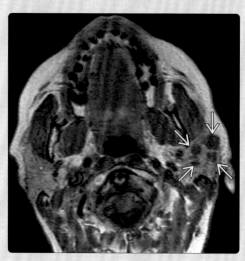
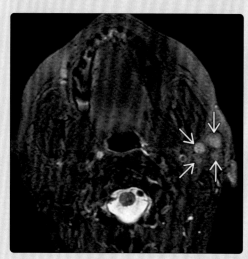

(Left) Axial T1WI MR reveals numerous small masses ➡ in the left parotid gland. These regional metastases are clearly visible on unenhanced images because of the contrast with the surrounding fat. (Right) Axial T2WI FS MR shows numerous masses ➡ in the left parotid gland with mildly increased T2 signal. Metastases may be more conspicuous on STIR images than on T2 images. These are regional metastases from lymphoepithelial carcinoma of the base of tongue.

TERMINOLOGY

Definitions

- Lymphangitic or hematogeneous tumor spread to intraparotid lymph nodes (systemic metastases)
- Parotid and periparotid nodes = **1st-order nodal station** for skin squamous cell carcinoma (SCCa) and melanoma from **scalp**, **auricle**, **and face** (regional metastatic disease)

IMAGING

General Features

- Best diagnostic clue
  - Multiple parotid masses in setting of known H&N malignancy
  - 1 or more focal masses in superficial or deep lobe of parotid gland
    - Often with associated preauricular ± cervical nodal masses
- Location
  - Intraparotid ± periparotid
- Size
  - 5 mm to 4 cm, usually 1-3 cm
- Morphology
  - Ovoid or round
  - Usually well defined but infiltrative if extranodal spread

CT Findings

- CECT
  - 1 or more intraparotid masses with sharp margins (early) or invasive margins (late, extranodal spread)
    - If extranodal, check for perineural tumor on CNVII
    - See if fat in stylomastoid foramen replaced with tumor
  - Nodes may be homogeneous or heterogeneous with central necrosis
  - Preauricular ± cervical nodal metastases may also be present
  - Periauricular or scalp skin thickening (primary skin malignancy)

MR Findings

- T1WI
  - Single or multiple intermediate signal masses
- T2WI
  - Uniform high signal or heterogeneous signal (necrosis)
- T1WI C+
  - Enhancing solid or cystic (central nodal necrosis) intraparotid nodal masses
  - If extranodal spread, may appear invasive

Ultrasonographic Findings

- Diagnostic features on US not characteristic enough to avoid biopsy
- US is useful to guide fine-needle aspiration of parotid masses

Nuclear Medicine Findings

- PET
  - If used in staging of primary tumor, may show intraparotid activity

Imaging Recommendations

- Best imaging tool
  - PET/CT most sensitive for identification of small nodes
  - MR most sensitive for extranodal spread and perineural tumor spread on CNVII
- Protocol advice
  - Image primary site, parotid, and remainder of neck nodal chains to clavicles
- MR is best tool to evaluate uncertain parotid masses
  - Deep tissue spread and perineural tumor are better defined by MR
  - T1 non-FS, unenhanced images often best delineate mass (inherent contrast between mass and fatty gland)
- All patients with invasive skin SCCa or melanoma on skin of face, scalp, and auricle should undergo staging PET/CT for intraparotid nodes ± nodes in cervical neck
  - MR obtained if PET/CT is positive

DIFFERENTIAL DIAGNOSIS

Benign Lymphoepithelial Lesions (BLEL-HIV)

- HIV or AIDS patient
- Multiple small, bilateral parotid cystic, and solid lesions

Parotid Sjögren Disease

- Autoimmune disease affecting salivary tissue
- Enlarged salivary glands
- Cystic dilatation of intraglandular ducts + lymphoid aggregates
- Punctate intraglandular Ca^{++} characteristic

Warthin Tumor

- Male smokers with painless cheek mass
- Often cystic on CT or MR
- 20% multifocal

Parotid Non-Hodgkin Lymphoma

- Patient usually has systemic non-Hodgkin lymphoma (NHL)
- Bilateral, multiple intraparotid nodes
- Very difficult to distinguish from metastases if no known primary

Recurrent Parotid Benign Mixed Tumor

- History of benign mixed tumor (BMT) surgical removal
- Multifocal masses; cluster of grapes appearance

PATHOLOGY

General Features

- Etiology
  - Skin of face, external ear, and scalp accounts for 75% of primary tumors
  - Lymphangitic or hematogeneous spread of tumor
    - Systemic metastases to parotid nodes rare
  - Regional spread of upper aerodigestive tract primary SCCa to parotid uncommonly occurs
- Parotid has intraglandular lymph nodes (unlike submandibular and sublingual glands)
  - Normal parotid: ~ 20 intraglandular nodes
- Embryology-anatomy
  - Parotid undergoes late encapsulation, incorporating nodes within its parenchyma

○ Parotid is "**forgotten nodal station**"

Gross Pathologic & Surgical Features

- Nodes may remain encapsulated or undergo extracapsular spread
- SCCa node: Tan-yellow nodules within parotid
- Melanoma node: Black, brown, or white rubbery mass

Microscopic Features

- Most common skin carcinomas
  ○ **SCCa (60%)**
    - **Metastatic SCCa is 2nd most common parotid malignancy**
  ○ Melanoma (15%)
- SCCa: Lymph node is partially or entirely replaced by epithelial-lined structure ± central cystic change
  ○ Epithelium lining of cystic spaces is composed of hypercellular and pleomorphic cell population, with loss of polarity and ↑ mitotic activity
- Melanoma: Diffuse proliferation of epithelioid ± spindle cells with abundant eosinophilic cytoplasm and prominent nucleoli
  ○ Immunochemistry: S100 protein and HMB-45 present
- Systemic metastases. Lung, breast primaries most common

CLINICAL ISSUES

Presentation

- Most common signs/symptoms
  ○ External ear, scalp, upper face skin cancer with enlarging parotid mass
  ○ CNVII dysfunction
  ○ Facial pain
  ○ Nonhealing sore (skin SCCa or melanoma) on skin of face, scalp, or auricle-external auditory canal associated with cheek mass

Demographics

- Age
  ○ 7th decade most frequent
- Gender
  ○ M:F = 2:1
- Epidemiology
  ○ Occurs in 1-3% of patients with H&N SCCa
  ○ Metastases = 4% of all parotid neoplasms
  ○ Intraparotid nodes more common in geographic regions of ↑ sun exposure

Natural History & Prognosis

- Prognosis depends heavily on presence of **extracapsular spread (8% vs. 79% local recurrence)**
- 5-year parotid control = 78%, but overall survival = 54%
- Metastatic SCCa involving parotid gland and neck nodes is aggressive form of SCCa with tendency for infiltrative growth pattern and multiple recurrences
- Some primary subsites (e.g., external ear) have worse prognosis
- Melanoma: Poor prognosis; rare long-term survivors

Treatment

- Parotidectomy, neck dissection + radiation therapy
  ○ Elective neck dissection in N0 neck improves disease-specific survival

- SCCa: Parotidectomy and neck dissection dictated by imaging and physical exam
  ○ Postoperative radiotherapy
- Melanoma: Parotidectomy and neck dissection dictated by lymphatic mapping and sentinel node identification
  ○ Adjuvant radiotherapy ± chemotherapy depends on context

DIAGNOSTIC CHECKLIST

Consider

- When imaging parotid nodal metastases from skin cancer, also scan cervical nodes to clavicle
- If SCCa or melanoma found in parotid nodes, check external ear and scalp for primary
  ○ Patients may not recall prior history of skin cancer
  ○ Skin cancer may be hidden above hairline at time of presentation of parotid node

Image Interpretation Pearls

- Multifocal unilateral disease is most suggestive of 1st-order nodal disease from adjacent skin sites
  ○ Solitary intraparotid nodal metastasis mimics primary parotid neoplasm
- Presence of bilateral nodes suggests systemic disease or hematogeneous metastatic spread

Reporting Tips

- Differential diagnosis for multifocal unilateral parotid masses with cervical adenopathy: Regional metastases, local NHL
- Differential diagnosis for multifocal unilateral parotid masses without cervical adenopathy: Warthin tumor, recurrent BMT, regional metastases, local NHL
- Differential diagnosis for multifocal bilateral parotid masses: Systemic metastases, systemic NHL, Warthin tumors, BLEL of HIV, Sjögren disease

SELECTED REFERENCES

1. Chen MM et al: Prognostic factors for squamous cell cancer of the parotid gland: an analysis of 2104 patients. Head Neck. 37(1):1-7, 2015
2. Pfisterer MJ et al: Squamous cell carcinoma of the parotid gland: a population-based analysis of 2545 cases. Am J Otolaryngol. 35(4):469-75, 2014
3. Sandu I et al: Misleading appearance in cervical lymph node US diagnosis - a report on sarcoidosis, Warthin tumor and squamous cell carcinoma metastases. Med Ultrason. 16(2):182-5, 2014
4. Peiffer N et al: Patterns of regional metastasis in advanced stage cutaneous squamous cell carcinoma of the auricle. Otolaryngol Head Neck Surg. 144(1):36-42, 2011
5. Lee SK et al: Parotid incidentaloma identified by combined 18F-fluorodeoxyglucose whole-body positron emission tomography and computed tomography: findings at grayscale and power Doppler ultrasonography and ultrasound-guided fine-needle aspiration biopsy or core-needle biopsy. Eur Radiol. 19(9):2268-74, 2009
6. Ch'ng S et al: Parotid and cervical nodal status predict prognosis for patients with head and neck metastatic cutaneous squamous cell carcinoma. J Surg Oncol. 98(2):101-5, 2008
7. Hinerman RW et al: Cutaneous squamous cell carcinoma metastatic to parotid-area lymph nodes. Laryngoscope. 118(11):1989-96, 2008
8. Veness MJ et al: Cutaneous head and neck squamous cell carcinoma metastatic to parotid and cervical lymph nodes. Head Neck. 29(7):621-31, 2007
9. Ch'ng S et al: Parotid metastasis--an independent prognostic factor for head and neck cutaneous squamous cell carcinoma. J Plast Reconstr Aesthet Surg. 59(12):1288-93, 2006

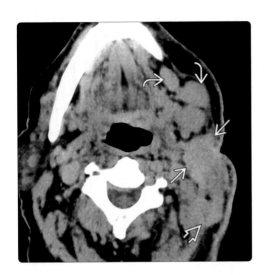

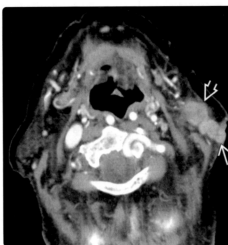

(Left) *Axial CECT shows a confluent mass* ⮕ *replacing the tail of the left parotid. Extensive level I* ⮕ *and level II* ⮕ *metastases are also seen. This patient had squamous cell carcinoma of the lateral scalp.* (Right) *Axial CECT demonstrates aggressive primary skin squamous cell carcinoma* ⮕ *spreading into deep subcutaneous soft tissues. Note that the 1st-order parotid tail lymph node* ⮕ *is affected.*

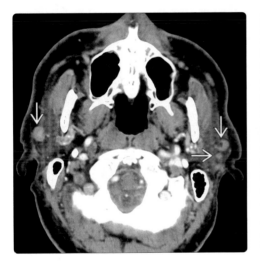

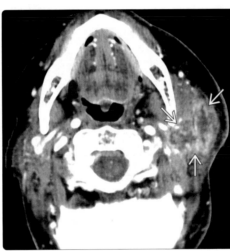

(Left) *Axial CECT reveals bilateral enhancing parotid masses* ⮕. *These represent systemic metastatic disease from chronic lymphocytic leukemia. They were accompanied by extensive cervical adenopathy (not shown).* (Right) *Axial CECT shows an ill-defined, heterogeneously enhancing mass* ⮕ *in the left parotid gland. The central necrosis and ill-defined margins are indicative of extracapsular spread. These are regional metastases from an angiosarcoma of the scalp.*

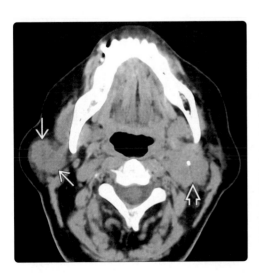

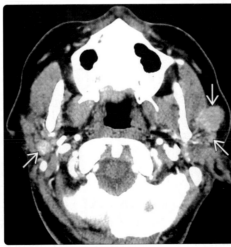

(Left) *Axial NECT shows a large, well-defined mass* ⮕ *in the right parotid gland representing hematogenous metastasis from lung cancer. A large regional metastasis* ⮕ *is also seen in contralateral level II, but no ascending cervical adenopathy was present on the right.* (Right) *Axial CECT demonstrates numerous bilateral, well-defined, uniformly enhancing parotid masses* ⮕ *in a patient with known breast cancer. These masses represent hematogeneous metastases.*

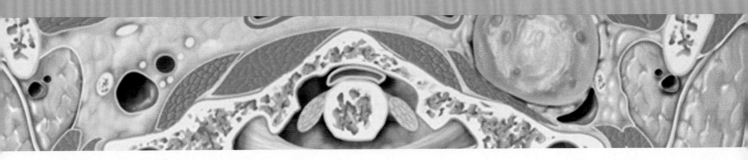

Summary Thoughts: Carotid Space

The carotid spaces (CS) are paired tubular spaces that traverse the suprahyoid neck (SHN) and infrahyoid neck (IHN) just lateral to the retropharyngeal space (RPS). The CS is enveloped by the **carotid sheath**, which is made up of all **3 layers of deep cervical fascia**. The SHN CS contains the internal carotid artery (ICA), internal jugular vein (IJV), and cranial nerves (CN) IX-XII. The IHN CS has within it only the common carotid artery (CCA), IJV, and the vagus nerve (CNX) trunk.

SHN CS mass displaces the anterior parapharyngeal space (PPS) fat anteriorly as it enlarges. Often the ICA is also displaced anteriorly by an enlarging SHN CS mass. An **IHN CS mass** engulfs the CCA or splays the carotid bifurcation (carotid body paraganglioma).

Important **CS tumors** include paraganglioma, schwannoma, neurofibroma, and sympathetic chain schwannoma. The internal jugular nodal chain is in close proximity to the superficial margin of the CS. As a result, when squamous cell carcinoma (SCCa) metastatic nodes undergo extranodal spread, they may injure the adjacent carotid artery and vagus nerve.

Imaging Techniques and Indications

CECT (+ CTA ± CTV) or MR (+ MRA ± MRV) easily identify most CS lesions. Certainly the CS mass lesions are readily seen using either technique. When using CT, CTA gives a multiplanar vascular-phase view of the intrinsic carotid diseases. CECT that allows contrast to penetrate into the soft tissues of the neck is better for delineation of CS mass lesions.

When using MR, remember to acquire T1 without contrast (to look for high-velocity flow void signature of paraganglioma). MRA & MRV may be helpful in defining a vascular CS lesion (ICA dissection, pseudoaneurysm, or IJV thrombosis).

Imaging Anatomy

The important **anatomic relationships** of the CS can be examined at the SHN and IHN level. At the SHN level the CS has the RPS medial, the perivertebral space (PVS) posterior, the deep lobe of the parotid space (PS) lateral, and the parapharyngeal space anterior. At the IHN level, the CS is bounded by the visceral space (VS) & RPS medially, PVS posteriorly, anterior cervical space anteriorly, and posterior cervical space laterally.

The CS extends from the skull base to the aortic arch. At its superior skull base margin, the **ICA** enters the **carotid canal** just as the **IJV** emerges from the floor of the **jugular foramen** (JF). The sympathetic plexus leaves its position on the medial surface of the nasopharyngeal CS to ascend in the ICA adventitia as the carotid plexus along the ICA course through the temporal bone. At the CS inferior margin, the **common carotid arteries** enter the **aortic arch**, and the **IJVs** merge with the **brachiocephalic veins**. The CS has nasopharyngeal, oropharyngeal, cervical, and mediastinal segments.

The **carotid sheath** surrounds the CS throughout its passage through the soft tissues of the neck. A unique aspect of the carotid sheath is that it is made up of **all three layers of deepcervical** (superficial, middle, and deep) **fascia**. In the SHN, the carotid sheath is a considerably less substantial fascia than in the IHN. In the IHN, the sheath is a well-defined, tenacious fascia. This is fortunate as it is in the cervical neck

that the CS suffers injury from trauma and spreading extranodal SCCa.

Important **CS internal structures** are best viewed from the perspective of what can be found in the SHN & IHN CS. The **SHN CS** contains the ICA & IJV along with the glossopharyngeal (CNIX), vagus (CNX), spinal accessory (CNXI), and hypoglossal (CNXII) CNs. Foci of normal neural crest derivative **glomus bodies** are found in the nodose ganglion of the vagus nerve approximately 2 cm below the floor of the JF of the skull base. They are also located in the JF above and the carotid bifurcation below. Along the medial border of the SHN CS is the sympathetic plexus.

All CNs but the vagus nerve have exited the SHN CS by the time it reaches the hyoid bone. **Normal internal structures** of the **IHN CS** include the vagus nerve, the CCA, and IJV. The **internal jugular nodal chain** is loosely wound into the external fascial layers along the surface of the CS. As such, this nodal chain is considered closely associated but **not** within the CS.

Approaches to Imaging Issues of Carotid Space

The answer to the question, "What **imaging findings** define a **CS mass**?" varies depending on the level of the lesion. If the lesion is in the **nasopharyngeal CS**, it displaces the PPS fat anteriorly and lifts the styloid process anterolaterally. At the level of the **oropharyngeal CS**, the PPS is again pushed anteriorly, but an important additional clue is the displacement of the posterior belly of the digastric muscle anterolaterally. At either the nasopharyngeal or oropharyngeal level, lesions in the posterior CS (vagal schwannoma, neurofibroma, paraganglioma) will bow the ICA anteriorly as they enlarge. A mass of the **infrahyoid CS** engulfs the CCA or splays the bifurcation (carotid body paraganglioma).

When CS lesion is identified on imaging, matching its radiologic findings to common CS lesions is often very rewarding as many of the lesions have distinctive imaging findings. If the lesion is intrinsic to the carotid artery, ICA tortuosity, dissection, pseudoaneurysm, and thrombosis should all be considered. Intrinsic IJV lesions should suggest IJV asymmetry, thrombophlebitis, and thrombosis. Tumors within the space include paraganglioma (MR high-velocity flow voids), schwannoma (tubular lesions with intramural cysts), and neurofibroma (target appearance on MR; low density on CECT).

Nasopharyngeal CS tumors may "**dumbbell**" inferiorly from the **JF** above. A careful inspection of the JF for imaging signs of simultaneous involvement is in order. If the JF is abnormal, the main differential diagnosis of the CS mass is glomus jugulare paraganglioma, JF schwannoma (CNIX-XI), or JF meningioma. **Bone CT** imaging clues that may be helpful include permeative-destructive changes along the margin of the JF (glomus jugulare), smooth, expansile JF with sclerotic margins (schwannoma), and permeative-sclerotic or hyperostotic changes (meningioma).

MR clues to consider for a **JF mass** extending into nasopharyngeal CS are plentiful. If the tumor has low-signal, high-velocity flow voids with vector of spread through the floor of the middle ear cavity, glomus jugulare is the first diagnostic consideration. A fusiform mass with intramural cystic change and a vector of spread that projects upward and medial toward the lateral medulla suggests schwannoma. JF

Differential Diagnosis of Carotid Space Lesion

Pseudolesions	CCA or ICA aneurysm
Ectatic CCA or ICA	ICA pseudoaneurysm
Carotid bulb ectasia	Fibromuscular dysplasia
Asymmetric IJV	Takayasu arteritis
Congenital	**Benign tumor**
2nd branchial cleft cyst variant	Carotid body paraganglioma
Inflammation or infection	Glomus vagale paraganglioma
CS cellulitis	Glomus jugulare paraganglioma, inferior extension
CS abscess	CNIX-XII schwannoma
Acute idiopathic carotidynia	Sympathetic chain schwannoma
Vascular	CNIX-XII neurofibroma
IJV thrombophlebitis	Jugular foramen meningioma, inferior extension
IJV thrombosis	**Malignant tumor**
CCA or ICA atherosclerosis	SCCa primary tumor invasion, perifascial spread
CCA or ICA thrombosis	SCCa extranodal tumor invasion
ICA dissection	Extranodal NHL, internal jugular nodal chain

Above is an exhaustive list of all lesions that can be found in the carotid space. The table is organized by general pathology category. CCA = common carotid artery; ICA = internal carotid artery; IJV = internal jugular vein; SCCa = squamous cell carcinoma; NHL = non-Hodgkin lymphoma.

meningioma lacks high-velocity signal voids and spreads centrifugally away from the JF.

Vascular lesions in the CS arise within the IJV or carotid artery. IJV thrombophlebitis mimics neck abscess clinically and is easily diagnosed because of the tubular luminal clot and surrounding soft tissue inflammatory changes. The more chronic IJV thrombosis clinically mimics a neck tumor, lacking the soft tissue inflammatory changes on imaging. Important carotid artery lesions include atherosclerosis, dissection with or without pseudoaneurysm, and fibromuscular dysplasia (FMD). This lesion group can be readily diagnosed with CTA with the exception of FMD, which may require angiography to diagnose.

Perhaps the most common image interpretation pitfall associated with CS lesions is the tendency to confuse SHN CS mass with lateral retropharyngeal nodal mass. **Lateral RPS mass** lesions displace the ICA-IJV in the CS posterolaterally whereas SHN CS mass lesions push the ICA anteriorly or anteromedially. As there are no nodes within the CS, if the imaging appearance suggests nodal disease, check to see if the ICA is pushed laterally. If so, you are looking at a lateral RPS lesion.

Clinical Implications

Lesions of the CS often present first with **hoarseness**. Endoscopy determines which vocal cord is paralyzed. **Left** vocal cord paralysis requires imaging from the posterior fossa to the aortopulmonic window, while **right** vocal cord paralysis only requires the scan to reach the clavicle inferiorly.

Proximal vagal neuropathy often includes other CN injury (CNIX, XI, or XII). Because the pharyngeal plexus branch of the vagus nerve is injured, the ipsilateral soft palate and superior constrictor muscles fasciculate in the acute phase and become patulous in the chronic phase of injury. In the chronic phase of proximal vagal neuropathy, imaging will show fatty infiltration of the ipsilateral soft palate and a patulous lateral pharynx due to constrictor muscle atrophy. Lesions causing proximal vagal neuropathy can be found involving the brainstem medulla, basal cistern, JF, or suprahyoid CS.

Distal vagal neuropathy is defined as isolated vagal neuropathy without the nasopharyngeal & oropharyngeal findings described above. In this setting, lesions are sought in the infrahyoid CS. Left-sided lesions may include diseases of the mediastinum, such as lung cancer. Right-sided lesions causing distal vagal neuropathy are usually clinically palpable at the time of imaging.

Postganglionic **Horner syndrome** presents with ptosis (droop of upper eyelid), miosis (decrease in pupil size), and anhydrosis (absence of sweat). The lesion causing Horner syndrome is sought along the segment of oculosympathetic pathway between superior cervical ganglion and eye. Much of this pathway is found between the supraclavicular and nasopharyngeal CS. Remember the sympathetic chain passes with the ICA up the skull base carotid canal. The radiologist must interrogate the cervical, oropharyngeal, and nasopharyngeal CS, the carotid canal in the skull base, cavernous sinus, & the orbit. In particular, ICA dissection must be excluded.

Selected References

1. Chong VF et al: The suprahyoid neck: normal and pathological anatomy. J Laryngol Otol. 113(6):501-8, 1999
2. Chong VF et al: Pictorial review: radiology of the carotid space. Clin Radiol. 51(11):762-8, 1996
3. Fruin ME et al: The carotid space of the infrahyoid neck. Semin Ultrasound CT MR. 12(3):224-40, 1991

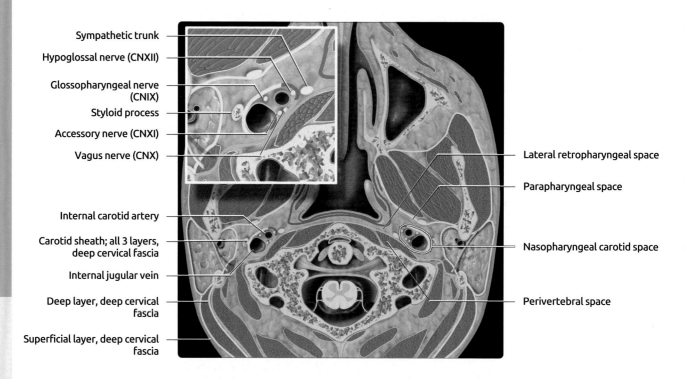

Sympathetic trunk

Hypoglossal nerve (CNXII)

Glossopharyngeal nerve (CNIX)

Styloid process

Accessory nerve (CNXI)

Vagus nerve (CNX)

Internal carotid artery

Carotid sheath; all 3 layers, deep cervical fascia

Internal jugular vein

Deep layer, deep cervical fascia

Superficial layer, deep cervical fascia

Lateral retropharyngeal space

Parapharyngeal space

Nasopharyngeal carotid space

Perivertebral space

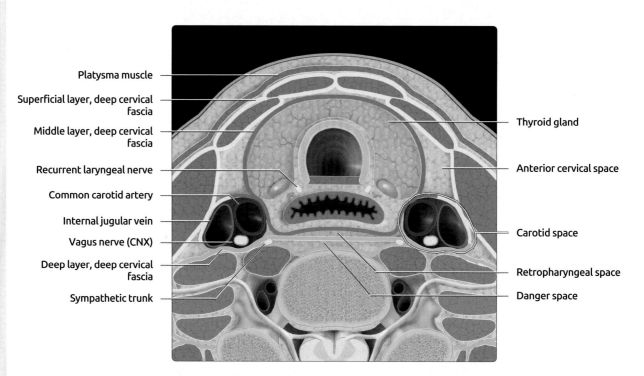

Platysma muscle

Superficial layer, deep cervical fascia

Middle layer, deep cervical fascia

Recurrent laryngeal nerve

Common carotid artery

Internal jugular vein

Vagus nerve (CNX)

Deep layer, deep cervical fascia

Sympathetic trunk

Thyroid gland

Anterior cervical space

Carotid space

Retropharyngeal space

Danger space

(Top) *Axial graphic of the suprahyoid neck (SHN) at the level of C1 vertebral body with insert shows magnified carotid space (CS). The suprahyoid CS contains CNIX-XII, the internal carotid artery (ICA), and the internal jugular vein (IJV). The carotid sheath is made up of components of all 3 layers of deep cervical fascia (tricolor line around CS). In the SHN, the carotid sheath is less substantial than in the infrahyoid neck (IHN). The sympathetic trunk runs just medial to the CS. **(Bottom)** Axial graphic shows the CS in the IHN. Note that the carotid sheath contains all 3 layers of the deep cervical fascia (tricolor line). In the IHN, the carotid sheath is tenacious throughout its length. The infrahyoid CS contains the common carotid artery (CCA), IJV, and only the vagus cranial nerve.*

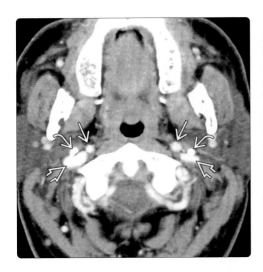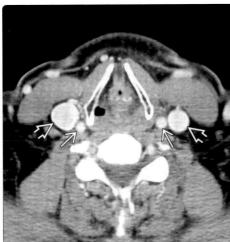

(Left) Axial CECT at the level of C1 vertebral body shows the nasopharyngeal CS contains the ICA ➡, IJV ➡, and CNIX-XII (not visible). Note that the CS is posterior to the styloid process ➡. (Right) Axial CECT at the level of the glottic larynx shows that the infrahyoid CS contains the CCA ➡, IJV ➡, and vagus nerve (not visible). Notice that the carotid sheath is also not visible on imaging.

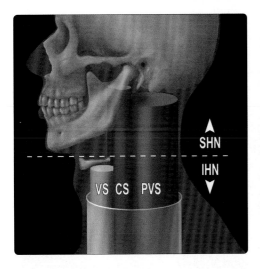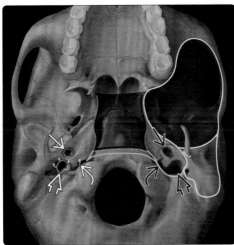

(Left) Lateral graphic of the cervical neck shows the tubular CS extending from the skull base [carotid canal and jugular foramen (JF)] to the aortic arch. (Right) Axial graphic of the skull base viewed from below shows the CS abutting the skull base. The ICA ➡ enters the carotid canal ➡, while the IJV ➡ emerges from the JF ➡. CNIX-XI is exiting the JF. CNXII ➡ is more medial as it enters the CS from the hypoglossal canal ➡.

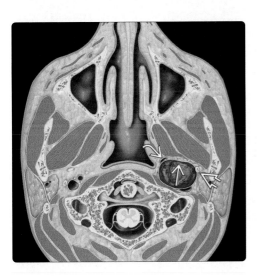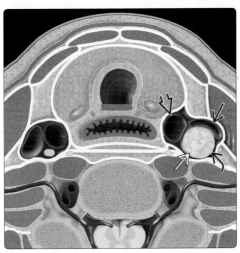

(Left) Axial graphic reveals a generic nasopharyngeal CS mass. As the CS mass enlarges, it pushes the parapharyngeal space fat anteriorly ➡ as well as lifts the styloid process anterolaterally ➡. Often the ICA is also lifted anteriorly ➡ by a CS mass. (Right) Axial graphic of an infrahyoid CS mass ➡ shows that the CCA ➡ and the IJV ➡ are displaced anteriorly. Note the vagus nerve ➡ is visible in the posterolateral aspect of this vagal schwannoma.

Tortuous Carotid Artery in Neck

TERMINOLOGY

- Synonyms: Retropharyngeal carotid, carotid transposition, kissing carotids, medialized carotid

IMAGING

- **CTA or MRA** easily establishes diagnosis
- CTA/CECT shows enhancing carotid artery (CA) in retropharyngeal space (RPS)
  - Round (axial) or tubular (coronal) vessel
  - Contiguous axial images reveal contiguous nature
- **Coronal reconstructions** best depict RPS CA

TOP DIFFERENTIAL DIAGNOSES

- CA pseudoaneurysm
- CA dissection
- Carotid body paraganglioma

PATHOLOGY

- CA pushes medially from carotid space, bows ± violates **lateral slip of deep cervical fascia** to enter RPS

CLINICAL ISSUES

- Incidental finding on neck CT or MR
- If symptomatic, pulsatile retropharyngeal or retrotonsillar mass
  - Globus sensation
  - May potentiate obstructive sleep apnea
- Common pseudolesion of older population
- Correct imaging diagnosis prevents treatment

DIAGNOSTIC CHECKLIST

- Tortuous CA in differential diagnosis of prevertebral soft tissue widening on lateral plain film
- Radiologist must recognize as **nonsurgical** lesion
- Key is recognizing **tubular nature** of ectatic CA
- **Must report in patients undergoing pharyngeal surgery**

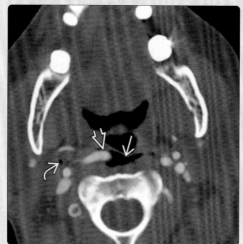
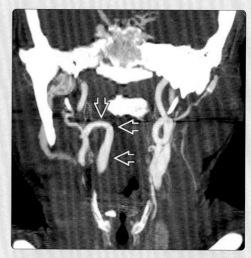

(Left) Axial CTA in a 62-year-old woman who suffered a stab wound to the right neck with a pharyngeal laceration demonstrates gas in the retropharyngeal ➡ and carotid spaces ➡. Medialized tortuous right internal carotid artery ➡ in the retropharyngeal space is incidentally seen. (Right) Coronal CTA demonstrates far medial course of the right internal carotid artery ➡ as it arches into the retropharyngeal space. Coronal images often best illustrate the serpiginous vascular nature of this variant.

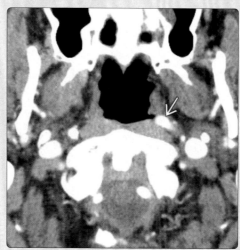
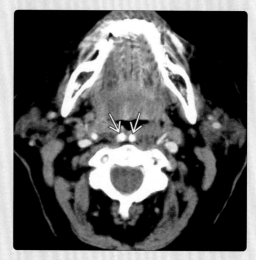

(Left) Axial CECT demonstrates medial deviation of the left internal carotid artery ➡. Note its exposed position near the mucosal surface at the level of the nasopharynx. Reporting this variant is important to avoid iatrogenic injury if pharyngeal intervention is planned. (Right) Axial NECT demonstrates a classic example of kissing carotids as bilateral ectatic internal carotid arteries contacting in the midline ➡ retropharyngeal space.

TERMINOLOGY

Synonyms

- Retropharyngeal carotid, carotid transposition, medialized carotid, kissing carotids

Definitions

- 1 or both carotid arteries (CAs) protrude medially into retropharyngeal space (RPS)

IMAGING

General Features

- Best diagnostic clue
  - **CTA shows enhancing CA running in RPS**
- Location
  - Retropharyngeal space
- Morphology
  - Tortuous CA

CT Findings

- CECT
  - Round (axial) or tubular (coronal) enhancing RPS structure
  - Contiguous axial images reveal structure as CA
  - Unilateral or bilateral
    - **Bilateral = kissing carotids**
- CTA
  - **Coronal reconstructions** best define nature of RPS CA
  - Tortuous vessel often is distal common CA + proximal internal CA

MR Findings

- T1WI
  - Round, low-signal retropharyngeal CA
- T2WI
  - Round, low-signal CA secondary to high-velocity flow void
- MRA
  - Coronal MPR best delineates retropharyngeal artery as CA

Imaging Recommendations

- Best imaging tool
  - CTA or MRA easily establishes diagnosis
  - Angiography not necessary to confirm diagnosis
- Protocol advice
  - CTA differentiates ectatic CA from other causes of pulsatile tonsillar or RPS mass

DIFFERENTIAL DIAGNOSIS

Carotid Artery Pseudoaneurysm

- Clinical: History of trauma or CA dissection; pulsatile mass
- Imaging: Complex carotid space mass

Carotid Artery Dissection

- Clinical: Sympathetic neuropathy ± vagal neuropathy ± TIA ± stroke
- Imaging: MR shows abnormal signal in CA wall; angio shows narrowed or occluded vessel

Carotid Body Paraganglioma

- Clinical: Pulsatile angle of mandible mass
- Imaging: Enhancing mass at carotid bifurcation

PATHOLOGY

General Features

- Etiology
  - Atherosclerosis causes fusiform enlargement & tortuosity of CA
    - Association with chronic hypertension
    - CA migrates with progressive ectasia
  - May be due to failure of complete descent of dorsal aortic root into chest with persistent embryologic angulation of carotids in children
- Associated abnormalities
  - Can be component of **velocardiofacial syndrome**
- Relevant anatomy
  - As CA pushes medially from normal position within carotid space, bows or violates **lateral slip of deep cervical fascia** (cloison sagittale) to reach RPS

CLINICAL ISSUES

Presentation

- Most common signs/symptoms
  - Incidental finding on neck CT or MR
  - If symptomatic, pulsatile retropharyngeal or retrotonsillar mass
- Other signs/symptoms
  - May potentiate obstructive sleep apnea
  - Globus sensation

Natural History & Prognosis

- CA may protrude further into RPS with advancing age
- Important implications for anesthesiologist when performing transoral block of glossopharyngeal nerve in pharynx or in difficult tracheal intubation
- Risk for CA injury during pharyngeal surgeries: TORS, tonsillectomy, adenoidectomy, & velopharyngeal narrowing

DIAGNOSTIC CHECKLIST

Consider

- Ectatic CA in differential diagnosis of prevertebral soft tissue widening on lateral plain film
- Big difference between clinical suspicion (suspect vascular tumor) & radiologic impression (tortuous CA)
  - Radiologist must recognize **nonsurgical nature** of lesion

Image Interpretation Pearls

- Key is recognizing tubular nature of ectatic CA

Reporting Tips

- Important to **report in patients undergoing pharyngeal surgery** to avoid iatrogenic carotid injury

SELECTED REFERENCES

1. Lukins DE et al: The moving carotid artery: a retrospective review of the retropharyngeal carotid artery and the incidence of positional changes on serial studies. AJNR Am J Neuroradiol. 37(2):336-41, 2016
2. Davis WL et al: The normal and diseased infrahyoid retropharyngeal, danger, and prevertebral spaces. Semin Ultrasound CT MR. 12(3):241-56, 1991

Carotid Artery Dissection in Neck

TERMINOLOGY

- Internal carotid artery dissection (ICAD)
- ICAD: Tear in internal carotid artery wall allows blood to enter & delaminate wall layers

IMAGING

- Pathognomonic findings of dissection: **Intimal flap** or **double lumen** (seen in < 10%)
- Aneurysmal dilatation seen in 30%
  - Commonly in distal subcranial segment of ICA
  - Focal pseudoaneurysm unusual
- Flame-shaped ICA occlusion (acute phase)
- ICAD most commonly originates in ICA 2-3 cm distal to carotid bulb & variably involve distal ICA
- Stops before petrous ICA
- Long-segment irregularity of vessel
- CTA & MRA emerging as superior technologies to image intramural & extraluminal dissection components
  - T1 FS MR best demonstrates **hyperintense mural hematomas**

TOP DIFFERENTIAL DIAGNOSES

- Fibromuscular dysplasia
- Atheromatous plaque
- Traumatic ICA pseudoaneurysm
- Carotid artery fenestration
- Reversible cerebral vasoconstrictive syndrome

CLINICAL ISSUES

- Ipsilateral pain in face, jaw, head, or neck
- Oculosympathetic palsy (miosis & ptosis, partial Horner syndrome)
- Ischemic symptoms (cerebral or retinal TIA or stroke)
- Bruit (40%)
- Lower cranial nerve palsies (especially CNX)
- Pulsatile tinnitus

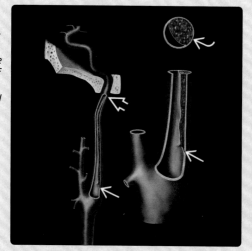
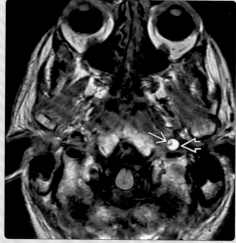

(Left) *Lateral graphic depicts typical internal carotid artery (ICA) dissection. Note that the dissection begins above bifurcation* ➡ *and ends at the skull base* ➡. *Cross section of a subintimal hematoma* ➡ *is also shown.* (Right) *Axial T1WI MR in a 47-year-old man who fell skiing 3 weeks prior to developing left frontotemporal headache shows T1 shortening within the crescentic subacute clot* ➡ *in the false lumen of the dissected left ICA. Note the high-signal thrombus* ➡ *within the true lumen of the vessel, which was occluded.*

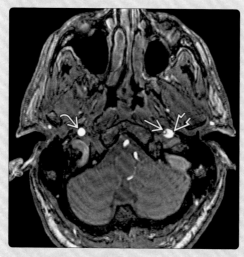
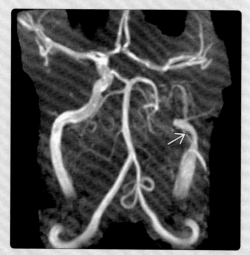

(Left) *Axial MRA source image in the same patient shows the high-signal thrombus in the false lumen* ➡ *as well as the thrombosed true lumen* ➡. *Note that there is a subtle difference in the signal of the thrombosed vessel on the left compared to the patent flow signal of the right ICA* ➡. (Right) *Coronal MRA reconstruction demonstrates projection of the T1 shortening from the thrombus onto the time of flight MIP image* ➡. *This is thrombus, not vascular flow. Distally, there is a lack of flow-related signal.*

TERMINOLOGY

Abbreviations

- Carotid artery dissection (CAD), internal carotid artery dissection (ICAD)

Definitions

- ICAD: Tear in internal carotid artery wall allows blood to enter & delaminate wall layers

IMAGING

General Features

- Best diagnostic clue
  o Pathognomonic findings of dissection: **Intimal flap** or **double lumen** (seen in < 10%)
  o **Aneurysmal dilatation** seen in 30%, commonly in distal subcranial segment of ICA
  o **Flame-shaped ICA occlusion** (acute phase)
- Location
  o ICADs most commonly originate in ICA 2-3 cm distal to carotid bulb & variably involve distal ICA
- Size
  o ICAD extends variable length along distal ICA
  o Stops before petrous ICA
- Morphology
  o ICA luminal narrowing ± focal aneurysmal dilatation

CT Findings

- CECT
  o **Narrowing** of dissected artery ± aneurysmal dilatation
  o May show **dissection flap** ± double lumen
- CTA
  o Shows narrowing of ICA lumen ± aneurysmal dilatation
  o May show intramural thrombus as low-attenuation crescent
  o May show dissection flap ± double lumen
  o Long-segment irregularity (alternating caliber) of vessel

MR Findings

- T1WI
  o T1 MR with fat saturation: Intramural hematoma (**hyperintense crescent** adjacent to ICA lumen)
  o Aneurysmal ICAD: Laminated stages of thrombosis (with intervening layers of methemoglobin & hemosiderin)
- T2WI
  o Aneurysmal form: Laminated stages of thrombosis (with intervening layers of methemoglobin & hemosiderin)
- FLAIR
  o Brain: Intracranial sequela of ischemia/stroke in ICA distribution
- T2* GRE
  o Hemorrhagic products in vessel wall/aneurysm may cause blooming susceptibility artifact
- DWI
  o Brain: Intracranial acute sequelae of ischemia/stroke show restricted diffusion
- MRA
  o Vessel tapering ± aneurysmal dilatation of dissected ICA

Ultrasonographic Findings

- Abnormal pattern of flow identified > 90% of cases

- Intimal flap or intramural hematoma seen in < 33% of cases
- Dissection site usually not seen

Angiographic Findings

- Pathognomonic: Intimal flap + double lumen (true & false)
- ICA lumen stenosis with slow flow
- Abrupt reconstitution of lumen
- Dissecting aneurysm or pseudoaneurysm
- Flame-shaped, tapered occlusion is usually acute
- Fibromuscular dysplasia changes in 15% of patients
- Spares carotid bulb; ends at extracranial opening of carotid canal

Imaging Recommendations

- Best imaging tool
  o Angiography remains gold standard for ICAD
  o CTA & MRA emerging as superior technologies to image intramural & extraluminal dissection components
    – Frequently 1st step in imaging evaluation
- Protocol advice
  o T1 MR with fat suppression best sequence for hyperintense mural hematomas

DIFFERENTIAL DIAGNOSIS

Carotid Fibromuscular Dysplasia

- Clinical: Young female patient with TIA
- Imaging: "String of beads" & long segment stenosis
  o May have associated ICAD

Atheromatous Plaque

- Clinical: Frequently history of hypertension
- Imaging: MRA/CTA may show prestenotic dilatation, narrowing of vessel due to plaque ± calcification in vessel wall

Traumatic ICA Pseudoaneurysm

- Clinical: History of recent or remote trauma
- Imaging: Dissecting aneurysm may be indistinguishable from traumatic pseudoaneurysm

Carotid Artery Fenestration

- Clinical: Asymptomatic, normal variant
- Imaging: Short segment fenestration often at C1/C2 level

Reversible Cerebral Vasoconstrictive Syndrome

- Associated with ICAD & vertebral artery dissections
- Clinical: Thunderclap headache presentation
- Imaging: Intracranial stenoses mimicking vasculitis

Vasospasm

- Clinical: ICA vasospasm can occur adjacent to neck infections and with trauma or arterial catheterization
- Often related to adjacent retropharyngeal neck infections, most commonly in children
  o No treatment needed; typically self-limited
- Imaging: Smooth narrowing without luminal flap or irregularity

Glomus Vagale Paraganglioma

- Clinical: Slowly growing painless mass
- Imaging: Nasopharyngeal carotid space mass with "salt & pepper" on T1 & avid enhancement CECT & T1 C+ MR

Carotid Space Schwannoma

- Clinical: Slowly enlarging painless mass; neurological symptoms often absent
- Imaging: Carotid space mass without high-velocity flow voids on T1; hyperintense on T2

PATHOLOGY

General Features

- Etiology
  - Dissections usually arise from intimal tear, blood enters artery wall, **intramural hematoma** forms (false lumen)
  - 2 types of associated aneurysm
    - **Dissecting aneurysm**: Some normal arterial wall layers present in wall of this aneurysm
    - **Pseudoaneurysm**: Subadventitial dissection causes pseudoaneurysm
      - □ Arterial wall contains no normal layers, just organized clot
  - 3 types of ICAD
    - **Spontaneous dissection**: Most common; etiology unknown
    - **Posttraumatic**: Vertebral artery dissection > ICAD
    - **Predisposed**: Dissection from arteriopathy (fibromuscular dysplasia, genetic syndromes)
- Associated abnormalities
  - Fibromuscular dysplasia
  - Ehlers-Danlos type IV
  - Marfan syndrome
  - Osteogenesis imperfecta type I
  - Autosomal dominant kidney disease
  - Reversible cerebral vasoconstrictive syndrome
- ICA most common cervical artery to dissect
  - Extracranial ICA more likely to dissect than intracranial
- Pharyngeal portion of extracranial ICA is mobile (carotid bulb to skull base)

Staging, Grading, & Classification

- Biffl grading scale
  - Grade I: Intimal irregularity with < 25% narrowing
  - Grade II: Dissection > 25% narrowing
  - Grade III: Arterial pseudoaneurysm
  - Grade IV: Arterial occlusion
  - Grade V: Transection with extravasation

CLINICAL ISSUES

Presentation

- Most common signs/symptoms
  - Ipsilateral pain in face, jaw, head, or neck
  - Oculosympathetic palsy (miosis & ptosis, partial Horner syndrome)
  - Ischemic symptoms (cerebral or retinal TIA or stroke)
  - Bruit (40%)
- Other signs/symptoms
  - Lower cranial nerve palsies (especially CNX)
  - Pulsatile tinnitus
  - Hyperextension or neck rotation (yoga, vigorous exercise, cough, vomiting, sneezing, resuscitation, neck manipulation)
  - Congenital Horner syndrome with traumatic delivery

- Clinical profile
  - H&N pain, partial Horner syndrome, TIA stroke triad (~ 33%)

Demographics

- Age
  - 30- to 55-year-old adults
  - Average age: 40 years old
- Epidemiology
  - Annual incidence 2.5-3 per 100,000
  - Extracranial ICAD > > intracranial ICAD or common carotid artery dissection
  - 20% of ICADs bilateral or involve vertebral arteries

Natural History & Prognosis

- 90% of stenoses resolve
- 66% of occlusions are recanalized
- 33% of pseudoaneurysms decrease in size
- Risk of recurrent dissection = 2% (1st month), then 1% per year (usually in another vessel)
- Risk of stroke due to thromboembolic disease ↑; related to severity of initial ischemic insult
- Death from ICAD < 5%

Treatment

- Intravenous heparin + oral warfarin (Coumadin) (unless contraindicated by hemorrhagic stroke)
- Antiplatelet therapy in asymptomatic patients & stable imaging findings for 6 months
- Endovascular stent placement rarely used
- Surgical treatment now rare option
  - Used when refractory to maximal medical & endovascular therapy
  - Interposition graft
  - Relatively high morbidity and mortality

DIAGNOSTIC CHECKLIST

Image Interpretation Pearls

- ICAD may present as luminal occlusion, stenosis, or aneurysmal dilatation (pseudoaneurysm)

SELECTED REFERENCES

1. Provenzale JM et al: Comparison of test performance characteristics of MRI, MR angiography, and CT angiography in the diagnosis of carotid and vertebral artery dissection: a review of the medical literature. AJR Am J Roentgenol. 193(4):1167-74, 2009
2. Chandra A et al: Spontaneous dissection of the carotid and vertebral arteries: the 10-year UCSD experience. Ann Vasc Surg. 21(2):178-85, 2007
3. Wu HC et al: Spontaneous bilateral internal carotid artery dissection with acute stroke in young patients. Eur Neurol. 56(4):230-4, 2006
4. Kono Y et al: Carotid arteries: contrast-enhanced US angiography-- preliminary clinical experience. Radiology. 230(2):561-8, 2004
5. Dziewas R et al: Cervical artery dissection--clinical features, risk factors, therapy and outcome in 126 patients. J Neurol. 250(10):1179-84, 2003
6. Logason K et al: Duplex scan findings in patients with spontaneous cervical artery dissections. Eur J Vasc Endovasc Surg. 23(4):295-8, 2002
7. Zuccoli G et al: Carotid and vertebral artery dissection: Magnetic Resonance findings in 15 cases. Radiol Med (Torino). 104(5-6):466-71, 2002
8. Brandt T et al: Pathogenesis of cervical artery dissections: association with connective tissue abnormalities. Neurology. 57(1):24-30, 2001

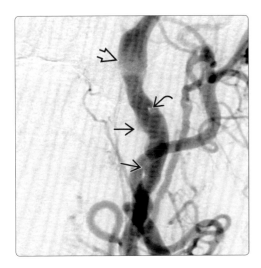
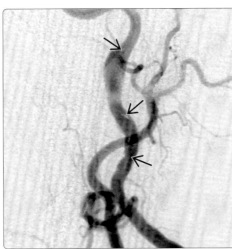

(Left) *Anteroposterior angiography in a 64-year-old man who presented with left hemisphere stroke demonstrates long-segment irregularity of the left ICA that is consistent with dissection ➡. A short segment of the intimal flap is visible ➡. There is also aneurysmal change distally ➡.* (Right) *Lateral angiography in the same patient reveals a long-segment lucency within the contrast column representing an intimal flap ➡ that is separating true and false lumina, both of which are patent.*

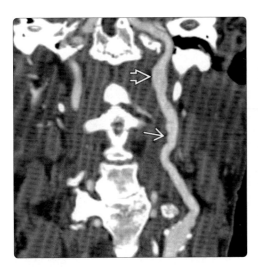
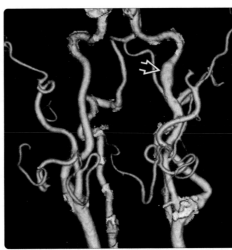

(Left) *Coronal CTA curved reconstruction in the same patient performed 2 years after the previous angiograms demonstrates persistent changes of dissection with residual wall irregularity ➡ and distal aneurysmal change ➡. The intimal flap is no longer visible.* (Right) *Coronal CTA oblique volume-rendered image in the same patient better demonstrates the residual aneurysmal change in the distal left internal carotid artery ➡.*

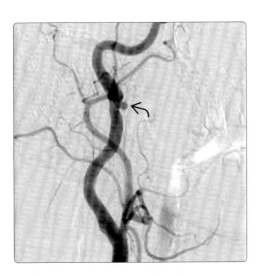
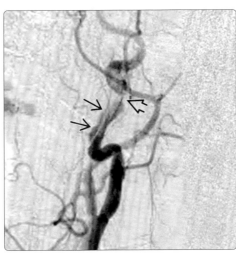

(Left) *Longitudinal oblique angiography in a 49-year-old woman involved in a motor vehicle head-on collision shows focal wall irregularity of the upper cervical right ICA, representing dissection. A focal pseudoaneurysm is present ➡.* (Right) *Lateral angiography in the same patient shows wall irregularity in the contralateral left ICA, which is also dissected ➡. The dissection has resulted in focal high-grade stenosis ➡.*

Carotid Artery Pseudoaneurysm in Neck

TERMINOLOGY

- Carotid artery pseudoaneurysm (CAPA)
- Synonyms: Carotid artery false aneurysm
- CAPA: Outpouching lacking part or all of carotid wall

IMAGING

- **CTA/CECT: Focal ↑ internal carotid artery (ICA) wall-lumen diameter**
- MR: Enlarged ICA with complex wall signal (stages of thrombosis with methemoglobin & hemosiderin)
  - Partly thrombosed CAPA may require enhanced MRA
- ICA lumen outpouching with extraluminal CAPA
- Associated dissection often present
- **Conventional angiography gold standard** for detection of CAPA ± ICA dissection
- **CECT & CTA show aneurysm size, extent of intraluminal thrombus, & flow**

TOP DIFFERENTIAL DIAGNOSES

- Carotid bulb ectasia; tortuous or looping carotid artery in neck; carotid artery dissection in neck

PATHOLOGY

- **Posttraumatic (with dissection or direct injury)**
- Sporadic subadventitial ICA dissection
- Atherosclerotic disease (frequently bilateral)
- Iatrogenic: Radiation, carotid endarterectomy
- Infection: Mycotic CAPA
- Congenital arterial wall anomaly

CLINICAL ISSUES

- Pulsatile neck mass
- Smaller CAPA + ICA dissection
  - Anticoagulation + observation ± aspirin
- Larger CAPA: Endovascular stent graft treatment of choice
  - Consider surgical repair or vessel sacrifice (endovascular occlusion) if other techniques fail

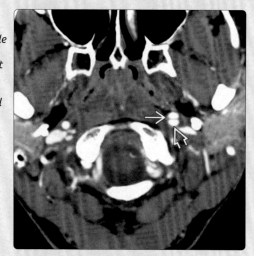
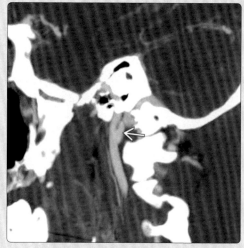

(Left) Axial CTA in a 29-year-old patient with cervical fractures following motorcycle crash shows abnormality involving the high cervical left internal carotid artery (ICA) with evidence of dissection with intimal flap ➡ and focal outpouching along posterior wall of vessel ➡. (Right) Sagittal CTA reformatted image in the same patient clearly demonstrates the pseudoaneurysm related to the ICA dissection ➡. Note that the reformatted image allows clear morphologic characterization while the axial image does not.

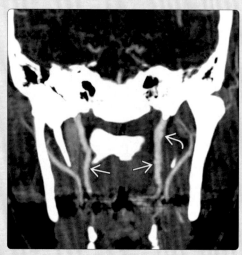
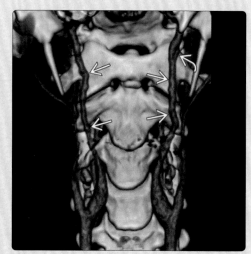

(Left) Coronal CTA in a 44-year-old woman with fibromuscular dysplasia (FMD) shows diffuse irregularity of both internal carotid arteries ➡, consistent with FMD. There is focal dissection with pseudoaneurysm involving the high cervical left internal carotid artery ➡. (Right) Coronal CTA volume-rendered image in the same patient more clearly demonstrates the left internal carotid artery pseudoaneurysm ➡. Diffuse vessel irregularity related to FMD is again seen ➡.

Carotid Artery Pseudoaneurysm in Neck

TERMINOLOGY

Abbreviations
- Carotid artery pseudoaneurysm (CAPA)

Synonyms
- Carotid artery false aneurysm
- May be indistinguishable from carotid blow out (in postradiotherapy setting)

Definitions
- CAPA: **Focal carotid artery outpouching**

IMAGING

General Features
- Best diagnostic clue
  - CTA/CECT: Focal ↑ ICA wall/lumen diameter
  - MR: Enlarged ICA with complex wall signal (stages of thrombosis with methemoglobin & hemosiderin)
- Location
  - Carotid space
  - Common sites = distal cervical ICA just below skull base & CCA
- Size
  - 1-3 cm
- Morphology
  - Saccular or fusiform

CT Findings
- NECT
  - Wall **calcification** if chronic
- CECT
  - Enhancement of central or eccentric lumen of partially thrombosed aneurysm
  - Enhancement irregular with intraluminal thrombus
- CTA
  - CAPA seen as **focal ICA or CCA outpouching**

MR Findings
- T1WI
  - Flow void in patent portion of lumen & residual aneurysm lumen
- T2WI
  - Complex flow in CAPA lumen
- T2* GRE
  - Thrombus may **bloom** (susceptibility effect)
- T1WI C+
  - Luminal enhancement from slow, complex flow
- MRA
  - CAPA seen as ICA outpouching
  - Be aware, partly thrombosed CAPA may **not** be seen without contrast-enhanced MRA

Angiographic Findings
- ICA luminal outpouching with extraluminal CAPA
- Associated ICA dissection often present

Imaging Recommendations
- Best imaging tool
  - Conventional angiography gold standard for detecting CAPA ± ICA dissection
    - Underestimates CAPA size
  - CECT & CTA show aneurysm size, extent of intraluminal thrombus & flow

DIFFERENTIAL DIAGNOSIS

Carotid Bulb Ectasia
- Imaging: Prominent CA bifurcation without thrombus

Tortuous Carotid Artery in Neck
- Imaging: Tortuous or looping CA mimics aneurysm

Carotid Artery Dissection in Neck
- Clinical: Sporadic or posttraumatic
- Imaging: Narrowed or occluded ICA

PATHOLOGY

General Features
- Etiology
  - Multiple categories
    - **Trauma (with dissection or direct injury)**
    - **Sporadic subadventitial ICA dissection**
    - Atherosclerotic disease (frequently bilateral)
    - Iatrogenic: Radiation, carotid endarterectomy
    - Infection: Mycotic CAPA
    - Congenital arterial wall anomaly: **Fibromuscular dysplasia**, cystic medial necrosis, Ehlers-Danlos, Marfan syndrome, Behçet disease

Gross Pathologic & Surgical Features
- CAPA lacks **normal arterial wall layers**
  - CAPA wall contained by adventitial sleeve, surrounding hematoma or soft tissues
  - Adventitia may be disrupted in penetrating trauma or irradiated necks

CLINICAL ISSUES

Presentation
- Most common signs/symptoms
  - Pulsatile neck mass
  - Lower cranial nerve palsy (CNIX-XII)
  - Ischemic symptoms ± stroke
  - Hemorrhage (particularly head & neck cancer patients)

Natural History & Prognosis
- CAPA thrombus may cause TIA-CVA
- Acute hemorrhage in setting of radiated head & neck SCCa often life threatening, requiring emergent treatment

Treatment
- Smaller & CAPA + ICA dissection may be treated conservatively with anticoagulation & observation ± aspirin
  - Heparin → warfarin (Coumadin)
- Larger CAPA: Endovascular stent graft treatment of choice
  - Surgical repair or vessel sacrifice if other techniques fail

SELECTED REFERENCES

1. Bodanapally UK et al: Vascular injuries to the neck after penetrating trauma: diagnostic Performance of 40- and 64-MDCT Angiography. AJR Am J Roentgenol. 205(4):866-72, 2015
2. Chokshi FH et al: 64-MDCT angiography of blunt vascular injuries of the neck. AJR Am J Roentgenol. 196(3):W309-15, 2011

TERMINOLOGY

- Fibromuscular dysplasia (FMD)
  - Arterial disease of unknown etiology
  - Overgrowth of smooth muscle, fibrous tissue
  - Affecting medium & large arteries

IMAGING

- Renal artery most common overall site (~ 75%)
- Cervicocranial FMD CTA/MRA findings
  - Vessel beading/irregularities: **String of beads**
  - **Arterial stenosis** without mural Ca++ (cf. ASVD)
  - FMD associations: Dissection, pseudoaneurysm, intracranial aneurysms
- DSA: Gold standard; 3 appearances
  - **Type 1 (85%)**: Typical string of beads; medial fibroplasia
  - **Type 2 (10%)**: Long tubular stenosis; intimal fibroplasia
  - **Type 3 (5%)**: Asymmetric outpouching along 1 side of artery
    - Periadventitial or periarterial fibroplasia

TOP DIFFERENTIAL DIAGNOSES

- Atherosclerosis
- Nonatherosclerotic vasculopathies
- Standing waves on DSA
- MRA motion artifact

PATHOLOGY

- 3 principal histopathologic varieties
  - **Medial fibroplasia**: Medial layer involvement (type 1)
  - **Intimal fibroplasia**: Intimal involvement (type 2)
  - **Perimedial fibroplasia**: Involvement of adventitia adjacent to media (type 3)
- Alternating zones of hyperplasia & weakening

CLINICAL ISSUES

- Treatment: Antiplatelet ± anticoagulant therapy
- Balloon angioplasty
- Covered stenting

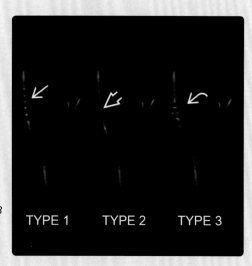

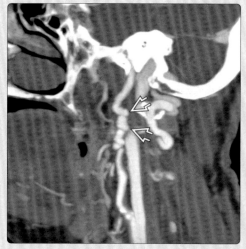

(Left) *Carotid bifurcation graphic shows the principal subtypes of fibromuscular dysplasia (FMD). Type 1 appears as alternating areas of constriction and dilatation* ➡, *type 2 as tubular stenosis* ➡, *and type 3 as focal corrugations ± a diverticulum* ➡. **(Right)** *Sagittal CTA reformation shows internal carotid artery string of beads. However, closer evaluation also shows focal outpouching* ➡ *along the course of both arteries, indicating that type 3 fibromuscular dysplasia is present.*

TYPE 1   TYPE 2   TYPE 3

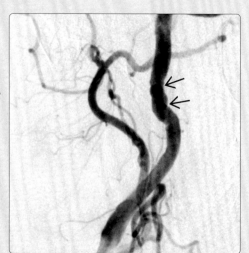

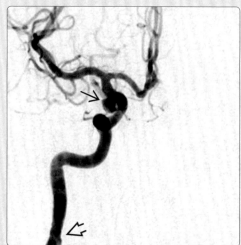

(Left) *Oblique right common carotid artery DSA shows irregular outpouchings* ➡ *in the cervical ICA consistent with FMD.* **(Right)** *Anteroposterior right internal carotid artery DSA in the same patient shows a 6-mm posterior communicating artery aneurysm* ➡, *which ruptured with resultant subarachnoid hemorrhage. Changes of FMD are again noted in the cervical ICA* ➡.

TERMINOLOGY

Abbreviations

- Fibromuscular dysplasia (FMD)

Definitions

- Arterial disease of unknown etiology affecting medium & large arteries
  - Arteriopathy with dysplastic arterial wall with overgrowth of smooth muscle & fibrous tissue

IMAGING

General Features

- Best diagnostic clue
  - Multifocal ± bilateral cervical carotid or vertebral artery irregularity on CTA/MRA/DSA
    - Appears like **string of beads** ± long segment stenosis
- Location
  - H&N: Lesions most commonly at C1-C2 levels
  - Craniocervical arteries (70%)
    - ICA (30-50%) > ECA > vertebral arteries
    - > 50% bilateral
    - Spares carotid bifurcation
  - Intracranial rare (supraclinoid ICA, MCA)
  - Peripheral vascular
    - **Renal arteries** affected 75% (40% bilateral)

CT Findings

- CTA
  - Morphological changes of FMD in carotid & vertebral artery circulations
    - Vessel beading/irregularities: **String of beads**
    - **Arterial stenosis** without mural Ca^{++} (cf. ASVD)
    - FMD associations: Dissection, pseudoaneurysm, intracranial aneurysms

MR Findings

- MRA
  - String of beads ± long segment stenosis

Angiographic Findings

- DSA: Gold standard; 3 appearances
  - **Type 1 (85%)**: Typical string of beads; medial fibroplasia
  - **Type 2 (10%)**: Long tubular stenosis; intimal fibroplasia
  - **Type 3 (5%)**: Asymmetric outpouching along 1 side of artery; periadventitial fibroplasia

DIFFERENTIAL DIAGNOSIS

Atherosclerosis, Extracranial

- ASVD affects older vasculopaths
- Typically short segment stenosis at or above carotid bifurcation with mural Ca^{++}

Carotid Dissection

- Irregular stenosis ± outpouching from associated pseudoaneurysm

PATHOLOGY

General Features

- Etiology

  - Unknown; thought to be dysplastic rather than degenerative or inflammatory
- Associated abnormalities
  - **Intracranial saccular aneurysms** (10%)
  - Spontaneous dissection (20%, ICA)
  - Thromboembolic sequela due to disturbed flow → thrombus formation
- May affect other medium-sized arteries (peripheral, abdominal, cephalic)
- Histopathology
  - Overgrowth of smooth muscle cells & fibrous tissue within arterial wall

CLINICAL ISSUES

Presentation

- Most common signs/symptoms
  - Hypertension (renal artery involvement → stenosis)
- Other signs/symptoms
  - Craniocervical FMD
    - Stenosis → TIA/stroke
    - ICA dissection ± stroke
    - Aneurysm → mass effect on adjacent structures; rupture (rare)

Demographics

- Age
  - Onset of symptoms: 25-50 yr
- Gender
  - M:F = 1:9 (medial subtype)
- Epidemiology
  - **Renal artery** > > **carotid** > vertebral > other arteries (lumbar, mesenteric, celiac, hepatic, iliac arteries)

Natural History & Prognosis

- Slowly progressive disorder

Treatment

- Antiplatelet ± anticoagulant therapy = conservative management for stroke prevention with cervical FMD
- Balloon angioplasty of stenoses
- Covered stenting
- Arterial reconstruction for aneurysm

SELECTED REFERENCES

1. Persu A et al: European consensus on the diagnosis and management of fibromuscular dysplasia. J Hypertens. 32(7):1367-78, 2014
2. Olin JW et al: The United States registry for fibromuscular dysplasia: results in the first 447 patients. Circulation. 125(25):3182-90, 2012
3. Cohen JE et al: Petrous carotid artery pseudoaneurysm in bilateral carotid fibromuscular dysplasia: treatment by means of self-expanding covered stent. Surg Neurol. 68(2):216-20; discussion 220, 2007
4. Nerantzis CE et al: Post-mortem angiographic and histologic findings of coronary artery fibromuscular dysplasia. Int J Cardiol. 122(3):e32-5, 2007
5. Beregi JP et al: Fibromuscular dysplasia of the renal arteries: comparison of helical CT angiography and arteriography. AJR Am J Roentgenol. 172(1):27-34, 1999

Acute Idiopathic Carotidynia

TERMINOLOGY

- Synonyms
  - Idiopathic or sclerosing (inflammatory) pseudotumor
  - Idiopathic carotiditis
  - Fay syndrome
- Controversial diagnosis: Syndrome vs. entity
- International Headache Society Classification Committee (IHSCC) criteria for diagnosis: Self-limited illness with ≥ 1 of following: Tenderness to palpation, swelling, ↑ pulsations over carotid
  - Imaging to exclude structural abnormality

IMAGING

- **Circumferential thickening of carotid wall**
  - Distal common carotid or carotid bifurcation area
  - Usually **no** luminal narrowing
- Contrast-enhanced MR better exam than CECT
  - **Markedly enhancing tissue only seen with MR**
  - CECT enhancement is poor

- Ultrasound: **Hypoechoic** soft tissue around distal common carotid artery and bifurcation

TOP DIFFERENTIAL DIAGNOSES

- Carotid artery dissection in neck
- Extracranial atherosclerosis
- Miscellaneous vasculitis
- SCCa extranodal tumor

CLINICAL ISSUES

- Tenderness to palpation over carotid
- Pulsatile neck mass, may be indurated
- Repeat clinical/imaging assessment after course of antiinflammatories to exclude other pathology
- Typical symptomatic resolution in days to weeks

DIAGNOSTIC CHECKLIST

- **Diagnosis of exclusion**
  - If early conservative management fails, histologic confirmation is important

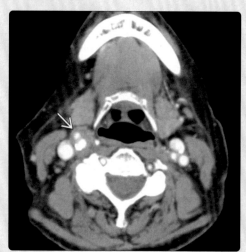
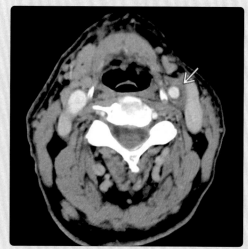

(Left) *Axial CECT of the neck reveals circumferential thickening of the common carotid wall ➡ at the carotid bifurcation. This patient was treated with steroids for presumptive diagnosis of carotidynia with symptoms resolving within 36 hours of treatment.* (Right) *Typical axial CECT of acute idiopathic carotidynia shows homogeneous soft tissue encasing the left distal common carotid artery ➡. There is no significant luminal narrowing.*

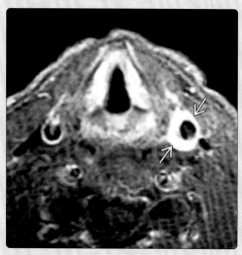
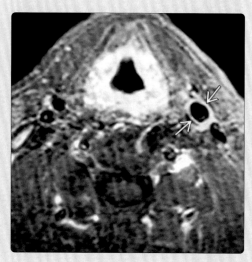

(Left) *Axial T1WI C+ FS MR in a patient with painful palpation in the left neck shows a thickened, intensely enhancing common carotid wall ➡ consistent with the diagnosis of carotidynia. Note the lack of luminal narrowing. (Courtesy G. W. Petermann, MD.)* (Right) *Axial T1 C+ FS MR in carotidynia post steroid therapy reveals mild residual wall thickening and enhancement involving the left common carotid wall ➡. (Courtesy G. W. Petermann, MD.)*

TERMINOLOGY

Synonyms

- Idiopathic or sclerosing (inflammatory) pseudotumor
- Idiopathic carotiditis
- Fay syndrome

Definitions

- International Headache Society Classification Committee (IHSCC) diagnostic criteria for carotidynia
  - Self-limited illness with ≥ 1 of following: Tenderness, swelling, ↑ pulsations over carotid
    - Image to exclude other structural abnormality
- Controversial diagnosis: Syndrome vs. entity
- Some consider it subset of vasculitis

IMAGING

General Features

- Best diagnostic clue
  - Tender mass surrounding carotid near bifurcation
- Location
  - Distal common carotid artery and bifurcation
  - Vessel wall involved **without** lumen narrowing
- Size
  - Craniocaudal extent 1.5-3.5 cm; 6- to 8-mm thick wall
- Morphology
  - **Circumferential thickening of carotid wall**

Imaging Recommendations

- Best imaging tool
  - Enhanced neck MR/MRA or ultrasound
    - MR demonstrates intense enhancement
      □ CECT enhancement is poor
    - Ultrasound can evaluate site of tenderness
- Protocol advice
  - Enhanced neck MR or ultrasound

CT Findings

- Homogeneous thickening of carotid wall
- Poorly or nonenhancing
- Thrombosed carotid dissection of soft plaque can appear similar

MR Findings

- Enhanced T1 fat-saturated MR
  - **Markedly enhancing tissue involving carotid wall**
  - Smoothly marginated without invasion
- T2: Increased intensity of thickened wall
  - Fibrous forms might have hypointense signal
- MRA: Absent or mild lumen stenosis; no irregularity

Ultrasonographic Findings

- Exact region of tenderness can be imaged
- **Hypoechoic** soft tissue around distal common carotid artery and bifurcation
- Increased vessel wall thickness
- **No significant lumen narrowing** or velocity elevation

DIFFERENTIAL DIAGNOSIS

Carotid Artery Dissection in Neck

- Lumen narrowing ± occlusion
- Axial T1 MR: High-signal subintimal hematoma
- Involves internal carotid artery above bifurcation

Extracranial Atherosclerosis

- Lumen narrowing ± calcification
- Carotid bulb or internal carotid

Miscellaneous Vasculitis

- Serum markers; angiography to confirm

Squamous Cell Carcinoma Extranodal Tumor

- Suspect if conservative therapy fails; biopsy indicated
- Entire carotid space involved; not just carotid wall

PATHOLOGY

General Features

- Etiology
  - Unknown; probably inflammatory

Staging, Grading, & Classification

- IHSCC diagnostic criteria noted above

Microscopic Features

- Nonspecific chronic inflammation
- Rarely biopsied

CLINICAL ISSUES

Presentation

- Most common signs/symptoms
  - Tenderness to palpation over carotid
- Other signs/symptoms
  - Pulsatile neck mass

Natural History & Prognosis

- Self-limited inflammatory condition

Treatment

- May respond to NSAID ± corticosteroids

DIAGNOSTIC CHECKLIST

Consider

- Enhanced MR or ultrasound best exams
- Repeat clinical/imaging assessment after course of antiinflammatories to exclude other pathology
  - Typical symptomatic resolution in days to weeks

Image Interpretation Pearls

- **Diagnosis of exclusion**
- If early conservative management fails, histologic confirmation is important

SELECTED REFERENCES

1. Behar T et al: Comparative evolution of carotidynia on ultrasound and magnetic resonance imaging. J Mal Vasc. 40(6):395-8, 2015
2. Kosaka N et al: Imaging by multiple modalities of patients with a carotidynia syndrome. Eur Radiol. 17(9):2430-3, 2007
3. Burton BS et al: MR imaging of patients with carotidynia. AJNR Am J Neuroradiol. 21(4):766-9, 2000

TERMINOLOGY

- Jugular vein thrombosis (JVT)
- **JVT**: Chronic internal jugular vein (IJV) thrombosis (> 10 days after acute event) in which clot persists within lumen after soft tissue inflammation is gone
- **JV thrombophlebitis**: Acute-subacute thrombosis of IJV with associated adjacent tissue inflammation

IMAGING

- Luminal clot (**filling defect**) in IJV on CECT with (thrombophlebitis) or without (thrombosis) associated soft tissue inflammatory changes
- **Tubular** vascular lesion of cervical neck
- US shows **noncompressible thrombus** and no flow

TOP DIFFERENTIAL DIAGNOSES

- Slow or turbulent flow in IJV (pseudothrombosis)
- Suppurative adenopathy
- Cervical neck abscess

- Squamous cell carcinoma malignant adenopathy

PATHOLOGY

- JVT pathogenesis: 3 mechanisms for thrombosis
  - **Endothelial damage** from indwelling line or infection, altered blood flow, and hypercoagulable state
  - **Venous stasis** from neck IJV compression (nodes) or mediastinum (superior vena cava syndrome) incites JVT
  - Migratory IJV thrombophlebitis (Trousseau syndrome) associated with **malignancy** (pancreas, lung, and ovary)
- **Lemierre syndrome**: IJV thrombosis associated with postanginal sepsis/necrobacillosis
  - Young healthy patients, unlike many other causes of JVT

CLINICAL ISSUES

- Aggressive intravenous antibiotics treat infection

DIAGNOSTIC CHECKLIST

- Do not mistake JVT with retropharyngeal space (RPS) edema for RPS abscess

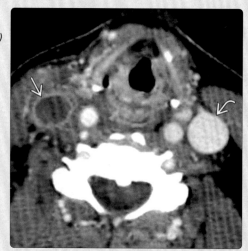
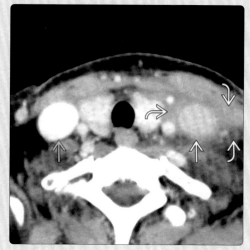

(Left) Axial CECT in a 58-year-old woman with renal failure, right internal jugular vein (IJV) hemodialysis catheter presented with right neck pain. Chronic right IJV thrombosis is seen ➡. Thin-wall enhancement of IJV venae vasorum and normal enhancement in patent left IJV ➡ are seen. (Right) Axial CECT in a 69-year-old woman with malignancy shows acute hyperdense thrombophlebitis involving the left IJV ➡. Note lower density compared with contrast-enhancing normal right IJV ➡ and surrounding tissue edema ➡.

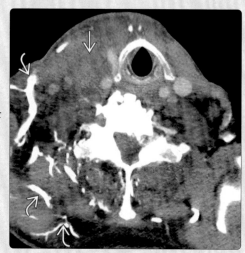
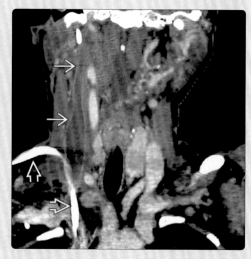

(Left) Axial CECT shows low-density nonenhancing acute thrombophlebitis of the right IJV ➡. Note surrounding edema and extensive contrast reflux into small collateral veins ➡. (Right) Coronal CT reconstruction shows IJV catheter ➡ and long-segment tubular thrombus within the right IJV ➡. Cervical region indwelling venous catheters predispose to JVT.

TERMINOLOGY

Abbreviations

- Jugular vein thrombosis (JVT)

Definitions

- JVT: Chronic internal jugular vein (IJV) thrombosis (> 10 days after acute event) in which clot persists within lumen after soft tissue inflammation is gone
- Jugular vein thrombophlebitis: Acute to subacute thrombosis of IJV with associated adjacent tissue inflammation (myositis and fasciitis)

IMAGING

General Features

- Best diagnostic clue
  - Luminal clot in IJV with (thrombophlebitis) or without (thrombosis) associated soft tissue inflammatory changes
- Location
  - IJV of extracranial H&N
- Size
  - IJV may be smaller than normal in chronic phase or enlarged in acute-subacute phase
- Morphology
  - Ovoid to round IJV luminal filling defect

Radiographic Findings

- Radiography
  - Central venous catheters in neck region increase JVT risk

CT Findings

- NECT
  - Acute thrombus is hyperdense
- CECT
  - **Acute-subacute IJV thrombophlebitis** (< 10 days)
    - Nonenhancing central **filling defect** (central low attenuation) within IJV
    - Acute thrombus can be hyperdense and may mimic patent IJV on CECT
    - Inflammation-induced loss of soft tissue planes surrounding thrombus-filled IJV
    - Enlarged vein diameter
    - Peripheral enhancement of (thickened) vessel wall (venae vasorum)
    - Increased density in fat surrounding carotid space (CS) secondary to edema cellulitis
    - Edema fluid may be present in retropharyngeal space (RPS) as secondary sign
  - **Chronic IJV thrombosis** (> 10 days)
    - Well-marginated, tubular thrombus fills IJV without adjacent inflammation
    - Tubular/linear enhancement of prominent **collateral veins** bypassing thrombosed IJV
- CTA
  - Filling defect in IJV
  - Large venous collaterals may be seen in chronic phase

MR Findings

- T1WI
  - IJV thrombus signal intensity depends on composition of clot (age)
  - Fat-suppressed sequences show acute thrombus as isointense
    - **Subacute clot** often **high signal** (methemoglobin)
  - Flow voids in collateral veins remain dark
- T2WI
  - Acute thrombus (early hours of acute event) in IJV lumen bright
  - Subacute IJV thrombus low signal
  - High-signal RPS edema may be present
- T2* GRE
  - Luminal thrombus may display susceptibility artifact (blooming) with low signal appearing larger than IJV
- T1WI C+
  - **Acute-subacute IJV thrombophlebitis**
    - Low-signal clot fills enlarged IJV
    - IJV wall enhancement with inhomogeneous enhancement of soft tissues surrounding CS
  - **Chronic JVT**
    - Filling defect in normal-sized IJV
    - Partial recanalization may allow contrast to outline clot in IJV
    - Venous collaterals around clotted IJV will be low signal or enhance depending on flow rate
    - No surrounding inflammation or edema
- MRV
  - Acute-subacute jugular vein thrombophlebitis: Clotted IJV is absent
  - Chronic jugular vein thrombosis
    - IJV on thrombosed side absent or small and irregular (partially recanalized)
    - Mature venous collaterals may be prominent

Ultrasonographic Findings

- **Noncompressible thrombus**
- Intraluminal clot appears as solid mass with midamplitude echoes
- Decreased dynamics: Decrease in venous pulsations and distension on Valsalva maneuvers
- Pulsed Doppler: **Absent flow** in affected vessel
- Spectral Doppler: Partial/complete loss of cardiac pulsatility ± respiratory phasicity
- US limitation
  - Nonvisualization of vessel cephalad to mandible and caudal to clavicle
  - Fresh clot has little inherent echogenicity
- US advantage: Noninvasive means for serial follow-up imaging during treatment of JVT

Angiographic Findings

- Retrograde catheter venography
  - High risk of dislodging infected thrombus or IJV perforation

Imaging Recommendations

- CECT/CTA in sick patient permits rapid diagnosis

DIFFERENTIAL DIAGNOSIS

Slow or Turbulent Internal Jugular Vein Flow (Pseudothrombosis)

- High signal intensity on T1 MR may be seen
- Look at all sequences; usually 1 will show flow void
  - If not, consider MRV or CTA (CT venogram) for further evaluation
- Beware nonopacified IJV on CTA, which can occur from technically early imaging post injection or more central venous obstruction

Suppurative Adenopathy

- Multiple focal cystic masses along internal jugular nodal chain

Cervical Neck Abscess

- Focal walled-off fluid collection in any neck space

Squamous Cell Carcinoma Metastatic Nodes

- Multiple focal, necrotic, and nonnecrotic masses
- Along internal jugular nodal chain

PATHOLOGY

General Features

- Etiology
  - JVT pathogenesis: 3 mechanisms for thrombosis
    - Endothelial damage from indwelling line (or IV drug use) or infection, altered blood flow, and hypercoagulable state
    - Venous stasis from compression of IJV in neck (nodes) or mediastinum (superior vena cava syndrome) can incite JVT
    - Migratory IJV thrombophlebitis (Trousseau syndrome) associated with malignancy (pancreas, lung, and ovary)
      - □ Elevated factor VIII and accelerated generation of thromboplastin cause hypercoagulable state
- **Lemierre syndrome**: IJV thrombosis associated with postanginal sepsis/necrobacillosis
  - *Fusobacterium necrophorum* = most common causal microorganism
  - Anaerobic oropharyngeal infection → **septic thrombophlebitis**
  - Septic thrombophlebitis of ipsilateral IJV
  - Subsequent septicemia, **septic embolization**, and metastatic abscesses (pulmonary septic emboli most common)
  - Uncommon complication: Pulmonary embolism
  - Young, previously healthy demographic
  - Consider possible genetic predisposing hypercoagulable state
    - Anticoagulation should be considered in high-risk patients

Microscopic Features

- JVT different from intraparenchymal hematoma
  - JVT: **Lamination** of thrombus occurs
    - No hemosiderin deposition
    - Delay in evolution of blood products (especially methemoglobin)

CLINICAL ISSUES

Presentation

- Most common signs/symptoms
  - **Acute-subacute thrombophlebitis** phase (< 10 days)
    - Swollen, hot, tender neck mass with fever
    - Radiology request may read "**rule out abscess**"
  - Chronic JVT phase
    - Palpable tender cord in peripheral neck
    - Radiology request may read "**evaluate tumor extent**"
  - Possible patient histories
    - May be spontaneous clinical event
    - Previous neck surgery, central venous catheterization, drug abuse, trauma, recent infection, hypercoagulable state, or malignancy

Demographics

- Age
  - Typically older, sicker patient population
  - **Lemierre is young healthy** population

Natural History & Prognosis

- IJV thrombophlebitis gives way to thrombosis over 7- to 14-day period with decreased soft tissue swelling
- Prognosis related to cause of IJV thrombosis
- IJV thrombosis itself is self-limited
  - Venous collaterals form to circumvent occluded IJV

Treatment

- Aggressive intravenous antibiotics given to treat any underlying infection
- Anticoagulant therapy only used in severe cases
  - Significant thromboembolism to lungs is rare

DIAGNOSTIC CHECKLIST

Consider

- Do not mistake JVT with RPS edema for RPS abscess
  - JVT with RPS edema 1 cause of **nonabscess RPS fluid**
- Do not mistake acute-subacute IJV thrombophlebitis as tumor
  - Biggest challenge comes with MR; CECT straightforward

Image Interpretation Pearls

- **Tubular** nature of JVT is key

SELECTED REFERENCES

1. Behpour-Oskooee M et al: Lemierre's syndrome with double heterozygote status in the methylenetetrahydrofolate reductase gene. World J Pediatr. 10(3):281-3, 2014
2. Galyfos G et al: Septic internal jugular vein thrombosis caused by Fusobacterium necrophorum and mediated by a broken needle. Scand J Infect Dis. 46(12):911-5, 2014
3. Ridgway JM et al: Lemierre syndrome: a pediatric case series and review of literature. Am J Otolaryngol. 31(1):38-45, 2010
4. Ascher E et al: Morbidity and mortality associated with internal jugular vein thromboses. Vasc Endovascular Surg. 39(4):335-9, 2005
5. Lin D et al: Internal jugular vein thrombosis and deep neck infection from intravenous drug use: management strategy. Laryngoscope. 114(1):56-60, 2004
6. Gong J et al: Lemierre's syndrome. Eur Radiol. 9(4):672-4, 1999
7. Provenzale JM et al: Systemic thrombosis in patients with antiphospholipid antibodies: lesion distribution and imaging findings. AJR Am J Roentgenol. 170(2):285-90, 1998

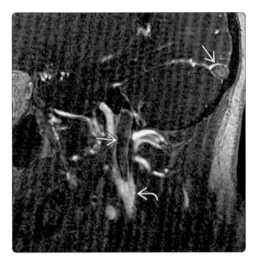

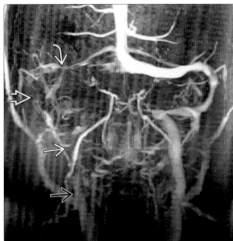

(Left) *Sagittal MRV source image in a 38-year-old woman with dural venous thrombosis with extension into the right IJV shows low-signal acute thrombus ➡ visible with patent enhancing portion of IJV noted more inferiorly ➡.* (Right) *Coronal MRV shows right transverse ➡ and sigmoid ➡ sinus thrombosis. Notice that the IJV in the nasopharyngeal carotid space is also thrombosed ➡. The IJV is patent ➡ inferiorly.*

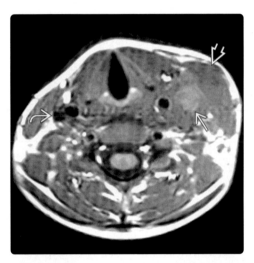

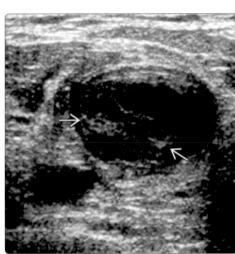

(Left) *Axial T1WI MR shows high-signal clot ➡ in swollen left IJV, indicating acute thrombophlebitis. Adjacent soft tissue planes are obscured by inflammation, including sternocleidomastoid edema ➡. Flow void is visible in the contralateral IJV ➡, although venous signal is variable on MR.* (Right) *Axial sonographic image shows mixed echogenicity within the IJV, consistent with intraluminal thrombus ➡. The IJV was also incompressible with the ultrasound probe, a key ultrasound clue to diagnosis.*

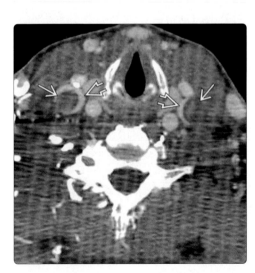

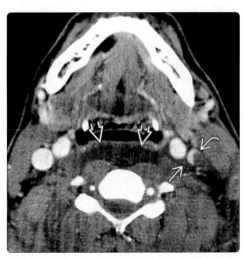

(Left) *Axial CECT in a dialysis patient with history of prior bilateral IJV catheter placement shows intraluminal low-density clot ➡ in both IJVs. Thin crescentic enhancement in the patent portion of both IJVs is visible ➡, indicating partial thrombosis.* (Right) *Axial CECT of acute left IJV thrombosis shows low-density IJV thrombus ➡. Edema is seen around the left carotid sheath ➡. Extensive retropharyngeal edema is also present without peripheral enhancement ➡. This should not be mistaken for retropharyngeal abscess*

Postpharyngitis Venous Thrombosis (Lemierre)

TERMINOLOGY

- Postanginal sepsis or septicemia, necrobacillosis
- Opportunistic infection causing septic thrombophlebitis & metastatic infection

IMAGING

- CECT: Ipsilateral tonsillar fullness, edema; abscess atypical
  - Internal jugular vein (IJV) ± tributary thrombophlebitis
  - Septic pulmonary emboli

TOP DIFFERENTIAL DIAGNOSES

- Jugular vein thrombosis
- Lung metastases

PATHOLOGY

- Usual agent is *Fusobacterium necrophorum*
  - Commensal anaerobic oral cavity bacillus
  - Many other agents possible, including *S. aureus*
- Historical features
  - Common diagnosis in preantibiotic era
  - Reemergence due to antibiotic resistance
- **Preceding pharyngitis in 90%** (less frequently after sinusitis, otitis, dental infection)

CLINICAL ISSUES

- Typical demographic: Teenagers and young adults
  - Usually healthy immunocompetent patients
- **4-12% mortality** despite aggressive treatment
- **Radiologist may be 1st to suggest diagnosis**
  - Often missed clinically & radiologically

DIAGNOSTIC CHECKLIST

- Classic imaging triad
  - **Pharyngitis + neck vein thrombosis + cavitary pulmonary nodules**
  - Other sites of metastatic infection may occur
- Making this diagnosis is key to accurate antimicrobial therapy and anticoagulation

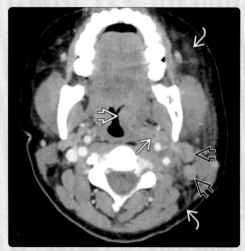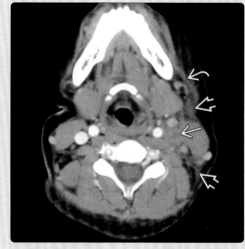

(Left) Axial CECT shows tonsil edema ⇨ and ipsilateral clot in venous tributaries ➡. Inflammatory changes of fat stranding ⬈ and reactive lymph nodes ⇨ are noted. (Right) Axial CECT shows nonopacification of the left IJV consistent with thrombosis ➡. Acute inflammation is evidenced by stranding within regional fat pads ⇨ and thickening of the platysma muscle ➡.

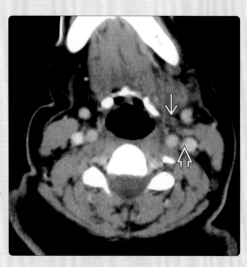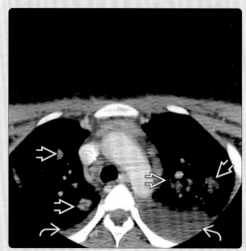

(Left) Axial CECT shows an earlier, more subtle case with few findings of neck inflammation. There is clot identified in the left facial vein ➡. Note that the IJV has suggestion of subtle, early intraluminal clot ➡. (Right) Axial CECT shows multiple pulmonary nodules ⇨ due to septic emboli. There are bilateral pleural effusions ➡. Although the differential diagnosis may include metastatic disease, the clinical picture of sepsis establishes the correct diagnosis.

Postpharyngitis Venous Thrombosis (Lemierre)

TERMINOLOGY

Synonyms

- Postanginal sepsis, necrobacillosis

Definitions

- Opportunistic infection causing septic thrombophlebitis & metastatic infection
  - Complication of recent pharyngotonsillitis or other upper respiratory infection (sinus, ear)

IMAGING

General Features

- Best diagnostic clue
  - Ipsilateral tonsillar fullness, edema; abscess atypical
  - Internal jugular vein (IJV) ± tributary thrombophlebitis
  - Multiple cavitary pulmonary nodules
- Location
  - **Tonsil** most common **primary source**
  - IJV or venous tributary thrombosis
  - **Metastatic infection** may occur anywhere, but **lungs** & joints most common

CT Findings

- CECT
  - Tonsil fullness, edema, or less commonly abscess
  - Ipsilateral vein thrombosis, usually IJV, but other small venous tributaries often involved
  - Neck inflammatory changes
    - Fat stranding, edema, retropharyngeal effusion, reactive adenopathy
  - Metastatic seeding: **Pulmonary nodules** (80%) > septic joint (15%) > elsewhere
    - Pulmonary septic emboli classically cavitary

MR Findings

- CECT best screening exam
- MR best for intracranial & orbital complications
  - Meningitis, abscess, cavernous sinus thrombosis

Imaging Recommendations

- Best imaging tool
  - CECT: Best for vein thrombosis & pulmonary nodules
  - MR: For suspected intracranial & orbital involvement
  - CT chest for pulmonary septic embolic

DIFFERENTIAL DIAGNOSIS

Jugular Vein Thrombosis

- Secondary to indwelling catheter, tumor compression/invasion, pro-thrombotic syndromes
- Other causes of septic thrombophlebitis

Lung Metastases

- Primary tumor often known
- Sepsis not part of clinical picture

PATHOLOGY

General Features

- Etiology

  - Usual agent is *Fusobacterium necrophorum* (commensal anaerobic oral cavity bacillus)
    - Pathogenic with altered host defenses
    - Pharyngitis → direct or venolymphatic spread → parapharyngeal & carotid spaces
    - **Preceding pharyngitis** in **90%** (less frequently after sinusitis, otitis, dental infection)
    - Preceding viral infection associated: EBV, CMV, H1N1
      - May induce transient immunosuppression predisposing secondary bacterial infection
  - Polymicrobial bacteremia common (33%)
- Historical features
  - Reemergence today due to antibiotic resistance

CLINICAL ISSUES

Presentation

- Most common signs/symptoms
  - Antecedent upper respiratory tract infection
    - Pharyngitis > peritonsillar abscess > otitis media
- Other signs/symptoms
  - Sore throat, fever, dyspnea, myalgias
  - Tender swollen neck
  - Sepsis ~ 7 days post resolved pharyngitis
- Clinical profile
  - Most common in 15- to 24-yr-old healthy patients
    - Rare > 40 yr old

Demographics

- Age
  - Most commonly seen in teenagers & young adults
    - Usually healthy, immunocompetent patients
  - M:F = 2:1

Natural History & Prognosis

- **High mortality**, even with treatment **(4-12%)**
- **Radiologist may be 1st to suggest diagnosis**
  - Not recognized in 1/3 of cases, or diagnosed late

Treatment

- Antimicrobial therapy
  - Broad-spectrum antibiotics may not cover *Fusobacteria*
- Anticoagulation often used but controversial
- Rare ligation of involved veins & abscess drainage

DIAGNOSTIC CHECKLIST

Image Interpretation Pearls

- Classic imaging triad: **Pharyngitis + ipsilateral neck vein thrombosis + cavitary pulmonary nodules**

Reporting Tips

- Consider this diagnosis with unexplained neck vein thrombosis to allow early treatment

SELECTED REFERENCES

1. Kim BY et al: Thrombophlebitis of the internal jugular vein (Lemierre syndrome): clinical and CT findings. Acta Radiol. 54(6):622-7, 2013
2. Hagelskjaer Kristensen L et al: Lemierre's syndrome and other disseminated Fusobacterium necrophorum infections in Denmark: a prospective epidemiological and clinical survey. Eur J Clin Microbiol Infect Dis. 27(9):779-89, 2008
3. Goyal M et al: Unusual radiological manifestations of Lemierre's syndrome: a case report. Pediatr Radiol. 25 Suppl 1:S105-6, 1995

Carotid Body Paraganglioma

TERMINOLOGY

- **Carotid body tumor**; glomus caroticum
- Chemodectoma; nonchromaffin paraganglioma

IMAGING

- Vascular mass splaying external and internal carotid arteries
- Rapid dynamic enhancement on CT and MR
- Serpentine or punctate vascular **flow voids** ("pepper") on MR, particularly in large lesions
- Hypoechoic vascular mass on duplex ultrasound
- Arteriovenous shunting on angiography

TOP DIFFERENTIAL DIAGNOSES

- Carotid space schwannoma or neurofibroma
- Carotid artery pseudoaneurysm or ectasia
- Glomus vagale paraganglioma
- Jugulodigastric lymph node

PATHOLOGY

- Multiple gene mutations (familial and sporadic)
  - Paraganglioma syndromes
  - Multiple endocrine neoplasia syndromes
  - von Hippel-Lindau syndrome
- Staging: **Shamblin grouping** (types I, II, III, IIIb)

CLINICAL ISSUES

- Slow-growing, painless, pulsatile mass
- Catecholamine-secreting carotid body paraganglioma is rare
- Related to chronic hypoxia in some patients
- Surgical excision is treatment of choice
- Preoperative embolization of larger lesions

DIAGNOSTIC CHECKLIST

- CT and MR appearances are diagnostic
- Imaging surveillance with MR for familial disease

(Left) Lateral graphic depicts a carotid body paraganglioma at the carotid bifurcation ➡, splaying the internal carotid artery (ICA) ➡ and external carotid artery (ECA) ➡. The main arterial feeder is the ascending pharyngeal artery ➡. The vagus ➡ and hypoglossal ➡ nerves are in close proximity. (Right) Axial CECT shows a classic carotid body paraganglioma ➡ with avid, fairly uniform enhancement. Notice the clear definition of the tumor sitting in the notch between the ICA ➡ and ECA ➡.

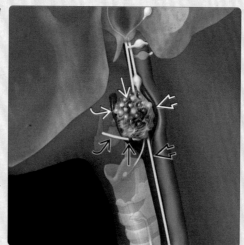
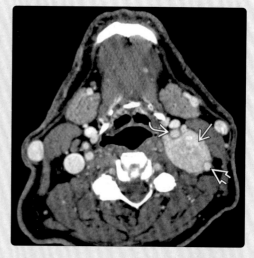

(Left) Axial T1WI MR shows a rounded mass in the left carotid space ➡, between 2 flow voids representing the ICA and ECA ➡. Small internal foci of signal void ("pepper") represent vascular flow of feeding vessels ➡. (Right) Axial T1WI C+ FS MR in the same patient shows intense enhancement of a solid mass ➡ between the splayed branches of the carotid artery ➡. The internal jugular vein is compressed at the lateral aspect of the mass ➡.

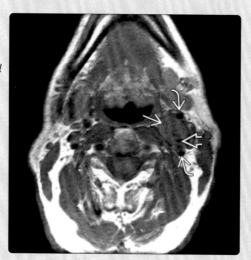
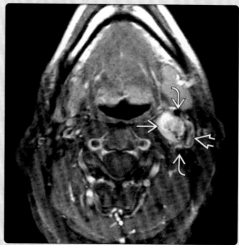

TERMINOLOGY

Abbreviations

- Carotid body paraganglioma (CBP)

Synonyms

- Carotid body tumor, glomus caroticum
- Chemodectoma, nonchromaffin paraganglioma

Definitions

- Benign vascular tumor arising in **carotid glomus** body located at carotid bifurcation

IMAGING

General Features

- Best diagnostic clue
  - Vascular mass **splaying external carotid artery (ECA) and internal carotid artery (ICA)**
- Location
  - Mass centered in **carotid bifurcation**
  - Typically unilateral; bilateral in 5-10%
- Size
  - Variable, usually 1-6 cm
- Morphology
  - Ovoid mass with broad, lobular surface contour
  - **Circumferential contact** of tumor to ICA predicts surgical classification
    - Type I: < 180°
    - Type II: > 180° and < 270°
    - Type III: > 270°

CT Findings

- NECT
  - Lobular mass splaying ECA and ICA
  - Density similar to muscles
- CECT
  - **Avidly enhancing** mass at bifurcation between ECA and ICA
  - Extends cephalad from carotid bifurcation
  - Dynamic enhancement is rapid compared to nerve sheath tumors and other masses
- CTA
  - Oblique sagittal reconstruction shows enhancing tumor in "Y" of carotid bifurcation

MR Findings

- T1WI
  - Mass signal similar to muscle
  - **Salt & pepper** appearance in larger legions
    - "Salt"
      - □ Secondary to subacute hemorrhage
      - □ **Uncommon finding** of limited diagnostic value
    - "Pepper"
      - □ Hypointense serpentine or punctate vascular channels show **flow void**
      - □ Expected finding in tumors > 2 cm
      - □ May be seen on tumor margin or within fibrous matrix of tumor parenchyma
- T2WI
  - Mildly hyperintense compared to muscle with salt & pepper heterogeneity
- T1WI C+
  - Intense, **rapid dynamic enhancement**
  - Larger high-velocity flow voids still visible

Ultrasonographic Findings

- **Hypoechoic** mass at carotid artery bifurcation
- Extensive vascularity on color Doppler images
- **Low-resistance** waveform on duplex scan

Angiographic Findings

- Splaying of ICA & ECA on early arterial images
- Prolonged, intense **tumor blush**
- Arteriovenous shunting creates "early vein" phenomenon
- **Ascending pharyngeal** artery is typical arterial feeder
- Angle of bifurcation predicts resectability
  - Splaying > 90° indicates less easily resected

Imaging Recommendations

- Best imaging tool
  - CECT or MR + angiography prior to surgery
- Protocol advice
  - Angiography useful preoperatively
    - Provide vascular **roadmap** for surgeon
    - Embolization for prophylactic hemostasis

DIFFERENTIAL DIAGNOSIS

Carotid Space Schwannoma

- Clinical
  - Sporadic or associated with neurofibromatosis type 2
- Imaging
  - Fusiform enhancing mass in carotid space
  - Does not splay carotid bifurcation

Carotid Space Neurofibroma

- Clinical
  - Sporadic or associated with neurofibromatosis type 1
- Imaging
  - Low-density, circumscribed mass in carotid space
  - Does not splay carotid bifurcation

Glomus Vagale Paraganglioma

- Clinical
  - Posterolateral high oropharyngeal mass
- Imaging
  - Mass centered higher, few cm below skull base
  - Similar high-velocity flow voids ("pepper")

Carotid Artery Pseudoaneurysm

- Clinical
  - History of trauma or dissection; pulsatile mass
- Imaging
  - Carotid artery mass with complex signal

Ectatic or Tortuous Carotid Artery

- Clinical
  - Older patient with atherosclerosis or hypertension
- Imaging
  - Enlarged, ectatic, tortuous, calcified carotid bulb

Jugulodigastric Lymph Node

- Clinical
  - Asymptomatic "pulsatile" mass

- Imaging
  - Enlarged node lateral to carotid space vessels

PATHOLOGY

General Features

- Etiology
  - Arise from carotid glomus bodies (paraganglia)
- Genetics
  - Multiple **gene mutations** identified in familial and sporadic types
    - *SDH* gene: Paraganglioma syndromes
      - □ *SDHB* subtype has higher risk of malignant transformation
    - *RET* protooncogene: Multiple endocrine neoplasia (MEN) syndromes
    - *VHL* gene: von Hippel-Lindau syndrome
- Associated abnormalities
  - **Paraganglioma syndromes**
    - Multiple head & neck paragangliomas
    - Adrenal pheochromocytoma in some subtypes
  - **MEN** type 2 syndromes
    - Medullary thyroid carcinoma
    - Adrenal pheochromocytoma
  - **von Hippel-Lindau** syndrome
    - Hemangioblastoma, endolymphatic sac tumor
    - Renal and pancreatic tumors and cysts

Staging, Grading, & Classification

- **Shamblin grouping**
  - Type I: Small tumor, easily dissected within periadvential plane
  - Type II: Larger tumor, adherent to and partially encasing carotid arteries
  - Type III: Large tumor, intimately adherent to and completely encasing carotid arteries
  - Type IIIb: Modification of original description; includes adherent tumors of smaller size

Gross Pathologic & Surgical Features

- Lobulated, reddish-purple mass with fibrous pseudocapsule

Microscopic Features

- **Chief cells** form characteristic nests (**zellballen**)
- Electromicroscopy shows neurosecretory granules

CLINICAL ISSUES

Presentation

- Most common signs/symptoms
  - Slow-growing, **painless**, **pulsatile** mass
- Other signs/symptoms
  - Vagal ± hypoglossal neuropathy in 20%
  - Catecholamine-secreting CBP is rare
    - May include paroxysmal hypertension, palpitations, flushing, and irritability
- Clinical profile
  - **Sporadic**
    - Most common presentation (80-90%)
    - Slow-growing, painless angle of mandible mass
    - Multicentric paragangliomas in 2-10%
  - **Familial**

- Variably reported between 10-50%
- Younger patients, 2nd to 4th decade
- Multiple tumors reported (25-75%)
  - **Hypoxic**/hyperplastic
    - Physiologic response due to chronic hypoxia
    - Cyanotic heart disease, COPD, high altitude

Demographics

- Age
  - Most common in **4th and 5th decade**
  - Can occur in children
- Gender
  - Overall slight male predilection
  - **Hypoxic type 8x** more common in **males**
- Epidemiology
  - Rare: 1-2 per 100,000
  - CBP is most common site for head & neck paragangliomas
  - Accounts for 70% of extraadrenal paragangliomas

Natural History & Prognosis

- Surgical outcome related to Shamblin classification
  - Cure without complication in lower group
  - Vagal and other neuropathies in higher group
- Malignant transformation uncommon (5-10%)
  - Histology is unreliable; diagnosed if metastasis seen

Treatment

- Surgical **excision** is treatment of choice
- Follow smaller lesions with "wait and scan" approach
- Preoperative **embolization** of larger lesions
  - Reduce blood loss and operation time
- Radiotherapy in poor surgical candidates

DIAGNOSTIC CHECKLIST

Consider

- CT and MR appearances are diagnostic
- Screening in familial patient group
  - Imaging surveillance with MR
    - Beginning in early adulthood
    - Avoid repeated CT due to radiation
  - Genetic screening of family members

Image Interpretation Pearls

- Arterial velocity flow voids ("pepper") are suggestive
- When CBP is suspected, look for **multiple lesions**
  - Contralateral carotid bifurcation (CBP)
  - High carotid space (glomus vagale)
  - Jugular foramen (glomus jugulare)

Reporting Tips

- Recommend surveillance in familial disease

SELECTED REFERENCES

1. Mourad M et al: Evaluating the role of embolization and carotid artery sacrifice and reconstruction in the management of carotid body tumors. Laryngoscope. ePub, 2016
2. Griauzde J et al: Imaging of vascular lesions of the head and neck. Radiol Clin North Am. 53(1):197-213, 2015
3. Arya S et al: Carotid body tumors: objective criteria to predict the Shamblin group on MR imaging. AJNR Am J Neuroradiol. 29(7):1349-54, 2008

Carotid Body Paraganglioma

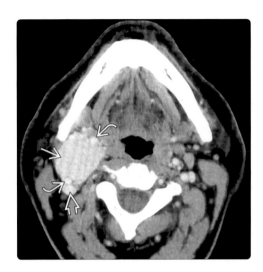
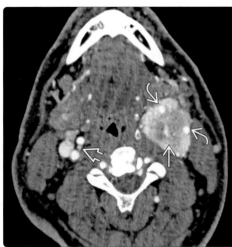

(Left) *Axial CECT shows a homogeneously enhancing mass at the right carotid bifurcation ➡ between the carotid artery branches ➡. The jugular vein is displaced posteriorly ➡.* **(Right)** *Axial CECT with early arterial phase contrast shows a heterogeneously enhancing mass at left carotid bifurcation ➡. The mass partially encases the carotid arteries ➡, indicating a Shamblin group II or III tumor. A tiny carotid bifurcation paraganglioma is seen on the right ➡. Patient likely has familial paragangliomas.*

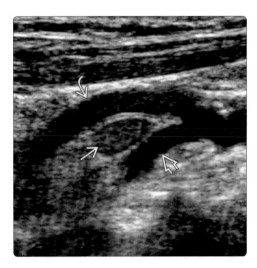
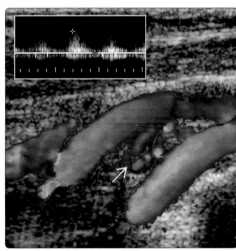

(Left) *Grayscale ultrasound shows a well-defined, hypoechoic mass ➡ located at the carotid bifurcation between the ICA ➡ and ECA ➡. This small lesion was found incidentally on CT performed for a patient with traumatic neck injuries.* **(Right)** *Duplex imaging in the same patient shows the highly vascular nature of the paraganglioma ➡ located in the crux of the bifurcation. Waveform analysis (inset) shows low-resistance characteristics.*

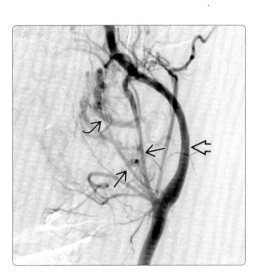
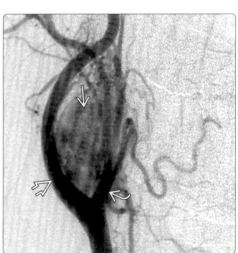

(Left) *Lateral common carotid artery catheter angiogram shows enlarged feeding vessels on the arterial phase ➡ with arteriovenous shunting resulting in an early enlarged draining vein ➡. The ICA is displaced posteriorly ➡.* **(Right)** *Lateral common carotid angiogram in the late arterial phase demonstrates intense carotid body paraganglioma blush ➡ between the EAC ➡ and IAC ➡.*

Glomus Vagale Paraganglioma

TERMINOLOGY

- Glomus vagale paraganglioma (GVP), vagal paraganglioma

IMAGING

- Avidly enhancing mass in nasopharyngeal carotid space centered ~ 2 cm below jugular foramen
  - Displaces carotid anteromedially
  - Displaces jugular vein posterolaterally
  - Displaces parapharyngeal fat anterolaterally
  - Displaces styloid process laterally
- Serpentine or punctate flow voids ("**pepper**") on MR
- Hyperintense on T2WI and STIR

TOP DIFFERENTIAL DIAGNOSES

- Carotid space schwannoma
- Carotid space neurofibroma
- Carotid space meningioma
- Carotid body paraganglioma

PATHOLOGY

- Arises from glomus bodies in nodose ganglion
- Multiple gene mutations (familial and sporadic)
  - Paraganglioma, multiple endocrine neoplasia-2, & von Hippel Lindau syndromes

CLINICAL ISSUES

- Painless, pulsatile lateral cervical mass
- Vagal neuropathy most common
- CNIX, CNXI, & CNXII neuropathies (larger tumors)
- Multicentric paragangliomas fairly common
- Surgical excision vs. observation
  - Certain loss of vagal function after surgery

DIAGNOSTIC CHECKLIST

- MR and CT appearances are diagnostic
- When GVP is suspected, look for multiple lesions
- Imaging surveillance with MR in familial disease

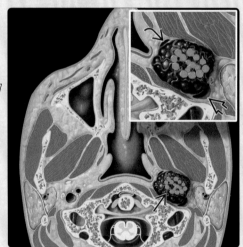
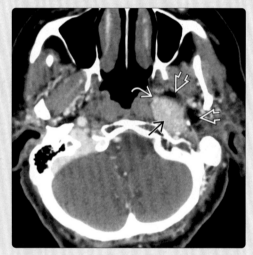

(Left) Axial graphic depicts a glomus vagale paraganglioma ➡, located in the nasopharyngeal carotid space. The mass is interposed between and displacing the internal carotid artery (ICA) ➡ and jugular vein ➡ (inset). (Right) Axial CECT shows a large, ovoid, diffusely enhancing mass adjacent to the skull base ➡, centered high in the left carotid space medial to styloid process. Note displacement of ICA ➡ anteromedially and parapharyngeal fat ➡ anterolaterally.

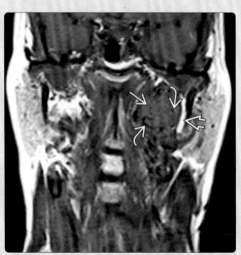
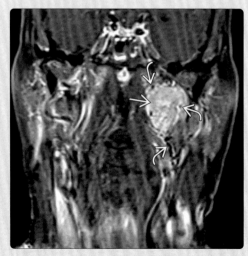

(Left) Coronal T1WI MR shows a solid, isointense mass high in left carotid space ➡. Small internal punctate and serpentine flow voids ➡ indicate the vascular nature of this lesion. Note the lateral displacement of the parapharyngeal fat ➡ adjacent to the carotid space. (Right) Coronal T1WI C+ FS MR in the same patient shows intense, homogeneous enhancement of the mass ➡, except for prominent vascular structures seen as focal flow voids ➡, despite the presence of intravascular contrast.

TERMINOLOGY

Abbreviations

- Glomus vagale paraganglioma (GVP)

Synonyms

- Vagal paraganglioma (PGL)

Definitions

- Benign vascular tumor arising in glomus bodies associated with **nodose ganglion** of vagus nerve

IMAGING

General Features

- Best diagnostic clue
  - Avidly enhancing mass high in **carotid space**
  - Between internal carotid artery (ICA) and jugular vein
- Location
  - Upper (nasopharyngeal) aspect of carotid space
    - Displaces **carotid anteromedially**
    - Displaces **jugular posterolaterally**
    - Displaces **parapharyngeal fat anterolaterally**
    - Displaces **styloid process laterally** and to lesser extent anteriorly
  - Arises from glomus bodies (paraganglia)
    - Vagus nerve nodose ganglion
    - 1-2 cm below floor of jugular foramen in nasopharyngeal carotid space
  - Large tumors may extend caudad toward carotid bifurcation or cephalad into jugular foramen
  - **Does not splay** carotid bifurcation
    - Consider multifocal PGL with carotid body tumor if splaying of carotid is seen
  - More common on right side of neck
- Size
  - Variable, usually 2-8 cm
  - Often large at diagnosis
- Morphology
  - Ovoid, lobulated, well marginated
  - Often **elongated** and **fusiform** in craniocaudal direction on coronal or sagittal images

CT Findings

- NECT
  - Soft tissue density similar to muscle
  - Permeative bone change if extension to skull base
- CECT
  - **Avidly enhancing** mass in upper carotid space
  - Bulk of tumor extracranial but may extend into jugular foramen
- CTA
  - Early enhancing mass just below skull base that displaces internal carotid anteromedially

MR Findings

- T1WI
  - Fusiform mass with signal similar to muscle
  - **Salt & pepper** appearance in larger lesions
    - "Salt": High T1 signal foci within GVP
      - □ Secondary to subacute hemorrhage
      - □ Uncommon finding, limited diagnostic value
    - "Pepper": Low T1 signal foci with GVP
      - □ Serpentine or punctate **flow voids**
      - □ Expected finding in tumors > 2 cm
- T2WI
  - Mildly hyperintense, with flow voids
- STIR
  - Moderately hyperintense, with flow voids
- T1WI C+
  - Intense, **rapid dynamic enhancement**
  - Larger high-velocity flow voids still visible
- MRA
  - Displaces ICA anteromedially

Angiographic Findings

- Anteromedial **displacement of ICA** without widening of carotid bifurcation
- Tortuous dilated feeding vessels
- Ascending pharyngeal artery is main arterial feeder
- Early, prolonged, intense **tumor blush**
- Arteriovenous shunting creates "early vein" phenomenon
- Angiographic goals
  - Search for multicentric tumors
  - Provide vascular **road map** for surgeon
  - Evaluate cervicocerebral circulation in case sacrifice of major vessel necessary
  - **Embolization** for prophylactic hemostasis

Nuclear Medicine Findings

- Somatostatin receptor scintigraphy (In-111 octreotide)
  - Confirmation of indeterminate lesions
  - Detection of multiple lesions

Imaging Recommendations

- Best imaging tool
  - Contrast-enhanced MR or CT
- Protocol advice
  - Field of view to cover from from skull base to carotid bifurcation on MR and CT

DIFFERENTIAL DIAGNOSIS

Carotid Space Schwannoma

- Clinical: Lateral neck mass
- Imaging: Fusiform mass, uniform enhancement
  - Cystic changes in larger lesions

Carotid Space Neurofibroma

- Clinical: Sporadic or associated with neurofibromatosis type 1
- Imaging: Fusiform mass, irregular if plexiform
  - Low-density T2 and STIR hyperintensity
  - Variable enhancement, less conspicuous on CT

Carotid Space Meningioma

- Clinical: Lower cranial neuropathies
- Imaging: Extension of jugular foramen mass

Carotid Body Paraganglioma

- Clinical: Pulsatile neck mass
- Imaging: Splaying of internal and external carotid

Carotid Artery Pseudoaneurysm

- Clinical: History of trauma or dissection

- Imaging: Carotid artery mass with complex signal

Jugular Vein Thrombosis

- Clinical: Tender mass, history of injury
- Imaging: Nonenhancing thrombus with edema

PATHOLOGY

General Features

- Etiology
  - Arises from **glomus bodies** (paraganglia)
    - Located in nodose ganglion of vagus nerve
    - Composed of chemoreceptor cells derived from neuroectoderm of primitive **neural crest**
- Genetics
  - Multiple **gene mutations** identified in familial and sporadic types
  - **PGL** syndromes
    - SDH genes; *SDHD* and *SDHB* subtypes
  - Multiple endocrine neoplasia (**MEN-2**) syndromes
    - *RET* protooncogene (10q11.2)
  - von Hippel-Lindau (**VHL**) syndrome
    - *VHL* gene (3p25-26)
- Associated abnormalities
  - Multiple head & neck PGL
  - Adrenal pheochromocytomas (PGL & MEN-2)
  - Medullary thyroid carcinoma (MEN-2)
  - Hemangioblastomas, endolymphatic sac tumors, renal and pancreatic tumors and cysts (VHL)

Staging, Grading, & Classification

- AJCC exclusion; use NCI-SEER summary staging
  - Peripheral/autonomic nerves of neck schema
  - SEER code C47.0

Gross Pathologic & Surgical Features

- Lobulated, reddish-purple mass with fibrous pseudocapsule

Microscopic Features

- Chief cells form characteristic nests (**zellballen**)
- Surrounding fibromuscular stroma
- Electromicroscopy shows neurosecretory granules

CLINICAL ISSUES

Presentation

- Most common signs/symptoms
  - **Painless, pulsatile** lateral cervical mass (85%)
    - Near angle of jaw, between cranial base and hyoid
    - Mobile in lateral directions
- Other signs/symptoms
  - Lower cranial nerve symptoms in 20-50%
  - **Vagal neuropathy** by far most common
    - Vocal cord paralysis with hoarseness
    - Variable, reported up to 50%
  - CNIX, CNXI, CNXII injury (10-20%)
    - Particularly larger tumors
  - Horner syndrome uncommon (5%)
  - Pulsatile tinnitus
  - Rarely hormonally active
- Clinical profile
  - **Sporadic**

- Majority of patients (50-80%)
- Multicentric PGLs in 5-20%
  - **Familial**
    - Positive family history common (20-50%)
    - Multicentric PGLs in 50-90%
    - Younger age at presentation

Demographics

- Age
  - Most common in **4th and 5th** decade
  - Younger presentation in familial cases
- Gender
  - **Female** predominance, M:F ~ 2:1
- Epidemiology
  - **Least common** of head & neck PGLs
    - Carotid body > jugulare/tympanicum > vagale
    - Vagale: **5%** of head & neck PGLs
  - Annual incidence ~ 1:100,000

Natural History & Prognosis

- Progressive vagal dysfunction as tumor grows
- Natural morbidity of cranial neuropathies may be less than that following surgery, particularly in older patients
- Malignant tumors uncommon (5-10%)

Treatment

- Options, risks, complications
  - **Surgical excision** vs. **observation**
    - Vagal neuropathy generally indicates surgery
    - Larger or growing tumors may indicate surgery
    - Older patients may not tolerate surgical morbidity
  - Surgical morbidity is unavoidable
    - **100% loss of vagal function**
    - Adjunctive procedures mitigate vagal dysfunction
    - Variable risk to CNIX, CNXI, & CNXII
  - Radiotherapy for lesion control in poor surgical candidates
- Bilateral GVP
  - Requires special consideration
  - Important to **preserve at least unilateral** vagus function

DIAGNOSTIC CHECKLIST

Consider

- MR and CT appearances are diagnostic
- Screening in familial patient group
  - Beginning in early adulthood

Image Interpretation Pearls

- MR arterial flow voids ("**pepper**") are highly suggestive
- When GVP is suspected, look for **multiple lesions**
  - Contralateral carotid space (GVP)
  - Carotid bifurcations (carotid body PGL)
  - Temporal bones (glomus jugulare/tympanicum)

Reporting Tips

- Recommend **surveillance** with MR in familial disease

SELECTED REFERENCES

1. Moore MG et al: Head and neck paragangliomas: an update on evaluation and management. Otolaryngol Head Neck Surg. 154(4):597-605, 2016

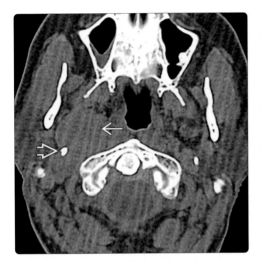
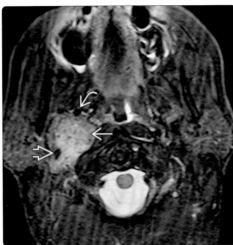

(Left) Axial NECT shows an isodense mass centered in high right carotid space ➡. The styloid process is displaced laterally ⮕. Although the styloid is generally described as located anterior to the carotid space, vagale tumors tend to displace the styloid laterally rather than anteriorly. (Right) Axial T2WI STIR MR in the same patient shows mass is moderately hyperintense ➡. The ICA is displaced anteromedially ↗, and the styloid process is displaced laterally ➡.

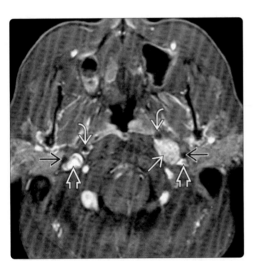
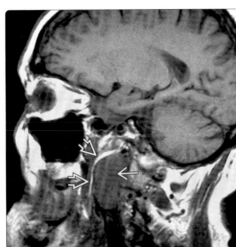

(Left) Axial T1WI C+ FS MR shows a relatively small vagale tumor on the left ➡. Note the positions of the ICAs ↗, jugular veins ⮕, and styloid processes ➡ on the affected and unaffected sides. (Right) Sagittal T1WI MR shows a well-circumscribed, intermediate-intensity mass ➡. Note the fusiform shape oriented along the long axis of the carotid space. On sagittal imaging, the parapharyngeal fat can be seen displaced anteriorly ⮕.

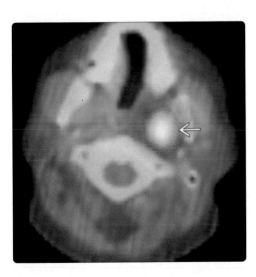
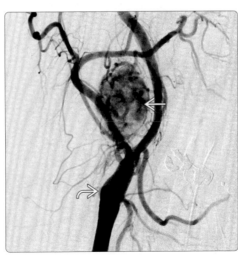

(Left) Axial SPECT/CT at 24 hours following In-111 octreotide injection shows a large region of activity in the high left carotid space ➡. This radionuclide targets the somatostatin receptors that are expressed by paragangliomas. (Right) Catheter angiogram in the arterial phase of common carotid injection shows an early, intense tumor blush ➡ with multiple prominent feeding vessels. The mass is above the common carotid artery bifurcation ↗, which is not splayed.

Carotid Space Schwannoma

TERMINOLOGY

- **Benign tumor** of **Schwann cells** that wrap around cranial nerve in **carotid space** (CS)
- Nerve of origin: **9-12 cranial nerves**; CNX (vagus nerve) most common

IMAGING

- Fusiform, enhancing CS mass
  - Larger schwannoma: Intramural cystic change
  - **MR: No high-velocity flow voids** characteristic
- Displacement pattern is characteristic
  - Nasopharyngeal CS schwannoma: Displaces PPS anteriorly and styloid process anterolaterally
  - Oropharyngeal CS schwannoma: Displaces PPS fat anteriorly and posterior belly of digastric laterally
  - Infrahyoid neck CS schwannoma: Displaces to contralateral neck, common carotid artery anteromedially, & posterior cervical space posterolaterally

TOP DIFFERENTIAL DIAGNOSES

- Carotid body paraganglioma
- Glomus vagale paraganglioma
- Carotid space neurofibroma
- Carotid space meningioma
- Vascular lesions (pseudoaneurysm or thrombosis)

PATHOLOGY

- Vagal schwannoma more common than other CN origins

CLINICAL ISSUES

- Typical presentation
  - Asymptomatic palpable mass
  - May present with dysphagia, IJV occlusion, Horner syndrome, vocal cord paralysis, sleep apnea, sore throat
- Age range: 20-60 years (average: 45)
- **Suprahyoid** CS schwannoma > > infrahyoid
- Preferred treatment: Gross total resection without sacrifice of nerve

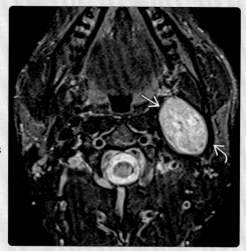
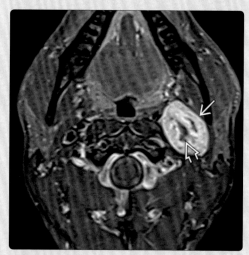

(Left) *Axial T2WI FS MR shows a circumscribed, hyperintense carotid space mass* ➡ *with lateral displacement of the posterior belly of the digastric muscle* ➡. *The lack of flow voids help differentiate this schwannoma from a paraganglioma.* (Right) *Axial T1WI C+ FS MR in the same patient reveals enhancement of the CS mass* ➡ *with regions of cystic change* ➡, *typical of a large schwannoma. CS schwannomas may arise from CNIX-XII or the cervical sympathetic chain, but most commonly arise from the vagus nerve (CNX).*

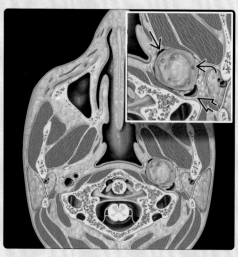
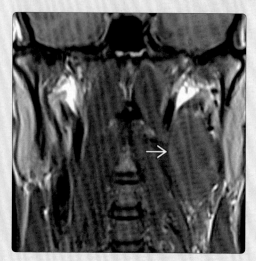

(Left) *Axial graphic depicts a typical nasopharyngeal carotid space schwannoma. Tumor is seen between the anteromedial internal carotid artery* ➡ *and the posterolateral internal jugular vein* ➡. *Carotid space schwannomas are typically fusiform, enhancing masses and may contain cystic, nonenhancing areas* ➡. (Right) *Coronal T1WI MR shows a carotid space fusiform mass* ➡ *predominantly isointense to muscle. The lack of flow voids is characteristic of schwannoma.*

TERMINOLOGY

Synonyms

- Neuroma, neurilemmoma

Definitions

- Benign tumor of Schwann cells that wrap around cranial nerve in carotid space (CS)

IMAGING

General Features

- Best diagnostic clue
  - **Fusiform**, enhancing CS mass (CT or MR) **without** flow voids (MR)
- Location
  - Carotid space from nasopharynx above to aortic arch below
- Size
  - Lesions are usually large when clinically detected
  - Range: 2-8 cm
- Morphology
  - Ovoid to fusiform
  - Tumor margins are smooth, sharply circumscribed
- Suprahyoid neck CS schwannoma displacement pattern is characteristic
  - **Nasopharyngeal CS schwannoma**: Displaces **parapharyngeal space (PPS) anteriorly** and styloid process anterolaterally
    - Internal carotid artery (ICA) is usually bowed over anteromedial surface
    - Internal jugular vein (IJV) is often posterolateral and commonly effaced
  - In oropharyngeal CS schwannoma: Displaces PPS fat anteriorly and posterior belly digastric muscle laterally
- Infrahyoid neck CS schwannoma displacement pattern: Thyroid-trachea displaced to contralateral neck, common carotid artery anteromedially and posterior cervical space posterolaterally
- **Lack of high-velocity flow voids** within tumor allows correct identification of nerve sheath tumor

CT Findings

- NECT
  - Well-circumscribed CS soft tissue density mass
  - Mass density similar to adjacent neck muscles
- CECT
  - Uniform enhancement is rule on CECT
    - Minority are low density even with enhancement
  - Focal areas of absent enhancement seen on CECT if **intramural cystic** change present
- CTA: ICA bowed over anterior surface of schwannoma

MR Findings

- T1WI
  - Variable T1 signal ranging from low to high
    - **No high-velocity flow voids**, even when large
- T2WI
  - Tumor hyperintense compared with muscle
  - **Intramural cysts**, if present, are high-signal foci within tumor
- T1WI C+

- Dense, homogeneous enhancement is typical
  - Intratumoral nonenhancing cysts often present in larger lesions
- MRA: Anteromedial displacement of ICA, without visible arterial supply
  - CS schwannoma itself not visualized on MRA
- MRV: Jugular vein may be flattened or occluded

Angiographic Findings

- Angiography is usually unnecessary unless tumor histopathology in doubt
- Scattered contrast "puddles" typical of schwannoma
- No dominant feeding arteries seen
- No arteriovenous shunting or vascular encasement

Imaging Recommendations

- Best imaging tool
  - Enhanced MR best starting exam

DIFFERENTIAL DIAGNOSIS

Carotid Body Paraganglioma

- Mass center: Nestled in common carotid artery bifurcation
- Splays apart external and internal carotid arteries
- MR: High-velocity flow voids in > 2-cm tumor

Glomus Vagale Paraganglioma

- Mass center: Nasopharyngeal CS, ~ 2 cm below skull base
- MR: High-velocity flow voids in > 2-cm tumor
- CT: Permeative-erosive bone margins

Carotid Space Neurofibroma

- Mass center: Carotid space
- CECT: Low-density, well-circumscribed CS mass
- MR: Cannot differentiate from vagal schwannoma
- Look for NF1 association (50%)

Carotid Space Meningioma

- Mass location: Emanates from jugular foramen above into nasopharyngeal CS
- Jugular foramen bony margins on bone CT: Permeative-sclerotic to hyperostotic
- T1WI C+ MR: Centrifugal spread pattern with dural "tails"

Carotid Artery Pseudoaneurysm in Neck

- Ovoid outpouching of carotid artery
- CECT: Lumen connected to carotid artery lumen
- MR: Complex, ovoid mass in carotid space

Internal Jugular Vein Thrombosis

- History of IJV instrumentation usually present
- Tubular lesion with central IJV filling defect on enhanced imaging

Sympathetic Chain Schwannoma

- Mass center: Posterior to carotid artery and IJV
- Displacement pattern: Pushes both carotid artery and IJV anteriorly
- MR: No high-velocity flow voids

PATHOLOGY

General Features

- Etiology

○ Arises from Schwann cells wrapping around cranial nerve in carotid space of extracranial H&N
○ Nerve of origin
  – Nasopharyngeal carotid space: **9-12 cranial nerves** possible
  – Oropharyngeal carotid space to aortic arch: **Vagus nerve**
  – Vagal schwannoma more common than other cranial nerve origins
• Associated abnormalities
  ○ Neurofibromatosis type 2

Gross Pathologic & Surgical Features

• White-tan, smooth, encapsulated, sausage-shaped mass

Microscopic Features

• Spindle cells with elongated nuclei
  ○ Alternating areas of organized, compact cells (Antoni A) and loosely arranged, relatively acellular tissue (Antoni B)
  ○ Both cell types present in all tumors
• Differentiated neoplastic Schwann cells
  ○ Malignant transformation is exceedingly rare
  ○ Melanotic malignant schwannomas have been described as distinct entity
    – May have intrinsic T1 hyperintensity as diagnostic feature
• Immunochemistry
  ○ Strong, diffuse, immunostaining for S100 protein
    – S100 protein: Neural-crest marker antigen present in supporting cell of nervous system

CLINICAL ISSUES

Presentation

• Most common signs/symptoms
  ○ Asymptomatic palpable mass
    – Nasopharyngeal and oropharyngeal CS schwannoma: Posterolateral pharyngeal wall mass
    – Cervical CS schwannoma: Anterolateral neck mass
  ○ Other signs/symptoms
    – Large suprahyoid schwannoma: May cause dysphagia or IJV occlusion
    – Horner syndrome
    – Vocal cord paralysis (hoarseness)
    – Sleep apnea
    – Sore throat
• Clinical profile
  ○ Healthy 45-year-old man with asymptomatic suprahyoid lateral retropharyngeal or infrahyoid lateral neck mass

Demographics

• Age
  ○ Range: 20-60 years
  ○ Average at presentation: 45 years
• Gender
  ○ Male predominance
• Epidemiology
  ○ Rare tumor of extracranial H&N
  ○ Suprahyoid CS schwannoma > > infrahyoid CS schwannoma

Natural History & Prognosis

• Delay in diagnosis is frequent due to nonspecific symptoms
• Slow but persistent tumor growth until airway compromise or cosmetic issues supervene
• Vagus nerve preservation is not always possible at surgery
  ○ If vagus nerve resection required, partial vagal neuropathy is present even if successful reconnection completed

Treatment

• Gross total resection without sacrifice of vagus nerve is treatment of choice
  ○ Enucleation of tumor with CNX preservation possible in most cases
  ○ Infrequently, nerve resection occurs at time of tumor removal
    – End-to-end anastomosis of vagus nerve used if short segment removed
    – Nerve graft interposition used if long segment vagus nerve is removed
  ○ Severe transient bradycardia may occur during removal
  ○ Postoperative symptoms in ~ 20% of patients
• Radiation therapy considered for patients who are poor surgical candidates

DIAGNOSTIC CHECKLIST

Consider

• If schwannoma localized to suprahyoid CS, look at jugular foramen (JF) for evidence of involvement
  ○ If JF involved, imaging findings are characteristic
    – Bone CT: Expanded jugular foramen with sharp, scalloped margins
    – T1WI C+ MR: Enhancing ovoid jugular foramen mass ± intramural cystic change
• Vascular schwannoma may mimic paraganglioma

Image Interpretation Pearls

• Fusiform, sharply circumscribed CS mass **without** high-velocity flow voids = schwannoma/neurofibroma
• Carotid and jugular vessel displacement often predicts likely nerve of origin of CS schwannoma
  ○ Vagal nerve schwannomas typically splay CCA or ICA away from IJV
  ○ Sympathetic chain schwannomas displace vessels together (typically anteriorly) and do not separate vein and arteries

SELECTED REFERENCES

1. Shinohara Y et al: Neurilemmoma of the Vagus Nerve in the Poststyloid Parapharyngeal Space. J Clin Diagn Res. 10(1):ZD17-9, 2016
2. Cavallaro G et al: A literature review on surgery for cervical vagal schwannomas. World J Surg Oncol. 13:130, 2015
3. Yafit D et al: An algorithm for treating extracranial head and neck schwannomas. Eur Arch Otorhinolaryngol. 272(8):2035-8, 2015
4. Kitazume Y et al: Diffusion-weighted magnetic resonance neurography for parapharyngeal schwannomas: preoperative determination of the originating nerves. J Comput Assist Tomogr. 38(6):930-5, 2014
5. Langerman A et al: Tumors of the cervical sympathetic chain—diagnosis and management. Head Neck. 35(7):930-3, 2013
6. Saito DM et al: Parapharyngeal space schwannomas: preoperative imaging determination of the nerve of origin. Arch Otolaryngol Head Neck Surg. 133(7):662-7, 2007
7. Som PM et al: Lesions of the parapharyngeal space. Role of MR imaging. Otolaryngol Clin North Am. 28(3):515-42, 1995

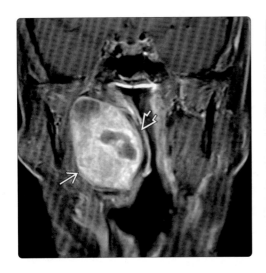

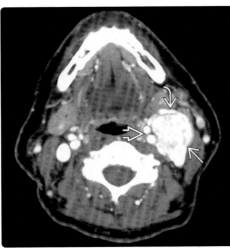

(Left) Coronal T1C+ FS MR shows an enhancing carotid space ➡ mass with cystic change, commonly seen in schwannomas. Medial displacement of the internal carotid artery is typical ➡. (Right) Axial CECT shows an avidly enhancing, suprahyoid carotid space mass ➡. The internal and external carotid arteries ➡ are displaced medially, typical of schwannoma. Anterior displacement of the internal jugular vein ➡ is unusual. When schwannomas are hypervascular, they may mimic a paraganglioma.

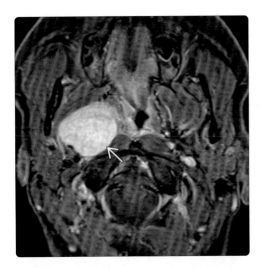

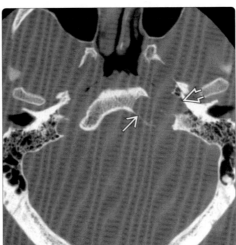

(Left) Axial T1WI C+ FS MR shows a large, homogeneously enhancing CS mass ➡, typical of a carotid space schwannoma. In this location, the schwannoma may arise from CNIX-XII. Vagal schwannomas are the most common. (Right) Axial bone CT in a patient with a carotid space mass shows a scalloped appearance within the clivus ➡, typical of a schwannoma. Nasopharyngeal CS schwannoma remodels the adjacent skull base ➡. In contrast, a paraganglioma would result in permeative bone changes.

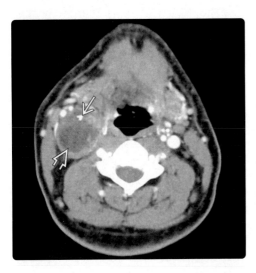

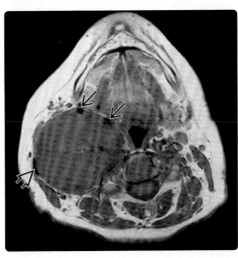

(Left) Axial CECT reveals a mostly cystic schwannoma in the carotid space just above the hyoid bone. Intramural cystic change ➡ is a common finding in larger schwannomas. Note the rare calcification ➡ seen in the anterior tumor wall. (Right) Axial T1WI MR shows a large CS mass with anteromedial displacement of the carotid vessels ➡ and posterolateral displacement of the internal jugular vein ➡. This enlarging neck mass was found to be a malignant peripheral nerve sheath tumor at resection.

Sympathetic Schwannoma

TERMINOLOGY

- Benign, slow-growing tumor of Schwann cells investing cervical sympathetic chain

IMAGING

- Most common appearance
  - Fusiform enhancing carotid space (CS) mass that displaces both carotid artery & jugular vein anteriorly
- Tumor location
  - Posterior to CS vessels (sympathetic chain lies posterior in CS)
- CECT or enhanced MR findings
  - Ovoid to fusiform enhancing mass in posterior CS
  - Small lesion: Homogeneous enhancement
  - Large lesion: Intratumoral (intramural) nonenhancing cysts may be seen
- CECT often 1st exam for neck mass

TOP DIFFERENTIAL DIAGNOSES

- Carotid space schwannoma
- Glomus vagale paraganglioma
- Carotid body paraganglioma
- Nodal SCCa in retropharyngeal space
- Carotid space neurofibroma

PATHOLOGY

- Solitary, well-encapsulated tumor arising from peripheral nerve
- Arises from cervical sympathetic chain Schwann cell sheath
- Associated with neurofibromatosis type 2 (multiple schwannomas, meningiomas, & ependymomas)

CLINICAL ISSUES

- Asymptomatic, palpable neck mass
- **Horner syndrome**, headache

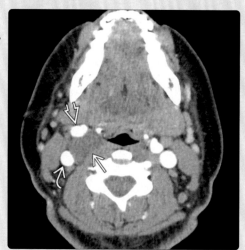
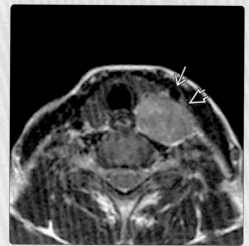

(Left) Axial CECT image shows ovoid mass ➡ posteromedial within carotid space (CS). Note the carotid artery on anterior surface ➡ with jugular vein along lateral surface of mass ➡. Minimal enhancement is atypical of schwannoma and may mimic neurofibroma. (Right) Axial T2WI MR shows a heterogeneous intermediate signal ovoid soft tissue mass displacing common carotid artery ➡ anteriorly. Internal jugular vein is displaced with carotid artery ➡. Compression of jugular vein may make it difficult to identify.

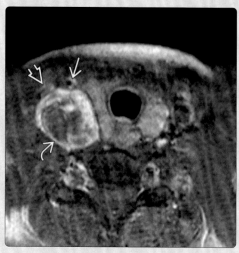
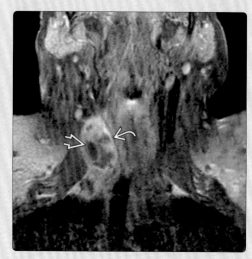

(Left) Axial T1WI C+ FS MR reveals an ovoid mass in posterior infrahyoid CS ➡. The sympathetic schwannoma displaces both the internal jugular vein ➡ and common carotid artery ➡ anteriorly. The simultaneous displacement of both CS vessels suggests the diagnosis of sympathetic schwannoma. (Right) Coronal T1WI C+ FS MR demonstrates a sympathetic schwannoma in carotid space. The tumor is heterogeneously enhancing mass ➡ posterior to CS. Intramural cystic change ➡ is common in large schwannomas.

Sympathetic Schwannoma

TERMINOLOGY

Synonyms

- Cervical sympathetic chain schwannoma, sympathetic neurilemmoma or neuroma

Definitions

- Benign, slow-growing tumor of **Schwann cells** investing **cervical sympathetic chain**

IMAGING

General Features

- Best diagnostic clue
  - Fusiform enhancing carotid space mass that displaces both carotid artery & internal jugular vein anteriorly
- Location
  - Arises from cervical sympathetic chain in posterior carotid space (CS)
    - Sympathetic chain normally lies posterior to both CS vessels
- Morphology
  - Ovoid, occasionally fusiform lesion

Imaging Recommendations

- Best imaging tool
  - CECT often 1st exam for neck mass

CT Findings

- CECT
  - Ovoid to fusiform mass displacing both carotid artery & internal jugular vein anteriorly
  - Smaller lesions may enhance uniformly
  - Intratumor (intramural) **cystic change** in larger lesions with nonenhancing areas

MR Findings

- T2WI
  - Posterior CS mass with intermediate signal intensity, higher than muscle
  - Intratumor cysts, if present, are hyperintense & sharply marginated
- T1WI C+
  - Homogeneous enhancement in small lesions
  - Cystic change in larger lesions demonstrated as nonenhancing areas

DIFFERENTIAL DIAGNOSIS

Carotid Space Schwannoma

- Typical and more common vagal schwannoma will separate carotid artery and jugular vein

Glomus Vagale Paraganglioma

- Heterogeneous enhancement with flow voids in larger lesions

Carotid Body Paraganglioma

- Classic location at carotid bifurcation
- Splays internal and external carotid

Nodal SCCa in Retropharyngeal Space

- Lateral retropharyngeal space (RPS) nodal disease may mimic sympathetic schwannoma

Neurofibroma, Carotid Space

- Low density on CECT

PATHOLOGY

General Features

- Etiology
  - Arise from Schwann cells of CS sympathetic plexus
- Associated abnormalities
  - Neurofibromatosis type 2 (multiple schwannomas, meningiomas, & ependymomas)

Staging, Grading, & Classification

- Benign tumor with rare malignant transformation

Gross Pathologic & Surgical Features

- Solitary, well-encapsulated tumor arising from peripheral nerve

Microscopic Features

- Spindle-shaped cells with elongated nuclei
  - Organized, compact cellular regions (Antoni A) and loose, relatively acellular tissue (Antoni B)
  - Both areas invariably present in tumors

CLINICAL ISSUES

Presentation

- Most common signs/symptoms
  - Asymptomatic, palpable neck mass
- Other signs/symptoms
  - **Horner syndrome**, headache

Demographics

- Epidemiology
  - Very rare tumor of carotid space
  - Much less common than vagal schwannoma

Treatment

- Surgical excision is curative
  - Postoperative Horner syndrome is common

DIAGNOSTIC CHECKLIST

Image Interpretation Pearls

- Evaluation of position of carotid artery and jugular vein is critical
  - Should both be displaced anteriorly
- Lack of **flow voids** in CS mass on MR suggests schwannoma or neurofibroma
  - If flow voids, paraganglioma most likely diagnosis

SELECTED REFERENCES

1. Navaie M et al: Diagnostic approach, treatment, and outcomes of cervical sympathetic chain schwannomas: a global narrative review. Otolaryngol Head Neck Surg. 151(6):899-908, 2014
2. Anil G et al: Imaging characteristics of schwannoma of the cervical sympathetic chain: a review of 12 cases. AJNR Am J Neuroradiol. 31(8):1408-12, 2010
3. Tomita T et al: Diagnosis and management of cervical sympathetic chain schwannoma: a review of 9 cases. Acta Otolaryngol. 129(3):324-9, 2009
4. Saito DM et al: Parapharyngeal space schwannomas: preoperative imaging determination of the nerve of origin. Arch Otolaryngol Head Neck Surg. 133(7):662-7, 2007
5. Bocciolini C et al: Schwannoma of cervical sympathetic chain: assessment and management. Acta Otorhinolaryngol Ital. 25(3):191-4, 2005

Carotid Space Neurofibroma

TERMINOLOGY

- Benign nerve sheath tumor in carotid space, arising from vagus nerve, sympathetic chain, or hypoglossal nerve

IMAGING

- Ovoid or fusiform mass centered in carotid space with mild or patchy enhancement
- Interposed between carotid and jugular
  - Displaces carotid anteromedially
  - Displaces jugular posterolaterally
- Infrahyoid lesions typically posterior to vessels
  - Displaces carotid and jugular anterolaterally
- Hypodense and poorly enhancing on CT
- Hyperintense with target sign on STIR or T2WI MR
- Homogeneous or patchy mild enhancement on MR

TOP DIFFERENTIAL DIAGNOSES

- Glomus vagale paraganglioma
- Carotid body paraganglioma
- Carotid space schwannoma
- Carotid artery pseudoaneurysm

PATHOLOGY

- Benign spindle cell neoplasm
- World Health Organization (WHO) grade 1 tumors

CLINICAL ISSUES

- Asymptomatic solitary or multiple neck masses
- Lower cranial nerve palsies in larger lesions
- Solitary NF: Isolated soft tissue neck mass
- Plexiform NF: Multinodular "bag of worms"
- 50% associated with NF1, 50% solitary
- Surgical removal of symptomatic isolated lesions
- Excision much more difficult for plexiform lesions

DIAGNOSTIC CHECKLIST

- Most conspicuous on STIR/fat-suppressed T2WI
- Often less conspicuous post contrast enhancement

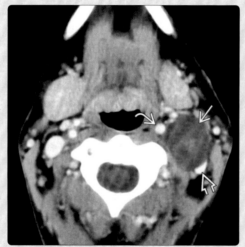
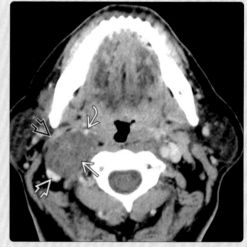

(Left) Axial CECT demonstrates a low-density mass with faint internal enhancement ➡ located in the left carotid space. The internal carotid artery (ICA) ➡ is displaced anteromedially, while the internal jugular vein (IJV) ➡ is displaced posterolaterally. (Right) Axial CECT shows a carotid space neurofibroma ➡ with density similar to the cervical spinal cord and minimal enhancement. Note the ICA pushed anteromedially ➡, the IJV posterolaterally ➡, and the posterior belly digastric muscle laterally ➡.

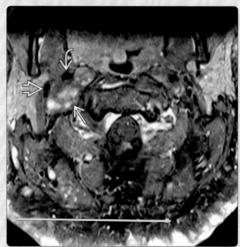
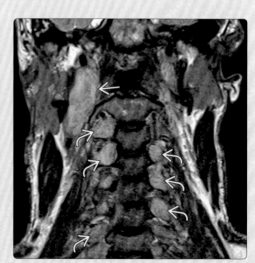

(Left) Axial T1 C+ FS MR in a patient with NF1 demonstrates an ovoid carotid space mass ➡ with patchy enhancement. The lesion displaces the ICA anteriorly ➡ and flattens and displaces the jugular vein anterolaterally ➡. (Right) Coronal T2 MR in the same patient demonstrates the typical elongated, oval contour and heterogeneous T2 hyperintensity of a vagal neurofibroma ➡. Stigmata of NF1 with multiple cervical nerve sheath tumors are evident ➡.

TERMINOLOGY

Abbreviations
- Neurofibroma (NF), neurofibromatosis type 1 (NF1)

Definitions
- **Benign nerve sheath tumor** in carotid space
- Arises from **vagus nerve** or **sympathetic** chain; superior lesions may arise from **hypoglossal** nerve

IMAGING

General Features
- Best diagnostic clue
  - **Ovoid** or **fusiform** mass centered in carotid space
- Location
  - Interposed **between carotid and jugular**
    - Displaces carotid **anteromedially**
    - Displaces jugular **posterolaterally**
  - Infrahyoid lesions typically **posterior** to vessels
    - Displaces carotid and jugular **anterolaterally**
- Size
  - Sporadic NF: Typically 2-5 cm in diameter
  - Plexiform NF1: Confluent masses up to 10 cm
- Morphology
  - Sporadic NF: **Ovoid or fusiform** shape
  - Plexiform NF: Poorly circumscribed, **multilobulated**

CT Findings
- CECT
  - Hypodense, **poorly enhancing** mass within carotid space

MR Findings
- T1WI
  - Isointense, relatively homogeneous mass
- T2WI
  - Very **hyperintense**, darker centrally (**target sign**)
- T1WI C+
  - Homogeneous or patchy **mild enhancement**

Imaging Recommendations
- Best imaging tool
  - Contrast-enhanced fat-suppressed MR
- Protocol advice
  - Most conspicuous on STIR or fat-suppressed T2

DIFFERENTIAL DIAGNOSIS

Glomus Vagale Paraganglioma
- Clinical: Asymptomatic or vagal neuropathy
- Imaging: Avidly enhancing mass with flow voids

Carotid Body Paraganglioma
- Clinical: Asymptomatic or pulsatile neck mass
- Imaging: Splaying of internal and external carotid

Carotid Space Schwannoma
- Clinical: Lateral neck mass
- Imaging: Fusiform, uniform enhancement

Carotid Artery Pseudoaneurysm
- Clinical: History of trauma or dissection
- Imaging: Carotid artery mass with complex signal

PATHOLOGY

General Features
- Etiology
  - Benign **spindle cell** neoplasm
- Genetics
  - Chromosome 17q11.2 in NF1 phenotype

Staging, Grading, & Classification
- World Health Organization (WHO) **grade 1** tumors

Gross Pathologic & Surgical Features
- Solitary NF: Ovoid, **circumscribed** nodule
- Plexiform NF: Infiltrative **"bag of worms"** texture

Microscopic Features
- Monotonous spindle cell proliferation
- "Wavy" or "buckled" nuclear shapes

CLINICAL ISSUES

Presentation
- Most common signs/symptoms
  - Asymptomatic **solitary** or **multiple** neck masses
- Other signs/symptoms
  - Lower cranial nerve **palsies** in larger lesions
- Clinical profile
  - Solitary NF: Isolated soft tissue neck mass
  - Plexiform NF: Multinodular **"bag of worms"** with associated NF1 stigmata

Demographics
- Age
  - Variable, average of 35 years
- Gender
  - **Female** predominance in carotid space lesions
- Epidemiology
  - 50% associated with NF1, 50% solitary

Natural History & Prognosis
- 5-10% **malignant degeneration** in NF1

Treatment
- Surgical removal of symptomatic isolated lesions
- Excision much more difficult for plexiform lesions

DIAGNOSTIC CHECKLIST

Consider
- Assess patient for other **signs of NF1**

Image Interpretation Pearls
- Most conspicuous on **STIR** or fat-suppressed **T2WI**

Reporting Tips
- Consider dedicated imaging of spine, brain, & orbits

SELECTED REFERENCES

1. Latham K et al: Neurofibromatosis of the head and neck: classification and surgical management. Plast Reconstr Surg. 135(3):845-55, 2015
2. Marocchio LS et al: Sporadic and multiple neurofibromas in the head and neck region: a retrospective study of 33 years. Clin Oral Investig. 11(2):165-9, 2007
3. Pang KP et al: Parapharyngeal space tumours: an 18 year review. J Laryngol Otol. 116(3):170-5, 2002

Carotid Space Meningioma

IMAGING

- Enhancing carotid space (CS) mass with **connection to jugular foramen (JF)** above
  - Enhancing, thickened dura around JF
  - ICA pushed anteriorly by CS mass
- Bone CT: JF margins show **permeative-sclerotic** or **hyperostotic** bone changes
- Protocol: Skull base focused MR with fat-saturated T1 C+
  - Bone CT of skull base to evaluate bones around JF

TOP DIFFERENTIAL DIAGNOSES

- Carotid body or glomus vagale paraganglioma
- Carotid space schwannoma
- Internal carotid artery (ICA) pseudoaneurysm

PATHOLOGY

- Carotid space meningioma originates from arachnoid cap cells in JF
- JF meningioma herniates inferiorly into nasopharyngeal CS

- Typically WHO grade I (> 90%)

CLINICAL ISSUES

- Patients 40-60 years; M:F = 1:2
- Gradual symptom progression (slow-growing, benign tumor)
- Treatment: Surgical resection ± radiation therapy
- Surgical resection limited by degree of ICA & lower cranial nerve involvement
- Radiotherapy for incomplete resection, extensive skull base invasion, or high morbidity patient

DIAGNOSTIC CHECKLIST

- If nasopharyngeal CS mass is associated with JF component, bony margins of JF may predict histology
- CS meningioma: **Permeative-sclerotic** or **hyperostotic**
- CS extension of glomus jugulare paraganglioma: **Permeative-destructive** JF margins
- CS schwannoma: **Smooth JF enlargement**

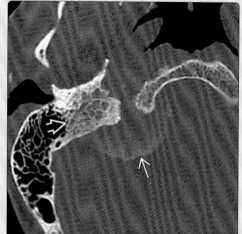
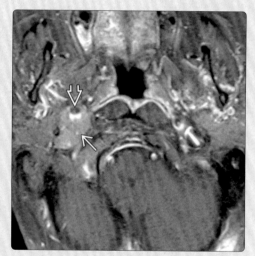

(Left) *Axial bone CT shows the typical mixed permeative-sclerotic pattern ➦ seen in meningiomas of the skull base and jugular foramen. Note the partially calcified ➥ intracranial portion of the tumor.* (Right) *Axial T1WI C+ FS MR shows the inferior extension of a jugular foramen meningioma into the carotid space ➥. Note the anterior location of the carotid artery ➦. These meningiomas originate from arachnoid cap cells within the jugular foramen. As the meningioma enlarges, it may herniate into the carotid space.*

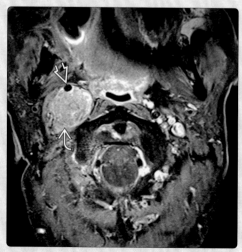
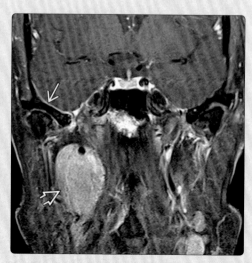

(Left) *Axial T1WI C+ FS MR shows a large enhancing right carotid space mass ➥ displacing the carotid artery anteriorly ➦. Note the lack of flow voids, which can help differentiate this meningioma from the more common paraganglioma.* (Right) *Coronal T1 C+ FS MR in the same patient shows the large carotid space meningioma ➥, which originated in the jugular foramen. Note the associated intracranial dural tail ➥, commonly seen in patients who have intracranial extension of a skull base meningioma.*

TERMINOLOGY

Abbreviations

- Carotid space meningioma (CSM)

Definitions

- Meningioma of nasopharyngeal carotid space (CS) emanating from jugular foramen (JF) above

IMAGING

General Features

- Best diagnostic clue
  - Connection to JF above with JF margins showing **permeative-sclerotic** or **hyperostotic** bone changes
  - Enhancing CS mass with lack of flow voids
- Location: Nasopharyngeal CS
- Morphology: Dumbbell-shaped (JF ↔ CS)

CT Findings

- NECT
  - Meningioma may be high density from psammomatous calcifications
- CECT
  - Moderately enhancing CS mass
  - ICA pushed anteriorly by CS mass
- Bone CT
  - JF margins: **Permeative-sclerotic** or **hyperostotic** bone changes

MR Findings

- T1WI
  - Muscle intensity ovoid JF-CS mass
  - Larger lesions may display occasional high-velocity flow voids
- T2WI: Low to intermediate intensity 2° to calcification
- T2* GRE: Susceptibility effect (blooming) possible
- T1WI C+: Mild to moderate enhancement
  - Enhancing, thickened dura around JF
  - May see dural tail
- MRA: ICA draped anteriorly over CSM

Angiographic Findings

- Prolonged capillary tumor blush without arteriovenous shunting or "early" vein appearance

Imaging Recommendations

- Protocol advice
  - Skull base focused MR with fat-saturated T1 C+ axial & coronal sequences
  - Bone CT of skull base to evaluate bones around JF

DIFFERENTIAL DIAGNOSIS

Carotid Body Paraganglioma

- Mass splays ECA & ICA at carotid bifurcation
- T1 MR shows parenchymal high-velocity flow voids

Glomus Vagale Paraganglioma

- Enhancing CS mass centered ~ 2 cm below skull base
- T1 MR shows parenchymal high-velocity flow voids

Carotid Space Schwannoma

- Well-circumscribed enhancing fusiform CS mass ± intramural cysts

ICA Pseudoaneurysm

- Narrowed ICA lumen with focal luminal outpouching

ICA Dissection

- CTA shows linear intraluminal intimal flap or crescent

PATHOLOGY

General Features

- Etiology
  - CSM originates from arachnoid cap cells in JF
  - JF meningioma herniates inferiorly into nasopharyngeal CS

Microscopic Features

- Clustered whorls & lobules of psammomatous calcifications & meningothelial cells

CLINICAL ISSUES

Presentation

- Most common signs/symptoms
  - Lateral posterior pharyngeal mass
  - Other signs/symptoms
    - Complex lower cranial neuropathy (CNIX-XII)

Demographics

- Age: Patients 40-60 years
- Gender: M:F = 1:2
- Epidemiology: Rare manifestation of rare tumor location (JF meningioma)

Natural History & Prognosis

- Gradual symptom progression (slow-growing tumor)
- Surgical treatment often complicated by increased cranial neuropathy ± stroke

Treatment

- Surgical resection limited by degree of ICA & lower cranial nerve involvement
- Radiotherapy for incomplete resection, extensive skull base invasion, or high morbidity patient
- Preoperative embolization may ↓ vascularity of tumor

DIAGNOSTIC CHECKLIST

Consider

- If nasopharyngeal CS mass is associated with JF component, bony margins of JF may predict histology
  - CS meningioma: Permeative-sclerotic or hyperostotic JF margins
  - CS extension of glomus jugulare paraganglioma: Permeative-destructive JF margins
  - CS schwannoma: Smooth JF enlargement

SELECTED REFERENCES

1. Thomas AJ et al: Nonparaganglioma jugular foramen tumors. Otolaryngol Clin North Am. 48(2):343-59, 2015
2. Battaglia P et al: Endoscopic endonasal transpterygoid transmaxillary approach to the infratemporal and upper parapharyngeal tumors. Otolaryngol Head Neck Surg. 150(4):696-702, 2014

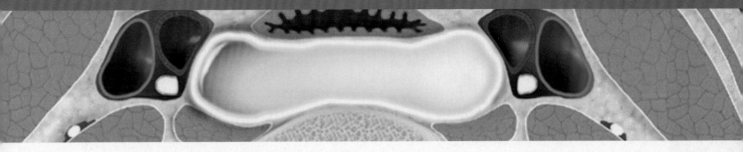

Summary Thoughts: Retropharyngeal Space

The retropharyngeal space (RPS) spans the length of the neck from the skull base to the mediastinum. As its name indicates, it lies posterior to the pharynx. More inferiorly in the neck, it lies posterior to the esophagus. It is located anterior to the cervical and upper thoracic spine and the prevertebral muscles. Anatomically, an additional fascia divides the RPS into 2 components: (1) An anterior true RPS and (2) a posterior danger space (DS). With imaging, it is rare to be able to delineate a lesion as residing in only 1 of these 2 spaces, so for most purposes the 2 are considered as 1 RPS.

The RPS contains only **medial** and **lateral** RPS **lymph nodes** and **fat**. This results in a very short differential diagnosis for pathology in this space, primarily a tumor or infection affecting the nodes. While this makes diagnosing easier, the RPS is actually an imaging and clinical "blind spot," with RPS nodes being inaccessible to direct observation or physical examination. Additionally, nonnecrotic nodes often appear isodense to prevertebral muscles on CECT and frequently lie far lateral in the RPS and medial to the internal carotid arteries. Therefore, it is critical that the radiologist methodically searches the RPS for adenopathy, particularly in patients with head and neck (H&N) malignancies.

After nodal disease, the next most common pathology is a frequently seen but poorly understood process known as retropharyngeal edema. While this process does not require treatment, it is a clue to other pathology in the H&N. Most importantly, it may pose a diagnostic challenge as it mimics the appearance of retropharyngeal abscess, which often requires surgical intervention.

Imaging Approaches and Indications

The presence of fat in the RPS makes this space readily identifiable on CT (due to its low density) and MR (due to its intrinsic T1 and T2 hyperintensity). As CECT is the imaging technique of choice for evaluation of H&N infections, it is often the initial modality for detection of RPS pathology. Imaging of any RPS process must cover from the skull base to the mediastinum because of the potential for craniocaudal and mediastinal spread of disease. Intravenous contrast is important to determine enhancement characteristics of an RPS collection that suggests an abscess, and for evaluation of nodal disease and nodal necrosis. It is also important for the evaluation of other neck structures, which may be responsible for RPS infection or edema. Review of the cervical spine for discitis-osteomyelitis as a potential infectious source is important during analysis of the neck CT or MR images.

MR allows excellent delineation of RPS contours but is less often used in evaluation of infection, except for discitis-osteomyelitis. MR is more sensitive than CT for detecting retropharyngeal adenopathy, which is important for the staging of many H&N tumors (particularly nasopharyngeal carcinoma).

Imaging Anatomy

The anterior margin of the RPS is delineated by the posterior pharyngeal wall and inferiorly by the posterior aspect of the esophagus. These structures are enveloped by a middle layer of deep cervical fascia (ML-DCF), also known as the **buccopharyngeal** and **visceral fascia**, respectively. The posterior margin of the RPS is defined by the **prevertebral fascia**, which is a deep layer of deep cervical fascia (DL-DCF).

Superiorly, the ML-DCF and DL-DCF insert on the central skull base, forming the superior boundary of the RPS. Inferiorly, the posterior margin of the RPS is the prevertebral fascia and blends with the anterior longitudinal ligament of the upper thoracic spine.

A second layer of prevertebral fascia (DL-DCF), known as the **alar fascia**, extends in a coronal orientation and divides the RPS into 2 compartments: The more anterior true RPS and the posterior DS. At approximately the T3 level, the alar fascia merges with the visceral fascia on the posterior aspect of the esophagus to form the inferior boundary of the true RPS. The DS extends more inferiorly in the posterior mediastinum and typically reaches the diaphragm. It is usually impossible on imaging to delineate 2 distinct spaces, so for all intents and purposes the RPS and DS are considered 1 RPS. It is important, however, to remember the potential for posterior mediastinal extension of an RPS process to the inferior aspect of the thorax.

The lateral limits of the RPS are defined by sagittally oriented slips of the DL-DCF that are called alar fascia or cloison sagittale (sagittal partition). This fascia separates the RPS contents from the carotid sheath, and generally appears less resistant to the spread of pathology within and from the RPS than the prevertebral and visceral fascia. As a consequence, RPS edema frequently extends laterally to the carotid sheaths. Similarly, RPS and DS often appear to communicate freely inferiorly despite the alar fascia.

Pseudolesions of the RPS include medial deviation of the carotid arteries and thyroid gland enlargement due to goiter or malignancy. Both the carotid arteries and thyroid tissue may present in a near midline location in the RPS, which likely occurs from laxity or disruption of this lateral alar fascia. Medial deviation of the carotid arteries is important to report, since iatrogenic injury can occur during transoral robotic surgery if this anatomic variant is not recognized.

Approaches to Imaging Issues of the Retropharyngeal Space

The answer to the question, "What imaging findings define a **RPS mass**?" varies slightly depending on the level in the neck. Throughout most of the neck, and particularly the infrahyoid neck, an RPS mass is clearly evident as a lesion posterior to the pharynx &/or esophagus and anterior to the prevertebral muscles and spine. The pharynx and the esophagus may be deviated anteriorly, and there may by flattening of prevertebral muscles against the spine. These findings help to clarify an RPS location.

In the suprahyoid neck, and particularly just below the skull base, the retropharyngeal space contains little fat and frequently appears to be more of a **potential space** with the prevertebral muscles and the pharynx closely opposed. Retropharyngeal nodes are located in the far lateral aspect of the RPS, immediately medial to the internal carotid arteries (ICAs). With a very thin RPS and prominent bellies of the prevertebral muscles, these RPS nodes appear to lie **lateral** to the prevertebral muscles. This is most evident in children, where large nonnecrotic RPS nodes, in association with prominent adenoidal tissue, are normal findings.

Nasopharyngeal or oropharyngeal infection, such as tonsillitis or pharyngitis, will result in reactive enlargement of these already prominent nodes in children. The presence of nonenhancing foci within RPS nodes in a child with infectious

Differential Diagnosis of Retropharyngeal Space

Pseudolesion	Congenital	Inflammatory	Infectious	Vascular	Treatment Related	Benign Tumor	Malignant Tumor
Tortuous carotid artery	Venous malformation	Reactive or inflammatory RPS node (suprahyoid neck)	Cellulitis/ phlegmon from adjacent infection	Edema associated with IJV thrombosis	Edema from radiation	Lipoma	Direct invasion by SCCa
Thyroid enlargement (goiter or malignancy)	Lymphatic malformation	RPS edema from longus colli tendonitis	RPS abscess from adjacent infection	Edema from Kawasaki disease	Edema from neck dissection	Schwannoma	RPS nodal spread of systemic metastasis or NHL
	Ectopic parathyroid adenoma (infrahyoid)		Suppurative adenopathy (suprahyoid neck)		Edema, seroma or CSF leak from spine surgery	Neurofibroma	Primary or invasive sarcoma

IJV = internal jugular vein; NPC = nasopharyngeal carcinoma; RPS = retropharyngeal space; SCCa = squamous cell carcinoma.

symptoms indicates **suppuration**. This is sometimes described as an intranodal abscess but does not typically require surgical intervention.

In adults, normal RPS nodes are less frequently found, and when seen are typically ≤ 5 mm. **Reactive enlargement** of RPS nodes may be found in adults with pharyngeal infection, although reactive nodal enlargement to 1 cm is unusual. RPS reactive adenopathy is distinctly less common in adults, which in part reflects the decreased frequency of pharyngeal infections in adults compared to children.

Enlarged RPS nodes in an adult > 8 mm are concerning for the possibility of **metastatic disease**. This is a 1st-order lymphatic drainage site for nasopharyngeal carcinoma, where unilateral or bilateral RPS metastases are designated as N1 disease. Other H&N tumors also drain to RPS nodes, either primarily or secondarily. Oropharyngeal squamous cell carcinoma (SCCa), sinonasal malignancies, middle ear malignancies, and thyroid carcinoma drain directly to RPS nodes. Other malignancies, such as posterior wall hypopharyngeal SCCa, invade the RPS and then drain through the lymphatic system to the RPS nodes. Non-Hodgkin lymphoma in the H&N frequently involves RPS nodes and may become particularly large without necrosis. Since RPS nodes are not detectable on clinical examination, it is important for imagers to pay particular attention to this area. One effective method is carefully searching along the medial aspect of the suprahyoid ICAs.

The differential diagnosis for a **well-defined, ovoid mass** in the suprahyoid RPS includes **carotid space (CS)** lesions that mimic RPS nodes by their location medial to the ICA. Schwannoma of the sympathetic chain typically lies medial to the ICA and vagal paragangliomas may be medial or posterior to the ICA. The absence of other adenopathy in the neck, or the clear demonstration of location in the CS, favors 1 of these 2 other entities.

If an RPS abnormality is **diffuse** rather than a focal mass, the diagnostic approach is quite different and can be defined as collections or masses. **Collections** have fluid density (CT) or intensity (MR) and tend to enlarge the entire RPS into either a "bow-tie" or rectangular contour. Whenever a fluid-distended RPS is found, the first consideration is to exclude an **RPS abscess**, which is typically rim-enhancing rectangular

distension of the RPS. More frequently evident in neck studies, however, is **RPS edema**, which is nonenhancing and tends to result in less marked RPS enlargement, with a lower volume rectangular contour. Once this diagnosis is suspected, the neck must be searched for an infectious source (typically of pharyngeal origin in children and spinal origin in adults), a vascular source (IJV thrombosis), inflammation (longus colli tendonitis), or evidence of recent treatment (spine or neck surgery, radiation).

Diffuse masses of the RPS may be lipomatous lesions, such as lipoma or liposarcoma, with fat density/signal on CT or MR imaging, other rare sarcomas, or congenital lesions, such as venous or lymphatic malformations, which share imaging characteristics with such lesions elsewhere in the H&N. These lesions are typically transspatial involving adjacent H&N spaces, as are plexiform neurofibromas, which are characteristic of NF1.

Clinical Implications

Small lesions of the RPS are typically **not** evident on clinical examination. It is only when lesions become significantly enlarged that bulging of a posterior pharyngeal wall is evident. It cannot be emphasized enough that the radiologist must consider the possibility of RPS metastatic nodal disease in **all H&N cancer patients** and must methodically search along the medial aspect of the cervical ICA. Nonnecrotic RPS nodes are more difficult to discern on CECT than MR, so vigilance is key.

Toxic patients with H&N infections, such as pharyngitis or tonsillitis, may be imaged to exclude the development of a, RPS abscess. This is a difficult clinical diagnosis because physical examination may not be fruitful. Thus, clinicians must rely largely on a high degree of clinical suspicion. The radiologist must exclude RPS abscess, or, if 1 is found, must delineate the entire craniocaudal extent and specifically exclude mediastinal involvement. Large abscesses may result in airway compromise, though it is rare that a patient presents with airway symptoms secondary to an RPS mass.

Selected References

1. Hoang JK et al: Multiplanar CT and MRI of collections in the retropharyngeal space: is it an abscess? AJR Am J Roentgenol. 196(4):W426-32, 2011

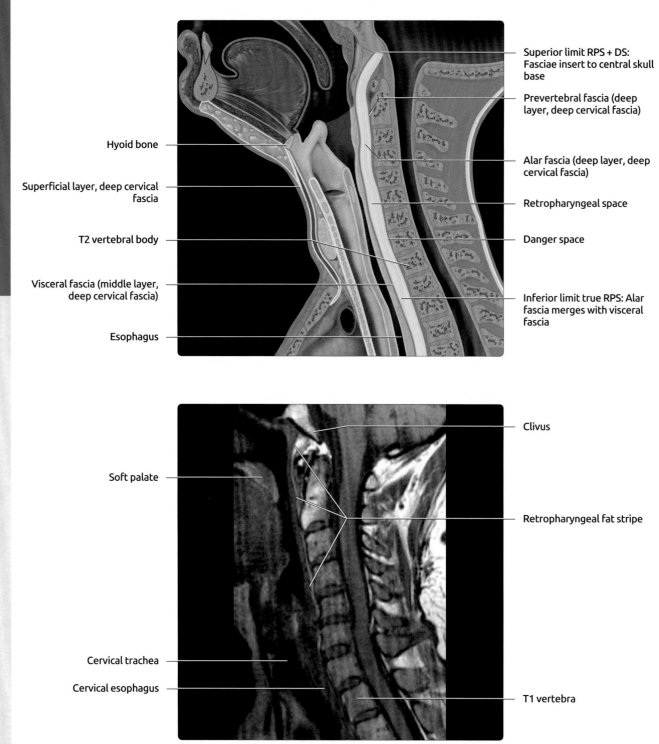

Hyoid bone

Superficial layer, deep cervical fascia

T2 vertebral body

Visceral fascia (middle layer, deep cervical fascia)

Esophagus

Superior limit RPS + DS: Fasciae insert to central skull base

Prevertebral fascia (deep layer, deep cervical fascia)

Alar fascia (deep layer, deep cervical fascia)

Retropharyngeal space

Danger space

Inferior limit true RPS: Alar fascia merges with visceral fascia

Soft palate

Cervical trachea

Cervical esophagus

Clivus

Retropharyngeal fat stripe

T1 vertebra

(Top) *Sagittal graphic shows the deep cervical fascia (DCF) layers, which determine and delineate the contours of the retropharyngeal space (RPS). The anterior contour of the RPS is defined by the visceral fascia, the middle layer DCF, which separates the RPS from the pharyngeal mucosal space of SHN and visceral space of the IHN. The posterior contour is formed by the prevertebral fascia (deep layer DCF). The alar fascia (also deep layer DCF) anatomically defines an anterior true RPS and more posterior danger space (DS), although this delineation is not typically evident at imaging. Inferiorly, the alar fascia blends with the visceral fascia at approximately T3, while superiorly the middle and deep layers of the DCF insert to the central skull base.* (Bottom) *Sagittal T1 MR shows thin, hyperintense signal corresponding to normal fat within the retropharyngeal space. Contents include this thin fat stripe and the retropharyngeal lymph nodes in the lateral suprahyoid neck. It can be considered as a potential space that is most visible when distended by disease.*

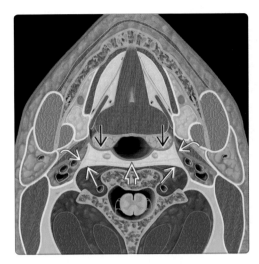 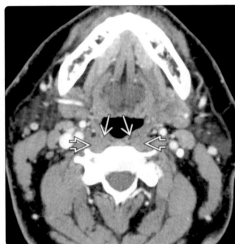

(Left) *Axial graphic at level of oropharynx illustrates predominantly fat-filled RPS. The anterior contour is delineated by middle layer DCF ⊡ and the posterior contour by prevertebral fascia (deep layer DCF) ➡. Alar fascia forms lateral margins ➡ and divider ➡ of RPS into anterior true RPS and posterior danger space.* (Right) *Axial CECT shows the typical appearance of RPS in a suprahyoid neck as a thin, low-density fat stripe ➡ anterior to prevertebral muscles ➡.*

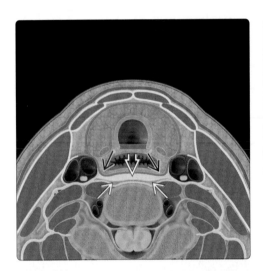 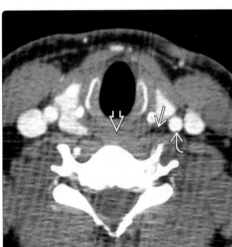

(Left) *Axial graphic at level of thyroid gland shows infrahyoid continuation of fat-filled RPS, now posterior to esophagus and again delineated anteriorly by visceral fascia (middle layer DCF) ⊡. Posterior DS ➡ separates true RPS ➡ from prevertebral muscles and cervical vertebrae.* (Right) *Axial CECT shows RPS as an almost imperceptible fat stripe anterior to PVS and posterior to hypopharynx ➡. Laterally, RPS has a triangular contour ➡ immediately medial to internal carotid artery ➡.*

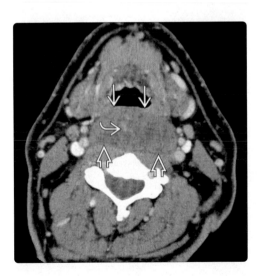 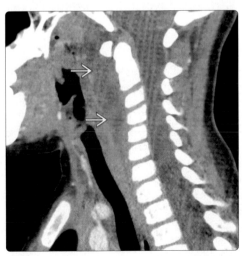

(Left) *Axial CECT shows a rare primary sarcoma of the RPS. Small areas of vascular enhancement are noted ➡. Note comparatively lower density relative to the pharynx anteriorly ➡ and prevertebral muscles ➡ posteriorly that helps correctly localize this mass.* (Right) *Midline sagittal CECT MPR demonstrates a RPS abscess ➡ in a child. Infected & noninfected fluid collections are the most common source of RPS lesions. Infections are most often due to suppurative nodal disease in children and spread of spinal infection in adults.*

Reactive Adenopathy of Retropharyngeal Space

TERMINOLOGY

- Benign enlargement of nodes in response to antigen
- Lateral retropharyngeal space (RPS) nodes known as nodes of Rouvière

IMAGING

- Retropharyngeal nodes found from skull base to hyoid bone
- May be difficult to detect on CT if no mass effect as isodense to prevertebral muscles
  - CECT aids in detection of RPS node & intranodal suppurative change
- Often elongate in craniocaudal direction so may appear round on axial CT
  - Coronal/sagittal reformats show oval shape
- If large or associated with inflammatory change, may deform pharyngeal contour, narrowing airway
- RPS nodes found from skull base to hyoid bone

TOP DIFFERENTIAL DIAGNOSES

- Suppurative RPS node
- Squamous cell carcinoma (SCCa) metastasis to RPS node
- Non-SCCa metastasis to RPS node
- Ectatic internal carotid artery

PATHOLOGY

- Most often in response to infectious agent

CLINICAL ISSUES

- Reactive RPS nodes common in children because of oral exposure to antigens

DIAGNOSTIC CHECKLIST

- Look for primary infection: Pharyngitis, tonsillitis
- Look for suppurative change/early abscess formation
- Consider metastatic disease in patients > 30 yr

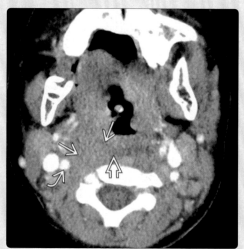
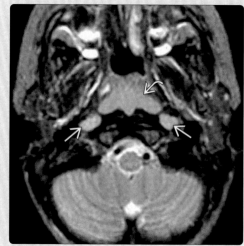

(Left) Axial CECT in a child with pharyngitis illustrates the difficulty in finding isodense RPS nodes on CT. Subtle mass effect is noted ➡ from the large right RPS node displacing ICA ➡. Low-density linear retropharyngeal edema ➡ delineates medial margin of reactive node. (Right) Axial T2 MR in a 2 year old shows prominent homogeneous retropharyngeal nodes ➡ and adenoid tissue ➡. Retropharyngeal nodes are much more evident on MR than CT; however, this is a normal finding in young children.

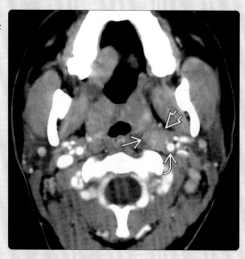
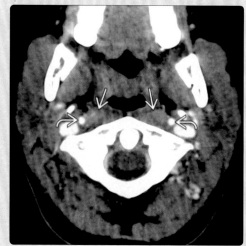

(Left) Axial CECT in a teenage patient with pharyngitis shows large reactive left retropharyngeal node ➡ medial to ICA ➡ and lateral to prevertebral muscle. There is no suppurative change or necrosis, but subtle linear intranodal enhancement is seen ➡. (Right) Axial CECT in a young woman with clinical and radiographic evidence of tonsillitis reveals bilateral, mildly enhancing homogeneous nodes ➡ medial to ICAs ➡. Subtle linear intranodal enhancement is evident on the right side.

TERMINOLOGY

Abbreviations

- Retropharyngeal space (**RPS**) nodes

Synonyms

- Reactive lymphoid hyperplasia, nodal hyperplasia; lateral RPS nodes: Nodes of Rouvière

Definitions

- Benign enlargement of nodes in response to antigen

IMAGING

General Features

- Best diagnostic clue
  - Prominent, mildly enlarged node in RPS; evidence of pharyngeal inflammation as source
- Location
  - RPS nodes found from skull base to hyoid bone; lateral nodes located medial to high cervical internal carotid arteries (ICA)
- Size
  - Uncommonly > 1 cm without suppurative change
- Morphology
  - Well-defined node medial to ICA, in RPS

CT Findings

- CECT
  - Variable enhancement, usually mild
  - Tend to be isodense to muscle so difficult to detect
  - Often elongate in craniocaudal direction so may appear round on axial CT; coronal/sagittal reformats show oval shape

MR Findings

- T1WI
  - Homogeneous low to intermediate signal
- T2WI
  - Homogeneous, intermediate signal intensity
- T1WI C+
  - Variable, usually mild enhancement

Ultrasonographic Findings

- RPS nodes not readily visible by ultrasound

Nuclear Medicine Findings

- PET
  - Mild FDG uptake may be seen

Imaging Recommendations

- Best imaging tool
  - CECT is study of choice for H&N infection
- Protocol advice
  - Contrast helps to detect node & suppurative change

DIFFERENTIAL DIAGNOSIS

Suppurative RPS Node

- Low-density RPS node with peripheral enhancement

Squamous Cell Carcinoma Metastasis to RPS Node

- Nasopharynx, posterior pharynx wall, sinus primary

Nonsquamous Cell Carcinoma Metastasis to RPS Node

- Differentiated thyroid carcinoma, sinus malignancies

Ectatic Internal Carotid Artery

- Common: ICA bows into RPS

PATHOLOGY

General Features

- Etiology
  - Most often in response to infectious agent
    - Often H&N source, such as pharyngitis, tonsillitis; generalized systemic viral infection
- Associated abnormalities
  - If large or associated with inflammatory change may deform pharyngeal contour, narrowing airway
  - When associated with extensive RPS inflammation may see narrowed adjacent ICA

Gross Pathologic & Surgical Features

- Retropharyngeal nodes rarely excised

Microscopic Features

- Histologic features of nodal hyperplasia: Follicular, sinus, diffuse or mixed patterns described

CLINICAL ISSUES

Presentation

- Most common signs/symptoms
  - Symptoms from primary infection source; nodes usually not palpable or disabling
- Clinical profile
  - Young patient with pharyngeal or systemic viral infection

Demographics

- Age
  - Usually < 30 yr
- Epidemiology
  - Common in children from oral exposure to antigens

Natural History & Prognosis

- Node may suppurate (form pus collection)
- Suppurative node can rupture, forming RPS abscess

Treatment

- Primary infectious source should be treated
- Patient monitored clinically for progression of symptoms and reimaged if concern for abscess or malignancy

DIAGNOSTIC CHECKLIST

Consider

- Look for primary infection: Pharyngitis, tonsillitis
- Look for suppurative change/early abscess formation
- Consider metastatic disease in patients > 30 yr
  - Particularly if no clinical signs of infection
  - Look for pharyngeal, thyroid, or sinus primary

SELECTED REFERENCES

1. Chong VF et al: Radiology of the retropharyngeal space. Clin Radiol. 55(10):740-8, 2000

Suppurative Adenopathy of Retropharyngeal Space

TERMINOLOGY

- Retropharyngeal adenitis, intranodal abscess
- Formation of pus in RPS node draining H&N infection

IMAGING

- CECT is 1st-line tool for evaluation of H&N infection
  - CECT best demonstrates suppuration
- RPS node lies medial to internal carotid artery
- Low density within enlarged node
- RPS cellulitis ± internal carotid narrowing
  - Vasospasm more common in kids, usually self-limited
- Node may show prominent peripheral enhancement
- Lateral RPS, does not cross midline like abscess
- MR: Restricted diffusion in suppurative node

TOP DIFFERENTIAL DIAGNOSES

- RPS reactive adenopathy
- RPS abscess
- RPS nodal squamous cell carcinoma

- RPS schwannoma
- RPS edema

PATHOLOGY

- H&N infection seeds RPS nodes
- Node draining infection enlarges = reactive node
- If untreated, progresses to suppurative node
- If still untreated, ruptures = RPS abscess

CLINICAL ISSUES

- More common in children and teens
- Sore throat, odynophagia, fever, neck pain

DIAGNOSTIC CHECKLIST

- Evaluate retropharynx for suppurative change with any H&N infection
- RPS nodes nonpalpable, can rapidly progress to abscess, sepsis, & airway compromise
- Consider metastatic disease if no inflammatory change or clinical infection, or if patient > 40 yr

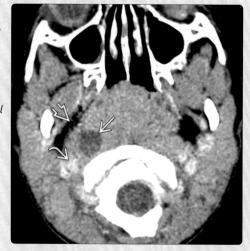
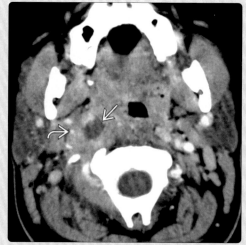

(Left) Axial CECT in a young child demonstrates a well-defined, low-density lesion ➡ anteromedial to right internal carotid artery ➡. This represents pus within right retropharyngeal lymph node and is associated with effacement of parapharyngeal fat ➡. (Right) Axial CECT in a different patient shows central low density within enlarged retropharyngeal space (RPS) node ➡. Extensive inflammatory change involves right carotid sheath and is associated with narrowing of distal cervical internal carotid artery ➡.

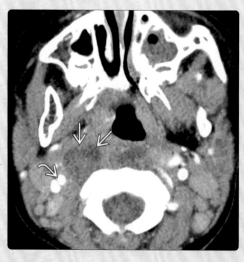
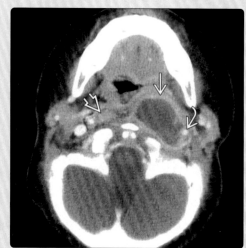

(Left) Axial CECT reveals lateral displacement of right internal carotid artery (ICA) ➡ by a heterogeneous rounded mass ➡. Retropharyngeal node is enlarged, and low density indicates early suppurative change. (Right) Axial CECT demonstrates a large suppurative node in the RPS ➡. Rim-enhancing fluid partly surrounds the left ICA, which is narrowed due to spasm ➡. Although worrisome on imaging, ICA spasm is usually self-limited. Note reactive adenopathy in right RPS ➡.

TERMINOLOGY

Abbreviations

- Retropharyngeal space (RPS)

Synonyms

- Retropharyngeal adenitis, intranodal abscess

Definitions

- Formation of pus in RPS node draining H&N infection

IMAGING

General Features

- Best diagnostic clue
  - Central cystic change within enlarged RPS node
  - Surrounding RPS ± pharyngeal inflammatory changes
- Location
  - RPS between skull base & hyoid bone
    - Medial to internal carotid arteries (ICA)
    - Lateral RPS, does not cross midline like abscess
- Size
  - Typically > 1 cm

CT Findings

- NECT
  - Prevertebral soft tissue fullness
  - May be difficult to identify node
- CECT
  - Low density within enlarged node
  - Node may show peripheral enhancement
  - RPS cellulitis ± ICA vasospasm
    - Vasospasm more common in kids, usually self-limited

MR Findings

- T2WI
  - Diffuse or focal central high intensity in RPS node
  - ↑ signal intensity of surrounding soft tissues
- DWI
  - Restricted diffusion in suppurative node
- T1WI C+
  - Peripheral node & adjacent soft tissue enhancement

Imaging Recommendations

- Best imaging tool
  - CECT is 1st-line tool for evaluation of H&N infection
  - CECT allows identification of initiating infection
- Protocol advice
  - Contrast allows appreciation of suppuration

DIFFERENTIAL DIAGNOSIS

RPS Reactive Adenopathy

- Incidental finding or upper respiratory tract infection
- Homogeneous nodal enlargement, no cystic change

RPS Abscess

- Toxic patient
- Fluid fills retropharyngeal space, wall enhancement

RPS Nodal Squamous Cell Carcinoma

- Solid or cystic RPS nodal mass without perinodal inflammatory change

- Sinonasal or naso-, oro-, or hypopharyngeal primary

RPS Schwannoma

- Ovoid mass in RPS, mimics node

RPS Edema

- Noninfected fluid without rim enhancement

PATHOLOGY

General Features

- Etiology
  - H&N infection seeds RPS nodes
    - Most commonly bacterial pharyngitis
    - Particularly *Staphylococcus aureus* & *Streptococcus*
  - Node draining infection enlarges = reactive node
    - If untreated, progresses to suppuration
    - If still untreated, ruptures = RPS abscess

CLINICAL ISSUES

Presentation

- Most common signs/symptoms
  - Sore throat, odynophagia
- Other signs/symptoms
  - Fever, poor oral intake, neck pain
  - Elevated WBC and ESR
- Clinical profile
  - Young sick patient, upper respiratory infection

Demographics

- Age
  - More common in children and teens
- Gender
  - M = F
- Epidemiology
  - Uncommon > 30 yr

Natural History & Prognosis

- If RPS cellulitis is extensive, can narrow airway
- Untreated suppurative node can result in RPS abscess

Treatment

- Antibiotics orally; if poor response then intravenously
- Incision & drainage (I&D) if progression to abscess

DIAGNOSTIC CHECKLIST

Consider

- Consider malignancy in patient > 40 yr
  - Especially if no inflammatory change or clinical infection

Image Interpretation Pearls

- Evaluate RPS carefully for suppurative change
  - RPS infection can rapidly progress to abscess, sepsis, & airway compromise

SELECTED REFERENCES

1. Shefelbine SE et al: Pediatric retropharyngeal lymphadenitis: differentiation from retropharyngeal abscess and treatment implications. Otolaryngol Head Neck Surg. 136(2):182-8, 2007
2. Davis WL et al: Retropharyngeal space: evaluation of normal anatomy and diseases with CT and MR imaging. Radiology. 174(1):59-64, 1990

Retropharyngeal Space Abscess

TERMINOLOGY

- Extranodal purulent fluid collection in retropharyngeal space (RPS)

IMAGING

- Lateral plain radiograph: Wide prevertebral distance
- CECT: RPS distended by low-density collection
- Convex anterior contour
- Enhancement of wall suggests abscess

TOP DIFFERENTIAL DIAGNOSES

- Retropharyngeal space edema
- Suppurative adenopathy in RPS
- Hypopharynx squamous cell carcinoma
- Lymphatic malformation
- Neurofibroma

PATHOLOGY

- Rupture of suppurative RPS node → RPS abscess

- Most commonly: *Staphylococcus aureus*, *Haemophilus*, *Streptococcus*
- Other less common causes
  - Ventral spread of discitis and prevertebral infection
  - Pharyngeal penetrating foreign body
  - Mediastinal abscess spreading cranially

CLINICAL ISSUES

- Septic patient: Fever, chills, elevated WBC and ESR
- Most < 6 years old, increasing incidence in adults
- Must evaluate for full craniocaudad extent
- CECT best evaluates vascular complications
  - Jugular vein thrombosis or thrombophlebitis
  - Internal carotid artery (ICA) pseudoaneurysm rare, suggests methicillin-resistan *S. aureus*
  - Narrowing of ICA caliber common, usually no clinical consequence
- Narrowing of pharyngeal lumen → stridor

(Left) *Axial graphic illustrates the location and typical contour of a retropharyngeal space (RPS) abscess* ➡ *displacing the pharynx or cervical esophagus* ➡ *anteriorly and flattening the prevertebral muscles.* (Right) *Axial CECT in a 10 month old with a 5-day history of febrile illness reveals a large, low-density ovoid collection distending the retropharyngeal space* ➡ *with anterior displacement of the pharynx and splaying of the carotid sheaths. Minimal enhancement of the wall is evident.*

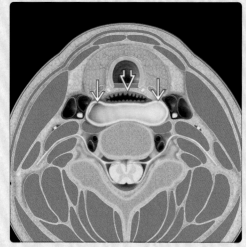 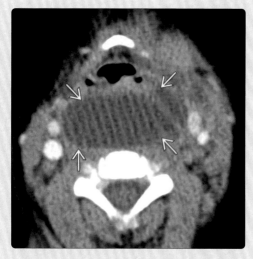

(Left) *Sagittal reformatted CECT in the same infant reveals an abscess* ➡ *displacing the pharynx and esophagus anteriorly and extending inferiorly to involve the superior mediastinum* ➡. (Right) *Axial CECT reveals the inferior extent of methicillin-resistant Staphylococcus aureus (MRSA) abscess to the superior mediastinum* ➡, *which was drained following a cervical approach to the abscess collection. There is no stridor or other signs of airway compromise, despite a displaced and narrowed airway.*

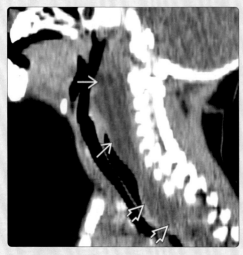 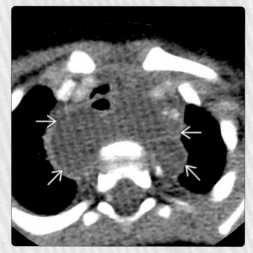

TERMINOLOGY

Abbreviations

- Retropharyngeal space (RPS)

Definitions

- RPS: Midline space posterior to pharyngeal mucosa and cervical esophagus from skull base to T3 vertebral level in mediastinum
- Extranodal purulent fluid collection in RPS = RPS abscess

IMAGING

General Features

- Best diagnostic clue
  - **Midline RPS fluid collection with mass effect** in toxic patient
- Location
  - Distends RPS, posterior to pharynx and anterior to prevertebral muscles
- Size
  - Variable, may extend skull base to mediastinum
- Morphology
  - Axial plane: Oval shape, convex anterior margin

Radiographic Findings

- Radiography
  - Lateral plain radiograph
    - **In children: Must perform during inspiration and with neck extension**
      - Neck flexion may → pseudothickening of prevertebral soft tissues in young children
      - Lateral fluoroscopy helpful to determine true vs. pseudothickening
    - Limited utility for defining extent and differentiating cellulitis/phlegmon from abscess
  - **Widened prevertebral soft tissue thickness**
  - Rarely RPS air, diagnostic of abscess if no history of trauma
  - Normal prevertebral soft tissue
    - C2: ≤ 7 mm at any age
    - C6: ≤ 14 mm if < 15 years, ≤ 22 mm in adults

CT Findings

- CECT
  - RPS markedly **distended** by fluid collection with **enhancing wall**
    - In early stages, enhancement may be subtle
    - Thick enhancing wall suggests mature abscess
    - Prevertebral muscles may also appear edematous
    - Gas rarely present
  - **Assess for complications**
    - Airway compromise
    - Internal carotid artery (ICA) frequently narrowed
    - ICA pseudoaneurysm rare, suggests methicillen-resistant *Staphylococcus aureus* (MRSA)
    - Internal jugular vein (IJV) thrombosis
    - Mediastinal extension

MR Findings

- Rarely utilized in septic patient
  - Tenuous airway, patient monitoring problematic

- May aid in differentiating danger space from RPS collection
  - Danger space is posterior to RPS, extends into mediastinum

Ultrasonographic Findings

- Not able to assess full craniocaudad and deep extent of disease
- Severely limited by operator experience, patient tolerance
- Helpful for evaluating jugular vein patency

Imaging Recommendations

- Best imaging tool
  - **CECT: Rapid imaging; see abscess and complications**
- Protocol advice
  - Helical axial CT from skull base to carina
  - Contrast loading bolus before IV infusion improves soft tissue contrast with rapid helical scanning

DIFFERENTIAL DIAGNOSIS

Retropharyngeal Space Edema

- Venous or lymphatic obstruction
  - IJV thrombosis or resection, XRT
- Regional inflammation
  - Pharyngitis, tonsillitis, longus colli tendinitis
- RPS fluid without definable wall or rim enhancement
  - In axial plane, bow tie in shape, concave anterior margin
- RPS vessels may traverse "collection"
- Drainage not required

Suppurative Adenopathy in RPS

- Central hypodense node in lateral RPS with adjacent cellulitis on CECT
- Pus formation in reactive node (suppuration) = intranodal abscess
- May progress to extranodal RPS abscess with inadequate medical therapy

Hypopharynx Squamous Cell Carcinoma

- Older nonseptic patient ± adenopathy
- Solid enhancing soft tissue mass invading deeply
- Also may occur with posterior oropharyngeal squamous cell carcinoma

Lymphatic Malformation

- Uni- or multilocular, nonenhancing cystic neck mass with nonenhancing wall (unless infected)

Neurofibroma

- May be low attenuation on CT
- Multiple and plexiform in neurofibromatosis type 1

PATHOLOGY

General Features

- Etiology
  - H&N infection (pharyngitis, tonsillitis) seeds RPS lymph node
    - Reactive node → suppurative intranodal abscess
    - **Nodal rupture → RPS abscess**
    - Most common organisms: *S. aureus, Haemophilus, Streptococcus*

- Ventral spread of discitis/osteomyelitis and prevertebral infection
  - More frequent cause of RPS abscess in adults
  - Pyogenic or tuberculous
- Pharyngeal penetrating foreign body
  - Child running with penetrating object in mouth
    - Sucker, toothbrush, toy
- Mediastinal abscess spreading cranially
  - Esophageal rupture and mediastinitis with danger space (DS) abscess

CLINICAL ISSUES

Presentation

- Most common signs/symptoms
  - Septic patient: Fever, chills, elevated WBC and ESR
  - Dysphagia, sore throat, poor oral intake, dehydration
- Other signs/symptoms
  - Posterior pharyngeal wall edema or bulge
  - Reactive cervical adenopathy
- Clinical profile
  - Toxic-appearing child with marked neck pain and limited movement, especially in extension
  - Uncommonly presents with airway compromise (stridor)

Demographics

- Age
  - Most often children **< 6 years old**
  - **Increasing frequency in adult population**
    - Immunocompromised states: Diabetes, HIV, alcoholism, malignancy
    - Discitis/osteomyelitis with perivertebral infection
    - Trauma with foreign body impaction
    - Following anterior cervical spine surgery
- Gender
  - M:F = 2:1
- Epidemiology
  - Reported increase in frequency over the last decade
  - Decrease incidence of abscess when infection detected and treated in earlier cellulitic stage

Natural History & Prognosis

- Prognosis generally excellent if early diagnosis, aggressive management
- Complications may result from infection spread
  - Narrowing of pharyngeal lumen → airway compromise and stridor
  - Inferior spread via danger space to mediastinum → mediastinitis
    - Up to 50% mortality (much less in infants)
  - Carotid space involvement
    - Jugular vein thrombosis or thrombophlebitis
    - Narrowing of ICA caliber often found; neurological sequelae infrequent
    - Rarely ICA pseudoaneurysm &/or rupture; described with MRSA infection
  - Perivertebral space abscess may → epidural abscess
  - Aspiration pneumonia
  - Grisel syndrome rare
    - Inflammatory, nontraumatic atlantoaxial subluxation

- Distension or loosening of atlantoaxial ligaments after H&N inflammation

Treatment

- **Early ENT consultation**
- IV antibiotics, airway management, fluid resuscitation
- Surgical intervention (incision and drainage) if significant or complex abscess present

DIAGNOSTIC CHECKLIST

Consider

- Lateral plain film: Often 1st-line screening tool
- CECT is study of choice
  - Determine RPS vs. perivertebral space
  - Distinguish RPS abscess from edema
  - Evaluate full craniocaudad extent
  - Evaluate for vascular/airway complications
  - Consider contrast prebolus before infusion to maximize wall enhancement

Image Interpretation Pearls

- Distinction from RPS edema sometimes difficult
- Convex anterior margin or oval-shaped collection suggests abscess
- Rim enhancement suggests abscess, though may be minimal initially or may not be evident due to rapid scanning techniques
- Important to evaluate for full extent of abscess and presence of complications
- **ENT consultation imperative**

SELECTED REFERENCES

1. Novis SJ et al: Pediatric deep space neck infections in U.S. children, 2000-2009. Int J Pediatr Otorhinolaryngol. 78(5):832-6, 2014
2. Schott CK et al: A pain in the neck: non-traumatic adult retropharyngeal abscess. J Emerg Med. 44(2):329-31, 2013
3. Abdel-Haq N et al: Retropharyngeal abscess in children: the rising incidence of methicillin-resistant Staphylococcus aureus. Pediatr Infect Dis J. 31(7):696-9, 2012
4. Baker KA et al: Use of computed tomography in the emergency department for the diagnosis of pediatric peritonsillar abscess. Pediatr Emerg Care. 28(10):962-5, 2012
5. Debnam JM et al: Retropharyngeal and prevertebral spaces: anatomic imaging and diagnosis. Otolaryngol Clin North Am. 45(6):1293-310, 2012
6. Maroldi R et al: Emergency imaging assessment of deep neck space infections. Semin Ultrasound CT MR. 33(5):432-42, 2012
7. Reilly BK et al: Retropharyngeal abscess: diagnosis and treatment update. Infect Disord Drug Targets. 12(4):291-6, 2012
8. Virk JS et al: Analysing lateral soft tissue neck radiographs. Emerg Radiol. 19(3):255-60, 2012
9. Wong DK et al: To drain or not to drain - management of pediatric deep neck abscesses: a case-control study. Int J Pediatr Otorhinolaryngol. 76(12):1810-3, 2012
10. Hoang JK et al: Multiplanar CT and MRI of collections in the retropharyngeal space: is it an abscess? AJR Am J Roentgenol. 196(4):W426-32, 2011
11. Elsherif AM et al: Indicators of a more complicated clinical course for pediatric patients with retropharyngeal abscess. Int J Pediatr Otorhinolaryngol. 74(2):198-201, 2010
12. Byramji A et al: Fatal retropharyngeal abscess: a possible marker of inflicted injury in infancy and early childhood. Forensic Sci Med Pathol. 5(4):302-6, 2009
13. Hudgins PA et al: Internal carotid artery narrowing in children with retropharyngeal lymphadenitis and abscess. AJNR Am J Neuroradiol. 19(10):1841-3, 1998

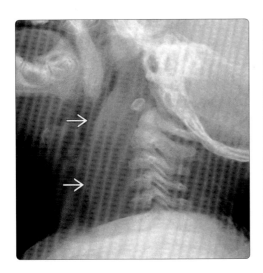
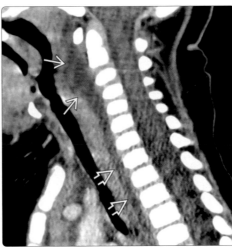

(Left) *Lateral radiograph in a 12-month-old boy with sepsis shows significant thickening of the prevertebral soft tissues* ➡. **(Right)** *Sagittal reformatted CECT in the same child clearly shows the cause of the prominent soft tissues as a convex anterior retropharyngeal abscess* ➡ *with extension of fluid into the posterior mediastinum* ➡.

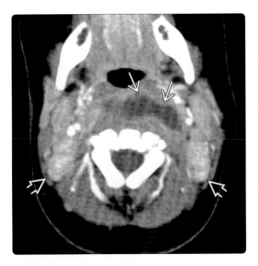
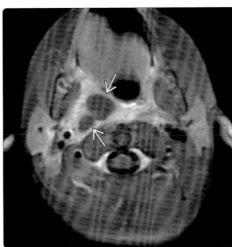

(Left) *Axial postcontrast CECT in a 5-month-old boy shows an irregular-shaped RPS fluid collection* ➡ *in the midline and to the left of midline, most likely an extranodal spread of the suppurative left lateral RP lymph node. Notice bilateral nonsuppurative cervical adenopathy* ➡.
(Right) *Axial T1 C+ FS MR in a child allergic to iodinated contrast demonstrates a well-defined abscess* ➡ *in the right lateral RPS with significant surrounding contrast enhancement.*

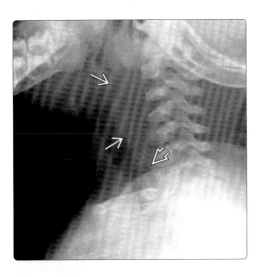
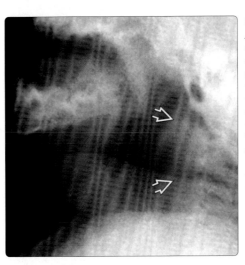

(Left) *Lateral radiograph in a 3 year old obtained with the neck in a neutral position shows prominence of the prevertebral soft tissues* ➡. *In addition, the film is exposed during expiration as evidenced by superior extension of the aerated cupula of the lung* ➡.
(Right) *Lateral spot fluoroscopic image exposed during deep inspiration in the same child demonstrates normal prevertebral soft tissues* ➡.

Retropharyngeal Space Edema

KEY FACTS

TERMINOLOGY

- Retropharyngeal space (RPS) effusion, benign retropharyngeal fluid
- Accumulation of sterile fluid, effacing RPS fat

IMAGING

- Clear demarcation from pharynx and prevertebral muscles
- NECT: Smooth expansion of RPS with **water density fluid**
- MR: Linear to lenticular ↓ T1 and ↑ T2 (**water signal**) in RPS
- CECT/MR C+: **No wall enhancement**

TOP DIFFERENTIAL DIAGNOSES

- RPS abscess
- Prominent normal retropharyngeal fat
- RPS lipoma
- Hypopharyngeal squamous cell carcinoma

PATHOLOGY

- Different inciting factors result in RPS transudate, cellulitis, or lymphatic fluid accumulation

CLINICAL ISSUES

- Self-limited or limited by course of causative process

DIAGNOSTIC CHECKLIST

- Key is to **differentiate from RPS abscess** 1st
  - ○ Rim-enhancing collection distending RPS
  - ○ Requires urgent ENT consultation
- Look for underlying cause; may be treatable
  - ○ Venous occlusive disease
  - ○ Recent chemotherapy or radiation therapy
  - ○ Current infection: Pharynx, teeth, sinus
  - ○ Longus colli tendinitis
  - ○ Kawasaki disease

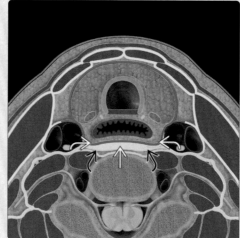
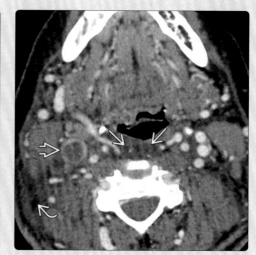

(Left) *Axial graphic illustrates retropharyngeal space (RPS) distension with edema ➡. Note fascial delineation of RPS by middle layer of deep cervical fascia (DCF) anteriorly ➡ and deep layer of DCF posteriorly ➡. (Right) Axial CECT reveals retropharyngeal space low-density fluid ➡ without peripheral enhancement due to right internal jugular vein (IJV) thrombosis ➡. Edematous changes are seen in the surrounding right carotid space and ipsilateral posterior cervical space deep fat ➡.*

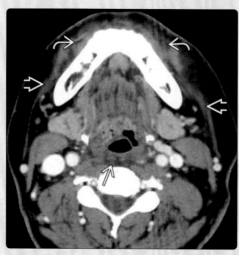
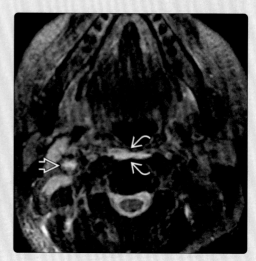

(Left) *Axial CECT shows bland RPS fluid without rim enhancement ➡. Note evidence of source: Cellulitis overlying the mandible ➡ and thickened platysma ➡ from nearby dental infection. (Right) Axial T2WI FS MR reveals RPS distension with thin, symmetric effusion ➡ of similar intensity to CSF. Source of RPS fluid is due to right IJV thrombosis. Note loss of IJV flow void with high signal intensity ➡.*

TERMINOLOGY

Abbreviations

- Retropharyngeal space (RPS)

Synonyms

- Retropharyngeal effusion, benign retropharyngeal fluid

Definitions

- Accumulation of sterile fluid, effacing RPS fat

IMAGING

General Features

- Best diagnostic clue
  - Thin collection of fluid in retropharyngeal space without enhancing wall
- Location
  - Retropharyngeal space
    - Anterior to prevertebral muscles (prevertebral portion of perivertebral space)
    - Posterior to pharynx (pharyngeal mucosal space)
    - RPS stretches from skull base superiorly to upper mediastinum inferiorly
- Size
  - Several millimeters anteroposterior dimension
  - Variable craniocaudal length of edema
- Morphology
  - Smooth expansion of RPS with fluid
  - Sharp demarcation from pharynx and prevertebral muscles

Radiographic Findings

- Radiography
  - Lateral plain film
    - Variably widened prevertebral tissues
    - Cannot distinguish RPS and perivertebral space
    - Cannot distinguish between infected and noninfected RPS collections
  - If caused by longus colli tendinitis, may see calcification at C1-2 level

CT Findings

- CECT
  - Uniform low (water) density fluid collection in RPS without rim enhancement
  - Look for possible causative factors
    - **Neck infection** or inflammatory changes
      - □ Focal rim-enhancing fluid (abscess)
      - □ Focal area of amorphous enhancing tissue (phlegmon)
    - **Venous thrombosis** or internal jugular vein (IJV) resection
      - □ IJV distension with luminal clot
    - Distended veins from **SVC syndrome**
    - Acute calcific **longus colli tendinitis**
      - □ C1-2 level calcifications present acutely
      - □ Calcifications may **not** be present in chronic cases (symptoms > 1 month)

MR Findings

- T1WI

  - Linear to lenticular low (water) signal intensity bland fluid collection between pharynx and prevertebral muscles
- T2WI
  - High signal intensity similar to CSF
- DWI
  - DWI helps distinguish between abscess (restricted) vs. edema (facilitated)
- T1WI C+
  - No rim enhancement of fluid collection
  - May see subtle enhancement of edematous tissues or enhancing vessels through fluid

Imaging Recommendations

- Best imaging tool
  - CECT readily evaluates retropharyngeal tissues, assesses contours and contrast enhancement
  - CECT also evaluates neck for possible causes
- Protocol advice
  - Contrast essential; must image from skull base to superior mediastinum
    - Allows detection of enhancement that might suggest RPS cellulitis/abscess
    - Allows evaluation of adjacent soft tissues and vessels for cause

DIFFERENTIAL DIAGNOSIS

Retropharyngeal Space Abscess

- Distension of RPS by fluid collection with **convex** margins
- **Rim enhancement** particularly in mature abscess
- Gas + fluid in RPS suggest abscess or necrotizing fasciitis if no history of prior instrumentation
- Prevertebral muscles or pharynx often difficult to delineate from collection
- Septic patient, neck pain, sore throat

Prominent Normal Retropharyngeal Fat

- Incidental finding
- More often in pediatric or Cushingoid patients
- No distension of RPS
- NECT/CECT: Fat density; negative Hounsfield units
- MR: T1 and T2 hyperintense, signal loss with T1/T2 FS

Retropharyngeal Space Lipoma

- Retropharyngeal lipoma distends RPS
- NECT/CECT: Fat density; negative Hounsfield unit measurement
  - Uniform fat density; may be unilateral
- MR: T1 hyperintensity, signal loss with T1 FS

Hypopharyngeal Squamous Cell Carcinoma

- Posterior pharyngeal wall squamous cell carcinoma (SCCa may infiltrate deeply
- Also possible with posterior oropharyngeal wall SCCa
- **Solid, enhancing** ill-defined infiltrative mass
- May also invade prevertebral muscles of perivertebral space

PATHOLOGY

General Features

- Etiology

- May be due to accumulation of lymphatic fluid, transudate, cellulitis, or CSF leak (pseudomeningocele)
- H&N inflammatory and infectious processes (**cellulitis** or **transudate**)
  - Pharyngitis, dental infection, sinusitis
  - Angioedema (anaphylaxis, ACE inhibitors)
  - Acute calcific longus colli tendinitis
    - Calcium hydroxyapatite deposition in longus colli muscle insertions
    - Self-limited inflammation that responds to steroids ± NSAIDs
  - Kawasaki disease (idiopathic acute self-limited vasculitis in infants and young children) may cause RPS effusion
    - Additional findings: RPS adenopathy ± palatine tonsil enlargement
- Current or recent chemotherapy or radiation therapy (**lymphedema**)
- Altered venous flow in neck (**transudate**)
  - IJV resection with radical or modified neck dissection
  - IJV thrombosis
  - Superior vena cava syndrome
  - Postpharyngitis venous thrombosis (Lemierre syndrome)
  - Neoplasm with venous compression or occlusion
- Pseudomeningocele post ACDF (CSF leak)
- Trauma (whiplash injury)

Microscopic Features

- Should not be aspirated as self-limited or limited by causative factors

CLINICAL ISSUES

Presentation

- Most common signs/symptoms
  - RPS fluid is asymptomatic though patient may have symptoms from primary cause
    - Radiation therapy, superior vena cava syndrome, recent H&N surgery, H&N inflammatory process
    - Longus colli tendinitis: Neck stiffness, sore throat, low-grade fever

Demographics

- Age
  - Any age; dependent on primary cause
- Gender
  - Male = female

Natural History & Prognosis

- Self limited or limited by course of causative process
  - Venous compromise: IJV thrombosis, IJV resection, or superior vena cava syndrome
    - Effusion improves spontaneously or with resolution of thrombosis
  - Radiation-induced RPS fluid typically appears at 4-6 weeks
    - Resolves spontaneously by 8-12 weeks
  - If due to adjacent H&N infection, will resolve with antibiotic therapy or surgical therapy
    - Some cases can become secondarily infected; imaging may be required for surveillance

- With calcific longus colli tendinitis, will resolve with treatment of acute inflammation

Treatment

- Does **not** require drainage
- No specific treatment necessary for fluid
- Try to identify primary cause that can be treated
  - Treat venous thrombosis with anticoagulants
  - Treat H&N infection with antibiotics or surgery as needed
  - Treat longus colli tendinitis with steroids ± NSAIDs

DIAGNOSTIC CHECKLIST

Consider

- Relatively common lesion seen on CECT in setting of complex neck disease
- Important to **differentiate from RPS abscess**
  - Abscess in RPS
    - **Mass effect** with distension of RPS with convex contours
    - Fluid collection **wall enhances**
    - Gas in RPS without history of recent instrumentation suggests abscess and/or necrotizing fasciitis
    - RPS abscess associated with adjacent cellulitis
    - ENT consultation if RPS abscess suspected

Image Interpretation Pearls

- Once RPS abscess excluded, look for cause of edema
  - Neck inflammatory/infectious process
  - Calcification at insertion site of prevertebral muscles (longus colli tendinitis)
  - Venous compromise: IJV thrombosis, resection, or superior vena cava syndrome
  - Recent chemotherapy or radiation therapy

Reporting Tips

- Report should reflect bland fluid without mass effect or rim enhancement
- Do not offer RPS abscess in differential diagnosis as may prompt surgical intervention

SELECTED REFERENCES

1. Al-Natour MS et al: Superior vena cava syndrome with retropharyngeal edema as a complication of ventriculoatrial shunt. Clin Case Rep. 3(10):777-80, 2015
2. Katsumata N et al: Characteristics of cervical computed tomography findings in kawasaki disease: a single-center experience. J Comput Assist Tomogr. 37(5):681-5, 2013
3. Paik NC et al: Tendinitis of longus colli: computed tomography, magnetic resonance imaging, and clinical spectra of 9 cases. J Comput Assist Tomogr. 36(6):755-61, 2012
4. Hoang JK et al: Multiplanar CT and MRI of collections in the retropharyngeal space: is it an abscess? AJR Am J Roentgenol. 196(4):W426-32, 2011
5. Kurihara N et al: Edema in the retropharyngeal space associated with head and neck tumors: CT imaging characteristics. Neuroradiology. 47(8):609-15, 2005
6. Chong VF et al: Radiology of the retropharyngeal space. Clin Radiol. 55(10):740-8, 2000
7. Mukherji SK et al: Radiologic appearance of the irradiated larynx. Part I. Expected changes. Radiology. 193(1):141-8, 1994
8. Glasier CM et al: CT and ultrasound imaging of retropharyngeal abscesses in children. AJNR Am J Neuroradiol. 13(4):1191-5, 1992
9. Davis WL et al: The normal and diseased infrahyoid retropharyngeal, danger, and prevertebral spaces. Semin Ultrasound CT MR. 12(3):241-56, 1991
10. Davis WL et al: Retropharyngeal space: evaluation of normal anatomy and diseases with CT and MR imaging. Radiology. 174(1):59-64, 1990

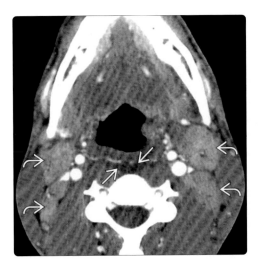
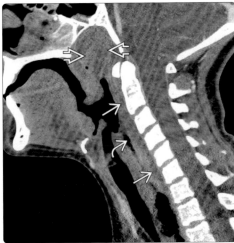

(Left) *Axial CECT reveals expansion of retropharyngeal space by low-density, nonenhancing fluid* ➡. *Prevertebral muscles and pharyngeal contours remain sharply defined. Bilateral reactive adenopathy* ➡ *also in patient with Streptococcus throat infection.* (Right) *Sagittal CECT MPR shows nonenhancing edema fluid in the RPS* ➡ *in a patient with tonsillar infection. Note enlarged hypodense adenoids* ➡. *Gas is present within the hypopharynx* ➡, *anterior to the RPS collection.*

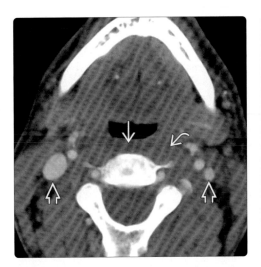
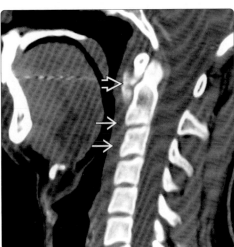

(Left) *CECT in patient with neck pain shows mild distension of RPS with low-density fluid* ➡ *in longus colli tendinitis. Note subtle enlargement, decrease in density, and less sharply defined left longus colli muscle* ➡, *though this is often difficult to detect on CT. No evidence of jugular vein* ➡ *thrombosis or edema of fat of deep neck spaces is seen.* (Right) *CECT reformat shows amorphous calcifications* ➡ *ventral to C1-C2 joint, diagnostic of acute calcific longus colli tendonitis. Subtle low-density edema in RPS* ➡.

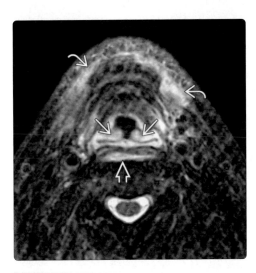
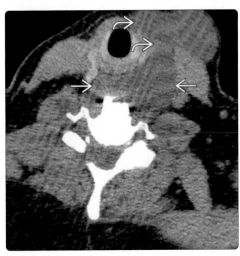

(Left) *Axial T2WI FS MR performed as a baseline study 8 weeks after chemoradiation for tonsil squamous cell carcinoma shows RPS fluid* ➡. *Extensive hyperintense edema is evident in subcutaneous* ➡ *and deep neck fat. Aryepiglottic folds* ➡ *are also edematous.* (Right) *Axial CECT demonstrates water density fluid in the RPS* ➡ *in a patient recently post anterior cervical discectomy and fusion who developed pseudomeningocele (CSF leak). Fluid extends anteriorly along the surgical tract into the anterior neck* ➡.

Nodal Squamous Cell Carcinoma of Retropharyngeal Space

KEY FACTS

TERMINOLOGY

- Malignant retropharyngeal space (RPS) nodes: Squamous cell carcinoma (SCCa) RPS nodes from nasopharyngeal or posterior wall pharyngeal primary SCCa

IMAGING

- Location
  - Only present in suprahyoid neck
  - Anterior to prevertebral strap muscles, medial to ICA
- Oval to round, ± centrally necrotic mass > 0.8 cm in RPS
- Ill-defined margins ± stranding of surrounding fat are features of extracapsular spread
- CECT findings
  - Nodes difficult to identify on CT, especially if small
  - Nodal necrosis: Central low density with variably thick, irregular enhancing wall
- MR more sensitive to detect RPS nodes than CT
- PET has role in staging & follow-up of H&N SCCa
  - Cystic/necrotic nodes may be PET negative

TOP DIFFERENTIAL DIAGNOSES

- Reactive RPS nodes
- Suppurative RPS nodes
- Direct RPS invasion by pharyngeal SCCa
- Non-Hodgkin lymphoma RPS nodes
- Thyroid RPS nodal metastasis
- Systemic RPS nodal metastasis

PATHOLOGY

- RPS nodes = primary drainage for posterior nasal cavity, ethmoid & sphenoid sinus, palate, nasopharynx & posterior wall of oro- & hypopharynx

CLINICAL ISSUES

- RPS malignant adenopathy is often clinically occult
- If large, bulging of posterolateral pharyngeal wall
- 75% of NPCa have RPS adenopathy at presentation
- 8-20% of oro- & hypopharyngeal wall SCCa have RPS nodes
  - Highest risk in posterior wall hypopharynx cancers (24%)

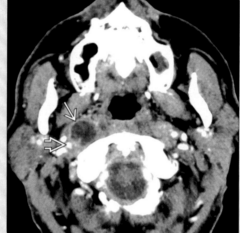
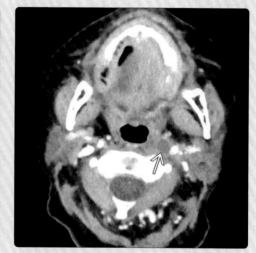

(Left) Axial CECT through the nasopharynx shows a large, necrotic lateral retropharyngeal node ➡ just medial to the internal carotid artery (ICA) ➡. In an adult, squamous cell carcinoma from the pharynx is the most likely primary site for this suspected malignant retropharyngeal node. (Right) Axial CECT demonstrates a cystic left retropharyngeal nodal metastasis ➡ in a patient with oropharyngeal SCCa. Corresponding PET showed no FDG uptake. Cystic nodes are a potential source of false-positive FDG PET studies.

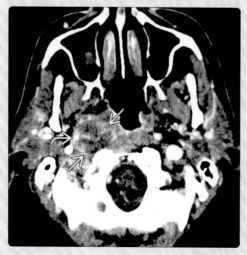
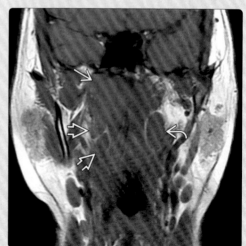

(Left) Axial CECT in a 63-year-old man treated with surgery & radiation therapy 1 year ago for oropharyngeal SCCa shows a large, clinically silent recurrent retropharyngeal space (RPS) nodal mass with irregular rim enhancement ➡. Note its location medial to the narrowed and encased right ICA ➡. (Right) Coronal T1WI MR in a patient with a mass in the upper pharynx ➡ shows a predominantly right-sided nasopharyngeal carcinoma with 2 right RPS ➡ nodes and 1 large left RPS node ➡.

TERMINOLOGY

Definitions

- Malignant retropharyngeal space (RPS) nodes: Squamous cell carcinoma (SCCa) RPS nodes from nasopharyngeal or posterior wall oropharyngeal primary SCCa

IMAGING

General Features

- Best diagnostic clue
  o Oval to round, ± centrally necrotic mass **> 0.8 cm** in RPS, medial to internal carotid artery (ICA)
- Location
  o RPS nodes are only present in suprahyoid neck
  o RPS nodes located anterior to prevertebral strap muscles, medial to ICA
- Size
  o Pathologic markers of RPS nodes
    – Size: > 0.8 cm minimum diameter in lateral RPS
    – Any node in medial RPS
    – **Necrosis ± extracapsular spread**, any size

CT Findings

- CECT
  o Often difficult to identify on CT, especially if small
  o Round/oval, mildly enhancing soft tissue density mass in RPS
  o Necrosis appears as central low density with variably thick, irregular enhancing wall
  o Ill-defined margins ± stranding of surrounding fat are features of extracapsular spread

MR Findings

- T1WI
  o Nodes isointense to muscle
- T2WI
  o Nodes hyperintense
- T1WI C+
  o Enhancing lateral or medial RPS node
  o If nodal necrosis, central low intensity with peripheral wall enhancement

Nuclear Medicine Findings

- PET
  o PET has role in staging & follow-up of H&N SCCa
    – Cystic/necrotic nodes may be PET(-)
  o Increased metabolic activity may diagnose metastatic SCCa in small, nonnecrotic RPS node

Imaging Recommendations

- Best imaging tool
  o MR best for detection of RPS nodes
    – On CECT, RPS nodes may be missed

DIFFERENTIAL DIAGNOSIS

RPS Reactive Adenopathy

- Typically in younger patients (< 30 yr old)
- Homogeneous RPS mass < 1 cm
- Multiple other reactive-appearing nodes & adenoidal & palatine tonsillar hyperplasia associated

RPS Suppurative Adenopathy

- Younger patient (< 30 yr old), pharyngitis, sepsis
- Intranodal abscess: Centrally necrotic, peripherally enhancing node ± RPS edema
- If suppurative node ruptures → RPS abscess

SCCa Direct RPS Invasion

- Posterior oro- or hypopharynx wall SCCa
- Direct, contiguous invasion into RPS

Non-Hodgkin Lymphoma RPS Nodes

- Usually large (> 2 cm), homogeneous, solid nodes
- Nodes involving multiple other H&N locations

Nodal Differentiated Thyroid Carcinoma (DTCa)

- CECT: Nodes may be cystic, heterogeneous, calcified
- MR: T1 hyperintense nodes characteristic

Metastatic Node, Non-SCCa, RPS

- Widespread metastatic disease usually present
- Metastatic nodal melanoma, breast, lung, other

PATHOLOGY

General Features

- Critical RPS nodal anatomy
  o RPS nodes = primary drainage for posterior nasal cavity, ethmoid & sphenoid sinus, palate, nasopharynx & posterior wall of oro- & hypopharynx

CLINICAL ISSUES

Presentation

- Most common signs/symptoms
  o If large, bulging of posterolateral pharyngeal wall
  o RPS malignant nodes are **often clinically occult**

Demographics

- Epidemiology
  o 75% of nasopharyngeal carcinoma has RPS adenopathy at presentation
  o 8-20% of oro- & hypopharyngeal wall SCCa have RPS nodes
    – Risk in hypopharynx highest for posterior wall cancers (24%)

Natural History & Prognosis

- Poor prognosis with RPS metastatic SCCa nodes
- NPCa N0 with RPS adenopathy has same prognostic implication as N1 disease

Treatment

- For NPCa, nodes included in radiation boost field
- For oro- & hypopharyngeal SCCa, surgical nodal dissection

SELECTED REFERENCES

1. Chu HR et al: Additional diagnostic value of (18)F-FDG PET-CT in detecting retropharyngeal nodal metastases. Otolaryngol Head Neck Surg. 141(5):633-8, 2009
2. Kaplan SL et al: The role of MR imaging in detecting nodal disease in thyroidectomy patients with rising thyroglobulin levels. AJNR Am J Neuroradiol. 30(3):608-12, 2009
3. King AD et al: Neck node metastases from nasopharyngeal carcinoma: MR imaging of patterns of disease. Head Neck. 22(3):275-81, 2000

Nodal Non-Hodgkin Lymphoma in Retropharyngeal Space

TERMINOLOGY

- NHL is lymphoreticular system malignancy
- Retropharyngeal space (RPS) from skull base to hyoid contains lateral & medial nodal groups
  - Lateral group = nodes of Rouvière
- Head & neck NHL has multiple forms
  - Nodal, non-nodal lymphatic or extralymphatic

IMAGING

- Oval-round, solid mass > **0.8 cm** (axial) in RPS
  - RPS nodes are medial to internal carotid arteries, at or above hyoid
- **Typically associated with other neck adenopathy**
  - May have enlargement of Waldeyer ring
- Necrosis ± extranodal spread suggest high-grade, aggressive NHL
- MR more sensitive than CT for detecting RPS nodes
- CT & MR cannot differentiate normal size, nonnecrotic NHL nodes from reactive nodes

- **Most NHL are FDG avid**; PET typically performed

TOP DIFFERENTIAL DIAGNOSES

- RPS reactive adenopathy
- RPS suppurative adenopathy
- RPS nodal SCCa or systemic metastasis
  - Pharyngeal SCCa > NHL > thyroid carcinoma > melanoma

CLINICAL ISSUES

- Increasing incidence of NHL
- Median age: 50-55 yr
- RPS nodes usually clinically occult
  - If large may see bulging of posterior pharyngeal wall
- Other manifestations of NHL in H&N
  - Extranodal, lymphatic disease in Waldeyer ring
  - Extranodal, extralymphatic site involvement

DIAGNOSTIC CHECKLIST

- Large, nonnecrotic node more likely NHL than SCCa

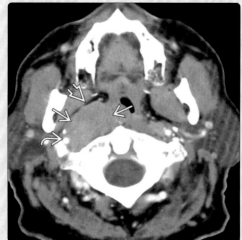 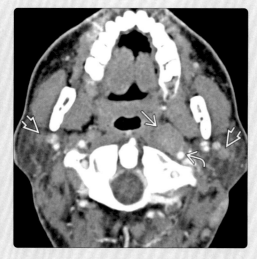

(Left) Axial CECT in a patient with non-Hodgkin lymphoma (NHL) shows a large homogeneously enhancing mass ➡ medial to internal carotid artery ➦. Right retropharyngeal node displaces parapharyngeal fat ➡ anterolaterally. (Right) Axial CECT in a different patient shows a large, oval, homogeneous, nonnecrotic left retropharyngeal node ➡ displacing the left internal carotid ➡ posterolaterally. Mildly prominent parotid nodes are also noted ➡ in this patient with NHL.

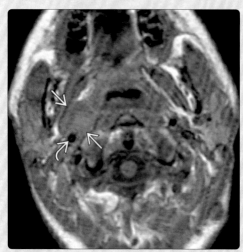 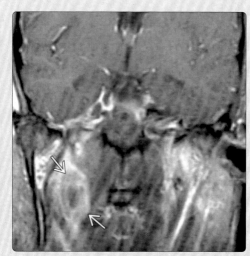

(Left) Axial T1WI MR reveals soft tissue mass ➡ medial to internal carotid artery ➦, representing abnormally enlarged lateral retropharyngeal node. Note that despite size, this node does not deform the pharyngeal lumen enough to be clinically evident. Patient had history of aplastic anemia & bone marrow transplant. (Right) Coronal T1WI C+ MR in same patient shows rim enhancement of the retropharyngeal node ➡ & central necrosis. Patient was found to have posttransplant NHL.

TERMINOLOGY

Abbreviations

- Non-Hodgkin lymphoma (NHL) in retropharyngeal space (RPS)

Definitions

- NHL is lymphoreticular system malignancy
  - Head & neck NHL has multiple forms
    - Nodal, non-nodal lymphatic (tonsils & adenoids), extralymphatic (e.g., thyroid, sinuses)
- RPS skull base to hyoid contains lateral & medial nodes
  - Lateral group = nodes of Rouvière

IMAGING

General Features

- Best diagnostic clue
  - Oval-round, solid mass > **0.8 cm** (axial) in RPS, **typically associated with other neck adenopathy**
- Location
  - RPS nodes only present in suprahyoid RPS
    - **Medial to internal carotid arteries** from skull base to hyoid
- Size
  - RPS nodes pathologic if > **0.8 cm (axial)**, necrotic, or infiltrative
- Morphology
  - Typically solid, rounded nodes
  - Necrosis ± extracapsular spread → high-grade NHL

CT Findings

- CECT
  - May be difficult to identify on CT, especially if small
  - Ovoid mildly enhancing soft tissue mass in RPS
    - Less enhancing compared to normal nodes (before treatment)

MR Findings

- T1WI
  - Nodes isointense to muscle
- T2WI
  - High-signal nodal masses
- STIR
  - High-signal nodal masses
- T1WI C+
  - Diffuse, mild to moderate enhancement

Nuclear Medicine Findings

- PET
  - Useful in staging & follow-up of most types of NHL, because of FDG avidity

Imaging Recommendations

- Best imaging tool
  - MR more sensitive for detecting RPS nodes than CT
  - FDG PET typically used for staging and surveillance in most types of NHL

DIFFERENTIAL DIAGNOSIS

RPS Reactive Adenopathy

- Homogeneous ovoid RPS mass ≤ 10 mm
- Multiple other reactive nodes ± tonsillar hyperplasia
- Typically pediatric patients

RPS Suppurative Adenopathy

- Usually < 30 yr old, septic with pharyngitis
- Central necrosis, peripheral enhancement
- Often associated with RPS edema

RPS Nodal Squamous Cell Carcinoma

- Most common cause of malignant RPS nodes
- Nodes are round ± central necrosis & features of extranodal extension

PATHOLOGY

General Features

- Associated abnormalities
  - Other manifestations of NHL in H&N
    - Extranodal, lymphatic disease in Waldeyer ring
    - Extranodal, extralymphatic site involvement

Staging, Grading, & Classification

- **World Health Organization (WHO)** is favored classification (2008)
  - Based on immunophenotype & morphology
  - More than 30 different types of NHL
    - B-cell neoplasms (80-85%)
    - T-cell & putative NK-cell neoplasms (15-20%)

CLINICAL ISSUES

Presentation

- Most common signs/symptoms
  - RPS nodes usually clinically occult
    - May see bulging of posterior pharyngeal wall
  - Other cervical nodes typically present
  - May have enlargement of Waldeyer ring

Demographics

- Epidemiology
  - Increasing incidence of NHL
  - Pharyngeal squamous cell carcinoma > NHL > thyroid carcinoma > melanoma metastases
- Age: Median 50-55 yr
- Gender: M:F = 1.5:1

Treatment

- Treatment depends on stage, cell type, patient age
- Chemo, XRT, or combined modality therapy (CMT)

DIAGNOSTIC CHECKLIST

Image Interpretation Pearls

- Large, nonnecrotic nodes suggests NHL, not squamous cell carcinoma
- Necrosis &/or extranodal spread or diffuse infiltration suggest high-grade, aggressive NHL

SELECTED REFERENCES

1. Hagtvedt T et al: Enhancement characteristics of lymphomatous lymph nodes of the neck. Acta Radiol. 51(5):555-62, 2010
2. Aiken AH et al: Imaging Hodgkin and non-Hodgkin lymphoma in the head and neck. Radiol Clin North Am. 46(2):363-78, ix-x, 2008

KEY FACTS

TERMINOLOGY

- Definition: Malignant retropharyngeal space (RPS) nodes of non-squamous cell carcinoma (SCCa) origin

IMAGING

- Best diagnostic clue: Oval to round ± centrally necrotic mass > **0.8 cm** in RPS, **medial to internal carotid artery**
  - Suprahyoid neck RPS **only**
- MR more sensitive for detecting RPS nodes
  - Small nodes may be unseen on CECT
- MR findings
  - Nodes usually isointense to muscle (T1)
  - DTCa or melanoma may be hyperintense on T1
  - High signal on T2
- CECT findings
  - Oval to round, mildly enhancing soft tissue density mass in RPS ± necrosis
  - Nodal necrosis: Central low density with irregular wall enhancement

- Extracapsular spread: Ill-defined margins ± stranding of surrounding fat
- DTCa nodes: Cystic or solid, heterogeneous ± calcified
- FDG avid nodes on PET

TOP DIFFERENTIAL DIAGNOSES

- RPS reactive adenopathy
- RPS suppurative adenopathy
- RPS nodal SCCa

CLINICAL ISSUES

- RPS malignant nodes **often clinically occult**
- If large, bulging of posterolateral wall of pharynx

DIAGNOSTIC CHECKLIST

- RPS non-SCCa nodes prompt search for primary
  - Posterior nasopharynx & skull base: Esthesioneuroblastoma, SNUC, other
  - Neck search for primary thyroid carcinoma in neck
  - Systemic tumor search for melanoma, NHL, other

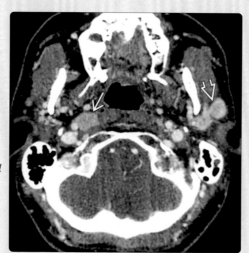
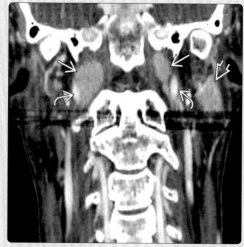

(Left) Axial CECT in a 44-year-old man who had undergone craniofacial resection, radiation, & chemotherapy for esthesioneuroblastoma 8 years prior shows a right lateral retropharyngeal space (RPS) nodal metastasis ➡. There is also a metastasis to the intraparotid nodes on the left ➡. (Right) Coronal CT reconstruction in the same patient demonstrates bilateral RPS nodal metastases ➡ just medial to the internal carotid arteries (ICAs) ➡. The intraparotid nodal disease ➡ is visible on the left.

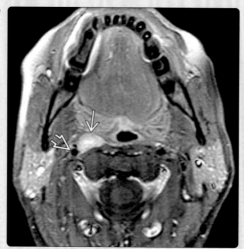
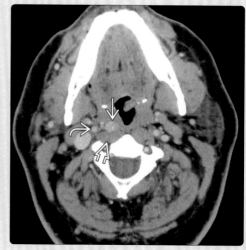

(Left) Axial T1WI C+ FS MR in a patient with recurrent medullary thyroid carcinoma demonstrates an enhancing metastatic node in the right RPS ➡ just medial to the right ICA ➡. (Right) Axial CECT shows an intensely enhancing medial RPS lymph node ➡, anterior to the prevertebral muscles ➡ and medial to the internal carotid artery ➡, in this biopsy-proven metastatic papillary thyroid cancer.

Non-Squamous Cell Carcinoma Metastatic Nodes in Retropharyngeal Space

TERMINOLOGY

Abbreviations
- Non-squamous cell carcinoma (SCCa) metastatic nodes in retropharyngeal space (RPS)

Definitions
- Malignant RPS nodes of non-SCCa origin
  - Differentiated thyroid carcinoma (DTCa), melanoma, esthesioneuroblastoma (ENB), NHL

IMAGING

General Features
- Best diagnostic clue
  - Oval to round ± centrally necrotic mass > **0.8 cm in RPS**, medial to ICA
- Location
  - Suprahyoid neck RPS **only**
  - Anterior to prevertebral strap muscles, medial to ICA
- Size
  - RPS nodes designated pathologic if > **0.8 cm** minimum diameter in lateral RPS + any node in medial RPS except in children
  - Children may have reactive medial & lateral RPS nodes

Imaging Recommendations
- Best imaging tool
  - MR more sensitive for detecting RPS nodes
    - Small nodes may be unseen on CECT
  - MR & CT unable to differentiate normal-sized, nonnecrotic nodes without extracapsular spread from reactive nodes

CT Findings
- CECT
  - Oval to round, mildly enhancing soft tissue density mass in RPS ± necrosis
  - Nodal necrosis: Central low density with irregular wall enhancement
  - Extracapsular spread: Ill-defined margins ± stranding of surrounding fat
  - DTCa nodes: Cystic or solid, heterogeneous ± calcification

MR Findings
- T1WI
  - Nodes isointense to muscle
  - DTCa node may be hyperintense (thyroglobulin or colloid content)
  - Melanoma node may be hyperintense (T1 shortening caused by melanin)
- T2WI
  - Nodes hyperintense
- T1WI C+
  - Nodal necrosis: Central low intensity with wall enhancement

Nuclear Medicine Findings
- PET
  - FDG PET useful to confirm nodal metastases in DTCa
    - Highest sensitivity & specificity in treated patients with rising thyroglobulin & negative radioiodine scan
  - FDG melanoma uptake varies with histology

DIFFERENTIAL DIAGNOSIS

RPS Reactive Adenopathy
- Homogeneous RPS mass < 1 cm in young
- Multiple other reactive-appearing nodes & adenoidal & tonsillar hyperplasia associated

RPS Suppurative Adenopathy
- Septic patient with pharyngitis
- Intranodal abscess: Centrally necrotic, peripherally enhancing node ± RPS edema

RPS Nodal Squamous Cell Carcinoma
- Most common cause of malignant RPS nodes
- Round nodes ± central necrosis

PATHOLOGY

General Features
- Etiology
  - Non-SCCa cancers from skull base, posterior nasal cavity, palate
    - ENB, sinonasal undifferentiated carcinoma (SNUC), sarcoma, other
  - Non-SCCa neck malignancy metastases: DTCa
    - Retrograde lymphatic spread via paratracheal chain to RPS chain
  - Systemic cancer with RPS nodal metastases: Melanoma, NHL

CLINICAL ISSUES

Presentation
- Most common signs/symptoms
  - RPS malignant nodes **often clinically occult**
- Other signs/symptoms
  - If large, bulging of posterolateral wall of pharynx

Natural History & Prognosis
- Prognosis on non-SCCa metastasis unknown

Treatment
- Extended radiation field or surgical excision

DIAGNOSTIC CHECKLIST

Consider
- RPS non-SCCa nodes prompt search for primary
  - Posterior nasopharynx & skull base: Esthesioneuroblastoma, SNUC, other
  - Neck search for primary thyroid carcinoma in neck
  - Systemic tumor search for melanoma, NHL, other

SELECTED REFERENCES

1. Kato H et al: Metastatic retropharyngeal lymph nodes: comparison of CT and MR imaging for diagnostic accuracy. Eur J Radiol. 83(7):1157-62, 2014
2. Kaplan SL et al: The role of MR imaging in detecting nodal disease in thyroidectomy patients with rising thyroglobulin levels. AJNR Am J Neuroradiol. 30(3):608-12, 2009
3. Zollinger LV et al: Retropharyngeal lymph node metastasis from esthesioneuroblastoma: a review of the therapeutic and prognostic implications. AJNR Am J Neuroradiol. 29(8):1561-3, 2008

SECTION 8
Perivertebral Space

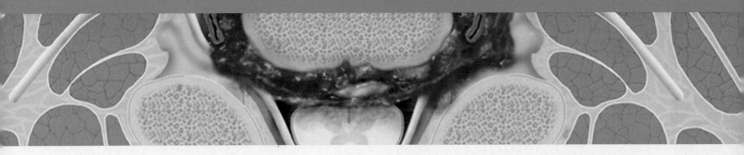

Summary Thoughts: Perivertebral Space

The perivertebral space (PVS) is a cylindrical space surrounding the vertebral column, extending from the skull base to the superior mediastinum. The **deep layer of the deep cervical fascia** (DL-DCF) completely encircles the PVS, which is subdivided into **prevertebral** (prevertebral-PVS) and **paraspinal** (paraspinal-PVS) portions or spaces.

A **prevertebral-PVS mass** will displace the prevertebral muscles **anteriorly**, distinguishing it from a retropharyngeal space (RPS) mass, which pushes the muscles posteriorly. A **paraspinal-PVS mass** bows the posterior cervical space (PCS) fat away from the posterior elements of the spine.

The DL-DCF serves as a tenacious barrier to the spread of malignancy or infection, and it will redirect extension of PVS disease to the **epidural space**.

The vast majority of PVS lesions originate in the **vertebral body** with **metastatic disease** and **infection** topping the list. Therefore, the vertebral body is usually diseased when a PVS lesion is found.

An imaging interpretation pitfall is mistaking a **hypertrophic levator scapulae muscle** for a mass. The hypertrophy is due to CNXI injury, usually from previous neck dissection. Ipsilateral atrophy of the trapezius and sternocleidomastoid muscles help in making the correct diagnosis.

Imaging Techniques & Indications

A lateral cervical plain film provides a quick check for prevertebral soft tissue swelling and for cervical vertebral body integrity. **CECT** with soft tissue and bone algorithm along with coronal & sagittal reformations is the best exam to evaluate the **cervical soft tissues** and **bones**. Contrast-enhanced cervical spine **MR** is the exam of choice to evaluate for **epidural extension** of disease.

Imaging Anatomy

The name PVS nicely describes the anatomy. It is a cylindrical space that is quite literally around (or peri-) the vertebral column. This helpful naming system was not always the case as the entire region, including portions **beside** and **behind** the vertebrae, was historically called the **pre**vertebral space. Since it seemed counterintuitive to use **pre**vertebral to describe structures posterolateral to the vertebrae, the old terminology was upgraded to the new.

The PVS is bounded by the DL-DCF and extends from the skull base to the superior mediastinum T4 level. It consists of **2 major components**: The **prevertebral**-PVS and **paraspinal**-PVS portions or spaces. The attachments of the DL-DCF to the vertebral transverse processes mark the division, with the prevertebral-PVS lying anterior and the paraspinal-PVS lying posterior.

Important anatomic relationships can be examined as they relate to these 2 subdivisions. Directly in front of the **prevertebral-PVS** throughout the extracranial head and neck are the retropharyngeal and danger spaces. Anterolateral are the paired carotid spaces and lateral lie the anterior aspects of the posterior cervical spaces. The **paraspinal-PVS** lies deep to the posterior cervical spaces and posterior to the cervical spine transverse processes.

The **DL-DCF** completely encircles the PVS. Its anterior portion (**anterior DL-DCF**) arches in front of the prevertebral muscles from 1 cervical spine transverse process to the opposite

transverse process. The posterior portion (**posterior DL-DCF**) arches over the paraspinal muscles to attach to the nuchal ligament of the vertebral body spinous processes.

The **anterior DL-DCF** is often referred to as the "**carpet**" by surgeons because surgical approach reveals a smooth, carpet-like surface on which the pharynx slides up and down. The "carpet" is extremely tenacious and serves as a 2-way barrier to the spread of disease. Therefore, expanding **tumor or infection** of the prevertebral-PVS will be redirected by this tough fascia along the path of least resistance to the **epidural space**. Coming from the other direction, pharyngeal malignancy is usually blocked from accessing the PVS.

Only the **brachial plexus** roots pierce the tough DL-DCF. The C1-C5 roots exit the neural foramina, pass between the anterior & middle scalene muscles in the prevertebral-PVS, then out through an opening in the DL-DCF. From there, they traverse the posterior cervical space on their way to the axilla. This creates a bidirectional highway for perineural spread of malignancy.

A working knowledge of important **PVS internal structures** is key to understanding the pathology & pathology mimics (pseudolesions) found within. The prevertebral-PVS contains the prevertebral muscles (longus colli and capitis), scalene muscles (anterior, middle, and posterior), brachial plexus roots, phrenic nerve (C3-C5), vertebral artery and vein, and vertebral body. The paraspinal-PVS contains the paraspinal muscles and the posterior elements of the vertebrae.

Approaches to Imaging Issues of Perivertebral Space

When trying to define a lesion in the H&N as in the PVS, one must 1st answer the question, "What **imaging findings** define a mass or lesion as **primary to the PVS**?" A lesion originates from the **prevertebral-PVS** if it is centered within the prevertebral muscles or vertebral body. Also, a mass that causes **anterior lifting** of the **prevertebral muscles** is arising from the prevertebral-PVS. In most cases, this feature clearly distinguishes a PVS mass from a RPS mass, which pushes the muscles posteriorly.

A mass is primary to the **paraspinal-PVS** if it is within the substance of the paraspinal musculature or if it bows the posterior cervical space fat away from the vertebral posterior elements.

When prevertebral-PVS disease is noted, one should always check for **epidural extension**. Remember that infection or malignancy that breaks out of the vertebral body into the PVS will be blocked by the tough DL-DCF. As a result the path of least resistance is deep spread into the epidural space through the neural foramen, possibly leading to **spinal cord compression**.

A possible route of disease travel into or out of the PVS is along the **brachial plexus**. Extranodal tumor from the axilla (most frequently breast carcinoma) may access the PVS by retrograde perineural spread along the brachial plexus. Conversely, a PVS invasive malignancy may spread antegrade along this pathway to the axillary apex.

Once a lesion has been identified as originating in the PVS, the differential diagnosis unique to the PVS should be reviewed. Identifying characteristic imaging findings of common PVS lesions often yields a short list of possible diagnoses. By far, the **most common lesions** of the PVS originate in the

Perivertebral Space Lesion Differential Diagnosis

Pseudolesions	Vertebral body osteomyelitis, pyogenic
Levator scapulae hypertrophy	Vertebral body osteomyelitis, tuberculous
Cervical rib	**Benign tumor**
Large transverse process	Brachial plexus schwannoma
Degenerative	Brachial plexus neurofibroma
Anterior disc herniation	Vertebral body benign bony tumors
Hypertrophic facet joint	**Malignant tumor/metastatic tumor**
Vertebral body osteophyte	Vertebral body metastasis
Vascular	Epidural metastasis
Vertebral artery dissection	Chordoma
Vertebral artery aneurysm	Non-Hodgkin lymphoma
Vertebral artery pseudoaneurysm	Direct invasion, squamous cell carcinoma posterior pharyngeal wall
Inflammatory/infectious	Vertebral body primary malignant tumors
Longus colli tendonitis	

Above is an exhaustive list of lesions that can be found in the perivertebral space. The table is organized by general pathology category.

vertebral body, with infection and metastatic disease at the top of the list. Therefore, when a PVS lesion is identified, the vertebral body should be evaluated, as it is usually diseased.

Vertebral body osteomyelitis can be differentiated from other entities on the differential diagnosis list by noting destructive changes of adjacent vertebral endplates with increased T2 signal and enhancement of the intervertebral disc on MR. The disc space will be spared in metastatic disease or non-Hodgkin lymphoma, which are more likely to involve multiple bones than to be solitary. Epidural disease can be seen in either metastatic disease or non-Hodgkin lymphoma.

An inflammatory lesion that may be confusing to the radiologist is longus colli tendonitis. Neck pain that may be accompanied by fever may be imaged with CECT. Prevertebral soft tissue swelling secondary to RPS edema with focal prevertebral soft tissue calcification at the C1/2 level must not be confused with RPS abscess. The lesion is due to foreign body inflammatory reaction to deposited crystals of calcium hydroxyapatite, but its pathophysiology is not further understood.

Diagnosis of chordoma is suggested by a destructive mass centered at the sphenooccipital junction in the clivus or upper cervical vertebral body associated with a large, T2 hyperintense soft tissue mass, commonly with perivertebral & epidural extension. When epidural extension occurs in the neck, cord compression is an early & severe consequence.

Benign neurogenic PVS tumors include brachial plexus schwannoma & neurofibroma. Both appear as circumscribed, fusiform, enhancing masses situated between the anterior & middle scalene muscles.

PVS vascular lesions involve the vertebral arteries, including vertebral artery dissection, aneurysm, or pseudoaneurysm. While all can be usually diagnosed by CTA, axial fat-saturated T1 MR may help in cases of dissection, showing intramural hematoma as a hyperintense crescent.

With most PVS pseudolesions (cervical rib, large transverse process) and degenerative changes (anterior disc herniation, hypertrophic facet joint, and vertebral body osteophyte) there is little diagnostic dilemma on cross-sectional imaging. Probably the biggest potential imaging pitfall when evaluating a PVS lesion is to mistake a hypertrophic levator scapulae muscle (LSM) for an enhancing mass or recurrent tumor. This "pseudolesion" is secondary to spinal accessory nerve (CNXI) injury, usually from previous neck dissection. The levator scapulae hypertrophies to help lift the arm to compensate for the atrophy of the sternocleidomastoid (SCM) and trapezius caused by spinal accessory neuropathy. On imaging, the LSM will be enlarged and may enhance. Look for small, fatty infiltrated ipsilateral trapezius and SCM muscles to confirm the diagnosis.

Clinical Implications

Clinical history provides important clues to differentiating PVS lesions. Fever, neck pain, and tenderness herald the onset of **vertebral body osteomyelitis** with possible progression to quadriparesis, if there is epidural pus. Patients with **metastatic disease** usually have a known primary and those with **non-Hodgkin lymphoma** have known systemic disease when PVS disease is found. Both can present with neck pain, radiculopathy, or myelopathy.

Brachial plexus **schwannomas** may be seen sporadically or in the setting of neurofibromatosis type 2 (multiple schwannomas). **Neurofibromas** may also be sporadic but are most commonly found in the setting of neurofibromatosis type 1. Typically, both are painless, slow-growing masses.

Vertebral artery injuries can be from minor (chiropractic manipulation) or major trauma and may present with delayed **stroke**, possibly with a lateral medullary (Wallenberg) syndrome if the posterior inferior cerebellar artery is involved.

Longus colli tendonitis is associated with 2-7 days of neck pain and odynophagia. A history of previous surgical neck dissection can usually be elicited in patients with a **hypertrophic levator scapulae muscle**.

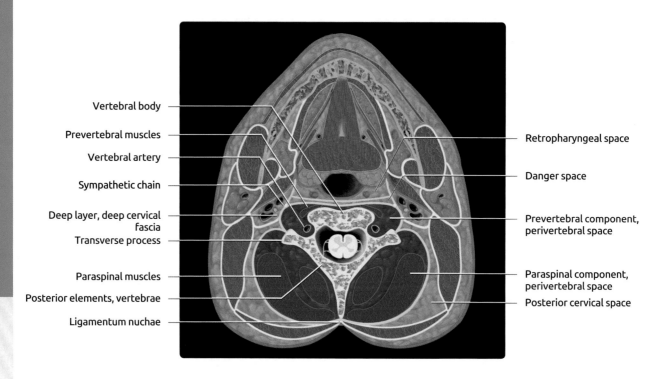

Vertebral body
Prevertebral muscles
Vertebral artery
Sympathetic chain
Deep layer, deep cervical fascia
Transverse process
Paraspinal muscles
Posterior elements, vertebrae
Ligamentum nuchae

Retropharyngeal space
Danger space
Prevertebral component, perivertebral space
Paraspinal component, perivertebral space
Posterior cervical space

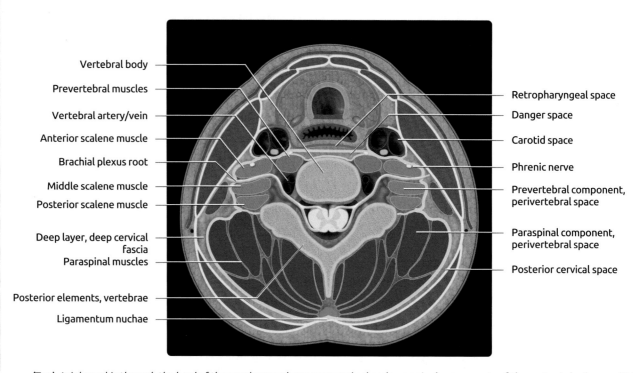

Vertebral body
Prevertebral muscles
Vertebral artery/vein
Anterior scalene muscle
Brachial plexus root
Middle scalene muscle
Posterior scalene muscle
Deep layer, deep cervical fascia
Paraspinal muscles
Posterior elements, vertebrae
Ligamentum nuchae

Retropharyngeal space
Danger space
Carotid space
Phrenic nerve
Prevertebral component, perivertebral space
Paraspinal component, perivertebral space
Posterior cervical space

(Top) *Axial graphic through the level of the oropharynx shows prevertebral and paraspinal components of the perivertebral space (PVS) beneath the deep layer of deep cervical fascia (DL-DCF). Notice this fascia curves medially to touch the transverse processes of the vertebra, dividing the PVS into prevertebral and paraspinal components. The danger and retropharyngeal spaces are anterior to the PVS, while the posterior cervical space is lateral and posterior.* **(Bottom)** *Axial graphic through the thyroid bed shows prevertebral & paraspinal components of the PVS beneath the DL-DCF. The DL-DCF is a tenacious barrier to the spread of infection or malignancy, which will be redirected to the epidural space. The brachial plexus roots pass between the anterior and middle scalene muscles in the prevertebral-PVS and serve as a 2-way highway for perineural spread of malignancy between the PVS and axillary apex.*

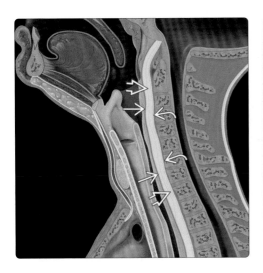

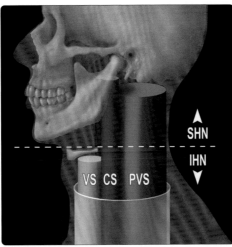

(Left) Sagittal graphic depicts midline spacial relationships of the infrahyoid neck. Just anterior to the PVS (purple) are the danger space ⇨ and retropharyngeal space ⇨. The tenacious DL-DCF ⇨ will usually redirect the spread of PVS disease to the epidural space. (Right) Lateral graphic of the extracranial head and neck shows the tubular PVS extending from the skull base to the mediastinum. DL-DCF completely encircles the PVS.

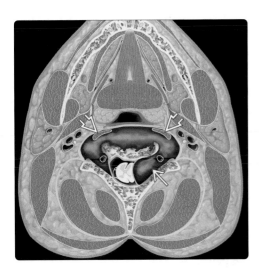

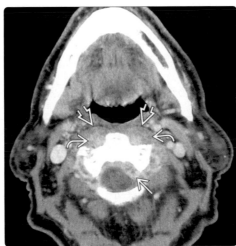

(Left) Axial graphic at the suprahyoid neck oropharyngeal level shows a generic PVS mass that elevates prevertebral muscles ⇨ & destroys vertebral body. Note DL-DCF (blue line) confines the mass and "forces" it into the epidural space ⇨. (Right) Axial CECT at the same level reveals enhancing phlegmon-abscess in the prevertebral portion of the PVS ⇨. Epidural abscess is seen on the left ⇨. Note the anteriorly lifted prevertebral muscles ⇨.

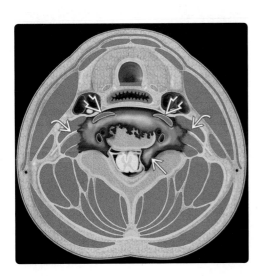

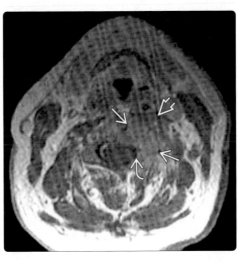

(Left) Axial graphic at thyroid level demonstrates a generic infrahyoid PVS mass arising from the vertebral body and elevating the prevertebral muscles ⇨. Brachial plexus ⇨ & vertebral arteries are engulfed, & epidural disease ⇨ is present. (Right) Axial T1WI MR shows an enhancing metastatic tumor involving the vertebral body and its posterior elements on the left ⇨ with extensive epidural tumor visible ⇨. Note the anteriorly displaced prevertebral muscle ⇨.

Levator Scapulae Muscle Hypertrophy

TERMINOLOGY

- Levator scapulae muscle hypertrophy (LSMH) in response to trapezius and sternocleidomastoid (SCM) muscle atrophy
- CNXI injury causes denervation atrophy of ipsilateral trapezius and SCM muscles

IMAGING

- CECT: LSMH with normal density of enlarged muscle
- T2WI MR: If acute, LSM may demonstrate ↑ signal
- T1WI C+ MR: If subacute, LSM may enhance slightly more than normal
- If associated with other cranial neuropathies (IX-XII), evaluate for possible skull base mass
- Findings of previous neck dissection (i.e., absence of ipsilateral jugular vein, loss of fat planes contiguous with carotid sheath and occasional absence of SCM) also present

TOP DIFFERENTIAL DIAGNOSES

- Contralateral LSM atrophy

- Levator scapulae muscle mass
  - Inflammatory or infectious lesion
  - Benign tumor: Lipoma, schwannoma, etc.
  - Malignant tumor: Invasive squamous cell carcinoma (SCCa), sarcoma, etc.

PATHOLOGY

- Damage to spinal accessory nerve leads to denervation atrophy of trapezius muscle with compensatory hypertrophy of LSM

CLINICAL ISSUES

- Palpable "mass" in perivertebral space
- Previous history of radical neck dissection for SCCa
- "Pseudolesion" recognition avoids potential needle biopsy

DIAGNOSTIC CHECKLIST

- If no previous neck surgery, look for lesion at skull base or brainstem for cause of CNXI neuropathy

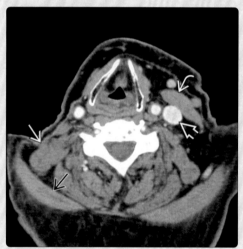

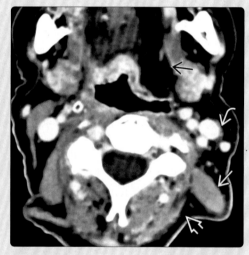

(Left) Axial CECT many months after right radical neck dissection shows levator scapulae muscle hypertrophy ➡ on the right. The internal jugular vein ➡ and sternocleidomastoid muscle ➡ are normal on the left. The trapezius ➡ is also atrophic. (Right) Axial CECT demonstrates hypertrophy of levator scapulae ➡ with atrophy of the trapezius ➡ and sternomastoid ➡ muscles secondary to jugular foramen paraganglioma (not shown). Tongue atrophy ➡ with fatty replacement is also present.

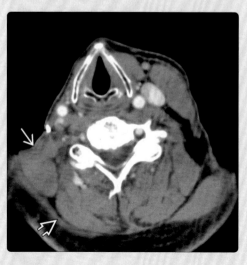

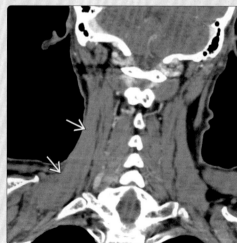

(Left) Axial CECT reveals a right hypertrophic levator scapulae muscle ➡. Note the absence of the right sternocleidomastoid muscle and IJV from previous right radical neck dissection. The trapezius muscle is atrophic ➡ as a result of injury to the spinal accessory cranial nerve at the time of surgery. (Right) Coronal CECT reformation in the same patient shows the hypertrophic levator scapulae muscle along its entire length ➡. The muscle otherwise appears normal in density on CT.

Levator Scapulae Muscle Hypertrophy

TERMINOLOGY

Abbreviations

- Levator scapulae muscle hypertrophy (LSMH)

Definitions

- CNXI (spinal accessory nerve) injury causes denervation atrophy of ipsilateral trapezius and sternocleidomastoid (SCM) muscles
- LSMH: Functional hypertrophy of levator scapulae muscle (LSM) in response to trapezius and SCM muscle atrophy

IMAGING

General Features

- Best diagnostic clue
  - Asymmetric LSM enlargement with denervated trapezius and SCM muscles
    - Findings of previous neck dissection also present (i.e., absence of ipsilateral jugular vein, loss of fat planes contiguous with carotid sheath and occasional absence of SCM)
- Morphology
  - LSM enlarged with convex margins

Radiographic Findings

- Radiography
  - Chest x-ray
    - Demonstrates soft tissue atrophy of trapezius muscle, with increased prominence of LSM shadow

CT Findings

- CECT
  - Chronic phase: LSM hypertrophy with normal density
  - Findings of underlying cause
    - Ipsilateral radical neck dissection most common
      □ Internal jugular vein (IJV), SCM, and spinal accessory nerve removed
      □ Atrophy of ipsilateral trapezius muscle from denervation
    - Less common causes: Ipsilateral jugular foramen mass (paraganglioma, schwannoma, meningioma, metastasis)
      □ CNX injury: Ipsilateral vocal cord paralysis
      □ CNXI injury: Ipsilateral trapezius and SCM muscle atrophy
      □ CNXII injury: Ipsilateral tongue muscle atrophy with fatty infiltration

MR Findings

- T1WI
  - Enlarged LSM in presence of atrophic trapezius muscle
  - If radical neck dissection, SCM muscle and IJV absent
- T2WI
  - Acute: LSM may demonstrate ↑ signal
  - Chronic: Enlarged LSM with normal signal intensity
- T1WI C+
  - Subacute: LSM may enhance slightly more than normal
  - Chronic: Enlarged LSM with convex margins

Imaging Recommendations

- Best imaging tool
  - Post radical neck dissection

- Follow-up of patients with previously treated squamous cell carcinoma (SCCa) of aerodigestive tract
  - Common method for follow-up is CECT
- Skull base mass
  - If associated with other cranial neuropathies (9-12), evaluate for possible skull base mass
  - MR with contrast enhancement and fat saturation combined with NECT of skull base is optimal

DIFFERENTIAL DIAGNOSIS

Contralateral LSM Atrophy

- Secondary to denervation
  - C3, C4, ± C5 nerve root compression secondary to cervical spondylosis, disc disease

Levator Scapulae Muscle Mass

- Inflammatory mass
- Benign neoplasm: Lipoma, schwannoma, other
- Malignant tumor: Invasive SCCa, sarcoma, other

PATHOLOGY

General Features

- Etiology
  - Damage to spinal accessory nerve, leads to denervation atrophy of trapezius muscle with compensatory hypertrophy of LSM

CLINICAL ISSUES

Presentation

- Most common signs/symptoms
  - Palpable "mass" in perivertebral space
  - Previous history of radical neck dissection for SCCa
- Other signs/symptoms
  - With skull base lesion, may have denervation changes of CNIX-XII

Demographics

- Epidemiology
  - Less commonly seen with more conservative node dissection approaches
  - Should not be seen if CNXI was spared in prior neck dissection

Treatment

- "Pseudolesion" recognition avoids potential needle biopsy

DIAGNOSTIC CHECKLIST

Consider

- If no previous neck surgery, look for lesion at skull base or brainstem for cause of CNXI neuropathy

Image Interpretation Pearls

- Observing IJV and SCM muscle absence allows radiologist to diagnose radical neck dissection as cause of hypertrophy

SELECTED REFERENCES

1. Shpizner BA et al: Levator scapulae muscle asymmetry presenting as a palpable neck mass: CT evaluation. AJNR Am J Neuroradiol. 14(2):461-4, 1993

KEY FACTS

TERMINOLOGY

- Acute calcific prevertebral tendonitis, longus colli tendonitis
- Inflammatory condition due to calcium hydroxyapatite deposition in longus colli tendon

IMAGING

- Process produces 3 distinct findings
  - **Calcifications** in prevertebral muscles at C1-C2
  - Inflammation with swelling of prevertebral muscles
  - Retropharyngeal space (RPS) edema
- These features best identified with CECT

TOP DIFFERENTIAL DIAGNOSES

- RPS effusion
- RPS abscess
- Perivertebral space infection

PATHOLOGY

- Deposition of **calcium hydroxyapatite crystals** with secondary inflammatory reaction
- Involves superior oblique fibers of longus colli that insert on C1 anterior tubercle

CLINICAL ISSUES

- Subacute neck pain, odynophagia, dysphagia
- Low-grade fever
- Self-limiting condition, although treat pain
- Analgesics & antiinflammatory medications

DIAGNOSTIC CHECKLIST

- Must differentiate from retropharyngeal infection
- 2 key features for diagnosis
  - Calcification at C1-C2 is pathognomonic
  - RPS edema is smoothly expansile, nonenhancing

(Left) Axial CECT (bone window) demonstrates pathognomonic focal central and left parasagittal amorphous calcification ➡ anteroinferior to C1 arch within prevertebral portion of perivertebral space, corresponding to longus colli tendon. (Right) Axial T1 C+ FS MR demonstrates focal low signal intensity representing calcification ➡, longus colli muscle enhancement ➡, and enhancing inflammatory change in retropharyngeal space ➡.

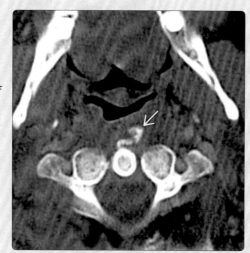
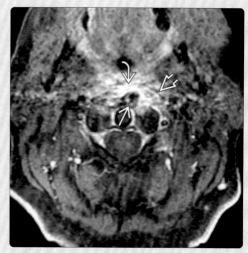

(Left) Axial T2 MR reveals extensive edema ➡ in retropharyngeal space associated with longus colli tendonitis. Fluid is anterior to the prevertebral muscles ➡ posteriorly and posterior to pharyngeal mucosal space. (Right) Sagittal T2 MR reveals marked focal hypointensity of calcification in longus colli muscle at mid-C2 level ➡. Note also hyperintense T2 signal of swollen prevertebral and retropharyngeal soft tissues ➡. There are no disc space changes that might reflect spondylodiscitis, an important exclusion.

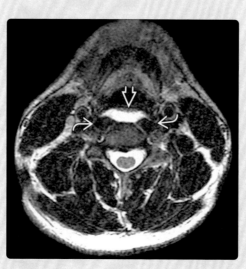
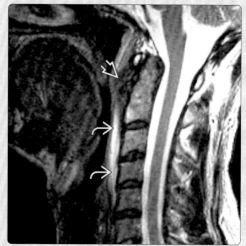

TERMINOLOGY

Synonyms

- Acute calcific prevertebral tendonitis, longus colli tendonitis

Definitions

- Inflammatory condition due to calcium hydroxyapatite deposition in longus colli tendon

IMAGING

General Features

- Best diagnostic clue
  - Focal C1-C2 prevertebral calcification with retropharyngeal edema
- Location
  - Calcifications in prevertebral space at C1-C2
  - Edema in muscles and retropharyngeal space (RPS)

Radiographic Findings

- Radiography
  - Lateral neck: Widening of prevertebral space
  - May see calcification anterior to C1-C2

CT Findings

- CECT
  - Prevertebral **calcification(s)** at C1-C2
  - Variable appearance of calcification(s)
    - Cloud-like (milk of calcium) → coarse & dense
  - Smooth, mild expansion of RPS without peripheral enhancement

MR Findings

- T2WI
  - Inflammation of prevertebral muscles better appreciated than with CT
  - RPS edema also hyperintense
  - ± C1-C2 joint fluid or vertebral body edema
- T2* GRE
  - Hypointense signal of longus colli insertions
- T1WI C+ FS
  - Diffuse prevertebral enhancement
  - No rim enhancement of RPS edema

Imaging Recommendations

- Best imaging tool
  - CT most sensitive to pathognomonic calcification
- Protocol advice
  - CECT with bone and soft tissue algorithm
  - Helps differentiate from retropharyngeal or perivertebral infection

DIFFERENTIAL DIAGNOSIS

RPS Effusion

- Often feature of longus colli tendonitis
- Also found with pharyngitis, jugular vein thrombosis, neck radiation

RPS Abscess

- Fluid collection distending RPS
- Peripheral enhancement of collection ± gas
- No prevertebral calcification

Perivertebral Space Infection

- Most commonly due to spondylodiscitis
- Vertebral body endplate erosions
- Often epidural/prevertebral phlegmon or abscess
- No prevertebral calcification

PATHOLOGY

General Features

- Etiology
  - Deposition of **calcium hydroxyapatite crystals** with secondary inflammatory reaction
  - Involves superior oblique fibers of longus colli
    - Tendons insert on C1 anterior tubercle

CLINICAL ISSUES

Presentation

- Most common signs/symptoms
  - Subacute neck pain, odynophagia, dysphagia
  - Low-grade fever
- Other signs/symptoms
  - ± mild elevation of ESR & WBC
  - Limitation of motion

Demographics

- Age
  - Most common 30-60 years

Natural History & Prognosis

- Self-limiting condition, although treat pain
- As symptoms resolve, calcifications resolve

Treatment

- Analgesics and antiinflammatory medications

DIAGNOSTIC CHECKLIST

Consider

- C1-C2 calcifications should be sought when RPS edema is present
- RPS edema must be distinguished from RPS infection, which might similarly present with neck pain

Image Interpretation Pearls

- Calcifications at C1-C2 are pathognomonic
- RPS edema is smoothly expanding, nonenhancing

SELECTED REFERENCES

1. Silva CF et al: Acute prevertebral calcific tendinitis: a source of non-surgical acute cervical pain. Acta Radiol. 55(1):91-4, 2014
2. Paik NC et al: Tendinitis of longus colli: computed tomography, magnetic resonance imaging, and clinical spectra of 9 cases. J Comput Assist Tomogr. 36(6):755-61, 2012
3. Offiah CE et al: Acute calcific tendinitis of the longus colli muscle: spectrum of CT appearances and anatomical correlation. Br J Radiol. 82(978):e117-21, 2009
4. Harnier S et al: Retropharyngeal tendinitis: a rare differential diagnosis of severe headaches and neck pain. Headache. 48(1):158-61, 2008
5. Eastwood JD et al: Retropharyngeal effusion in acute calcific prevertebral tendinitis: diagnosis with CT and MR imaging. AJNR Am J Neuroradiol. 19(9):1789-92, 1998
6. Artenian DJ et al: Acute neck pain due to tendonitis of the longus colli: CT and MRI findings. Neuroradiology. 31(2):166-9, 1989

KEY FACTS

TERMINOLOGY

- Perivertebral space infection (PVS) phlegmon, PVS abscess
- Deep neck infection centered on prevertebral muscles, disc space, vertebral body (VB)
- Most often due to spondylodiscitis
- Uncommonly follows neck or spine surgery
- Rarely direct seeding of PVS muscles

IMAGING

- Heterogeneously enhancing prevertebral muscles or rim-enhancing low-intensity collection
- Anterior displacement of retropharyngeal fat or retropharyngeal fluid
- Large collections more often seen with atypical organisms, especially TB
- Look for epidural phlegmon/abscess
- Bone destruction on CECT and bone CT
- MR C+ for bone and epidural changes

TOP DIFFERENTIAL DIAGNOSES

- Retropharyngeal space abscess
- VB metastasis, PVS
- Lymphoma
- Chordoma

PATHOLOGY

- Spondylodiscitis most often hematogenous infection
- Most common pyogenic organism is *Staphylococcus aureus*
- Worldwide, tuberculosis is most common cause

DIAGNOSTIC CHECKLIST

- Differentiate prevertebral space process from retropharyngeal space
- Search for spondylodiscitis as cause
- Must carefully evaluate for epidural extension ± cord compression
- T1 C+ FS MR best evaluates epidural involvement

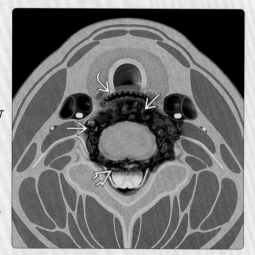
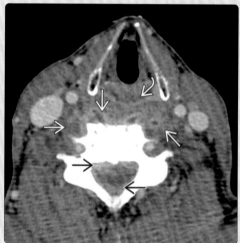

(Left) Axial graphic depicts typical findings of perivertebral space infection. Phlegmonous soft tissue ➡ surrounds vertebral body, displacing esophagus ➡ anteriorly and producing epidural phlegmon/abscess dorsally ➡. (Right) Axial CECT shows heterogeneously enhancing tissue ➡ abutting and surrounding vertebral body. Hypopharynx ➡ is displaced anteriorly. Careful evaluation of spinal canal reveals densely enhancing tissue ➡ around cervical cord indicating epidural phlegmon.

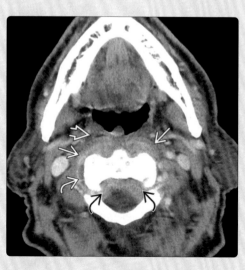
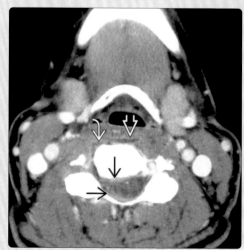

(Left) Axial CECT at C2 level shows collar of heterogeneously enhancing tissue ➡ abutting vertebral body, directly posterior to thin stripe of retropharyngeal fat ➡. Note intraspinal epidural component ➡. A small area of early abscess is present ➡. (Right) Axial CECT reveals heterogeneously enlarged prevertebral tissues with focal pool of rim-enhancing pus ➡. Inflamed tissues extend from epidural phlegmon ➡. Small retropharyngeal fluid collection is also noted ➡.

TERMINOLOGY

Abbreviations
- Perivertebral space (PVS) infection

Synonyms
- PVS phlegmon, PVS abscess

Definitions
- Deep neck infection centered at prevertebral muscles, disc space, vertebral body (VB)
  - Most often due to cervical spondylodiscitis
- Phlegmon = inflammation from diffuse tissue infection
- Abscess = marginated collection of pus

IMAGING

General Features
- Best diagnostic clue
  - Prevertebral muscle swelling or collection with destruction or signal change in adjacent VB/disc
- Location
  - Within or posterior to prevertebral muscles, posterior to retropharyngeal space (RPS)
  - Cervical spondylodiscitis most common at C5-C6 level
- Size
  - Variable
    - Phlegmon results in distended PVS muscles
    - Pyogenic infection more commonly phlegmon with small abscesses
    - Atypical organisms, especially TB, may form large (several cm) collections
- Morphology
  - PVS infection most often due to **spondylodiscitis**
    - Spread of infection into prevertebral ± paraspinal components
      - □ Cellulitis with phlegmon → focal then coalescent abscess
    - Infection may simultaneously involve epidural space
      - □ May result in cord compression ± infarction
      - □ Common in cervical spondylodiscitis
      - □ Extensive spinal involvement may be seen
  - **Pyogenic spondylodiscitis**
    - Typically involves disc and adjacent end plates
    - More acute disease presentation and symptoms than TB spondylitis
    - Presents with severe pain, fever ± neurologic deficit
  - **Tuberculous spondylitis**
    - Selectively involves VB with relative sparing of endplates and disc
    - May spread under anterior longitudinal ligament to involve multiple VB levels
    - Reactive sclerosis less common
    - Perivertebral soft tissue involvement common, may result in multiple abscesses ± calcification
    - VB collapse with deformity more often than neurologic deficit as presentation
    - Kyphotic deformity may result
  - Atypical infections (e.g., fungus, blastomycosis) usually behave similar to TB

- Spondylodiscitis uncommonly follows neck or cervical spine surgery
- PVS infection usually from osseous or disc infection, rarely from direct muscle seeding

Radiographic Findings
- Radiography
  - Plain films may reveal pyogenic discitis
    - < 7 days: Prevertebral soft tissue swelling
      - □ Cannot distinguish prevertebral from RPS mass
    - 7-10 days: Erosion of VB endplate
    - > 2 weeks: Narrow disc space, endplate destruction
    - > 3 weeks: Reactive sclerosis
  - Chronic infection: VB collapse, ± tissue calcifications

CT Findings
- CECT
  - Enhancing, heterogeneous enlarged prevertebral muscles
  - Anteriorly displaced RPS and posterior pharyngeal wall
  - May see rim-enhancing abscess
  - Look for intraspinal epidural phlegmon/abscess
- Bone CT
  - Endplate erosion → frank VB destruction
  - Sagittal reformats illustrate spine alignment

MR Findings
- T1WI
  - Heterogeneously enlarged prevertebral muscles
  - Loss of T1 signal in VB
- T2WI
  - Hyperintensity of prevertebral muscles, disc, and VB
  - Abscess typically markedly hyperintense
  - May also see RPS edema
- DWI
  - Infected disc space often restricts diffusion
- T1WI C+
  - Heterogeneously enhancing prevertebral muscles or rim-enhancing low-intensity collection
  - Diffuse, ill-defined enhancement of prevertebral muscles, disc, VB, and epidural space
  - Look for epidural phlegmon/abscess
  - Enhancement may involve adjacent spaces: CS, RPS

Nuclear Medicine Findings
- Bone scan
  - Sensitive, but nonspecific for spondylodiscitis
  - Arterial hyperemia with progressive focal uptake
  - TB infection cold in 35-40%
- PET
  - Usually FDG avid, but nonspecific

Imaging Recommendations
- Best imaging tool
  - CECT frequently initial study for neck pain, fever
  - Either CECT or MR good for delineating and distinguishing RPS and PVS processes
  - CT best for bone changes and aspiration guidance
  - MR best for epidural extent ± cord compromise
- Protocol advice
  - If uncertain about epidural involvement on CECT, recommend MR C+

o Add fat saturation to T1 C+ MR for complete evaluation of epidural extent

DIFFERENTIAL DIAGNOSIS

Retropharyngeal Space Abscess

- Collection between pharynx and prevertebral space
- Flattens anterior aspect of prevertebral muscles
- Most often secondary to pharyngeal infection
- Normal VB and disc spaces

Vertebral Body Metastasis, PVS

- VB destruction that typically spares disc space
- Soft tissue extension anteriorly mimics PVS phlegmon, but no edema
- Epidural extension ± cord compromise as well
- Other VB lesions may be evident

Lymphoma

- Centered in VB or posterior elements
- May result in associated PVS or epidural mass
- Intermediate to low T2 signal, solid enhancement

Chordoma

- In cervical spine, most often located at C2
- VB mass with lobulated PVS components
- Markedly intense on T2 MR (like CSF signal), but solid enhancement

Ewing Sarcoma

- Rarely arises in VB or sacrum
- Destructive VB soft tissue mass ± PVS and epidural mass
- Disc typically spared

PATHOLOGY

General Features

- Etiology
  - PVS infection most often secondary to **cervical spondylodiscitis**
    - Cervical spine is least common site of spondylodiscitis
  - Wide variety of causative organisms
    - Most common pyogenic organism is *Staphylococcus aureus*
    - Most common worldwide is tuberculosis
      - □ Uncommon in cervical spine
  - Predisposing conditions
    - Diabetes, IV drug use, transplant or other immunocompromised patients
    - Unwell patients: Elderly, pneumonia, urinary tract infection, skin infection
  - Spondylodiscitis uncommonly follows neck or cervical spine surgery
  - PVS infection rarely due to direct muscle seeding

CLINICAL ISSUES

Presentation

- Most common signs/symptoms
  - Cervical spondylodiscitis
    - Localized severe progressive neck pain and stiffness
    - Fever, malaise, torticollis
    - 20% present with myelopathy from epidural mass

- Other signs/symptoms
  - Prevertebral abscess
    - Dysphagia, odynophagia, and shortness of breath

Demographics

- Age
  - Any
  - Highest incidence 6th and 7th decades
- Epidemiology
  - Spondylodiscitis represents 2-7% of all osteomyelitis

Natural History & Prognosis

- Epidural spread of PVS infection/spondylodiscitis may result in neurologic compromise
  - PVS infection is confined by deep cervical fascia
  - Fascia may direct infection into epidural space

Treatment

- Initial treatment
  - Aspiration/decompression of abscess collections
  - Long-term intravenous antibiotics
- Other surgical treatment
  - Debridement of dead bone
  - Supportive bony fusion if VB collapse or kyphosis

DIAGNOSTIC CHECKLIST

Image Interpretation Pearls

- In adult patient with prevertebral muscle inflammation/abscess, carefully assess spine for spondylodiscitis
- Differentiate prevertebral space from RPS process
- Search for spondylodiscitis or VB mass
  - Distinguish typical pyogenic spondylodiscitis from atypical or tuberculous spondylitis
- Look for epidural collection, cord compression

Reporting Tips

- Must evaluate for epidural component ± cord compression
  - Recommend MR C+ if unsure of epidural extent
  - Useful to image entire spine if epidural abscess is present

SELECTED REFERENCES

1. Mills MK et al: Imaging of the perivertebral space. Radiol Clin North Am. 53(1):163-80, 2015
2. Gonzalez-Beicos A et al: Imaging of acute head and neck infections. Radiol Clin North Am. 50(1):73-83, 2012
3. Rana RS et al: Head and neck infection and inflammation. Radiol Clin North Am. 49(1):165-82, 2011
4. Holmgaard R et al: Cervical spondylodiscitis–a rare complication of palatopharyngeal flap surgery. Cleft Palate Craniofac J. 45(6):674-6, 2008
5. Karadimas EJ et al: Spondylodiscitis. A retrospective study of 163 patients. Acta Orthop. 79(5):650-9, 2008
6. Curry JM et al: Cervical discitis and epidural abscess after tonsillectomy. Laryngoscope. 117(12):2093-6, 2007
7. Acosta FL Jr et al: Diagnosis and management of adult pyogenic osteomyelitis of the cervical spine. Neurosurg Focus. 17(6):E2, 2004
8. Ledermann HP et al: MR imaging findings in spinal infections: rules or myths? Radiology. 228(2):506-14, 2003
9. Longo M et al: Contrast-enhanced MR imaging with fat suppression in adult-onset septic spondylodiscitis. Eur Radiol. 13(3):626-37, 2003
10. Stabler A et al: Imaging of spinal infection. Radiol Clin North Am. 39(1):115-35, 2001

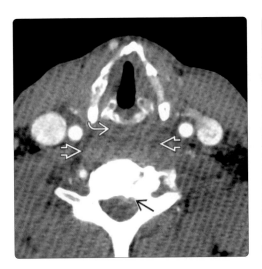
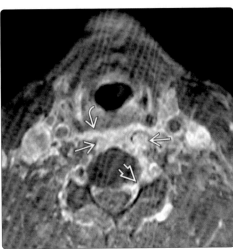

(Left) Axial CECT in a patient with septicemia, history of drug abuse, and neck pain shows marked prevertebral soft tissue thickening ➔ displacing hypopharynx ➔ anteriorly. Subtle epidural phlegmon is also evident ➔. (Right) Axial T1WI C+ FS MR in same patient demonstrates extensive soft tissue enhancement in prevertebral space ➔, with infiltration of longus colli muscles as well as involvement of retropharyngeal space ➔. Subtle left foraminal and epidural enhancement is also evident ➔.

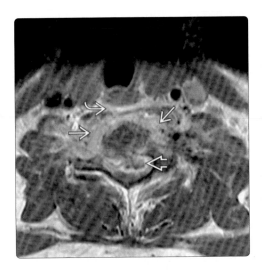
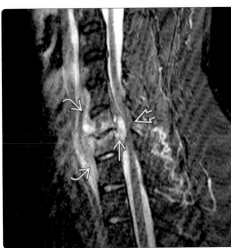

(Left) Axial T1WI C+ MR demonstrates extensive prevertebral muscle solid enhancement ➔ and enlargement, displacing retropharyngeal fat ➔ anteriorly. Abnormal epidural enhancement is also noted with rim-enhancing epidural abscess ➔. (Right) Sagittal STIR MR illustrates spondylodiscitis at C6-7 with loss of disc space, abnormally high vertebral body signal, prevertebral phlegmon ➔, and epidural abscess ➔. There is significant resulting cord compression ➔.

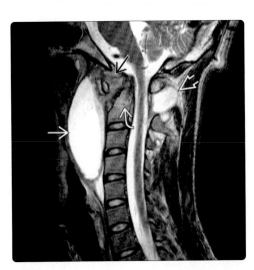
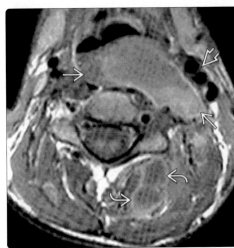

(Left) Sagittal T2 MR shows C1-2 subluxation. Note C2 marrow edema ➔ with tuberculous phlegmon anterior to the odontoid ➔ and large prevertebral space subligamentous abscess ➔. Note posterior left paraspinal space abscess ➔ within paraspinal musculature. (Right) Axial T1 C+ MR, same patient, shows a large heterogeneous tuberculous abscess ➔. Well-defined collection displaces pharynx and carotid vessels ➔ without significant inflammation. Patient also has left posterior paraspinal abscess ➔.

Vertebral Artery Dissection in Neck

TERMINOLOGY

- Vertebral artery (VA) dissection
- Narrowing &/or occlusion of VA secondary to intimal tear and subadventitial hematoma

IMAGING

- 2 typical forms of VA dissection
- **Steno-occlusive dissection**
  - Dissection to subintimal plane with vessel luminal narrowing or occlusion
- **Dissecting aneurysm**
  - Dissection into subadventitial plane with dilatation of outer wall
- Intramural hematoma is pathognomonic
  - Best seen as **bright crescent** on T1 FS MR
- CTA source images show contour changes of lumen
- Conventional angiography is gold standard

TOP DIFFERENTIAL DIAGNOSES

- Extracranial atherosclerosis
- Fibromuscular dysplasia
- Miscellaneous vasculitis

PATHOLOGY

- **Traumatic** VA dissection
  - Direct or indirect arterial injury
- **Spontaneous** VA dissection
  - Many associations and predisposing factors

CLINICAL ISSUES

- Age: Majority < 45 yr

DIAGNOSTIC CHECKLIST

- Check other vessels carefully for 2nd dissection
- Evaluate carefully for the suboccipital rind sign
- Report degree of luminal narrowing

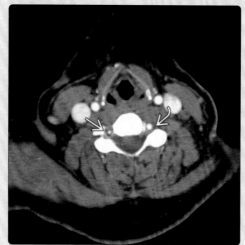
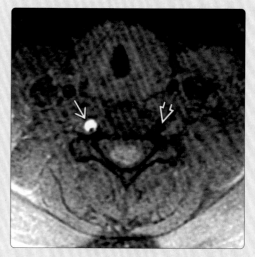

(Left) Axial CTA shows a normal symmetric appearance of the common carotid arteries with adjacent jugular veins. The left vertebral artery (VA) is patent ➘ and normal in caliber. Right VA shows markedly diminished lumen caliber ➘ and wall thickening representing mural hematoma. (Right) Axial T1WI FS MR in a patient with vertebral dissection reveals hyperintense crescent within wall of right VA ➘ significantly narrowing VA lumen. This is typical of an intramural hematoma. Note normal left VA flow void ➘.

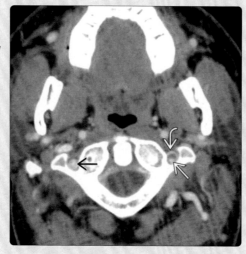
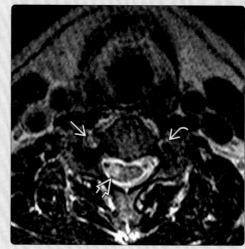

(Left) Axial CTA shows rim enhancement of left VA ➘ with low-density mural hematoma and contrast filling narrowed lumen ➘. Subtle linear lucency in right VA proved not to be dissection flap ➘. (Right) Axial T2 MR in a different patient with neck trauma and cervical fractures reveals traumatic VA dissection as loss of right vertebral flow void ➘, as compared to normal left side ➘. Note right cervical hemicord hyperintensity from infarction ➘.

TERMINOLOGY

Abbreviations

- Vertebral artery (VA) dissection

Definitions

- Narrowing &/or occlusion of VA secondary to intimal tear and subadventitial hematoma

IMAGING

General Features

- Best diagnostic clue
  - Key cross-sectional finding is **crescentic hyperintensity** on T1 FS MR
- Morphology
  - 2 typical forms of VA dissection
  - **Steno-occlusive dissection**
    - Long segment stenosis → string sign
  - **Dissecting aneurysm**
    - Focal or fusiform aneurysmal dilatation ± stenosis
    - Usually involves intradural VA
    - May present with subarachnoid hemorrhage

CT Findings

- CTA
  - Axial source images show contour changes of lumen
  - **Suboccipital rind sign**
    - Normally opacified VA lumen with mural hematoma

MR Findings

- T1WI
  - Mural hematoma signal varies with time
    - Hyperacute & acute blood
      - Oxy-/deoxyhemoglobin: Iso- → hyperintense
    - Subacute blood (~ 2-3 days)
      - Methemoglobin intrinsically bright on T1 MR
- T1WI FS
  - FS makes mural methemoglobin more conspicuous
  - Inferior presaturation to create black blood imaging also very useful
- T2WI
  - Loss of normal flow void
- MRA
  - Reveals lumen caliber changes
    - Aneurysmal dilatation & stenosis/occlusion

Angiographic Findings

- Vessel contour changes, including aneurysmal dilatation & stenosis/occlusion
- Intimal flap/double lumen are specific

Imaging Recommendations

- Best imaging tool
  - **Intramural hematoma** is **pathognomonic**
    - Best seen with T1 FS MR
  - Conventional angiography is gold standard
    - May miss dissection if subtle change in lumen diameter
- Protocol advice
  - Black blood MR, MRA, or CTA for VA evaluation
  - Brain imaging to evaluate for infarctions

DIFFERENTIAL DIAGNOSIS

Extracranial Atherosclerosis

- Multiple vessels involved with eccentric, irregular stenoses

Fibromuscular Dysplasia

- Multiple, focal web-like strictures (string of beads) or long-segment stenosis

Miscellaneous Vasculitis

- Stenoses involving multiple, variably sized vessels

PATHOLOGY

General Features

- Etiology
  - **Traumatic VA dissection**
    - Direct arterial injury (penetrating trauma)
    - Indirect injury ± cervical fractures
  - **Spontaneous VA dissection**
    - Multiple associations and predisposing factors
      - Hypertension
      - Vascular abnormality: Fibromuscular dysplasia (FMD), Marfan syndrome, collagen vascular disease, homocystinuria

CLINICAL ISSUES

Presentation

- Most common signs/symptoms
  - Neck pain, headache, or posterior circulation stroke

Demographics

- Age
  - Majority < 45 yr
- Epidemiology
  - Dissection → 5-20% of strokes in young patients

Treatment

- Steno-occlusive dissection → anticoagulation
- Dissecting aneurysm → ligation or coil embolization
- Complete resolution of lumen abnormality in ~ 80%

DIAGNOSTIC CHECKLIST

Image Interpretation Pearls

- Evaluate axial CTA carefully for suboccipital rind sign if normal lumen but high clinical suspicion

SELECTED REFERENCES

1. Ben Hassen W et al: Imaging of cervical artery dissection. Diagn Interv Imaging. 95(12):1151-61, 2014
2. Lum C et al: Vertebral artery dissection with a normal-appearing lumen at multisection CT angiography: the importance of identifying wall hematoma. AJNR Am J Neuroradiol. 30(4):787-92, 2009
3. Provenzale JM et al: Comparison of test performance characteristics of MRI, MR angiography, and CT angiography in the diagnosis of carotid and vertebral artery dissection: a review of the medical literature. AJR Am J Roentgenol. 193(4):1167-74, 2009
4. Provenzale JM: MRI and MRA for evaluation of dissection of craniocerebral arteries: lessons from the medical literature. Emerg Radiol. 16(3):185-93, 2009
5. Tan MA et al: Late complications of vertebral artery dissection in children: pseudoaneurysm, thrombosis, and recurrent stroke. J Child Neurol. 24(3):354-60, 2009
6. Rodallec MH et al: Craniocervical arterial dissection: spectrum of imaging findings and differential diagnosis. Radiographics. 28(6):1711-28, 2008

TERMINOLOGY

- Benign Schwann cell neoplasm that **arises from brachial plexus** (BP) in perivertebral space (PVS)

IMAGING

- Well-circumscribed, **fusiform mass** along course of BP
- Occur along course of BP in any segment
- Intra- & extradural and neural foramen
- In PVS between anterior & middle scalene muscles
- 3D STIR to produce MR neurography increasing in utilization to depict BP normal anatomy and schwannomas

TOP DIFFERENTIAL DIAGNOSES

- Systemic nodal metastases
- Neurofibroma
- Lateral meningocele
- Malignant peripheral nerve sheath tumor

PATHOLOGY

- Cystic degeneration & hemorrhage common
- Firm, encapsulated, fusiform mass
- Attaches to and displaces nerve
- Multiple schwannomas occur with multiple inherited schwannomas, meningiomas, ependymomas, & schwannomatosis

CLINICAL ISSUES

- 5% of benign soft tissue neoplasms
- Malignant degeneration rare, more common with multiple schwannoma syndromes
- Development of pain should raise suspicion for malignancy

DIAGNOSTIC CHECKLIST

- Determination that lesion is along course of BP is key
- Roots of BP (C5-T1) emerge into scalene triangle, between anterior and middle scalene muscles

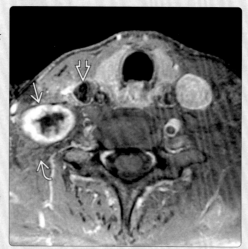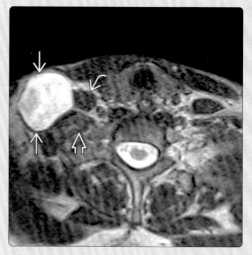

(Left) Axial T1WI C+ FS MR demonstrates large schwannoma ➔ in lower right neck overlying middle scalene muscle ➔ with intense, irregular peripheral enhancement. Central nonenhancement represents cystic degeneration. Lesion is more lateral in location than expected for lower cervical nodes, which typically abut the internal jugular vein ➔. (Right) Axial T2WI MR shows heterogeneously hyperintense schwannoma in lower neck ➔ splaying & deforming anterior ➔ & middle ➔ scalene muscles in perivertebral space.

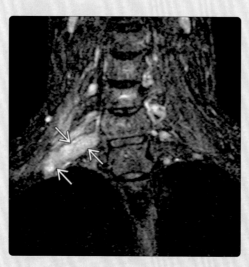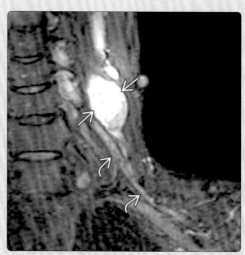

(Left) Coronal STIR MR (MR neurography technique) demonstrates asymmetrically enlarged right CNVIII nerve root ➔ extending from CNVII-T1 neural foramen. (Right) Coronal STIR MR in a different patient shows fusiform, heterogeneously hyperintense schwannoma ➔ of lower neck. Note marked hyperintensity as compared to adjacent brachial plexus elements ➔ that lesion parallels. Needle biopsy caused arm twitching but did confirm diagnosis.

TERMINOLOGY

Abbreviations

- Brachial plexus (BP) schwannoma

Definitions

- Benign Schwann cell neoplasm that arises from BP in perivertebral space (PVS)

IMAGING

General Features

- Best diagnostic clue
  - Well-circumscribed, fusiform mass along course of BP
- Location
  - Occur along course of BP in any segment
    - Intra- & extradural and neural foramen
    - In PVS between anterior & middle scalene muscles
- Morphology
  - Fusiform or dumbbell-shaped mass

CT Findings

- NECT
  - Typically isodense to muscle; calcification uncommon
  - When paraspinal, bony neural foramen shows **smooth enlargement**
- CECT
  - Mild to moderate enhancement

MR Findings

- T1WI
  - **Fusiform mass**, isointense to muscle
- T2WI
  - Heterogeneously hyperintense
  - **Target sign**: Central hypointense, peripheral hyperintense signal
  - **Fascicular sign**: Multiple, irregular, central hypointense foci
- STIR
  - 3D STIR to produce MR neurography increasing in utilization to depict BP normal anatomy and schwannomas
- T1WI C+
  - Moderate heterogeneous enhancement
    - **Intramural cysts** common
  - More uniform enhancement when small

Imaging Recommendations

- Protocol advice
  - T1WI with FS and STIR improve conspicuity

DIFFERENTIAL DIAGNOSIS

Systemic Nodal Metastases

- Supraclavicular nodes are metastatic site for chest and abdominal disease
- Lower cervical nodes medial to anterior scalene muscle, adjacent to internal jugular vein

Neurofibroma

- May be indistinguishable from schwannoma on MR
- Typically lower density on NECT, approaching water density
- Cystic degeneration & hemorrhage uncommon

Lateral Meningocele

- Fusiform cystic mass follows CSF density/intensity
- Contiguous with spinal canal

Malignant Peripheral Nerve Sheath Tumor

- Progressively enlarging, irregular, heterogeneous mass
- Typically associated with pain

PATHOLOGY

Gross Pathologic & Surgical Features

- Firm, encapsulated, well-circumscribed, gray-tan, fusiform mass attached to & displacing nerve
- Cystic degeneration & hemorrhage common

Microscopic Features

- Tumor arises from Schwann cells of nerve sheath
- Alternating regions of high cellularity (Antoni A) & loose, myxoid component (Antoni B)

CLINICAL ISSUES

Presentation

- Most common signs/symptoms
  - Painless, slow-growing mass in lateral neck ± radiculopathy

Demographics

- Age
  - Peaks at 20-30 years

Natural History & Prognosis

- Slow-growing lesion
- Malignant degeneration rare, more common with multiple schwannoma syndromes
- Development of **pain** should raise suspicion for **malignancy**

DIAGNOSTIC CHECKLIST

Image Interpretation Pearls

- Determination that lesion is along course of BP is key
- Roots of BP (C5-T1) emerge into scalene triangle, between anterior and middle scalene muscles

Reporting Tips

- When describing any low neck lesion, always describe relationship of lesion to BP course

SELECTED REFERENCES

1. Lutz AM et al: MR imaging of the brachial plexus. Neuroimaging Clin N Am. 24(1):91-108, 2014
2. Chhabra A et al: High-resolution 3T MR neurography of the brachial plexus and its branches, with emphasis on 3D imaging. AJNR Am J Neuroradiol. 34(3):486-97, 2013
3. Guerrissi JO: Solitary benign schwannomas in major nerve systems of the head and neck. J Craniofac Surg. 20(3):957-61, 2009
4. Siqueira MG et al: Management of brachial plexus region tumours and tumour-like conditions: relevant diagnostic and surgical features in a consecutive series of eighteen patients. Acta Neurochir (Wien). 151(9):1089-98, 2009
5. Gupta G et al: Malignant peripheral nerve sheath tumors. Neurosurg Clin N Am. 19(4):533-43, v, 2008
6. Binder DK et al: Primary brachial plexus tumors: imaging, surgical, and pathological findings in 25 patients. Neurosurg Focus. 16(5):E11, 2004
7. Wittenberg KH et al: MR imaging of nontraumatic brachial plexopathies: frequency and spectrum of findings. Radiographics. 20(4):1023-32, 2000

Chordoma in Perivertebral Space

TERMINOLOGY

- Rare low-grade primary malignant tumor of notochord origin

IMAGING

- Cervical spine: C2-5 most often
- Lytic vertebral body (VB) lesion without collapse
- CT: Lobulated low-density soft tissue mass
  - Coarse, amorphous calcifications in 30%
- MR: Marked T2 hyperintensity, similar to CSF
  - Typically heterogeneous enhancement
- FDG PET: Heterogeneous, increased uptake

TOP DIFFERENTIAL DIAGNOSES

- VB metastasis, perivertebral space (PVS)
- PVS infection
- Brachial plexus schwannoma
- Vertebral chondrosarcoma

PATHOLOGY

- Arises from embryonic notochord
- Lobulated, soft, grayish mass with pseudocapsule
- 3-7% all chordomas arise in cervical spine
- Myxoid stroma & characteristic **physaliphorous cells**

CLINICAL ISSUES

- 3rd-6th decade, peaks in 5th decade
- Presents from local pressure effects on cord or prevertebral structures
- May present with nonspecific neck pain
- Treat primarily with surgery, then follow with radiotherapy
- Slow-growing lesion, tendency for local recurrence

DIAGNOSTIC CHECKLIST

- Marked T2 hyperintensity is key to diagnosis

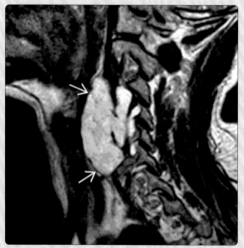
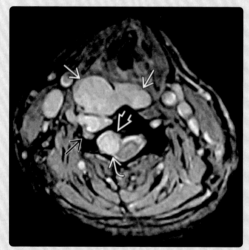

(Left) Sagittal T2 MR in a patient with neck swelling & palpable mass demonstrates large, multilevel, markedly hyperintense chordoma arising from cervical vertebral body (VB) with a large soft tissue component extending into perivertebral space (PVS) ➡. (Right) Axial T2* image demonstrates cervical chordoma that erodes VB ➡, extends into epidural space & spinal canal ➡, with bulky tumor in PVS ➡. Tumor is contiguous with right vertebral artery ➡. Lobulated configuration is well shown.

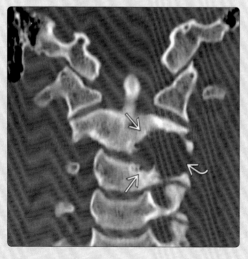
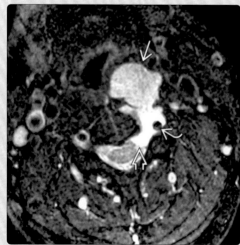

(Left) Coronal CT reformat demonstrates cervical chordoma involving contiguous C2 and C3 levels. The mass has extensive bone destruction with relatively well-defined margins ➡ & with no discernible matrix. The lesion extends into & involves the neural foramen ➡. (Right) Axial T2WI MR of typical cervical chordoma with PVS extension ➡ without vertebral body destruction is shown. The mass extends into the neural foramen with epidural extension ➡ & nearly encases the left vertebral artery ➡.

TERMINOLOGY

Definitions

- Rare low-grade primary malignant tumor of notochord origin

IMAGING

General Features

- Best diagnostic clue
  - Destructive vertebral body (VB) lesion with well-defined, T2 hyperintense, & enhancing perivertebral mass
- Location
  - Cervical spine: C2-5 most often
- Morphology
  - VB mass spares posterior elements
  - Associated lobulated soft tissue mass
  - On occasion, may involve adjacent vertebra mimicking spondylodiscitis

Radiographic Findings

- Radiography
  - Lytic, destructive lesion without VB collapse

CT Findings

- NECT
  - Coarse, amorphous calcifications in 30%
- CECT
  - Lobulated soft tissue mass typically low density

MR Findings

- T1WI
  - Low to intermediate signal intensity
- T2WI
  - **Markedly hyperintense**, similar to CSF
  - May have T2 hypointense fibrous septations
- T1WI C+
  - Typically heterogeneous enhancement

Nuclear Medicine Findings

- PET
  - Heterogeneous, increased FDG uptake

Imaging Recommendations

- Best imaging tool
  - CT & MR are complementary
    - Bone CT best shows VB lysis & occasional calcifications
    - MR for soft tissue extent; T2 hyperintensity of lesion suggests diagnosis

DIFFERENTIAL DIAGNOSIS

VB Metastasis, Perivertebral Space

- Destructive VB soft tissue mass
- Variable signal intensity on T2WI MR

Perivertebral Space Infection

- Disc space narrowing, endplate destruction
- Diffuse marrow, disc, epidural, & perivertebral space enhancement

Brachial Plexus Schwannoma, Perivertebral Space

- Intermediate to high T2 signal follows nerve root
- Smoothly scallops neural foramen

Chondrosarcoma

- Destructive VB ± posterior element lesion
- CT shows chondroid matrix mineralization
- Very high signal intensity on T2WI MR

PATHOLOGY

General Features

- Etiology
  - Arise from embryonic notochord
  - Location parallels distribution of notochordal rests
    - 50% sacrococcygeal region
    - 35% sphenooccipital region
    - 15% spine: Cervical > lumbar > thoracic

Microscopic Features

- Myxoid stroma & characteristic **physaliphorous cells**
  - Large cells with eosinophilic cytoplasm containing multiple vacuoles & central nuclei

CLINICAL ISSUES

Presentation

- Most common signs/symptoms
  - Typically presents from local mass effect
  - Gradual onset neck pain, numbness

Demographics

- Gender
  - M:F = 2:1
- Epidemiology
  - 3-7% all chordomas arise in cervical spine

Natural History & Prognosis

- Slow-growing lesion, tendency for local recurrence
- Metastatic disease in 5-43%

Treatment

- Surgery & complete resection is treatment of choice
- Proton beam is favored radiotherapy after surgery

DIAGNOSTIC CHECKLIST

Image Interpretation Pearls

- Marked T2 hyperintensity with heterogeneous enhancement is key to diagnosis
- Carefully evaluate for vascular encasement

SELECTED REFERENCES

1. Lau CS et al: Pediatric chordomas: a population-based clinical outcome study involving 86 patients from the surveillance, epidemiology, and end result (SEER) Database (1973-2011). Pediatr Neurosurg. ePub, 2016
2. Yasuda M et al: Chordomas of the skull base and cervical spine: clinical outcomes associated with a multimodal surgical resection combined with proton-beam radiation in 40 patients. Neurosurg Rev. 35(2):171-82; discussion 182-3, 2012
3. Brennan PM et al: Chordoma masquerading as a nerve root tumour – a clinical lesson. Br J Radiol. 82(983):e231-4, 2009
4. Jiang L et al: Upper cervical spine chordoma of C2-C3. Eur Spine J. 18(3):293-298; discussion 298-300, 2009
5. Zhou H et al: Cervical chordoma in childhood without typical vertebral bony destruction: case report and review of the literature. Spine (Phila Pa 1976). 34(14):E493-7, 2009
6. Smolders D et al: Value of MRI in the diagnosis of non-clival, non-sacral chordoma. Skeletal Radiol. 32(6): 343-50, 2003

TERMINOLOGY

- Metastatic tumor to cervical vertebral body (VB) ± invasion of perivertebral space (PVS)

IMAGING

- Spinal metastases proportionate to red marrow
- Lumbar > thoracic > cervical spine
- > 50% have multiple level involvement
- Destructive VB mass
- Expanded, infiltrated, or displaced prevertebral muscles

TOP DIFFERENTIAL DIAGNOSES

- PVS infection
- Longus colli tendinitis
- PVS chordoma

PATHOLOGY

- Vertebral metastases may be confined by **prevertebral fascia**, directing tumor to **epidural space**

- Most VB metastases from hematogenous spread
- Adults most often lung, breast, prostate, kidney, GI
- Children most often hematologic malignancies & neuroblastoma
- Rarely tumor directly penetrates PVS from posterior pharyngeal wall

CLINICAL ISSUES

- Vertebral metastasis is most common malignant spine lesion
- Vertebra is most common site of bone metastasis
- Treatment depends on tumor type, symptomatology, and neurological complications
  - Radiation therapy ± stereotactic radiotherapy, endovascular tumor embolization, vertebroplasty, surgical resection for cord decompression ± spine stabilization
- Ongoing bone destruction leads to fracture, instability, deformity, & neurological compromise

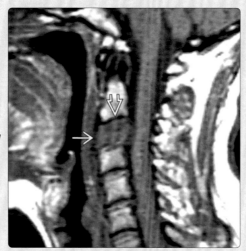
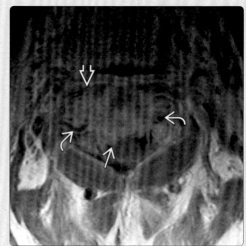

(Left) *Sagittal T1WI MR reveals C3 vertebral body (VB) replaced by renal cell carcinoma metastasis. There is anterior extension into perivertebral space (PVS) ➡. Note diffusely hypointense VB marrow with preservation of adjacent disc space ➡.* (Right) *Axial T1WI C+ MR in a patient with upper limb symptoms and past history of breast cancer shows enhancing C2 vertebra with epidural ➡ and prevertebral ➡ extension. Note tumor abuts and partially surrounds vertebral arteries ➡.*

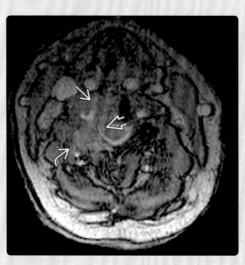
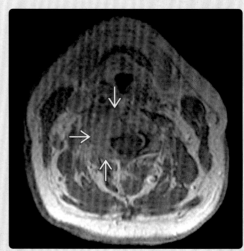

(Left) *Axial T2 GRE image shows high signal intensity of osseous metastases involving VB, posterior elements, and extending into prevertebral ➡ and paraspinal ➡ portions of PVS. Minimal epidural tumor ➡ is present.* (Right) *Postcontrast axial T1 MR image shows diffuse enhancement throughout C4 lesion ➡ with better depiction of tumor interface with muscle and subarachnoid space.*

Vertebral Body Metastasis in Perivertebral Space

TERMINOLOGY

Abbreviations
- Vertebral body (VB) metastasis in perivertebral space (PVS)

Definitions
- Metastatic tumor to cervical VB ± invasion of PVS

IMAGING

General Features
- Best diagnostic clue
  - Destructive mass of VB ± PVS ± epidural extension
  - Often involves multiple VB and multiple spine segments
- Location
  - Cervical VB ± adjacent pre- and perivertebral and epidural tissues
  - Spinal metastases proportionate to red marrow
    - Lumbar > thoracic > cervical spine
  - > 50% have multiple level involvement
- Morphology
  - Destructive VB mass
  - Expanded or displaced prevertebral muscles

Radiographic Findings
- Radiography
  - Increased prevertebral soft tissues
  - Variable destruction of VB ± VB collapse
  - Lytic or sclerotic or mixed destructive changes of VB

CT Findings
- CECT
  - Enhancing irregular soft tissue involving or displacing prevertebral muscles
  - **Epidural tumor**: Solid intraspinal enhancement posterior to VB
    - May be subtle on CECT
- Bone CT
  - Loss of normal bone trabeculae ± cortex
  - Variable **VB collapse** on sagittal/coronal reformats
  - Irregular sclerosis ± lytic change

MR Findings
- T1WI
  - Focal or diffuse hypointense VB lesion(s)
  - **Disc space** usually **preserved**
    - Appear brighter than marrow when diffuse disease
- T2WI
  - Most metastases iso- to hyperintense; sclerotic metastases hypointense
  - Perivertebral component usually hyperintense
  - Look for flow void of vertebral arteries
- STIR
  - Usually hyperintense with normal fat marrow suppressed
- DWI
  - Low ADC value favors tumor over benign VB edema
- T1WI C+
  - Enhancing VB lesion with soft tissue extension into PVS ± intraspinal epidural space
  - Perivertebral involvement has variable appearance but usually solid enhancement

- Irregular enhancement of tissues mimicking phlegmon
- Enhancing tissue displacing/invading prevertebral muscles

Nuclear Medicine Findings
- Bone scan
  - Usually seen as focal increased uptake
  - May be negative when metastasis is small and within medullary cavity
- PET
  - FDG uptake in bone and soft tissue metastases

Imaging Recommendations
- Best imaging tool
  - Different modalities have different strengths
  - Bone scintigraphy
    - Cost-effective & readily available whole-body screening test
    - May show other bony metastatic foci
    - Underestimates spine metastases compared to MR
  - Bone CT
    - Helpful for clarifying suspicious MR, bone scan, or PET lesions
    - Useful in guiding needle biopsy
    - Useful in planning spinal stabilization surgery when fusion is contemplated
  - MR imaging
    - Direct evaluation of vertebral, PVS, & epidural involvement
    - Optimal demonstration of cord compromise ± cord signal abnormality
    - Early, noncortical VB metastases may only be seen with MR
- Protocol advice
  - Important to evaluate entire spine especially when surgery or radiation is considered
    - Ensures treatment of all lesions with potential neurological compromise
  - MR: Fat-saturation sequences (T2, STIR, and T1 C+) distinguish bone metastases from fatty marrow
    - DWI sequences also helpful in problematic cases

DIFFERENTIAL DIAGNOSIS

PVS Infection
- Pyogenic discitis: Disc and VB endplate edema and destruction
- Atypical infections (fungal, TB): Centered in VB
- Phlegmon ± abscess in adjacent soft tissues
- Posterior VB elements usually not involved

Longus Colli Tendinitis
- Benign inflammation at insertion of longus colli muscle
- Small calcifications at longus colli origin
- Prevertebral and retropharyngeal edema

PVS Chordoma
- Markedly hyperintense on T2 MR
- In PVS tends to have lobulated contour
- VB height usually preserved

PATHOLOGY

General Features

- Etiology
  - Most VB metastases from hematogenous spread
  - Adults with PVS metastasis
    - Most often lung, breast, prostate, kidney, GI
    - 15-25% unknown primary
  - Children with PVS metastasis
    - Leukemia, neuroblastoma, Ewing sarcoma
  - Rarely tumor directly penetrates PVS from posterior pharyngeal wall (squamous cell carcinoma)
  - Vertebral metastases may be confined by **prevertebral fascia**, directing tumor to **epidural space**

Staging, Grading, & Classification

- Tomita surgical classification system for metastases; estimates potential risk for spine instability
  - Type 1: VB
  - Type 2: Pedicle extension
  - Type 3: Body and into lamina
  - Type 4: Epidural extension
  - Type 5: Perivertebral extension
  - Type 6: Extension to adjacent vertebra(e)
  - Type 7: Multiple separate vertebral bodies
- This classification useful for radiological description of spine metastases
- Tomita grading score for metastases
  - To estimate patient survival with treatment
  - Points given for speed of tumor growth, presence of visceral and bone metastases
  - Final score in range 2-10 (2 = best prognosis)
- Tomita score & classification probably best used together & in conjunction with neurological symptoms to plan surgery, radiation/chemotherapy

Gross Pathologic & Surgical Features

- Softened, eroded bone ± adjacent soft tissue mass

CLINICAL ISSUES

Presentation

- Most common signs/symptoms
  - 90-95% present with **pain**
    - Local, radicular, or referred
  - Neurological compromise from cord or nerve root compression
- Other signs/symptoms
  - Fever, sepsis not in clinical picture
- Clinical profile
  - Adult patient with known primary tumor presenting with spine pain & neurological compromise

Demographics

- Age
  - Most often > 50 yr
- Gender
  - M = F
- Epidemiology
  - Vertebral column most common site of bone metastasis

- Vertebral metastasis is most common malignant spine lesion
- 10-40% prevalence with systemic cancer

Natural History & Prognosis

- Ongoing bone destruction leads to fracture, instability, deformity, & neurological compromise
- Untreated, potential for epidural involvement and cord compression
  - Neurologic deficits rarely recover after treatment

Treatment

- Treatment depends on tumor type, symptomatology, and neurological complications
- Treatment options include
  - Radiation therapy ± stereotactic radiotherapy, endovascular tumor embolization, vertebroplasty, surgical resection for cord decompression ± spine stabilization
- Intravenous corticosteroid administration when cord compression

DIAGNOSTIC CHECKLIST

Consider

- VB metastasis mimics infectious spondylodiscitis
  - Especially atypical infections
    - Fungal and TB tend to also be found in VB center with disc sparing

Image Interpretation Pearls

- Important to obtain and carefully review bone CT images for trabecular loss, cortical destruction
- Carefully evaluate epidural space and spinal cord
- Obtain MR with any neurological symptoms or when epidural aspect not well evaluated
- Evaluate vertebral arteries for compression or occlusion
- Assess fracture risk

SELECTED REFERENCES

1. Mesfin A et al: Management of metastatic cervical spine tumors. J Am Acad Orthop Surg. 23(1):38-46, 2015
2. Prince EA et al: Interventional management of vertebral body metastases. Semin Intervent Radiol. 30(3):278-81, 2013
3. Grankvist J et al: MRI and PET/CT of patients with bone metastases from breast carcinoma. Eur J Radiol. 81(1):e13-8, 2012
4. Eleraky M et al: Management of metastatic spine disease. Curr Opin Support Palliat Care. 4(3):182-8, 2010
5. Kim DS et al: Magnetic resonance imaging diagnoses of bone scan abnormalities in breast cancer patients. Nucl Med Commun. 30(9):736-41, 2009
6. Laufer I et al: The accuracy of [(18)F]fluorodeoxyglucose positron emission tomography as confirmed by biopsy in the diagnosis of spine metastases in a cancer population. Neurosurgery. 64(1):107-13; discussion 113-4, 2009
7. Cascini G et al: Whole-body magnetic resonance imaging for detecting bone metastases: comparison with bone scintigraphy. Radiol Med. 113(8):1157-70, 2008
8. Tokuhashi Y et al: A revised scoring system for preoperative evaluation of metastatic spine tumor prognosis. Spine (Phila Pa 1976). 30(19):2186-91, 2005
9. Bauer H et al: Surgical strategy for spinal metastases. Spine (Phila Pa 1976). 27(10):1124-6, 2002
10. Mehta RC et al: MR evaluation of vertebral metastases: T1-weighted, short-inversion-time inversion recovery, fast spin-echo, and inversion-recovery fast spin-echo sequences. AJNR Am J Neuroradiol. 16(2):281-8, 1995

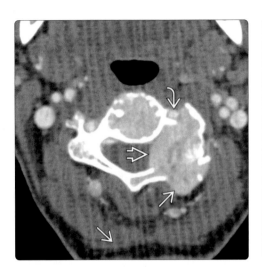

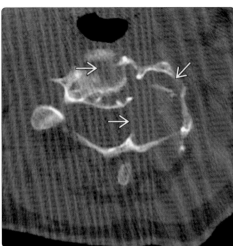

(Left) *Axial CECT demonstrates large, enhancing mass involving C3 vertebra, left facet and lamina. Note extension into paraspinal component of PVS* ➡. *Intraspinal tumor* ➡ *has smooth interface with dura. Tumor is around left vertebral artery* ➡. (Right) *Axial bone CT better illustrates the lesion* ➡ *as predominately lytic and expansile. This destructive lesion was a thyroid carcinoma metastasis and was embolized prior to surgical resection.*

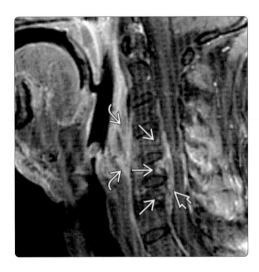

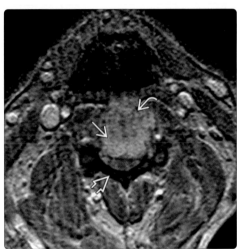

(Left) *Sagittal T1WI C+ FS MR reveals multilevel tumor* ➡ *and extensive epidural* ➡ *and prevertebral extraosseous tumor* ➡. *Posterior elements are also diffusely infiltrated. Involvement of multiple adjacent vertebrae is type 6 in the Tomita classification.* (Right) *Axial STIR image shows suppression of normal marrow signal in posterior elements* ➡ *of VB compared to intrinsically bright metastasis involving VB* ➡ *and extending into prevertebral tissues* ➡.

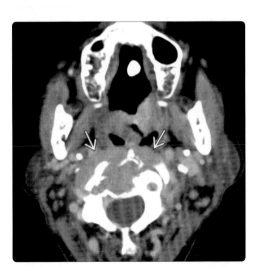

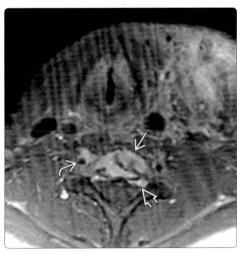

(Left) *Axial CECT shows cervical metastasis destroying 2 VBs. Note that despite destructive nature of lesion, soft tissue component does not traverse deep layer, deep cervical fascia* ➡, *remaining confined to PVS.* (Right) *Axial T1 enhanced fat-saturated MR reveals enhancement of metastatic tumor in the VB* ➡ *spreading anterolaterally to engulf the right vertebral artery* ➡. *There is also posterolateral spread into the left epidural space* ➡.

SECTION 9
Posterior Cervical Space

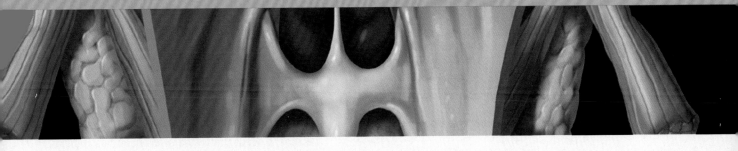

Summary Thoughts: Posterior Cervical Space

The posterior cervical space (PCS) lies in the lateral neck deep to the sternocleidomastoid (SCM) and trapezius muscles and includes the triangle of fat between them. This triangle of fat is superficial to the paraspinal muscles and is known clinically as the **posterior triangle** of the neck. The PCS is small superiorly, encompassing just a region of tissue around the mastoid tip, but it expands inferiorly to encompass most of the lateral neck.

The most frequent pathology to affect the PCS is inflammatory or malignant **lymphadenopathy** in the spinal accessory chain. Identifying the likely source of the primary tumor is of great importance. Other pathology in the PCS is often related to CNXI, which runs obliquely across the PCS, or the brachial plexus, which traverses the lower PCS.

Imaging Approaches and Indications

Masses and inflammation of the PCS may be imaged either with CECT or MR of the neck, depending on regional preferences. Be sure to include the entire PCS, from the mastoid tip through the clavicles.

Imaging Anatomy

Superficial PCS **anatomic boundaries** include the SCM and trapezius muscles and the superficial space (platysma and subcutaneous fat). Deep to the PCS lies the prevertebral (more anteriorly) and paraspinal (more posteriorly) portions of the perivertebral space (PVS). Anteromedial to the PCS, the carotid space (CS) is found.

The PCS has complex **fascial boundaries**. The deep margin of the PCS is separated from the PVS by the deep layer of the deep cervical fascia (DCF); the superficial margin of the PCS is separated from the SCM and trapezius, as well as from the superficial space, by the superficial (investing) layer of the DCF. The PCS is separated from the CS by all 3 layers of the DCF that make up the carotid sheath.

The main **PCS contents** are fat, lymph nodes, and the spinal accessory nerve (CNXI). The nerve lies along the floor of the space, running obliquely from anterosuperior to posteroinferior. The nodes included are predominantly from the **spinal accessory chain**, along with portions of the transverse cervical chain. This corresponds to **level V** if the nodes are strictly posterior to the posterior border of the SCM or **levels IIB, III, and IV** if the nodes are deep to the SCM.

Segments of the **brachial plexus** run through the PCS. After the trunks of the brachial plexus emerge from the scalene triangle between the anterior and middle scalene muscles, they ramify into divisions and then cords within the PCS before continuing into the axilla.

The dorsal scapular nerve and segmental cervical nerve roots also traverse the PCS, as does the 3rd portion of the subclavian artery, but the bulk of the PCS is filled with **fat**.

While radiologists divide the neck into fascial-lined spaces, clinicians divide the neck into muscular triangles. The triangle that corresponds to the PCS is the **posterior triangle** of the neck, between the SCM and trapezius muscles. The posterior triangle can be subdivided into the occipital and subclavian triangles using the inferior belly of the omohyoid muscle as the dividing line. The occipital triangle is superior to the omohyoid, whereas the subclavian triangle is inferior.

- Occipital triangle contains fat, CNXI, dorsal scapular nerve, and spinal accessory nodes
- Subclavian triangle contains 3rd portion of subclavian artery and brachial plexus

Approaches to Imaging Issues of Posterior Cervical Space

Multiple imaging findings help answer the question, "What defines a mass as being in the PCS?" First, the lesion should arise within the PCS fat. Larger PCS masses will displace the CS anteromedially, elevate the SCM (aggressive malignancies may invade into SCM, obliterating the intervening fat), and flatten the deeper prevertebral and paraspinal muscles.

The PCS contains nodes from both level V and levels II through IV. This situation yields the question, "How can these nodal stations be distinguished?" Draw an imaginary line from the posterior border of one SCM to the posterior border of the other SCM. If the center of the affected node is posterior to this line, the node is assigned to level V. If it is anterior to this line, it is a level II-IV internal jugular node. The level II-IV nodes are sorted by horizontal landmarks. If the node is above the hyoid bone, it belongs to level II. If it is below the cricoid cartilage, it belongs to level IV, while between these landmarks lies level III.

Clinical Implications

PCS masses can affect function of CNXI, but the most frequent source of CNXI dysfunction is prior surgery in the PCS. When CNXI is injured or resected, the SCM and trapezius muscles atrophy. Acutely, the muscles may enlarge and enhance, but chronically, the muscles shrink and undergo fatty infiltration. In postsurgical patients, the SCM has often been resected, so atrophy of the trapezius muscle may be the only radiologic clue to prior CNXI injury.

When the trapezius muscle is dysfunctional, the **levator scapulae muscle** takes over its function in elevating the scapula. The levator scapulae muscle is one of the lateral paraspinal muscles. When it hypertrophies, it may be mistaken for a pathologic mass (such as recurrent tumor) both clinically and radiologically.

Differential Diagnosis

PCS Differential Diagnosis by Pathology Category
- Pseudolesion: Cervical rib
- Congenital: Lymphatic malformation, 3rd branchial cleft cyst
- Inflammatory: Reactive or sarcoid adenopathy
- Infectious: TB adenitis, suppurative adenitis, abscess
- Benign tumor: Lipoma, CNXI or brachial plexus schwannoma or neurofibroma
- Malignant primary tumor: Sarcoma, primary non-Hodgkin lymphoma (NHL) of PCS nodes
- Metastatic nodes: H&N squamous cell carcinoma, NHL, differentiated thyroid cancer, melanoma

Selected References

1. Parker GD et al: Radiologic evaluation of the normal and diseased posterior cervical space. AJR Am J Roentgenol. 157(1):161-5, 1991

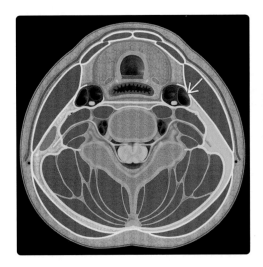

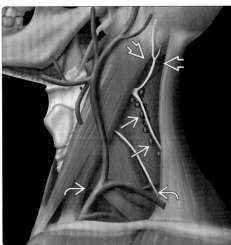

(Left) *Axial graphic depicts the normal posterior cervical space (PCS) (blue-green shading) below the level of the hyoid bone. Complex fascial margins include the superficial layer of the deep cervical fascia (DCF) (yellow line), the deep layer of the DCF (blue line), and the tricolored carotid sheath ➡ (containing all 3 layers of DCF).* (Right) *Lateral graphic shows that the spinal accessory nodal chain ➡ follows the general course of the spinal accessory nerve (CNXI). The PCS is smaller superiorly ➡ than inferiorly ➡.*

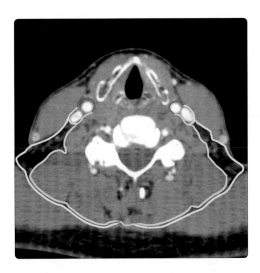

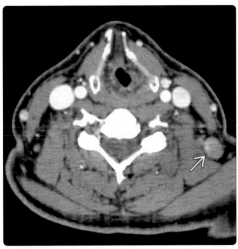

(Left) *Normal axial CECT has the PCS fascial boundaries drawn onto it. The portions of the superficial (yellow) and deep (light blue) layers of the DCF that surround the PCS are depicted.* (Right) *Axial CECT of the infrahyoid neck shows a typical PCS mass. This enlarged lymph node ➡ lies strictly posterior to the posterior margin of the sternocleidomastoid, so it is classified as level V. Clinically, this mass would be within the posterior triangle.*

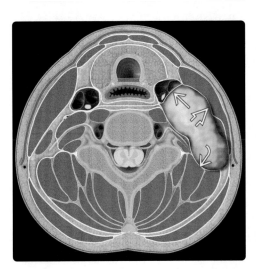

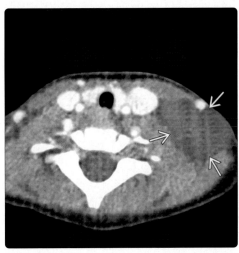

(Left) *Axial graphic of a generic PCS mass reveals compression of the deep paraspinal muscles ➡, elevation of the sternocleidomastoid muscle ➡, and anteromedial displacement of the carotid sheath ➡.* (Right) *Axial CECT demonstrates an ill-defined, low-density mass ➡ filling the infrahyoid PCS. The conformational configuration, uniform low density (fluid), and lack of enhancement are strongly suggestive of the diagnosis lymphatic malformation.*

TERMINOLOGY

- Synonyms: Neuroma, neurinoma, neurilemmoma, nerve sheath tumor
- Schwannoma in PCS primarily from 3 sites
  - Distal brachial plexus root or trunk
  - Cervical sensory nerve
  - CNXI

IMAGING

- CT: Well-delineated, solitary, fusiform mass
  - Isodense to hypodense mass
- MR: Modality of choice for presurgical evaluation
  - Contrast-enhanced images critical
  - Large schwannomas often have **cystic** component
- US: Hypoechoic mass with posterior acoustic enhancement
  - Marked hypervascularity on color Doppler

TOP DIFFERENTIAL DIAGNOSES

- Spinal accessory reactive node
- Spinal accessory squamous cell carcinoma metastatic node
- Spinal accessory non-Hodgkin lymphoma node
- Lymphatic malformation

CLINICAL ISSUES

- Rapid enlargement suggests malignant degeneration
- Core biopsy needed for diagnosis
- Treatment is surgical enucleation
  - Excellent long-term results
  - Aim to preserve nerve function (frequently impossible)
  - Conservative imaging surveillance another option

DIAGNOSTIC CHECKLIST

- **Look for nerve or foramen of origin**
  - In upper neck from jugular foramen (CNXI), in lower neck from brachial plexus (C5-T1)
  - Mass pointing between anterior and middle scalene indicates brachial plexus origin
- Main differential is solitary PCS nodal mass

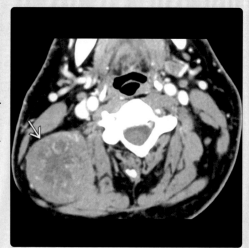
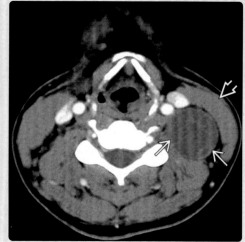

(Left) Axial CECT demonstrates a large, well-defined mass ➡ in the posterior cervical space (PCS) with heterogeneous enhancement. This schwannoma arises from CNXI, which traverses the PCS. (Right) Axial CECT shows a round, well-defined, poorly enhancing mass ➡ in the PCS. Schwannomas in this location will sometimes be entirely cystic. Note lateral displacement of the overlying sternocleidomastoid muscle (SCM) ➡ but sparing of the surrounding fat planes.

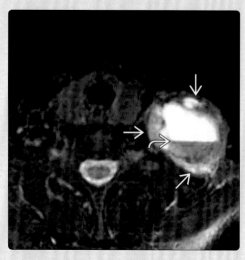
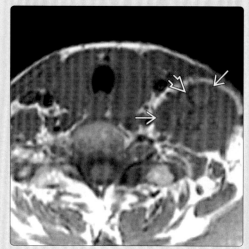

(Left) Axial T2 FS MR shows a large mass ➡ in the PCS with well-defined margins. It is unusual for a schwannoma to have a fluid level ➡, but it does occur occasionally, and this lesion shows internal hemorrhage. (Right) Axial T1 MR shows a large, well-defined mass ➡ with predominantly uniform intermediate signal in the PCS, with intact surrounding fat planes. Flow voids ➡ within the mass are suggestive of paraganglioma, but may also rarely be seen with schwannoma.

TERMINOLOGY

Abbreviations

- Schwannoma of posterior cervical space (PCS)

Synonyms

- Neuroma, neurinoma, neurilemmoma, nerve sheath tumor

Definitions

- Benign, slow-growing Schwann cell neoplasm arising in PCS from CNXI, brachial plexus, or cervical sensory nerve

IMAGING

General Features

- Best diagnostic clue
  - Solitary, fusiform, enhancing PCS mass
  - Schwannoma of CNXI: Displaces jugular vein anteriorly and medially
- Location
  - Suprahyoid PCS: Between paraspinous and sternocleidomastoid muscles, posterior to jugular vein
  - Infrahyoid PCS: Between scalene and sternocleidomastoid muscles, lateral to jugular vein
    - May emerge along branchial plexus from between anterior and middle scalene into PCS
- Size
  - Variable, may be > 14 cm
- Morphology
  - Well-delineated, solitary, fusiform mass

CT Findings

- NECT
  - Isodense or **hypodense** to muscle
- CECT
  - Homogeneous enhancement of solid component
  - Large schwannomas often have nonenhancing **cystic component**

MR Findings

- T1WI
  - Homogeneous signal, isointense to muscle
- T2WI
  - Hyperintense compared to muscle
  - Occasionally, fluid level present in cystic component
- T1WI C+
  - Homogeneous enhancement of solid component
  - Cystic components best appreciated post contrast as nonenhancing foci
  - Occasionally, signal voids present (mimics paraganglioma)

Ultrasonographic Findings

- Grayscale ultrasound
  - Solitary, oval, hypoechoic mass with posterior acoustic enhancement
  - Lacks echogenic hilum of lymph node
- Color Doppler
  - Marked hypervascularity on color Doppler
  - Can be obliterated with transducer pressure

Angiographic Findings

- Angiography not routinely used for diagnosis or management
- Hypovascular ± venous puddling

Nuclear Medicine Findings

- PET
  - Variable FDG avidity

Image-Guided Biopsy

- Schwannomas infamous for poor cellularity on FNA
- **Core biopsy** needed for diagnosis
  - Nerve damage very unlikely in lesions > 1 cm

Imaging Recommendations

- Best imaging tool
  - **MR is technique of choice** for presurgical evaluation
    - Extent of lesion
    - Nerve of origin
- Protocol advice
  - Contrast-enhanced images with fat suppression critical

DIFFERENTIAL DIAGNOSIS

Spinal Accessory Reactive Node

- Reniform configuration (central fatty hilum)
- Uniform mild enhancement
- Well-defined margins

Spinal Accessory Squamous Cell Carcinoma Metastatic Node

- Rim-enhancing or solid mass with thick walls, mural nodularity
- Usually multiple, as level V unusual site for solitary regional metastasis

Spinal Accessory Non-Hodgkin Lymphoma Node

- Uniformly enhancing ovoid mass
- Usually multiple
- Systemic non-Hodgkin lymphoma may not be known

Spinal Accessory Suppurative Node

- Tender posterior triangle masses
- Ovoid, rim-enhancing mass
- Surrounding fat stranding
- If solitary, may mimic schwannoma

Lymphatic Malformation

- **Multilocular cystic spaces** without perceptible wall
- May have solid components if mixed venolymphatic malformation
- Multiloculated high T2 signal intensity ± fluid levels

3rd Branchial Cleft Anomaly

- Young adult
- Ovoid, unilocular, cystic PCS mass

Subclavian Artery Aneurysm

- **Pulsatile lower neck mass** contiguous with subclavian artery
- Enhancement identical to adjacent artery
  - Thrombus unlikely to completely fill aneurysm

- Complex MR signal due to turbulent flow and luminal thrombus

PATHOLOGY

General Features

- Etiology
  - Benign Schwann cell neoplasm **arising from CNXI, brachial plexus, or cervical sensory nerve**
- Genetics
  - Usually sporadic and isolated
  - 1/3 to 1/2 of patients with sporadic schwannomas have deletion at NF2 locus on chromosome 22
- Associated abnormalities
  - **Neurofibromatosis type 2: Multiple schwannomas** with bilateral acoustic schwannomas, meningiomas, and ependymomas
    - Chromosome 22 mutation
  - Schwannomatosis: Multiple schwannomas without acoustic schwannomas or other manifestations of NF2
    - Mutation of NF2 locus found in schwannomas but not in peripheral blood
- Arises focally from nerve sheath fascicle as eccentric mass displacing nerve
- Schwannoma in PCS primarily from 3 sites
  - Distal brachial plexus root or trunk
  - Cervical sensory nerve
  - CNXI
- Brachial plexus > cervical sensory nerve > CNXI schwannoma

Gross Pathologic & Surgical Features

- Lobulated but smooth, encapsulated, fusiform mass arising eccentrically from nerve
- Gray-tan on cut section; firm, rubbery texture
  - Small intramural cysts may be seen
- Variant: Plexiform schwannoma: Gross plexiform pattern mimicking plexiform neurofibroma
  - Not associated with neurofibromatosis
- Variant: Melanocytic schwannoma: Pigmented, poorer prognosis

Microscopic Features

- Encapsulated, benign spindle cell tumor
- Differentiated neoplastic Schwann cells in collagenous matrix
- Antoni A areas: Compact cells
  - Rows of parallel nuclei around acellular areas = Verocay bodies
- Antoni B areas: More myxoid, less cellular
- Thick-walled vessels and scattered inflammatory cells also present
- Nerve axons may be seen at periphery but not within tumor
- Strongly positive for S100 protein stain

CLINICAL ISSUES

Presentation

- Most common signs/symptoms
  - **Slow-growing** posterior neck mass; may be incidental finding
    - Rapid enlargement suggests malignant degeneration

- Other signs/symptoms
  - May be exacerbated by pressure on lesion
  - Recurring mild neck pain with muscle spasm
  - Denervation atrophy of trapezius and sternocleidomastoid muscles (CNXI)

Demographics

- Age
  - Peak (without phakomatosis): 20-50 years
  - 10% < 21 years
- Gender
  - No gender predilection
- Epidemiology
  - < 1% of all head and neck neoplasms
  - Schwannoma is **most common solitary neurogenic tumor in neck**
  - 25-45% of schwannomas arise in head and neck

Natural History & Prognosis

- **Malignant degeneration very rare** in isolated lesions
  - Malignant peripheral nerve sheath tumor (MPNST) usually arises sporadically or in association with NF1
  - Rapidly enlarging mass near cervical sensory nerve ± pain or nerve dysfunction
- Melanocytic schwannomas very rare
  - 25% metastasize
- Incompletely excised schwannoma may locally recur

Treatment

- Surgical enucleation
  - Excellent long-term results
  - Aim to preserve nerve fibers and neural function, though frequently impossible
    - Conservative imaging surveillance another option
  - Complete resolution of symptoms expected
  - Initial neurapraxia is most common complication

DIAGNOSTIC CHECKLIST

Consider

- If multiple schwannomas or child, consider NF2

Image Interpretation Pearls

- Look for nerve or foramen of origin
  - In upper neck from jugular foramen (CNXI), in lower neck from brachial plexus (C5-T1)
  - Look for mass pointing between anterior and middle scalene to indicate brachial plexus origin
- Evaluate full extent of mass (axillary, intrathoracic, skull base)
- Main differential is reactive, inflammatory, or neoplastic level V (spinal accessory) lymph node

SELECTED REFERENCES

1. Sinkkonen ST et al: Experience of head and neck extracranial schwannomas in a whole population-based single-center patient series. Eur Arch Otorhinolaryngol. 271(11):3027-34, 2014
2. Kato H et al: "Flow-void" sign at MR imaging: a rare finding of extracranial head and neck schwannomas. J Magn Reson Imaging. 31(3):703-5, 2010
3. Kato H et al: Fluid-fluid level formation: a rare finding of extracranial head and neck schwannomas. AJNR Am J Neuroradiol. 30(7):1451-3, 2009
4. Biswas D et al: Extracranial head and neck schwannomas--a 10-year review. Auris Nasus Larynx. 34(3):353-9, 2007

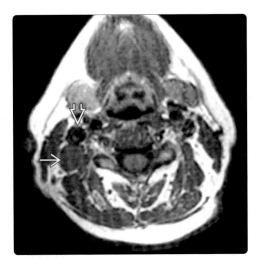

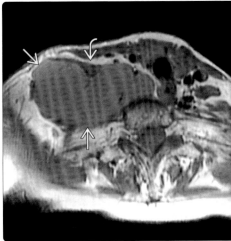

(Left) *Axial T1 MR shows a well-defined, intermediate-signal ovoid mass ➡ in the PCS, just posterior to the internal jugular vein ➡. Based on location and imaging characteristics, this schwannoma might be mistaken for an enlarged lymph node.* (Right) *Axial PD FSE MR shows a lobulated mass ➡ in the lower right neck. The mass narrows as it passes posterior to the anterior scalene muscle ➡. This indicates that the mass has arisen from the brachial plexus.*

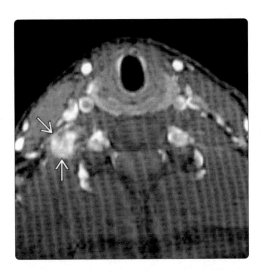

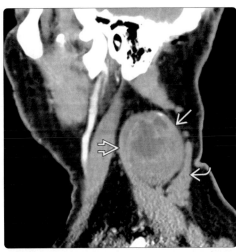

(Left) *Axial T1 C+ FS MR shows a well-defined, heterogeneously enhancing mass ➡ along the medial aspect of the PCS. This is a typical location for a schwannoma of the sensory cervical nerve roots.* (Right) *Sagittal CECT reformat shows a heterogeneously enhancing, well-defined, ovoid mass ➡ in the PCS between the sternocleidomastoid ➡ and trapezius ➡ muscles, with intact surrounding fat planes. This is a characteristic location for a schwannoma of CNXI.*

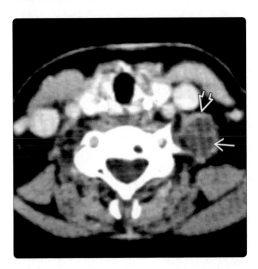

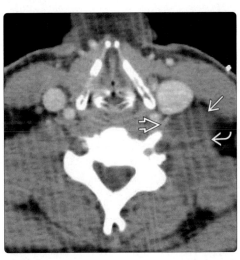

(Left) *Axial CECT shows heterogeneous distal brachial plexus schwannoma protruding from between scalene muscles into medial PCS. Note intramural cystic change ➡ and displacement of the anterior scalene muscle anteriorly ➡.* (Right) *Axial CECT shows relatively hypodense posterior cervical space schwannoma ➡. Note characteristic location between the anterior ➡ and middle ➡ scalene muscles, indicating brachial plexus origin.*

Squamous Cell Carcinoma in Spinal Accessory Node

TERMINOLOGY

- Nodal chain accompanying spinal accessory nerve (CNXI)
- Spinal accessory chain divided into level IIB & level V nodes

IMAGING

- **Cervical nodes** concerning for **malignancy** if
  - ○ **Necrosis**
  - ○ Ill-defined margins ± stranding of surrounding fat = extracapsular spread (most specific sign)
  - ○ Shape: **Round** node more likely pathologic; reniform nodes likely benign
  - ○ Number: Groups of **≥ 3** borderline enlarged nodes more likely pathologic
  - ○ Size: **> 1 cm** in diameter (least specific sign)
- US- or CT-guided biopsy for equivocal nodes
- CECT best 1st tool for indeterminate neck mass
- PET/CT most appropriate for unknown primary or for staging once SCCa diagnosis established
  - ○ Can change nodal stage of disease

TOP DIFFERENTIAL DIAGNOSES

- Reactive adenopathy
- Suppurative adenopathy
- Non-Hodgkin lymphoma nodes
- Thyroid cancer node metastasis
- Skin cancer nodal metastasis from scalp/face
- Posterior cervical space schwannoma

PATHOLOGY

- Nasopharyngeal, oropharyngeal, & hypopharyngeal primaries often present with CNXI nodal mets

CLINICAL ISSUES

- Single nodal metastasis ↓ survival by 50%
- Treatment depends on primary site & nodal stage

DIAGNOSTIC CHECKLIST

- **Identification of 1° tumor is important**
- Large (> 2 cm) nonnecrotic nodes suggest NHL, not SCCa

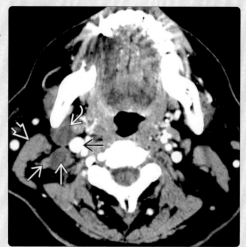
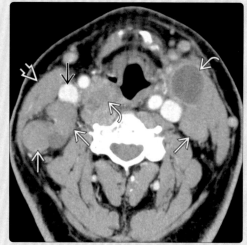

(Left) Axial CECT shows spinal accessory metastases ➡ from SCCa in zone IIB. Note that the nodes are deep to the sternocleidomastoid muscle (SCM) ➡ and posterior to the internal jugular vein (IJV) ➡. Zone IIA nodes ➡ are also present, but they are not part of the spinal accessory chain. Central necrosis gives the nodes a cystic appearance. (Right) Axial CECT shows solidly enhancing nodes ➡ in the spinal accessory chain (zone IIB, deep to the SCM ➡ and posterior to the IJV ➡). Other nodal stations are also represented ➡.

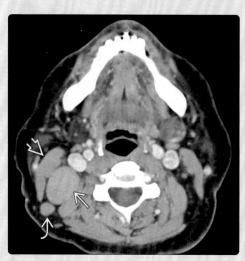
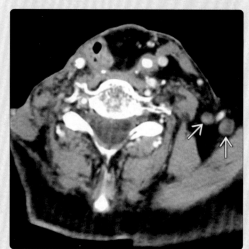

(Left) Axial CECT shows SCCa in the spinal accessory chain, involving both zone IIB ➡ and zone V ➡. Note that the zone V node lies strictly posterior to the SCM ➡, while the zone IIB node is deep to the muscle. (Right) Axial CECT shows recurrent contralateral spinal accessory nodes ➡ after laryngectomy and right neck dissection. These nodes are low in the neck, such that the spinal accessory nerve is along the posterior aspect of the posterior cervical space.

Squamous Cell Carcinoma in Spinal Accessory Node

TERMINOLOGY

Abbreviations

- Squamous cell carcinoma (SCCa)
- Posterior cervical space (PCS)

Definitions

- Spinal accessory node: Nodal chain accompanying spinal accessory nerve (CNXI)
- Spinal accessory chain divided between 2 surgical levels
  - **Level IIB** for upper spinal nodes deep to sternocleidomastoid muscle (SCM) but posterior to internal jugular vein
  - **Level V** for PCS; strictly posterior to SCM

IMAGING

General Features

- Best diagnostic clue
  - Single or multiple, round/oval, ± **centrally necrotic** soft tissue masses along course of CNXI
  - Cervical nodes concerning for malignancy if
    - **Necrosis** or **extracapsular spread** (most specific sign)
    - Shape: Round node more likely pathologic; reniform nodes likely benign
    - Number: Groups of ≥ 3 borderline enlarged nodes more likely pathologic
    - Size: > 1-cm diameter (least specific sign)

CT Findings

- CECT
  - **Necrosis** appears as foci of low density with variably thick, irregular peripheral enhancement
  - Ill-defined margins ± stranding of surrounding fat = **extracapsular spread**

MR Findings

- T1WI
  - Nodes isointense to muscle
- T2WI
  - Nodes hyperintense
- T1WI C+ FS
  - Best demonstrates nodal necrosis as central low intensity with peripheral wall enhancement

Ultrasonographic Findings

- Grayscale ultrasound
  - Typically hypoechoic, with loss of hilar definition
  - Poorly defined borders = extracapsular spread

Nonvascular Interventions

- Ultrasound- or CT-guided biopsy for equivocal nodes

Nuclear Medicine Findings

- PET/CT
  - Can detect nodal metastases that are negative on CT/MR
  - Can change nodal stage of disease

Imaging Recommendations

- Best imaging tool
  - CECT initially for indeterminate neck mass
  - PET/CT most appropriate for unknown primary or for staging once SCCa diagnosis established

DIFFERENTIAL DIAGNOSIS

Reactive Adenopathy

- **Nonnecrotic** reniform nodes < 2 cm
- Associated adenoidal & tonsillar hypertrophy

Suppurative Adenopathy

- Centrally low density, peripherally enhancing nodes with stranding of surrounding fat
- Patient usually septic with tender neck masses

Non-Hodgkin Lymphoma Lymph Nodes

- Large **homogeneous** lymph nodes
- Bilateral & multispatial typically

Differentiated Thyroid Carcinoma Lymph Nodes

- Avidly enhancing nodes ± Ca++, cystic change

Skin Cancer Nodal Metastasis

- Skin cancers of scalp & face

Posterior Cervical Space Schwannoma

- Well-circumscribed **solitary** mass within PCS
- Enhancing ovoid mass ± internal cyst formation

PATHOLOGY

General Features

- Nasopharyngeal, oropharyngeal, & hypopharyngeal cancers may present with spinal accessory metastases

CLINICAL ISSUES

Presentation

- Most common signs/symptoms
  - Palpable mass in "posterior triangle"
  - Extranodal tumor spread results in "fixed" node

Demographics

- Epidemiology
  - Most common malignant neck nodes (> 80%)

Natural History & Prognosis

- Single nodal SCCa metastasis ↓ survival by 50%
- Extracapsular spread = poorer prognosis

Treatment

- Surgery vs. chemoradiation depends on primary site & nodal stage

DIAGNOSTIC CHECKLIST

Consider

- Identification of primary tumor of paramount importance

Image Interpretation Pearls

- Large nonnecrotic nodes suggest NHL, not SCCa

SELECTED REFERENCES

1. Curtin HD et al: Comparison of CT and MR imaging in staging of neck metastases. Radiology. 207(1):123-30, 1998
2. Parker GD et al: Radiologic evaluation of the normal and diseased posterior cervical space. AJR Am J Roentgenol. 157(1):161-5, 1991

TERMINOLOGY

- Non-Hodgkin lymphoma (NHL)
- Spinal accessory nodes also known as posterior triangle or posterior cervical space nodes
  - Level IIB: Posterior to jugular vein
  - Level V: Posterior to sternocleidomastoid muscle

IMAGING

- Nodal NHL may be multiple 1- to 3-cm nodes or dominant large node may be > 5 cm
- May involve multiple neck nodal groups
- Typically homogeneous, nonnecrotic nodes
- Necrosis/extracapsular spread suggests high-grade, aggressive NHL
- Calcification may be seen post treatment
- Generally FDG avid though some variability
- Standard NHL staging relies on CT/MR & FDG PET

TOP DIFFERENTIAL DIAGNOSES

- Reactive lymph nodes
- Suppurative lymph nodes
- Spinal accessory squamous cell carcinoma (SCCa) node
- Posterior cervical space schwannoma
- Differentiated thyroid carcinoma nodes

CLINICAL ISSUES

- Painless posterior triangle masses ± other nodes
- Increased risk in immunocompromised patients

DIAGNOSTIC CHECKLIST

- NHL 2nd most common H&N tumor after SCCa
- Some imaging features favor NHL over SCCa
  - Large solid nodes
  - Posterior triangle nodes in isolation
  - Posterior triangle + superior mediastinum nodes

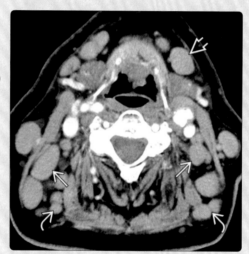
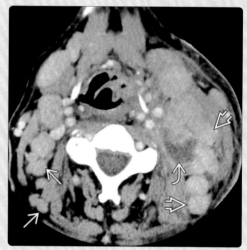

(Left) Axial CECT shows homogeneous solid node enlargement in levels IIB ➡ and VA ➡. Multiple enlarged nodes are evident in other groups including IB ➡. (Right) Axial CECT demonstrates extensive adenopathy. Right spinal accessory chain ➡ and jugular chain have multiple enlarged solid nodes. Left side shows multiple solid ➡ and necrotic ➡ nodes in spinal accessory chain with extranodal spread. Necrosis suggests high-grade non-Hodgkin lymphoma.

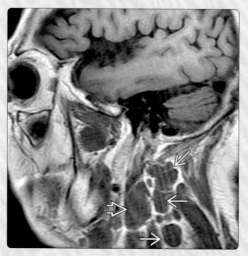
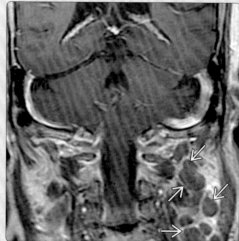

(Left) Sagittal T1 MR demonstrates a cluster of prominent nodes in high posterior triangle ➡ and high jugular chain ➡ in a patient presenting with a nasopharyngeal mass. Pathology showed lymphoma. (Right) Coronal T1 C+ MR shows well-defined, minimally enhancing nodes ➡ in posterior cervical fat. Note that nodes are only mildly enlarged, show no necrosis, but appear round. Asymmetric cluster of nodes also suggests pathologic nature. This proved to be diffuse large B-cell lymphoma.

TERMINOLOGY

Abbreviations
- Non-Hodgkin lymphoma (NHL)

Definitions
- Spinal accessory nodes also known as **posterior triangle** or **posterior cervical space** nodes
  - **Level IIB** deep to sternocleidomastoid muscles (SCM), posterior to jugular vein
  - **Levels VA & VB** posterior to SCM

IMAGING

General Features
- Best diagnostic clue
  - Multiple **homogeneous**, round, enlarged nodes in posterior triangle
- Location
  - Unilateral or bilateral ± other nodal groups or superior mediastinum
- Size
  - Nodal NHL may be
    - Multiple 1- to 3-cm solid nodes
    - Dominant large node up to 5 cm
- Morphology
  - Typically homogeneous, nonnecrotic
  - Necrosis or extracapsular spread (ECS) uncommon, suggests high-grade NHL

CT Findings
- CECT
  - Homogeneous, slightly higher density than muscle
  - Loss of hilar fat & vessels
  - Calcification may be seen post treatment

MR Findings
- T1WI
  - Nodes isointense to muscle
- T2WI
  - Nodes homogeneously hyperintense
- T1WI C+
  - Uniform mild enhancement

Nuclear Medicine Findings
- PET/CT
  - Generally FDG avid though some variability
    - ↑ avidity → ↑ tumor aggressivity
  - Useful for both staging & surveillance

Imaging Recommendations
- Best imaging tool
  - CECT best modality for evaluation of neck mass
  - Standard staging for NHL is CT/MR & FDG PET

DIFFERENTIAL DIAGNOSIS

Reactive Lymph Nodes
- Nonnecrotic oval nodes < 2 cm
- Adenoidal & tonsil hypertrophy or active infection

Suppurative Lymph Nodes
- Central low density with peripheral enhancement

- Patient usually septic with tender neck mass

Spinal Accessory Squamous Cell Carcinoma Node
- Central necrosis & ECS findings favor squamous cell carcinoma (SCCa)
- Pharyngeal SCCa often presents with level IIB nodes
- Level V SCCa nodes uncommon in absence of internal jugular chain nodes

Posterior Cervical Space Schwannoma
- Ovoid or tubular well-circumscribed, solitary mass

Differentiated Thyroid Carcinoma Nodes
- Cystic, heterogeneous, calcified nodes more typical
- Uncommon in absence of level III/IV nodes

PATHOLOGY

Staging, Grading, & Classification
- **World Health Organization classification (2008)**
  - Based on immunophenotype & morphology
  - More than 30 different types of NHL
    - **80-85%: B-cell neoplasms**
    - 15-20%: T-cell & putative NK-cell neoplasms
- **Modified Ann Arbor staging system** for clinical staging, treatment, & prognosis
  - Determined by location of disease sites & symptoms

CLINICAL ISSUES

Presentation
- Most common signs/symptoms
  - Painless posterior triangle masses ± other nodes
- Other signs/symptoms
  - Systemic: Night sweats, fevers, weight loss

Demographics
- Age
  - Median 50-55 years
- Epidemiology
  - Increased risk in immunocompromised patients

Natural History & Prognosis
- May be indolent, progressive but not curable, or aggressive but often curable

Treatment
- Depends on stage, cell type, patient age
- Chemo, XRT, or combined modality therapy

DIAGNOSTIC CHECKLIST

Image Interpretation Pearls
- NHL 2nd most common H&N tumor after SCCa
- Some imaging features favor NHL over SCCa
  - Large (> 2 cm) solid nodes
  - Posterior triangle without jugular chain nodes
  - Posterior triangle & superior mediastinum nodes
- Nodal necrosis &/or ECS suggests high-grade NHL

SELECTED REFERENCES

1. Cronin CG et al: Clinical utility of PET/CT in lymphoma. AJR Am J Roentgenol. 194(1):W91-W103, 2010

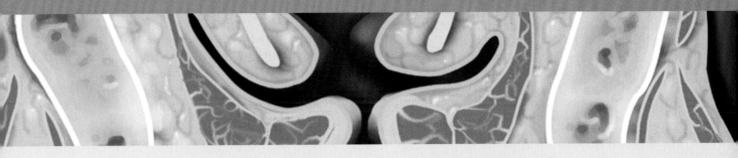

SECTION 10
Visceral Space

Summary Thoughts: Visceral Space

The visceral space (VS) is a tubular space that occupies the midline anterior aspect of the infrahyoid neck. Extending to the superior mediastinum, the VS lies between the laterally placed carotid spaces (CSs) and is completely encircled by the middle layer of deep cervical fascia (ML-DCF), also known as the **visceral fascia**.

While the largest VS components are the hypopharynx-larynx, trachea, and esophagus, the **thyroid gland** most often necessitates imaging of this space. The other key anatomic elements of the VS are not normally identifiable on routine imaging; the **parathyroid glands** are only evident if hyperplastic or neoplastic, and the **recurrent laryngeal nerves** (RLNs) cannot be seen, although their course through the VS must be carefully evaluated whenever vocal cord paralysis is present. The larynx and hypopharynx are covered elsewhere.

Imaging Techniques & Indications

Both CT or MR are excellent modalities for demonstrating the **thyroid** and its relationship to other VS and neck structures. As there is no inferior fascial limit to the VS, any cross-sectional imaging should continue into the superior mediastinum and preferably to the level of the left pulmonary artery. This will encompass the entire course of the left RLN and all of the superior mediastinal nodes. CT is preferred for evaluation of the left RLN, as it allows better review of any pulmonary pathology.

If there is clinical suspicion of **thyroid neoplasia**, iodinated contrast should not be administered for CT. **Iodinated contrast** is taken up by differentiated thyroid carcinoma (DTCa) and **may delay therapeutic ^{131}I for up to 6 months**.

Ultrasound (US) allows excellent high-resolution evaluation of the thyroid, its adjacent nodes, and, when enlarged, the parathyroid glands. **Color Doppler** should always be used when evaluating a thyroid nodule, as increased vascularity is a frequent finding in malignant lesions. It is also important when searching for hypervascular parathyroid adenomas.

Tc-99m-sestamibi is the most sensitive and specific **nuclear medicine** technique for localizing **parathyroid adenomas** and is often supplemented with preoperative US. When these studies are equivocal or discordant, or in a postoperative patient with recurrent hyperparathyroidism, MR or multidetector CECT techniques may be useful to identify ectopic adenomas. Several different CECT protocols have been described, aiming to capitalize on the arterial phase enhancement of parathyroid adenomas. Some protocols advocate imaging from the skull base to the left pulmonary artery, although suprahyoid ectopic adenomas are rare.

Imaging Anatomy

The VS is the anterior tubular space in the midline of the infrahyoid neck. It is completely encircled by the ML-DCF. The VS shares a common fascial wall with the retropharyngeal space, which is immediately posterior and contains only fat in the infrahyoid neck. The VS is surrounded anteriorly and anterolaterally by the strap muscles, sternocleidomastoid muscles, and the anterior cervical fat. Both muscle groups are enclosed by the superficial layer of DCF (SL-DCF). The CSs are at the lateral margin of the VS, with the ML-DCF contributing to the **carotid sheaths**.

The **larynx** and **hypopharynx** are infrahyoid continuations of the oropharynx, and these structures are contiguous with the **trachea** and **esophagus**, respectively, which then traverse the VS to the mediastinum.

The paired thyroid lobes are joined by a midline isthmus. The **thyroid** lobes "cup" the cricoid cartilage and first tracheal rings. It is this intimate relation that allows thyroid tumors to invade the trachea.

There are 2 pairs of **parathyroid glands**. The superior glands are consistently found at the posterosuperior aspect of the thyroid, in the lateral aspect of the tracheoesophageal groove (TEG). The inferior lobes are in a similar position near the inferior aspect of the thyroid; however, they are less reliably found in this location. They are often found lower in the neck or within the superior mediastinum.

Paratracheal nodes are found in the TEG and are commonly referred to as **level VI nodes**.

Also located in the TEG, the **RLNs** ascend in the neck to the level of the cricothyroid joint, where they enter the larynx to supply the vocal cords. The **right RLN** arises from the vagus nerve in the low neck, then loops around the subclavian artery to enter the inferior VS. The **left RLN** arises more inferiorly, looping beneath the aortic arch before ascending to the VS.

Approaches to Imaging Issues of Visceral Space

Infrahyoid neck lesions differ from suprahyoid masses in that their **space of origin** is typically not an imaging dilemma. The VS has carotid sheaths on either side but is not otherwise surrounded by sources of pathological processes in the same way that the suprahyoid neck spaces are. The VS does, however, have several common diagnostic dilemmas.

The **"nonspecific" thyroid mass** incidentally found on CT or MR is the most common imaging dilemma in the VS. This type of lesion is a well-defined round or oval mass within the thyroid gland, with or without calcifications, cystic change, or hemorrhage, and is not associated with adenopathy. Sharply delineated contours are found with benign colloid cysts and thyroid adenomas; however, they may also be seen with DTCa (papillary and follicular) and with medullary thyroid carcinoma.

- **Calcifications** are not an uncommon feature in **adenomas**, whereas fine, speckled calcifications are a frequent finding in DTCa, particularly the papillary type. Coarse calcifications may be found in **medullary thyroid carcinoma. Hemorrhage** or **cystic degeneration** within a thyroid adenoma results in a very heterogeneous appearance of a mass, which mimics malignant necrotic change. Finally, size of thyroid lesion does not indicate any particular pathology. Benign thyroid adenomas can grow to many centimeters in size, whereas malignant thyroid papillary carcinomas may only be several millimeters but already metastatic to nodes.
- Clearly there is a large overlap of benign and malignant features with **CT** and **MR**. The most concerning characteristics on these modalities are invasive features, such as extrathyroidal extension with infiltration of adjacent tissues or associated neck adenopathy. Such cases do not pose a significant imaging dilemma and should all be referred for **fine-needle aspiration** (FNA).
- **US** is able to identify unique imaging features that are most concerning for malignancy and hence is often the second-line study after a lesion is found on CT or MR. Thyroid US will frequently identify characteristics of a

Differential Diagnosis: Visceral Space

Pseudolesion	Metabolic
Thyroid pyramidal lobe	Multinodular goiter
Patulous cervical esophagus	**Benign tumor**
Inflammatory	Thyroid adenoma
Chronic lymphocytic thyroiditis (Hashimoto)	Parathyroid adenoma
Infectious	Recurrent laryngeal nerve schwannoma
Suppurative thyroiditis	**Malignant tumor**
Congenital	Differentiated thyroid carcinoma (DTCa)
Infrahyoid thyroglossal duct cyst	Paratracheal node from DTCa
Degenerative	Thyroid anaplastic carcinoma
Colloid cyst of thyroid	Thyroid non-Hodgkin lymphoma
Parathyroid cyst	Systemic metastasis to thyroid
Esophagopharyngeal diverticulum (Zenker)	Parathyroid carcinoma
Lateral cervical esophageal diverticulum	Tracheal adenoid cystic carcinoma
Tracheal diverticulum	Cervical esophageal carcinoma

multinodular goiter when only 1 nodule was originally evident on clinical or CECT evaluation. US also allows differentiation between **cystic**, and therefore benign, thyroid lesion from a **solid lesion** and allows image-guided FNA of the latter.

- On **PET/CT** imaging, diffuse thyroid uptake is not an uncommon finding and may be due to **thyroiditis**. Thyroid function tests can determine whether the patient has subclinical hypothyroidism. **Focal** thyroid FDG **uptake** has ~ **20%** chance of **malignancy**. FNA should be obtained if this is incidentally found during PET imaging.

TEG lesions may also prove to be a VS diagnostic dilemma. TEG lesions reside in or efface the triangle of fat between the posterior wall of the trachea and the anterior margin of the esophagus. Well-defined nodules (< 1 cm and clearly distinct from the thyroid, trachea, and esophagus) may be **level VI lymph nodes**. These are a drainage site for thyroid malignancies but also squamous cell carcinoma of the larynx, hypopharynx, and esophagus and are often involved in non-Hodgkin lymphoma. Searching for other nodes and a primary source is helpful in making this diagnosis. **Parathyroid adenomas** may mimic nodes unless arterial-phase imaging is performed, in which most appear **hypervascular** with distinctive avid enhancement. **Schwannomas** here are rare and are difficult to diagnose prospectively. The differential for these well-defined lesions is an exophytic thyroid or esophageal mass, such as an adenoma or diverticulum, respectively. Multiplanar imaging may clarify these relationships.

- When soft tissue **infiltrates the TEG** and effaces its fat triangle, the differential favors a **malignant process**, such as thyroid, parathyroid, or esophageal carcinoma or thyroid lymphoma. These neoplastic processes more often present clinically with disruption of the RLN and **vocal cord paralysis**.

Clinical Implications

Patients may be referred for cross-sectional imaging with either a **midline neck mass ± lateral neck mass(es)** from **adenopathy**. When protocoling such a study, it is important to remember that, if DTCa is a possible cause, consideration should be given to US, MR, or even NECT rather than CECT. Iodinated contrast can delay therapeutic ^{131}I up to 6 months. Clinical indicators of possible thyroid cancer include young women with neck masses, particularly low neck masses and/or cystic lymph nodes, and masses associated with vocal cord paralysis.

There are 3 main considerations for a **rapidly growing VS mass**: (1) Hemorrhage or cystic degeneration of thyroid adenoma, (2) anaplastic thyroid carcinoma, and (3) thyroid lymphoma. The latter 2 lesions can appear quite similar on imaging, although lymphoma is more frequently a homogeneous lesion. Calcifications, cystic change, and hemorrhage are much less common in lymphoma than anaplastic carcinoma, which is typically heterogeneous and has a greater tendency to invade the trachea.

When imaging is required for preoperative evaluation of the complete extent of a **multinodular goiter (MNG)**, 2 considerations must be kept in mind: (1) The scan is performed with the patient's arms by his or her side so as not to exaggerate the substernal extension that occurs with the patient's arms positioned over their head, and (2) up to 5% of MNGs harbor a focus of DTCa. While most often these are small foci that have not metastasized, the neck should be carefully evaluated for adenopathy and any invasive features of the thyroid contours that might make surgery complex.

Selected References

1. Loevner LA et al: Cross-sectional imaging of the thyroid gland. Neuroimaging Clin N Am. 18(3):445-61, vii, 2008
2. Parker EE et al: MR imaging of the thoracic inlet. Magn Reson Imaging Clin N Am. 16(2):341-53, x, 2008
3. Babbel RW et al: The visceral space: the unique infrahyoid space. Semin Ultrasound CT MR. 12(3):204-23, 1991

Visceral Space Overview

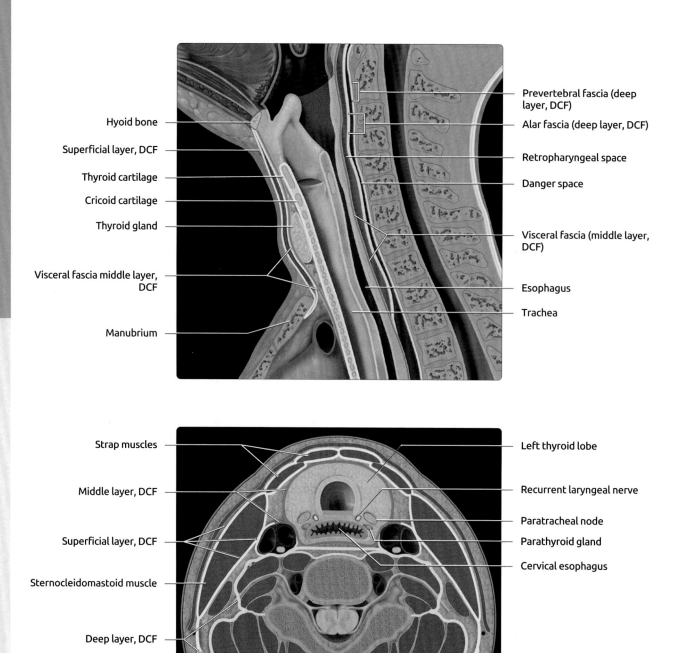

Hyoid bone

Superficial layer, DCF

Thyroid cartilage

Cricoid cartilage

Thyroid gland

Visceral fascia middle layer, DCF

Manubrium

Prevertebral fascia (deep layer, DCF)

Alar fascia (deep layer, DCF)

Retropharyngeal space

Danger space

Visceral fascia (middle layer, DCF)

Esophagus

Trachea

Strap muscles

Middle layer, DCF

Superficial layer, DCF

Sternocleidomastoid muscle

Deep layer, DCF

Left thyroid lobe

Recurrent laryngeal nerve

Paratracheal node

Parathyroid gland

Cervical esophagus

(Top) Sagittal graphic illustrates the craniocaudal extent of the visceral space (VS) in the anterior aspect of the neck. At the hyoid bone, the superficial and middle layers of deep cervical fascia (DCF) insert. The superficial layer encloses the strap muscles of the anterior neck and sternocleidomastoid muscles of the lateral neck. These muscles surround but are separate from the VS. The middle layer of DCF surrounds the VS. The larynx and cervical trachea and the hypopharynx and cervical esophagus form longitudinal columns within this space from the hyoid to the mediastinum. (Bottom) Axial graphic depicts the anterior central location of the VS in the infrahyoid neck, between the carotid sheaths. Other important VS structures surround the larynx/trachea and the hypopharynx/esophagus, such as the thyroid gland, superior and inferior parathyroid glands, and level VI lymph nodes. The recurrent laryngeal nerves course superiorly to the larynx in the tracheoesophageal grooves.

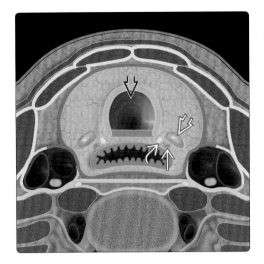

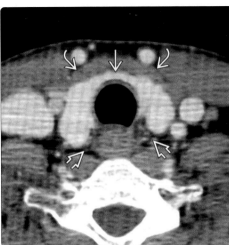

(Left) *Axial graphic depicts the thyroid gland in anterior VS wrapping around the trachea. Graphic also illustrates 3 key structures found in tracheoesophageal groove: Recurrent laryngeal nerve (RLN), paratracheal lymph nodes, and parathyroid gland.* (Right) *Axial CECT at the level of thyroid gland isthmus (which crosses the anterior surface of trachea beneath strap muscles) shows normal fat, small vessels, and tiny lymph nodes in the tracheoesophageal groove.*

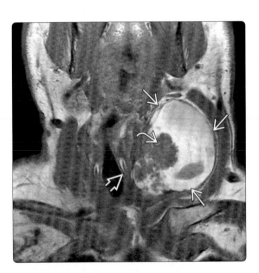

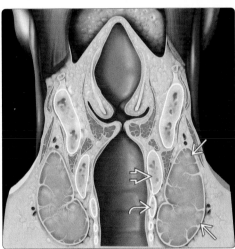

(Left) *Coronal T1 MR shows heterogeneous solid and cystic infrahyoid neck mass arising from the left thyroid. Note the intrinsic hyperintensity within the cystic component from thyroglobulin. This was found to be papillary thyroid carcinoma, displacing larynx without cricoid invasion.* (Right) *Coronal graphic shows the relationship of thyroid to cricoid cartilage and the 1st tracheal ring. It is important to carefully examine cricoid and proximal trachea for invasion of malignant thyroid tumor.*

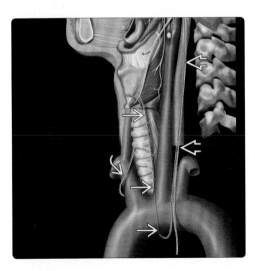

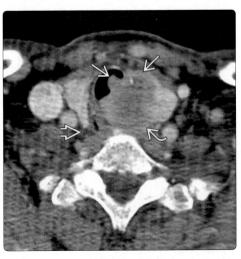

(Left) *Lateral graphic illustrates ascending course of RLNs in the tracheoesophageal groove of the VS. Left RLN arises from left vagus in superior mediastinum. Right RLN arises from vagus at level of subclavian artery.* (Right) *Axial CECT in a patient with left RLN paralysis shows heterogeneous mass within the left thyroid lobe that invades trachea and is inseparable from esophagus. Fat of left tracheoesophageal groove appears infiltrated, compared with normal right side.*

TERMINOLOGY

- Hashimoto thyroiditis, chronic/sclerosing lymphocytic thyroiditis

IMAGING

- Best imaging modality is ultrasound for diagnosis & monitoring
  - US: Early stage shows enlarged lobulated thyroid, decreased echogenicity, & marked hypervascularity
  - US: Late stage shows small echogenic fibrosed gland with absent flow signals
- CECT: Diffuse moderately **enlarged**, **low-density thyroid** without calcifications, cysts, or necrosis

TOP DIFFERENTIAL DIAGNOSES

- Multinodular goiter
- Invasive fibrous (Riedel) thyroiditis
- Thyroid non-Hodgkin lymphoma (NHL)
- Thyroid anaplastic carcinoma

PATHOLOGY

- Some CLT occurs in setting of isolated or systemic **Immunoglobulin G4 (IgG4)** related disease
- Antithyroid autoantibodies in serum
- Micro: Atrophic follicles, Hürthle cell metaplasia, fibrosis, lymphocyte & plasma cell infiltration
- 60-80x risk of thyroid **NHL**
- > 90% of patients with primary thyroid NHL have CLT

CLINICAL ISSUES

- Most commonly in women 30-50 years old
- Gradual painless enlargement of thyroid
- Patients most often euthyroid
- Most important complication is increased incidence of thyroid malignancy

DIAGNOSTIC CHECKLIST

- Rapid enlargement of thyroid in patient with history of CLT: NHL until proven otherwise

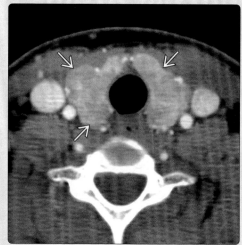
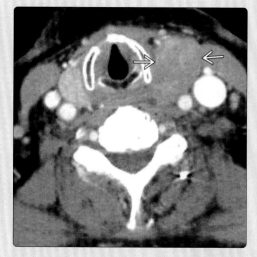

(Left) Axial CECT in a patient with CLT shows an enlarged thyroid gland ➡ with inhomogeneous hypodense enhancement & lobulated texture. Heterogeneity & moderate enlargement mimic small multinodular goiter; however, there are no calcifications, hemorrhage, or cystic changes evident. (Right) CECT in a 68 year-old woman with a rapidly enlarging left neck mass shows an ill-defined hypodense left thyroid mass ➡, which was a large B-cell lymphoma developing in the background of preexisting CLT at histopathology.

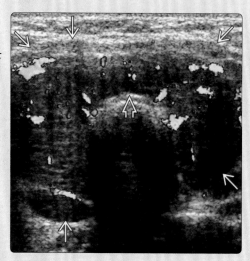
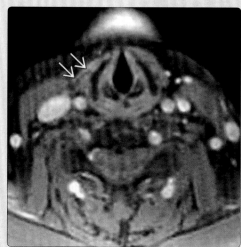

(Left) Transverse color Doppler ultrasound in the early phase of C shows diffusely enlarged, hypoechoic left and right ➡ thyroid lobes and thyroid isthmus ➡. Moderate parenchymal hypervascularity is evident. (Right) Axial T1WI C+ MR in a patient with a long history of hypothyroidism and biopsy-proven CLT reveals chronic phase changes with markedly atrophic thyroid so that only the right lobe is evident ➡. This has little appreciable contrast enhancement.

TERMINOLOGY

Abbreviations
- Chronic lymphocytic thyroiditis (CLT)

Synonyms
- Hashimoto thyroiditis, sclerosing lymphocytic thyroiditis

Definitions
- Chronic, autoimmune-mediated lymphocytic inflammation of thyroid gland

IMAGING

General Features
- Best diagnostic clue
  - CECT: Diffuse moderately **enlarged, low-density thyroid** without calcifications or necrosis
- Size
  - Early phase: Moderate thyroid enlargement
  - Late phase: Diffusely atrophic gland
- Morphology
  - Heterogeneous texture with accentuation of lobular architecture by fibrosis

CT Findings
- CECT
  - Diffusely decreased density typical
  - No necrosis, cysts, or calcification

MR Findings
- T2WI FS
  - May see increased intensity with lower intensity fibrotic bands

Ultrasonographic Findings
- Grayscale ultrasound
  - Early stages
    - Enlarged lobulated thyroid with heterogeneous, **diffusely decreased echogenicity**
  - Later stages
    - Small, heterogeneous, & echogenic thyroid
- Color Doppler
  - Early phases: Marked parenchymal hypervascularity
  - Later phases: Blood flow signals are absent

Nuclear Medicine Findings
- PET
  - CLT may show thyroidal uptake
- **Tc-99m-pertechnetate & iodine 123**
  - Early: Diffuse uniform increased activity
  - Later: Coarse patchy activity

Imaging Recommendations
- Best imaging tool
  - Ultrasound for diagnosis & monitoring

DIFFERENTIAL DIAGNOSIS

Multinodular Goiter
- Diffuse heterogeneous enlargement of thyroid
- Cystic degeneration, calcification, or hemorrhage

Invasive Fibrous (Riedel) Thyroiditis
- Benign fibrosis with diffuse thyroid enlargement
- Fibrosis extends beyond gland to neck soft tissues

Thyroid Non-Hodgkin Lymphoma
- Infiltrative mass diffusely enlarges gland
- Nonnecrotic adenopathy frequently also present

Thyroid Anaplastic Carcinoma
- Heterogeneous, infiltrative thyroid mass
- Necrotic adenopathy frequently present

PATHOLOGY

General Features
- Etiology
  - **Antithyroid autoantibodies**
  - Variants of CLT
    - Reidel &/or fibrous thyroiditis &/or **immunoglobulin G4 (IgG4)-related disease**
- Associated abnormalities
  - **Thyroid non-Hodgkin lymphoma (NHL)**
    - 60-80x risk of developing thyroid NHL

CLINICAL ISSUES

Presentation
- Most common signs/symptoms
  - Gradual painless enlargement of thyroid
    - Patients most often **euthyroid** with normal T3 & T4 hormones ("subclinical thyroiditis")
  - Other signs/symptoms
    - 20% present with hypothyroidism
    - 5% have early "hashitoxicosis": Thyrotoxicosis with excess T3/T4 release
- Clinical profile
  - Women > 40 years with gradual thyroid enlargement

Demographics
- Age
  - Peak incidence: 4th-5th decades
  - Juvenile form predominantly in adolescents
- Gender
  - M:F = 1:9

Natural History & Prognosis
- **Increased incidence of thyroid malignancy**
  - Most often NHL

DIAGNOSTIC CHECKLIST

Consider
- **Rapid enlargement** of thyroid in patient with history of CLT: **NHL until proven otherwise**

SELECTED REFERENCES

1. Fujita A et al: IgG4-related disease of the head and neck: CT and MR imaging manifestations. Radiographics. 32(7):1945-58, 2012
2. Anderson L et al: Hashimoto thyroiditis: Part 2, sonographic analysis of benign and malignant nodules in patients with diffuse Hashimoto thyroiditis. AJR Am J Roentgenol. 195(1):216-22, 2010
3. Kim HC et al: Primary thyroid lymphoma: CT findings. Eur J Radiol. 46(3):233-9, 2003

KEY FACTS

TERMINOLOGY

- Diffuse, multinodular enlargement of thyroid gland in response to chronic TSH stimulation

IMAGING

- Diffuse enlargement of thyroid gland with heterogeneous, nodular appearance
- **40%** have **retrosternal extension**
- CT findings
  - Calcifications, degenerative cysts, & hemorrhage
  - Clear delineation from displaced structures
- MR: Heterogeneous signal and enhancement

TOP DIFFERENTIAL DIAGNOSES

- Thyroid colloid cyst
- Thyroid adenoma
- Thyroid differentiated carcinoma
- Thyroid anaplastic carcinoma

PATHOLOGY

- **Sporadic goiter**: Etiology usually unknown, rarely drug induced
- **Endemic goiter**: Associated with iodine deficiency
- 5% have malignant focus at surgery
- Anaplastic thyroid carcinoma may arise from MNG

CLINICAL ISSUES

- Most patients euthyroid, rarely hypothyroid
- Toxic goiter = MNG + hyperthyroidism; uncommon
- Plummer disease = toxic adenoma within MNG

DIAGNOSTIC CHECKLIST

- Well-defined contour of thyroid despite bizarre imaging appearance is key to diagnosis
- Perform presurgical CT with arms by patient's side
- Ensure neck CT covers to inferior limit of MNG

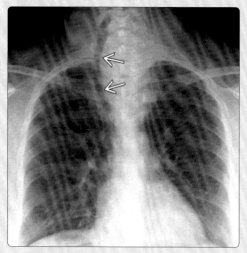
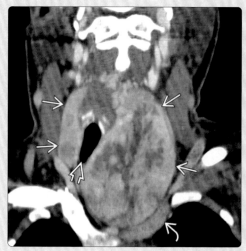

(Left) Posteroanterior chest radiograph demonstrates marked displacement of cervical and thoracic trachea ➡ by a large, left-sided neck & superior mediastinum mass. (Right) Coronal reformatted CECT in the same patient illustrates craniocaudad extent of the MNG ➡ with heterogeneous thyroid tissue bilaterally, but more marked left lobe enlargement. Marked displacement of the subglottic larynx and trachea is evident ➡. The left brachiocephalic vein ➡ is displaced inferiorly but not compressed by the left lobe.

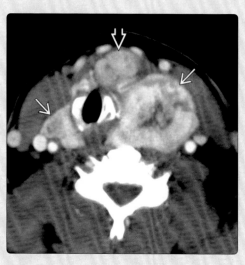
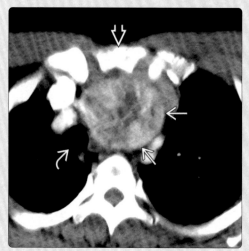

(Left) Axial CECT at level of cricoid shows markedly heterogeneous, lobulated, and enlarged thyroid lobes ➡ as well as thyroid isthmus ➡. No calcifications or frank cysts are evident. Despite heterogeneity of thyroid, gland margins are well defined and adjacent structures merely displaced. (Right) Axial CECT through cervicothoracic junction in the same patient reveals inferior extension of enlarged left lobe ➡ into superior mediastinum, posterior to manubrium ➡. The trachea is displaced to the right ➡.

TERMINOLOGY

Abbreviations
- Multinodular goiter (MNG)

Synonyms
- Simple nodular goiter, nontoxic goiter

Definitions
- Diffuse, multinodular enlargement of thyroid gland in response to chronic TSH stimulation
- Retrosternal goiter: MNG extends to mediastinum

IMAGING

General Features
- Best diagnostic clue
  - Well-marginated, diffuse enlargement of thyroid gland with heterogeneous, nodular appearance
  - Often **calcifications**, **degenerative cysts**, and **hemorrhage**
- Location
  - Visceral space, thyroid bed
  - **Retrosternal** extension in **40%**
    - Most anterior mediastinum, rarely posterior
    - Retrosternal MNG = most common cause anterior mediastinal mass
- Size
  - May become very large (> 15 cm)
- Morphology
  - Well-marginated, diffuse thyroid enlargement
    - Carotid vessels displaced away from midline
    - Trachea compressed ± displaced

Radiographic Findings
- Radiography
  - Chest x-ray findings
    - If all suprasternal: Normal CXR or tracheal deviation/narrowing
    - If **retrosternal**: Superior mediastinal mass + **tracheal deviation & narrowing**

CT Findings
- NECT
  - **Low-density** areas of **degenerative** & **colloidal cysts**
  - Intermediate-density solid nodules & fibrosis
  - **High-density** foci from **hemorrhage** & **calcification**
    - **90% Ca⁺⁺**: Amorphous, ring-like, curvilinear
- CECT
  - Thyroid parenchyma replaced with multiple, variably sized, heterogeneous solid & cystic masses
  - Clear delineation from adjacent displaced structures
  - Diffuse, inhomogeneous enhancement
  - No associated lymphadenopathy
  - Coronal reformats
    - Brachiocephalic vessels "cradle" inferior MNG

MR Findings
- T1WI
  - Generally low intensity, isointense to muscles
  - Focal high signal intensity with fine calcifications or hemorrhage
  - Low signal intensity with cystic degeneration or coarse calcifications
- T2WI
  - Heterogeneous intermediate to high intensity
  - Low signal with fibrosis & coarse calcifications
  - Focal high signal with cystic degeneration & hemorrhage
- DWI
  - Preliminary data: ADC of malignant nodules < ADC of normal tissue < ADC of benign nodules
- T1WI C+
  - Diffuse heterogeneous enhancement

Ultrasonographic Findings
- Grayscale ultrasound
  - Multiple nodules, bilateral diffuse thyroid involvement
  - Solid nodules usually **isoechoic**, small portions hypoechoic (5%)
  - Nodules unencapsulated but sharply defined, "haloed"
  - Mass has heterogeneous internal echo pattern with debris, septa, solid/cystic portions
    - Ca⁺⁺ seen as hyperechoic foci with dense shadowing
    - Cystic, hypoechoic regions from hemorrhage, degeneration, or colloid within nodule

Nuclear Medicine Findings
- PET
  - Heterogeneous uptake common
  - Focal uptake within gland requires biopsy
- Tc-99m pertechnetate or I-123
  - No role in initial evaluation of nontoxic goiter
  - Determines mediastinal mass is thyroid in nature
  - Heterogeneously iodine avid, with suppression of surrounding parenchyma

Imaging Recommendations
- Best imaging tool
  - CECT is exam of choice for evaluation of MNG
    - Extent & severity of airway compression
    - Presence & extent of retrosternal MNG
    - Unusual extensions of MNG (e.g., retroesophageal, suprahyoid)
  - US used to guide needle biopsy of solid nodules
  - If malignancy suspected, MR imaging stages nodal extent without compromising I-131 therapy
- Protocol advice
  - Important to perform neck CT with arms by side
  - Arms elevated, as with chest CT, falsely exaggerates retrosternal extent

DIFFERENTIAL DIAGNOSIS

Thyroid Colloid Cyst
- Variable size cystic mass within thyroid
- Adjacent normal thyroid tissue

Thyroid Adenoma
- Solitary intrathyroidal mass without local invasion or adenopathy
- Adjacent normal thyroid tissue seen

Thyroid Differentiated Carcinoma
- Tumor may occupy all or part of thyroid gland

- Thyroid gland margins may be invasive

Thyroid Anaplastic Carcinoma

- Rapidly enlarging, heterogeneous, invasive tumor originating from thyroid gland

Thyroid Non-Hodgkin Lymphoma

- Large, solid, occasionally invasive tumor originating from thyroid gland
- Typically multiple cervical lymph nodes

PATHOLOGY

General Features

- Etiology
  - **Sporadic goiter**
    - Etiology usually unknown
    - Generally adequate dietary iodine intake
    - Rarely drug induced: Lithium, aminoglutethimide
  - **Endemic goiter**
    - Environmental iodine deficiency → TSH elevation
    - Results in gradual, diffuse thyroid hyperplasia
    - Involution + fibrosis + focal hyperplasia→ nodules
- Associated abnormalities
  - 5% have malignant focus at surgery
    - Same incidence as single thyroid nodule
  - Differentiated thyroid carcinoma most common
    - Anaplastic thyroid carcinoma may arise from MNG

Gross Pathologic & Surgical Features

- Aggregate of multiple, partially encapsulated, variably sized colloid & adenomatous nodules

Microscopic Features

- Distended follicles with colloid & hyperplasia
- Follicle degeneration leads to infarction, hemorrhage, fibrosis, cyst formation, & calcification

CLINICAL ISSUES

Presentation

- Most common signs/symptoms
  - Large, multinodular lower neck mass
  - MNG most common cause of asymmetric thyroid enlargement
- Other signs/symptoms
  - Airway compression (55%), hoarseness (15%), dysphagia & superior vena cava syndrome (10%)
- Clinical profile
  - Most euthyroid
  - Toxic MNG = hyperthyroidism + MNG
    - Either multiple hyperfunctioning areas in MNG or toxic adenoma in MNG (Plummer disease)
    - Iodinated drug (e.g., amiodarone) can induce hyperthyroidism in nontoxic MNG

Demographics

- Age
  - Sporadic goiter has no specific age
  - Endemic goiter occurs during childhood
    - Continues to increase in size with age
- Gender
  - F:M = 2-4:1

- Epidemiology
  - Sporadic
    - 3-5% of population in developed countries
  - Endemic
    - > 13% of world population affected
    - Mild iodine deficiency: Goiter prevalence 5-20%
    - Moderate iodine deficiency: Goiter 20-30%
    - Severe iodine deficiency: Goiter > 30%

Natural History & Prognosis

- Growth & nodule production → functional autonomy
- Functional autonomy rarely results in thyrotoxicosis
- Spontaneous regression vs. gradually increasing size with development of multiple nodules, local compression symptoms ± cosmetic complaints

Treatment

- No treatment for asymptomatic, nonpalpable MNG identified on neck imaging done for other reasons
- Patients with prominent, growing, hard nodule may have aspiration to exclude malignancy
- Large, nontoxic, compressive MNG: Surgical removal
  - Postoperative thyroid hormone replacement
  - Hypoparathyroidism or recurrent laryngeal nerve injury rare complications
  - Radioiodine if significant comorbidities prohibit surgery
- Toxic MNG: Surgery or radioiodine therapy

DIAGNOSTIC CHECKLIST

Consider

- **Well-defined thyroid contour** despite **bizarre imaging appearance** is **key** to diagnosis

Image Interpretation Pearls

- Always perform presurgical CT evaluation with arms by patient's side, not above head
- Ensure neck CT covers to inferior limit of MNG

SELECTED REFERENCES

1. Bombil I et al: Incidental cancer in multinodular goitre post thyroidectomy. S Afr J Surg. 52(1):5-9, 2014
2. Brito JP et al: Prevalence of thyroid cancer in multinodular goiter versus single nodule: a systematic review and meta-analysis. Thyroid. 23(4):449-55, 2013
3. Erdem G et al: Diffusion-weighted images differentiate benign from malignant thyroid nodules. J Magn Reson Imaging. 31(1):94-100, 2010
4. Moalem J et al: Treatment and prevention of recurrence of multinodular goiter: an evidence-based review of the literature. World J Surg. 32(7):1301-12, 2008
5. Pollard DB et al: Preoperative imaging of thyroid goiter: how imaging technique can influence anatomic appearance and create a potential for inaccurate interpretation. AJNR Am J Neuroradiol. 26(5):1215-7, 2005
6. Hedayati N et al: The clinical presentation and operative management of nodular and diffuse substernal thyroid disease. Am Surg. 68(3): 245-51; discussion 251-2, 2002
7. Yousem DM et al: Clinical and economic impact of incidental thyroid lesions found with CT and MR. AJNR Am J Neuroradiol. 18(8): 1423-8, 1997
8. Bashist B et al: Computed tomography of intrathoracic goiters. AJR Am J Roentgenol. 140(3):455-60, 1983

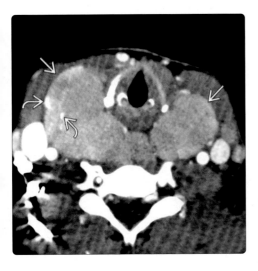
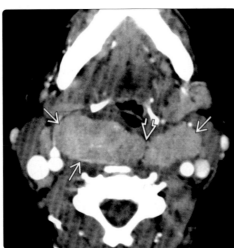

(Left) *Axial CECT through level of the infraglottic larynx in a patient with MNG shows symmetric enlargement of thyroid lobes ➡, which appear hyperdense with patchy areas of low density and small focal calcifications ➡. The gland remains sharply demarcated with no evidence of invasion of adjacent soft tissues.* (Right) *Axial CECT more superiorly at level of hyoid in the same patient shows unusual cranial growth, with MNG extending posteriorly and medially around pharynx ➡ so that lobes meet in midline ➡.*

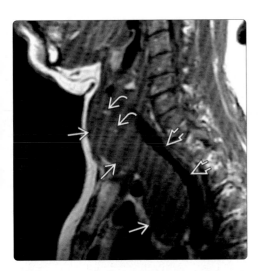
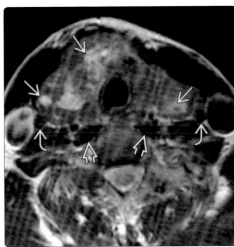

(Left) *Sagittal T1WI MR demonstrates narrowing and displacement of the trachea ➡ posteriorly as goiter ➡ extends from lower neck to superior mediastinum. Focal areas of T1 shortening ➡ within enlarged thyroid represent calcifications or hemorrhage.* (Right) *Axial T2WI MR in the same patient shows nodular goiter with heterogeneous texture and areas of hyperintense cystic degeneration ➡. T2 better demonstrates clear delineation of thyroid from adjacent strap muscles ➡ and carotid arteries ➡.*

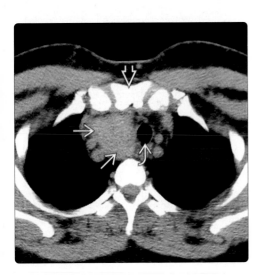
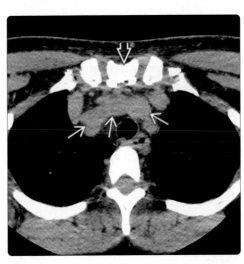

(Left) *Axial NECT for a large, multinodular goiter shows inferior aspect of enlarged right thyroid lobe ➡, posterior to manubrium ➡ & displacing the trachea ➡ medially. Study was performed as chest CT with arms above head.* (Right) *Axial NECT in the same patient, same day, at same level ➡, performed as a neck study with arms at patient's side, shows no retrosternal extension of MNG. Only great vessels ➡ are evident. This illustrates the importance of arms at side technique for preoperative evaluation.*

TERMINOLOGY

- 2 benign categories that present as thyroid nodule
  - True adenoma and adenomatous nodule

IMAGING

- Thyroid adenoma
  - Well-defined nodule compresses adjacent gland
- Adenomatous nodule
  - Less distinct lesion contours; ± multiple lesions
- Calcifications or cystic change may be seen
- Large adenomas often have heterogeneous enhancement with degeneration
- No invasive features or neck adenopathy
- FDG uptake may be seen in adenomas
- Nuclear scintigraphy
  - Hot nodules are usually benign adenomas
  - 20% cold nodules are malignant

TOP DIFFERENTIAL DIAGNOSES

- Thyroid colloid cyst
- Multinodular goiter
- Parathyroid adenoma
- Thyroid differentiated carcinoma

PATHOLOGY

- Adenomatous nodule > follicular adenoma
- Hürthle cell adenoma least common
- While FNA can suggest adenoma, only resection can distinguish from carcinoma

CLINICAL ISSUES

- Typically nonfunctioning, most commonly incidental imaging finding
- Do not evaluate suspected thyroid mass with CECT
  - Iodinated contrast delays iodine treatment of malignant thyroid tumor

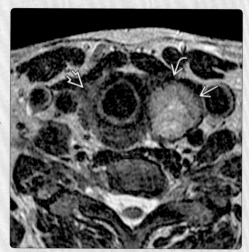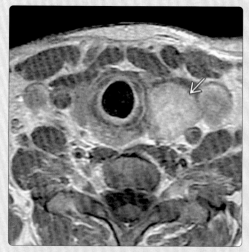

(Left) Axial T2WI MR reveals mildly hyperintense mass ➡ replacing much of left thyroid lobe, with only thin rim of normal gland evident at anterior margin ➡. Mass is well circumscribed and clearly delineated from strap muscles and adjacent carotid artery and jugular vein. Right thyroid lobe appears small ➡. (Right) Axial T1WI C+ MR in the same patient reveals diffusely homogeneous enhancement of mass ➡. There is no neck adenopathy. At resection, lesion was determined to be follicular adenoma.

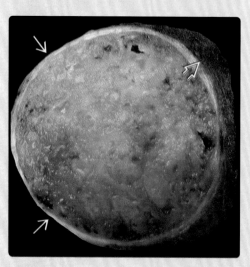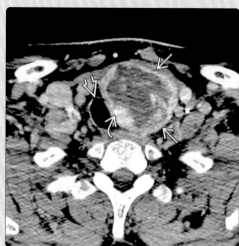

(Left) Gross pathology shows follicular adenoma. There is a thick, well-formed fibrous connective tissue capsule ➡ separating the adenoma from the surrounding thyroid parenchyma. There is compression of the adjacent thyroid ➡, which is more beefy red. (Right) Axial CECT shows a large, heterogeneous mass ➡ with central low density arising within left thyroid lobe. Focal calcification is evident ➡. Mass abuts trachea ➡, but there is no evidence of invasion.

TERMINOLOGY

Definitions

- **True adenoma**: Benign neoplasm of thyroid glandular epithelium with fibrous encapsulation
  - Follicular adenoma and Hürthle cell adenoma
- **Adenomatous nodule**: Focal adenomatous hyperplasia with incomplete capsule
  - Also known as colloid nodule

IMAGING

General Features

- Best diagnostic clue
  - Thyroid adenoma
    - Well-defined nodule compresses adjacent gland
  - Adenomatous nodule
    - Less distinct lesion contours; multiple lesions often present
  - No imaging characteristic highly specific for benign adenoma
- Location
  - Intrathyroidal, though may be exophytic
- Size
  - Usually < 4 cm; palpable if > 1 cm
- Morphology
  - Adenoma: Well-defined encapsulated small nodule
  - Adenomatous nodule: Incomplete capsule, less sharp demarcation from adjacent gland

CT Findings

- CECT
  - Findings nonspecific
  - No invasive features or adenopathy
  - Heterogeneous enhancement with degenerative changes
  - Coarse calcifications may be seen

MR Findings

- T1WI
  - Typically iso- or hypointense
  - Foci of increased signal intensity from hemorrhage or calcification
- T2WI
  - Typically hyperintense
- T1WI C+
  - Homogeneous or heterogeneous enhancement

Ultrasonographic Findings

- Grayscale ultrasound
  - Usually **isoechoic**; may be hyper or hypoechoic
  - Adenoma: Smooth peripheral echo-poor halo
  - Adenomatous nodule: Often incomplete halo
  - Ultrasound features suggesting benign lesion
    - Thin, well-defined halo, regular margin, coarse calcifications
    - "Comet tail" artifact within nodule
    - No neck adenopathy
- Color Doppler
  - Thyroid adenoma: Spoke-wheel pattern; peripheral blood vessels extending toward center of lesion
  - Adenomatous nodule has more diffuse vascularity

Nuclear Medicine Findings

- PET
  - FDG uptake can be seen in adenomas
    - Biopsy recommended to exclude malignancy
- Thyroid scintigraphy (Tc-99m pertechnetate or iodine-123)
  - **Hot nodule**: Focally increased activity
    - Most often hyperfunctioning thyroid adenoma
    - 50% are autonomous adenoma
    - **< 1% are malignant lesions**
  - **Cold nodule**: Absence of activity
    - Most often adenoma/adenomatous nodule or cyst
    - **20% are malignant lesions**

Imaging Recommendations

- Best imaging tool
  - Thyroid nodule common **incidental** CT or MR finding
    - Recommend US if invasive appearance or abnormal lymph nodes
    - If **< 35 years of age**, recommend US for **≥ 1 cm** in size
    - If **≥ 35 years of age**, recommend US for **≥ 1.5 cm** in size
  - Ultrasound helpful for differentiating benign and malignant
    - Also allows FNA guidance and evaluation of nodes
  - Thyroid scintigraphy can determine if hot nodule; likely benign
- Protocol advice
  - Do not evaluate new thyroid mass with CECT
    - Iodinated contrast delays iodine treatment of malignant thyroid tumor

DIFFERENTIAL DIAGNOSIS

Thyroid Colloid Cyst

- Cystic degeneration of nodule
- Variable MR T1 signal intensity from colloid or hemorrhage

Multinodular Goiter

- Multiple nodules in diffusely enlarged thyroid
- Heterogeneous thyroid texture and coarse calcifications common

Parathyroid Adenoma

- Delineated by fat plane from posterior aspect of thyroid gland
- Rarely ectopic intrathyroidal parathyroid adenoma; diagnosis made by FNA

Thyroid Differentiated Carcinoma

- Focal intrathyroidal mass, may have invasive margins
- Calcifications often seen with papillary type
- Cervical lymphadenopathy frequently found

PATHOLOGY

General Features

- Etiology
  - No inducing factors known
- While FNA can suggest adenoma, lobectomy only can differentiate from carcinoma

- FNA showing "follicular lesion" has 10-20% chance of malignancy

Gross Pathologic & Surgical Features

- Thyroid adenoma: Circumscribed, encapsulated lesions of varying color (gray to white to tan)
  - Compress adjacent normal thyroid tissue
  - Hemorrhage, fibrosis, calcification, and cyst formation may be seen
  - FNA can suggest diagnosis but cannot determine malignant capsular or vascular invasion
- Adenomatous nodules: Circumscribed but only partially encapsulated; more often multiple

Microscopic Features

- Several histologic types of adenoma
- Different types may be present in same gland
  - Follicular (simple), macrofollicular (colloid), microfollicular (fetal), trabecular-solid (embryonal)
  - Hürthle cell (oncocytic) adenoma: Granular cells with pink cytoplasm
- Degenerative changes, such as hemorrhage, cyst formation, fibrosis, and calcification may be present
- Significant mitotic activity or necrosis not common in absence of prior FNA or trauma
  - Raises concern for malignancy, though not diagnostic of carcinoma

CLINICAL ISSUES

Presentation

- Most common signs/symptoms
  - Slow-growing solitary palpable neck nodule
- Clinical profile
  - Usually asymptomatic as nonfunctioning
    - Hyperthyroidism is uncommon presentation ("toxic adenoma")
    - Functional adenomas commonly ≥ 3 cm
  - Clinical factors favoring benign diagnosis
    - Family history of autoimmune disease (Hashimoto), benign nodules or goiter
    - Thyroid hyper- or hypofunction; multinodular goiter without dominant nodule
    - Soft, smooth, mobile nodule; painful or tender
  - Clinical factors favoring malignancy
    - Age < 20 years or > 60 years; male patients
    - History of thyroid carcinoma, prior radiation, family history of multiple endocrine neoplasia
    - Firm, hard, immobile nodule; neck adenopathy

Demographics

- Age
  - May be found in all age groups
- Gender
  - M:F = 1:4
- Epidemiology
  - Thyroid nodules common
    - 25% by ultrasound
    - 30-60% at autopsy
  - Adenomatous nodules more common than adenomas

Natural History & Prognosis

- Follicular adenoma: Slow growing; rarely associated with malignancy
  - Rapid enlargement may occur with spontaneous hemorrhage
  - May degenerate to form thyroid cyst
- Hürthle cell adenoma: Slow growing, may spontaneously infarct
- Adenomatous hyperplasia: More likely to have degenerative changes

Treatment

- Those nodules with "suspicious" or "malignant" features from US criteria should be excised surgically
- Hot nodules followed clinically and with US
- **Cold nodules** have **20%** risk of malignancy
  - FNA by palpation or ultrasound-guided
  - Nondiagnostic FNA → repeat aspiration or resection
- Autonomous hyperfunctioning nodules can be treated by several methods
  - I-131 ablation with risk of hypothyroidism
  - Ethanol injection with risk of recurrent laryngeal nerve injury
  - Surgical resection

DIAGNOSTIC CHECKLIST

Consider

- Thyroid nodules common; frequently incidental imaging finding
- 95% benign, clinically not important: Adenomatous nodules, adenomas, thyroid cysts, focal thyroiditis
- Diagnosis of adenoma may be suggested by FNA but not proven without surgical resection

Image Interpretation Pearls

- Imaging cannot differentiate between adenoma and low-grade neoplasm
- Evaluation of suspected thyroid mass with CECT may delay radioactive iodine treatment
- US can determine whether single or multiple, cystic or solid
- Thyroid scintigraphy: < 1% hot nodules malignant; 20% cold nodules malignant

SELECTED REFERENCES

1. Hoang JK et al: Managing incidental thyroid nodules detected on imaging: white paper of the ACR Incidental Thyroid Findings Committee. J Am Coll Radiol. 12(2):143-50, 2015
2. Yoon JH et al: Malignancy risk stratification of thyroid nodules: comparison between the thyroid imaging reporting and data system and the 2014 American Thyroid Association Management Guidelines. Radiology. 150056, 2015
3. Kamran SC et al: Thyroid nodule size and prediction of cancer. J Clin Endocrinol Metab. 98(2):564-70, 2013
4. Baier ND et al: Fine-needle aspiration biopsy of thyroid nodules: experience in a cohort of 944 patients. AJR Am J Roentgenol. 193(4):1175-9, 2009
5. Lee EW et al: How diagnostic is ultrasound-guided neck mass biopsy (fine-needle capillary sampling biopsy technique)?: evaluation of 132 nonthyroid neck mass biopsies with pathologic analysis over 7 years at a single institution. J Ultrasound Med. 28(12):1679-84, 2009
6. Liu Y: Clinical significance of thyroid uptake on F18-fluorodeoxyglucose positron emission tomography. Ann Nucl Med. 23(1):17-23, 2009
7. Desser TS et al: Ultrasound of thyroid nodules. Neuroimaging Clin N Am. 18(3):463-78, vii, 2008
8. Loevner LA et al: Cross-sectional imaging of the thyroid gland. Neuroimaging Clin N Am. 18(3):445-61, vii, 2008

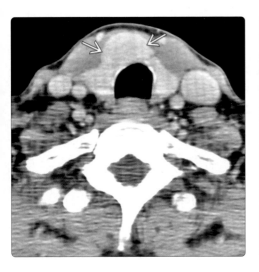 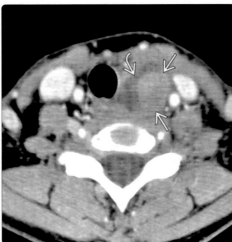

(Left) *Axial CECT demonstrates exophytic homogeneous mass ➡ arising from isthmus of thyroid. The mass is almost isodense to remaining thyroid gland, has no calcifications, and is not associated with adenopathy.* **(Right)** *Axial CECT through lower neck shows a well-defined but heterogeneous mass ➡ in left lower neck, which displaces carotid artery and jugular vein laterally. Heterogeneous nature with eccentric low density ➡ is due to cystic degeneration with infarction of adenoma.*

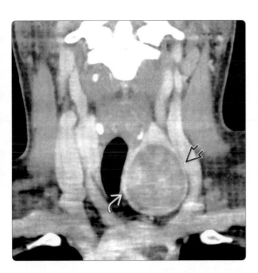 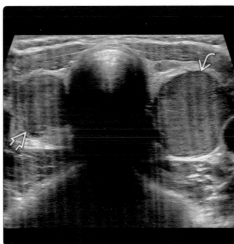

(Left) *Coronal CECT reveals a follicular thyroid adenoma. The adenoma is seen as a low-density, heterogeneously enhancing intrathyroidal mass ➡. Notice the well circumscribed margins and mass effect on the trachea without invasive features ➡.* **(Right)** *Midline transverse US shows bilateral thyroid nodules. The left nodule reveals a well-defined capsule ➡ and was a follicular adenoma on excision. The right nodule shows slightly ill-defined lateral margin ➡ and was a follicular carcinoma on excision.*

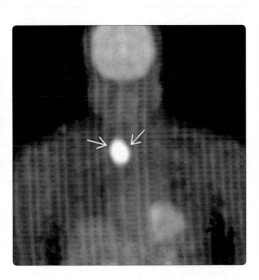 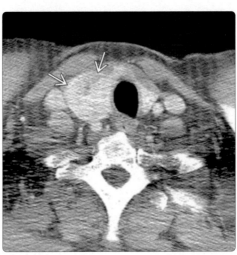

(Left) *Anteroposterior PET reveals focal intense uptake in right lower neck of patient with cutaneous T-cell lymphoma ➡; the image was taken to help determine the extent of metastatic disease.* **(Right)** *Axial CECT through lower neck demonstrates enlarged heterogeneous nodule ➡ in right thyroid gland without evidence of extrathyroidal extension. No adenopathy is evident. FDG uptake may be seen in both benign and malignant thyroid nodules. FNA is typically performed to exclude malignancy.*

Parathyroid Adenoma in Visceral Space

TERMINOLOGY

- Benign neoplasm of parathyroid gland producing excess parathyroid adenoma, resulting in hypercalcemia

IMAGING

- Adenoma 10-30 mm; normal gland 5 x 3 x 1 mm
- Round or oval, well-circumscribed solid mass best characterized on cross-sectional imaging by hypervascular nature
- Nuclear scintigraphy: Usual 1st-line imaging study
- **Tc-99m sestamibi** > 90% sensitive and > 90% specific
  - **Focal increased uptake** on early and **delayed** images
  - May perform as SPECT ± CT to localize
- Nuclear subtraction scans helpful if thyroid mass
- US: Homogeneous, **hypoechoic, hypervascular**
  - Dependent on operator experience
- CECT: **Arterial-phase** (30 sec) avid enhancement helps distinguish from lymph node
- MR: T2 iso- to hyperintense compared to thyroid

TOP DIFFERENTIAL DIAGNOSES

- Reactive lymph nodes
- Thyroid adenoma
- Multinodular goiter
- Parathyroid cyst
- Parathyroid carcinoma

CLINICAL ISSUES

- Most patients have asymptomatic hypercalcemia
- Hypercalcemia may have wide range of symptoms
  - "Stones, bones, groans, and psychic moans"

DIAGNOSTIC CHECKLIST

- Preoperative imaging role and optimal modality remain controversial
- Paratracheal node, esophagus, or exophytic thyroid mass may be mistaken for parathyroid adenoma
  - Compare scintigraphy and US/CT/MR to avoid these mistakes

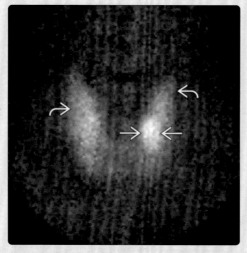
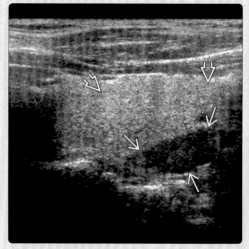

(Left) Anteroposterior delayed Tc-99m sestamibi scan demonstrates parathyroid adenoma with persistent focal uptake ➡ in lower aspect left thyroid. Only faint residual tracer is evident in thyroid ➡. (Right) Longitudinal ultrasound in the same patient reveals a hypoechoic, solid ovoid lesion ➡ that measures 15 x 9 x 7 mm posterior to left thyroid lobe ➡. Color Doppler also showed lesion to be hypervascular. Parathyroid adenoma was resected with normalization of parathyroid hormone levels and resolution of hypercalcemia.

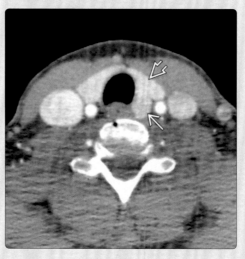
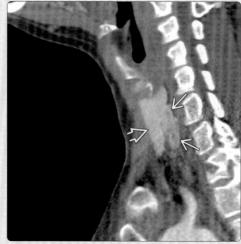

(Left) Axial CECT in a patient with acute hoarseness shows a well-defined round lesion ➡ in left tracheoesophageal groove. Mass is distinct from posterior aspect left thyroid lobe ➡ and appears slightly less enhancing than thyroid on this delayed scan. (Right) Sagittal CECT shows a heterogeneous oval mass ➡ immediately posterior to left thyroid ➡. There is internal heterogeneity from degeneration, which led to adenoma enlargement. Vocal cord paralysis resolved postoperatively.

TERMINOLOGY

Abbreviations
- Parathyroid adenoma (PT Ad)

Definitions
- Benign neoplasm of parathyroid gland producing excess parathyroid hormone (PTH), resulting in **hypercalcemia**

IMAGING

General Features
- Best diagnostic clue
  - Nuclear scintigraphy shows focal uptake of sestamibi or thallium
  - Hypoechoic mass with ↑ vascularity on ultrasound
  - Intensely enhancing mass on arterial-phase CECT with washout on delayed CECT
- Location
  - Upper parathyroid glands
    - Posterior to upper-mid pole of thyroid
    - Rarely posterior to pharynx or esophagus
  - Lower parathyroid glands
    - 65% at inferior thyroid, lateral to lower pole
    - **35%** lower parathyroids **ectopic**, from angle of mandible to lower anterior mediastinum
  - Ectopic location ≤ 20%
    - Hyoid, carotid sheath, mediastinum, intrathyroid
- Size
  - Adenoma typically 1-3 cm in size
    - Normal gland 5 x 3 x 1 mm
- Morphology
  - Round or oval, well-circumscribed solid mass
  - Usually homogeneous, but cystic degeneration and hemorrhage may occur

CT Findings
- CECT
  - Parathyroid protocol best accomplished with multiphase technique using early **arterial** (CTA) and delayed (venous) phase CT
    - Many centers include NECT ± additional late delayed scan; down side is added radiation dose
    - NECT helps distinguish lower density parathyroid tissue from normally radiodense thyroid
    - Usually 2nd-line imaging modality after prior indeterminate localization &/or to improve anatomical localization for surgical planning
  - Circumscribed soft tissue mass; mimics lymph node on delayed CECT
  - **Early intense enhancement > > lymph node** (30 sec post injection)
    - Washout on delayed (90 sec) CECT
    - ± central low density or cystic change

MR Findings
- T1WI
  - Iso- to hypointense compared to thyroid
- T2WI
  - Iso- to hyperintense compared to thyroid
- T1WI C+
  - Often enhance avidly

Ultrasonographic Findings
- Grayscale ultrasound
  - Homogeneous, well-defined, **hypoechoic** solid mass
  - Typically adjacent to thyroid gland, medial to common carotid artery
  - Inferior for ectopic retrovisceral and mediastinal adenomas
- Color Doppler
  - Usually **hypervascular**

Nuclear Medicine Findings
- Tc-99m sestamibi alone
  - Lipid-soluble myocardial perfusion tracer, taken up by thyroid **and** parathyroids
  - Rapid washout from thyroid, retention in parathyroids
  - Focal ↑ uptake on early and **delayed** images
  - Advantages: Single radiotracer, dual-phase acquisition, able to perform SPECT
- Subtraction techniques
  - Tl-201/Tc-99m pertechnetate
  - Tc-99m sestamibi/I-123
  - Tc-99m sestamibi/Tc-99m pertechnetate
    - Tl-201 and sestamibi taken up by thyroid **and** parathyroid glands
    - Tc-99m pertechnetate and I-123 **only** taken up by thyroid gland
    - Subtraction studies remove thyroid uptake, left with parathyroid uptake
  - Helpful technique if multinodular goiter, thyroid masses

Imaging Recommendations
- Best imaging tool
  - Tc-99m sestamibi scintigraphy has high sensitivity (> 90%) and specificity (> 90%)
    - Useful for ectopic glands: Upper neck, mediastinum, intrathyroid
  - US, multiphase CT or MR for discordant localization and postoperative neck
- Protocol advice
  - **Scintigraphy usual 1st exam** for initial evaluation
  - **Ultrasound** complimentary to scintigraphy
    - Excellent for **perithyroid location** adenoma
    - Limited in mediastinum and postoperative neck
    - Operator experience is important
  - **CECT** or MR usually reserved for discordant scintigraphy and ultrasound or postoperative neck
  - Parathyroid arteriography and venous sampling when noninvasive studies nondiagnostic

DIFFERENTIAL DIAGNOSIS

Reactive Lymph Nodes
- Paratracheal node in tracheoesophageal groove
- Typically not hypervascular

Thyroid Adenoma
- May be exophytic, extend to tracheoesophageal groove
- US, CT, and MR may misinterpret
- Intrathyroid PT Ad misinterpreted as thyroid adenoma

Multinodular Goiter

- Any hypermetabolic thyroid disease may retain sestamibi → false-positive
- Exophytic nodules mimic PT Ad

Parathyroid Cyst in Visceral Space

- Cystic lesion in parathyroid location

Parathyroid Carcinoma

- Invasive mass in parathyroid location

PATHOLOGY

General Features

- Normal parathyroid distribution
  - 83% of patients have 2 superior and 2 inferior glands
  - 13% of patients have > 4 glands, ~ 3% only 3 glands
- Superior parathyroid glands
  - Arise from 4th branchial pouch with thyroid
  - Short descent, close relation to thyroid gland result in relatively fixed location
  - Rarely ectopic
- Inferior parathyroid glands
  - Arise from 3rd branchial pouch with thymus
  - Long descent results in more variable position
  - **35% ectopic**, along thymopharyngeal duct course
    - Locations: Near hyoid, within carotid sheath, intrathyroid, intrathymic, and mediastinal
    - Parathyroid gland may be covered by or attached to thyroid capsule causing intrathyroid location

Gross Pathologic & Surgical Features

- Lobulated mass with glistening capsule
- Occasional calcification, cystic degeneration, fatty deposition

Microscopic Features

- Hypercellular collection of chief cells with follicular architecture

CLINICAL ISSUES

Presentation

- Most common signs/symptoms
  - Most patients have asymptomatic hypercalcemia
- Other signs/symptoms
  - **Hypercalcemia** may have wide range of symptoms
    - Bone pain related to osseous demineralization
    - Abdominal pain from renal calculi, constipation, peptic ulcer disease, pancreatitis
    - Lethargy, depression, less often psychosis
      - □ **"Stones, bones, groans, and psychic moans"**

Demographics

- Age
  - Adults; not pediatric neoplasm
- Gender
  - F > M (3:1)
- Epidemiology
  - Primary hyperparathyroidism: 1 in 700 adults
    - 75-85% parathyroid adenoma
    - 10-15% parathyroid hyperplasia

- 2-3% multiple parathyroid adenoma
- < 1% parathyroid carcinoma
- Secondary hyperparathyroidism
  - More common; from chronic renal failure

Natural History & Prognosis

- Surgical excision curative

Treatment

- Surgical excision
  - No preoperative imaging: Bilateral neck exploration
    - 90-95% cure rate with experienced surgeons
  - Preoperative imaging: Unilateral neck exploration
    - Decreased morbidity, improved success rates
    - High surgical risk patients and recurrent/persistent elevated PTH
- Minimally invasive radioguided parathyroidectomy
  - Patients with clearly localizing sestamibi scan
  - Preoperative injection of Tc-99m sestamibi
  - Handheld gamma ray detecting probe guides surgeon to parathyroid adenoma
- Percutaneous injection of absolute ethanol
  - High-risk surgical patients
  - Ultrasound guidance required

DIAGNOSTIC CHECKLIST

Consider

- Imaging role and modality choice remain controversial
  - Many surgeons report fewer complications, higher success rates using preoperative imaging
  - **Imaging required** if **persistent or recurrent postoperative disease** and with **ectopic PT ad**

Image Interpretation Pearls

- Paratracheal lymph node, protruding esophagus, or exophytic thyroid mass may be mistaken for PT Ad
- Cross correlate nuclear scintigraphy and US/CT/MR to avoid this error

SELECTED REFERENCES

1. Bahl M et al: Parathyroid adenomas and hyperplasia on four-dimensional CT scans: three patterns of enhancement relative to the thyroid gland justify a three-phase protocol. Radiology. 277(2):454-62, 2015
2. Raghavan P et al: Dynamic CT for parathyroid disease: are multiple phases necessary? AJNR Am J Neuroradiol. 35(10):1959-64, 2014
3. Patel CN et al: Clinical utility of ultrasound and 99mTc sestamibi SPECT/CT for preoperative localization of parathyroid adenoma in patients with primary hyperparathyroidism. Clin Radiol. 65(4):278-87, 2010
4. Harari A et al: Negative preoperative localization leads to greater resource use in the era of minimally invasive parathyroidectomy. Am J Surg. 197(6):769-73, 2009
5. Levine DS et al: Hybrid SPECT/CT imaging for primary hyperparathyroidism: case reports and pictorial review. Clin Nucl Med. 34(11):779-84, 2009
6. Randall GJ et al: Contrast-enhanced MDCT characteristics of parathyroid adenomas. AJR Am J Roentgenol. 193(2):W139-43, 2009
7. Thomas DL et al: Single photon emission computed tomography (SPECT) should be routinely performed for the detection of parathyroid abnormalities utilizing technetium-99m sestamibi parathyroid scintigraphy. Clin Nucl Med. 34(10):651-5, 2009
8. Zald PB et al: The role of computed tomography for localization of parathyroid adenomas. Laryngoscope. 118(8):1405-10, 2008
9. Rodgers SE et al: Improved preoperative planning for directed parathyroidectomy with 4-dimensional computed tomography. Surgery. 140(6):932-40; discussion 940-1, 2006
10. Weber AL et al: The thyroid and parathyroid glands. CT and MR imaging and correlation with pathology and clinical findings. Radiol Clin North Am. 38(5):1105-29, 2000

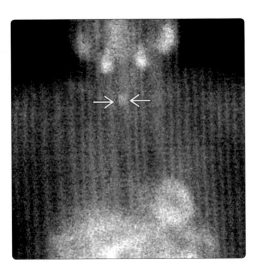

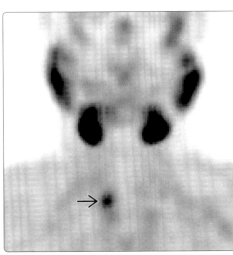

(Left) *Anteroposterior planar image of neck and chest following injection of Tc-99m sestamibi shows only small focus tracer uptake in neck* ➡. *Sestamibi is taken up by thyroid and parathyroid glands; however, patient had prior thyroidectomy. Persistent uptake was also found at this site on delayed images.* (Right) *Anterior delayed Tc-99m sestamibi scan demonstrates uptake in the inferior right thyroid region* ➡, *compatible with parathyroid adenoma.*

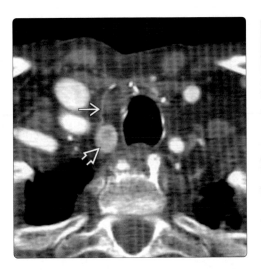

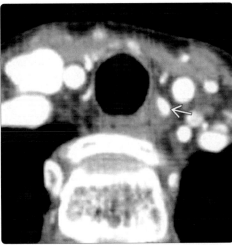

(Left) *Axial arterial-phase CECT demonstrates a typical "polar artery"* ➡ *supplying a parathyroid adenoma* ➡ *inferior to the thyroid gland in the upper mediastinal fat.* (Right) *Axial arterial-phase CECT demonstrates a typical intensely enhancing parathyroid adenoma* ➡, *missed on prior ultrasound and sestamibi imaging. This adenoma was relatively inconspicuous on delayed (venous-phase) CT due to density similar to esophagus, highlighting the importance of the arterial phase for best detection.*

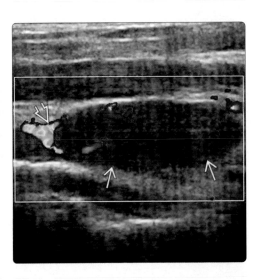

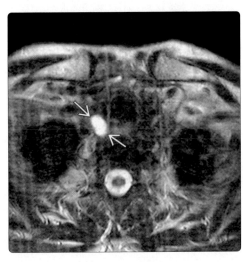

(Left) *Longitudinal color Doppler US shows hypoechoic parathyroid adenoma* ➡ *with typical increased vascularity at the pole* ➡. *(Courtesy B. Foster, MD.)* (Right) *Axial T2 MR shows an ovoid mass* ➡ *to be of uniform high signal intensity, higher than thyroid or nodes. Heterogeneous solid enhancement was evident with gadolinium administration (not shown). Sharp contours of mass suggest benign lesion.*

Differentiated Thyroid Carcinoma

TERMINOLOGY

- 2 types of differentiated thyroid carcinoma (DTCa): Papillary & follicular carcinoma

IMAGING

- Most often focal thyroid mass ± extracapsular invasion ± metastatic nodes
  - Rarely in ectopic thyroid, thyroglossal duct cyst
- CT: Variable size, texture, Ca++, invasive features
  - Nodal metastases **cystic** or solid, small or large, ± **Ca++**
- **Do not give iodinated contrast if suspected DTCa**
  - Delays I-131 therapy up to 6 months
- MR: Variable signal reflects intrinsic T1 signal of Tg &/or hemorrhage
- US: Concerning features: Hypoechoic, ill defined, microcalcification, taller than wide, hypervascular
- PET/CT: Use if tumor does not take up I-131

TOP DIFFERENTIAL DIAGNOSES

- Thyroid colloid cyst
- Thyroid follicular adenoma
- Multinodular goiter
- Thyroid medullary carcinoma
- Thyroid anaplastic carcinoma
- Thyroid non-Hodgkin lymphoma

PATHOLOGY

- **Papillary = 80%, follicular = 10%** of thyroid cancers
- **Papillary** prefers **nodal** spread; **follicular** prefers **hematogenous** spread

CLINICAL ISSUES

- 3x more common in women; peaks in 20s to 30s
- 5-year survival: Stages I & II > 90%, stage IV 40%
- **Rising serum thyroglobulin** is indicator of recurrence

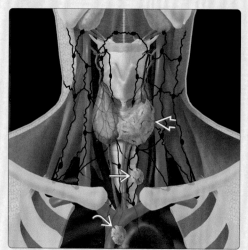
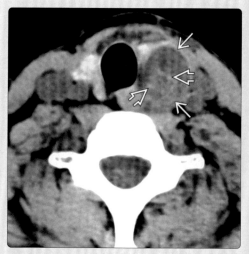

(Left) Coronal graphic illustrates a left thyroid lobe differentiated thyroid carcinoma (DCTa) primary tumor ➡ with metastatic nodal disease in the left paratracheal chain ➡ and superior mediastinum ➡. (Right) Axial NECT shows a well-defined mass ➡ arising from the left thyroid lobe with fine, speckled microcalcifications ➡ centrally. Small calcifications such as these are a suspicious finding for DTCa and especially papillary carcinoma. Intrathyroid tumor is < 4 cm = T2.

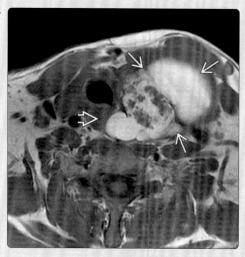
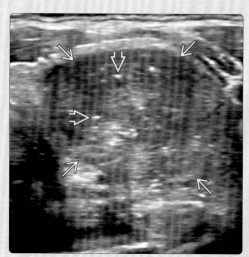

(Left) Axial T1 MR in a 49-year-old man with an enlarging neck mass shows a heterogeneous solid and cystic mass arising in left thyroid lobe ➡, displacing esophagus ➡. Note the intrinsic hyperintensity from thyroglobulin. This feature is also present in multiple nodes. Tumor determined to be papillary thyroid carcinoma. (Right) Longitudinal thyroid ultrasound in a different patient reveals a well-defined mass ➡ with multiple tiny, hyperechoic microcalcifications ➡, found to be a papillary carcinoma.

TERMINOLOGY

Abbreviations

- Differentiated thyroid carcinoma (DTCa)

Definitions

- Malignancy arising from epithelial thyroid cells with well-defined histology
  o Papillary or follicular, with multiple variants

IMAGING

General Features

- Best diagnostic clue
  o **Ultrasound** is main modality for DTCa diagnosis
  o Focal intrathyroidal mass ± extracapsular invasion ± metastatic nodes
  o Microcalcifications suggest papillary carcinoma
- Location
  o Primary tumor arises within thyroid gland
    – Rarely ectopic thyroid, thyroglossal duct cyst wall
  o Nodal metastases most often found at levels VI, IV, & superior mediastinum
- Size
  o Variable: From lesion of several millimeters found at thyroidectomy to tumor replacing whole lobe
- Morphology
  o Variable: Well-defined, solid mass mimicking benign lesion to heterogeneous, invasive mass

CT Findings

- CECT
  o Primary tumor findings highly variable
    – Single or multiple nodules or diffuse infiltration
    – Small, well-circumscribed to large, ill-defined, heterogeneous invasive mass
    – Solid, cystic, or mixed
    – ± calcifications; typically tiny, speckled
  o Lymph node findings highly variable, often bilateral
    – Small, solid, reactive-appearing but rounded
    – Large, heterogeneous, high-density cystic nodes
    – Focal calcification may be seen in solid nodes
- **If CT ordered with suspected DTCa, do not give contrast**

MR Findings

- Variable
  o High T1 signal reflects thyroglobulin (Tg) &/or hemorrhage (methemoglobin)
- Primary tumor: Intrathyroidal mass, focal, multinodular, or diffusely infiltrating
  o Typically heterogeneous signal and enhancement
  o Evaluate neck for invasion, especially trachea
- Nodes: Small, round, solid to large, cystic or mixed
  o Cystic nodes may be **T1 and T2 hyperintense**; difficult to see without fat saturation
  o DWI: Low ADC suggests metastases

Ultrasonographic Findings

- Grayscale ultrasound
  o May exactly mimic benign adenoma
  o Findings suggesting malignancy: Hypoechoic, ill-defined margins, microcalcifications, taller-than-wide shape
- Color Doppler
  o **High vascularity** suggests malignancy

Nuclear Medicine Findings

- PET/CT
  o Not useful for DTCa, which is I-131 avid
    – Useful in I-131-negative (dedifferentiated) disease
- I-131 scintigraphy
  o Diagnostic scan 4-6 weeks following thyroidectomy
    – Patient will be hypothyroid (TSH > 50)
  o If thyroid remnant or metastasis detected, ablative dose of I-131 administered
- Tc-99m pertechnetate or I-123 no longer used

Imaging Recommendations

- Best imaging tool
  o Sonography useful for lesion characterization, biopsy guidance, & surveillance
    – Distinguishes solid & cystic masses, facilitates biopsy
  o Cross-sectional imaging used to stage large thyroid tumors (MR preferred over CECT/NECT)
- Protocol advice
  o **Do not give iodinated contrast if suspect DTCa**
    – Delays I-131 therapy up to 6 months
  o Cross-sectional imaging must include **superior mediastinal nodes**
  o For detection of recurrent disease
    – I-131 scan ± ultrasound
    – PET/CT if ↑ serum Tg but negative I-131 scan

DIFFERENTIAL DIAGNOSIS

Thyroid Colloid Cyst

- Simple cyst; may be hemorrhagic
- Ultrasound clarifies cystic nature of lesion

Thyroid Follicular Adenoma

- Solitary intrathyroidal mass without local invasion or adenopathy

Multinodular Goiter

- Multiple nodules in enlarged thyroid gland

Thyroid Medullary Carcinoma

- May exactly mimic DTCa when imaged

Thyroid Anaplastic Carcinoma

- Rapidly enlarging, invasive thyroid tumor

Thyroid Non-Hodgkin Lymphoma

- Rapidly enlarging, invasive thyroid mass
- Associated lymphadenopathy rarely necrotic

PATHOLOGY

General Features

- Etiology
  o Most often sporadic but associated with radiation
  o DTCa arises from endodermally derived follicular cells that are TSH sensitive

Staging, Grading, & Classification

- AJCC 2010, 7th edition
  o Primary tumor (T)

DTCa Staging (AJCC 2010)

Patient Under 45 Years of Age	Patient Aged 45 Years or Older
Stage I	Stage I
Any T, any N, M0	T1, N0, M0
Stage II	Stage II
Any T, any N, M1	T2, N0, M0
	Stage III
	T3, N0, M0 **or** T1-3, N1a, M0
	Stage IV
	IVA: T4a, any N, M0 **or** T1-T3, N1b, M0
	IVB: T4b, any N, M0 **and IVC:** Any T, any N, M1

Adapted from 7th edition AJCC Staging Forms.

- T1a: Intrathyroidal **≤ 1 cm**, T1b: **> 1 cm & ≤ 2 cm**
- T2: Intrathyroidal **> 2 cm & ≤ 4 cm**
- T3: Intrathyroidal **> 4 cm or minimal extrathyroidal extension**
- T4a: **Marked extrathyroid extension**
  - □ Invades larynx, trachea, esophagus, recurrent laryngeal nerve, subcutaneous tissue
- T4b: **Very advanced disease**
  - □ Invades prevertebral fascia, surrounds carotid or mediastinal vessels
- Regional lymph nodes (N)
  - N1a: Level VI (pretracheal, paratracheal, prelaryngeal nodes)
  - N1b: Any other cervical nodes or superior mediastinum
- **Overall staging (AJCC 2010) reflects patient age**

Microscopic Features

- ± calcification, necrosis, fibrosis, cysts, & hemorrhage
- Papillary carcinoma
  - 50% have calcific psammoma bodies
- Follicular carcinoma

CLINICAL ISSUES

Presentation

- Most common signs/symptoms
  - Painless, palpable, solitary thyroid nodule
- Other signs/symptoms
  - May present with neck mass from metastatic nodes
  - Rapidly growing thyroid mass, hoarseness
- Clinical profile
  - Female patient with firm thyroid nodule

Demographics

- Age
  - Peak incidence 3rd & 4th decade
- Gender
  - M:F = 1:3
- Epidemiology
  - Thyroid tumors: Papillary 80%, follicular 10%, medullary 7%, anaplastic 2%, non-Hodgkin lymphoma 1%

Natural History & Prognosis

- Patterns of spread
  - Local invasion of adjacent structures (T3-T4)
  - **Nodes: 50% papillary**, 10% follicular at presentation
    - Paratracheal, deep cervical, spinal accessory, retropharyngeal, superior mediastinal
  - Distant spread: 20% follicular, ≤ 10% papillary
    - Typically to lungs, bones, & brain
- Overall good prognosis
  - 5-year survival rate: Stages I & II > 90%, stage IV 40%
- **Follicular** worse prognosis than papillary
- **Tall cell variant of papillary** much worse prognosis
- **Rising serum Tg** indicates recurrence

DIAGNOSTIC CHECKLIST

Consider

- Vast majority of thyroid lesions are benign
- Thyroid lesion biopsy recommended if
  - Solid lesion ≥ 1-cm diameter (< 35 years)
  - Solid lesion ≥ 1.5-cm diameter (> 35 years)
  - Clear malignant features, such as extracapsular spread
  - Cervical adenopathy
- If worrisome solitary thyroid nodule seen on any modality, go directly to image-guided biopsy

Image Interpretation Pearls

- Suspect DTCa when
  - Nodal mass(es) in **young female patient**
  - **Cystic** or mixed cystic/solid neck nodes
  - **Calcified** (CT) or **T1-hyperintense** (MR) nodes
  - Bilateral low neck (level IV, VB, VI) nodes
- Avoid iodinated contrast if patient is candidate for ablative I-131; may stun residual disease up to 6 months

SELECTED REFERENCES

1. Hoang JK et al: Managing incidental thyroid nodules detected on imaging: white paper of the ACR Incidental Thyroid Findings Committee. J Am Coll Radiol. 12(2):143-50, 2015
2. Aiken AH: Imaging of thyroid cancer. Semin Ultrasound CT MR. 33(2):138-49, 2012
3. Wu LM et al: The accuracy of ultrasonography in the preoperative diagnosis of cervical lymph node metastasis in patients with papillary thyroid carcinoma: A meta-analysis. Eur J Radiol. 81(8):1798-805, 2012

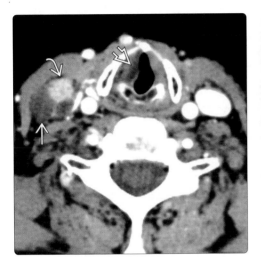

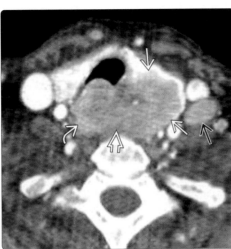

(Left) *Axial CECT shows a partially cystic node* ➡️ *in right level III. Walls are imperceptible, but a large, enhancing mural nodule* ➡️ *and septations are evident, typical imaging findings of metastatic DTCa. Note the right vocal cord* ➡️ *is paralyzed, another sign of thyroid cancer.* (Right) *Axial CECT in a patient with left vocal cord paralysis due to a papillary thyroid carcinoma* ➡️ *invading the tracheoesophageal groove* ➡️ *is shown. Tumor is inseparable from the esophagus* ➡️. *Note associated adenopathy* ➡️.

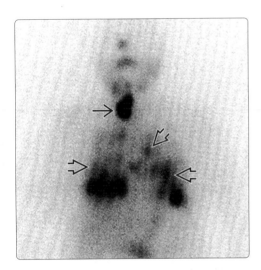

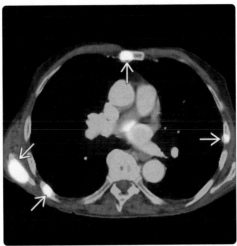

(Left) *Anteroposterior projection from a diagnostic I-131 scan in a patient with thyroid follicular carcinoma shows a large area of uptake in the thyroid bed* ➡️ *as well as extensive areas of uptake throughout both lungs* ➡️. (Right) *Axial PET/CT reveals numerous bone metastases* ➡️ *from follicular thyroid carcinoma. While papillary carcinoma prefers nodal spread, follicular carcinoma is more prone to hematogenous metastases to bone or lung.*

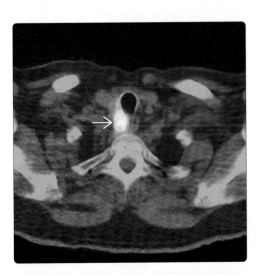

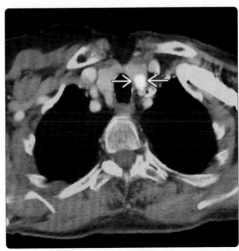

(Left) *Axial PET/CT in a patient previously treated for DTCa with rising thyroglobulin but negative I-131 scan shows FDG uptake in the right tracheoesophageal groove* ➡️, *consistent with recurrent disease.* (Right) *Axial PET/CT performed for staging of pharyngeal SCCa reveals incidental high uptake in left thyroid* ➡️. *Diffuse thyroid uptake is usually benign; focal uptake is associated with malignancy in 20% of cases, so incidental masses must be biopsied. This was found to be DTCa.*

TERMINOLOGY

- Medullary thyroid carcinoma (MTCa)
- Rare neuroendocrine malignancy arising from thyroid parafollicular C cells that produce calcitonin
- Most MTCa sporadic; 15-25% MTCa inherited

IMAGING

- Heterogeneous, well-circumscribed thyroid mass
- Most have similar-appearing nodal metastases
- ± calcifications in tumor &/or nodes
- Intravenous iodine not contraindicated for MTCa
- Inherited forms: Often younger patient with multifocal, infiltrative tumors
- Ultrasound shows hypoechoic, irregular mass
- Color Doppler hypervascularity evident
- PET/CT not used, as not reliably FDG avid
- I-131 MIBG or octreotide scintigraphy for metastases

TOP DIFFERENTIAL DIAGNOSES

- Multinodular goiter
- Thyroid adenoma
- Thyroid differentiated carcinoma
- Thyroid non-Hodgkin lymphoma

PATHOLOGY

- Type 2 multiple endocrine neoplasia (MEN) syndromes
  - MEN2B: Younger, more aggressive disease
- Familial medullary thyroid carcinoma
  - Later onset, more indolent course than MEN

CLINICAL ISSUES

- Usually present with thyroid mass
- Serum calcitonin and CEA usually elevated
- Treatment primarily surgical ± XRT
- Prophylactic thyroidectomy if RET mutation

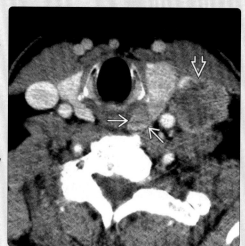
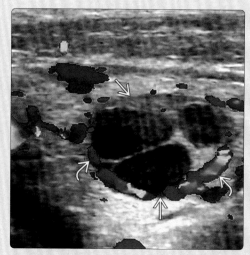

(Left) Axial CECT shows small left thyroid mass ➡ in tracheoesophageal groove with heterogeneous ipsilateral adenopathy ➥. Appearance suggests primary thyroid neoplasm, which is most commonly differentiated carcinoma; however, this was sporadic form of medullary carcinoma. (Right) Longitudinal color Doppler US through thyroid shows a mixed cystic and solid mass ➡ with peripheral vascularity ➥. Ultrasound features of medullary carcinoma are variable, but increased vascularity is typical.

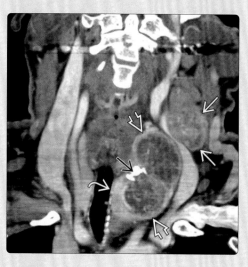
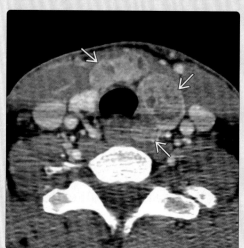

(Left) Coronal CECT shows a heterogeneous but well-defined thyroid mass ➥ with coarse calcifications ➥ and ipsilateral similarly heterogeneous adenopathy ➡. At surgery, tumor was found to have infiltrated tracheal wall ➥. (Right) Axial CECT shows multiple left thyroid and isthmus lesions ➥ found to be multifocal medullary thyroid carcinoma (MTCa). Lesions are all similarly heterogeneous but well defined and not calcified. Iodinated contrast is not contraindicated with MTCa.

Medullary Thyroid Carcinoma

TERMINOLOGY

Abbreviations
- Medullary thyroid carcinoma (MTCa)

Synonyms
- Thyroid neuroendocrine carcinoma

Definitions
- Rare neuroendocrine malignancy arising from thyroid parafollicular C cells that produce calcitonin
- Inherited forms of MTCa
  - Multiple endocrine neoplasia (MEN) syndromes
  - Familial medullary thyroid carcinoma (FMTC)

IMAGING

General Features
- Best diagnostic clue
  - Solid lesion in thyroid with ipsilateral nodal metastases
- Location
  - Within thyroid gland
  - Nodal metastasis: Level VI and superior mediastinum
    - Less commonly: Levels III & IV, retropharyngeal nodes
- Size
  - 2-25 mm; < 1 cm considered microcarcinoma
  - May be multifocal, particularly inherited forms
- Morphology
  - Solid, usually well-circumscribed mass
  - **Infiltrative variant seen with familial forms**

CT Findings
- CECT
  - Low-density, heterogeneous, well-circumscribed mass in thyroid
  - May be multifocal, especially with inherited forms
  - ± calcifications in tumor &/or nodal metastases
    - Fine or coarse calcifications
      - □ Fine suggest papillary thyroid carcinoma (PTC)
  - Nodal metastases typically solid

MR Findings
- Usually well-defined mass with ipsilateral nodes
- May see irregular margins and extraglandular extension
- Nodes less often cystic or T1 intense like PTC

Ultrasonographic Findings
- Grayscale ultrasound
  - Hypoechoic, irregular intrathyroidal mass
- Color Doppler
  - Hypervascularity with irregular arrangement of vessels

Nuclear Medicine Findings
- PET
  - **MTCa not reliably FDG avid**
    - Frequent false-negative scans
    - Consider only when elevated tumor markers but normal cross-sectional imaging
- **I-131 MIBG**
  - Allows whole-body imaging for metastases
- **Octreotide scintigraphy (In-111 pentreotide)**
  - May miss liver metastases due to physiological hepatic uptake
- **C-11 methionine** may prove to have utility

Imaging Recommendations
- Best imaging tool
  - US most often used for initial evaluation of thyroid nodule
    - FNA can be performed at same time
    - Core biopsy preferable due to higher sensitivity
  - CECT required for thorough evaluation of neck and mediastinum for nodes
    - Iodinated contrast not contraindicated as it is with differentiated thyroid carcinoma (DTCa)
- Protocol advice
  - CECT extending to carina to evaluate mediastinal nodes

DIFFERENTIAL DIAGNOSIS

Multinodular Goiter
- Enlarged gland with multiple nodules, coarse calcifications

Thyroid Adenoma
- Focal mass without evidence of invasion
- No neck adenopathy

Thyroid Differentiated Carcinoma
- Most common thyroid tumor
- Solid or cystic nodal metastases

Thyroid Non-Hodgkin Lymphoma
- Diffuse enlargement of gland with infiltrative mass
- Rarely see calcifications or necrosis

PATHOLOGY

General Features
- Etiology
  - **75-85% sporadic MTCa**
    - No identified exogenous cause
    - Not related to preexisting thyroid conditions
  - **15-25% inherited MTCa**
    - More often multifocal &/or infiltrative
  - **Type 2 MEN syndromes**
    - Autosomal dominant inherited syndrome
    - **MEN2A**: Multifocal MTCa, pheochromocytoma, parathyroid hyperplasia, hyperparathyroidism
    - **MEN2B**: MEN2A plus mucosal neuromas of lips, tongue, GI tract, and conjunctiva
      - □ Younger patients, more aggressive tumors
  - **FMTC**
    - Autosomal dominant, only neoplasm is MTCa
    - Later onset, more indolent course than MEN
- Genetics
  - Associated with **mutations of *RET* proto-oncogene** on chromosome 10q11.2
    - 100% of familial and 40-60% of sporadic cases
    - Screen for *RET* mutations in family of MTCa patients

Staging, Grading, & Classification
- AJCC staging (7th edition, 2010)
  - TNM follows that for DTCa
  - **When multifocal tumor, use largest component**

MTCa Staging (AJCC 2010)

Tumor Staging (T)	Nodal Staging (N)	Metastases (M)
T1a: Intrathyroidal ≤ 1 cm	**N1a**: Level VI (pretracheal, paratracheal, prelaryngeal nodes)	**M0**: No distant metastasis
T1b: Intrathyroidal > 1 cm and ≤ 2 cm	**N1b**: Any other cervical nodes or superior mediastinum	**M1**: Distant metastasis
T2: Intrathyroidal > 2 cm and ≤ 4 cm		
T3: Intrathyroidal > 4 cm or minimal extrathyroidal extension		
T4a: Marked extrathyroid extension to larynx, trachea, esophagus		
T4b: Invades prevertebral fascia or surrounds carotid vessels		

Adapted from 7th edition AJCC Staging Forms.

Microscopic Features

- Proliferation of large, atypical round to polygonal cells with granular cytoplasm
- **Stains strongly for calcitoninin in 80%**

CLINICAL ISSUES

Presentation

- Most common signs/symptoms
  - Painless thyroid nodule
  - Less commonly dysphagia, hoarseness, pain
  - **Elevated serum calcitonin**
    - Used as screening tool for estimation of extent of disease and for posttreatment surveillance
- Other signs/symptoms
  - Diarrhea from elevated calcitonin
  - Paraneoplastic syndromes uncommon: Cushing or carcinoid syndromes
  - Other serum markers may also be elevated
    - Carcinoembryonic antigen (CEA)
    - Chromogranin A
- Clinical profile
  - Middle-aged patient with low neck mass or family history of MEN with tumor found on screening exam

Demographics

- Age
  - Mean: Sporadic = 50 years; inherited = 30 years
  - Pediatric MTCa usually inherited, especially MEN2B
- Gender
  - F > M in Caucasians and in children
- Epidemiology
  - 5-10% of all thyroid gland malignancies
  - 14% of thyroid cancer deaths
  - 10% of pediatric thyroid malignancies (MEN2)

Natural History & Prognosis

- May metastasize by local invasion, lymphatics, or hematogenously
- Up to 75% have lymphadenopathy at presentation
- Distant metastasis to lungs, liver, bones
- Lung metastases frequently miliary, mimics TB
- **Overall 5-year survival = 72%; 10-year = 56%**

- Indicators of better prognosis
  - Female patients, younger age at surgery
  - FMTC and MEN2A syndromes
  - Tumor < 10 cm, no nodes, early stage disease
  - Normal preoperative CEA levels, complete surgical resection

Treatment

- Resection of primary tumor and regional nodal disease
  - Total thyroidectomy, level VI ± superior mediastinal lymph nodes
  - Levels II-V resected if positive lateral neck nodes
- Adjuvant radiation therapy if extensive soft tissue invasion or extracapsular nodal spread
- Prophylactic thyroidectomy performed if familial *RET* mutation detected
  - FMTC and MEN2A: Thyroidectomy at age 5-6
  - MEN2B: Thyroidectomy during infancy

DIAGNOSTIC CHECKLIST

Consider

- Consider familial syndromes with young patient or multifocal tumors

Image Interpretation Pearls

- Imaging appearance may mimic DTCa
  - Nodes not often cystic like DTCa
  - Intrinsic T1 hyperintensity not typical as with DTCa
  - MTCa calcifications may be coarser
  - MTCa more often multifocal

Reporting Tips

- CT/MR important for detection of nodal disease
  - Image to carina for superior mediastinum nodes
  - Look for distant metastases
- PET/CT not recommended, as FDG avidity variable

SELECTED REFERENCES

1. Delorme S et al: Medullary thyroid carcinoma: imaging. Recent Results Cancer Res. 204:91-116, 2015
2. Ganeshan D et al: Current update on medullary thyroid carcinoma. AJR Am J Roentgenol. 201(6):W867-76, 2013

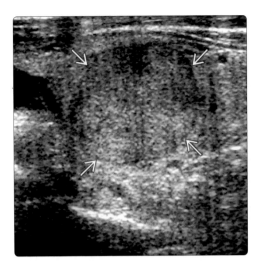

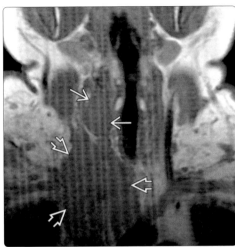

(Left) Longitudinal ultrasound shows a well-defined, solid mass ➡ within thyroid gland with hypoechoic halo. No specific features distinguish this from adenoma or differentiated carcinoma. (Right) Coronal T1WI MR in a patient with prior thyroidectomy for sporadic medullary carcinoma shows focal recurrence in right thyroid bed ➡ and a large, infiltrating mass in superior mediastinum ➡ surrounding the vessels and compressing right jugular vein. This was also shown to be recurrent medullary carcinoma.

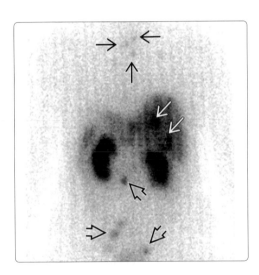

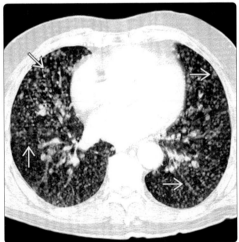

(Left) Posterior view of octreotide scan shows multifocal medullary uptake within thyroid bed ➡ from MTCa. Multiple foci of uptake within lower spine and sacrum ➡ represent bony metastases, and there are probable liver metastases ➡. (Right) Axial NECT shows innumerable tiny nodules ➡ scattered throughout both lungs. Both MTCa and differentiated thyroid carcinoma can produce a miliary pattern of lung metastases that should be distinguished from miliary tuberculosis.

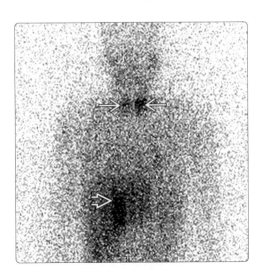

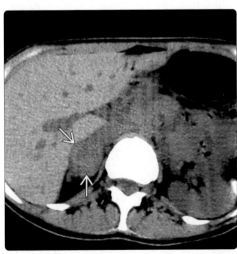

(Left) Frontal view of MIBG scan shows bilateral uptake with thyroid bed ➡, representing multifocal primary MTCa. There is also uptake in the right adrenal gland ➡ consistent with pheochromocytoma in this patient proven to have multiple endocrine neoplasm type syndrome. (Right) Axial NECT of abdomen in the same patient shows a heterogeneous mass ➡ replacing right adrenal gland, consistent with adrenal pheochromocytoma.

TERMINOLOGY

- Abbreviation: Anaplastic thyroid carcinoma (ATCa)
- Synonym: Undifferentiated thyroid tumor
- Often arises from differentiated thyroid carcinoma or multinodular goiter (MNG)

IMAGING

- General findings
  - Large, heterogeneous, infiltrating thyroid mass
  - Necrosis, hemorrhage, calcifications
  - Invades surrounding structures and spaces
  - Common to have nodal metastases at presentation
- CECT for suspected ATCa
  - Iodinated contrast not an issue with ATCa
- US: Inadequate for staging purposes
- PET/CT: FDG avid but considered unnecessary tool
- Bone scan: Bone metastases evaluation for staging
- I-123 and I-131 scintigraphy not useful due to lack of iodine concentration

TOP DIFFERENTIAL DIAGNOSES

- Thyroid non-Hodgkin lymphoma
- Thyroid differentiated carcinoma
- Thyroid medullary carcinoma
- MNG
- Thyroid adenoma

PATHOLOGY

- 50% distant metastasis: Lungs, bone, brain
- Automatically staged as T4, stage IV tumors

CLINICAL ISSUES

- Tumor of elderly; mean age: 71 years
- Rapidly growing, large, painful neck mass
- 1-2% of thyroid malignancies 39% of thyroid deaths
- Lethal tumor; mean survival: 6 months
- Aggressive treatment early, late presentation typically palliative

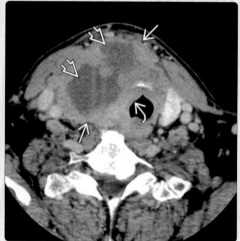
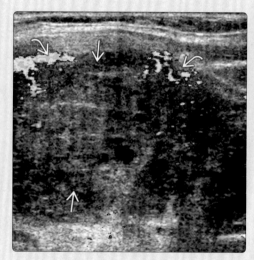

(Left) Axial CECT demonstrates large, heterogeneous, predominantly right-sided thyroid mass ➡ with large pools of low-density necrosis ➡. Mass cannot be separated from strap muscles and infiltrates cricothyroid membrane to tracheal lumen ➡. (Right) Doppler US shows right thyroid lobe appearing completely replaced by large heterogeneous lobulated solid mass ➡ with irregular margins. No internal calcifications are evident; however, color Doppler shows prominent peripheral vascularity ➡.

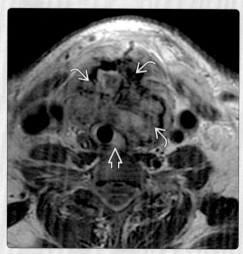
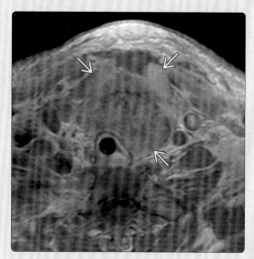

(Left) Axial T2WI MR in a patient with stridor imaged after tracheostomy shows extensive areas of marked signal loss ➡ suggesting either fibrosis, calcifications (which were not evident on CT), or hemosiderin deposition. T2 signal surrounding tube represents both secretions and infiltrative tumor ➡. (Right) Axial T1WI C+ MR in the same patient illustrates infiltrative nature of this aggressive, heterogeneously enhancing neoplasm ➡, which involves strap muscles and other extrathyroidal tissues.

TERMINOLOGY

Abbreviations

- Anaplastic thyroid carcinoma (ATCa)

Synonyms

- Undifferentiated thyroid carcinoma

Definitions

- Aggressive, lethal thyroid malignancy
  - **Arises** from **differentiated thyroid carcinoma** (DTCa), **multinodular goiter** (MNG), or de novo

IMAGING

General Features

- Best diagnostic clue
  - Elderly woman with heterogeneous invasive mass arising from thyroid
- Location
  - Begins in thyroid gland but frequently transspatial
- Size
  - Typically > 5 cm at presentation
- Morphology
  - Large, heterogeneous, infiltrating thyroid mass

CT Findings

- CECT
  - Heterogeneous, diffusely infiltrating mass
  - Up to 75% have necrosis and hemorrhage
  - Many demonstrate calcifications; typically dense, amorphous
    - Probably from underlying **MNG**
  - Invades adjacent infrahyoid neck spaces
    - Larynx, trachea, recurrent laryngeal nerve, esophagus
  - Cervical lymphadenopathy very common
    - Up to 50% of metastatic nodes are necrotic

MR Findings

- T1WI
  - Heterogeneous invasive tumor with adenopathy
  - Hemorrhage, necrosis, and calcification may result in heterogeneous mixed signal
- T2WI
  - Variable, typically diffuse iso- to hyperintense
- T1WI C+
  - Heterogeneous enhancement

Ultrasonographic Findings

- Grayscale ultrasound
  - Poorly defined, invasive, hypoechoic mass

Nuclear Medicine Findings

- Bone scan
  - Initial staging for bone metastases
- PET/CT
  - High FDG avidity
  - No benefit for staging over CT/MR
- I-123 and I-131 scintigraphy
  - Not used in evaluation or treatment of ATCa
  - Does **not** concentrate iodine because of highly undifferentiated cells

Imaging Recommendations

- Best imaging tool
  - If ATCa diagnosis suspected, then CECT adequate
  - When diagnosis unknown, MR of neck and mediastinum is exam of choice for staging
- Protocol advice
  - Image down to carina for nodal metastases

DIFFERENTIAL DIAGNOSIS

Thyroid Non-Hodgkin Lymphoma

- Homogeneous mass, rarely calcified or necrotic
- Associated with Hashimoto thyroiditis

Thyroid Differentiated Carcinoma

- Unilateral thyroid mass ± fine calcifications ± cystic adenopathy

Thyroid Medullary Carcinoma

- May mimic morphology of early ATCa
- Often smaller and more well defined than ATCa

Multinodular Goiter

- Multiple nodules in enlarged thyroid gland
- No invasive features or adenopathy

Thyroid Adenoma

- Noninvasive intrathyroidal mass without adenopathy
- May hemorrhage and rapidly increase in size

PATHOLOGY

General Features

- Etiology
  - Often occurs in iodine-deficient areas and in setting of preexisting thyroid pathology
    - 33% MNG
    - 25% DTCa
    - Possibly arises by prolonged stimulation with thyroid-stimulating hormone
  - Rarely can develop de novo
  - Thought to arise from endodermally derived follicular cells
    - **Does not concentrate iodine or express thyroglobulin**
- Associated abnormalities
  - Distant metastasis present in 50% or greater
    - Lungs, bones, and brain

Staging, Grading, & Classification

- Adapted from American Joint Committee on Cancer (AJCC) 7th edition
- **All anaplastic thyroid staged as T4 tumors**
  - T4a: Confined to thyroid gland
  - T4b: Gross extrathyroidal extension
- **All anaplastic thyroid considered stage IV**
  - Stage IVA: T4a
  - Stage IVB: T4b
  - Stage IVC: M1

Gross Pathologic & Surgical Features

- Invasive mass that extends through thyroid gland capsule

Anaplastic Thyroid Carcinoma Staging

Tumor staging (T)
All anaplastic thyroid carcinomas considered T4
T4a: Intrathyroidal anaplastic carcinoma
T4b: Anaplastic carcinoma with gross extrathyroidal extension
Adapted from 7th edition AJCC Staging Forms.

Microscopic Features

- High degree of mitotic activity with substantial infiltration
- Commonly hemorrhagic and necrotic
- Squamoid, spindle cell, and giant cell histologic variants
- 25% have concomitant **DTCa**
- Some pathologists distinguish between anaplastic and undifferentiated carcinoma
  - AJCC considers them to be synonymous

CLINICAL ISSUES

Presentation

- Most common signs/symptoms
  - **Rapidly growing**, large, painful neck mass
  - Symptoms from local invasion
    - Larynx or trachea: Dyspnea
    - Recurrent laryngeal nerve: Hoarseness
    - Esophagus: Dysphagia
- Other signs/symptoms
  - Predisposing factors: Preexisting MNG, neck radiation
  - On examination: Firm thyroid mass, typically > 5 cm
    - Nodal disease frequently present at presentation

Demographics

- Age
  - Older individuals
  - Mean age: 70 years
- Gender
  - F:M = 3:1
- Epidemiology
  - Rare; 1-2% of thyroid malignancies
  - 39% of thyroid cancer deaths

Natural History & Prognosis

- ATCa is 1 of most aggressive tumors
  - **Mean survival: 6 months**
  - Mortality: 70% at 6 months, 80% at 12 months
- Less grave prognosis
  - Age < 60 years, intrathyroidal tumor, use of combined surgery and radiotherapy
- Death usually from airway obstruction or complications of pulmonary metastases

Treatment

- Aggressive treatment if early diagnosis and tumor not spread outside thyroid
- Multimodality with surgery ± radiotherapy & chemotherapy
- **Late-stage treatment usually palliative**

DIAGNOSTIC CHECKLIST

Consider

- If large neck mass, always consider DTCa 1st; should not use iodinated contrast during CT
  - Image with NECT, MR, or ultrasound
- Iodinated contrast is not contraindicated with anaplastic carcinoma

Image Interpretation Pearls

- Rapidly enlarging thyroid mass: ATCa, thyroid non-Hodgkin lymphoma (NHL), or hemorrhagic adenoma
  - NHL more often homogeneous than ATCa
  - ATCa more often has hemorrhage, calcifications
  - ATCa tends to be in older patients

Reporting Tips

- Anaplastic carcinoma is always T4 tumor
  - Intrathyroidal disease: T4a = stage IVA
  - Gross extrathyroidal extension: T4b = stage IVB
  - Metastatic disease: M1 = stage IVC

SELECTED REFERENCES

1. Dibelius G et al: Noninvasive anaplastic thyroid carcinoma: report of a case and literature review. Thyroid. 24(8):1319-24, 2014
2. Mohebati A et al: Anaplastic thyroid carcinoma: a 25-year single-institution experience. Ann Surg Oncol. 21(5):1665-70, 2014
3. Saindane AM: Pitfalls in the staging of cancer of thyroid. Neuroimaging Clin N Am. 23(1):123-45, 2013
4. Smallridge RC et al: American Thyroid Association guidelines for management of patients with anaplastic thyroid cancer. Thyroid. 22(11):1104-39, 2012
5. Chen J et al: Surgery and radiotherapy improves survival in patients with anaplastic thyroid carcinoma: analysis of the surveillance, epidemiology, and end results 1983-2002. Am J Clin Oncol. 31(5):460-4, 2008
6. Neff RL et al: Anaplastic thyroid cancer. Endocrinol Metab Clin North Am. 37(2):525-38, xi, 2008
7. Volante M et al: Poorly differentiated thyroid carcinoma: diagnostic features and controversial issues. Endocr Pathol. 19(3):150-5, 2008
8. Kebebew E et al: Anaplastic thyroid carcinoma. Treatment outcome and prognostic factors. Cancer. 103(7):1330-5, 2005
9. Wiseman SM et al: Anaplastic transformation of thyroid cancer: review of clinical, pathologic, and molecular evidence provides new insights into disease biology and future therapy. Head Neck. 25(8):662-70, 2003
10. Vini L et al: Management of thyroid cancer. Lancet Oncol. 3(7):407-14, 2002
11. Haigh PI et al: Completely resected anaplastic thyroid carcinoma combined with adjuvant chemotherapy and irradiation is associated with prolonged survival. Cancer. 91(12):2335-42, 2001
12. Lind P et al: The role of F-18FDG PET in thyroid cancer. Acta Med Austriaca. 27(2):38-41, 2000
13. Weber AL et al: The thyroid and parathyroid glands. CT and MR imaging and correlation with pathology and clinical findings. Radiol Clin North Am. 38(5):1105-29, 2000
14. Takashima S et al: CT evaluation of anaplastic thyroid carcinoma. AJNR Am J Neuroradiol. 11(2):361-7, 1990

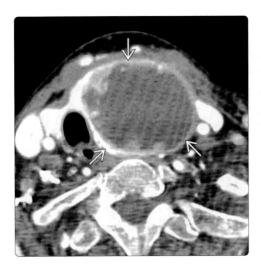

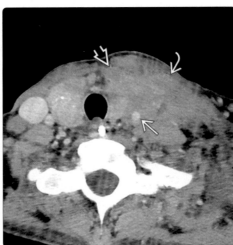

(Left) *Axial CECT shows a well-defined mass* ➡ *confined to thyroid gland with cystic degeneration and peripheral enhancement, mimicking colloid cyst. Anaplastic thyroid carcinoma confined to thyroid gland is unusual and staged as T4a. It has slightly better prognosis.* (Right) *Axial CECT demonstrates large infiltrating left thyroid and neck mass* ➡. *There is involvement of the sternocleidomastoid muscle* ➡ *and encasement of the left common carotid artery* ➡.

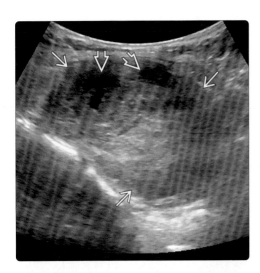

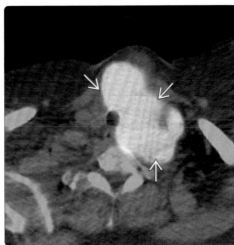

(Left) *Longitudinal oblique ultrasound shows well-defined mass* ➡ *with heterogeneous echotexture and small focal areas of necrosis* ➡. *Ultrasound findings, such as these, are nonspecific but are concerning for tumor and should lead to recommendation for fine-needle aspiration.* (Right) *Axial fused PET/CT demonstrates large markedly FDG-avid mass* ➡ *extending from left thyroid into surrounding tissues. PET/CT not typically used, as all tumors are T4, stage IV disease.*

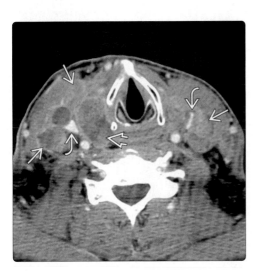

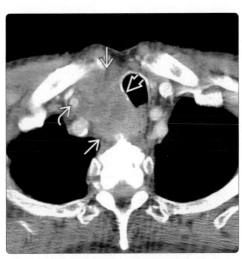

(Left) *Axial CECT demonstrates extensive bilateral necrotic nodes* ➡, *inseparable from deep aspect of sternocleidomastoid muscles, and compressing jugular veins* ➡. *The nodal mass is seen on the right contiguous with the similarly heterogeneous and low-density thyroidal infiltrative mass* ➡. (Right) *Axial CECT shows large heterogeneous and low-density mass* ➡ *in right superior mediastinum, subtly infiltrating wall of trachea* ➡ *and encasing right common carotid artery* ➡.

Non-Hodgkin Lymphoma of Thyroid

TERMINOLOGY

- Thyroid non-Hodgkin lymphoma (NHL)
  - Lymphoma arising in thyroid gland

IMAGING

- Rapidly enlarging, solid, noncalcified thyroid mass in elderly woman with history of chronic lymphocytic thyroiditis
- 80% solitary homogeneous thyroid mass
- 20% multiple masses or diffuse infiltration
- CECT: Necrosis and calcification uncommon
- US: Well-defined, homogeneous, hypoechoic
- PET/CT generally useful except if MALT lymphoma

TOP DIFFERENTIAL DIAGNOSES

- Anaplastic thyroid carcinoma
- Multinodular goiter
- Chronic lymphocytic (Hashimoto) thyroiditis
- Thyroid differentiated carcinoma

PATHOLOGY

- Most often diffuse large **B-cell lymphoma**
- 40-80% of cases occur in patients with **chronic lymphocytic (Hashimoto) thyroiditis**
  - Hashimoto has 70x increased risk of thyroid NHL

CLINICAL ISSUES

- Presents as rapidly enlarging neck mass
- 2-5% of all thyroid malignancies
- 5-yr survival: 75-95%
  - Extrathyroidal spread: ↓ 5-yr survival to 35%
- Nonsurgical disease, unless acute relief of airway obstruction is required

DIAGNOSTIC CHECKLIST

- Main differential is **anaplastic thyroid carcinoma**
- NHL more homogeneous; no necrosis, hemorrhage
- NHL less likely to invade tissues such as trachea

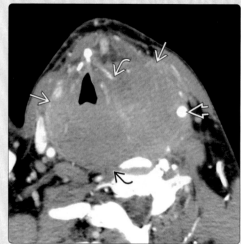
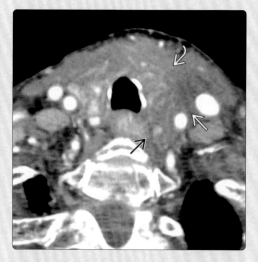

(Left) Axial CECT shows large, minimally enhancing mass ➡ centered in thyroid gland. Mass invades laryngeal cartilages ➡ and prevertebral muscles ➡ and surrounds carotid artery ➡. Homogeneous density of mass suggests lymphoma, but anaplastic thyroid cancer is main differential. (Right) Axial CECT shows infiltrative non-Hodgkin lymphoma of left thyroid with invasion of carotid sheath ➡, esophagus ➡, and overlying strap muscles ➡.

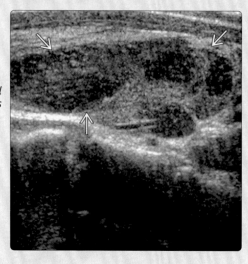
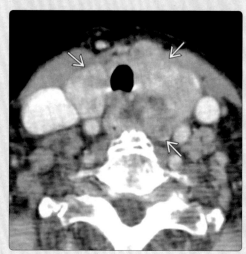

(Left) Longitudinal ultrasound of thyroid gland shows low echogenicity lobular mass ➡. Uniform nature of lymphoma can result in low echogenicity on ultrasound, which may be mistaken for cyst. (Right) Axial CECT shows multifocal masses ➡ in thyroid. Although this primary lymphoma might be mistaken for a multinodular goiter, focal loss of definition of thyroid margins and absence of calcification suggest alternate diagnosis. Loss of clarity of borders is particularly suspicious for malignancy.

TERMINOLOGY

Abbreviations

- Non-Hodgkin lymphoma (NHL)

Definitions

- Extranodal, extralymphatic lymphoma originating from thyroid gland
  - Excludes systemic NHL that secondarily involves thyroid

IMAGING

General Features

- Best diagnostic clue
  - Rapidly enlarging, solid, noncalcified thyroid mass in elderly woman with history of chronic lymphocytic thyroiditis
- Size
  - Often large at presentation; 5-10 cm
- Morphology
  - Diffuse, homogeneous, enlarged thyroid
  - 80% present as solitary thyroid mass, remainder as multiple masses or diffuse infiltration

CT Findings

- CECT
  - Most often homogeneous, solid, hypodense mass
  - Necrosis, hemorrhage, or calcification uncommon

MR Findings

- T1WI
  - Hypointense to normal surrounding thyroid gland
- T2WI
  - Hyperintense to normal surrounding thyroid gland
- T1WI C+
  - Primary tumor lower signal than surrounding residual thyroid gland

Ultrasonographic Findings

- Pseudocystic: Well-defined, homogeneous, markedly hypoechoic mass

Nuclear Medicine Findings

- PET/CT
  - Generally useful in lymphoma
  - MALT subtype often has low FDG avidity

Imaging Recommendations

- Best imaging tool
  - PET/CT for staging after diagnosis established
  - CECT alone if MALT-type lymphoma

DIFFERENTIAL DIAGNOSIS

Anaplastic Thyroid Carcinoma

- Rapidly enlarging, invasive thyroid mass
- Calcification, necrosis, & hemorrhage common

Multinodular Goiter

- Multiple nodules in enlarged thyroid gland
- No adenopathy

Chronic Lymphocytic (Hashimoto) Thyroiditis

- Most often chronic, diffuse thyromegaly
- No adenopathy

Thyroid Differentiated Carcinoma

- Poorly marginated thyroid mass ± calcifications
- Adenopathy solid or cystic

PATHOLOGY

General Features

- Etiology
  - In 40-80% of cases, NHL complicates **chronic lymphocytic (Hashimoto) thyroiditis (CLT)**
    - CLT has 70x increased risk of thyroid NHL

Staging, Grading, & Classification

- Anatomic staging (Ann Arbor staging)
  - Localized to thyroid classified as stage IE
  - Regional lymph nodes changes to stage IIE

Microscopic Features

- 3 main types involve thyroid gland primarily
  - Diffuse large B-cell lymphoma
    - Most common; poorly differentiated NHL
  - Marginal zone B-cell MALT lymphoma
  - Follicular lymphoma
- Rarely, Hodgkin, Burkitt, & T-cell lymphomas

CLINICAL ISSUES

Presentation

- Most common signs/symptoms
  - Rapidly enlarging thyroid mass, frequently with associated neck adenopathy
- Other signs/symptoms
  - Symptom from local mass effect or invasion

Demographics

- Age
  - Range: 50-80 yr; peak: Late 60s
- Gender
  - F:M = 3:1
- Epidemiology
  - 2-5% of all thyroid malignancies
  - 1-2% of all extranodal lymphomas occur in thyroid

Natural History & Prognosis

- MALT has best prognosis: 5-yr survival > 95%
- Follicular NHL: 5-yr survival = 87%
- Diffuse B-cell has worst prognosis: 5-yr survival = 75%
- Extrathyroidal spread reduces 5-yr survival to 35%

Treatment

- Rituximab + chemotherapy ± radiation
- Nonsurgical, unless airway compromised

SELECTED REFERENCES

1. Wang Z et al: Primary thyroid lymphoma has different sonographic and color Doppler features compared to nodular goiter. J Ultrasound Med. 34(2):317-23, 2015
2. Xia Y et al: Sonographic appearance of primary thyroid lymphoma-preliminary experience. PLoS One. 9(12):e114080, 2014
3. Stein SA et al: Primary thyroid lymphoma: a clinical review. J Clin Endocrinol Metab. 98(8):3131-8, 2013
4. Walsh S et al: Thyroid lymphoma: recent advances in diagnosis and optimal management strategies. Oncologist. 18(9):994-1003, 2013

TERMINOLOGY

- Parathyroid carcinoma (PTCa)
- Low-grade malignancy arising from 1 of parathyroid glands

IMAGING

- Typically posterior to thyroid gland, > 3 cm
- **Large size, thick capsule suggest carcinoma**
- Often indistinguishable from PT adenoma
- PTCa may be larger lesion ± invasion; younger patient than adenoma
- Tc-99m sestamibi, sonography, and CECT useful
- Tc-99m sestamibi localizes source of hyperparathyroidism
- US most sensitive after scintigraphy
- US: Hypoechoic, well defined
- CECT/MR: Useful for ectopic gland tumors & evaluating extent of invasive disease

TOP DIFFERENTIAL DIAGNOSES

- Parathyroid adenoma
- Thyroid adenoma
- Thyroid differentiated carcinoma

PATHOLOGY

- 80% well differentiated

CLINICAL ISSUES

- Patients present with severe hypercalcemia
- Most often in 4th-5th decade, F = M
- 5-yr survival = 70-85%

DIAGNOSTIC CHECKLIST

- PTCa rare and mimics PT adenoma clinically & radiographically
- Large presumed PT adenoma with invasive margins suggests PTCa diagnosis

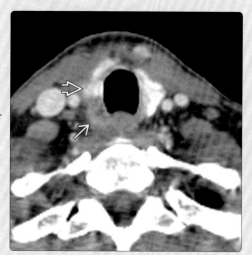
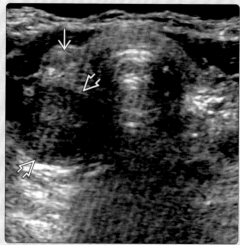

(Left) Axial CECT shows an ill-defined mass ⇨ in right tracheoesophageal groove displacing thyroid gland ⇨ anteriorly, representing parathyroid carcinoma. The differential for this lesion is parathyroid adenoma, exophytic thyroid adenoma, or carcinoma. (Right) Axial ultrasound at level of thyroid isthmus shows homogeneous hypoechoic mass ⇨ posterior to right thyroid lobe ⇨, displacing thyroid gland anteriorly. Lesion has well-defined contours but was found to be parathyroid carcinoma.

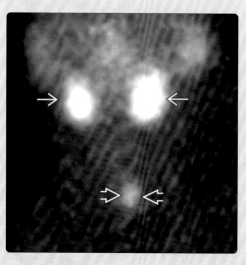
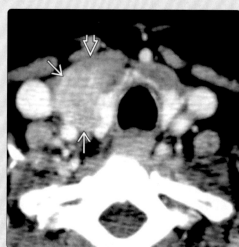

(Left) Frontal scintigraphy from late phase of Tc-99m sestamibi shows normal submandibular gland uptake ⇨ but abnormal focus ⇨ in lower left neck, representing parathyroid carcinoma. Parathyroid adenoma would appear identical. (Right) Axial CECT shows large intrathyroidal mass ⇨ with ill-defined borders invading strap muscles ⇨. Although most parathyroid carcinomas arise posterior to thyroid, they may also be intrathyroidal and indistinguishable from primary thyroid carcinoma.

TERMINOLOGY

Abbreviations
- Parathyroid carcinoma (PTCa)

Definitions
- Low-grade malignancy arising from parathyroid gland

IMAGING

General Features
- Best diagnostic clue
  - Uniform mass displacing thyroid gland anteriorly, with focal areas of **soft tissue invasion**
- Location
  - Usually posterior to thyroid gland; may be within
  - Rarely arises from ectopic parathyroid gland
- Size
  - Usually > 3 cm; typically larger than adenoma at presentation
- Morphology
  - Usually well defined; may have invasion of surrounding structures

Nuclear Medicine Findings
- Tc-99m sestamibi
  - Localizes source of hyperparathyroidism
  - SPECT/CT fusion useful

Ultrasonographic Findings
- Grayscale ultrasound
  - Ovoid, well-marginated mass posterior to thyroid
  - Similar to adenomas in sonographic appearance
    - **Large size, thick capsule suggest carcinoma**
  - Sonography most sensitive **after** sestamibi
- Color Doppler
  - High vascularity more suggestive of carcinoma than adenoma

CT Findings
- CECT
  - Useful for carcinoma arising in ectopic glands, especially mediastinum
  - Adjacent soft tissue invasion highly suggestive of PTCa diagnosis

Imaging Recommendations
- Best imaging tool
  - Tc-99m sestamibi 1st, sonography or CECT
  - Often 2 modalities utilized prior to surgery

DIFFERENTIAL DIAGNOSIS

Parathyroid Adenoma
- Often indistinguishable from PTCa

Thyroid Adenoma
- Well-defined intrathyroidal mass

Thyroid Differentiated Carcinoma
- Poorly defined intrathyroidal mass ± nodes
- Usually appears more aggressive than PTCa

PATHOLOGY

General Features
- Trabecular pattern, mitotic figures, thick fibrous bands, capsular &/or vascular invasion

Staging, Grading, & Classification
- 80% well differentiated

CLINICAL ISSUES

Presentation
- Most common signs/symptoms
  - Severe hypercalcemia often greater than other causes of hyperparathyroidism
    - Fatigue, bone & joint pain, headache, depression, digestive symptoms, calculi
- Other signs/symptoms
  - Associated with hyperparathyroidism-jaw tumor syndrome
    - Autosomal dominant disease, chr1q25-q31
    - Parathyroid tumors + jaw fibroosseous tumors

Demographics
- Age
  - Usually 4th-5th decade; range: 8-85 yr old
    - Younger on average than PT adenoma
- Gender
  - F = M; note that F > > M for adenomas
- Epidemiology
  - Very rare with < 1,000 cases in English literature
  - < 1% of hyperparathyroidism

Natural History & Prognosis
- Slow, indolent growth
- 5-yr survival = 70-85%
- Nodes not predictive of outcome
- Death more likely from hypercalcemia than tumor

Treatment
- En bloc resection is mainstay of treatment
  - Level VI dissection usually included

DIAGNOSTIC CHECKLIST

Image Interpretation Pearls
- Parathyroid carcinoma is rare and mimics adenoma clinically and radiographically; it is usually not suspected until pathologic evaluation

Reporting Tips
- Brown tumors of hyperparathyroidism should not be mistaken for bone metastases

SELECTED REFERENCES

1. Asare EA et al: Parathyroid carcinoma: an update on treatment outcomes and prognostic factors from the national cancer data base (NCDB). Ann Surg Oncol. 22(12):3390-5, 2015
2. Sadler C et al: Parathyroid carcinoma in more than 1,000 patients: a population-level analysis. Surgery. 156(6):1622-9; discussion 1629-30, 2014
3. Owen RP et al: Parathyroid carcinoma: a review. Head Neck. 33(3): 429-36, 2011
4. Dudney WC et al: Parathyroid carcinoma. Otolaryngol Clin North Am. 43(2):441-53, xi, 2010

Thyroglossal Duct Cyst Carcinoma

TERMINOLOGY

- Malignant tumor arising from remnants of embryologic thyroglossal duct (TGD)

IMAGING

- CECT or MR: Most often occurs as solid component ± calcifications within TGD cyst
- May occur as tumor within solid ectopic thyroid tissue from tongue base to lower neck
- CECT more likely to show calcifications
- US: Look for solid components ± calcifications with thyroglossal duct cyst
- PET: Carcinoma may be FDG avid

TOP DIFFERENTIAL DIAGNOSES

- Thyroglossal duct cyst
- Lingual thyroid
- Oral cavity dermoid and epidermoid

PATHOLOGY

- < 95% TGD carcinoma (TGDCa) are papillary thyroid
- < 5% are squamous carcinoma; more aggressive

CLINICAL ISSUES

- Enlarging midline neck mass; no symptoms to distinguish from benign TCD
- Most commonly adults; mean = 40 years
- < 2% of TGD cysts have carcinoma

DIAGNOSTIC CHECKLIST

- Presence of calcification is supportive of TGDCa
- Presence of solid components in TGD cyst can be due to prior inflammation
- Report either & consider FNA prior to TCD resection
- Always comment on presence/absence of normal thyroid tissue

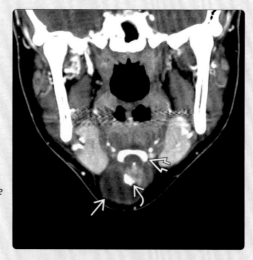
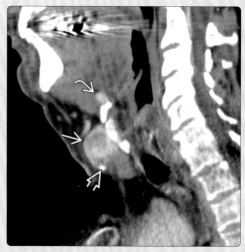

(Left) Coronal CECT reveals a midline neck cystic mass ➡ that is intimately related to the hyoid bone ➡. At the superior aspect of the cyst, there is enhancing soft tissue and dense calcifications ➡. (Right) Sagittal reformatted CECT of TGDCa shows a solid heterogeneous mass ➡ just below the hyoid bone, which contains focal calcification at the inferior aspect ➡. An additional small solid rest of ectopic tissue is present above the hyoid ➡. There was no normal-appearing thyroid in the lower neck.

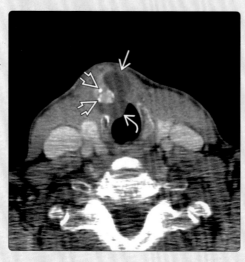
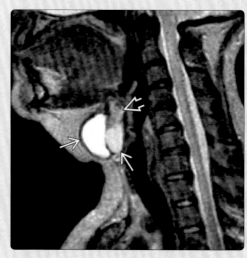

(Left) Axial CECT shows a subglottic paramedian complex cystic TGDCa ➡ within infrahyoid strap muscles. The cystic component of the mass is submucosal in the subglottic endolarynx ➡. Within the extralaryngeal cystic mass, an enhancing nodule with punctate calcifications is visible ➡. (Right) Sagittal T2WI MR shows an infrahyoid hyperintense multilobulated cystic mass ➡ with intermediate to low intensity of the superior solid nodule ➡. This nodule is enhanced with contrast and was TGDCa.

TERMINOLOGY

Abbreviations

- Thyroglossal duct carcinoma (TGDCa)

Definitions

- Malignant tumor arising from remnants of embryologic thyroglossal duct (TGD)
  - Most often occurs within TGD

IMAGING

General Features

- Best diagnostic clue
  - Solid ± calcified components within TGD cyst
  - Heterogeneous ectopic thyroid tissue ± calcifications
- Location
  - Tongue base (foramen cecum) to lower neck
  - 50% of TGD cysts are around hyoid level
    - 25% suprahyoid, 25% infrahyoid
- Size
  - Cystic component variable in size
  - Neoplastic component most often small (~ 1 cm)

CT Findings

- CECT
  - Midline hyoid-suprahyoid or paramedian infrahyoid cystic mass
    - Look for solid components ± calcification
    - May see frankly invasive solid tumor
  - Tumor may be within solid ectopic thyroid
    - Look for more heterogeneous component ± calcifications
  - Calcification uncommon with inflammation alone

MR Findings

- Solid component within TGD
- TGD cyst has variable T1 and T2 signal
  - Depends on thyroglobulin, inflammation, hemorrhage

Ultrasonographic Findings

- Grayscale ultrasound
  - Anechoic or hypoechoic midline neck mass
    - Look for solid component ± echoes from calcifications

Nuclear Medicine Findings

- PET/CT
  - FDG uptake may be found within TGD
    - Not specific for malignancy

Imaging Recommendations

- Best imaging tool
  - CECT may show calcifications associated with carcinoma
  - Both CT and MR show solid and cystic components
- Protocol advice
  - CECT: Evaluate cyst on soft tissue and bone windows for calcifications

DIFFERENTIAL DIAGNOSIS

Thyroglossal Duct Cyst

- Midline congenital mass
- Cystic, ± multiloculated; ± solid components

Lingual Thyroid

- Congenital failure of thyroid gland descent
- Thyroid gland absent or abnormally high in neck
- Rarely complicated by carcinoma

Oral Cavity Dermoid and Epidermoid

- Cystic or fat-containing mass in floor of mouth or submandibular region
- Not associated with hyoid bone

PATHOLOGY

Microscopic Features

- < 95% of TGDCa are papillary thyroid (PTC)
- < 5% are squamous carcinoma; more aggressive
- PTC often contains psammoma bodies, which can result in calcifications evident on CT

CLINICAL ISSUES

Presentation

- Most common signs/symptoms
  - Enlarging midline neck mass; no symptoms to distinguish from benign TGD
  - Most diagnosed on pathologic review of TGD cyst

Demographics

- Age
  - Most commonly **adults**; mean = 40 years
  - Pediatric cases rare; mean = 13 years
- Gender
  - Carcinoma slightly more common in female patients
- Epidemiology
  - **< 2% of TGD cysts have carcinoma**
    - 1 adult series reported 6.5% incidence of TGDCa

Treatment

- Complete resection of TGD (Sistrunk procedure)
- TGDCa treatment often necessitates thyroidectomy

DIAGNOSTIC CHECKLIST

Consider

- Presence of calcification is more supportive of TGDCa
- Presence of solid components in TGD cyst may be due to prior inflammation
  - Consider FNA prior to resection

Image Interpretation Pearls

- Any imaging study of TGD cysts should be carefully evaluated for solid and calcified components
- Always comment on presence/absence of normal thyroid tissue

SELECTED REFERENCES

1. Shah S et al: Squamous cell carcinoma in a thyroglossal duct cyst: a case report with review of the literature. Am J Otolaryngol. 36(3):460-2, 2015
2. Wei S et al: Pathology of thyroglossal duct: an institutional experience. Endocr Pathol. 26(1):75-9, 2015
3. Carter Y et al: Thyroglossal duct remnant carcinoma: beyond the Sistrunk procedure. Surg Oncol. 23(3):161-6, 2014
4. Forest VI et al: Thyroglossal duct cyst carcinoma: case series. J Otolaryngol Head Neck Surg. 40(2):151-6, 2011
5. Glastonbury CM et al: The CT and MR imaging features of carcinoma arising in thyroglossal duct remnants. AJNR Am J Neuroradiol. 21(4):770-4, 2000

Cervical Esophageal Carcinoma

TERMINOLOGY

- Cervical esophageal carcinoma (CECA)
- > 95% CECa are squamous cell carcinoma (SCCa)

IMAGING

- Cervical esophagus = lower cricoid to thoracic inlet
- **Posterior midline** visceral space focal or invasive mass
- CECT/MR: Both adequate to evaluate invasive extent of tumor
  - Esophageal wall thickened + ill-defined margin
  - Frequent extension to hypopharynx, larynx, thyroid
  - Cord paralysis from recurrent laryngeal nerve involvement
  - Look for level VI and mediastinal nodes
- PET/CT best tool for staging, monitoring, and surveillance

TOP DIFFERENTIAL DIAGNOSES

- Hypopharyngeal SCCa
- Thyroid anaplastic carcinoma

- Thyroid non-Hodgkin lymphoma

PATHOLOGY

- Strong association with tobacco & alcohol abuse
- AJCC staging as for all esophagus
  - **T1-T3**: Depth of wall invasion
  - **T4**: Invasion of adjacent structures
- Nodal disease present in 70% at diagnosis

CLINICAL ISSUES

- Typically presents with dysphagia, weight loss
- Frequently detected late with poor prognosis
- 5-year survival = 10%
- Definitive chemoradiotherapy preferred with advanced presentation

DIAGNOSTIC CHECKLIST

- Many H&N SCCa patients are smokers, alcoholics
  - Increased risk of 2nd primary malignancy must be considered when imaging these patients

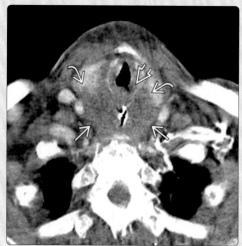
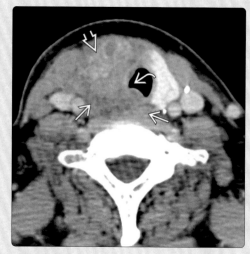

(Left) CECT shows infiltrative, aggressive-appearing midline mass ➡ in the posterior visceral space invading the thyroid gland ➡ and cricoid cartilage ➡. A nasogastric tube is in the center of this posterior midline esophageal SCCa. (Right) Axial CECT shows a heterogeneous mass ➡ filling posterior & right side of visceral space. Right thyroid lobe is replaced ➡, & trachea ➡ is invaded. This esophageal SCCa mimics anaplastic thyroid carcinoma or thyroid lymphoma. This primary tumor is T4 due to invasion of adjacent structures.

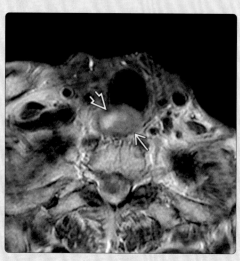
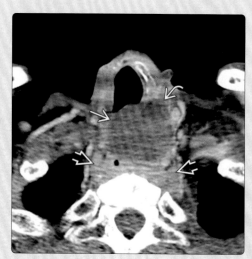

(Left) Axial T2WI MR in a 62-year-old man who had chemoradiation for tongue base SCCa 7 years prior shows eccentric thickening of cervical esophageal wall ➡, outlined by hyperintense obstructed secretions ➡. This was proven to be a small esophageal SCCa. (Right) Axial CECT at the level of the cervical thoracic junction shows a large posterior midline esophageal SCCa ➡. Anterior invasion on the left ➡ is visible with retropharyngeal-danger space invasion seen posteriorly ➡.

TERMINOLOGY

Abbreviations

- Cervical esophageal carcinoma (CECa)

Definitions

- Malignancy of lining epithelium of cervical esophagus
  o > 95% are squamous cell carcinoma (SCCa)

IMAGING

General Features

- Best diagnostic clue
  o **Concentric or eccentric esophageal thickening** with ill-defined outer margins
  o Infiltrative mass in posterior midline visceral space
- Location
  o Cervical esophagus defined from lower border cricoid to thoracic inlet (suprasternal notch)

Fluoroscopic Findings

- Barium swallow
  o Mucosal-based, irregular filling defect
  o Luminal narrowing with larger lesions

CT Findings

- CECT
  o Ill-defined enhancing circumferential or eccentric esophageal mass
  o May be enhancing infiltrative mass of **posteromedial visceral space**
  o Frequent extension to hypopharynx, larynx, or thoracic esophagus

MR Findings

- T2 hyperintense and enhancing midline posterior visceral space mass

Nuclear Medicine Findings

- PET/CT
  o SCCa consistently FDG avid

Imaging Recommendations

- Best imaging tool
  o PET/CT is best imaging tool for staging, monitoring, and surveillance
    – Local disease extent with CT
    – Regional and distant disease with PET
- Protocol advice
  o Must image to **carina** to ensure coverage of mediastinal nodes
  o MR helpful for prevertebral invasion by loss of fat planes

DIFFERENTIAL DIAGNOSIS

Hypopharyngeal Squamous Cell Carcinoma

- Arises at or above cricoid level
- May extend into esophagus

Thyroid Anaplastic Carcinoma

- Elderly patient with rapidly enlarging neck mass
- Heterogeneous, infiltrative thyroid mass

PATHOLOGY

General Features

- Etiology
  o Strong association with tobacco & alcohol abuse
  o Increased incidence with caustic stricture, achalasia, prior radiation
  o Association with **Plummer-Vinson syndrome**
- Associated abnormalities
  o 15% have synchronous or metachronous tumors
    – Especially H&N SCCa, lung carcinoma

Staging, Grading, & Classification

- American Joint Committee on Cancer staging as for all esophagus
  o T1-T3 defined by depth of invasion of wall
  o T4a tumor invades resectable structures
  o T4b tumor invades nonresectable structures

CLINICAL ISSUES

Presentation

- Most common signs/symptoms
  o Early stages asymptomatic
  o Dysphagia, weight loss
- Other signs/symptoms
  o Sensation of fullness, retrosternal pain
  o Hoarseness: Recurrent laryngeal nerve involvement

Demographics

- Age
  o Peak age: 55-65 years
- Gender
  o M:F = 4:1

Natural History & Prognosis

- Tendency to invade local visceral space or hypopharynx
- Frequently detected late with poor prognosis
  o 70% have level VI node involvement at diagnosis
- Distant metastases to liver, lung, pleura, & bones
- Overall 5-year survival = 10%

Treatment

- Definitive chemoradiotherapy preferred
- Radical resection of esophagus & hypopharynx with jejunal interposition or gastric pull-up

DIAGNOSTIC CHECKLIST

Consider

- Many patients with H&N SCCa are smokers, alcoholics
  o Be aware risk of 2nd primary malignancy on follow-up scan

Image Interpretation Pearls

- Look for paratracheal & superior mediastinum nodes

SELECTED REFERENCES

1. Grass GD et al: Cervical esophageal cancer: a population-based study. Head Neck. 37(6):808-14, 2015
2. Hong SJ et al: New TNM staging system for esophageal cancer: what chest radiologists need to know. Radiographics. 34(6):1722-40, 2014
3. Ng T et al: Advances in the surgical treatment of esophageal cancer. J Surg Oncol. 101(8):725-9, 2010

KEY FACTS

TERMINOLOGY

- Mucosa-lined outpouching of posterior hypopharynx
- Posterior pulsion diverticulum **above** cricopharyngeus

IMAGING

- Sac arising from posterior pharynx at C5-6 level
- Extends posteroinferiorly and to **left** side
- **Barium esophagram** is best imaging tool
  - Confirms diagnosis and shows diverticular neck
  - Evaluates associated reflux and hiatal hernia
- On CT/MR usually incidental finding
- CECT: Well-defined mass posterior and to left of esophagus
  - Nonenhancing mass with air, fluid, ± food debris
- MR: Sagittal plane best delineates sac
  - May have air-fluid level
  - Food debris results in heterogeneous signal
  - May see linear enhancement of mucosa

TOP DIFFERENTIAL DIAGNOSES

- Lateral cervical esophageal diverticulum
- Paratracheal air cyst
- Parathyroid cyst
- Thyroid carcinoma nodal metastasis

PATHOLOGY

- Herniation occurs at Killian dehiscence
- Multiple causes proposed; likely multifactorial
- Almost all have hiatal hernia
- Many have reflux esophagitis

CLINICAL ISSUES

- As diverticulum enlarges, symptoms increase
- Complications mostly related to obstruction and aspiration of retained ingested material
- Squamous cell carcinoma is rare complication

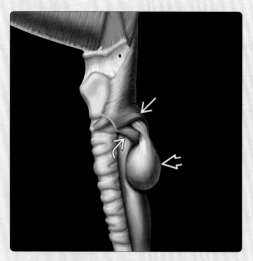

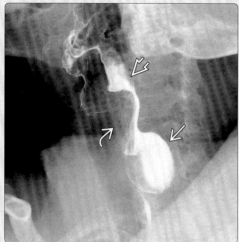

(Left) Graphic depicts Zenker diverticulum ⮕ with herniation at Killian dehiscence between thyropharyngeal ⮕ and cricopharyngeal ⮕ fibers of inferior constrictor muscle. (Right) Barium esophagram demonstrates a large diverticulum with retained layering contrast ⮕ from the posterior lateral junction of the hypopharynx ⮕ and the cervical esophagus ⮕. The posterior lateral projection confirms this lesion as an esophagopharyngeal (Zenker) diverticulum.

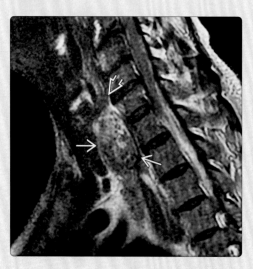

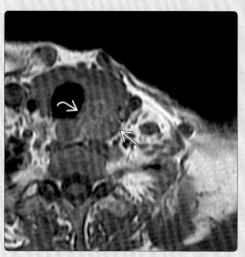

(Left) Parasagittal T2WI MR shows a saccular well-circumscribed collection of heterogenous signal ⮕ just below the cricoid cartilage ⮕ at the level of C5-C6. (Right) Axial T1WI MR of brachial plexus in the same patient shows an incidental finding of a left Zenker diverticulum ⮕. Image demonstrates the mouth of the diverticulum through Killian dehiscence in the posterior esophagus that is flattened anterior to the diverticulum ⮕.

TERMINOLOGY

Synonyms

- Pharyngeal pouch, pharyngoesophageal diverticulum, posterior hypopharyngeal diverticulum

Definitions

- Mucosa-lined outpouching of posterior hypopharynx
- Posterior pulsion diverticulum **above** cricopharyngeus

IMAGING

General Features

- Best diagnostic clue
  - Well-defined mass posterior and to **left** of esophagus
  - **Air** on cross-sectional images is **key finding**
- Location
  - Arises from posterior pharynx just above C5-6 level
- Size
  - Variable, small to several centimeters
- Morphology
  - Sac-like outpouching descending behind cervical esophagus

Fluoroscopic Findings

- Barium-filled sac extends caudally posterior and to **left** of cervical esophagus
- Distended sac partially obstructs esophagus
- Cricopharyngeus may indent posterior esophagus
- Associated hiatal hernia and reflux esophagitis possible
- Irregularity of diverticular contour suggests inflammation or neoplasia

CT Findings

- CECT
  - Nonenhancing thin wall mass with air, fluid, or debris

MR Findings

- T2WI
  - Signal depends on contents, often heterogeneous
- T1WI C+
  - May see linear enhancement of mucosa

Imaging Recommendations

- Best imaging tool
  - Barium esophagram best illustrates diverticulum
- Protocol advice
  - Oblique and lateral barium swallow images reveal diverticular neck

DIFFERENTIAL DIAGNOSIS

Lateral Cervical Esophageal Diverticulum

- Lateral outpouching of proximal cervical esophagus
- **Below** cricopharyngeus muscle
- Barium swallow differentiates from esophagopharyngeal (Zenker) diverticulum

Paratracheal Air Cyst

- Air-filled structure posterior and to **right** of cervical or proximal trachea

Parathyroid Cyst

- Degenerative or congenital along parathyroid tract

Thyroid Carcinoma Nodal Metastasis

- Level VI node from differentiated thyroid carcinoma
- Does not contain air

PATHOLOGY

General Features

- Etiology
  - Herniation occurs at Killian dehiscence
  - Multiple causes proposed, likely multifactorial
- Associated abnormalities
  - Almost all have hiatal hernia
  - Many have reflux esophagitis

Staging, Grading, & Classification

- 2 descriptive classifications based on size alone
- Van Overbeek & Groote
  - Small < 1 vertebra in size, large > 3 vertebra
- Morton & Bartley
  - Small < 2 cm, medium 2-4 cm, large > 4 cm

CLINICAL ISSUES

Presentation

- Most common signs/symptoms
  - Dysphagia as pouch compresses esophagus
  - Regurgitation of contents
  - Respiratory symptoms due to chronic aspiration

Demographics

- Age
  - Usually > 60 years, rarely < 40 years

Natural History & Prognosis

- As diverticulum enlarges, symptoms increase
- Squamous cell carcinoma is rare complication (0.3%)

Treatment

- Elderly patients with minimal symptoms are frequently treated by observation alone
- Symptomatic diverticula can be treated by endoscopic or external surgical techniques

DIAGNOSTIC CHECKLIST

Consider

- Barium esophagram is standard
  - Confirm diagnosis and demonstrate diverticular neck
  - Evaluate for hiatal hernia and reflux esophagitis
  - Suspect carcinoma if irregular mucosa

Image Interpretation Pearls

- Heterogeneous mass on CT/MR can be confusing
- Posterolateral **left** location and **presence of air** are key

SELECTED REFERENCES

1. Mantsopoulos K et al: Clinical relevance and prognostic value of radiographic findings in Zenker's diverticulum. Eur Arch Otorhinolaryngol. 271(3):583-8, 2014
2. Prisman E et al: Zenker diverticulum. Otolaryngol Clin North Am. 46(6):1101-11, 2013

TERMINOLOGY

- Synonym: Colloid nodule
- Definition: Fluid lesion of thyroid containing stored form of thyroid hormone (colloid)

IMAGING

- Typically 1-4 cm; when large, usually hemorrhagic
- Sharply defined, fluid-filled lesion
- CECT: Low-density, round to oval lesion
  - Thyroid tissue "beaks" around cyst
- MR: T2 hyperintense, well-defined lesion
  - T1 frequently hyperintense, may be iso- or hypointense to thyroid
- Ultrasound is key modality for determining nature
  - Shows **thin wall with smooth margins**
  - Typically anechoic, ↑ through transmission
  - Colloid crystals may be suspended in fluid with **posterior comet-tail artifact**

TOP DIFFERENTIAL DIAGNOSES

- Thyroid adenoma
- Simple thyroid cyst
- Thyroid differentiated carcinoma
- Thyroglossal duct cyst

CLINICAL ISSUES

- 15-25% thyroid nodules
- May rapidly enlarge from hemorrhage
- Often incidental imaging finding
  - Smaller cysts commonly seen during thyroid ultrasound
- Benign lesion without malignant potential

DIAGNOSTIC CHECKLIST

- Important to carefully evaluate "cystic" lesion on ultrasound
- Complex thyroid "cyst" may be malignant degenerating lesion

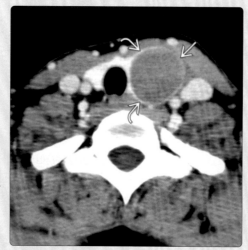
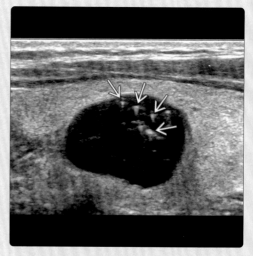

(Left) Axial CECT demonstrates ovoid, sharply defined, low-density mass ➡ in left thyroid lobe with thyroid tissue "beaking" around anterior and posterior margins of mass ➡. Needle aspiration of lesion revealed a hemorrhagic colloid cyst. (Right) Longitudinal grayscale ultrasound demonstrates a typical colloid nodule with multiple characteristic echogenic foci and comet-tail artifacts suspended in the cyst ➡. These represent colloid particles in viscous fluid concentrated with thyroglobulin.

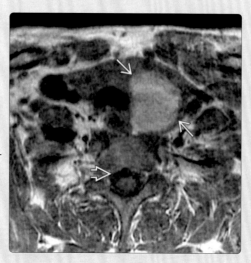
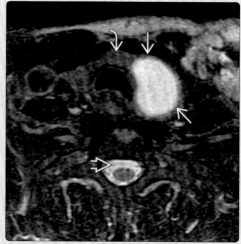

(Left) Axial T1 MR demonstrates a large well-defined mass ➡ within left thyroid lobe that is hyperintense to CSF ➡. Mass abuts and displaces left strap muscles anteriorly, but there are no aggressive features to suggest an invasive mass. (Right) Axial T2 FS MR shows mass ➡ to be uniformly & markedly hyperintense, similar to intensity of CSF ➡. Lesion clearly resides within the left thyroid lobe and is sharply demarcated from normal adjacent thyroid isthmus ➡. No adenopathy is evident in neck.

TERMINOLOGY

Synonyms

- Colloid nodules

Definitions

- Fluid lesion of thyroid containing stored form of thyroid hormone (colloid)

IMAGING

General Features

- Best diagnostic clue
  - Ultrasound demonstrates thin rim lesion with anechoic contents ± colloid crystals
- Location
  - Within thyroid gland
- Size
  - Typically 1-4 cm; when large, usually hemorrhagic
- Morphology
  - Round cystic lesion

Imaging Recommendations

- Best imaging tool
  - Ultrasound best evaluates thyroid nodules to determine whether truly cystic

CT Findings

- CECT
  - Low density, round to oval lesion

MR Findings

- T1WI
  - Signal intensity varies with concentration of fluid
  - Frequently hyperintense; may be hypo- or isointense
- T2WI
  - Hyperintense, uniform
- T1WI C+
  - No significant enhancement of lesion

Ultrasonographic Findings

- Grayscale ultrasound
  - Thin wall with smooth margins
  - Anechoic with increased through transmission
  - Colloid crystals may be suspended in fluid with **posterior comet-tail artifact**
- Color Doppler
  - No significant vascularity of wall

DIFFERENTIAL DIAGNOSIS

Thyroid Adenoma

- Hemorrhagic degeneration mimics colloid cyst
- Echogenic fluid on ultrasound
- Color or power Doppler shows vascularity of thickened wall

Simple Thyroid Cyst

- Uncommon; true cyst with epithelial lining
- Ultrasound: Anechoic with thin, smooth wall

Thyroid Differentiated Carcinoma

- Rarely predominantly cystic mass
- Solid components on imaging

- Focal calcification may be evident

Thyroglossal Duct Cyst

- Congenital, developmental anomaly
- Can occur anywhere from tongue base to thyroid

PATHOLOGY

Microscopic Features

- Rarely true cyst with epithelial lining
- Usually degenerated macronodule with accumulated serous fluid, colloid substance, or blood

CLINICAL ISSUES

Presentation

- Most common signs/symptoms
  - May be detected as palpable nodule
  - May present with rapid increase in size from hemorrhage
  - Often incidental imaging finding
- Other signs/symptoms
  - When very large may displace or distort larynx

Demographics

- Epidemiology
  - 15-25% thyroid nodules

Natural History & Prognosis

- Benign lesions without malignant potential

DIAGNOSTIC CHECKLIST

Image Interpretation Pearls

- Ultrasound is key modality for determining if lesion is truly cyst and for differentiating from other lesions, including rare cystic papillary carcinoma
- Important to carefully evaluate cystic lesion on ultrasound
  - Solid components may harbor malignancy

SELECTED REFERENCES

1. Virmani V et al: Sonographic patterns of benign thyroid nodules: verification at our institution. AJR Am J Roentgenol. 196(4):891-5, 2011
2. Kabala JE: Computed tomography and magnetic resonance imaging in diseases of the thyroid and parathyroid. Eur J Radiol. 66(3):480-92, 2008
3. Loevner LA et al: Cross-sectional imaging of the thyroid gland. Neuroimaging Clin N Am. 18(3):445-61, vii, 2008

Lateral Cervical Esophageal Diverticulum

TERMINOLOGY

- Synonym: Killian-Jamieson diverticulum
- **Lateral outpouching** from **proximal cervical esophagus below cricopharyngeus muscle**

IMAGING

- Small, smoothly marginated lateral sac
- **Usually unilateral, left sided**
- Bilateral in 25%; rarely unilateral, right sided
- Diameter: 0.2-5.0 cm; average: 1.4 cm
- Barium swallow (frontal & lateral) best imaging tool
  - Lateral sac; overlaps anterior esophageal wall
- Incidental finding on CECT/MR
  - Round or oval mass lateral to esophagus
  - Abuts and may displace left thyroid lobe &/or common carotid artery anteriorly
  - Contents may be air, fluid, food debris, or mixed

TOP DIFFERENTIAL DIAGNOSES

- Esophago-pharyngeal (Zenker) diverticulum
- Thyroid carcinoma nodal metastasis
- Parathyroid cyst

PATHOLOGY

- Protrusion through **Killian-Jamieson triangle** in **anterolateral wall** of cervical esophagus
  - Zenker at posterior midline Killian dehiscence

CLINICAL ISSUES

- Less common than Zenker diverticulum
- **Usually asymptomatic**, incidental imaging finding
- May have dysphagia from pharyngeal dysmotility
- Respiratory symptoms uncommon as cricopharyngeus prevents reflux to hypopharynx
- Most not surgically treated due to asymptomatic nature

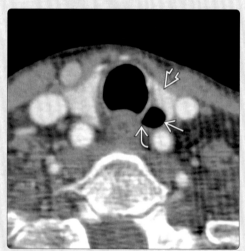
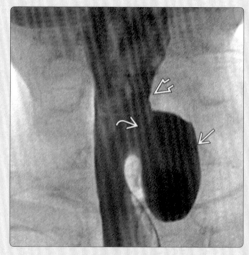

(Left) Axial CECT shows air-filled diverticulum ➡ interposed between cervical esophagus, left thyroid lobe ➡, and common carotid. Note the air "points" ➡ toward esophagus, a clue to its origin. (Right) Frontal esophagram shows a prominent diverticular outpouching ➡ from the left lateral cervical esophageal wall ➡ compatible with a lateral cervical esophageal diverticulum (Killian-Jamieson). This lesion is below the level of the indentation from the cricopharyngeus muscle ➡.

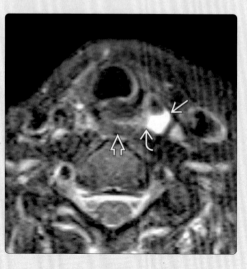
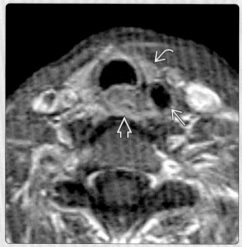

(Left) Axial T2 FS MR shows an irregular mass ➡ lateral to cervical esophagus ➡. Mass has air-fluid level with hyperintense fluid layering posteriorly and subtly points toward cervical esophagus ➡, suggesting its organ of origin. (Right) Axial T1 C+ FS MR reveals esophageal diverticulum as an air-filled hypointense structure ➡ in lower neck posterior to left thyroid lobe ➡ and lateral to cervical esophagus ➡. Left common carotid artery is also displaced anteriorly, lateral to thyroid.

TERMINOLOGY

Synonyms

- Killian-Jamieson diverticulum, proximal lateral cervical esophageal diverticulum
- Lateral pharyngoesophageal diverticulum

Definitions

- Lateral outpouching from proximal cervical esophagus

IMAGING

General Features

- Location
  - **Usually unilateral, left sided**
  - Bilateral up to 25%
  - Rarely unilateral, right sided
- Size
  - Average diameter: 1.4 cm
  - Range: 0.2-5.0 cm
- Morphology
  - Smoothly marginated round-oval sac

Imaging Recommendations

- Best imaging tool
  - Barium swallow best for confirming diagnosis
- Protocol advice
  - True lateral and frontal views should be obtained

Radiographic Findings

- Barium swallow findings
  - Frontal view: Small outpouching from proximal cervical esophagus
  - Lateral view: Arises below cricopharyngeus impression
    - Diverticulum overlaps anterior esophageal wall
- Aspiration rare as cricopharyngeus closes above diverticulum preventing reflux to larynx

CT Findings

- CECT
  - Well-defined round or oval mass lateral to proximal esophagus
  - May see air "pointing" toward esophagus
  - Abuts and may displace anteriorly, left thyroid lobe and common carotid artery
  - Density may be air, fluid, food debris, or mixed

MR Findings

- T2WI
  - Signal varies depending on luminal contents
  - Well-defined mass lateral to cervical esophagus
    - Abuts/displaces left thyroid and common carotid artery

DIFFERENTIAL DIAGNOSIS

Esophagopharyngeal (Zenker) Diverticulum

- Arises from **posterior midline above cricopharyngeus**

Thyroid Carcinoma Nodal Metastasis

- Level VI adenopathy from differentiated carcinoma
- Variable density (CT) or intensity (MR)
- Does not contain air

Parathyroid Cyst

- Degenerative or congenital along parathyroid tract
- Fluid density/intensity
- Does not contain air

PATHOLOGY

General Features

- Etiology
  - Protrusion through muscular gap (Killian-Jamieson triangle) in anterolateral wall of cervical esophagus
    - Inferior to cricopharyngeus and lateral to longitudinal muscle of esophagus just below insertion on posterior cricoid cartilage
    - Note Zenker diverticulum through Killian dehiscence in posterior portion of cricopharyngeus
  - Develops from refluxed pressure against competent cricopharyngeus
- Associated abnormalities
  - May see in association with esophageal-pharyngeal (Zenker) diverticulum

CLINICAL ISSUES

Presentation

- Most common signs/symptoms
  - Vast majority asymptomatic, incidental imaging finding
  - Dysphagia from pharyngeal dysmotility
- Other signs/symptoms
  - Respiratory symptoms uncommon as diverticulum below cricopharyngeus, preventing reflux to hypopharynx and larynx

Demographics

- Age
  - Usually > 60 years
- Epidemiology
  - Uncommon diverticulum
  - Less common than esophagopharyngeal (Zenker) diverticulum

Treatment

- Typically not treated if asymptomatic
- Diverticulectomy ± esophagomyotomy if symptomatic

DIAGNOSTIC CHECKLIST

Consider

- Arises from lateral cervical esophagus **below cricopharyngeus**
  - Zenker arises just above cricopharyngeus in midline

Image Interpretation Pearls

- Lateral barium swallow best for distinguishing from Zenker
  - On lateral swallow overlaps anterior esophageal wall

Reporting Tips

- Less common than Zenker and more likely to be asymptomatic

SELECTED REFERENCES

1. Bock JM et al: Clinical conundrum: Killian-Jamieson diverticulum with paraesophageal hernia. Dysphagia. 31(4):587-91, 2016

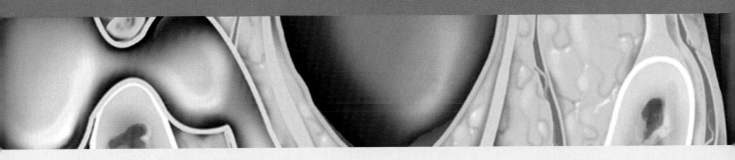

SECTION 11
Hypopharynx, Larynx, and Cervical Trachea

Summary Thoughts: Hypopharynx & Larynx

The hypopharynx and larynx both begin at the lower margin of the oropharynx and end at the lower margin of the cricoid cartilage. The **hypopharynx** is part of the digestive tract, carrying food and liquids to the esophagus. The **larynx** is part of the respiratory tract, connecting to the trachea, creating speech, and preventing aspiration.

Imaging of the **hypopharynx** and **larynx** is commonly performed for evaluation and staging of **squamous cell carcinoma (SCCa)**. Other common pathologies requiring imaging include laryngocele, thyroglossal duct cyst, and trauma. **Important tracheal lesions** include iatrogenic stenosis from intubation or tracheostomy, extrinsic compression or invasion by mass, and, less commonly, tracheal inflammatory diseases.

The **larynx** and **hypopharynx** are intimately related anatomically, sharing 2 common walls. This means that pathology in one location readily involves the other. One should be able to distinguish the 2 sites and define their anatomical subsites, particularly when **staging SCCa**.

Imaging Techniques & Indications

CECT with sagittal and coronal reformations is the study of choice for the hypopharynx, larynx, and trachea. A standard protocol covers from the alveolar mandible to the clavicles at 2.5- to 3.0-mm intervals during quiet respiration, 90 seconds after contrast bolus. For hypopharyngeal or laryngeal SCCa, a **2nd pass** may help assess vocal cord motion. This is performed from the hyoid to cricoid during a breath hold, which opens the pyriform sinuses while the cords adduct.

MR is less commonly used because of breathing artifacts, but it is a useful adjunctive modality for staging of SCCa because it is more sensitive in the detection of laryngeal **cartilage invasion**.

FDG-PET/CT can help identify 2nd primary malignancies of the lung and upper aerodigestive tract in SCCa patients. It is useful for evaluation of recurrent or residual SCCa but is subject to false-positive results in the 2-3 months after radiation therapy. It increases nodal detection in advanced T tumors but does not consistently identify subcentimeter nodes due to camera resolution limitations.

Embryology

The **laryngeal ventricle** marks the division of 2 embryologically distinct laryngeal components. The **supraglottic larynx** forms from primitive buccopharyngeal anlage and the **glottic** and the **subglottic larynx** form from tracheobronchial buds. The buccopharyngeal anlage has a much richer lymphatic network compared with the tracheobronchial buds. As a result, **supraglottic SCCa** has a much higher incidence of **nodal metastases** at presentation compared with **glottic** and **subglottic SCCa**.

Imaging Anatomy

The **hypopharynx** is part of the digestive tract, connecting the oropharyngeal mucosal space to the esophagus. At its superior limit, the hyoid bone, the glossoepiglottic fold, and the pharyngoepiglottic fold demarcate the valleculae, which are part of the oropharynx. The cricopharyngeus muscle defines the inferior limit of the hypopharynx, just below the cricoid cartilage.

The **3 major hypopharyngeal subsites** are the pyriform sinus, posterior wall, and postcricoid region. The **pyriform sinuses** are symmetric pouches hanging behind the larynx. The anteromedial margins of the pyriform sinuses are the posterolateral walls of the supraglottic **aryepiglottic (AE) folds**. The pyriform sinus inferior tip, or pyriform apex, is at the level of the true vocal cords (TVC).

The **posterior hypopharyngeal wall** is the inferior continuation of the posterior oropharyngeal wall, extending from the hyoid to the inferior cricoid margin. Mucosa covering the posterior surface of the cricoid cartilage is the **postcricoid region**. This is 1 of the "shared walls" of the hypopharynx and larynx but is considered hypopharyngeal.

As part of the respiratory tract and the junction between the upper and lower airways, the **larynx** lies between the oropharynx and the trachea. The thyroid, cricoid, and arytenoid cartilages make up the framework over which the laryngeal soft tissues are draped.

As the largest of the laryngeal cartilages, the **thyroid cartilage** "shields" the larynx. Two laminae meet anteriorly at an acute angle in the midline to form an inverted V appearance on axial images. The posteriorly located **superior cornua** attach to the thyrohyoid membrane, and **inferior cornua** articulate medially with the cricoid cartilage sides, forming the cricothyroid joint. This is a useful imaging landmark for the entry of the recurrent laryngeal nerve to the larynx.

The **cricoid cartilage** provides structural integrity to the larynx as the only complete ring. It has a **signet ring** shape with a shorter anterior arch and the quadrate lamina forming the signet posteriorly. Paired pyramidal **arytenoid cartilages** perch atop the posterior lamina with true synovial cricoarytenoid articulations. The arytenoid **vocal processes** project anteriorly and are attachments for the posterior margins of the **TVC**. The inferior limit of the cricoid marks the junction between the larynx and the trachea.

There are **3 areas** of the **larynx** with components that become important when staging SCCa. These are the supraglottic, glottic, and subglottic larynx. The **supraglottic larynx** (supraglottis) extends from the tip of the epiglottis above to the laryngeal ventricles below. **Important components** include the vestibule (supraglottic airway), epiglottis, preepiglottic space, arytenoid cartilages, false vocal cords, and paraglottic (paralaryngeal) spaces.

- The **epiglottis** is a leaf-shaped cartilage that serves as a lid to the endolaryngeal "box," which closes to prevent aspiration during swallowing. It has a superior **free margin** that projects above the hyoid bone and inferiorly is fixed to the thyroid cartilage by the thyroepiglottic ligament, just below the midline notch. Anterior to the epiglottis and posterior and inferior to the hyoid bone lies the fat-filled, preepiglottic space, a clinical blind spot for submucosal tumor.
- The **false vocal cords** are the mucosal surfaces of the laryngeal vestibule. Deep to the false vocal cords are the paired **paraglottic spaces**. These fat-filled spaces merge superiorly into the preepiglottic space and extend inferiorly deep to the TVC in the glottis.
- The **AE folds** extend from the cephalad tips of the arytenoid cartilages to the inferolateral free margin of the epiglottis. The AE folds form the superolateral borders of the supraglottis and also form the anteromedial margin of the pyriform sinuses (part of the

Hypopharynx, Larynx, & Trachea Lesion Differential Diagnosis

Congenital	Trauma
Laryngomalacia	Arytenoid cartilage dislocation
Laryngeal web	Cricoid or thyroid cartilage fracture
Thyroglossal duct cyst	Hematoma
Degenerative/acquired	Laceration
Laryngocele (saccular cyst)	**Benign neoplasms**
Retention cyst	Hemangioma
Infectious/inflammatory	Chondroma
Laryngotracheobronchitis (croup)	Lipoma
Epiglottitis/supraglottitis	Squamous papilloma
Tuberculosis	**Malignant neoplasms**
Sarcoid	Squamous cell carcinoma (SCCa)
Rheumatoid arthritis	Sarcoma (chondrosarcoma)
Amyloid	Minor salivary gland tumor
Wegener granulomatosis	Lymphoma

hypopharynx). They are the 2nd "shared wall." An AE fold SCCa is called a "marginal supraglottic laryngeal tumor."

The **glottic larynx** (glottis) essentially consists of the TVC and their mucosal covering. The **TVC** are comprised of thyroarytenoid muscle, with medial fibers called the "vocalis muscle." Medially, there are thick elastic bands known as the vocal ligaments. TVC meet in the midline anteriorly at the **anterior commissure**, which is only adequately imaged during quiet respiration. The **posterior commissure** is the mucosal surface between the arytenoid cartilages anterior to the cricoid. The mucosa over these areas normally measures ≤ 1 mm in thickness.

The **subglottic larynx** (subglottis) includes the undersurface of the TVC to the lower border of the cricoid cartilage. Its lateral walls are formed by the **conus elasticus**, a fibroelastic membrane extending from the vocal ligaments above to the cricoid below, which is not visible on imaging. Similar to the commissures of the glottis, the mucosa of the subglottis is normally < 1 mm in thickness.

The **trachea** connects the larynx to the lungs, beginning just below the cricoid and ending in the chest at the carina. Each "imperfect" cartilaginous ring surrounds the anterior 2/3 of the trachea, with a fibromuscular membrane covering the flat posterior portion. **Important anatomic relationships** include the thyroid lobes laterally, thyroid isthmus anteriorly from the 2nd-4th tracheal rings, and esophagus posteriorly. Posterolaterally, the tracheoesophageal grooves contain the recurrent laryngeal nerves, paratracheal nodes, and parathyroid glands.

Approaches to Imaging Issues of Hypopharynx, Larynx, & Trachea

It is important to be able to distinguish laryngeal and hypopharyngeal anatomical structures when evaluating pathology in this region, especially when **staging SCCa**. Two key "shared walls" are the **postcricoid region**, which is part of the hypopharynx, and the **AE folds**, which are considered supraglottic larynx.

There are **clinical blind spots** in the hypopharynx and larynx where imaging plays a critical role in tumor detection. In the hypopharynx, the **pyriform sinus apex** is a major site to search in patients presenting with "unknown primary" adenopathy.

In the larynx, the normally fat-filled preepiglottic and paraglottic spaces are clinical blind spots for submucosal spread of SCCa. As no fascia divides these spaces, SCCa can travel freely from one to the other.

Cartilage involvement with SCCa is an important clinical blind spot and also an area of imaging complexity. Irregular cartilage ossification makes determination of cartilage involvement difficult. The diagnosis of invasion should not be made lightly, as it is an indicator for total laryngectomy, as opposed to voice conservation surgery or chemoradiation. Cartilage invasion can only be determined when there is clear medullary invasion, cartilage destruction, or tumor mass on the outer extralaryngeal side of cartilage.

The clinical endoscopic exam provides useful information that may be essential for imaging evaluation, particularly for early T-stage glottic tumors. Conversely, imaging is very important for staging SCCa and especially important for guiding surgeons to biopsy sites when a patient presents with an unknown primary tumor.

Clinical Implications

Hoarseness is a common presentation for tumors of the **larynx**. Glottic SCCa usually presents at an early stage with hoarseness. Subglottic SCCa is often discovered at an advanced stage with extralaryngeal spread. Supraglottic SCCa is often diagnosed in an advanced stage because hoarseness does not develop until the tumor grows down to the vocal cords. Supraglottic and hypopharyngeal SCCa often present with or from nodal metastases. Other symptoms include sore throat, dysphagia, and referred otalgia.

Tracheal lesions present with **shortness of breath** and **stridor** and may carry the diagnosis of "asthma." Primary tracheal tumors are rare; one is more likely to see displacement, compression, or invasion of the trachea by an extrinsic mass.

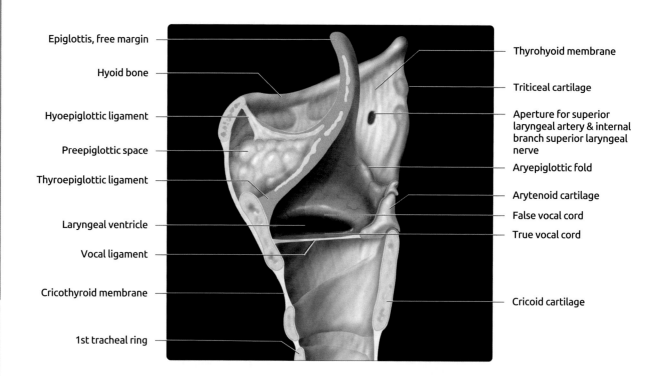

Epiglottis, free margin

Hyoid bone

Hyoepiglottic ligament

Preepiglottic space

Thyroepiglottic ligament

Laryngeal ventricle

Vocal ligament

Cricothyroid membrane

1st tracheal ring

Thyrohyoid membrane

Triticeal cartilage

Aperture for superior laryngeal artery & internal branch superior laryngeal nerve

Aryepiglottic fold

Arytenoid cartilage

False vocal cord

True vocal cord

Cricoid cartilage

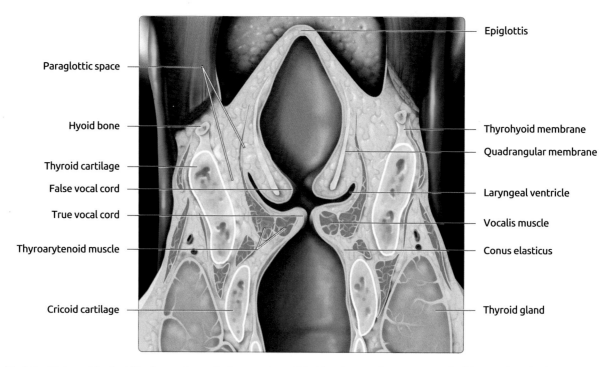

Paraglottic space

Hyoid bone

Thyroid cartilage

False vocal cord

True vocal cord

Thyroarytenoid muscle

Cricoid cartilage

Epiglottis

Thyrohyoid membrane

Quadrangular membrane

Laryngeal ventricle

Vocalis muscle

Conus elasticus

Thyroid gland

(Top) Sagittal graphic of midline larynx shows the laryngeal ventricle, the airspace that separates the false vocal cords above and true vocal cords below. Aryepiglottic (AE) folds project from the tip of arytenoid cartilage to inferolateral margin of epiglottis and represent a junction between the supraglottic larynx and hypopharynx. The epiglottis attaches to thyroid cartilage by thyroepiglottic ligament and to hyoid bone by hyoepiglottic ligament. Note the aperture in the thyrohyoid membrane for passage of superior laryngeal vessels and the internal branch of the superior laryngeal nerve. (Bottom) Coronal graphic posterior view of larynx shows false and true vocal cords separated by laryngeal ventricle. Quadrangular membrane is fibrous membrane that extends from upper arytenoid and corniculate cartilages to lateral epiglottis. Conus elasticus is a fibroelastic membrane that extends from the vocal ligament of true vocal cord to cricoid. These membranes represent a relative barrier to tumor spread but are not seen on routine imaging.

Hypopharynx, Larynx, and Trachea Overview

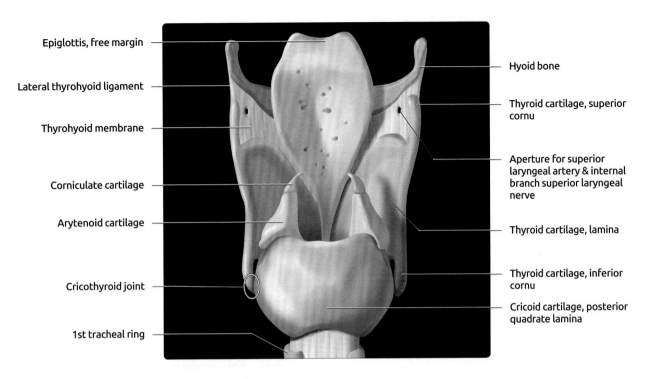

Epiglottis, free margin

Lateral thyrohyoid ligament

Thyrohyoid membrane

Corniculate cartilage

Arytenoid cartilage

Cricothyroid joint

1st tracheal ring

Hyoid bone

Thyroid cartilage, superior cornu

Aperture for superior laryngeal artery & internal branch superior laryngeal nerve

Thyroid cartilage, lamina

Thyroid cartilage, inferior cornu

Cricoid cartilage, posterior quadrate lamina

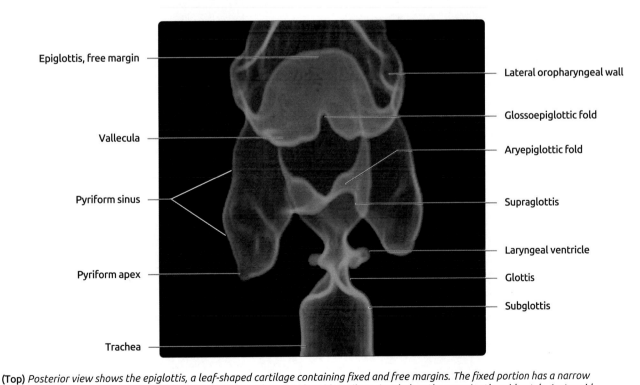

Epiglottis, free margin

Vallecula

Pyriform sinus

Pyriform apex

Trachea

Lateral oropharyngeal wall

Glossoepiglottic fold

Aryepiglottic fold

Supraglottis

Laryngeal ventricle

Glottis

Subglottis

(Top) *Posterior view shows the epiglottis, a leaf-shaped cartilage containing fixed and free margins. The fixed portion has a narrow stem that attaches by thyroepiglottic ligament to internal aspect thyroid cartilage, just below the superior thyroid notch. Arytenoid cartilages perch on and articulate with the superior aspect of posterior cricoid cartilage. Inferior thyroid cornu articulates with cricoid in synovial-lined cricothyroid joint. Cricoid cartilage is the only complete ring in endolarynx and provides structural integrity. It is comprised of the anterior arch and taller posterior quadrate lamina. Lower border of cricoid represents junction between larynx and trachea. Thyroid, cricoid, and most of arytenoids are hyaline cartilage and ossify with age. Epiglottis, corniculate, and vocal process of arytenoid are yellow fibrocartilage and do not tend to ossify.* (Bottom) *Frontal view of 3D surface-rendered CT shows normal mucosal surfaces of oropharynx, hypopharynx, larynx, and trachea when distended during phonation.*

(Left) *Axial graphic at the level of hyoid bone through the roof of hypopharynx shows anterior preepiglottic space filled with fat ⇨. Midline glossoepiglottic fold ➡, free margin of epiglottis ⇨, and lateral pharyngoepiglottic folds ⇨ delineate contours of valleculae.* (Right) *Axial CECT at the same level reveals a hypodense fat-filled preepiglottic space ⇨ and the anterior margin of the glossoepiglottic fold ➡, which separates valleculae. The free margin of the epiglottis ⇨ is visible.*

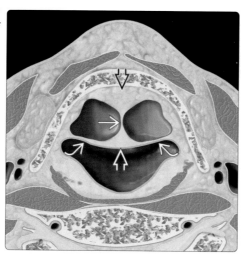 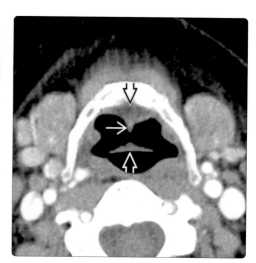

(Left) *Axial graphic at the midsupraglottic level shows the hyoepiglottic ligament ⇨ to the fixed portion of the epiglottis ⇨. AE folds ➡ are part of the supraglottic larynx but also form the anterior wall of the pyriform sinuses ⇨ and therefore form a junction between larynx and hypopharynx.* (Right) *Axial CECT at the same level shows the hyoepiglottic ligament ➡ and the fixed portion of the epiglottis ⇨ anteriorly. The posterior wall of the AE folds ⇨ forms the anterior wall of the pyriform sinuses ➡.*

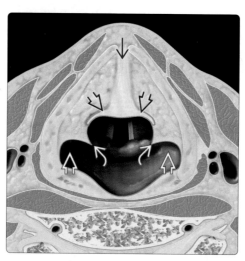 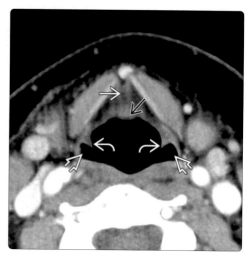

(Left) *Axial graphic depicts glottis or true vocal cord (TVC) level where vocalis ➡ and thyroarytenoid ⇨ muscles are evident deep to vocal ligaments ⇨. Pyriform sinus apex ⇨ reaches the level of TVC and cricoarytenoid joints ⇨.* (Right) *Axial CECT shows cricoarytenoid joints ⇨, indicating that the scan is at the level of the glottis. TVC ➡ are abducted as the study was performed during quiet respiration. Note the thin normal anterior commissure ➡ during this phase.*

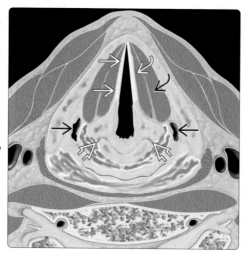 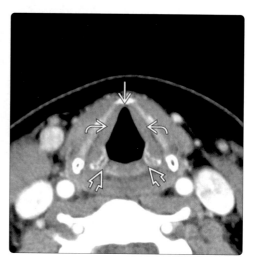

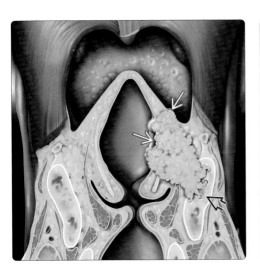

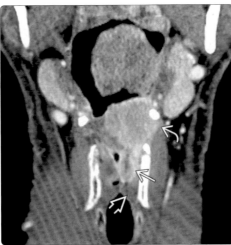

(Left) Coronal graphic depicts supraglottic squamous cell carcinoma (SCCa) ➡ centered in the left AE fold and false cord, laterally invading thyroid cartilage ➡. (Right) Coronal CECT reformatted image demonstrates a large enhancing mass arising in the left supraglottic larynx and extending inferiorly down paraglottic fat to false cord ➡. There is no evidence of extension to true cord ➡. Superiorly, the mass extends up to the valleculae, and laterally, it protrudes through the thyrohyoid membrane ➡.

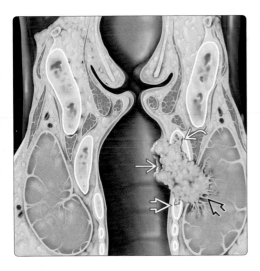

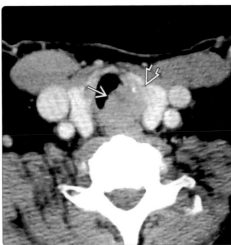

(Left) Coronal graphic depicts subglottic SCCa ➡ invading laterally through cricoid cartilage ➡ into thyroid gland ➡. First tracheal ring cartilage is also involved ➡. Nodal drainage for subglottic tumors is to levels IV and VI nodes initially. (Right) Axial CECT through the lower neck reveals the inferior aspect of subglottic SCCa ➡ as it invades laterally into the left thyroid gland ➡. Approximately 50% of subglottic tumors present at this T4 stage.

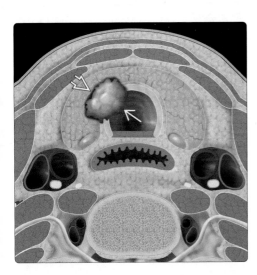

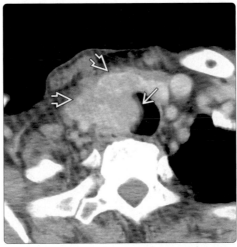

(Left) Axial graphic through the thyroid bed illustrates a tracheal wall mass protruding into tracheal lumen ➡ and laterally invading the thyroid gland ➡. Cervical tracheal wall lesions are rare, but diagnosis is often delayed due to nonlocalizing symptoms that may be misinterpreted as asthma. (Right) Axial CECT shows a tracheal wall carcinoma invading laterally and anteriorly into the thyroid gland ➡. Patient presented with stridor from tumor encroachment on tracheal lumen ➡.

Croup

TERMINOLOGY

- Benign, self-limited viral inflammation of upper airway
- Symmetric subglottic edema results in stridor & characteristic "barky" cough

IMAGING

- Radiographs used to exclude more serious causes of stridor (rather than diagnosing croup)
- Frontal view: Often more revealing than lateral view
  - Gradual, symmetric tapering of subglottic trachea from inferior to superior
    - Steeple, pencil tip, or inverted V configuration
    - Loss of normal "shoulders" (focal lateral convexities) of subglottic trachea secondary to edema
- Lateral view: Best for excluding other diagnoses
  - Relatively mild narrowing of AP dimension
  - Haziness with loss of subglottic tracheal wall definition
  - ± hypopharyngeal overdistention

TOP DIFFERENTIAL DIAGNOSES

- Foreign body
- Epiglottitis
- Exudative tracheitis
- Angioedema
- Infantile hemangioma
- Iatrogenic subglottic stenosis

CLINICAL ISSUES

- Acute clinical syndrome characterized by "barky" or seal-like ("croupy") cough, inspiratory stridor, hoarseness
  - Age range: 6 months to 3 years; peak: 1 year
- ± prodrome of low-grade fever, mild cough, rhinorrhea
- Affected child usually well otherwise
- Most cases successfully treated with corticosteroids ± nebulized epinephrine with < 4-hour observation
- Recurrent episodes or atypical age suggest alternate diagnosis

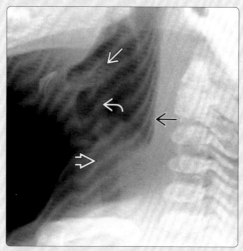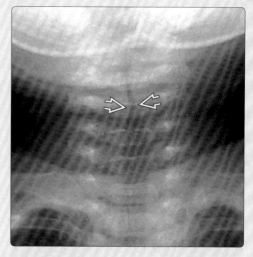

(Left) Lateral radiograph in a 9 month old with stridor shows haziness of the subglottic airway ➡. Overdistention (ballooning) of the hypopharynx is noted ➡. The epiglottis ➡ & aryepiglottic folds ➡ are normal. (Right) AP radiograph in the same patient shows symmetric narrowing of the subglottic trachea ➡, typical of croup. The loss of the normal abrupt subglottic/glottic shouldering with gradual tapering of the subglottic airway lumen from inferior to superior is referred to as the steeple sign.

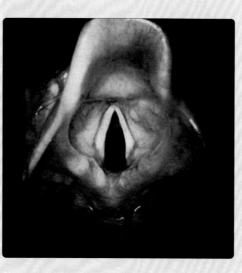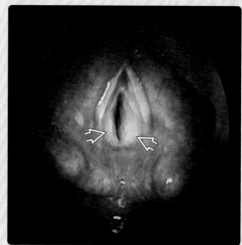

(Left) Endoscopic photograph shows a normal appearance of the subglottic airway. The subglottis is widely patent such that the mucosa is actually hidden beneath the vocal cords. (Right) Endoscopic photograph in a child with viral croup shows edematous subglottic mucosa ➡, which is visualized through the vocal cords. There is marked narrowing of the subglottic airway lumen, predominantly in the transverse dimension.

TERMINOLOGY

Synonyms

- Acute laryngotracheitis

Definitions

- Croup: Self-limited viral inflammation of subglottic trachea causing stridor & characteristic cough
- Acute laryngotracheobronchitis: Croup plus lower airway involvement
- Spasmodic croup: Recurrent episodes, typically without viral prodrome or fever
- Atypical croup: Recurrent episodes or croup outside expected age range

IMAGING

General Features

- Best diagnostic clue
  - Symmetric subglottic airway narrowing with gradual tapering from inferior to superior on anteroposterior (AP)/frontal radiograph
  - Loss of normal focal "shoulders" of subglottis/glottis
- Morphology
  - Normal
    - Uniform caliber of cervical & thoracic trachea from subglottis to carina
    - Normal "shoulders" at subglottis/glottis: Symmetric, focal convex/angular lateral margins of airway
      - More horizontal than vertical
  - Croup shows gradual tapering of subglottic trachea from inferior to superior
    - Affected vertical length variable; most commonly upper 1/2-1/3
    - Edema effaces normal subglottic "shoulders"

Radiographic Findings

- Radiography
  - AP/Frontal view
    - Steeple, pencil tip, or inverted V configuration of subglottic trachea
      - Loss of normal "shoulders" (lateral convexities) of subglottic trachea secondary to subglottic edema
      - Narrowing extends inferior to pyriform sinuses
  - Lateral view
    - Mild narrowing of subglottic trachea in AP dimension
      - In contrast to moderate to marked narrowing of transverse dimension on frontal view
    - Haziness with poor definition of subglottic tracheal wall
    - ± hypopharyngeal overdistention
      - Hypopharynx may be collapsed with distension of lower cervical trachea on expiratory image
    - Normal epiglottis, aryepiglottic folds, retropharyngeal soft tissues
    - No foreign body

Imaging Recommendations

- Best imaging tool
  - Diagnosis of croup primarily clinical, not imaging-based
    - Radiographs primarily used to exclude more serious causes of stridor
  - Frontal radiograph most useful view to confirm croup
  - Lateral radiograph helps exclude other diagnoses
- Protocol advice
  - Ensure that neck is extended with adequate inspiration on lateral view
    - Decreases crowding of airway structures that may simulate disease in young child
  - Avoid image acquisition while child swallows

DIFFERENTIAL DIAGNOSIS

Foreign Body

- Minority of foreign bodies radiopaque
  - May appear as soft tissue density but with straight, irregular, or pointed margins
- Can lodge virtually anywhere in airway from nasal/oral cavities to bronchi
  - Right main bronchus most common lower airway site
    - Causes asymmetric lung aeration on chest radiographs
  - Tracheal foreign bodies uncommon
- Symptoms depend on location of object
- Esophageal foreign bodies may also cause edema of adjacent trachea, especially in subacute/chronic setting

Epiglottitis

- Typically occurs in older children
  - Historical mean age (pre-Hib vaccine) = 3 years
  - Now teenagers more common
- Severe, life-threatening condition
- Marked enlargement of epiglottis & aryepiglottic folds
- May cause symmetric subglottic narrowing on frontal view

Exudative Tracheitis

- Toxic-appearing child, typically 6-10 years old
- Intraluminal filling defects (pseudomembranes)
- Plaque-like irregularity &/or poor definition of tracheal wall
- Asymmetric subglottic narrowing

Thermal Injury

- History of smoke inhalation, burns

Angioedema

- Rapid swelling of facial soft tissues & upper airway
  - ± itching, pain, hives
- May be due to allergic reaction or hereditary angioedema

Infantile Hemangioma

- Asymmetric airway narrowing with focal convex mass bulging from tracheal wall into lumen
  - Often not visible radiographically
- Associated with cutaneous infantile hemangiomas of face/neck in "beard" distribution
- Develops in 1st few weeks of life & grows rapidly over 6-12 months before beginning slow spontaneous regression

Iatrogenic Subglottic Stenosis

- History of prolonged intubation
- Predisposes to recurrent croup-like episodes

PATHOLOGY

General Features

- Etiology
  - Benign, self-limited condition secondary to viral illness
  - Infectious agents
    - Most cases: **Parainfluenza viruses** types 1-3
    - Less frequently: Rhinovirus, enterovirus, respiratory syncytial virus, influenza, measles; bacterial forms uncommon (consider *Corynebacterium diphtheria* & *Mycoplasma pneumoniae*)
  - Leads to inflammation & edema of subglottic airway
    - Redundant mucosa predisposes to edema & narrowing
      □ Loose mucosal attachment of conus elasticus
    - Swelling of vocal cords leads to hoarseness
    - Characteristic (but not specific) "barking/barky" cough results from inflammation of larynx & trachea
    - Inspiratory stridor due to proportionately small subglottic trachea in young children
      □ Same viral infections & edema do not compromise adult-sized airway
- Associated abnormalities
  - With atypical or spasmodic croup
    - 20-64% incidence of large airway lesions: Subglottic hemangioma, stenosis, laryngeal cleft, tracheomalacia, laryngomalacia, papillomatosis, laryngeal web, or vocal cord paralysis
    - Additional common disorders in this group: Gastroesophageal reflux, asthma, sleep-disordered breathing, allergies, chronic cough, prematurity

Staging, Grading, & Classification

- Clinical staging
  - Mild: Stridor at rest or when agitated
  - Moderate: Stridor plus mild tachypnea, mild retractions
  - Severe: Stridor plus respiratory distress, severe retractions, ± altered mental status

CLINICAL ISSUES

Presentation

- Most common signs/symptoms
  - Acute clinical syndrome characterized by "barking" or seal-like ("croupy") cough, inspiratory stridor, hoarseness, respiratory distress
- Other signs/symptoms
  - ± prodrome of low-grade fever, mild cough, rhinorrhea
  - Affected child usually well otherwise & able to manage secretions
  - More severe cases: Intercostal retractions, tachypnea, pallor, cyanosis, tachycardia, altered mental status
  - Symptoms worse at night or with agitation
  - May occur with other symptoms of lower respiratory tract infection (wheezing, cough, etc.)

Demographics

- Age
  - Range: 6 months to 3 years; peak: 1 year
  - If > 3 years, consider other acute causes of stridor
    - Mean of atypical croup: 2.7-4.8 years
  - If < 6 months, consider predisposing abnormality

- Gender
  - M:F = 3:2
- Epidemiology
  - Most common cause of acute upper airway obstruction in young children
    - Affects 5% of children by age 2 years
    - Affects 3% of children per year
  - Seasonal occurrence with viral disease
    - Most prevalent in fall-winter

Natural History & Prognosis

- Benign, self-limited disease
- 75% of mild cases resolve within 3 days
- 11% of mild & 49% of moderate cases of croup worsen
- 53% of severe cases require endotracheal intubation
- Overall: 8% hospitalized, 1% admitted to intensive care unit
- 5% return to emergency department < 1 week after initial evaluation
  - Consider other causes with recurrence, persistence

Treatment

- Most frequently managed supportively as outpatient
  - Mild croup: Systemic or nebulized corticosteroids, 2-hour observation
  - Moderate croup: Above + nebulized epinephrine, 4-hour observation
  - Severe croup: Above (can repeat epinephrine), admission to hospital
- Parents reassured, instructed to monitor for worsening course
- Endoscopy/bronchoscopy rarely needed if
  - Foreign body suspected
  - Superimposed exudative tracheitis suggested by clinical & imaging features
    - Requires membrane stripping, IV antibiotics, ± intubation
  - Assistance required for intubation in severe croup

DIAGNOSTIC CHECKLIST

Consider

- Alternate diagnosis with recurrent episodes or atypical age

SELECTED REFERENCES

1. Darras KE et al: Imaging acute airway obstruction in infants and children. Radiographics. 35(7):2064-79, 2015
2. Delany DR et al: Role of direct laryngoscopy and bronchoscopy in recurrent croup. Otolaryngol Head Neck Surg. 152(1):159-64, 2015
3. Duval M et al: Role of operative airway evaluation in children with recurrent croup: a retrospective cohort study. Clin Otolaryngol. 40(3):227-33, 2015
4. Hodnett BL et al: Objective endoscopic findings in patients with recurrent croup: 10-year retrospective analysis. Int J Pediatr Otorhinolaryngol. 79(12):2343-7, 2015
5. Johnson DW: Croup. BMJ Clin Evid. 2014
6. Petrocheilou A et al: Viral croup: diagnosis and a treatment algorithm. Pediatr Pulmonol. 49(5):421-9, 2014
7. Choi J et al: Common pediatric respiratory emergencies. Emerg Med Clin North Am. 30(2):529-63, x, 2012
8. Huang CC et al: Images in clinical medicine. Steeple sign of croup. N Engl J Med. 367(1):66, 2012
9. Virk JS et al: Analysing lateral soft tissue neck radiographs. Emerg Radiol. 19(3):255-60, 2012
10. Zoorob R et al: Croup: an overview. Am Fam Physician. 83(9):1067-73, 2011

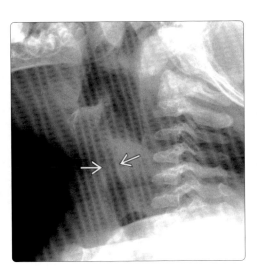

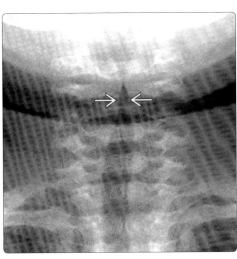

(Left) Lateral radiograph in a 7-month-old child with stridor shows symmetric narrowing of the subglottic airway ➡. (Right) AP radiograph of the same child shows the steepled appearance ➡ of symmetric subglottic airway narrowing that is typical of viral croup.

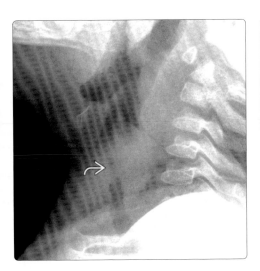

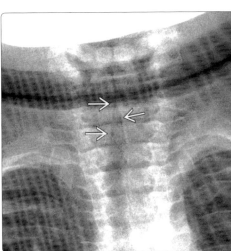

(Left) Lateral radiograph in an 8-month-old child with fever & a "barky" cough shows poor definition & haziness of the subglottic airway ➡, a common finding in viral croup. (Right) AP radiograph in the same patient shows severe narrowing of the subglottic trachea ➡, which gradually tapers from inferior to superior.

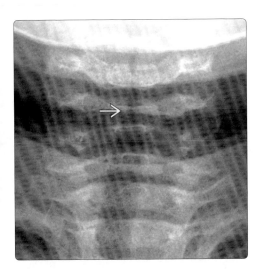

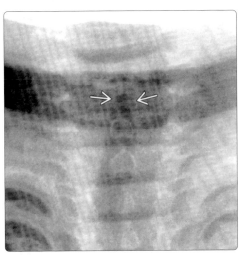

(Left) AP radiograph in a 16-month-old child with stridor shows symmetric subglottic airway narrowing ➡, typical of viral croup. (Right) AP radiograph in a normal child shows the typical shouldering ➡ of the subglottic airway, which is more focal & horizontal than the long, gradual, vertical "steepling" seen in croup.

KEY FACTS

TERMINOLOGY

- Infectious inflammation of epiglottis and supraglottic larynx → airway obstruction

IMAGING

- Lateral radiograph
  - Enlarged epiglottis (**thumb sign**)
  - Aryepiglottic folds thick and convex superiorly
  - Ballooning of hypopharynx
- Frontal radiograph
  - May see symmetric subglottic narrowing
- CECT usually not required
  - Rarely see phlegmon or abscess

TOP DIFFERENTIAL DIAGNOSES

- Croup
- Exudative tracheitis
- Retropharyngeal abscess

PATHOLOGY

- Most often *Haemophilus influenzae* type b (Hib)
- Decreased incidence after Hib vaccination

CLINICAL ISSUES

- **Acute life-threatening disease**, often requires emergent intubation
- **Toxic child** with difficulty breathing and swallowing
- Mean age 14.6 years after Hib vaccine introduced
- May also occur in adults

DIAGNOSTIC CHECKLIST

- Life-threatening emergency, so may not be imaged
- For radiograph: Child should be upright, comfortable
  - Do not agitate or place in supine position
  - Have physician escort with equipment to secure airway if necessary

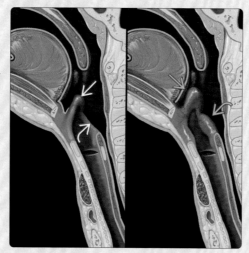
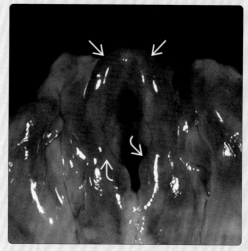

(Left) Lateral graphic shows normal supraglottic larynx on left with sharply defined epiglottis ➡ and straight or slightly concave aryepiglottic (AE) folds ➡. Graphic on right shows epiglottitis with thick, swollen epiglottis ➡ and convex, inflamed AE folds ➡. (Right) Gross pathology specimen shows markedly swollen, reddened epiglottis ➡ and similarly inflamed AE folds ➡, narrowing supraglottic lumen.

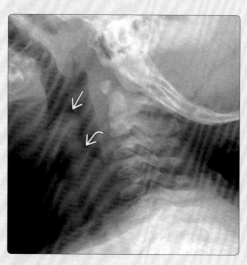
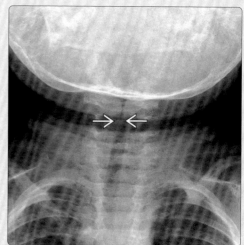

(Left) Lateral radiograph in a 6-month-old infant with epiglottitis shows diffuse swelling of epiglottis ➡, resulting in thumb sign. AE folds ➡ are thick, with a convex contour indicating supraglottic inflammation. (Right) AP radiograph in different child with epiglottitis demonstrates mildly steepled appearance of subglottic trachea ➡, which on AP radiograph alone is indistinguishable from croup. With epiglottitis, this appearance is due to accompanying subglottic edema.

Supraglottitis

KEY FACTS

TERMINOLOGY

- Synonym: Adult epiglottitis
- Definition: Relatively uncommon, potentially life-threatening infection/inflammation of supraglottic larynx in adult with sore throat & dysphagia

IMAGING

- CECT: Thickened epiglottis, aryepiglottic folds, obliterated preepiglottic fat
  o + mucosal enhancement
  o Often involves tonsils and base of tongue
- CECT not for diagnosis but to evaluate complications or patients with difficult clinical exam
  o Contraindicated if airway compromise

TOP DIFFERENTIAL DIAGNOSES

- Supraglottic squamous cell carcinoma
- Radiated larynx
- Epiglottitis in child

- Laryngeal trauma
- Caustic or thermal laryngeal injury

PATHOLOGY

- Adult epiglottitis now more common than pediatric
- Etiology: Usually *Streptococcus* or *Staphylococcus* species

CLINICAL ISSUES

- Presentation: Sore throat and dysphagia
- Most resolve with IV antibiotics ± steroids
- Airway management: Observation, intubation, or tracheostomy (15%)
  o Less likely to require airway intervention than children with epiglottitis

DIAGNOSTIC CHECKLIST

- Inflammation affects entire supraglottic larynx ± posterior oropharynx & tongue base, **not** just epiglottis
- Comment if complicated by abscess (ring-enhancing fluid collection) or emphysematous changes (multiple air dots)

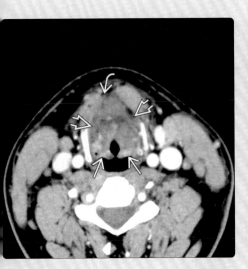

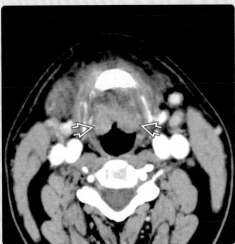

(Left) *Axial CECT in an adult patient with sore throat and dysphagia reveals the typical findings of supraglottitis. There are thickening and enhancement of the epiglottis* ➡ *with soft tissue obliteration of the preepiglottic* ➡ *and superior paraglottic fat* ➡. **(Right)** *Axial CECT in the same patient shows enlargement and enhancement of the lingual tonsils* ➡. *Supraglottitis can also involve the soft palate, base of tongue, valleculae, uvula, and prevertebral soft tissues.*

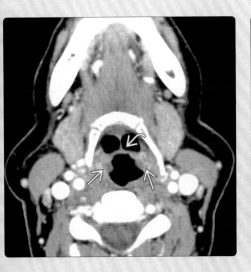

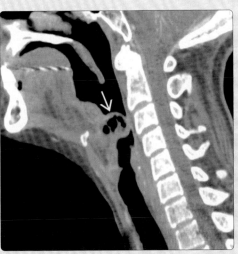

(Left) *Axial CECT shows a variant case of supraglottitis with thickening and enhancement of the aryepiglottic folds* ➡, *with relative sparing of the epiglottis* ➡. *Variable involvement of the epiglottis decreases the sensitivity of plain films in making the diagnosis.* **(Right)** *Sagittal CECT reformat demonstrates epiglottic enlargement with central air density* ➡, *characteristic of emphysematous supraglottitis. Emphysematous supraglottitis is more common in AIDS patients.*

KEY FACTS

TERMINOLOGY

- Mucosal injury, fracture, or dislocation of larynx
- External blunt trauma or penetrating injury
- Internal iatrogenic injury from intubation or endoscopy

IMAGING

- CT soft tissue windows best evaluate cartilage
- CECT if penetrating injury to evaluate vessels
- May see 1 or multiple cartilage abnormalities
- Hematoma can be clue to fracture or dislocation
- Airway may be deformed from fracture or narrowed from hematoma

TOP DIFFERENTIAL DIAGNOSES

- Vocal cord paralysis
- Radiated larynx
- Relapsing polychondritis

PATHOLOGY

- Blunt trauma, especially motor vehicle crashes
- Strangulation or hanging
- Penetrating injury, such as knife or gunshot wound
- Iatrogenic injury secondary to intubation

CLINICAL ISSUES

- Best outcome with early definitive treatment
- Most important initial aim is to stabilize airway

DIAGNOSTIC CHECKLIST

- Arytenoid dislocation can mimic paralyzed cord
- Injury may be subtle, requires high degree of suspicion
- Look for hematoma as clue to fracture/dislocation
- Look for deformity/narrowing of airway
- Always check larynx on trauma C-spine CT
- Soft tissue algorithm/window best for poorly ossified cartilage

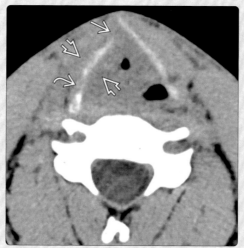
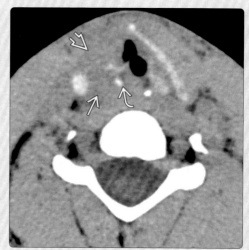

(Left) Axial NECT through the supraglottic larynx shows step-off at the superior thyroid notch ➡. There is a subtle fracture of the right thyroid lamina with internal rotation ➡ of fractured cartilage and diffuse edema ➡ of larynx and extralaryngeal tissues. (Right) Axial NECT more inferiorly in same patient, just above the cricoarytenoid joints, shows the anteromedial displacement of the right arytenoid cartilage ➡ and widening of right cricothyroid space ➡. Extensive laryngeal and paralaryngeal edema ➡ is evident.

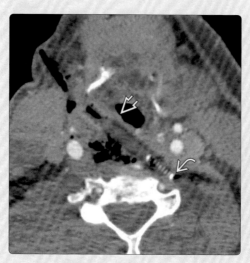
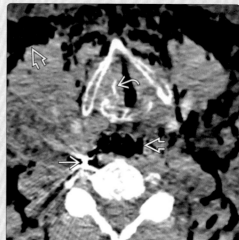

(Left) Axial CTA performed for a pen stabbing through the supraglottic larynx shows displaced edematous right aryepiglottic fold ➡. The pen tip ➡ terminates adjacent to the left vertebral artery, illustrating importance of CTA in penetrating injuries. (Right) Axial CTA from gunshot victim shows diffuse soft tissue emphysema ➡ and shrapnel ➡ adjacent to the cervical vertebra. There are comminuted fractures of cricoid cartilage and the right arytenoid with displaced fragment into the right true vocal cord ➡.

TERMINOLOGY

Definitions

- Mucosal injury, fracture, or dislocation of laryngeal cartilages

IMAGING

General Features

- Best diagnostic clue
  - Edema or hematoma of soft tissues and laryngeal cartilage deformity
- Location
  - Fractures occur to thyroid or cricoid cartilages; hyoid and arytenoid rare
  - Dislocation of cricoarytenoid or cricothyroid joint

Radiographic Findings

- Radiography
  - Deformity of larynx, narrowing of airway
  - Extraluminal gas with mucosal laceration

CT Findings

- NECT
  - May see 1 or multiple abnormalities
  - Extraluminal gas with mucosal laceration
  - Hematoma can be clue to fracture or dislocation
    - Vocal cord, paraglottic, subglottic swelling
  - Airway may be deformed from fracture or narrowed from hematoma
  - **Thyroid cartilage fracture**
    - Vertical: Midline or paramedian, alar splaying
    - Horizontal: Best depicted on coronal images
  - **Cricoid ring fracture**: Usually multiple, disrupt ring and may lead to airway collapse
  - **Hyoid fracture (rare)**: Separation of hyoid
  - **Cricothyroid joint dislocation**: Widened cricothyroid gap
  - **Arytenoid cartilage dislocation**: Typically anterior
  - **Epiglottic injury**: Soft tissue swelling, avulsion at petiole, epiglottic tear
  - **Laryngotracheal separation**: Horizontal tracheal tear, often acutely fatal
    - Associated with bilateral recurrent laryngeal nerve injury
- CECT
  - Important with penetrating neck injury to evaluate vessels

Imaging Recommendations

- Best imaging tool
  - CT demonstrates soft tissue and cartilage injury best
- Protocol advice
  - Thin axial helical CT slices with multiplanar reformats
  - Soft tissue algorithm/window best for poorly ossified cartilage
  - Penetrating injuries require CECT/CTA to evaluate vessels

DIFFERENTIAL DIAGNOSIS

Vocal Cord Paralysis

- Arytenoid displaced anteromedially
- Enlarged ipsilateral pyriform sinus and ventricle
- Atrophy of ipsilateral cricoarytenoid muscle
- May find causative lesion along course of recurrent laryngeal nerve

Radiated Larynx

- Sclerosis, fragmentation of cartilage
- Evidence of radiation to adjacent tissues

Relapsing Polychondritis

- Autoimmune cartilage destruction associated with collagen vascular diseases (especially SLE)
- Affects ear, nose, articular cartilage, larynx, tracheobronchial tree
- Laryngeal edema, sclerosis, enlargement or demineralization of cartilage

PATHOLOGY

General Features

- Etiology
  - Number of different mechanisms of laryngeal injury
    - Blunt neck trauma or external penetrating injury
    - Iatrogenic laryngeal injury
  - Blunt trauma, especially motor vehicle crashes
    - Larynx compressed against cervical spine, splitting thyroid cartilage and crushing cricoid
    - Soft tissue injuries due to shearing forces
  - Strangulation or hanging
    - Laryngeal fractures without mucosal lacerations
  - Clothesline injury when victim's neck collides with horizontal barrier
    - Laryngeal fractures, laryngotracheal separation
    - High incidence of recurrent laryngeal nerve injury
    - Especially epiglottic injury
  - Penetrating injury, such as knife or gunshot wound
  - Iatrogenic injury from intubation or endoscopy
    - Mucosal injury with abrasions or lacerations
    - Arytenoid cartilage dislocation
    - Left side more often than right
- Associated abnormalities
  - **Often associated with intracranial injuries, cervical spine or esophageal injuries**
  - Laryngeal injury may not be apparent initially

Staging, Grading, & Classification

- Schaefer system of classifying laryngeal injury
  - Determined by CT and clinical examination
- Directs management and predicts morbidity
  - Group I: Minor hematoma/laceration, no fracture
    - Minor airway symptoms, requires observation
  - Group II: Edema/hematoma, minor mucosal injury, no cartilage exposure, nondisplaced fracture
    - Airway compromise ± tracheostomy
  - Group III: Massive edema, mucosal tear, exposed cartilage, cord immobility
    - Above treatment ± exploration

- o Group IV: Group III + > 2 fracture lines, massive mucosal trauma
  - – Above treatment ± stent
- o Group V: Laryngotracheal separation
  - – Often fatal, requires surgical repair

- o From level of false cord to 1st tracheal ring
- o Helps prevent luminal stenosis, preserve normal shape of endolarynx
- Primary repair or supraglottic hemilaryngectomy for epiglottic injuries

CLINICAL ISSUES

Presentation

- Most common signs/symptoms
  - o Respiratory distress, stridor, cough, hemoptysis, anterior neck pain
  - o Hoarseness, dysphonia, vocal cord paralysis
- Other signs/symptoms
  - o Subcutaneous emphysema, ecchymosis
  - o Loss of tracheal protuberance (Adam's apple), tracheal deviation
- Clinical profile
  - o Patient with anterior neck trauma, stridor, change in voice, neck ecchymosis, subcutaneous emphysema

Demographics

- Age
  - o Laryngeal cartilage injury less common in children
    - – Higher riding larynx sheltered by mandible
- Epidemiology
  - o 1-6 patients per 15,000-42,500 trauma victims
  - o Incidence decreasing in seat belt era
  - o Up to 6% intubated patients

Natural History & Prognosis

- Early definitive surgical treatment associated with better outcome
- Adverse outcomes from laryngeal trauma
  - o Granulation tissue with airway compromise (early), laryngotracheal stenosis (late)
  - o Vocal cord immobility with loss or alteration of voice
    - – Vocal cord paralysis or arytenoid dislocation
  - o Disordered swallowing ± aspiration

Treatment

- Most important initial aim is to stabilize airway: Grade II or higher injury usually requires tracheostomy
- Endoscopy &/or surgical exploration to evaluate
  - o Mucosal tears and cartilage exposure
    - – Mucosal tears are risk for infection
    - – Cartilage exposure predisposes to chondronecrosis, fibrosis, and granulation tissue formation
  - o Cricoid fractures, multiple or displaced fractures, displaced cricoarytenoid joint
  - o Vocal cord immobility or laceration, hemorrhage
- Nonoperative management
  - o Patients with only minor mucosal lacerations sparing free margin of vocal cord and anterior commissure
  - o Hyoid fracture managed conservatively
  - o Single nondisplaced thyroid cartilage fracture, no exposed cartilage
- Endoscopic reduction
  - o Arytenoid cartilage dislocation requires early reduction
- Open reduction and internal fixation
  - o Displaced, comminuted laryngeal fractures
- Airway stenting may be required for grade IV injury

DIAGNOSTIC CHECKLIST

Consider

- Arytenoid dislocation can mimic paralyzed vocal cord clinically and on imaging
- **CECT or CTA** should be performed in penetrating injuries to evaluate vessels

Image Interpretation Pearls

- Cartilage best evaluated with soft tissue windows
- Look for hematoma as clue to fracture/dislocation
- Subtle deformity of airway may mean cricoid fracture
- Incomplete cartilage ossification can mimic fracture

Reporting Tips

- Trauma history is key for differential diagnosis
- Injury may be subtle, requires **high degree of suspicion**
  - o Evaluate each cartilage and joint in turn
- Always check larynx on trauma C-spine CT
  - o Look for deformity/narrowing of airway

SELECTED REFERENCES

1. Jain U et al: Management of the traumatized airway. Anesthesiology. 124(1):199-206, 2016
2. Schweiger C et al: Post-intubation acute laryngeal injuries in infants and children: a new classification system. Int J Pediatr Otorhinolaryngol. 86:177-82, 2016
3. Becker M et al: MDCT in the assessment of laryngeal trauma: value of 2D multiplanar and 3D reconstructions. AJR Am J Roentgenol. 201(4):W639-47, 2013
4. Robinson S et al: Multidetector row computed tomography of the injured larynx after trauma. Semin Ultrasound CT MR. 30(3):188-94, 2009
5. Bell RB et al: Management of laryngeal trauma. Oral Maxillofac Surg Clin North Am. 20(3):415-30, 2008
6. Juutilainen M et al: Laryngeal fractures: clinical findings and considerations on suboptimal outcome. Acta Otolaryngol. 128(2):213-8, 2008
7. McCrystal DJ et al: Cricotracheal separation: a review and a case with bilateral recovery of recurrent laryngeal nerve function. J Laryngol Otol. 120(6):497-501, 2006
8. Scaglione M et al: Acute tracheobronchial injuries: impact of imaging on diagnosis and management implications. Eur J Radiol. 59(3):336-43, 2006
9. Verschueren DS et al: Management of laryngo-tracheal injuries associated with craniomaxillofacial trauma. J Oral Maxillofac Surg. 64(2):203-14, 2006
10. Bhojani RA et al: Contemporary assessment of laryngotracheal trauma. J Thorac Cardiovasc Surg. 130(2):426-32, 2005
11. Hwang SY et al: Management dilemmas in laryngeal trauma. J Laryngol Otol. 118(5):325-8, 2004
12. Kuttenberger JJ et al: Diagnosis and initial management of laryngotracheal injuries associated with facial fractures. J Craniomaxillofac Surg. 32(2):80-4, 2004
13. de Mello-Filho FV et al: The management of laryngeal fractures using internal fixation. Laryngoscope. 110(12):2143-6, 2000
14. Brosch S et al: Clinical course of acute laryngeal trauma and associated effects on phonation. J Laryngol Otol. 113(1):58-61, 1999
15. LeBlang SD et al: Helical CT of cervical spine and soft tissue injuries of the neck. Radiol Clin North Am. 37(3):515-32, v-vi, 1999
16. Hoover CA et al: Vocal fold hemorrhage following laryngeal trauma. Ear Nose Throat J. 77(5):364-6, 1998
17. Duda JJ Jr et al: MR evaluation of epiglottic disruption. AJNR Am J Neuroradiol. 17(3):563-6, 1996
18. Meglin AJ et al: Three-dimensional computerized tomography in the evaluation of laryngeal injury. Laryngoscope. 101(2):202-7, 1991
19. Priest RE et al: Laryngotracheal injuries. Ann Otol Rhinol Laryngol. 76(4):786-92, 1967

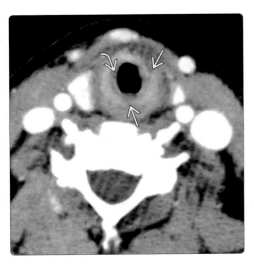

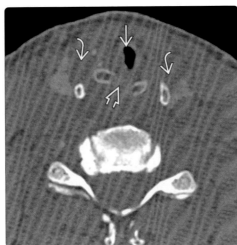

(Left) *Axial CECT depicts 2 fractures of the cricoid ring* ➡. *Soft tissue windows best evaluate poorly ossified cartilages. Circumferential density internal to the cricoid ring from mucosal hematoma and edema* ➡ *is a clue to subtle fractures.* (Right) *Axial NECT in a different patient demonstrates a more obvious displaced posterior midline cricoid fracture* ➡ *with marked airway deformity and narrowing* ➡. *Notice subtle but extensive perilaryngeal hematoma and edema displacing thyroid lobes* ➡.

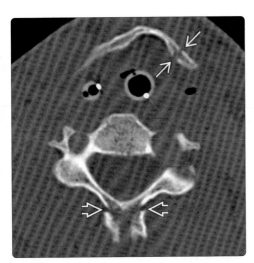

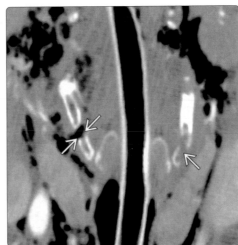

(Left) *Axial NECT shows a rare, minimally displaced hyoid fracture* ➡. *Note the spinous process fractures* ➡ *present in this intubated patient who also has extensive edema of neck soft tissues.* (Right) *Coronal CECT reformat in a different patient reveals bilateral horizontal thyroid alar fractures* ➡. *Extensive soft tissue emphysema may be due to pneumomediastinum, but air at the right alar fracture suggests a laryngeal mucosal injury. This requires surgical evaluation.*

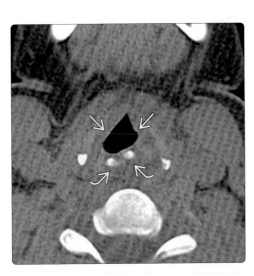

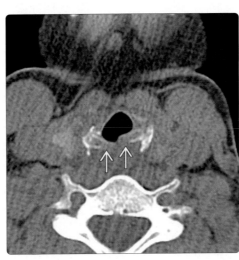

(Left) *Axial NECT of a patient previously in a motor vehicle crash, now presenting with complete aphonia, shows both arytenoid cartilages are dislocated and appear medially rotated* ➡. *The airway is deformed, and both vocal cords appear atrophic* ➡. (Right) *Axial NECT in the same patient reveals chronic fracture of posterior midline cricoid cartilage* ➡ *with splaying of fragments and deformity of airway contour. Mucosal irregularity suggests granulation tissue more commonly seen after cartilage exposure.*

TERMINOLOGY

- Hemangioma involving subglottic airway

IMAGING

- **Asymmetric** subglottic narrowing in young child
  - Classically subglottic, may be transglottic
- **Enhancing submucosal mass** on CT/MR
  - May be circumferential, bilateral, or unilateral
  - Usually asymmetric or affecting only 1 side, L > R

TOP DIFFERENTIAL DIAGNOSES

- Congenital subglottic-tracheal stenosis
  - **Symmetric** tracheal narrowing
- Iatrogenic subglottic-tracheal stenosis
  - Prior history of intubation or tracheostomy
- Croup
  - **Symmetric** subglottic tracheal narrowing
- Tracheomalacia
  - Abnormal **dynamic collapse** of intrathoracic trachea

- Exudative tracheitis
  - **Intraluminal filling defects**/inflammatory exudates

PATHOLOGY

- Benign **vascular neoplasm**
- **PHACES** syndrome
- 3 phases of growth and regression
  - Proliferative phase begins few weeks after birth
  - Involuting phase shows gradual regression
  - Involuted phase complete by late childhood
- **GLUT1 positive** in all phases

CLINICAL ISSUES

- **Inspiratory stridor** in infants < 6 months
- Usually symptomatic prior to 6 months of age
- Treatment
  - Conservative monitoring, propranolol, corticosteroids, laser therapy, surgical excision rarely required
  - Combination of therapies used in 75% of children

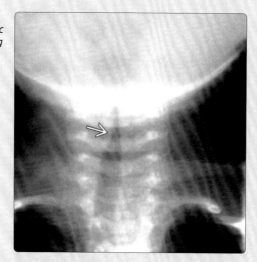
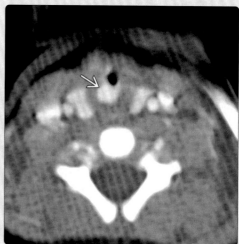

(Left) *Anteroposterior radiograph shows asymmetric subglottic tracheal narrowing* ➡ *in a 2-week-old infant presenting with stridor. Asymmetric narrowing is always concerning for hemangioma, as opposed to symmetric subglottic narrowing that is typical of croup.* (Right) *Axial CECT in the same patient shows a well-defined, enhancing hemangioma* ➡ *along the dorsolateral aspect of the subglottic airway.*

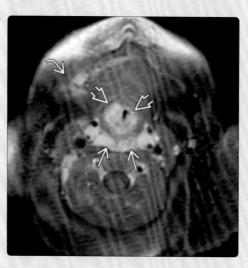
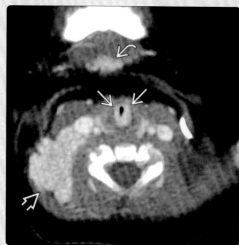

(Left) *Axial T1WI C+ FS MR in a child with PHACES syndrome demonstrates multiple enhancing hemangiomas in the retropharyngeal space* ➡, *surrounding the subglottic trachea* ➡ *and in the right submental space* ➡. (Right) *Axial CECT in an 11-week-old girl demonstrates a circumferential, well-defined subglottic hemangioma* ➡. *Notice also the posterior cervical space* ➡ *and submental infantile hemangiomas* ➡, *which should raise the question of PHACES syndrome.*

TERMINOLOGY

Definitions

- Hemangioma involving subglottic airway

IMAGING

General Features

- Best diagnostic clue
  o **Asymmetric** subglottic narrowing in young child
    – **Enhancing submucosal mass** on CT/MR
- Location
  o Classically **subglottic**; may be transglottic
  o Usually asymmetric or affecting only 1 side, L > R

Radiographic Findings

- Asymmetric subglottic tracheal narrowing on anteroposterior radiograph

CT Findings

- Usually solitary, enhancing subglottic mass

MR Findings

- Intermediate T1/hyperintense T2, + + enhancement

Imaging Recommendations

- Best imaging tool
  o 3D CT helps define mass and tracheal compression
    – Quicker than MR and may not need sedation
  o Adjust CT technique for pediatric patient
  o MR more sensitive, but sedation usually needed

DIFFERENTIAL DIAGNOSIS

Congenital Subglottic-Tracheal Stenosis

- **Symmetric** tracheal narrowing
  o Complete tracheal rings
    – Round tracheal configuration on axial images
- ± pulmonary sling or congenital heart disease

Iatrogenic Subglottic-Tracheal Stenosis

- Prior history of intubation or tracheostomy

Croup

- **Symmetric** subglottic tracheal narrowing
- Most common in children 8 months to 3 years

Tracheomalacia

- Abnormal **dynamic collapse** of intrathoracic trachea

Exudative Tracheitis

- **Intraluminal filling defects**/inflammatory exudates
- Children usually older than those with viral croup

PATHOLOGY

General Features

- Etiology
  o Benign **vascular neoplasm** of proliferating endothelial cells
  o **Not** vascular malformation
- Genetics
  o Majority sporadic
- Associated abnormalities

  o Cutaneous hemangiomas in 50%
  o **PHACES** syndrome: **P**osterior fossa brain malformations, **h**emangiomas of face, **a**rterial anomalies, **c**ardiac anomalies, **e**ye abnormalities, **s**ternal clefts or **s**upraumbilical raphe
    – 7% have subglottic hemangiomas

Staging, Grading, & Classification

- Mulliken and Glowacki classification of hemangiomas and vascular malformations
  o Reflects cellular kinetics and clinical behavior
- 3 phases of growth and regression
  o **Proliferative phase** begins few weeks after birth and continues for 1-2 years
  o **Involuting phase** shows gradual regression over next several years
  o **Involuted phase** usually complete by late childhood

Microscopic Features

- **GLUT1** immunohistochemical marker: **Positive** in all phases of infantile hemangioma

CLINICAL ISSUES

Presentation

- Most common signs/symptoms
  o **Inspiratory stridor** in infants < 6 months
- Other signs/symptoms
  o **Cutaneous hemangiomas** in **50%**
  o Hoarseness or abnormal cry

Demographics

- Age
  o Usually symptomatic prior to 6 months of age

Natural History & Prognosis

- Majority of lesions have progressive airway obstruction during proliferative phase
- Symptoms resolve after involution
- Benign condition but can have fatal outcome
- Diagnosis made at endoscopy

Treatment

- General principles
  o Combination of therapies used in 75% of children
- Conservative monitoring
- Propranolol: Considered 1st-line treatment in recent years
- Systemic corticosteroids
  o ± rebound growth when steroids tapered
- Intralesional corticosteroids
- CO2 laser therapy
- Laryngotracheoplasty: Direct excision of small masses, usually not required with current medical therapies

SELECTED REFERENCES

1. Vivas-Colmenares GV et al: Analysis of the therapeutic evolution in the management of airway infantile hemangioma. World J Clin Pediatr. 5(1):95-101, 2016
2. Wang CF et al: Treatment of infantile subglottic hemangioma with oral propranolol. Pediatr Int. 58(5):385-388, 2016
3. Mulliken JB et al: Hemangiomas and vascular malformations in infants and children: a classification based on endothelial characteristics. Plast Reconstr Surg. 69(3):412-22, 1982

TERMINOLOGY

- Laryngeal CSa: Cartilage-producing chondrocytic neoplasm with cellular atypia, bone destruction, or local invasion

IMAGING

- **Expansile mass within laryngeal cartilage** with intact mucosal surfaces, chondroid matrix
- Most arise in cricoid > thyroid cartilage
- CT: **Ring-like or "popcorn" calcifications** (chondroid matrix) in expansile intracartilage mass
  - Noncalcific component of mass hypodense to muscle
  - Cartilage/bone destruction or local invasion
- MR: **T2-hyperintense** mass, best seen with T2 FS, STIR
  - T1WI C+: Heterogeneous enhancement

TOP DIFFERENTIAL DIAGNOSES

- Chondroma
  - Cannot be reliably differentiated from CSa with imaging; particularly noncalcified lesions

- Other sarcomas: Osteosarcoma bone forming
  - Synovial cell sarcoma, fibrosarcoma, malignant fibrous histiocytoma: No calcified matrix
- Metastasis to laryngeal cartilage

PATHOLOGY

- Arise from hyaline cartilage: Cricoid (72%), thyroid (20%), and, very rarely, arytenoid cartilage
- CSa of elastic cartilage (epiglottis) exceedingly rare

CLINICAL ISSUES

- Dysphagia or palpable neck mass (with exophytic growth pattern), dysphonia, stridor
- Symptoms often present for long duration, suggesting indolent process
- Submucosal mass on endoscopy

DIAGNOSTIC CHECKLIST

- If expansile mass arises from laryngeal cartilage, look for arc or ring-like Ca++

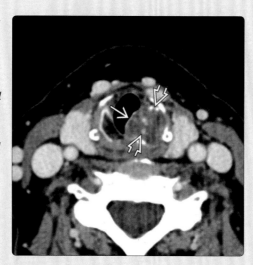
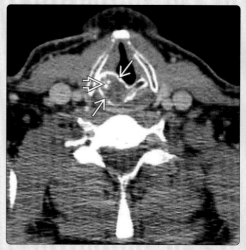

(Left) *Axial CECT in a 55-year-old woman with hoarseness shows a predominantly hypodense chondrosarcoma (CSa)* ➡ *arising from the left cricoid cartilage with internal calcifications* ⇨. **(Right)** *Axial CECT shows a well-defined, expansile mass involving the right cricoid cartilage* ➡. *Small foci of internal calcified chondroid matrix are present* ⇨ *in this grade I CSa.*

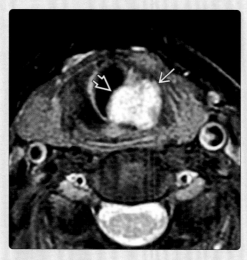
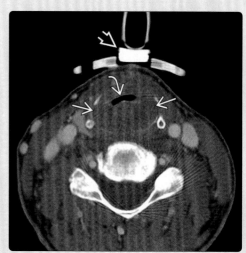

(Left) *Axial T2 FS MR shows this CSa as a homogeneously hyperintense mass* ➡ *impinging on the subglottic lumen* ⇨. **(Right)** *Axial bone CT shows a noncalcified, low-grade CSa* ➡. *In such a case, imaging cannot differentiate CSa and benign chondroma. Note the tracheostomy apparatus* ⇨, *necessitated by airway compromise* ➡ *caused by the tumor.*

Laryngeal Chondrosarcoma

TERMINOLOGY

Abbreviations

- Chondrosarcoma (CSa)

Definitions

- Laryngeal CSa: Cartilage-producing chondrocytic neoplasm with cellular atypia, bone destruction, or local invasion

IMAGING

General Features

- Best diagnostic clue
  - Expansile mass arising within laryngeal cartilage with intact mucosal surfaces, arc or ring-like calcification
- Location
  - In larynx, most arise in cricoid lamina (posterior or posterolateral) > thyroid cartilage (inferolateral)
    - Cricoid cartilage: 72%, thyroid cartilage: 20%
  - Rare in arytenoid cartilage or epiglottis
  - Typically subglottic in location
- Size
  - 1-6 cm
  - Often large at presentation if airway is spared
    - Tumor growing away from laryngeal lumen
- Morphology
  - Bulky, lobular mass centered in cartilage
  - Chondroid matrix typical

Radiographic Findings

- Radiography
  - Mass of variable density may be exophytic from laryngeal cartilage or grow inward thereby narrowing laryngeal air column
  - Stippled calcifications

CT Findings

- NECT
  - **Ring-like or "popcorn" calcifications** (chondroid matrix) in expansile mass arising from cricoid or thyroid cartilage with smooth mucosal covering
  - Not all tumors are calcified
    - Noncalcific (soft tissue) tumor component hypodense to muscle
  - Cartilage/bone destruction or local invasion may be seen in aggressive lesions
  - Presence of soft tissue mass or osteocartilaginous destruction suggests higher grade CSa
  - Often causes airway narrowing
- CECT
  - Modest if any enhancement

MR Findings

- T1WI
  - Intermediate signal intensity; isointense to muscle
- T2WI
  - **Hyperintense** mass; heterogeneity most common with more heavily calcified lesions
- STIR
  - Hyperintense mass
- T1WI C+
  - Heterogeneous enhancement

Imaging Recommendations

- Best imaging tool
  - CT best shows calcified chondroid matrix of tumor
- Protocol advice
  - High-resolution axial helical CECT with thin (1.5- to 2.5-mm) collimation
  - Multiplanar reformations help surgical planning

DIFFERENTIAL DIAGNOSIS

Chondroma

- Cannot be reliably differentiated from CSa with imaging
  - Particularly true in noncalcified lesions
- CT: Mass with chondroid matrix
- MR: T2-hyperintense mass

Other Sarcomas

- Includes osteo-, fibro-, synovial cell sarcomas & malignant fibrous histiocytoma
- Osteosarcoma associated with sunburst pattern of calcification
- Other sarcomas not usually calcified

Tracheopathia Osteochondroplastica

- Submucosal calcified cartilaginous ± osseous nodules
- Usually involves inferior 1/3 of trachea

Relapsing Polychondritis

- Immune-mediated inflammatory destruction of type II collagen in cartilage
  - Typically in many sites: Ear, nose, articular cartilage, larynx, & tracheobronchial tree
- Occurs in patients with vasculitides, collagen vascular diseases (including SLE), other autoimmune diseases
- May cause edema, sclerosis, enlargement or demineralization of cartilage in larynx

Nodular Chondrometaplasia, Larynx

- Posttraumatic condition
- Fibrocartilage (not hyaline cartilage)
- Can be challenging histologically

Metastasis to Laryngeal Cartilage

- Destructive mass centered in laryngeal cartilage

Squamous Cell Carcinoma, Larynx

- Mucosal mass evident endoscopically
- Not arising in, or expanding, cartilage

PATHOLOGY

General Features

- Etiology
  - May arise from pluripotential mesenchymal cells involved in hyaline cartilage ossification
  - Possible role of ischemic change in benign chondroma causing CSa
- Arises from hyaline cartilage: Cricoid (72%), thyroid (20%), and, very rarely, arytenoid cartilage
- CSa of elastic cartilage (epiglottis) exceedingly rare

Staging, Grading, & Classification

- Well differentiated (grade I)

- o Small, dark nuclei, scant-absent mitoses
- o Variable matrix, chondroid & myxoid components resembling hyaline cartilage
- o Calcification common
- Moderately differentiated (grade II)
  - o Larger nuclei with greater cellularity
  - o More prominent myxoid matrix, occasional mitoses (< 2 per 10 HPF)
- Poorly differentiated (grade III)
  - o Still greater cellularity, mitoses common (≥ 2 per 10 HPF)
  - o Prominent nucleoli
  - o Matrix may contain fusiform spindle cells
  - o Necrosis

Gross Pathologic & Surgical Features

- Lobular surface with gritty/crunchy consistency
- White to blue-gray, semitranslucent, with myxoid-mucinous matrix
- Submucosal mass with intact mucosa typical
- Rarely, mucosal erythema ± ulceration in advanced tumors

Microscopic Features

- Hypercellularity, enlarged hyperchromatic (acidophilic) nuclei, multinucleation
- Malignant areas may be localized within more benign-appearing lesion (chondroma)
  - o May be missed on limited sampling
- Even on complete microscopic review, it may be difficult to differentiate benign from malignant lesion

CLINICAL ISSUES

Presentation

- Most common signs/symptoms
  - o Progressive hoarseness & dyspnea
  - o Submucosal mass on endoscopy
  - o Other symptoms: Dysphagia or palpable neck mass, pain
    - − Symptoms often present for long duration, suggesting indolent process

Demographics

- Age
  - o Mean: 64 years
- Gender
  - o M:F = 3.6:1
- Epidemiology
  - o Laryngeal CSa accounts for ~ 0.5% of laryngeal malignancies
  - o Represents < 0.2% of all H&N malignancies

Natural History & Prognosis

- Most CSa are low grade with good prognosis
- No significant difference in outcome based on grade, location, or treatment method
  - o Outcome worse in patients with myxoid CSa
- May dedifferentiate, often to malignant fibrous histiocytoma or fibrosarcoma, with poor prognosis
- Metastases are extremely rare

Treatment

- Surgical resection is treatment of choice

- o Voice conservation surgery with complete lesion removal
- Surgical approach is same for benign and low-grade malignant lesions
- Partial resection associated with recurrences in ≤ 20% of cases
  - o Patients often do well with salvage laryngectomy
- Total laryngectomy may be required
  - o For extensive cricoid involvement
  - o For large or recurrent tumors
  - o When tumor-free margin cannot be obtained with partial laryngectomy
- Cricoid resection with thyroid-tracheal anastomosis over stent for large cricoid tumors

DIAGNOSTIC CHECKLIST

Consider

- Determine if mass arises from laryngeal cartilage
- Assess if involved laryngeal cartilage is expanded or eroded/destroyed
- History of prior laryngeal trauma may suggest alternative chondrometaplasia

Image Interpretation Pearls

- If **T2-hyperintense mass** seen on MR arises from laryngeal cartilage, do CT to look for chondroid matrix
- **Arc- or ring-like calcifications** are pathognomonic for laryngeal cartilaginous neoplasms

Reporting Tips

- Report laryngeal cartilage of origin
- If on benign end of spectrum, report inability to differentiate chondroma from CSa by imaging

SELECTED REFERENCES

1. Bathala S et al: Chondrosarcoma of larynx: review of literature and clinical experience. J Laryngol Otol. 122(10):1127-9, 2008
2. Becker M et al: Imaging of the larynx and hypopharynx. Eur J Radiol. 66(3):460-79, 2008
3. Leclerc JE: Chondrosarcoma of the larynx: case report with a 14-year follow-up. J Otolaryngol Head Neck Surg. 37(5):E143-7, 2008
4. Sauter A et al: Chondrosarcoma of the larynx and review of the literature. Anticancer Res. 27(4C):2925-9, 2007
5. Baatenburg de Jong RJ et al: Chondroma and chondrosarcoma of the larynx. Curr Opin Otolaryngol Head Neck Surg. 12(2):98-105, 2004
6. Rinaggio J et al: Dedifferentiated chondrosarcoma of the larynx. Oral Surg Oral Med Oral Pathol Oral Radiol Endod. 97(3):369-75, 2004
7. Cohen JT et al: Hemicricoidectomy as the primary diagnosis and treatment for cricoid chondrosarcomas. Laryngoscope. 113(10):1817-9, 2003
8. Jones DA et al: Cartilaginous tumours of the larynx. J Otolaryngol. 32(5):332-7, 2003
9. Orlandi A et al: Symptomatic laryngeal nodular chondrometaplasia: a clinicopathological study. J Clin Pathol. 56(12):976-7, 2003
10. Windfuhr JP: Pitfalls in the diagnosis and management of laryngeal chondrosarcoma. J Laryngol Otol. 117(8):651-5, 2003
11. Palacios E et al: Chondrosarcoma of the larynx. Ear Nose Throat J. 81(2):83, 2002
12. Thompson LD et al: Chondrosarcoma of the larynx: a clinicopathologic study of 111 cases with a review of the literature. Am J Surg Pathol. 26(7):836-51, 2002
13. Thome R et al: Long-term follow-up of cartilaginous tumors of the larynx. Otolaryngol Head Neck Surg. 124(6):634-40, 2001
14. Wang SJ et al: Chondroid tumors of the larynx: computed tomography findings. Am J Otolaryngol. 20(6):379-82, 1999
15. Wippold FJ 2nd et al: Chondrosarcoma of the larynx: CT features. AJNR Am J Neuroradiol. 14(2):453-9, 1993

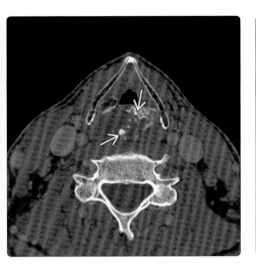
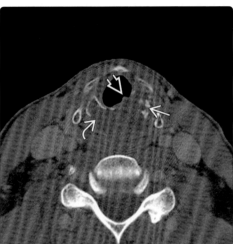

(Left) *Axial bone CT in a patient with CSa arising from the upper margin of the cricoid cartilage shows the internal chondroid calcifications* ➔ *characteristic of CSa.* (Right) *Subglottic axial bone CT reveals characteristic chondroid calcifications* ➔ *of the chondrosarcoma. The tumor is narrowing the subglottic airway* ➔. *Note the loss of the posterior margin of the cricoid cartilage* ➔.

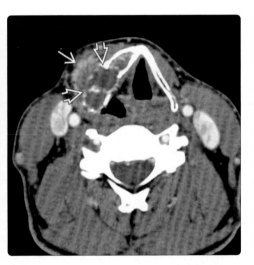
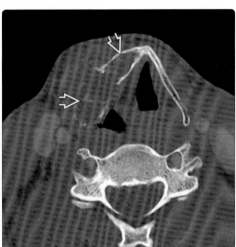

(Left) *Axial CECT in a patient with CSa of the thyroid cartilage demonstrates a lesion that clearly arises with and widens the right side of the thyroid cartilage. Notice that the tumor has extended laterally into the superficial soft tissues* ➔ *beyond the destroyed outer cortex of the cartilage* ➔. (Right) *Axial bone CT shows subtle internal chondroid-type calcifications* ➔ *typical of chondrosarcoma.*

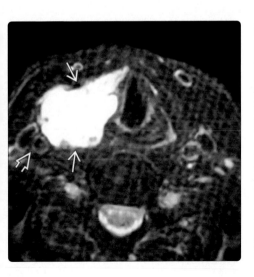
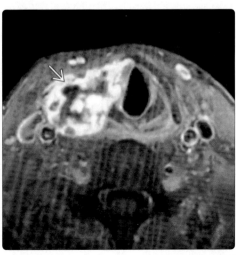

(Left) *Axial T2 FS MR shows a hyperintense thyroid cartilage mass* ➔ *growing away from the laryngeal lumen & displacing the carotid space laterally* ➔. *T2 hyperintensity would be atypical for carcinoma. Imaging suggests a chondroid lesion, first thought to be a CSa. Chondroma was found at resection.* (Right) *Axial T1 C+ FS MR reveals heterogeneous enhancement* ➔ *in this exophytic chondroma. This maging appearance could represent chordoma or CSa.*

KEY FACTS

TERMINOLOGY

- Spectrum of soft tissue and cartilage changes following radiation therapy (XRT) for H&N tumors
- Changes may be XRT **effects** or **complications**
  - XRT effects seen in all patients
  - Complications seen in minority

IMAGING

- Radiation effects
  - Acute-subacute: Submucosal edema, increased linear mucosal enhancement
  - Chronic: Fibrosis and atrophy
- Radiation complications
  - Persistent edema > 6 months
  - **Chondronecrosis**: Cartilage fragmentation/collapse, sclerosis, adjacent gas
- Treatment failure
  - Persistent mass, solid enhancement, deep ulcer

TOP DIFFERENTIAL DIAGNOSES

- Transglottic squamous cell carcinoma
- Supraglottitis
- Laryngeal trauma

CLINICAL ISSUES

- Patient symptoms variable, may be minimal
- Higher XRT dose increases severity of XRT effects and increases complication rates
- Baseline CT/MR should be done ~ 8 weeks post XRT

DIAGNOSTIC CHECKLIST

- Submucosal edema and prominent mucosal enhancement are expected findings post XRT
- Chondronecrosis and persistent edema represent XRT complications
- Persistent or enlarged mass on baseline posttreatment scan indicates treatment failure

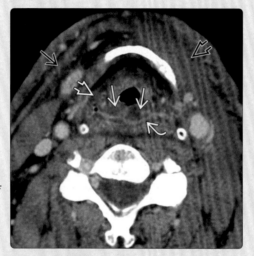
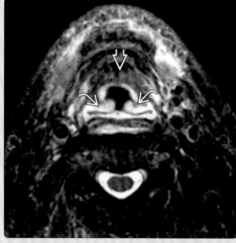

(Left) *Axial CECT in a patient radiated after left modified neck dissection shows marked edema of both aryepiglottic (AE) folds* ➡ *with thin, linear enhancement of mucosa* ➡. *Note hazy edema of paraglottic* ➡ *and preepiglottic fat and subcutaneous soft tissues* ➡ *with platysma thickening* ➡. (Right) *Axial T2WI FS MR 8 weeks following chemoXRT for tonsillar SCCa reveals extensive symmetric edema of all soft tissues. Hyperintense, edematous, thick AE folds* ➡ *efface pyriform sinuses. Note hazy preepiglottic fat* ➡.

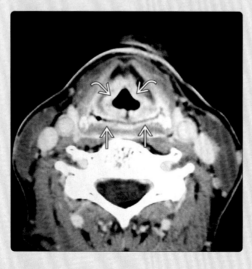
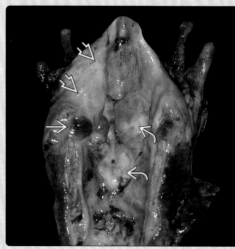

(Left) *Following XRT for laryngeal SCCa, there is particularly prominent mucositis, manifested as thick but regular enhancement of the mucosal surfaces of the larynx* ➡ *and hypopharynx* ➡. *Absence of nodularity or discrete mass is reassuring.* (Right) *Gross pathology following laryngectomy with larynx opened from midline posterior incision demonstrates diffuse laryngeal swelling* ➡, *particularly affecting aC fold* ➡. *Note focal hemorrhagic necrosis at left cricothyroid joint* ➡.

TERMINOLOGY

Definitions

- Spectrum of soft tissue and cartilage changes following radiation therapy (XRT) for H&N tumors
  - **Radiation effects**
    - Acute-subacute: Diffuse edema and inflammation
    - Chronic: Evolves to fibrosis and atrophy
  - **Radiation complications**
    - Persistent laryngeal edema ≥ 6 months
    - Laryngeal chondronecrosis

IMAGING

General Features

- Best diagnostic clue
  - Diffuse laryngeal edema without discrete mass plus radiation changes in neck
- Location
  - **All tissues** in radiation field show XRT changes
    - Supraglottic edema often most prominent
- Morphology
  - Acute-subacute effects: Diffuse edema and mucosal enhancement without discrete mass
  - Chronic effects: Generalized tissue and fat atrophy

CT Findings

- CECT
  - Typical XRT effects: **Acute-subacute**
    - Diffuse laryngeal and pharyngeal **low-density submucosal edema**
      - ▫ Thickened epiglottis, aryepiglottic and false folds
      - ▫ Effaced pyriform sinuses
      - ▫ Anterior and posterior commissure thickening
      - ▫ Haziness of paraglottic and preepiglottic fat
    - Mucosa generally shows **increased thin linear enhancement**
    - Mucosal ulceration not uncommon
      - ▫ Deep ulcer, solid enhancement suggests tumor
  - Typical XRT effects: **Chronic**
    - Fibrosis + atrophy with ↓ volume all neck tissues
    - Decreased low-density edema and enhancement
  - Radiation complications: **Chondronecrosis**
    - Laryngeal cartilage fragmentation/collapse, adjacent gas
    - Cartilage sclerosis concerning for necrosis if not present pre XRT
    - Osteoradionecrosis of hyoid has been reported with similar findings
- CT perfusion
  - Shorter mean transit time in tumor than XRT changes

MR Findings

- MR changes reflect same pathological stages as CT
- **Acute-subacute** XRT effects
  - Submucosal edema → marked T2 hyperintensity
  - Haziness of fat: ↓ T1 signal, ↑ T2 signal
  - Prominent diffuse, thin mucosal enhancement
  - DWI: Lower ADC values in tumor compared to XRT change
- **Chronic** XRT effects

- o T2 hyperintensity gradually resolves
- o Fat returns to more normal signal; decreased fat bulk
- o Mucosal enhancement diminishes
- Radiation complications: **Chondronecrosis**
  - o Increased T2 signal and enhancement of cartilage
  - o Focal gas may be subtle: Low signal on all sequences
  - o Fragmentation of cartilage often subtle on MR

Nuclear Medicine Findings

- PET/CT
  - o No FDG uptake in normal treated larynx
    - Negative predictive value: 91%
  - o Pitfall: False-positive from infection, recent biopsy

Imaging Recommendations

- Best imaging tool
  - o Any imaging can be complex in early phase
  - o CECT usually significantly easier for patient, as fewer swallowing problems from poorly handled secretions
  - o FDG PET may help clarify indeterminate findings
- Protocol advice
  - o **Baseline CT or MR** should be obtained ~ **8 weeks post XRT/chemoradiation**
    - Persistent or enlarging mass indicates treatment failure
    - If using CECT, allow delay after contrast injection to maximize enhancement of soft tissue mass

DIFFERENTIAL DIAGNOSIS

Transglottic Squamous Cell Carcinoma

- Solid, enhancing, irregular mass spanning cords
- May see infiltration of paraglottic fat and cartilage
- Frequently see adenopathy as well

Supraglottitis

- Submucosal edema of supraglottic tissues
- In adults, may form small abscesses
- Remaining neck tissues appear normal

Larynx Trauma

- May see cartilage fracture, joint subluxation
- Submucosal altered density from hematoma, edema
- More focal laryngeal changes

PATHOLOGY

General Features

- Etiology
  - o Higher dose increases XRT effects and complications
  - o Concurrent chemoradiation improves results but increases severity of acute XRT effects
    - Probably increases frequency of severe late effects
  - o Underlying vascular disease, continued smoking, and infection increase complication rates

Gross Pathologic & Surgical Features

- Thickening and induration of mucosa and submucosa

Microscopic Features

- Acute-subacute: Endothelial damage with increased permeability and interstitial edema, inflammatory infiltrate

- Chronic: Fibrosis, collagen deposition, blood vessel endarteritis, lymphatic fibrosis
  - New blood and lymphatic channels may form with edema resolution
  - Collagen and muscle disorganization, ↑ collagen and fibronectin
- Decreased perfusion to cartilage may cause ischemic injury, leading to chondritis, possibly chondronecrosis

CLINICAL ISSUES

Presentation

- Most common signs/symptoms
  - May be minimally symptomatic
  - Hoarseness, mucosal dryness, dysphagia
  - Pain and dyspnea with more severe changes
- Other signs/symptoms
  - Patients with chondronecrosis may have respiratory distress, pain, odynophagia, weight loss
- Clinical profile
  - Patient with history of XRT ± chemotherapy presenting with hoarseness and dysphagia

Natural History & Prognosis

- **Radiation effect**
  - XRT edema and inflammation improve over time
  - Marked symptomatology may necessitate gastrostomy feeding
- **Radiation complications**
  - **~ 10% have persistent late (> 6 months) edema**
    - Increasing incidence with increasing XRT dose
  - **≤ 5% have chondronecrosis**
    - Peaks in 1st year, may occur > 10 years post XRT
    - More common if large tumor, cartilage invasion, or perichondrial disruption
    - Also more common if ongoing smoking, vascular disease, or infection
    - May lead to laryngeal collapse and death

Treatment

- Supportive therapy: Humidifier, voice rest, smoking cessation, reflux treatment
- Severe dysphagia/odynophagia may require temporary gastrostomy
- Radiation chondronecrosis may necessitate laryngectomy or tracheostomy
  - Hyperbaric oxygen therapy may be offered for chondronecrosis

DIAGNOSTIC CHECKLIST

Consider

- Important to become thoroughly familiar with expected XRT effects
  - Enables detection of tumor or complication
- Any imaging can be complex in early phase

Image Interpretation Pearls

- Radiation treatment → tissue edema and inflammation → fibrosis, scarring, and atrophy
- Check cartilage for fragmentation, gas, or new sclerosis
- All tissues in radiation field show XRT changes

- Chondronecrosis shows cartilage fragmentation and gas
- Persistent or enlarged mass on baseline posttreatment scan indicates treatment failure
- Mucosal ulcers common; deep ulcer or solid enhancement suggests tumor

SELECTED REFERENCES

1. Yang L et al: Nasopharyngeal granulomatous mass after radiotherapy for nasopharyngeal carcinoma. Auris Nasus Larynx. 43(3):330-5, 2016
2. Saito N et al: Posttreatment CT and MR imaging in head and neck cancer: what the radiologist needs to know. Radiographics. 32(5):1261-82; discussion 1282-4, 2012
3. Berg EE et al: Pathologic effects of external-beam irradiation on human vocal folds. Ann Otol Rhinol Laryngol. 120(11):748-54, 2011
4. Bisdas S et al: Perfusion CT in squamous cell carcinoma of the upper aerodigestive tract: long-term predictive value of baseline perfusion CT measurements. AJNR Am J Neuroradiol. 31(3):576-81, 2010
5. Faggioni L et al: CT perfusion of head and neck tumors: how we do it. AJR Am J Roentgenol. 194(1):62-9, 2010
6. Yoo JS et al: Osteoradionecrosis of the hyoid bone: imaging findings. AJNR Am J Neuroradiol. 31(4):761-6, 2010
7. Debnam JM et al: Benign ulceration as a manifestation of soft tissue radiation necrosis: imaging findings. AJNR Am J Neuroradiol. 29(3):558-62, 2008
8. Abdel Razek AA et al: Role of diffusion-weighted echo-planar MR imaging in differentiation of residual or recurrent head and neck tumors and posttreatment changes. AJNR Am J Neuroradiol. 28(6):1146-52, 2007
9. Sanguineti G et al: Dosimetric predictors of laryngeal edema. Int J Radiat Oncol Biol Phys. 68(3):741-9, 2007
10. Mukherji SK et al: Imaging of the post-treatment larynx. Eur J Radiol. 44(2):108-19, 2002
11. Nömayr A et al: MRI appearance of radiation-induced changes of normal cervical tissues. Eur Radiol. 11(9):1807-17, 2001
12. Filntisis GA et al: Laryngeal radionecrosis and hyperbaric oxygen therapy: report of 18 cases and review of the literature. Ann Otol Rhinol Laryngol. 109(6):554-62, 2000
13. Baron-Hay S et al: Life threatening laryngeal toxicity following treatment with combined chemoradiotherapy for nasopharyngeal cancer: a case report with review of the literature. Ann Oncol. 10(9):1109-12, 1999
14. De Vuysere S et al: CT findings in laryngeal chondroradionecrosis. JBR-BTR. 82(1):16-8, 1999
15. Fitzgerald PJ et al: Delayed radionecrosis of the larynx. Am J Otolaryngol. 20(4):245-9, 1999
16. Hermans R et al: CT findings in chondroradionecrosis of the larynx. AJNR Am J Neuroradiol. 19(4):711-8, 1998
17. Schmalfuss IM et al: Arytenoid cartilage sclerosis: normal variations and clinical significance. AJNR Am J Neuroradiol. 19(4):719-22, 1998
18. Greven KM et al: Can positron emission tomography distinguish tumor recurrence from irradiation sequelae in patients treated for larynx cancer? Cancer J Sci Am. 3(6):353-7, 1997
19. Greven KM et al: Positron emission tomography of patients with head and neck carcinoma before and after high dose irradiation. Cancer. 74(4):1355-9, 1994
20. Mukherji SK et al: Radiologic appearance of the irradiated larynx. Part I. Expected changes. Radiology. 193(1):141-8, 1994
21. Mukherji SK et al: Radiologic appearance of the irradiated larynx. Part II. Primary site response. Radiology. 193(1):149-54, 1994
22. Tart RP et al: Value of laryngeal cartilage sclerosis as a predictor of outcome in patients with stage T3 glottic cancer treated with radiation therapy. Radiology. 192(2):567-70, 1994
23. Tartaglino LM et al: Imaging of radiation changes in the head and neck. Semin Roentgenol. 29(1):81-91, 1994
24. Briggs RJ et al: Laryngeal imaging by computerized tomography and magnetic resonance following radiation therapy: a need for caution. J Laryngol Otol. 107(6):565-8, 1993
25. Bronstein AD et al: Soft-tissue changes after head and neck radiation: CT findings. AJNR Am J Neuroradiol. 10(1):171-5, 1989

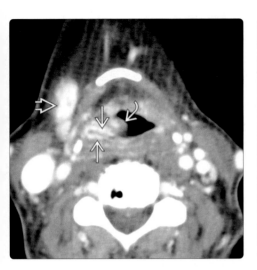
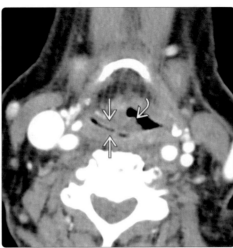

(Left) *Early posttreatment CECT in a patient with left supraglottic SCCa demonstrates marked enhancement of mucosa of right pyriform sinus* ⮕ *and thickening of Ea fold* ⮕. *Note pronounced enhancement of right submandibular gland* ⮕, *an expected XRT effect.* (Right) *Three years later, mucosal enhancement has normalized* ⮕, *though the AE fold remains thickened* ⮕. *Persistent supraglottic thickening is common following resolution of other XRT effects.*

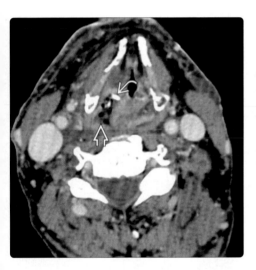
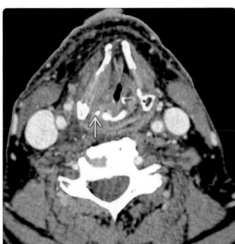

(Left) *Axial CECT in a patient 4 months following chemotherapy and XRT for hypopharyngeal SCCa shows air* ⮕ *and soft tissue posterior to sclerotic right arytenoid cartilage* ⮕. (Right) *Axial CECT in the same patient 3 months later reveals autoamputation of right arytenoid with only small osseous remnant* ⮕. *Hypopharyngeal swelling has markedly diminished, confirming nontumoral radionecrosis of arytenoid and hypopharynx. Chondronecrosis represents radiation complication.*

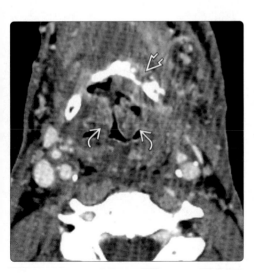
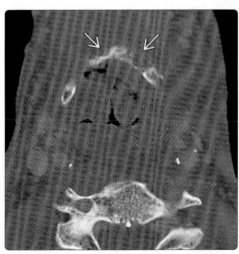

(Left) *Axial CECT in a patient radiated for supraglottic SCCa demonstrates marked swelling of both AE folds* ⮕, *resulting in considerable airway narrowing. There is a fragmented appearance to the hyoid bone* ⮕, *concerning for osteoradionecrosis or tumor erosion. There is no adjacent solid soft tissue mass.* (Right) *Axial bone CT in the same patient more clearly depicts fragmented appearance of the hyoid* ⮕ *subsequently proven to represent osteoradionecrosis, a more unusual form of laryngeal radionecrosis.*

KEY FACTS

TERMINOLOGY

- Internal laryngocele: Dilated, air- or fluid-filled laryngeal saccule; located in paraglottic region of supraglottis
- Mixed laryngocele: Extends laterally through thyrohyoid membrane to low submandibular space
- Pyolaryngocele: Pus-containing superinfected laryngocele
- Secondary laryngocele: Glottic or inferior supraglottic lesion obstructs laryngeal ventricle (15% all laryngoceles)

IMAGING

- Best diagnostic clue
  - Internal laryngocele: Thin-walled, air- or fluid-filled cystic lesion communicating with laryngeal ventricle
  - Mixed laryngocele: Internal + extralaryngeal extension through thyrohyoid membrane
  - Pyolaryngocele: Pus-filled laryngocele with thick, enhancing walls
  - Secondary laryngocele: Glottic or inferior supraglottic lesion causal

TOP DIFFERENTIAL DIAGNOSES

- Thyroglossal duct cyst
- 2nd branchial cleft cyst
- Vallecular cyst
- Lateral hypopharyngeal pouch
- Supraglottitis with abscess
- Laryngeal saccule (normal ventricular appendix)

CLINICAL ISSUES

- Caused by chronic increase in intraglottic pressure
- Seen in glass blowers, wind instrument players, and chronic coughers

DIAGNOSTIC CHECKLIST

- Comment in report if extralaryngeal extension is present
  - If so, mixed laryngocele requires open surgical approach
- Evaluate for infiltrating endolaryngeal mass
  - 5% are secondary laryngoceles
  - SCCa of glottis or low supraglottis is major culprit

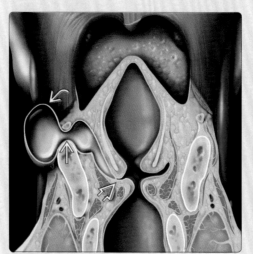
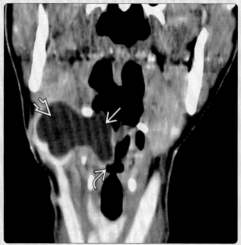

(Left) Coronal graphic shows a laryngocele with extralaryngeal extension. There is an isthmus ➡ where the lesion squeezes through the thyrohyoid membrane to the low submandibular space ➡. Note stenosis at the laryngeal ventricle ➡. (Right) Coronal CECT reformat shows a similar lesion. This is also known as a "mixed" laryngocele because it contains internal ➡ (intralaryngeal) and external ➡ (extralaryngeal) portions. It can be followed to the laryngeal ventricle ➡.

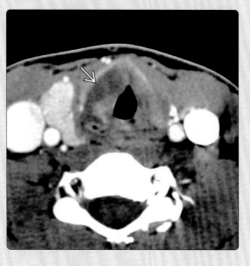
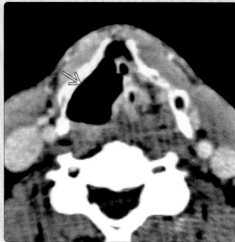

(Left) Axial CECT demonstrates the typical findings of a fluid-filled, internal (simple) laryngocele. There is a nonenhancing, fluid density lesion ➡ confined to the right paraglottic region of the supraglottis, lateral to the false vocal cord. (Right) Axial CECT in a professional trumpet player shows an air-filled sac confined to the right paraglottic region ➡. Findings are typical of an air-filled, internal (simple) laryngocele.

Laryngocele

TERMINOLOGY

Synonyms

- Internal laryngocele = simple laryngocele
- Mixed (combined, external) laryngocele: Laryngocele with extralaryngeal extension
- Saccular cyst: Currently, term best reserved for congenital laryngocele

Definitions

- **Laryngeal saccule**: Normal mucosal outpouching projecting superiorly from **laryngeal ventricle**
  - Contains numerous mucous glands
  - Some think saccule's function is lubrication of true cords
- **Internal laryngocele**: Dilated, air- or fluid-filled laryngeal saccule
  - Located in paraglottic space of supraglottis
  - Synonym: Simple laryngocele
- **Mixed laryngocele**: Extends from paraglottic space through thyrohyoid membrane to low submandibular space (SMS)
  - Synonym: Mixed laryngocele
  - Contains internal (intralaryngeal) & external (extralaryngeal) components
- **Pyolaryngocele**: Pus-containing superinfected laryngocele
- **Secondary laryngocele**: Glottic or inferior supraglottic SCCa obstructs laryngeal ventricle
  - 15% of all laryngoceles

IMAGING

General Features

- Best diagnostic clue
  - Thin-walled, fluid- or air-filled cystic lesion communicating with laryngeal ventricle, ± extralaryngeal extension through thyrohyoid membrane
- Location
  - Internal laryngocele: Supraglottic paraglottic space
  - Mixed laryngocele: Paraglottic space → through thyrohyoid membrane → SMS
- Size
  - Variable; may enlarge with Valsalva maneuver
- Morphology
  - Circumscribed, thin walled
  - Mixed lesions have isthmus when passing outside larynx through thyrohyoid membrane
  - If pyolaryngocele, thickened walls with adjacent inflammation
  - If secondary, infiltrating mass seen in low supraglottis or glottis

Radiographic Findings

- Radiography
  - Air pocket seen in upper cervical soft tissues
  - Soft tissue/fluid density projects against air column in supraglottic region

CT Findings

- CECT
  - Internal laryngocele
    - Circumscribed, thin-walled, fluid or air density within **paraglottic space** of supraglottis

- Absent to minimal peripheral enhancement
- Paraglottic lesion connects to laryngeal ventricle
  - Coronal plane shows this connection best
  - Mixed laryngocele
    - Paraglottic cyst passes through thyrohyoid membrane into SMS
      - **Isthmus** (waist) at thyrohyoid membrane
      - Coronal plane shows paraglottic-SMS connection
  - Pyolaryngocele: Thick enhancing walls
  - Secondary laryngocele: Enhancing, infiltrative glottic or low supraglottic lesion
    - Most commonly from SCCa
    - Amyloid infiltration rare cause

MR Findings

- T1WI
  - Low T1, thin walled, fluid intensity
- T2WI
  - High T2, thin walled, fluid intensity
- T1WI C+
  - Thin walled; absent to minimal linear peripheral enhancement
  - Thick enhancing walls if pyolaryngocele

Imaging Recommendations

- Best imaging tool
  - CECT of cervical soft tissues
- Protocol advice
  - Coronal reformatted images best demonstrate relationship to laryngeal ventricle, thyrohyoid membrane, & SMS

DIFFERENTIAL DIAGNOSIS

Thyroglossal Duct Cyst

- Midline cystic mass adjacent to mid-portion of hyoid bone
- Extralaryngeal, embedded in infrahyoid strap muscles
- May project into preepiglottic space

2nd Branchial Cleft Cyst

- Cystic mass posterior to submandibular gland at angle of mandible
- Displaces submandibular gland anteromedially, carotid space medially, & sternocleidomastoid muscle posterolaterally
- No connection to larynx

Laryngeal Saccule (Ventricular Appendix)

- Normal structure; a pseudolesion when air-filled
- Causes no submucosal deformity

Vallecular Cyst

- Cyst typically displaces epiglottis posteriorly
- Lies anterior to epiglottis, unilateral or bilateral
- Congenital lesion

Lateral Hypopharyngeal Pouch

- Air- or fluid-filled outpouching off lateral hypopharyngeal wall

Supraglottitis With Abscess

- Peripherally enhancing mass with central low density

- No connection to laryngeal ventricle or thyrohyoid membrane

PATHOLOGY

General Features

- Etiology
  - Commonly acquired; rarely congenital
  - Increased intraglottic pressure creates "ball-valve phenomenon" at communication of laryngeal ventricle with saccule
    - Saccule (appendix of laryngeal ventricle) expands
    - Causes: Glass blowing, playing a wind instrument, excessive coughing
  - Secondary laryngoceles from proximal saccular obstruction are less common (15%)
    - From **SCCa**, post-inflammatory stenosis, trauma, surgery, or amyloid

Gross Pathologic & Surgical Features

- Smooth-surfaced, sac-like specimen

Microscopic Features

- Lined by respiratory epithelium (ciliated, columnar) with fibrous wall

CLINICAL ISSUES

Presentation

- Most common signs/symptoms
  - Principal presenting symptom
    - Internal laryngocele: Larger lesions present with hoarseness or stridor
      □ When small, often incidental and asymptomatic
    - Mixed laryngocele: Anterior neck mass, low submandibular space just below angle of mandible
      □ May expand with modified Valsalva
- Other signs/symptoms
  - Sore throat, dysphagia, stridor, airway obstruction
- Clinical profile
  - Glass blowers, wind instrument players, chronic coughers

Demographics

- Age
  - Age at presentation: > 50 years old
- Gender
  - More common in male patients
- Ethnicity
  - More common in Caucasians
- Epidemiology
  - Bilateral laryngoceles: 30%
  - Internal laryngocele 2x as common as mixed laryngocele

Natural History & Prognosis

- Gradual enlargement over time
- With continued growth, laryngocele penetrates thyrohyoid membrane to enter neck in lower submandibular space
- Excellent prognosis after removal

Treatment

- 1st endoscopically exclude an underlying lesion of true or false cords obstructing laryngeal ventricle

- Isolated internal laryngocele: Microlaryngoscopic CO2 laser resection
- Mixed laryngocele: External transthyrohyoid membrane approach

DIAGNOSTIC CHECKLIST

Consider

- Does lesion change size with Valsalva?
- Is patient a glass blower, wind instrument player, or chronic cougher?

Image Interpretation Pearls

- Best diagnostic clue: Fluid- or air-filled, thin-walled lesion communicating with laryngeal ventricle
- Do not forget to look for occult SCCa in low supraglottis or glottic larynx
- Coronal plane best to show relationships to laryngeal ventricle & thyrohyoid membrane

Reporting Tips

- Extension through thyrohyoid membrane into SMS?
  - Yes: Mixed laryngocele
  - No: Internal laryngocele
- Thickening/prominent enhancement of laryngocele wall?
  - Yes: Pyolaryngocele
- Mass in low supraglottis or glottis?
  - Yes: Secondary laryngocele (accounts for ~ 15%)
  - Remember, endoscopy necessary to fully exclude obstructing mass

SELECTED REFERENCES

1. Zelenik K et al: Treatment of Laryngoceles: what is the progress over the last two decades? Biomed Res Int. 2014:819453, 2014
2. Dursun G et al: Current diagnosis and treatment of laryngocele in adults. Otolaryngol Head Neck Surg. 136(2):211-5, 2007
3. Akbas Y et al: Asymptomatic bilateral mixed-type laryngocele and laryngeal carcinoma. Eur Arch Otorhinolaryngol. 261(6):307-9, 2004
4. Ling FT et al: Is there a role for conservative management for symptomatic laryngopyocele? Case report and literature review. J Otolaryngol. 33(4):264-8, 2004
5. Ettema SL et al: Laryngocele resection by combined external and endoscopic laser approach. Ann Otol Rhinol Laryngol. 112(4):361-4, 2003
6. Harney M et al: Laryngocele and squamous cell carcinoma of the larynx. J Laryngol Otol. 115(7):590-2, 2001
7. Thabet MH et al: Lateral saccular cysts of the larynx. Aetiology, diagnosis and management. J Laryngol Otol. 115(4):293-7, 2001
8. Cassano L et al: Laryngopyocele: three new clinical cases and review of the literature. Eur Arch Otorhinolaryngol. 257(9):507-11, 2000
9. Nazaroglu H et al: Laryngopyocele: signs on computed tomography. Eur J Radiol. 33(1):63-5, 2000
10. Aydin O et al: Laryngeal amyloidosis with laryngocele. J Laryngol Otol. 113(4):361-3, 1999
11. Alvi A et al: Computed tomographic and magnetic resonance imaging characteristics of laryngocele and its variants. Am J Otolaryngol. 19(4):251-6, 1998
12. Celin SE et al: The association of laryngoceles with squamous cell carcinoma of the larynx. Laryngoscope. 101(5):529-36, 1991
13. Glazer HS et al: Computed tomography of laryngoceles. AJR Am J Roentgenol. 140(3):549-52, 1983

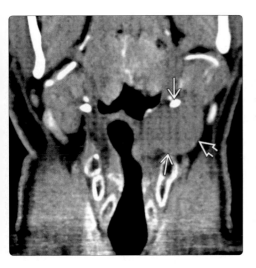
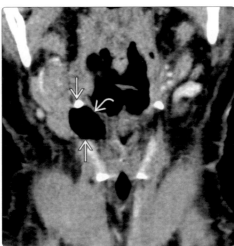

(Left) *Coronal CECT reformat in a patient with an anterior neck mass that enlarged with Valsalva reveals a left-sided, fluid-filled laryngocele with extralaryngeal extension (mixed). The lesion passes through the thyrohyoid membrane ➡ to the low submandibular space ➡.* (Right) *Coronal CECT reformat in another patient shows an air-filled sac ➡ traversing the thyrohyoid membrane ➡. An open surgical approach is required to treat this type of mixed laryngocele.*

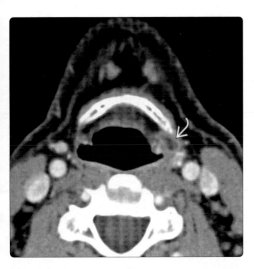
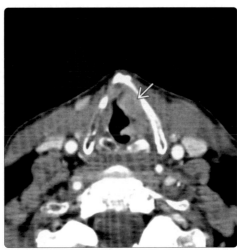

(Left) *Axial CECT shows a fluid density lesion in the left paraglottic region of the supraglottis ➡. On this image alone, findings suggest an internal (simple) laryngocele.* (Right) *Axial CECT of the same patient at the level of the true cords shows an infiltrative left glottic mass ➡, which obstructs the laryngeal ventricle and causes the secondary laryngocele seen on the previous image. About 15% of all laryngoceles are secondary.*

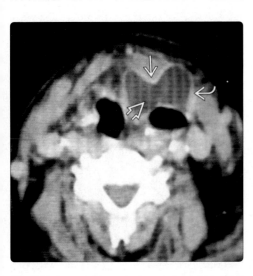
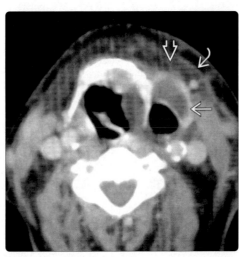

(Left) *Axial CECT in a patient with fevers & neck mass shows an air- & fluid-filled laryngocele with extralaryngeal extension (mixed) ➡. The walls are thick and enhancing ➡. Note lesion isthmus ➡ as it passes through thyrohyoid membrane.* (Right) *Axial CECT in the same patient reveals inflammatory stranding of adjacent subcutaneous fat ➡ & thickening of the platysma ➡, in addition to wall thickening & enhancement ➡. These are the typical findings of a pyolaryngocele.*

TERMINOLOGY

- Vocal cord paralysis, true vocal cord paralysis, recurrent laryngeal nerve paralysis
- Immobilization of true vocal cord by ipsilateral vagus (CNX) or recurrent laryngeal nerve dysfunction

IMAGING

- Constellation of unilateral laryngeal findings
  - Paramedian position of affected true vocal cord
  - Ballooning of laryngeal ventricle = sail sign
  - Anteromedial rotation of arytenoid cartilage
  - Medially displaced, thickened aryepiglottic fold
  - Enlarged pyriform sinus

TOP DIFFERENTIAL DIAGNOSES

- Laryngeal trauma
- Laryngocele
- Glottic (laryngeal) squamous cell carcinoma

PATHOLOGY

- Injury to or lesion compressing CNX anywhere from medulla to recurrent laryngeal nerve
- Most common etiologies: Neoplasm, trauma, idiopathic & nonmalignant thoracic pathology
- Can also group by location: Jugular foramen, carotid space, mediastinum, & tracheoesophageal groove

CLINICAL ISSUES

- Hoarseness, dysphonia, "breathy voice"

DIAGNOSTIC CHECKLIST

- Evaluate entire course of CNX and recurrent laryngeal nerve
- **Right** recurrent laryngeal nerve arises from CNX at **subclavian artery**
- **Left** recurrent laryngeal nerve arises from CNX at **aortopulmonary window**

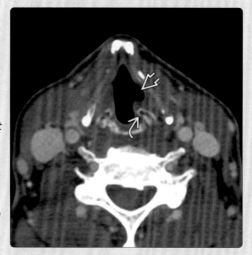
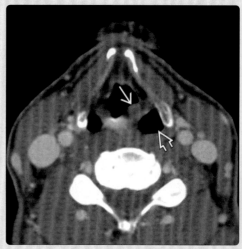

(Left) CECT in a patient with new-onset hoarseness shows slightly medially rotated left arytenoid cartilage ➡ & a more prominent dilated left laryngeal ventricle ➡. This is sometimes referred to as the sail sign, as it mimics the spinnaker of a boat. (Right) Axial CECT in the same patient demonstrates asymmetrically enlarged left pyriform sinus ➡ and a medial position of the left aryepiglottic fold ➡, which also appears thickened. Imaging features are consistent with clinical finding of left vocal cord paralysis (VCP).

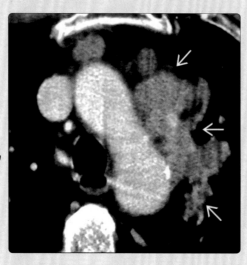
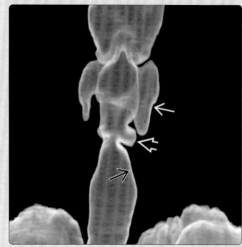

(Left) Axial CECT in same patient stresses the importance of scanning the aortopulmonary window for left VCP. A mediastinal mass (lung carcinoma) ➡ involves the left recurrent laryngeal nerve as it courses under the aortic arch. (Right) Anteroposterior 3D volume rendering of the airway in a patient with left VCP shows an enlarged ipsilateral laryngeal ventricle ➡ and pyriform sinus ➡ with flattening of the subglottic arch ➡.

TERMINOLOGY

Abbreviations

- Vocal cord paralysis (VCP), true vocal cord paralysis (TVCP), recurrent laryngeal nerve paralysis (RLNP)

Definitions

- Immobilization of true vocal cord by ipsilateral vagus (CNX) or recurrent laryngeal nerve dysfunction

IMAGING

General Features

- Best diagnostic clue
  - Paramedian vocal cord & **ipsilateral** findings
    - Ballooning of laryngeal ventricle sail sign
    - Enlarged pyriform sinus
    - Medially displaced aryepiglottic fold
- Location
  - Primary imaging findings are in larynx
  - Causative lesions can be anywhere from medulla (CNX origin) to recurrent laryngeal nerve
    - CNX traverses **jugular foramen**, descends neck in **carotid space**
    - **Right** CNX extends to clavicle, **recurs around right subclavian artery**
    - **Left** CNX extends into mediastinum, **recurs via aortopulmonary window**
    - Recurrent laryngeal nerves ascend to larynx in **tracheoesophageal grooves**
- Morphology
  - Affected cord is flaccid, paramedian in location

Radiographic Findings

- Radiography
  - Chest radiograph is less sensitive than CT but is often 1st test ordered if left TVCP
    - Pancoast tumor, mediastinal mass/adenopathy, cardiomegaly, enlarged aorta

CT Findings

- CECT
  - Paramedian position of affected true vocal cord with ipsilateral ancillary findings
    - Ballooning of laryngeal ventricle = **sail sign**
    - Anteromedial rotation of arytenoid cartilage
    - Medially displaced, thick aryepiglottic fold
    - Enlarged pyriform sinus
    - Cricoarytenoid muscle atrophy
  - If mass along CNX course from brainstem to jugular foramen
    - CNIX, CNXI dysfunction often also evident
      - CNIX injury → loss of ipsilateral pharynx sensation
      - CNXI injury → ipsilateral trapezius & sternocleidomastoid denervation
  - If mass along CNX in superior carotid space to level of hyoid
    - CNIX, CNXI + CNXII dysfunction often evident
      - CNXII injury → ipsilateral tongue denervation
  - Be aware of post thyroplasty vocal cord appearance
    - Procedures add bulk to paralyzed cord, improves voice
    - Vocal cord more midline, no longer patulous

      - Low density = fat injected to cord
      - High density = Silastic or Gore-Tex implants or Teflon injection
- CTA
  - Helpful to determine internal carotid artery (ICA) dissection

MR Findings

- MR shows same anatomic findings as CT
  - Medialized cord with patulous enlarged ventricle
  - Ipsilateral medial aryepiglottic fold and large pyriform sinus
- **Pitfall** in MR is acute-subacute denervation
  - T2 hyperintense & enhancing vocal cord muscle
  - May be erroneously interpreted as tumor

Nuclear Medicine Findings

- PET
  - Absent FDG uptake in denervated cord
    - Contralateral normal cord has asymmetric uptake
    - **Pitfall** if normal side interpreted as abnormal uptake
  - Teflon injection thyroplasty incites granulomatous reaction that may take up FDG

Imaging Recommendations

- Best imaging tool
  - CECT is 1st-line imaging tool for evaluation of hoarseness or known VCP
- Protocol advice
  - CECT from skull base to carina
  - Evaluate entire course of both CNX & recurrent laryngeal nerves

DIFFERENTIAL DIAGNOSIS

Laryngeal Trauma

- Arytenoid dislocation may occur with intubation
- Mimics VCP clinically and on imaging
- Look for other signs of trauma; clinical history is key
- Successful treatment requires early reduction

Laryngocele

- Air-filled internal laryngocele may be misinterpreted as enlarged laryngeal ventricle
- Normal arytenoid and aryepiglottic fold location maintained
- No pyriform sinus dilation

Glottic (Laryngeal) Squamous Cell Carcinoma

- Primary tumor may result in reduced cord mobility (T2 tumor)
- Direct extension or nodal metastases can cause VCP if injure vagus or recurrent laryngeal nerve

PATHOLOGY

General Features

- Etiology
  - Injury to or lesion compressing CNX anywhere from medulla to recurrent laryngeal nerve
  - Most common etiologies: Neoplasm, trauma, idiopathic pathology

- o **Neoplastic infiltration** of recurrent laryngeal nerve or CNX
  - Chest: Lung carcinoma, mediastinal adenopathy
  - Neck: Thyroid carcinoma, neck adenopathy
  - Jugular foramen: Meningioma, glomus jugulare, metastases
- o **Traumatic** (including **iatrogenic**) **injury** to nerve
  - Stabbing injury to neck
  - Carotid artery dissection
  - Thyroidectomy, carotid endarterectomy, anterior cervical spine fusion
- o **Idiopathic**
  - Many probably toxic, inflammatory (viral, postviral), or ischemic
  - No causative finding on imaging
  - Toxicity: Vincristine, alcohol
  - Other neuropathies: Radiation-induced, myasthenia gravis, vitamin B12 deficiency
- o **Nonmalignant thoracic causes**
  - Also known as cardiovocal (Ortner) syndrome
  - Atrial septal defect, Eisenmenger complex, patent ductus arteriosus, primary pulmonary hypertension, and aortic aneurysm with stretching of recurrent laryngeal nerve

CLINICAL ISSUES

Presentation

- Most common signs/symptoms
  - o Hoarseness, dysphonia, "breathy voice"
- Other signs/symptoms
  - o Uncommonly patients may be asymptomatic, with normal voice
  - o Aspiration (especially liquids), insufficient cough
  - o Foreign body sensation in larynx
  - o Shortness of breath sensation, air wasting
- Clinical profile
  - o Adult presenting with hoarseness

Demographics

- Gender
  - o No known gender predilection in adults
  - o M > F in pediatric age group
- Epidemiology
  - o Fewer "idiopathic" cases in CT era

Natural History & Prognosis

- VCP due to recurrent nerve or CNX injury rarely recovers
- Toxic or infectious VCP often self-limited
  - o > 80% resolve within 6 months
- Recovery uncommon if no improvement by 9 months

Treatment

- Initially conservative, many "idiopathic" cases will spontaneously improve
- Voice therapy
- **Vocal cord augmentation**: Material injected to paraglottic space
  - o Temporary: Resorbable materials (Gelfoam, hyaluronic acid, collagen)
  - o Permanent: Fat, calcium hydroxylapatite, Teflon

- Teflon reserved for terminal patients, as > 50% develop granuloma
- **Laryngeal framework surgery**
  - o Medialization thyroplasty with Silastic or Gore-Tex implant
  - o Arytenoid adduction
  - o Laryngeal reinnervation (hypoglossal nerve, ansa cervicalis)

DIAGNOSTIC CHECKLIST

Consider

- If vocal cord paralysis evident
  - o Determine whether vagal neuropathy or RLNP
  - o Evaluate for signs of additional cranial neuropathies: CNIX, XI, XII
  - o Regardless, evaluate brainstem, jugular foramen, then entire neck ± chest, along entire course of vagus and recurrent laryngeal nerve
- Right recurrent laryngeal nerve arises from CNX at subclavian artery
- Left recurrent laryngeal nerve arises from CNX at aortopulmonary window

Imaging Pitfalls

- MR: Acute-subacute denervation results in T2 hyperintense & enhancing cord
  - o May be misinterpreted as vocal cord tumor
- FDG PET: Denervated cord does not take up FDG
  - o Contralateral cord may be misinterpreted as tumor
- CECT: Dense medialized cord following thyroplasty
  - o Mimics cord tumor with cord paralysis
  - o Teflon granuloma will also take up FDG

SELECTED REFERENCES

1. Carneiro-Pla D et al: Impact of vocal cord ultrasonography on endocrine surgery practices. Surgery. 159(1): 58-63, 2016
2. Chen DW et al: Routine computed tomography in the evaluation of vocal fold movement impairment without an apparent cause. Otolaryngol Head Neck Surg. 152(2):308-13, 2015
3. Siu J et al: A comparison of outcomes in interventions for unilateral vocal fold paralysis: A systematic review. Laryngoscope. ePub, 2015
4. Wear VV et al: Evaluating "eee" phonation in multidetector CT of the neck. AJNR Am J Neuroradiol. 30(6):1102-6, 2009
5. Kumar VA et al: CT assessment of vocal cord medialization. AJNR Am J Neuroradiol. 27(8):1643-6, 2006
6. Ardito G et al: Revisited anatomy of the recurrent laryngeal nerves. Am J Surg. 187(2):249-53, 2004
7. Myssiorek D: Recurrent laryngeal nerve paralysis: anatomy and etiology. Otolaryngol Clin North Am. 37(1):25-44, 2004
8. Richardson BE et al: Clinical evaluation of vocal fold paralysis. Otolaryngol Clin North Am. 37(1):45-58, 2004
9. Chin SC et al: Using CT to localize side and level of vocal cord paralysis. AJR Am J Roentgenol. 180(4):1165-70, 2003
10. Schneider B et al: Concept for diagnosis and therapy of unilateral recurrent laryngeal nerve paralysis following thoracic surgery. Thorac Cardiovasc Surg. 51(6):327-31, 2003
11. Yeretsian RA et al: Teflon-induced granuloma: a false-positive finding with PET resolved with combined PET and CT. AJNR Am J Neuroradiol. 24(6):1164-6, 2003
12. Zeitels SM et al: Laryngology and phonosurgery. N Engl J Med. 349(9):882-92, 2003
13. Hughes CA et al: Unilateral true vocal fold paralysis: cause of right-sided lesions. Otolaryngol Head Neck Surg. 122(5):678-80, 2000
14. Romo LV et al: Atrophy of the posterior cricoarytenoid muscle as an indicator of recurrent laryngeal nerve palsy. AJNR Am J Neuroradiol. 20(3):467-71, 1999

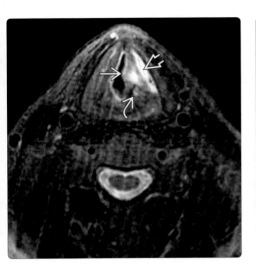
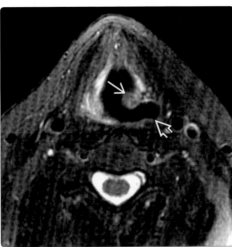

(Left) *Axial T2WI FS MR shows marked T2 hyperintensity of the left true cord* ⇒ *in acute/subacute VCP. This represents thyroarytenoid denervation change, a potential pitfall in the acute/subacute setting, where it can be misinterpreted as a neoplasm. Note the typical medial cord location* ⇒ *and anteromedial arytenoid rotation* ⇒. *(Right) Axial T2 FS MR in the same patient depicts additional findings of left VCP with a medially displaced, thickened left aryepiglottic fold* ⇒ *and dilated left pyriform sinus* ⇒.

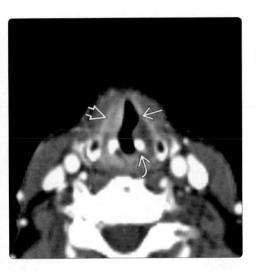
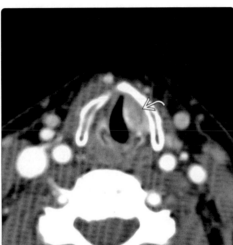

(Left) *Axial PET/CT in a patient with left VCP, as indicated by anteromedial arytenoid rotation* ⇒ *and ballooning of the laryngeal ventricle* ⇒, *is shown. There is asymmetric uptake in the normal right cord* ⇒, *not to be mistaken for tumor. (Right) Axial CECT shows the vocal cords with amorphous high density in the left true vocal cord* ⇒. *History revealed prior Teflon injection for left VCP. It is important not to mistake this for malignancy. Note: Teflon can also cause granulomatous reaction, resulting in a false-positive PET scan.*

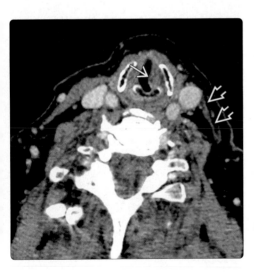
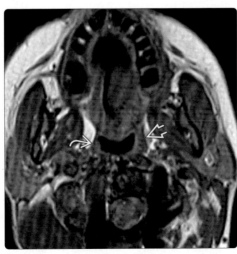

(Left) *Axial CECT demonstrates the medial position of the left cord* ⇒. *Note atrophy of the left sternocleidomastoid muscle* ⇒, *indicating concurrent CNXI denervation. VCP, plus CNIX and CNXI involvement, points to a skull base lesion, as seen in this patient with skull base glomus jugulotympanicum. (Right) Axial T1WI MR shows the soft palate with atrophy of the right superior pharyngeal constrictor muscles* ⇒ *(compare to normal side* ⇒) *due to pharyngeal plexus injury, indicating a vagus nerve lesion above the palate level.*

KEY FACTS

TERMINOLOGY

- Synonyms: Subglottic or laryngotracheal stenosis
- Definition: Nondevelopmental narrowing of cervical airway below vocal cords
  - Due to intrinsic pathology or extrinsic process compressing or invading airway

IMAGING

- **Intrinsic stenosis** usually iatrogenic from intubation or tracheostomy
  - Soft tissue narrows lumen
  - May see irregular, fragmented cartilage
- **Extrinsic stenosis** usually due to thyroid mass
  - Multinodular goiter: Enlarged heterogeneous lobes, ± calcifications, hemorrhage, cysts
  - Thyroid carcinoma or non-Hodgkin lymphoma: May compress or invade airway

TOP DIFFERENTIAL DIAGNOSES

- Subglottic infantile hemangioma
- Vascular rings and slings
- Congenital subglottic-tracheal stenosis

CLINICAL ISSUES

- **50%** stenosis before dyspnea on exertion
- **> 75%** airway narrowing before symptoms at rest

DIAGNOSTIC CHECKLIST

- For intrinsic subglottic/tracheal pathology
  - Evaluate degree and length of stenosis
  - Evaluate for cartilaginous deformity
  - 2D and 3D reconstructed images may help define extent and degree of stenosis
- If tracheal invasion, measure length of airway involvement
  - Determine whether cricoid cartilage involved

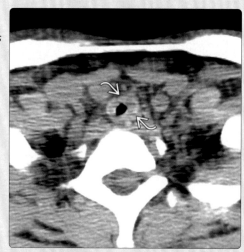
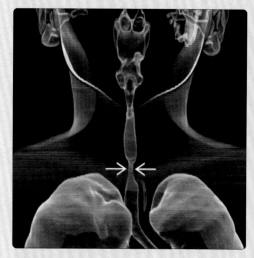

(Left) Axial NECT at thoracic inlet in a patient with history of prolonged intubation shows smooth, noncalcified, circumferential thickening ➡ of cervical tracheal wall with significant narrowing of airway lumen. (Right) Volume-rendered 3D image from axial helical NECT demonstrates tracheal stenosis at thoracic inlet related to cuffed tube injury. Note abrupt shelf of stenosis but with smooth edges ➡.

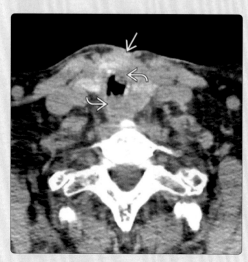
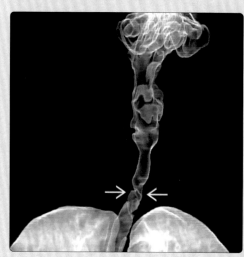

(Left) Axial NECT in a patient with previous tracheostomy reveals subglottic-tracheal narrowing with marked luminal irregularity due to exuberant granulation tissue ➡. Note skin thickening with increased density of subcutaneous fat from scarring along tracheostomy tract ➡. (Right) Volume-rendered 3D image from axial helical NECT demonstrates irregular subglottic tracheal stenosis over multiple centimeters due to granulation tissue at prior tracheostomy site ➡.

TERMINOLOGY

Synonyms

- Subglottic stenosis
- Laryngotracheal stenosis

Definitions

- Nondevelopmental narrowing of cervical airway below vocal cords
  - Due to intrinsic pathology or extrinsic process compressing or invading airway

IMAGING

General Features

- Best diagnostic clue
  - Narrowing of airway below vocal cords
- Location
  - Most commonly subglottic larynx and proximal cervical trachea
- Size
  - Length of stenosis varies with etiology
- Morphology
  - Circumferential or eccentric narrowing, smooth or irregular

Radiographic Findings

- Radiography
  - Narrowing of tracheal air column
  - Trachea may be displaced if asymmetric or unilateral thyroid mass

CT Findings

- Imaging findings depend on cause of stenosis
- **Intrinsic stenosis**: Most often due to **prior intubation** or **tracheostomy**
  - Concentric or eccentric soft tissue internal to cricoid/trachea
  - May be smooth or irregular soft tissue
  - Stenosis from tracheostomy more often irregular and longer segment than stenosis from intubation
- Evaluate carefully for cricoid or tracheal ring deformity or destruction
  - Cartilage necrosis in iatrogenic stenosis
  - Cartilage fracture following trauma
  - Cartilage collapse with relapsing polychondritis, Wegener granulomatosis
  - Cartilage invasion with squamous cell carcinoma (SCCa)
- May see calcification of submucosal tissues
  - Relapsing polychondritis, amyloidosis
- **Extrinsic stenosis**: Most common cause is **thyroid mass**
  - Multinodular goiter: Enlarged heterogeneous lobes, ± calcifications, hemorrhage, cysts
  - Thyroid carcinoma or non-Hodgkin lymphoma (NHL): May compress or invade trachea
    - Evaluate carefully for soft tissue in lumen, cartilage destruction
    - Differentiated carcinoma: ± calcifications
    - Anaplastic: Infiltrates, often necrosis, neck nodes
    - Thyroid NHL: Infiltrates, rarely necrosis, often nodes

Imaging Recommendations

- Best imaging tool
  - CT allows best evaluation of airway and cartilage contour and caliber
- Protocol advice
  - Thin-section (1-2 mm) helical imaging allows 2D and 3D reformations
    - Volume rendering and "virtual endoscopy" views
  - Contrast important for evaluation of tumors and exclusion of vascular rings
  - Inspiratory and expiratory scans helpful if tracheomalacia suspected

DIFFERENTIAL DIAGNOSIS

Subglottic Infantile Hemangioma

- Intensely enhancing submucosal mass internal to cricoid ring
- May be circumferential or eccentric
- Symptomatic in infancy with proliferative growth phase

Vascular Rings and Slings

- Vascular rings, pulmonary sling, or innominate artery compression of trachea
- CECT, CTA, or MRA displays vascular anomaly

Congenital Subglottic-Tracheal Stenosis

- Complete tracheal ring(s); no membranous portion
- Trachea develops round contour on axial images
- May be associated with tracheoesophageal fistula

PATHOLOGY

General Features

- Etiology
  - Due to **intrinsic** or **extrinsic** pathology
  - **Intrinsic subglottic or cervical tracheal pathology**
    - Iatrogenic stenosis post tracheostomy or prolonged intubation
      - Most common cause of acquired stenosis **(90%)**
      - Pressure/ischemic necrosis of mucosa and underlying tracheal wall by balloon or tube
    - Laryngeal trauma
      - Acute fracture of cricoid with hematoma
      - Cricoid fracture may heal with distorted contour, fibrosis
    - Laryngeal SCCa
      - Subglottic primary SCCa or transglottic tumor
    - Granulomatous diseases
      - Sarcoidosis, Wegener granulomatosis
    - Cartilage or mucosal inflammatory diseases
      - SLE, relapsing polychondritis, amyloid
      - Inflammation, fibrosis, ± calcifications
    - Tracheopathia osteochondroplastica
  - **Extrinsic compression or invasion of subglottis/cervical trachea**
    - Thyroid pathology
      - Multinodular goiter compresses and may displace airway
      - Differentiated or anaplastic thyroid carcinomas invade airway
      - Thyroid NHL more commonly compresses airway

- Neck adenopathy
  - □ Lymphoma or thyroid carcinoma nodes compress airway

Gross Pathologic & Surgical Features

- Intubation- or tracheostomy-related stenosis
  - Circumferential scarring with loss of integrity of tracheal cartilage rings and dense fibrosis
  - Mucosal ulceration

Microscopic Features

- Intubation- or tracheostomy-related stenosis
  - Destruction of cartilage rings with loss of type I collagen and aggrecan, dense fibrosis, plasma cell infiltrates
  - Calcification in cartilage rings, ± interruption of elastic fibers, loss of integrity of mucosal basal membrane
  - Hypertrophy of mucosal and submucosal layers, loss of ciliated mucosal epithelium

CLINICAL ISSUES

Presentation

- Most common signs/symptoms
  - Dyspnea, stridor
    - Typically several weeks post intubation
    - May be months to years later
  - 50% airway narrowing required to produce dyspnea on exertion
  - > 75% airway narrowing required before symptoms occur at rest
- Other signs/symptoms
  - Hemoptysis, wheezing, cough
  - Recurrent respiratory infections
- Clinical profile
  - Dyspnea and stridor arising in patient with history of intubation

Demographics

- Epidemiology
  - Post intubation, up to 20% incidence
    - Risk of stenosis declines with softer, more compliant, and low-pressure intubation balloons
  - Post tracheostomy, up to 20% incidence
    - Risk of stenosis declines with good tracheostomy hygiene and frequent tube changes

Natural History & Prognosis

- Depends largely on cause of stenosis
  - Iatrogenic stenosis may slowly progress
  - Multinodular goiter causes slow, gradual stenosis
    - Often minimal airway symptoms
  - Thyroid carcinoma and NHL are rapidly enlarging tumors
    - Secure airway is 1st priority

Treatment

- Treatment may be either endoscopic or open surgery
- Endoscopic treatment options
  - Balloon dilatation
  - Stenting
  - Laser resection
- Open surgery options
  - Resection of stenotic segment with reanastomosis

- Slide tracheoplasty
- Cartilage grafts
- Endoscopic treatment has lower morbidity but may require multiple sessions
- Lesions involving subglottic larynx more difficult to treat than pure tracheal lesions
- Longer and multiple stenoses more difficult to treat

DIAGNOSTIC CHECKLIST

Consider

- Most common cause is iatrogenic, prior subglottic/tracheal injury
- Extrinsic masses most commonly thyroid or nodal

Image Interpretation Pearls

- For intrinsic subglottic/tracheal pathology
  - Evaluate degree and length of stenosis
  - Evaluate for cartilaginous deformity
  - 2D and 3D reconstructed images may help define extent and degree of stenosis
- If tracheal invasion, measure length of airway involvement
  - Determine whether cricoid cartilage involved

SELECTED REFERENCES

1. D'Andrilli A et al: Subglottic tracheal stenosis. J Thorac Dis. 8(Suppl 2):S140-7, 2016
2. Young E et al: Tracheal stenosis following percutaneous dilatational tracheostomy using the single tapered dilator: an MRI study. Anaesth Intensive Care. 42(6):745-51, 2014
3. Melkane AE et al: Management of postintubation tracheal stenosis: appropriate indications make outcome differences. Respiration. 79(5):395-401, 2010
4. Herrington HC et al: Modern management of laryngotracheal stenosis. Laryngoscope. 116(9):1553-7, 2006
5. Berrocal T et al: Congenital anomalies of the tracheobronchial tree, lung, and mediastinum: embryology, radiology, and pathology. Radiographics. 24(1):e17, 2004
6. Grenier PA et al: Multidetector-row CT of the airways. Semin Roentgenol. 38(2):146-57, 2003
7. Lorenz RR: Adult laryngotracheal stenosis: etiology and surgical management. Curr Opin Otolaryngol Head Neck Surg. 11(6):467-72, 2003
8. Mostafa BE: Endoluminal stenting for tracheal stenosis. Eur Arch Otorhinolaryngol. 260(9):465-8, 2003
9. Wain JC: Postintubation tracheal stenosis. Chest Surg Clin N Am. 13(2):231-46, 2003
10. Grenier PA et al: New frontiers in CT imaging of airway disease. Eur Radiol. 12(5):1022-44, 2002
11. Hoppe H et al: Multidetector CT virtual bronchoscopy to grade tracheobronchial stenosis. AJR Am J Roentgenol. 178(5):1195-200, 2002
12. Lee KH et al: Benign tracheobronchial stenoses: long-term clinical experience with balloon dilation. J Vasc Interv Radiol. 13(9 Pt 1):909-14, 2002
13. Prince JS et al: Nonneoplastic lesions of the tracheobronchial wall: radiologic findings with bronchoscopic correlation. Radiographics. 22 Spec No:S215-30, 2002
14. Rea F et al: Benign tracheal and laryngotracheal stenosis: surgical treatment and results. Eur J Cardiothorac Surg. 22(3):352-6, 2002
15. Zagalo C et al: Morphology of trachea in benign human tracheal stenosis: a clinicopathological study of 20 patients undergoing surgery. Surg Radiol Anat. 24(3-4):160-8, 2002
16. Faust RA et al: Real-time, cine magnetic resonance imaging for evaluation of the pediatric airway. Laryngoscope. 111(12):2187-90, 2001
17. Gluecker T et al: 2D and 3D CT imaging correlated to rigid endoscopy in complex laryngo-tracheal stenoses. Eur Radiol. 11(1):50-4, 2001
18. Berdon WE: Rings, slings, and other things: vascular compression of the infant trachea updated from the midcentury to the millennium–the legacy of Robert E. Gross, MD, and Edward B. D. Neuhauser, MD. Radiology. 216(3):624-32, 2000
19. Tsunezuka Y et al: Tracheobronchial involvement in relapsing polychondritis. Respiration. 67(3):320-2, 2000

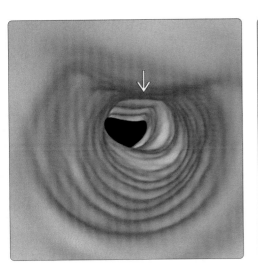
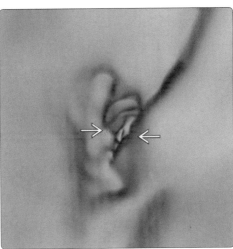

(Left) CT virtual bronchoscopy shows normal tracheal lumen. Note the membranous portion of the trachea ➡. This image is oriented so that the viewer is looking caudally toward the carina. (Right) CT virtual bronchoscopy demonstrates markedly irregular tracheal luminal stenosis ➡ due to granulation tissue at prior tracheostomy site.

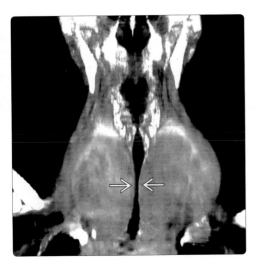
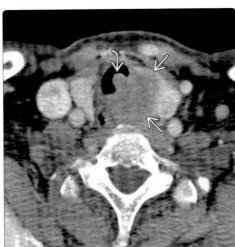

(Left) Coronal 3D rendering of a large thyroid multinodular goiter shows long-segment, smooth, side-to-side subglottic tracheal stenosis ➡ from extrinsic compression. (Right) Axial CECT in a patient presenting with shortness of breath and hoarseness shows homogeneous papillary carcinoma ➡ arising in left thyroid and invading cervical trachea. Intraluminal tumor nodule ➡ narrows airway.

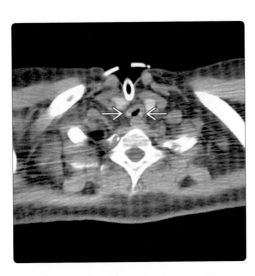
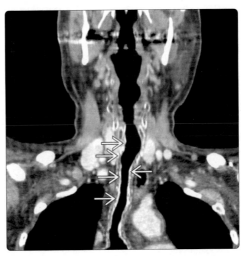

(Left) Axial NECT shows narrowing of tracheal lumen with thickening and deformity of tracheal wall ➡ in a patient with relapsing polychondritis. This finding involved most of the trachea. (Right) Coronal CECT curved 2D reconstruction shows irregular narrowing of trachea with prominent submucosal calcified nodules ➡ due to tracheopathia osteochondroplastica.

Lymph Nodes

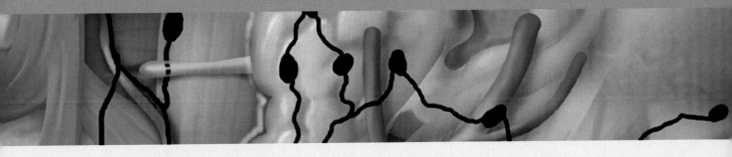

Summary Thoughts: Cervical Nodes

Cervical lymph nodes can be classified based on anatomic distribution or surgical levels used for neck dissection.

The key decision when assessing a lymph node is deciding whether it is **abnormal**. Traditionally, size criteria have been employed, but a multifactorial approach (size, homogeneity, morphology, enhancement, and borders) is more useful.

If a lymph node appears abnormal, one must decide whether it harbors inflammation (reactive), infection (suppurative), or tumor [usually squamous cell carcinoma (SCCa)]. This distinction is often quite difficult, especially with uncommon inflammatory diseases.

It is important for radiologists to understand the typical patterns of nodal spread of disease. Particular attention must be paid to subclinical lymph nodes (e.g., retropharyngeal).

Imaging Anatomy

Anatomically, the cervical lymph nodes are organized into groups (submental, submandibular, parotid, facial, occipital, and retropharyngeal) and chains (internal jugular, spinal accessory, transverse cervical, paratracheal, and external jugular).

- **Submental** group: Midline, between anterior bellies of digastric muscles
- **Submandibular** group: Anterior to posterior margin of submandibular gland, lateral to anterior belly of digastric
- Parotid group: Within parotid gland itself
- Facial group: Scattered across face (includes mandibular, buccal, infraorbital, malar, and retrozygomatic)
- Occipital group: Posterior and inferior to calvarium
- Retropharyngeal group: In retropharyngeal space
- **Internal jugular** chain (IJC): Surrounding IJ vein from skull base to thoracic inlet
- **Spinal accessory** chain (SAC): Along course of CNXI across posterior cervical space of neck
- **Transverse cervical** chain (TCC): Along transverse cervical artery, in supraclavicular fossa; connects inferior aspects of IJC and SAC
- Paratracheal (juxtavisceral) chain: Anterior (midline, overlying strap muscles) and lateral to trachea (tracheoesophageal groove)
- External jugular chain: Superficial to sternocleidomastoid (SCM)
- Major chains (IJC, SAC, TCC) form triangle of nodes in lateral neck

Surgically, the cervical lymph nodes are organized into **6 levels** (or zones) based on surgical landmarks. Radiologic landmarks are used to approximate the surgical boundaries on imaging.

- Level I: Submental (level Ia) and submandibular (level Ib) clusters, located inferior to mandible; receives drainage from lips, floor of mouth, and oral tongue; drains into level II
- Level II: Upper portions of IJC (level IIa) and SAC (level IIb); anterior or deep to SCM, superior to **hyoid bone**; receives drainage from all nodal clusters and from pharynx; drains into level III
- Level III: Mid 1/3 of IJC; anterior or deep to SCM, inferior to hyoid but superior to bottom of **cricoid cartilage**; receives drainage from larynx and level II; drains into level IV

- Level IV: Bottom of IJC and medial half of TCC; anterior or deep to SCM, inferior to cricoid cartilage; receives drainage from level III and chest and abdomen
- Level V: Bottom of SAC (level Va) and posterior half of TCC (level Vb); lies in posterior cervical space, strictly posterior to back edge of SCM; receives drainage from occipital, retropharyngeal, periauricular, and parotid regions; drains into level IV and mediastinum
- Level VI: Paratracheal chain; superficial to strap muscles, between carotid arteries and lateral to trachea in tracheoesophageal groove; receives drainage from visceral space (especially thyroid gland), drains into level IV, mediastinum
- In radiation oncology, "supraclavicular nodes" are considered distinct entity, but, in radiology scheme, they are part of levels IV and V
- Numerous sonographic classification schemes are available, only some of which correspond to formal radiologic classification

Many nodes found in anatomic classification scheme are not included in the surgical scheme because they are not included in routine neck dissections. These may be overlooked clinically and merit particular attention from radiologists.

- **Retropharyngeal nodes**, in particular, cannot be palpated or clinically visualized, thus relying on radiologic identification of pathology; lesions of sinonasal tract and nasopharynx drain to these nodes, which may also harbor metastatic thyroid carcinoma
- **Parotid nodes** receive drainage from periauricular region and scalp; most common tumors involved here are skin SCCa or melanoma
- **Facial and occipital** metastases are less frequent but still important when they occur

A few cervical lymph nodes have been singled out and named because of clinical importance or radiologic appearances.

- **Signal (Virchow) node**: Lowest node in IJC; if no primary tumor evident in neck, consider chest or abdomen primary, with metastasis carried via thoracic duct; left > right
- **Rouvière node**: Highest node in retropharyngeal group; lies within 2 cm of skull base; site of spread for nasopharyngeal carcinoma, esthesioneuroblastoma
- **Jugulodigastric (sentinel) node**: Lies within IJC just above hyoid bone; larger than surrounding nodes

Imaging Techniques and Indications

CECT is the 1st-line imaging modality to evaluate an adult patient with a neck mass of uncertain etiology. In children, US or MR should be considered first in order to minimize ionizing radiation. If the mass turns out to be metastatic, CECT usually can identify the primary site of origin. In the setting of a known malignancy, CECT or MR can be used to stage the nodes or to search for recurrence. However, whole-body FDG PET/CT is the preferred modality for oncologic imaging, particularly the assessment of regional and distant disease.

Advanced imaging techniques, such as quantitative diffusion imaging (DWI), dynamic contrast-enhanced (DCE) MR perfusion, and dual-energy CT, show promise for improving the sensitivity and specificity of detecting nodal metastatic disease. While advanced imaging of cervical nodes has increased, larger multicenter studies are needed to establish reproducible diagnostic thresholds and imaging protocols. In

Lymph Nodes Differential Diagnosis

Inflammatory	Infectious	Regional metastases
Reactive nodes	Viral upper respiratory infection	Squamous cell carcinoma
Castleman disease	Tuberculosis	NHL
Kimura disease	Atypical *Mycobacterium* species	Melanoma
Kikuchi disease	Cat scratch disease	Salivary neoplasms
Rosai-Dorfman disease	HIV adenopathy	Thyroid carcinoma
Inflammatory pseudotumor	**Malignant primary tumor**	Lung cancer
	Hodgkin lymphoma	
	Non-Hodgkin lymphoma (NHL)	**Systemic metastases**

current practice, these techniques remain investigational and are not yet considered standard of care.

Approaches to Lymph Node Imaging Issues

Deciding whether a mass arises within a lymph node can be difficult in a few specific locations. In the submandibular space, nodal masses lie anterior to the facial vein, whereas glandular masses lie posterior to the vein. In the lower left neck, the signal node and the distal thoracic duct have a similar location, so a dilated distal thoracic duct may mimic an enlarged node, particularly on T2WI MR. However, the duct is purely cystic and can be followed proximally into the superior mediastinum. In level II, 2nd branchial cleft anomalies and lymph nodes have a similar location, and metastatic disease from the oral cavity is often purely cystic. In adults, metastatic SCCa should be considered the diagnosis until proven otherwise. In children, basal cell carcinoma is more likely in this location.

Deciding whether a lymph node harbors malignancy is one of the most difficult (and important) issues in head and neck imaging. Traditionally, size criteria have been employed, but, when used in isolation, size criteria have poor accuracy. Furthermore, there is limited agreement on which axis of the node to measure and appropriate size thresholds. Instead, a multifactorial approach including other imaging findings should be used in addition to size criteria to improve the accuracy of assessment. None of these findings on its own is a perfect distinguishing characteristic, and all should be taken into consideration.

- **Homogeneity**: Central necrosis in untreated lymph node is highly suspicious for cancer; caveat: Do not mistake normal fatty hilum for necrosis when seen with partial volume averaging artifact
- **Morphology**: Normal nodes are reniform (i.e., kidney-shaped) with central hilum containing fat and vessels; malignant nodes are ovoid, round, or show focal cortical expansion
- **Enhancement**: Node that enhances more than its counterparts is worrisome
- **Borders**: Irregular borders with infiltration of surrounding fat are indicative of cancer and suspicious for **extracapsular spread**

Understanding the usual **patterns of lymphatic spread** from various primary sites is critical for several reasons: (1) Particular attention can be given to areas of likely spread (e.g., retropharyngeal space nodes in nasopharyngeal carcinoma or lower cervical nodes in lung cancer), (2) equivocal lymph nodes that are outside the usual pattern are less suspicious, (3) likely locations of the primary tumor can be suspected in patients presenting with a nodal mass, and (4) nodal disease outside the usual pattern can prompt a search for a 2nd primary.

The enhancement pattern of a lymph node can help to predict the site of origin. **Necrotic nodes** with a thick enhancing wall are most likely secondary to tonsillar or tongue base SCCa. **Cystic nodes** with imperceptible walls are associated with papillary thyroid carcinoma. Large, uniformly enhancing nodes are suggestive of lymphoma. Additionally, nodal **microcalcifications** or intrinsic **bright T1 signal** are suspicious for differentiated thyroid carcinoma, often showing a similar appearance to the primary thyroid malignancy.

Clinical Implications

One of the most vexing clinical problems in H&N oncology is the **unknown primary tumor**. This occurs when a patient presents with a nodal mass that proves to be metastatic SCCa. Because SCCa does not arise within a lymph node, a mucosal primary must be sought. There are different definitions regarding how thorough the search must be before declaring the primary to be unknown; usually, the patient must undergo physical examination, panendoscopy, conventional imaging (CECT or MR), and blind biopsies of likely sites of origin.

Unknown primary tumors are important because patients must undergo irradiation to all mucosal surfaces to ensure that the unseen primary is included. This is extremely morbid because of xerostomia and dry mouth. However, patients with unknown primary tumors have a relatively good prognosis. **FDG PET/CT** identifies the primary tumor in ~ 25% of patients who fit the definition of an unknown primary tumor and should be considered as routine work-up in these patients.

Patients with enlarged upper neck nodes and enlargement of Waldeyer lymphatic ring usually have an upper respiratory infection. Unfortunately, lymphoma and HIV adenopathy can have an identical appearance, so clinical or radiologic follow-up is needed to exclude these more troubling diseases.

The **signal node**, located at the medial neck base, has particular clinical significance. Although it is sometimes affected by metastatic disease from the neck or upper mediastinum, it may also receive metastatic disease from abdominal primaries without intervening nodes in the chest (presumably via the thoracic duct). Thus, when patients present with nodal disease in the signal node, whole-body imaging is warranted to discover the primary tumor.

Selected References

1. Eisenmenger LB et al: Imaging of head and neck lymph nodes. Radiol Clin North Am. 53(1):115-32, 2015

Lymph Node Overview

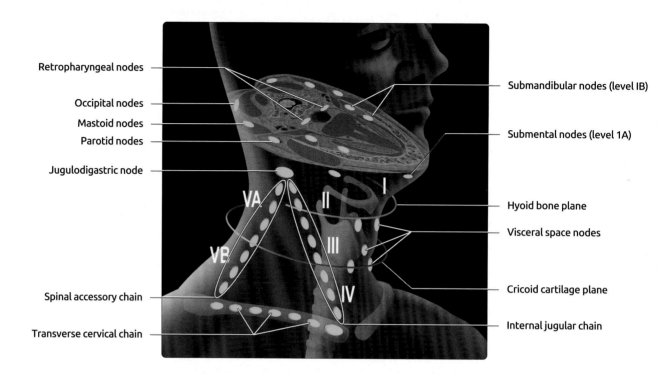

Retropharyngeal nodes

Occipital nodes

Mastoid nodes

Parotid nodes

Jugulodigastric node

Spinal accessory chain

Transverse cervical chain

Submandibular nodes (level IB)

Submental nodes (level 1A)

Hyoid bone plane

Visceral space nodes

Cricoid cartilage plane

Internal jugular chain

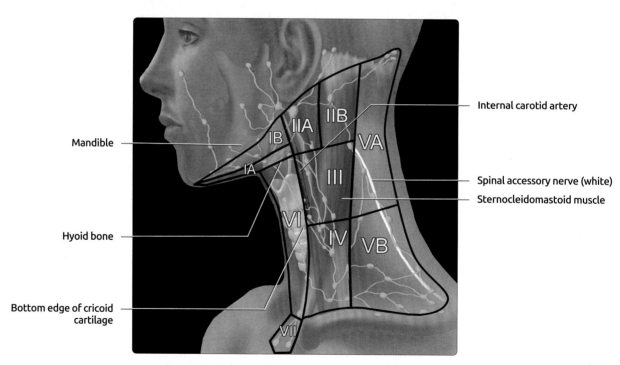

Mandible

Hyoid bone

Bottom edge of cricoid cartilage

Internal carotid artery

Spinal accessory nerve (white)

Sternocleidomastoid muscle

(Top) *Lateral oblique graphic of the cervical neck depicts an axial slice through the suprahyoid neck. Note that the major node chains [internal jugular chain (IJC), spinal accessory chain (SAC), transverse cervical chain] form a triangle in the lateral neck. The planes of the hyoid bone (blue arc) and cricoid cartilage (orange circle) divide the IJC and SAC into surgical levels. **(Bottom)** Lateral neck graphic shows the boundaries of the surgical levels. The chains and groups in this image are divided up not by their anatomic groups, as in the previous image, but by surgical landmarks. The hyoid bone separates level Ia from level VI and level II from level III. The inferior margin of the cricoid cartilage separates level III from level IV and level Va from level Vb. The posterior edge of the sternocleidomastoid muscle (SCM) separates levels II, III, and IV from level V. The carotid artery separates level VI from levels III and IV. The inferior margin of the mandible separates level Ib from the facial lymph nodes.*

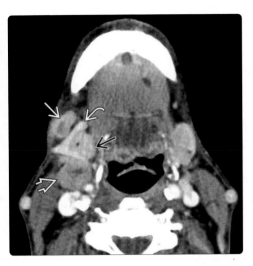

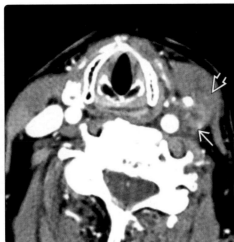

(Left) Axial CECT shows an abnormal submandibular space mass ➡ anterior to the facial vein ➡, indicating it is a level Ib lymph node. The submandibular gland ➡ lies posterior to the vein. Nodes that lie posterior to the gland ➡ are in level II. (Right) Axial CECT shows a left lateral neck mass ➡ deep to the SCM muscle. Irregular margins and loss of the normal fat plane ➡ between the mass and the SCM indicate extracapsular spread, a definitive sign of malignancy.

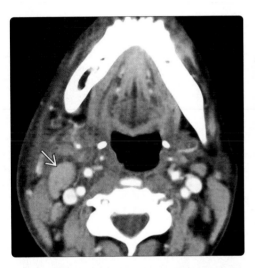

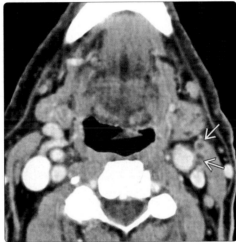

(Left) Axial CECT shows a markedly enlarged level II lymph node ➡. By size criteria, this node would be considered malignant, but its kidney-shaped configuration is indicative of its benign nature (reactive node). (Right) Axial CECT shows multiple heterogeneously enhancing 2- to 4-mm level II lymph nodes ➡. By size criteria, this node would be normal. The presence of central necrosis, however, is a definitive sign of malignancy if seen prior to treatment.

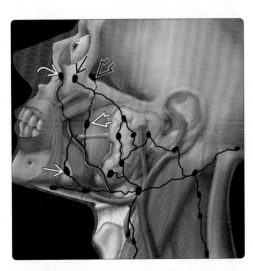

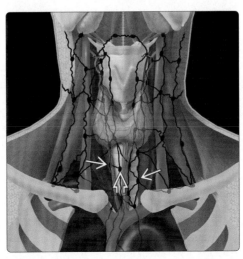

(Left) Lateral graphic shows facial lymph nodes. Anteriorly note the mandibular ➡ and infraorbital nodes ➡. The buccinator node ➡ is along the anterior margin of the buccinator muscle. The malar node ➡ and retrozygomatic node ➡ are superior. (Right) Frontal graphic reveals nodal drainage of anterior neck. The thyroid gland drains into visceral space nodes (level VI), known as the pretracheal ➡ and paratracheal ➡ nodes.

Reactive Lymph Nodes

TERMINOLOGY

- Reactive nodes: Benign, reversible enlargement of nodes in response to antigen stimulus
- Nodal involvement may be acute or chronic, localized or generalized

IMAGING

- Multiple well-defined oval-shaped or reniform nodes
- Nodes of normal size or mildly enlarged
  - Size alone is relatively poor predictor of benignity
  - In children, reactive nodes may be ≥ 2 cm
- CECT is 1st-line imaging modality
  - Enhancement minimal to mild, homogeneous
  - Linear enhancement within node is characteristic
- Increasing role of US elastography in differentiating benign, reactive nodes from malignancy

TOP DIFFERENTIAL DIAGNOSES

- Squamous cell carcinoma nodal metastases

- Systemic nodal metastases
- Non-Hodgkin lymphoma nodes
- Tuberculous adenitis
- Sarcoid nodes

PATHOLOGY

- Node reaction seen as specific histologic patterns of hyperplasia: Follicular, sinus, diffuse, or mixed

CLINICAL ISSUES

- Common clinical problem in pediatric age group
- Less common in adults
  - Always consider malignancy or HIV infection

DIAGNOSTIC CHECKLIST

- Reactive nodes typically oval-shaped or reniform, clustered
- Adjacent cellulitis suggests bacterial infection
- Focal nonenhancement suggests suppuration or necrosis
- Supraclavicular and posterior cervical location more concerning for malignancy

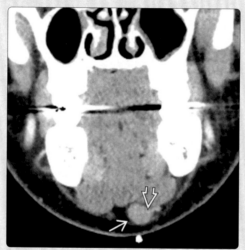
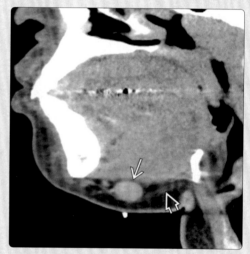

(Left) Coronal CECT in a teenager with a palpable lump shows a solid, ovoid left IA lymph node ➡ subjacent to skin marker. Note subtle intranodal linear enhancement ➡, an imaging feature commonly seen in reactive adenopathy. The enlarged node resolved with short course of antibiotics. (Right) Sagittal CECT (same patient) shows benign, ovoid morphology of the reactive node ➡. Reactive nodes show homogeneous density without necrosis and can be followed clinically to resolution. Note bowed platysma muscle ➡.

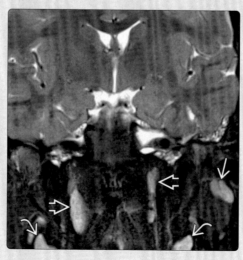
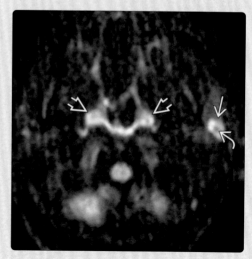

(Left) Coronal T2 FS MR in child with left otitis externa and media shows reactive adenopathy, including enlarged parotid ➡, retropharyngeal ➡, and high deep cervical ➡ nodes. Reactive nodes are solid, homogeneous, and reniform in shape. (Right) Axial DWI trace in same patient is sensitive for identifying lymph nodes, which are bright relative to adjacent structures. An enlarged, reactive left parotid node ➡ maintains a dark, fatty hilum ➡. Note associated adenoidal hyperplasia ➡.

TERMINOLOGY

Synonyms

- Reactive adenopathy, reactive lymphoid hyperplasia, nodal hyperplasia

Definitions

- Benign, reversible enlargement of nodes in response to antigen stimulus
  - Nodal involvement may be acute or chronic, localized or generalized
- "Reactive" implies benign etiology

IMAGING

General Features

- Best diagnostic clue
  - Multiple well-defined, kidney-shaped (reniform) nodes
    - Nodes of normal size or mildly enlarged
- Location
  - Any of nodal groups of H&N
- Size
  - Wide size range
    - Adult: Often up to 1.5 cm
    - Child: Reactive node may be ≥ 2 cm
  - Size is relatively poor predictor of benignity if considered in isolation
- Morphology
  - Reactive node is typically oval or reniform
    - Rounded morphology, cortical expansion concerning for malignancy

CT Findings

- NECT
  - Homogeneous well-defined nodes, isodense or hypodense to muscle
  - Stranding of adjacent fat frequently associated when acute infectious cause
- CECT
  - Enhancement minimal to mild, homogeneous
  - Linear enhancement within node characteristic
  - Hyperplasia of pharyngeal lymphoid tissue (Waldeyer ring) often associated

MR Findings

- T1WI
  - Homogeneous low to intermediate signal intensity
- T2WI
  - Homogeneous intermediate to high signal intensity
  - Cystic change suggests suppuration or tumoral necrosis
- DWI
  - Benign nodes tend to have higher ADC values than neoplastic nodes
    - Optimal ADC thresholds remain undefined
- T1WI C+
  - Variable enhancement, usually mild & homogeneous
  - Linear central enhancement favors benign node
  - Tonsillar enlargement (Waldeyer ring) may be found

Ultrasonographic Findings

- Reniform nodes with echogenic vascular hilus
- US elastography is promising tool for differentiating reactive nodes from metastatic adenopathy
  - Malignant nodes demonstrate higher stiffness than benign lymph nodes

Nuclear Medicine Findings

- PET
  - Mild FDG uptake may be seen
  - Marked uptake more likely with active granulomatous disease or tumor

Imaging Recommendations

- Best imaging tool
  - CECT is 1st-line tool for evaluation of adenopathy
    - Differentiates reactive from suppurative nodes and cellulitis from abscess
    - Allows determination of node extent and evaluation for potential malignant cause
- Protocol advice
  - Contrast enhancement important to detect cystic or suppurative intranodal change

DIFFERENTIAL DIAGNOSIS

Squamous Cell Carcinoma Nodal Metastases

- Enlarged round node or cluster of nodes
- Necrosis suggests nonreactive, malignant node
- Primary pharyngeal lesion should be sought

Systemic Nodal Metastases

- Supraclavicular node suggests infraclavicular primary

Non-Hodgkin Lymphoma Nodes

- Multiple large nodes, often ≥ 1.5 cm
- Enlargement of Waldeyer ring may be seen
- Homogeneous mild contrast enhancement

Tuberculous Adenitis

- Suppurative TB adenopathy in multiple neck nodes
- Rupture with adjacent phlegmon & fistula possible
- Positive chest x-ray common

Sarcoid Nodes

- Homogeneous, well-defined nodes, often > 2 cm
- Intraparotid nodes often involved
- Positive thoracic nodes common

PATHOLOGY

General Features

- Etiology
  - Response to infectious agent, chemical, drug, or foreign antigen
    - Includes viruses, bacteria, parasites, and fungi
- Associated abnormalities
  - Hyperplasia of pharyngeal lymphoid tissue (Waldeyer ring) often with viral infections
  - Inflammation of same lymphoid tissue (e.g., tonsillitis) may be cause of adenopathy
  - Associated findings may suggest causative agent
    - Stranding of adjacent fat common with bacteria, rare with atypical mycobacteria

- **Generalized adenopathy** suggests viral infection, collagen vascular disease, or malignancy
- Parotid lymphoepithelial lesions ± adenoidal hypertrophy suggests **HIV adenopathy**
- Parotid adenopathy frequently seen with **sarcoid**

Gross Pathologic & Surgical Features

- Firm, rubbery, mobile, enlarged nodes

Microscopic Features

- Node reaction with different histologic patterns of **hyperplasia**
  - **Follicular**: Follicles increase in size and number
    - e.g., idiopathic, HIV adenopathy, rheumatoid arthritis
  - **Sinus**: Sinuses enlarge and fill with histiocytes
    - e.g., sinus histiocytosis
  - **Diffuse**: Node infiltrated by sheets of cells
    - e.g., viral adenitis
  - **Mixed**: Combination of follicular, sinus, and diffuse
    - e.g., TB, cat scratch
- Culture or staining may reveal infectious agent
- Granulomatous pattern shows histiocyte aggregation ± necrotic material
  - Response to irritant that histiocytes cannot digest or T-cell-mediated immune response
  - Mycobacteria: Acid-fast bacilli with Ziehl Neelsen stain in 25-56%
  - Cat scratch: *Bartonella henselae* or *Bartonella quintana*
  - Sarcoid: Nonnecrotizing granulomas
  - Sarcoid-like: Epithelioid cell granulomas in reaction to tumors
    - Mimic metastases at diagnosis, during treatment, or after treatment completed

CLINICAL ISSUES

Presentation

- Most common signs/symptoms
  - Firm, sometimes fluctuant, freely mobile subcutaneous nodal masses
  - Other signs/symptoms
    - Bacterial adenitis and cat scratch usually painful
    - Nontuberculous mycobacteria (NTM) usually nontender
- Clinical profile
  - Pediatric or teenage presentation with nodal enlargement
  - Patient with known primary neoplasm may have "borderline" size nodes that are only reactive

Demographics

- Age
  - Any age but most common in pediatric age group
    - Neonatal neck nodes not palpable
  - Children: Organisms have predilection for specific ages
    - < 1 year: *Staphylococcus aureus*, group B *Streptococcus*, Kawasaki disease
    - 1-5 years: *S. aureus*, group A β-hemolytic *Streptococcus*, atypical mycobacteria
    - 5-15 years: Anaerobic bacteria, toxoplasmosis, cat-scratch disease, tuberculosis
- Ethnicity

- High incidence of *Mycobacterium tuberculosis* in developing countries
- Epidemiology
  - Common clinical problem in pediatric age group
    - Pediatric nodes not often imaged
    - Most children have lymphadenopathy at some time
    - Most adenopathy is result of infection, though organism may not be identified
  - Less common in adults
    - Most important differential considerations are malignancy or HIV infection

Natural History & Prognosis

- Bacterial infection, non-TB *Mycobacterium*, and cat scratch frequently progress to necrotic nodes
- Chronic inflammation may result in fatty metaplasia
  - Low-density nodal hilus mimics necrosis

Treatment

- Many reactive nodes resolve spontaneously, including cat scratch
- Antibiotics, if bacterial cause suspected
- Nodal aspiration or biopsy may be necessary
  - Failed response to antibiotics
  - Rapid increase in nodal size
  - Associated systemic adenopathy or unexplained fever & weight loss
  - Features concerning for malignancy
    - Nodes feel hard &/or matted to examination
    - Supraclavicular or posterior cervical node location
- If needle aspiration shows nonspecific reactive changes, follow clinically for 3-6 months
- Persistent adenopathy requires repeat needle aspiration to rule out lymphoma, metastasis, or TB

DIAGNOSTIC CHECKLIST

Consider

- Adjacent cellulitis suggests bacterial infection
- Always consider metastatic disease, non-Hodgkin lymphoma (NHL), and HIV in nonpediatric age group
- Certain locations should raise concern
  - Postauricular nodes in child > 2 years likely clinically significant
  - Supraclavicular nodes are neoplastic in ~ 60%
  - Posterior cervical nodes suggest NHL, skin nodal metastases, or nasopharyngeal carcinoma

Image Interpretation Pearls

- Imaging findings often nonspecific with multiple homogeneous mildly enlarged or normal-sized nodes
- Oval-shaped nodes more likely benign and reactive
- Central linear vascular enhancement is characteristic
- Focal nonenhancement within node suggests suppuration or necrosis

SELECTED REFERENCES

1. Al Kadah B et al: Cervical lymphadenopathy: study of 251 patients. Eur Arch Otorhinolaryngol. 272(3):745-52, 2015
2. Choi YJ et al: Ultrasound elastography for evaluation of cervical lymph nodes. Ultrasonography. 34(3):157-64, 2015
3. Eisenmenger LB et al: Imaging of head and neck lymph nodes. Radiol Clin North Am. 53(1):115-32, 2015

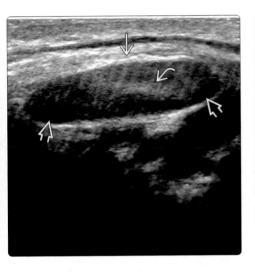

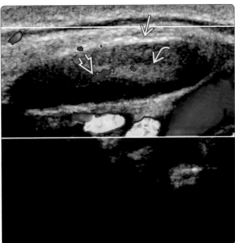

(Left) *Transverse grayscale ultrasound demonstrates the typical appearance of a reactive submandibular node ➡. Note the low internal echogenicity ➡ with echogenic fatty hilum ➡.* (Right) *Transverse color Doppler ultrasound of the same reactive submandibular node ➡ shows typical vascularity ➡ associated with the echogenic hilum ➡.*

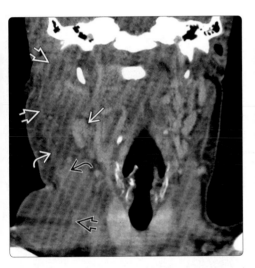

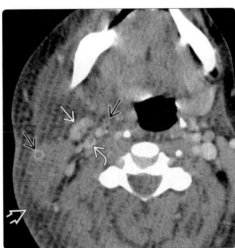

(Left) *Coronal CECT in an IV drug user shows the typical appearance of reactive level II node ➡. Reactive nodes are enlarged but maintain an ovoid or reniform morphology. Note additional diffuse edema ➡, platysma thickening ➡, rim-enhancing early abscess ➡, & septic thrombophlebitis in the external jugular vein ➡.* (Right) *Axial CECT in the same patient shows a kidney bean-shaped reactive level II node ➡ in a patient with extensive cellulitis ➡ & septic thrombophlebitis. Note filling defects in IJV ➡ & tributary veins ➡ from thrombus.*

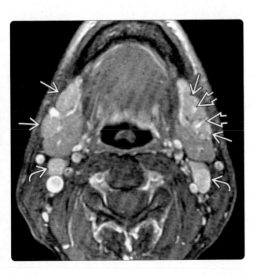

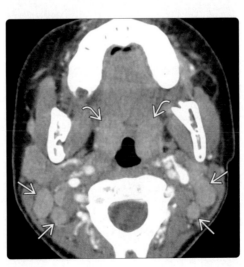

(Left) *Axial T1WI C+ FS MR shows prominent bilateral homogeneously enhancing reactive nodes in the upper cervical ➡ and submandibular ➡ chains. Note linear enhancement of the central vessel in some nodes ➡.* (Right) *Axial CECT in patient with nonsuppurative tonsillopharyngitis shows bilateral enlarged, ovoid reactive nodes ➡ without fat stranding or suppuration. Palatine tonsillar enlargement and hyperemia are evident ➡.*

Suppurative Lymph Nodes

TERMINOLOGY

- Adenitis, acute lymphadenitis, intranodal abscess
- Pus formation within nodes from bacterial infection

IMAGING

- Enlarged node with intranodal fluid and surrounding inflammation (cellulitis)
- Most often jugulodigastric, submandibular, retropharyngeal nodes
- Contrast should be administered to best appreciate extent of suppurative changes
- Consider CT or US-guided aspiration for diagnosis and minimally invasive therapy

TOP DIFFERENTIAL DIAGNOSES

- Squamous cell carcinoma nodes
- 2nd branchial cleft anomaly
- Nontuberculosis *Mycobacterium* nodes
- Tuberculosis nodes

- Fatty nodal metaplasia

PATHOLOGY

- *Staphylococcus* and *Streptococcus* most frequent causative organisms
- Pediatric infections show clustering of organisms by age range
- Dental infections are typically polymicrobial and predominantly anaerobic

DIAGNOSTIC CHECKLIST

- If no significant cellulitic changes around node
  - In children consider nontuberculosis mycobacteria
  - In adults consider squamous cell carcinoma or thyroid carcinoma nodal metastases
- Look for primary infectious source on images
  - Pharyngitis, dental infection, salivary gland calculi
- With any neck infection, must evaluate for airway compromise, thrombophlebitis, and pseudoaneurysm

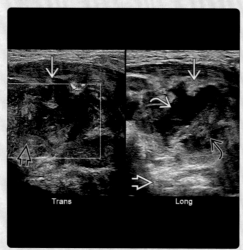
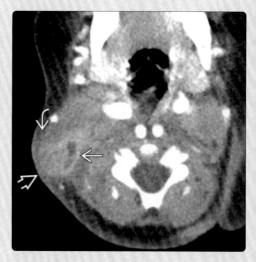

(Left) Transverse (left) and longitudinal (right) color Doppler and grayscale US of an infant with suppurative adenopathy show enlarged, heterogeneous echogenicity level II node ➡ with complex, cystic contents ➡, internal debris ➡, posterior acoustic enhancement ➡, and peripheral hyperemia ➡. (Right) Axial CECT in the same patient shows a rim-enhancing, centrally cystic/necrotic right level II suppurative lymph node ➡. Note overlying cellulitis with skin thickening ➡ and edema ➡.

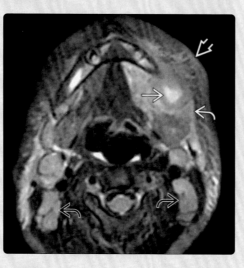
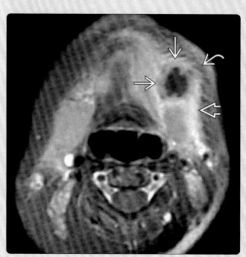

(Left) Axial T2 FS MR shows an enlarged cystic/necrotic submandibular lymph node with central bright T2 signal ➡. Note additional features of infection/inflammation, including edema in the left submandibular space ➡ and overlying cellulitis ➡. Multiple solid reactive nodes ➡ are present. (Right) Axial T1 C+ FS MR in the same patient shows thick peripheral enhancement of the suppurative node ➡. Note adjacent inflammatory changes with stranding of subcutaneous fat ➡ and thickened platysma ➡.

TERMINOLOGY

Synonyms

- Adenitis, acute lymphadenitis, intranodal abscess

Definitions

- Pus formation within nodes from bacterial infection

IMAGING

General Features

- Best diagnostic clue
  - Enlarged node with intranodal fluid and surrounding inflammation (cellulitis)
- Location
  - Any of nodal groups of H&N
    - Most often: Jugulodigastric, submandibular, retropharyngeal
  - Unilateral or bilateral
- Size
  - Typically enlarged node or confluence of nodes
  - 1- to 4-cm range
- Morphology
  - Ovoid to round, large node with cystic changes
  - Often poorly defined margins
  - Additional solid or suppurative nodes typically present

CT Findings

- CECT
  - Enhancing nodal wall with central hypodensity/lack of enhancement
  - Stranding of adjacent fat and subcutaneous tissues
  - If progresses to abscess: Irregular, ill-defined, peripherally enhancing, low-density collection

MR Findings

- T1WI
  - Node with central low signal intensity
  - Surrounding fat has hazy signal intensity
- T2WI
  - Node with diffuse or central high signal intensity
  - Fat saturation best demonstrates surrounding hyperintense tissues
- DWI
  - Complimentary to routine pulse sequences
  - Suppurative, necrotic nodes have reduced diffusivity (bright DWI trace, dark ADC signal)
  - May show higher DWI trace and lower ADC signal relative to metastatic necrotic nodes
    - Optimal ADC thresholds remain undefined
- T1WI C+
  - Marked peripheral enhancement with poorly defined margin
  - Absent central enhancement

Ultrasonographic Findings

- Central decreased echogenicity with increased through transmission
- Color Doppler shows increased peripheral vascularity
  - Very low resistance and pulsatility indices

Nuclear Medicine Findings

- PET
  - Node has increased FDG uptake
  - Absent central uptake usually beyond PET resolution

Imaging Recommendations

- Best imaging tool
  - CECT usually 1st-line imaging modality with neck infections
    - To determine site of infection and adenopathy
    - Localizing for aspiration or surgical planning
  - CECT has excellent spatial and contrast resolution
    - Allows determination of focal absence of enhancement indicating pus
  - Carefully evaluate bone CT images
    - Exclude dental infection and salivary gland calculus disease as cause
- Protocol advice
  - Contrast should be administered to best appreciate extent of suppurative changes

DIFFERENTIAL DIAGNOSIS

Squamous Cell Carcinoma Nodes

- Usually painless, hard nodes; no hot overlying skin
- On imaging may have nodularity of enhancing wall
- Typically no adjacent inflammation unless extracapsular spread
- Primary tumor mass often evident

2nd Branchial Cleft Anomaly

- 2nd branchial cleft cyst mimics suppurative or metastatic level II node
- Solitary unilateral mass, posterior to submandibular gland
- No inflammation of surrounding tissues unless secondarily infected

Nontuberculosis *Mycobacterium* Lymph Nodes

- Asymmetric enlarged nodes with adjacent subcutaneous necrotic ring-enhancing masses
- Minimal or absent subcutaneous fat stranding
- Purified protein derivative (PPD) skin test weakly reactive in ~ 55%, interferon-γ release assay usually negative
- Pediatric age group; usually ≤ 5 years of age

Tuberculosis Lymph Nodes

- Painless, low jugular and posterior cervical low-density nodes
- Calcification may be present
- Strongly reactive tuberculosis (PPD) skin test, positive interferon-γ release assay
- Systemically unwell with pulmonary infection

Fatty Nodal Metaplasia

- Chronic inflammation results in fatty change of nodal hilus
- Fat density on CT; fat intensity on MR
- Well-defined node, no inflammatory change

PATHOLOGY

General Features

- Etiology
  - Primary H&N infection

– Adjacent lymph nodes enlarge in reaction to pathogen: **Reactive nodes**
– Intranodal exudate forms containing protein-rich fluid with dead neutrophils (pus): **Suppurative nodes**
– If untreated or incorrectly treated, suppurative nodes rupture, then interstitial pus is walled-off by immune system: **Abscess** in soft tissues
○ Reactive nodes from viral pathogen may have 2° bacterial superinfection creating suppurative nodes
- Associated abnormalities
  ○ Primary causes of H&N infection include pharyngitis, salivary gland ductal calculus, dental decay ± mandibular osteomyelitis

Gross Pathologic & Surgical Features

- Fluctuant neck mass with erythematous, warm skin
- Aspiration of pus is diagnostic

Microscopic Features

- Acute inflammatory cell infiltrate in necrotic background
  ○ Presence of neutrophils and macrophages
  ○ Negative staining for acid-fast bacilli
- *Staphylococcus* and *Streptococcus* most frequent organisms
  ○ Increasing incidence of MRSA
- Pediatric infections show clustering of organisms by age
  ○ Infants < 1 year: *Staphylococcus aureus*, group B *Streptococcus*
  ○ Children 1-4 years: *S. aureus,* group A β-hemolytic *Streptococcus*, atypical mycobacteria
  ○ 5-15 years: Anaerobic bacteria, toxoplasmosis, cat scratch disease, tuberculosis
- Dental infections: Typically polymicrobial; predominantly anaerobic organisms

CLINICAL ISSUES

Presentation

- Most common signs/symptoms
  ○ Painful neck mass(es)
    – Often reddened, hot overlying skin
  ○ Fever, poor oral intake
  ○ Elevated WBC and ESR
- Other signs/symptoms
  ○ Other symptoms referable to primary source of infection
    – Pharyngeal/laryngeal infection: May have drooling, respiratory distress
    – Peritonsillar infection: May have trismus
    – Retropharyngeal or paravertebral infection: May have neck stiffness
- Clinical profile
  ○ Young patient presents with acute/subacute onset of tender neck mass and fever

Demographics

- Age
  ○ Most commonly seen in pediatric and young adult population
  ○ Odontogenic neck infections: Adults > > children

Natural History & Prognosis

- Conglomeration of suppurative nodes or rupture of node results in abscess formation

○ Superficial neck abscesses: Anterior or posterior cervical space, submandibular space
○ Deep neck abscesses: Retropharyngeal or parapharyngeal space
- Deep space abscesses can rapidly progress with airway compromise

Treatment

- Antibiotics only for small suppurative nodes and primary infection
- Incision and drainage for large suppurative nodes, abscesses, or poor response to antibiotics
  ○ Role for CT and US-guided aspiration for minimally invasive management
- Nodes from atypical mycobacteria should be excised to prevent recurrence or fistula/sinus tract

DIAGNOSTIC CHECKLIST

Consider

- Pediatric patient
  ○ Consider nontuberculous mycobacterial adenitis if no significant inflammatory changes
- Adult patient
  ○ Consider metastatic squamous cell carcinoma or thyroid carcinoma with necrotic or cystic nodes
    – Especially if inflammatory history or signs are absent
  ○ Look for tooth infection ± mandibular osteomyelitis if no other cause

Image Interpretation Pearls

- Fatty metaplasia with chronic infection can mimic pus formation
  ○ Look for fat in node
  ○ No surrounding cellulitis present
- Look for primary infectious source on images
  ○ Pharyngitis, dental infection, salivary gland calculi
- Evaluate airway for compromise with any neck infection
  ○ Bigger problem in deep infections
- Evaluate vascular structures for thrombophlebitis

SELECTED REFERENCES

1. Eisenmenger LB et al: Imaging of head and neck lymph nodes. Radiol Clin North Am. 53(1):115-32, 2015
2. Worley ML et al: Suppurative cervical lymphadenitis in infancy: microbiology and sociology. Clin Pediatr (Phila). 54(7):629-34, 2015
3. Georget E et al: Acute cervical lymphadenitis and infections of the retropharyngeal and parapharyngeal spaces in children. BMC Ear Nose Throat Disord. 14:8, 2014
4. Martin CA et al: Contribution of CT scan and CT-guided aspiration in the management of retropharyngeal abscess in children based on a series of 18 cases. Eur Ann Otorhinolaryngol Head Neck Dis. 131(5):277-82, 2014
5. Kato H et al: Necrotic cervical nodes: usefulness of diffusion-weighted MR imaging in the differentiation of suppurative lymphadenitis from malignancy. Eur J Radiol. 82(1):e28-35, 2013
6. Sauer MW et al: Acute neck infections in children: who is likely to undergo surgical drainage? Am J Emerg Med. 31(6):906-9, 2013
7. Hegde AN et al: Imaging in infections of the head and neck. Neuroimaging Clin N Am. 22(4):727-54, 2012
8. Koç O et al: Role of diffusion weighted MR in the discrimination diagnosis of the cystic and/or necrotic head and neck lesions. Eur J Radiol. 62(2):205-13, 2007
9. Ahuja A et al: An overview of neck node sonography. Invest Radiol. 37(6):333-42, 2002
10. Hudgins PA: Nodal and nonnodal inflammatory processes of the pediatric neck. Neuroimaging Clin N Am. 10(1):181-92, ix, 2000

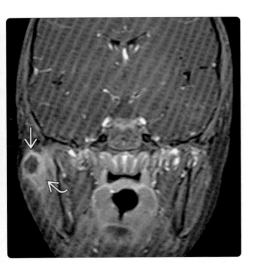

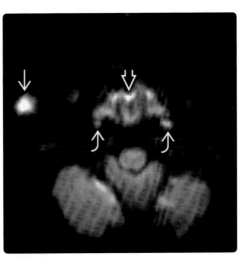

(Left) *Coronal T1 C+ FS MR in an 8-year-old boy with right cheek swelling shows a peripherally enhancing, centrally necrotic intraparotid mass ➡ with adjacent inflammatory stranding ➡. Fine-needle aspiration revealed suppurative adenitis.* **(Right)** *Axial DWI trace in the same patient shows the parotid mass ➡ to have central reduced diffusivity, typical of suppurative adenitis. Note reactive enlargement of the nasopharyngeal lymphoid tissue ➡ and reactive retropharyngeal lymph nodes ➡.*

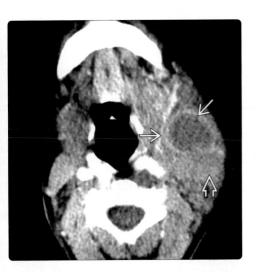

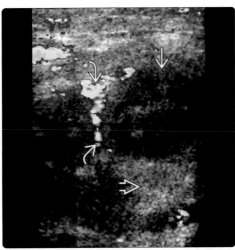

(Left) *Axial CECT demonstrates a well-defined, low-density submandibular mass with thin peripheral rim enhancement ➡. Suppurative node is associated with extensive inflammation of left neck tissues, sternocleidomastoid muscle, and solid reactive adenopathy ➡.* **(Right)** *Longitudinal ultrasound of suppurative IB node shows hypoechoic rounded mass ➡ with increased through transmission ➡, indicating cystic contents. Color Doppler reveals increased vascularity at periphery ➡.*

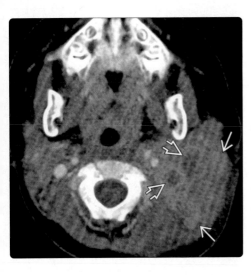

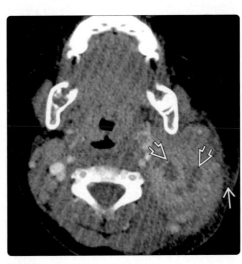

(Left) *Axial CECT in a young child shows a conglomerate transspatial upper neck mass with focal areas of low density ➡, indicating suppurative changes. Conglomerate mass additionally contains solid, reactive nodes ➡.* **(Right)** *Axial CECT more inferiorly in the same patient reveals further focal areas of pus ➡ in this conglomeration of nodes. Stranding of subcutaneous fat ➡ superficial to mass suggests infectious cause. Aspirated pus revealed Staphylococcus aureus.*

Tuberculous Lymph Nodes

TERMINOLOGY

- Cervical TB adenitis
- Adenopathy due to *Mycobacterium tuberculosis* infection

IMAGING

- Conglomerate nodal mass most commonly with **thick** enhancing rim and central necrosis
- Inflammatory changes often seen
- Obtain CXR if TB suspected

TOP DIFFERENTIAL DIAGNOSES

- Non-TB *Mycobacterium* nodes
- Cat-scratch disease
- Suppurative nodes
- Kikuchi-Fujimoto disease

PATHOLOGY

- **Caseating granulomas**, smear for acid-fast bacilli
- Excisional biopsy more sensitive than FNA

CLINICAL ISSUES

- Cervical nodes #1 site of extrapulmonary TB adenopathy
- Most common cause of adenopathy worldwide
- Increasing incidence in USA
  - Increasing prevalence of AIDS, immunosuppressive drugs, immigrants from endemic countries
- Systemically unwell patients with pulmonary disease
- 80-100% strongly **reactive skin test (PPD)**, interferon-γ release assay more sensitive
- PPD may be negative with immunodeficiency
- Treat with 4-drug regimen

DIAGNOSTIC CHECKLIST

- Consider when inflammatory changes associated with necrotic nodal masses
- Rim enhancement most commonly thick and irregular
- Must consider if patient may be immunosuppressed
- Suspicion for TB warrants **immediate** call to ordering physician

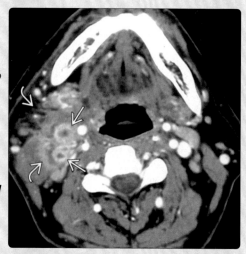
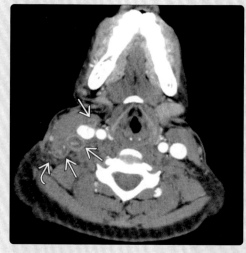

(Left) Axial CECT shows multiple necrotic cervical nodes ➡ with thick rim enhancement, typical of TB. Marked extranodal inflammatory changes are also evident ⬈. (Right) Axial CECT in a Sudanese woman with tuberculous lymphadenitis unresponsive to medical therapy demonstrates multiple necrotic cervical lymph nodes ➡. Note adjacent stranding/edema in the posterior cervical space ➡ related to active inflammation.

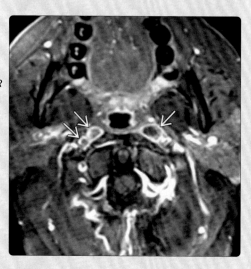
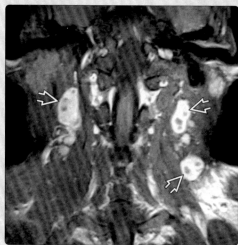

(Left) Axial T1WI C+ FS demonstrates bilateral intensely enhancing, but centrally necrotic, retropharyngeal nodes ➡. (Right) Coronal T1WI C+ FS MR in the same patient shows markedly enhancing nodes ➡ in posterior cervical chains bilaterally but without significant surrounding inflammatory changes. Large nodes have focal areas of low signal intensity representing caseation necrosis. Patient was otherwise asymptomatic, but biopsy revealed granulomas and M. tuberculosis infection.

TERMINOLOGY

Abbreviations

- Tuberculosis (TB) lymph nodes

Definitions

- Adenopathy due to *Mycobacterium tuberculosis* infection

IMAGING

General Features

- Best diagnostic clue
  - Most commonly **thick rim-enhancing nodal mass** with central necrosis & inflammatory changes
- Location
  - Cervical nodes #1 site of extrapulmonary TB adenopathy

Imaging Recommendations

- Best imaging tool
  - CECT for nodal necrosis ± calcifications

Radiographic Findings

- Radiography
  - Obtain CXR if TB suspected

CT Findings

- CECT
  - Node or nodal cluster with cystic changes
  - Rim enhancement typically **thick** and irregular
  - **Nodal calcification** may be evident
  - Adjacent inflammatory changes typical

MR Findings

- T1WI C+ FS
  - Centrally necrotic nodal mass or multiple nodes
  - Thick, irregularly enhancing nodal periphery

Ultrasonographic Findings

- Grayscale ultrasound
  - Cluster of predominantly hypoechoic nodes with adjacent inflammation
- Color Doppler
  - Vascular resistance: Reactive nodes < TB nodes < malignant nodes

Nuclear Medicine Findings

- PET/CT
  - Increased FDG uptake in active disease; may be valuable for monitoring disease status in HIV patients

DIFFERENTIAL DIAGNOSIS

Non-TB *Mycobacterium* Nodes

- Systemically well child, usually < 5 yr
- Persistent preauricular or submandibular node(s)

Cat-Scratch Disease

- Reactive adenopathy in nodes draining skin lesion
- Occurs 1-2 weeks following scratch incident

Suppurative Lymph Nodes

- Typically stranding of fat and adjacent structures
- Systemically unwell with fever, painful mass

PATHOLOGY

General Features

- Etiology
  - Transmission by aerosolized droplets
- Associated abnormalities
  - Concurrent inguinal/axillary adenopathy more common in HIV-positive patients

Gross Pathologic & Surgical Features

- Nodes rubbery or firm and matted with induration of overlying skin
  - ~ 10% have fistula

Microscopic Features

- Caseating granulomas, smear for acid-fast bacilli (AFB)
- Gold standard: AFB culture with sensitivity
- Excisional biopsy more sensitive than FNA

CLINICAL ISSUES

Presentation

- Most common signs/symptoms
  - Painless enlargement of cervical node(s)
  - Systemically unwell with pulmonary disease
    - Fever, night sweats, weight loss, cough
- Other signs/symptoms
  - 80-100% strongly reactive tuberculin skin test with purified protein-derivative (PPD)
  - PPD may be negative with immunodeficiency
  - Newer interferon-γ release assays more sensitive (> 95%) than PPD

Demographics

- Age
  - Peak: 20-30 yr, M < F
- Epidemiology
  - Most common cause of adenopathy worldwide
  - Increasing incidence in USA
    - Increasing prevalence of AIDS
  - Increasing multidrug resistance

Treatment

- Medical therapy with 4-drug regimen
- Surgery reserved for residual enlarged nodes, inadequate response to medical therapy

DIAGNOSTIC CHECKLIST

Consider

- Patients typically unwell, ± immunosuppressed, abnormal CXR, abnormal PPD or interferon-γ release assay

Image Interpretation Pearls

- Necrotic nodes most commonly with thick, irregular rim enhancement
- Associated inflammatory changes favor infection

SELECTED REFERENCES

1. Oishi M et al: Clinical study of extrapulmonary head and neck tuberculosis: a single-institute 10-year experience. Int Arch Otorhinolaryngol. 20(1):30-3, 2016
2. Vorster M et al: Advances in imaging of tuberculosis: the role of ¹⁸F-FDG PET and PET/CT. Curr Opin Pulm Med. 20(3):287-93, 2014

Non-TB *Mycobacterium* Nodes

TERMINOLOGY

- Non-TB *Mycobacterium* (NTM) nodes: Chronic neck infection with NTM
- Most often *Mycobacterium avium* **complex**

IMAGING

- Unilateral submandibular or preauricular painless mass in afebrile young child
- CXR: No pulmonary disease
- Ultrasound for neck mass evaluation and FNA
- CECT: Rim-enhancing, cystic-appearing node(s)
  - Minimal surrounding inflammatory changes

TOP DIFFERENTIAL DIAGNOSES

- Suppurative lymph nodes
- Tuberculosis lymph nodes
- Cat scratch disease
- 2nd branchial cleft anomaly

PATHOLOGY

- Necrotizing granulomatous inflammation with acid-fast bacilli (Z-N stain)
- NTM creates fistula to skin surface if untreated

CLINICAL ISSUES

- Increasing incidence in immunosuppressed patients
- PPD test may be weakly reactive; **interferon γ release assay** usually negative (may effectively rule out TB)
- Complete excision has > 90% success rate
- Antimycobacterial agents as adjuvant therapy
- I and D alone has 16-27% recurrence rate

DIAGNOSTIC CHECKLIST

- Always consider when cervical nodal mass not responding to standard treatment
- Consider if necrotic node with minimal surrounding inflammation
- Especially afebrile child < 5 years with painless mass

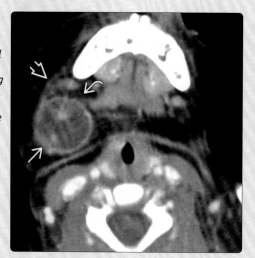
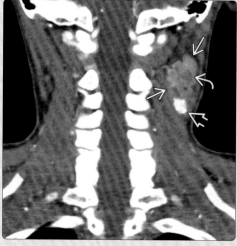

(Left) *Axial CECT of a child with non-TB Mycobacterium (NTM) adenitis shows a large, necrotic, submandibular nodal mass →. Stranding of adjacent fat ➦ and thickening of the platysma ⇨ is minimal. When history is of short duration, fat stranding may be more conspicuous. Nodal calcification is not evident.* (Right) *Coronal CECT in a different child with chronic NTM adenitis shows a conglomerate nodal mass → with internal cystic/necrotic regions ➦ and coarse calcification ⇨.*

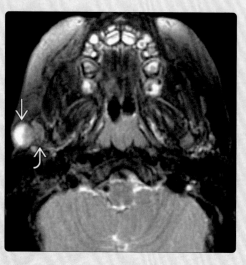
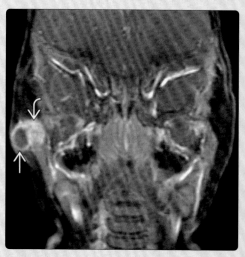

(Left) *Axial T2 FS MR in an 11 month old with right preauricular mass demonstrates a well-defined, predominantly hyperintense lesion → in subcutaneous tissues of right cheek, abutting superficial lobe of right parotid gland ➦. There is no evidence of infiltration of surrounding subcutaneous fat.* (Right) *Coronal T1 C+ FS MR in the same child reveals lesion → to be cystic with peripheral enhancement and shows inflammation of adjacent superficial parotid lobe ➦. FNA revealed Mycobacterium avium complex.*

Sarcoidosis Lymph Nodes

KEY FACTS

TERMINOLOGY

- **Noncaseating granulomatous** inflammatory disease of unknown etiology

IMAGING

- Nonnecrotic, homogeneous, smoothly enlarged lymph nodes
- Nodal calcification may be present on CT
- Mild nodal enhancement with CT or MR
- PET/CT may be useful for assessing extent of systemic disease or determining site for biopsy
  - SUV frequently > 3.0; up to 15
- DWI may be of some value in differentiating FDG-avid sarcoidosis nodes from malignancy
  - Typically higher ADC value than malignant nodes; **CAUTION**: Appropriate thresholds not defined

TOP DIFFERENTIAL DIAGNOSES

- Reactive lymph nodes

- Non-Hodgkin lymphoma nodes
- Histiocytic necrotizing lymphadenitis (Kikuchi-Fujimoto)
- Kimura disease

PATHOLOGY

- Unknown cause; probably result of immune response to various environmental triggers

CLINICAL ISSUES

- Usually develops < 50 years, peak at 20-39 years
- F > M
- > 90% of patients have thoracic nodes, pulmonary, skin, ± ocular sarcoid
- Fatigue, night sweats, and weight loss are common

DIAGNOSTIC CHECKLIST

- Diagnosis of exclusion
- Include in differential diagnosis when "reactive" or lymphoma-like nodes seen
- Search upper thorax on neck CT for pulmonary disease

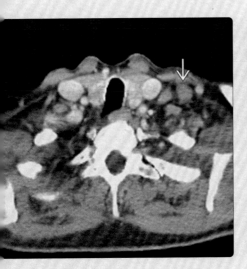

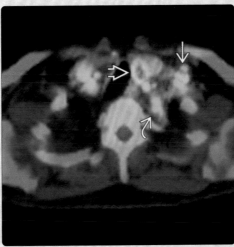

(Left) Axial CECT shows nonspecific enlargement of left supraclavicular lymph node ➡ without necrosis. Other enlarged cervical and mediastinal nodes (not shown) raise concern for lymphoma versus sarcoidosis. (Right) Fused axial FDG-PET/CT in the same patient shows increased FDG uptake in left supraclavicular node ➡, as well as other mildly FDG-avid nodes ➡. Biopsy revealed noncaseating granulomas, confirming sarcoidosis. Diffuse thyroid FDG uptake ➡ reflects thyroiditis, not uncommon in sarcoidosis.

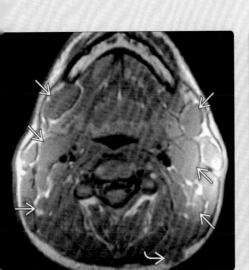

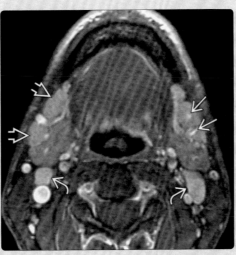

(Left) Axial T1WI MR reveals diffuse smoothly enlarged cervical lymph nodes ➡ bilaterally without evidence of necrosis. A left suboccipital node is evident ➡. Imaging differential of this appearance is non-Hodgkin lymphoma, reactive adenopathy, and less commonly sarcoidosis. (Right) Axial T1WI C+ FS MR reveals bilateral enlarged, ovoid submandibular ➡ and upper jugular nodes ➡ in a patient with sarcoidosis. Central linear intranodal enhancement ➡, typically found in reactive nodes, is evident in multiple lymph nodes.

Giant Lymph Node Hyperplasia (Castleman Disease)

TERMINOLOGY

- Castleman disease (CD)
- Multicentric Castleman disease (MCD)
- Uncommon benign idiopathic hypervascular polyclonal lymphoid hyperplasia
- Clinical subtypes: **Unifocal** (90%) and **multicentric**
- Histologic subtypes
  - Hyaline vascular (90%)
  - Plasma cell (< 10%)
  - Human herpesvirus 8 (HHV-8) related
  - MCD not otherwise specified

IMAGING

- Most often mediastinum (70%), then H&N (15%)
- > 90% of H&N lesions are unifocal disease
- Moderate to markedly enhancing nodal mass
- CECT: Central **nonenhancing scar**; uncommon
- T2 MR: Hypointense **striations** described; uncommon
- Hypoechoic on US with intense peripheral vascular flow

TOP DIFFERENTIAL DIAGNOSES

- Non-Hodgkin lymphoma lymph nodes
- Reactive lymph nodes
- Differentiated thyroid carcinoma
- Carotid body paraganglioma

PATHOLOGY

- Unclear etiology, likely related to interleukin-6
- Most often unifocal, hyaline vascular type, asymptomatic
- Multifocal form rare, plasma cell type, symptomatic
- Diagnosis requires core biopsy or node excision

CLINICAL ISSUES

- Unifocal CD: Surgery curative
- MCD: Variable, aggressive course

DIAGNOSTIC CHECKLIST

- CT and MR often nonspecific
- Consider with strongly enhancing nodal mass

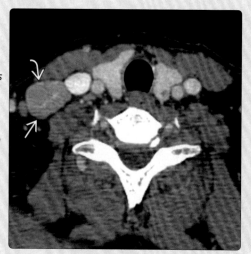
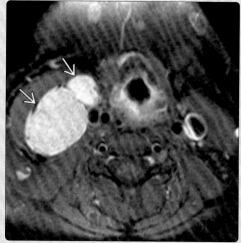

(Left) *Axial CECT for palpable neck mass shows a solitary, mildly enlarged lymph node ➡. There is homogeneous enhancement with associated prominent vessels ➡. This was unifocal hyaline vascular variant of Castleman disease (CD) cured with surgical resection.* (Right) *Axial T1 C+ FS MR in a different adult with hyaline vascular type of CD reveals right internal jugular chain nodes ➡ with uniform enhancement. The more posterior node is markedly enlarged. This is not evidence of extracapsular spread or inflammation.*

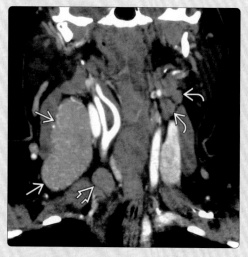
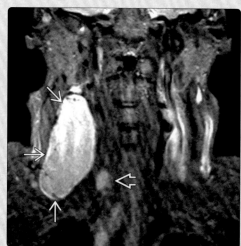

(Left) *Coronally reformatted CECT shows a large, homogeneous, moderately enhancing node ➡ along the right internal jugular chain. Also seen are additional smaller, less enhancing nodes in low-level VI ➡ and along contralateral jugular chain ➡.* (Right) *Coronal T2WI FS MR in the same patient shows a large node ➡ to be markedly homogeneously hyperintense with no intranodal necrosis or inflammatory changes surrounding node. A smaller, moderately hyperintense node ➡ is also evident.*

TERMINOLOGY

Abbreviations

- Castleman disease (CD)
- Multicentric Castleman disease (MCD)

Synonyms

- Angiofollicular lymphoid hyperplasia, follicular lymphoreticuloma, angiomatous lymphoid hamartoma, lymph nodal hamartoma

Definitions

- Uncommon benign hypervascular nonclonal lymphoproliferative disorder
  - Clinical subtypes: **Unifocal** and **multicentric** (MCD)
  - Histologic classification
    - Hyaline vascular (90%)
    - Plasma cell (< 10%)
    - Human herpesvirus 8 (HHV-8) related
    - MCD not otherwise specified

IMAGING

General Features

- Best diagnostic clue
  - Solitary, **moderate to markedly enhancing** nodal mass
- Location
  - Most frequently chest (70%), H&N (15%)
  - Single node or adjacent nodes (unifocal) or multiple nodal groups (multicentric)
    - > 90% H&N lesions are **unifocal** disease
  - Rare extranodal neck locations reported
    - Parotid, submandibular gland, palate, larynx, parapharyngeal space, and floor of mouth
- Size
  - Variable: 5-10 cm
- Morphology
  - Ovoid neck mass

CT Findings

- NECT
  - Well-circumscribed, homogeneous oval mass, isodense to muscle
  - Calcifications uncommon in neck
- CECT
  - Moderate to marked homogeneous contrast enhancement
  - Prominent adjacent vessels are common
  - Central nonenhancing scar described, not often seen

MR Findings

- T1WI
  - Hypointense or isointense to muscle
- T2WI
  - Hyperintense ovoid nodal mass or masses
  - Branching T2 hypointense **striations** described but not often found
- T1WI C+
  - Moderate to marked homogeneous contrast enhancement

Ultrasonographic Findings

- Grayscale ultrasound
  - Homogeneous hypoechoic mass
  - Posterior acoustic enhancement
- Color Doppler
  - Intense peripheral vascular flow, small scattered foci centrally

Nuclear Medicine Findings

- PET
  - Mild to moderate FDG uptake in unifocal CD
  - Higher FDG uptake in MCD

Imaging Recommendations

- Best imaging tool
  - CT usually initial modality for evaluation of neck mass
  - PET/CT helpful in evaluation of MCD
- Protocol advice
  - Contrast administration essential for CT
  - Evaluate MR carefully for striations on T2WI

DIFFERENTIAL DIAGNOSIS

Non-Hodgkin Lymphoma Nodes

- Usually multiple enlarged nodes, frequently bilateral
- Homogeneous, mild contrast enhancement

Reactive Lymph Nodes

- More often multiple moderate-sized nodes
- Variable enhancement, ± inflammation

Differentiated Thyroid Carcinoma

- May be enhancing nodal mass ± cystic change ± calcifications
- Primary intrathyroidal tumor may be small

Carotid Body Paraganglioma

- Splays internal and external carotid arteries
- CECT: Enhances to same degree as adjacent vessels
- T1WI MR: Flow voids present

PATHOLOGY

General Features

- Etiology
  - Poorly understood, likely exaggerated immune response similar to process with normal antigenic stimuli
  - Related to excessive interleukin-6 (IL-6) production
    - Inappropriate immune response to chronic antigenic stimulation or infectious agent
    - Induces vascular endothelial growth factor production
  - Multicentric form has been associated with HHV-8 and AIDS
    - HHV-8-infected cells secrete viral encoded IL-6

Staging, Grading, & Classification

- Unifocal form most common, most often hyaline vascular histology
- Multifocal form rare, frequently plasma cell histology

Gross Pathologic & Surgical Features

- Smooth to nodular well-circumscribed mass
- Firm, rubbery texture

Microscopic Features

- Diagnosis requires core biopsy or node excision
- **Hyaline vascular (90%)**
  - Most often unifocal and asymptomatic
  - Irregularly shaped, enlarged nodes with radially arranged capillaries penetrating germinal center
    - So-called lollipop pattern
  - Germinal centers enveloped by concentric layers of mature lymphocytes
  - Interfollicular stroma with prominent hyalinized vascular network
- **Plasma cell (9%)**
  - Most often multicentric form
  - > 50% systemic symptoms and serologic abnormalities
  - Dense perisinusoidal and interfollicular plasmacytosis
  - Less prominent vascular network and less hyalinization
- Flow cytometry in both types shows polyclonal B-cell lymphocyte expansion
- **Mixed (hyaline vascular + plasma cell) < 1%**

CLINICAL ISSUES

Presentation

- Most common signs/symptoms
  - Most often unifocal form, usually asymptomatic or palpable mass
  - Multicentric form ± plasma cell type frequently symptomatic
    - Fever, diaphoresis, fatigue, weight loss, and hepatosplenomegaly
  - Multicentric form ± plasma cell type often abnormal serology
    - Anemia, hyperglobulinemia, polyclonal gammopathy, leukocytosis, plasmacytosis, hypoalbuminemia
    - Elevated or reduced platelet count
  - 50% plasma cell types have elevated ESR
- Clinical profile
  - Patients usually present with asymptomatic neck mass

Demographics

- Age
  - Occurs in all age groups, though H&N disease rare in children
  - Peak incidence: 2nd to 4th decades
  - Older age for MCD: 5th and 6th decades
- Gender
  - M = F
- Epidemiology
  - Rare cause of neck mass
  - Usually unifocal form in neck
    - 98% are hyaline vascular type

Natural History & Prognosis

- Enlargement of masses may result in compression of adjacent structures
- **Unifocal: Benign** course, surgery curative
- **Multicentric**: Variable course, most poor prognosis
  - More rapid progression and poor outcomes in AIDS and HHV-8
  - Not uncommon for multicentric form to have malignant transformation

- Transform into non-Hodgkin lymphoma (10-15%) or Kaposi sarcoma (13%)

Treatment

- Unifocal form
  - Surgical excision treatment of choice
    - 100% cure with complete resection
    - Preoperative embolization can reduce blood loss and facilitate total excision
  - If unresectable, surgical debulking followed by systemic therapy
  - Limited indication for radiation therapy
- Multicentric form
  - Chemotherapy then steroids to prevent relapse
  - Radiotherapy for palliation of obstructive or compressive symptoms
  - Careful observation for recurrence and malignant transformation

DIAGNOSTIC CHECKLIST

Consider

- **Unifocal form** usually hyaline vascular, asymptomatic, and cured with excision
- **Multicentric form** usually plasma cell type, often symptomatic, and aggressive disease course
- FNA usually not diagnostic, core biopsy or nodal excision required

Image Interpretation Pearls

- While CT or MR may be suggestive, findings are often nonspecific
- Consider with moderate to markedly enhancing mass along jugular nodal chain with prominent adjacent vessels
- Rare findings of focal **nonenhancing scar** (CECT) or **hypointense striations** (T2 MR) suggest diagnosis
- Also consider when focal, possibly transspatial, large, moderate to markedly enhancing neck mass

SELECTED REFERENCES

1. Hill AJ et al: Multimodality imaging and clinical features in Castleman disease: single institute experience in 30 patients. Br J Radiol. 20140670, 2015
2. Jiang XH et al: Castleman disease of the neck: CT and MR imaging findings. Eur J Radiol. 83(11):2041-50, 2014
3. Chen YF et al: Clinical features and outcomes of head and neck castleman disease. J Oral Maxillofac Surg. 70(10):2466-79, 2012
4. Bonekamp D et al: Castleman disease: the great mimic. Radiographics. 31(6):1793-807, 2011
5. Barker R et al: FDG-PET/CT imaging in the management of HIV-associated multicentric Castleman's disease. Eur J Nucl Med Mol Imaging. 36(4):648-52, 2009
6. Cronin DM et al: Castleman disease: an update on classification and the spectrum of associated lesions. Adv Anat Pathol. 16(4):236-46, 2009
7. Gupta A et al: Multicentric hyaline-vascular type Castleman disease presenting as an epidural mass causing paraplegia: a case report. Clin Lymphoma Myeloma. 9(3):250-3, 2009
8. Ozgursoy OB et al: Castleman disease in the parapharyngeal space: unusual presentation and differential diagnostic imaging features of the disease. J Otolaryngol Head Neck Surg. 38(5):E118-20, 2009
9. Rao HG et al: Unusual location for Castleman's disease. J Laryngol Otol. 123(1):e3, 2009
10. Barker R et al: Imaging in multicentric Castleman's disease. J HIV Ther. 13(3):72-4, 2008
11. Souza KC et al: Cervical Castleman's disease in childhood. J Oral Maxillofac Surg. 66(5):1067-72, 2008

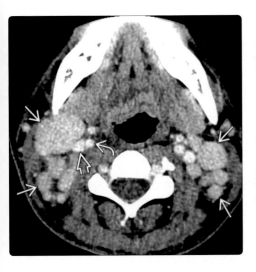
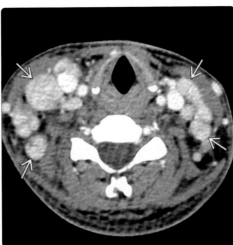

(Left) Axial CECT in a teenage girl with extensive bilateral cervical adenopathy shows multiple cervical nodes ➡ of varying size, with enhancement nearly as intense as internal carotid artery ➡ and jugular vein ➡. (Right) Axial CECT in the same patient shows additional adenopathy ➡ without evidence of necrosis, calcification, or surrounding inflammatory changes. Lymph node biopsy proved CD of mixed hyaline vascular and plasma cell type. This is the rarest form of CD.

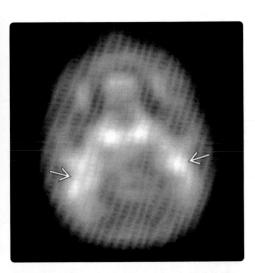
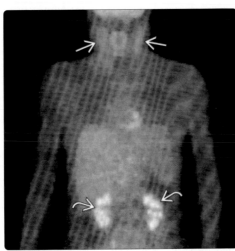

(Left) Axial FDG PET study performed 2 days after CT in the same patient reveals mild uptake in the neck ➡. (Right) Anteroposterior PET in the same patient demonstrates no evidence of significant FDG uptake through the rest of the body and only mild uptake in the neck ➡. Renal activity was normal ➡.

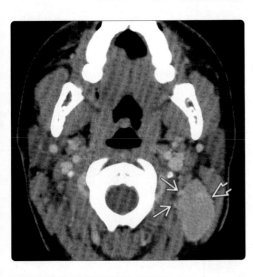
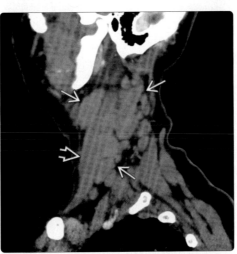

(Left) Axial CECT in a teenage girl demonstrates an enlarged, avidly enhancing, left level IIB lymph node ➡. Notice the prominent adjacent vessels ➡. This was the hyaline vascular variant of unicentric CD. (Right) Parasagittal CECT of the neck shows diffuse enlarged lymph nodes ➡ surrounding the sternocleidomastoid ➡. These do not demonstrate the avid enhancement of previous cases. This patient has the plasma cell variant of CD as well as multicentric disease.

Histiocytic Necrotizing Lymphadenitis (Kikuchi-Fujimoto)

KEY FACTS

TERMINOLOGY

- Histiocytic necrotizing lymphadenitis
- Synonym: Kikuchi-Fujimoto disease
- Benign idiopathic necrotizing cervical adenitis of **young Asian adults**

IMAGING

- **Unilateral**, homogeneous, mildly enlarged nodes with **inflammatory stranding**
- Posterior cervical and jugular chain
- Nodes appear solid or rim enhancing, but not necessarily necrotic on imaging

TOP DIFFERENTIAL DIAGNOSES

- Non-Hodgkin lymphoma lymph nodes
- Systemic nodal metastases
- Cat scratch disease
- Tuberculosis lymph nodes

PATHOLOGY

- Cortical and paracortical coagulative necrosis
- Cellular infiltrate of histiocytes and immunoblasts
- Possibly exuberant T-cell-mediated immune response to variety of nonspecific stimuli
- Associated with increased incidence of systemic lupus erythematosus
- Higher **Japanese** and other **Asian** incidence may be due to *HLA* genes

CLINICAL ISSUES

- Most commonly in Asian women in 3rd decade
- Tender unilateral posterior neck nodes and high fever
- 30-50% have other systemic symptoms
- Usually resolves without treatment in 1-4 months

DIAGNOSTIC CHECKLIST

- Symptoms, imaging, & histology mimic lymphoma
- Diagnosis requires excisional biopsy

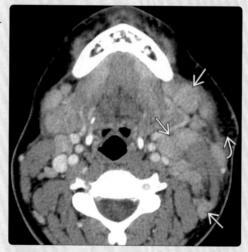
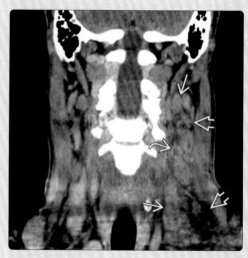

(Left) Axial CECT shows predominantly left-sided, well-defined, noncalcifying nodes ➡. Nodes have homogeneous moderate enhancement. Nodes appear somewhat matted, and there is adjacent stranding of subcutaneous fat ➡. (Right) Coronal CECT depicts numerous enlarged left jugular chain lymph nodes ➡. Some demonstrate rim enhancement ➡. Inflammatory fat stranding is present adjacent to the nodes ➡.

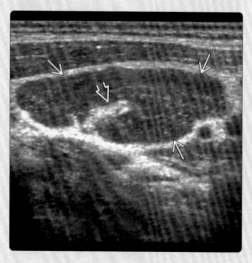
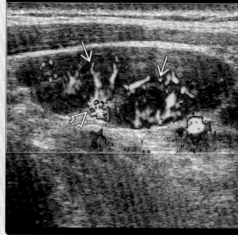

(Left) Longitudinal US obtained in posterior neck shows a hypoechoic enlarged node ➡ with a hypertrophied cortex but normal hilar architecture ➡ in a patient with histiocytic necrotizing lymphadenitis (Kikuchi-Fujimoto disease). Note the absence of associated soft tissue edema, intranodal necrosis, or matting of nodes. (Right) Power Doppler US in the same patient reveals prominent vascularity of the perihilar cortex ➡ and hilum ➡. This is a classic appearance of histiocytic necrotizing lymphadenitis.

TERMINOLOGY

Abbreviations

- Histiocytic necrotizing lymphadenitis (HNL)

Synonyms

- Kikuchi-Fujimoto disease

Definitions

- Benign idiopathic necrotizing cervical adenitis of **young Asian adults**

IMAGING

General Features

- Best diagnostic clue
  - Unilateral, homogeneous, mildly enlarged nodes, levels 2-5, with inflammatory stranding
- Location
  - Posterior cervical and jugular chain
  - Unilateral > bilateral
  - Mediastinal/abdominal nodes less common
- Size
  - Nodes usually 0.5-4.0 cm

CT Findings

- CECT
  - Mildly enlarged **nodes** with variable appearance
    - Homogeneously solid or rim-enhancing hypodense
  - Perinodal inflammatory changes

MR Findings

- T2WI
  - Central nonenhancing areas are not hyperintense
- T1WI C+ FS
  - Solidly enhancing or peripherally enhancing nodes

Ultrasonographic Findings

- Grayscale ultrasound
  - Homogeneous hypoechoic enlarged nodes with echogenic hilum
- Power Doppler
  - **Hypervascularity** of hilum

Nuclear Medicine Findings

- PET/CT
  - **Increased FDG uptake** in enlarged nodes

DIFFERENTIAL DIAGNOSIS

Non-Hodgkin Lymphoma Nodes

- Non-Hodgkin lymphoma (NHL) nodes often larger than HNL nodes
- Perinodal inflammation rare in NHL

Systemic Nodal Metastases

- Viral-like illness with HNL, uncommon with mets
- Necrosis in metastatic nodes hyperintense on T2

Cat Scratch Disease

- Regional adenopathy following scratch incident

Tuberculosis Lymph Nodes

- Typically accompanied by thoracic TB

PATHOLOGY

General Features

- Etiology
  - Unknown but probably infectious or autoimmune
- Genetics
  - Higher **Japanese** and other **Asian** incidence may be due to *HLA* genes
- Associated abnormalities
  - Well-reported increased incidence of systemic lupus erythematosus
  - Associated with other autoimmune disorders

Microscopic Features

- Excisional biopsy required for definitive diagnosis
- Necrosis is microscopic, not often macroscopic

CLINICAL ISSUES

Presentation

- Most common signs/symptoms
  - Tender unilateral posterior neck nodes & high fever
- Other signs/symptoms
  - 30-50% have extranodal involvement
    - Upper respiratory symptoms, malaise, headache
    - Mouth ulcers, hepatosplenomegaly, arthritis
  - Most laboratory tests are normal
    - May have leukopenia, raised ESR & CRP

Demographics

- Age
  - Adults < 30 years
- Gender
  - Female predominance
- Epidemiology
  - Most commonly in Asians, especially Japanese

Natural History & Prognosis

- Usually benign, self-limited over 1-4 months
- Uncommonly complicated course with poor outcome

Treatment

- Symptomatic: Nonsteroidal antiinflammatory drugs or oral steroids

DIAGNOSTIC CHECKLIST

Consider

- Symptoms, imaging, and histology mimic lymphoma
- Definitive diagnosis requires excisional biopsy

Image Interpretation Pearls

- Some features that should raise possibility of HNL
  - Young Japanese/Asian woman
  - Unilateral, homogeneous, moderately enlarged nodes, levels 2-5
  - Inflammatory changes with nodes

SELECTED REFERENCES

1. Dumas G et al: Kikuchi-fujimoto disease: retrospective study of 91 cases and review of the literature. Medicine (Baltimore). 93(24):372-82, 2014
2. Ludwig BJ et al: Imaging of cervical lymphadenopathy in children and young adults. AJR Am J Roentgenol. 199(5):1105-13, 2012

TERMINOLOGY

- Kimura disease (KD): Angiolymphoid proliferation with **serum eosinophilia** and elevated **IgE**
  - Inflammatory disorder with multiple H&N masses

IMAGING

- Classic triad
  - Subcutaneous and deep tissue masses of H&N
  - Salivary gland masses: Parotid > submandibular
  - Solid cervical lymphadenopathy
- CT or MR findings
  - Variable enhancement (CT) and signal (MR)
  - Due to varying vascularity and fibrosis

TOP DIFFERENTIAL DIAGNOSES

- Nodal non-Hodgkin lymphoma
- Parotid mucoepidermoid carcinoma
- Nodal sarcoidosis
- Parotid metastatic nodal disease

PATHOLOGY

- Unknown etiology; allergic and autoimmune theories favored
- ~ 50% have renal dysfunction

CLINICAL ISSUES

- Chronic, slowly progressive course over years
- Benign, can be self-limiting

DIAGNOSTIC CHECKLIST

- KD is great mimicker, like lymphoma
- Most common in **young Asian male patients**
- Diagnostic triad
  - Painless subcutaneous H&N masses with regional adenopathy
  - Blood and tissue eosinophilia
  - Markedly elevated serum IgE
- Recommend renal function tests

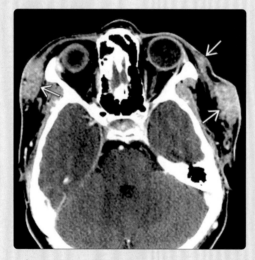
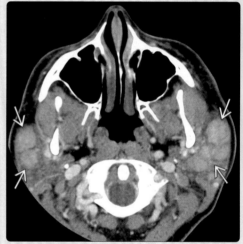

(Left) Axial CECT in a young Asian female patient with 9-year history of slowly enlarging forehead nodules reveals multiple bilateral subcutaneous plaque-like lesions ➡, with significant deformity of scalp and facial contours. (Right) Axial neck CECT in the same patient shows multiple bilateral enhancing intraparotid nodules ➡. Numerous enlarged cervical nodes were also present bilaterally (not shown). Biopsy of forehead lesion was revealed to be Kimura disease (KD).

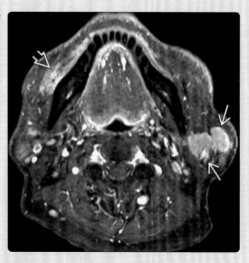
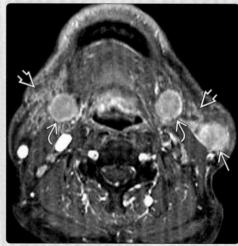

(Left) Axial T1WI C+ FS MR in a patient with KD demonstrates intensely enhancing left intraparotid masses ➡ within the left parotid gland. Ill-defined, enhancing infiltration of right cheek deep soft tissues ➡ is evident on contralateral side as well. (Right) More inferior axial T1WI C+ FS MR in the same patient shows bilateral enhancing submandibular lesions ➡ in addition to hazy, infiltrated appearance of deep and subcutaneous fat ➡ around them. Tail of parotid enhancing node is evident on left ➡.

TERMINOLOGY

Abbreviations
- Kimura disease (KD)

Synonyms
- Eosinophilic hyperplastic lymphogranuloma, eosinophilic lymphogranuloma, eosinophilic folliculosis

Definitions
- **Angiolymphoid proliferation with peripheral eosinophilia and elevated IgE**
- Benign chronic inflammatory disorder resulting in multiple masses of H&N
  - Primarily in **young Asian male patients**

IMAGING

General Features
- Best diagnostic clue
  - Imaging triad
    - Subcutaneous nodules, salivary gland masses, lymphadenopathy
  - Clinical triad
    - Painless firm nodes/nodules, blood and tissue eosinophilia, markedly elevated serum IgE
- Location
  - Subcutaneous and deep tissues of H&N
    - Rare sites: Orbit, lacrimal gland, hard palate, larynx, dura
  - Salivary gland: Parotid > submandibular
    - Less often minor salivary glands
  - Cervical lymphadenopathy very common (60-100%)
    - Occasionally axillary, inguinal, or antecubital fossa nodes
- Size
  - Average lesion: 3 cm (range: 2-11 cm)
- Morphology
  - Variable due to variation in vascular elements and fibrosis
  - Subcutaneous masses: Variable, commonly ill-defined borders
  - Salivary gland involvement may be diffuse infiltration, ill-defined mass, or intraparotid nodes
  - Enlarged nodes well defined, nonnecrotic

CT Findings
- CECT
  - **Subcutaneous masses**: Ill defined, plaque-like > focal, well defined
    - Plaque-like lesions have moderate or poor enhancement
      - May have overlying tissue atrophy
    - Well-defined lesions typically have intense enhancement
  - Nodes rounded, solid, with moderate-intense enhancement
    - Nodal enhancement tends to mirror lesion enhancement

MR Findings
- T1WI

- Isointense or hypointense nodal masses compared to parotid glands
- T2WI
  - Usually hyperintense
    - Chronic fibrotic lesions may be hypointense
- T1WI C+
  - Solidly enhancing nodes and masses characteristic
  - Less enhancement with chronic, fibrotic lesions

Ultrasonographic Findings
- Grayscale ultrasound
  - Poorly marginated subcutaneous masses
    - Hypoechoic with hyperechoic bands creates woolly appearance
  - Enlarged nodes solid and hypoechoic with homogeneous internal echoes
    - Preserved echogenic hilum
- Power Doppler
  - Prominent intranodal or intralesional vessels with low resistance

Nuclear Medicine Findings
- PET
  - Increased uptake of FDG
- Other nuclear medicine studies
  - Uptake of 111 In-pentetreotide, Tc-99m-labeled autologous granulocytes
  - Uptake of Tl-201 SPECT on early and delayed images

Imaging Recommendations
- Best imaging tool
  - CT or MR demonstrates nodes and masses
- Protocol advice
  - Contrast important for extent of nodal involvement and parotid evaluation

DIFFERENTIAL DIAGNOSIS

Nodal Non-Hodgkin Lymphoma
- Usually bilateral adenopathy
- No subcutaneous masses
- May also have involvement of Waldeyer ring

Parotid Mucoepidermoid Carcinoma
- Intraparotid or neck nodes associated
- No subcutaneous masses
- More subacute time course of onset
- Facial nerve palsy may be found clinically

Nodal Sarcoidosis
- Primary manifestation is multiple enlarged nodes
- Can involve entire parotid gland or intraparotid nodes
- Chest x-ray usually shows mediastinal adenopathy
- No subcutaneous masses

Parotid Metastatic Nodal Disease
- Multiple intraparotid nodes, often with necrosis
- Frequently squamous cell carcinoma or melanoma from local skin primary malignancy

PATHOLOGY

General Features

- Etiology
  - Unknown, though allergic and autoimmune theories favored because of elevated serum IgE
    - Altered T-cell immunoregulation or IgE-mediated type 1 hypersensitivity
    - Excessive production of eosinophilic cytokines, such as IL-4
  - Perhaps follows arthropod bites or infection: Virus, parasite, *Candida*
- Associated abnormalities
  - 15-60% have renal dysfunction including nephrotic syndrome
    - Can precede development of subcutaneous lesions
  - Associations with asthma, Loeffler syndrome, and connective tissue diseases reported

Gross Pathologic & Surgical Features

- Tumorous masses of subcutaneous tissues, salivary glands, and adenopathy
- Vascular, rubbery, fibrotic masses
- Nodes may form confluent mass ± adherent to overlying dermis

Microscopic Features

- Abnormal proliferation of lymphoid follicles and vascular endothelium with dense eosinophilic infiltrate
- Lymphoid hyperplasia with germinal centers containing cellular, vascular, and fibrous components
  - **Dense eosinophilic infiltrates** and eosinophilic microabscesses with central necrosis
  - Abundant plasma cells and lymphocytes (proliferation of HLA-DR CD4 cells)
  - Vascular proliferation and variable fibrosis around and within lesion
- Immunofluorescence studies
  - Germinal centers contain heavy **IgE deposits**
  - Variable IgG, IgM, and fibrinogen
- Previously considered 1 entity with angiolymphoid hyperplasia with eosinophilia (ALHE)
  - ALHE differs from KD clinically and histologically
    - H&N dermal nodules in middle-aged Caucasian women
    - Rarely adenopathy, 20% blood eosinophilia
  - Vascular proliferation and atypia suggest neoplasia more than inflammation

CLINICAL ISSUES

Presentation

- Most common signs/symptoms
  - Insidious onset of solitary or multiple painless swellings of H&N
    - Predominantly preauricular and submandibular
  - 60-100% cervical adenopathy
  - Laboratory
    - Peripheral eosinophilia and elevated serum IgE
- Other signs/symptoms
  - ~ 50% have renal disease
    - Most often extramembranous glomerulonephritis

- Proteinuria → nephrotic syndrome
- Evaluate for renal dysfunction with creatinine, BUN, and urinary protein
  - Occasional localized or generalized pruritus
  - Facial nerve palsy not reported with parotid involvement
- Clinical profile
  - 30-year-old Asian man with painless neck masses

Demographics

- Age
  - Onset peaks in 3rd decade
  - Rarer sites of occurrence tend to be older patients
- Gender
  - M:F = 3-10:1
- Ethnicity
  - Endemic in Asians, particularly Chinese and Japanese
  - Uncommon in Caucasians, rare in Africans

Natural History & Prognosis

- Chronic, slowly progressive course over years
- Potentially disfiguring
  - Large (≥ 5 cm) subcutaneous lesions may ulcerate
- Spontaneous resolution reported
- No malignant potential

Treatment

- Resection of mass lesion(s)
  - Up to 25% recur
- Intralesional or oral steroids may temporize, though not cure
- Cyclosporine A reported to induce remission
- Consider radiotherapy for persistent/problematic lesions
- Observation alone if not symptomatic or disfiguring

DIAGNOSTIC CHECKLIST

Consider

- KD is great mimicker, like lymphoma
- KD should be distinguished clinically and histologically from ALHE
- Recommend serology for IgE, eosinophil count, and renal function tests

Image Interpretation Pearls

- KD is difficult diagnosis to make by imaging alone
- Chronicity of masses or abnormal serology findings helpful
- Look for **triad of imaging findings**, particularly in Asian male patients
  - Subcutaneous enhancing nodules
  - Salivary gland masses or nodes
  - Cervical adenopathy

SELECTED REFERENCES

1. Lin YY et al: Kimura's disease: clinical and imaging parameters for the prediction of disease recurrence. Clin Imaging. 36(4):272-8, 2012
2. Park SW et al: Kimura disease: CT and MR imaging findings. AJNR Am J Neuroradiol. 33(4):784-8, 2012
3. Horikoshi T et al: Head and neck MRI of Kimura disease. Br J Radiol. 84(1005):800-4, 2011
4. Gopinathan A et al: Kimura's disease: imaging patterns on computed tomography. Clin Radiol. 64(10):994-9, 2009
5. Sun QF et al: Kimura disease: review of the literature. Intern Med J. 38(8):668-72, 2008

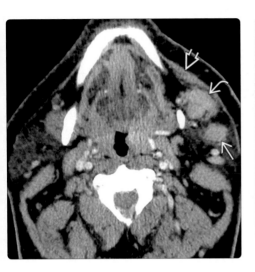
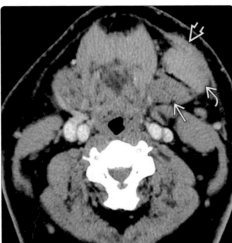

(Left) *Axial CECT in a patient with KD demonstrates a solid, mildly enhancing mass within tail of left parotid gland ➡ and additional smaller, mildly enhancing, and ill-defined left submandibular mass ➡. Infiltration and thickening of platysma ➡ is evident.* (Right) *A more inferior axial CECT in the same patient reveals the true size of submandibular space plaque-like mass ➡, displacing the submandibular gland ➡ posteriorly. Platysma muscle ➡ is thickened and ill defined. Mild enhancement suggests the more fibrotic form of KD.*

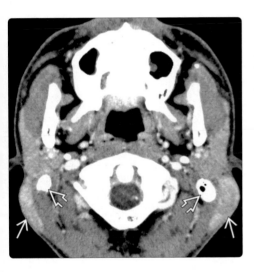
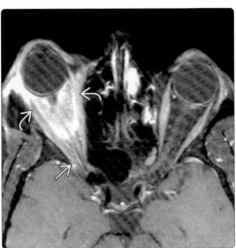

(Left) *Axial CECT in a teenage Asian boy presenting with left postauricular "cyst" shows bilateral subcutaneous heterogeneously enhancing plaques ➡ posterior to mastoid tips ➡. No parotid masses or significant adenopathy were evident in this pathology-proven case of KD.* (Right) *Axial T1WI C+ FS MR shows uncommon variant of KD. Infiltrating intensely enhancing homogeneous tissue ➡ involves entire right orbit extending to but not beyond the orbital apex ➡, resulting in proptosis.*

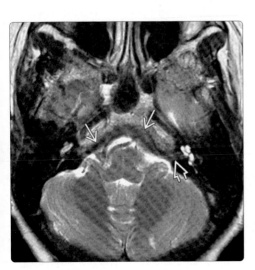
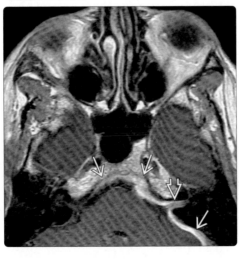

(Left) *Axial T2WI MR shows rare manifestation of KD. This patient with sensorineural hearing loss has subtle T2 hypointensity ➡ along the cranial surface of the clivus. Note the filling of the left internal auditory canal (IAC) ➡ with low-signal material.* (Right) *Axial T1WI C+ MR in the same patient shows intensely enhancing and thickened dura ➡ overlying the clivus and within the IAC ➡. KD may mimic other entities like sarcoid and idiopathic inflammatory pseudotumor.*

Nodal Hodgkin Lymphoma in Neck

TERMINOLOGY

- Hodgkin lymphoma (HL)
- Characterized by presence of **Reed-Sternberg cells**

IMAGING

- Most HL patients present due to **neck adenopathy**
- Single nodal group or contiguous groups
- Mediastinal nodes frequently involved at presentation
- Head and neck HL is rarely extranodal
- CECT: Homogeneous solid nodal masses
  o Necrosis or calcification uncommon
- CECT and FDG PET are basic staging modalities
- FDG PET shows **marked activity**
- Persistently positive PET during treatment has high sensitivity for prediction of relapse
- FDG PET differentiates posttreatment inactive scar from residual tumor

TOP DIFFERENTIAL DIAGNOSES

- Reactive lymph nodes
- Nodal differentiated thyroid carcinoma
- Nodal non-HL
- Nodal squamous cell carcinoma

PATHOLOGY

- Neoplastic cells are Reed-Sternberg cells
- Most of tumor bulk is reactive inflammatory cells, not neoplastic cells
- 95% classic HL; more aggressive type
- 5% nodular lymphocyte-predominant HL

CLINICAL ISSUES

- Young adult with enlarging, painless neck mass
- 40% have **B symptoms**: Fever, sweats, weight loss
- HL is potentially curable
- 5-year survival: Stages I-III (≥ 85%), stage IV (80%)

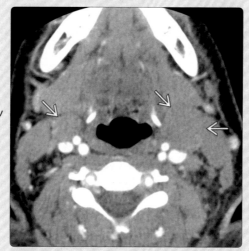
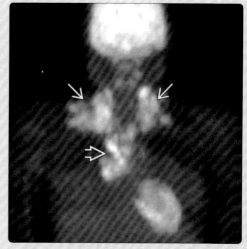

(Left) *Axial CECT in a teen girl with palpable neck masses demonstrates bilateral adenopathy* ➡, *larger on the left. Nodes are homogeneous and isodense to muscle without necrosis or calcifications.* (Right) *Coronal projection from FDG PET study in the same patient demonstrates marked nodal uptake in lower neck bilaterally* ➡ *and superior mediastinum* ➡. *PET study showed no evidence of infradiaphragmatic disease although focal nodular lung disease was demonstrated (extranodal disease).*

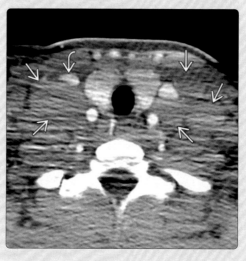
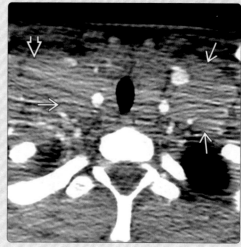

(Left) *Axial CECT more inferiorly demonstrates multiple solid large nodal masses isodense to muscle. On both sides, nodes splay common carotid* ➡ *& internal jugular vein (IJV). The right IJV* ➡ *is flattened.* (Right) *Axial CECT at the cervicothoracic junction shows additional bilateral nodal masses* ➡ *abutting carotid sheaths, with supraclavicular nodes* ➡ *also evident. This was nodular sclerosing Hodgkin lymphoma (HL), determined to be stage IV. It was successfully treated with chemoradiation, without relapse at 4 years.*

TERMINOLOGY

Abbreviations

- Hodgkin lymphoma (HL)
  - Classic Hodgkin lymphoma (CHL)
  - Nodular lymphocyte-predominant Hodgkin lymphoma (NLPHL)

Synonyms

- Hodgkin disease

Definitions

- HL: Classic or nodular lymphocyte-predominant
  - Characterized by presence of **Reed-Sternberg (RS) cells**
- CHL: Most common type of HL

IMAGING

General Features

- Best diagnostic clue
  - Young patient with neck and mediastinal adenopathy
- Location
  - HL most commonly cervical and mediastinal nodes
    - **Involves contiguous nodal groups**
  - Rarely involves Waldeyer ring or other extranodal neck sites (< 1%)
- Size
  - Variable nodal size: 2-10 cm
  - No strict size criteria, but nodes usually large and asymmetric
- Morphology
  - Single nodal chain ± spread to contiguous chain
  - 60-80% present with neck/supraclavicular nodes

CT Findings

- NECT
  - Homogeneous lobulated round masses
  - Calcification uncommon except after treatment
- CECT
  - Variable enhancement
  - Necrosis may be seen as low-density center

MR Findings

- T1WI
  - Enlarged iso- to hypointense round nodes
- T2WI
  - Nodes hyperintense compared with muscle
- T1WI C+
  - Variable, usually homogeneous nodal enhancement

Ultrasonographic Findings

- Grayscale ultrasound
  - Well-defined enlarged round nodes with homogeneous internal echoes
- Power Doppler
  - Increased flow centrally and peripherally

Nuclear Medicine Findings

- PET
  - FDG PET shows **marked activity**
  - Persistently positive scan during and after treatment has high sensitivity for prediction of relapse

Imaging Recommendations

- Best imaging tool
  - CECT is basic staging tool for assessment of disease
  - FDG PET for staging and assessing treatment response
- Protocol advice
  - CECT neck with chest, abdomen, and pelvis at initial evaluation

DIFFERENTIAL DIAGNOSIS

Reactive Lymph Nodes

- Multiple nodes; not as large as HL nodes

Nodal Differentiated Thyroid Carcinoma

- Favors lower neck and superior mediastinum
- Mediastinal nodes not usually bulky
- Variable MR signal: Thyroglobulin, cystic change

Non-Hodgkin Lymphoma in Lymph Nodes

- Imaging cannot distinguish HL and non-HL (NHL) nodes
- NHL more frequently extranodal (30%)

Nodal Squamous Cell Carcinoma

- Central nodal necrosis, extranodal spread common
- Primary tumor usually known

PATHOLOGY

General Features

- Etiology
  - Unknown
  - **Up to 50% Epstein-Barr virus (EBV)(+)**
    - Almost 100% of HIV-associated HL are EBV(+)
- Genetics
  - Familial association
    - 2-9x increased risk for siblings
- Associated abnormalities
  - Increased incidence with HIV infection though not AIDS-defining malignancy
    - Tends to be aggressive form with poorer prognosis

Staging, Grading, & Classification

- **World Health Organization** (WHO) is favored classification system
  - Rests on final pathological evaluation
  - HL either classic (95%) or nodular lymphocyte predominant (5%)
- **Ann Arbor staging system** is for clinical staging, treatment, and prognosis
  - Determined by location of disease sites in body and clinical symptoms

Gross Pathologic & Surgical Features

- Node described as firm and rubbery
- Image-guided core needle biopsy may make diagnosis and obviate lymphadenectomy

Microscopic Features

- RS cell = multinucleate giant cell; neoplastic B-lymphocyte clonal proliferation
  - Large lymphocytes with > 1 nucleus
- Most of tumor bulk is reactive mixed inflammatory cells, not neoplastic cells

Hodgkin Lymphoma

WHO Classification (2008)	Ann Arbor Staging System
Classical Hodgkin lymphoma (95%)	Stage I: Single nodal region; IE single extralymphatic organ or site
Nodular sclerosing (60-80%)	Stage II: ≥ 2 node regions; IIE extralymphatic site plus node region on same side of diaphragm
Mixed cellularity (15-30%)	Stage III: Nodes on both sides of diaphragm; IIIE plus extralymphatic site; IIIS plus spleen; IIIE, S both involved
Lymphocyte rich (5%)	Stage IV: Disseminated ≥ 1 extralymphatic tissues ± nodes, or isolated extralymphatic organ with distant nodes
Lymphocyte depleted (< 1%)	Category A and B
Nodular lymphocyte-predominant Hodgkin lymphoma (5%)	Category A: No systemic symptoms
Different immunophenotype, behaves like low-grade non-Hodgkin lymphoma	Category B: Fever, 10% weight loss or night sweats

- NLPHL
  - Few or no RS cells but "popcorn" lymphocytic and histiocytic cells

CLINICAL ISSUES

Presentation

- Most common signs/symptoms
  - Painless, enlarged, "rubbery" nodes
  - 25-40% have category **B symptoms**
    - Fever, night sweats, > 10% body weight loss
  - NLPHL rarely extranodal disease or B symptoms
    - Usually presents as early-stage disease (stage I, II)
- Other signs/symptoms
  - Fatigue, pruritus, anemia
  - Mediastinal adenopathy may present as cough, shortness of breath, and chest pain
  - 25% Pel-Ebstein fever: 1-2 weeks high fever, 1-2 weeks afebrile
  - < 10% have alcohol-induced pain in nodal disease
    - Uncommon but pathognomonic for HL
- Clinical profile
  - 20-year-old patient presents with enlarging, painless neck mass ± category B symptoms

Demographics

- Age
  - Median age = 27 years
  - CHL: Peak = 20-24 years; smaller peak > 50 years
  - NLPHL: Peaks in childhood and 4th decade
- Gender
  - M > F
- Ethnicity
  - Less common in Asians and African Americans
- Epidemiology
  - 14% of all lymphomas
  - EBV infection or mononucleosis has small ↑ risk of HL

Natural History & Prognosis

- Potentially curable
  - Most relapses occur within 3 years of treatment
- 5-year survival: Stage I-III (≥ 85%)
- 5-year survival: Stage IV (80%)
- Overall 15-year survival (68%)

- Poor prognostic features
  - Large mediastinal mass, > 50 years, ↑ ESR, ↑ white blood cell count, ↓ red blood cell count, > 4 areas involved
- NLPHL usually stage I, II and behaves like low-grade NHL

Treatment

- Chemotherapy, radiation, or combined-modality therapy (CMT)
- New regimens currently being developed to modify long-term toxicity
  - Because RS cells relatively sparse, could target those cells directly
- Chemotherapy
  - ABVD (Adriamycin, bleomycin, vinblastine, dacarbazine) is standard regimen
- Radiation therapy (XRT)
  - 30-45 Gy to involved nodes plus contiguous chain
- Early-stage CHL: CMT (ABVD + XRT)
- Early-stage NLPHL: Radiation
- Advanced stage HL: High-dose chemotherapy + XRT
- Relapses: High-dose chemotherapy and bone marrow transplantation

DIAGNOSTIC CHECKLIST

Consider

- Residual masses after treatment may not represent active disease
  - FDG PET differentiates persistent disease from inactive scar or sterile treated tumor

Image Interpretation Pearls

- CT and FDG PET are basic staging modalities for HL
  - After node biopsy ± bone marrow biopsy
- Imaging cannot distinguish nodal HL and NHL
  - Neck adenopathy is common presentation of both
  - HL is less common than NHL, rarely extranodal
  - HL presents at younger age

SELECTED REFERENCES

1. Skelton E et al: Image-guided core needle biopsy in the diagnosis of malignant lymphoma. Eur J Surg Oncol. 41(7):852-8, 2015
2. Chiaravalloti A et al: Initial staging of Hodgkin's disease: role of contrast-enhanced 18F FDG PET/CT. Medicine (Baltimore). 93(8):e50, 2014

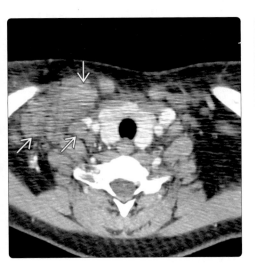

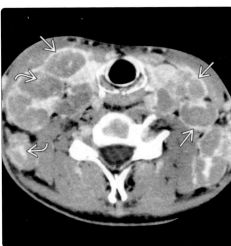

(Left) *Axial CECT through lower neck in a young adult shows multiple enlarged nodes ➡ forming a matted mass. Nodes are generally isodense to muscle and show no calcifications. This was determined to be stage IIA nodular sclerosing (classic) Hodgkin disease.* (Right) *Axial CECT through neck in a different patient reveals multiple large bilateral neck nodes ➡. Nodes are isodense to muscle; however, there is unusual marked peripheral enhancement with some internal nodal enhancement ➡.*

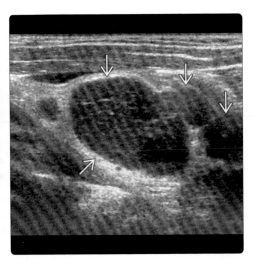

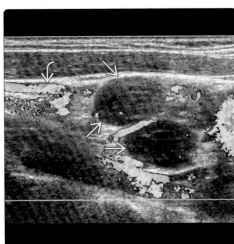

(Left) *Longitudinal ultrasound through lower right neck shows level IV lymphadenopathy ➡. Nodes are variable in size with heterogeneity of internal echogenicity but appear predominantly solid. A normal hilar contour could not be seen with any of these nodes, and calcifications were not evident. The largest lymph node measured 3 cm x 2 cm.* (Right) *Power Doppler ultrasound reveals partial compression of veins with slowed flow ➡ above moderately enlarged, rounded, solid nodes ➡.*

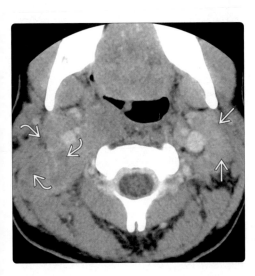

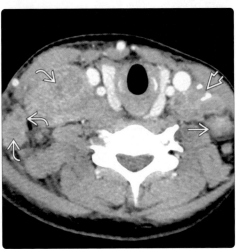

(Left) *Axial CECT shows a young adult previously treated with chemoXRT for nodular sclerosing HL. Bilateral adenopathy is evident with both homogeneous solid nodes ➡, typical of HL and other more heterogeneous nodes with cystic changes ➡.* (Right) *Axial CECT more inferiorly reveals additional heterogeneous ➡ and homogeneous solid nodes ➡. Focal calcifications ➡ are unusual in HL and probably reflect previously treated nodes from chemoXRT 18 months prior.*

KEY FACTS

TERMINOLOGY

- Non-Hodgkin lymphoma (NHL) is lymphoreticular system malignancy
- Multiple different NHL subtypes
- Multiple forms of NHL in H&N
  - Nodal, nonnodal lymphatic, nonnodal extralymphatic NHL

IMAGING

- Multiple bilateral, enlarged nodes involving multiple nodal chains
- Typically **large, solid**, round, or oval nodes
- Enhancement may be variable, even in same patient
- **Necrosis/extranodal spread** suggests **aggressive NHL**
- May see different patterns of nodes
  - Multiple mildly enlarged, 1- to 3-cm nodes
  - Dominant, markedly enlarged node
- FDG PET shows variable avidity
  - High in aggressive NHL, lower in more indolent NHL

TOP DIFFERENTIAL DIAGNOSES

- Reactive adenopathy
- Tuberculosis lymph nodes
- Sarcoidosis lymph nodes
- Hodgkin lymphoma nodes
- Nodal metastases from systemic primary

PATHOLOGY

- 80-85% B-cell tumors, most common diffuse large B-cell lymphoma
- Often associated with AIDS

CLINICAL ISSUES

- Adult with painless neck masses
- May be indolent & progressive but not curable, or aggressive but often curable
- Treat with XRT, chemotherapy, or both
- 5-year survival: Stages I-II (85%), stages III-IV (50%)

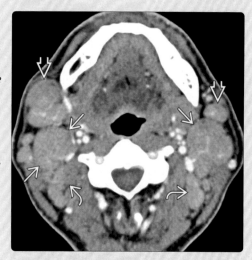
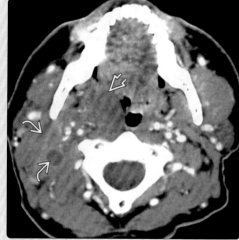

(Left) *Axial CECT shows multiple large, round, solid lymph nodes in every chain of the suprahyoid neck. Bilateral nodes are evident in levels IIA ➡, IIB ➡, and IB ➡. Absence of necrosis with such large nodes suggests that these are not metastases from H&N squamous cell carcinoma.* (Right) *Axial CECT in a different patient shows nodal and tonsillar lymphoma. Level II nodal mass is partially necrotic ➡, with extranodal infiltration of fat and paraspinal muscles. Right tonsil is homogeneously enlarged ➡.*

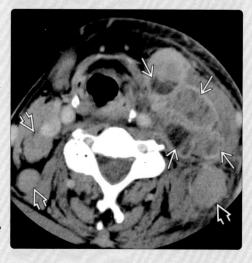
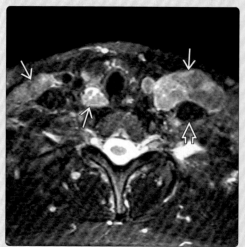

(Left) *Axial CECT demonstrates massive left nodal conglomerate, some with necrosis ➡. Surrounding induration and stranding of fat in left neck suggests inflammatory response. Other large nonnecrotic nodes ➡ are seen bilaterally.* (Right) *Axial T2WI FS MR reveals multiple heterogeneous and predominantly hyperintense nodal masses ➡. Despite large size, nodes insinuate around structures with little mass effect and no arterial compression. Largest node wraps around anterior scalene muscle ➡.*

TERMINOLOGY

Abbreviations
- Non-Hodgkin lymphoma (NHL)

Definitions
- NHL is lymphoreticular system malignancy, thought to arise from lymphocytes & derivatives
- Multiple different NHL subtypes
  - Most common (> 30%): Diffuse large B-cell lymphoma (DLBCL)
- H&N NHL has multiple forms
  - Nodal, nonnodal lymphatic (tonsils, lingual lymphoid, adenoids), nonnodal extralymphatic (e.g., thyroid)

IMAGING

General Features
- Best diagnostic clue
  - Bilateral, enlarged nodes involving multiple nodal chains
- Location
  - All cervical nodal chains may be involved
  - Levels II, III, IV, superficial & parotid nodes often involved
- Size
  - Different patterns of nodes
    - Multiple mildly enlarged, 1- to 3-cm nodes
    - Dominant node 3-5 cm in size; may be ≤ 10 cm
- Morphology
  - Round or oval enlarged nodes, typically **solid**
  - **Nodal necrosis ± extranodal tumor** spread suggests **aggressive NHL**
    - AIDS-associated NHL often aggressive: Necrosis & surrounding induration

CT Findings
- NECT
  - Nodal density similar to muscle
- CECT
  - Bulky ovoid masses bilaterally in multiple cervical node chains
  - Enhancement may be variable, even in same patient

MR Findings
- T1WI
  - Nodes isointense to muscle
- T2WI
  - Nodes usually iso- or slightly hyperintense to muscle
- DWI
  - Initial enthusiasm regarding whole-body DWI but cannot replace PET/CT
- T1WI C+
  - Minimal homogeneous nodal enhancement
  - Necrotic adenopathy enhances peripherally

Ultrasonographic Findings
- Typically diffuse, homogeneous, decreased echogenicity

Nuclear Medicine Findings
- PET
  - FDG PET/CT is best staging & treatment assessment modality
  - **FDG PET** shows **variable avidity**
    - Higher in aggressive, lower in more indolent NHL

Imaging Recommendations
- Best imaging tool
  - CECT often initial imaging tool, but FDG PET/CT critical for staging
  - US used to guide biopsy if nodes are smaller or deeper
    - Pass should be sent for flow cytometry to detect monoclonal population
    - Core biopsy recommended for nodal architecture
- Protocol advice
  - PET/CT critical to determine extent of disease
  - Bidimensional measurements should be reported on cross-sectional imaging
    - Choose 3 nodes for size measurements, & measure same nodes on follow-up imaging

DIFFERENTIAL DIAGNOSIS

Reactive Adenopathy
- Patient usually < 20 years of age with viral infection
- Diffuse, nonnecrotic adenopathy, usually < 2 cm

Tuberculosis Lymph Nodes
- Systemically ill patient; strongly positive PPD & abnormal chest x-ray
- Diffuse adenopathy; heterogeneous nodes

Sarcoidosis Lymph Nodes
- Diffuse cervical lymphadenopathy that may exactly mimic NHL
- Calcifications may be seen

Hodgkin Lymphoma Nodes
- Nodal NHL cannot be differentiated from Hodgkin lymphoma (HL) on imaging

Nodal Metastases From Systemic Primary
- Known primary tumor (lung, breast, etc.)
- Often unilateral

PATHOLOGY

General Features
- Etiology
  - Malignant monoclonal unregulated proliferation of lymphocytes
  - Evidence suggests **viral** cause but yet to be proven
    - Association with EBV or HTLV-1, especially African Burkitt & AIDS-associated lymphomas
- Genetics
  - Lymphoma may be classified by gene expression & rearrangement
- Associated abnormalities
  - Often associated with AIDS in children or adults
    - 2nd most common cancer in AIDS patients
  - Disseminated disease common

Staging, Grading, & Classification
- **WHO** is current classification as of 2008
- Based on pathological evaluation
  - B-cell neoplasms (80-85%)
    - Precursor B-lymphoblastic leukemia/lymphoma

Ann Arbor Staging Classification

Stage I	Single nodal region or lymphatic structure (Waldeyer ring) or single extralymphatic organ or site (IE)
Stage II	≥ 2 node regions on same side of diaphragm (II) or localized contiguous involvement of 1 extranodal organ or site and its regional nodes ± other node regions on same side of diaphragm (IIE)
Stage III	Node regions on both sides of diaphragm (III); may have spleen (IIIS) or localized contiguous involvement of only 1 extranodal site (IIIE) or both (IIISE)
Stage IV	Disseminated disease: ≥ 1 extranodal organ or tissue, ± associated nodes or isolated extralymphatic disease with distant nodal involvement
Additional Designations	
A	No symptoms
B	Fever, night sweats, unexplained weight loss > 10% of body weight in 6 months
X	Bulky disease: > 10-cm long axis nodal mass or mediastinal mass > 1/3 of chest diameter at T5/6 on PA chest x-ray

- Peripheral B-cell neoplasms
  - T-cell & putative NK-cell neoplasms (15-20%)
    - Precursor T-lymphoblastic leukemia/lymphoma
    - Peripheral T-cell & NK-cell neoplasms
- **Modified Ann Arbor staging system** (1989) is for clinical staging, treatment, & prognosis
  - Determined by location of disease sites in body & clinical symptoms

Gross Pathologic & Surgical Features

- Nodes firm & "rubbery"

Microscopic Features

- Microscopic features depend on cell of origin
  - B- & T-cell lymphomas composed of precursor (lymphoblastic) cells or mature lymphocytes
- Flow cytometry is positive for monoclonal population

CLINICAL ISSUES

Presentation

- Most common signs/symptoms
  - Painless large or multiple small "rubbery" neck masses
  - Systemic symptoms: Night sweats, recurrent fever, weight loss, fatigue, & pruritic skin rash
- Other signs/symptoms
  - Superior vena cava syndrome due to mass effect may cause facial & neck swelling from edema
- Clinical profile
  - Adult with painless neck mass/masses

Demographics

- Age
  - Median: 53 years
- Gender
  - M:F = 1.5:1.0
- Epidemiology
  - Increasing incidence of NHL
  - ~ 5% of all H&N cancers
  - 5% of cancer cases in USA

Natural History & Prognosis

- May be indolent, progressive but not curable, or aggressive but often curable
- 5-year survival: Stages I, II (85%)
- 5-year survival: Stages III, IV (50%)

- Predictors of poorer prognosis
  - Age > 60 years, > 1 extranodal site, stage III or IV, AIDS-related

Treatment

- Exact treatment of NHL depends on stage, cell type, & patient age
- Treated with XRT, chemotherapy, or combined modality therapy
  - H&N NHL may be treated with XRT alone (stages I, II)
  - Disseminated NHL (stages III, IV) treated with chemotherapy ± XRT
  - Bone marrow transplant may be performed

DIAGNOSTIC CHECKLIST

Consider

- Range of presentations suggestive of NHL
  - Diffuse cervical nodes with variable texture in adult
  - Multiple 1- to 3-cm nodes in multiple nodal chains
  - Large nonnecrotic node without H&N primary
  - Retropharyngeal, occipital, parotid, & submandibular nodes
  - AIDS patient with neck mass
- Imaging cannot distinguish nodal NHL from HL
  - NHL more common
  - NHL tends to present in older patients
  - Extranodal disease suggests NHL

Image Interpretation Pearls

- Successful posttreatment CT or MR scans
  - **≥ 50% ↓ in nodal size with ↓ number of nodes**
- Controversy regarding what is imaging equivalent of "treatment response"
- Fused PET/CT likely to aid defining complete vs. partial response

Reporting Tips

- Consider reporting bidimensional measurements of 3 index nodes on initial & follow-up imaging

SELECTED REFERENCES

1. American Joint Committee on Cancer: AJCC Cancer Staging Manual. 7th ed. New York: Springer. 599-615, 2010
2. Shinya T et al: Dual-time-point F-18 FDG PET/CT for evaluation in patients with malignant lymphoma. Ann Nucl Med. 26(8):616-21, 2012

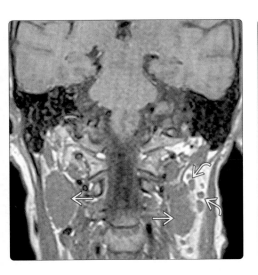

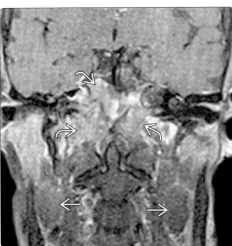

(Left) Coronal T1WI MR demonstrates large, bulky, bilateral, hypointense level IIB lymph nodes ➜, with scattered small nodes ➱ around dominant nodes. Note the lack of surrounding induration with these symmetric nodes. (Right) Coronal T1WI C+ FS MR in the same patient reveals minimal enhancement of nodes ➜ without features to suggest nodal necrosis. Patient also had nonnodal, extralymphatic non-Hodgkin lymphoma (NHL) with infiltrative, mildly enhancing tumor involving osseous skull base ➱.

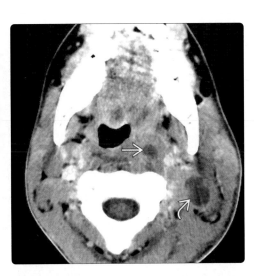

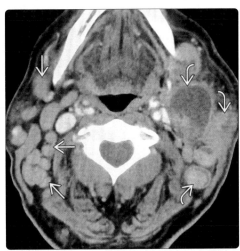

(Left) Axial CECT in a teenage boy with Burkitt-type NHL shows necrotic retropharyngeal node ➜ deforming pharyngeal lumen. Necrotic left high jugular chain node ➱ is evident. (Right) Axial CECT in an immunocompromised patient shows multiple small solid right nodes ➜; the biopsy proved positive for NHL. On the left side, note the large, necrotic nodal masses with surrounding induration & extracapsular extension ➱. The left-side nodal tumor was found to be squamous cell carcinoma from H&N primary.

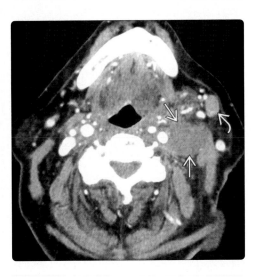

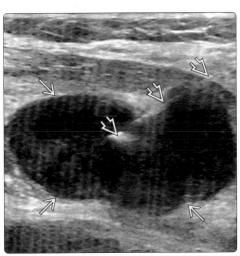

(Left) Axial CECT shows nonenhancing low-density left level II node ➜ displacing carotid artery and jugular vein medially. A smaller enhancing node ➱ is evident lateral to submandibular gland. FNA revealed high-grade NHL in both nodes. Variable appearance of nodes is not uncommon. (Right) Longitudinal oblique ultrasound demonstrates markedly hypoechoic, large, ovoid, well-defined node ➜ with absent hilus. Echogenic biopsy needle track ➱ shows needle tip in central portion of node.

KEY FACTS

TERMINOLOGY

- Differentiated thyroid carcinoma (DTC)
- Metastatic node(s) from papillary or follicular thyroid carcinoma

IMAGING

- US: Look for cystic change, hyperechoic calcifications, loss of hilar architecture
- Peripheral vascularization on power Doppler
- CECT may be done but delays ^{131}I-radioablation
- Nodes heterogeneous: Solid, cystic, calcified
- MR: Nodes heterogeneous in size and signal
- FDG PET: Not useful for DTC
  - Best for **recurrence** when ↑ **thyroglobulin** with negative iodide scan
- I-123 & I-131 scans show low sensitivity, high specificity

TOP DIFFERENTIAL DIAGNOSES

- Nodal squamous cell carcinoma
- Nodal non-Hodgkin lymphoma
- Nodal tuberculosis
- Systemic nodal metastases

PATHOLOGY

- Extranodal extension may be poor prognostic characteristic

CLINICAL ISSUES

- Nodal metastases common; however, prognostically significant only if > 45 yr of age
- Slow-growing nodal mass may be tumor presentation

DIAGNOSTIC CHECKLIST

- If nodal mass is presentation, some features highly suggestive of DTC
  - Heterogeneous nodes
  - **Calcifications** on CT or US
  - Variable T1 intensity on MR
- Thyroid primary may not be evident on CT/MR

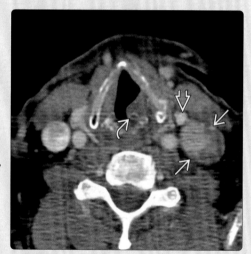
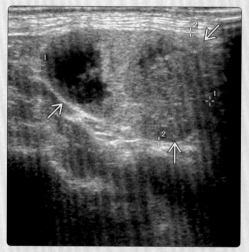

(Left) Axial CECT shows a large, heterogeneous, left level III lymph node ➡ displacing jugular vein ➡ anteriorly. Calcifications were present more inferiorly in this node. Note medially rotated left arytenoid cartilage ➡ indicating left vocal cord paralysis, which was secondary to invasive left thyroid mass. (Right) Longitudinal ultrasound in the same patient shows marked internal heterogeneity of enlarged level III node ➡, which on fine-needle aspiration revealed papillary thyroid carcinoma.

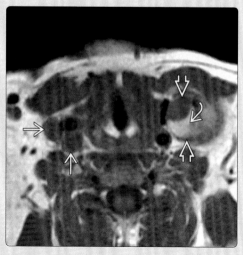
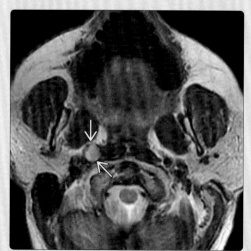

(Left) Axial T1WI MR through lower neck shows a cluster of round, minimally enlarged homogeneous nodes on right at level III ➡ and a more complex cystic and solid mass in lower left neck ➡. T1 hyperintensity within posterior cystic component ➡ makes papillary thyroid carcinoma most likely primary. (Right) Axial T2WI MR more superiorly in the same patient shows an enlarged, round, right retropharyngeal node ➡. Thyroidectomy revealed thyroid papillary carcinoma in nonenlarged heterogeneous gland.

Nodal Differentiated Thyroid Carcinoma

TERMINOLOGY

Abbreviations

- Differentiated thyroid carcinoma (DTC)

Definitions

- Metastatic node(s) from papillary or follicular thyroid carcinoma

IMAGING

General Features

- Best diagnostic clue
  - **Heterogeneous solid** and **cystic enlarged nodes**
  - Focal calcifications (CT/US) or T1 hyperintensity (MR) highly suggestive of DTC
- Location
  - Central compartment or level VI most common
  - Level II, III, IV, supraclavicular occur secondarily
    - Bilateral nodal metastases common
  - Retropharyngeal nodal metastases occur especially when lateral cervical nodes present
- Size
  - Variable between patients and in single patient
    - Nodes may be 2-3 cm, but commonly < 1 cm

Imaging Recommendations

- Best imaging tool
  - Ultrasound often 1st-line tool for nonpalpable metastases
  - MR useful for retropharyngeal, deep cervical, or mediastinal metastases
- Protocol advice
  - Consider thyroid carcinoma in young female patient with neck mass
    - Ultrasound excellent nodal screening tool
    - CECT can be done but will need to wait 6 weeks before diagnostic ^{123}I or therapeutic ^{131}I

CT Findings

- CT
  - Overall sensitivity poor, as nodal metastases often small
  - **Nodes heterogeneous: Solid, cystic, calcified, variable in size & enhancement**

MR Findings

- T1WI
  - Frequently bright from thyroglobulin or colloid
- T2WI
  - Variable, most often hyperintense

Ultrasonographic Findings

- Grayscale ultrasound
  - Generally enlarged, round, hypoechoic nodes
  - 3 features concerning for malignancy
    - Cystic appearance, hyperechoic calcifications, loss of hilar architecture
  - Allows guided fine-needle aspiration
- Power Doppler
  - Peripheral vascularization highly suggestive of malignancy

Nuclear Medicine Findings

- PET/CT
  - Not useful for differentiated thyroid carcinoma
  - Best for nodal recurrence when ↑ thyroglobulin with negative iodide scan
- ^{123}I & ^{131}I scans
  - Poor sensitivity, near 100% specificity

DIFFERENTIAL DIAGNOSIS

Nodal Sqaumous Cell Carcinoma

- May be heterogeneous, cystic, or solid
- Rarely have calcifications

Nodal Non-Hodgkin Lymphoma

- Usually multiple large homogeneous nodes
- Calcifications rare except post treatment

Nodal Tuberculosis

- Thick rim of enhancement with central necrosis
- Calcifications may be evident

Systemic Nodal Metastases

- Adenocarcinoma metastases may have calcifications

PATHOLOGY

General Features

- Etiology
  - Metastatic disease from primary thyroid papillary or follicular carcinoma

Staging, Grading, & Classification

- < 45 yr: Nodal disease does not alter staging
- > 45 yr: Higher locoregional recurrence
  - N1A = level VI
  - N1B = I-V, retropharynx or superior mediastinum
- Extranodal extension may be poor prognostic characteristic

CLINICAL ISSUES

Demographics

- Age
  - Most patients 25-65 yr
- Gender
  - F > M
- Epidemiology
  - Papillary nodal metastases > 50% at presentation
    - Up to 64% of patients have primary tumor < 1 cm

Natural History & Prognosis

- Nodes prognostically significant only if > 45 yr old

DIAGNOSTIC CHECKLIST

Image Interpretation Pearls

- Heterogeneous nodes are common
- CT/US calcifications or MR T1 hyperintensity suggest DTC
- Thyroid primary carcinoma may not be evident on CT/MR

SELECTED REFERENCES

1. Yeh MW et al: American Thyroid Association statement on preoperative imaging for thyroid cancer surgery. Thyroid. 25(1):3-14, 2015

TERMINOLOGY

- Cervical metastatic adenopathy from infraclavicular primary tumor
- Virchow node is left supraclavicular nodal metastasis

IMAGING

- Nodes generally in lower neck, especially on left
- Variable size nodes, often > 1.5 cm
- May be cluster of small nodes
- May form conglomerate mass > 5-6 cm
- Calcification on CT when primary tumor is adenocarcinoma

TOP DIFFERENTIAL DIAGNOSES

- Reactive lymph nodes
- Sarcoidosis nodes
- Squamous cell carcinoma (SCCa) metastatic nodes
- Non-Hodgkin lymphoma nodes

PATHOLOGY

- Esophageal, breast, and lung malignancies are most common primary tumors
- May be unknown primary tumor
- Focal nonenhancement on CT/MR corresponds to nest of tumor cells or necrosis

CLINICAL ISSUES

- Systemic neck metastases less common than H&N SCCa nodes

DIAGNOSTIC CHECKLIST

- If patient presents with nodal mass, 1st look for H&N primary tumor
- If infrahyoid nodal metastasis, suspect systemic primary tumor
- When neck nodes are calcified, suspect thyroid primary or systemic adenocarcinoma

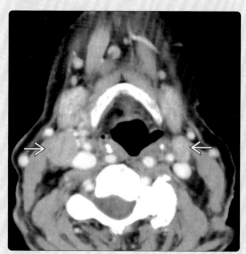
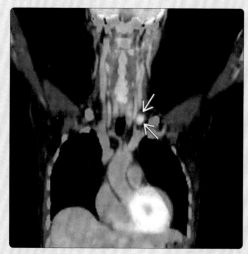

(Left) Axial CECT shows enlarged, noncalcified, solidly enhancing bilateral level IIA neck nodes ➡. No primary source was present in H&N, but the patient was found to have primary lung carcinoma. (Right) Coronal PET/CT in a patient with ovarian carcinoma reveals a single enlarged left supraclavicular node ➡ with FDG avidity. The patient had been previously treated for abdominal metastases and had known pulmonary metastases at the time of study.

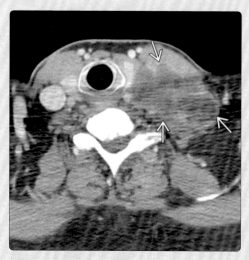
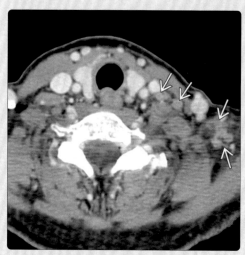

(Left) Axial CECT shows large complex conglomerate left supraclavicular nodal mass ➡ with extensive necrosis & infiltration of scalene and sternocleidomastoid muscles. Patient had neural deficits from invasion of brachial plexus. Fine-needle aspiration revealed metastatic colonic adenocarcinoma. (Right) Axial CECT reveals multiple small nodes ➡ in lower left neck in a patient with known metastatic breast carcinoma. Nodes are heterogeneous, many with focal eccentric low density, indicating necrosis.

TERMINOLOGY

Definitions

- Cervical metastatic adenopathy from infraclavicular primary tumor
- **Virchow node** is left supraclavicular nodal metastasis
  - Usually abdominal or pelvic primary malignancy

IMAGING

General Features

- Best diagnostic clue
  - Enlarged &/or necrotic cervical node or nodal cluster in patient with systemic malignancy
- Location
  - Most often lower neck
  - Frequently unilateral
- Size
  - Variably sized nodes, often > 1.5 cm
  - May be cluster of small nodes
  - May form conglomerate mass > 5-6 cm

CT Findings

- NECT
  - Calcification seen when primary tumor is adenocarcinoma
- CECT
  - Round node > 1.5 cm or cluster of nodes
  - Nodes generally clustered toward lower neck, especially on left
  - Homogeneous or heterogeneous enhancement
  - Coronal reformations help differentiate enhancing node from subclavian vein

MR Findings

- T1WI
  - Cervical nodal mass usually isointense to muscle
- T2WI
  - Nodes slightly hyperintense compared to muscle
- T1WI C+
  - Minimal enhancement common; peripherally when nodes necrotic

Ultrasonographic Findings

- Grayscale ultrasound
  - Enlarged round node, absent echogenic hilus, nodal necrosis

Imaging Recommendations

- Best imaging tool
  - CECT best modality for assessing palpable cervical nodes

DIFFERENTIAL DIAGNOSIS

Reactive Lymph Nodes

- Nodes more commonly in suprahyoid neck

Sarcoidosis Lymph Nodes

- Lower neck and mediastinal adenopathy common
- Nodes may be calcified

Squamous Cell Carcinoma Metastatic Nodes

- Known H&N primary squamous cell carcinoma (SCCa)

- Nodal metastases most commonly ipsilateral to lesion, involving levels II and III

Non-Hodgkin Lymphoma Nodes

- Large, usually nonnecrotic nodes throughout neck

PATHOLOGY

General Features

- Associated abnormalities
  - Esophageal, breast, and lung malignancies most common
    - May be unknown primary

Staging, Grading, & Classification

- Cervical adenopathy from infraclavicular tumor represents distant metastatic disease

Gross Pathologic & Surgical Features

- Nodal mass > 3 cm = confluent metastatic nodes
- Left > right lower neck, probably because thoracic duct is on left

Microscopic Features

- Neoplastic cells first localize in subcapsular sinus, then proliferate into body of node
- Focal nonenhancement on CT/MR corresponds to nest of tumor cells or necrosis

CLINICAL ISSUES

Presentation

- Most common signs/symptoms
  - Low cervical neck mass in patient with systemic malignancy

Demographics

- Epidemiology
  - Systemic neck metastases less common than H&N SCCa nodes

Natural History & Prognosis

- Disseminated disease associated with poor prognosis

Treatment

- Selective neck dissection may be performed for nodes
- Most patients undergo chemotherapy
- Radiation less frequently performed as systemic disease

DIAGNOSTIC CHECKLIST

Consider

- If patient presents with nodal mass 1st, then look for H&N primary SCCa
- Extend imaging through chest for esophageal or lung primary or other metastases
- If infrahyoid nodal metastasis, suspect systemic primary
- When nodes are calcified, suspect thyroid carcinoma or systemic adenocarcinoma

SELECTED REFERENCES

1. Giridharan W et al: Lymph node metastases in the lower neck. Clin Otolaryngol. 28(3):221-6, 2003
2. Ahuja A et al: An overview of neck node sonography. Invest Radiol. 37(6):333-42, 2002

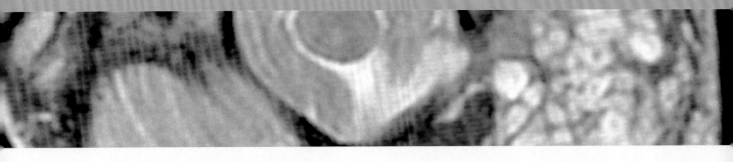

SECTION 13
Transspatial and Multispatial

Summary Thoughts: Trans- and Multispatial Lesions

Transspatial and multispatial terms are used to describe specific subsets of lesions found in the head and neck. The **transspatial** descriptor is used to describe a lesion that involves multiple **contiguous** spaces or areas of the extracranial head and neck. **Multispatial** is applied to a lesion that is found in multiple **noncontiguous** spaces or areas.

Approaches to Imaging Issues in Trans- and Multispatial Lesions

Transspatial Lesions

Transspatial lesions are defined as involving multiple contiguous spaces or areas in the neck. In the soft tissues of the suprahyoid neck, infrahyoid neck, and oral cavity, where the anatomy can be defined by fascia-circumscribed spaces, this term is directly applicable. In the skull base, sinuses, nose, and orbit where the anatomic areas are distinct but not fascia defined, the term can still be used to describe lesions that involve multiple contiguous areas.

Transspatial lesions generally fall into 4 major pathologic categories: Congenital, inflammatory-infectious, benign tumor, and malignant tumor.

- **Congenital lesions** form at the same time or prior to fascia in extracranial head and neck. As a result, they do not always stay within spatial boundaries and are often transspatial. Congenital lesions, such as venous and lymphatic malformation, commonly appear transspatial when first imaged.
- **Inflammatory-infectious lesions** fall within the transspatial group when cellulitis, phlegmon, or abscess involves multiple contiguous spaces. In the case of abscess, defining each space involved for the surgeon ensures that each space is entered with either a probe or a drain.
- **Benign tumors**, such as infantile hemangioma and schwannoma, often involve multiple contiguous spaces. In the case of schwannoma, this is because the nerves that they form from normally run through multiple spaces as they course through head and neck.
- **Malignant tumors** invade contiguous spaces as they enlarge; in fact, squamous cell carcinoma (SCCa) of pharynx and oral cavity initially arises from mucosal space/surface and immediately invades deeply into surrounding soft tissue spaces. Larger SCCa primary tumors are almost always transspatial at presentation. Along with perineural tumor, the exact spaces invaded by primary SCCa determine tumor resectability and radiation ports.

Multispatial Lesions

The term **multispatial** is helpful in describing lesions of the head and neck that occupy multiple noncontiguous spaces or areas. These lesions generally are identified as 1 of 3 pathologic categories: Congenital, inflammatory-infectious, and malignant neoplasms.

- **Congenital lesions** that may be multispatial include neurofibromatosis types 1 and 2, PHACES syndrome, and other syndromes that have multiple noncontiguous manifestations.
- **Inflammatory-infectious nodal lesions** are commonly multispatial at presentation; reactive nodes may progress to suppurative nodes (intranodal abscesses);

tuberculous adenopathy may also be multispatial; any of the many rarer nodal diseases of head and neck may also present as multispatial.

- **Malignant tumors** of head and neck are often transspatial in their primary site and multispatial in their nodal spread; oral cavity and pharyngeal SCCas and non-Hodgkin lymphoma (NHL) (of Waldeyer lymphatic ring) are both prone to this behavior; Hodgkin lymphoma neck nodes and systemic nodal metastases may also be multispatial in head and neck.

Transspatial Diseases of H&N

Congenital Lesions
- Venous malformation
- Lymphatic malformation
- Branchial cleft cysts
- Thyroglossal duct cyst
- Thymic cyst
- Neurofibromatosis type 1 (plexiform neurofibroma)

Inflammatory and Infectious Lesions
- Cellulitis
- Phlegmon
- Abscess
- Invasive fungal sinusitis
- Sinonasal Wegener granulomatosis
- Fibromatosis

Benign Tumors
- Schwannoma
- Neurofibroma
- Infantile hemangioma
- Hemangiopericytoma

Malignant Tumors
- Pharyngeal SCCa
- NHL, extranodal
- Rhabdomyosarcoma
- Anaplastic carcinoma of thyroid
- Sinonasal SCCa
- Sinonasal undifferentiated carcinoma
- Esthesioneuroblastoma of nose
- Chondrosarcoma of skull base
- Chordoma of skull base

Multispatial Diseases of H&N

Congenital Lesions
- Neurofibromatosis type 1
- Neurofibromatosis type 2
- PHACES association

Inflammatory and Infectious Lesions
- Reactive adenopathy
- Suppurative adenopathy
- Tuberculous adenopathy

Malignant Tumors
- Pharyngeal SCCa + malignant nodes
- NHL extranodal + nodal
- Systemic metastases
- Metastatic neuroblastoma

Selected References

1. Aiken AH et al: Imaging Hodgkin and non-Hodgkin lymphoma in the head and neck. Radiol Clin North Am. 46(2):363-78, ix-x, 2008
2. Vogelzang P et al: Multispatial and transpatial diseases of the extracranial head and neck. Semin Ultrasound CT MR. 12(3):274-87, 1991

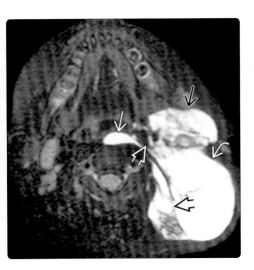

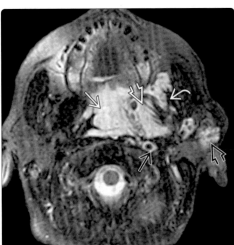

(Left) *Axial T2WI FS MR demonstrates a large, hyperintense lymphatic malformation of the neck, which is multilocular and transspatial. Multiple contiguous space involvement includes the retropharyngeal ➡, carotid ⮕, posterior cervical ➡, submandibular ➡, and perivertebral ➡ spaces.* (Right) *Axial T2WI FS MR in a patient with a large venous malformation shows transspatial involvement of the pharyngeal mucosal ➡, parapharyngeal ⮕, masticator ➡, carotid ➡, and parotid ⮕ spaces.*

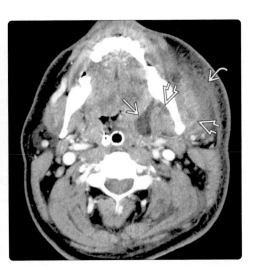

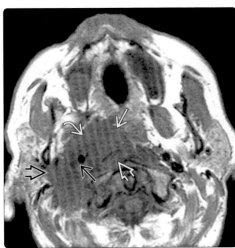

(Left) *Axial CECT in a septic patient with trismus reveals a transspatial infection in the deep face. Abscess in the parapharyngeal ➡ and masticator ⮕ spaces are accompanied by contiguous, superficial space cellulitis ➡.* (Right) *Axial T1WI MR demonstrates an invasive, transspatial nasopharyngeal carcinoma. This nasopharyngeal mucosal space carcinoma ➡ has directly invaded the parapharyngeal ⮕, perivertebral ⮕, carotid ➡, and parotid ⮕ spaces.*

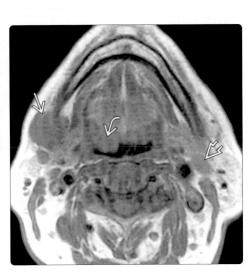

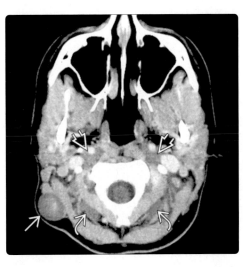

(Left) *Axial T1WI MR in a patient with multiple H&N lesions shows abnormal lymph node in the submandibular ➡ and parotid ⮕ spaces accompanied by a focal mass in the pharyngeal mucosal space ➡ (lingual tonsil). This example of multispatial disease is caused by NHL.* (Right) *Axial CECT in a 31-year-old woman with neurofibromatosis type 1 reveals multispatial low-density neurofibromas. In this image, the neurofibromas can be identified in the superficial ➡, carotid ⮕, and perivertebral ➡ spaces.*

Prominent Thoracic Duct in Neck

TERMINOLOGY

- a.k.a. left lymphatic duct
- Normal anatomical structure draining lymph and chyle from abdomen and left chest

IMAGING

- Tubular structure with same density/intensity as CSF
- Average diameter: 4-5 mm
- Courses cranially in **left** lower neck posterior to common carotid artery
- Laterally drains to junction of internal jugular vein & subclavian vein

TOP DIFFERENTIAL DIAGNOSES

- Squamous cell carcinoma node
- Differentiated thyroid carcinoma node
- Nodal metastasis from systemic disease
- Lymphocele
- 4th branchial anomaly

PATHOLOGY

- Drains lymph and chyle from abdomen and left chest to venous circulation
- Right-sided thoracic duct uncommonly also found, ends in right subclavian vein

CLINICAL ISSUES

- Incidental normal finding
- Obstruction results in pleural effusion
- Probable source of metastasis to left supraclavicular node (Virchow node)

DIAGNOSTIC CHECKLIST

- Key imaging features
  - Tubular structure in left neck
  - Isointense/isodense to CSF
- May be mistaken for cystic level IV or VI node
- May be mistaken for 4th branchial anomaly

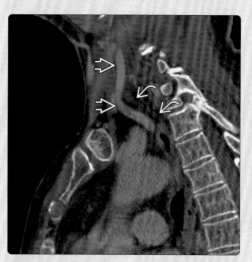
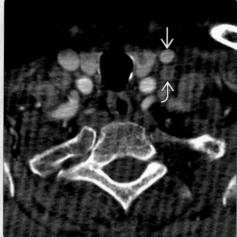

(Left) Sagittal reformat CECT demonstrates a tubular, low-density thoracic duct ➔ ascending from the chest posterior to the left carotid artery ➔, which may be mistaken for a thrombosed vessel. (Right) Axial CECT shows a more lateral location of the thoracic duct ➔ as it courses toward the terminus at the junction of the internal jugular vein (IJV) and subclavian vein ➔. The thoracic duct mimics a node in its axial cross section contour.

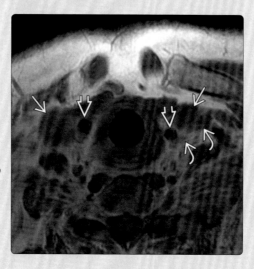
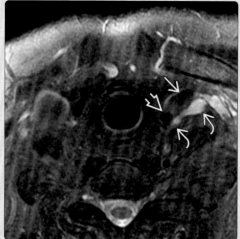

(Left) Axial T1 MR shows normal carotid arterial flow voids ➔ and mixed signal in the IJVs ➔, as is frequently seen on MR. The right jugular vein is dominant in this patient. The thoracic duct is evident at the subtle tubular structure posterior to the left jugular vein ➔. (Right) Axial T2 FS MR shows the thoracic duct ➔ as markedly intense varicose structure posterior to the left carotid artery ➔ and IJV ➔. The thoracic duct appears isointense to CSF on all sequences.

Prominent Thoracic Duct in Neck

TERMINOLOGY

Synonyms
- Enlarged left lymphatic duct

Definitions
- Thoracic duct: Normal anatomical structure draining lymph from abdomen and left chest

IMAGING

General Features
- Best diagnostic clue
  - Tubular structure with same density/intensity as CSF coursing superiorly, posterior to common carotid artery, then laterally to insert to junction of internal jugular vein and subclavian vein
- Location
  - Left lower neck posterior to carotid sheath
- Size
  - Average diameter: 4-5 mm
  - Thoracic duct length in adult: 38-45 cm
  - In neck, courses 3-4 cm above clavicle
- Morphology
  - Tubular structure
  - Appears varicose with many dilating just prior to terminus

Imaging Recommendations
- Best imaging tool
  - Evident on 55% CT exams
  - Most readily seen on T2 MR, especially when FS used

CT Findings
- CECT
  - Nonenhancing, tubular structure
  - On axial slices, may be mistaken for node

MR Findings
- Always follows signal intensity similar to CSF
  - T1 low intensity, T2 hyperintensity

DIFFERENTIAL DIAGNOSIS

Squamous Cell Carcinoma Nodes
- Squamous cell carcinoma (SCCa) nodes not infrequently necrotic (or cystic)
- Level IV or VI are drainage sites from larynx/hypopharynx or from SCCa nodes more superiorly
- Other nodes usually present

Differentiated Thyroid Carcinoma Nodes
- Thyroid carcinoma nodes may be cystic
- Variable signal intensity on MR due to colloid or hemorrhage
  - May be bright on T1 prior to contrast
- Other nodes usually present
- Differentiated thyroid carcinoma nodes can have variable MR appearances even in same case

Nodal Metastasis From Systemic Disease
- Supraclavicular fossa is well-known site for metastatic disease from chest and abdomen
  - So-called "Virchow node"

Lymphocele
- Idiopathic or postsurgical lymph-filled neck cyst
- Supraclavicular fossa, L > R

4th Branchial Anomaly
- More anterior in neck at level of or within thyroid gland
- Responsible for recurrent suppurative left thyroiditis

PATHOLOGY

General Features
- Etiology
  - Normal anatomical structure
  - Drains lymph from abdomen and left chest to venous circulation

Gross Pathologic & Surgical Features
- Valves present to prevent backflow
- Valves at terminus prevent venous backflow to duct
- May divide into 2 branches with right ending in right subclavian vein

CLINICAL ISSUES

Presentation
- Most common signs/symptoms
  - Asymptomatic; incidental imaging finding

Demographics
- Age
  - Increases in diameter slightly with age
- Gender
  - M = F

Natural History & Prognosis
- Obstruction may result in pleural effusion
- Probable source of metastases to left supraclavicular nodes

DIAGNOSTIC CHECKLIST

Consider
- Incidental normal finding
- May be mistaken for necrotic (cystic) level IV or VI node
  - Especially in setting of known systemic malignancy or differentiated thyroid carcinoma

Image Interpretation Pearls
- Key imaging features are tubular nature and isointense/isodense to CSF

SELECTED REFERENCES

1. Bang JH et al: Anatomic variability of the thoracic duct in pediatric patients with complex congenital heart disease. J Thorac Cardiovasc Surg. 150(3):490-5, 2015
2. Chen JM: The thoracic duct: Predictably unpredictable? J Thorac Cardiovasc Surg. 150(3):497, 2015
3. Ebada AH et al: Retroperitoneal intranodal contrast agent injection for lymphangiographic imaging of the thoracic duct in view of percutaneous intervention. J Vasc Interv Radiol. 26(9):1403-5, 2015
4. Phang K et al: Review of thoracic duct anatomical variations and clinical implications. Clin Anat. 27(4):637-44, 2014
5. Liu ME et al: Normal CT appearance of the distal thoracic duct. AJR Am J Roentgenol. 187(6):1615-20, 2006

KEY FACTS

TERMINOLOGY

- Benign neoplasm composed of mature fat

IMAGING

- 15% of lipomas occur in H&N
- 5% are multiple, more often in female patients
- May occur in any H&N space & may be transspatial
- Well-circumscribed, homogeneous mass composed of fat and displacing normal structures
- Homogeneous fat with minimal internal stranding
  - 8% have small nonfatty soft tissue component
- CT: Homogeneous, well-defined, low-density mass
- MR: Homogeneous signal of subcutaneous fat
- CT or MR: Any enhancement or soft tissue raises concern for liposarcoma
- FDG PET: No uptake in bland benign lipoma
  - Uptake suggests sarcoma or lipoma variant

TOP DIFFERENTIAL DIAGNOSES

- Dermoid
- Teratoma
- Lymphatic malformation
- Liposarcoma

CLINICAL ISSUES

- Asymptomatic lump in neck, more often in male patients
- Clinical differential is lymphatic malformation
- Most often found in 5th-6th decade

DIAGNOSTIC CHECKLIST

- CT: Measure density to determine fat content
- MR: Use chemical-selective fat saturation techniques, not STIR, to prove fat content
- If lipoma has soft tissue or enhancement, cannot distinguish from well-differentiated liposarcoma

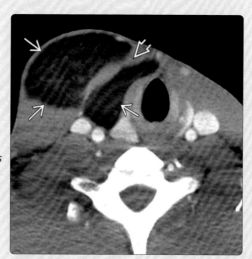

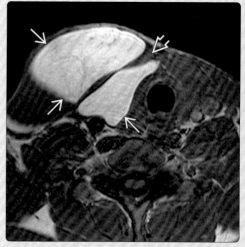

(Left) *Axial CECT through the lower neck of a young adult with a prominent neck mass demonstrates a well-defined low-density right neck mass ➡. Mass herniates around anterior portion of omohyoid muscle ➡, displaces tissues with no evidence of infiltration.* (Right) *Axial T1WI MR 6 weeks later shows intrinsically hyperintense mass ➡, enveloping omohyoid ➡ without invasion of adjacent tissues. Mass was thought to have enlarged clinically.*

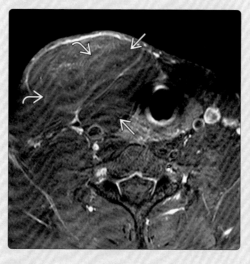

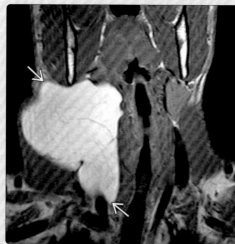

(Left) *Axial T1WI C+ FS MR reveals suppression of the high-intensity fat within the mass ➡, while also showing mildly complicated fibrous internal architecture ➡.* (Right) *Coronal T1WI MR illustrates craniocaudal extent of the mass ➡. Scan also shows mass effect on larynx, which was deviated to a greater extent across midline than on prior CT, raising concern for liposarcoma rather than lipoma. Resection of mass showed mature adipose tissue of benign lipoma.*

TERMINOLOGY

Definitions

- Benign neoplasm composed of mature fat

IMAGING

General Features

- Best diagnostic clue
  - Well-circumscribed, homogeneous mass composed of fat, displacing normal structures
- Location
  - 15% of lipomas occur in H&N
  - 5% are multiple, more often in female patients
  - May occur in any H&N space; may be transspatial
  - Most common sites in H&N
    - Posterior cervical, submandibular space
    - Anterior cervical, parotid spaces
- Size
  - Highly variable; may become massive
- Morphology
  - Well-defined mass with thin capsule and smooth contours
  - Majority have homogeneous fat content with **minimal internal stranding**
  - 8% of benign lipomas have small nonfatty soft tissue component
    - **Cannot be distinguished from well-differentiated liposarcoma** by imaging

CT Findings

- NECT
  - Homogeneous, well-defined, low-attenuation mass
    - Fat density in Hounsfield units = -65 to -120
- CECT
  - Well-defined, low-density, nonenhancing mass
  - Any significant enhancement raises concern for liposarcoma

MR Findings

- T1WI
  - Homogeneous hyperintense mass; follows signal of subcutaneous fat
  - Uniform signal loss on fat-suppressed images
- T2WI
  - Follows signal intensity of subcutaneous fat
- T1WI C+
  - No enhancement on T1WI C+ FS
  - Any significant matrix enhancement raises concern for liposarcoma

Ultrasonographic Findings

- Well-defined, compressible mass
- Multiple echogenic lines oriented parallel to skin
- 75% hyperechoic, 25% iso-/hypoechoic relative to muscle
- No deep acoustic enhancement or attenuation

Imaging Recommendations

- Best imaging tool
  - CT or MR both clearly determine fat content
  - Imaging is diagnostic, defines deep extent and pertinent anatomic relations

- Protocol advice
  - Use **chemical-selective fat saturation** rather than STIR to prove lipid content

Nuclear Medicine Findings

- PET/CT
  - Typically no uptake in benign lipoma
  - FDG uptake suggests liposarcoma
  - Uptake may be seen in (benign) hibernoma
  - Mild uptake in angiolipoma also described

DIFFERENTIAL DIAGNOSIS

Dermoid

- In H&N, most often floor of mouth, less commonly submandibular
- Thin-walled unilocular cyst with enhancing rim
- Contents usually heterogeneous mixture of fat & fluid
  - Uniform fat, globules of fat, or fat-fluid levels

Teratoma

- Neoplasm arising from all 3 embryonic germ cell layers
- Typically multiloculated large masses with complex imaging; may contain fat

Lymphatic Malformation

- Key clinical differential diagnosis for lipoma
- Thin-walled, uni- or multilocular cystic mass

Liposarcoma

- Solid mass typically with some fat component; usually enhances
- Well-differentiated liposarcoma may exactly mimic lipoma with stranding
- Plasma D-dimer levels may help differentiate lipoma from liposarcoma

PATHOLOGY

General Features

- Etiology
  - Most common benign mesenchymal tumor
  - Fat in lipoma is unavailable for systemic metabolism
    - Lipoma responds minimally to systemic weight changes
    - Lipoma may become more prominent after systemic weight loss
- Genetics
  - 80% of solitary lipomas have genetic aberration: 12q, 6p, 13q
- Associated abnormalities
  - Several syndromes associated with lipomas/lipomatosis
    - **Benign symmetric lipomatosis (Madelung disease)**
      - Diffuse, symmetric, unencapsulated fatty accumulation
      - Most commonly neck & upper back
      - Posterior superficial, posterior cervical, anterior cervical, & perivertebral spaces
      - Middle-aged men of Mediterranean descent; history of alcohol abuse
    - **Familial multiple lipomatosis**
      - Multiple small, well-demarcated, encapsulated lipomas

□ Commonly extremities, sparing neck & shoulders
□ Strong familial component
− **Dercum disease**
  □ Rare condition with multiple, painful lipomas
  □ Typically on extremities of obese postmenopausal women
− **Gardner syndrome**
  □ Osteomas, soft tissue tumors, & colonic adenomatous polyps
  □ Soft tissue tumors: **Lipoma**, fibroma, leiomyoma, neurofibroma, & desmoid tumors

Gross Pathologic & Surgical Features

- Typically encapsulated, smooth or lobulated, soft yellow masses
- **Benign pathologic variants of lipoma**
  o **Fibrolipoma**
    − Mature fibrous tissue associated with lipoma
  o **Infiltrating lipoma** (intramuscular lipoma)
    − Unencapsulated mature adipose tissue that infiltrates adjacent tissues
    − High risk of recurrence if intramuscular extensions not meticulously dissected
    − Uncommon in H&N region
  o **Angiolipoma**
    − Fatty tumor separated by enhancing small vessels
    − Often painful, may be multiple
    − Rare in H&N region, usually extremities
    − Tend to be found around puberty
  o **Spindle cell lipoma**
    − Variable proportions of mature fat & fibroblast-like spindle cells
    − Typically subcutaneous tissues of posterior neck
    − Indistinguishable from liposarcoma
    − 4th-6th decade, M > > F
  o **Hibernoma**
    − Benign encapsulated tumor consisting of brown fat, usually mixed with mature adipose tissue
    − Imaging depends on proportion of mature fat vs. brown fat
    − Brown fat has imaging characteristics similar to muscle ± enhancement
    − FDG uptake reported; may see variable uptake over time
  o **Lipoblastoma**
    − Focal fatty tumor or diffuse lipoblastomatosis
    − Benign pediatric lesion, almost all patients < 5 years age
    − Rarely in H&N, usually in extremities

Microscopic Features

- Composed of mature adipocytes that are uniform in size & shape
  o No necrosis, atypia, or increased mitotic rate
- Occasional fibrous connective tissue septations

CLINICAL ISSUES

Presentation

- Most common signs/symptoms
  o Asymptomatic lump in neck

− Clinically may be mistaken for lymphatic malformation
  o Stable size after initial period of discernible growth
- Other signs/symptoms
  o Large masses may present with symptoms attributable to compression of surrounding structures
- Clinical profile
  o Male patient with asymptomatic compressible neck mass

Demographics

- Age
  o Most often found in 5th-6th decade
- Gender
  o M > F

Natural History & Prognosis

- Benign, slowly enlarging mass
- Recurrence after excision suggests liposarcoma or inadequately resected infiltrating lipoma

Treatment

- Typically not resected unless compressing structures, such as airway, or for cosmetic reasons

DIAGNOSTIC CHECKLIST

Consider

- Carefully evaluate for presence of internal nodularity, enhancement, or stranding
  o These features raise possibility of liposarcoma
  o Be sure to articulate this in report

Image Interpretation Pearls

- Contrast-enhancing components suggest liposarcoma
- CT: Measure Hounsfield units to prove fat content
- MR: Use **chemical-selective fat saturation** techniques, not STIR, to confirm fat content

Reporting Tips

- Define full extent of lesion, specifically all spaces involved and tissues displaced

SELECTED REFERENCES

1. Tadisina KK et al: Syndromic lipomatosis of the head and neck: a review of the literature. Aesthetic Plast Surg. 39(3):440-8, 2015
2. Yoshiyama A et al: D-dimer levels in the differential diagnosis between lipoma and well-differentiated liposarcoma. Anticancer Res. 34(9):5181-5, 2014
3. Choi JW et al: Spindle cell lipoma of the head and neck: CT and MR imaging findings. Neuroradiology. 55(1):101-6, 2013
4. Kok KY et al: Lipoblastoma: clinical features, treatment, and outcome. World J Surg. 34(7):1517-22, 2010
5. Cappabianca S et al: Lipomatous lesions of the head and neck region: imaging findings in comparison with histological type. Radiol Med. 113(5):758-70, 2008
6. Dalal KM et al: Diagnosis and management of lipomatous tumors. J Surg Oncol. 97(4):298-313, 2008
7. Smith CS et al: False-positive findings on 18F-FDG PET/CT: differentiation of hibernoma and malignant fatty tumor on the basis of fluctuating standardized uptake values. AJR Am J Roentgenol. 190(4):1091-6, 2008
8. Zhang XY et al: Madelung disease: manifestations of CT and MR imaging. Oral Surg Oral Med Oral Pathol Oral Radiol Endod. 105(5):e57-64, 2008
9. Hameed M: Pathology and genetics of adipocytic tumors. Cytogenet Genome Res. 118(2-4):138-47, 2007
10. Gritzmann N et al: Sonography of soft tissue masses of the neck. J Clin Ultrasound. 30(6):356-73, 2002
11. Tien RD et al: Improved detection and delineation of head and neck lesions with fat suppression spin-echo MR imaging. AJNR Am J Neuroradiol. 12(1):19-24, 1991

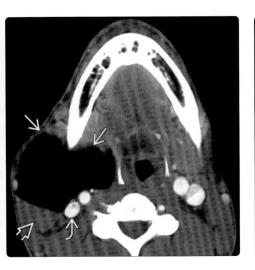

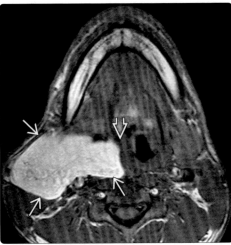

(Left) *Axial CECT shows a very low-density, uniform, well-defined lesion ➡ in right neck that presented as "parotid mass." The mass displaces sternocleidomastoid muscle ➡ and carotid & jugular ➡ vessels posteriorly, with no aggressive invasive features.* **(Right)** *Axial T1WI MR without gadolinium reveals uniform hyperintensity of the mass ➡ abutting pharyngeal wall ➡ and displacing the pharynx to left. Fat-saturated T2 and postcontrast T1 images displayed complete suppression of signal.*

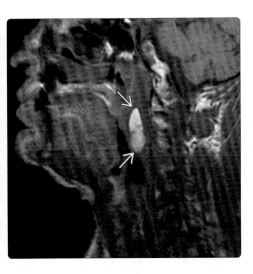

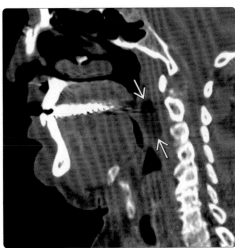

(Left) *Sagittal T1WI MR without gadolinium shows a slightly lobulated, intrinsically hyperintense, well-defined mass ➡ in the retropharyngeal space. Mass was evident on clinical examination as fullness of right posterior oropharyngeal wall.* **(Right)** *Sagittal reformatted CECT in the same patient 5 years later shows no evidence of change in size or contour of mass ➡, which shows homogeneous fat density and no evidence of enhancement within or surrounding it. Stability favors benign lipoma.*

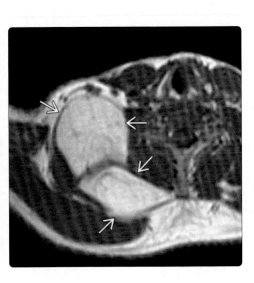

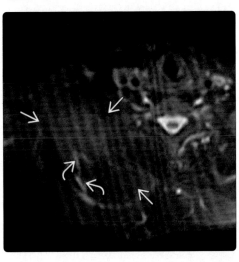

(Left) *Axial T1WI MR in a 53-year-old man with prior history of coccyx liposarcoma and now shoulder mass shows a lobulated mass ➡ in the right supraclavicular, paraspinal region. The mass is intrinsically hyperintense.* **(Right)** *Axial T2WI FS MR shows almost complete suppression of signal intensity, but for normal vessels ➡ associated with mass. No abnormal gadolinium enhancement or other features to suggest sarcomatous lesion are evident. Resected mass ➡ proved to be benign lipoma.*

Hemangiopericytoma of Head and Neck

TERMINOLOGY

- Hemangiopericytoma (HPC)
- Uncommon, slow-growing vascular neoplasm of varying malignancy

IMAGING

- Most HPCs occur in lower extremities, pelvis
- 15% occur in H&N
  - Intracranial/meningeal: Parasellar & paraclival
  - Orbit, cervical soft tissues, sinonasal cavity
- CT findings
  - Well circumscribed, lobular, avidly enhancing; more invasive behavior if high grade (CECT)
  - May see bone erosion or remodeling (bone CT)
- MR findings
  - Intermediate T1, high T2 signal
  - Vascular **flow voids** common
  - Prominent enhancement, typically uniform

TOP DIFFERENTIAL DIAGNOSES

- Skull base meningioma
- Skull base metastasis
- Skull base trigeminal schwannoma
- Clivus chordoma
- Orbital cavernous hemangioma
- Sinonasal angiomatous polyp

PATHOLOGY

- **50%** malignant, typically low grade
- Histologic similarities to solitary fibrous tumor

CLINICAL ISSUES

- Resection is treatment of choice ± XRT
- Local recurrence ≤ 50%; 30% metastases < 10 years
- HPC mimics many more common tumors
- Consider HPC if avidly enhancing, well-circumscribed mass
- Signs and symptoms depend on tumor location

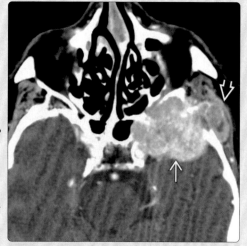
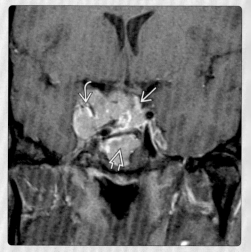

(Left) Axial CECT shows skull base hemangiopericytoma (HPC) with bone destruction and extension into the middle fossa ➡ and masticator space ➡. Absence of hyperostosis is clue that this is not a meningioma, though distinction from other destructive masses is difficult. (Right) Coronal T1WI C+ FS MR reveals parasellar HPC with intrasellar ➡ and infrasellar ➡ components and prominent internal flow voids ➡. Preoperative diagnosis was meningioma; these lesions may be indistinguishable on imaging.

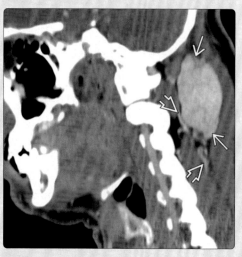
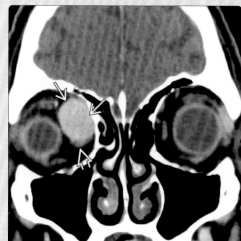

(Left) Sagittal reconstructed CECT reveals a densely enhancing mass ➡ in the suboccipital musculature with prominent vasculature adjacent to the lesion ➡. Paraspinal soft tissues are a characteristic location of cervical HPC. (Right) Coronal CECT shows a prominently enhancing, well-circumscribed HPC ➡ abutting a distorted medial rectus muscle ➡ and obscuring the superior oblique muscle. Cavernous hemangiomas are considerably more common and may demonstrate identical imaging features.

TERMINOLOGY

Abbreviations

- Hemangiopericytoma (HPC)

Synonyms

- Sinonasal HPC, a.k.a. **glomangiopericytoma**

Definitions

- Uncommon, slow-growing vascular neoplasm with variable degree of malignant potential

IMAGING

General Features

- Best diagnostic clue
  - Nonspecific appearance: Well-circumscribed, avidly enhancing solid mass
    - Mimics many different tumors depending on site
- Location
  - Most common in lower extremities, retroperitoneum/pelvis
  - 15% in H&N
    - Intracranial/meningeal: Parasellar & paraclival
    - Retrobulbar orbit
    - Cervical paraspinal soft tissues
    - Sinonasal: Nasal cavity, maxillary sinus
- Size
  - Variable
- Morphology
  - Well circumscribed, invasive when high grade

CT Findings

- CECT
  - Lobular, exophytic mass
  - May erode or remodel bone
  - Prominent enhancement is characteristic
    - Uniform > heterogeneous

MR Findings

- T1WI
  - Intermediate T1 signal
- T2WI
  - High T2 signal
  - Vascular flow voids common
- T1WI C+
  - Prominent enhancement is characteristic
    - Uniform > heterogeneous

DIFFERENTIAL DIAGNOSIS

Skull Base Meningioma

- Meningioma more frequently sessile with dural tail, calcification, hyperostosis

Skull Base Metastasis

- Destructive bone lesion with soft tissue component

Skull Base Trigeminal Schwannoma

- Centered in Meckel cave

Clivus Chordoma

- Midline destructive clival lesion

- Typically T2 hyperintense

Orbital Cavernous Hemangioma

- Soft, distensible retrobulbar masses

Sinonasal Angiomatous Polyp

- Intensely enhancing, noninvasive nasal mass

PATHOLOGY

Staging, Grading, & Classification

- **50% malignant**, typically **low grade**
- Wide path range from benign to malignant
  - Malignant HPC has been called low-grade sarcoma

Microscopic Features

- Arise from pericytes of Zimmerman
- Histologic and immunohistochemical overlap with **solitary fibrous tumor (SFT)**
- Sinonasal HPC likely represents similar but distinct entity
  - Best termed **"glomangiopericytoma"**

CLINICAL ISSUES

Presentation

- Most common signs/symptoms
  - Presentation depends on site of tumor
    - Skull base: Cranial neuropathy, ophthalmoplegia
    - Orbit: Painless proptosis
    - Cervical soft tissue: Painless mass
    - Sinonasal: Nasal obstruction, epistaxis

Demographics

- Age: Wide range (peaks in 4th decade)
- Epidemiology: Rare tumor

Natural History & Prognosis

- Local recurrence in 50%; 30% metastasizes < 10 years
- Metastases, most frequently to lung
- Sinonasal lesions have more indolent course

Treatment

- Wide local excision is main treatment
- Radiation used for high-grade tumor, positive surgical margins, or recurrence
- Monitor for recurrence for > 10 years

DIAGNOSTIC CHECKLIST

Consider

- Include HPC in differential for **avidly enhancing, well-circumscribed masses**
  - **Mimicker** of many more common lesions

SELECTED REFERENCES

1. Shaigany K et al: A population-based analysis of head and neck hemangiopericytoma. Laryngoscope. 126(3):643-50, 2016
2. Wallace KM et al: Endovascular preoperative embolization of orbital hemangiopericytoma with n-butyl cyanoacrylate glue. Ophthal Plast Reconstr Surg. 30(4):e97-100, 2014
3. Bignami M et al: Endoscopic, endonasal management of sinonasal haemangiopericytoma: 12-year experience. J Laryngol Otol. 124(11):1178-82, 2010
4. Bonde VR et al: Two patients with intracavernous haemangiopericytoma. J Clin Neurosci. 16(2):330-3, 2009

TERMINOLOGY

- Plexiform neurofibroma (PNF): Architecturally complex neurofibroma involving multiple nerve fascicles
  - **Pathognomonic** for **neurofibromatosis type 1 (NF1)**

IMAGING

- **Lobular, serpiginous infiltrative transspatial mass**
- CECT has nonspecific infiltrative appearance
  - Mild contrast enhancement
- MR best characterizes and delineates complete extent
  - Lobulated T2 hyperintensity
  - Central T2 hypointense foci: **Target sign**

TOP DIFFERENTIAL DIAGNOSES

- Venous malformation
- Lymphatic malformation
- Sarcoma

PATHOLOGY

- Deletion in *NF1* gene on long arm of **chromosome 17**
- Autosomal dominant inheritance
- Decreased production of neurofibromin (tumor suppressor) protein

CLINICAL ISSUES

- Present at birth or develops with age
- "Bag of worms" on clinical exam
- PNFs in **~ 30% of NF1**
- 5-10% risk of malignant transformation

DIAGNOSTIC CHECKLIST

- On CECT appears as infiltrative solid mass
- On MR may mimic venous malformation; distinguish with target sign
- Look for other manifestations of NF1

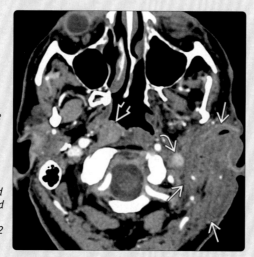
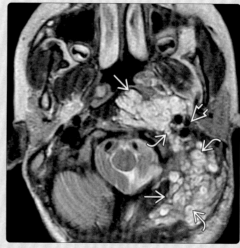

(Left) Axial CECT demonstrates a minimally enhancing infiltrative soft tissue mass ➡ involving subcutaneous and deep tissues. The mass abuts and surrounds the left internal jugular vein ➡. Notice the mildly enhancing lesion of the right prevertebral muscle ➡. (Right) Axial T2WI MR reveals characteristic MR findings of plexiform neurofibroma ➡ in prevertebral and paraspinous tissues and around the carotid sheath ➡. The multilobulated mass is hyperintense except for the central areas of low T2 signal ➡.

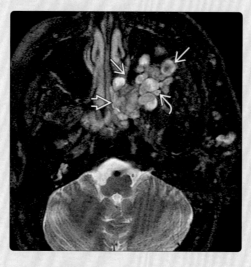
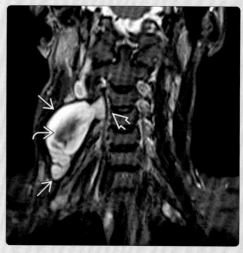

(Left) Axial T2WI FS MR in a patient with neurofibromatosis type 1 shows a multilobulated mass ➡ distending left pterygopalatine fossa & extending into the posterior nasal cavity ➡ through the sphenopalatine foramen. The target sign of focal low signal ➡ suggests plexiform neurofibroma. (Right) Coronal STIR MR shows a large right neck plexiform neurofibroma ➡ from the right C3-C4 neuroforamen ➡. This multilobulated mass shows the classic target sign of central T2 hypointensity ➡.

TERMINOLOGY

Abbreviations

- Neurofibromatosis type 1 (NF1)
- Plexiform neurofibroma (PNF)

Definitions

- PNF: Architecturally complex neurofibroma involving multiple nerve fascicles
  o Often found in areas of branched nerves
  o Pathognomonic for NF1

IMAGING

General Features

- Best diagnostic clue
  o T2 FS MR shows lobular, **serpiginous contour** of **transspatial mass** with **focal target signs**
- Location
  o Trunk, limbs, or H&N most common
  o May be superficial cutaneous, subcutaneous, or deep
- Morphology
  o Lobular mass infiltrating through tissues along nerve branches

Imaging Recommendations

- Best imaging tool
  o MR best characterizes and delineates complete extent
- Protocol advice
  o Multiplanar imaging best for delineating full extent
    - Fat saturation sequences helpful for T2 and T1 C+

CT Findings

- CECT
  o Mildly enhancing infiltrative solid mass

MR Findings

- T1WI
  o Isointense to muscle
- T2WI FS
  o Hyperintense lobulated transspatial mass
  o Central low signal foci are characteristic: **Target sign**
- T1WI C+ FS
  o Mild to moderately enhancing

DIFFERENTIAL DIAGNOSIS

Venous Malformation

- Close mimic on imaging
- Phleboliths evident in this lesion; best seen on CT

Lymphatic Malformation

- Nonenhancing, cystic transspatial mass

Sarcoma

- Infiltrative malignant tumor, anywhere in H&N
- Rapid growth, ± adenopathy

PATHOLOGY

General Features

- Genetics
  o Deletion in *NF1* gene on long arm of chromosome 17
    - Results in decreased production of **neurofibromin** (tumor suppressor) protein
    - Autosomal dominant inheritance
- Associated abnormalities
  o NF1 has many spine, neck, & brain findings
    - Circumscribed dermal neurofibromas
    - Sphenoid wing dysplasia with cephalocele
    - Vascular stenoses and aneurysms
    - Optic nerve glioma
    - Brain and spinal cord astrocytomas
    - Cervical spine neurofibromas
    - Scoliosis

Staging, Grading, & Classification

- World Health Organization (WHO) grade 1 tumors

Gross Pathologic & Surgical Features

- Diffuse tortuosity, enlargement of nerve & branches

Microscopic Features

- Schwann cells, axons, and endoneural fibroblasts enclosed by perineurium

CLINICAL ISSUES

Presentation

- Most common signs/symptoms
  o Superficial lesions palpable, disfiguring
    - "Bag of worms" on clinical exam
- Other signs/symptoms
  o Specific to tissues infiltrated

Demographics

- Age
  o Variable: Present at birth or develops with age
- Epidemiology
  o NF1 incidence: 1 in 3,000
  o PNFs found in ~ **30% of NF1**

Natural History & Prognosis

- **5-10% risk** of **malignant transformation** (usually to malignant peripheral nerve sheath tumor)
  o Progressive enlargement/pain suggest degeneration

Treatment

- Impossible to completely resect
- Debulking may be performed for cosmetic or functional reasons

DIAGNOSTIC CHECKLIST

Image Interpretation Pearls

- CECT: Appears as infiltrative solid mass
- MR: May mimic venous malformation; distinguish with target sign
- Evaluate for other manifestations of NF1

SELECTED REFERENCES

1. Latham K et al: Neurofibromatosis of the head and neck: classification and surgical management. Plast Reconstr Surg. 135(3):845-55, 2015
2. Setabutr D et al: Neurofibromatosis of the larynx causing stridor and sleep apnea. Am J Otolaryngol. 35(5):631-5, 2014
3. Jett K et al: Clinical and genetic aspects of neurofibromatosis 1. Genet Med. 12(1):1-11, 2010

KEY FACTS

TERMINOLOGY

- Posttransplantation lymphoproliferative disorder (PTLD)
- Uncontrolled lymphoid growth in transplant recipient on immunosuppressive therapy
- Disease spectrum ranges from hyperplasia to malignancy
  - Reactive hyperplasia → polymorphic PTLD → monomorphic PTLD → Hodgkin disease & non-Hodgkin lymphoma-like PTLD

IMAGING

- Mimics H&N lymphoma seen in nontransplant patients
- May also mimic pharyngeal infection and abscesses
- Consider when history of transplant plus any nodal or extranodal enlargement, or H&N mass
  - Adenotonsillar &/or nodal enlargement
  - Sinonasal masses or infiltrating tissue to skull base
  - Orbital or oral cavity mass
- Increased FDG uptake on PET/CT

TOP DIFFERENTIAL DIAGNOSES

- Tonsillar inflammation
- Tonsillar/peritonsillar abscess
- Reactive lymph nodes
- Invasive fungal sinusitis

PATHOLOGY

- Therapeutic T-cell suppression allows proliferation of B cells infected with EBV

CLINICAL ISSUES

- Solid organ transplant > > bone marrow transplant
- More common in pediatric transplant patients
- Up to 80% 1st year post transplant

DIAGNOSTIC CHECKLIST

- Consider PTLD with every transplant patient when imaging suggests infection or lymphoma-like lesions

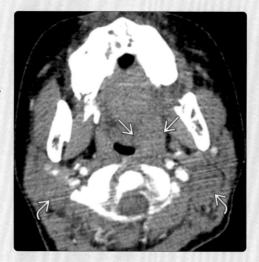

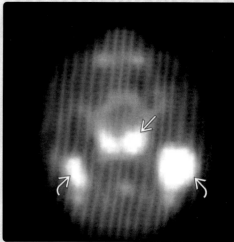

(Left) *Axial CECT shows asymmetrically enlarged left palatine tonsil* ➡ *but no abnormal enhancement or peritonsillar collection. Multiple enlarged, homogeneous neck nodes are apparent* ➡ *in high jugular chains.* (Right) *Axial PET in same patient reveals marked FDG avidity in bilateral neck nodes* ➡ *with asymmetric FDG uptake in left palatine tonsil* ➡. *PTLD can mimic tonsillitis with reactive adenopathy, but transplant history is key. Biopsy distinguishes these processes.*

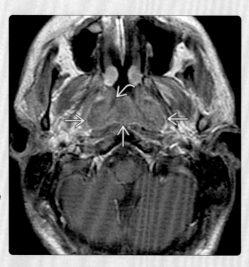

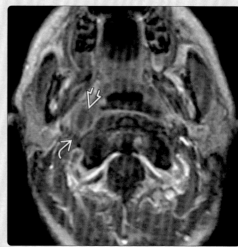

(Left) *Axial T1 C+ MR shows enlarged enhancing nasopharyngeal adenoidal tissue* ➡. *Tonsil has endophytic growth and irregular mucosal margin* ➡. (Right) *Inferiorly, note enlarged right retropharyngeal node* ➡ *anteromedial to right internal carotid artery* ➡. *Retropharyngeal node is centrally necrotic with peripheral enhancement. No retropharyngeal edema is seen as might be expected with suppurative node and tonsillitis.*

TERMINOLOGY

Abbreviations

- Posttransplantation lymphoproliferative disorder (PTLD)

Definitions

- Uncontrolled lymphoid growth in transplant recipient on immunosuppressive therapy
- Spectrum of disease: Hyperplasia to malignancy

IMAGING

General Features

- Best diagnostic clue
  - History of transplant plus any nodal, extranodal enlargement, or H&N mass
- Location
  - Anywhere in H&N: Extranodal or nodal
  - Waldeyer ring, sinonasal, orbit, or oral cavity
  - Nodal involvement seen as 2 forms
    - Large nodal masses
    - Clusters of normal-sized nodes

Imaging Recommendations

- Best imaging tool
  - Either CT or MR adequate for delineating H&N mass
  - FDG PET for staging and response to treatment
- Protocol advice
  - Postcontrast imaging best shows necrosis & nodes

CT Findings

- CECT
  - Markedly enhancing enlarged adenoids or tonsils
    - More often deeply invasive than exophytic
  - H&N mass or infiltrating soft tissue at skull base

MR Findings

- T1WI C+ FS
  - Intensely enhancing, aggressive-appearing masses
  - Necrotic or solid nodes

Nuclear Medicine Findings

- PET/CT
  - Increased FDG uptake in PTLD

DIFFERENTIAL DIAGNOSIS

Tonsillar Inflammation

- Enlarged, heterogeneously enhancing tonsil

Tonsillar/Peritonsillar Abscess

- Rim-enhancing, low-density focus in or around tonsil

Reactive Lymph Nodes

- Common in children and teens

Invasive Fungal Sinusitis

- Infiltration of perisinus fat, deep facial fat planes

PATHOLOGY

General Features

- Etiology

- Therapeutic T-cell suppression allows proliferation of B cells infected with EBV
- Greatest risk factors
  - EBV-naïve recipient of EBV-infected donor organ

Staging, Grading, & Classification

- World Health Organization (WHO) categories (2008)
  - Early lesions
    - Plasmacytic hyperplasia
    - Infectious mononucleosis-like lesion
  - Polymorphic PTLD
  - Monomorphic PTLD (classify according to lymphoma resembled)
    - B-cell neoplasms
    - T-cell neoplasms
  - Classic Hodgkin lymphoma-type PTLD

Gross Pathologic & Surgical Features

- Predilection for extranodal sites of disease

Microscopic Features

- EBV detectable in tissues

CLINICAL ISSUES

Presentation

- Most common signs/symptoms
  - H&N: Adenopathy, nasal obstruction, sinusitis, sore throat
  - Less common: Oral mucosal ulcer or mass
  - Generalized: Fever, ↓ weight, night sweats

Demographics

- Age
  - Pediatric patients have 4x incidence of adults
- Epidemiology
  - 2-3% of adult transplant recipients
  - Up to 8% of pediatric transplant patients

Natural History & Prognosis

- Most often after solid organ transplant, less often after bone marrow or stem cell transplant
- Up to 80% in 1st year post transplant
  - Highest incidence: Heart-lung, lung, or small bowel
  - Lowest incidence: Kidney transplant
- Prognosis determined by tumor burden at diagnosis and PTLD category

Treatment

- Reduction of immunosuppression is key
- Anti-CD20 monoclonal antibody
- Surgery, radiation, chemotherapy, EBV-specific cytotoxic lymphocytes, anti-EBV peptides

DIAGNOSTIC CHECKLIST

Consider

- Consider PTLD when transplant patient has imaging findings of infection or lymphoma

SELECTED REFERENCES

1. Rosenberg AS et al: Hodgkin lymphoma post-transplant lymphoproliferative disorder: a comparative analysis of clinical characteristics, prognosis, and survival. Am J Hematol. 91(6):560-5, 2016

KEY FACTS

TERMINOLOGY

- Synonyms: Extraosseous or nasopharyngeal chordoma
- Extraosseous atypical H&N chordoma instead of usual clival origin
- Rare extraosseous locally aggressive tumor of notochordal origin

IMAGING

- CT findings
  - Lobular heterogeneous minimally enhancing nasopharyngeal mass
  - Dystrophic calcifications common
  - Anterior clival scalloping with well-defined **midline tract** to medial basal canal
- MR findings
  - Lobular heterogeneous nasopharyngeal mass with midline clival tract along course of notochordal remnant
  - Heterogeneous ↑ ↑ T2 signal intensity present
  - ↑ ↑ T2 signal intensity helps differentiate from ↓ T2 signal in other nasopharyngeal malignancies
- Heterogeneous enhancement pattern most common

TOP DIFFERENTIAL DIAGNOSES

- Tornwaldt cyst
- Nasopharyngeal carcinoma
- Non-Hodgkin lymphoma

DIAGNOSTIC CHECKLIST

- Consider extraosseous chordoma when ↑ ↑ T2 signal nasopharyngeal mass extends from midline clival cleft
- Preoperative report must note extension along midline clival tract, so complete resection is performed

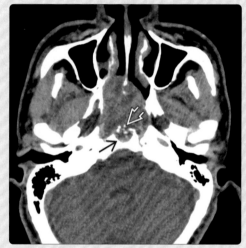
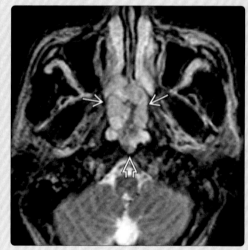

(Left) Axial CECT demonstrates a large nasopharyngeal extraosseous chordoma filling the airway. Notice the anterior clival midline scalloping in the area of the medial basal canal ➡. Characteristic bone fragments ➡ are visible in the posterior midline of the tumor. (Right) Axial T2 MR in the same patient reveals the high signal chordoma ➡ in the posterior nose and nasopharyngeal airway. The midline scalloping of the anterior clivus is visible ➡.

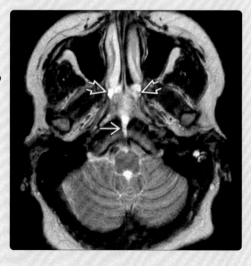
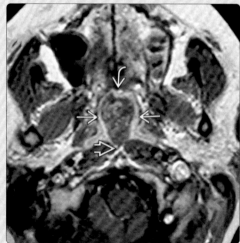

(Left) Axial T2 MR reveals focal midline anterior clival defect ➡, representing path of the primitive notochord. Tract must be resected with nasopharyngeal component to avoid local recurrence. Note hyperintense mass obstructs posterior nasal cavity bilaterally ➡. (Right) Axial T1WI C+ MR shows an ovoid, rim-enhancing midline extraosseous chordoma ➡ that extends through prevertebral muscles ➡ to the posterior margin of the hard palate ➡.

TERMINOLOGY

Synonyms

- Nasopharyngeal chordoma

Definitions

- Rare extraosseous locally aggressive tumor of notochordal origin
  - Location & presenting signs differ from classic clival chordoma

IMAGING

General Features

- Best diagnostic clue
  - Submucosal nasopharyngeal mass with **midline clival tract** along course of notochordal remnant
- Location
  - Nasopharynx with connection to midline clival bony defect
  - Extraosseous atypical H&N chordoma instead of usual clival origin
  - Extension to nasal cavity or maxillary sinus rarely reported
- Size
  - Variable, from 1-7 cm in maximum diameter
- Morphology
  - Lobulated, often bulky

Imaging Recommendations

- Best imaging tool
  - T2 MR best shows **hyperintense** mass with **sinus tract** extending from mass to midline clival defect

CT Findings

- CECT
  - Lobular heterogeneous minimally enhancing nasopharyngeal mass
    - Dystrophic calcifications common
- Bone CT
  - Anterior clival scalloping with well-defined **midline tract** to medial basal canal
    - **Medial basal canal**: Cephalad exit tract of notochord, extending from intraclival location into nasopharyngeal soft tissues

MR Findings

- T1WI
  - Hypointense with rare scattered regions of ↑ signal from intratumoral hemorrhage
- T2WI
  - Heterogeneous ↑ ↑ signal intensity present
    - ↑ ↑ T2 signal helps differentiate from ↓ T2 signal in other nasopharyngeal malignances
- T1WI C+
  - Heterogeneous enhancement pattern most common

DIFFERENTIAL DIAGNOSIS

Tornwaldt Cyst

- Small central cyst without discrete clival sinus tract

Nasopharyngeal Carcinoma

- Paramedian mass usually iso - to hypointense on T2
- Skull base destruction usually off midline, without discrete clival cleft

Pharyngeal Mucosal Space Non-Hodgkin Lymphoma

- Bulky nasopharyngeal mass usually iso- to hypointense on T2
- Associated retropharyngeal, cervical adenopathy common

PATHOLOGY

General Features

- Etiology
  - Notochordal remnant with tumor extending from nasopharynx to medial basal canal of clivus

Gross Pathologic & Surgical Features

- Lobular bulky mass with fibrous pseudocapsule

Microscopic Features

- Heterogeneous mass with regions of necrosis, mucoid material, old blood products, & dystrophic calcification
- Oval **physaliphorous cells** predominate

CLINICAL ISSUES

Presentation

- Most common signs/symptoms
  - Nasopharyngeal fullness or nasal obstruction when nasal cavity extension present
  - Mastoid & middle ear opacification if tumor obstructs eustachian tube

Demographics

- Age
  - Ranges from 1st decade to 70 yr
  - Mean age at presentation: 42 yr

Natural History & Prognosis

- Prognosis generally better for younger patients

Treatment

- Complete surgical extirpation is treatment of choice
- Tumor in midline clival tract must be resected to bone to prevent recurrence

DIAGNOSTIC CHECKLIST

Consider

- Extraosseous chordoma when ↑ ↑ T2 nasopharyngeal mass is present extending to midline bony clival cleft

Reporting Tips

- Preoperative report must note extension along midline clival tract, so complete resection is performed

SELECTED REFERENCES

1. Sajisevi M et al: Nasopharyngeal masses arising from embryologic remnants of the clivus: a case series. J Neurol Surg Rep. 76(2):e253-e257, 2015
2. Yan ZY et al: Primary chordoma in the nasal cavity and nasopharynx: CT and MR imaging findings. AJNR Am J Neuroradiol. 31(2):246-50, 2010
3. Nguyen RP et al: Extraosseous chordoma of the nasopharynx. AJNR Am J Neuroradiol. 30(4):803-7, 2009

KEY FACTS

TERMINOLOGY

- **N**on-**H**odgkin **l**ymphoma (NHL)
- Heterogeneous lymphoreticular system malignancy
- H&N NHL has multiple forms
  - Nodal, nonnodal lymphatic (tonsils, lingual lymphoid, & adenoids), extralymphatic (e.g., skull base, thyroid, sinuses)

IMAGING

- **Nodal NHL**
  - Multiple 1- to 3-cm solid nodes
  - Dominant large node up to 5 cm
  - Aggressive NHL may have necrosis
- **Nonnodal lymphatic NHL**
  - Enlarged, homogeneously enhancing tonsils &/or adenoids ± enlarged ipsilateral nodes
  - May be heterogeneous & infiltrative
- **Extralymphatic NHL**
  - Focal or infiltrative mass in any tissue in neck

TOP DIFFERENTIAL DIAGNOSES

- Wide differential diagnosis depending on form of NHL: Nodal, nonnodal lymphatic, extralymphatic
- Lymphoma is one of great mimickers

PATHOLOGY

- WHO is favored classification (2008)
- Modified Ann Arbor staging system is for clinical staging, treatment, and prognosis
- Lugano classification also used to assess interim and treatment response

CLINICAL ISSUES

- Treatment depends on cell type, stage, patient age
- Chemo, XRT, or combined modality therapy
- May be indolent, progressive but not curable, or aggressive but often curable
- 5-year survival: Stage I/II 85%, III/IV 50%

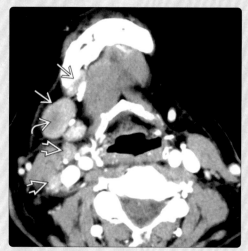

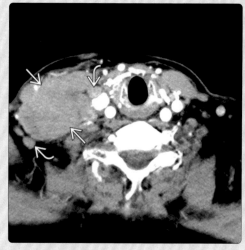

(Left) Axial CECT in 66-year-old patient shows multiple nodal masses in right levels IB ➡ and IIA ➡ nodal locations. Submandibular nodes are heterogeneous with eccentric low density ➡, suggesting necrosis, and posterior IIA node is irregular and poorly defined. (Right) Axial CECT in infrahyoid neck demonstrates homogeneous mass ➡ inseparable from the right sternocleidomastoid muscle, with multiple smaller abnormal nodes ➡. Biopsy showed diffuse large B-cell lymphoma.

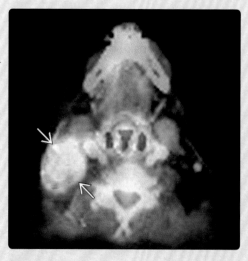

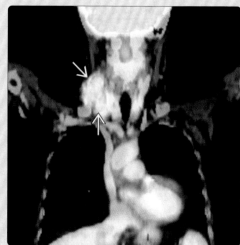

(Left) Axial PET/CT, same patient, demonstrates marked FDG uptake in level IIA node ➡. Baseline PET is critical, as change in SUV after treatment determines treatment response. (Right) Coronal PET/CT shows nodal mass ➡, with an SUV of 21.2. Patient was treated with radiation and chemotherapy, but the lymphoma recurred the following year and did not respond to salvage therapy.

TERMINOLOGY

Abbreviations

- Non-Hodgkin lymphoma (NHL)

Definitions

- Lymphoma is heterogeneous lymphoreticular system malignancy
  - Over 50 types of lymphoma have been described based on histologic & molecular criteria
- All lymphomas designated Hodgkin (HL) or NHL
  - HL: Neoplastic Reed-Sternberg cells with mixed inflammatory cell mass
  - NHL: Multiple subtypes of **B-cell, T-cell,** or **NK-cell** lymphomas/leukemias
    - Diffuse large B-cell lymphoma most common (30%)
- **H&N NHL has multiple forms**
  - **Nodal, nonnodal lymphatic** (tonsils, adenoids, lingual lymphoid), **extralymphatic** (e.g., thyroid, sinuses)

IMAGING

General Features

- Best diagnostic clue
  - Enlarged, nonnecrotic nodes ± tonsillar mass
  - Extralymphatic form appears as infiltrative mass in almost any H&N area
  - Image-guided core biopsy often required to confirm and assign subtype
    - Flow cytometry confirms monoclonal population of lymphocytes

CT Findings

- **Nodal NHL**
  - Multiple 1- to 3-cm solid nodes
  - Dominant large node up to 5 cm
  - Aggressive NHL shows necrosis or extranodal spread
- **Nonnodal lymphatic NHL**
  - Enlarged, homogeneously enhancing tonsils ± adenoids
  - May be confined to 1 tonsillar structure, multiple structures, or entire Waldeyer ring
    - Nasopharyngeal **(adenoids), palatine, lingual tonsil**
  - ± enlarged ipsilateral nodes
  - Aggressive NHL
    - Often more heterogeneous enhancement with necrosis
- **Extralymphatic NHL**
  - Appears as focal or infiltrative mass
  - Involves almost any tissue or site in neck
    - Skull base, cranial nerves, lacrimal gland, extraocular muscles, sinonasal, facial bones (especially premaxillary soft tissues), masticator space, parotid or thyroid gland

MR Findings

- T1WI
  - Typically iso- or slightly hyperintense to muscle
- T2WI
  - Intermediate intensity, hyperintense to muscle
  - More aggressive tumors are heterogeneous
- DWI
  - **Low ADC values** (dark) in solid components
  - Necrotic areas show high ADC values
- T1WI C+ FS
  - Intermediate homogeneous enhancement
  - More aggressive tumors heterogeneous

Nuclear Medicine Findings

- PET/CT
  - PET/CT used for initial staging of all NHL
  - FDG PET shows **variable avidity**
    - Higher in aggressive, lower in more indolent NHL
  - Interim PET/CT, obtained during treatment, assesses response
    - Patients with limited response during treatment will have change in therapy
  - Posttherapy PET/CT used to assess treatment response

Imaging Recommendations

- Best imaging tool
  - Standard staging is FDG PET/CT or PET/CECT

DIFFERENTIAL DIAGNOSIS

Nodal NHL

- Squamous cell carcinoma (SCCa) metastatic nodes
- HL nodes
- Reactive lymph nodes

Nonnodal Lymphatic NHL

- SCCa oropharynx (base of tongue lingual tissue, palatine tonsils)
- Nasopharyngeal carcinoma
- Tonsillar lymphoid hyperplasia
- Minor salivary gland malignancy pharyngeal mucosal space

Extralymphatic NHL

- Idiopathic extraorbital inflammation (pseudotumor)
- Orbital idiopathic inflammation (pseudotumor)
- SCCa sinonasal
- Esthesioneuroblastoma
- Rhabdomyosarcoma
- Anaplastic thyroid carcinoma
- Invasive fibrous thyroiditis (Riedel)
- Fibromatosis

PATHOLOGY

General Features

- Etiology
  - Multiple varying risk factors: Immunesuppression, infectious agents, genetic mutations
    - Viral infection: EBV, HIV, human T-cell leukemia lymohoma virus-1, hepatitis C
    - Chronic immune system suppression/stimulation: Sjogren syndrome, celiac sprue, rheumatoid arthritis
    - History of prior ionizing radiation
- Genetics
  - Increased incidence in 1st-degree relatives
    - Variable heritability by subtypes

Staging, Grading, & Classification

- **WHO** is favored classification (2008)
  - Based on immunophenotype & morphology
  - More than 30 different types of NHL

Ann Arbor Staging Classification

Stage	Distribution of Disease
Stage I	Involvement of single lymph node region or lymphoid structure (e.g., spleen, thymus, Waldeyer ring) or single IE
Stage II	Involvement of ≥ 2 lymph node regions on same side of diaphragm (II) or localized contiguous involvement of only 1 extranodal organ or site and its regional nodes ± other node regions on same side of diaphragm (IIE)
Stage III	Involvement of node regions on both sides of diaphragm (III); may have spleen (IIIS) or localized contiguous involvement of only 1 extranodal site (IIIE) or both (IIIE, IIIS)
Stage IV	Disseminated disease: ≥ 1 extranodal organ or tissue, ± associated nodes or isolated extralymphatic disease with distant nodal involvement
Additional Designations	
A	No symptoms
B	Fever, night sweats, unexplained weight loss > 10% of body weight in 6 months
X	Bulky disease: > 10-cm long axis nodal mass or mediastinal mass > 1/3 chest diameter at T5/6 on PA CXR

IE = extralymphatic site.

- **B-cell** neoplasms (80-85%)
  - ☐ Precursor B-lymphoblastic leukemia/lymphoma
  - ☐ Peripheral B-cell neoplasms
- **T-cell** & putative **NK-cell** neoplasms (15-20%)
  - ☐ Precursor T-lymphoblastic leukemia/lymphoma
  - ☐ Peripheral T-cell and NK-cell neoplasms
- 8 most common NHL types
  - **DLBCL: 30%**
    - Aggressive NHL; multiple subtypes
  - **Follicular lymphoma: 20%**
    - Usually indolent, may be high grade
  - **Small lymphocytic lymphoma of chronic lymphocytic leukemia type: < 10%**
    - Nodal form of chronic lymphocytic leukemia
  - **Marginal zone lymphoma (MZL): < 10%**
    - Splenic MZL: Elderly patients, no nodes
  - **Mucosa-associated lymphoid tissue: 5%**
    - Indolent NHL; **lacrimal gland, thyroid**
  - **Mantle cell lymphoma: 7%**
    - Waldeyer ring in H&N; usually presents stage IV
  - **Peripheral T-cell lymphoma: 5-10%**
    - Indolent to aggressive; variable response to treatment
    - Leukemia-like, cutaneous, and nodal forms
    - **Nasal NK T-cell lymphoma** previously known as "lethal midline granuloma"
  - **Burkitt lymphoma**
    - Rare, highly aggressive, strong male preponderance
      - ☐ **Endemic (Africa): Tumor mass of face/jaw**
      - ☐ Sporadic (USA): Bulky abdominal disease
- **Modified Ann Arbor staging system** is for clinical staging, treatment, and prognosis
- **Lugano classification** now commonly used to assess response

CLINICAL ISSUES

Presentation

- Most common signs/symptoms
  - **Nodal**: Presentation with neck mass
  - **Nonnodal lymphatic**: Naso- or oropharyngeal mass, but associated neck adenopathy may be presenting symptom
  - **Extralymphatic**: Mass, pain, cranial neuropathy
- Other signs/symptoms
  - **Systemic B symptoms, such as fevers, night sweats, weight loss**

Demographics

- Age
  - Median: 53 years (range: 18-70)
- Gender
  - M:F = 1.5:1.0
- Epidemiology
  - Increasing incidence of NHL
  - 5% of cancer cases in USA; ~ 5% of H&N cancers

Natural History & Prognosis

- Variable prognosis, from curable to indolent to rapidly aggressive
- 5-year survival: Stage I/II 85%, III/IV 50%
- Predictors of poor treatment outcome
  - Age > 60 years, > 1 extranodal site, stage III/IV, ↑ lactate dehydrogenase, poor performance status

Treatment

- Treatment depends on cell type, stage, patient age
- Chemo, XRT, or combined modality therapy
- Bone marrow transplant may be performed for recurrent or refractory disease

DIAGNOSTIC CHECKLIST

Image Interpretation Pearls

- Necrosis ± extranodal spread or diffuse infiltration suggests high-grade, aggressive NHL
- NHL, especially extralymphatic, is great mimicker
- Image-guided core biopsies, if requested, should be sent for flow cytometry and nodal architecture

SELECTED REFERENCES

1. Johnson SA et al: Imaging for staging and response assessment in lymphoma. Radiology. 276(2):323-38, 2015
2. Cheson BD et al: Recommendations for initial evaluation, staging, and response assessment of Hodgkin and non-Hodgkin lymphoma: the Lugano classification. J Clin Oncol. 32(27):3059-68, 2014

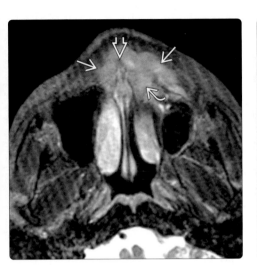

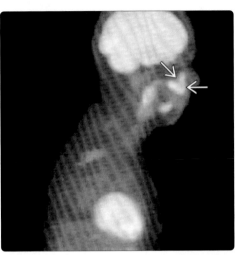

(Left) *Axial T2WI FS MR shows a young adult with several weeks of maxillary pain that prompted a root canal before biopsy revealed diffuse large B-cell lymphoma. Lobulated hyperintense mass ➡ involves anterior aspect of left maxilla, crossing midline at anterior nasal spine ➡. Premaxillary mass with bone invasion ➡ is classic for extranodal NHL.* (Right) *Lateral projection from FDG PET shows high uptake in maxillary mass ➡ but no abnormal uptake elsewhere. No B symptoms were present. Patient was treated with combined modality therapy.*

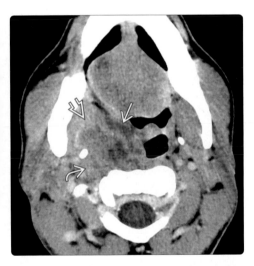

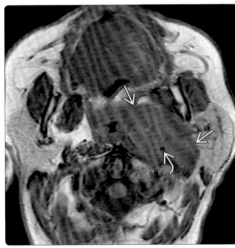

(Left) *Axial CECT in HIV(+) patient with facial pain shows large necrotic right tonsillar mass ➡ infiltrating masticator ➡, parapharyngeal, retropharyngeal, and carotid spaces ➡. Biopsy showed atypical Burkitt lymphoma.* (Right) *Axial T1WI MR in patient with diffuse large B-cell lymphoma shows a large transspatial deep facial and skull base mass ➡. Note mass surrounds & narrows the left internal carotid artery ➡ within the carotid space.*

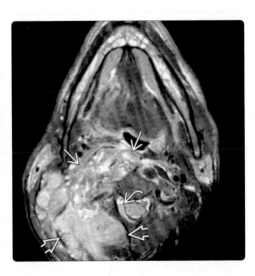

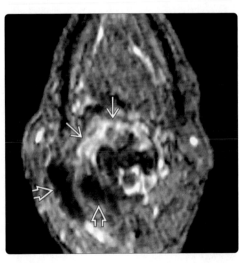

(Left) *Axial T2WI MR in an HIV(+) patient with a rapidly enlarging mass shows extensive infiltrating mass in right prevertebral ➡ and paraspinous ➡ muscles. The prevertebral component is heterogeneous and necrotic, whereas the posterior component is solid and homogeneous. There is intraspinal epidural extension ➡.* (Right) *Axial ADC map, same patient, shows restricted diffusion ➡ in multifocal solid posterior component but not in prevertebral tumor ➡. The biopsy showed Burkitt lymphoma.*

Transspatial and Multispatial

TERMINOLOGY

- Soft tissue malignancy arising from fat tissue
- Heterogeneous tumor with variable pathology; therefore, variable imaging
- Well-differentiated, intermediate (myxoid), and poorly differentiated types (round cell, pleomorphic, & dedifferentiated)

IMAGING

- Well-differentiated liposarcoma
  - Lobulated mass, > 75% fat, septations > 2 mm, enhancing nodules, ± Ca++
  - May mimic complex benign lipoma
- Poorly differentiated liposarcoma
  - Heterogeneous, enhancing infiltrative mass ± amorphous fatty foci
  - May not see macroscopic fat on CT or MR
- FDG PET uptake in solid, nonfatty components

TOP DIFFERENTIAL DIAGNOSES

- Lipoma
- Sarcoma
- Teratoma

PATHOLOGY

- Develop de novo, rarely from benign lipoma
- **T1** = tumor ≤ 5 cm, T2 = tumor > 5 cm
- Nodal disease rare; **N1** = any node = stage III

CLINICAL ISSUES

- Painless enlarging soft palpable mass
- Posterior cervical space is most common in H&N
- Peak age range: 50-65 yr
- Local recurrence common
- 5-year survival: Low grade ≤ 90%, high grade 50%
- Wide local resection ± radiation ± chemotherapy

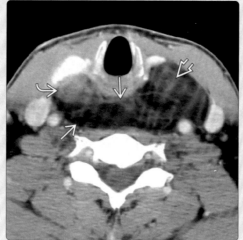

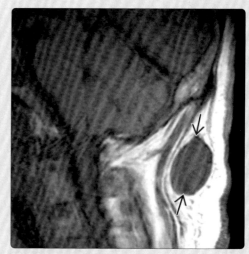

(Left) Axial CECT demonstrates a large complex mass ⇒ distending retropharyngeal space. Mass is mostly fat density; however, fat stranding is present on the left ⇒, & note enhancement ⇒ on the right. Well-differentiated liposarcoma is otherwise fatty density. (Right) Sagittal T1WI MR shows a well-defined solid mass ⇒ (grade 1 myxoid liposarcoma) in midline posterior neck fat, superficial to paraspinous muscles. Mass shows no intrinsic T1 high signal but enhanced intensely with contrast.

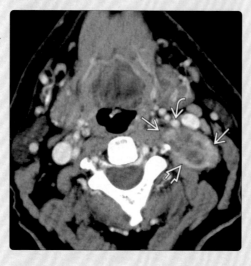

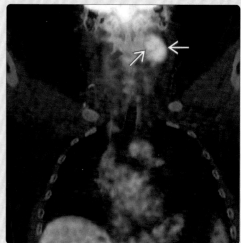

(Left) Axial CECT demonstrates irregular, heterogeneous mass ⇒ in left neck with infiltration of paraspinous muscle ⇒ and anterior displacement of jugular vein and internal carotid artery ⇒. There is no discernible low-density fat in mass. (Right) Coronal PET/CT in the same patient reveals moderately intense uptake in paravertebral mass ⇒. Lesion was found to be round cell (myxoid) liposarcoma and was resected after induction chemotherapy.

Liposarcoma of Head and Neck

TERMINOLOGY

Definitions

- Soft tissue malignancy arising from fat tissue

IMAGING

General Features

- Best diagnostic clue
  - Soft tissue mass with **variable appearance**
    - From well-defined, predominantly fatty mass with tissue stranding ± nodules
    - To ill-defined, heterogeneous, nonfatty solid mass mimicking any sarcoma
- Location
  - Posterior cervical space is most common in H&N
  - Liposarcoma more commonly in extremities, retroperitoneum
- Size
  - Variable
    - Size is important for staging; tumor > 5 cm is highest stage = T2
- Morphology
  - Well differentiated: Circumscribed, lobulated mass
  - Poorly differentiated: Infiltrating, amorphous mass

CT Findings

- CECT
  - Well differentiated: Lobulated mass, > 75% fat, septations > 2 mm, enhancing nodules, ± Ca^{++}
  - Poorly differentiated: Heterogeneous, enhancing infiltrative mass ± amorphous fatty foci

MR Findings

- MR appearance **variable**, similar to CECT
  - Well differentiated
    - > 75% intrinsically T1 hyperintense fatty component that suppresses with fat saturation
    - Thick septations, enhancing solid nodules
  - Poorly differentiated
    - Predominantly solid soft tissue mass, ± fat foci
    - Heterogeneous enhancement, ill-defined contours

Nuclear Medicine Findings

- FDG PET uptake in solid, nonfatty components

Imaging Recommendations

- Best imaging tool
  - MR best demonstrates soft tissue extent

DIFFERENTIAL DIAGNOSIS

Lipoma

- 8% benign lipomas have soft tissue component
- Exactly mimics well-differentiated liposarcoma

Sarcoma

- May be indistinguishable from fat-poor liposarcoma

Teratoma

- Rare neoplasm arising from all 3 germ cell layers
- Usually during infancy or childhood, rarely in adults
- Multiloculated mass with complex imaging ± fat

PATHOLOGY

General Features

- Etiology
  - Develop de novo, rarely from benign lipoma

Staging, Grading, & Classification

- **All soft tissue sarcomas staged** with **same** AJCC system (2010)
  - **T1** = tumor ≤ 5 cm
  - **T2** = tumor > 5 cm
  - Nodal disease rare; **N1** = any node = stage III
- **FNCLCC** system for **histologic tumor grading**
  - Grade determined by sum score of: Differentiation (1-3) + mitosis (1-3) + necrosis (0-2)

Gross Pathologic & Surgical Features

- Varies depending on histology, vascularity, necrosis, proportions of mature fat and fibrous tissue

Microscopic Features

- Well-differentiated liposarcoma
  - 20-30% of cases
- Myxoid liposarcoma
  - 30-50% of cases
- Round cell liposarcoma
  - Poorly differentiated variant of myxoid
- Pleomorphic liposarcoma
  - Highly undifferentiated
- Dedifferentiated liposarcoma: Rare

CLINICAL ISSUES

Presentation

- Most common signs/symptoms
  - Painless enlarging palpable mass

Demographics

- Age
  - Adult tumor: Peak ages 50-65 yr
- Epidemiology
  - 3-6% of liposarcomas occur in H&N

Natural History & Prognosis

- Local recurrence common
- Lung metastases seen in 85-90% of poorly differentiated sarcomas

Treatment

- Wide local resection ± radiation ± chemotherapy

DIAGNOSTIC CHECKLIST

Image Interpretation Pearls

- **Imaging appearances are variable**
  - Well differentiated with > 75% fat: Complex lipoma
  - May be solid, invasive mass with no evidence of fat, mimicking any other sarcoma

SELECTED REFERENCES

1. Gerry D et al: Liposarcoma of the head and neck: analysis of 318 cases with comparison to non-head and neck sites. Head Neck. 36(3):393-400, 2014
2. O'Neill JP et al: Head and neck sarcomas: epidemiology, pathology, and management. Neurosurg Clin N Am. 24(1):67-78, 2013

KEY FACTS

TERMINOLOGY

- Synovial sarcoma (SSa): Malignant soft tissue tumor with epithelial and mesenchymal components

IMAGING

- Lobular **nonnodal, nonmucosal** soft tissue mass in H&N
- CT/MR: Lobular enhancing mass, ± cysts, Ca⁺⁺, hemorrhage
- Locations
  - Hypopharynx > > > masticator space, parapharyngeal space, paranasal sinuses, infratemporal fossa

TOP DIFFERENTIAL DIAGNOSES

- Rhabdomyosarcoma
- Malignant fibrous histiocytoma
- Hemangiopericytoma
- Nerve sheath tumor, benign and malignant
- Pleomorphic adenoma

PATHOLOGY

- Dual epithelial and mesenchymal differentiation
  - Biphasic: Classic form; mesenchymal and epithelial components
  - Monophasic: Mesenchymal component predominates
  - Poorly differentiated: Epithelioid morphology

CLINICAL ISSUES

- **Young adult** presenting with solitary nonnodal, nonmucosal H&N mass
- Prognosis for H&N SSa
  - ↓ prognosis if poorly differentiated
  - ↓ prognosis in older (> 30 years) patients, larger SSa with bony invasion, hemorrhage, or paraspinal
  - ↓ prognosis for upper aerodigestive tract lesions
  - ↑ prognosis if calcification present
- Preferred treatment: Complete excision and postoperative radiation

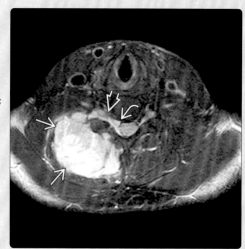
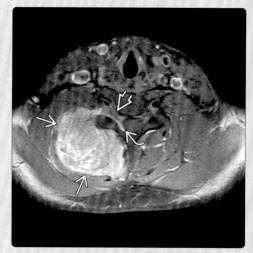

(Left) *Axial T2WI FS MR demonstrates a well-defined, hyperintense mass in right paraspinal component of the perivertebral space* ➡ *with deep extension via the neural foramen* ➡ *to the epidural area* ➡. *Differential diagnosis would be nerve sheath tumor.* (Right) *Axial T1WI C+ FS MR shows avid enhancement of paraspinal synovial sarcoma* ➡. *Notice the cervical nerve root* ➡ *is seen as a low-intensity line surrounded by tumor. Epidural tumor* ➡ *is again seen.*

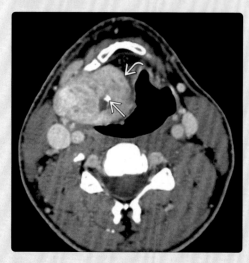
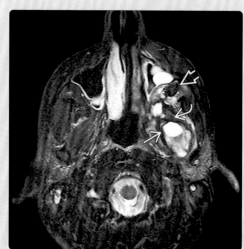

(Left) *Axial CECT at the hyoid level shows a well-defined, heterogeneously enhancing, submucosal lesion in paraglottic space of supraglottic larynx* ➡ *with focal Ca⁺⁺* ➡. (Right) *Axial T2WI FS MR demonstrates "triple signal" in a heterogeneous, well-defined mass with Ca⁺⁺ or hemorrhage* ➡, *cystic component* ➡, *and intervening solid component* ➡. *Final pathology revealed synovial sarcoma.*

TERMINOLOGY

Abbreviations

- Synovial sarcoma (SSa)

Definitions

- Malignant soft tissue tumor with epithelial and mesenchymal components

IMAGING

General Features

- Best diagnostic clue
  - Heterogeneous, well-defined, **nonnodal, nonmucosal** soft tissue mass
- Location
  - Hypopharynx > > > masticator space, parapharyngeal space, paranasal sinuses, infratemporal fossa
- Size
  - Variable, 2-8 cm

CT Findings

- CECT
  - Well-defined lobular mass
  - Mild heterogeneous enhancement ± cysts, Ca^{++}, hemorrhage
  - Bone invasion extremely rare

MR Findings

- T1WI
  - Iso- to slightly hyperintense to muscle
- T2WI
  - Hyperintense relative to muscle
  - Often heterogeneous with iso-, hypo-, & hyperintense foci from solid, cystic, Ca^{++} &/or hemorrhage
- T1WI C+
  - Heterogeneous enhancing mass ± septations

Imaging Recommendations

- Best imaging tool
  - Contrast-enhanced MR

DIFFERENTIAL DIAGNOSIS

Rhabdomyosarcoma

- Middle ear, sinus, nasopharynx, and adjacent spaces
- Aggressive soft tissue mass ± nodes
- Intermediate signal all MR sequences

Malignant Fibrous Histiocytoma (Formerly Fibrosarcoma)

- Most common sarcoma of H&N in adults
- Low to intermediate signal all MR sequences

Hemangiopericytoma

- Sinonasal, dural, perivertebral space
- Locally aggressive mass; prominent vasculature; bone invasion common

Nerve Sheath Tumors

- Benign > > malignant
- Generally well-defined mass, T2 hyperintense

Pleomorphic Adenoma

- Commonly T2-hyperintense, lobulated mass
  - Carcinoma ex pleomorphic adenoma typically heterogeneously T2 hyperintense

PATHOLOGY

General Features

- Genetics
  - Translocation t(X;18)(p11.2;q11.2) specific for SSa
  - Misnomer; named for cellular appearance rather than cell of origin
  - Dual epithelial and mesenchymal cell differentiation
    - Biphasic: Classic form; mesenchymal and epithelial components

Gross Pathologic & Surgical Features

- Areas of necrosis, hemorrhage, and cysts common

CLINICAL ISSUES

Presentation

- Most common signs/symptoms
  - Palpable mass
  - May have lymph node metastases

Demographics

- Age
  - Adolescents and young adults; typical range: 15-35 years
- Epidemiology
  - 7-10% of all sarcomas (4th most common)
    - 3% of SSa arise in H&N
    - Far more common in extremities

Natural History & Prognosis

- Prognosis for SSa in H&N more favorable than in extremity
  - ↓ prognosis if poorly differentiated
  - ↓ prognosis in older (> 30 years) patients, larger SSa with bony invasion, hemorrhage, or paraspinal
  - ↓ prognosis for upper aerodigestive tract lesions
  - ↑ prognosis if calcification present

Treatment

- Complete excision with negative margins
- Postoperative XRT
  - Systemic therapy for disseminated disease

DIAGNOSTIC CHECKLIST

Consider

- SSa unique among sarcomas; well-defined soft tissue mass with heterogeneous SI on T2WI MR

Reporting Tips

- Ca^{++}, hemorrhage, septations, mixed solid cystic components
- Lymph node metastases

SELECTED REFERENCES

1. Hu PA et al: Clinical, pathological and unusual MRI features of five synovial sarcomas in head and neck. Br J Radiol. 88(1050):20140843, 2015
2. O'Sullivan PJ et al: Radiological features of synovial cell sarcoma. Br J Radiol. 81(964):346-56, 2008

Malignant Peripheral Nerve Sheath Tumor of Head and Neck

TERMINOLOGY

- Malignant tumor of Schwann cell or other nerve sheath cell origin

IMAGING

- CECT findings
  - Infiltrating soft tissue mass associated with peripheral nerve
- NECT findings
  - Bone erosion or regressive remodeling/foraminal enlargement
- MR findings
  - Irregular mass with heterogeneous signal; no target sign on T2
  - May see flow voids
- FDG PET
  - In neurofibromatosis type 1 (NF1), ↑ SUV may differentiate known neurofibroma from malignant peripheral nerve sheath tumor (MPNST)

TOP DIFFERENTIAL DIAGNOSES

- Neurofibroma
- Schwannoma
- Hemangiopericytoma
- Malignant fibrous histiocytoma

PATHOLOGY

- Majority arise de novo in normal peripheral nerve
- **30-50%** occur in **NF1** patients

CLINICAL ISSUES

- "Schwannoma recurrence" should suggest MPNST
- Mixed sensory & motor symptoms are clues: Neurologic deficit rare with benign tumor
- Wide en bloc surgical resection ± radiation therapy
- Distant metastases common: Lung > liver & bone
- Overall poor prognosis

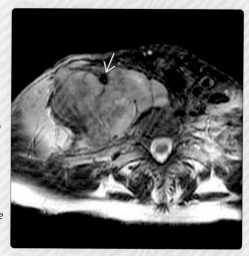
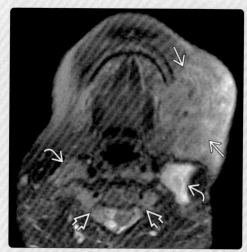

(Left) Axial T2WI MR shows heterogeneous T2 hyperintense signal in a well-defined lesion between the right anterior ➡ scalene muscle & middle scalene muscle in location of the brachial plexus. There are no specific imaging findings to differentiate this MPNST from a benign NST. (Right) Axial T2WI MR shows an ill-defined, left cheek MPNST ➡ infiltrating adjacent soft tissues. Note the multiple well-defined neurofibromas in the neck bilaterally ➡ & in the cervical neural foramina ➡ in this patient with NF1.

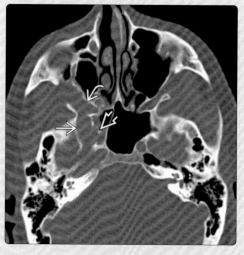
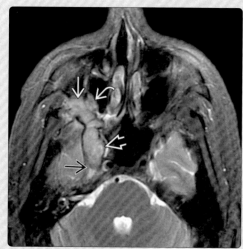

(Left) Axial bone CT shows an MPNST affecting the 2nd division of trigeminal nerve (CNV2) causing regressive remodeling & widening of pterygopalatine fossa ➡ & foramen rotundum ➡ & destruction of right lateral sphenoid sinus wall ➡. (Right) Axial T2WI FS MR in the same patient reveals heterogeneous CNV2 MPNST invading soft tissues of the pterygopalatine fossa ➡ & right maxillary sinus ➡, indicating aggressive behavior. Mass involves infraorbital nerve, cavernous sinus ➡, & Meckel cave ➡.

Malignant Peripheral Nerve Sheath Tumor of Head and Neck

TERMINOLOGY

Abbreviations

- Malignant peripheral nerve sheath tumor (MPNST)

Synonyms

- Neurogenic sarcoma, malignant schwannoma, malignant neurolemmoma, neurofibrosarcoma

Definitions

- Malignant tumor of Schwann cell or other nerve sheath cell origin

IMAGING

General Features

- Best diagnostic clue
  - Infiltrating soft tissue mass associated with peripheral nerve
- Location
  - Rare in head & neck region
    - Brachial plexus, sympathetic chain, CNV
    - May arise from preexisting neurofibromas
- Size
  - Larger in neurofibromatosis type 1 (NF1)

CT Findings

- CECT
  - Heterogeneously enhancing mass with no Ca^{2+}
- Bone CT
  - Bone erosion, remodeling, foraminal enlargement

MR Findings

- T1WI
  - Tumor is isointense to muscle
- T2WI
  - Heterogeneous signal; no target sign
  - Irregular margins & peritumor edema strongly suggest MPNST over benign PNST
- DWI
  - ↑↑ restricted DWI; low ADC (< 1.0-1.1×10^{-3} mm²/s)
- T1WI C+
  - Heterogeneous enhancement

Nuclear Medicine Findings

- PET
  - In NF1, may differentiate known neurofibroma from MPNST
    - SUV generally higher in MPNST

Imaging Recommendations

- Best imaging tool
  - Enhanced MR ± bone CT if affecting bone (e.g., skull base)
  - PET + MR = highest specificity differentiating benign PNST from MPNST

DIFFERENTIAL DIAGNOSIS

Neurofibroma

- May have target sign on T2 ± central enhancement

Schwannoma

- Heterogeneous appearance; cannot distinguish from MPNST
- May have central enhancement (never in MPNST)

Hemangiopericytoma

- Heterogeneous signal mass commonly with flow void; no bone destruction
- May have Ca^{2+}; never present in MPNST

Malignant Fibrous Histiocytoma

- Cannot distinguish from MPNST on imaging

PATHOLOGY

General Features

- Etiology
  - Majority arise de novo in normal peripheral nerve
  - **30-50%** occur in **NF1** patients
    - Deeper plexiform neurofibromas at higher risk
  - **10%** of MPNST associated with **radiation exposure**

Staging, Grading, & Classification

- No accepted staging system

Microscopic Features

- Unencapsulated spindle cell tumor
- Histologic diagnosis difficult

CLINICAL ISSUES

Presentation

- Most common signs/symptoms
  - Enlarging soft tissue mass
- Other signs/symptoms
  - Mixed sensory & motor symptoms
    - Neurologic deficit rare in benign tumors

Demographics

- Age
  - 20-50 years (10 years earlier in NF1)

Natural History & Prognosis

- "Schwannoma recurrence" often signals presence of MPNST
- Nodal metastases rare
- Distant metastases common: Lung (33%) > > liver & bone
- Poor prognosis

Treatment

- Wide en bloc resection ± postoperative radiation therapy

DIAGNOSTIC CHECKLIST

Image Interpretation Pearls

- Infiltrative fusiform tumor along peripheral nerve
- Never see target sign on T2 in NF1 setting

SELECTED REFERENCES

1. Broski SM et al: Evaluation of (18)F-FDG PET and MRI in differentiating benign and malignant peripheral nerve sheath tumors. Skeletal Radiol. 45(8):1097-105, 2016
2. Soldatos T et al: Advanced MR imaging of peripheral nerve sheath tumors including diffusion imaging. Semin Musculoskelet Radiol. 19(2):179-90, 2015

Transspatial and Multispatial

TERMINOLOGY

- Benign lymph-filled cyst due to leaking lymphatic channels
- Lymphatic cyst, lymphocyst, chylocele, chyloma, chylous cyst, (distal) thoracic duct cyst

IMAGING

- Best imaging tools are CECT and ultrasound
- Characteristic location is low posterior cervical space in **supraclavicular fossa**
  - Between scalene and sternocleidomastoid muscles
- Unilocular, well-circumscribed cyst with **no visible cyst wall**, enhancement, or septa
  - Cyst wall thickened ± enhancing if complicated by infection/treatment
  - Fluid density (CT HU usually 0-20) or signal (MR)

TOP DIFFERENTIAL DIAGNOSES

- Congenital neck cysts
  - Lymphatic malformation
  - 3rd branchial cleft
  - Thymic cyst
- Postoperative seroma, hematoma, or pseudomeningocele
- Systemic nodal metastases
- Suppurative lymph nodes

PATHOLOGY

- Endothelial-lined cyst with acellular fluid and **fat droplets**

CLINICAL ISSUES

- Growing painless neck mass without signs of infection
- Treatment options
  - Complete surgical removal is curative
  - Percutaneous sclerotherapy if surgery not possible

DIAGNOSTIC CHECKLIST

- Consider lymphocele in **postoperative** patient with low posterior cervical space supraclavicular cyst pointing toward confluence of internal jugular and subclavian veins
- FNA to confirm ± imaging surveillance if atypical

(Left) *Gross specimen of a lymphocele shows its typical encapsulated appearance. These masses are usually easy to remove surgically, with subsequent cure.* (Right) *Sagittal CECT MPR demonstrates the typical CT characteristics of a lymphocele: A unilocular nonseptated round or ovoid water density cyst in the supraclavicular fossa with no perceptible cyst wall ➡ or enhancement.*

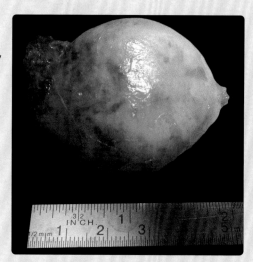
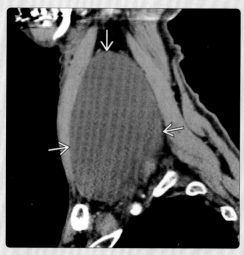

(Left) *Axial CECT shows bilateral lymphoceles ➡ in a patient post thyroid resection for cancer. Clips from prior node dissection ➡ are a clue to postsurgical origin from lymphatic duct iatrogenic injury.* (Right) *Coronal T1 MR shows a spontaneously occurring, lobulated, unilocular, fluid signal intensity lymphocele in the right supraclavicular fossa just above the subclavian ➡ and internal jugular ➡ venous confluence.*

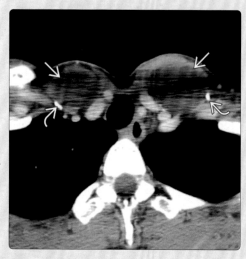
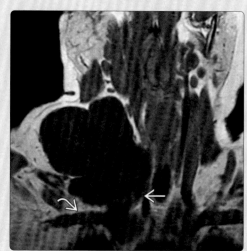

TERMINOLOGY

Synonyms

- Lymphatic cyst, lymphocyst, chylocele, chyloma, chylous cyst, (distal) thoracic duct cyst

Definitions

- Benign lymph-filled cyst formed from leaking disrupted lymphatic channels

IMAGING

General Features

- Best diagnostic clue
  - Nonenhancing unilocular fluid density/signal intensity cyst in supraclavicular fossa
- Location
  - **Posterior cervical space**
  - **Left side** more common
  - **Supraclavicular fossa** most common
    - Found anywhere along course of jugular lymph trunks, either side of neck, or distal thoracic duct on left
    - Rarely high in neck along course of jugular trunks
    - Distal thoracic duct cyst may be mediastinal &/or cervical
  - Between scalene and sternocleidomastoid muscles
  - Posterior ± lateral to carotid space, pointing toward confluence of internal jugular and subclavian veins
- Morphology
  - Round, oval, ± lobulations

CT Findings

- NECT
  - Unilocular fluid density cyst
    - HU usually 0-20
  - Well circumscribed
  - No soft tissue nodularity
  - Lack of perceptible cyst wall
    - Lack of septations and surgical history help distinguish from lymphatic malformation
- CECT
  - Nonenhancing cyst wall unless complicated by infection or prior treatment

MR Findings

- T1WI C+
  - No enhancement unless complicated
- Fluid signal intensity on all MR sequences

Ultrasonographic Findings

- Grayscale ultrasound
  - Anechoic or hypoechoic; ↑ through transmission
  - Septa and debris uncommon unless complicated

Imaging Recommendations

- Best imaging tool
  - CECT
  - Sonography useful, particularly for FNA guidance
- Protocol advice
  - Contrast to exclude infectious or neoplastic causes

DIFFERENTIAL DIAGNOSIS

Congenital Neck Cysts

- Lymphatic malformation
  - Usually transspatial with septa and fluid levels
- 3rd branchial cleft cyst
  - Pediatric age group without surgical history
  - Thin cyst wall; rim enhancing if infected
- Thymic cyst
  - Left cervical-thoracic dumbbell cyst when large

Postoperative Seroma or Hematoma

- Found within surgical bed
- Seroma is CSF signal
- Subacute hematoma is hyperdense on NECT, T1 hyper- and T2 hypointense

Pseudomeningocele (CSF Leak)

- CSF density/signal all sequences
- Enlarging over time with postural headache clinically

Systemic Nodal Metastases

- Cystic nodal metastases usually have perceptible cyst wall with rim enhancement

Suppurative Lymph Nodes

- Enhancing cyst wall with irregular shape or nodularity

PATHOLOGY

Gross Pathologic & Surgical Features

- Bland, acellular fluid with **lipid droplets**
- **Endothelial-lined cyst** ± lymph channel adventitial capsule

CLINICAL ISSUES

Presentation

- Most common signs/symptoms
  - Painless enlarging supraclavicular neck mass
  - Spontaneous or acquired (postoperative or posttraumatic)

Treatment

- Surgical resection curative
- Percutaneous sclerotherapy if not surgical candidate or surgery unsuccessful

DIAGNOSTIC CHECKLIST

Consider

- Ultrasound, CECT, MR show bland fluid without cyst wall
- FNA diagnostic with acellular fluid having lipid droplets

Image Interpretation Pearls

- Consider lymphocele in postoperative patient with low posterior cervical space cyst pointing toward confluence of internal jugular and subclavian veins

SELECTED REFERENCES

1. Hamilton BE et al: Characteristic imaging findings in lymphoceles of the head and neck. AJR Am J Roentgenol. 197(6):1431-5, 2011
2. Moesgaard L et al: Cervical thoracic duct cyst: a differential diagnosis of left supraclavicular swelling. Eur Arch Otorhinolaryngol. 264(7):797-9, 2007

Sinus Histiocytosis (Rosai-Dorfman) of Head and Neck

KEY FACTS

TERMINOLOGY

- Sinus histiocytosis: Benign pseudolymphomatous clinicopathologic entity of unknown etiology

IMAGING

- **Massive, bilateral cervical lymphadenopathy**
- H&N extranodal sites ~ **50%**
  - Skin, sinonasal area, orbit, eyelids, bone, salivary glands, & dura
- Rare other extranodal sites
  - Oral cavity, pharynx, trachea, bronchi, & mediastinal lymph nodes
- CT or MR findings
  - Homogeneously enhancing large lymph nodes
  - Enhancing extranodal infiltrates
  - **T2 low signal** of nodal or extranodal lesions common

TOP DIFFERENTIAL DIAGNOSES

- Non-Hodgkin lymphoma

- Reactive lymph nodes
- Skull base meningioma
- Langerhans cell histiocytosis

PATHOLOGY

- Unknown pathophysiology

CLINICAL ISSUES

- Clinical presentation
  - Painless neck masses
- Age at presentation
  - < 20 years old (80%)
- Natural history
  - Long history of benign disease involvement common
  - ↑ morbidity when immunologic dysfunction present (arthritis, circulating autoantibodies)
- Treatment
  - Clinical observation preferred
  - Surgical debulking if vital structure compression

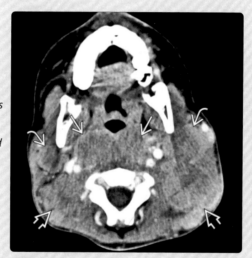
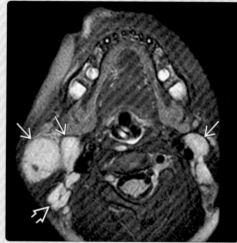

(Left) Axial CECT shows very large bilateral retropharyngeal nodes ➡ in association with massive adenopathy in the internal jugular ➡ and spinal accessory nodal chains ➡. Non-Hodgkin lymphoma nodes were suspected before biopsy revealed sinus histiocytosis. (Right) Axial STIR MR in a child reveals large jugulodigastric ➡ and spinal accessory ➡ lymph nodes. Notice the right parotid tail large nodal focus as well. Nodal biopsy showed sinus histiocytosis.

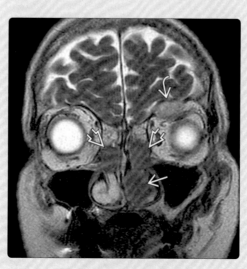
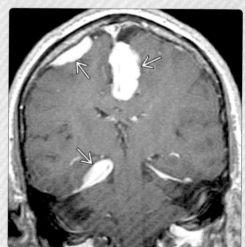

(Left) Coronal T2 MR shows multifocal low-signal nasal ➡ and ethmoid sinus ➡ masses. Note also the slightly higher signal left extraconal orbital ➡ sinus histiocytosis lesion. (Right) Coronal T1 C+ MR demonstrates multiple dural-based, strongly enhancing masses ➡ originally thought to be multiple meningiomatosis. Surgical pathology revealed sinus histiocytosis.

TERMINOLOGY

Abbreviations

- Sinus histiocytosis (SH)

Synonyms

- SH with massive lymphadenopathy, Rosai-Dorfman disease

Definitions

- Benign pseudolymphomatous clinicopathologic entity of unknown etiology

IMAGING

General Features

- Best diagnostic clue
  - Massive, bilateral cervical lymphadenopathy in patient < 20 years of age
- Location
  - **Bilateral cervical lymphadenopathy**
  - Extranodal sites ~ 50%: Skin, sinonasal area, orbit, eyelids, bone, salivary glands, & dura
  - Rare other extranodal sites: Oral cavity, pharynx, trachea, bronchi, & mediastinal lymph nodes

Imaging Recommendations

- Best imaging tool
  - CECT or enhanced MR
  - If suprahyoid lesions, enhanced MR

CT Findings

- CECT
  - Homogeneously enhancing large lymph nodes
    - Bilateral & very large in children
  - Enhancing extranodal infiltrates
    - **Skin, sinuses, nose, orbit, eyelids, bone, salivary glands, & dura**
    - Parotid glands: Low-density foci reported

MR Findings

- T1WI
  - Low signal intensity relative to muscle
- T2WI
  - Relatively **low signal** intensity compared to muscle
    - May help differentiate SH from other causes of lymph node enlargement & extranodal infiltrates
- T1WI C+
  - Homogeneous enhancing large neck nodes
  - Enhancing extranodal infiltrating masses

Ultrasonographic Findings

- Grayscale ultrasound
  - Nonspecific hypoechoic nodes/extranodal infiltrates

DIFFERENTIAL DIAGNOSIS

Non-Hodgkin Lymphoma

- May exactly mimic

Reactive Lymph Nodes

- Large, diffuse adenopathy common in children

Skull Base Meningioma

- SH of dura may mimic meningioma

Langerhans Cell Histiocytosis

- Nodal disease rare

PATHOLOGY

General Features

- Etiology
  - Unknown pathophysiology
  - Postulated etiologies: Infectious cause, immunodeficiency, autoimmune disease, neoplastic process
- Associated abnormalities
  - Increased morbidity & mortality when associated immunologic abnormality exists
    - Examples: Arthritis, circulating autoantibodies

Microscopic Features

- "Sinusal" lymph node architecture with clustering of lymphocytes simulating germinal centers
- Emperipolesis: Histiocytes phagocytize lymphocytes, plasma cells, erythrocytes, or polymorphonuclear leukocytes
- Immunohistochemical (IHC) analysis
  - SH histiocyte-positive IHC stains: S100 protein positivity; CD68, CD163
  - SH histiocyte-negative IHC stain: CD1a
- Intracytoplasmic eosinophilic globules (Russell bodies) in plasma cells

CLINICAL ISSUES

Presentation

- Most common signs/symptoms
  - Painless neck masses, fevers
  - Elevated erythrocyte sediment rate positive (90%)

Demographics

- Age
  - < 20 years old (80%)
    - < 10 years old (66%)
- Epidemiology
  - More common in African & West Indian heritage

Natural History & Prognosis

- Long history of benign disease involvement common
- ↑ morbidity when immunologic dysfunction present

Treatment

- Most patients do not require treatment
- Surgical debulking in cases of vital structure compression
- Radiation, chemotherapy, and steroids not proven efficacious

SELECTED REFERENCES

1. Dalia S et al: Rosai-Dorfman disease: tumor biology, clinical features, pathology, and treatment. Cancer Control. 21(4):322-7, 2014
2. La Barge DV 3rd et al: Sinus histiocytosis with massive lymphadenopathy (Rosai-Dorfman disease): imaging manifestations in the head and neck. AJR Am J Roentgenol. 191(6):W299-306, 2008
3. Ottaviano G et al: Extranodal Rosai-Dorfman disease: involvement of eye, nose and trachea. Acta Otolaryngol. 126(6):657-60, 2006

Fibromatosis of Head and Neck

TERMINOLOGY

- Aggressive fibromatosis, extraabdominal desmoid, infantile fibromatosis
- Rare infiltrative mass of benign monoclonal fibroblast proliferation

IMAGING

- Ill-defined, nonnecrotic transspatial enhancing mass in any H&N space
- Variable appearance: May be sharply circumscribed or infiltrative
- CT: No tumor matrix calcification or ossification
- MR: T1 iso- to hypointense compared to muscle
- T2 hyperintense ± hypointense bands
- Generally avid enhancement on MR
- Contrast-enhanced MR is study of choice, as it best shows relationship to critical structures
- If image-guided biopsy performed, always get core sample for histology and stains

TOP DIFFERENTIAL DIAGNOSES

- Non-Hodgkin lymphoma, especially nonnodal
- Rhabdomyosarcoma
- Soft tissue fibrosarcoma
- Soft tissue metastases

PATHOLOGY

- Infiltrative unencapsulated growth with uniform spindle cells and collagenous stroma
- In adults, more likely to be associated with Gardner syndrome, familial adenomatous polyposis
- Infantile fibromatosis differs in demographics, genetics, behavior, and treatment

CLINICAL ISSUES

- No nodal or distant metastatic potential but high local recurrence rate
- Complete resection is treatment of choice
- Radiation ± chemotherapy as adjuvant treatment

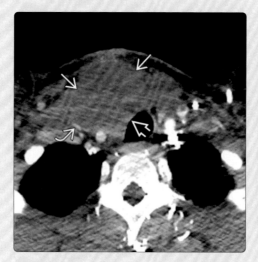
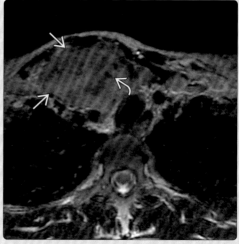

(Left) Axial CECT through the low neck in a young adult shows a homogeneous, nonenhancing mass ➡️ isodense to and indistinguishable from neck muscles. The mass abuts and displaces the trachea ➡️ and displaces and compresses the right jugular vein ➡️. (Right) Axial T2WI MR in the same patient better delineates the hyperintense mass ➡️ from adjacent strap and sternocleidomastoid muscles and shows focal and linear areas of low signal ➡️. The mass is clearly separate from the trachea and vessels.

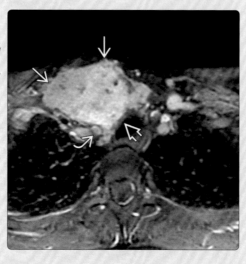
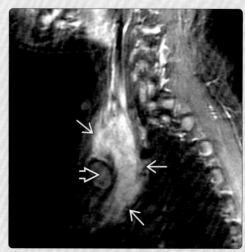

(Left) Axial T1WI C+ FS MR shows diffuse marked enhancement of the mass ➡️. Fibromatosis abuts trachea ➡️ in superior mediastinum but does not infiltrate the tracheal wall. Note clear plane between mass and right common carotid artery ➡️. (Right) Sagittal T2WI FS MR best illustrates craniocaudal extent of mass ➡️, from infrahyoid neck, posterior to clavicle ➡️, into the superior mediastinum. At resection, it was distinct from the thymus and thyroid but encased the right recurrent laryngeal nerve, which was sacrificed.

Fibromatosis of Head and Neck

TERMINOLOGY

Synonyms

- Aggressive fibromatosis, extraabdominal desmoid, infantile fibromatosis

Definitions

- Rare infiltrative mass lesion of benign monoclonal fibroblast proliferation
  - In H&N, these are deep fibromatoses
  - Superficial fibromatoses most often in extremities

IMAGING

General Features

- Best diagnostic clue
  - Ill-defined, infiltrative, nonnecrotic transspatial enhancing mass
- Location
  - Any space of extracranial H&N; often transspatial
  - Most commonly: Supraclavicular area, masticator space
- Size
  - Most often 3-10 cm
  - < 15% cases are multiple lesions
- Morphology
  - May have well-circumscribed margin
  - More aggressive lesions have irregular margins with local muscle and bone invasion
  - May see both well-demarcated and infiltrative margins in same lesion

CT Findings

- CECT
  - May appear sharply circumscribed or infiltrative
  - Mild to moderate contrast enhancement
  - No tumor matrix calcification or ossification
- Bone CT
  - May erode or invade bone

MR Findings

- T1WI
  - Iso- to hypointense compared to muscle
- T2WI
  - Generally hyperintense
  - Hypointense bands corresponding to collagen bundles often seen
- T1WI C+
  - Variable, but generally avid enhancement
- MRA
  - Larger neck lesions may encircle and compress vessels
- **Recurrent tumor**
  - After excision, recurrence often has more poorly defined, infiltrative margins
  - Following radiation, tumor decreases in T1 and T2 signal, becomes more well defined

Imaging Recommendations

- Best imaging tool
  - Contrast-enhanced MR is study of choice
    - Best demonstrates lesion extent and relationship to neural and vascular structures
    - Best study for evaluating response to treatment and recurrence
- Protocol advice
  - Near skull base both MR and bone CT recommended
    - Contrast-enhanced MR defines soft tissue extent
    - Bone CT identifies bone invasion or erosion
- If image-guided biopsy performed, core sample essential so histomorphology and special stains can be performed

Nuclear Medicine Findings

- PET/CT
  - Preliminary reports describe heterogeneous mild to moderate FDG uptake

DIFFERENTIAL DIAGNOSIS

Non-Hodgkin Lymphoma

- May infiltrate multiple spaces when in extranodal, extralymphatic site
- Usually associated with pathologic adenopathy in addition to nonnodal mass

Rhabdomyosarcoma

- Children or young adults, often with cranial neuropathy
- Most often temporal bone, orbit, sinonasal; less often deep face

Soft Tissue Fibrosarcoma

- Very rare malignant tumor of deep face
- If in masticator space, difficult to distinguish from aggressive fibromatosis

Soft Tissue Metastases

- Typically older patient with known primary tumor
- Multiple enhancing nodular lesions ± nodes

PATHOLOGY

General Features

- Etiology
  - Arises from connective tissue, fascia, and muscle aponeurotic structures
    - Unclear whether **reactive** or **neoplastic growth**
  - Unknown cause but various factors proposed: Trauma, surgery, and endocrine
    - Rare fibromatoses after cervical spine surgery
    - Abdominal fibromatoses can occur after pregnancy in anterior abdominal wall
- Genetics
  - Mutations found in β-catenin protein or adenomatous polyposis coli gene
    - Fibromatoses accumulate excess intranuclear β-catenin protein
    - Mutations not always found in infantile fibromatoses
- Associated abnormalities
  - Most infantile and adult cases are sporadic
  - In adults more likely to be associated with polyposis syndromes
    - Familial adenomatous polyposis
    - Gardner syndrome
      - □ Autosomal dominant: Polyposis coli, osteomas, fibromas, and epidermoid cysts

□ Aggressive fibromatosis may be 1st presentation of Gardner syndrome in child

Staging, Grading, & Classification

- No accepted staging system
- Does not metastasize to nodes or distant sites

Gross Pathologic & Surgical Features

- Whitish, firm, fibrous mass ± adjacent bone and skeletal muscle invasion

Microscopic Features

- Infiltrative unencapsulated growth with uniform spindle cells and collagenous stroma
- Bland microscopic appearance: No necrosis or abnormal mitoses
- Spindle cell nuclei stain diffusely for β-catenin

CLINICAL ISSUES

Presentation

- Most common signs/symptoms
  - Painless, firm, growing, fixed mass
- Other signs/symptoms
  - Other symptoms depend on tissues involved
    - Lower neck: Radiculopathy, brachial plexopathy
    - Deep face: Trismus, dysphagia, airway obstruction
    - Below skull base: Cranial neuropathies
    - Orbit: Proptosis
- Clinical profile
  - Young adult with firm, painless neck mass
  - Adult with prior history of cervical spine surgery

Demographics

- Age
  - Any age, but peaks 15-40 years
  - Infantile fibromatosis: < 6 years
- Gender
  - More common in female patients after puberty
  - Infantile fibromatosis: M = F
- Epidemiology
  - Rare entity accounting for 0.03% of all neoplasms in human body
  - H&N lesions account for 12-15% of all fibromatoses

Natural History & Prognosis

- Unpredictable clinical behavior
  - Teen and adult fibromatosis usually more aggressive than childhood fibromatosis
- Locally aggressive, causing morbidity by invading tissues
- No metastatic potential but high local recurrence rate
  - 10-80% recurrence rate
  - Most recurrences within 2-3 years, up to 6 years
- Cases of spontaneous regression without treatment reported
- Fibromatosis is rarely cause of death in afflicted patients

Treatment

- **Surgery is treatment of choice**
  - Aim is to achieve microscopically negative margin
  - Functional considerations in H&N may limit complete resection

- Radiation for incomplete resection, recurrent tumor, or if lesion not safely resectable
  - Generally not advocated in pediatric patients
- Chemotherapy may be with noncytotoxic or cytotoxic drugs
  - Noncytotoxics: Tamoxifen (antiestrogen) and nonsteroidal antiinflammatory drugs
  - Cytotoxic agents: Vinblastine and methotrexate
    - Reserved for refractory or severely morbid disease
- For recurrent but stable lesions, clinical observation alone may be considered

DIAGNOSTIC CHECKLIST

Consider

- Fibromatosis of H&N when large painless transspatial mass present
- Adult fibromatosis may rarely be associated with prior cervical spine surgery/instrumentation
- Infantile fibromatosis behaves somewhat differently
  - Less aggressive, less often associated with gene mutations, polyposis syndromes

Image Interpretation Pearls

- Think of aggressive fibromatosis if malignant-appearing mass in neck of young adult
- Main differential is sarcoma of deep tissues
- Image-guided biopsy should be core so histomorphology and special stains can be performed

Reporting Tips

- MR is imaging study of choice to delineate complete extent of lesion
- **Determine relationship of lesion to critical structures**
  - Nerves, vessels, trachea, esophagus, skull base, vertebrae

SELECTED REFERENCES

1. Lacayo EA et al: Deep neck fibromatosis after diskectomy and cervical fusion: case series and review of the literature. AJR Am J Roentgenol. 1-5, 2016
2. Otero S et al: Desmoid-type fibromatosis. Clin Radiol. 70(9):1038-45, 2015
3. Collin M et al: Ossifying fibroma of the middle turbinate revealed by infection in a young child. Eur Ann Otorhinolaryngol Head Neck Dis. 131(3):193-5, 2014
4. Wang W et al: Age-based treatment of aggressive fibromatosis in the head and neck region. J Oral Maxillofac Surg. 72(2):311-21, 2014
5. Rhim JH et al: Desmoid-type fibromatosis in the head and neck: CT and MR imaging characteristics. Neuroradiology. 55(3):351-9, 2013
6. Soto-Miranda MA et al: Surgical treatment of pediatric desmoid tumors. A 12-year, single-center experience. Ann Surg Oncol. 20(11):3384-90, 2013
7. Dinauer PA et al: Pathologic and MR imaging features of benign fibrous soft-tissue tumors in adults. Radiographics. 27(1):173-87, 2007
8. Goodwin RW et al: MRI appearances of common benign soft-tissue tumours. Clin Radiol. 62(9):843-53, 2007
9. Tolan S et al: Fibromatosis: benign by name but not necessarily by nature. Clin Oncol (R Coll Radiol). 19(5):319-26, 2007
10. Okuno S: The enigma of desmoid tumors. Curr Treat Options Oncol. 7(6):438-43, 2006
11. Abikhzer G et al: Aggressive fibromatosis of the head and neck: case report and review of the literature. J Otolaryngol. 34(4):289-94, 2005
12. Collins BJ et al: Desmoid tumors of the head and neck: a review. Ann Plast Surg. 54(1):103-8, 2005

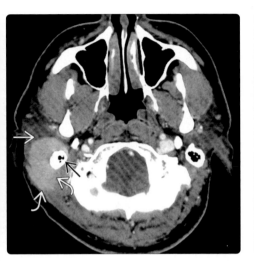

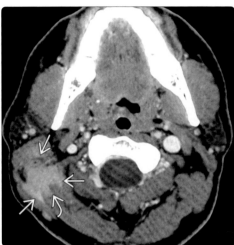

(Left) *Axial CECT shows an enhancing mass at right skull base, encircling the mastoid tip ➡. Fibromatosis appears sharply circumscribed from posterior superficial parotid gland ➡ but has a more ill-defined posterior paraspinous margin ➡.* (Right) *Axial CECT, more inferior, demonstrates ill-defined inferior aspect of enhancing fibromatosis ➡. Note infiltrative mass-like appearance, with irregular margin at interface with paraspinal muscles ➡, suggesting malignant infiltration.*

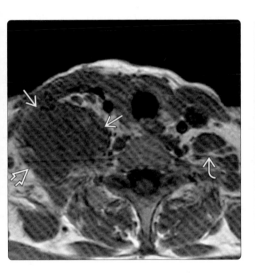

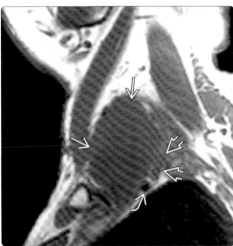

(Left) *Axial T1WI MR in a man reveals a solid mass ➡ in lower neck isointense to muscle, with ill-defined posterior margin ➡. Note normal left brachial plexus trunk posterior to anterior scalene muscle ➡.* (Right) *Sagittal T1WI MR shows intimate relationship of the mass ➡ to subclavian artery ➡. Brachial plexus trunks ➡ are displaced at dorsal aspect of mass. At resection, plexus and phrenic nerve involvement by fibromatosis precluded complete excision, necessitating adjuvant radiation.*

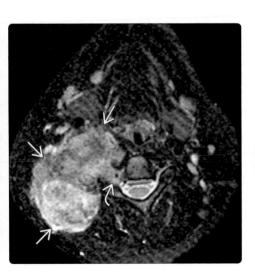

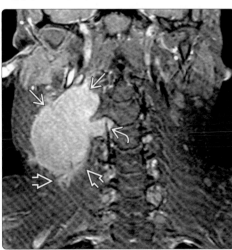

(Left) *Axial T2WI FS MR in a teenage girl with enlarging right neck mass demonstrates heterogeneously hyperintense lesion ➡ infiltrating paraspinous muscles. The lesion extends into right C3-4 neural foramen ➡ and encircles vertebral artery.* (Right) *Coronal T1WI C+ FS MR shows homogeneous enhancement of right paraspinous mass ➡, with both well-defined and more ill-defined ➡ contours. The latter feature raised concern for malignancy. Note the patent but encircled right vertebral artery ➡.*

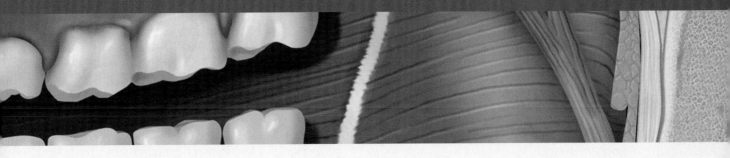

SECTION 14
Oral Cavity

Summary Thoughts: Oral Cavity

The oral cavity (OC) is the area of the suprahyoid neck anterior to the oropharynx and inferior to the sinonasal region. Imaging indications for the OC are usually highly refined because the referring physician can see all mucosal surfaces and palpate most lesions found here. The radiologist's role is to assess the deep tissue extent of OC tumors and space-based differential diagnoses when a deep tissue lesion is discovered. Three indications drive the vast majority of CT and MR exams of the OC: (1) Staging OC squamous cell carcinoma (SCCa), (2) evaluating for abscess and its etiology, and (3) differentiating submandibular nodal and gland mass.

Imaging Techniques & Indications

Tumor Assessment

Both CECT and enhanced MR are used to stage SCCa. Primary tumor and nodal metastases are assessed simultaneously in either case. CT is often compromised by dental amalgam artifact. MR is less affected by dental amalgam and better delineates soft tissue extent of tumor and perineural tumor. As a result, enhanced fat-saturated MR is considered a superior tool for staging OC SCCa.

Infection Assessment

In the clinical setting of suspected OC infection, CECT with mandible and maxilla bone windows is the preferred imaging exam. Abscess of any OC space is easily assessed with CECT. Infectious causes like **mandibular teeth decay** with associated apical cyst or mandibular osteomyelitis and submandibular duct **stone** are more easily seen on bone CT images.

Imaging Anatomy

The OC is the area above the hyoid bone, anterior to the oropharynx and inferior to the sinuses and nose. Its borders are defined superiorly as the hard palate and maxillary alveolar ridge, laterally by the cheek, posteriorly by the oropharyngeal lingual tonsil and soft palate, and inferiorly by the platysma. The OC contains the oral tongue, mandible body and teeth, maxillary ridge and teeth, and the hard palate. The mandible and maxilla and their associated teeth will be covered in the mandible and maxilla overview module.

The OC can be subdivided into 4 distinct imaging areas: (1) **Oral mucosal space/surface** (OMS), (2) **sublingual space** (SLS), (3) **submandibular space** (SMS), and (4) **root of tongue** (ROT). Each area contains unique structures and provides its own space-specific differential diagnosis.

The **OMS** is covered by a continuous mucosal sheet of nonkeratinized stratified squamous epithelium. Since primary SCCa tumors arise within the OMS, the mucosal components are defined according to **SCCa subsites**. These include the mucosa overlying the oral tongue, floor of mouth (FOM), alveolar ridge, retromolar trigone (RMT), buccal (cheek), and hard palate. Subepithelial collections of **minor salivary glands** are most commonly located in the inner surface of the lip, buccal mucosa, and palate.

The **SLS** is an area within the deep oral tongue superomedial to mylohyoid muscles and lateral to the genioglossus muscle that is **not** encapsulated by fascia. Anteriorly, the SLS runs into the mandible. The SLS is horseshoe-shaped, with the 2 sides communicating anteriorly under the frenulum of the tongue. Posteriorly, the SLS empties into the superior SMS and the inferior parapharyngeal space (PPS). No fascia separates the

posterior SLS from the SMS and inferior PPS. All 3 spaces communicate at the posterior edge of the mylohyoid muscle.

- The SLS contains multiple oral tongue structures. SLS nerves include the **lingual nerve** (sensory branch of CNV3 + chorda tympani branch of CNVI with taste fibers from anterior 2/3 of tongue) and distal **CNIX** and **CNXII**. The tongue's vascular pedicle (lingual artery and vein) passes through the SLS. The sublingual glands and ducts as well as the deep portion of the submandibular gland and submandibular gland duct are all found in the SLS. Finally, the anterior margin of the hyoglossus muscle projects into the posterior SLS from below.

The **SMS** (surgical synonym is submaxillary space) is located inferolateral to the mylohyoid muscle, superior to the hyoid bone, and deep to the platysma muscle. It is the only fascia-lined OC space. The superficial layer of deep cervical fascia lines its deep and superficial surfaces. The deep slip of fascia is found along the external surface of the mylohyoid muscle, and the superficial slip of fascia lines the deep margin of the platysma muscle. Posteriorly, no fascia separates the SMS from the inferior PPS or posterior SLS spaces.

- The SMS can be conceptualized as a horseshoe-shaped space between the mylohyoid above and the hyoid bone below. There is no fascia blocking the spread of disease from side to side in the SMS.
- The SMS contains the **submandibular gland** and submental (level IA) and submandibular (level IB) **nodes**. These 2 structures are responsible for most SMS masses. Other critical structures within the SMS include the facial vein and artery, the caudal loop of CNXII, the anterior belly of the digastric muscle, and fat.

The **ROT** is a term used by surgeons to describe the deep midline oral tongue above the mylohyoid sling and below the extrinsic tongue muscles. The ROT ends anteriorly at the mandibular symphysis. It is made up of the **genioglossus muscle** and the fibrofatty **lingual septum**.

There are 4 additional structures that require specific mention when reviewing the OC anatomy: The **mylohyoid** and **geniohyoid muscles**, the **oral tongue**, and the **RMT**. The **mylohyoid** and **geniohyoid** muscles form the **FOM**. The mylohyoid muscle arises from the mylohyoid line of the medial mandibular body. Anterior and middle fibers insert into median fibrous raphe extending from the symphysis menti to the hyoid bone to its posterior margin. Posterior mylohyoid fibers pass inferomedially to insert into the hyoid bone body. The mylohyoid muscle has been described as the **muscular "sling"** separating the SLS or SMS.

- The OC component of the tongue is referred to as the **oral tongue** and represents the anterior 2/3 of the entire tongue. The posterior 1/3 is called the **base of tongue (lingual tonsil)** and is part of the oropharynx. The **extrinsic tongue muscles** of the oral tongue include the genioglossus, hyoglossus, styloglossus, and palatoglossus. The **genioglossus** is the large, fan-shaped muscle arising anteriorly from the superior mental spine on the inner surface of the symphysis menti of the mandible. It inserts along the entire length of the undersurface of the intrinsic tongue muscles. The **hyoglossus** is a thin, quadrilateral-shaped muscle arising from the body and cornu of the hyoid bone, from there passing vertically upward to insert into the side of the tongue. The **styloglossus** arises from the styloid process and stylomandibular ligament and passes

Differential Diagnosis: Oral Cavity

Pseudolesion	Congenital	Inflammatory-Infectious	Benign Tumor	Malignant Tumor
CNXII atrophy (SLS, ROT)	Lymphatic malformation (SLS, SMS, ROT)	Phlegmon or abscess (SLS, SMS, ROT)	BMT, sublingual gland (SLS)	SCCa (OMS)
CNV3 atrophy (SMS)	Venous malformation (SLS, SMS, ROT)	Dilated submandibular duct + stone (SLS)	BMT, submandibular gland (SMS)	Oral tongue SCCa
Accessory salivary gland (SMS)	Dermoid/epidermoid (SLS, SMS, ROT)	Submandibular gland sialadenitis (SMS)	BMT, hard palate (OMS)	Floor of mouth SCCa
	Lingual thyroid (ROT, SMS, PMS-BOT)	Sublingual gland sialadenitis (SLS)	Lipoma (SMS)	Retromolar trigone SCCa
	Thyroglossal duct cyst (ROT, SMS, PMS-BOT)	Submandibular gland mucocele (SMS)		Alveolar ridge SCCa
	Cellulitis (SLS, SMS, ROT)	Chronic sclerosis sialadenitis (SMS)		Hard palate SCCa
	2nd branchial cleft cyst (SMS)	Simple (SLS) or diving (SLS-SMS) ranula		Buccal mucosa SCCa
		Sialocele (SLS)		Submandibular gland (SMS) or sublingual gland (SLS) carcinoma
		Reactive or suppurative nodes (SMS)		Nodal SCCa or NHL nodes (SMS, levels IA or IB)

OMS = oral mucosal space; PMS = pharyngeal mucosal space; SLS = sublingual space; SMS = submandibular space; ROT = root of tongue; BOT = base of tongue (lingual tonsil); BMT = benign mixed tumor; SCCa = squamous cell carcinoma; NHL = non-Hodgkin lymphoma.

anteroinferiorly between the external and internal carotid arteries to insert into the side of the tongue. Finally, the **palatoglossus** is a thin muscle arising from the anterior surface of the soft palate. From there, it passes anteroinferiorly in front of the palatine tonsil to insert into the side of the tongue. The palatoglossus underlies the anterior tonsillar pillar, which serves as the dividing line between the OC and the oropharynx.

- The **RMT** is a small, triangular-shaped region of OC mucosa behind the last mandibular molar. SCCa of the RMT can spread early into critical proximal locations, such as the masticator space and PPS. Since the **pterygomandibular raphe** (fibrous band at the intersection of the buccinator muscle and the superior constrictor muscle) extends from the hamulus of the medial pterygoid plate above to the medial aspect of the RMT below, RMT SCCa can spread readily in a superior direction along this perifascial route.

Approaches to Imaging Issues in the Oral Cavity

There are 3 main OC imaging indications: (1) Staging of primary SCCa and nodes, (2) searching for abscess and its cause, and (3) evaluating an SMS mass to determine if the mass is nodal or glandular. Knowing the clinical context can affect the type of exam (CECT vs. MR) and facilitate the creation of a highly relevant radiology report. Without clinical history, assigning a lesion to a space of origin (OMS, SLS, ROT, SMS) and comparing its radiologic features to those of the **space-specific differential diagnoses** is an alternative approach to analyzing OC images.

OMS SCCa is known at the time of imaging. The mucosal extent of the SCCa is best determined by the clinician. Imaging is critical to evaluate deep soft tissue extent, bone involvement, perineural tumor, and nodal spread. Small tumors may be extremely subtle or even occult to imaging,

and for this reason it is very helpful to know the primary subsite when reading OMS SCCa scans. This allows careful evaluation for features that are key to surgical management, such as cortical bone erosion. Each OC primary SCCa subsite has its own set of imaging questions that should be considered at the time of primary tumor staging. Refer to the module on each of these primary sites in the SCCa content area to review these imaging questions.

SMS masses usually arise from either the submandibular gland or the submandibular nodal chain (level IA and IB). Making this distinction allows the imager to develop a differential diagnosis based on glandular disease or nodal disease. Note that a smaller submandibular gland tumor may be difficult to see on CECT. US or MR may be used in the cases where the clinician is certain a lesion is present and CECT is equivocal.

ROT lesions are rare. The differential diagnosis of ROT lesions is short, as can be seen by the global differential diagnosis table. If a lesion appears to bow the genioglossus muscles laterally away from each other, then it should be considered primary to the ROT.

Differential Diagnosis

When there is no history available and a lesion is found within the OC, assigning it a space of origin and reviewing that space-specific differential diagnosis can be a very useful strategy for evaluating the imaging exam findings. Review of the global differential diagnosis table provided here shows the space or spaces where the OC lesions are found. This global differential diagnosis can be subdivided into 4 distinct differential diagnoses lists based on the 4 major OC anatomic areas (OMS, SLS, SMS, and ROT).

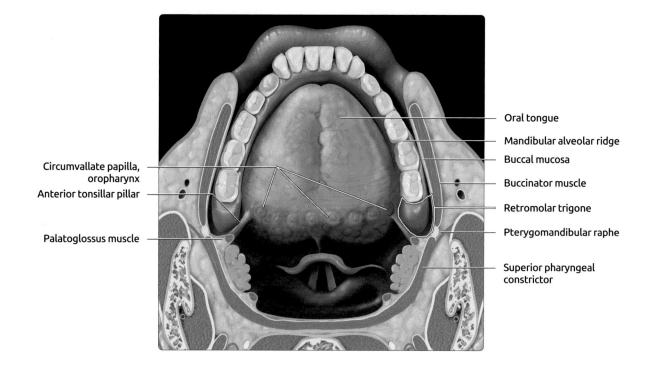

Oral tongue

Mandibular alveolar ridge

Buccal mucosa

Buccinator muscle

Retromolar trigone

Pterygomandibular raphe

Superior pharyngeal constrictor

Circumvallate papilla, oropharynx

Anterior tonsillar pillar

Palatoglossus muscle

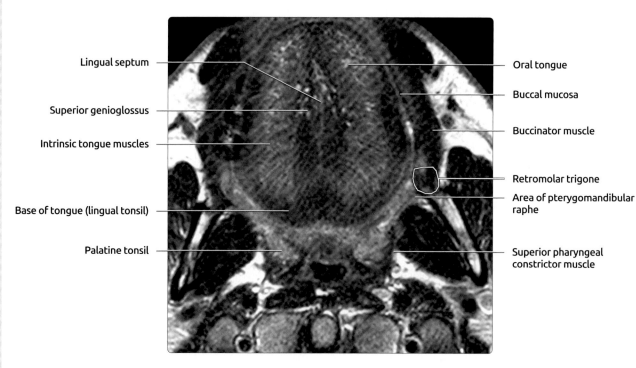

Lingual septum

Superior genioglossus

Intrinsic tongue muscles

Base of tongue (lingual tonsil)

Palatine tonsil

Oral tongue

Buccal mucosa

Buccinator muscle

Retromolar trigone

Area of pterygomandibular raphe

Superior pharyngeal constrictor muscle

(Top) *Axial graphic shows oral mucosal space &/or surface (OMS) shaded in blue. Notice that the circumvallate papilla, a superficial line of taste buds, divides anterior oral cavity (OC) from posterior oropharynx. The lingual tonsil is part of oropharynx, not the OC. Four of the 6 squamous cell carcinoma (SCCa) subsites are labeled on the right, including the oral tongue, alveolar ridge, buccal mucosa, and retromolar trigone (RMT). The floor of mouth (FOM) and hard palate subsites are not shown. Note that the pterygomandibular raphe (PMR) connects the posterior margin of buccinator muscle to anterior margin of the superior pharyngeal constrictor muscle. The RMT represents a key route of perifascial spread of SCCa of the RMT.* **(Bottom)** *Axial T2 MR through the superior tongue shows the mucosal subsites on the right along with the buccinator, PMR, and superior constrictor adjacent to the RMT. Note the oropharyngeal palatine and lingual tonsils labeled on the left.*

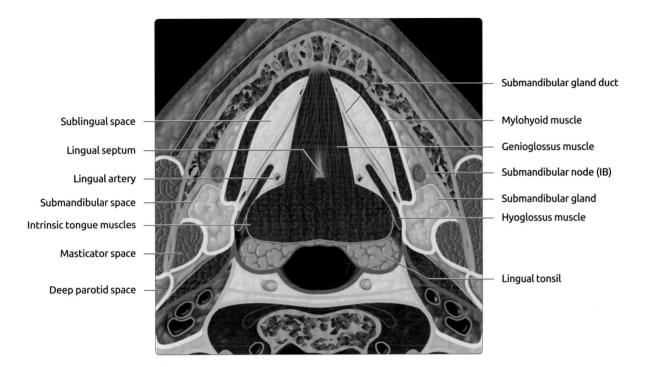

Sublingual space
Lingual septum
Lingual artery
Submandibular space
Intrinsic tongue muscles
Masticator space
Deep parotid space

Submandibular gland duct
Mylohyoid muscle
Genioglossus muscle
Submandibular node (IB)
Submandibular gland
Hyoglossus muscle
Lingual tonsil

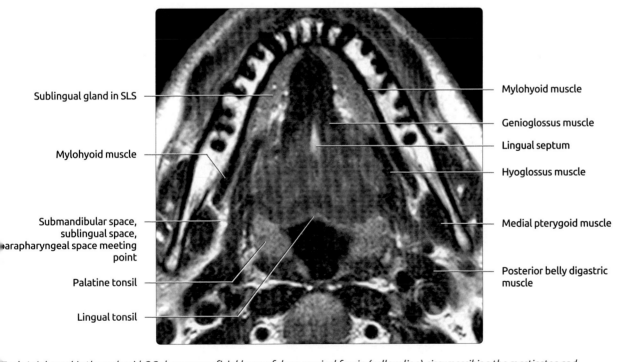

Sublingual gland in SLS
Mylohyoid muscle
Submandibular space, sublingual space, parapharyngeal space meeting point
Palatine tonsil
Lingual tonsil

Mylohyoid muscle
Genioglossus muscle
Lingual septum
Hyoglossus muscle
Medial pterygoid muscle
Posterior belly digastric muscle

Top) *Axial graphic through mid-OC shows superficial layer of deep cervical fascia (yellow line) circumscribing the masticator and parotid spaces posteriorly and defining deep margin of submandibular space (SMS) (colored in blue). Notice the principal occupants of SMS are submandibular gland and level I nodes. The green sublingual space (SLS) has many structures within it, including the sublingual gland, submandibular duct, lingual artery, and the anterior margin of hyoglossus muscle.* **(Bottom)** *Axial T2 MR shows the structures of the FOM and root of tongue (ROT). Notice the symmetric paired genioglossus muscles separated by a fatty lingual septum. The hyoglossus muscles insert into the lateral aspect of the tongue and delineate the location of the submandibular duct, which courses between hyoglossus and mylohyoid and terminates in oral anterior aspect of the FOM. The sublingual glands are nestled anteriorly in the FOM also.*

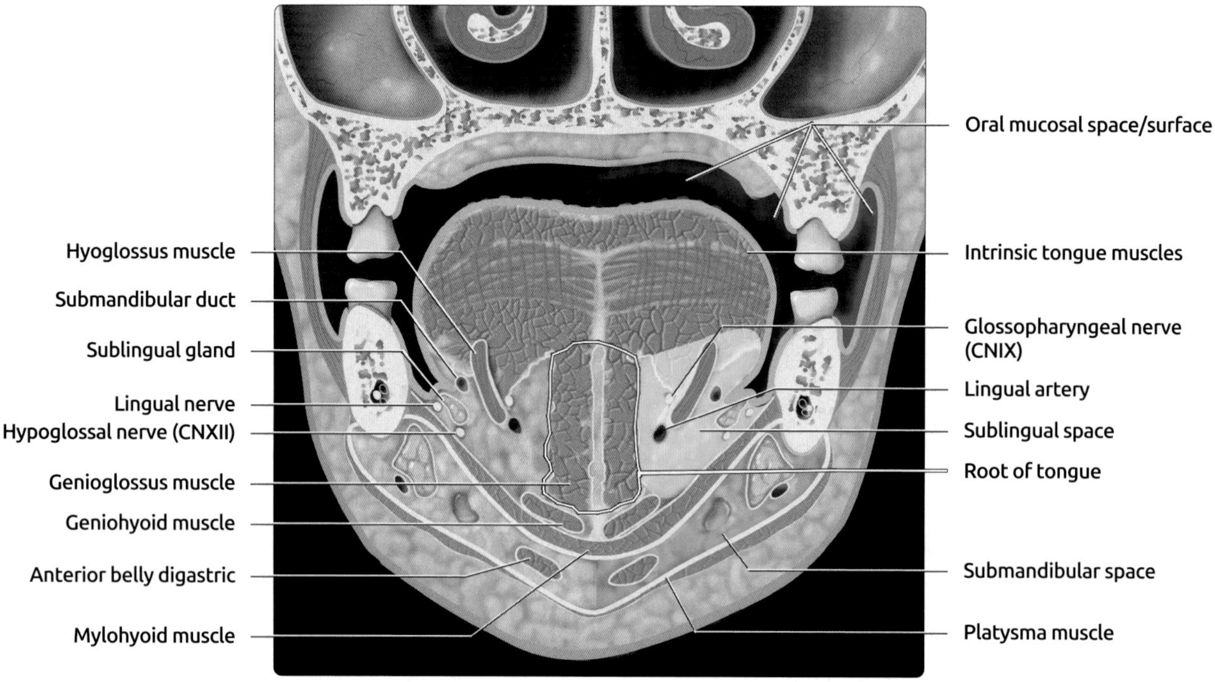
Oral mucosal space/surface
Hyoglossus muscle
Intrinsic tongue muscles
Submandibular duct
Glossopharyngeal nerve (CNIX)
Sublingual gland
Lingual artery
Lingual nerve
Hypoglossal nerve (CNXII)
Sublingual space
Root of tongue
Genioglossus muscle
Geniohyoid muscle
Submandibular space
Anterior belly digastric
Platysma muscle
Mylohyoid muscle

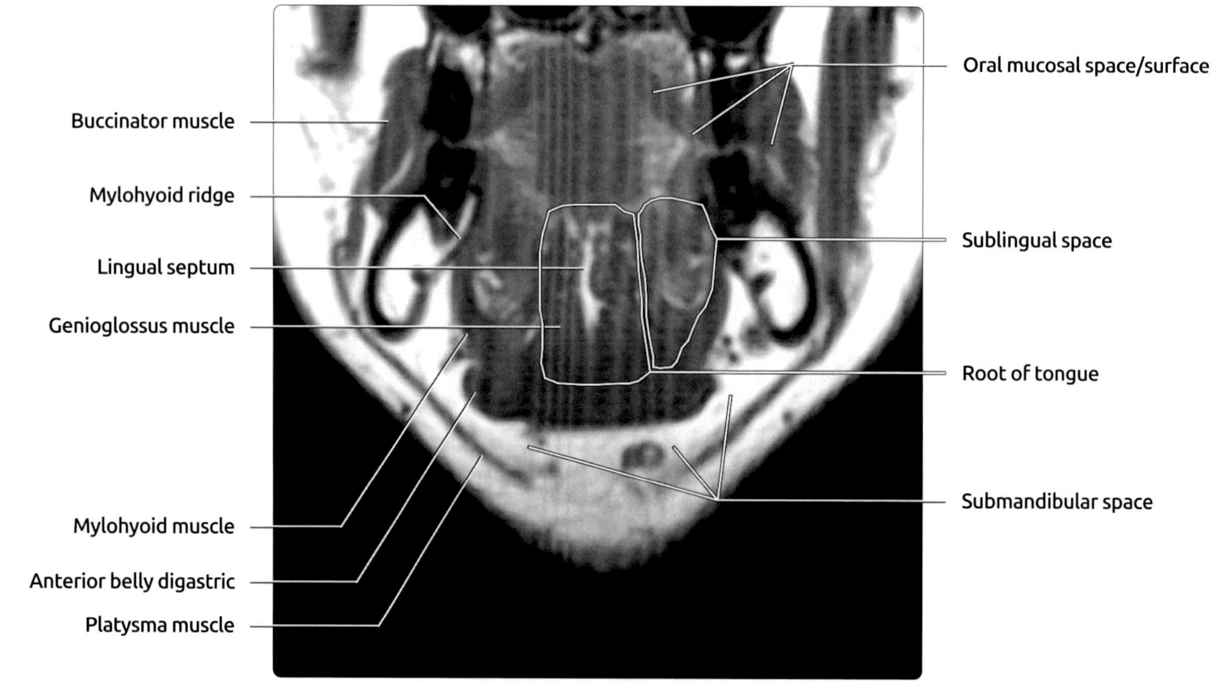
Oral mucosal space/surface
Buccinator muscle
Mylohyoid ridge
Sublingual space
Lingual septum
Genioglossus muscle
Root of tongue
Submandibular space
Mylohyoid muscle
Anterior belly digastric
Platysma muscle

(Top) *Coronal graphic through OC shows the mylohyoid muscle inserting on each side of the OC along the mylohyoid ridges of the medial mandible. This muscle separates the superomedial SLS (green) from inferolateral SMS (blue). The SLS contains the lingual nerve and artery, submandibular duct, CNIX, CNXII, and sublingual gland. The SMS contains the submandibular gland, facial vein and artery, level I nodes, and anterior belly of the digastric muscle. Genioglossus and the lingual septum form the ROT. The OMS lines the surface of the OC (purple).* **(Bottom)** *Coronal T1 MR depicts the mylohyoid muscular sling (FOM) "strung" between the mylohyoid ridges of the mandible. The OMS is difficult to identify on a closed-mouth image, while the SLS, SMS, and ROT are all well delineated. Notice that the neurovascular contents of the SLS and SMS cannot be identified.*

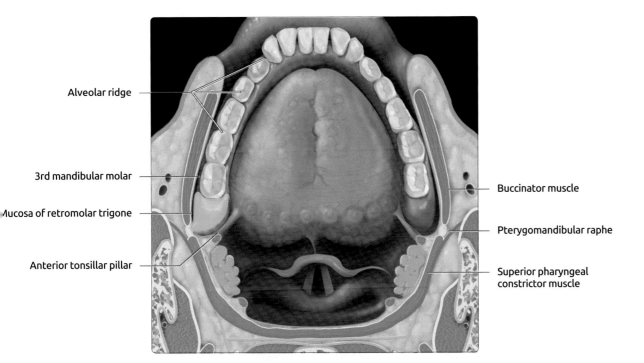

Alveolar ridge

3rd mandibular molar

Mucosa of retromolar trigone

Anterior tonsillar pillar

Buccinator muscle

Pterygomandibular raphe

Superior pharyngeal constrictor muscle

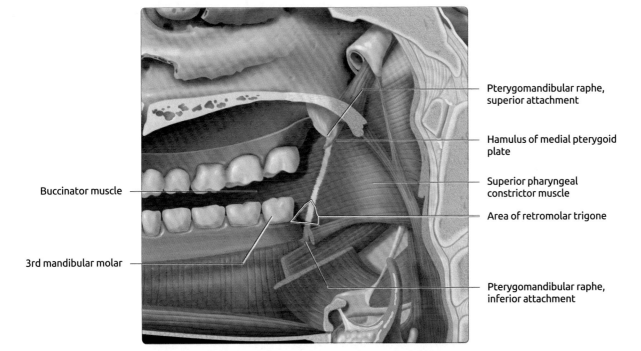

Buccinator muscle

3rd mandibular molar

Pterygomandibular raphe, superior attachment

Hamulus of medial pterygoid plate

Superior pharyngeal constrictor muscle

Area of retromolar trigone

Pterygomandibular raphe, inferior attachment

(Top) Axial graphic highlights the RMT (shaded in light blue on the left) and the PMR. Notice that the mucosal surface of the RMT is found directly behind the mandibular 3rd molar. The RMT is designated as its own OC subsite for SCCa, but it is really just the most posterior portion of the alveolar ridge. The proximity to the PMR (fascial band connecting buccinator and superior constrictor muscles) is important when SCCa occurs in the RMT because it gives the tumor access to the pterygoid plate above via this perifascial spread route. (Bottom) Sagittal graphic viewed from inside the mouth delineates the full extent of the PMR. Note the cephalad PMR attachment to the hamulus of the medial pterygoid plate and its inferior attachment to the posterior aspect of the mylohyoid ridge on the inner mandibular cortex. The PMR "connects" the buccinator muscle to the superior pharyngeal constrictor muscle.

KEY FACTS

TERMINOLOGY

- Hypoglossal nerve (CNXII)
- Loss of nerve supply to muscles of 1/2 tongue

IMAGING

- Asymmetry of tongue appearance with linear demarcation of abnormality; varies over time
- CT density and MR signal intensity vary over time
- Acute (typically < 1 month)
  - 1/2 tongue initially swollen, then atrophies
  - Enhancement variable
- Subacute (typically 1-20 months)
  - Loss of volume and fatty change of 1/2 tongue
  - Decreasing enhancement
- Chronic (typically > 20 months)
  - Fatty atrophy, no enhancement
- Image course of CNXII from skull base to hyoid

TOP DIFFERENTIAL DIAGNOSES

- Lingual tonsil squamous cell carcinoma (SCCa)
- Oral tongue SCCa
- Oral cavity lymphatic malformation
- Oral cavity venous malformation

PATHOLOGY

- Many causes; may be isolated or with CNIX-XI

DIAGNOSTIC CHECKLIST

- Frequent source of mistaken identity
- Flaccid 1/2 of tongue hangs posteriorly into oropharynx, mistaken for (ipsilateral) tongue base tumor
- Contralateral larger 1/2 of tongue may be mistaken for tongue tumor
- No FDG uptake may be called contralateral tumor
- Sharp line delineating unilateral changes is key

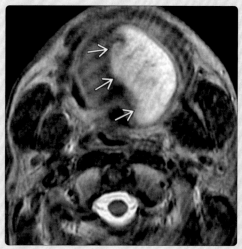
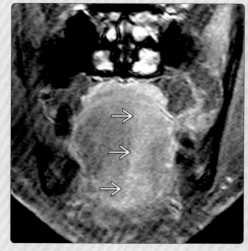

(Left) Axial T2 MR shows acute stage of tongue denervation with swollen left hemitongue and markedly increased T2 signal from edema ➡. Note sharp delineation of abnormality. Denervation was due to perineural tumor spread along CNXII. (Right) Coronal T1 C+ FS MR shows subacute denervation changes with heterogeneous enhancement of unilateral left tongue musculature ➡. Note sharp demarcation of changes. Finding was secondary to skull base metastatic focus involving hypoglossal canal.

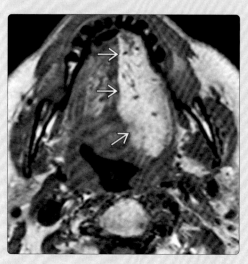
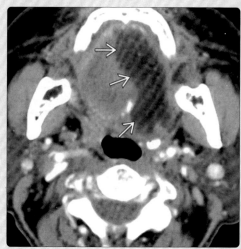

(Left) Axial T1 MR shows chronic changes of tongue denervation with markedly increased signal ➡ in left hemitongue, consistent with fatty replacement. Hypoglossal denervation was due to jugular foramen paraganglioma (not shown). (Right) Axial CECT shows fatty atrophy from chronic left hypoglossal nerve denervation ➡. Right 1/2 of tongue appears larger than left and can be mistaken for tongue tumor. Denervation found to be secondary to destructive bone lesion at hypoglossal canal.

TERMINOLOGY

Synonyms

- Hypoglossal nerve (CNXII) palsy, hypoglossal nerve paralysis, tongue denervation

Definitions

- Loss of nerve supply to muscles supplying tongue
  - Note palatoglossus supplied by CNX

IMAGING

General Features

- Best diagnostic clue
  - Asymmetry of tongue appearance with linear demarcation of abnormality
- Location
  - Unilateral tongue musculature
- Morphology
  - Varies over time
    - Initially swollen, then atrophies
    - Flaccidity of ipsilateral tongue muscles

CT Findings

- CECT
  - Initial: Unilateral swelling of tongue
    - Ipsilateral tongue flaccidity
  - Later: Loss of volume and decreased density of 1/2 of tongue

MR Findings

- Signal intensity varies over time following denervation
- Acute (typically < 1 month)
  - Tongue swollen, flaccid
  - Increased T2 intensity of 1/2 of tongue, subtly decreased T1 signal
  - Enhancement variable in acute phase
- Subacute (typically 1-20 months)
  - Swelling resolves, fatty atrophy
  - Increasing T1 hyperintensity, decreasing enhancement
- Chronic (typically > 20 months)
  - Atrophy of hemitongue
  - Marked T1 hyperintensity, enhancement resolves

Nuclear Medicine Findings

- PET/CT
  - Denervated 1/2 of tongue has decreased FDG uptake

Imaging Recommendations

- Best imaging tool
  - Either CECT or MR evaluates CNXII course well
- Protocol advice
  - Must image skull base to hyoid along course of CNXII

DIFFERENTIAL DIAGNOSIS

Lingual Tonsil Squamous Cell Carcinoma (SCCa)

- Enhancing tumor at base of tongue

Oral Tongue SCCa

- Enhancing lesion most commonly arising from lateral margin

Oral Cavity Lymphatic Malformation

- Multiloculated septated transspatial lesion

Oral Cavity Venous Malformation

- Enhancing, irregular lesion involving multiple spaces

PATHOLOGY

General Features

- Etiology
  - Lesion along course of CNXII
  - If isolated CNXII neuropathy, most commonly due to skull base lesion
    - Bone lesion: Metastasis or direct tumor invasion, osteomyelitis
    - Postoperative: Injury at endarterectomy, neck dissection
    - Vascular: Carotid dissection, vascular malformation
    - Postradiation: Fibrosis
    - Rarely brainstem or CPA lesion
  - With other cranial nerves: CNIX-XI
    - Upper carotid sheath lesion, skull base lesion to jugular foramen

CLINICAL ISSUES

Presentation

- Most common signs/symptoms
  - Tongue deviation to side of denervation on protrusion
  - Tongue paralysis, fasciculations, loss of tone
- Other signs/symptoms
  - Other cranial nerves may be involved: CNIX-XI
- Clinical profile
  - Most often older patient with skull base lesion or head & neck tumor

DIAGNOSTIC CHECKLIST

Consider

- Frequent source of mistaken identity
  - Flaccid 1/2 of tongue hangs posteriorly into oropharynx mimicking (ipsilateral) tongue base tumor
  - Contralateral tongue may be mistaken as abnormally enlarged secondary to tongue tumor
  - Loss of FDG uptake may be mistaken for contralateral tumor on PET/CT

Image Interpretation Pearls

- Key imaging feature is sharp line delineating unilateral tongue changes

Reporting Tips

- Carefully review course of CNXII to find cause

SELECTED REFERENCES

1. Timbang MR et al: Hypoglossal nerve paralysis results in hypermetabolic activity on positron emission tomography/computed tomography in the contralateral tongue. Laryngoscope. 125(6):1382-4, 2015
2. Murakami R et al: MR of denervated tongue: temporal changes after radical neck dissection. AJNR Am J Neuroradiol. 19(3):515-8, 1998
3. Murakami R et al: CT and MR findings of denervated tongue after radical neck dissection. AJNR Am J Neuroradiol. 18(4):747-50, 1997
4. Harnsberger HR et al: Major motor atrophic patterns in the face and neck: CT evaluation. Radiology. 155(3):665-70, 1985

Submandibular Space Accessory Salivary Tissue

TERMINOLOGY

- Accessory salivary tissue in mylohyoid boutonnière
- Normal salivary tissue in abnormal position within submandibular space (SMS)

IMAGING

- Benign-appearing SMS mass, with density/intensity following normal salivary glands
- SMS; inferior to mylohyoid, most commonly anterior to submandibular gland

TOP DIFFERENTIAL DIAGNOSES

- SMS reactive nodal disease
- SMS lymphatic malformation
- SMS abscess
- Diving ranula
- Submandibular gland mucocele

PATHOLOGY

- Ectopic sublingual or submandibular gland tissue in SMS

CLINICAL ISSUES

- Most commonly **incidental** & discovered on imaging for unrelated indications
- May occasionally present as SMS mass
- Subject to same spectrum of disease as other salivary tissue, including sialadenitis and sialolithiasis, though these occur only rarely

DIAGNOSTIC CHECKLIST

- Include diagnosis of accessory salivary tissue when evaluating submandibular masses
- Accessory SMS salivary tissue focus, when discovered, is "leave alone" lesion
- Look for density/intensity that follows normal submandibular gland parenchyma

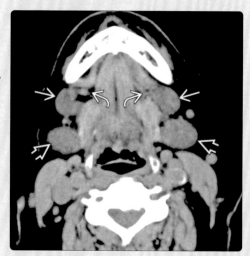
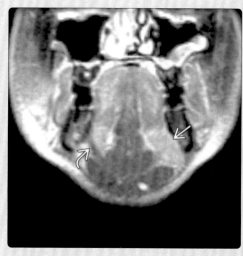

(Left) Axial NECT demonstrates bilateral accessory salivary tissue in submandibular space ➡. Bilateral mylohyoid dehiscence is evident ➡. Note density of accessory salivary tissue is identical to that of native submandibular glands ➡. (Right) Coronal T1 postcontrast MR reveals the left sublingual gland ➡ extending into the submandibular space through a defect in the left mylohyoid. The right mylohyoid is intact ➡.

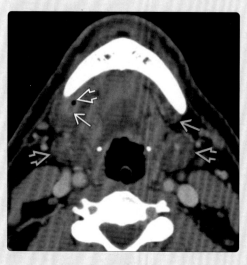
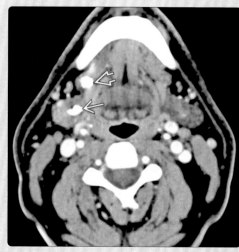

(Left) Axial CECT image shows relative enhancement of inflamed right accessory salivary tissue, particularly of its duct ➡, which contains gas ➡. Compare to normal density of left accessory tissue ➡. Note normal submandibular glands ➡. (Right) Axial CECT shows a calcified mass in hyperdense right submandibular gland ➡. Accessory salivary tissue is present anteriorly & medially with an additional stone ➡. This appearance is consistent with sialolithiasis within both native & accessory salivary tissue.

TERMINOLOGY

Synonyms

- Accessory salivary tissue in mylohyoid boutonnière

Definitions

- Normal salivary tissue in abnormal position in submandibular space (SMS)

IMAGING

General Features

- Best diagnostic clue
  - Benign-appearing SMS mass, with density/intensity following normal salivary glands
- Location
  - SMS; inferior to mylohyoid, most commonly anterior to submandibular gland (SMG)
- Size
  - Variable, usually small, < 2 cm
- Morphology
  - Ovoid to lobulated
  - Pear-shaped when projects into mylohyoid defect

CT Findings

- NECT
  - SMS mass with density similar to normal SMG
  - Mylohyoid defect may be visible
- CECT
  - Enhances similar to normal SMG
    - Increased density common, indicative of inflammation

MR Findings

- T1WI
  - SMS mass with signal similar to SMG
- T2WI
  - Signal parallels SMG
- T1WI C+
  - Enhancement similar to SMG

Imaging Recommendations

- Best imaging tool
  - CECT
- Protocol advice
  - Thin sections with multiplanar reformations, especially coronal

DIFFERENTIAL DIAGNOSIS

SMS Reactive Nodal Disease

- SMS mass distinct from SMG
  - Nodal morphology will vary based on underlying disease

SMS Abscess

- Rim-enhancing cystic mass with extensive cellulitis

Diving Ranula

- Comet-shaped unilocular mass with tail in collapsed SLS (tail sign) & head in posterior SMS
- May dive through mylohyoid defect

SMS Lymphatic Malformation

- Multilocular transspatial cystic mass

SMG Mucocele

- Well-circumscribed SMG cystic mass

PATHOLOGY

General Features

- Etiology
  - Ectopic sublingual or SMG tissue in SMS
    - Present in about 1/3 of individuals
  - Occurs in association with congenital defect in mylohyoid boutonnière
    - Defects occur in about 75% of individuals
      - May contain fat, blood vessels, salivary tissue
    - Occasionally, entire sublingual glands may herniate through defect & lie completely below mylohyoid

Gross Pathologic & Surgical Features

- Normal salivary gland parenchyma

Microscopic Features

- Normal salivary gland cellular makeup

CLINICAL ISSUES

Presentation

- Most common signs/symptoms
  - Most commonly **incidental imaging finding**
  - Other signs/symptoms
    - May occasionally present as SMS mass

Treatment

- Imaging diagnosis allows avoidance of intervention
- When accessory tissue involved with salivary disease, treatment is determined by pathological process

DIAGNOSTIC CHECKLIST

Consider

- Include diagnosis of accessory salivary tissue when evaluating submandibular masses
- Accessory SMS salivary tissue focus, when discovered, is "leave alone" lesion

Image Interpretation Pearls

- Look for density/intensity that follows normal SMG parenchyma
- Susceptible to same pathology as orthotopic glands

SELECTED REFERENCES

1. Harrison JD et al: Postmortem investigation of mylohyoid hiatus and hernia: aetiological factors of plunging ranula. Clin Anat. 26(6):693-9, 2013
2. Kiesler K et al: Incidence and clinical relevance of herniation of the mylohyoid muscle with penetration of the sublingual gland. Eur Arch Otorhinolaryngol. 264(9):1071-4, 2007
3. du Toit DF et al: Salivary glands: applied anatomy and clinical correlates. SADJ. 59(2):65-6, 69-71, 73-4, 2004
4. Hopp E et al: Mylohyoid herniation of the sublingual gland diagnosed by magnetic resonance imaging. Dentomaxillofac Radiol. 33(5):351-3, 2004
5. White DK et al: Accessory salivary tissue in the mylohyoid boutonniere: a clinical and radiologic pseudolesion of the oral cavity. AJNR Am J Neuroradiol. 22(2):406-12, 2001
6. Koybasioglu A et al: Submandibular accessory salivary gland causing Warthin's duct obstruction. Head Neck. 22(7):717-21, 2000
7. Engel JD et al: Mylohyoid herniation: gross and histologic evaluation with clinical correlation. Oral Surg Oral Med Oral Pathol. 63(1):55-9, 1987

Oral Cavity Dermoid and Epidermoid

TERMINOLOGY

- Cystic oral cavity (OC) lesion resulting from congenital epithelial inclusion or rest
- Dermoid: Epithelial elements plus dermal adnexa
- Epidermoid: Epithelial elements only

IMAGING

- Dermoid and epidermoid appear as well-demarcated cysts in OC
- Dermoid more often midline
- Dermoid: Complex cystic mass, often with fat &/or calcification
- MR best reveals foci of fat with chemical shift artifact
  o Fat also bright on T1WI and low signal with fat saturation
- Epidermoid: Fluid contents only
- Both dermoid and epidermoid may have restricted diffusion on DWI

TOP DIFFERENTIAL DIAGNOSES

- Ranula
- Lymphatic malformation of OC
- Submandibular cystic metastatic squamous cell carcinoma node
- Thyroglossal duct cyst
- OC abscess

CLINICAL ISSUES

- Average age at presentation: 30 years
- Painless subcutaneous or submucosal mass (85-90%)
- Often grows rapidly during puberty when sebaceous glands activated
- Surgical resection curative

DIAGNOSTIC CHECKLIST

- OC dermoid, epidermoid, ranula, and lymphatic malformation may appear indistinguishable

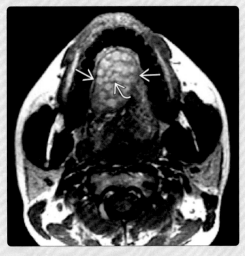
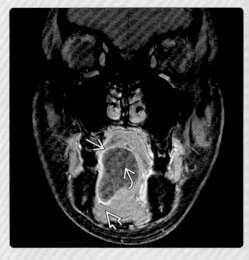

(Left) Axial T1WI MR through floor of mouth shows an ovoid, well-circumscribed mass ➡. There are internal hyperintense globules with chemical shift artifact ➡ that indicate fatty content, consistent with dermoid cyst. (Right) Coronal T1WI C+ FS MR shows a well-circumscribed mass with thin rim enhancement ➡ superior to the mylohyoid muscle ➡, consistent with sublingual location. Internal fat globules ➡ are markedly hypointense with fat saturation technique and confirm dermoid cyst.

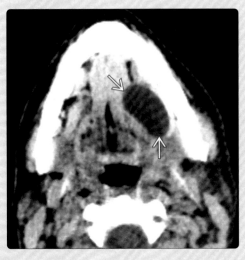
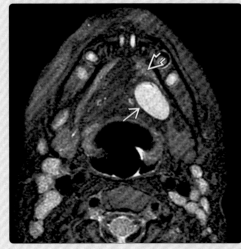

(Left) Axial NECT shows a well-circumscribed cystic mass in the left sublingual space ➡, pathologically proven to be dermoid. Sublingual space dermoid, without visible complex elements, mimics epidermoid, simple ranula, and lymphatic malformation. (Right) Axial STIR MR in a different patient reveals a well-circumscribed, hyperintense epidermoid in the left sublingual space ➡, posterior to the sublingual gland ➡. With simple fluid content, epidermoid is indistinguishable from ranula or lymphatic malformation.

TERMINOLOGY

Synonyms

- Developmental oral cavity (OC) cyst, ectodermal inclusion cyst, dermoid cyst

Definitions

- Cystic OC lesion resulting from congenital epithelial inclusion or rest
  - **Dermoid**: Epithelial elements plus dermal adnexa
  - **Epidermoid**: Epithelial elements only
- Rarer entity is teratoid cyst
  - Epithelial elements plus other tissue, such as bone, cartilage, or muscle

IMAGING

General Features

- Best diagnostic clue
  - Dermoid and epidermoid appear as well-demarcated cysts in OC
  - Dermoid: Fatty, fluid, or mixed contents
  - Epidermoid: Fluid only
- Location
  - Submandibular space (SMS), sublingual space (SLS), or root of tongue (ROT)
  - Dermoid cyst more frequently midline
- Size
  - Typically < 4 cm
- Morphology
  - Ovoid or tubular
    - Most show thin definable wall (75%)
    - 20% have nodular soft tissue in wall or on periphery of cyst

CT Findings

- NECT
  - Low-density, unilocular, well-circumscribed mass
    - Dermoid: Fatty internal material, mixed-density fluid, calcification (< 50%)
    - Epidermoid: Fluid density without complex features
- CECT
  - May see subtle enhancement of wall
  - If dermoid has minimal complex elements, can be indistinguishable from epidermoid

MR Findings

- T1WI
  - Well-circumscribed mass in OC
  - Dermoid: Complex fluid signal is characteristic
    - Focal or diffuse high signal suggests fat
      - Fat proven by chemical shift artifact or fat-saturation techniques
  - Epidermoid: Homogeneous fluid signal
    - Diffuse high signal may reflect protein content
- T2WI
  - Dermoid: Heterogeneous high signal
    - Intermediate signal if fat
    - Focal areas of low signal if calcifications
  - Epidermoid: Homogeneous high signal
- DWI
  - Either dermoid or epidermoid may show restricted diffusion
- T1WI C+
  - Thin rim enhancement often evident

Ultrasonographic Findings

- May be useful for evaluation of superficial lesions
- Dermoid: Mixed internal echoes from fat; echogenic foci with dense shadowing if calcifications
- Epidermoid: Pseudosolid appearance with uniform internal echoes
  - Cellular material within cyst creates pseudosolid appearance
  - Posterior wall echo enhancement is clue to cystic nature

Imaging Recommendations

- Best imaging tool
  - CECT or MR for localization
  - MR best for distinguishing dermoid and epidermoid
    - If complex signal, then lesion most likely represents dermoid
- Protocol advice
  - CT: Thin section with multiplanar reconstructions aids in specific OC localization
  - MR: Include fat-suppression sequences to prove presence of fat

DIFFERENTIAL DIAGNOSIS

Ranula

- Simple ranula may exactly mimic SLS epidermoid
  - Unilateral thin-walled SLS cystic mass
- Diving ranula may also mimic SLS-SMS epidermoid
  - Comet-shaped unilocular mass with "tail" in collapsed SLS and "head" in posterior SMS

OC Lymphatic Malformation

- Transspatial cystic mass
- May hemorrhage, resulting in fluid levels
- Infected lymphatic malformation may have complex proteinaceous contents

Squamous Cell Carcinoma Nodes

- Cystic metastatic nodal disease
- Submandibular nodes (level IB)
- Most often from OC primary including lip

Thyroglossal Duct Cyst

- Midline cystic neck mass between hyoid and foramen cecum
- In posterior tongue root mimics epidermoid

OC Abscess

- Clinical setting of septic patient with painful OC mass is distinctive
- Rim-enhancing cystic mass often with extensive tongue and soft tissue cellulitis-edema

PATHOLOGY

General Features

- Etiology
  - 2 theories: Congenital and acquired

– Congenital inclusion of dermal elements at site of embryonic 1st and 2nd branchial arches
  □ Sequestration of trapped surface ectoderm during midline fusion in 3rd-4th embryonic weeks
– Acquired traumatic implantation of epithelial elements within OC mucosa

Staging, Grading, & Classification

- Meyer classification (pathological)
  o Dermoid: Epithelium-lined cyst containing skin appendages, such as sebaceous and sweat glands, and hair follicles in cyst wall
  o Epidermoid: Lined with simple squamous epithelium and surrounding connective tissue
  o Teratoid: Epithelium-lined cyst containing mesodermal or endodermal elements, such as muscle, bones, teeth, & mucous membranes

Gross Pathologic & Surgical Features

- Oily or cheesy material; tan, yellow, or white
- May contain blood or chronic blood products
- Cyst wall is 2- to 6-mm-thick fibrous capsule

Microscopic Features

- Dermoid
  o Contains dermal structures including sebaceous glands, hair follicles, blood vessels, **fat** ± collagen
    – Sweat glands in minority (20%)
    – Lined by keratinizing squamous epithelium
  o Dermoid diagnosis can be difficult for pathologist if full cyst lining not available
- Epidermoid
  o Simple squamous cell epithelium with fibrous wall
- Teratoid cyst
  o Contains elements from all 3 germ cell layers
    – Dermoid features plus other contents, such as bone, muscle, and cartilage

CLINICAL ISSUES

Presentation

- Most common signs/symptoms
  o Painless subcutaneous or submucosal mass (85-90%)
  o Other signs/symptoms
    – Dysphagia, globus oral sensation
    – Airway encroachment when large
    – Uncommonly acute presentation with cyst rupture and inflammation
- Clinical profile
  o Young man with painless SMS/SLS mass

Demographics

- Age
  o Most often in late teens to 20s
    – Average age at presentation: 30 years
- Gender
  o M:F = 3:1
- Epidemiology
  o Dermoid and epidermoid are least common of congenital neck lesions
  o < 25 % of H&N dermoids occur in OC

o 90% of OC/oropharynx masses are squamous cell carcinoma

Natural History & Prognosis

- Benign lesion with slow growth
- Present during childhood but small and dormant
- May enlarge, become symptomatic when sebaceous glands activated during adolescence
- Sudden growth may also indicate cyst rupture
  o Significant inflammation and increased size

Treatment

- Surgical resection curative
  o Entire cyst must be removed to prevent recurrence
- Extracapsular excision can be performed by intraoral or external approach
- Surgical approach may be decided by lesion position relative to mylohyoid muscle
  o SLS: Superomedial to mylohyoid muscle
    – Intraoral approach with good cosmetic and functional results
  o SMS: Inferolateral to mylohyoid
    – Submandibular approach
- Postoperative complications rare
- Steroids or nonsteroidal drugs calm inflammation in ruptured lesions

DIAGNOSTIC CHECKLIST

Consider

- OC dermoid, epidermoid, ranula, and lymphatic malformation often seem indistinguishable

Image Interpretation Pearls

- Presence of fat ± calcium characterizes dermoid
- When hemorrhagic fluid levels are present, consider lymphatic malformation
- Comet shape with components in SLS and SMS supports diving ranula

SELECTED REFERENCES

1. Sahoo NK et al: Dermoid cysts of maxillofacial region. Med J Armed Forces India. 71(Suppl 2):S389-94, 2015
2. Baliga M et al: Epidermoid cyst of the floor of the mouth. Natl J Maxillofac Surg. 5(1):79-83, 2014
3. Al-Khateeb TH et al: Cutaneous cysts of the head and neck. J Oral Maxillofac Surg. 67(1):52-7, 2009
4. Beil CM et al: Oral and oropharyngeal tumors. Eur J Radiol. 66(3):448-59, 2008
5. Fujimoto N et al: Dermoid cyst with magnetic resonance image of sack-of-marbles. Br J Dermatol. 158(2):415-7, 2008
6. Kandogan T et al: Sublingual epidermoid cyst: a case report. J Med Case Reports. 1:87, 2007
7. Göl IH et al: Congenital sublingual teratoid cyst: a case report and literature review. J Pediatr Surg. 40(5):e9-e12, 2005
8. Din SU: Dermoid cyst of the floor of mouth. J Coll Physicians Surg Pak. 13(7):416-7, 2003
9. Ho MW et al: Simultaneous occurrence of sublingual dermoid cyst and oral alimentary tract cyst in an infant: a case report and review of the literature. Int J Paediatr Dent. 13(6):441-6, 2003
10. Longo F et al: Midline (dermoid) cysts of the floor of the mouth: report of 16 cases and review of surgical techniques. Plast Reconstr Surg. 112(6):1560-5, 2003
11. Mathews J et al: True lateral dermoid cyst of the floor of the mouth. J Laryngol Otol. 115(4):333-5, 2001

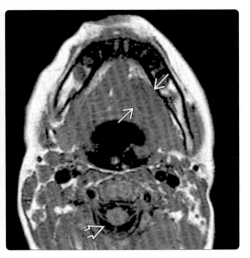

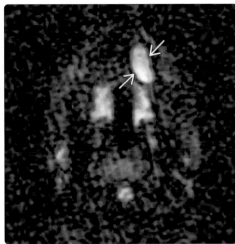

(Left) *Axial T1WI MR reveals sublingual space epidermoid ➡. Lesion signal is only minimally hypointense relative to skeletal muscle and considerably hyperintense to CSF ➡. Appearance is consistent with increased protein content and suggests prior infection or possibly hemorrhage.* (Right) *Axial DWI MR in the same patient demonstrates intrinsic high signal ➡ within sublingual lesion, representing restricted diffusion. Both dermoids and epidermoids may exhibit this appearance.*

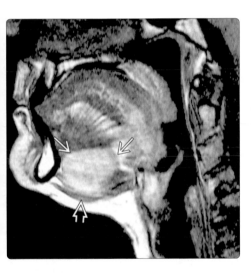

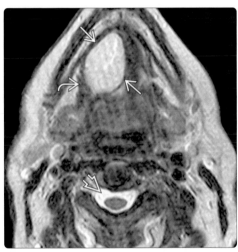

(Left) *Sagittal T1WI MR depicts hyperintense, well-defined epidermoid ➡ arising in the anterior root of tongue and depressing the floor of mouth muscles ➡. Diffuse high signal suggests increased protein content.* (Right) *Axial T2WI MR in the same patient reveals mildly heterogeneous high signal within epidermoid ➡ in the right floor of mouth. Signal is lower intensity than CSF ➡, again reflecting proteinaceous content. Attenuated mylohyoid muscle is seen along the lateral aspect of the lesion ➡.*

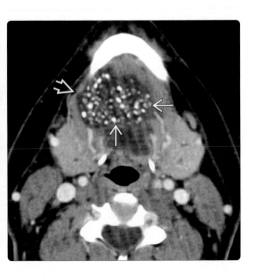

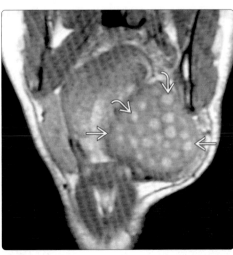

(Left) *Axial CECT reveals well-circumscribed paramedian sublingual space mass ➡, medial to the attenuated mylohyoid muscle ➡. Multiple stippled calcifications and otherwise heterogeneous low attenuation are evident, consistent with dermoid cyst.* (Right) *Coronal T1WI MR shows a large sublingual dermoid ➡, stretching the mylohyoid muscle laterally. Internal round hyperintense foci ➡ are fat and distinguish dermoid from other sublingual cysts, such as epidermoid, ranula, or lymphatic malformation.*

Oral Cavity Lymphatic Malformation

TERMINOLOGY

- Lymphangioma, cystic hygroma
- Distinguishing lympathic malformation (LM) from venous malformation has treatment implications

IMAGING

- Macrocystic (uni- or multilocular) or microcystic
- Microcystic LM more often transspatial
- Submandibular space involvement common
- Typical cystic imaging features on CT/MR
  o Fluid-fluid levels indicate prior hemorrhage
- LM have relative paucity of mass effect given size
- Cysts + solid enhancement or phleboliths suggest venous or mixed venolymphatic malformation

TOP DIFFERENTIAL DIAGNOSES

- Ranula
- Oral cavity abscess
- Dermoid & epidermoid, oral cavity
- Thyroglossal duct cyst

PATHOLOGY

- 1 type of slow-flow vascular malformation
- Classified into macrocystic & microcystic forms

CLINICAL ISSUES

- Diffuse microcystic malformations often have significant functional/cosmetic impairment
  o Potential for airway obstruction
- Intralesional hemorrhage common & may result in dramatic enlargement
- Enlargement may occur with upper respiratory infection

DIAGNOSTIC CHECKLIST

- Contrast-enhanced MR best for characterization
- Rim enhancement only
- Fluid-fluid levels in transspatial cystic mass highly characteristic

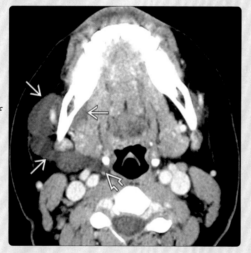
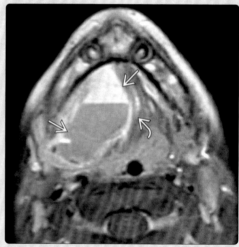

(Left) Axial CECT reveals a multilobulated cystic mass ➡ predominantly in right submandibular space but insinuating around posterior margin of submandibular gland & into parapharyngeal space ➡. Note no perceptible soft tissue, wall, or evidence of contrast enhancement. (Right) T1WI C+ FS MR in a different patient depicts well-demarcated, path-proven lymphatic malformation (LM) ➡ in right sublingual space displacing genioglossus muscles medially ➡. Complex signal with fluid-fluid level indicates prior hemorrhage.

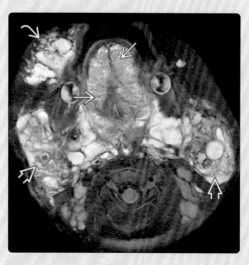
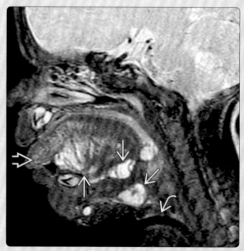

(Left) Axial T2WI FS MR illustrates extensive diffuse microcystic & macrocystic LM involving many spaces of neck & oral cavity. Hyperintense components are evident in tongue ➡, parapharyngeal, carotid, retropharyngeal, parotid ➡, & buccal ➡ spaces. (Right) Sagittal STIR MR delineates LM infiltration ➡ of root & base of tongue, through to submandibular space. Sagittal MR assesses degree of tongue protrusion ➡, which is useful for assessing therapy response. Note tracheotomy ➡ for airway management.

TERMINOLOGY

Abbreviations
- Lymphatic malformation (LM)

Synonyms
- Lymphangioma, cystic hygroma

Definitions
- Congenital malformation with lymphatic features
- May be part of venolymphatic (mixed) malformation

IMAGING

General Features
- Location
  - Uni- or transspatial
  - Microcystic more frequently transspatial
  - In oral cavity, submandibular space (SMS) involvement common
- Size
  - Variable
- Morphology
  - Soft, invaginating lesion with relative paucity of mass effect given size

CT Findings
- NECT
  - Low-density cystic mass
    - Macrocystic form appears well delineated
    - Microcystic form may appear more infiltrative
    - Fluid-fluid levels indicate prior hemorrhage
  - Phleboliths indicate venous or mixed malformation
- CECT
  - Minimal enhancement of thin peripheral rim

MR Findings
- T1WI
  - Primarily hypointense
  - Fluid-fluid levels & high signal indicate prior hemorrhage
- T2WI
  - Hyperintense
  - Microcystic forms have only moderate T2 hyperintensity; may appear solid
- T1WI C+
  - Mild enhancement of thin peripheral rim
  - Central enhancement supports venous (or mixed venolymphatic) malformation

Ultrasonographic Findings
- Primarily hypo- or anechoic transspatial mass
  - Blood products alter echogenicity of cyst

Imaging Recommendations
- Best imaging tool
  - Contrast-enhanced MR for characterization
  - T2WI best to evaluate macrocystic vs. microcystic appearance: Useful in treatment planning
- Protocol advice
  - T2 FS MR best delineates lesion extent

DIFFERENTIAL DIAGNOSIS

Ranula
- Unilocular simple (sublingual space) or diving (sublingual space-SMS) cyst

Abscess, Oral Cavity
- Rim-enhancing low-density mass with cellulitis

Dermoid & Epidermoid, Oral Cavity
- Unilocular cystic mass with fluid or complex signal

Thyroglossal Duct Cyst
- Unilocular cyst in root or base of tongue

PATHOLOGY

General Features
- Etiology
  - Localized defect of vascular morphogenesis; 1 type of slow-flow vascular malformation
- Genetics
  - Usually sporadic but may be seen in Turner, Noonan, & fetal alcohol syndromes

Staging, Grading, & Classification
- Classified into macrocystic & microcystic forms
  - Microcystic LM respond poorly to intralesional therapy

CLINICAL ISSUES

Presentation
- Most common signs/symptoms
  - Soft, doughy mass
  - May present with airway obstruction
- Other signs/symptoms
  - Intralesional hemorrhage common (may result in dramatic enlargement)
  - May rapidly enlarge with upper respiratory infection

Demographics
- Age
  - Present at birth, grow with child

Natural History & Prognosis
- High local recurrence rate with incomplete resection

Treatment
- Percutaneous sclerosing agents of macrocystic LM include OK-432, alcohol, & doxycycline
- Surgical resection if lesion is isolated, unilocular, & not associated with major vessels or nerves
- CO_2 laser useful for tongue lesions

DIAGNOSTIC CHECKLIST

Image Interpretation Pearls
- Fluid-fluid levels in transspatial mass
- Thin peripheral rim enhancement only

SELECTED REFERENCES

1. Gloviczki P et al: Vascular malformations: an update. Perspect Vasc Surg Endovasc Ther. 21(2):133-48, 2009
2. Koeller KK et al: Congenital cystic masses of the neck: radiologic-pathologic correlation. Radiographics. 19(1):121-46; quiz 152-3, 1999

Lingual Thyroid

TERMINOLOGY

- Thyroid tissue in abnormal location in base of tongue (BOT) or floor of mouth
- Ectopic thyroid tissue

IMAGING

- Well-circumscribed rounded midline BOT mass
  - Usually at site of foramen cecum
- Less commonly in sublingual space or tongue root
- Imaging features similar to normal thyroid tissue
- High density on NECT due to iodine content
- Usually avid homogeneous enhancement

TOP DIFFERENTIAL DIAGNOSES

- Venous malformation
- Hemangioma, upper airway
- Tonsillar tissue, prominent/asymmetric
- Non-Hodgkin lymphoma, lingual tonsil

PATHOLOGY

- Arrest of thyroid precursor descent in 1st trimester

CLINICAL ISSUES

- Most common location of ectopic thyroid (90%)
- Lingual thyroid more common in female patients
- In 75% lingual thyroid is only functioning tissue
- Thyroid hormone production may be insufficient, resulting in ectopic thyroid gland enlargement
- Goiter in ectopic gland reported with obstructive symptoms
- Differentiated thyroid carcinoma in lingual thyroid is rare but serious potential complication

DIAGNOSTIC CHECKLIST

- Diagnosis suggested by well-defined, ovoid or round mass in tongue base or floor of mouth
- Intrinsic high density on CT characteristic
- Must check for additional cervical thyroid tissue

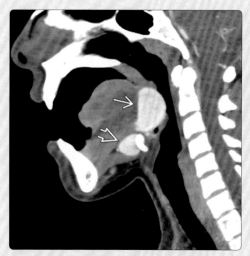
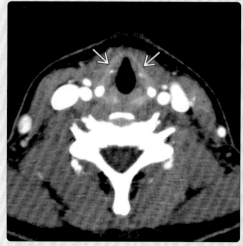

(Left) Sagittal CECT shows a young woman with a tongue base mass. Multifocal midline hyperdense mass is consistent with lingual thyroid ➡. Additional component of ectopic thyroid anterior to the hyoid body ➡ is shown. (Right) Axial CECT of a patient with lingual thyroid, at the level of thyroid cartilage ➡, shows no visible thyroid tissue on either side.

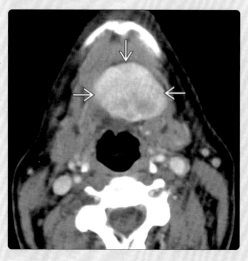
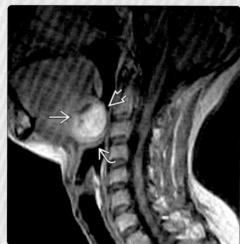

(Left) Axial CECT demonstrates a sharply defined submucosal mass ➡ in the midline floor of the mouth. Heterogeneous density suggests development of a goiter. (Right) Sagittal T1 MR shows a heterogeneous hyperintense mass ➡ in the midline base of the tongue. Note the narrowing of the oropharyngeal airway ➡ and posterior and inferior displacement of the epiglottis ➡.

TERMINOLOGY

Synonyms

- Ectopic thyroid tissue

Definitions

- Thyroid tissue in abnormal location in base of tongue (BOT) or floor of mouth

IMAGING

General Features

- Best diagnostic clue
  - Well-circumscribed midline BOT mass
  - Imaging characteristics similar to normal thyroid
- Location
  - Midline BOT at level of foramen cecum
  - Less commonly in sublingual space or tongue root
- Size
  - 1-3 cm
- Morphology
  - Well circumscribed, round or ovoid

CT Findings

- NECT
  - Sharply marginated rounded mass
  - High density secondary to iodine accumulation
- CECT
  - Avid homogeneous enhancement

MR Findings

- T1WI
  - Isointense to mildly hyperintense relative to tongue
- T2WI
  - Mildly to strikingly hyperintense relative to tongue
- T1WI C+
  - Variable; most often homogeneous enhancement greater than tongue

Nuclear Medicine Findings

- Tc-99m pertechnetate or radioiodine scan to confirm diagnosis

Imaging Recommendations

- Best imaging tool
  - NECT: High-density rounded mass at midline BOT
- Protocol advice
  - Continue imaging through infrahyoid neck to determine if thyroid tissue is in normal location

DIFFERENTIAL DIAGNOSIS

Venous Malformation

- Vasoformative anomaly demonstrates prominent T2 hyperintensity and contrast enhancement

Infantile Hemangioma, Upper Airway

- Cavernous more common than capillary (infantile)

Tonsillar Tissue, Prominent/Asymmetric

- Prominent lingual lymphoid tonsils at entire width of BOT

Non-Hodgkin Lymphoma, Lingual Tonsil

- Isolated or in association with nodal or tonsillar lymphoma

PATHOLOGY

General Features

- Etiology
  - Arrest of thyroid anlage migration within tongue base between 3rd and 7th week of gestation
    - Complete arrest: No cervical thyroid in thyroid bed (75%)
    - Partial arrest: High cervical thyroid (25%)
- Associated abnormalities
  - May occur in association with other thyroid migration anomalies, such as thyroglossal duct cyst

CLINICAL ISSUES

Presentation

- Most common signs/symptoms
  - Dysphagia, dysphonia, dyspnea, obstructive sleep apnea
  - Most patients hypothyroid (60%) or euthyroid
- Other signs/symptoms
  - 25% of infants with congenital hypothyroidism will have ectopic gland

Demographics

- Gender
  - Females more often than males (M:F = 1:4)
- Epidemiology
  - Lingual location most common site of ectopic thyroid (90%)
  - Extremely rare with estimated incidence (1:10,000 to 1:100,000)

Natural History & Prognosis

- Lingual thyroid may expand rapidly during puberty
  - Goiter in lingual thyroid has been reported
- Carcinoma of lingual thyroid rare
  - Most often follicular thyroid carcinoma, in contradistinction to orthotopic gland, which is most commonly papillary

Treatment

- Thyroid hormone replacement 1st to shrink gland at BOT
- Surgical resection if obstructive symptoms
- Some advocate radioiodine ablation

DIAGNOSTIC CHECKLIST

Consider

- When lingual thyroid identified, must comment on status of infrahyoid thyroid tissue in thyroid bed
  - Only functioning thyroid tissue in 75%

Image Interpretation Pearls

- Well-defined midline tongue base mass with intrinsic high density on NECT

SELECTED REFERENCES

1. Prisman E et al: Transoral robotic excision of ectopic lingual thyroid: case series and literature review. Head Neck. 37(8):E88-91, 2015
2. Zander DA et al: Imaging of ectopic thyroid tissue and thyroglossal duct cysts. Radiographics. 34(1):37-50, 2014
3. Hari CK et al: Follicular variant of papillary carcinoma arising from lingual thyroid. Ear Nose Throat J. 88(6):E7, 2009

Ranula

TERMINOLOGY

- Simple ranula (SR), diving ranula (DR)
- Ranula: Sublingual gland (SLG) or sublingual space (SLS) minor salivary gland retention cyst
- SR: True cyst confined to SLS
- DR: SR ruptured to submandibular space (SMS)

IMAGING

- **SR**: Unilocular SLS cyst
  - Unilateral oval or bilateral horseshoe shape
- **DR**: Comet-shaped unilocular cyst
  - "Body" in SMS and "tail" in SLS
  - **Tail sign** = collapsed SLS portion
- Posterior: Tail medial to mylohyoid, body medial to SMG
- Lateral: Tail in anterior SLS & body anterior to SMG
- CECT: Unilocular water density cyst, thin wall enhancement
- C+ MR: Signal intensity follows CSF
- US: Hypoechoic cysts of SLS ± SMS
  - SLG herniation through mylohyoid defect in DR common

TOP DIFFERENTIAL DIAGNOSES

- Oral cavity lymphatic malformation
- Oral cavity dermoid & epidermoid
- 2nd branchial cleft anomaly
- Suppurative lymph nodes

PATHOLOGY

- Retention cyst resulting from trauma or inflammation of SLG or SLS minor salivary gland
- Herniated SLG in DR supports trauma concept

CLINICAL ISSUES

- Simple more common than DR
- Lateral DR more common than posterior DR

DIAGNOSTIC CHECKLIST

- Many imaging and clinical mimics
- Tail is key to determining DR
- **T2 FS MR** best sequence to show subtle tail sign

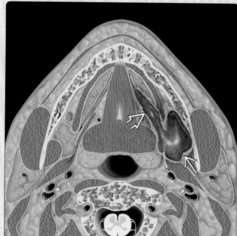 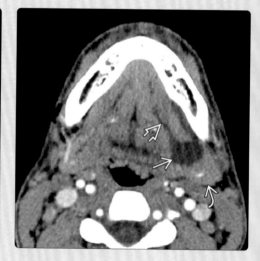

(Left) Axial graphic depicts a diving ranula herniating posteriorly from the sublingual space (SLS) into the submandibular space ➡. The tail sign ➡ is the collapsed portion of the cyst in the SLS. (Right) Axial CECT demonstrates a rounded cystic mass ➡ in the submandibular space abutting the posterior margin of the mylohyoid muscle and displacing the submandibular gland ➡ posterolaterally. A linear, low-density tail ➡ extends anteriorly within the left SLS representing the tail sign of collapsed ranula cyst.

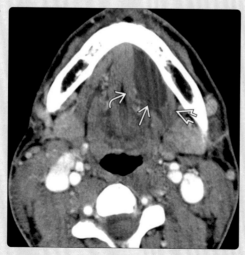 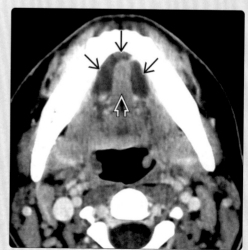

(Left) Axial CECT shows simple unilateral ranula as an ovoid, low-density lesion in left anterior SLS ➡. There is no perceptible thickening or enhancement of wall. Mylohyoid is displaced posterolaterally ➡ and genioglossus ➡ bowed medially. (Right) Axial CECT demonstrates a cystic, horseshoe-shaped lesion ➡ in anterior SLS, curving around and above genioglossus muscle ➡ insertion on mandible. This is a characteristic simple ranula involving both sides of the SLS.

TERMINOLOGY

Abbreviations

- Simple ranula (SR), diving ranula (DR)

Synonyms

- SR: Sublingual gland (SLG) mucocele, SLG mucous retention cyst
- DR: Plunging ranula

Definitions

- SLG or minor salivary gland retention cyst
  o Simple: True cyst confined to sublingual space (SLS)
  o Diving: Extravasation pseudocyst; ruptured SR extending into submandibular space (SMS)
- Term ranula derives from Latin "rana," meaning "frog"
  o Sublingual blebs in mouth of frog resemble SR

IMAGING

General Features

- Best diagnostic clue
  o Simple: Well-defined, thin-walled SLS cyst
  o Diving: Thin-walled SMS cyst with **SLS "tail"**
- Location
  o SR: SLS (i.e., above mylohyoid muscle)
  o DR: SMS & SLS
- Size
  o Simple usually < 3 cm as limited to SLS
  o Diving may be large; usually ≤ 10 cm
- Morphology
  o SR
    – Unilateral oval or lenticular unilocular SLS cyst
    – Bilateral horseshoe-shaped unilocular SLS cyst
  o DR
    – Comet-shaped unilocular SMS cyst, "tail" in SLS
    – If large may involve parapharyngeal space (PPS)

CT Findings

- CECT
  o SR
    – Unilocular low-density SLS cystic mass with subtle or no linear wall enhancement
    – May extend to contralateral SLS (horseshoe shape)
  o DR
    – **Tail sign**: Collapsed SLS portion
    – **Posteriorly** over back of mylohyoid: Tail medial to mylohyoid & body often medial to submandibular gland (SMG)
    – **Laterally** through mylohyoid muscle defect (more common): Tail in anterior SLS & body often anterior to SMG
  o Infected ranula (current or recent)
    – Distended cyst with thick, enhancing wall

MR Findings

- T1WI
  o Diffuse low fluid signal intensity (similar to CSF)
- T2WI
  o Markedly high fluid signal intensity (similar to CSF)
- T1WI C+
  o Thin linear or nonenhancement of wall if not infected
  o Current or recent infection → thicker wall; may alter T1 & T2 signal also

Ultrasonographic Findings

- Hypoechoic, well-defined cystic mass within SLS (± SMS if DR)
- SLG herniation through mylohyoid defect very common in DR
  o May predispose to trauma & DR

Imaging Recommendations

- Best imaging tool
  o CECT is best study for defining extent of ranula
- Protocol advice
  o Multiplanar reformats aid delineation of diving component
  o T2 FS MR best sequence for demonstrating subtle tail sign along SLS

DIFFERENTIAL DIAGNOSIS

Oral Cavity Lymphatic Malformation

- Multilocular transspatial cystic mass
- Lobulation, septation, and heterogeneity suggest LM
  o May involve several spaces when transspatial
  o Peripheral linear wall enhancement may be present

Oral Cavity Dermoid & Epidermoid

- Unilateral low-density/signal mass in SLS with thin, nonenhancing wall
- In SLS, epidermoid can look identical to SR
  o Fat density (CT) or high signal (T1 MR) diagnostic of dermoid
  o Diffusion restriction characteristic of epidermoid

2nd Branchial Cleft Anomaly

- Ovoid unilocular mass in posterior SMS
- No tail sign to SLS
- Tends to displace SMG anteriorly, not laterally

Suppurative Lymph Nodes

- Multiple cystic-appearing SMS nodes
- Separate suppurative/reactive nodes suggest diagnosis
- Associated inflammation & clinical history are key

Oral Cavity Abscess

- Patient usually septic with tender oral cavity
- Single or multiple collections with enhancing wall(s)
- Associated inflammatory changes in fat

Submandibular Gland Mucocele

- Cyst "bubbles" off margin of submandibular gland
- No tail sign to SLS

Oral Cavity Sialocele

- True sialocele: Distended submandibular duct
- False sialocele: Extravasated saliva contained within fibrous pseudocapsule

PATHOLOGY

General Features

- Etiology

- Retention cyst resulting from trauma or inflammation of SLG or SLS minor salivary gland
- Congenital ranula from imperforate salivary duct or ostial adhesion
- SR ruptures → pseudocyst without epithelial lining (DR)
  - Ruptures posteriorly over posterior margin of mylohyoid to posterior SMS
  - Ruptures laterally through mylohyoid button hole (boutonnière) defect, anterior to SMG (most common)
  - Extension to parapharyngeal space in < 10%

Staging, Grading, & Classification
- SR develops 1st in SLS
  - May enlarge to fill entire unilateral SLS
  - May extend to contralateral SLS above mandibular insertion of genioglossus muscle
- DR secondary to rupture of SR
  - Rupture of retention cyst into subjacent SMS

Gross Pathologic & Surgical Features
- Simple: Fluctuant sublingual mass, often with bluish color
- Diving: Fluctuant mass of extravasated mucus

Microscopic Features
- SR has squamous, cuboidal, or columnar epithelial lining
  - Cyst contains mucus-saliva
- DR is pseudocyst with no epithelial lining but fibrous and granulation tissue, dense connective tissue, chronic inflammatory cells
  - Contains mucus pools

CLINICAL ISSUES
Presentation
- Most common signs/symptoms
  - Painless swelling of floor of mouth (SR)
  - DR typically present as submandibular mass, which is displaced SMG
    - Displaced SMG may have partially obstructed duct ± inflammatory changes
  - Either can present as waxing and waning masses
- Other signs/symptoms
  - 50% have history of prior neck or oral cavity trauma
- Clinical profile
  - 30 year old with painless floor of mouth mass

Demographics
- Age
  - Pediatric to adults; median: 30 years
  - Congenital ranula in infant
- Gender
  - M slightly > F
- Ethnicity
  - Increased incidence of DR in Maori of New Zealand and Pacific Island Polynesians (Polynesia, Melanesia, Micronesia)
- Epidemiology
  - SR more common than DR
  - Lateral extension through meyloid defect most common type of DR
  - Congenital ranula is rare

Natural History & Prognosis
- Large SR can fill unilateral SLS, may involve contralateral side
- Children: May spontaneously resolve in 6 months
- Adults: Tend to rupture to SMS as DR
- Recurrence may occur depending on surgical treatment

Treatment
- Controversial: Multiple options described
  - Transoral excision of SLG & evacuation of cyst
    - Fewest complications and lowest recurrence rate
    - Biopsy of pseudocyst wall important to confirm diagnosis
  - Transoral excision of SLG & cyst
    - Sialendoscopy-assisted transoral SLG resection
  - Transcervical excision of SMG, SLG, and cyst
  - Marsupialization
    - Associated with high recurrence rate
  - Laser excision & vaporization
- Nonsurgical options
  - Sclerotherapy with intracystic OK-432 & bleomycin
  - Cyst aspiration alone; highest recurrence rate

DIAGNOSTIC CHECKLIST
Consider
- Many imaging and clinical mimics

Image Interpretation Pearls
- DR is suspected based on "tail" observation
  - If behind posterior margin of mylohyoid muscle, SMS cyst often medial to SMG
  - If laterally through mylohyoid defect, SMS cystic component often anterior to SMG
- While helpful, direction of SMG displacement not diagnostic of lateral or posterior DR
  - Must demonstrate "tail"
- **T2 FS MR** best sequence and modality for delineating subtle tail sign

SELECTED REFERENCES
1. Lee JY et al: Plunging ranulas revisited: a CT study with emphasis on a defect of the mylohyoid muscle as the primary route of lesion propagation. Korean J Radiol. 17(2):264-70, 2016
2. Lee DH et al: Treatment outcomes of the intraoral approach for a simple ranula. Oral Surg Oral Med Oral Pathol Oral Radiol. 119(4):e223-5, 2015
3. Owens DJ et al: Orthodontics: A traumatic cause of ranula. Br Dent J. 219(5):194-5, 2015
4. Li J et al: Correct diagnosis for plunging ranula by magnetic resonance imaging. Aust Dent J. 59(2):264-7, 2014
5. Yang Y et al: Surgical results of the intraoral approach for plunging ranula. Acta Otolaryngol. 134(2):201-5, 2014
6. Harrison JD et al: Postmortem investigation of mylohyoid hiatus and hernia: aetiological factors of plunging ranula. Clin Anat. 26(6):693-9, 2013
7. Jain P et al: Plunging ranulas: high-resolution ultrasound for diagnosis and surgical management. Eur Radiol. 20(6):1442-9, 2010
8. Macdonald AJ et al: Giant ranula of the neck: differentiation from cystic hygroma. AJNR Am J Neuroradiol. 24(4):757-61, 2003

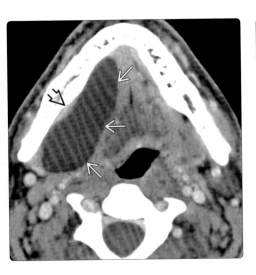

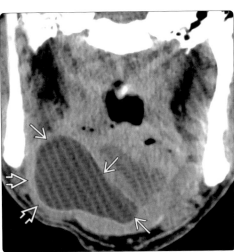

(Left) *Axial CECT shows a large simple ranula ➡ distending the right sublingual space and bowing the mylohyoid muscle ⬌ laterally. There is no appreciable enhancement or thickening of cyst wall or adjacent inflammatory changes.* **(Right)** *Coronal delayed CECT shows inferolateral bowing of the mylohyoid muscle ⬌ by a large, thin-walled unilocular cyst ➡. Simple ranula appears identical to sublingual space epidermoid, and definitive diagnosis requires pathology or clear congenital history.*

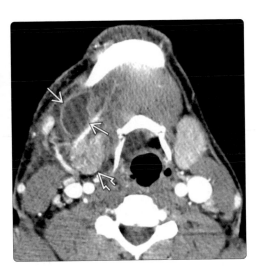

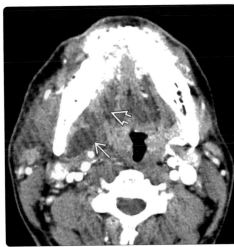

(Left) *Axial CECT in a young adult patient with marked pain and swelling shows a rim-enhancing, low-density mass ➡ in the right submandibular space anterolateral to the submandibular gland ⬌ with extensive adjacent inflammatory changes.* **(Right)** *Axial CECT shows posterosuperior aspect of ranula ➡ extending toward posterior margin of mylohyoid muscle, suggesting diagnosis of diving ranula, which has become acutely secondarily infected. Note swelling of right floor of mouth ⬌.*

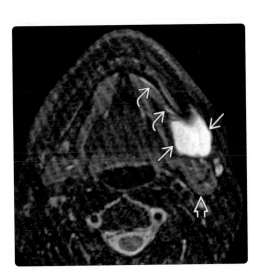

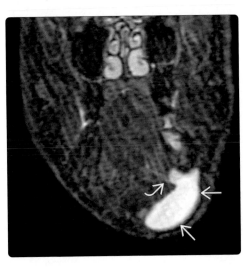

(Left) *Axial T2 FS MR in a young adult with recurrent submandibular mass and 2 prior cyst aspirations shows a well-defined, markedly hyperintense mass ➡ anterior to the submandibular gland ⬌ and lateral to mylohyoid muscle. T2 FS MR best shows subtle tail sign ➡ from laterally diving ranula.* **(Right)** *Coronal T2 FS MR shows laterally diving ranula as a large submandibular space cystic mass ➡ and subtle tail sign ➡ through boutonnière defect of mylohyoid muscle.*

TERMINOLOGY

- Definition: Ruptured submandibular duct (SMD) extravasates saliva into sublingual space (SLS)

IMAGING

- CECT findings
  - SLS fluid density lesion ± enhancing adjacent inflammatory soft tissues
  - Rarely extends into posterior submandibular space (SMS)
  - If associated with SMD calculus, SMD enlargement with enhancing, enlarged submandibular gland
  - Fluid collection is distinct from SMD
- CECT best delineates sialocele & calculus if present

TOP DIFFERENTIAL DIAGNOSES

- Ranula
- SLS epidermoid
- SLS abscess
- SLS lymphatic malformation

PATHOLOGY

- Etiology: **SMD injury** with leakage of saliva into SLS
  - SMD calculus with rupture > > rupture from trauma or surgery

CLINICAL ISSUES

- Common presentation: Fluctuant, soft, painless sublingual mass
  - Patient with SMD stone, recent oral cavity surgery, or trauma presents with new SLS mass
- Sialocele cause: Obstructing SMD calculus > > posttraumatic or postoperative
- Sialocele location: Parotid space > > SLS > SMS

DIAGNOSTIC CHECKLIST

- When cystic SLS lesion is identified, look closely for possible obstructing calculi

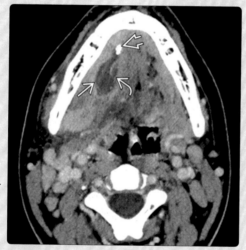
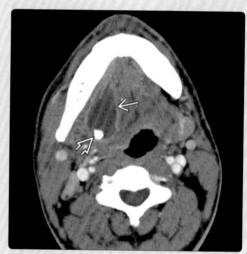

(Left) *Axial CECT shows a calculus obstructing the submandibular duct ➡ at the terminal papilla, causing the submandibular duct to dilate ➡. Duct rupture has occurred with sialocele ➡ visible in the medial sublingual space.* **(Right)** *Axial CECT reveals an ovoid cystic lesion in the right sublingual space ➡. Dependent calculus is seen posteriorly ➡. This patient most likely began with a stone obstructing the submandibular duct. When the duct ruptured, the stone fell into the sialocele.*

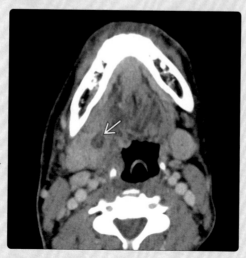
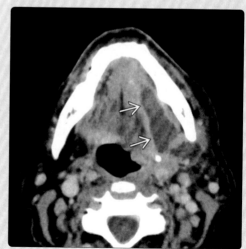

(Left) *Axial CECT demonstrates a small cystic mass in the posterior sublingual space ➡. Ranula, sialocele, and epidermoid were all considered. At surgery, a small pocket of saliva with a fibrous pseudocapsule was found.* **(Right)** *Axial CECT in a patient with history of facial trauma and floor of mouth swelling shows a cystic lesion in the left sublingual space ➡. Both ranula and sialocele were considered; sialocele was found at surgery. History of facial trauma supported sialocele diagnosis.*

TERMINOLOGY

Abbreviations

- Oral cavity (OC)

Synonyms

- Floor of mouth, sublingual, lingual, or submandibular duct (SMD) sialocele

Definitions

- Ruptured SMD extravasates saliva into sublingual space (SLS)

IMAGING

General Features

- Best diagnostic clue
  - Cystic SLS lesion along course of SMD
- Location
  - SLS ± submandibular space (SMS)
- Size
  - Variable, usually < 3 cm
- Morphology
  - Ovoid to lenticular

CT Findings

- CECT
  - SLS fluid density lesion ± enhancing adjacent inflammatory soft tissues
    - Rarely extends into posterior SMS
  - If associated with SMD calculus, SMD enlargement with enhancing and enlarged submandibular gland (SMG)
  - Fluid collection is distinct from SMD
    - SMD may or may not be dilated

MR Findings

- T1WI
  - Low (fluid) signal lesion in SLS ± dilated SMD
- T2WI
  - High (fluid) signal lesion in SLS ± dilated SMD
- T1WI C+
  - Rim-enhancing fluid signal lesion

Imaging Recommendations

- Best imaging tool
  - CECT best delineates sialocele & calculus if present
- Protocol advice
  - Multislice CT scanners can reformat volumetric data sets in oblique planes
    - Oblique reformations can also be obtained around dental amalgam, without repeat scanning acquisitions

DIFFERENTIAL DIAGNOSIS

Ranula

- Unilateral smoothly marginated fluid collection in SLS; no calculus

Sublingual Space Epidermoid

- Ovoid fluid collection in SLS
- DWI shows restricted diffusion

Oral Cavity Abscess in Sublingual Space

- Rim-enhancing SLS fluid collection

Sublingual Space Lymphatic Malformation

- SLS-SMS multilocular transspatial cystic lesion
- No perceptible wall visible unless infected

PATHOLOGY

General Features

- Etiology
  - **SMD injury** with leakage of saliva into SLS
    - SMD calculus with rupture > > rupture from trauma or surgery

Gross Pathologic & Surgical Features

- Saliva outside SMD but contained within **fibrous pseudocapsule**

Microscopic Features

- Fibrous granulation tissue capsule surrounding saliva pocket

CLINICAL ISSUES

Presentation

- Most common signs/symptoms
  - Fluctuant, soft, painless sublingual mass
- Clinical profile
  - Patient with SMD stone or recent OC surgery or trauma presents with new SLS mass

Demographics

- Epidemiology
  - Obstructing SMD calculus > > posttraumatic or postoperative
  - Parotid space sialocele > > SLS sialocele > SMS sialocele

Natural History & Prognosis

- If left alone, sialocele may continue to enlarge

Treatment

- Propantheline bromide
- Local injection of botulinum toxin type A (30-50 U)
  - Used for parotid sialoceles

DIAGNOSTIC CHECKLIST

Consider

- Simple ranula, SLS epidermoid, & sialocele without SMD calculus have similar appearances
  - Simple ranula: Ovoid SLS retention cyst
  - SLS epidermoid: DWI shows restricted diffusion
  - SLS sialocele: Saliva-filled cystic SLS collection
    - History of OC surgery, trauma, or SMD calculus

SELECTED REFERENCES

1. Torre-León C et al: A novel approach in the treatment of a posttraumatic sialocele. Otolaryngol Head Neck Surg. 148(3):529-30, 2013
2. Ang AH et al: Idiopathic submandibular sialoceles in the neck. Otolaryngol Head Neck Surg. 132(3):517-9, 2005
3. Cholankeril JV et al: Post-traumatic sialoceles and mucoceles of the salivary glands. Clin Imaging. 17(1):41-5, 1993

Submandibular Gland Sialadenitis

TERMINOLOGY

- Inflammation of submandibular gland (SMG)

IMAGING

- Most often **acute inflammation** + obstructed duct
  - **Duct calculus** or stenosis, floor-of-mouth tumor
  - 90% calculi opaque on occlusal view x-ray
  - Submandibular sialography rarely used
- **CECT** recommended to evaluate gland ± calculus
  - Ductal dilatation ± calculus, stenosis, or tumor
  - Ipsilateral enlarged SMG + cellulitis
- NECT unnecessary; calculus & vessel densities differ
- **Chronic recurrent sialadenitis** less common
  - Ipsilateral atrophic SMG, ± fatty change
- Autoimmune disease (Sjögren) uncommon in SMG
- Fibroinflammatory disease (Küttner tumor) rare
- MR more sensitive for gland parenchymal changes

TOP DIFFERENTIAL DIAGNOSES

- Dental infection
- Squamous cell carcinoma nodal metastases
- SMG carcinoma
- SMG benign mixed tumor

CLINICAL ISSUES

- SMG calculi more often within duct than gland
- SMG sialadenitis only 10% major gland sialadenitis

DIAGNOSTIC CHECKLIST

- Most often results from ductal calculus or stenosis
- Determine where in duct stones are located
- Beware: Calculi may be obscured by dental amalgam
- Look carefully for obstructing floor-of-mouth tumor
- If no calculi, consider duct stenosis or gland disease
  - Sjögren syndrome, sialadenosis, Küttner tumor

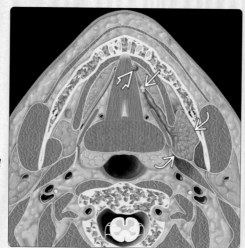

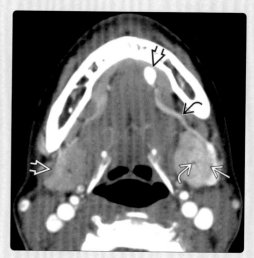

(Left) Axial graphic depicts submandibular duct calculus ➡ in distal duct just proximal to papilla ➡. Proximal duct and intraductal radicles are enlarged. The submandibular gland (SMG) is inflamed and enlarged ➡. (Right) Axial CECT demonstrates an asymmetrically enhancing, enlarged left SMG ➡ compared to the right ➡. Calculus is evident in the distal submandibular duct at the level of the ductal papilla ➡. Only mild prominence of the duct at hilum is evident ➡. A prominent vessel in floor of mouth is also noted ➡.

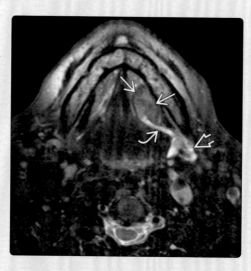

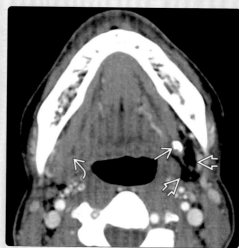

(Left) Axial T2 FS MR demonstrates a well-circumscribed mass in the left floor of mouth ➡ in a patient with mucosal SCCa. The mass is obstructing the left submandibular duct ➡, and there is secondary inflammation of the left SMG ➡, which is hyperintense. (Right) Axial CECT through floor of mouth in a patient with right submandibular "mass" shows dense calculus ➡ in proximal duct at SMG hilus. Note marked fatty atrophy with left chronic sialadenitis ➡. Right "mass" was normal SMG ➡.

TERMINOLOGY

Abbreviations

- Submandibular gland (SMG) sialadenitis

Definitions

- Inflammation of SMG from any cause
- **Acute sialadenitis**: Usually with duct calculus
  - Most often *Staphylococcus aureus* infection
- **Chronic sialadenitis**: Recurrent SMG inflammation with reduced saliva flow
- **Secondary SMG sialadenitis**
  - Ductal obstruction from floor-of-mouth SCCa
- **Sialolithiasis**: Concretions within SMG ductal system
- **Autoimmune sialadenitis**
  - Sjögren syndrome
  - **Chronic sclerosing sialadenitis**: Küttner tumor
    - Fibrosis & inflammation with IgG4-related systemic disease; SMG > > parotid
- **Sialadenosis**: Noninflammatory SMG swelling
  - Causes include diabetes, cirrhosis, and hypothyroidism

IMAGING

General Features

- Best diagnostic clue
  - Ductal dilatation ± calculus or stenosis
    - Acute: Ipsilateral enlarged SMG + cellulitis
    - Chronic: Ipsilateral atrophic SMG
- Location
  - SMG stones can be divided by location
    - Distal: Ductal opening in anterior floor of mouth
    - Proximal: Towards SMG hilum
  - Calculi typically within duct, not SMG parenchyma
- Size
  - Acute-subacute inflammation: SMG enlarged
  - Chronic: SMG small, ± fatty replacement

Radiographic Findings

- Radiography
  - Occlusal views: 90% calculi radiopaque

CT Findings

- CECT
  - **Acute sialadenitis** secondary to **calculus**
    - Duct calculus with dilated duct and enlarged enhancing SMG
    - Reactive nodes, ± floor-of-mouth cellulitis
  - Chronic sialadenitis ± calculus
    - Atrophic, fatty replaced ± intraductal calculus
  - **Secondary SMG sialadenitis**
    - Anterior floor-of-mouth invasive, enhancing mass
    - Dilated SMG duct and enlarged, enhancing SMG
    - Look for erosion of mandible

MR Findings

- MR typically not obtained in acute inflammation
  - MR sialography may show calculus as low signal
- Chronic sialadenitis, including autoimmune disease
  - Heterogeneous gland, prominent T2-intense ducts
  - May have fatty gland with T1 & T2 hyperintensity

Ultrasonographic Findings

- With calculus: Duct dilatation in enlarged gland
  - Ability to visualize calculus operator dependent

Imaging Recommendations

- Best imaging tool
  - CECT to evaluate gland ± calculus
  - NECT unnecessary: Calculus & vessel densities differ

DIFFERENTIAL DIAGNOSIS

SCCa Nodal Metastases

- Submandibular space (SMS) mass distinct from SMG

Submandibular Gland Carcinoma

- Infiltrating mass arising in SMG

Submandibular Gland Benign Mixed Tumor

- Well-circumscribed SMG mass, ± calcifications

PATHOLOGY

General Features

- Etiology
  - Most commonly SMG duct (Wharton) obstruction
    - Calculi, duct stenosis, rarely floor-of-mouth tumor
  - Less common: Chronic recurrent inflammation
  - Rarely: Primary gland inflammation
    - Sjögren syndrome, chronic sclerosing sialadenitis, sialadenosis, bacterial or viral infection

CLINICAL ISSUES

Presentation

- Other signs/symptoms
  - 30% of calculi present with painless mass
  - 80% of painful SMS masses due to calculus disease

Demographics

- Epidemiology
  - Gland calculi: 85% SMG ducts, 15% parotid
  - SMG only 10% major gland sialadenitis

DIAGNOSTIC CHECKLIST

Consider

- Most common cause is ductal calculus or stenosis

Reporting Tips

- Determine where in duct stones are located
  - Beware: Calculi may be obscured by dental amalgam
- Look carefully for obstructing floor-of-mouth tumor
- If no calculi, may be duct stenosis or **gland disease**
  - Sjögren, sialadenosis are bilateral
  - Chronic sclerosing sialadenitis usually unilateral

SELECTED REFERENCES

1. Schwartz N et al: Combined approach sialendoscopy for management of submandibular gland sialolithiasis. Am J Otolaryngol. 36(5):632-5, 2015
2. Wei TW et al: Chronic sclerosing sialadenitis of the submandibular gland: an entity of IgG4-related sclerosing disease. Int J Clin Exp Pathol. 8(7):8628-31, 2015
3. Sumi M et al: The MR imaging assessment of submandibular gland sialoadenitis secondary to sialolithiasis: correlation with CT and histopathologic findings. AJNR Am J Neuroradiol. 20(9):1737-43, 1999

Oral Cavity Abscess

TERMINOLOGY

- Oral cavity (OC) abscess
- Synonyms: Sublingual space (SLS), tongue, lingual, submandibular space (SMS), root of tongue (ROT), or OC transspatial abscess
- OC abscess: Focal collection of pus within OC space(s)
- May be in 1 space or multiple contiguous spaces (transspatial)

IMAGING

- CECT findings
  - Abscess: Rim-enhancing, fluid collection in OC space(s)
  - Found within anatomic spaces (SMS, SLS, &/or ROT)
  - Phlegmon: Enhancing inflammatory tissue without focal fluid/pus
  - Cellulitis: Adjacent soft tissue stranding ± dermal thickening
  - Reactive or suppurative nodes
- CECT = best exam for OC abscess examination

TOP DIFFERENTIAL DIAGNOSES

- Oral tongue squamous cell carcinoma (SCCa)
- Simple or diving ranula
- OC dermoid/epidermoid
- Sialocele of submandibular duct

CLINICAL ISSUES

- Sublingual or submandibular swelling
- Painful tongue with dysphagia, dysphonia
- Treatment: Surgical drainage + antibiotics

DIAGNOSTIC CHECKLIST

- Consider abscess mimics: Primary OC SCCa, ranula, epidermoid/dermoid, sialocele
- Define space(s) with abscess: SLS, SMS, ROT
- Find underlying cause: Tooth abscess ± mandibular osteomyelitis, submandibular duct calculus, pharyngitis + suppurative node

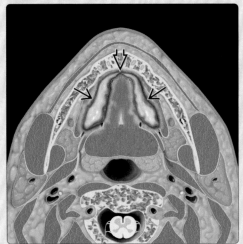
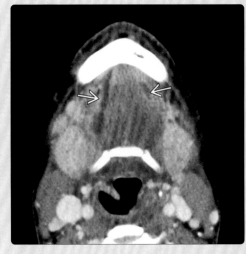

(Left) Axial graphic depicts a bilateral sublingual space abscess ⊡. The walled-off infected fluid collection is seen superomedially to the mylohyoid muscles and has a characteristic midline isthmus ⊡ anteriorly at the midline. (Right) Axial CECT demonstrates an axial plane horseshoe-shaped sublingual space abscess with a fluid collection with surrounding enhancement within both ⊡ sublingual spaces. The sublingual spaces connect anteriorly under the frenulum of the tongue (not seen).

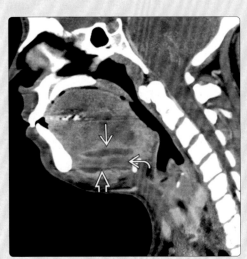
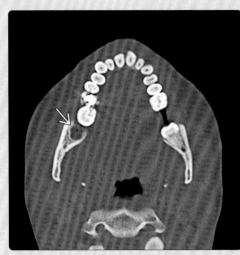

(Left) Sagittal CECT through the midline demonstrates an unusual oral cavity abscess with fluid tracking both above ⊡ and below ⊡ the mylohyoid muscle ⊡. (Right) Axial bone CT through the mandible demonstrates an empty molar tooth socket on the right ⊡ at the site of a recently removed tooth, which was the origin of the oral cavity abscess infection in this case.

TERMINOLOGY

Abbreviations

- Oral cavity (OC)

Synonyms

- Sublingual space (SLS) abscess, submandibular space (SMS) abscess, tongue abscess, root of tongue (ROT) abscess, oral abscess, lingual abscess

Definitions

- OC abscess: Focal collection of pus within OC space(s)
  - May be in 1 space or multiple contiguous spaces (transspatial)

IMAGING

General Features

- Best diagnostic clue
  - CECT shows rim-enhancing, focal fluid collection in OC space(s)
- Location
  - OC space(s)
    - SLS
    - SMS
    - ROT in lingual septum between SLSs
- Size
  - May become large in deep OC spaces
- Morphology
  - Conform to surrounding anatomic landscape/spaces (mandible, SMS, SLS, ROT)

Radiographic Findings

- Plain film may show soft tissue swelling & empty tooth socket
- Dental x-ray or Panorex
  - Periapical tooth abscess
  - Mandibular cortex dehiscence secondary to pus draining from tooth

CT Findings

- CECT
  - Abscess: Rim-enhancing fluid collection
  - **SLS abscess**
    - Unilateral: Fluid collection superomedial to mylohyoid muscle
    - Bilateral: Axial horseshoe-shaped fluid collection with anterior "isthmus"
  - **SMS abscess**: Fluid collection inferolateral to mylohyoid muscle
    - Bilateral: Coronal horseshoe-shaped fluid collection with inferior "isthmus"
  - **ROT abscess**: Midline fluid collection between SLSs in low lingual septum
  - Associated phlegmon, cellulitis, or myositis
    - Phlegmon: Enhancing inflammatory tissue without focal fluid/pus
    - Cellulitis: Adjacent soft tissue stranding
      - □ Dermal thickening
    - Myositis: Enhancing, enlarged muscle
  - Submandibular, high internal jugular chain reactive or suppurative adenopathy

- Bone CT
  - Often underlying **tooth infection**
    - Tooth or teeth with periapical lucency/abscess
    - Mandibular cortex focal dehiscence possible
  - **Mandibular osteomyelitis**
    - Permeative mandibular bone changes
    - Focal bone destruction possible
    - Periosteal reaction common

MR Findings

- T1WI
  - Low signal in fatty marrow of mandible at site of infected tooth
- T2WI
  - Abscess: High signal focal fluid collection
- DWI
  - Diffusion restriction in abscess
- T1WI C+
  - Rim-enhancing fluid collection(s)
  - Coronal plane helps define SLS (superomedial to mylohyoid muscle) from SMS (inferolateral to mylohyoid muscle) abscesses

Ultrasonographic Findings

- Hypoechoic collection within OC musculature is diagnostic in septic clinical setting
- Needle aspiration for diagnosis done simultaneously

Nuclear Medicine Findings

- Bone scan
  - Increased uptake in regions of mandibular osteomyelitis
  - 3-phase bone scan very sensitive for osteomyelitis

Imaging Recommendations

- Best imaging tool
  - CECT
- Protocol advice
  - Routine cervical soft tissue neck CECT study
  - Dental amalgam may obscure OC abscess
- CECT is study of choice for OC infectious processes
  - Soft tissue windows: Identify abscess location
  - Bone window: Identify tooth infection, mandible osteomyelitis, or submandibular duct calculus
- Panorex CT often helpful in evaluating mandible & possible dental sources of infection
  - 1-mm axial acquisition series through entire mandible, with oblique coronal curved reformations
  - Simulates plain film Panorex views with improved resolution

DIFFERENTIAL DIAGNOSIS

Oral Tongue Squamous Cell Carcinoma

- Clinical: Mucosal squamous cell carcinoma (SCCa) lesion usually obvious
- CT-MR findings
  - Enhancing invasive oral tongue mass
  - Cystic-necrotic neoplasm may mimic OC abscess

Simple or Diving Ranula

- Clinical
  - Simple ranula: Sublingual bluish translucent mass

- o Diving ranula: Compressible angle of mandible mass
- CT-MR findings
  - o Simple ranula: Nonenhancing low-density, low T1/high T2 SLS lesion
    - − By imaging, may mimic SLS epidermoid
  - o Diving ranula: Nonenhancing low signal, low T1/high T2 SMS lesion with SLS "tail"

Oral Cavity Dermoid & Epidermoid

- Clinical: Floor of mouth or SMS slow-growing mass
- CT findings
  - o Epidermoid: Unilateral low-density, nonenhancing SMS or SLS mass
  - o Dermoid: Unilateral fluid ± fat density, nonenhancing SMS or SLS mass
  - o No associated cellulitis-edema with either
- MR findings
  - o Epidermoid: Low T1, high T2, DWI restriction (DWI can mimic abscess, but clinical presentation different)
  - o Dermoid: If fat macroscopic, high T1 within mass
    - − **Bag of marbles** appearance classic

Sialocele of Submandibular Duct

- True sialocele: Enlarged proximal submandibular duct ± obstructing calculus
- False sialocele: Fluid collection adjacent to duct in SLS without enhancing wall

PATHOLOGY

General Features

- Etiology
  - o OC abscess: Most common cause = dental decay of mandibular premolar, canine, or incisor tooth with root abscess leading to mandibular osteomyelitis
    - − SLS abscess: Tooth root abscess breaks out **above** (superior to) mylohyoid line of medial mandible with pus then walled off in SLS
    - − SMS abscess: Tooth root abscess breaks out **below** (inferior to) mylohyoid line of medial mandible with pus then walled off in SMS
  - o Other causes of OC abscess
    - − Submandibular duct calculus: SLS abscess
    - − Pharyngitis + suppurative SMS nodes: SMS abscess
    - − Penetrating trauma: SLS, SMS, or ROT abscess
    - − Intravenous drug abuse: SLS, SMS, or ROT abscess
  - o Up to 20% of deep neck infections have no identifiable source

Gross Pathologic & Surgical Features

- Putrid-smelling abscess pocket entered with surgical drain

Microscopic Features

- Oral flora predominate: *Streptococcus*, *Staphylococcus*
- Abscess is mixed culture of aerobic & anaerobic organisms

CLINICAL ISSUES

Presentation

- Most common signs/symptoms
  - o Sublingual or submandibular swelling
- Other signs/symptoms
  - o Painful tongue with dysphagia, dysphonia

- o Elevation & backward displacement of tongue may compromise airway
- o History of recent oral antibiotic treatment common
- Clinical profile
  - o Older patients with bad dentition

Demographics

- Age
  - o Elderly
- Epidemiology
  - o Tooth abscess/mandibular osteomyelitis > > all other causes

Natural History & Prognosis

- Prognosis for full recovery excellent

Treatment

- Extraction of infected tooth (if present)
- Root canal therapy
- Surgical drainage of abscess cavity
  - o Approach varies depending on location(s) involved
- Intravenous antibiotics
  - o Penicillin or amoxicillin effective against most aerobic & anaerobic bacteria
  - o When penicillin-resistant organisms present
    - − Use amoxicillin-clavulanate, clindamycin, or combination of metronidazole plus amoxicillin or macrolide

DIAGNOSTIC CHECKLIST

Consider

- Mimics of abscess in OC
  - o Cystic-necrotic OC primary SCCa
  - o Ranula, epidermoid/dermoid: No inflammatory changes
  - o False sialocele: May be superinfected

Image Interpretation Pearls

- 1st define abscess space(s): SLS, SMS, &/or ROT
- Comment on unilateral or bilateral, unispatial or transspatial nature of abscess
- Search for underlying cause
  - o Review mandible bone window images for **tooth abscess ± mandibular osteomyelitis**
  - o If teeth normal, check for **submandibular duct stone**
  - o In children, look for **pharyngitis with suppurative SMS node**

Reporting Tips

- Report both abscess location(s) and probable cause

SELECTED REFERENCES

1. Capps EF et al: Emergency imaging assessment of acute, nontraumatic conditions of the head and neck. Radiographics. 30(5):1335-52, 2010. Erratum in: Radiographics. 31(1):316, 2011
2. Fang WS et al: Primary lesions of the root of the tongue. Radiographics. 31(7):1907-22, 2011
3. Kim HJ et al: Tongue abscess mimicking neoplasia. AJNR Am J Neuroradiol. 27(10):2202-3, 2006
4. Ozturk M et al: Tongue abscesses: MR imaging findings. AJNR Am J Neuroradiol. 27(6):1300-3, 2006
5. Branstetter BF 4th et al: Infection of the facial area, oral cavity, oropharynx, and retropharynx. Neuroimaging Clin N Am. 13(3):393-410, ix, 2003

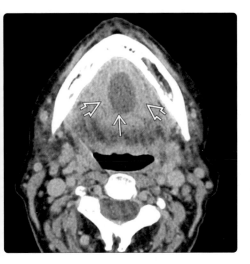

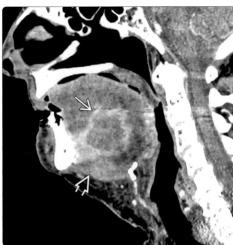

(Left) *Axial CECT shows a midline oral cavity abscess as an oval fluid density collection* ➡ *located centrally within the root of the tongue, bowing the genioglossus muscles* ➡ *laterally.* (Right) *Sagittal CECT shows a root of tongue abscess* ➡ *above the mylohyoid muscle* ➡ *in the midline deep tongue. This appearance can mimic invasive squamous cell carcinoma but has a different clinical presentation and appearance.*

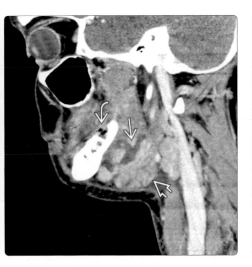

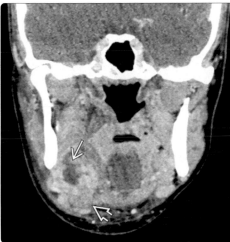

(Left) *Sagittal CECT reveals an infected mandibular tooth socket* ➡ *with pus* ➡ *extending inferiorly into the submandibular space. The inflamed submandibular gland* ➡ *is displaced inferiorly by the abscess.* (Right) *Coronal CECT shows the posterior submandibular space abscess* ➡ *displacing the enlarged, inflamed submandibular gland* ➡ *inferiorly. Sialoadenitis in this case is secondary to an adjacent infected socket and abscess.*

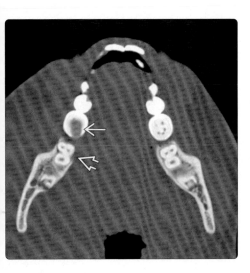

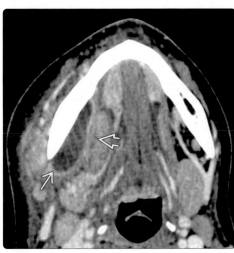

(Left) *Axial bone CT through the mandibular teeth shows dental decay* ➡ *with mandibular cortex loss* ➡*, suggesting that both tooth abscess and mandibular osteomyelitis are present.* (Right) *Axial CECT shows rim-enhancing fluid collection of pus leaking out inferiorly into the submandibular space. The submandibular space abscess* ➡ *displaces the mylohyoid muscle* ➡ *medially as a result.*

Submandibular Gland Benign Mixed Tumor

TERMINOLOGY

- Synonym: Pleomorphic adenoma

IMAGING

- CECT
  - Enlarged submandibular gland (SMG) with focal or diffuse heterogeneous mass ± calcification
  - Isodense lesions may be "invisible"
  - Dual-phase CECT improves conspicuity
- MR
  - Small lesion: Low T1, high T2 intensity, homogeneous enhancement
  - Large lesion: More heterogeneous, ± focal areas of very high T2 signal, signal loss with calcification
  - Variable low T2 intensity "capsule"
- US
  - Well-defined, solid, intraglandular lesion
  - Large lesion may show focal cysts, calcification
- Best imaging tool

- **MR > CECT** (some masses poorly seen on CECT)
- **US affords excellent SMG evaluation**

TOP DIFFERENTIAL DIAGNOSES

- SMG sialadenitis
- SMG mucocele
- SMG carcinoma
- Submandibular space lymphadenopathy
- Chronic sclerosing sialadenitis (Kuttner tumor)

PATHOLOGY

- Epithelial, myoepithelial, and stromal components

CLINICAL ISSUES

- Most common neoplasm of SMG

DIAGNOSTIC CHECKLIST

- If patient presents with palpable submandibular mass
  - Determine if mass is in SMG or extrinsic (node)
  - If no mass found on CECT, recommend US or MR

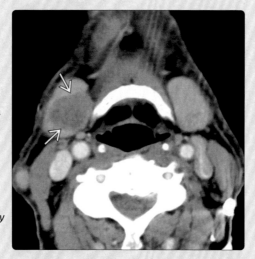
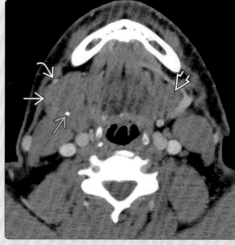

(Left) Axial CECT shows a hypodense focal mass ➡ enlarging the right submandibular gland (SMG). This lesion is well defined, favoring benign nature, but requires pathology confirmation. (Right) Axial CECT shows an enlarged right SMG ➡ compared to the left gland ➡. The displaced anterior facial vein ➡ confirms intraglandular mass origin. This benign mixed tumor was nearly "invisible" due to isodensity, except for mass-related gland asymmetry and a focal calcification ➡.

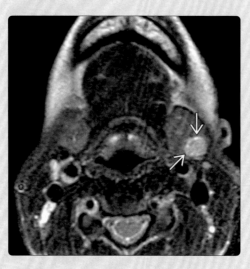
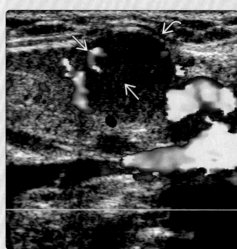

(Left) Axial T2WI MR in a young woman with a palpable submandibular mass shows a well-circumscribed and hyperintense oval lesion within the left SMG ➡ with no evidence of extension outside of gland. (Right) Longitudinal oblique color Doppler ultrasound in the same patient shows a well-defined solid structure within the left SMG, distorting its external contour ➡. No internal calcifications or cystic change are evident. Vascular flow is evident at the periphery and internal aspect of this solid lesion ➡.

Submandibular Gland Benign Mixed Tumor

TERMINOLOGY

Abbreviations

- Submandibular gland (SMG) benign mixed tumor (BMT)

Synonyms

- Pleomorphic adenoma

Definitions

- Benign heterogeneous salivary gland primary tumor

IMAGING

General Features

- Best diagnostic clue
  - Enlarged SMG with focal or diffuse heterogeneous mass ± calcification
- Location
  - Submandibular space (SMS)
- Size
  - Variable: 1-4 cm
- Morphology
  - Small: Ovoid, well-demarcated SMG mass
  - Large: Lobulated heterogeneous mass ± calcification

CT Findings

- CECT
  - Small lesion is usually well defined; may deform external contour
  - Large lesion usually heterogeneous density and texture
  - Isodense lesions may be inseparable from normal gland
    - Asymmetric size is clue to underlying mass
    - Dual-phase CECT improves conspicuity
  - Variable calcification, cystic changes in larger BMT
  - Mild to moderate enhancement

MR Findings

- Findings largely determined by BMT size
  - Small lesion: Low T1, high T2 intensity, homogeneous enhancement
  - Large lesion: More heterogeneous, ± focal areas of very high T2 signal, signal loss with calcification
  - Variable low T2 intensity "capsule"

Ultrasonographic Findings

- Grayscale ultrasound
  - Well-defined, solid, intraglandular lesion
  - Large lesion may show focal cysts, calcification

Nuclear Medicine Findings

- Marked FDG avidity on PET/CT mimics malignancy

Imaging Recommendations

- Best imaging tool
  - **MR > CECT** (some SMG masses are poorly seen on CECT)
  - **US affords excellent SMG evaluation**

DIFFERENTIAL DIAGNOSIS

Submandibular Gland Sialadenitis

- Acute: Enlarged gland that completely enhances
  - Predisposing sialoliths ± sialectasis may be present
- Chronic: Atrophic gland with little enhancement

Submandibular Gland Mucocele

- Fluid collection within SMG

Submandibular Gland Carcinoma

- Enhancing, invasive mass arising from SMG

Reactive Lymph Nodes

- Ovoid mass with fat plane separating it from SMG
- Anterior facial vein separates nodes from SMG

Nodal Squamous Cell Carcinoma in Submandibular Space

- Nodal mass separate from SMG, ± necrosis

Chronic Sclerosing Sialadenitis (Kuttner Tumor)

- Inflammatory etiology mimics neoplasm
- Some cases are IgG4 related

PATHOLOGY

Microscopic Features

- Interspersed epithelial, myoepithelial, and stromal cellular components
  - Calcification, hyalinization, and rarely ossification

CLINICAL ISSUES

Presentation

- Most common signs/symptoms
  - Slow-growing, painless SMS mass

Demographics

- Age
  - Most commonly present > 40 years
- Epidemiology
  - BMT is most common neoplasm of SMG

Natural History & Prognosis

- Untreated, 5-25% degenerate to malignant tumor
- Usually occurs 15-20 years after initial diagnosis

Treatment

- Complete excision of intact gland and tumor
- Operative rupture of BMT capsule seeds surgical bed
- Results in multifocal recurrence; surgically challenging

DIAGNOSTIC CHECKLIST

Consider

- Fine-needle aspiration has variable success
  - Sampling and interpretation errors common

Image Interpretation Pearls

- If patient presents with palpable submandibular mass
  - Determine if mass is in SMG or extrinsic (node)
  - If no mass found on CECT, recommend US or MR

SELECTED REFERENCES

1. Kashiwagi N et al: Conventional MRI findings for predicting submandibular pleomorphic adenoma. Acta Radiol. 54(5):511-5, 2013
2. Kei PL et al: CT "invisible" lesion of the major salivary glands a diagnostic pitfall of contrast-enhanced CT. Clin Radiol. 64(7):744-6, 2009

Palate Benign Mixed Tumor

TERMINOLOGY

- Palate benign mixed tumor (BMT)
- Synonym: Palate pleomorphic adenoma
- Definition: Benign minor salivary gland tumor of palate

IMAGING

- General imaging findings
  - Most commonly found at soft-hard palate juncture
  - Small BMT: Well-defined palatal mass with homogeneous avid enhancement
  - Large BMT: Lobulated with heterogeneous enhancement
- Bone CT: Larger BMT remodels bony hard palate
- MR findings
  - Intermediate-high T2 signal ovoid palatal mass
  - Very high T2 signal suggests BMT
  - Larger BMT often with inhomogeneous signal (necrosis, blood products, calcification)

- Sagittal and coronal plane T2 and T1 C+ FS MR sequences best (orthogonal to palate)

TOP DIFFERENTIAL DIAGNOSES

- Palatal minor salivary gland neoplasms
- Palatal squamous cell carcinoma

PATHOLOGY

- Arise in minor salivary glands of palate
- Interspersed epithelial, myoepithelial, and stromal cellular components must be identified to diagnose BMT

CLINICAL ISSUES

- Typical presentation is painless palatal mass
- Most common minor salivary gland neoplasm (~ 40%)
- Most common site, minor salivary gland BMT (~ 10%)
- Risk factors for malignant transformation (carcinoma ex pleomorphic adenoma) are longevity and recurrence (~ 3-4%)
  - Palatal neuropathy suggests malignancy

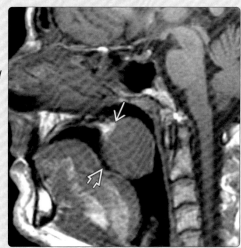
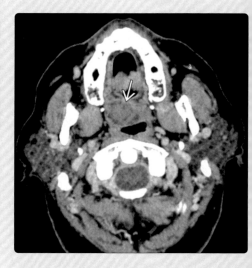

(Left) Midline sagittal T1 MR shows a large ovoid mass at the junction of the soft and hard palate ⇒ causing mild remodeling of the osseous hard palate ⇒, with preserved normal T1 hyperintensity (indicating no invasion). This is the most common location for oral cavity benign mixed tumor (BMT). (Right) Axial CECT demonstrates a well-circumscribed, somewhat heterogeneous, mildly enhancing soft tissue mass ⇒ in the soft palate. Surgical removal revealed this to be a BMT.

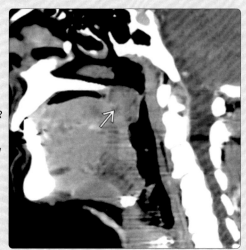
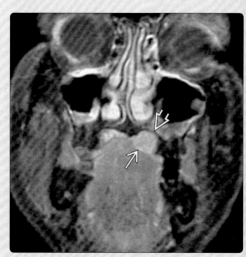

(Left) Sagittal CECT near the midline reveals a well-circumscribed, mildly enhancing heterogeneous mass ⇒ in the soft palate. BMT and dermoid were both initially considered in the imaging differential diagnosis. (Right) Coronal T1WI C+ FS MR shows a moderately enhancing, well-circumscribed left hard palate mass ⇒. Hard palate bone is remodeled by this BMT ⇒.

TERMINOLOGY

Abbreviations
- Palate benign mixed tumor (BMT)

Synonyms
- Palate pleomorphic adenoma

Definitions
- Benign tumor arising from palate minor salivary glands

IMAGING

General Features
- Best diagnostic clue
  - Small palate BMT: Well-defined palatal mass with avid enhancement
  - Large BMT: Often lobulated mass with heterogeneous enhancement
- Location
  - Soft-hard palate junction
- Size
  - Variable: < 2 cm most commonly

CT Findings
- CECT
  - Small palate BMT: Well-defined, homogeneously enhancing ovoid mass
  - Large palate BMT: Lobulated mass with heterogeneous enhancement
    - Dystrophic calcifications uncommon
    - Low-attenuation areas of degenerative necrosis
    - Old blood products possible
- Bone CT
  - Larger lesions cause remodeling of hard palate

MR Findings
- T1WI
  - Small BMT: Homogeneous low-intermediate signal mass
  - Large BMT: Lobulated heterogeneous mass
    - Hyperintense signal foci if blood products
    - Focal low signal areas if necrosis present
- T2WI
  - Small BMT: Uniform intermediate-high signal mass
  - Large BMT: Heterogeneous high signal mass
    - Low signal tumor capsule often visible
  - **Very high T2 signal** suggests **BMT**
- STIR
  - High signal may be more conspicuous than T2 sequence
- DWI
  - May have ↑ ADC values compared to malignant palatal tumor
    - DWI signal intensity nonspecific
- T1WI C+
  - Variable heterogeneous or avid homogeneous enhancement

Imaging Recommendations
- Best imaging tool
  - Enhanced MR with thin sections through palate
  - Bone CT helps define tumor bony margins
- Protocol advice
  - Sagittal and coronal plane T2 and T1 C+ FS MR sequences best (axial suboptimal given parallel to palate)

DIFFERENTIAL DIAGNOSIS

Palatal Minor Salivary Gland Neoplasms
- Malignant minor salivary gland neoplasms
  - Invasive tumor with osseous destruction
  - Perineural tumor CNV2 likely
- Other benign minor salivary neoplasms

Palatal Squamous Cell Carcinoma
- Aggressive tumor + osseous destruction
- May mimic palatal BMT when small

PATHOLOGY

General Features
- Etiology
  - Benign tumor arising from palate minor salivary gland tissue

Microscopic Features
- Interspersed epithelial, myoepithelial, and stromal cellular components must be seen to diagnose BMT
- May have components of calcification, necrosis, blood products, and hyalinization

CLINICAL ISSUES

Presentation
- Most common signs/symptoms
  - Painless palatal mass
    - Most common minor salivary gland neoplasm (~ 40%)
    - Most common site, minor salivary gland BMT (~ 10%)
  - Risk factors for malignant transformation (carcinoma ex pleomorphic adenoma) are longevity and recurrence (~ 3-4%)
- Other signs/symptoms
  - Palatal neuropathy suggests malignancy

Demographics
- Age
  - Age range ~ 30-60 years

Natural History & Prognosis
- Slow-growing, painless palatal mass
  - Rapid enlargement concerning for malignant degeneration
- Rare potential for metastasis in benign BMT

Treatment
- Complete surgical resection of encapsulated mass
  - Adequate soft tissue margins critical to avoid cellular "spillage" and future seeding of surgical bed

SELECTED REFERENCES

1. Kato H et al: CT and MR imaging findings of palatal tumors. Eur J Radiol. 83(3):e137-46, 2014
2. Lingam RK et al: Pleomorphic adenoma (benign mixed tumour) of the salivary glands: its diverse clinical, radiological, and histopathological presentation. Br J Oral Maxillofac Surg. 49(1):14-20, 2011

Sublingual Gland Carcinoma

TERMINOLOGY

- Primary salivary malignancy of sublingual gland (SLG)

IMAGING

- CECT: Well-defined or invasive sublingual space (SLS) mass
  - Mild to moderately enhancing; may be subtle
  - Look for evidence of mandible erosion
- MR: Variable signal and contrast enhancement
  - Well-differentiated tumors may have ↑↑ T2 signal
  - FS & STIR improve conspicuity
- Look for invasion of extrinsic tongue muscles
- PET: Generally low FDG avidity unless high grade

TOP DIFFERENTIAL DIAGNOSES

- Floor of mouth squamous cell carcinoma
- Ranula
- Oral cavity abscess
- Oral cavity lymphatic malformation

PATHOLOGY

- Adenoid cystic carcinoma (ACCa)
  - Strong propensity for perineural spread
  - Tends to hematogenously spread to lungs
  - Slow-growing; may metastasize many years later
- Mucoepidermoid carcinoma (MECa)
  - Tends to spread to lymph nodes
- Malignant degeneration of benign mixed tumor

CLINICAL ISSUES

- Painless, hard anterior floor of mouth mass on palpation
- 30-60 years of age, M:F = 1:1
- 80% of SLG masses are malignant
- Prognosis depends on stage > histologic grade
- Treatment primarily surgical ± XRT

DIAGNOSTIC CHECKLIST

- Aggressive-appearing lesions within SLS should be considered malignant until proven otherwise

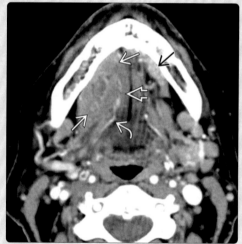
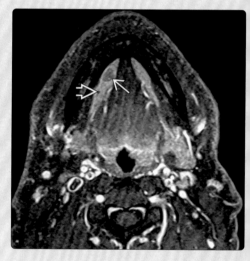

(Left) Axial CECT shows the asymmetric floor of the mouth from a large infiltrative ACCa ➡ in the right sublingual gland (SLG). Tumor extends into the genioglossus muscle ➡ and neurovascular bundle ➡, allowing ready access to CNV3 and CNX. Note normal left SLG ➡. (Right) Axial T1WI C+ FS MR shows a well-defined small mass ➡ in right SLG representing early MECa. The tumor is hypointense to the normal SLG ➡ but can have variable enhancing characteristics. There is no evidence of mandible invasion.

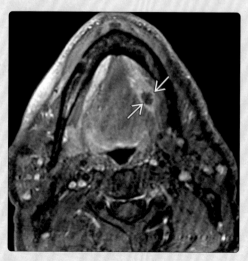
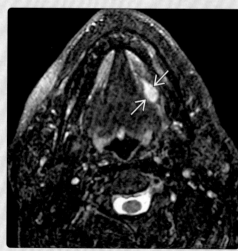

(Left) Axial T1WI C+ FS MR demonstrates a small heterogeneous left SLG mass ➡ with ill-defined borders. The irregular contours suggest this mass may be malignant; however, even well-defined lesions are statistically more likely to be malignant in SLG. (Right) Axial T2WI FS MR in the same patient shows the mass ➡ to be markedly hyperintense. More differentiated salivary malignancies produce fluid/mucin and have high signal. This was found to be MECa.

TERMINOLOGY

Abbreviations

- Sublingual gland (SLG) carcinoma
- Adenoid cystic carcinoma (ACCa)
- Mucoepidermoid carcinoma (MECa)

Definitions

- Primary salivary malignancy in SLG
  - ACCa > MECa > others

IMAGING

General Features

- Best diagnostic clue
  - Well-defined or invasive sublingual space (SLS) mass
- Location
  - SLS: Potential space superomedial to mylohyoid muscle
- Size
  - Usually < 2 cm

CT Findings

- CECT
  - Mild to moderately enhancing SLS mass
  - May be subtle lesion on imaging
  - Look for invasion of extrinsic tongue muscles
- Bone CT
  - Look for evidence of mandible erosion

MR Findings

- T1WI
  - Isointense to muscle
- T2WI
  - Variable: Well-differentiated, may be high signal
  - FS or STIR improves mass conspicuity
- T1WI C+
  - Variable contrast enhancement

Nuclear Medicine Findings

- PET
  - Generally low FDG avidity, unless high grade

Imaging Recommendations

- Best imaging tool
  - CECT is useful 1st-line tool
  - Enhanced MR has less dental amalgam artifacts
- Protocol advice
  - Thin-section CECT with bone and soft tissue algorithm

DIFFERENTIAL DIAGNOSIS

Floor of Mouth Squamous Cell Carcinoma

- Not able to distinguish from SLG carcinoma

Ranula

- Unilocular fluid-filled lesion without enhancement

Oral Cavity Abscess

- Rim-enhancing cystic mass with cellulitis

Oral Cavity Lymphatic Malformation

- Multilocular nonenhancing cystic mass

PATHOLOGY

General Features

- Etiology
  - ACCa & MECa most common neoplasms
  - MECa associated with radiation exposure

Staging, Grading, & Classification

- Adapted from 7th edition AJCC Staging Forms (2010)
  - **T1**: ≤ 2 cm without extraparenchymal extension
  - **T2**: > 2 & ≤ 4 cm, no extraparenchymal extension
  - **T3**: > 4 cm &/or extraparenchymal extension
  - **T4a**: Invades mandible or skin
  - **T4b**: Invades skull base, pterygoid plates, encases carotid

Microscopic Features

- **Adenoid cystic carcinoma**
  - Unencapsulated; cribriform, tubular, & solid variants
- **Mucoepidermoid carcinoma**
  - Epidermoid, intermediate, & mucus-secreting cells

CLINICAL ISSUES

Presentation

- Most common signs/symptoms
  - Painless, hard mass in anterior floor of mouth on palpation
- Other signs/symptoms
  - Numbness suggests lingual nerve perineural tumor

Demographics

- Age
  - 30-60 years old
- Epidemiology
  - 80% of primary SLG masses are malignant

Natural History & Prognosis

- ACCa: Slow-growing tumor
  - Strong propensity for perineural tumor spread
  - Metastasizes to lungs; may be delayed (> 10 years)
- MECa: Less indolent tumor
  - Greater likelihood of node metastases
- Prognosis depends on **stage** > **histologic grade**

Treatment

- En bloc resection of anterior floor of mouth
- Postoperative radiotherapy for high stage, high grade

DIAGNOSTIC CHECKLIST

Image Interpretation Pearls

- Aggressive-appearing lesions within SLS should be considered malignant until proven otherwise

Reporting Tips

- Must search for bone invasion & perineural tumor

SELECTED REFERENCES

1. Asaumi J et al: Assessment of carcinoma in the sublingual region based on magnetic resonance imaging. Oncol Rep. 9(6):1283-7, 2002

Submandibular Gland Carcinoma

TERMINOLOGY

- Primary malignancy arising in submandibular gland (SMG)
- Most commonly adenoid cystic (ACCa), mucoepidermoid (MECa), adenocarcinoma (AdCa)

IMAGING

- Focal or irregular SMG mass ± adjacent soft tissue invasion
- CECT: Asymmetric &/or heterogeneous SMG
  - Well-defined or ill-defined mass
  - Gland may be focally or diffusely hypodense
  - Mild to moderate contrast enhancement
- MR: Intermediate to high mixed T2 signal
  - Heterogeneous gadolinium enhancement
  - MR: Use fat saturation (FS) on T2 & T1 C+
- PET/CT: Low FDG avidity, unless high grade
- US: Ill-defined, hypoechoic lesion

TOP DIFFERENTIAL DIAGNOSES

- SMG sialadenitis

- SMG benign mixed tumor
- SMG mucocele
- Reactive lymph nodes
- Nodal squamous cell carcinoma in submandibular space

PATHOLOGY

- Beware FNA sampling & interpretive errors

CLINICAL ISSUES

- Painless submandibular swelling or focal mass
- **45%** SMG neoplasms are **malignant**
- ACCa: Spreads via nerves, also to lungs
- MECa & AdCa: Nodal & hematogenous spread

DIAGNOSTIC CHECKLIST

- 1st determine whether mass is **within SMG or extrinsic**, such as node
- **Beware subtle or occult SMG mass** on CECT
  - If none found on CECT, recommend US or MR

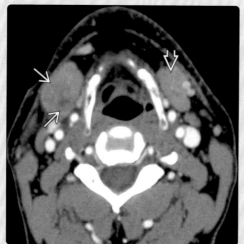
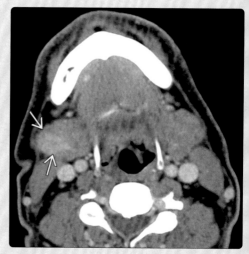

(Left) Axial CECT shows asymmetric enlargement of the right submandibular gland (SMG) compared to the left ➡ with hypodense ill-defined mass ➡ in posterior aspect. On resection, the mass was found to be adenocarcinoma confined to the SMG. (Right) Axial CECT in an adult with fluctuating neck fullness shows asymmetric fullness and poorly marginated enhancement in the lateral right SMG ➡. The image was interpreted as vascular malformation, but patient age and MR did not support this. FNA revealed ACCa.

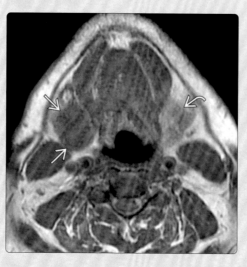
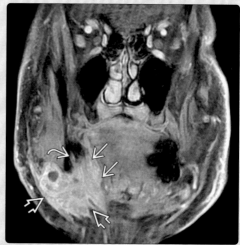

(Left) Axial T1 MR demonstrates a fuller and more hypointense right SMG ➡ compared to the left ➡ in a patient with palpable abnormality; this was misinterpreted as gland asymmetry. No adenopathy is present. (Right) Coronal T1 C+ FS MR in the same patient 2 years later reveals ill-defined, heterogeneous right SMG ➡ with infiltration of the tumor medially through mylohyoid muscle ➡. Note involvement of the mandible and inferior alveolar nerve ➡. Tumor was found to be adenocarcinoma with metastatic nodes.

TERMINOLOGY

Abbreviations

- Submandibular gland (SMG) carcinoma

Definitions

- Primary malignancy arising in SMG

IMAGING

General Features

- Best diagnostic clue
  - Well-defined or invasive mass arising from SMG
- Location
  - Most often superficial aspect of SMG
- Size
  - Usually < 3 cm
- Morphology
  - Well-defined or invasive SMG mass
  - May have homogeneous, enlarged SMG

CT Findings

- CECT
  - Asymmetric &/or heterogeneous SMG
  - Mild to moderately enhancing SMG mass
- Bone CT
  - Bone erosion and calcifications (uncommon)

MR Findings

- T1WI
  - Isointense to muscle, hypointense to gland
- T2WI
  - Intermediate to high mixed signal intensity
  - **High grade** tends to be **intermediate to low signal**
- T1WI C+
  - Variable contrast enhancement

Nuclear Medicine Findings

- PET/CT
  - Generally low FDG avidity, unless high grade

Ultrasonographic Findings

- Grayscale ultrasound
  - Typically ill-defined, hypoechoic lesion

Imaging Recommendations

- Best imaging tool
  - Multiplanar CECT often 1st-line tool
  - US: Excellent for superficial portion SMG
  - MR offers best delineation of contours
- Protocol advice
  - Thin-section CECT: Bone & soft tissue algorithm
  - MR: Use fat saturation (FS) on T2 and T1 C+

DIFFERENTIAL DIAGNOSIS

Submandibular Gland Sialadenitis

- Enlarged, diffusely enhancing SMG ± stone ± sialectasis
- Chronic disease leads to atrophic SMG
- Chronic sclerosing sialadenitis mimics malignancy

Submandibular Gland Mucocele

- Unilocular, fluid-filled intraglandular lesion

- Usually no enhancement

Submandibular Gland Benign Mixed Tumor

- Well-demarcated, ovoid SMG mass

Reactive Lymph Nodes

- Ovoid lesion adjacent to normal SMG

Nodal Squamous Cell Carcinoma in Submandibular Space

- Enlarged node adjacent to SMG

PATHOLOGY

Staging, Grading, & Classification

- Adapted from American Joint Committee on Cancer 7th edition staging (2010)
  - **T1**: ≤ 2 cm without extraparenchymal extension
  - **T2**: > 2 & ≤ 4 cm, no extraparenchymal extension
  - **T3**: > 4 cm &/or extraparenchymal extension
  - **T4a**: Invades skin, mandible, ear canal, ± facial nerve
  - **T4b**: Invades skull base ± pterygoid plates ± encases carotid artery

Microscopic Features

- 3 main pathologies: **Adenoid cystic adenocarcioma (ACCa), mucoepidermoid carcinoma (MECa), adenocarcinoma (AdCa)**
- Beware FNA sampling & interpretive errors
  - Biopsy may be necessary to resolve

CLINICAL ISSUES

Presentation

- Most common signs/symptoms
  - Painless submandibular swelling or focal mass
- Other signs/symptoms
  - Chin or lower lip numbness suggests infiltration of inferior alveolar nerve
  - Lower lip weakness suggests facial nerve branch invasion

Demographics

- Age
  - 40-70 years old
- Epidemiology
  - **45%** of SMG tumors are **malignant**
  - **40%** of malignant SMG tumors are **ACCa**

Treatment

- En bloc complete resection of tumor
- Postoperative radiotherapy for high stage, high grade

DIAGNOSTIC CHECKLIST

Image Interpretation Pearls

- **If presentation of mass or fullness**
  - 1st determine if mass is **SMG or extrinsic**, such as node
  - Recommend US or MR if CECT negative

SELECTED REFERENCES

1. Weon YC et al: Salivary duct carcinomas: clinical and CT and MR imaging features in 20 patients. Neuroradiology. 54(6):631-40, 2012

TERMINOLOGY

- Abbreviation: Minor salivary gland malignancy (MSGM)
- Most common MSGM: Adenoid cystic carcinoma (ACCa) & mucoepidermoid carcinoma (MECa)

IMAGING

- MSGM location: Submucosa of upper aerodigestive tract
  - Hard-soft palate junction > > buccal mucosa
- Oral cavity well defined, smooth submucosal mass
- Bone CT findings
  - Bone erosion: Palate, mandible
  - Greater and lesser palatine foramen enlargement
- MR findings
  - T1: Low signal tumor replaces hard palate marrow fat
  - T1 C+ FS for PNT spread
- PET imaging best for staging/restaging

TOP DIFFERENTIAL DIAGNOSES

- Squamous cell carcinoma
- Benign mixed tumor of palate
- Dermoid & epidermoid
- Dentigerous cyst
- Nasopalatine duct cyst

PATHOLOGY

- Prognosis depends on **stage > histologic grade**

CLINICAL ISSUES

- **ACCa**: Tendency for **PNT**, lung metastases
- **MECa**: Tendency for regional malignant **nodes**
- Treatment: Surgical resection ± postoperative radiation

DIAGNOSTIC CHECKLIST

- Long-term (> 10 year) imaging follow-up recommended given **tendency to recur late**
- Check for PNT in MSGM
- Remove FS on T1 C+ MR if susceptibility obscures anatomy
- Noncontrast T1 MR may offer best inherent contrast

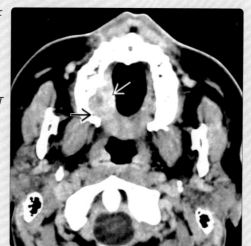
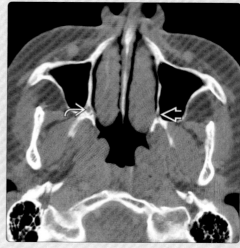

(Left) Axial CECT shows classic example of an adenoid cystic carcinoma (ACCa) in the right hard palate ➡ invading adjacent bone & thus gaining access to the greater palatine nerve in the greater palatine canal ⮕. (Right) Axial bone CT shows widening of the right greater palatine canal ➡, indicating perineural tumor spread along the greater palatine nerve. Note normal left canal ⮕. Tumor can now spread to the pterygopalatine fossa giving access to V2, vidian nerve, orbit, nasal cavity, & infratemporal fossa.

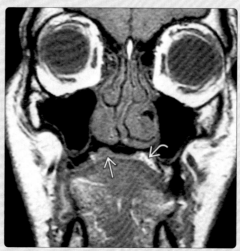
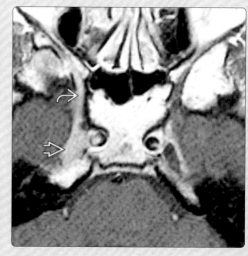

(Left) Coronal T1WI MR shows dark tumor ➡ infiltration of the hard palate marrow in this patient with ACCa. Note normal fat signal ➡ in the contralateral hard palate. Noncontrast T1 MR may offer better inherent tumor contrast in areas with fat. (Right) Axial T1 C+ MR in different patient with hard palate ACCa shows perineural tumor along the maxillary division of trigeminal nerve (V2) in foramen rotundum ➡ and cavernous sinus ⮕, from contiguous greater palatine nerve and pterygopalatine fossa invoement (not shown).

TERMINOLOGY

Abbreviations

- Oral cavity minor salivary gland malignancy (MSGM)

Definitions

- Primary minor salivary gland malignancy
  - Located in submucosa upper aerodigestive tract

IMAGING

General Features

- Best diagnostic clue
  - Oral cavity well defined, smooth submucosal mass
- Location
  - Hard palate > > buccal mucosa > other oral cavity sites
- Size
  - Small (< 2 cm), visible on physical exam

CT Findings

- CECT
  - Homogeneously enhancing mass
- Bone CT
  - Bone erosion (palate, mandible)
  - Greater & lesser palatine foramen enlargement

MR Findings

- T1WI
  - Tumor isointense to muscle
  - Excellent inherent contrast
- T2WI
  - High signal lesion compared to muscle
- T1WI C+
  - Homogeneously enhancing tumor
  - Best delineates perineural tumor (PNT) spread

Nuclear Medicine Findings

- PET imaging best for staging/restaging

Imaging Recommendations

- Best imaging tool
  - MR less affected by dental amalgam artifacts than CT
    - T1 C+ FS MR visualizes PNT best
      - □ Remove FS if susceptibility obscures anatomy

DIFFERENTIAL DIAGNOSIS

Squamous Cell Carcinoma

- May mimic minor salivary gland malignancy

Benign Mixed Tumor of Palate

- Well-circumscribed oral mucosal mass

Dermoid or Epidermoid

- Well-defined oral cavity mass with fatty ± fluid contents

Dentigerous Cyst

- Maxillary cystic mass ± unerupted tooth

Nasopalatine Duct Cyst

- Anterior, midline hard palate cyst

PATHOLOGY

General Features

- Etiology
  - Mucoepidermoid carcinoma (MECa): Associated with radiation exposure

Staging, Grading, & Classification

- MSGM uses same TNM staging as squamous cell carcinoma in each anatomic site
- TNM staging system
  - T1: ≤ 2 cm
  - T2: > 2 but ≤ 4 cm
  - T3: Tumor > 4 cm
  - T4a: Cortical bone, CNV3, extrinsic tongue muscles, skin
  - T4b: Masticator space, pterygoid plates, or skull base, ± encases interal carotid artery
- Prognosis depends on stage > histologic grade

Microscopic Features

- Adenoid cycstic carcinoma (ACCa): Unencapsulated neoplasm with varied growth patterns (cribriform, tubular, & solid)
- MECa: Epidermoid, intermediate, & mucus-secreting cells

CLINICAL ISSUES

Presentation

- Most common signs/symptoms
  - Painless, slowly enlarging submucosal mass
    - MSGM in adults unless proven otherwise
  - Other signs/symptoms
    - Facial numbness signifies PNT along CNV2

Demographics

- Age
  - 30-60 years old
- Epidemiology
  - MSGM: 0.5-1.5% of all H&N carcinoma
    - **ACCa = 40%** of malignancies in MSG

Natural History & Prognosis

- **ACCa**: Tendency for **PNT** + lung metastases
- **MECa**: Tendency for regional malignant **nodes**

Treatment

- Tumor resection including perineural extension
- Postoperative radiotherapy for high grade/high stage

DIAGNOSTIC CHECKLIST

Consider

- Long-term (> 10 year) imaging follow-up recommended given **tendency to recur late**

Image Interpretation Pearls

- Hard palate MSGM: Check for CNV PNT
- Remove FS on T1 C+ MR if susceptibility obscures anatomy
- Noncontrast T1 MR may offer better inherent contrast

SELECTED REFERENCES

1. Aydil U et al: Neoplasms of the hard palate. J Oral Maxillofac Surg. 72(3):619-26, 2014

Submandibular Space Nodal Non-Hodgkin Lymphoma

KEY FACTS

TERMINOLOGY

- Submandibular space (SMS) nodal non-Hodgkin lymphoma (NHL)
- NHL develops in lymphoreticular system

IMAGING

- CECT findings
  - Multiple, bilateral, nonnecrotic enlarged level I SMS nodes
  - May see only dominant, single large node
  - Usually large, solid, round nodes
  - Necrosis/extranodal spread indicate aggressive NHL
- PET/CT increasingly used to determine disease extent

TOP DIFFERENTIAL DIAGNOSES

- Reactive lymph nodes
- Nodal squamous cell carcinoma of SMS
- Nodal metastases from systemic primary
- Sarcoidosis lymph nodes

- Tuberculosis lymph nodes

PATHOLOGY

- Unregulated malignant monoclonal lymphocytes in lymphoreticular system
- Multiple different NHL subtypes
  - Most common (> 30%) diffuse large B-cell lymphoma
  - Multiple other subtypes

CLINICAL ISSUES

- Presentation: Painless multiple SMS masses
- Treatment: Radiotherapy, chemotherapy, or both
- 5% all H&N cancers
- Prognosis
  - 5-year survival: Stage I-II (85%), stage III-IV (50%)

DIAGNOSTIC CHECKLIST

- Consider NHL if imaging reveals multiple 1- to 3-cm cervical nodes in multiple nodal chains, especially if nonnecrotic

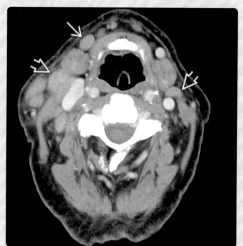
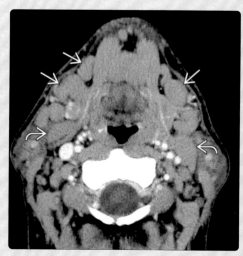

(Left) Axial CECT at the level of the hyoid bone in a patient with non-Hodgkin lymphoma (NHL) demonstrates diffuse adenopathy in the upper neck, with a prominent right submandibular IB node ➡ and bilateral level II nodes ➡. (Right) Axial CECT reveals multiple smoothly marginated, enlarged level IB nodes in the submandibular space bilaterally ➡ along with large, solid level II nodes ➡ in a patient with NHL.

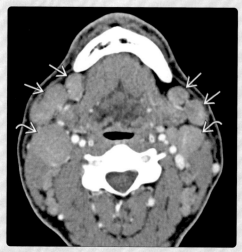
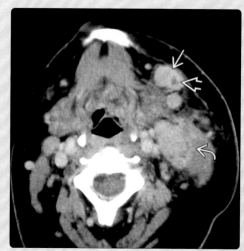

(Left) Axial CECT at the level of the inferior mandible shows large nonnecrotic NHL nodes in the level IB submandibular chain ➡ and bilateral level II jugulodigastric group ➡. (Right) Axial CECT in this HIV(+) patient with NHL shows a prominent left level IB submandibular space node ➡ with a small focus of cystic change ➡. A larger level II jugulodigastric node appears to invade the adjacent sternocleidomastoid muscle ➡. Nodal necrosis and extranodal NHL spread usually indicate a high-grade NHL is present.

TERMINOLOGY

Abbreviations

- Submandibular space (SMS) nodal non-Hodgkin lymphoma (NHL)

Definitions

- NHL = lymphoreticular system malignancy, postulated to arise from lymphocytes & derivatives

IMAGING

General Features

- Best diagnostic clue
  - Multiple, bilateral, large nodes involving multiple nodal chains
- Location
  - Any nodal chain may be affected, including level I
- Size
  - Multiple 1- to 3-cm nodes common
  - Dominant node may reach 3-5 cm in size
- Morphology
  - Nodes round or oval, typically solid

CT Findings

- CECT
  - Multiple bilateral round nodes; multiple nodal chains
  - Enhancement pattern variable
    - From isodense to muscle to diffuse enhancement

MR Findings

- T1WI
  - Nodes isointense to muscle
- T2WI
  - Nodes iso- or slightly hyperintense to muscle
- T1WI C+
  - Mild homogeneous nodal enhancement
  - Necrotic nodes enhance peripherally

Imaging Recommendations

- Best imaging tool
  - CECT usually initial imaging exam
- Protocol advice
  - PET/CT increasingly used to determine disease extent

DIFFERENTIAL DIAGNOSIS

Reactive Lymph Nodes

- Patient < 20-30 years with viral infection
- Diffuse, nonnecrotic nodes; usually < 2 cm

Nodal Squamous Cell Carcinoma of SMS

- Known oral cavity, anterior face or skin squamous cell carcinoma
- Level IA & IB nodes > 1.5 cm ± central nodal necrosis

Nodal Metastases From Systemic Primary

- Known primary tumor (lung, breast, etc.)
- Often unilateral

Sarcoidosis Lymph Nodes

- Diffuse cervical nodes may exactly mimic NHL
- Calcifications may be seen

Tuberculosis Lymph Nodes

- Systemically ill patient with strongly positive PPD + abnormal chest x-ray
- Diffuse heterogeneously enhancing nodes

PATHOLOGY

General Features

- Etiology
  - Unregulated malignant monoclonal lymphocytes in lymphoreticular system
  - Evidence suggests viral cause but yet to be proven
- Associated abnormalities
  - Often associated with AIDS in children & adults
    - 2nd most common cancer in AIDS patients
- Multiple different NHL subtypes
  - Most common (> 30%) diffuse large B-cell lymphoma

Microscopic Features

- Microscopic features depend on cell of origin
  - B- & T-cell lymphomas composed of precursor (lymphoblastic) cells or mature lymphocytes

CLINICAL ISSUES

Presentation

- Most common signs/symptoms
  - Painless multiple small rubbery SMS masses
- Other signs/symptoms
  - Systemic symptoms include night sweats, recurrent fevers, weight loss, fatigue, rash

Demographics

- Age
  - Median: 50-55 years
- Epidemiology
  - NHL incidence ↑ with age; ↑ in immunocompromised patients
  - 5% all H&N cancers

Natural History & Prognosis

- May be indolent, progressive but not curable, or aggressive but curable
- Predictors of poorer prognosis
  - Age > 60 years, > 1 extranodal site, stage III or IV, AIDS related

Treatment

- Depends on cell type, stage, & patient age
- Usually treated with XRT ± chemotherapy
  - Stage I and II: H&N NHL, XRT alone
  - Stage III and IV: Disseminated NHL, chemotherapy ± XRT

DIAGNOSTIC CHECKLIST

Consider

- NHL: If imaging reveals multiple 1- to 3-cm cervical nodes in multiple nodal chains, especially if nonnecrotic

SELECTED REFERENCES

1. Harnsberger HR et al: Non-Hodgkin's lymphoma of the head and neck: CT evaluation of nodal and extranodal sites. AJR Am J Roentgenol. 149(4):785-91, 1987

KEY FACTS

TERMINOLOGY

- Submandibular space (SMS), nodal squamous cell carcinoma (SCCa)

IMAGING

- SMS level IA & IB nodes
  - Level IA: Suprahyoid node(s) between anterior belly of digastric muscles
  - Level IB: Suprahyoid node(s) located lateral, & immediately anterior to a line tangent to posterior border of submandibular glands
- CECT or MR findings
  - CECT generally preferred over MR for nodal staging
  - CECT improves N staging accuracy over clinical staging
  - SMS nodes **> 1.5 cm** considered malignant in context of H&N SCCa
  - **Central nodal necrosis** considered sign of malignant involvement in any size node
  - Irregular enhancing margin invades adjacent soft tissues implies **extracapsular spread**
- PET/CT
  - Superior to CT/MR in clinical N0 neck
- Ultrasonographic findings
  - Round node with loss of hilar echogenicity
  - Main limitation is some nodes are inaccessible

TOP DIFFERENTIAL DIAGNOSES

- Suppurative lymph nodes
- Nodal non-Hodgkin lymphoma

CLINICAL ISSUES

- Treatment: Primary tumor resection vs. chemoradiotherapy ± nodal dissection
- Prognostic implication of malignant adenopathy
  - Single unilateral node ↓ prognosis by 50%
  - Bilateral nodes ↓ prognosis by 75%
  - Extracapsular spread ↓ prognosis by further 50%

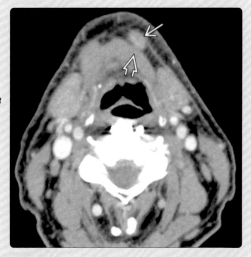
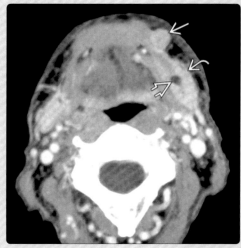

(Left) Axial CECT in a patient with a lower lip sqaumous cell carcinoma (SCCa) shows a single pathologic (subtle low-density center) SMS node ➡. The node is lateral to the anterior belly of the digastric muscle ➡, making it a level IB node. (Right) Axial CECT through the suprahyoid neck reveals an enlarged, round, enhancing metastatic level IB SCCa node ➡. The left submandibular gland (SMG) ➡ is enlarged & enhancing with dilated hilar duct ➡. Anterior floor of mouth SCCa (not shown) has obstructed the submandibular duct.

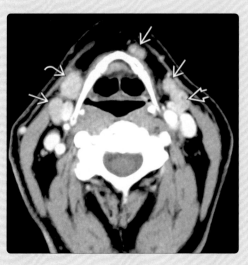
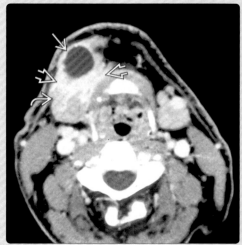

(Left) Axial CECT in a patient with anterior floor of mouth primary SCCa shows multiple level IB nodes. A few enhance ➡, but not all are malignant by CT criteria. Two nodes meet criteria for malignancy: One on right based on size > 1.5 cm ➡, and one on left due to central low density ➡. (Right) Axial CECT reveals a large cystic level IB SMS nodal mass ➡ in a patient with lateral tongue SCCa. Enhancing spreading nodal margins ➡ inseparable from surrounding tissues suggest extracapsular extension. The SMG ➡ is engulfed by spreading tumor.

TERMINOLOGY

Abbreviations

- Submandibular space (SMS), squamous cell carcinoma (SCCa)

Definitions

- Submandibular level I nodal metastasis from primary H&N SCCa

IMAGING

General Features

- Best diagnostic clue
  - Enlarged (> 1.5 cm), abnormally rounded, or centrally necrotic SMS node(s)
- Location
  - SMS level IA & IB nodes
    - Level IA nodes: Between anterior bellies of digastric muscles
    - Level IB nodes: Anterior, lateral, & anterior to posterior border of submandibular glands
- Size
  - SMS nodes > 1.5 cm considered malignant in context of H&N SCCa
    - Central nodal necrosis in any size node considered pathologic
- Morphology
  - Round contour + loss of fatty hilum: Suspicious for malignant involvement
  - Node with enhancing, irregular margins: Suspicious for extracapsular tumor spread

CT Findings

- CECT
  - Enhancing level IA or IB nodal mass > 1.5 cm ± central necrosis
  - Irregular enhancing margin invades adjacent soft tissues: Extranodal spread
  - High prevalence of positive nodes in clinically N0 necks in oral cavity SCCa, especially tongue

MR Findings

- T1WI C+
  - Enhancing level IA or IB nodal mass > 1.5 cm ± central low signal

Ultrasonographic Findings

- Grayscale ultrasound
  - Round node with loss of hilar echogenicity
  - Main limitation is nodes too deep for visualization (e.g., retropharyngeal nodes)

Nuclear Medicine Findings

- PET/CT
  - FDG: Focal areas of ↑ uptake matching SMS node indicates malignant nature
    - Superior to CT/MR in clinically N0 neck

DIFFERENTIAL DIAGNOSIS

Suppurative Lymph Nodes

- Sick or septic patient
- Central fluid density within nodes
- Can mimic SCCa nodes

Nodal Non-Hodgkin Lymphoma of SMS

- Multiple bilateral, large, usually nonnecrotic nodes
- No primary SCCa on clinical exam

PATHOLOGY

General Features

- Etiology
  - Lymphatic spread of primary SCCa to SMS nodes
  - Common drainage pathways for SCCa SMS nodes
    - All oral cavity sites
    - Anterior facial structures, lips, and skin
    - Oropharynx & hypopharynx SCCa can spread to SMS nodes if N2 disease (1 or more nodes in levels II-IV already involved)

Microscopic Features

- Metastases 1st lodge in subcapsular sinus → spread through node
- Characterized by squamous differentiation frequently with keratinizing morphology
- Necrosis, edema, or tumor cells in nodes may appear as nodal low density on CECT

CLINICAL ISSUES

Presentation

- Most common signs/symptoms
  - Painless, firm SMS mass
    - May be fixed to mandible ± adjacent tissues

Demographics

- Age
  - Most commonly > 40 yr

Natural History & Prognosis

- **Nodal metastasis** is single **most important prognostic factor** for H&N SCCa
  - Single unilateral node ↓ prognosis by 50%
  - Bilateral nodes reduce prognosis by 75%
  - Extranodal spread reduces prognosis by further 50%
    - Risk of recurrence ↑ 10x

Treatment

- Surgical resection ± chemoradiotherapy ± node dissection

DIAGNOSTIC CHECKLIST

Consider

- Nodal size (> 1.5 cm) or parenchymal inhomogeneity key to labeling malignant based on imaging

SELECTED REFERENCES

1. Furukawa M et al: The prevalence of lymph node metastases in clinically N0 necks with oral cavity squamous cell carcinoma: is CT good enough for nodal staging? Acta Radiol. 55(5):570-8, 2014
2. Ahuja AT et al: Ultrasound of malignant cervical lymph nodes. Cancer Imaging. 8:48-56, 2008
3. King AD et al: Necrosis in metastatic neck nodes: diagnostic accuracy of CT, MR imaging, and US. Radiology. 230(3):720-6, 2004

SECTION 15
Mandible-Maxilla and Temporomandibular Joint

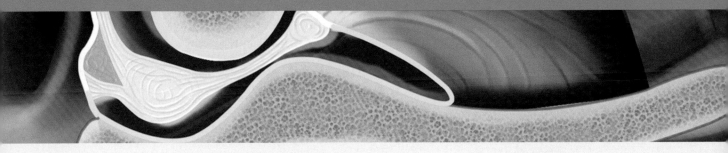

Imaging Techniques & Indications

Mandible and Maxilla

The study of choice for evaluating the mandible and maxilla is **thin-section bone algorithm CT** and **CECT**. A standard protocol consists of coverage from the orbits to the hyoid at ≤ 1-mm intervals following contrast administration and postprocessing with both bone and soft tissue algorithm. Axial images should be acquired parallel to the inferior border of the mandible. Acquiring the maxilla and mandible angled separately so as to avoid artifact from dental restorations assists in evaluation of the alveolar ridge and adjacent structures. Multiplanar reformats should be performed in the coronal and sagittal planes. In addition, it is frequently helpful to the referring clinician to reformat in a panoramic view.

MR of the maxillofacial complex is used to assess marrow changes, involvement of the inferior alveolar nerve, and soft tissue involvement of adjacent structures. T1-/T2-weighted and contrast-enhanced images should be acquired from the orbits to the hyoid at 3 mm and ideally should be acquired with high-resolution/small-FOV techniques. As with CT, axial images should be acquired parallel to the inferior border of the mandible. STIR or T2 fat-saturation sequences along with contrast enhancement are sensitive for marrow/nerve changes associated with inflammation or neoplastic involvement.

TMJ

MR is the tool of choice for evaluating the TMJ. Small surface, circular (3 inch) or TMJ coils are ideally used, although multichannel coils (12 channels or greater) provide adequate signal. Sagittal images are acquired perpendicular to the long axis of the condyle ("corrected sagittal oblique") at 3-mm intervals. T1-weighted or proton density sagittal images are acquired in the closed- and open-mouth positions. Cine images provide the most accurate assessment of condylar rotation and translation and the associated disc function. Sagittal T2-weighted images are acquired to assess for joint effusion. Coronal T1-weighted images in the closed-mouth position are used to assess medial or lateral disc displacements as well as multiplanar views of the condyle. Contrast-enhanced images are generally reserved for the evaluation of synovitis or tumors.

CT imaging of the TMJ is generally reserved for the evaluation of **trauma**, assessment of bony abnormalities or **calcified masses**, or **joint reconstruction** with metallic prosthesis. Thin-section bone algorithm images are acquired at 1-mm intervals from the sella to the hyoid and reformatted in the coronal and sagittal planes.

Imaging Anatomy

Mandible and Maxilla

The **maxilla** consists of a **body** containing the maxillary sinus and 4 processes: **Zygomatic, frontal, alveolar,** and **palatine**. The maxilla forms the boundaries of 3 cavities: The roof of the oral cavity, the floor and lateral wall of the nasal cavity, and the floor of the orbit. In addition, the maxilla forms the anterior boundary of the infratemporal and pterygopalatine fossae and contributes to the formation of the infraorbital and pterygomaxillary fissures. The zygomatic (**malar**) process contributes to the inferior pillar of the zygomatic buttress. The frontal (nasal) process articulates with the nasal bones on the lateral surface, with the medial surface forming the lateral wall of the nasal cavity and articulating with the ethmoid bone to enclose the agger nasi cells and anterior ethmoidal cells.

The posterior border of the frontal process forms the lacrimal fossa and the anterior lacrimal crest. The **alveolar process** is the thickest and most spongy part of the maxilla and forms the alveolar arches containing the dentition and their supporting periodontal structures. The 3D U-shaped configuration of the maxillary alveolus is such that benign expansile inflammatory or neoplastic processes will typically expand it concentrically. Innervation of the teeth and gingiva is via the anterior and posterior superior alveolar nerves.

The **maxillary tuberosity** is the rounded most posterior eminence of the alveolar arch, which articulates with the pyramidal process of the palatine bone. The palatine process is a relatively thick horizontal bone that forms the roof of the mouth and the floor of the nasal cavity. The incisive foramen lies in the anterior midline of the premaxilla and transmits the nasopalatine nerves and descending palatine artery. The premaxillary suture, posterior to the incisive foramen, separates the anterior premaxilla from the more posterior palatine process, which forms the anterior 75% of the hard palate. The remainder of the hard palate is formed by the horizontal plate of the palatine bone and contains foramina for the **greater and lesser palatine nerves**. The blood supply to the palate is formed from the descending palatine artery emerging through the greater palatine foramen and running in a shallow groove along the lateral aspect of the palate to the incisive foramen. The blood supply to the maxillary alveolus is via the posterior superior alveolar artery, which supplies the gingiva, premolar, and molar teeth. The incisors and canines are supplied by the anterior &/or middle superior alveolar arteries, which are branches of the infraorbital artery.

The **mandible** consists of a horseshoe-shaped body and vertical rami joining in the anterior midline symphysis. On the external surface of the mandible, at roughly the level of the 1st premolar, is the mental foramen for the mental nerve and vessels. Emerging anterosuperiorly from the ramus is the triangular eminence of the coronoid process to which the temporalis and masseter muscles attach. At the posterior-superior termination of the ramus is the condyloid process consisting of the condyle supported by the more constricted neck. On the medial (lingual) surface of the ramus is the **mandibular foramen** for intraosseous passage of the neurovascular supply, namely the inferior alveolar nerve and artery. The mandibular foramen is bounded by a small bony spine, the lingula. The coronoid process and condyle are separated by a depression, the mandibular (coronoid) notch, through which the masseteric vessels and nerves pass.

Permanent dentition consists of 32 teeth: 2 central incisors, 2 lateral incisors, 2 canines, 4 premolars, and 6 molars in each jaw. These are numbered 1-16 in the maxilla right to left and 17-32 in the mandible left to right. **Primary dentition** consists of 20 teeth: 2 central incisors, 2 lateral incisors, 2 canines, and 4 molars in each jaw. These are numbered A-J in the maxilla and K-T in the mandible. Dental infection in the form of dental caries or periodontal disease spreads into the alveolus through the root apex or through the **periodontal ligament** (PDL) space. The PDL is a potential conduit for development of infection following alveolar fracture as well as direct intraosseous extension of gingival squamous cell carcinoma.

TMJ

The **TMJ complex** consists of the diarthrodial osseous articulation between the mandibular condyle and the glenoid fossa and articular eminence of the temporal bone. The TMJ is the only joint in which articulating surfaces are covered by

Mandible-Maxilla Differential Diagnosis

Inflammatory/infectious	Cysts	Malignant neoplasms
Apical rarefying osteitis	**Odontogenic**	**Nonodontogenic**
Radicular cyst	Dentigerous cyst	Gingival squamous cell carcinoma
Osteomyelitis	Glandular odontogenic cyst	Osteosarcoma/chondrosarcoma
Osteonecrosis	Calcifying epithelial odontogenic cyst	Multiple myeloma or metastasis
Osteoradionecrosis	**Benign neoplasms**	**Odontogenic**
Congenital/developmental	**Nonodontogenic**	Odontogenic carcinoma
Solitary median maxillary central incisor	Osteoma	Odontogenic sarcoma
Acquired	Ossifying fibroma	**Fibroosseous lesions**
Stafne bone cavity	**Odontogenic**	Periapical osseous dysplasia
Simple bone cyst	Odontoma	Florid osseous dysplasia
Central giant cell granuloma	Keratocystic odontogenic tumor	Fibrous dysplasia
Cysts	Ameloblastoma	Cherubism
Nonodontogenic	Odontogenic myxoma	**Other**
Nasopalatine duct cyst	Adenomatoid odontogenic tumor	Neurofibroma, schwannoma
Nasolabial cyst	Calcifying epithelial odontogenic tumor	Eosinophilic granuloma

TMJ Differential Diagnosis

Meniscal dislocation	Anterior, medial, lateral, or (rarely) posterior displacement of articular disc
Juvenile idiopathic arthritis	Bilateral flattened, deformed mandibular condyles, joint effusion, synovial enhancement
Synovial chondromatosis	Multiple calcified small nodules in superior joint space
Pigmented villonodular synovitis	Locally destructive mass with peripheral hypointense rim on MR
Calcium pyrophosphate dihydrate deposition disease	Chunky, diffuse, calcified mass

fibrocartilage. The articular disc is a biconcave, dense, avascular fibrous connective tissue with 3 segments: The anterior band, which is attached to the capsule and fibers of the superior belly of the lateral pterygoid muscle, the thin intermediate zone, and the posterior band. The bilaminar zone or retrodiscal tissues attach to the posterior band and provide neurovascular innervation.

Approaches to Imaging Issues of Mandible & Maxilla

As lesions of the mandible and maxilla may arise from a myriad of odontogenic and nonodontogenic tissues, it is best to use a systematic approach to evaluate lesions of the jaw. The 1st step is to try to determine whether the lesion is odontogenic or nonodontogenic in origin. Infectious and inflammatory lesions usually have a dental origin, even if remote. **Odontogenic** cysts and benign and malignant neoplasms usually arise from, or are centered within, tooth-bearing areas of the alveolus. The major exception to this is gingival squamous cell carcinoma extending through the gingiva or PDL space. **Nonodontogenic lesions** often arise at the tooth root apices or superior (maxilla) or inferior (mandible) to them.

Once an assessment of odontogenic vs. nonodontogenic is achieved, an evaluation of lesion features, such as location, cystic vs. solid, presence of internal calcification, loculation, bony expansion or erosion, and enhancement, will narrow the differential. Most odontogenic lesions are cystic, cystic-appearing, or relatively hypodense on CT. They are distinguished by their location, loculation, presence of internal

calcification, and expansion/erosion of bone. Most dentigerous cysts and keratocystic odontogenic tumors do not become loculated until large; most ameloblastomas demonstrate multiple loculations. The only odontogenic lesions with internal calcification are the odontoma, calcifying epithelial cyst/tumor, and adenomatoid odontogenic tumor. Malignant neoplasms generally demonstrate more enhancement than benign lesions.

There are 3 **key pieces of information** the referring clinician needs to know:
- Does lesion or fracture involve lamina dura & PDL space or tooth roots?
- Does lesion or fracture in mandible involve inferior alveolar canal?
- Does lesion extend to adjacent structures or spaces, including maxillary sinus, orbit, pterygopalatine fossa, buccal vestibule and space, masticator space, or sublingual or submandibular space?

Selected References
1. Mosier KM: Lesions of the jaw. Semin Ultrasound CT MR. 36(5):444-50, 2015
2. Mosier KM: Magnetic resonance imaging of the maxilla and mandible: signal characteristics and features in the differential diagnosis of common lesions. Top Magn Reson Imaging. 24(1):23-37, 2015
3. Aiken A et al: MR imaging of the temporomandibular joint. Magn Reson Imaging Clin N Am. 20(3):397-412, 2012
4. Curé JK et al: Radiopaque jaw lesions: an approach to the differential diagnosis. Radiographics. 32(7):1909-25, 2012

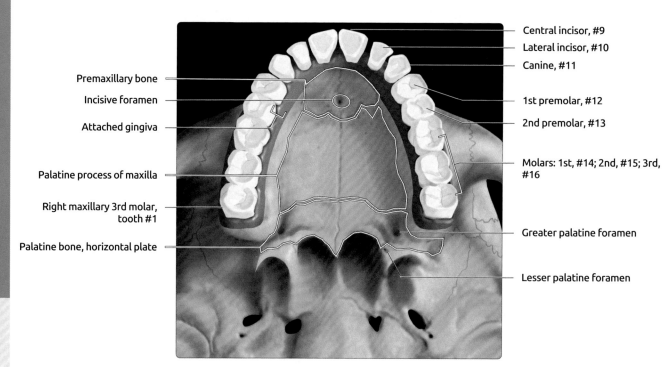

Premaxillary bone

Incisive foramen

Attached gingiva

Palatine process of maxilla

Right maxillary 3rd molar, tooth #1

Palatine bone, horizontal plate

Central incisor, #9

Lateral incisor, #10

Canine, #11

1st premolar, #12

2nd premolar, #13

Molars: 1st, #14; 2nd, #15; 3rd, #16

Greater palatine foramen

Lesser palatine foramen

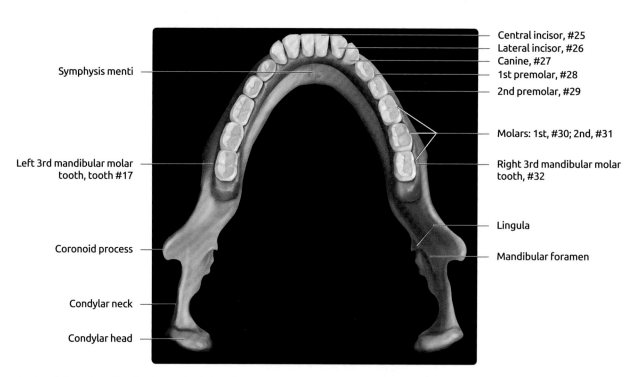

Symphysis menti

Left 3rd mandibular molar tooth, tooth #17

Coronoid process

Condylar neck

Condylar head

Central incisor, #25

Lateral incisor, #26

Canine, #27

1st premolar, #28

2nd premolar, #29

Molars: 1st, #30; 2nd, #31

Right 3rd mandibular molar tooth, #32

Lingula

Mandibular foramen

(Top) *Axial graphic of hard palate and maxillary alveolar ridge viewed from below shows the anterior premaxillary bone and the larger palatine process of the maxillary bone. Posteriorly is the horizontal plate of the palatine bone. Note the anterior midline incisive canal and the posterolateral greater and lesser palatine foramina. The alveolus is covered by attached gingiva, which is the oral mucous membrane bound to the tooth and the alveolus. The maxilla has 16 permanent teeth; numbering begins with the right 3rd molar.*
(Bottom) *Axial graphic of mandible seen from above demonstrates the cephalad condylar head and neck leading to the more inferior ramus. The mandibular foramen is seen on the inner surface of the mandibular ramus. The cephalad projecting coronoid processes attach to the temporalis muscle tendons. The U-shaped mandibular bodies fuse in the midline at the symphysis menti. There are 16 permanent teeth, numbered beginning at the left 3rd molar from 17 to 32 (right 3rd molar tooth).*

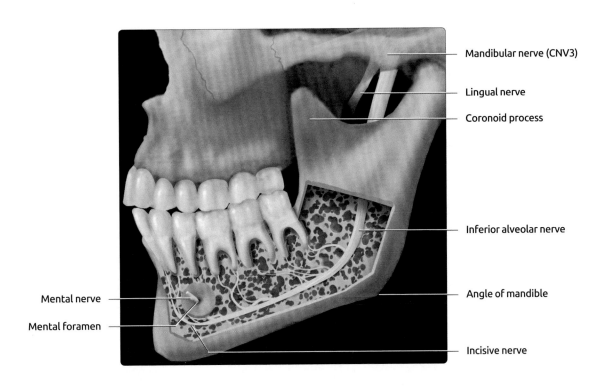

Mandibular nerve (CNV3)

Lingual nerve

Coronoid process

Inferior alveolar nerve

Angle of mandible

Incisive nerve

Mental nerve

Mental foramen

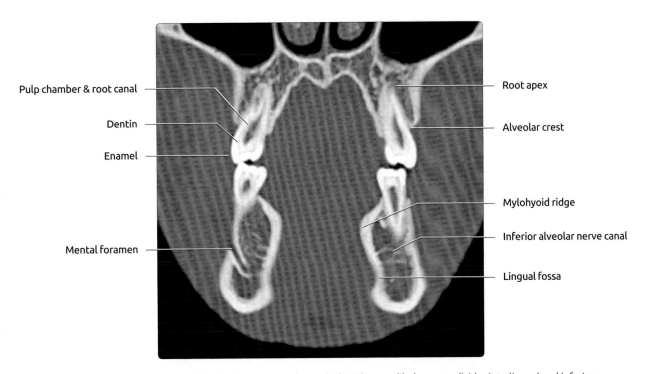

Pulp chamber & root canal

Dentin

Enamel

Mental foramen

Root apex

Alveolar crest

Mylohyoid ridge

Inferior alveolar nerve canal

Lingual fossa

(Top) *Lateral drawing of mandible with its lateral cortex removed reveals that the mandibular nerve divides into lingual and inferior alveolar nerves. The inferior alveolar nerve divides distally into mental and incisive branches. The mental nerve branch reaches the superficial chin through the mental foramen.* (Bottom) *Coronal bone CT through the anterior mandible is shown. The most common lesion of the maxilla and mandible is dental infection, primarily through carious lesions involving the enamel and dentin with or without extension to the pulp. Lesions at the root apex typically result from infection transgressing the pulp. Apical lesions may also arise from infection of the periodontium with loss of bone at the alveolar crest. The jaws are the only bones with direct exposure to the external environment via the teeth. Infection from teeth may extend through the buccal or lingual cortex to adjacent spaces. The proximity of the lingual fossa to premolar or molar roots predisposes to involvement of the sublingual and submandibular space.*

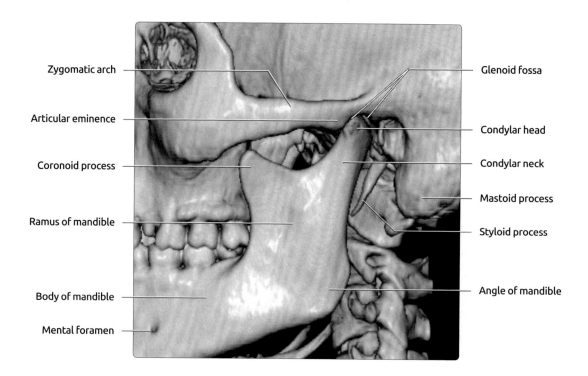

Zygomatic arch

Articular eminence

Coronoid process

Ramus of mandible

Body of mandible

Mental foramen

Glenoid fossa

Condylar head

Condylar neck

Mastoid process

Styloid process

Angle of mandible

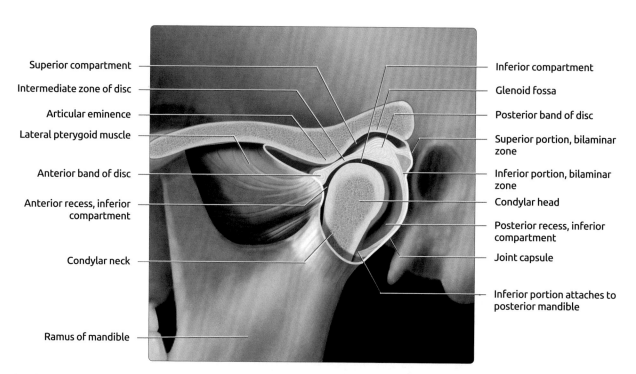

Superior compartment

Intermediate zone of disc

Articular eminence

Lateral pterygoid muscle

Anterior band of disc

Anterior recess, inferior compartment

Condylar neck

Ramus of mandible

Inferior compartment

Glenoid fossa

Posterior band of disc

Superior portion, bilaminar zone

Inferior portion, bilaminar zone

Condylar head

Posterior recess, inferior compartment

Joint capsule

Inferior portion attaches to posterior mandible

(Top) *Sagittal 3D VRT image shows the osseous anatomy of TMJ. The condylar head is situated in the glenoid fossa deep to the posterior zygomatic arch. The zygomatic arch provides some protection laterally for the TMJ in the setting of trauma. The TMJ must be fully evaluated on all mandibular trauma cases to ensure that no dislocation of the mandibular condyle has occurred.* (Bottom) *Magnified lateral graphic of the TMJ shows the articular disc with its anterior and posterior bands. The thinner part of the disc connecting these bands is called the intermediate zone. The disc separates the joint into a superior and an inferior compartment. Note the lateral pterygoid muscle inserting anteriorly on the joint capsule and anterior band. The posterior margin of the posterior band is referred to as the bilaminar zone, with the superior strut attaching to the posterior mandibular fossa, while the inferior strut attaches to the posterior margin of the mandibular condyle.*

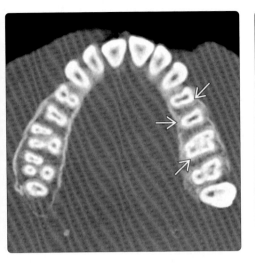

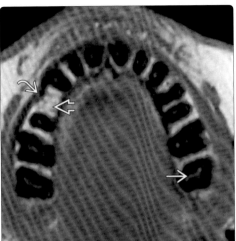

(Left) *Axial bone CT shows normal adult maxilla. Each tooth is surrounded by the periodontal ligament space containing fibers of the periodontal ligament and the lamina dura (cortical bone forming the tooth socket)* ➡. (Right) *Axial T1 MR shows the normal adult maxilla. Note the slightly hyperintense vascular tissue of the pulp chamber* ➡, *the normal yellow marrow* ➡, *and the attached gingiva* ➡.

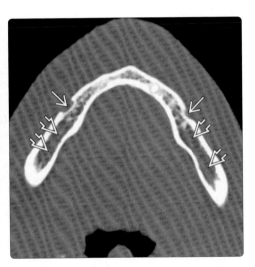

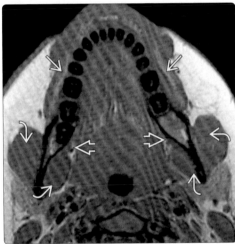

(Left) *Axial bone CT of the mandible shows bilateral mental foramen* ➡ *with inferior alveolar canals* ➡ *containing inferior alveolar nerves and arteries. The mandible is an end-artery system with ↑ risk relative to the maxilla for development of osteomyelitis, osteonecrosis, or osteoradionecrosis.* (Right) *Axial T1 MR shows the relationship of the mandible to the buccal vestibule/space* ➡, *masticator space* ➡, *and submandibular space* ➡, *all routes for spread of infection or tumor.*

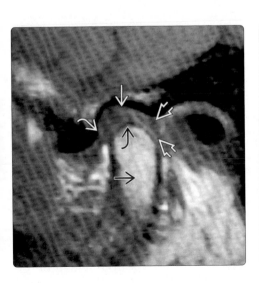

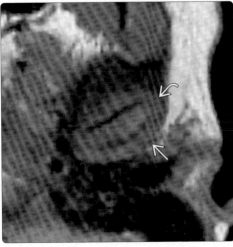

(Left) *Sagittal T1 MR shows the posterior band in normal position at about the 11 to 12 o'clock position relative to the condyle* ➡, *the intermediate zone* ➡, *and the superior and inferior struts of the bilaminar zone (retrodiscal tissue)* ➡. *Note the normal marrow signal* ➡ *and intact cortex* ➡. (Right) *Axial T1 MR through the left TMJ demonstrates the joint capsule surrounding the joint* ➡. *Note the auriculotemporal nerve exiting the joint space posterolaterally* ➡.

Solitary Median Maxillary Central Incisor

TERMINOLOGY

- Solitary median maxillary central incisor (SMMCI) syndrome

IMAGING

- Small, **triangle-shaped hard palate**
- **Single maxillary central incisor** in midline
- Congenital nasal pyriform aperture stenosis (CNPAS), midnasal stenosis, or choanal atresia in 90%
- ± **holoprosencephaly (HPE)**

TOP DIFFERENTIAL DIAGNOSES

- Congenital nasal pyriform aperture stenosis
  ○ Solitary central maxillary incisor in 60%
- Choanal atresia
  ○ Rarely with solitary central maxillary incisor
- Mesiodens
  ○ Supernumerary midline tooth develops between 2 maxillary central incisors

PATHOLOGY

- Associated with mutations in human sonic hedgehog (*SHH*) gene & deletions on chromosomes 7 & 18
- *SHH* mutations are most frequent etiology of HPE
  ○ SMMCI can be considered predictor or risk factor for HPE or gene carrier status

CLINICAL ISSUES

- Respiratory distress during feeding
- Hypotelorism, microcephaly, short stature, hypopituitarism

DIAGNOSTIC CHECKLIST

- Look for SMMCI, CNPAS, or choanal atresia when imaging neonates with feeding/breathing difficulties
- If SMMCI diagnosed, be sure to check for findings of HPE

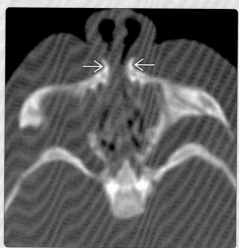
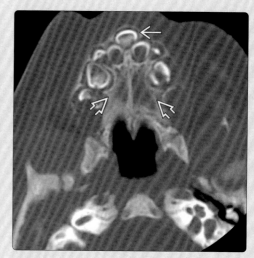

(Left) Axial bone CT at the level of the anterior nasal inlet demonstrates pyriform aperture stenosis ➡. (Right) Axial bone CT in the same patient at the level of the hard palate shows a solitary median maxillary central incisor ➡ and a small, triangle-shaped hard palate ➡. Brain MR in this child was normal.

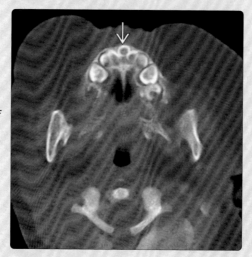
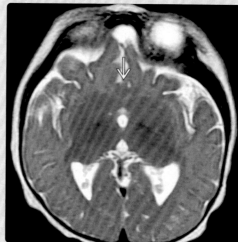

(Left) Axial bone CT shows a single midline maxillary central incisor ➡ in a patient who also had congenital pyriform aperture stenosis. (Right) Axial T2WI brain MR in the same infant shows very mild lobar holoprosencephaly with incomplete separation of hemispheres ➡.

Solitary Median Maxillary Central Incisor

TERMINOLOGY

Abbreviations

- Solitary median maxillary central incisor (SMMCI) syndrome
  - o Favored term

Synonyms

- Monosuperoincisivodontic dwarfism: Original term (1976)
- Solitary median maxillary central incisor, short stature, choanal atresia/midnasal stenosis syndrome
- Shortened to SMMCI syndrome, as other features not necessarily present in all cases
- Single central incisor, single maxillary central incisor syndrome, & single incisor syndrome
  - o These terms do not adequately describe peculiarly formed central incisor tooth

IMAGING

General Features

- Best diagnostic clue
  - o Triangle-shaped hard palate with solitary central maxillary incisor tooth located in midline

CT Findings

- Narrow anterior palate, **triangular shape**
- **Single maxillary central incisor** in midline
  - o May be unerupted
  - o Primary and permanent dentition
- + **congenital nasal obstruction** in **90%**
  - o Congenital nasal pyriform aperture stenosis (CNPAS) > midnasal stenosis & choanal atresia
- ± **holoprosencephaly** (HPE)

MR Findings

- Findings often more confusing on MR
  - o Tooth buds appear more crowded
- Prenatal MR diagnosis has been reported
- ± HPE

Imaging Recommendations

- Best imaging tool
  - o Bone CT
- Protocol advice
  - o Look for associated stenosis of pyriform aperture, midnasal cavity, or choanal atresia
  - o Consider **MR** to evaluate brain for **midline anomalies**

DIFFERENTIAL DIAGNOSIS

Congenital Nasal Pyriform Aperture Stenosis

- Solitary central maxillary incisor in 60%

Choanal Atresia

- Most common congenital abnormality of nasal cavity
  - o 1:5,000-8,000 births

Mesiodens

- Supernumerary midline tooth develops between 2 maxillary central incisors

PATHOLOGY

General Features

- Genetics
  - o Associated with mutations in human sonic hedgehog (*SHH*) gene & deletions on chromosomes 7 & 18
    - – *SHH* mutations are most frequent etiology of HPE
    - – SMMCI can be considered predictor or risk factor for HPE or gene carrier status
- Associated abnormalities
  - o CHARGE (ocular **c**oloboma, **h**eart defects, choanal **a**tresia, developmental **r**etardation, **g**enital/urinary anomalies, **e**ar abnormalities)
  - o VACTERL (**v**ertebral defects, **a**nal atresia, **c**ardiovascular defects, **t**rache**o**esophageal fistula, **r**adial ray or renal anomalies, **l**imb defects)
  - o Velocardiofacial, Duane retraction, Goldenhar & DiGeorge syndromes
  - o Clavicle hypoplasia, HPE, pituitary insufficiency, microcephaly, oromandibular-limb hypogenesis syndrome type I, ectodermal dysplasia, congenital cardiac anomalies, spine abnormalities

Gross Pathologic & Surgical Features

- Absent labial frenulum and incisive papilla

CLINICAL ISSUES

Presentation

- Most common signs/symptoms
  - o Respiratory distress during feeding
    - – When associated with CNPAS, midnasal stenosis, or choanal atresia/stenosis, nasal obstruction hampers breathing when infant feeds
    - – Clinical mimic of nasolacrimal duct mucocele → nasal obstruction
- Other signs/symptoms
  - o Hypotelorism, microcephaly, short stature, hypopituitarism

Demographics

- ~ 1:50,000 live births

Treatment

- Directed toward relief of associated nasal stenosis
  - o Surgical enlargement and stenting

DIAGNOSTIC CHECKLIST

Image Interpretation Pearls

- Look for SMMCI, CNPAS, or choanal atresia when imaging neonates with feeding/breathing difficulties
- Be sure to check for findings of HPE

SELECTED REFERENCES

1. Giannopoulou EZ et al: Solitary median maxillary central incisor. J Pediatr. 167(3):770.e1, 2015
2. Ginat DT et al: CT and MRI of congenital nasal lesions in syndromic conditions. Pediatr Radiol. 45(7):1056-65, 2015
3. Poelmans S et al: Genotypic and phenotypic variation in six patients with solitary median maxillary central incisor syndrome. Am J Med Genet A. 167A(10):2451-8, 2015

KEY FACTS

TERMINOLOGY

- Rare, benign, developmental cyst in nasal ala
- Synonyms: Nasoalveolar cyst, Klestadt cyst

IMAGING

- Typically < 2 cm; ≤ 10% bilateral
- Pyriform rim, between upper lip & nasal vestibule
- CT: Nonenhancing hyperdense ± dense fluid levels
  - May cause bone remodeling of maxilla as enlarges
- MR: T2 hyperintense cyst with variable T1 intensity
  - No contrast enhancement of lesion

TOP DIFFERENTIAL DIAGNOSES

- Nasopalatine duct cyst
- Nasolacrimal duct mucocele
- Periapical (radicular) cyst
- Dermoid and epidermoid of oral cavity

PATHOLOGY

- Developmental; 2 theories of pathogenesis
  - Persistence of anlage of nasolacrimal duct or inclusion cyst from formation of facial skeleton
  - Former is favored theory

CLINICAL ISSUES

- Mean age: 40 years; M:F = 1:3
- Presents as facial swelling ± nasal obstruction
- Smooth fluctuant mass, loss of nasolabial fold
- 30% present with infection: Swelling, pain, erythema
- Surgical excision is definitive treatment

DIAGNOSTIC CHECKLIST

- Extraosseous origin distinguishes from odontogenic lesions
- Look for bone erosion, extension to turbinate, or nasolacrimal duct obstruction

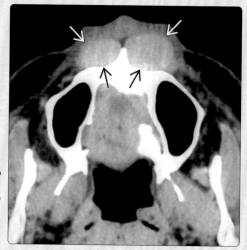
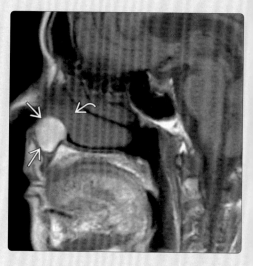

(Left) Axial NECT demonstrates bilateral, well-demarcated, hyperdense rounded lesions ➡ anterior to premaxilla. Lesions result in subtle, left greater than right, remodeling of the maxilla ➡. Fewer than 10% of nasolabial cyst cases are bilateral. (Right) Sagittal T1 MR shows a sharply marginated, diffusely hyperintense nasolabial cyst ➡. Note the proximity of the superior aspect of the lesion to the inferior turbinate ➡ and floor of the nasal vestibule. On exam, these were submucosal masses.

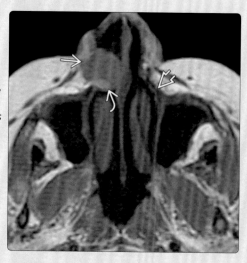
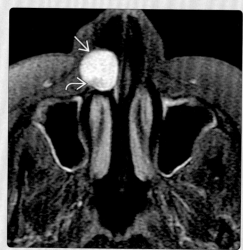

(Left) Axial T1 MR shows a well-defined mass ➡ at the pyriform rim that extends into the nasal vestibule. Mass appears slightly increased in signal compared to the muscle with more focal hyperintensity ➡, reflecting proteinaceous debris. Note that lesion nestles into maxilla with subtle bone erosion compared to contralateral side ➡. (Right) Axial T2 FS MR reveals typical homogeneous round T2 hyperintensity of the nasolabial cyst ➡, with subtly hypointense proteinaceous debris ➡.

TERMINOLOGY

Synonyms
- Nasoalveolar cyst, Klestadt cyst

Definitions
- Rare, benign, developmental cyst in nasal ala

IMAGING

General Features
- Best diagnostic clue
  - **Extraosseous** cystic mass in paramedian location at nares
- Location
  - Submucosal, anterior nasal floor
  - Pyriform rim, between upper lip & nasal vestibule
- Size
  - Typically < 2 cm; < 10% bilateral

CT Findings
- CECT
  - Iso- to hyperdense nonenhancing soft tissue mass
  - May have dense dependent fluid levels from calcium oxalate crystals
- Bone CT
  - May cause bone remodeling of maxilla as enlarges

MR Findings
- T1WI
  - Slightly **hyperintense** from proteinaceous debris
- T2WI
  - Homogeneously hyperintense
- T1WI C+
  - No contrast enhancement of lesion

Imaging Recommendations
- Best imaging tool
  - CT is adequate for delineation of lesion
- Protocol advice
  - CECT confirms absence of solid component
  - Bone CT images for remodeled bone change

DIFFERENTIAL DIAGNOSIS

Nasopalatine Duct Cyst
- Occurs in nasopalatine duct/incisive foramen → intraosseous midline maxillary alveolus
- Uniform corticated expansion of incisive foramen and nasopalatine canal
- Typically no extraalveolar extension to nasolabial unless very large

Nasolacrimal Duct Mucocele
- Failure of canalization of nasolacrimal duct
- Typically appear in infancy
- Usually accompanying dacryocystitis, epiphora, or intranasal mass

Periapical (Radicular) Cyst
- Intraosseous alveolar location
- Associated with root apex of tooth having caries or periodontal disease

Dermoid and Epidermoid of Oral Cavity
- Usually presents in infancy, childhood
- Very rare in nasolabial area

PATHOLOGY

General Features
- Etiology
  - Developmental; 2 theories of pathogenesis
    - Persistence of anlage of nasolacrimal duct
      - □ Favored theory of formation
    - Inclusion cyst from formation of facial skeleton
      - □ After fusion of medial & lateral nasal processes and maxillary prominence

Gross Pathologic & Surgical Features
- Gray-blue color; thick fibrous capsule
- Contains mucoid or serous fluid

Microscopic Features
- Pseudostratified, stratified, or mixed respiratory and squamous epithelium with mucous goblet cells

CLINICAL ISSUES

Presentation
- Most common signs/symptoms
  - Swelling of nasolabial fold, upper lip
  - ± nasal obstruction

Demographics
- Age
  - Lesions present in adults; mean age: 40 years
- Gender
  - M:F = 1:3
- Ethnicity
  - More prevalent in African American & Hispanic populations

Natural History & Prognosis
- May grow toward nasolabial fold or vestibule of mouth or nose
- 30% present with infection of cyst

Treatment
- Surgical excision is definitive treatment
  - Sublabial approach; recurrence rare

DIAGNOSTIC CHECKLIST

Image Interpretation Pearls
- **Extraosseous origin** distinguishes from odontogenic lesions
  - Prevents unnecessary maxillary surgical/dental intervention

SELECTED REFERENCES

1. Sumer AP et al: Nasolabial cyst: case report with CT and MRI findings. Oral Surg Oral Med Oral Pathol Oral Radiol Endod. 109(2):e92-4, 2010
2. Iida S et al: Spheric mass beneath the alar base: MR images of nasolabial cyst and schwannoma. AJNR Am J Neuroradiol. 27(9):1826-9, 2006
3. Cure JK et al: MR of nasolabial cysts. AJNR Am J Neuroradiol. 17(3):585-8, 1996

Periapical Cyst (Radicular)

TERMINOLOGY

- Synonym = radicular cyst
- **Most common odontogenic cyst**
- Periapical rarefying osteitis = newer term to include periapical cyst, periapical granuloma, and periapical abscess

IMAGING

- **Ovoid cyst at apex of nonvital tooth**
- Millimeters to ≤ 1 cm usually
- CT: Ovoid to round corticated lucency associated with tooth apex
- May see dental caries: Enamel ± crown erosion

TOP DIFFERENTIAL DIAGNOSES

- Lateral periodontal cyst
- Keratocystic odontogenic tumor
- Dentigerous (follicular) cyst

PATHOLOGY

- Develops after inflammation and necrosis of pulp ("nonvital" tooth)
  - Most often from dental caries, periodontal disease
  - Less often posttraumatic
- Pulp necrosis → growth of epithelial rests of Malassez in periodontal ligament

CLINICAL ISSUES

- Most commonly found on dental radiographs
- Usually asymptomatic unless secondary infection
- Infection → intermittent intense jaw pain
- May progress to periapical abscess ± cellulitis
- Most prevalent in 3rd-5th decade

DIAGNOSTIC CHECKLIST

- Report relationship of lesion to important structures
  - Maxillary teeth: Maxillary sinus
  - Mandible: Inferior alveolar nerve canal

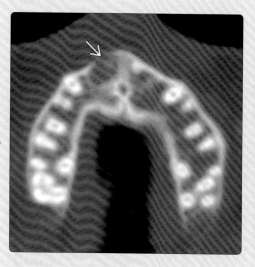
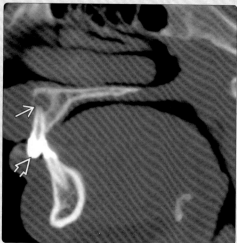

(Left) Axial bone CT demonstrates a small periapical radicular cyst ➡ associated with the right maxillary central incisor, without periosteal reaction or extraosseous soft tissue mass. (Right) Sagittal reformatted bone CT in the same patient shows the periapical cyst ➡ and dental amalgam ⊋ in the same tooth.

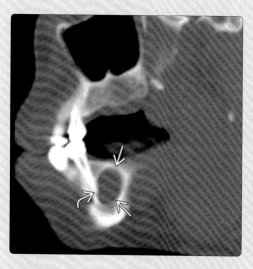
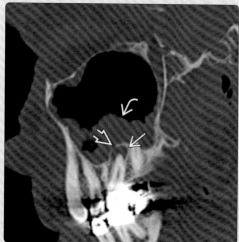

(Left) Sagittal reformatted bone CT shows a well-corticated unilocular cyst ➡ at the root apex of the right mandibular 1st premolar tooth. The cyst is contiguous with lamina dura and periodontal ligament space ⊅, indicating it is likely of inflammatory origin. (Right) Sagittal reformatted bone CT shows a moderate-sized maxillary periapical cyst ➡ with a focal dehiscence ⊋ in the cyst roof and associated inferior maxillary sinus odontogenic sinusitis ⊅.

TERMINOLOGY

Synonyms

- Radicular cyst

Definitions

- Focal cyst at apex of nonvital tooth
- Periapical rarefying osteitis = newer term to include periapical cyst, periapical granuloma, and periapical abscess

IMAGING

General Features

- Best diagnostic clue
  - **Ovoid cyst at apex of tooth with dental caries**
- Location
  - Tooth apex (= tip of root)
- Size
  - Millimeters to ≤ 1 cm usually
  - May enlarge to multiple centimeters if neglected
- Morphology
  - Ovoid to round

Imaging Recommendations

- Best imaging tool
  - **Primary imaging modality dental radiographs**
  - Bone CT best shows lesion for H&N radiologist
- Protocol advice
  - Thin-section bone CT with 3-plane reformats

CT Findings

- Bone CT
  - Ovoid to round corticated lucency associated with **tooth apex**
    - Increased lucency of pulp
    - May see dental caries: Enamel ± crown erosion
  - Often multiple in cases of extremely poor dentition
  - Maxillary lesions may be associated with maxillary sinus opacification
    - When present, called "odontogenic sinusitis"

Radiographic Findings

- See best with dental radiographs
  - Corticated cyst at root apex
  - Loss of lamina dura
  - Widening of periodontal ligament space
- Nonvital tooth associated with caries, periodontal disease, root resorption

MR Findings

- Nonenhancing lesion at root apex
  - T1 hypointense and T2 hyperintense

DIFFERENTIAL DIAGNOSIS

Lateral Periodontal Cyst

- Developmental cyst from dental lamina remnants
- Usually associated with lateral root surface of mandibular premolar **vital** teeth

Keratocystic Odontogenic Tumor (Odontogenic Keratocyst)

- Large expansile cystic mass, usually within alveolus of posterior mandible
- Small keratocystic odontogenic tumor may be **adjacent to root apex**

Dentigerous (Follicular) Cyst

- Developmental lesion around **crown** of unerupted or impacted teeth
- Unilocular cyst, most often mandibular 3rd molar

PATHOLOGY

General Features

- Etiology
  - **Develops after inflammation and necrosis of pulp ("nonvital" tooth)**
    - Most often from dental caries, periodontal disease
    - Less often posttraumatic
  - Pulp necrosis → growth of epithelial rests of Malassez in periodontal ligament
  - Central liquefaction necrosis of epithelial rests → cyst formation

CLINICAL ISSUES

Presentation

- Most common signs/symptoms
  - Usually **asymptomatic** unless secondary infection
- Other signs/symptoms
  - Intermittent intense jaw pain or pain with chewing

Demographics

- Age
  - Any age; most prevalent 3rd-5th decade
- Epidemiology
  - **Most common odontogenic cyst**
  - ~ 15% of all periapical lesions

Natural History & Prognosis

- May progress to periapical abscess ± cellulitis

Treatment

- Treatment depends on degree of inflammation
  - Endodontic therapy (root canal)
  - Tooth extraction with antibiotics if destruction of tooth severe and tooth is nonrestorable

DIAGNOSTIC CHECKLIST

Reporting Tips

- Report relationship of lesion to adjacent, important structures
  - Maxillary teeth: Maxillary sinus
  - Mandible: Inferior alveolar nerve canal

SELECTED REFERENCES

1. Chapman MN et al: Periapical lucency around the tooth: radiologic evaluation and differential diagnosis. Radiographics. 33(1):E15-32, 2013
2. Curé JK et al: Radiopaque jaw lesions: an approach to the differential diagnosis. Radiographics. 32(7):1909-25, 2012

Dentigerous Cyst

TERMINOLOGY

- Benign developmental jaw cyst associated with crown of unerupted tooth
- Synonym = follicular cyst

IMAGING

- Well-circumscribed, expansile cyst **surrounding crown of unerupted or impacted tooth**
- Sclerotic border spares osseous cortex
- Typically displaces teeth, rarely resorbs
- 75% found in mandible
- Mandibular 3rd molars > maxillary 3rd molars > maxillary canines

TOP DIFFERENTIAL DIAGNOSES

- Keratocystic odontogenic tumor
- Ameloblastoma
- Periapical (radicular) cyst

PATHOLOGY

- Arises after developmental anomaly during formation of enamel (amelogenesis)
- Slow-growing benign cyst
- 20% of all odontogenic cysts

CLINICAL ISSUES

- Most patients asymptomatic
- Symptomatic if cyst infection or fracture
- Recurrence rare following complete resection
- Ameloblastomas may develop in cyst wall
- Malignant transformation to carcinoma is rare

DIAGNOSTIC CHECKLIST

- When reviewing odontogenic cysts distinguishing lesions can be difficult
  - Cyst always related to unerupted tooth crown
  - Typically remains unilocular even when large

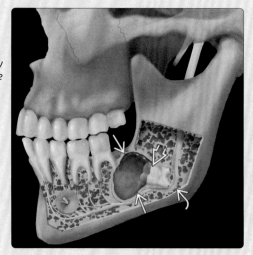
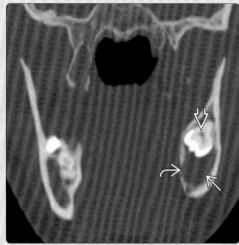

(Left) Lateral graphic of mandible with the lateral cortical surface removed depicts a classic unilocular dentigerous cyst ➡ intimately related to the crown ➡ of the unerupted 3rd mandibular molar tooth. The inferior alveolar canal ➡ is displaced by the molar. (Right) Coronal bone CT demonstrates an impacted left 3rd mandibular molar ➡ associated with the smooth-walled cyst ➡ that expands the mandible and thins the lingual cortex ➡. The cyst abuts the crown and has no calcifications or periosteal reaction.

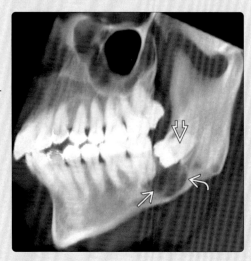
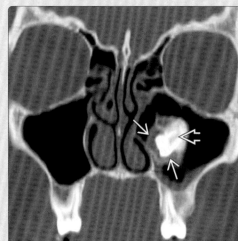

(Left) Ray-sum CT rendering depicts the appearance of a classic dentigerous cyst. The impacted mandibular molar ➡ has a well-defined unilocular cyst ➡ adjacent to the crown. The cyst and molar displace the inferior alveolar canal ➡ inferiorly. (Right) Coronal bone CT demonstrates an impacted maxillary 3rd molar tooth ➡ displaced into the maxillary sinus. A small cyst is evident ➡, arising from around the crown. Dentigerous cysts typically displace the tooth in the direction opposite of the vector of the cyst.

Dentigerous Cyst

TERMINOLOGY

Synonyms
- Follicular cyst

Definitions
- Benign developmental jaw cyst associated with crown of unerupted tooth
- Dentigerous means "having teeth"; lesion is intimately associated with tooth

IMAGING

General Features
- Best diagnostic clue
  o Well-circumscribed, expansile cyst surrounding **crown of unerupted or impacted tooth**
- Location
  o **75% found in mandible**
  o Mandibular 3rd molars > maxillary 3rd molars > maxillary canines
- Size
  o Variable; ≥ 1 cm
- Morphology
  o Unilocular cyst; rarely multilocular

Radiographic Findings
- Radiography
  o Well-demarcated cyst surrounding crown of unerupted tooth
    – Typically displaces teeth
    – Less commonly resorbs apical tooth structures

CT Findings
- Bone CT
  o Thin-walled, well-circumscribed cyst surrounding crown of unerupted tooth
  o Sclerotic border spares osseous cortex
  o Maxilla lesion may extend into sinus
  o Tendency to displace tooth in opposite direction of cyst

MR Findings
- T1WI
  o Low to intermediate signal intensity cyst
    – May contain proteinaceous material or cholesterol crystals; ↑ T1 signal
- T2WI
  o Homogeneously hyperintense signal in cyst
  o Thin corticated rim is hypointense
- T1WI C+ FS
  o No solid enhancement within cyst; cyst wall thin rim of uniform enhancement

Imaging Recommendations
- Best imaging tool
  o Thin-slice bone CT
- Protocol advice
  o **Bone algorithm** thin-section CT of face with axial & coronal reformats

DIFFERENTIAL DIAGNOSIS

Keratocystic Odontogenic Tumor (Odontogenic Keratocyst)
- Uni- or multilocular cystic mass
- Envelops entire unerupted tooth, does **not** arise from crown
- More likely to have aggressive bone changes

Ameloblastoma
- May be unilocular, exactly mimicking dentigerous cyst
- May be unilocular with enhancing nodule
- May be multilocular expansile mass

Periapical (Radicular) Cyst
- Small cyst at root of tooth (tooth apex)
- Associated with caries or periodontal disease

PATHOLOGY

General Features
- Etiology
  o Developmental anomaly occurring during formation of enamel (amelogenesis)
  o Fluid accumulates between reduced enamel epithelium & surface → cyst surrounding crown

CLINICAL ISSUES

Presentation
- Most common signs/symptoms
  o Most patients **asymptomatic**
- Other signs/symptoms
  o Symptomatic if cyst infection or fracture

Demographics
- Age
  o 2nd-4th decade
- Epidemiology
  o 2nd most common jaw cyst after radicular cysts

Natural History & Prognosis
- Slow-growing benign cyst
- Recurrence rare following complete resection
- Mural ameloblastomas may occur
- Malignant transformation to carcinoma is rare

Treatment
- Enucleation of cyst & extraction of unerupted tooth
- Marsupialization or fenestration of cyst may preserve permanent tooth in children

DIAGNOSTIC CHECKLIST

Reporting Tips
- Describe bone remodeling secondary to lesion
  o Displacement of inferior alveolar canal
  o Bowing of floor of maxillary sinus, extension to orbit

SELECTED REFERENCES

1. Mosier KM: Lesions of the jaw. Semin Ultrasound CT MR. 36(5):444-50, 2015
2. Mosier KM: Magnetic resonance imaging of the maxilla and mandible: signal characteristics and features in the differential diagnosis of common lesions. Top Magn Reson Imaging. 24(1):23-37, 2015

Simple Bone Cyst (Traumatic)

KEY FACTS

TERMINOLOGY

- Solitary bony cavity; "cyst" designation is misnomer

IMAGING

- CT: Solitary well-corticated, lucent area in body, ramus, or condyle of mandible
  - Homogeneously iso- to hypodense with no internal calcification or matrix
- T2 MR: Hyperintense; no fluid-fluid levels
- T1 C+ MR: Delayed enhancement key

TOP DIFFERENTIAL DIAGNOSES

- Aneurysmal bone cyst
- Periapical (radicular) cyst
- Giant cell granuloma of mandible-maxilla
- Keratocystic odontogenic tumor
- Unicystic ameloblastoma

PATHOLOGY

- Cystic cavity with connective tissue membrane; no epithelial lining
- "Traumatic" designation misnomer; < 1/2 associated with prior trauma
- May be found adjacent to osteomas, fibroosseous lesions, hypercementosis

CLINICAL ISSUES

- Incidental finding on imaging
- 10-30 years
- Variable but low recurrence rate reported
- Treatment: Surgical exploration to exclude other odontogenic lesions

DIAGNOSTIC CHECKLIST

- Look for association with teeth, cortical thinning and erosion, enhancement pattern to exclude other odontogenic lesions

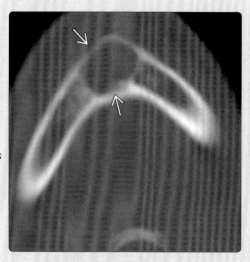

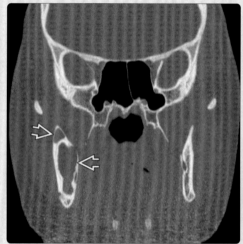

(Left) Axial bone CT shows a unilocular simple bone cyst in the symphyseal mandible with a well-defined, corticated cortex ➡. Despite the size, there is no significant bony expansion. (Right) Coronal bone CT demonstrates a lucent ➡ right mandibular lesion involving/expanding the posterior mandibular body, angle, and ramus. The cortex is thinned over the lucent component but intact over the sclerotic component. There is a thin lucent zone surrounding the sclerotic component.

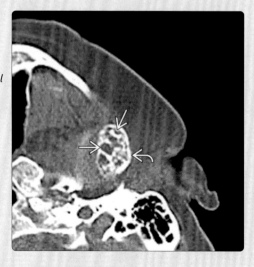

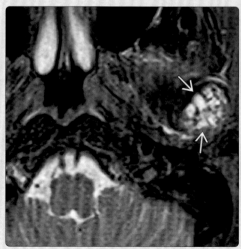

(Left) Axial bone CT shows multiple cystic foci in the mandibular condyle ➡ with thickened and intact septations. Note the cortex is also intact ➡. The differential for this appearance necessarily includes aneurysmal bone cyst and central giant cell granuloma. (Right) Axial T2WI FS MR in the same patient shows the typical hyperintensity of the cystic cavities ➡ without fluid-fluid levels. At surgical exploration, the diagnosis of simple bone cyst was made.

Simple Bone Cyst (Traumatic)

TERMINOLOGY

Abbreviations

- Simple bone cyst (SBC)

Synonyms

- Solitary or traumatic bone cyst

Definitions

- SBC: Solitary bony cavity; "cyst" designation is misnomer

IMAGING

General Features

- Best diagnostic clue
  - Single corticated lucent area in body, ramus, or condyle of mandible
- Location
  - Anywhere in mandible; most common in posterior molar regions, ramus
  - Maxillary lesions rare; more common in female patients
- Size
  - Typically 1 cm or larger
- Morphology
  - Nonexpansile; very well defined

Radiographic Findings

- Intraoral plain film
  - Well-defined, unilocular radiolucency superimposed over or below root apices
  - Lamina dura and periodontal ligament space of involved teeth intact

CT Findings

- CECT
  - Mildly enhancing at periphery
- Bone CT
  - Solitary well-corticated, lucent area in body, ramus, or condyle of mandible
  - Typically **nonexpansile**; if present, very mild
    - Bone margins uniform, not scalloped
  - Sclerotic margins or osteophytic reaction at cortical surface possible
    - No internal septations
  - No association with teeth

MR Findings

- T2WI
  - Homogeneous hyperintensity without fluid-fluid levels
- T1WI C+
  - Mildly enhancing
  - Dynamic contrast: Enhancement from margin to center on delayed images

DIFFERENTIAL DIAGNOSIS

Aneurysmal Bone Cyst

- More prevalent in maxilla than SBC
- Bone CT appearance often identical to SBC
- Fluid-fluid levels on T2 MR

Periapical (Radicular) Cyst

- Associated with caries and periodontal disease

- Lucent or lytic lesion at tooth root apex
- Lamina dura and periodontal ligament space is lost in associated tooth

Giant Cell Granuloma of Mandible-Maxilla

- Large lesions usually have septations
- Tend to be expansile

Keratocystic Odontogenic Tumor

- Older patients (> 30 years of age)
- Bone margin not as well defined or corticated
- Large lesions expand longitudinally or concentrically

Unicystic Ameloblastoma

- Older patients (> 30 years of age)
- Bone margin not as well defined or corticated
- Enhancement throughout lesion on CT, MR

PATHOLOGY

General Features

- Etiology
  - Unknown; hypothesized etiologies include
    - Medullary infarct following trauma but < 1/2 associated with prior trauma
    - Disturbance in osteoblast differentiation or altered bone metabolism

Gross Pathologic & Surgical Features

- Empty/partially empty bone cavity with straw-colored fluid or old necrosis

Microscopic Features

- Cystic cavity with connective tissue membrane; **no epithelial lining**
- Some have dysplastic bone at margins

CLINICAL ISSUES

Presentation

- Most common signs/symptoms
  - Incidental finding on imaging
- Other signs/symptoms
  - Pain, swelling if associated with trauma

Demographics

- Age
  - 10-30 years

Natural History & Prognosis

- Recurrence rate variable (~ 2-26%); higher with multiple lesions (~ 70%)
- Account for ~ 1% of jaw cysts

Treatment

- Surgery to exclude other odontogenic lesions

SELECTED REFERENCES

1. Harmon M et al: A radiological approach to benign and malignant lesions of the mandible. Clin Radiol. 70(4):335-50, 2015
2. Suei Y et al: Radiographic findings and prognosis of simple bone cysts of the jaws. Dentomaxillofac Radiol. 39(2):65-71, 2010
3. Matsuzaki H et al: MR imaging in the assessment of a solitary bone cyst. Eur J Radiol. 45(1): 37-42, 2003

KEY FACTS

TERMINOLOGY

- Definition: Developmental cyst arising from nasopalatine duct

IMAGING

- Bone CT findings
  - Well-circumscribed, rounded enlargement of maxillary incisive canal
  - Incisive canal with diameter **> 1 cm** is presumed nasopalatine duct cyst
  - Lamina dura and periodontal ligament space of adjacent teeth intact
- MR findings
  - Homogeneously iso- to hyperintense T1, hyperintense T2 signal
  - Typically nonenhancing

TOP DIFFERENTIAL DIAGNOSES

- Periapical (radicular) cyst
- Residual cyst
- Apical periodontitis
- Median palatal cyst
- Keratocystic odontogenic tumor
- Dentigerous (follicular) cyst

CLINICAL ISSUES

- Most common nonodontogenic fissural cyst
- Clinical presentation
  - Incidental finding on CT or MR
  - Less commonly pain, swelling of anterior maxilla
- Treatment: Enucleation via palatine or buccal approach
  - Recurrence rate very low

DIAGNOSTIC CHECKLIST

- Single rounded corticated lucent cyst in midline maxilla
- Look for widening along paired nasopalatine ducts
- Report extension to nasal cavity or displacement of teeth by larger lesions

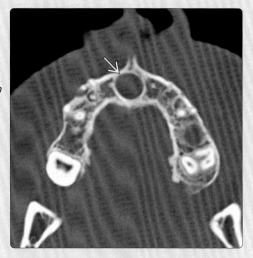 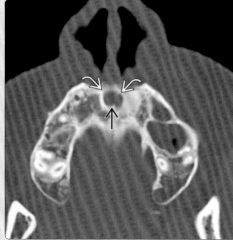

(Left) *Axial bone CT shows a corticated uniform and concentric expansion of the incisive canal in the midline maxillary alveolus* ➡, *typical of nasopalatine duct cyst.* (Right) *Axial bone CT shows an expansile nasopalatine duct cyst extending superiorly along the paired nasopalatine ducts* ➡, *which are seen separated here by a very thin bony septation* ➡.

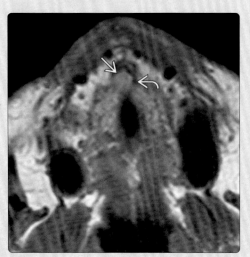 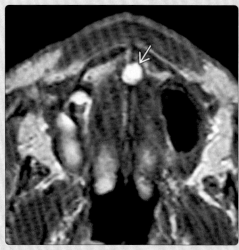

(Left) *Axial T1 MR shows an intermediate to slightly T1-hyperintense expansion of the incisive canal* ➡ *by a nasopalatine duct cyst. Note the thin but preserved cortex* ➡. (Right) *Axial T2 MR shows the classic MR appearance of a nasopalatine duct cyst. Note the uniformly round, homogeneously T2 hyperintense area in the midline maxilla* ➡.

TERMINOLOGY

Abbreviations

- Nasopalatine duct cyst (NPDC)

Synonyms

- Incisive canal cyst

Definitions

- Developmental cyst arising from nasopalatine duct
- **Most common** nonodontogenic fissural cyst

IMAGING

General Features

- Best diagnostic clue
  - Well-circumscribed, rounded enlargement of incisive canal in maxilla
- Location
  - Incisive canal lingual (posterior) to maxillary central incisor teeth
- Size
  - ≥ 1 cm
    - Incisive canal with diameter **> 1 cm** is presumed NPDC

Imaging Recommendations

- Best imaging tool
  - Thin-section bone algorithm CT
- Protocol advice
  - Thin-section facial bone CT with axial, coronal, sagittal reformations

CT Findings

- NECT
  - Lesion is hypodense
- Bone CT
  - **Smooth, rounded enlargement of incisive canal of > 1 cm**
  - May cause thinning and dehiscence of lingual cortex of maxilla
  - Larger lesions will extend to nasal cavity
  - Lamina dura and periodontal ligament (PDL) space of adjacent teeth intact

MR Findings

- Homogeneously iso- to hyperintense T1, hyperintense T2 signal
- Typically nonenhancing
  - May enhance with inflammatory component

DIFFERENTIAL DIAGNOSIS

Periapical (Radicular) Cyst

- Cyst arising from infected tooth
- Associated with caries/periodontal disease in maxillary teeth
- **Not** centrally located within incisive canal but may involve it secondarily

Residual Cyst

- Persistent radicular cyst remaining after extraction or loss of infected tooth
- Adjacent to, **not** centrally located within incisive canal

Apical Periodontitis

- Infection at apex of tooth root associated with caries/periodontal disease
- Loss of lamina dura and widening of PDL space at/around root apex
- Lytic area millimeters to centimeters in size; noncorticated
- May extend into incisive canal secondarily

Median Palatal Cyst

- Developmental cyst of newborn
- Located at junction of hard and soft palate

Keratocystic Odontogenic Tumor (Odontogenic Keratocyst)

- Unilocular cystic mass ± associated teeth
- When large, expands and may erode maxilla
- Typically arises in canine region in maxilla, molars in mandible; rare in midline maxilla

Dentigerous (Follicular) Cyst

- Most common odontogenic cyst
- Arises from around **crown** of unerupted or impacted teeth

PATHOLOGY

General Features

- Etiology
  - Fissural cyst arising from embryological remnants of incisive canal between oral & nasal cavities

Microscopic Features

- Cyst lined by respiratory ± stratified squamous epithelium

CLINICAL ISSUES

Presentation

- Most common signs/symptoms
  - Incidental finding on CT or MR
- Other signs/symptoms
  - Pain, swelling of anterior maxilla

Demographics

- Age
  - Typically diagnosed at 30-40 years of age
- Gender
  - Males slightly > females

Natural History & Prognosis

- Recurrence rate very low; < 2% when enucleated

Treatment

- Surgical enucleation via palatine or buccal approach

SELECTED REFERENCES

1. Gohel A et al: Benign jaw lesions. Dent Clin North Am. 60(1):125-41, 2016
2. Sane VD et al: Role of cone-beam computed tomography in diagnosis and management of nasopalatine duct cyst. J Craniofac Surg. 25(1):e92-4, 2014
3. Sirotheau Corrêa Pontes F et al: Nonendodontic lesions misdiagnosed as apical periodontitis lesions: series of case reports and review of literature. J Endod. 40(1):16-27, 2014
4. Chapman MN et al: Periapical lucency around the tooth: radiologic evaluation and differential diagnosis. Radiographics. 33(1):E15-32, 2013
5. Hisatomi M et al: MR imaging of epithelial cysts of the oral and maxillofacial region. Eur J Radiol. 48(2):178-82, 2003
6. Swanson KS et al: Nasopalatine duct cyst: an analysis of 334 cases. J Oral Maxillofac Surg. 49(3):268-71, 1991

TMJ Juvenile Idiopathic Arthritis

TERMINOLOGY

- Juvenile idiopathic arthritis (JIA)
- **Autoimmune** musculoskeletal synovial inflammatory disease of childhood

IMAGING

- Bone CT best demonstrates contours of TMJ
  - Flat, deformed mandibular condyles & wide, flat condylar fossae
  - Condyle concavity or bifid
  - Bilateral disease more common than unilateral
  - May have secondary osteoarthritis with osteophytes
- MR may show joint space enhancement & early inflammation before joint destruction
  - TMJ discs thin, perforated, or absent
- In cervical spine, may see atlantoaxial subluxation, vertebral fusion, & ↓ AP vertebral body dimension

TOP DIFFERENTIAL DIAGNOSES

- TMJ condylar hypoplasia
- TMJ degenerative disease
- TMJ synovitis/capsulitis

CLINICAL ISSUES

- JIA affects 1-22 per 1,000 children worldwide
- TMJ involved in 20-90% of children with JIA
  - More likely if systemic disease, young age at diagnosis, & long duration of activity
- TMJ and masticator muscle pain, decreased range of jaw motion, retrognathia, micrognathia
- **70% asymptomatic** when MR shows acute arthritis
- Treat with either or both local &/or systemic therapy
  - Local: Occlusal devices, arthrocentesis, intraarticular injections
  - Systemic: NSAIDs, methotrexate, sulfasalazine

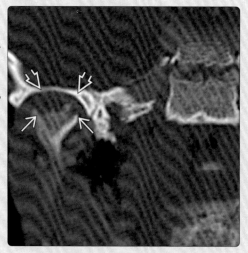
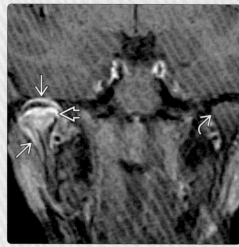

(Left) Coronal bone CT in a 4-year-old girl with juvenile idiopathic arthritis (JIA) demonstrates irregular chronic erosion of right mandibular condyle ➡. Note also wide, flattened condylar fossa ➡. (Right) Coronal T1WI C+ FS MR in the same child with JIA reveals marked inflammatory enhancement involving joint ➡ and marrow space of right mandibular condyle ➡. Left TMJ ➡ shows no inflammatory change, normal condyle, and normal condylar fossa.

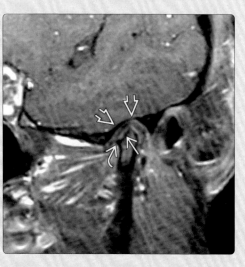
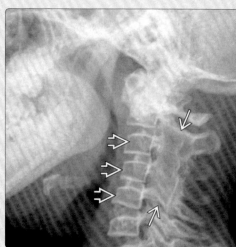

(Left) Sagittal oblique T1WI C+ FS MR in a 21-year-old woman with longstanding JIA reveals small mandibular condyle with irregular, low-intensity sclerotic margins ➡ and widened, flat condylar fossa ➡. There is no inflammatory enhancement, but note the small anterior osteophyte ➡ from secondary osteoarthritis. (Right) Lateral radiograph in a 13-year-old girl with JIA demonstrates classic fusion of posterior elements of C2-5 ➡ and decreased AP dimension of corresponding vertebral bodies ➡.

TERMINOLOGY

Abbreviations

- Juvenile idiopathic arthritis (JIA)

Synonyms

- Juvenile rheumatoid/chronic arthritis

Definitions

- **Autoimmune** musculoskeletal synovial inflammatory disease of childhood
- Begins < 16 years of age

IMAGING

General Features

- Best diagnostic clue
  - Bilateral flat, deformed mandibular condyles with wide condylar fossae
- Location
  - Primarily large joints: Knees, wrists, ankles
  - Head & neck: TMJ, craniovertebral junction, & cervical spine

CT Findings

- Bone CT
  - Flat & deformed mandibular condyles + wide, flat condylar fossae
  - Bilateral > unilateral
  - May have secondary osteoarthritis with joint space narrowing & osteophyte formation
  - In cervical spine, may see **atlantoaxial subluxation**
    - Fusion & ↓ AP vertebral body dimension

MR Findings

- T1WI
  - Flat & deformed mandibular condyles + wide, flat condylar fossae
- T2WI
  - Hyperintense joint effusion, bone marrow edema, &/or subchondral cysts less common
  - TMJ discs thin, perforated, or absent
- T1WI C+
  - **Joint space enhancement**
  - May see early inflammation before joint destruction
  - May be abnormal without symptoms
- **Dynamic imaging**: Decreased condyle translation
- **Cervical spine & craniovertebral junction**
  - Atlantoaxial subluxation
  - Cranial settling, basilar invagination
  - Fusions → ankylosis and ↓ AP dimension vertebral bodies

DIFFERENTIAL DIAGNOSIS

TMJ Condylar Hypoplasia

- Bilateral: Pierre Robin & Treacher Collins
- Unilateral: Hemifacial microsomia

TMJ Degenerative Disease

- Articular disc displaced anterior in position

TMJ Synovitis/Capsulitis

- Enhancing synovium/capsule

PATHOLOGY

Staging, Grading, & Classification

- International League of Associations for Rheumatology (ILAR) is most wisely used classification
  - 7 subtypes based on clinical features during first 6 months of disease
    - Oligoarticular JIA (50-60%)
    - Polyarticular JIA rheumatoid factor positive & negative (30-35%)
    - Systemic JIA (10-20%)
    - Juvenile psoriatic arthritis (2-15%)
    - Enthesitis-related arthritis (1-7%)
    - Undifferentiated arthritis

CLINICAL ISSUES

Presentation

- Most common signs/symptoms
  - In children with MR findings of acute TMJ arthritis, **70% asymptomatic**
  - TMJ and masticator muscle pain
- Other signs/symptoms
  - **Retrognathia**
  - Mandibular growth disturbance → **micrognathia**
  - Facial asymmetry
  - Unilateral mandibular hypoplasia
  - Chewing difficulties & decreased mouth opening (decreased maximal incisor opening)
  - Posterior rotation of mandible

Demographics

- Epidemiology
  - Most common childhood autoimmune musculoskeletal inflammatory disease
    - TMJ involved in 20-90% of children & ≤ 70% adults with longstanding JIA
    - TMJ involvement more likely if systemic disease, young age at diagnosis, & long duration of activity
  - F >> M

Treatment

- Systemic therapy
  - NSAIDs, corticosteroids, methotrexate, sulfasalazine, biologic agents (monoclonal antibodies or soluble receptors)
- Local therapy
  - Arthrocentesis
  - Occlusal devices and functional appliances
  - Intraarticular injections

SELECTED REFERENCES

1. Kristensen KD et al: Clinical predictors of temporomandibular joint arthritis in juvenile idiopathic arthritis: a systematic literature review. Semin Arthritis Rheum. 45(6):717-32, 2016
2. von Kalle T et al: Early detection of temporomandibular joint arthritis in children with juvenile idiopathic arthritis - the role of contrast-enhanced MRI. Pediatr Radiol. 45(3):402-10, 2015

Mandible-Maxilla Osteomyelitis

TERMINOLOGY

- Definition: Polymicrobial bacterial infection, usually odontogenic, of mandible > maxilla

IMAGING

- CECT/bone CT findings
  - Acute osteomyelitis: Bone destruction, tooth/socket abnormality ± associated soft tissue abscess
  - Chronic osteomyelitis: Bone sclerosis with periosteal reaction ± sequestrum
- Enhanced MR findings
  - MR sensitive for acute and chronic osteomyelitis
  - Shows full extent of mandible marrow involvement
  - If dental amalgam obscures CT, MR may show subtle abscess formation not seen by CT
- Serial exams may be necessary to confirm osteomyelitis & document positive clinical response

TOP DIFFERENTIAL DIAGNOSES

- Mandible-maxilla osteoradionecrosis
- Mandible-maxilla bisphosphonate osteonecrosis
- Infiltrative neoplasm invading mandible
  - Alveolar ridge or other perimandibular squamous cell carcinoma
  - Mandibular non-Hodgkin lymphoma
  - Mandibular metastasis
- Primary chronic osteomyelitis
- Langerhans histiocytosis, mandible-maxilla

DIAGNOSTIC CHECKLIST

- Identify source of infection
  - Infected tooth ± periapical abscess by far most common source
  - Other sources: Posttraumatic or postsurgical site
- Interrogate soft tissues of masticator & submandibular spaces for abscess & fistulous tract

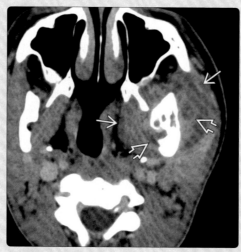 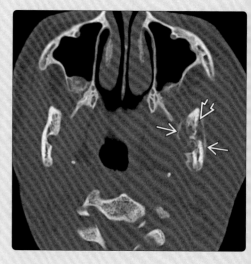

(Left) Axial CECT in a 15 yr old with previous surgical repair of a mandibular fracture, now with swelling & pain in the left cheek, reveals marked inflammation of left masticator space ➡. The foci of low density represent early transformation of phlegmon to abscess ➡. (Right) Axial bone CT in the same patient shows periosteal reaction along the cortex of the mandibular ramus ➡ and both permeative and sclerotic bone changes centrally ➡. Findings suggest osteomyelitis.

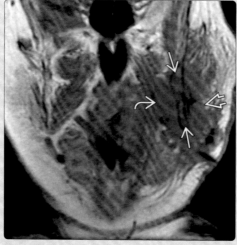 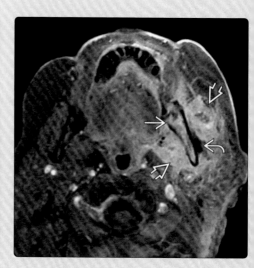

(Left) Coronal T1WI MR shows 79 yr old with recurrent masticator space abscess 12 weeks after initial diagnosis and drainage. Normal high signal marrow fat has been replaced ➡ in left hemimandible, consistent with osteomyelitis. Note edema in medial pterygoid ➡ and masseter ➡ muscles. (Right) Axial T1WI C+ FS MR in the same patient reveals diffuse enhancement of the left marrow space ➡ with masticator space enhancement (phlegmon) ➡ and small lateral compartment abscess ➡.

TERMINOLOGY

Synonyms

- Acute osteomyelitis or secondary chronic osteomyelitis

Definitions

- Polymicrobial bacterial infection, usually odontogenic, of mandible > maxilla

IMAGING

General Features

- Best diagnostic clue
  - CECT/bone CT
    - Acute: Lytic, permeative changes in mandible with soft tissue inflammation
    - Chronic: Sclerotic or permeative-sclerotic changes with periosteal reaction & sequestrum

Imaging Recommendations

- Best imaging tool
  - CECT: Use both soft tissue and bone algorithms

Radiographic Findings

- Acute: Ill-defined lucency of bone
- Chronic: Sclerotic or sclerotic-permeative pattern; periosteal reaction

CT Findings

- CECT
  - Phlegmon/frank abscess often present in perimandibular, submandibular, sublingual, & masticator spaces
  - Transspatial induration/enhancement common
- Bone CT
  - Acute: Destruction of cancellous & cortical bone
    - Associated soft tissue edema, phlegmon, or abscess
  - Chronic: Bony sclerosis, laminar periosteal reaction, sequestrum

MR Findings

- T1WI
  - Loss of T1 signal as marrow fat replaced by edema and exudate (acute) or fibrosis/sclerosis (chronic)
- STIR
  - Acute: Marked marrow hyperintensity
  - Chronic: Variable, depending on degree of fibrosis & sclerosis
- T1WI C+ FS
  - Acute: Marked marrow space enhancement
  - Chronic: Variable enhancement

Nuclear Medicine Findings

- 3-phase bone scan with Tc-99m MDP is sensitive/specific

DIFFERENTIAL DIAGNOSIS

Mandible-Maxilla Osteoradionecrosis

- Bone loss with intraosseous gas 6-12 months post radiation

Mandible-Maxilla Bisphosphonate Osteonecrosis

- Bone loss occurring with current/previous bisphosphonate therapy

Infiltrative Neoplasm Invading Mandible

- Can produce invasive soft tissue mass & bone destruction
- Alveolar ridge squamous cell carcinoma
- Mandibular non-Hodgkin lymphoma
- Mandibular metastasis
- Sclerotic metastasis can mimic chronic osteomyelitis

Primary Chronic Osteomyelitis

- More insidious course, with greater involvement of mandible
- May present as manifestation of systemic disease
  - Chronic recurrent multifocal osteomyelitis
  - Synovitis, acne, pustulosis, hyperostosis, osteomyelitis

PATHOLOGY

General Features

- Etiology
  - Nonodontogenic: Trauma, postsurgical, hematogenous (rare)

Staging, Grading, & Classification

- Acute (signs/symptoms < 4 weeks); chronic (> 4 weeks)
- May need image-guided FNA of soft tissue or bony component for culture

Gross Pathologic & Surgical Features

- Acute: Purulent exudate
- Chronic: Devitalized bone, fibrosis, & chronic inflammation

Microscopic Features

- Acute: Marrow exudate with neutrophils, fibrin, necrotic debris, and microorganisms
- Chronic: Marrow fibrosis, periosteal reaction, osteoblastic sclerosis, sequestrum

CLINICAL ISSUES

Presentation

- Most common signs/symptoms
  - Pain, swelling, and tenderness of jaw

Natural History & Prognosis

- Inadequate treatment leads to bone destruction, abscess, & fistula

Treatment

- Acute: Oral ± IV antibiotics; abscess drainage
- Chronic: Surgical debridement, hyperbaric oxygen

DIAGNOSTIC CHECKLIST

Consider

- Consider malignancy if persistent soft tissue lesion with bone destruction
- Serial physical and CT exams may be necessary to confirm osteomyelitis & document positive clinical response

SELECTED REFERENCES

1. Schuknecht B et al: Osteomyelitis of the mandible. Neuroimaging Clin N Am. 13(3):605-18, 2003

TMJ Calcium Pyrophosphate Dihydrate Deposition Disease

KEY FACTS

TERMINOLOGY

- Calcium pyrophosphate deposition disease (**CPPD**)
- **Metabolic disease** resulting in peri- or intraarticular **chondrocalcinosis**
  - **Tophaceous (tumoral)** TMJ form most prevalent
- Synonym: Pseudogout

IMAGING

- Calcified TMJ lesion
  - May involve masticator or parotid space or adjacent skull base
- Bone CT
  - Mild/early CPPD: Subtle calcifications in TMJ
  - Late/severe CPPD →
    - Chunky **diffusely calcified** mass
    - Calcified mass may have **ground-glass** appearance
    - Associated remodeling, erosion, or mass effect on condyle
  - 50% have involvement of multiple joints

- MR
  - T1: **Low-** to intermediate-signal lesion; capsule & joint space expansion
  - T2: **Hypointense**, somewhat heterogeneous mass
  - T1 C+: Heterogeneously enhancing TMJ lesion

TOP DIFFERENTIAL DIAGNOSES

- Synovial chondromatosis
- Chondrosarcoma
- Chondroblastoma
- Pigmented villonodular synovitis

PATHOLOGY

- **CP crystals** in synovial fluid are diagnostic
  - In polarized light, crystals are **birefringent**

CLINICAL ISSUES

- Presenting symptoms: Preauricular pain & swelling
- Treatment: Surgical excision + arthrocentesis

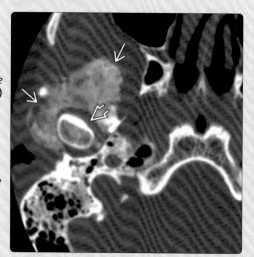
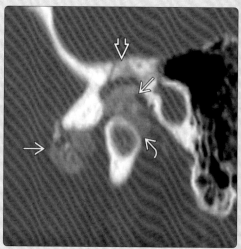

(Left) *Axial bone CT through the skull base reveals extensive calcific density surrounding the condyle and neck of the right mandible ➡. Note sparing of the joint space around the condyle ⇲. (Right) Sagittal bone CT reformation in the same patient better delineates the calcifications ➡ in relation to the TMJ. Note condylar fossa demineralization and erosion ⇲, resulting in a defect of the middle cranial fossa. The inferior joint space is compressed but spared ➡.*

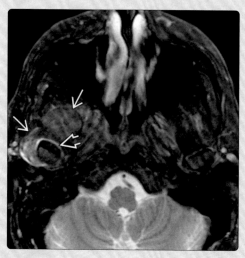
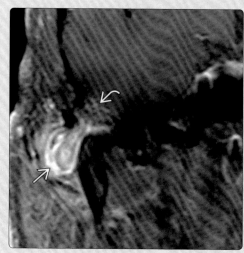

(Left) *Axial T2 FS MR in a patient with calcium pyrophosphate deposition disease in the right TMJ shows heterogeneous but predominantly low-signal intensity lesion ➡ along the margins of the TMJ. Note joint space fluid around the head of the mandibular condyle ⇲. (Right) Coronal T1 C+ FS MR shows enhancement of the inferolateral mass ➡. Note the glenoid fossa defect and mild dural enhancement ➡ without overt intracranial extension.*

TERMINOLOGY

Abbreviations

- Calcium pyrophosphate dihydrate deposition disease (CPPD)

Synonyms

- Pseudogout

Definitions

- **Metabolic disease** resulting in peri- or intraarticular **chondrocalcinosis**
  - **Tophaceous (tumoral) CPPD** form most prevalent in TMJ

IMAGING

General Features

- Best diagnostic clue
  - Calcified TMJ mass
- Location
  - Intracapsular > extracapsular
    - May involve masticator space (MS), parotid space (PS), adjacent skull base
- Size
  - Typically 1 cm or larger

CT Findings

- Bone CT
  - Mild/early CPPD: Subtle calcifications in TMJ
  - Late/severe CPPD
    - Chunky, **diffusely calcified** mass
    - Calcified mass may have **ground-glass** appearance
    - Associated degenerative changes with remodeling, erosion, or mass effect on condyle
    - May have associated demineralization/erosion of skull base, EAC
      - □ May mimic malignancy
  - **50% involve multiple joints**: Knee, hand, wrist, shoulder, spine

MR Findings

- T1WI
  - **Low-** to intermediate-signal TMJ lesion
  - Expansion of joint capsule & joint space
  - Remodeling or erosion of mandibular condyle
- T2WI
  - **Hypointense**, somewhat heterogeneous mass
- T1WI C+
  - Heterogeneously enhancing lesion

Imaging Recommendations

- Best imaging tool
  - Combination bone CT + TMJ MR
- Protocol advice
  - Thin-section bone CT, enhanced TMJ MR

DIFFERENTIAL DIAGNOSIS

Synovial Chondromatosis

- Multiple small, **calcified loose bodies** in superior joint space
  - Usually do not form contiguous solid mass

- Associated condylar osteoarthritis

Chondrosarcoma

- **Calcified** or partially calcified **TMJ mass**
- Tends to arise from or be intimately associated with condyle
- Condylar erosion, resorption
- T2 signal higher than with CPPD; more diffusely enhancing
- Often extends into MS, PS, skull base, temporal bone

Chondroblastoma

- Rare in TMJ
- Lytic condylar expansion ± calcified mass
- May infiltrate through disc & capsule
- 3rd decade; male predilection

Pigmented Villonodular Synovitis

- Intraarticular loose bodies T2 hypointense & noncalcified

PATHOLOGY

General Features

- Etiology
  - Exact pathophysiology unclear
    - Sporadic, familial, and secondary/metabolic forms
  - Unknown noxious event incites cascade that evolves toward hypertrophy & degeneration of chondrocytes
  - Rare in TMJ

Microscopic Features

- Calcium pyrophosphate **crystals** in synovial fluid is diagnostic
  - Crystals **birefringent** in polarized light
    - Gout = nonrefringent crystals of uric acid
- Metaplastic chondroid tissue; pleomorphic hyperchromatic nuclei

CLINICAL ISSUES

Presentation

- Most common signs/symptoms
  - Preauricular pain, swelling, trismus
  - Can cause hearing loss with temporal bone involvement
- Other signs/symptoms
  - Crepitus in TMJ

Treatment

- Surgical excision, arthrocentesis

SELECTED REFERENCES

1. Morales H et al: Imaging approach to temporomandibular joint disorders. Clin Neuroradiol. 26(1):5-22, 2016
2. Abdelsayed RA et al: Tophaceous pseudogout of the temporomandibular joint: a series of 3 cases. Oral Surg Oral Med Oral Pathol Oral Radiol. 117(3):369-75, 2014
3. Petscavage-Thomas JM et al: Unlocking the jaw: advanced imaging of the temporomandibular joint. AJR Am J Roentgenol. 203(5):1047-1058, 2014
4. Meltzer, DE at al: Extradiskal pathology of temporomandibular joint: MR imaging and CT manifestations. Neurographics. 3:185-193, 2013
5. Zweifel D et al: Tophaceuos calcium pyrophosphate dihydrate deposition disease of the temporomandibular joint: the preferential site? J Oral Maxillofac Surg. 70(1):60-7, 2012
6. Marsot-Dupuch K et al: Massive calcium pyrophosphate dihydrate crystal deposition disease: a cause of pain of the temporomandibular joint. AJNR Am J Neuroradiol. 25(5):876-9, 2004

TERMINOLOGY

- Pigmented villonodular synovitis (**PVNS**)
- Benign, locally aggressive, tumefactive disease of synovium

IMAGING

- CT: **Erosion** of mandibular **condyle** ± glenoid fossa
  - Lobulated, rounded lytic lesions
  - May extend to greater wing of sphenoid, temporal bone, intracranially
- T1 MR: **Hypointense** to isointense nodules with peripheral rim of low signal
- T2 MR: **Hypointense** lobulated nodules ± cystic areas of hyperintensity &/or joint effusion
  - Hypointensity due to **hemosiderin** deposition
    - Associated blooming artifact characteristic
- T1 C+ MR: Portions of mass may show mild enhancement
- Best imaging tool: Dedicated C+ MR & thin bone CT
- Interpretation pearl: T1/T2-hypointense joint nodules within TMJ joint are **noncalcified** on NECT

TOP DIFFERENTIAL DIAGNOSES

- Synovial chondromatosis
  - **Calcified nodules** in TMJ joint
- Giant cell tumor
- Chondrosarcoma
- Calcium pyrophosphate dihydrate deposition disease

PATHOLOGY

- Etiology: Unknown
  - Monarticular hyperplastic TMJ inflammation
- Plump histiocytes with **giant cells + hemosiderin**
- **Radiologic-pathologic correlation** important since histology may mimic sarcoma

CLINICAL ISSUES

- Presenting symptoms: Preauricular pain, swelling, trismus
- Age: 2nd-4th decades
- Gender: F:M = 3:1; recent data suggests F ~ M
- Treatment: Complete surgical resection

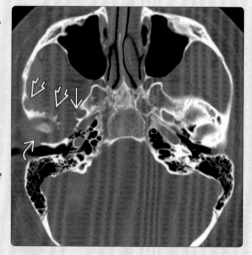
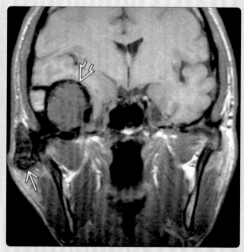

(Left) *Axial bone CT demonstrates widening of the right TMJ joint space* ➡ *and multiple rounded erosions of the adjacent skull base involving the internal aspect of the zygomatic arch* ➡ *and greater wing of the sphenoid up to the lateral margin of foramen ovale* ➡. **(Right)** *Coronal T1 MR shows a hypointense right TMJ mass* ➡ *with a periphery of lower signal intensity. A hypointense contiguous middle cranial fossa extraaxial mass* ➡ *is evident with similar markedly low-signal peripheral rim.*

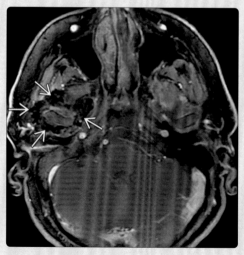
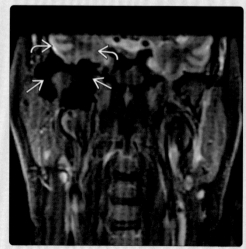

(Left) *Axial T1 C+ FS MR shows multiple nodular foci of hypointense signal* ➡ *in and surrounding the widened right TMJ joint space in this case of pigmented villonodular synovitis (PVNS). Note the minimal associated enhancement.* **(Right)** *Coronal STIR MR demonstrates nodular foci of markedly hypointense signal* ➡ *surrounding the right mandible condylar head in this case of PVNS. Note the "blooming" of the adjacent skull base from hemosiderin in these nodules* ➡, *a nearly pathognomonic finding.*

TERMINOLOGY

Abbreviations

- Pigmented villonodular synovitis (**PVNS**)

Definitions

- **Benign**, locally aggressive, **tumefactive disease of synovium**

IMAGING

General Features

- Best diagnostic clue
  - **Monarticular hyperplastic, inflammatory process involving TMJ**
- Location
  - Rare in TMJ
    - More common in knee, hip, shoulder, ankle, wrist
- Size
  - Typically 1 cm or > at diagnosis

Imaging Recommendations

- Best imaging tool
  - T2 & T1 C+ MR
- Protocol advice
  - TMJ & skull base enhanced MR & thin-section bone CT

CT Findings

- Bone CT
  - **Erosion** of mandibular condyle ± glenoid fossa
    - Lobulated, rounded **lytic** lesions
  - When large, erosive mass may extend to greater wing of sphenoid, temporal bone, & intracranially
  - **Joint nodules** are **noncalcified** (distinguishes from synovial chondromatosis)

MR Findings

- T1WI
  - Hypointense to isointense mass with **peripheral rim of low signal**
- T2WI
  - Hypointense, lobulated mass often with peripheral rim of low signal
    - Hypointensity due to **hemosiderin** deposition
  - Cystic areas of synovial fluid will be hyperintense ± joint effusion
- T1WI C+
  - Mild enhancement of portions of mass common

DIFFERENTIAL DIAGNOSIS

Synovial Chondromatosis

- Bone CT: **Calcified nodules** surrounding mandibular condyle
- MR: Multiple hypointense nodules in joint space (mimics PVNS)

Giant Cell Tumor

- Most commonly involves sphenoid & temporal bones in H&N
- Expansile mass with benign "eggshell" wall on bone CT
  - Multiple lytic lesions may have bubbly appearance

Chondrosarcoma

- Bone destruction on bone CT with variable chondroid calcified matrix
- Hypointense to isointense on T1, hyperintense to isointense on T2 MR
- Heterogeneously enhancing on CECT or T1 C+ MR

Calcium Pyrophosphate Dihydrate Deposition Disease

- Diffusely calcified mass involving TMJ on CT
- 50% involve multiple joints

PATHOLOGY

General Features

- Etiology
  - Unknown
    - Thought to represent inflammatory or reactive synovial infiltrate

Microscopic Features

- **Radiologic-pathologic correlation** important since histology may mimic sarcoma
- Plump histiocytes with **giant cells** + **hemosiderin**
- Erosion into surrounding bone; no atypia or mitoses
- Lymphoplasmacytic infiltrate and chondroid metaplasia

CLINICAL ISSUES

Presentation

- Most common signs/symptoms
  - Preauricular pain, swelling
- Other signs/symptoms
  - Trismus

Demographics

- Age
  - 2nd-4th decades
- Gender
  - F:M = 3:1; recent data suggests F ~ M

Natural History & Prognosis

- Low recurrence rate with complete resection

Treatment

- Complete surgical resection

DIAGNOSTIC CHECKLIST

Consider

- Both giant cell tumor & chondrosarcoma tend to enhance more than PVNS

Image Interpretation Pearls

- T1/T2-hypointense joint nodules within TMJ joint are noncalcified on NECT

SELECTED REFERENCES

1. Le WJ et al: Pigmented villonodular synovitis of the temporomandibular joint: CT imaging findings. Clin Imaging. 38(1):6-10, 2014
2. Murphey MD et al: Pigmented villonodular synovitis: radiologic-pathologic correlation. Radiographics. 28(5):1493-518, 2008
3. Kim KW et al: Pigmented villonodular synovitis of the temporomandibular joint: MR findings in four cases. Eur J Radiol. 49(3):229-34, 2004

KEY FACTS

TERMINOLOGY

- **Synovial metaplasia** with foci of **hyaline cartilage**

IMAGING

- **Calcified nodules** in superior joint space (SJS)
- Location: Most commonly found in SJS of TMJ
  - Rarely may have extracapsular extension
  - Locations: Masticator space, parotid space, intracranial
- Protocol: Thin-section multiplanar bone CT + MR TMJ
- Bone CT findings
  - **Calcified nodules** surround **mandibular condyle**
  - Degenerative changes involving condyle common
- T1/proton density MR findings
  - Multiple **hypo-** to **isointense nodules** in SJS
  - Separate from articular disc
- T2 MR: Superior joint space **effusion** ± expansion; fluid surrounds collection of hypointense nodules
- T1 C+ MR: Enhancing synovium

TOP DIFFERENTIAL DIAGNOSES

- Osteochondritis dissecans
- Calcium pyrophosphate dihydrate deposition disease
- Pigmented villonodular synovitis
- Osteochondroma
- Chondrosarcoma

PATHOLOGY

- **Synovial inflammation** with lymphocytes, macrophages, giant cells
- Milgram staging
  - Phase 1: Synovial metaplasia with no chondroid nodules
  - Phase 2: Active synovial metaplasia & chondroid nodules
  - Phase 3: Chondroid nodules with no active synovial disease

CLINICAL ISSUES

- Presenting symptoms: Preauricular pain, swelling
- Treatment: Arthroscopy, synovectomy, condylectomy

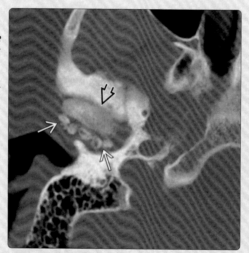
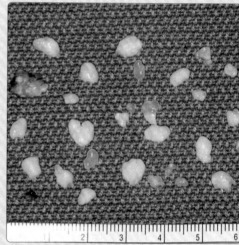

(Left) *Axial bone CT demonstrates multiple small, calcified nodules ➡ within the right temporomandibular joint (TMJ). The condyle is sclerotic and slightly irregular ➡ with anterior narrowing of the joint space due to degenerative change.* (Right) *Gross pathology specimen taken from TMJ affected by synovial chondromatosis shows calcified bodies exposed on a surgical towel. Notice the variable size of these nodules, from 2-10 millimeters.*

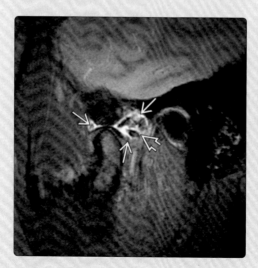
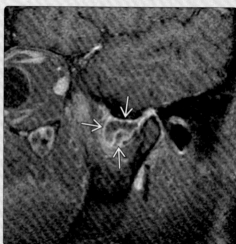

(Left) *Sagittal oblique T2 FS MR shows distension of the right TMJ capsule with hyperintense fluid ➡ surrounding the low-signal calcified loose bodies ➡.* (Right) *Sagittal T1 C+ FS MR reveals a rim-enhancing ➡ cystic lesion within the anterior aspect of the TMJ. The superior joint space is distended. The peripheral enhancement reflects enhancing synovium.*

TERMINOLOGY

Definitions

- **Synovial metaplasia** with formation of foci of **hyaline cartilage**

IMAGING

General Features

- Best diagnostic clue
  - Multiple **calcified nodules** ("loose bodies") in superior joint space (SJS)
- Location
  - Most commonly found in superior joint space of TMJ
  - Reported predilection for right TMJ
  - Rarely may have extracapsular extension
    - Most common areas of spread include masticator space, parotid space, or middle cranial fossa
- Size
  - Calcifications vary from millimeters to centimeters

Imaging Recommendations

- Best imaging tool
  - TMJ MR ± bone CT

CT Findings

- Bone CT
  - Multiple **calcified nodules** surrounding mandibular condyle
  - Condylar articular surface degenerative changes also commonly seen

MR Findings

- T1WI
  - Multiple **hypointense nodules** in superior joint space
  - Separate from articular disc
- T2WI
  - SJS > inferior joint space (IJS) effusion ± expansion
  - Fluid surrounds collection of hypointense nodules
- T1WI C+
  - Enhancing synovium

DIFFERENTIAL DIAGNOSIS

Osteochondritis Dissecans

- Results from transchondral fracture
  - Failure of healing & fragment displacement
- Condylar erosive defect with adjacent fragment

Calcium Pyrophosphate Dihydrate Deposition Disease

- Acute and chronic forms rare in TMJ
- Tophaceous pseudogout: Rare form of calcium pyrophosphate dihydrate most frequent in TMJ
  - Ca^{++} mass involving condyle or joint space; may mimic chondrosarcoma

Pigmented Villonodular Synovitis

- T2-hypointense nodules due to hemosiderin are **noncalcified** on CT

Osteochondroma

- Metaplasia of periosteum or osteochondral layer

- Produces cartilage → ossifies
- Characteristic cartilage cap
- Typically develops in & from tendinous attachment of pterygoid muscles
- Condylar head enlargement often present

Chondrosarcoma

- Lytic defects of condyle
- ~ 50% chondroid calcification
- Associated intra- &/or extracapsular enhancing mass

PATHOLOGY

General Features

- Etiology
  - Unknown
  - Typically secondary in TMJ to degenerative joint disease or prior trauma

Staging, Grading, & Classification

- Milgram staging
  - Phase 1: Synovial metaplasia with no chondroid nodules
  - Phase 2: Active synovial metaplasia & chondroid nodules
  - Phase 3: Chondroid nodules with no active synovial disease

Microscopic Features

- Synovial membrane **inflammation** with lymphocytes, macrophages, giant cells
- Cartilage metaplasia
- Fibroblast growth factor and TGFβ3 play role in genesis

CLINICAL ISSUES

Presentation

- Most common signs/symptoms
  - Preauricular pain, swelling
- Other signs/symptoms
  - Trismus; crepitus of joint

Demographics

- Age
  - Adults (mean: 4th decade)
- Gender
  - F:M = 4:1

Natural History & Prognosis

- Recurrence rate low
- Synovial chondrosarcoma arising within very rare but reported

Treatment

- Arthroscopy, synovectomy, condylectomy

SELECTED REFERENCES

1. Peyrot H et al: Synovial chondromatosis of the temporomandibular joint: CT and MRI findings. Diagn Interv Imaging. 95(6):613-4, 2014
2. Meng J et al: Clinical and radiologic findings of synovial chondromatosis affecting the temporomandibular joint. Oral Surg Oral Med Oral Pathol Oral Radiol Endod. 109(3):441-8, 2010
3. Wang P et al: Synovial chondromatosis of the temporomandibular joint: MRI findings with pathological comparison. Dentomaxillofac Radiol. 41(2):110-6, 2012
4. Murphey MD et al: Imaging of synovial chondromatosis with radiologic-pathologic correlation. Radiographics. 27(5):1465-88, 2007

KEY FACTS

TERMINOLOGY

- Giant cell reparative lesion of mandible > maxilla

IMAGING

- General imaging findings
  - Loculated, expansile mass with wavy septations
  - Anterior mandible ≥ body & ramus > maxilla
- Bone CT findings
  - **Expansile, multiloculated** midline mandibular lesion
  - Septations at **right angle** to cortex
  - Scalloping & cortical dehiscence common in large lesions
- Best imaging tool: CECT
  - Isodense (to muscle); **moderately enhancing** mass

TOP DIFFERENTIAL DIAGNOSES

- Aneurysmal bone cyst (ABC)
  - ~ 15% of central giant cell granulomas contain intralesional ABC
- Cherubism

- Ameloblastoma
- Ossifying fibroma
- Brown tumor of hyperparathyroidism

PATHOLOGY

- Unknown etiology; reactive granuloma vs. benign neoplasm
- Histopathology overlaps with giant cell tumor

CLINICAL ISSUES

- Presentation: Pain, swelling of mandible or maxilla
- Age at presentation: Adolescence to 3rd decade
- Treatment of choice: Surgical enucleation with peripheral ostectomy
- Large lesions may be treated with intralesional calcitonin or corticosteroids

DIAGNOSTIC CHECKLIST

- Expansile, septated, moderately enhancing mass in anterior mandible of young adult
- Report cortical perforation, root resorption

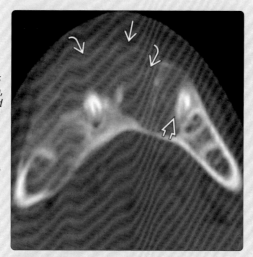

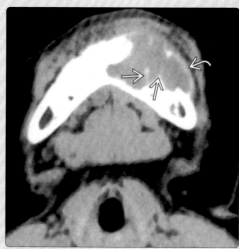

(Left) Axial bone CT shows a multiloculated, expansile central giant cell granuloma (CGCG) ➡ centered in the anterior mandible. Note the multiple thin, wavy septations ➡ characteristic of this lesion, giving the classically described soap bubble appearance. The lamina dura and roots of adjacent teeth ➡ are preserved. (Right) Axial NECT reveals an isodense, expansile, parasymphyseal mandibular CGCG. Septations spanning the lesion are subtle ➡. The buccal cortex is thinned but intact ➡ with no soft tissue extension.

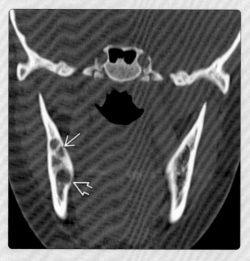

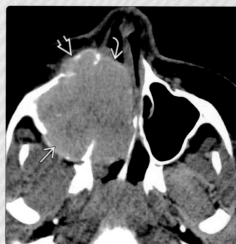

(Left) Coronal bone CT shows a loculated, radiolucent CGCG of the mandibular ramus without internal calcifications that thins mandibular cortex ➡ and is distinct from inferior extraction socket ➡. (Right) Axial CECT demonstrates a large, enhancing, expansile mass filling the right maxillary sinus ➡. This maxillary CGCG dehisces the anterior wall maxillary sinus ➡. Also note obstruction of the right nasal passage ➡ with deviation of the nasal septum.

TERMINOLOGY

Abbreviations

- Central giant cell granuloma (CGCG)

Synonyms

- Giant cell reparative granuloma

Definitions

- Giant cell reparative lesion of mandible or maxilla

IMAGING

General Features

- Best diagnostic clue
  o **Expansile** mass with **"right angle" septations**
- Location
  o **Anterior midline mandible** ≥ body & ramus > maxilla
    - ~ 50% of lesions anterior to 1st molar in alveolus
    - ~ 35% cross midline
  o May be located anywhere in mandible or maxilla
  o Rarely multiple
    - Multiple lesions have been reported in Noonan syndrome and neurofibromatosis type 1
- Size
  o Typically > 1 cm; often large at diagnosis

Imaging Recommendations

- Best imaging tool
  o CECT
- Protocol advice
  o Thin-section CECT
  o Bone CT shows septations and relationship to teeth

CT Findings

- CECT
  o Isodense (to muscle) **moderately enhancing** mass
- Bone CT
  o **Loculated, expansile** mass with thin to coarse wavy **septations**
    - Septations often at **right angle** to cortex
    - Smaller lesions: Thicker, coarse septations
    - Large lesions: Thin, wavy septations
  o Center of mass of alveolar lesions typically inferior to root apices
  o May have internal areas of mineralization
  o Scalloping and cortical dehiscence common in large lesions

MR Findings

- T1WI
  o Hypo- to isointense
- T2WI
  o Hypo- to isointense
- T1WI C+
  o Heterogeneously mild to moderate enhancement

DIFFERENTIAL DIAGNOSIS

Aneurysmal Bone Cyst

- ~ 15% of CGCGs contain intralesional aneurysmal bone cyst
- Majority of lesions in molar region of mandibular ramus

- > 60% female; age < 20 years
- CT: Can appear identical to CGCG
- MR: Fluid-fluid levels on T2 sequence

Cherubism

- Mutations in chromosome 4p16.3
- Multifocal giant cell lesions in infants and children
- CT: Multiple CGCGs in posterior mandible and maxilla

Ameloblastoma

- Predominately 3rd-5th decade
- Most common in tooth-bearing molar regions, mandible > maxilla
- CT: Multiloculated lucent expansile mass
  o **Septations** tend to be **coarser than CGCG**

Ossifying Fibroma

- Most common in premolar region of mandible
- Lesions with fibrous component can mimic CGCG
- CT: Calcified/ossified mass with lucent capsule

Brown Tumor of Hyperparathyroidism

- Rare in jaws; occurs with 1° or 2° hyperparathyroidism
- ↑ serum Ca^{++}, ↑ PTH, ↑ alkaline phosphatase
- In jaws, CT and MR appearance often identical to CGCG

PATHOLOGY

General Features

- Etiology
  o Unknown: Controversy over reactive granuloma vs. benign neoplasm
    - Histopathology overlaps with giant cell tumor

Microscopic Features

- Vascular, fibroblastic, or myxoid stroma
- Heterogeneous **clumps of giant cells** + fibroblastic areas, new bone, hemorrhage
- No necrosis

CLINICAL ISSUES

Presentation

- Most common signs/symptoms
  o Pain, swelling of mandible > maxilla

Demographics

- Age
  o Adolescence to 3rd decade; mean: 25 years
- Gender
  o F:M = 2:1

Natural History & Prognosis

- Recurrence rate: ~ 5-15%

Treatment

- Surgical excision: Treatment of choice but potential damage to teeth

SELECTED REFERENCES

1. Triantafillidou K et al: Central giant cell granuloma of the jaws: a clinical study of 17 cases and a review of the literature. Ann Otol Rhinol Laryngol. 120(3):167-74, 2011
2. Nackos JS et al: CT and MR imaging of giant cell granuloma of the craniofacial bones. AJNR Am J Neuroradiol. 27(8):1651-3, 2006

KEY FACTS

TERMINOLOGY

- Benign but locally aggressive neoplasm originating from odontogenic epithelium
- Arises in tooth-bearing areas of mandibular or maxillary alveolus

IMAGING

- CT findings
  - **Expansile multiloculated** or multilobulated mixed cystic & solid posterior mandible mass, usually near 3rd molar
  - Lesions in maxilla usually arise within premolar-1st molar region
  - Typically associated with **unerupted tooth**
- MR findings
  - T2: ↑ signal intensity of cystic areas
  - Smaller tumors: **Enhancing mural nodule**

TOP DIFFERENTIAL DIAGNOSES

- Periapical (radicular) cyst
- Dentigerous cyst
- Keratocystic odontogenic tumor
- Odontogenic myxoma
- Ossifying fibroma
- Aneurysmal bone cyst

CLINICAL ISSUES

- 3rd-5th decade
- Slow-growing, expansile, painless mass
- Progressive loosening of teeth
  - Nonhealing "tooth abscess"

DIAGNOSTIC CHECKLIST

- Larger dentigerous cyst (DC) and keratocystic odontogenic tumor (KOT) may mimic ameloblastoma
  - Ameloblastomas expand mandible more concentrically than DC or KOT
- High T2 signal intensity suggests ameloblastoma, rather than more aggressive neoplasm

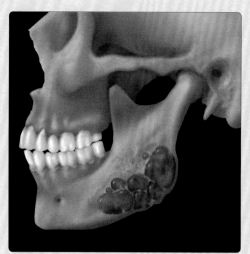
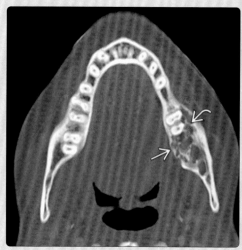

(Left) Lateral graphic shows mandibular ameloblastoma as a "bubbly," multilocular, expansile lesion. The location proximal to the 3rd molar is typical. (Right) Axial bone CT shows the classic appearance of solid/multicystic ameloblastoma as a multiloculated expansile mass in the 2nd-3rd molar region of the mandible ➡. Note the thinned overlying cortex and the characteristic multiple coarse septations ➡.

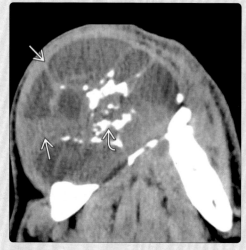
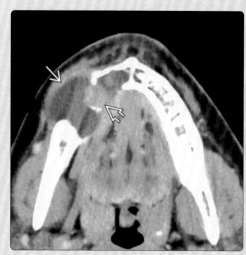

(Left) Axial NECT of a desmoplastic type reveals a multicystic mass with thick soft tissue septations ➡ and cortical fragments ➡. This type occurs largely in the anterior maxilla and mandible. (Right) Axial CECT of a unicystic ameloblastoma with a mural nodule shows the hypodense mass is nonenhancing and expansile ➡ with a central hyperdense and mildly enhancing nodule ➡. Note that the nodule lies adjacent to the eroded lingual cortex with potential for involvement of the sublingual space.

TERMINOLOGY

Synonyms

- Adamantoblastoma, adamantinoma (old, nonspecific terms; no longer used)

Definitions

- Locally aggressive, benign neoplasm arising from mandibular or maxillary odontogenic epithelium

IMAGING

General Features

- Best diagnostic clue
  - "Bubbly," multilocular, mixed cystic-solid mass in posterior mandible or maxilla associated with unerupted 3rd molar tooth
- Location
  - Mandible: Usually centered in 3rd molar, mandibular ramus region
  - Maxilla: Usually centered in premolar, 1st molar region
    - Affects maxillary sinus before nasal cavity
- Size
  - > 2 cm at discovery in most cases
- Morphology
  - Mandible: Tumor tends to be confined by thick cortex
  - Maxilla: Tumor more readily extends beyond bone into maxillary sinus and nasal cavity due to thin maxillary cortex
  - Imaging presentation reflects pathologic type: Solid-multicystic, desmoplastic, or unicystic ± mural nodule

Radiographic Findings

- Radiography
  - Unilocular or multilocular (80%) radiolucent mass with scalloped borders and expanded, thinned cortical margins
  - No calcifications in matrix

CT Findings

- CECT
  - Smaller lesions with marginal enhancement only
  - Larger lesions with extraosseous extension show moderate soft tissue enhancement mixed with cystic (low-density) areas
    - Extraosseous extension is uncommon
- Bone CT
  - Uni- (20%) or **multilocular (80%)** with scalloped borders
  - **"Bubbly" pattern** is typical; not pathognomonic
  - Unerupted molar tooth association common
  - Resorption of adjacent teeth
  - Extensive thinning of mandible or maxilla cortex
  - Low-density osteolytic lesion that does not mineralize its matrix

MR Findings

- T1WI
  - Mixed signal intensity
  - Low T1 signal intensity (cystic) typical but high signal occasionally seen
- T2WI
  - Mixed signal intensity

  - When large with extraosseous extension, high T2 signal helps differentiate from malignant tumors
- STIR
  - Increased signal intensity of cystic areas
- DWI
  - Solid areas show ↓ ADC
  - Cystic areas show ↑ ADC > keratocystic odontogenic tumor
- T1WI C+
  - Smaller tumors: **Enhancing mural nodule**
    - May represent "tumor growth center," which must be completely resected to achieve surgical cure
  - Enhancement of septations frequently seen
  - Solid regions show rapid enhancement on dynamic MR, reaching maximum contrast by 60 seconds
  - Cystic areas show no enhancement
  - Enhanced imaging may overestimate region of true tumor involvement
  - No evidence of perineural spread

Imaging Recommendations

- Best imaging tool
  - Contrast-enhanced thin-section CT with soft tissue and bone algorithm
- Enhanced thin-section CT best delineates both focal enhancing mural nodules as well as tumor-bone relationships
- Enhanced MR best defines extraosseous components and association with critical neurovascular structures
  - Especially true in maxilla: Relationships to sinus, nasal cavity, and orbit
- Both CT and MR may be required to differentiate from other cystic mandibular lesions

DIFFERENTIAL DIAGNOSIS

Periapical (Radicular) Cyst

- Clinically painful with carious lesion or periodontal disease
- Bone CT: Loss of lamina dura and widening of periodontal ligament space
  - Larger lesions are destructive, not expansile

Dentigerous Cyst

- Bone CT: Unilocular cystic lesion surrounding **tooth crown**
- No enhancing mural nodule
- Unilocular and smaller multilocular ameloblastoma may mimic dentigerous cysts

Keratocystic Odontogenic Tumor

- Bone CT: Unilocular or multilocular cystic lesion of mandible associated with **unerupted tooth**
  - Lesion envelops around or incorporates crown and tooth root
- Tendency for less buccal-lingual expansion than ameloblastoma
- No enhancing mural nodule
- Unilocular and smaller multilocular ameloblastoma may mimic keratocystic odontogenic tumor

Odontogenic Myxoma (Myxofibroma)

- Uncommon benign tumor arising from dental papilla

- Bone CT: Unilocular or multilocular cystic lesion posterior maxilla or mandible
  - Expansile mass with finer locular septations than typical ameloblastoma
- Myxomatous matrix results in ↑ HU on CT and ↓ T2 on MR relative to ameloblastoma or keratocystic odontogenic tumor

Mandible-Maxilla Ossifying Fibroma

- Bone CT: Fibrotic lytic phase appears as cystic, loculated, or "bubbly" expansile mass
  - Tends to scallop around tooth roots
  - Wispy septations in expanded cortical bone
- Central ossification, ↑ HU, ↓ T1 and T2

Mandible-Maxilla Aneurysmal Bone Cyst

- Children more common than adults
- Bone CT: Large, round, multilocular mass
- NECT or MR: Fluid-fluid levels
- No enhancing mural nodule

PATHOLOGY

General Features

- Etiology
  - Benign epithelial odontogenic tumor arising from ameloblast (epithelial cell in innermost layer of enamel organ)
- Associated abnormalities
  - 20% of ameloblastomas may arise from dentigerous cysts
- Mandible to maxilla ratio = 5:1
  - Molar and ramus area > premolar area > symphysis
  - Unerupted 3rd molar tooth often concurrent finding

Gross Pathologic & Surgical Features

- Expansile, multilobular mass in mandible or maxilla
- Mixed lesions, such as ameloblastic odontoma, ameloblastic fibroma, or ameloblastic fibroodontoma, are rare
  - Occur in children

Microscopic Features

- Unencapsulated
- Proliferating sheets or islands of odontogenic epithelium
- Odontogenic tumor of epithelial elements
  - Marginal, palisading, columnar cells with hyperchromatic, small nuclei arranged away from basement membrane
- Histologic types: Plexiform, desmoplastic, follicular, and granular cell
- Malignant variants: Ameloblastic carcinoma and malignant ameloblastoma (may metastasize)

CLINICAL ISSUES

Presentation

- Most common signs/symptoms
  - Hard, painless mandibular mass
  - Other signs/symptoms
    - Loose teeth, painless swelling
    - Bleeding, poorly healing tooth extraction
    - May be no early clinical symptoms
- Clinical profile
  - Adult with painless, slowly growing mandibular mass

Demographics

- Age
  - Most commonly presents in 30-50 year olds
  - Unilocular lesions often seen in younger age group
- Epidemiology
  - 2nd most common odontogenic tumor (35%)
  - 2nd most common benign mandibular tumor
  - 1% of all lesions of mandible and maxilla

Natural History & Prognosis

- Slow-growing, sometimes indolent, benign neoplasm
- Often takes years to become symptomatic
- Malignant transformation is rare (1%)
  - Referred to as ameloblastic carcinoma
- Tumor recurrence is common (33%)
  - Recurrence may require more aggressive 2nd en bloc resection
  - Unilocular tumor recurs much less frequently (15%) than multilocular group

Treatment

- Complete surgical excision when small
  - Curettement no longer acceptable therapy
- En bloc removal for larger lesions
- Chemotherapy and radiotherapy are contraindicated

DIAGNOSTIC CHECKLIST

Consider

- Larger dentigerous cyst and keratocystic odontogenic tumor most difficult to differentiate from ameloblastoma
- Key is relationship to teeth and absence of nodular enhancement in these 2 lesions compared to ameloblastoma

Image Interpretation Pearls

- Ameloblastomas often have resorption of adjacent tooth roots
- **High T2 signal** suggests ameloblastoma, rather than more aggressive neoplasm

Reporting Tips

- Relationship to, or involvement of, inferior alveolar nerve canal in mandible
- Extraalveolar extension to sublingual/submandibular space, buccal space, masticator space, maxillary sinus, pterygopalatine fissure, or orbit

SELECTED REFERENCES

1. Fujita M et al: Diagnostic value of MRI for odontogenic tumours. Dentomaxillofac Radiol. 42(5):20120265, 2013
2. Sumi M et al: Diffusion-weighted MR imaging of ameloblastomas and keratocystic odontogenic tumors: differentiation by apparent diffusion coefficients of cystic lesions. AJNR Am J Neuroradiol. 29(10):1897-901, 2008
3. Asaumi J et al: Application of dynamic MRI to differentiating odontogenic myxomas from ameloblastomas. Eur J Radiol. 43(1):37-41, 2002
4. Hayashi K et al: Dynamic multislice helical CT of ameloblastoma and odontogenic keratocyst: correlation between contrast enhancement and angiogenesis. J Comput Assist Tomogr. 26(6):922-6, 2002
5. Mosier KM: Lesions of the Jaw. Semin Ultrasound CT MR. 36(5):444-50, 2015
6. Mosier KM: Magnetic resonance imaging of the maxilla and mandible: signal characteristics and features in the differential diagnosis of common lesions. Top Magn Reson Imaging. 24(1):23-37, 2015

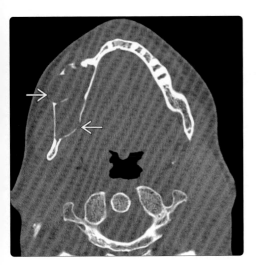

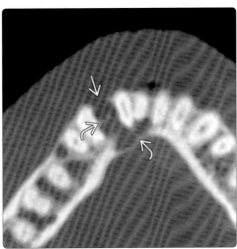

(Left) *Axial bone CT shows a large, expansile, multiloculated mass in the body of the mandible on the right. The aggressive character of these lesions is appreciated in the convex expansion of the buccal and lingual cortex, accompanied by marked thinning and focal dehiscence ➡. (Right) Axial bone CT shows a small solid/multicystic lesion enlarging between the lateral incisor and the canine teeth. Note the septations ➡ despite its small size and perforation of the buccal cortex ➡.*

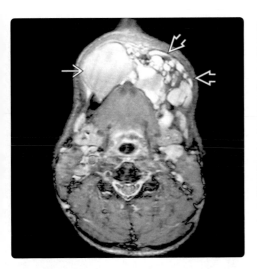

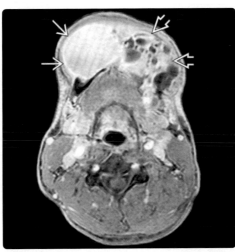

(Left) *Axial STIR MR of a large mandibular ameloblastoma suggests a fluid-fluid level in the large, right-sided, cystic component ➡. Note the multilocular, T2-hyperintense component on the left ➡. (Right) Axial T1WI C+ FS MR of the same mandibular ameloblastoma demonstrates prominent enhancement of the walls of both the large, right-sided, unilocular cyst ➡ and of the smaller, multilocular, left-sided, cystic components ➡.*

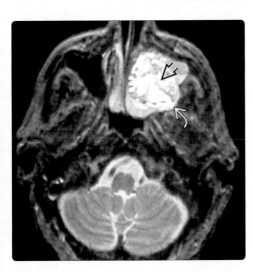

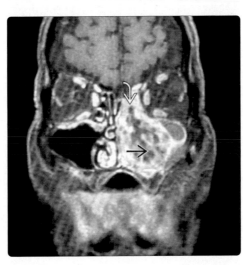

(Left) *Axial T2WI FS MR of a maxilla ameloblastoma shows both solid and cystic components in a multiloculated pattern. Note the typical bright T2 signal ➡ of the cystic components and the expansion of the posterior maxillary sinus walls ➡. (Right) Coronal T1WI C+ FS MR of the same ameloblastoma demonstrates the typical enhancement of the septations ➡. The locally aggressive nature of these lesions is likewise evident by the extension into the nasal cavity and ethmoid air cells ➡.*

KEY FACTS

TERMINOLOGY

- Keratocystic odontogenic tumor (KOT)
  - Previously known as odontogenic keratocyst
- Benign cystic neoplasm of jaw with aggressive behavior and high recurrence rate

IMAGING

- May displace developing teeth or resorb roots of erupted teeth
  - **Not** related to unerupted crown
- Bone CT: Unilocular cystic mass with sclerotic rim
  - Expansile solitary unilocular jaw lesion
    - Multilocular jaw cyst ↑ risk (12x) of KOT
  - 75% posterior mandible, often near 3rd molar
  - Extends longitudinally in mandible
- CECT: No solid enhancement
- C+ MR: Cystic with thin, enhancing rim
  - Greater enhancement with recurrent KOT

TOP DIFFERENTIAL DIAGNOSES

- Periapical (radicular) cyst
- Dentigerous (follicular) cyst
- Ameloblastoma

PATHOLOGY

- Thin-walled, friable cyst containing fluid and debris
- Viscosity of contents depends on keratinaceous debris
  - Straw-colored fluid → pus-like → "cheesy" mass

CLINICAL ISSUES

- 50% present with jaw swelling
- Rapid growth and high recurrence rate

DIAGNOSTIC CHECKLIST

- 7% of KOTs are multiple
- If multiple KOTs, consider **basal cell nevus syndrome**
- Look for dural calcifications on same CT scan

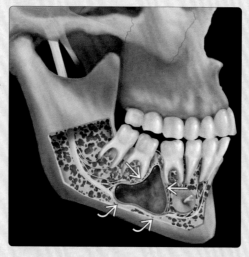
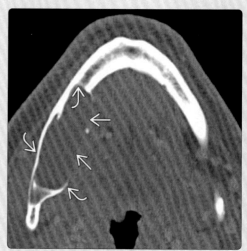

(Left) *Lateral graphic of the mandible with the buccal cortex removed illustrates features of classic keratocytic odontogenic tumor (KOT). A cystic lesion ➡ splays the roots of the 1st and 2nd molar teeth, enlarging the marrow space and displacing the inferior alveolar nerve ➡.* **(Right)** *Axial bone CT in a patient with confirmed KOT demonstrates an expansile, unilocular cystic mass ➡ extending along long axis of mandible. Cortex is smoothly scalloped ➡ along most margins but is imperceptible at the lingual aspect.*

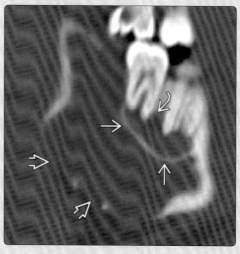
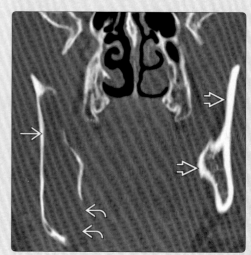

(Left) *Sagittal reconstruction of a mandible bone CT demonstrates an expansile mass with characteristic scalloping between roots of teeth ➡. Note that mylohyoid line of mandible is preserved ➡, despite marked thinning of the inferior mandibular cortex ➡.* **(Right)** *Coronal reconstruction of bone CT shows that KOT tends to expand through the ramus ➡. The cortex is diffusely thinned, but the lingual cortex ➡ is imperceptible. The degree of bony expansion is evident in comparison to the normal left side ➡.*

TERMINOLOGY

Abbreviations

- Keratocystic odontogenic tumor (KOT)

Synonyms

- Odontogenic keratocyst, primordial cyst

IMAGING

General Features

- Best diagnostic clue
  - Expansile, solitary, unilocular jaw lesion
- Location
  - **75% posterior mandible**, often near 3rd molar
  - In maxilla, most commonly near canine
- Size
  - 1-9 cm; average: 3 cm

Radiographic Findings

- Radiography
  - Expansile cystic mass; may have "cloudy" lumen
  - 50% unilocular, lucent with sclerotic rim
  - May displace developing teeth, resorb roots of erupted teeth, cause tooth extrusion

CT Findings

- CECT
  - No detectable enhancement
- Bone CT
  - Distinctly corticated **expansile cystic mass**, often with scalloped border
  - Typically extends longitudinally in mandible
  - May be near unerupted tooth but **not** crown
  - Density varies with viscosity of contents

MR Findings

- T1WI
  - Intermediate to high signal intensity due to ortho-/parakeratin &/or hemorrhage
- T2WI
  - Heterogeneous, low to high signal intensity
- T1WI C+
  - Thin or no enhancing rim, no solid mass
  - Greater enhancement seen with recurrent KOT

Imaging Recommendations

- Best imaging tool
  - CT allows complete evaluation for diagnosis
    - CECT determines no solid enhancement
    - Bone algorithm best delineates lesion
- Protocol advice
  - Thin-section CT with multiplanar reformats

DIFFERENTIAL DIAGNOSIS

Periapical (Radicular) Cyst

- Unilocular cyst associated with tooth root
- Associated with dental caries and infection

Dentigerous (Follicular) Cyst

- Developmental unilocular cyst
- Arises from unerupted tooth crown

Ameloblastoma

- Expansile, "bubbly" lesion
- Enhancing wall and nodules

PATHOLOGY

General Features

- Etiology
  - Arises from remnants of **dental lamina**
  - Now classified as cystic tumor
- Associated abnormalities
  - Associated with Marfan and Noonan syndromes
  - 7% of KOTs are multiple
    - **50%** have **basal cell nevus syndrome**

Gross Pathologic & Surgical Features

- Thin, friable cyst containing fluid and keratin debris
  - Straw-colored fluid → pus-like → "cheesy" mass

Microscopic Features

- Fibrous wall lined by squamous epithelium
- Microcysts or daughter cysts may be seen

CLINICAL ISSUES

Presentation

- Most common signs/symptoms
  - 50% present with jaw swelling
- Other signs/symptoms
  - Pain, paresthesia, trismus

Demographics

- Age
  - Wide range; peaks in 4th decade
- Epidemiology
  - 5-10% of jaw cysts
  - Since reclassification, one of most common odontogenic tumors

Natural History & Prognosis

- Rapid growth and high recurrence rate

Treatment

- Enucleation with aggressive curettage

DIAGNOSTIC CHECKLIST

Consider

- If multiple KOTs, consider basal cell nevus syndrome
  - Look for dural calcifications on same CT scan

Image Interpretation Pearls

- Classic appearance is unilocular mandibular cyst
  - No solid enhancing tissue
  - Often related to 3rd molar

SELECTED REFERENCES

1. Mosier KM: Magnetic resonance imaging of the maxilla and mandible: signal characteristics and features in the differential diagnosis of common lesions. Top Magn Reson Imaging. 24(1):23-37, 2015
2. Mosier KM: Lesions of the jaw. Semin Ultrasound CT MR. 36(5):444-50, 2015
3. Johnson NR et al: Frequency of odontogenic cysts and tumors: a systematic review. J Investig Clin Dent. 5(1):9-14, 2014

(Left) *Axial CECT shows a KOT as a diffusely low-density, expansile lesion* ➡ *involving the posterior mandibular body and ramus. No enhancement is evident. Lateral cortical dehiscence* ➡ *is present, but the lesion remains sharply defined, and there is no masseter muscle invasion. Asymmetry of cheek contour is evident.* (Right) *Coronal NECT shows mild expansion of angle of mandible by KOT* ➡ *but greater expansion as mass extends superiorly into ramus where there is marked thinning of cortex* ➡.

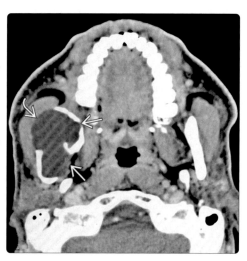 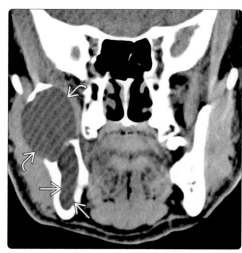

(Left) *Axial T1 MR shows a heterogeneous mass emanating from the mandible into the masticator muscles with disruption of the mandibular cortex* ➡. *Areas of high signal intensity* ➡ *within the mass, a feature of KOT, are due to keratinaceous debris.* (Right) *Coronal T2 MR shows T2-hyperintense signal within the lesion, consistent with fluid content in this KOT. This image also clarifies that, while the mass involves the masticator space medially* ➡ *and laterally* ➡, *there is no infiltration of adjacent tissues.*

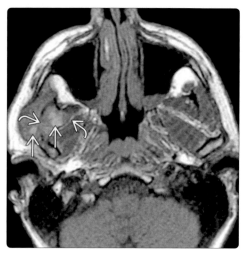 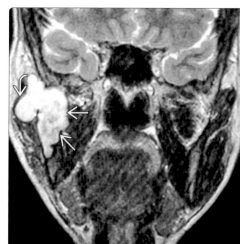

(Left) *Axial bone CT demonstrates a unilocular cystic lesion* ➡ *involving posterior body of right mandible. The lesion results in mild expansion of the mandible and some cortical scalloping but no dehiscence. An impacted contralateral left 3rd molar is evident* ➡. (Right) *Axial bone CT more inferiorly in the same patient shows that the cystic mass* ➡ *is associated with an unerupted right 3rd molar* ➡. *This finding is most often associated with dentigerous cyst; however, pathology proved the lesion to be a KOT.*

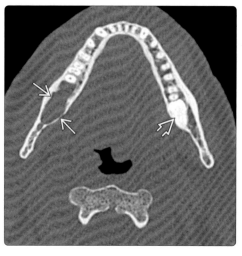 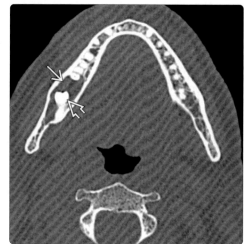

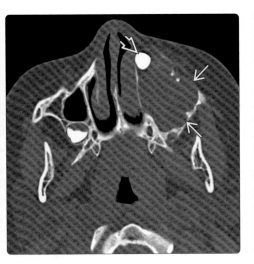

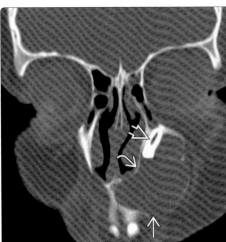

(Left) *Axial bone CT of a maxillary KOT demonstrates an expansile cystic mass filling the left maxillary sinus and smoothly scalloping and thinning walls ➡. The cyst erodes apices of maxillary teeth and displaces the unerupted left maxillary canine superiorly, medially, and anteriorly ⇨.* (Right) *Coronal bone CT of a maxillary KOT shows thinning and dehiscence of the maxillary alveolus ➡ and distortion of lateral nasal wall ➡. Coronal plane best demonstrates direction of displacement of canine tooth ⇨.*

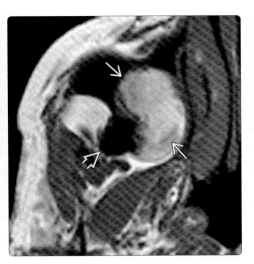

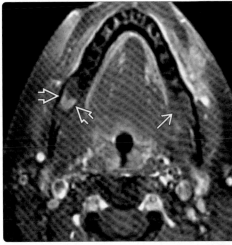

(Left) *Axial T1 MR shows an intrinsically hyperintense signal in this well-defined maxillary KOT ➡ filling the inferior aspect of the maxillary sinus. The mass is adjacent to an impacted or displaced maxillary molar tooth ⇨.* (Right) *Axial T1 C+ FS MR in a patient with basal cell nevus syndrome shows bilateral cystic masses adjacent to 3rd mandibular molars. The left-sided lesion ➡ shows no perceptible enhancement. The right side ⇨ shows a thick, enhancing rim, more common with recurrent lesions.*

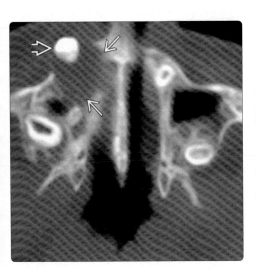

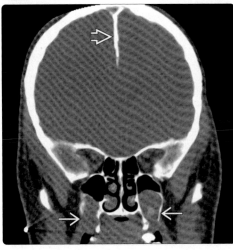

(Left) *Axial bone CT in a patient with basal cell nevus syndrome demonstrates a lytic, expansile right alveolus mass ➡ displacing tooth anteriorly ⇨. Bony margins of cystic lesion are less well defined than typically seen.* (Right) *Coronal NECT in a 19 year old with a prior resected mandibular KOT, pineoblastoma resected as infant, and basal cell nevi shows bilateral, expansile, heterogeneous maxillary lesions ⇨. Note the marked dural calcification ⇨ typically seen with basal cell nevus syndrome.*

Mandible-Maxilla Osteosarcoma

KEY FACTS

TERMINOLOGY

- Malignant tumor with ability to produce osteoid from neoplastic cells

IMAGING

- Bone CT: Bone destruction with aggressive periosteal reaction and osteoid formation
- MR best evaluates soft tissue component of tumor
  - Intramedullary and extraosseous soft tissues
- Bone scan or PET/CT: Increased tracer uptake

TOP DIFFERENTIAL DIAGNOSES

- Mandible-maxilla osteomyelitis
- Mandible-maxilla osteoradionecrosis
- Mandible-maxilla metastasis
- Ewing sarcoma
- Langerhans cell histiocytosis

PATHOLOGY

- Heterogeneous mass with ossified and nonossified components
- Chondroblastic > osteoblastic > fibroblastic

CLINICAL ISSUES

- Mean age: 35 years; M:F = 1.5:1
- Prognosis depends on pathologic type, size, location, and presence of metastases
- 5-year survival: 40%
- Complete resection affords best chance of survival

DIAGNOSTIC CHECKLIST

- **Aggressive periosteal reaction** suggests osteosarcoma
- If not present, consider infection or metastasis
- Consider XRT-induced sarcoma if patient had radiation years prior

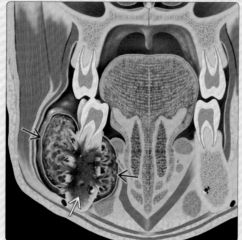
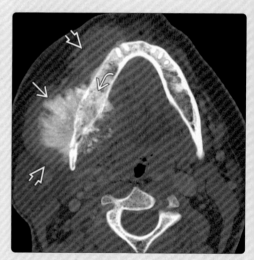

(Left) Coronal graphic shows right mandible osteosarcoma. Note soft tissue mass perforating through cortex ➡ and intramedullary tumor ➡. (Right) Axial bone CT demonstrates a large, dense mass arising from the right mandible ➡. Mass has both osteoid matrix and periosteal reaction. This is classic periosteal reaction associated with osteosarcomas where periosteum is lifted off perpendicular to bone. Marrow within involved portion of mandible is sclerotic ➡. Note associated soft tissue mass ➡.

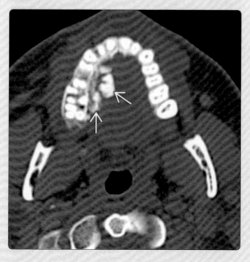
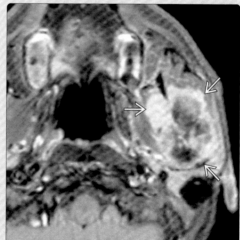

(Left) Axial bone CT through maxilla shows exophytic mass with amorphous immature new bone ➡ and cortical breakthrough. This is the parosteal form of osteosarcoma. Note absence of significant associated nonossified soft tissue mass. (Right) Axial T1WI C+ FS MR shows heterogeneous enhancement of soft tissue component of osteosarcoma arising in mandible. Note tumor has infiltrated the parotid gland, masseter, and pterygoid muscles ➡.

TERMINOLOGY

Synonyms

- Osteogenic sarcoma

Definitions

- Malignant tumor arising from bone with ability of neoplastic cells to produce osteoid

IMAGING

General Features

- Best diagnostic clue
  - Bone destruction with aggressive periosteal reaction and tumor bone formation
- Location
  - Mandible more common than maxilla
    - Angle, ramus, or body of mandible
- Size
  - Variable; usually < 10 cm
- Morphology
  - Destructive lesion with osteoid formation

Radiographic Findings

- Radiography
  - Poorly defined alveolar mass, ± tumoral calcification, with aggressive periosteal reaction
  - Unilateral symmetric widening of periodontal ligament space of teeth in absence of dental disease

CT Findings

- CECT
  - Moderate enhancement of solid components
- Bone CT
  - Expansile lesion with increased density, **aggressive periosteal reaction**
    - "Sunburst" periosteal reaction most typical

MR Findings

- Heterogeneous signal intensity on T1 & T2
  - Mineralized tumor = low T1, low T2
  - Solid nonmineralized tumor = intermediate T1, high T2
- Heterogeneous contrast enhancement

Nuclear Medicine Findings

- Bone scan
  - Increased tracer uptake
    - Useful for staging, detection of metastases ± skip lesions

Imaging Recommendations

- Best imaging tool
  - CT best for demonstrating osseous destruction, osteoid matrix
    - Thin-section bone algorithm NECT
  - MR best for soft tissue & intramedullary extent

DIFFERENTIAL DIAGNOSIS

Mandible-Maxilla Osteomyelitis

- Bony destruction without osteoid formation; ± sequestrum formation

- Garré sclerosing osteomyelitis: Lytic bone destruction with exuberant periosteal reaction

Mandible-Maxilla Osteoradionecrosis

- Peaks in 2 years following radiation
- Lytic and sclerotic destruction

Mandible-Maxilla Metastasis

- Aggressive bony destructive changes
- No periosteal reaction or tumoral calcification

Ewing Sarcoma

- Irregular, destructive lytic mass
- Does not produce osteoid matrix

Langerhans Cell Histiocytosis

- Punched-out lytic lesion
- May have soft tissue swelling but little enhancement

Fibromatosis

- Irregular lytic destructive lesion
- No osteoid matrix or periosteal reaction

PATHOLOGY

General Features

- Etiology
  - Primary etiology unknown in most cases
  - **May occur following radiation to face**
    - Typically > 10 years after XRT

Microscopic Features

- Highly pleomorphic, spindle-shaped tumor cells producing different forms of osteoid
- **Chondroblastic** > osteoblastic > fibroblastic

CLINICAL ISSUES

Presentation

- Most common signs/symptoms
  - Enlarging soft tissue mass over mandible with ↑ pain

Natural History & Prognosis

- Mandibular osteosarcomas less likely to metastasize than long bone tumors
- Prognosis depends on path type, size, location, metastases
- **5-year survival: ~ 65%**

Treatment

- Complete resection affords best chance of survival
- ± adjuvant chemotherapy, radiation

SELECTED REFERENCES

1. Mosier KM: Magnetic resonance imaging of the maxilla and mandible: signal characteristics and features in the differential diagnosis of common lesions. Top Magn Reson Imaging. 24(1):23-37, 2015
2. Wang S et al: Osteosarcoma of the jaws: demographic and CT imaging features. Dentomaxillofac Radiol. 41(1):37-42, 2012

Mandible-Maxilla Osteoradionecrosis

TERMINOLOGY

- Osteoradionecrosis
- Complication of XRT with necrosis of bone and failure to heal

IMAGING

- Mandible > > maxilla or skull base
- Associated soft tissue edema and induration common
- Difficult to exclude superinfection
- CT: Mixed lytic/sclerotic bone with sequestra
- MR: Diffuse low T1, high T2 signal from edema
- Diffuse enhancement common

TOP DIFFERENTIAL DIAGNOSES

- Osteomyelitis
- Bisphosphonate osteonecrosis
- Alveolar ridge squamous cell carcinoma (SCCa)
- Radiation-induced 2nd primary tumor

PATHOLOGY

- Radiation results in damage to small blood vessels, resulting in hypovascular marrow
- Impairs ability of bone to cope with stressors, such as infection or trauma
- May be precipitated by biopsy or tooth extraction
- Pathologic fracture through bone common

CLINICAL ISSUES

- Most often follows XRT for oral cavity SCCa
- Exposed bone from ulcerated mucosa usually present
- Incidence peaks 1st 6-12 months post-XRT
- May occur years after XRT

DIAGNOSTIC CHECKLIST

- Jaw pain, nonhealing mucosal ulceration, lytic/sclerotic CT changes
- Must exclude recurrent SCCa as source of changes

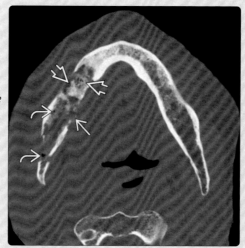
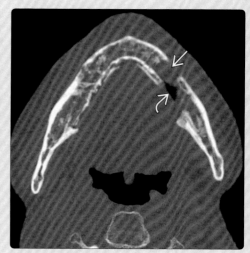

(Left) Axial bone CT demonstrates typical mixed lytic/sclerotic changes and cortical bone interruption ⇨ in the right hemimandible following XRT. Note the intraosseous gas bubbles ⇨ and evolving bone-within-bone appearance ⇨ due to intraosseous bone sequestra. (Right) Axial bone CT in a different patient shows a primarily lytic pattern of osteoradionecrosis (ORN) with interrupted cortex ⇨ and intraosseous gas ⇨. There is also pathologic fracture of the left mandibular body with offsetting of bone.

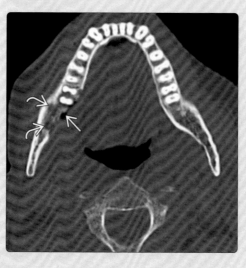
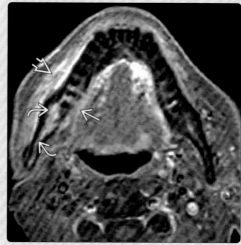

(Left) Axial bone CT shows mandibular extraction socket with a small bubble of gas ⇨ indicating mucosal erosion, with hazy lucency of the adjacent bone ⇨. Patient had exposed bone on the physical exam. (Right) Axial T1WI MR in the same patient shows enhancement in the mandible ⇨ and diffusely in lingual ⇨ and buccal ⇨ soft tissues around the mandible. With a history of prior XRT and now a swollen right face with exposed bone around the socket, imaging is most consistent with early ORN.

TERMINOLOGY

Abbreviations

- Osteoradionecrosis (ORN)

Definitions

- Complication of XRT with necrosis of bone and failure to heal

IMAGING

General Features

- Best diagnostic clue
  - Mixed lytic/sclerotic bone in patient previously treated with radiation therapy
    - Exposed bone through ulcerated skin or mucosa usually present
    - Often complicated by fracture; may have infection as well
    - Lack of discrete soft tissue mass helps differentiate from recurrent tumor
- Location
  - In H&N, most often seen in jaw and skull base
    - Mandible > > maxilla or other facial bones
    - Temporal or sphenoid bone of skull base
    - Also described in frontal and hyoid bones
- Size
  - May be focal or extensive
  - May be associated with necrosis of surrounding soft tissues

Imaging Recommendations

- Best imaging tool
  - Bone CT is best diagnostic modality
  - Soft tissue imaging shows diffuse inflammation but no mass
- Protocol advice
  - Thin bone algorithm CT slices with coronal and sagittal reformations
    - Multiplanar images help plan surgery and potential reconstruction
    - Oblique sagittal reformations parallel to plane of mandible angle essential
  - CECT if superimposed infection or recurrent tumor suspected clinically

Radiographic Findings

- Extraoral plain film
  - Mixed lytic/sclerotic bone
  - Extent of involvement and destruction often underestimated by radiography

CT Findings

- CECT
  - Soft tissue edema and induration common, even when no superinfection
  - Focal abnormal enhancement or small abscesses may be evident when infected
  - Fistulization to skin can occur
- Bone CT
  - Cortical bone disruption on background of mixed lysis and sclerosis

- Loss of trabeculation results in lytic appearance with superimposed sclerosis
  - Sequestered spicules of bone and fragmentation common
  - Bubbles of air often present within abnormal mandible or in adjacent necrotic tissues
  - Pathological fractures may be evident, may precipitate patient presentation
- PET/CT
  - Marked FDG uptake typically seen with ORN
    - Probably due to inflammatory component
  - CECT important to interpret with PET study to detect recurrent tumor
  - PET/CT and CECT may suggest recurrent tumor, but exposed bone in oral cavity or through skin strongly supports ORN

MR Findings

- T1WI
  - Diffuse low signal intensity of marrow space
  - Disrupted cortex may be evident
- T2WI
  - Diffuse high signal of marrow space
  - Adjacent tissues may appear edematous also
- T1WI C+ FS
  - Diffuse enhancement of marrow common
  - No adjacent solid mass

DIFFERENTIAL DIAGNOSIS

Osteomyelitis

- Mixed lytic/sclerotic bone in patient with infected tooth or extraction site and no history of XRT
- Osteomyelitis may be found with ORN; frequently difficult to differentiate

Bisphosphonate Osteonecrosis

- Mixed lytic/sclerotic bone in patient treated with intravenous bisphosphonates
- Patient has no radiation history

Alveolar Ridge Squamous Cell Carcinoma

- Primarily destructive bone changes with mucosal ulceration
- Solid soft tissue enhancing lesion
- Recurrent squamous cell carcinoma (SCCa) is main imaging differential when ORN is present

Radiation-Induced Second Primary Tumor

- Occurs many years after XRT; typically ≥ 8 years
- Sarcoma is most frequent; often associated with soft tissue mass

PATHOLOGY

General Features

- Etiology
  - Radiation results in damage to small blood vessels
    - Endothelial cells lining blood vessels are destroyed, resulting in obstructive arteriopathy
    - Impairs ability of bone to respond to stressors
  - ORN often precipitated by infection or trauma including tooth extraction or **tissue biopsy**
- Associated abnormalities

- o Bacterial infection in necrotic bone often present
  - – Current theory suggests osteomyelitis not primary event
  - – Gram-positive actinomycosis bacterial infection commonly associated with ORN

Staging, Grading, & Classification

- Various staging or clinical grading systems used
- **Store and Boysen staging for jaw**
  - o Stage 0: Mucosal defects only
  - o Stage I: Radiologic evidence of ORN + intact mucosa
  - o Stage II: Radiologic evidence of ORN + denuded bone
  - o Stage III: Exposed radionecrotic bone + orocutaneous fistulae

Gross Pathologic & Surgical Features

- Necrotic fragmented bone with sequestra and spicules
- Fragile, ulcerated mucosa with exposed bone

Microscopic Features

- **Bone necrosis primarily due to hypoxia**
  - o XRT results in obliteration of arteries, including inferior alveolar artery
- Bone is hypocellular and periosteum nonviable
- Biopsy specimen may be complicated with osteonecrosis, osteomyelitis, and recurrent/residual tumor

CLINICAL ISSUES

Presentation

- Most common signs/symptoms
  - o Ulcerated skin or mucosa with exposed necrotic bone in patient with prior history of H&N XRT
    - – Mandible is most common facial bone involved
    - – May be exposed through oral ulceration
- Other signs/symptoms
  - o Fistulization to skin
  - o Oral pain, trismus, dysesthesia, foul breath
  - o Masticator space infection with small abscesses

Demographics

- Epidemiology
  - o Multiple factors influence incidence of ORN
    - – Tumor: Risk increased with stage III/IV primary tumor
    - – XRT plan: Risk increased with higher dose, large field size, short treatment time
      - □ Intensity modulated XRT (IMRT) with lower bone exposure has lower incidence of ORN
    - – Treatment: Risk increased if surgery (mandibulectomy or other osteotomy) in addition to XRT
    - – Patient factors: Risk increased with poor oral hygiene, ongoing alcohol and tobacco exposure

Natural History & Prognosis

- Incidence of ORN is ≤ 6%
- Incidence peaks: 1st 6-12 months post XRT

Treatment

- **Prevention** most important **prior** to XRT
  - o Dental extractions and periodontal care prior to XRT
  - o Improved nutritional status prior and during XRT
  - o Cessation of tobacco and alcohol use

- Conservative treatment includes antibiotics and local irrigation
- Hyperbaric oxygen therapy to promote angiogenesis and aid in treating associated infection
  - o Essential to exclude residual/recurrent tumor prior to hyperbaric oxygen treatment
- Sequestrectomy and primary wound closure for early disease
- Bone resection and reconstruction for severe progressive disease

DIAGNOSTIC CHECKLIST

Consider

- ORN in any patient treated with XRT and new pain, nonhealing mucosal ulceration, lytic/sclerotic CT changes
- Essential to exclude **recurrent SCCa** as source of pain and cortical disruption
  - o Tumor favored when solid soft tissue mass present
- While ORN may occur several years after treatment, if ≥ 8 years, consider **XRT-induced sarcoma,** especially if soft tissue mass associated

Image Interpretation Pearls

- Check for local infection or pathologic fracture

Reporting Tips

- Describe extent of disease, cortical bone disruption, exposed bone spicules, and sequestrations

SELECTED REFERENCES

1. Deshpande SS et al: Osteoradionecrosis of the mandible: through a radiologist's eyes. Clin Radiol. 70(2):197-205, 2015
2. Schultz BD et al: Classification of mandible defects and algorithm for microvascular reconstruction. Plast Reconstr Surg. 135(4):743e-54e, 2015
3. Zaghi S et al: Changing indications for maxillomandibular reconstruction with osseous free flaps: a 17-year experience with 620 consecutive cases at UCLA and the impact of osteoradionecrosis. Laryngoscope. 124(6):1329-35, 2014
4. Cheriex KC et al: Osteoradionecrosis of the jaws: a review of conservative and surgical treatment options. J Reconstr Microsurg. 29(2):69-75, 2013
5. Armin BB et al: Brachytherapy-mediated bone damage in a rat model investigating maxillary osteoradionecrosis. Arch Otolaryngol Head Neck Surg. 138(2):167-71, 2012
6. Dholam KP et al: Dental implants in irradiated jaws: a literature review. J Cancer Res Ther. 8 Suppl 1:S85-93, 2012
7. Tchanque-Fossuo CN et al: Amifostine remediates the degenerative effects of radiation on the mineralization capacity of the murine mandible. Plast Reconstr Surg. 129(4):646e-55e, 2012
8. Cannady SB et al: Free flap reconstruction for osteoradionecrosis of the jaws–outcomes and predictive factors for success. Head Neck. 33(3):424-8, 2011
9. Nabil S et al: Incidence and prevention of osteoradionecrosis after dental extraction in irradiated patients: a systematic review. Int J Oral Maxillofac Surg. 40(3):229-43, 2011
10. O'Dell K et al: Osteoradionecrosis. Oral Maxillofac Surg Clin North Am. 23(3):455-64, 2011
11. Tamplen M et al: Standardized analysis of mandibular osteoradionecrosis in a rat model. Otolaryngol Head Neck Surg. 145(3):404-10, 2011
12. Thariat J et al: [Revisiting the dose-effect correlations in irradiated head and neck cancer using automatic segmentation tools of the dental structures, mandible and maxilla.] Cancer Radiother. 15(8):683-90, 2011
13. Bak M et al: Contemporary reconstruction of the mandible. Oral Oncol. 46(2):71-6, 2010
14. Chrcanovic BR et al: Osteoradionecrosis of the jaws–a current overview–part 1: Physiopathology and risk and predisposing factors. Oral Maxillofac Surg. 14(1):3-16, 2010
15. Jacobson AS et al: Reconstruction of bilateral osteoradionecrosis of the mandible using a single fibular free flap. Laryngoscope. 120(2):273-5, 2010

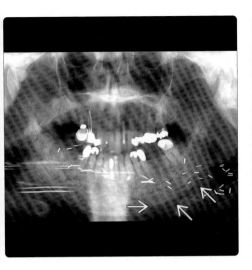

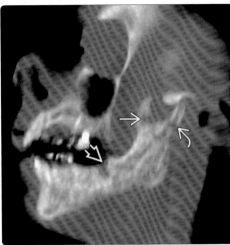

(Left) *Panorex from a patient with prior surgery and XRT to the oral cavity reveals diffuse thickening and sclerosis of the mandible with coarsened trabeculae and loss of definition of the cortical bone along the inferior left hemimandibular margin* ➡. (Right) *Sagittal oblique reconstruction shows heterogeneous multifocal lucency, cortical interruption, and trabecular and cortical thickening and sclerosis. Note deep molar extraction socket* ➡. *There is fragmentation of the coronoid process* ➡ *and condylar neck* ➡.

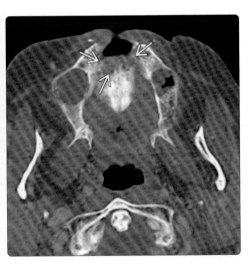

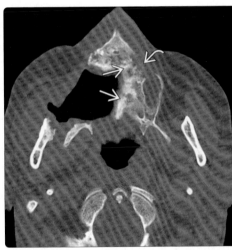

(Left) *Axial bone CT in a patient treated with XRT for nasal septal squamous cell carcinoma shows lytic process of the anterior maxilla with the discrete wedge of destroyed and missing bone* ➡. (Right) *Axial bone CT in a different patient shows right surgical palatectomy, but mixed sclerotic* ➡ *and lytic* ➡ *changes in the left maxilla, which was included in XRT field. The maxilla is relatively radioresistant, and ORN is rare. Imaging findings are identical as seen in the mandible and other facial and skull base bones.*

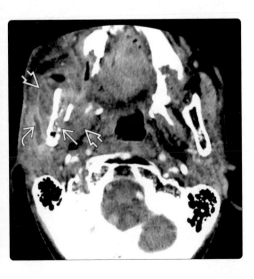

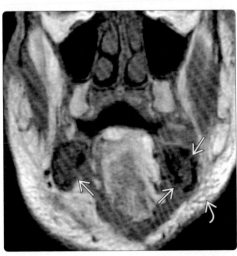

(Left) *Axial CECT shows ORN of the right mandible complicated by the infection of the masticator space. There is cortical interruption* ➡ *and diffuse severe edema of the parotid gland and muscles of mastication* ➡, *and dilated parotid duct* ➡ *filled with inflammatory debris.* (Right) *Coronal T1WI MR shows diffuse replacement of normal mandibular fatty marrow signal. There are multiple focal areas of interrupted cortical bone* ➡. *Induration and edema of subcutaneous tissues* ➡ *are common findings in ORN mandible.*

Mandible-Maxilla Osteonecrosis

TERMINOLOGY

- Necrosis of mandible or maxilla associated with medications, often **bisphosphonates**

IMAGING

- CT
  - Early: Nonhealing extraction socket
  - Late: Diffuse destructive changes in alveolar ridge
    - Widened periodontal ligament spaces
    - May be associated with pathologic fracture
- Tissue swelling if severe, infected, pathologic fracture
- MR: Variable signal from edema and bone changes
  - Enhancement common & does not imply infection
- Typically FDG avid

TOP DIFFERENTIAL DIAGNOSES

- Mandible-maxilla osteomyelitis
- Mandible-maxilla osteoradionecrosis
- Mandible-maxilla metastasis

CLINICAL ISSUES

- Nonhealing exposed bone, after 8 weeks, in patient with no prior craniofacial radiation
- Mimics dental infection & follows tooth extraction
- **Mandible much more common** than maxilla

DIAGNOSTIC CHECKLIST

- Diagnosis should be considered in patient with nonhealing extraction socket or jaw pain
- Often difficult or forgotten diagnosis in cancer patients: Metastasis vs. osteonecrosis
- Medication history (especially bisphosphonates) may be unknown to radiologist
- Typically mixed lytic-sclerotic mandible-maxilla with edema in surrounding tissues ± reactive adenopathy
- Look for pathologic fracture, extension of lytic process to inferior alveolar canal, abscess from secondary infection

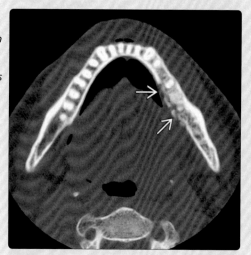
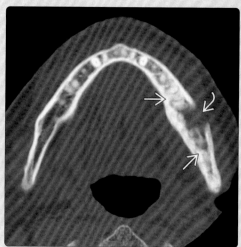

(Left) Axial bone CT demonstrates lytic cortical lesion ➡ of left mandible with periapical lucency of left mandibular molars. Findings are diagnostic of osteonecrosis in a patient with a nonhealing ulcer, exposed bone, and bisphosphonate exposure. (Right) Axial bone CT shows a typical case of mandibular osteonecrosis related to intravenous bisphosphonates. Note the mixed sclerotic ➡ and lytic ➡ lesion in left mandible body at site of recent tooth extraction.

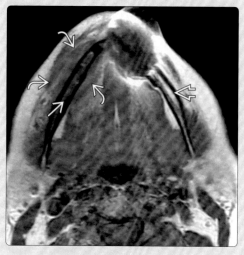
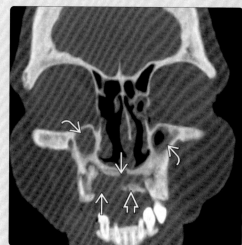

(Left) Axial T1WI MR in a patient on bisphosphonates for metastatic breast cancer and new jaw pain shows normal marrow on left ➡ but low-signal edema in right mandible ➡. Adjacent soft tissue inflammation ➡ is noted. Distinguishing metastasis from osteonecrosis can be very difficult. (Right) Coronal bone CT shows severe maxillary osteonecrosis with destruction ➡ in a patient with multiple myeloma and IV bisphosphonates. Note bone sequestrum ➡. Maxillary sinus opacification ➡ is probably not associated.

TERMINOLOGY

Abbreviations
- Mandible-maxilla (Md-Mx) osteonecrosis (ON)

Synonyms
- Medication-related osteonecrosis of jaws
- Bisphosphonate-related osteonecrosis of jaws

Definitions
- Necrosis of mandible or maxilla associated with **medication (often bisphosphonate)** use
  - Nonhealing exposed bone, after 8 weeks, in patient with no history of prior craniofacial radiation

IMAGING

General Features
- Best diagnostic clue
  - Bone CT showing mixed sclerotic & lytic destructive changes at extraction site
- Location
  - **Mandible** > > > **maxilla**
  - Often located on alveolar ridge with loss of teeth
  - Advanced disease extends into mandibular ramus
- Size
  - Varies: Focal to large area of bone destruction

Radiographic Findings
- Radiography
  - Mixed permeative & sclerotic changes with cortical destruction & periosteal reaction
  - Involvement of inferior alveolar canal by lytic process or pathologic fracture in severe cases

CT Findings
- Bone CT
  - Early: Nonhealing extraction socket
  - Late: Diffuse destructive changes in alveolar ridge
  - Widened periodontal ligament spaces
  - May be associated with **pathologic fracture**
  - Soft tissue swelling if destruction is severe, infected, or associated with pathologic fracture
  - After treatment: No new lytic changes, but sclerosis is permanent

MR Findings
- T2WI
  - Variable appearance
    - Acute: Bone edema shows high signal intensity
    - Healing phase: Variable or even low intensity if sclerotic
  - Surrounding soft tissues, especially muscles of mastication, often hyperintense due to edema
  - Nonnecrotic level I & II reactive adenopathy common
- T1WI C+ FS
  - **Enhancement** in healing bone & surrounding soft tissues common
    - Does not usually imply infection or tumor

Imaging Recommendations
- Best imaging tool
  - Radiography (panorex) usually 1st imaging utilized to confirm diagnosis
  - Bone CT; CECT if suspected infection
- Protocol advice
  - Bone CT with axial and coronal reformats to display full extent of disease, including loss of teeth

DIFFERENTIAL DIAGNOSIS

Mandible-Maxilla Osteomyelitis
- Infected tooth involves adjacent mandible
- Periosteal reaction, cortical sinus tract ± adjacent abscess

Mandible-Maxilla Osteoradionecrosis
- Prior radiation for oral cavity or oropharynx squamous cell carcinoma
- Focal permeative bone changes ± dissolution on CT

Mandible-Maxilla Metastasis
- Known primary malignancy present
- Destructive soft tissue mass in mandible

PATHOLOGY

General Features
- Etiology
  - Associated with new medications/bisphosphonates with antiresorptive and antiangiogenic properties
    - Treat metabolic & oncologic bone lesions: Paget disease, multiple myeloma, bone metastases
    - Mechanism of action: Suppress osteoclast activity, reduce bone resorption and osteolysis
  - Interval between medication exposure & Md-Mx ON may be **months to years**

Gross Pathologic & Surgical Features
- Ulcerated lesions in oral cavity, often with exposed nonviable bone
- Clinical exam **essential** for diagnosis as biopsy may exacerbate process

CLINICAL ISSUES

Presentation
- Most common signs/symptoms
  - Jaw pain and ulcers with loose teeth or nonhealing extraction socket
- Other signs/symptoms
  - Acute, severe pain: Check for pathologic fracture

Natural History & Prognosis
- Local debridement and discontinuation of medication/bisphosphonate should halt progression
- **Osteonecrosis is permanent**

Treatment
- Cease drug therapy & antibiotics if also infected
- Surgical debridement of necrotic bony sequestra or destroyed jaw

SELECTED REFERENCES

1. Bodem JP et al: Surgical management of bisphosphonate-related osteonecrosis of the jaw stages II and III. Oral Surg Oral Med Oral Pathol Oral Radiol. 121(4):367-72, 2016

Introduction and Overview of Squamous Cell Carcinoma

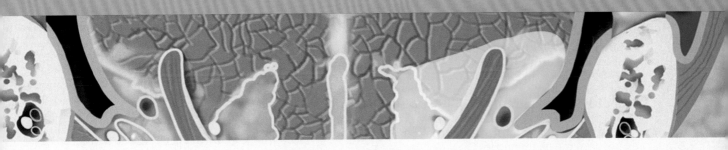

Summary Thoughts: Squamous Cell Carcinoma

Squamous cell carcinoma (SCCa) is, without question, the most common malignancy in the H&N. Recent developments in the understanding of the molecular nature and causes of SCCa now reveal it to be a heterogeneous malignancy.

In most sites of the H&N, **tobacco** is the most common causative agent in the development of mucosal dysplasia and neoplasia. **Alcohol** is a synergistic cofactor, while poor oral hygiene and genetics are also contributing risk factors. Paralleling the declining trend of smoking over the last 30 years, there has been an overall decline in the incidence of H&N SCCa, particularly in the oral cavity, larynx, and hypopharynx. Conversely, in the oropharynx there has been a rise in **base of tongue (BOT)** or **lingual** and **palatine tonsillar SCCa**, particularly in patients under 60 years, who may have a limited or no history of tobacco and alcohol use. This increasingly common group of SCCa tumors is positive for human papillomavirus (HPV), most commonly the HPV-16 subtype, which is also responsible for anogenital neoplasms. Currently in the United States, about 60% of oropharyngeal SCCa (especially tonsil and BOT) are due to HPV. HPV(+) SCCa appears to be more responsive to chemoradiation than HPV(-) SCCa, and patients have an overall better survival. Patients with HPV(+) tumors who are also smokers carry an intermediate prognosis.

Nasopharyngeal carcinoma (NPC) is a distinctly different neoplasm with the most common histopathological subtypes associated with **Epstein-Barr virus** infection. The least common and most aggressive form (keratinizing NPC) is related to tobacco and alcohol abuse, although some pathology literature has also suggested an association with HPV infection.

While our current understanding of SCCa is evolving through greater molecular interrogation of these tumors, the radiologists' roles remain largely unchanged. At the time of diagnosis, the radiologist must report details about the primary tumor to assign a **tumor stage**, including the **size** and **local extent** of the primary, detecting **PNT**, and assessing regional **nodes** and **distant** spread of disease. Following treatment, both **baseline** and **surveillance** imaging require careful evaluation to detect **residual** or **recurrent SCCa, treatment complications**, and **second primary neoplasms**.

Imaging Approaches and Indications

There is no definitive best imaging modality for all H&N sites when staging SCCa. Some specific tumor sites are better served by either **CECT or MR or PET/CECT**. A patient with copious secretions or pain may not tolerate long MR sequences, and, in that instance, CECT or PET combined with CECT is preferred. Excellent quality neck imaging is more readily reproducible from patient to patient using CT than MR. Also, large field of view, nonoptimized MR sequences, and lack of familiarity with basic neck anatomy make detection of key findings difficult. A poorly performed and inaccurately interpreted neck MR scan is an expensive, unsatisfactory alternative to CT imaging.

MR does offer specific utility in certain areas. For example, it is the preferred staging tool for NPC because detection of skull base infiltration (T3) or intracranial disease (T4) is extremely important for staging and treatment planning. MR offers better soft tissue contrast for detecting small primary tonsillar tumors and evaluating the deep extent of a lesion when

planning surgical resection or **intensity-modulated radiation therapy (IMRT)**. For this reason, MR may be used in the oral cavity and oropharynx. In the larynx, MR is so affected by motion artifact that it is largely reserved for determination of cartilage penetration (T4a) when CECT is equivocal. Finally, nodal disease at any site is almost equally well evaluated with either CECT or MR, but PET is superior to both anatomic studies.

Given the complexity of neck anatomy, **FDG PET** in the H&N is best performed as a combined PET/CECT examination. There are variable degrees of normal FDG uptake in muscles, brown fat, salivary and lymphoid tissue, and recent biopsy sites. These all are potential false-positive pitfalls in PET imaging, but routine measurement and reporting of standardized uptake values can obviate the pitfalls. A potential false-negative finding is absence of uptake in a cystic/necrotic node, but correlation with neck CECT imaging will allow correct identification of cystic/necrotic nodal metastases.

Ultrasound (US) has a limited role in H&N SCCa. Skilled ultrasonographers claim US is highly accurate for determining extracapsular spread (ECS) of a nodal metastasis. US can also serve as imaging guidance for fine-needle aspiration.

Imaging Anatomy

SCCa arises from the mucosal surface of the upper airway and digestive tract, the pharynx and larynx. The pharynx is really a muscular tube encased by the middle layer of deep cervical fascia (DCF) and attached to the skull base by the pharyngobasilar fascia. The **pharyngeal mucosal space** is a continuous sheet of tissue on the airway side of the DCF. It is divided into separate sites anatomically. Staging of mucosal SCCa is individualized to each site or subsite.

The **nasopharynx**, posterior to the nasal cavity, extends from the most cranial pharynx at the skull base to the soft palate. Inferiorly, it is contiguous with the **oropharynx**, which extends caudally to the hyoid bone. The anterior tonsillar pillars and the circumvallate papillae of the tongue define the anterior limit of the oropharynx. The anterior 2/3 of the tongue lies in the oral cavity and is known as the oral tongue. The posterior 1/3 is called the tongue base and is part of the oropharynx.

Below the hyoid bone, the pharynx divides to form the **larynx**, which is continuous with the trachea, and the hypopharynx, which joins the cervical esophagus. The posterior wall of the hypopharynx is a continuation of the posterior wall of the oropharynx. Lateral "pockets" of the hypopharynx form the pyriform sinuses and are separated from the larynx by the aryepiglottic (AE) folds. Nearly 2/3 of hypopharyngeal SCCa arise in the pyriform sinuses. The larynx is anterior in the neck and has 3 subsites: The supraglottic larynx, which includes the epiglottis, AE folds, and false cords; the glottis, or true vocal cords; and the subglottis, which is contiguous with the cervical trachea. More than 1/2 of all laryngeal SCCa are glottic in origin.

Approaches to Imaging Issues in H&N SCCa

Staging a SCCa is performed using the American Joint Committee on Cancer classification system, currently in its 7th edition (2010). Referral to the site-specific tumor (T) and nodal (N) features at the time of film review greatly enhances an imaging report. When the size of a T or N is important for tumor or nodal stage, respectively, the longest diameter is measured. Some superficial oral cavity tumors are best measured on clinical examination. The key role of cross-sectional imaging is to evaluate features that are not evident on exam, such as deep extent or bone infiltration, which may upstage a tumor or alter treatment options.

The detection of a **perineural tumor** (PNT) may significantly alter the surgical resection &/or the radiation treatment field. Both mucosal and skin SCCa exhibit neurotropism, as do some salivary gland tumors and lymphomas. PNT is usually more evident on MR but may be detected on CT with careful evaluation of skull base foramina and known routes of spread.

Metastatic **nodal disease** is the most important prognostic factor in H&N SCCa. For all sites but the nasopharynx, a single node < 3 cm in diameter is staged as N1, which is stage III disease. A larger node or multiple or bilateral nodes define N2 and stage IV disease. NPC commonly has extensive, large nodal metastases; therefore, this tumor has separate, distinct nodal staging criteria. With any H&N SCCa, the neck should be evaluated for enlarged, heterogeneous, or frankly necrotic nodes. ECS, while not formally upstaging the nodal disease, may change the treatment approach, as it is usually associated with a poorer prognosis and higher rate of tumor recurrence.

At the time of a staging neck CECT scan, the lung apices and the bones should also be evaluated for **metastases**. Finally, many SCCa H&N cancer patients have increased risk of a **second primary neoplasm**. Second primary tumors are most frequently found with hypopharyngeal SCCa, and 1/3 are synchronous with the initial SCCa.

Following surgery, radiation, &/or chemotherapy, a **posttreatment baseline** imaging study should be obtained to confirm absence of **residual disease**. This also serves as a roadmap of an anatomically changed neck to aid in detection of **recurrent disease**. At our institution, the initial posttreatment study for almost all SCCa is a PET/CECT. PET/CECT should be delayed around 10-12 weeks to minimize false-positive FDG uptake from posttreatment inflammatory changes. A baseline CECT study may be obtained at 8-10 weeks following chemoradiation, while postsurgical studies are often obtained at 10-12 weeks.

The **posttreatment baseline** scan following radiation &/or chemotherapy should show no evidence of residual disease. The presence of enlarged nodes or residual primary mass following treatment is of concern and is typically surgically resected. Posttreatment neck dissections are ideally performed before 10 weeks to minimize the complexity of surgery that results with neck fibrosis. So-called borderline soft tissue at baseline CT/MR may be carefully watched, may undergo US-guided aspiration, or may be resected.

Radiation therapy has changed enormously over the last 2 decades with increasing use of **IMRT** for H&N cancers. IMRT maximizes dose to the tumor, minimizes radiation to normal surrounding tissues, and requires accurate delineation of tumor margins. Greater input from radiologists to ensure accurate treatment volumes may be needed, with MR, PET/CECT, or CECT alone. Radiation ± **chemotherapy** results in significant changes in appearance of neck soft tissues. Radiation results in acute inflammation and edema of all tissues in the radiation field. Over time, this changes to fibrosis, atrophy, and altered appearances on CECT and MR. Both acute and chronic expected radiation changes can be confusing on CECT or MR.

Surgical resection of a primary tumor &/or cervical neck nodes also results in changes to normal neck contours.

Familiarity with the types of nodal **neck dissections** and common **flap reconstructions** helps to evaluate both complications and recurrence. Knowledge of what surgical procedure was performed prior to evaluating posttreatment imaging is critical. Some resections, such as selective neck dissections, can be subtle on imaging, while large resections with flap reconstructions can be quite complex. MR is less affected by hardware artifact and more sensitive for recurrent tumors; however, the muscular component of a flap reconstruction undergoes denervation changes resulting in variable MR signal intensity and enhancement. On the baseline scan following neck reconstruction, residual or progressive tumors should be described.

Recurrent SCCa most often occurs during the first 2 years following initial treatment. The frequency of **surveillance imaging** during this time is variable and may be performed in 3- to 6-month intervals, depending on the initial tumor stage, prognostic features, and the clinical course, including physical findings. At the follow-up imaging examination, the possibility of a **second primary tumor** must be considered. Remember to look for **residual, recurrent, and new** tumors on every follow-up study.

How to Stage New Tumor With CT or MR

- Determine site of primary; open TNM staging table for specific primary site
- Evaluate size and local extent of tumor; what is deep extent; is there bone marrow infiltration; is there PNT; how far does it go in each direction; primary is best described in dedicated paragraph in report
- Evaluate regional drainage nodes and contralateral node(s); are there retropharyngeal nodes
- Evaluate included lungs and bones for metastases
- In our experience, having access to PET or PET/CECT greatly increases staging accuracy

Clinical Implications

When a patient presents with a new neck mass that is nodal SCCa, an initial clinical examination is performed in the ENT surgeon's office. If a primary site is not evident, it is considered to be an **unknown primary tumor**, and imaging has an important role in finding the primary so that biopsy can be directed. There are 4 key sites to consider first when evaluating a neck CECT or MR in search of an unknown primary tumor: (1) nasopharynx: **Fossa of Rosenmüller**, (2) oropharynx: **Palatine tonsil**, (3) oropharynx: **BOT or lingual tonsil**, and (4) hypopharynx: **Apex of pyriform sinus**. The fossa of Rosenmüller and pyriform sinus apex may be clinical "blind spots," either at the in-office examination or, if very small, even at the direct endoscopy. The palatine and lingual tonsils may harbor a tumor in the depths of crypts, so the mucosal tumor may not be evident visually or on palpation. In all 4 locations, asymmetric soft tissue on cross-sectional imaging is key.

The changing demographics of tonsillar and BOT lingual SCCa, due to the rising incidence of HPV(+) oropharyngeal SCCa, make it imperative that the radiologist is vigilant when evaluating a younger, nonsmoking subset of patients presenting with a new neck mass, which may be a cystic/necrotic or solid metastatic node. **A new neck mass in an adult, unless obviously a thyroid goiter, should be assumed to be neoplastic until proven otherwise.**

Sites and Subsites of Head and Neck Squamous Cell Carcinoma

Nasopharynx	Oral cavity	Hypopharynx
Fossa of Rosenmüller	Oral tongue	Pyriform sinus
	Floor of mouth	Postcricoid region
Oropharynx	Alveolar ridge: Maxilla	Posterior hypopharyngeal wall
Palatine tonsil	Buccal mucosa	**Larynx**
Posterior oropharyngeal wall	Hard palate	Supraglottis
Soft palate	Lip	Glottis
Lingual tonsil/base of tongue	Retromolar trigone	Subglottis
	Alveolar ridge: Mandible	

Nasopharynx (AJCC 2010)

Anatomic Stage/Prognostic Groups

Stage 0	Tis (in situ)	N0	M0
Stage I	T1	N0	M0
Stage II	T2	N0	M0
	T1-T2	**N1**	M0
Stage III	**T3**	N0-N2	M0
	T1-T3	**N2**	M0
Stage IVA	**T4**	N0-N2	M0
Stage IVB	Any T	**N3**	M0
Stage IVC	Any T	Any N	**M1**

Adapted from 7th edition AJCC Staging Forms.

All Other Head and Neck Sites (AJCC 2010)

Anatomic Stage/Prognostic Groups

Stage 0	Tis (in situ)	N0	M0
Stage I	T1	N0	M0
Stage II	T2	N0	M0
Stage III	T3	N0	M0
	T1-T3	**N1**	M0
Stage IVA	**T4a**	N0-N1	M0
	T1-T4a	**N2**	M0
Stage IVB	**T4b**	Any N	M0
	Any T	**N3**	M0
Stage IVC	Any T	Any N	**M1**

Adapted from 7th edition AJCC Staging Forms.

Selected References

1. Landry D et al: Squamous cell carcinoma of the upper aerodigestive tract: a review. Radiol Clin North Am. 53(1):81-97, 2015
2. Hudgins PA et al: Introduction to the imaging and staging of cancer. Neuroimaging Clin N Am. 23(1):1-7, 2013
3. Genden EM et al: Human papillomavirus and oropharyngeal squamous cell carcinoma: what the clinician should know. Eur Arch Otorhinolaryngol. 270(2):405-16, 2012
4. Srinivasan A et al: Biologic imaging of head and neck cancer: the present and the future. AJNR Am J Neuroradiol. 33(4):586-94, 2012
5. Yoshizaki T et al: Current understanding and management of nasopharyngeal carcinoma. Auris Nasus Larynx. 39(2):137-44, 2012
6. Trotta BM et al: Oral cavity and oropharyngeal squamous cell cancer: key imaging findings for staging and treatment planning. Radiographics. 31(2):339-54, 2011
7. Ang KK et al: Human papillomavirus and survival of patients with oropharyngeal cancer. N Engl J Med. 363(1):24-35, 2010
8. Subramaniam RM et al: Fluorodeoxyglucose-positron-emission tomography imaging of head and neck squamous cell cancer. AJNR Am J Neuroradiol. 31(4):598-604, 2010

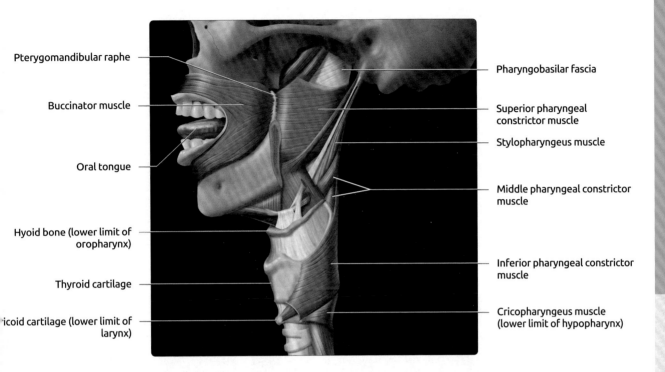

Pterygomandibular raphe

Buccinator muscle

Oral tongue

Hyoid bone (lower limit of oropharynx)

Thyroid cartilage

Cricoid cartilage (lower limit of larynx)

Pharyngobasilar fascia

Superior pharyngeal constrictor muscle

Stylopharyngeus muscle

Middle pharyngeal constrictor muscle

Inferior pharyngeal constrictor muscle

Cricopharyngeus muscle (lower limit of hypopharynx)

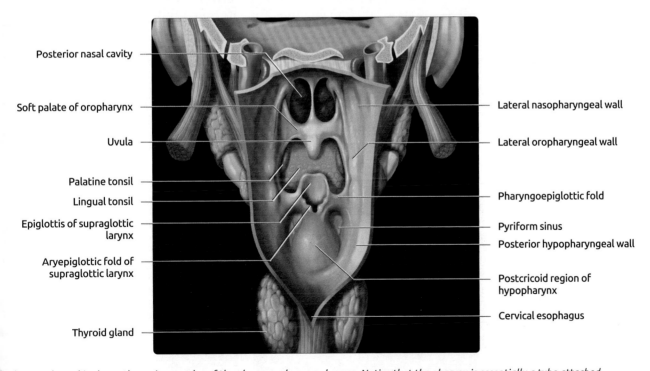

Posterior nasal cavity

Soft palate of oropharynx

Uvula

Palatine tonsil

Lingual tonsil

Epiglottis of supraglottic larynx

Aryepiglottic fold of supraglottic larynx

Thyroid gland

Lateral nasopharyngeal wall

Lateral oropharyngeal wall

Pharyngoepiglottic fold

Pyriform sinus

Posterior hypopharyngeal wall

Postcricoid region of hypopharynx

Cervical esophagus

(Top) *Lateral graphic shows the major muscles of the pharyngeal mucosal space. Notice that the pharynx is essentially a tube attached superiorly to the skull base and formed from the superior, middle, and inferior pharyngeal constrictor muscles. The nasopharynx, oropharynx, and hypopharynx are contiguous segments of this tube, with the oral cavity contiguous anteriorly with the oropharynx. The larynx is intimately related to the hypopharynx and originates at the lower aspect of the oropharynx.* **(Bottom)** *Graphic of the pharyngeal mucosal space/surface as if opened from behind shows that this space can be divided into nasopharyngeal, oropharyngeal, and hypopharyngeal areas. The lymphatic ring of the pharyngeal mucosal space (Waldeyer) contains the nasopharyngeal adenoids and the oropharyngeal palatine and lingual tonsils or base of tongue.*

(Left) *Axial graphic of the nasopharyngeal mucosal space (blue) shows superior pharyngeal constrictor* ➡ *and levator veli palatini muscles* ➡ *within the space. The middle layer of deep cervical fascia (pink line) provides a deep margin to the space.* (Right) *Axial T1WI C+ FS MR in a 32-year-old Asian woman with trismus shows a large, mildly enhancing mass* ➡ *arising in the right nasopharynx & infiltrating the masticator space & clivus* ➡*. Involvement of cranial nerves found T4N2, stage IV NPC. Note the levator veli* ➡*.*

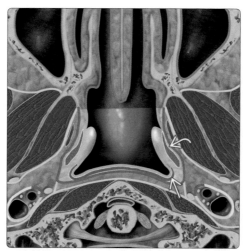
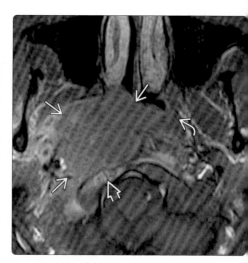

(Left) *Axial graphic of the oropharyngeal mucosal space (blue) viewed from above reveals distinction from a more anterior oral cavity. Anterior* ➡ *and posterior tonsillar pillars, palatine tonsils* ➡*, and lingual tonsil* ➡*, a.k.a. base of tongue, are most common primary SCCa sites.* (Right) *Axial T1WI C+ FS MR in a 66 year old with asymmetry noted by dentist on examination shows a moderately enhancing mass* ➡ *in the tonsillar fossa. This case is unusual for the absence of adenopathy and is T1N0, stage I SCCa.*

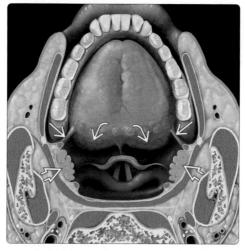
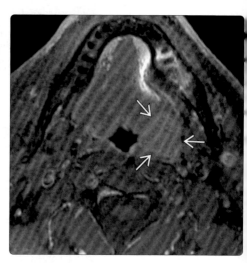

(Left) *Axial graphic shows the hypopharyngeal aspect of the pharyngeal mucosal space. At the level of the supraglottis, the hypopharynx is made up of the pyriform sinus* ➡ *& posterior wall* ➡*. AE folds* ➡ *are part of the supraglottis & separate the larynx from the hypopharynx.* (Right) *Axial CECT in a patient presenting with extensive matted bilateral adenopathy* ➡ *demonstrates an irregular, superficially spreading mass arising from posterior hypopharyngeal wall* ➡*. This is T3N2c, stage IVA SCCa. Note the AE fold* ➡*.*

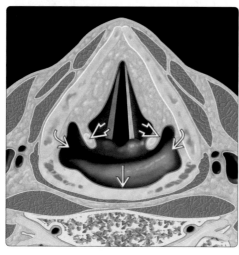
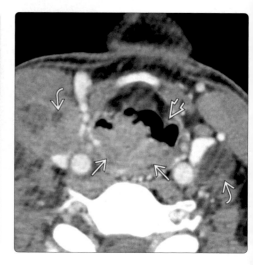

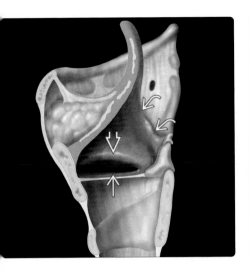

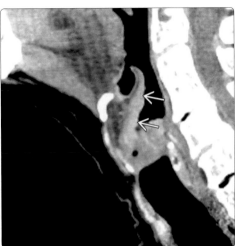

(Left) *Sagittal graphic of larynx shows true the vocal cord* ➡ *of the glottic larynx. False cord* ➡ *lies above and parallels this, while the AE fold* ➡ *projects from the tip of arytenoid cartilage to the inferolateral margin of the epiglottis. Subglottis extends from below the true cords to the inferior cricoid margin.* (Right) *Sagittal CECT reconstructed image in a 73-year-old woman demonstrates abnormal thickening of the laryngeal surface of the epiglottis* ➡. *This is T2N2c, stage IVA SCCa.*

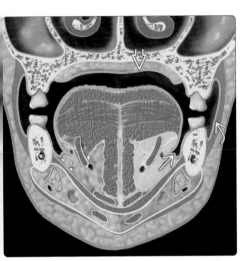

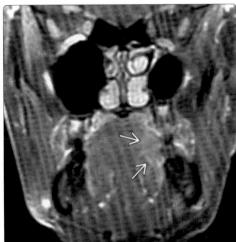

(Left) *Coronal graphic shows the oral mucosal space/surface (blue) on the left. Hard palate* ➡, *oral tongue, upper and lower alveolar ridge, buccal* ➡, *and floor of mouth* ➡ *mucosal surfaces are seen. Coronal plane is helpful for deep involvement of BOT, floor of mouth, and mandible.* (Right) *Coronal T1WI C+ FS MR in a 32-year-old woman with a remote history of cigarette and marijuana use shows a heterogeneous, mildly enhancing lesion of lateral tongue* ➡. *This is T2N2b, stage IVA SCCa.*

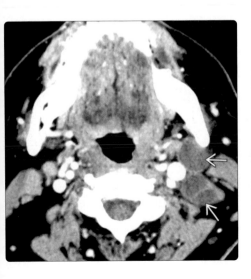

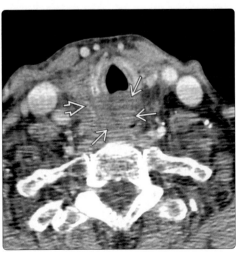

(Left) *CECT in a 46-year-old woman with neck masses shows multiple necrotic/cystic nodes* ➡. *There was no primary on clinical exam or imaging, although tonsillectomy revealed a small primary tumor. This is T1N2b, stage IVA SCCa.* (Right) *Axial CECT in a 78-year-old man with new hoarseness 7 months following completion of radiation for T1 glottic SCCa shows ill-defined esophageal mass* ➡ *infiltrating the right tracheoesophageal groove* ➡. *Lesion was found to be a 2nd primary tumor (esophageal SCCa).*

SECTION 17
Primary Sites, Perineural Tumor and Nodes

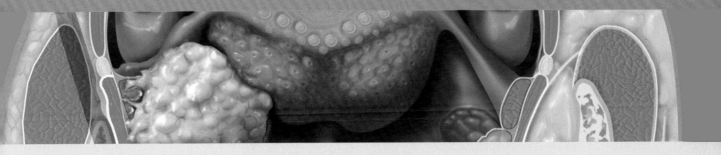

Nasopharyngeal Carcinoma

TERMINOLOGY

- Nasopharyngeal carcinoma (NPC)
- Mucosal tumor of lateral pharyngeal recess (fossa of Rosenmüller), strongly associated with EBV infection

IMAGING

- MR best demonstrates parapharyngeal fat, skull base infiltration, and intracranial tumor
- Nodal disease in 90% at presentation: Retropharyngeal, levels II and V most common
- Metastatic nodes often large ± necrosis
- NPC is markedly FDG avid

TOP DIFFERENTIAL DIAGNOSES

- Adenoidal benign lymphoid hyperplasia
- Nasopharyngeal non-Hodgkin lymphoma
- Nasopharyngeal minor salivary gland malignancy
- Pituitary macroadenoma

PATHOLOGY

- **25%: Keratinizing NPC** (previously type I)
- **75%: Nonkeratinizing NPC** (NK NPC)
  - Strongly associated with EBV
  - **15% differentiated** (previously type II)
  - **60% undifferentiated** (previously type III)
- Rare: Basaloid squamous cell carcinoma

CLINICAL ISSUES

- Peak incidence: 40-60 years
- Pediatric NPC rare; most often undifferentiated NK
- Clinical presentations
  - Bloody nasal discharge or epistaxis
  - 50-70% present with mass from metastatic nodes
  - Serous otitis from eustachian tube obstruction
- NK NPC has 5-year survival ~ 75%
- Keratinizing NPC has 5-year survival 20-40%

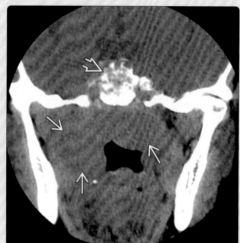
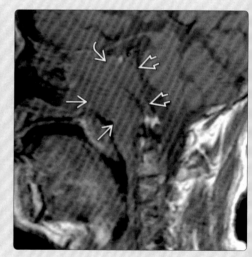

(Left) Coronal NECT of paranasal sinuses, performed in a 62-year-old Asian man for evaluation of nasal stuffiness and epistaxis, demonstrates an asymmetric bulky mass of nasopharynx ➡ with heterogeneous, mottled texture of clivus ⇗. (Right) Sagittal T1WI MR in the same patient reveals a large soft tissue mass in the nasopharynx ➡ extending superiorly to the sphenoid and sella ⇗. There is replacement of normally hyperintense fatty marrow of the clivus ⇗ without clival expansion.

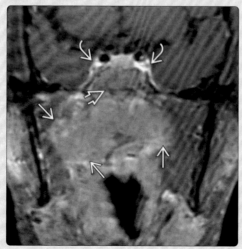
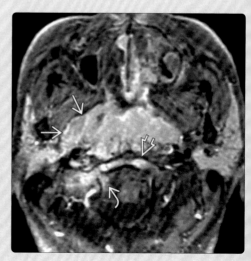

(Left) Coronal T1WI C+ FS MR reveals moderate enhancement of a bulky mass ➡ filling the nasopharynx with an indistinct right lateral margin. Enhancing tumor extends cranially to infiltrate the sphenoid bone ⇗. There is no abnormality of cavernous sinuses ⇗. (Right) Axial T1WI C+ FS MR shows infiltration of parapharyngeal fat ➡. There is abnormal enhancement of basisphenoid ⇗ consistent with marrow infiltration. More significantly, however, there is abnormal right hypoglossal nerve enhancement ⇗. This is a T4 tumor.

TERMINOLOGY

Abbreviations

- Nasopharyngeal carcinoma (NPC)

Definitions

- Primary mucosal malignancy arising in nasopharynx, most strongly associated with EBV infection

IMAGING

General Features

- Best diagnostic clue
  - Lateral pharyngeal recess mass with deep extension and cervical adenopathy
- Location
  - Arises in lateral pharyngeal recess, a.k.a. fossa of Rosenmüller
- Morphology
  - Poorly marginated mucosal mass with deep extension and invasion
  - Nodal disease in 90% at presentation

CT Findings

- CECT
  - Mildly enhancing off-midline nasopharyngeal mass
  - Metastatic nodes often large, ± necrosis
  - Retropharyngeal nodes often subtle on imaging, as they appear isodense to muscle
- Bone CT
  - May show destruction of clival cortex or pterygoid plates

MR Findings

- T1WI
  - Asymmetric mass, hypo- to isointense to muscle
  - Sensitive for infiltration of parapharyngeal fat and marrow involvement
- T2WI
  - Moderate hyperintensity of NPC compared with muscle
- T1WI C+ FS
  - Best illustrates infiltration of deep face, intracranial, and cavernous sinus disease
    - Coronal images aid in this evaluation
  - Mild homogeneous tumor enhancement

Nuclear Medicine Findings

- PET/CT
  - Markedly FDG-avid tumor, nodes, and metastases
  - If small primary, can miss with thick slices due to brain FDG uptake

Imaging Recommendations

- Best imaging tool
  - MR is recommended by American Joint Committee on Cancer (AJCC) for staging
    - Most sensitive for skull base and intracranial tumor spread
    - More sensitive than clinical exam/US/CT for detection of retropharyngeal nodes
    - CECT is alternative choice
  - PET/CT often obtained if N2/3 disease at staging or recurrent tumor

- Protocol advice
  - T1 MR best shows infiltration of skull base with loss of fat signal
  - Postcontrast axial and coronal images best demonstrate intracranial spread

DIFFERENTIAL DIAGNOSIS

Adenoidal Benign Lymphoid Hyperplasia

- Large adenoids seen in children, teens, and HIV patients
- Symmetric enlargement without infiltration of adjacent tissues

Nasopharyngeal Non-Hodgkin Lymphoma

- Midline symmetric mass, ± deep infiltration to prevertebral muscles
- In clivus, tends to expand rather than infiltrate

Nasopharyngeal Minor Salivary Gland Malignancy

- Uncommon primary tumor, nodal metastases uncommon
- May be small primary with extensive infiltration

Pituitary Macroadenoma

- Large sella mass extending through sphenoid to nasopharynx
- Expansion of sella is key imaging finding

Pharyngeal Mucosal Space Sarcoma

- Rare; more common differential in children
- Submucosal, aggressive mass

PATHOLOGY

General Features

- Etiology
  - **Nonkeratinizing (NK)** strongly associated with **prior EBV infection**
    - EBV DNA found in tumor cells and in premalignant (dysplastic, in situ) lesions
  - Other proposed factors
    - Carcinogens (nitrosamines) in food eaten as child
    - Genetic predisposition
      - □ Increased risk in 1st-degree relatives
      - □ HLA-A2 + HLA-Bsin2 → increased risk for NPC
    - Prior radiation
    - Tobacco and alcohol most associated with basaloid squamous cell carcinoma (BSCCa) and keratinizing NPC

Staging, Grading, & Classification

- **AJCC Classification, 2010**
  - TNM staging; NPC has **unique nodal staging**

Gross Pathologic & Surgical Features

- Pathological types classified by World Health Organization (WHO)
- **Keratinizing NPC** (previously type I)
  - Poorly, moderately, or well differentiated
- **NK NPC**
  - PCR for EBV positive 75-100%
    - Differentiated (previously type II)
    - Undifferentiated (previously type III)
- **BSCCa**

AJCC Nasopharynx Staging (2010)

Tumor or Metastatic Stage (T or M)	Nodal Stage (N)
T1: Confined to nasopharynx or extension to oropharynx or nasal cavity	**N1**: ≥ 1 unilateral metastasis ≤ 6 cm &/or unilateral/bilateral retropharyngeal nodes ≤ 6 cm
T2: Extension to parapharyngeal fat	**N2**: Bilateral nodal metastases ≤ 6 cm
T3: Clivus or paranasal sinus invasion	**N3a**: Nodal metastases > 6 cm
T4: Intracranial spread, cranial nerve, orbit, hypopharynx, masticator space	**N3b**: Nodal metastasis to supraclavicular fossa
M0: No distant metastasis	
M1: Distant metastasis	

Note: This nodal staging is unique to nasopharyngeal carcinoma. Adapted from 7th edition AJCC Staging Forms.

- ○ Typically EBV & HPV negative

CLINICAL ISSUES

Presentation
- Most common signs/symptoms
  - ○ Conductive hearing loss secondary to middle ear obstruction
    - − Obstruction or infiltration of eustachian tube
  - ○ Bloody nasal discharge or epistaxis
  - ○ 50-70% present with mass from metastatic nodes
- Other signs/symptoms
  - ○ Uncommonly presents with cranial neuropathies

Demographics
- Age
  - ○ Peak incidence: 40-60 years
  - ○ Pediatric NPC rare; most often undifferentiated NK
- Gender
  - ○ M:F = 2.5:1
- Ethnicity
  - ○ NK NPC endemic in southern China
    - − 800 cases per 1 million
    - − Most of rest of world < 10 per 1 million
  - ○ ↓ risk in 2nd- and 3rd-generation American-born Chinese
  - ○ In children in USA, ↑ risk in African Americans
- Epidemiology
  - ○ Worldwide, most common NP adult malignancy
    - − Most common cancer in Asian men
  - ○ NK NPC 75% > keratinizing NPC 25% > BSCCa rare

Natural History & Prognosis
- Keratinizing NPC: Poorest prognosis; 5-year survival 20-40%
- NK NPC: Radiosensitive, better prognosis; 5-year survival ~ 75%
- BSCCa: Generally poor
- Most NPC presents as **stage III** (T3 &/or N2), **stage IVA** (T4), or **stage IVB** (N3)
- ≥ 90% have nodal metastases at presentation, often bilateral
  - ○ Retropharyngeal nodes primary site
  - ○ Level II and V nodes next most common
- 5% have distant metastases at presentation, poorer prognosis
- ≤ 30% recur with distant metastases
  - ○ Bone: Sclerotic or lytic lesions

- ○ Chest and liver also common sites

Treatment
- Generally radiosensitive, especially NK NPC
  - ○ T1: XRT alone
  - ○ T2-T4: XRT + chemotherapy
  - ○ M1: Chemotherapy; XRT only if good response
- Neck dissection for residual disease post treatment

DIAGNOSTIC CHECKLIST

Consider
- Carefully evaluate nasopharynx whenever middle ear obstruction in adult
- Lymphoma is main differential with NP mass ± adenopathy
  - ○ More often midline and expands clivus

Image Interpretation Pearls
- T1 MR sensitive for parapharyngeal space and bone marrow invasion
- T1 C+ key for intracranial, perineural, and cavernous sinus invasion

Reporting Tips
- Certain key tumor findings should be sought
  - ○ Parapharyngeal fat infiltration (T2)
  - ○ Skull base invasion (T3)
  - ○ Intracranial or cranial nerve involvement (T4)
- Nodal disease is common; nodes often large
  - ○ Retropharyngeal, level II and V nodes most often
  - ○ Supraclavicular nodes = N3b
    - − Important, therefore, to describe any low neck nodes (IV or VB) as potentially supraclavicular

SELECTED REFERENCES

1. King AD et al: Detection of nasopharyngeal carcinoma by MR imaging: diagnostic accuracy of MRI compared with endoscopy and endoscopic biopsy based on long-term follow-up. AJNR Am J Neuroradiol. 36(12):2380-5, 2015
2. Lan M et al: Prognostic value of cervical nodal necrosis in nasopharyngeal carcinoma: analysis of 1800 patients with positive cervical nodal metastasis at MR imaging. Radiology. 276(2):536-44, 2015
3. Lee AW et al: Management of nasopharyngeal carcinoma: current practice and future perspective. J Clin Oncol. 33(29):3356-64, 2015
4. Zhang GY et al: Prognostic value of grading masticator space involvement in nasopharyngeal carcinoma according to MR imaging findings. Radiology. 273(1):136-43, 2014
5. Chan AT: Current treatment of nasopharyngeal carcinoma. Eur J Cancer. 47 Suppl 3:S302-3, 2011

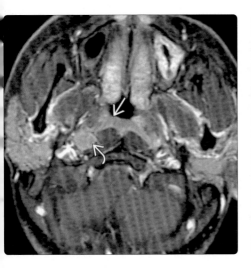

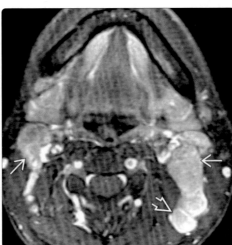

(Left) *Axial T1WI C+ FS MR in a 26-year-old Asian man presenting with neck masses demonstrates subtly asymmetric soft tissue fullness of nasopharynx mucosa* ➡, *though without infiltration of the prevertebral muscles. Enlarged right retropharyngeal node is evident* ➡. **(Right)** *Axial T1WI C+ FS MR in the same patient demonstrates bilateral enlarged level II* ➡ *and left level V* ➡ *nodes, which proved to be undifferentiated nonkeratinizing carcinoma, positive for EBV. This is staged as T1N2, stage III disease.*

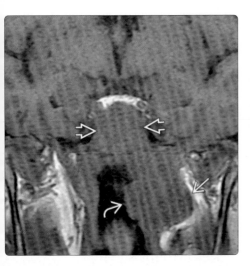

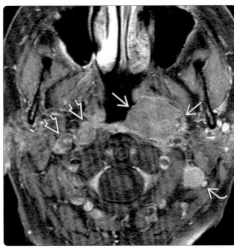

(Left) *Coronal T1 MR shows an infiltrative T1 hypointense mass in the superior lateral nasopharynx* ➡, *extending into the clivus* ➡ *and the left parapharyngeal space* ➡. *Endoscopic biopsy showed nonkeratinizing nasopharyngeal carcinoma (NPC).* **(Right)** *Axial T1 C+ FS in same patient shows NPC in left lateral nasopharyngeal recess extending in the parapharyngeal space* ➡. *Contralateral retropharyngeal* ➡ *and ipsilateral level IIB* ➡ *nodal metastases are well seen. This is staged as T3N2 or stage III.*

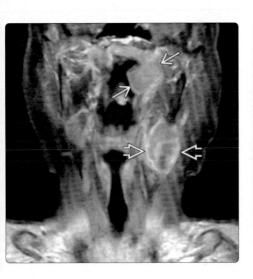

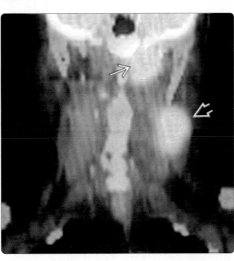

(Left) *Coronal T1WI C+ FS MR in a 65-year-old woman with newly diagnosed NPC demonstrates an ulcerated enhancing mass in the left nasopharynx* ➡ *associated with necrotic ipsilateral level II nodes* ➡. *Contralateral nodes were also found. Biopsy showed poorly differentiated keratinizing carcinoma.* **(Right)** *Coronal fused PET/CT shows intense FDG uptake in a left NPC* ➡ *and in level II node* ➡. *No distant metastases were found. This NPC was staged as T2N2M0, stage III disease.*

TERMINOLOGY

- Base of tongue oropharyngeal SCCa
- Tonsillar tissue at posterior 1/3 of tongue

IMAGING

- Primary tumor may be ulceroinfiltrative lesion or exophytic mass
- Nodal disease common even with subtle primary
- CECT most often used but MR more accurate for tumor extent
  - CECT: Scan ≥ 90 seconds after IV contrast to maximize tumor and mucosal enhancement
  - MR: Fat-sat enhances soft tissue contrast: T2 & T1 C+
- PET/CT: Staging, unknown primary search, posttreatment baseline scan
  - Beware of FDG-negative cystic nodal metastasis

TOP DIFFERENTIAL DIAGNOSES

- Lingual tonsil lymphoid hyperplasia

- Lingual tonsil non-Hodgkin lymphoma
- Palatine tonsil SCCa
- Lingual tonsil benign mixed tumor
- Lingual tonsil minor salivary gland malignancy

PATHOLOGY

- Oropharyngeal SCCa classically associated with tobacco + alcohol abuse
- Increasing incidence of HPV(+) oropharyngeal SCCa

CLINICAL ISSUES

- Most common presentation is sore throat
- Typically at least 1 node, even when small
- 30% present with bilateral adenopathy
- Demographics changing with increasing incidence of HPV(+) SCCa
  - Patients younger, more commonly nonsmokers
  - HPV is favorable prognostic biomarker
- Overall 5-yr survival = 50%

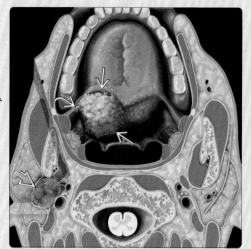
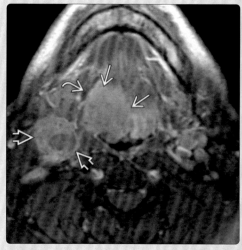

(Left) Axial graphic depicts lingual tonsil SCCa ➡ with ipsilateral adenopathy ➡. Tongue base tumor has predominantly exophytic growth but infiltrates inferior aspect of anterior tonsillar pillar ➡. (Right) Axial T1WI C+ FS MR in a 58-year-old alcoholic presenting with persistent right neck mass after dental procedure demonstrates enlarged, heterogeneous, right level II node ➡. Primary tumor is in ipsilateral lingual tonsil ➡ and infiltrates floor of mouth, medial to hyoglossus muscle ➡.

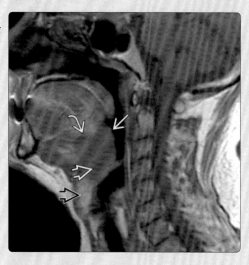
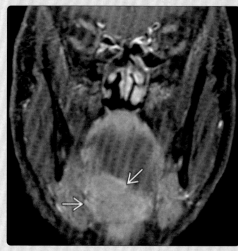

(Left) Sagittal T1WI MR in the same patient shows fullness at the right base of tongue ➡ with a tumor replacing the lingual tonsillar tissue and infiltrating into the floor of mouth ➡. Tumor extends inferiorly to valleculae ➡ but does not extend inferiorly into preepiglottic fat ➡. (Right) Coronal T1WI C+ FS MR shows an asymmetric mass ➡ at the right base of tongue in the same patient. This was found to be an invasive SCCa and staged T4a N2c, stage IVA, and received chemoradiation. Patient was well at 4-year follow-up.

Base of Tongue Squamous Cell Carcinoma

TERMINOLOGY

Abbreviations
- Base of tongue (BOT) squamous cell carcinoma (SCCa)

Synonyms
- Lingual tonsil SCCa

Definitions
- Epithelial tumor arising in **oropharyngeal** tonsillar tissue at tongue base
  - Extends from posterior 1/3 of tongue to valleculae
  - Distinct entity from oral tongue SCCa

IMAGING

General Features
- Best diagnostic clue
  - Asymmetric enlargement of lingual tonsil or invasive tongue base mass
  - Early nodal metastasis common
    - Most commonly levels II-IV
    - Complex lymph drainage and nodes often bilateral
- Location
  - Lymphoid tissue, posterior to circumvallate papilla of tongue, extending inferiorly to vallecula
- Size
  - Variable: May present from nodes while still < 2 cm, or be > 4 cm and minimally symptomatic
- Morphology
  - **Ulceroinfiltrative** lesion or **exophytic** mass filling airway

CT Findings
- CECT
  - Usually moderately enhances, as does lingual tonsil
  - Small lesion: Mucosal asymmetry; often subtle
  - Large lesion: Exophytic enhancing mass or ulceroinfiltrating lesion
  - Nodal disease solid, moderately enhancing, or cystic

MR Findings
- T1WI
  - Isointense to tongue musculature
- T2WI
  - Hyperintense to muscle in tongue & floor of mouth
- T1WI C+
  - Moderate to marked enhancement

Nuclear Medicine Findings
- PET
  - SCCa is reliably FDG avid; generally greater than normal lingual tonsillar tissue
  - Beware of FDG-negative cystic nodal metastasis

Imaging Recommendations
- Best imaging tool
  - CECT most commonly used: Cheaper, quicker
  - MR provides more accurate evaluation of tumor extent
    - Superior soft tissue contrast
    - Less affected by dental amalgam artifact
  - PET/CT: 3 main uses in oropharyngeal SCCa
    - Detection of primary tumor if otherwise occult

- Staging: For distant metastases if T3/T4 or extensive nodal disease
  - Baseline: 3 months post chemoXRT
    - High negative predictive value for residual SCCa
- Protocol advice
  - CECT: **Delay imaging ≥ 90 seconds after contrast**
    - Maximizes tumor and mucosal enhancement
  - MR: T2 FS & T1 C+ FS improves tissue contrast

DIFFERENTIAL DIAGNOSIS

Lingual Tonsil Lymphoid Hyperplasia
- Symmetric without deep invasion or discrete mass
- Other lymphoid tissues hyperplastic

Lingual Tonsil Non-Hodgkin Lymphoma
- Exophytic mass or diffusely enlarged tonsil
- Often large, nonnecrotic nodes

Palatine Tonsil SCCa
- Palatine & lingual tonsils meet at glossotonsillar sulcus
- May be difficult to discern from which SCCa arises

Lingual Tonsil Benign Mixed Tumor
- Sharply marginated mass in lingual tonsil
- Pedunculates into airway when large

Lingual Tonsil Minor Salivary Gland Malignancy
- Rare; may be indistinguishable from SCCa
- Nodal metastases much less common

PATHOLOGY

General Features
- Etiology
  - Oropharyngeal SCCa has 2 identified causes
  - **Tobacco and alcohol abuse**
    - Alcohol abuse is independent risk factor and potentiates tobacco effects
    - Results in mucosal metaplasia, dysplasia → neoplasia
    - Ongoing use during treatment reduces survival
  - **Human papilloma virus (HPV) infection**
    - Oncoproteins expressed that destabilize tumor suppressor proteins (p53 and pRB)
    - HPV-16 most prevalent subtype (~ 90%)
    - Typically younger patients, smaller primary, often nonsmokers
    - Overall improved prognosis
- Associated abnormalities
  - Increased incidence of oropharyngeal SCCa in patients with Fanconi anemia

Staging, Grading, & Classification
- American Joint Committee on Cancer staging forms 2010
  - Primary tumor (T) stage and nodal (N) stage criteria
    - All oropharyngeal tumors use same TNM criteria
  - Oropharyngeal SCCa nodal staging uses same criteria as oral cavity, larynx, and hypopharynx

Gross Pathologic & Surgical Features
- Tan or white in color
- Ulceroinfiltrative or exophytic growth pattern

AJCC Oropharynx Staging

Tumor (T): Size Measured in Greatest Dimension	Nodal Metastasis (N): Size in Greatest Dimension
T1: Tumor ≤ 2 cm	**N1:** Single ipsilateral node ≤ 3 cm
T2: Tumor < 2, ≤ 4 cm	**N2a:** Single ipsilateral node > 3 cm, ≤ 6 cm
T3: Tumor > 4 cm	**N2b:** Multiple ipsilateral nodes ≤ 6 cm
T4a: Invades larynx, medial pterygoid or extrinsic tongue muscles, hard palate, mandible	**N2c:** Bilateral or contralateral nodes ≤ 6 cm
T4b: Invades lateral pterygoid muscle, pterygoid plates, lateral nasopharynx, skull base, encases carotid	**N3:** Nodal metastasis > 6 cm
Distant metastasis (M): M0 = No distant metastasis; **M1** = Distant metastasis	

Adapted from 7th edition AJCC Staging Forms.

Microscopic Features

- Squamous differentiation with intracellular bridges or keratinization ± keratin pearls
- Further classified into well, moderately, or poorly differentiated
  - **Up to 60% poorly differentiated**

CLINICAL ISSUES

Presentation

- Most common signs/symptoms
  - Most common presentation is **sore throat**
  - May present with neck nodal mass without obvious primary tumor
- Other signs/symptoms
  - Feeling of fullness or mass in throat
  - Ipsilateral otalgia from referred pain
- Clinical profile
  - Classic: 50 yr old with history of heavy tobacco & alcohol use and new neck node mass
  - HPV(+): Middle-aged male nonsmoker with history of multiple sexual partners

Demographics

- Age
  - Adults; typically > 45 yr
  - Average age becoming younger with HPV(+) SCCa
- Gender
  - M > F
- Epidemiology
  - Incidence of traditional H&N SCCa is declining
    - Correlates with declining rates of tobacco use
  - **Rapid increase incidence of HPV(+) oropharyngeal carcinoma**

Natural History & Prognosis

- Even T1/2 tumors typically present with **at least 1 node**
  - 30% present with bilateral adenopathy
- 30-50% distant metastasis, particularly if poorly controlled local disease
  - Lungs > bones > liver
- **Overall 5-yr survival ~ 50%**
- Ulceroinfiltrative tends to have worse prognosis than exophytic SCCa
- **HPV is favorable prognostic factor biomarker**

Treatment

- Treatments changing with favorable HPV prognosis
- Chemoradiation is mainstay although resection may be performed for exophytic lesion in airway
- T1/T2 SCCa may be treated with surgery or definitive XRT alone
  - Transoral robotic surgery increasing in popularity ± nodal dissection
  - XRT: Intensity-modulated radiation therapy
- Postchemoradiation surveillance important
  - CECT/MR at 6-8 weeks &/or PET/CT at 3 months
  - Salvage surgery for residual disease

DIAGNOSTIC CHECKLIST

Image Interpretation Pearls

- SCCa may be very difficult to detect and delineate on CECT as both mucosa & tumor enhance
- Do not mistake cystic level II metastatic node as 2nd branchial cleft cyst in adult patient

Reporting Tips

- Measure **greatest diameter** of primary & **define full extent of tumor spread**
  - Anterior: Sublingual space, tongue root, & floor of mouth
  - Lateral: Medial pterygoid muscle, mandible
  - Posterior: Anterior tonsillar pillar, palatine tonsil
  - Inferior: Supraglottic larynx & preepiglottic space
- Look for ipsilateral **and** contralateral nodal disease
- Always consider **2nd primary neoplasm** at diagnosis and follow-up
  - 15% 2nd primary in tobacco-/alcohol-associated SCCa of H&N
  - H&N, esophageal, or lung carcinoma

SELECTED REFERENCES

1. Taghipour M et al: Use of 18F-Fludeoxyglucose-positron emission tomography/computed tomography for patient management and outcome in oropharyngeal squamous cell carcinoma: a review. JAMA Otolaryngol Head Neck Surg. 1-7, 2015
2. Corey A: Pitfalls in the staging of cancer of the oropharyngeal squamous cell carcinoma. Neuroimaging Clin N Am. 23(1):47-66, 2013
3. Loevner LA et al: Transoral robotic surgery in head and neck cancer: what radiologists need to know about the cutting edge. Radiographics. 33(6):1759-79, 2013
4. Trotta BM et al: Oral cavity and oropharyngeal squamous cell cancer: key imaging findings for staging and treatment planning. Radiographics. 31(2):339-54, 2011

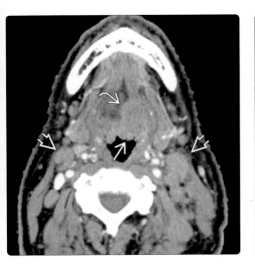
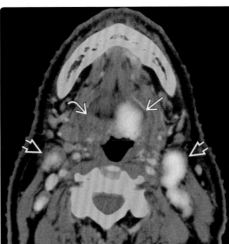

(Left) CECT in 62-year-old man demonstrates an infiltrative mass originating from the left base of tongue ➡ invading the tongue extrinsic muscles ➡. Bilateral prominent lymph nodes with ill-defined capsules are also present bilaterally ➡, suggestive of extracapsular spread. This was biopsy-proven BOT SCCa. (Right) FDG PET/CT in the same patient demonstrates elevated FDG uptake within the base of tongue SCCa ➡ compared to normal lingual tonsil ➡. FDG uptake is also present within the bilateral metastatic lymph nodes ➡.

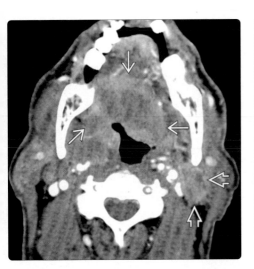
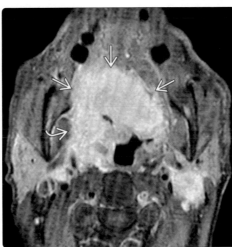

(Left) Axial CECT obtained in a 65 year old with a history of heavy tobacco and alcohol use and 25-lb weight loss associated with dysphagia and throat pain shows heterogeneous enlarged left level II node ➡ with large ulceroinfiltrative mass involving entire tongue base ➡. (Right) Axial T1WI C+ FS MR in the same patient better delineates extent of tumor infiltration into floor of mouth ➡ and medial pterygoid muscle ➡. This was staged as T4a N2c M1, stage IVC. Patient died 4 months later.

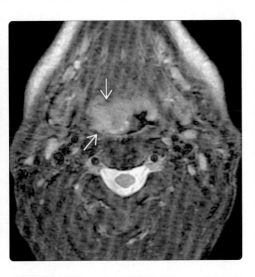
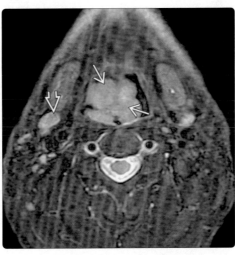

(Left) Axial T2WI FS MR in a patient presenting with sore throat and fullness demonstrates asymmetric enlargement of right lingual tonsil ➡, without evidence of deep infiltration. (Right) Axial T2WI FS MR more inferiorly shows bulky exophytic nature of mass ➡, which fills much of oropharyngeal airway above valleculae. Multiple ipsilateral enlarged heterogeneous nodes were also present at diagnosis ➡. Lesion was resected prior to chemoradiation and shown to be basaloid variant of SCCa.

TERMINOLOGY

- Palatine tonsil squamous cell carcinoma (SCCa)
  - Most common oropharyngeal SCCa subsite

IMAGING

- Variable appearance and presentation of primary tumor
- Small lesion may be occult on clinical ± imaging
- Larger lesions often exophytic or deeply invasive
- Adenopathy common, most often ipsilateral level II
  - Nodes solid, cystic, or mixed
- PET/CECT, CECT alone, or MR used to stage primary and nodal extent
- PET/CECT: Confirms primary, detects smaller metastatic nodes, distant mets
- MR: Improves detection of small primary and delineation of tumor extent

TOP DIFFERENTIAL DIAGNOSES

- Tonsillar lymphoid hyperplasia
- Tonsillar/peritonsillar abscess
- Palatine tonsil non-Hodgkin lymphoma
- Palatine tonsil benign mixed tumor

PATHOLOGY

- **HPV** associated with tonsil SCCa, especially HPV-16
- Tobacco + alcohol abuse also associated with tonsil SCCa
- HPV typically younger patient, smaller primary, overall better treatment response and survival

CLINICAL ISSUES

- Presentation: Ipsilateral ear pain, dysphagia, or new neck node
- **75-80%** have **adenopathy** at presentation
  - Primary tumor may be clinically and imaging occult
- Most patients > 45 years, but rising incidence in those < 45 years [HPV(+)]
- Treatment evolving with recognition that HPV(+) tumors have better prognosis

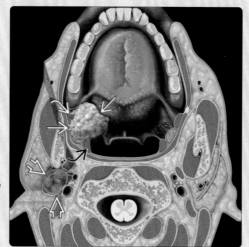
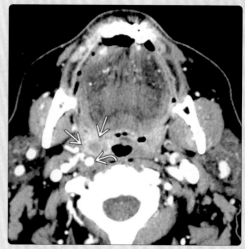

(Left) Axial graphic shows palatine tonsillar primary SCCa ➡ in the lateral wall of oropharynx with involvement of anterior tonsillar pillar ➡. Posterior tonsillar pillar is not infiltrated ➡. Note ipsilateral level II adenopathy ➡. (Right) Axial CECT (same patient) reveals 1.8 x 1.0 cm centrally hypodense tonsil mass ➡, found to be well-differentiated SCCa. Several ipsilateral enlarged nodes are also present, staging this as T1 N2b tumor, stage IVA disease. Patient received chemoradiation. Medialized right ICA ➡ precludes TORS.

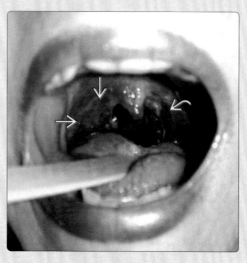
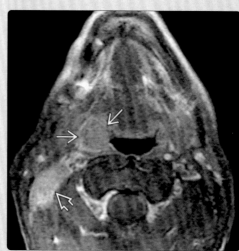

(Left) Clinical photograph in a woman with dysphagia and right throat and ear pain demonstrates indurated ulcerated right palatine tonsil ➡. Note effacement of anterior tonsillar pillar with normal comparison on the left ➡. (Right) Axial T1WI C+ FS MR in a patient presenting with right neck mass demonstrates superior aspect of nodal conglomerate ➡, FNA of which revealed SCCa. A well-defined primary palatine tonsillar tumor is evident ➡, measuring 2.2 x 1.8 cm. Tumor is staged as T2 N2b, stage IVA.

Palatine Tonsil Squamous Cell Carcinoma

TERMINOLOGY

Abbreviations

- Palatine tonsil squamous cell carcinoma (SCCa)

Definitions

- Epithelial tumors arising in lateral oropharynx in tonsillar fossa or pillars

IMAGING

General Features

- Best diagnostic clue
  - Asymmetrically enlarged heterogeneous palatine tonsil, usually with invasive deep margins
- Location
  - Tonsillar fossa > > anterior tonsillar pillar > posterior tonsillar pillar
- Size
  - Variable from small, clinically occult lesion to large, exophytic tonsil mass
- Morphology
  - Early small tumors may be mucosal only
  - Advanced lesions bulky with local invasion

CT Findings

- CECT
  - Small lesion may be difficult to delineate
  - Larger lesions may be exophytic or deeply invasive
    - Typically moderate or heterogeneous enhancement
  - Adenopathy most common at ipsilateral level II
    - Nodes enlarged, often round, ± central necrosis
    - Node may appear entirely cystic
    - Interrupted nodal capsule or surrounding induration suggests extranodal spread or extension
  - If transoral robotic surgery (TORS) considered, must exclude medialized ipsilateral internal carotid artery

MR Findings

- T1WI
  - Tonsil usually enlarged
  - Tumor mildly hypo- to isointense to normal tonsil
- T2WI FS
  - Slightly hyperintense to normal tonsil and muscle
  - Uncommonly small and T2 hypointense
- T1WI C+ FS
  - Tumor tends to enhance more than tonsil

Nuclear Medicine Findings

- PET
  - SCCa primary and metastatic nodes FDG avid
  - Tonsil normally has FDG uptake, making small lesions difficult to appreciate
  - Asymmetric physiologic FDG uptake may be seen
    - **SUV max ratio** of tonsils **> 1.48** suggests SCCa

Ultrasonographic Findings

- Grayscale ultrasound
  - Not useful for determination or evaluation of primary site

Imaging Recommendations

- Best imaging tool

- PET/CECT: Combination of 2 best stages primary, metastatic adenopathy, distant mets
  - May help to determine location of unknown primary when no lesion on clinical examination
- CECT or MR may also be used to stage tonsillar primary and nodal metastases
- MR: Better tissue contrast improves detection of small primary and delineation of tumor extent
- Protocol advice
  - PET/CECT: Best performed prior to mucosal biopsies, especially when searching for unknown primary tumor

DIFFERENTIAL DIAGNOSIS

Tonsillar Lymphoid Hyperplasia

- Enlarged tonsils without discrete mass or deep invasion
- Typically symmetrically enlarged, lingual tonsils, and adenoids also often enlarged

Tonsillar/Peritonsillar Abscess

- Young adult with acute febrile illness
- Intratonsillar or peritonsillar rim-enhancing fluid collection
- Reactive nodes ± retropharyngeal edema

Palatine Tonsil Benign Mixed Tumor

- Sharply marginated tonsillar mass
- Usually markedly hyperintense on T2 MR

Palatine Tonsil Non-Hodgkin Lymphoma

- Submucosal mass enlarges tonsil ± deep invasion
- Often associated with large, nonnecrotic neck nodes
- May be indistinguishable from SCCa

PATHOLOGY

General Features

- Etiology
  - 2 identified causes: Tobacco + alcohol, and HPV infection
  - **Tobacco + alcohol abuse** results in mucosal metaplasia and dysplasia
    - Dose dependent and synergistic effects
    - Continued use reduces survival despite treatment
  - **HPV(+)**
    - Expresses oncoproteins that destabilize tumor suppressor proteins (p53 and pRB)
    - HPV-16 most prevalent subtype (~ 90%)
    - Infection strongly associated with sexual behavior
    - Patients typically younger, smaller primary tumors, often nonsmokers
    - Overall prognosis better than tumors in smokers
- Associated abnormalities
  - Increased incidence with positive family history, especially if also tobacco/alcohol use

Staging, Grading, & Classification

- Adapted from **American Joint Committee on Cancer (AJCC) 2010** staging forms
- All oropharyngeal tumors use same TNM criteria
- Oropharyngeal nodal staging uses same criteria as oral cavity, larynx, and hypopharynx

Gross Pathologic & Surgical Features

- Ill-defined, ulcerative, indurated mucosal lesion

AJCC Oropharynx Staging (2010)

Tumor (T): Size Measured in Greatest Dimension	Nodal Metastasis (N): Size in Greatest Dimension
T1: Tumor ≤ 2 cm	**N1:** Single ipsilateral node ≤ 3 cm
T2: Tumor > 2, ≤ 4 cm	**N2a:** Single ipsilateral node > 3 cm, ≤ 6 cm
T3: Tumor > 4 cm	**N2b:** Multiple ipsilateral nodes ≤ 6 cm
T4a: Invades larynx, medial pterygoid or extrinsic tongue muscles, hard palate, mandible	**N2c:** Bilateral or contralateral nodes ≤ 6 cm
T4b: Invades lateral pterygoid muscle, pterygoid plates, lateral nasopharynx, skull base, encases carotid	**N3:** Nodal metastasis > 6 cm
Distant metastasis (M): M0 = no distant metastasis, **M1** = distant metastasis	

Adapted from 7th edition AJCC Staging Forms.

- Tan or white in color; exophytic or infiltrative

Microscopic Features

- Squamous differentiation with intracellular bridges or keratinization, ± keratin pearls
- Further classified by tumor differentiation: Well, moderately, or poorly
  - ~ 60% of tumors are moderately differentiated

CLINICAL ISSUES

Presentation

- Most common signs/symptoms
  - Ipsilateral ear pain, dysphagia
  - Level II ipsilateral metastatic node may be initial presentation
    - **75-80% have adenopathy at presentation**, 15% bilateral
- Other signs/symptoms
  - Location-specific symptoms
    - Anterior extension into posterior oral cavity: Tongue pain, obstructed submandibular duct with sialadenitis
    - Masticator space invasion: Trismus, V3 numbness
    - Mandibular invasion: Jaw pain, inferior alveolar nerve numbness
- Clinical profile
  - HPV(+): Middle-aged man, nonsmoker, ± multiple sexual partners
  - Classic: Older man with history of tobacco and alcohol use and new neck nodal mass

Demographics

- Age
  - Adult patients, typically > 45 years
  - Age of presentation decreasing with HPV(+) tumors
- Gender
  - M > F
- Epidemiology
  - **70-80% oropharyngeal tumors** are tonsil origin
  - Incidence increasing despite declining tobacco use
  - HPV-related cancers rapidly ↑ in USA since 1990

Natural History & Prognosis

- **HPV is favorable prognostic biomarker**: Overall better treatment response and survival

  - Disease-free survival for HPV(+) SCCa better for nonsmokers (80%) than smokers (55-65%)
- Nodal metastasis significantly reduces 5-year survival
  - Worse prognosis with extracapsular spread and distal nodal metastasis
- Locoregional recurrence mostly occurs within 24 months
- Distant metastatic disease: Lungs > skeletal > hepatic

Treatment

- Regimens changing with recognition of better prognosis for HPV(+) disease
  - Initially, HPV(+) tumors treated same as tonsillar SCCa in smokers
- TORS for tonsil primary becoming common, followed by neck dissection or radiation for nodal disease
- Smaller tumors, T1-2: 2 options
  - Chemotherapy and radiation to tumor and neck
  - TORS and nodal dissection or radiation to neck
- Larger tumors &/or extensive nodal disease
  - Chemoradiation main treatment regimen
- Posttreatment surveillance for residual disease important
  - PET/CECT at 3 months or CECT/MR at 8 weeks
  - Salvage surgery if residual disease present

DIAGNOSTIC CHECKLIST

Image Interpretation Pearls

- **In adult patient, cystic level II node should not be called 2nd branchial cleft cyst**
  - Palatine tonsil is common occult primary site

Reporting Tips

- **If nodal mass is presenting symptom, carefully describe size, asymmetry, enhancement in ipsilateral tonsil**
  - Tonsil SCCa often presents clinically as new neck node
- Then describe pathologic lymph nodes based on size, necrosis, or FDG avidity, especially level II

SELECTED REFERENCES

1. Chi AC et al: Oral cavity and oropharyngeal squamous cell carcinoma–an update. CA Cancer J Clin. 65(5):401-21, 2015
2. Corey A: Pitfalls in the staging of cancer of the oropharyngeal squamous cell carcinoma. Neuroimaging Clin N Am. 23(1):47-66, 2013
3. Loevner LA et al: Transoral robotic surgery in head and neck cancer: what radiologists need to know about the cutting edge. Radiographics. 33(6):1759-79, 2013

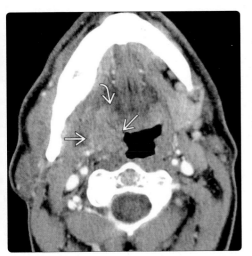
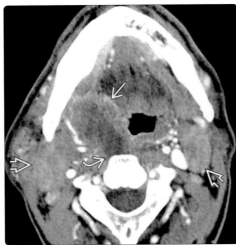

(Left) *Axial CECT in alcoholic smoker presenting with multiple right neck masses shows an enlarged right palatine tonsil mass (> 2 cm)* ➡, *extending into the posterior oral cavity* ➡. *Staging was T2 N2b. Patient was lost to follow-up.* (Right) *Axial CECT, same patient 1 year later, shows dramatic progression of disease. Stage is now T4a N2c M1. The tumor is much larger, extending into the oral cavity* ➡ *and likely into prevertebral tissues* ➡. *Note bilateral metastatic adenopathy* ➡.

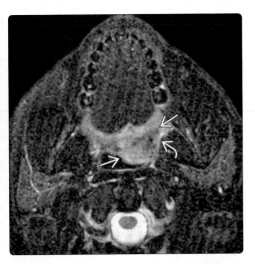
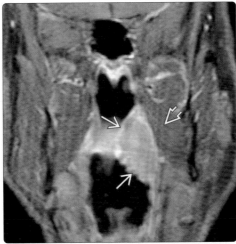

(Left) *Axial T2WI FS MR in a 50 year old presenting with a palatine tonsil mass shows heterogeneous exophytic left tonsillar tumor* ➡. *Well-defined lateral margin* ➡ *implies no deep invasion.* (Right) *Coronal T1WI C+ FS MR in the same patient shows the exophytic nature of large, > 4 cm, left palatine tonsillar SCCa* ➡. *MR clearly illustrates the absence of deep extension to medial pterygoid muscle* ➡. *This was staged as T3 N0 M0, stage III, and the patient received chemoradiation.*

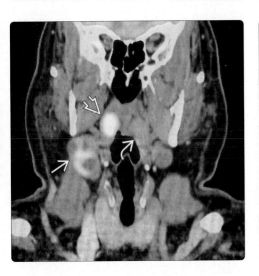
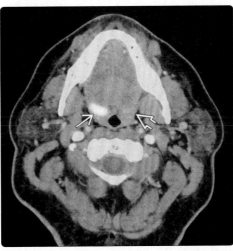

(Left) *Coronal PET/CT in a patient with new right palpable neck mass shows there is increased FDG uptake in large level II nodal conglomerate* ➡ *and asymmetric FDG uptake in right tonsillar SCCa* ➡. *Note the normal left tonsil* ➡. (Right) *Axial PET/CT in the same patient demonstrates asymmetric increased FDG uptake in the right palatine tonsil* ➡ *compared to the left* ➡. *CECT did not reveal a lesion in this area. Given an elevated SUV max ratio (> 1.48), the right tonsil was biopsied and revealed SCCa.*

Posterior Oropharyngeal Wall Squamous Cell Carcinoma

TERMINOLOGY

- Squamous cell carcinoma (SCCa) arising from posterior pharyngeal wall
  - **Soft palate** is superior limit; **hyoid** is inferior limit

IMAGING

- Lobulated posterior oropharyngeal wall mass
- CT: Mild to moderately enhancing soft tissue
- MR: Isointense to muscle on T1, moderate T2 signal
  - Moderate contrast enhancement
- Intact retropharyngeal fat plane on MR has high negative predictive value for tumor invasion
- SCCa reliably FDG avid

TOP DIFFERENTIAL DIAGNOSES

- Nasopharyngeal carcinoma
- Posterior hypopharyngeal wall SCCa
- Venous malformation

PATHOLOGY

- 85-90% of oropharyngeal cancers are SCCa
- Most posterior oropharyngeal SCCa are well differentiated

CLINICAL ISSUES

- Relatively rare; much less common than lingual & palatine tonsil SCCa
- Strong association with tobacco & alcohol abuse
- Typically relatively asymptomatic until late stage
- May extend posteriorly into retropharyngeal space &/or prevertebral space

DIAGNOSTIC CHECKLIST

- If primary surgery considered, suggest MR to determine if prevertebral invasion
- Nodal metastases should be carefully sought
  - Retropharyngeal, especially if prevertebral invasion
  - Bilateral nodes frequently found: N2c = stage IVA

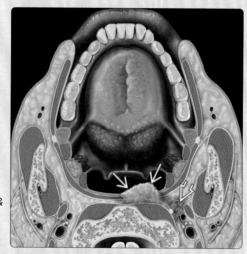
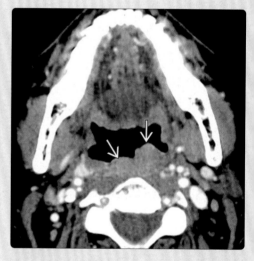

(Left) *Transverse graphic depicts irregular SCCa arising from the posterior oropharyngeal wall ➡ and invading the retropharyngeal fat. Invasion of prevertebral muscle indicates a T4b tumor. Note ipsilateral necrotic metastatic retropharyngeal node ➡ medial to the carotid artery.* (Right) *Axial CECT demonstrates a mildly enhancing soft tissue mass in the left paramedian posterior oropharyngeal wall ➡. Prevertebral muscle invasion & adenopathy are not evident. Patient had extensive tobacco and alcohol history.*

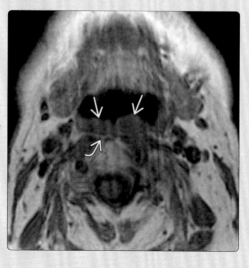
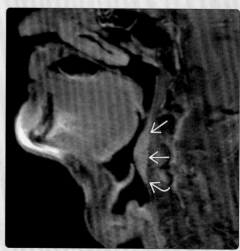

(Left) *Axial T1WI MR in a patient with dysphagia shows irregular bilobed thickening of the posterior oropharyngeal wall ➡. Hyperintense retropharyngeal fat is seen on right side ➡ but is indistinct on left side. No evidence of prevertebral muscle invasion, however.* (Right) *Sagittal T1WI C+ FS MR shows the left-sided component of a pharyngeal wall tumor that bulges into the posterior oropharynx ➡. Inferiorly, it reaches superior aspect of the hypopharynx ➡ but does not extend superiorly to the nasopharynx. This was a T2N0M0 tumor.*

TERMINOLOGY

Definitions

- Mucosal squamous cell carcinoma (SCCa) arising from **posterior pharyngeal wall** between soft palate & level of hyoid

IMAGING

General Features

- Location
  - Posterior wall of pharynx from soft palate to level of hyoid

CT Findings

- Lobulated posterior oropharyngeal wall mass
- Mild to moderately enhancing

MR Findings

- Posterior oropharyngeal wall, T1 isointense to muscle
- T2 moderately intense mass, moderate contrast enhancement
- Presence of intense retropharyngeal fat plane has high negative predictive value for tumor invasion
- Even with MR it is difficult to determine invasion; surgery often definitive study

Nuclear Medicine Findings

- PET/CT
  - SCCa reliably FDG avid

Imaging Recommendations

- Best imaging tool
  - Either CT or MR excellent cross-sectional tools
  - If surgical resection considered, MR should be obtained to search for preserved retropharyngeal fat
  - PET/CT for staging or baseline 3 months post treatment

DIFFERENTIAL DIAGNOSIS

Nasopharyngeal Carcinoma

- Typically grows in lateral nasopharyngeal recess
- Can extend inferiorly to oropharynx, still T1 tumor

Posterior Hypopharyngeal Wall SCCa

- Uncommon primary hypopharyngeal SCCa
- Can extend superiorly to oropharynx

Venous Malformation

- Heterogeneous mass with moderate to marked enhancement
- Often involves multiple adjacent spaces

PATHOLOGY

General Features

- Etiology
  - Strong association with tobacco & alcohol abuse

Staging, Grading, & Classification

- **Use same American Joint Committee on Cancer TNM (2010) staging system as for all oropharyngeal SCCa**

Microscopic Features

- 85-90% of oropharyngeal cancers are SCCa
- Rarely, basaloid-type SCCa

CLINICAL ISSUES

Presentation

- Most common signs/symptoms
  - Typically relatively asymptomatic until late stage
    - 70% present at T3 or T4
  - Dysphagia ± nodal mass
    - Unlike palatine & lingual tonsil SCCa, does not present as unknown primary

Demographics

- Age
  - Most patients > 45 yr
- Gender
  - M > F
- Epidemiology
  - Rare (≤ 5%); much less common than lingual & palatine tonsil SCCa

Natural History & Prognosis

- May extend posteriorly into retropharyngeal space &/or prevertebral space
  - Increases likelihood of retropharyngeal nodal metastases
- Because close to midline, often bilateral nodal metastases
  - Up to **30%** have retropharyngeal **nodal metastases**
- Overall 5-yr survival 30-40%

Treatment

- General guidelines
  - If small, N0: Radiation alone
  - Larger tumors, ≥ N1: Chemoradiation ± neck dissection
- Small tumors may undergo primary resection
  - Increase in transoral robotic surgery (TORS) or transoral laser microsurgery
- Prevertebral invasion indicates unresectable tumor

DIAGNOSTIC CHECKLIST

Image Interpretation Pearls

- If primary surgery considered, suggest MR to determine prevertebral invasion

Reporting Tips

- Nodal metastases should be carefully sought
  - Retropharyngeal, especially if prevertebral invasion
  - Bilateral nodes frequently found (N2c)

SELECTED REFERENCES

1. Canis M et al: Oncologic results of transoral laser microsurgery for squamous cell carcinoma of the posterior pharyngeal wall. Head Neck. 37(2):156-61, 2015
2. De Felice F et al: Treatment of squamous cell carcinoma of the posterior pharyngeal wall: Radiotherapy versus surgery. Head Neck. 38 Suppl 1:E1722-9, 2015
3. Corey A: Pitfalls in the staging of cancer of the oropharyngeal squamous cell carcinoma. Neuroimaging Clin N Am. 23(1):47-66, 2013
4. Tshering Vogel DW et al: Cancer of the oral cavity and oropharynx. Cancer Imaging. 10:62-72, 2010
5. Hsu WC et al: Accuracy of magnetic resonance imaging in predicting absence of fixation of head and neck cancer to the prevertebral space. Head Neck. 27(2):95-100, 2005

TERMINOLOGY

- Human papillomavirus-related [HPV(+)] oropharyngeal squamous cell carcinoma (SCCa)
  - Most often HPV type 16

IMAGING

- Imaging findings identical to oropharyngeal SCCa from tobacco & alcohol
- CECT/MR: Level II ± III adenopathy; single or multiple, solid or necrotic/cystic nodes
- Enhancing mass in palatine or lingual tonsil
- PET/CECT may be helpful to determine unknown primary site, as often small

TOP DIFFERENTIAL DIAGNOSES

- 2nd branchial cleft cyst
- Non-Hodgkin lymphoma nodes
- Pharyngeal mucosal space non-Hodgkin lymphoma
- Asymmetric lymphoid tissue

PATHOLOGY

- Staging is same as for all oropharyngeal SCCa
- No specific histologic characteristics distinguish HPV(+) SCCa from HPV(-) SCCa
- HPV causation determined by staining for HPV DNA or p16 kinase inhibitor

CLINICAL ISSUES

- Presentation: Unilateral neck mass, level IIA nodes
- Typically younger, mostly male, often nonsmokers
- Much better prognosis than oropharyngeal HPV(-) SCCa seen with tobacco & alcohol abuse
- Intermediate prognosis if smoker with HPV(+) SCCa
- Treat with concurrent radiation & chemotherapy

DIAGNOSTIC CHECKLIST

- Consider HPV(+) SCCa in adult with new neck mass, even if node looks like 2nd branchial cleft cyst

(Left) Axial CECT shows a normal base of tongue bilaterally ➡ and no high IIA adenopathy. (Right) Axial CECT, same patient, shows a cystic septated mass in right neck ➡. Fine-needle aspiration of node revealed SCCa, and the endoscopic biopsy showed primary HPV(+) SCCa in right base of tongue. Small tongue base primary neoplasms may be occult on cross-sectional imaging. HPV(+) oropharyngeal SCCas are notorious for small primary tumors but large and often cystic-appearing nodal metastases.

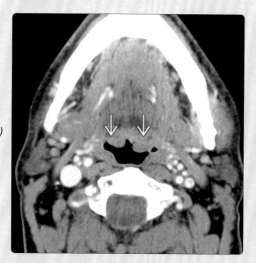
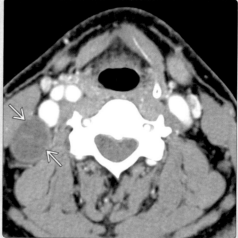

(Left) Axial CECT in patient with right ear pain and bulky cervical adenopathy shows small enhancing mass in right palatine tonsil ➡. This CECT would be interpreted as normal if there was no adenopathy. (Right) Axial CECT, same patient, shows large anterior right level IIA node ➡. Nodal necrosis is apparent as regions of low density ➡. In situ hybridization was + for HPV-16 infection. With metastatic level IIA nodes, primary tumor is usually in ipsilateral oropharynx, either tonsil or base of tongue.

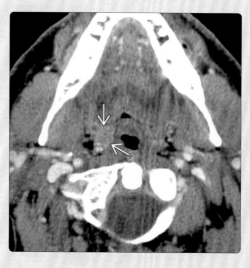
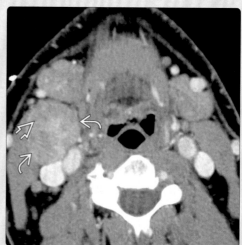

TERMINOLOGY

Abbreviations

- Human papillomavirus (HPV)

Definitions

- Subgroup of oropharyngeal squamous cell carcinoma (SCCa) caused by HPV infection
  - 87-96% HPV type 16

IMAGING

General Features

- Best diagnostic clue
  - Young male with level II adenopathy ± mass in palatine or lingual tonsil
  - Imaging appearance same as SCCa of oropharynx related to tobacco use
- Location
  - Nodes: Level II ± III, ipsilateral or bilateral
  - Primary SCCa: Tonsil or base of tongue
- Size
  - Primary tumor variable; no relationship between size and adenopathy
  - Primary often small or occult on imaging despite adenopathy
- Morphology
  - Adenopathy variable in number and size with no relationship to size of primary
  - Nodal met may be round and cystic in appearance

CT Findings

- CECT
  - Adenopathy variable: Range from single solid or cystic node to bulky multilevel adenopathy
    - Nodes usually level II and III; may be frankly cystic
    - Irregular nodal margins with "dirty" fat suggests extracapsular spread (ECS)
      □ Pathologic data suggests perinodal inflammatory changes may simulate ECS
  - Enhancing, variable-sized mass in tonsillar fossa or tongue base
    - Primary oropharyngeal tumor variable in size and stage, may be occult
    - Local extension to extrinsic tongue muscles of oral cavity, supraglottic larynx, medial pterygoid muscle, hard palate, or mandible upstages to T4a

MR Findings

- T1WI
  - Metastatic node: > 15-mm level II or III node ipsilateral to primary
  - Primary: Homogeneous, isointense mass (to muscle) in tonsil or base of tongue
- T2WI
  - Metastatic node: > 15-mm level II or III node, hyperintense to muscle or markedly ↑↑ SI if cystic/necrotic
  - Primary: Isointense or minimally hyperintense tonsil or base of tongue mass
- T1WI C+ FS

- Metastatic node: > 15-mm level II or III node enhances homogeneously if nonnecrotic or peripherally if centrally necrotic
- Primary: Enhancing mass in tonsil or base of tongue

Ultrasonographic Findings

- Levels II, III, ± IV cystic and solid enlarged nodes

Nuclear Medicine Findings

- PET/CT
  - HPV(+) SCCa primary & nodal mets will be FDG avid
  - Small lesions may be difficult to detect
    - Normal tonsillar tissue also FDG avid
  - Beware falsely FDG(-) "cystic" nodes

Imaging Recommendations

- Best imaging tool
  - PET/CECT best evaluates primary and metastatic adenopathy
  - PET/CECT may be only modality to find primary
- Protocol advice
  - CECT done with ≤ 3-mm slice thickness with adequate contrast bolus
  - IV contrast for best mucosal enhancement
  - Delay image acquisition ~ 90 seconds to guarantee mucosal enhancement

DIFFERENTIAL DIAGNOSIS

2nd Branchial Cleft Cyst

- In adult, 2nd branchial cleft cyst (BCC) is diagnosis of exclusion and much less likely than HPV-related nodal met from SCCa of oropharynx

Non-Hodgkin Lymphoma Nodes

- May be indistinguishable from nodal met from SCCa of oropharynx

Pharyngeal Mucosal Space Non-Hodgkin Lymphoma

- SCCa of oropharynx usually unilateral, whereas lymphoma often bilateral

Asymmetric Lymphoid Tissue of Pharyngeal Mucosal Space

- Should have no pathologic adenopathy

PATHOLOGY

Staging, Grading, & Classification

- Staging is same as for all oropharyngeal SCCa using AJCC staging system

Gross Pathologic & Surgical Features

- Primary tumor may be found at tonsillectomy in surgical specimen
- HPV(+) SCCa tends to arise from tonsillar crypts
- Tobacco-related HPV(-) SCCa tends to arise from surface epithelium

Microscopic Features

- No specific histologic characteristics distinguish HPV(+) from HPV(-) tumors
- General histological features include
  - Prominent basaloid-like morphology

- Infiltrating lymphocytes
- No dysplasia of surface epithelium
- No significant keratinization
- **HPV causation determined by staining for HPV DNA or p16 kinase inhibitor**
- Immunohistochemistry for **p16** kinase inhibitor
  - Sensitive, relatively cheap, easy to perform
  - Can be performed with FNA/core biopsy specimen
- In situ hybridization (**ISH**) or polymerase chain reaction (**PCR**) staining is direct test for **HPV DNA**
  - Both tests expensive and time consuming
  - PCR most sensitive test, very difficult to perform well
  - ISH less sensitive but most specific test

Human Papillomavirus

- Up to 200 different HPV genotypes determined
- 60% cutaneous HPV types; manifest as warts
- 40% mucosal HPV types; wider spectrum of disease
  - HPV-6 & -11 (low risk) cause benign mucosal and anogenital papillomas
  - HPV-16 & -18 (high risk) cause invasive cervical, anogenital, and oropharyngeal carcinomas
- HPV-16: E6 and E7 oncoproteins inactivate tumor suppressor protein p53 and retinoblastoma pRb protein
  - E6 protein degrades p53 tumor suppressor protein, which interferes with DNA repair and apoptosis
    - Tobacco & alcohol-related SCCa have p53 **mutation**
  - E7 protein inactivates pRb → further loss of cell cycle control
    - To restore control, host cell increases **p16, cyclin-dependent kinase inhibitor**
    - Staining for p16 in tumor cells is molecular indicator of HPV-induced malignancy

CLINICAL ISSUES

Presentation

- Most common signs/symptoms
  - New unilateral neck mass from level IIA metastatic adenopathy
- Other signs/symptoms
  - Ipsilateral ear pain, dysphagia

Demographics

- Age
  - Generally younger patient group than HPV(-) SCCa
  - Range: 31-78 years
- Gender
  - 85% male
- Ethnicity
  - > 90% white
- Epidemiology
  - 80% of oropharyngeal SCCa in USA are HPV-related
  - HPV is most common sexually transmitted infection worldwide
  - Risk directly correlates with number of sexual partners and oral sex practices

Natural History & Prognosis

- Overall **better prognosis** than patients with oropharyngeal HPV(-) smoking-related SCCa

- Better local and regional control, fewer 2nd primary tumors, patients generally in better health
  - Survival in advanced oropharyngeal tumors up to 2-3x that for HPV(-) SCCa
- Survival benefit less pronounced but still present if HPV(+) SCCa plus significant tobacco history
- HPV(+) SCCa and no smoking: Overall 90% 5-year survival
- HPV(-) SCCa and > 10 packs per year smoking: Overall 50% 5-year survival
- ECS of tumor from nodes may **not be poor prognostic indicator** for HPV(+) SCCa as it is for HPV(-) SCCa
  - Perinodal "dirty" fat may be inflammatory response and not ECS

Treatment

- Most often concurrent radiation therapy (XRT) and cisplatin-based chemotherapy
- Transoral robotic surgery (TORS) or transoral laser microsurgery ± XRT/chemoXRT
  - TORS approved for T1 and T2 SCCa, so imaging staging critical

DIAGNOSTIC CHECKLIST

Consider

- HPV(+) SCCa of oropharynx in any adult patient with new neck mass that looks like 2nd BCC
- HPV(+) SCCa tends to have more extensive nodal disease, but ECS may not be poor prognostic indicator

Image Interpretation Pearls

- 2nd BCC is diagnosis of exclusion in adult patient; nodal met should be 1st consideration
- Primary in tonsil or base of tongue lingual tonsils often very small or occult

Reporting Tips

- Dictation should include stage and description of primary oropharyngeal tumor and nodal stage
  - Tumor stage T1-T3 based on size of primary
  - T4a and T4b based on involvement of specific surrounding structures
- Nodal status should be reported using AJCC staging
- If dictating stage not done, be sure to include what findings need to be noted for stage
- For TORS: Note retropharyngeal internal carotid artery (ICA) and significant nodal ECS
  - TORS may not be done if ICA medialized or macroscopic nodal ECS

SELECTED REFERENCES

1. Horne ZD et al: Confirmation of proposed human papillomavirus risk-adapted staging according to AJCC/UICC TNM criteria for positive oropharyngeal carcinomas. Cancer. 122(13):2021-30, 2016
2. Subramaniam RM et al: PET/CT imaging and human papilloma virus-positive oropharyngeal squamous cell cancer: evolving clinical imaging paradigm. J Nucl Med. 55(3):431-8, 2014
3. Cantrell SC et al: Differences in imaging characteristics of HPV-positive and HPV-Negative oropharyngeal cancers: a blinded matched-pair analysis. AJNR Am J Neuroradiol. 34(10):2005-9, 2013
4. Loevner LA et al: Transoral robotic surgery in head and neck cancer: what radiologists need to know about the cutting edge. Radiographics. 33(6):1759-79, 2013
5. Corey AS et al: Radiographic imaging of human papillomavirus related carcinomas of the oropharynx. Head Neck Pathol. 6 Suppl 1:S25-40, 2012

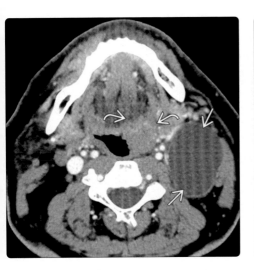

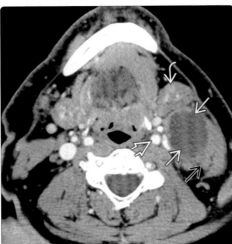

(Left) *Axial CECT demonstrates a large, unilocular cystic left neck mass ➡, which mimics 2nd branchial cleft cyst by location. Note mass in lower pole of left palatine tonsil ➡.* (Right) *Axial CECT more inferiorly shows cystic/necrotic mass ➡ lateral to carotid sheath ➡, posterior to submandibular gland ➡, and anteromedial to sternocleidomastoid muscle ➡, again mimicking 2nd branchial cleft cyst. This was a metastatic node from HPV(+) tonsil SCCa.*

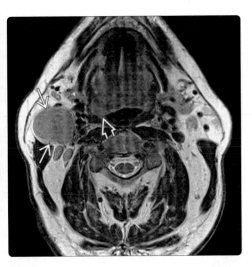

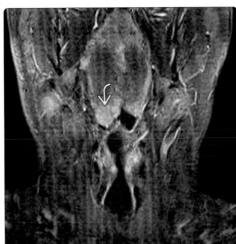

(Left) *Axial T2 MR shows a solid level IIA pathologic node ➡. Subtle asymmetric fullness of the tonsil ➡ is within normal limits although, if no other abnormality was found to explain adenopathy, biopsy would be recommended.* (Right) *Coronal T2 FS MR in the same patient shows hyperintensity of right lingual tonsil ➡. Even though this asymmetry can be within normal limits, presence of malignant adenopathy makes asymmetry significant. This proved to be HPV(+) lingual tonsil SCCa.*

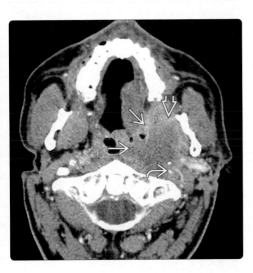

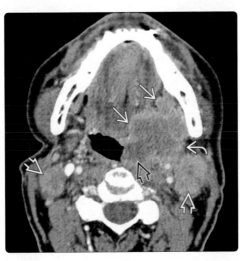

(Left) *Axial CECT shows infiltrative SCCa ➡ extending into the masticator space ➡ and surrounding and narrowing the left internal carotid artery ➡, indicating a stage T4b tumor. This was determined to be p16(+), indicating HPV infection.* (Right) *Axial CECT inferiorly shows tonsillar SCCa ➡ extending anteriorly into oral cavity ➡ and along posterior oropharyngeal wall ➡ to the midline. Bulky bilateral necrotic IIA nodes ➡ make nodal stage N2c.*

Soft Palate Squamous Cell Carcinoma

TERMINOLOGY

- Mucosal squamous cell carcinoma (SCCa) arising from soft palate (SP) and uvula (tip of SP)
- 5-25% of all oropharyngeal SCCa

IMAGING

- Best evaluated with sagittal and coronal plane rather than axial
- CECT: Mildly enhancing infiltrative mass; SP may just appear diffusely thickened
- MR: Focal or diffuse moderately enhancing lesion
- MR allows excellent evaluation of soft tissues, bone involvement, & perineural spread
- FDG PET: SCCa reliably FDG avid

TOP DIFFERENTIAL DIAGNOSES

- Palatine tonsil SCCa
- SP minor salivary gland malignancy
- Expected radiation changes

PATHOLOGY

- Oropharyngeal SCCa American Joint Committee on Cancer TNM staging system (2010)

CLINICAL ISSUES

- Patients may present with irritation at back of throat or be asymptomatic
- Strongly associated with tobacco and alcohol abuse
- 5-yr overall survival = 51%
- Up to 25% have 2nd primary H&N tumor

DIAGNOSTIC CHECKLIST

- May spread across midline and to palatine tonsil
- Look for submucosal spread of tumor and infiltration of parapharyngeal fat
- 60-70% T3/T4 present with nodal metastases
- Strong tendency for bilateral nodal metastases, especially with T4
- Check level 2 and retropharyngeal nodes carefully

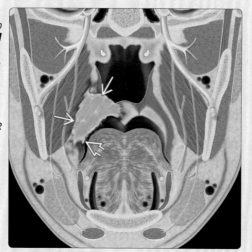
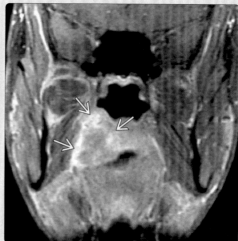

(Left) Coronal graphic illustrates location and growth pattern of soft palate SCCa ➡ that involves palatal arch and adjacent parapharyngeal fat & extends toward the midline. Laterally, it extends down the pharyngeal wall ➡, where it can involve the palatine tonsil. (Right) Coronal T1WI C+ FS MR in a young patient with heavy tobacco & alcohol use shows heterogeneously enhancing mass ➡ of right half of soft palate. This proved to be poorly differentiated SCCa with basaloid features (T4a from medial pterygoid invasion).

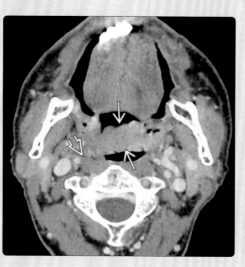
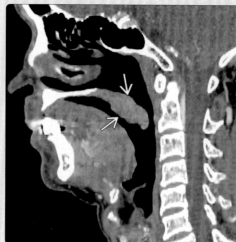

(Left) Axial CECT in a patient unable to be scanned by MR shows diffuse thickening and mild enhancement of the soft palate ➡ extending bilaterally toward the lateral pharyngeal walls. A subtly prominent right retropharyngeal node ➡ is evident, although not clearly necrotic. This tumor was staged as T2N1M0 (stage III) moderately to well-differentiated SCCa of the soft palate. (Right) Sagittal reformatted CECT best illustrates the contour of this bulky soft palate tumor ➡.

Soft Palate Squamous Cell Carcinoma

TERMINOLOGY

Definitions

- Mucosal squamous cell carcinoma (SCCa) arising from soft palate (SP) and uvula (tip of SP)

IMAGING

General Features

- Best diagnostic clue
  - Diffusely or asymmetrically thickened SP
- Location
  - SP; posterior border of hard palate to uvula
  - Tendency to spread across midline &/or to palatine tonsil of lateral oropharynx
- Size
  - Most present T1/T2, therefore < 4 cm
- Morphology
  - Mildly enhancing on CECT, moderately enhancing on MR; ill-defined mass
    - Tendency for submucosal infiltration

CT Findings

- CECT
  - **Often difficult to fully appreciate in axial plane**
    - Mildly enhancing infiltrative mass
    - SP may just appear diffusely thickened

MR Findings

- T1WI
  - Isointense to muscle, slightly hypointense to SP
- T2WI FS
  - Mildly hyperintense to normal SP
- T1WI C+ FS
  - Focal or diffuse moderately enhancing lesion

Nuclear Medicine Findings

- PET/CT
  - SCCa reliably FDG avid

Imaging Recommendations

- Best imaging tool
  - MR allows excellent evaluation of soft tissues, bone involvement, & perineural spread
    - Sagittal and coronal plane more helpful than axial
- Protocol advice
  - CECT: Thin slices with sagittal and coronal reformats
  - MR: Coronal T1, T2FS, and T1WI C+ FS important

DIFFERENTIAL DIAGNOSIS

Palatine Tonsil SCCa

- Tumor arising in tonsil may spread cephalad to SP
- May be difficult to determine primary site on imaging

Soft Palate Minor Salivary Gland Malignancy

- Focal or infiltrating lesion; can be entirely submucosal
- More commonly arises in hard palate

Expected Radiation Changes

- Diffuse SP thickening and enhancement are common findings post XRT
- Seen in association with other neck XRT changes

PATHOLOGY

Staging, Grading, & Classification

- Oropharyngeal SCCa American Joint Committee on Cancer TNM staging system (2010)

Microscopic Features

- Most often moderately to poorly differentiated SCCa
- Basaloid SCCa rarely reported

CLINICAL ISSUES

Presentation

- Most common signs/symptoms
  - Unusual sensation or irritation at back of throat
  - May be asymptomatic

Demographics

- Age
  - Most commonly 5th-7th decades
- Gender
  - M > F; likely reflecting tobacco use
- Epidemiology
  - 5-25% of all oropharyngeal SCCa

Natural History & Prognosis

- Strongly associated with tobacco and alcohol abuse
- 75% present with early stage disease T1/T2
- 69% N0 at presentation
- 5-yr overall survival = 51%
- 5-yr recurrence-free survival = 58%

Treatment

- Different schools of thought favor definitive radiation **versus** surgery ± XRT
- Later stage tumors probably require chemotherapy in addition to surgery/XRT

DIAGNOSTIC CHECKLIST

Consider

- Look for submucosal spread of tumor and infiltration of parapharyngeal fat, which may not be clinically evident
- May spread across midline and to ipsilateral/contralateral tonsil
- 60-70% of T3/T4 have nodal metastases at presentation
- Strong tendency for bilateral nodal metastases, especially with T4
  - Check level 2 and retropharyngeal nodes carefully
- Up to 25% have 2nd primary H&N tumor

Image Interpretation Pearls

- Sagittal and coronal images most helpful for evaluating primary site

SELECTED REFERENCES

1. Corey A: Pitfalls in the staging of cancer of the oropharyngeal squamous cell carcinoma. Neuroimaging Clin N Am. 23(1):47-66, 2013
2. Overton LJ et al: Squamous cell carcinoma of the uvula: an analysis of factors affecting survival. Laryngoscope. 123(4):898-903, 2013
3. Iyer NG et al: Surgical management of squamous cell carcinoma of the soft palate: Factors predictive of outcome. Head Neck. 34(8):1071-80, 2012
4. Cohan DM et al: Oropharyngeal cancer: current understanding and management. Curr Opin Otolaryngol Head Neck Surg. 17(2):88-94, 2009

TERMINOLOGY

- Oral tongue squamous cell carcinoma (SCCa) definition: Oral cavity mucosal malignancy arising from anterior 2/3 of tongue

IMAGING

- Imaging used to define deep extent and nodes
- Lateral margin > undersurface > > tip of tongue
- CECT/MR: Variably enhancing invasive lesion
- Superficial lesion may be occult to imaging
- MR better evaluates extent of primary than CT
- MR less affected by dental amalgam artifact

TOP DIFFERENTIAL DIAGNOSES

- Lingual tonsil SCCa
- Tongue schwannoma
- Venous malformation of tongue
- Oral cavity abscess
- Alveolar soft part sarcoma of tongue

PATHOLOGY

- Strong association with tobacco and alcohol
- Clinical assessment more accurate than imaging for mucosal size (T1-T3)
- Imaging important for deep extent and nodes
- 1st-order nodal drainage: Submandibular (IB), then jugulodigastric group (IIA)
- Beware of "skip nodes" where anterior tongue tumors drain directly to levels III or IV
- Up to 35% have ≥ N1 disease at diagnosis
- 30% "N0" necks have microscopic nodal metastases

CLINICAL ISSUES

- Painful nonhealing ulcer of oral tongue
- Median age: 61 years; M:F = 4:1
- Treatment primarily surgical resection ± radiation
- Overall 5-year survival: 60%

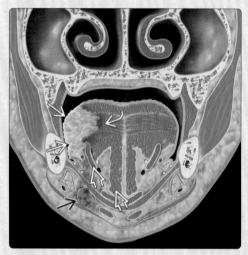
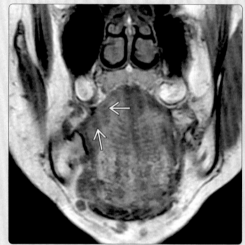

(Left) Coronal graphic illustrates lateral oral tongue squamous cell carcinoma (SCCa) ➡ infiltrating intrinsic tongue muscles ➡. Coronal plane allows scrutiny of extrinsic tongue muscles ➡, infiltration of which designates the tumor as T4a. Ipsilateral 1B node also shown ➡. (Right) Coronal T1WI MR in a woman with a painful right tongue ulcer shows subtle low signal intensity at the lateral tongue margin ➡. There is no evidence of involvement of extrinsic muscles or contralateral tumor spread.

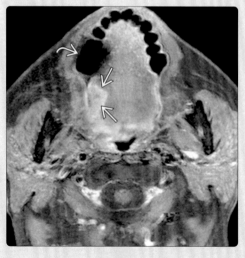
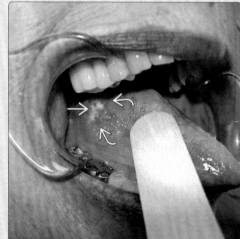

(Left) Axial T1WI C+ FS MR in the same patient shows marked enhancement a of wedge-shaped ulcer at posterolateral tongue surface ➡. No enlarged neck nodes are present. Note that despite amalgam ➡, the tumor is still well seen. (Right) Clinical photograph demonstrates a lateral tongue ulcer ➡ with indurated adjacent tissue ➡. Tumor was staged as T2 N0 by clinical exam and imaging and treated by hemiglossectomy with ipsilateral selective neck dissection (I-III). Final pathology concurred: pT2 N0 SCCa, stage II.

Oral Tongue Squamous Cell Carcinoma

TERMINOLOGY

Abbreviations
- Oral tongue squamous cell carcinoma (SCCa)

Definitions
- Oral cavity (OC) mucosal malignancy arising from anterior 2/3 of tongue
  - Distinct from base of tongue (oropharyngeal SCCa)

IMAGING

General Features
- Best diagnostic clue
  - Asymmetric enhancement ± ulcer of lateral aspect tongue
- Location
  - Oral tongue defined as freely mobile portion
    - Tip, lateral borders, dorsum, and undersurface
  - Most commonly arises from **lateral margin**
    - Next most common is undersurface
- Size
  - Variable, both in superficial and deep extent
    - Mucosal size best determined clinically
- Morphology
  - Irregular ulcer with variable deep invasion

CT Findings
- CECT
  - Variably enhancing oral tongue mucosal lesion
  - Superficial lesion may be occult to imaging
- Bone CT
  - If deep infiltration to floor of mouth, may invade mandible

MR Findings
- T1WI
  - Low signal intensity compared to tongue tissues
- T2WI
  - Typically increased signal intensity
  - Most readily observed with fat saturation
- T1WI C+
  - Variable enhancement, mild to moderate
  - Large tumors show ulceration with rim enhancement

Nuclear Medicine Findings
- PET/CT
  - SCCa is reliably FDG avid
  - Modality not often employed unless large primary or extensive nodal metastases

Imaging Recommendations
- Best imaging tool
  - MR preferred imaging modality in OC
    - Superior tissue contrast to identify primary and deep or contralateral extent of tumor
    - Less affected by dental amalgam artifact than CT
- Protocol advice
  - Fat saturation helps with tissue contrast for T2WI and T1WI C+
  - If CECT obtained, thin slices allow coronal reformats, which aid in evaluating deep extent

DIFFERENTIAL DIAGNOSIS

Lingual Tonsil SCCa
- Invasive tongue base tumor may extend into oral tongue
- More commonly invades floor of mouth, tongue root

Tongue Schwannoma
- Well-circumscribed mass within oral tongue
- Homogeneous enhancement

Venous Malformation of Tongue
- Congenital vascular lesion
- Calcified phleboliths virtually diagnostic

Oral Cavity Abscess
- Rim-enhancing cystic mass often with extensive cellulitis
- Typically associated with dental disease

Alveolar Soft Part Sarcoma of Tongue
- Aggressive enhancing tumor may involve body of tongue
- Typically women < 35 years

PATHOLOGY

General Features
- Etiology
  - Strong link with smoking, chewing tobacco, and alcohol
    - Also, chewing betel nut, paan
  - Conflicting evidence for alcohol-containing mouthwash and OC cancer
    - Some advise use of mouthwash without alcohol
  - Fruit and vegetable consumption appears to reduce risk of OC SCCa
- Genetics
  - Squamous cell carcinoma-related oncogene (*DCUN1D1*)
    - May play role in pathogenesis of oral tongue SCCa through amplification of chromosome 3q26
    - May be predictor of regional metastases and marker for aggressiveness and outcome

Staging, Grading, & Classification
- **American Joint Committee on Cancer (AJCC) staging forms (2010)**
- Note that clinical assessment is more accurate than imaging for mucosal size
- Imaging is important for determination of **deep extent: Must look for features that make tumor T4**
  - T4a: Tumor invades through cortical bone, deep muscles of tongue, maxillary sinus, skin of face
  - T4b: Tumor invades masticator space, pterygoid plates, skull base, or encases carotid
  - Contralateral spread important for surgical resection
- Anterior tongue SCCa
  - More often involves floor of mouth
- **Malignant nodes common at presentation**
  - Up to 35% have ≥ N1 disease preoperatively
  - 30% "N0" necks have microscopic nodal metastases
- 1st-order nodal drainage: Submandibular (IB), then jugulodigastric group (IIA)
  - Occasionally, anterior tumors drain directly to midjugular (III) or low jugular (IV): **"Skip nodes"**
  - Midline tumor more likely to have **bilateral** nodes

AJCC Oral Cavity Staging (2010)

Tumor (T): Clinical assessment of mucosal extent more accurate than imaging	Nodal stage (N)
Tis: Carcinoma in situ	**N1**: Ipsilateral node ≤ 3 cm
T1: Tumor ≤ 2 cm	**N2a**: Ipsilateral node > 3 cm, ≤ 6 cm
T2: Tumor > 2, ≤ 4 cm	**N2b**: Multiple ipsilateral nodes ≤ 6 cm
T3: Tumor > 4 cm	**N2c**: Bilateral or contralateral ≤ 6 cm
T4a: Tumor invades deep tongue muscles (genioglossus, hyoglossus, palatoglossus, styloglossus), maxillary sinus, skin of face, through cortical bone	**N3**: Nodal mass > 6 cm
T4b: Tumor invades masticator space, pterygoid plates, skull base, or encases carotid	**Distant metastasis (M)**
	M0: No distant metastasis
	M1: Distant metastasis

Adapted from 7th edition AJCC Staging Forms.

T = tumor, N = nodal, M = metastasis.

- o Tongue tip tumors may drain to submental (I)
- Lower nodes more likely to have distant mets
  - o Lungs > bones or liver

Gross Pathologic & Surgical Features

- Red or red and white well-demarcated areas of roughness and induration
- Ulcerated areas clearly indurated, hard on palpation with pain

Microscopic Features

- Squamous differentiation with intracellular bridges or keratinization, ± keratin pearls
- Further classified by amount of differentiation
  - o Well, moderately, poorly, or undifferentiated

CLINICAL ISSUES

Presentation

- Most common signs/symptoms
  - o Pain; occurs with smaller size than many OC tumors
  - o Nonhealing ulcer of oral tongue mucosa
    - – Ulcer older than 3 weeks is suspicious
- Other signs/symptoms
  - o Tongue mass + neck masses from regional nodes
  - o Bleeding

Demographics

- Age
  - o Median: 61 years
- Gender
  - o M:F = 4:1
- Epidemiology
  - o > 90% of OC malignancies are SCCa
    - – Most common sites: Tongue and floor of mouth
  - o Rising incidence of tongue SCCa

Natural History & Prognosis

- Survival significantly impacted by ongoing tobacco and alcohol abuse
- Invasion of adjacent structures significantly reduces prognosis
- **Overall 5-year survival: 60%**
  - o If no nodal metastases ~ 77%

Treatment

- Treatment primarily surgical resection ± radiation
  - o Local resection
  - o Hemiglossectomy
    - – If large tumor not crossing midline
    - – Midline determined by fatty lingual septum
  - o Total glossectomy
    - – Rarely performed, high morbidity
- To minimize recurrence, 1.5-2 cm margin required
  - o Hence preoperative (imaging) determination of **deep** extent may be **crucial** to surgeon
- Some programs advocate elective selective neck dissection for OC SCCa due to high risk of occult nodal metastases

DIAGNOSTIC CHECKLIST

Consider

- Clinical assessment of **mucosal extent** more accurate than imaging
  - o Superficial lesion may be occult on MR/CECT
- Imaging evaluation of **deep extent and nodes** better than clinical
  - o MR typically evaluates extent better than CECT
  - o Nodes frequently present, often occult to clinical exam and imaging

Reporting Tips

- Determine if tumor crosses to contralateral side, as this prohibits hemiglossectomy
- Look for deeply invasive features that upstage tumor to T4a/b
- Evaluate for ipsilateral and contralateral IB and IIA nodes
- Beware "skip nodes" (III or IV without higher levels), especially with anterior tongue tumors

SELECTED REFERENCES

1. Mücke T et al: Tumor thickness and risk of lymph node metastasis in patients with squamous cell carcinoma of the tongue. Oral Oncol. 53:80-4, 2016
2. Seki M et al: Histologic assessment of tumor budding in preoperative biopsies to predict nodal metastasis in squamous cell carcinoma of the tongue and floor of the mouth. Head Neck. 38 Suppl 1:E1582-90, 2016
3. Madana J et al: Computerized tomography based tumor-thickness measurement is useful to predict postoperative pathological tumor thickness in oral tongue squamous cell carcinoma. J Otolaryngol Head Neck Surg. 44:49, 2015

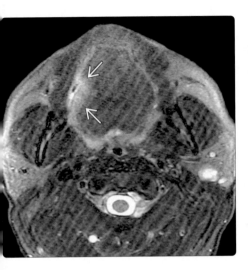

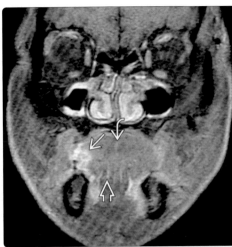

(Left) *Axial T2WI FS MR demonstrates a small right lateral tongue tumor, subtly evident as lenticular region of increased signal intensity ➡. Ill-defined margins are typical. The lesion does not approach the midline.* (Right) *Coronal T1WI C+ FS MR in the same patient demonstrates enhancement of lateral tongue ulcer ➡. The lesion does not extend inferiorly to genioglossus ➡ or other extrinsic tongue muscles and does not reach the midline lingual septum ➡. Hemiglossectomy and SND showed T1 N0 SCCa, stage I.*

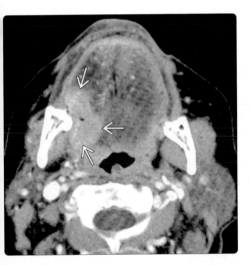

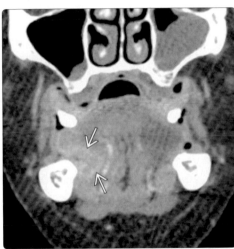

(Left) *Axial CECT in a 59-year-old smoker with a 5-month history of painful tongue lesion demonstrates avidly enhancing irregular ulcerative mass ➡ arising from lateral posterior margin of tongue. Single level II node is evident on inferior CT images.* (Right) *Coronal CECT reformatted image shows irregular enhancement of ulcer ➡. There is no evidence of deep infiltration of extrinsic tongue muscles, and tumor did not approach midline. Right hemiglossectomy and modified neck dissection revealed T2 N1 SCCa, stage III.*

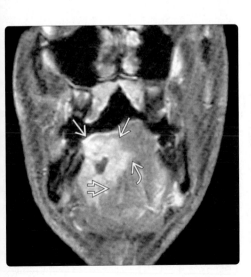

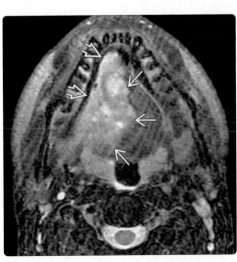

(Left) *Coronal T1WI C+ FS MR demonstrates a large, enhancing, but centrally necrotic irregular mass ➡ arising in the right lateral tongue, invading genioglossus ➡, & extending across the midline ➡.* (Right) *Axial T2WI FS MR through the floor of mouth (same patient) better illustrates tumor infiltration ➡ & extension up to the right mandible ➡, although no evidence of bone infiltration is present. Total glossectomy & floor of mouth resection was performed, as patient was only 31 years old; T4a N2b SCCa, stage IVA was proven.*

KEY FACTS

TERMINOLOGY

- Floor of mouth (FOM) squamous cell carcinoma (SCCa)
  - FOM mucosa overlies mylohyoid & hyoglossus muscles, and body of tongue rests on it

IMAGING

- CECT: Irregular mild to moderately enhancing mass
- MR: Loss of normal FOM anatomical planes on T1
  - Increased T2 signal intensity & enhancement
- SCCa reliably FDG avid; increasing role in current practice
- May exactly mimic sublingual gland carcinoma

TOP DIFFERENTIAL DIAGNOSES

- Sublingual gland carcinoma
- Oral tongue SCCa
- Venolymphatic malformation
- Ranula
- Oral cavity abscess

PATHOLOGY

- Strongly associated with tobacco (smoking & chewing) and alcohol abuse
- ≤ 35% have nodes at presentation: Levels I, II
- High incidence of occult nodal metastases

CLINICAL ISSUES

- Most commonly 50-70 years; M:F = 2:1
- Painful hard ulcer/lesion, ± loose teeth
- Overall 5-year survival = 60%

DIAGNOSTIC CHECKLIST

- May present as submandibular gland obstructive sialadenitis
- Clinical mucosal size more accurate than imaging
- Imaging important for deep extent & nodes
  - Genioglossus, mylohyoid, base of tongue
  - Cortical bone erosion, marrow infiltration

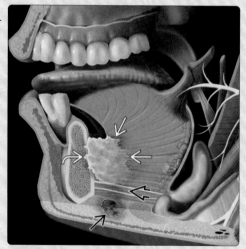
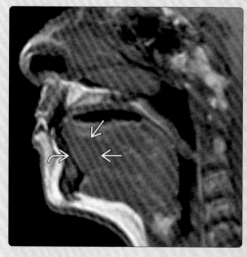

(Left) Graphic illustrates the most common location of floor of mouth (FOM) squamous cell carcinoma ➡, within 2 cm of the midline anterior FOM. It is important at imaging to evaluate for invasion inferiorly to genioglossus and mylohyoid ⊟ muscles, posteriorly to tongue base, and mandibular involvement anteriorly ➡ or laterally. This may require both MR & CT. Second aim of imaging is evaluation of nodal disease ➡. (Right) Sagittal T1WI MR demonstrates mass ➡ of low intensity compared to tongue muscles, abutting midline mandible ➡.

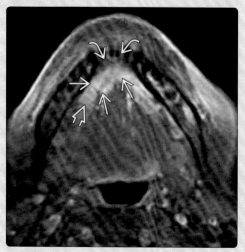
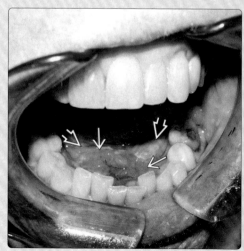

(Left) Axial T1WI C+ FS MR in the same patient shows a subtle anterior midline FOM lesion ➡ that involves the anterior aspect of the right sublingual gland ➡. Note the loss of low-intensity cortex of the adjacent mandible ➡. This was confirmed on bone CT. No abnormal nodes were found. (Right) Clinical photograph in same patient reveals a tumor ➡ in anterior FOM & shows relation to sublingual glands ➡. Composite resection & bilateral selective neck dissection (I-III) confirmed T4a N0 disease (mandible involvement).

Floor of Mouth Squamous Cell Carcinoma

TERMINOLOGY

Abbreviations

- Floor of mouth (FOM) squamous cell carcinoma (SCCa)

Definitions

- Oral cavity mucosal malignancy arising from FOM
  - Inner surface of mandibular alveolar ridges to undersurface of tongue

IMAGING

General Features

- Best diagnostic clue
  - Irregular enhancing mass in anterior FOM
- Location
  - Most within 2 cm of anterior midline FOM
- Size
  - Variable: Several mm to several cm

CT Findings

- CECT
  - Mild to moderately enhancing irregular FOM mass
  - May exactly mimic sublingual gland carcinoma
  - May obstruct drainage of 1 or both submandibular gland ducts → sialadenitis
- Bone CT
  - Must evaluate carefully for cortical erosion

MR Findings

- T1WI
  - Low signal mass in relation to FOM tissues
    - **Subtle loss of normal anatomical contours**
- T2WI
  - Increased signal intensity
    - Often easier to identify with fat saturation
- T1WI C+
  - Variable enhancement: Mild to moderate
  - Tumor infiltrating marrow typically enhances

Nuclear Medicine Findings

- PET/CT
  - SCCa reliably FDG avid; increasing role in current practice

Imaging Recommendations

- Best imaging tool
  - MR best for determining tumor extent
  - Bone CT important when tumor abuts mandible
  - Expanding role of PET/CT; highest sensitivity
- Protocol advice
  - CECT: Soft tissue and bone algorithm in 2 planes
    - "Puffed-cheek" scan improves mucosal assessment

DIFFERENTIAL DIAGNOSIS

Sublingual Gland Carcinoma

- May be impossible to distinguish by imaging

Oral Tongue Squamous Cell Carcinoma

- Anterior &/or large lesions may invade FOM

Venolymphatic Malformation

- Heterogeneous moderate to marked enhancement

- Calcified phleboliths essentially diagnostic

Ranula

- Rim-enhancing fluid mass in FOM

Oral Cavity Abscess

- Rim-enhancing collection(s) + FOM cellulitis

PATHOLOGY

General Features

- Etiology
  - Strongly associated with tobacco (smoking and chewing) and alcohol abuse
    - Chewing betel nut, paan in parts of Asia

Staging, Grading, & Classification

- American Joint Committee on Cancer (AJCC) (2010)
- Same classification for all oral cavity tumors
  - T1: ≤ 2 cm in greatest diameter
  - T2: > 2 & ≤ 4 cm in greatest diameter
  - T3: > 4 cm in greatest diameter
  - T4a: Tumor invades through cortical bone into extrinsic tongue muscles, skin of face
  - T4b: Tumor invades masticator space, pterygoid plates, skull base, or encases carotid
- Clinical **mucosal extent** more accurate than imaging
- Imaging important for **deep extent: Look for features that make tumor T4**
- Nodal staging: AJCC follows oropharyngeal & laryngeal nodal staging
- 1st-order drainage is **level I, then level II**
  - **Up to 35%** have nodes found at presentation
  - **30% occult nodal metastases** in oral cavity SCCa
- Metastatic disease: Absent = M0, present = M1
  - Lung metastases more common than bone & liver

CLINICAL ISSUES

Presentation

- Most common signs/symptoms
  - Painful hard ulcer/lesion in FOM
- Other signs/symptoms
  - Invasion of mandible may lead to loose teeth

Demographics

- Age
  - Most commonly 50-70 years

Natural History & Prognosis

- **Overall 5-year survival = 60%**

Treatment

- Primary resection ± reconstruction, ± neck dissection
- ± adjuvant radiation
- Future role of superselective intraarterial chemotherapy?

SELECTED REFERENCES

1. Arya S et al: Oral cavity squamous cell carcinoma: role of pretreatment imaging and its influence on management. Clin Radiol. 69(9):916-30, 2014
2. Hong HR et al: Clinical values of (18) F-FDG PET/CT in oral cavity cancer with dental artifacts on CT or MRI. J Surg Oncol. 110(6):696-701, 2014
3. American Joint Committee on Cancer: AJCC Cancer Staging Manual. 7th ed. New York: Springer, 2010

KEY FACTS

TERMINOLOGY

- SCCa arising from teeth-bearing bone of mandible, maxilla

IMAGING

- Small lesions may be occult to imaging
- Larger lesions: **Enhancing, infiltrating mass** ± underlying **bone destruction**
- Coronal plane useful for CT or MR evaluation
- Bone CT: Cortical destruction ± enlarged nerve canal
- MR: Marrow signal & enhancement similar to tumor
- PET/CT: Increasing role in clinical practice
  - Detection of nodal and distant metastases
  - Complimentary to MR for detecting marrow invasion (higher specificity, but lower sensitivity)

TOP DIFFERENTIAL DIAGNOSES

- Osteomyelitis
- Osteoradionecrosis
- Osteonecrosis
- Metastasis
- Osteosarcoma

CLINICAL ISSUES

- **10%** oral cavity SCCa
- Nonhealing ulcer of jaw, pain, swelling, bleeding, ill-fitting dentures
- Overall 5-year survival ~ 60%
- Surgical resection ± reconstruction ± radiation

DIAGNOSTIC CHECKLIST

- Evaluate local spread, bone infiltration, nodes
- Mandible: Buccal space, masticator space, floor of mouth
- Maxilla: Nasal cavity, maxillary sinus, palate
- Alveolar ridge mucosa attached to bone; allows early marrow infiltration: T4a
- If in bone, evaluate for perineural tumor spread
  - Inferior alveolar (mandible) or palatine (maxilla)
- Metastatic spread favors facial, level I & II nodes

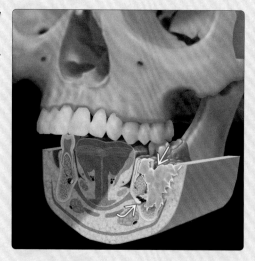
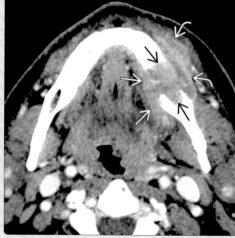

(Left) Graphic illustrates SCCa ➡ arising from mandibular alveolar ridge and invading mandible body, making it T4a. Note involvement of inferior alveolar nerve ➡, which is important for complete resection. (Right) Axial CECT demonstrates heterogeneous mass with destruction of left mandibular body ➡. Mass extends laterally to involve gingivobuccal sulcus and cheek ➡ and medially to involve floor of mouth ➡. Lesion was T4aN1 and completely excised with reconstruction by composite flap.

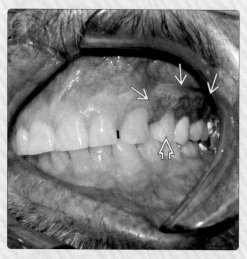
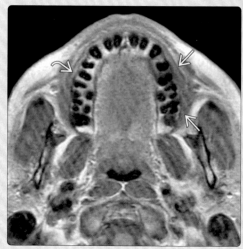

(Left) Clinical photograph of a 66-year-old man depicts an irregular red, indurated, ulcerated lesion ➡ of the left maxillary alveolar ridge, from the 1st premolar ➡. Biopsy revealed invasive SCCa, & the clinical examination suspected it to be T2N0. (Right) Axial T1 MR in the same patient shows markedly subtle soft tissue fullness ➡ lateral to maxillary alveolus, with a loss of normal fat planes compared to contralateral side ➡. No convincing marrow infiltration was apparent by imaging, & partial maxillectomy concurred.

Alveolar Ridge Squamous Cell Carcinoma

TERMINOLOGY

Abbreviations

- Alveolar ridge squamous cell carcinoma (SCCa)

Synonyms

- Alveolar gingival SCCa

Definitions

- Oral cavity malignancy arising from teeth-bearing bone of mandible or maxilla
  - SCCa of gingiva overlying alveolus
  - Primary SCCa of alveolar bone extremely rare

IMAGING

General Features

- Best diagnostic clue
  - **Enhancing, infiltrating jaw mass; bone destruction**
- Location
  - Mandibular or maxillary alveolar ridge
    - Alveolar ridge = teeth-bearing portion of jaw
- Size
  - Varies from mm to several cm
- Morphology
  - Poorly marginated mass

CT Findings

- CECT
  - Irregular, mild to moderately enhancing lesion
  - Small lesions may be occult to imaging
- Bone CT
  - Destruction of alveolar bone of mandible/maxilla
  - Enlarged inferior alveolar canal (mandible)/palatine canal (maxilla) suggest perineural tumor

MR Findings

- T1WI
  - Isointense to muscle
  - Bone infiltration suggested by loss of high signal
- T1WI C+
  - Moderately enhancing mass of jaw
  - Marrow enhancement suggests invasion
    - Evaluate entire length of nerve to brainstem

Imaging Recommendations

- Best imaging tool
  - MR preferred for complete tumor extent
    - Bone marrow and perineural tumor spread
    - Less affected by dental amalgam artifact
  - Bone CT or Panorex used for cortical destruction
- Protocol advice
  - MR: Axial & coronal planes, fat saturation on T1 C+
  - CECT: Bone & soft tissue algorithm, axial & coronal

Nuclear Medicine Findings

- PET/CT
  - SCCa reliably FDG avid
  - Increasing role in current practice
  - Complimentary to MR for detecting marrow invasion

DIFFERENTIAL DIAGNOSIS

Mandible-Maxilla Osteomyelitis

- Destructive focus ± adjacent soft tissue abscess

Mandible-Maxilla Osteoradionecrosis

- Destructive mandibular focus, prior XRT

Mandible-Maxilla Osteonecrosis

- Most commonly seen now with bisphosphonate

Mandible-Maxilla Metastasis

- Aggressive mandibular mass, known primary

Mandible-Maxilla Osteosarcoma

- Aggressive mandibular lesion with periosteal reaction

PATHOLOGY

General Features

- Etiology
  - Alcohol & tobacco → epithelial metaplasia → neoplasia

Staging, Grading, & Classification

- American Joint Committee on Cancer (AJCC) 2010
  - T1: Tumor ≤ 2 cm in greatest dimension
  - T2: Tumor > 2 & ≤ 4 cm in greatest dimension
  - T3: Tumor > 4 cm in greatest dimension
  - T4a: Tumor invades through cortical bone into extrinsic tongue muscles, skin of face
  - T4b: Tumor invades masticator space, pterygoid plates, skull base, or encases carotid
- **Imaging is critical for determination of T4 status**

CLINICAL ISSUES

Presentation

- Most common signs/symptoms
  - Nonhealing ulcer of jaw

Demographics

- Age
  - Mean: 65 years
- Epidemiology
  - **10%** of oral cavity SCCa

Natural History & Prognosis

- SCCa spreads locally to adjacent spaces
  - Maxilla: Medially to palate, maxillary sinus, nasal cavity
  - Mandible: Medially to floor of mouth, laterally to buccal & masticator spaces
- Some believe alveolar ridge SSCa has lower metastatic rate than other oral cavity SCCa: Facial nodes, levels I, II
- **Overall 5-year survival ~ 60%**

Treatment

- Surgical resection ± reconstruction
  - ± elective neck dissection, adjuvant radiation

SELECTED REFERENCES

1. Geetha P et al: Primary intraosseous carcinoma of the mandible: a clinicoradiographic view. J Cancer Res Ther. 11(3):651, 2015
2. Abd El-Hafez YG et al: Comparison of PET/CT and MRI for the detection of bone marrow invasion in patients with squamous cell carcinoma of the oral cavity. Oral Oncol. 47(4):288-95, 2011

TERMINOLOGY

- Retromolar trigone (RMT) squamous cell carcinoma (SCCa)
- RMT has complex shape: Mucosa over mandibular body and ramus posterior to molars, ascending to maxillary tuberosity

IMAGING

- RMT contiguous with anterior tonsillar pillar, buccal mucosa, & alveolar ridge mucosa
  - SCCa primary site may be difficult to determine
- CECT: Mildly enhancing mass, may be occult if small
  - Look for asymmetry of fat planes
  - Puffed-cheek technique may improve visualization of mucosal space tumor in RMT
  - Dental amalgam artifact may obscure primary tumor or tumor spreading via pterygomandibular raphe
- MR: Allows most accurate delineation of primary tumor, marrow infiltration, perineural & perifascial tumor
  - Less affected by dental amalgam artifact

- SCCa reliably FDG avid in PET-CT
  - Not often used unless extensive nodal disease

TOP DIFFERENTIAL DIAGNOSES

- Masticator space abscess
- Buccal mucosa SCCa
- Oral minor salivary gland malignancy

CLINICAL ISSUES

- Tumor often indolent with late presentation
- Bone/masticator muscle involvement → pain, trismus
  - Both indicate T4 disease; poorest prognosis
  - **Imaging key for determination of T4 disease**

DIAGNOSTIC CHECKLIST

- RMT site results in complex tumor spread patterns
  - Buccal & masticator spaces, oral cavity, & oropharynx
  - Mandible, maxilla, inferior alveolar nerve
  - Via **pterygomandibular raphe** to pterygoid plate
- Must evaluate for all potential spread sites

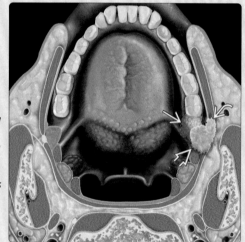
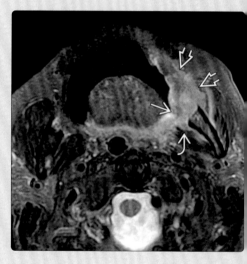

(Left) *Graphic illustrates squamous cell carcinoma (SCCa)* ➡ *arising posterior to the 3rd molar and extending superiorly along the pterygomandibular raphe and laterally onto the buccinator* ➡. *Tumor encroaches on the anterior tonsillar pillar* ➡ *of oropharynx.* (Right) *Axial T2WI FS MR in a patient with poorly healing socket following tooth extraction shows mildly hyperintense soft tissue mass* ➡ *from RMT, which infiltrates to medial pterygoid* ➡ *(T4b disease). SCCa also infiltrates laterally to masseter and cheek* ➡ *along buccinator.*

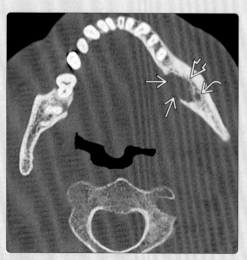
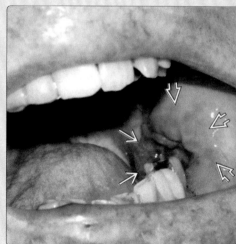

(Left) *Axial bone CT in the same patient shows large lytic defect* ➡ *in the left mandible with ill-defined lateral margin* ➡. *Note the proximity of defect to the inferior alveolar canal* ➡. *Imaging features stage this as T4b.* (Right) *Clinical photograph in the same patient shows mucosal well-differentiated SCCa* ➡ *in the retromolar trigone. Note fullness of the left cheek* ➡, *indicating submucosal infiltration of the tumor and correlating with MR findings.*

Retromolar Trigone Squamous Cell Carcinoma

TERMINOLOGY

Abbreviations

- Retromolar trigone (RMT) squamous cell carcinoma (SCCa)

Definitions

- Oral cavity mucosal malignancy
- RMT: Mucosa overlying ascending ramus of mandible posterior to molars, extending superiorly to maxillary tuberosity

IMAGING

General Features

- Best diagnostic clue
  - Focal enhancing lesion centered in RMT ± mandible or maxilla invasion
- Location
  - Mandibular angle, posterior to molars
  - RMT contiguous with anterior tonsillar pillar, buccal mucosa, & alveolar ridge mucosa, so primary site may be difficult to determine
- Size
  - Variable: < 2 cm (T1) to large mass infiltrating cheek and oropharynx

CT Findings

- CECT
  - Mildly enhancing infiltrative mass
- Bone CT
  - Important for cortical disruption, marrow infiltration

MR Findings

- T1WI
  - Isointense to muscle
    - Look for loss of marrow intensity
- T2WI
  - Hyperintense as compared to muscle
- T1WI C+ FS
  - Mild to moderately enhancing infiltrating mass
  - Evaluate for perineural tumor if mandible invaded

Nuclear Medicine Findings

- PET/CT
  - SCCa reliably FDG avid

Imaging Recommendations

- Best imaging tool
  - MR gives best delineation of tumor extent, marrow infiltration, perineural tumor
    - Small lesion may be occult on CECT
    - MR less affected by dental amalgam artifact
- Protocol advice
  - If CECT obtained, reformat in coronal plane also
    - Bone and soft tissue algorithm postprocessing

DIFFERENTIAL DIAGNOSIS

Masticator Space Abscess

- Heterogeneous enhancement, cellulitis

Buccal Mucosa SCCa

- Lesion arising from inner surface cheeks or lips

Oral Minor Salivary Gland Malignancy

- Often more focal mass but has perineural spread

PATHOLOGY

Staging, Grading, & Classification

- American Joint Committee on Cancer (AJCC) 2010
  - **T1**: ≤ 2 cm in greatest diameter
  - **T2**: > 2 & ≤ 4 cm in greatest diameter
  - **T3**: > 4 cm in greatest diameter
  - **T4a**: Tumor invades through cortical bone & into extrinsic tongue muscles, skin of face
  - **T4b**: Tumor invades masticator space, pterygoid plates, skull base, or encases carotid
- Clinical mucosal extent more accurate than imaging
- **Imaging key for determination of T4 disease**

CLINICAL ISSUES

Presentation

- Most common signs/symptoms
  - Often indolent: Late presentation, high T stage
  - Bone/masticator muscle involvement results in pain, trismus

Demographics

- Age
  - Mean age: 67 yr
- Epidemiology
  - 7% of oral cavity tumors

Natural History & Prognosis

- Site of RMT allows for **unique tumor spread patterns**
  - Anterolaterally to buccinator muscle & cheek
  - Posterolaterally to buccal fat & masticator space
  - Posteromedially to tongue
  - Posteriorly to anterior tonsillar pillar & oropharynx
  - Superiorly to maxilla via **pterygomandibular raphe**
  - Inferiorly into mandible ± inferior alveolar nerve
- Poor prognosis if bone or masticator space invasion
- 30% have nodal metastasis at diagnosis
- **Overall 5-year survival ~ 60%**

Treatment

- Typically surgical resection ± adjuvant radiation
  - Surgery + radiation = best 5-year survival
- Some advocate primary radiation for low T-stage

DIAGNOSTIC CHECKLIST

Reporting Tips

- Tumor has **complex potential spread patterns**; important that imaging studies evaluated for all

SELECTED REFERENCES

1. Hitchcock KE et al: Retromolar trigone squamous cell carcinoma treated with radiotherapy alone or combined with surgery: a 10-year update. Am J Otolaryngol. 36(2):140-5, 2015
2. Mazziotti S et al: Diagnostic approach to retromolar trigone cancer by multiplanar computed tomography reconstructions. Can Assoc Radiol J. 65(4):335-44, 2014
3. Binahmed A et al: Population-based study of treatment outcomes in squamous cell carcinoma of the retromolar trigone. Oral Surg Oral Med Oral Pathol Oral Radiol Endod. 104(5):662-5, 2007

TERMINOLOGY

- Buccal mucosa squamous cell carcinoma (SCCa)
- Oral cavity mucosal malignancy arising from inner lining of cheek and lips

IMAGING

- Typically difficult to identify with routine imaging
- Mild to moderately enhancing irregular lesion
- Look for asymmetrically infiltrated buccal fat
- CECT: "Puffed cheek" method works well to separate mucosal surfaces and see site of origin
- MR: Hypointense gauze padding works similarly and often better tolerated with long MR sequences
- FDG avid (reserved for advanced nodal disease)
  - Nodes are important prognostic factor

TOP DIFFERENTIAL DIAGNOSES

- Oral cavity infection
- Oral cavity minor salivary gland malignancy

PATHOLOGY

- Traditionally poorest prognosis of oral cavity SCCa
  - Recent studies suggest similar prognosis to cancers in other oral cavity sites once age at diagnosis, tumor stage, treatment, and race are taken into consideration
- Strong association with tobacco, alcohol, betel nut, & paan
- All oral cavity tumors use same TNM classification
- Imaging important for deep extent
  - Identifying buccal space invasion & T4 features
  - T4a: Tumor invades skin of face, through cortical bone, into extrinsic tongue muscles
  - T4b: Tumor invades masticator space, pterygoid plates, skull base, or encases carotid

DIAGNOSTIC CHECKLIST

- Clinical history indicating site of lesion important
- Look for infiltration of buccal space fat
  - If present, evaluate for masticator space infiltration
- 1st-order node drainage: Buccal & level I, II nodes

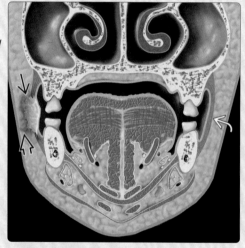
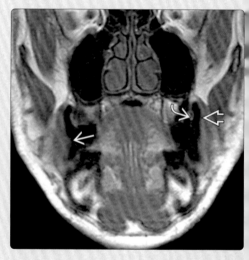

(Left) Coronal graphic depicts a T2 (2-4 cm size) buccal mucosal squamous cell carcinoma ➡ that has invaded the underlying buccinator muscle & subcutaneous fat ➡. If the lesion had involved the cheek skin, it would be staged as T4. Note the normal left buccinator ➡. (Right) Coronal T1WI MR performed with a patient using the "puffed cheek" method shows the cheek ➡ displaced from gingival mucosa ➡ and subtle nodularity of the right buccal mucosa ➡, representing SCCa. No evidence of deep infiltration is seen.

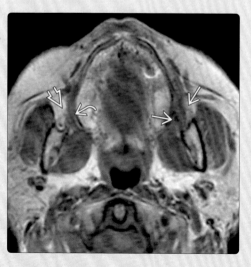
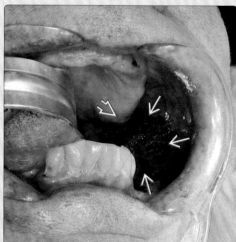

(Left) Axial T1WI MR demonstrates an ill-defined tissue filling the buccal fat pad ➡ from deep infiltration of buccal mucosal malignancy. Note the smooth contours on the contralateral side ➡ and the clean buccal fat ➡. Without a clear history of the primary site, buccal fat infiltration may only be a subtle imaging finding. (Right) Clinical photograph in the same patient shows buccal mucosal primary SCCa ➡ along the posterior aspect of the inner cheek, extending to the posterior margin maxillary (edentulous) alveolus ➡.

Buccal Mucosa Squamous Cell Carcinoma

TERMINOLOGY

Abbreviations

- Buccal mucosa squamous cell carcinoma (SCCa)

Definitions

- Mucosal malignancy arising from inner lining of cheek, lips

IMAGING

General Features

- Best diagnostic clue
  - May be very subtle, even when infiltrating buccal fat
- Location
  - Most often inner aspect of cheek
- Size
  - Variable: Several mm to several cm

CT Findings

- CECT
  - Often extremely difficult to see on routine imaging
  - Look for subtle asymmetry of buccal fat
  - Mild to moderately enhancing irregular lesion

MR Findings

- Hard to see primary lesion without clinical history
  - Isointense on T1, slightly hyperintense T2
  - Look for infiltration of buccal fat
- Variable enhancement: Mild to moderate

Nuclear Medicine Findings

- PET/CT
  - SCCa reliably FDG avid

Imaging Recommendations

- Best imaging tool
  - MR generally preferred in oral cavity with better tissue contrast for delineation of tumor extent
- Protocol advice
  - CECT: Soft tissue and bone algorithm in 2 planes
    - "Puffed cheek" method works well to separate opposed mucosal surfaces
  - MR: "Puffed cheek" method not often successful because of sequence time
    - Consider use of gauze padding in cheek instead

DIFFERENTIAL DIAGNOSIS

Oral Cavity Infection

- Superinfected traumatic ulcer may result in local inflammation ± cellulitis
- May have reactive buccal adenopathy

Oral Cavity Minor Salivary Gland Malignancy

- Uncommonly arises from buccal mucosa
- Indistinguishable from SCCa

PATHOLOGY

General Features

- Etiology
  - Strongly associated with tobacco (smoking and chewing) and alcohol abuse

- In oral cavity, the association with tobacco is strongest for floor of mouth and buccal mucosa
  - In central and Southeast Asia, associated with chewing betel nut and paan (tobacco + nut + lime)

Staging, Grading, & Classification

- American Joint Committee on Cancer (AJCC) 2010
- **Same classification for all oral cavity tumors**
  - T1: ≤ 2 cm in greatest diameter
  - T2: > 2 cm & ≤ 4 cm in greatest diameter
  - T3: > 4 cm in greatest diameter
  - T4a: Tumor invades skin of face, through cortical bone, into extrinsic tongue muscles
  - T4b: Tumor invades masticator space, pterygoid plates, skull base, or encases carotid
- **Nodal staging**: AJCC, follows oropharyngeal & laryngeal nodal staging
- **Metastatic disease**: Absent = M0, present = M1

CLINICAL ISSUES

Presentation

- Most common signs/symptoms
  - Mild discomfort; may "catch" in teeth

Demographics

- Age
  - Mean: 50-70 years
- Gender
  - M > F
- Epidemiology
  - In North America, represents 10% of oral malignancies
  - In Taiwan, represents up to 37% from chewing betel nut and paan

Natural History & Prognosis

- Tendency for submucosal spread, then laterally to skin
- Generally poor prognosis because of high recurrence rate and invasive spread
  - Overall prognosis: Up to 60% 5-year survival
- Poor prognostic factors: Positive surgical margin, **cervical nodal metastasis (especially if extracapsular spread)**, advanced tumor stage, tumor thickness > 7 mm

Treatment

- Surgical: Resection ± reconstruction ± nodal dissection
- ± adjuvant radiation

DIAGNOSTIC CHECKLIST

Image Interpretation Pearls

- Clinical history indicating site of lesion important
- Look for infiltration of buccal fat
  - If present, evaluate for masticator space infiltration
- Look for buccal and level I, II nodes

SELECTED REFERENCES

1. Camilon PR et al: Does buccal cancer have worse prognosis than other oral cavity cancers? Laryngoscope. 124(6):1386-91, 2014
2. Erdogan N et al: Puffed-cheek computed tomography: a dynamic maneuver for imaging oral cavity tumors. Ear Nose Throat J. 91(9):383-4, 386, 2012
3. Dillon JK et al: Gauze padding: a simple technique to delineate small oral cavity tumors. AJNR Am J Neuroradiol. 32(5):934-7, 2011

Hard Palate Squamous Cell Carcinoma

TERMINOLOGY

- Hard palate squamous cell carcinoma (SCCa)
- Oral cavity mucosal malignancy of roof of mouth

IMAGING

- Often extremely subtle, may be occult to imaging
- Variable size from several mm to several cm
- **Coronal plane** imaging **key** for either CT or MR
- CECT: Mild to moderately enhancing ill-defined lesion with associated bone erosion
  - Both soft tissue & bone algorithm important
- MR: Low T1 tumor signal contrasts against hyperintense palate marrow and mucosa
  - T1 C+ FS and T2 FS aid tumor delineation
  - Look at **greater palatine canal** and **pterygopalatine fossa** for CNV2 perineural tumor (PNT)

TOP DIFFERENTIAL DIAGNOSES

- Hard palate minor salivary gland carcinoma

- Palate benign mixed tumor
- Invasive sinonasal SCCa

CLINICAL ISSUES

- Ulcer ± mass on roof of mouth; often painful
- Clinically obvious lesion may be subtle on CT or MR
- Rare tumor; least common oral cavity site
- In this location, SCCa is less common than minor salivary malignancies
- Overall 5-year survival ~ 60%
- Treatment: Surgical resection ± neck dissection ± XRT
  - Elective neck dissection associated with lower recurrence rate, better overall survival

DIAGNOSTIC CHECKLIST

- Must evaluate bone for erosion ± infiltration
- MR better evaluates **greater palatine canal** & **pterygopalatine fossa** for CNV2 PNT
- Evaluate carefully for nodal metastases

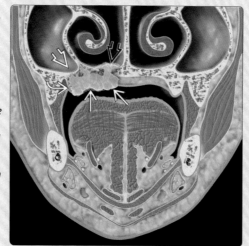

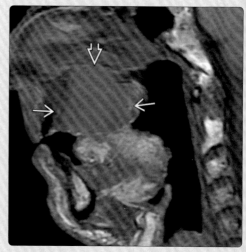

(Left) Coronal graphic illustrates oral cavity SCCa ➡ arising from mucosa of hard palate and infiltrating underlying bone. The tumor may extend through palatine portion of maxilla ➡ to floor of the nasal cavity, or through the alveolar bone ➡, or to the maxillary sinus ➡. Perineural tumor spread may occur along the 2nd division of trigeminal nerve, V2. (Right) Sagittal T1WI MR shows a patient with prior retromolar trigone SCCa and a new large oral cavity SCCa ➡ that destroys hard palate and extends into the nasal cavity ➡.

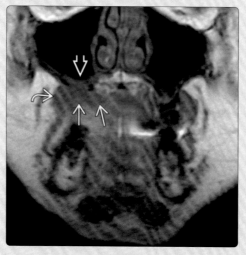

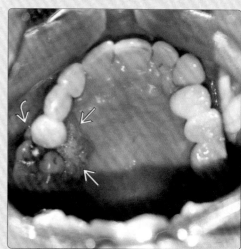

(Left) Coronal T1WI MR demonstrates subtle mucosal lesion ➡ of hard palate that extends through maxillary alveolus to both buccal mucosa ➡ and the maxillary sinus floor ➡. The tumor is T4aN0, stage IVA disease. Palatal lesions are often best seen on T1 precontrast and in coronal plane. (Right) Clinical photograph taken with an oral mirror demonstrates a clinically obvious maxillary mass involving the palatal mucosa ➡. The tumor was extremely subtle on imaging. Extension through to buccal surface is also evident ➡.

Hard Palate Squamous Cell Carcinoma

TERMINOLOGY

Abbreviations

- Hard palate squamous cell carcinoma (SCCa)

Definitions

- Oral cavity malignancy arising from mucosa overlying hard palate

IMAGING

General Features

- Location
  - Hard palate (best known as roof of mouth)
- Size
  - Variable: Several mm to several cm

CT Findings

- CECT
  - Often extremely subtle or occult to imaging
  - Mild to moderate enhancement
- Bone CT
  - Erosion of bone often found

MR Findings

- Low T1 signal contrasts against bright palate marrow
- Mild to moderate enhancement

Imaging Recommendations

- Best imaging tool
  - MR allows evaluation of marrow and perineural tumor spread along palatine canals
- Protocol advice
  - Coronal plane essential for either CT or MR
  - CECT: Obtain soft tissue and bone algorithm

DIFFERENTIAL DIAGNOSIS

Hard Palate Minor Salivary Gland Carcinoma

- Mucoepidermoid & adenoid cystic carcinoma most frequent and much more common than SCCa
- May be smooth bone erosion or aggressive destruction
- Perineural tumor frequently found

Palate Benign Mixed Tumor

- Well-circumscribed T2 intense round mass
- Typically smooth erosion of bone

Sinonasal SCCa

- Maxillary sinus tumor may extend into palate
- Clinically presents as submucosal mass

PATHOLOGY

General Features

- Etiology
  - Associated with tobacco and alcohol abuse but not as strong an association as other oral cavity SCCa sites
  - Fruits and vegetables appear to have protective effect

Staging, Grading, & Classification

- American Joint Committee on Cancer (AJCC) 2010
- All oral cavity malignancies use same TNM staging
- T1: ≤ 2 cm in greatest diameter

- T2: > 2 cm & ≤ 4 cm
- T3: > 4 cm
- T4a: Tumor invades maxillary sinus, skin of face, through cortical bone, deep tongue muscles
- T4b: Tumor invades masticator space, pterygoid plates, skull base, or encases carotid
- Size of mucosal component best evaluated clinically

Gross Pathologic & Surgical Features

- Red & white well-demarcated areas of induration
- Ulcerated areas indurated, tender upon palpation

Microscopic Features

- Squamous differentiation with intracellular bridges or keratinization, ± keratin pearls
- Further classified by degree of differentiation

CLINICAL ISSUES

Presentation

- Most common signs/symptoms
  - Painful ulcer on roof of mouth
- Other signs/symptoms
  - Bleeding, ill-fitting dentures, loose teeth
  - Facial tingling/pain → V2 perineural tumor

Demographics

- Age
  - Mean age: 70 yr
- Gender
  - M > F

Natural History & Prognosis

- Survival strongly correlates with T stage
  - Mean survival: T1 = 8 yr, T4 ~ 4 yr
- Nodal metastasis significantly impacts survival
  - Levels I, II are 1st-order drainage sites
- Overall 5-year survival ~ 60%

Treatment

- Surgical resection ± neck dissection ± adjuvant radiation

DIAGNOSTIC CHECKLIST

Consider

- Often very subtle lesion at imaging, though typically clinically apparent

Image Interpretation Pearls

- Coronal plane imaging is key for either CT or MR

Reporting Tips

- Must evaluate bone for erosion &/or infiltration
- MR better evaluates palatine canals for greater palatine nerve (CNV2) perineural tumor
- Evaluate carefully for nodal metastases

SELECTED REFERENCES

1. Givi B et al: Impact of elective neck dissection on the outcome of oral squamous cell carcinomas arising in the maxillary alveolus and hard palate. Head Neck. 38 Suppl 1:E1688-94, 2016
2. Arya S et al: Oral cavity squamous cell carcinoma: role of pretreatment imaging and its influence on management. Clin Radiol. 69(9):916-30, 2014
3. Kato H et al: CT and MR imaging findings of palatal tumors. Eur J Radiol. 83(3):e137-46, 2014

KEY FACTS

TERMINOLOGY

- Mucosal malignancy of hypopharyngeal subsite
  - 2/3 of all hypopharyngeal squamous cell carcinoma (SCCa) arise in pyriform sinus

IMAGING

- Pharyngoepiglottic fold to postcricoid region
- Variable tumor size/appearance at presentation
  - May present as small unknown primary with metastatic nodes
  - Or, presents as large T3-4 tumor, minimal symptoms, metastatic adenopathy
- Mild to moderately enhancing irregular mass
- Arises from apex or anterior, posterior, or lateral wall
- May fill pyriform sinus &/or circumferentially involve walls
- Note that AE fold SCCa considered supraglottic laryngeal SCCa, with different staging
- FDG PET/CECT efficient modality to anatomically stage primary pyriform sinus mass, nodes, and metastatic disease

TOP DIFFERENTIAL DIAGNOSES

- Vocal cord paralysis
- Supraglottitis
- 4th branchial cleft cyst
- Hypopharyngeal minor salivary gland malignancy

PATHOLOGY

- Strong association with tobacco & alcohol abuse
- Prior radiation is also risk factor

CLINICAL ISSUES

- Often minimal symptoms: Sore throat, dysphagia, otalgia
- Up to 75% have adenopathy at presentation
- Nodes frequently bilateral (N2c)
- 20-40% develop distant metastases
- Overall 5-year survival: ~ 40%
- 16% have 2nd primary malignancies

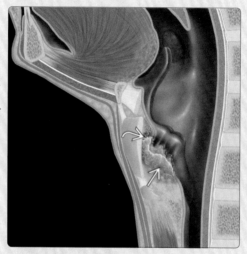
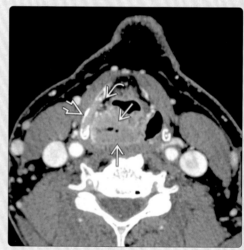

(Left) Lateral graphic illustrates pyriform sinus squamous cell carcinoma (SCCa) ➔ arising from anterior wall and extending toward paraglottic fat ➔. Tumor location does not result in airway or swallowing obstruction. (Right) Axial CECT in a 65-year-old man with extensive smoking history and sore throat demonstrates mass filling right pyriform sinus ➔. Mass appears superficially spreading, involving all walls of sinus but not spreading anteriorly to paraglottic fat ➔ or laterally into thyroid cartilage ➔.

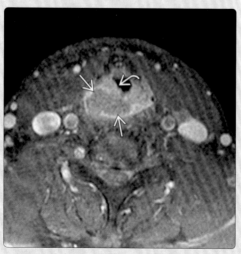
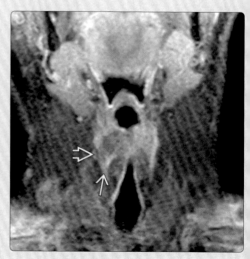

(Left) Axial T1WI C+ FS MR in the same patient shows relatively less enhancement of SCCa ➔ than of mucosa of larynx and hypopharynx. Right aryepiglottic (AE) fold is displaced anteriorly, but laryngeal surface ➔ is normal. (Right) Coronal T1WI C+ FS MR in the same patient shows lesion filling pyriform sinus ➔ apex. Tumor abuts cartilage ➔ but does not invade or extend laterally to soft tissues. PET/CT obtained due to suspicious bone lesions on CT was negative. This was T2 N1 M0, SCCa treated with chemoradiation.

TERMINOLOGY

Abbreviations

- Squamous cell carcinoma (SCCa)

Definitions

- Mucosal malignancy of hypopharyngeal subsite
- 2/3 of all hypopharyngeal SCCa arise in pyriform sinus

IMAGING

General Features

- Location
  - Pharyngoepiglottic fold to proximal esophagus
    - Lateral margin is lateral pharyngeal wall
    - Medial margin is lateral surface of aryepiglottic (AE) folds and cricoid and arytenoid cartilages
- Size
  - Variable: May be small "unknown primary" in patient presenting with adenopathy or T3-4 with minimal symptoms
- Morphology
  - Irregular infiltrating and ulcerative mass

CT Findings

- CECT
  - Mild to moderately enhancing, irregular, ulcerative mass
  - May fill pyriform sinus &/or circumferentially involve walls
  - May arise from apex or anterior, posterior, or lateral wall
    - Apex: Inferior extension can occur to postcricoid region
      □ If submucosal spread, then occult to clinical exam
    - Anterior: Spread into paraglottic fat of larynx
    - Lateral: Spreads to parapharyngeal tissues (T4a)
      □ May infiltrate through thyrohyoid membrane
      □ Look for thyroid cartilage invasion (T4a)
      □ Look for carotid involvement (T4b), suggested by > 270° encasement
    - Posterior: May invade prevertebral tissues (T4b); imaging can exclude this but is not accurate for confirming it
    - Superior extension often occurs to oropharynx
  - Note **AE fold SCCa** is considered **supraglottic laryngeal SCCa**, with different staging
- Bone CT
  - Look for cartilage erosion, destruction, or sclerosis
    - Sclerosis is sensitive but has poor specificity, as sclerosis alone often represents perichondritis
    - Erosion/destruction more accurate for invasion

MR Findings

- Primary tumor features
  - Low to intermediate T1, intermediate to high T2 signal intensity
  - Heterogeneous gadolinium enhancement
- Cartilage penetration (T4a) on MR
  - Cartilage hyperintensity alone on T2 suggests edema/perichondritis
  - **Penetration = tumor through cartilage**
  - Cartilage involved if
    - T2 SI of cartilage = T2 tumor, and

    - T1 C+ FS SI of cartilage = same SI of primary tumor
- Adenopathy may be solid or necrotic
  - Look for ill-defined margins suggesting extracapsular spread (ECS)

Nuclear Medicine Findings

- PET/CT
  - May be used when staging advanced hypopharyngeal SCCa to exclude contralateral adenopathy and M1 disease
  - May be useful when metastatic adenopathy present clinically but pyriform sinus tumor is occult

Imaging Recommendations

- Best imaging tool
  - PET/CECT together best stage pyriform sinus SCCa, confirm adenopathy, and detect distant metastases
  - CECT alone often done as 1st step
  - MR has adjunctive role for cartilage invasion
- Protocol advice
  - CECT: Imaging obtained in quiet respiration; 90-second delay after IV contrast for mucosal enhancement

DIFFERENTIAL DIAGNOSIS

Vocal Cord Paralysis

- Pyriform sinus of paralyzed side will be dilated, so contralateral pyriform sinus appears mass-like

Supraglottitis

- Inflammatory enlargement of AE folds

4th Branchial Cleft Cyst

- 3rd or 4th branchial cleft anomaly most common presentation in younger patient
- a.k.a. pyriform sinus fistula: From apex of pyriform sinus to lower neck

Hypopharyngeal Minor Salivary Gland Malignancy

- Extremely rare lesion in hypopharynx
- Often heterogeneously hyperintense on T2WI with cystic changes

PATHOLOGY

General Features

- Etiology
  - Strong association with tobacco & alcohol abuse
  - Prior radiation is also risk factor
- Associated abnormalities
  - 16% have 2nd primary tumors
    - 2/3 metachronous, 1/3 synchronous
    - 2/3 oral cavity, pharynx, esophagus
    - 1/3 lung, larynx

Staging, Grading, & Classification

- **All 3 subsites of hypopharynx** (pyriform sinus, postcricoid region, posterior hypopharyngeal wall) **use same staging system**
- American Joint Committee on Cancer (AJCC) 2010
- Same as nodal staging for oropharynx & oral cavity
- Pitfall: Invasion of prevertebral fascia cannot be predicted with 100% sensitivity with imaging

AJCC Hypopharynx Staging (2010)

Tumor Stage (T)	Nodal Stage (N)
T1: 1 subsite &/or ≤ 2 cm in greatest dimension	**N1**: Ipsilateral node ≤ 3 cm
T2: > 1 subsite or adjacent site **or** > 2 & ≤ 4 cm without hemilarynx fixation	**N2a**: Ipsilateral node > 3 cm, ≤ 6 cm
T3: > 4 cm **or** fixation of larynx **or** extension to esophagus	**N2b**: Multiple ipsilateral nodes ≤ 6 cm
T4: Moderately advanced (T4a) or very advanced (T4b) local disease	**N2c**: Bilateral or contralateral ≤ 6 cm
T4a: Invades cricoid/thyroid cartilage, hyoid, thyroid gland, central compartment soft tissue including strap muscles & subcutaneous fat	**N3**: Nodal mass > 6 cm
T4b: Invades prevertebral fascia, encases carotid, or involves mediastinum	**Distant Metastasis (M)**
	M0: No metastasis; **M1**: Distant metastasis

Adapted from 7th edition AJCC Staging Forms.

- o Preservation of retropharyngeal fat stripe: Fascia not invaded
- o Loss of fat stripe: Fascia may or may not be invaded

Gross Pathologic & Surgical Features
- Poorly marginated invasive and ulcerative or exophytic mass of hypopharynx

Microscopic Features
- Squamous differentiation with intracellular bridges or keratinization

CLINICAL ISSUES

Presentation
- Most common signs/symptoms
  - o Most common presentation is sore throat or dysphagia
  - o Otalgia as referred pain
    - – Internal laryngeal nerve & auricular nerve of CNX to external auditory canal & pinna
- Other signs/symptoms
  - o May present with palpable adenopathy and unknown primary site

Demographics
- Age
  - o > 50 years typically
- Gender
  - o M > F
- Epidemiology
  - o 65% of hypopharyngeal SCCa arise in pyriform sinus
    - – 20% postcricoid region, 15% posterior wall

Natural History & Prognosis
- Often presents as T3 or T4 as delay to diagnosis common; conversely may be unknown primary, T1, with adenopathy
- Up to 75% have adenopathy at presentation as rich vascular-lymphatic architecture
  - o Most often levels II, III, IV
  - o Nodes frequently bilateral (N2c)
- Anterior extension to larynx common as pyriform sinus apex at true vocal cord level
- 20-40% develop distant metastases
  - o Lungs > bones & liver
- Overall 5-year survival: ~ 40%
  - o Hypopharyngeal has poorest prognosis of H&N SCCa

- 16% have 2nd primary malignancies
  - o Significant impact on patient survival

Treatment
- Small tumors (T1, some T2): Open or endoscopic partial laryngopharyngectomy or radiation
- Large tumors: Laryngopharyngectomy ± chemo/radiation; however, trend to organ preservation with chemoradiation ± salvage surgery
- T4b tumors typically treated with chemotherapy &/or radiation for palliation

DIAGNOSTIC CHECKLIST

Consider
- When patient presents with **otalgia**, need to image pharynx, as pyriform sinus SCCa may have referred pain

Image Interpretation Pearls
- Small pyriform sinus apex SCCa may present as unknown primary
  - o Clinical examination blind spot
- Larger SCCa may fill sinus and extend to larynx; difficult to determine wall of origin
  - o Can distend sinus with CT Valsalva or phonation technique
- Look carefully for extrapharyngeal extension
  - o Anterior: Larynx
  - o Lateral: Thyrohyoid membrane, thyroid cartilage
  - o Posterior: Prevertebral invasion
  - o Inferior: Postcricoid subsite of hypopharynx and to esophagus
  - o Superior: Oropharynx extension common

Reporting Tips
- Hypopharyngeal SCCa patients have high incidence of 2nd primary tumor

SELECTED REFERENCES

1. Tanzler ED et al: Challenging the need for random directed biopsies of the nasopharynx, pyriform sinus, and contralateral tonsil in the workup of unknown primary squamous cell carcinoma of the head and neck. Head Neck. 38(4):578-81, 2016
2. Chen AY et al: Pitfalls in the staging squamous cell carcinoma of the hypopharynx. Neuroimaging Clin N Am. 23(1):67-79, 2013
3. Park YM et al: Feasiblity of transoral robotic hypopharyngectomy for early-stage hypopharyngeal carcinoma. Oral Oncol. 46(8):597-602, 2010

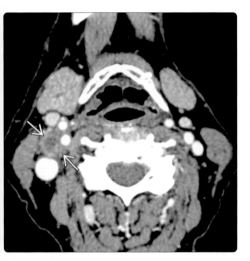

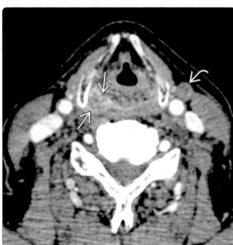

(Left) *Axial CECT in a 55-year-old man with long smoking & alcohol history presenting with a palpable right neck mass shows a necrotic, right level II nodal mass ➡ abutting carotid bifurcation. Aspiration revealed SCCa, but primary tumor was not evident on in-office examination.* (Right) *Axial CECT in the same patient reveals a subtle small area of asymmetric enhancement ➡ in the right pyriform sinus apex, which proved to be primary SCCa. Note contralateral necrotic metastatic node ➡.*

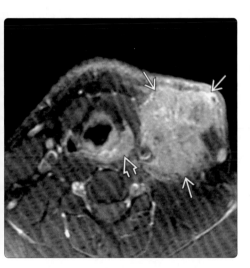

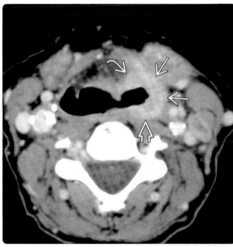

(Left) *Axial T1WI C+ FS MR shows a large, conglomerate nodal metastasis ➡ with extracapsular spread, and left pyriform sinus poorly differentiated SCCa ➡, T2 N2c. Patient had chemoXRT and dissection of residual nodes and was disease free at 4 years.* (Right) *Axial CECT in a patient with dysphagia and otalgia shows a moderately enhancing mass (involving all walls of pyriform sinus ➡) extending into paraglottic fat ➡. Tumor also spreads posteriorly to prevertebral muscles ➡, with loss of retropharyngeal fat.*

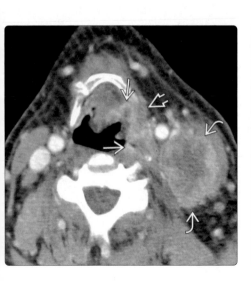

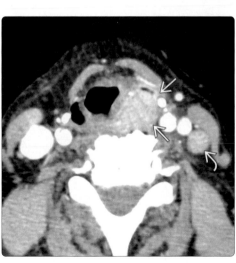

(Left) *Axial CECT in a man with 40-pound weight loss shows irregular, mildly enhancing SCCa ➡ arising in pyriform sinus and extending up to lateral oropharyngeal wall. Tumor extends out to soft tissues ➡. Large ipsilateral nodal metastasis has extracapsular spread ➡ (T4a N3).* (Right) *Axial CECT in an 82 year old shows SCCa arising in the posterolateral pyriform sinus wall ➡. Tumor was associated with left vocal cord paralysis, nodes ➡, and lung metastases. Staged as T3 N2b M1. Patient chose palliative care.*

KEY FACTS

TERMINOLOGY

- Squamous cell carcinoma (SCCa) arising from mucosa overlying posterior cricoid cartilage
  - 1 of 3 subsites of hypopharynx (HP)

IMAGING

- Often difficult scans to read
- Mass of lower HP with invasion anteriorly to larynx, superiorly and laterally in HP, or inferiorly to esophagus
- CECT: Mildly enhancing irregular mass
- MR: May better clarify cartilage invasion
- PET/CT: SCCa is reliably FDG avid

TOP DIFFERENTIAL DIAGNOSES

- Pharyngitis
- Posterior hypopharyngeal wall SCCa
- Cervical esophageal carcinoma

PATHOLOGY

- Strong association with tobacco and alcohol abuse
- Association with Plummer-Vinson syndrome
- Staged using American Joint Committee on Cancer TNM (2010) as for all hypopharyngeal SCCa

CLINICAL ISSUES

- Presents with sore throat, dysphagia
- Often presents late: T3 or T4
- 60% have nodes at diagnosis; often bilateral
- Poorest prognosis for all H&N SCCa with 5-year survival = 30%

DIAGNOSTIC CHECKLIST

- Key features to evaluate on scans
  - T3: > 4 cm or esophageal invasion
  - T4a: Cartilage or paralaryngeal invasion
  - T4b: Carotid encasement, mediastinal invasion

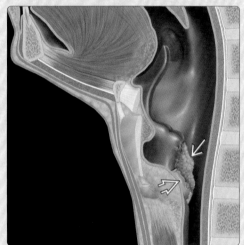
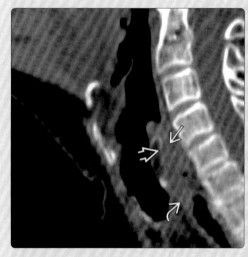

(Left) Lateral graphic of hypopharynx illustrates irregular tumor ➡ arising from mucosal surface covering posterior cricoid ring ➡. Cartilage erosion is depicted here. Note proximal cervical esophagus is just inferior to postcricoid hypopharynx. (Right) Sagittal CECT reformatted image shows exophytic mass ➡ distending lower hypopharynx, posterior to cricoid ➡, without cartilage destruction. Note extension below inferior cricoid cartilage to cervical esophagus ➡. This is staged as T3N0 SCCa.

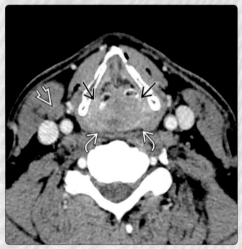
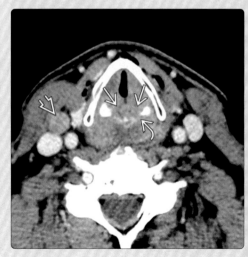

(Left) Axial CECT in a different patient shows soft tissue fullness of the lower hypopharynx. A mildly enhancing tumor infiltrates around the arytenoid cartilages ➡, while the retropharyngeal fat is clear posteriorly ➡. This feature helps to distinguish it from a posterior hypopharyngeal wall tumor. Right adenopathy is present ➡. (Right) Axial CECT inferiorly shows fullness of hypopharynx and irregular destruction of cricoid ➡ with tumor extension into posterior larynx ➡. Note the right neck node ➡. This is T4aN2c SCCa.

TERMINOLOGY

Definitions

- Squamous cell carcinoma (SCCa) arising from mucosa overlying posterior aspect of cricoid cartilage
  - 1 of 3 subsites of hypopharynx (HP)
    - 3 HP subsites: Pyriform sinus, posterior pharyngeal wall, postcricoid

IMAGING

General Features

- Best diagnostic clue
  - Irregular, moderately enhancing mass infiltrating into cricoid and larynx
- Location
  - Mucosa covering posterior aspect of cricoid cartilage
    - Anterior wall of lower HP
    - From arytenoid cartilages to inferior cricoid level

CT Findings

- CECT
  - Irregular, variably enhancing mass distending lower HP
  - Infiltrates anteriorly to cricoid cartilage and larynx

MR Findings

- T1 isointense to muscle, T2 moderately hyperintense
- Mild to moderate contrast enhancement

Imaging Recommendations

- Best imaging tool
  - CECT often best; patient may not tolerate long MR sequences
  - MR may be helpful for confirming cartilage invasion
- Protocol advice
  - CECT with sagittal and coronal reformations

Nuclear Medicine Findings

- PET/CT
  - SCCa primary and adenopathy are reliably FDG avid

DIFFERENTIAL DIAGNOSIS

Pharyngitis

- Infection/inflammation of mucosa most often with immunocompromised patients

Posterior Hypopharyngeal Wall SCCa

- Extension from postcricoid HP common
- May be difficult to differentiate from postcricoid SCCa in collapsed HP

Cervical Esophageal Carcinoma

- Uncommon primary tumor but may extend superiorly to HP

PATHOLOGY

General Features

- Etiology
  - Strong association with tobacco and alcohol abuse
  - 16% with Plummer-Vinson syndrome develop postcricoid region SCCa

Staging, Grading, & Classification

- American Joint Committee on Cancer (AJCC) 2010
- Staging for postcricoid region same as for all HP SCCa

CLINICAL ISSUES

Presentation

- Most common signs/symptoms
  - Sore throat, dysphagia
- Other signs/symptoms
  - May present with neck mass from adenopathy

Demographics

- Age
  - Peaks in 7th decade
- Gender
  - M >> F
- Epidemiology
  - **Postcricoid region** is uncommon hypopharyngeal site (20%)
    - Pyriform sinus 65%, posterior wall 15%
  - Tumors usually large at diagnosis

Natural History & Prognosis

- Postcricoid SCCa has tendency for submucosal spread
  - Especially inferiorly to esophagus (T3) or superiorly to oropharynx
- Often presents late with laryngeal invasion
- 60% nodes at presentation, levels III, IV; often bilateral
- **Poorest prognosis for all H&N SCCa**
  - Overall 5-year relative survival = 30%
  - 5-year relative survival: Stage I = 49%, stage IV = 23%

Treatment

- Small T1-2
  - Rare; partial pharyngectomy or radiation
- Larger T2 may be amenable to chemoradiation
- T3, T4a: Laryngopharyngectomy and neck dissection
  - Organ preservation: Chemoradiation is alternative
- T4b: Chemoradiation

DIAGNOSTIC CHECKLIST

Image Interpretation Pearls

- Imaging useful to evaluate for features that might upstage
  - T3: > 4 cm or esophageal invasion
  - T4a: Cartilage or paralaryngeal invasion
  - T4b: Carotid encasement, mediastinal or prevertebral invasion
- PET/CECT best for initial staging

Reporting Tips

- Often difficult scans to read
  - Mass located posterior to glottis/subglottis
  - Mass often invades larynx: Look for cricoid invasion

SELECTED REFERENCES

1. Chen AY et al: Pitfalls in the staging squamous cell carcinoma of the hypopharynx. Neuroimaging Clin N Am. 23(1):67-79, 2013
2. Hall SF et al: TNM-based stage groupings in head and neck cancer: application in cancer of the hypopharynx. Head Neck. 31(1):1-8, 2009

TERMINOLOGY

- Squamous cell carcinoma (SCCa) arising from mucosa of posterior wall of phárynx from hyoid bone to esophageal inlet
  - 15% are hypopharyngeal SCCa

IMAGING

- CECT: Irregular, mildly enhancing mass distending lower hypopharynx
- Often, superficial spread superiorly to oropharynx or inferiorly to esophagus
- May invade posteriorly into prevertebral muscles through prevertebral fascia
- SCCa is reliably FDG avid

TOP DIFFERENTIAL DIAGNOSES

- Postcricoid region SCCa
- Cervical esophageal carcinoma
- Pharyngitis

PATHOLOGY

- Strong association with tobacco and alcohol abuse
- Hypopharyngeal SCCa all use same AJCC TNM staging

CLINICAL ISSUES

- Often asymptomatic until late, stage III-IV
- ≤ 75% have nodes at diagnosis; often bilateral
- Up to 50% present with neck mass from nodes
- Poor prognosis; overall 5-year survival ~ 30%

DIAGNOSTIC CHECKLIST

- Commonly spreads superiorly to oropharynx (T2)
- Look for inferior spread to esophagus (T3)
- May infiltrate prevertebral muscles (T4b)
  - Imaging not accurate for predicting invasion
  - Preservation of retropharyngeal fat excludes this
- Carotid encasement or mediastinal invasion (T4b)

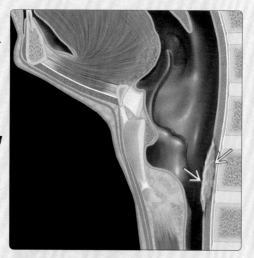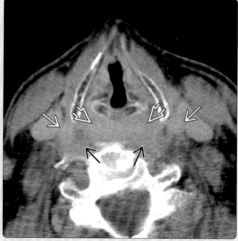

(Left) *Lateral graphic illustrates posterior hypopharyngeal wall SCCa ➡. These tumors often spread superiorly to oropharynx or caudally to esophagus. Invasion of prevertebral muscles designates T4b.* (Right) *Axial CECT at the level of the cricoarytenoid joints shows abnormal soft tissue ➡ posterior to cricoid. The mass has ill-defined margins. Poor definition of the prevertebral muscles ➡ is highly suspicious for invasion, and a tumor abuts both common carotid arteries ➡. This is T4bN1 SCCa.*

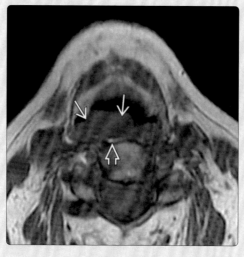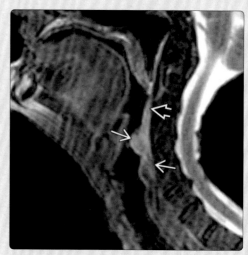

(Left) *Axial T1WI MR in an immunosuppressed woman with bilateral lung transplants shows a lobulated mass ➡ arising from the posterior pharyngeal wall. Retropharyngeal fat ➡ is not clearly defined; however, MR has limited accuracy in predicting prevertebral invasion.* (Right) *Sagittal T2WI FS MR in same patient shows superficial spreading nature of posterior hypopharyngeal wall SCCa ➡ extending superiorly to oropharynx ➡. Patient was asymptomatic, and lesion was only found on clinical examination. This is T2N1.*

TERMINOLOGY

Definitions

- Squamous cell carcinoma (SCCa) arising from posterior wall mucosa of pharynx from hyoid bone to esophageal inlet
  - Subsite of hypopharynx

IMAGING

General Features

- Best diagnostic clue
  - Irregular, moderately enhancing mass of posterior hypopharyngeal wall extending superiorly to oropharynx posterior wall
- Location
  - Posterior wall of hypopharynx from level of hyoid to inferior border of cricoid cartilage
    - Lateral limits are apex of pyriform sinuses
- Size
  - Variable; typically presents late
- Morphology
  - Irregular infiltrative mass

CT Findings

- CECT
  - Irregular, mildly enhancing mass distending lower hypopharynx
  - Tends to spread superiorly to oropharynx
  - May infiltrate posteriorly into prevertebral muscles

MR Findings

- T1 isointense to muscle, T2 moderately hyperintense
- Mild to moderate contrast enhancement

Nuclear Medicine Findings

- PET/CT
  - SCCa is reliably FDG avid

Imaging Recommendations

- Best imaging tool
  - CECT often best, as patient may not tolerate long MR sequences
  - MR may be helpful if resection planned, to evaluate suspected prevertebral fascia invasion
- Protocol advice
  - T1 MR best for infiltration of retropharyngeal fat
  - T2 helpful for prevertebral muscle invasion

DIFFERENTIAL DIAGNOSIS

Postcricoid Region SCCa

- Arises from anterior wall lower hypopharynx

Cervical Esophageal Carcinoma

- Uncommon tumor but may spread superiorly to hypopharynx

Pharyngitis

- Infection/inflammation often in immunocompromised patients

PATHOLOGY

General Features

- Etiology
  - Strong association with tobacco and alcohol abuse
  - Association with Plummer-Vinson syndrome

Staging, Grading, & Classification

- Uses same American Joint Committee on Cancer TNM (2010) staging as for all hypopharyngeal SCCa

CLINICAL ISSUES

Presentation

- Most common signs/symptoms
  - Dysphagia, sore throat
- Other signs/symptoms
  - Up to 50% present with neck mass from nodes
  - Weight loss, otalgia

Demographics

- Age
  - Peak incidence in 7th decade
- Gender
  - M >> F
- Epidemiology
  - Least common hypopharyngeal site (15%)
    - Pyriform sinus (65%), postcricoid region (20%)

Natural History & Prognosis

- Tendency to present late, stage III-IV
- ≤ 75% have **nodal metastases** at diagnosis
- Nodal drainage often bilateral
  - Levels III, IV, and VI
  - Superior spread to retropharyngeal nodes also
- Distant metastases develop in 20-40%
- **Hypopharyngeal SCCa has poorest prognosis of all H&N SCCa**
  - Overall 5-year survival ~ 30%

Treatment

- Small T1-T2 SCCa: Surgical resection ± radiation therapy (XRT)
- Some T2: ChemoXRT
- T3-T4a: Laryngopharyngectomy ± XRT or organ preservation chemoXRT
- T4b: Palliative chemoXRT

DIAGNOSTIC CHECKLIST

Image Interpretation Pearls

- May infiltrate posteriorly to prevertebral muscles (T4b)
  - Preservation of retropharyngeal fat excludes infiltration
  - Imaging not accurate for muscle invasion
- Look for carotid encasement, mediastinal invasion (both T4b)

SELECTED REFERENCES

1. Canis M et al: Oncologic results of transoral laser microsurgery for squamous cell carcinoma of the posterior pharyngeal wall. Head Neck. 37(2):156-61, 2015
2. Becker M et al: Imaging of the larynx and hypopharynx. Eur J Radiol. 66(3):460-79, 2008

KEY FACTS

TERMINOLOGY

- Mucosal squamous cell carcinoma (SCCa) arising in supraglottic (SG) larynx

IMAGING

- CECT: Enhancing mass arising from mucosa of supraglottis subsite
  - Epiglottis, aryepiglottic fold, or false vocal cord
- Look for preepiglottic & paraglottic space involvement with tumor = T3 disease
- Look for cartilage erosion; describe if inner cortex (T3) or through cartilage (T4)
- Cartilage sclerosis is nonspecific, may be perichondritis from adjacent tumor
- Look carefully for extralaryngeal extension to surrounding soft tissues (T4)
- Nodes frequent; 1st nodal station is level II
- Epiglottis SCCa frequently drains bilaterally

TOP DIFFERENTIAL DIAGNOSES

- Laryngocele
- Gastroesophageal reflux
- Rheumatoid larynx
- Laryngeal sarcoidosis
- Laryngeal adenoid cystic carcinoma

CLINICAL ISSUES

- Sore throat, dysphagia, referred ear pain
- May present with metastatic nodes as neck mass
- Typical patient is > 50-year-old man with history of tobacco & alcohol abuse
- 5-year survival rate = 75% for all SG-SCCa

DIAGNOSTIC CHECKLIST

- Always search for 2nd primary in patient with tobacco/alcohol history

(Left) Coronal graphic shows T4 supraglottic squamous cell carcinoma (SCCa) involving the left false vocal cord and aryepiglottic (AE) fold ➡ with invasion of thyroid cartilage ➡. Only mucosal portion ➡ of the tumor is visible on endoscopy. Submucosal extent and cartilage invasion, which are only seen on imaging, are key to staging. (Right) Axial CECT shows similar findings with invasion of bilateral paraglottic fat ➡ and left AE fold ➡. Tumor bulges through thyroid cartilage notch ➡. Pyriform sinus ➡ is normal.

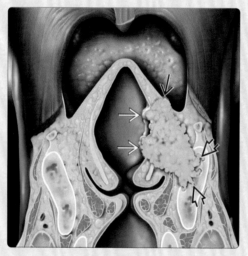
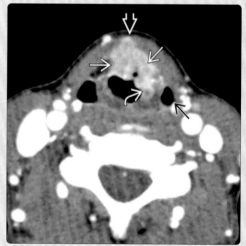

(Left) Axial CECT shows small epiglottic mass ➡, staged as T3 due to preepiglottic space invasion ➡. Mass is symmetric, making it hard to appreciate; however, epiglottis should never be this thick or enhancing. No nodes are evident, but search must be bilateral, especially with epiglottic tumors. (Right) Axial CECT shows small T1 posterior laryngeal SCCa with mass on left AE fold ➡. Left pyriform sinus is collapsed ➡, but no tumor is present in hypopharynx. Endoscopy critical to confirm lack of tumor in pyriform sinus.

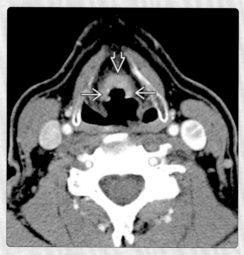
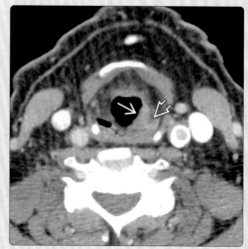

Supraglottic Laryngeal Squamous Cell Carcinoma

TERMINOLOGY

Abbreviations
- Supraglottic squamous cell carcinoma (SG-SCCa)

Synonyms
- SCCa of epiglottis, aryepiglottic (AE) folds, false vocal cords

Definitions
- SCCa originating on mucosa of any part of supraglottic larynx
  - SG subsites: Epiglottis, AE folds, & false cords
  - SG deep spaces: Preepiglottic space (PES) & paraglottic space (PGS)

IMAGING

General Features
- Best diagnostic clue
  - Moderately enhancing, infiltrating mass of epiglottis, AE fold, or false vocal cord, often with associated malignant adenopathy
- Location
  - Any portion of larynx from hyoid to laryngeal ventricle
- Size
  - Variable, larger than glottic or subglottic SCCa in most cases because detected later
- Morphology
  - Moderately enhancing mass invades deep tissues of larynx, including PES ± PGS
  - Advanced tumors: Laryngeal cartilage destruction ± malignant nodes

CT Findings
- CECT
  - Moderately enhancing mass involving epiglottis, AE fold, false vocal cord, PES, ± PGS
  - Epiglottic SCCa: Mass in suprahyoid epiglottis ("free margin") or body of epiglottis
    - Symmetry of bilateral lesion can "hide" lesion
    - PES involvement is clinically occult but denotes T3 stage
  - AE fold SCCa: Posterolateral spread to pyriform sinus (hypopharynx) or anterior to false cord
    - Tumor may extend over superior AE fold to pyriform sinus
  - False cord SCCa: Deep invasion into PGS should be sought
  - **PES spread** allows extension to **anterior commissure** and **true vocal cord (TVC)**
  - **PGS spread** allows **true cord** or **thyroid cartilage** involvement
  - **Extralaryngeal extension** = tumor in soft tissues outside larynx
    - Most often: Through thyrohyoid notch or thyrocricoid ligament
    - Less often: Directly through thyroid cartilage
    - Extralaryngeal extension = **T4a**
    - Generally treated with total laryngectomy
- Bone CT
  - Cartilage sclerosis, erosion, or destruction
    - Sclerosis alone sensitive but low specificity for tumor invasion; often perichondritis
    - Erosion &/or lysis most specific

MR Findings
- T1WI
  - Low- to intermediate-intensity mass
- T2WI
  - Intermediate-intensity soft tissue mass
  - Marked T2-hyperintense cartilage suggests cartilage edema/perichondritis
  - Isointense cartilage SI to tumor suggests invasion
- T1WI C+
  - Homogeneous solid tumor enhancement
  - Cartilage enhancement > tumor: Suggests cartilage invasion less likely
  - Cartilage enhancement = tumor: Suggests cartilage invasion more likely

Nuclear Medicine Findings
- PET/CT
  - Marked FDG uptake in SCCa tumor & nodes
  - Role for PET mainly for nodes and distant mets with advanced T stage, or recurrent tumor

Imaging Recommendations
- Best imaging tool
  - PET/CECT preferred imaging tool in staging SG-SCCa
    - Coronal reformats best delineate craniocaudal spread of SG-SCCa
    - Sagittal plane best delineates PES invasion
  - MR adjunctive when questionable cartilage invasion
- Protocol advice
  - CECT: Axial plane reconstructed at 2.5- to 3-mm slices
  - Wider windows essential to evaluate for cartilage invasion
    - Cartilage invasion/erosion: Erosion of inner cortex only (T3)
    - Cartilage penetration: Tumor through full thickness (T4)

DIFFERENTIAL DIAGNOSIS

Laryngocele
- Cystic mass in either paraglottic (internal or simple) or extralaryngeal space (external or mixed)
- Secondary laryngocele: Glottic or SG-SCCa obstructs laryngeal ventricle

Gastroesophageal Reflux
- Reversible edematous changes of posterior larynx, including AE folds and often TVC

Rheumatoid Larynx
- Cricoarytenoid swelling with history of rheumatoid arthritis

Laryngeal Sarcoidosis
- Glottic and SG thickening, usually without discrete laryngeal mass

Laryngeal Adenoid Cystic Carcinoma
- Very rare submucosal mass of larynx
- Mimics SG-SCCa but is less likely to invade cartilage

PATHOLOGY

General Features

- Etiology
  - Tobacco ± alcohol abuse
  - Larynx is divided embryologically into 2 parts
    - Supraglottis: Vascular & lymphatic rich
    - Glottis-subglottis: Vascular & lymphatic poor
- Genetics
  - Allelic loss or loss of heterozygosity (8p) frequent in H&N SCCa
  - SG-SCCa: Loss in p23 region of chromosome 8 is independent predictor of poor prognosis
  - HER2/neu (ERBB2) oncogene expression & positive nodes associated with distant metastasis

Staging, Grading, & Classification

- American Joint Committee on Cancer (AJCC) staging forms (2010)
- Accurate staging requires knowledge of true vocal cord (TVC) function, clinical & endoscopic finding
  - T1: Tumor in 1 supraglottic subsite with normal TVC mobility
  - T2: Tumor invading mucosa in > 1 supraglottic subsite without laryngeal fixation
    - Extension to mucosa of base of tongue, vallecula, medial wall of pyriform sinus = T2 lesion
  - T3: Endolaryngeal tumor with fixed TVC ± invasion of PES, PGS, postcricoid hypopharynx, or inner cortex of thyroid cartilage
  - T4a: Tumor invades through thyroid cartilage ± to other extralaryngeal tissues
    - e.g., trachea, cervical soft tissues, strap muscles, thyroid gland, esophagus
  - T4b: Tumor invades prevertebral space, encases carotid artery, or invades mediastinal structures

Gross Pathologic & Surgical Features

- Poorly marginated, ulcerative, &/or indurated mucosal lesion

Microscopic Features

- Usually nonkeratinizing, moderately or poorly differentiated SCCa
- Squamous differentiation with intracellular bridges or keratinization

CLINICAL ISSUES

Presentation

- Most common signs/symptoms
  - Sore throat, dysphagia, referred ear pain
  - May present as neck mass = metastatic nodal disease
- Other signs/symptoms
  - Hoarseness, aspiration if TVC involved
- Clinical profile
  - Male > 50 years of age with history of alcohol & tobacco use

Demographics

- Age
  - Usually over 50 years of age
- Gender
  - M:F = 9:1
- Epidemiology
  - 2.5% of all cancers in men; 0.5% in women
  - > 95% of malignant larynx tumors are SCCa
  - 30% of all laryngeal SCCa are supraglottic

Natural History & Prognosis

- Presents late with nodes, as SG itself is clinically silent
  - 35% have nodal metastases at presentation
  - **Level II** is most common 1st drainage site
  - Epiglottis, a midline structure, frequently drains bilaterally
- 5-year survival rate = 75% for all SG-SCCa
- Prognosis best for inferiorly located tumors
  - Involves TVC, thus presents early with hoarseness

Treatment

- **T1/T2** (smaller tumors): Laser surgery or XRT only
- **T3**: Small proportion may have laser resection or partial laryngectomy
- **T3/T4a** (larger tumors): XRT & chemotherapy
- **T4a**: Extralaryngeal extension or through thyroid cartilage = total laryngectomy
- **T4b**: Palliative nonsurgical treatment

DIAGNOSTIC CHECKLIST

Consider

- Combined endoscopic and imaging information needed for accurate stage
- **Always search for 2nd primary in patient with tobacco/alcohol history**

Image Interpretation Pearls

- Cartilage sclerosis nonspecific: Perichondritis or true cartilage invasion
  - T2 & T1 C+ MR best to confirm cartilage penetration
- SG larynx lymphatic-rich → frequent metastatic nodes
- Nodal metastases prevalence increases with T stage

Reporting Tips

- Describe: Bulk of tumor in SG larynx, but report full extent of mass
- Describe: Status of cartilage
  - Is cartilage normal?
  - Has tumor eroded inner cortex?
  - Is cartilage completely penetrated?
- Describe: Extralaryngeal tumor essential to report

SELECTED REFERENCES

1. Gómez Serrano M et al: Cartilage invasion patterns in laryngeal cancer. Eur Arch Otorhinolaryngol. 273(7):1863-9, 2016
2. Mor N et al: Functional anatomy and oncologic barriers of the larynx. Otolaryngol Clin North Am. 48(4):533-45, 2015
3. Hartl DM et al: CT-scan prediction of thyroid cartilage invasion for early laryngeal squamous cell carcinoma. Eur Arch Otorhinolaryngol. 270(1):287-91, 2013
4. Gilbert K et al: Staging of laryngeal cancer using 64-channel multidetector row CT: comparison of standard neck CT with dedicated breath-maneuver laryngeal CT. AJNR Am J Neuroradiol. 31(2):251-6, 2010
5. Becker M et al: Neoplastic invasion of laryngeal cartilage: reassessment of criteria for diagnosis at MR imaging. Radiology. 249(2):551-9, 2008

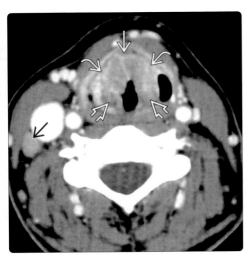

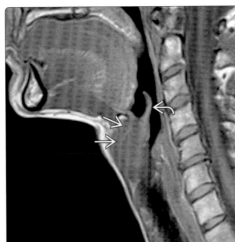

(Left) Axial CECT shows a large, bulky supraglottic SCCa that fills both paraglottic spaces ⇉, crosses at midline →, and involves both aryepiglottic folds ⇉. Note airway compromise and metastatic level III node on right ⇶. (Right) Sagittal T1WI MR shows a bulky supraglottic SCCa filling preepiglottic space ⇉ and replacing fat, but sparing the suprahyoid epiglottis ⇉. Sagittal MR or CECT reformations nicely show involvement of preepiglottic fat, which denotes at least T3 disease.

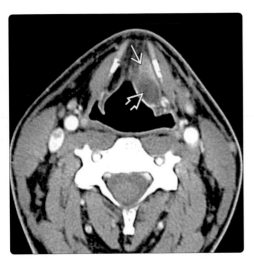

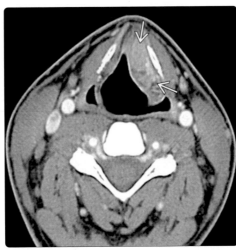

(Left) Axial CECT shows a mixed-density supraglottic mass distending paraglottic fat. The nonenhancing mucoid density portion of mass ⇉ is due to an internal laryngocele that developed from an obstruction of laryngeal ventricle by tumor ⇉. (Right) Axial CECT in the same patient, just inferior to previous image, shows SCCa involving entire paraglottic space ⇉. Thyroid ala is sclerotic but not destroyed. Left infrahyoid strap muscles are normal, without evidence of extralaryngeal spread. This is a T3 tumor.

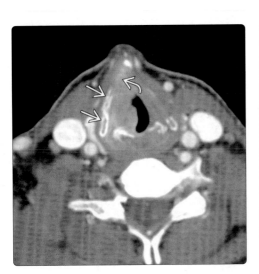

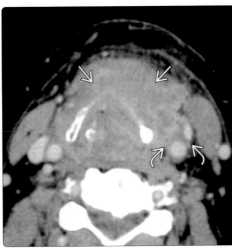

(Left) Axial CECT shows a large right false cord SCCa. Thyroid cartilage is sclerotic →, a nonspecific finding that cannot accurately predict cartilage invasion. Tumor penetration through inner & outer cortex is present anteriorly ⇉. This is a T4a tumor. (Right) Axial CECT shows a large T4a supraglottic SCCa with complete airway obstruction. The tumor has extended through thyroid cartilage, and bulky extralaryngeal SCCa invades strap muscles ⇉. Note the close proximity to the carotid sheath ⇉.

KEY FACTS

TERMINOLOGY

- Squamous cell carcinoma (SCCa) arising on mucosal surface of glottic larynx
- Vocal cord, anterior and posterior commissures

IMAGING

- Typically, diagnosis known at time of imaging
  - Imaging important to assess supra- or subglottic extension, cartilage invasion, nodes
- CECT/MR findings may be subtle if small tumor
- SCCa typically anterior true vocal cord &/or anterior commissure
- Metastatic nodes uncommon, typically late
- CECT: Enhancing infiltrative or exophytic mass
- CECT has fewer motion artifacts than MR; obtain during quiet respiration to best assess cords
- MR has adjunctive role for cartilage invasion if CECT not definitive
- FDG avid on PET; reserved for late-stage tumors

TOP DIFFERENTIAL DIAGNOSES

- Gastroesophageal reflux disease
- Laryngeal chondrosarcoma
- Rheumatoid larynx
- Laryngeal adenoid cystic carcinoma

PATHOLOGY

- Strongly associated with tobacco & alcohol abuse
- Keratinizing well- to moderately differentiated SCCa

CLINICAL ISSUES

- Much more common in male patients; usually > 50 years
- Often presents early with low T stage because of symptoms of hoarseness or change in voice
- T1: XRT or laser surgery; > 90% 5-year survival
- T4: Laryngectomy; 30-60% 5-year survival rate

(Left) Axial CECT shows an enhancing right TVC exophytic mass ➡. Anterior and posterior commissures are normal. Right arytenoid cartilage sclerosis ➡ is nonspecific, may be either perichondritis from edema or tumor invasion. Diagnosis was T1a tumor. (Right) Axial CECT reveals SCCa involving the entire left true TVC, anterior commissure ➡, and anterior 1/3 of right cord ➡. Left arytenoid ➡ and thyroid cartilages are sclerotic but without destruction or cartilage penetration. This is T1b tumor by imaging.

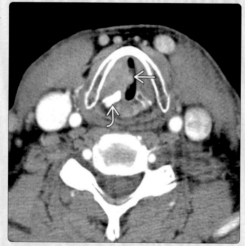
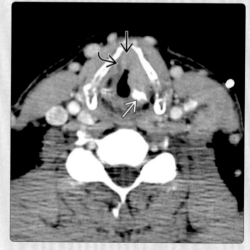

(Left) Axial CECT shows bulky, ulcerated anterior SCCa involving both vocal cords and anterior commissure ➡. Both anterior thyroid cartilages are sclerotic with erosion of inner cortex ➡, upstaging tumor to T3. (Right) Axial T1WI C+ FS MR in a patient previously treated for right TVC SCCa and biopsy-proven recurrence shows an enhancing tumor involving the right cricoid cartilage ➡, penetrating through thyroid cartilage ➡ to the right strap muscles ➡. Diagnosis was T4a tumor.

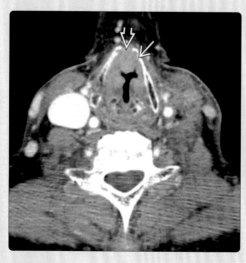
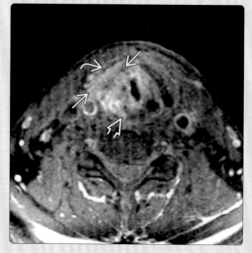

Glottic Laryngeal Squamous Cell Carcinoma

TERMINOLOGY

Abbreviations
- Glottic squamous cell carcinoma (G-SCCa)

Definitions
- SCCa arising on mucosal surface of glottic larynx
  - Vocal cord, anterior and posterior commissures

IMAGING

General Features
- Best diagnostic clue
  - Enhancing irregular true vocal cord (TVC)
- Location
  - Most often anterior TVC and anterior commissure

CT Findings
- CECT
  - Enhancing infiltrative or exophytic TVC mass
  - Imaging findings may be very subtle if small tumor
  - Metastatic nodes uncommon, typically late with large tumor

MR Findings
- T1WI
  - Low- to intermediate-intensity TVC mass
- T2WI
  - Intermediate-intensity TVC mass
- T1WI C+
  - Homogeneous enhancement

Nuclear Medicine Findings
- PET
  - Rarely obtained for G-SCCa, as nodal metastases unusual

Imaging Recommendations
- Best imaging tool
  - CECT obtained with quiet breathing has fewer motion artifacts than MR
  - MR has adjunctive role for cartilage invasion
- Protocol advice
  - CECT should be obtained during quiet respiration
  - < 1-mm slices allow coronal reformations
    - Supraglottic spread: Across laryngeal ventricle
    - Subglottic spread: > 1 cm below TVC

DIFFERENTIAL DIAGNOSIS

Gastroesophageal Reflux Disease
- Vocal cords edematous with mucosal enhancement

Rheumatoid Larynx
- Cricoarytenoid joint swelling

Laryngeal Chondrosarcoma
- T2-hyperintense submucosal mass of thyroid or cricoid cartilage

Laryngeal Adenoid Cystic Carcinoma
- Typically submucosal and more hyperintense on T2

PATHOLOGY

General Features
- Etiology
  - Strongly associated with tobacco & alcohol abuse

Staging, Grading, & Classification
- American Joint Committee on Cancer (AJCC) 2010
  - **T1**: Limited to cord(s) or commissures, with normal cord mobility
    - **T1a**: Tumor limited to 1 cord
    - **T1b**: Tumor involves both cords
  - **T2**: Supra- ± subglottic spread &/or impaired cord mobility
  - **T3**: Fixed vocal cord &/or paraglottic space invasion ± inner thyroid cartilage erosion
  - **T4a**: Tumor through outer cortex of thyroid cartilage ± extralaryngeal extension
  - **T4b**: Invades prevertebral muscles, encases carotid artery, or invades mediastinal soft tissues

CLINICAL ISSUES

Presentation
- Most common signs/symptoms
  - Typically presents with hoarseness, change in voice

Demographics
- Age
  - Patients typically > 50 years old
- Gender
  - M:F = 9:1
- Epidemiology
  - 60% of laryngeal SCCa are glottic tumors

Natural History & Prognosis
- Anterior cords are dense, avascular fibroelastic tissue without lymphatics
  - **Therefore nodal spread uncommon, late**
- Prognosis generally good for early tumors
  - T1: > 90% 5-year survival rate
  - T4: 30-60% 5-year survival rate

Treatment
- Small T1 tumors: Laser surgery or XRT alone
- Higher stage, larger tumor: Combination of XRT and partial or total laryngectomy

DIAGNOSTIC CHECKLIST

Consider
- Typically, diagnosis is known at time of imaging
- CECT to assess for supra or subglottic extension, cartilage involvement or nodal spread
- MR helpful to clarify cartilage penetration

Image Interpretation Pearls
- If anterior commissure > 1 mm thick, then likely involved with tumor

SELECTED REFERENCES

1. Wang CC et al: Transoral robotic surgery for early glottic carcinoma involving anterior commissure: preliminary reports. Head Neck. 38(6):913-8, 2016

KEY FACTS

TERMINOLOGY

- Mucosal squamous cell carcinoma (SCCa) originating from subglottic larynx
  - Inferior aspect of true vocal cord (TVC) to inferior cricoid cartilage

IMAGING

- Enhancing mass internal to cricoid ring that fills lumen or invades extralaryngeal tissues
- Local tumor spread patterns
  - May spread superiorly to TVC(s)
  - Cricoid cartilage invasion common (T4)
- Nodal metastases: Uncommon (20%) except for advanced stage
- 50% present as T4 tumor
- Thin-section CECT: Best shows tumor extent
  - Coronal reformats helpful for craniocaudal tumor
- MR: Intermediate T2, enhances with gadolinium
  - If cartilage signal = tumor signal, suggests invasion

- PET/CT: FDG-avid tumor and nodes

TOP DIFFERENTIAL DIAGNOSES

- Glottic larynx SCCa
- Larynx trauma
- Larynx adenoid cystic carcinoma
- Larynx chondrosarcoma
- Rheumatoid larynx

CLINICAL ISSUES

- < 5% of laryngeal SCCa are subglottic
- > 50-year-old male smoker &/or drinker
- Stridor, dyspnea, hoarseness if TVC involved
- Subglottic SCCa has long asymptomatic period
- Overall 5-year survival: 50%

DIAGNOSTIC CHECKLIST

- **Imaging critical**: Clinical & endoscopic staging more difficult than glottic or supraglottic SCCa

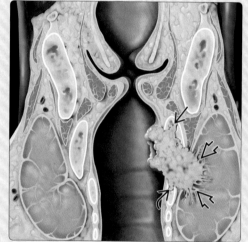
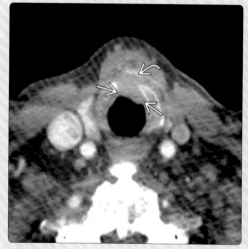

(Left) Coronal graphic depicts left subglottic SCCa tumor invading cricoid ➡, 1st tracheal ring ➡, and thyroid gland ➡. This is an AJCC stage T4a SCCa tumor. (Right) Axial CECT demonstrates typical subglottic SCCa ➡ in anterior subglottis. Note midline cricoid cartilage destruction with definite extralaryngeal extension into infrahyoid strap muscles ➡, designating T4a tumor. This is the most common pattern of extension. No soft tissue should be present between cartilage inner table and airway.

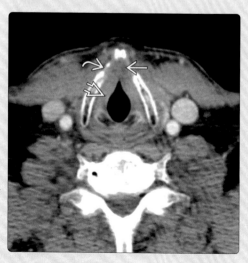
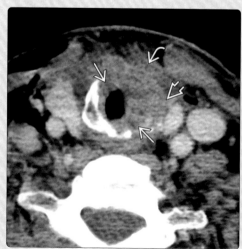

(Left) Axial CECT immediately below true vocal cord (TVC) ➡ reveals extremely subtle, symmetric, minimally enhancing subglottic SCCa ➡ in anterior airway. Image is below TVC, as arytenoid cartilages are not present. There is subtle erosion and sclerosis of right thyroid cartilage ➡. One must know if TVC mobility is normal to stage this tumor. (Right) Axial CECT of a T4a tumor shows a large mass destroying much of the cricoid cartilage ➡, with extralaryngeal spread ➡ and thyroid gland invasion ➡.

Subglottic Laryngeal Squamous Cell Carcinoma

TERMINOLOGY

Abbreviations

- Squamous cell carcinoma (SCCa)

Definitions

- Mucosal SCCa originating from subglottic larynx
- Inferior aspect of true vocal cord (TVC) to lower border of cricoid cartilage

IMAGING

General Features

- Best diagnostic clue
  - Enhancing mucosal mass narrows subglottic lumen
- Morphology
  - Bulky, intraluminal mass or infiltrative, focal mass invading cricoid cartilage

CT Findings

- CECT
  - Enhancing luminal mass; may spread to TVC
  - Cricoid cartilage invasion common
  - Nodes unusual due to limited lymphatic drainage
    - Pretracheal & paratracheal nodes most often

MR Findings

- T1WI
  - Low to intermediate signal intensity
- T2WI
  - Intermediate signal intensity
  - If cartilage signal = tumor signal, suggests invasion
- T1WI C+ FS
  - Usually homogeneous enhancement
  - If cartilage enhancement = tumor enhancement, indicates tumor invasion

Nuclear Medicine Findings

- PET
  - As with all SCCa, tumor is FDG avid

Imaging Recommendations

- Best imaging tool
  - CECT preferred because of motion on MR
  - MR more accurate for detection of cartilage invasion
- Protocol advice
  - Thin-section CECT best shows tumor extent
    - Coronal reformats helpful for craniocaudal tumor

DIFFERENTIAL DIAGNOSIS

Glottic Larynx SCCa

- Subglottic spread of glottic primary is difficult to distinguish from primary subglottic SCCa

Larynx Trauma

- Edema and hemorrhage around fractures

Larynx Adenoid Cystic Carcinoma

- Typically submucosal, T2 hyperintense, less locally aggressive

Larynx Chondrosarcoma

- Tumor centered in cartilage, chondroid calcifications

- T2-hyperintense submucosal mass on MR

Rheumatoid Larynx

- Cricoarytenoid and subglottic swelling in patient with rheumatoid arthritis

PATHOLOGY

General Features

- Etiology
  - Tobacco &/or alcohol abuse

Staging, Grading, & Classification

- American Joint Committee on Cancer (AJCC) 7th edition staging forms (2010)
- T stage
  - T1: Tumor limited to subglottis
  - T2: Tumor to TVC with normal or impaired mobility
  - T3: Tumor limited to larynx with fixed TVC
  - T4a: Tumor invades cricoid or thyroid cartilage ± invasion of extralaryngeal tissues
  - T4b: Tumor invades prevertebral space, encases carotid artery, or invades mediastinum

Gross Pathologic & Surgical Features

- Glottis & subglottis embryologically distinct from supraglottic larynx
  - Nodes & metastases occur late in disease course

CLINICAL ISSUES

Presentation

- Most common signs/symptoms
  - Stridor, dyspnea, hoarseness if TVC involved

Demographics

- Age
  - Typically > 50 years old
- Gender
  - M >> F
- Epidemiology
  - < 5% of laryngeal SCCa are subglottic

Natural History & Prognosis

- Subglottic SCCa has long asymptomatic period
  - 50% present as T4 tumor
- Overall 5-year survival: 50%

Treatment

- Large tumors (T4) require total laryngectomy + XRT
- Primary radiotherapy may allow laryngeal conservation
- Subglottic stomal recurrences common
  - Probably from unusual lymphatic spread to paratracheal nodes

DIAGNOSTIC CHECKLIST

Image Interpretation Pearls

- Any tissue internal to cricoid ring should be viewed as possible tumor

SELECTED REFERENCES

1. Marchiano E et al: Subglottic squamous cell carcinoma: a population-based study of 889 cases. Otolaryngol Head Neck Surg. 154(2):315-21, 2016

TERMINOLOGY

- Secondary laryngocele: Lesion obstructs laryngeal ventricle causing internal or mixed laryngocele
- Squamous cell carcinoma (SCCa) is most common cause of secondary laryngocele

IMAGING

- CECT with coronal reformats
  o Thin-walled air- or fluid-filled internal or mixed laryngocele with glottic &/or supraglottic soft tissue mass
  o Obstructing SCCa: Enhancing, infiltrative glottic or low supraglottic mass in area of ventricle
  o Paraglottic laryngocele extends to margin of SCCa
  o Internal laryngocele: Thin-walled fluid or air density paraglottic space cyst
  o Mixed laryngocele: Paraglottic cyst passes through thyrohyoid membrane into submandibular space

TOP DIFFERENTIAL DIAGNOSES

- Primary laryngocele
- 2nd branchial cleft cyst
- Thyroglossal duct cyst

PATHOLOGY

- Lesion obstructs laryngeal ventricle with consequent internal or mixed laryngocele
  o Laryngeal SCCa > > inflammation > trauma
  o 15% of all laryngoceles

CLINICAL ISSUES

- SCCa: Hoarseness, stridor from fixation of vocal cord

DIAGNOSTIC CHECKLIST

- If laryngocele is found in smoker, search for laryngeal SCCa in area of laryngeal ventricle
- Stage primary SCCa as if laryngocele not present

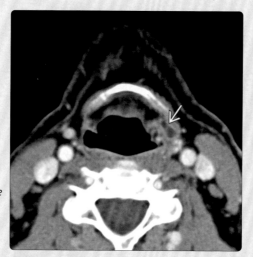
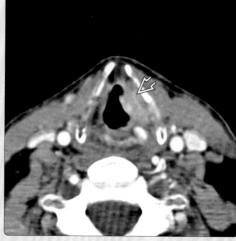

(Left) Axial CECT reveals a small, left-sided, secondary internal laryngocele ➡ in the high left paraglottic space. (Right) Axial CECT at the level of the glottis reveals an enhancing, infiltrative squamous cell carcinoma (SCCa) involving the left true vocal cord ➡. The endoscopic assessment suggests the tumor involves the superior false vocal cord, but the CECT demonstrated that a secondary internal laryngocele caused the submucosal mass effect in this area.

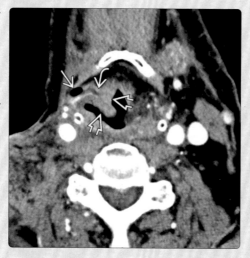
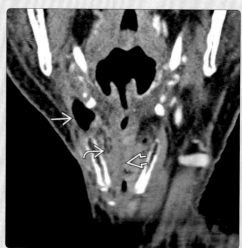

(Left) Axial CECT shows an air-filled mixed secondary laryngocele ➡ with a fluid-filled stalk ➡ obstructed by a supraglottic enhancing SCCa ➡. The SCCa in this image involves the false cord and enlarges the aryepiglottic fold. (Right) Coronal CECT in the same patient reveals the air-filled external secondary laryngocele ➡, the fluid-filled tubular saccule ➡, and supraglottic and glottic SCCa ➡. Remember to search for a laryngeal SCCa in all adults where CECT reveals a laryngocele.

Laryngeal Squamous Cell Carcinoma With Secondary Laryngocele

TERMINOLOGY

Abbreviations

- Squamous cell carcinoma (SCCa)

Definitions

- **Secondary laryngocele**: Obstruction of laryngeal ventricle causes internal or mixed laryngocele
  - Most common obstructing lesion: Laryngeal SCCa
- **Internal laryngocele**: Dilated air or fluid-filled laryngeal saccule within paraglottic space
- **Mixed laryngocele**: Paraglottic space internal laryngocele extends through thyrohyoid membrane into low submandibular space (SMS)
- **Pyolaryngocele**: Secondary infection of any laryngocele

IMAGING

General Features

- Best diagnostic clue
  - Thin-walled air- or fluid-filled internal or mixed laryngocele with ipsilateral glottic &/or supraglottic soft tissue mass (SCCa)
- Location
  - Causal SCCa: Glottis or low supraglottis lesion involving laryngeal ventricle

Radiographic Findings

- Radiography
  - Air pocket seen in upper cervical soft tissues

CT Findings

- CECT
  - Obstructing SCCa: Enhancing, infiltrative glottic, or low supraglottic mass
    - Involves area of laryngeal ventricle
    - Paraglottic laryngocele extends to margin of SCCa
  - Secondary laryngocele
    - Internal laryngocele: Thin-walled fluid- or air-density paraglottic space cystic mass
    - Mixed laryngocele: Paraglottic cyst passes through thyrohyoid membrane into SMS

MR Findings

- T2WI
  - Obstructing SCCa: Intermediate signal, infiltrative glottic &/or low supraglottic mass
  - Secondary laryngocele: High signal paraglottic space lesion ± SMS extension (mixed laryngocele)
- T1WI C+
  - Obstructing SCCa: Enhancing, infiltrative glottic &/or low supraglottic mass involving laryngeal ventricle
  - Secondary laryngocele: Rim enhancing only

Imaging Recommendations

- Best imaging tool
  - CECT often gives least motion-degraded images

DIFFERENTIAL DIAGNOSIS

Primary Laryngocele

- Laryngocele without obstructing lesion found

Thyroglossal Duct Cyst

- Midline cystic lesion embedded in infrahyoid strap muscles
- May project in midline to preepiglottic space

2nd Branchial Cleft Cyst

- Cystic lesion posterior to submandibular gland at angle of mandible
- No connection to larynx

PATHOLOGY

General Features

- Etiology
  - Lesion obstructs laryngeal ventricle with consequent internal or mixed laryngocele
    - Laryngeal SCCa > > inflammation > trauma
    - 15% of all laryngoceles

Microscopic Features

- Laryngocele: Lined by respiratory epithelium (ciliated, columnar) with fibrous wall

CLINICAL ISSUES

Presentation

- Most common signs/symptoms
  - SCCa: Hoarseness, stridor from fixation of vocal cord
- Other signs/symptoms
  - Laryngocele: Laryngoscopy shows submucosal supraglottic mass
    - SCCa may be difficult to see
  - Mixed laryngocele: Anterior neck mass at hyoid bone level

Natural History & Prognosis

- Laryngocele will continue to grow slowly until SCCa treated

Treatment

- Successful treatment of SCCa may or may not treat secondary laryngocele

DIAGNOSTIC CHECKLIST

Image Interpretation Pearls

- If laryngocele is found in smoker, search for laryngeal SCCa in area of laryngeal ventricle
- Stage obstructing SCCa primary tumor as if laryngocele not present
- Define secondary laryngocele as internal or mixed

SELECTED REFERENCES

1. Akdogan O et al: The association of laryngoceles with squamous cell carcinoma of the larynx presenting as a deep neck infection. B-ENT. 3(4):209-11, 2007
2. Akbas Y et al: Asymptomatic bilateral mixed-type laryngocele and laryngeal carcinoma. Eur Arch Otorhinolaryngol. 261(6):307-9, 2004
3. Harney M et al: Laryngocele and squamous cell carcinoma of the larynx. J Laryngol Otol. 115(7):590-2, 2001
4. Harvey RT et al: Radiologic findings in a carcinoma-associated laryngocele. Ann Otol Rhinol Laryngol. 105(5):405-8, 1996
5. Celin SE et al: The association of laryngoceles with squamous cell carcinoma of the larynx. Laryngoscope. 101(5):529-36, 1991
6. Close LG et al: Asymptomatic laryngocele: incidence and association with laryngeal cancer. Ann Otol Rhinol Laryngol. 96(4):393-9, 1987

TERMINOLOGY

- Perineural tumor (PNT)
- Malignant tumor spread along sheath of large nerves distant from 1° site

IMAGING

- Most often found along CNV branches & CNVII
- MR more sensitive than CECT for PNT
- CECT: May be extremely subtle
  - Enlarged nerve, ± mild enhancement
  - Smoothly widened foramina or canals
  - Muscular denervation atrophy (typically masticator from CNV3 PNT)
- MR: Nerve enlarged & enhancing, loss of normal fat signal along course of nerves
  - T1WI without fat saturation is mainstay of diagnosis, with contrast necessary for intracranial PNT

TOP DIFFERENTIAL DIAGNOSES

- Schwannoma
- Neurofibroma
- Skull base meningioma
- Invasive fungal sinusitis
- Lymphoma

PATHOLOGY

- Neurotropic tumors
  - Adenoid cystic, squamous cell carcinoma, melanoma, lymphoma
  - Skin, parotid, palate, nasopharynx
- Detection is critical for treatment planning (surgery &/or radiation)

DIAGNOSTIC CHECKLIST

- Examine nerve(s) at risk from end organ to nucleus
- PNT may spread anterograde & retrograde, may have skip lesions, and may cross between nerves

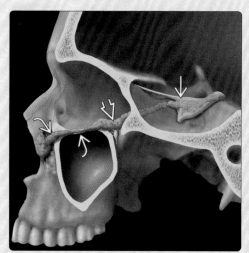 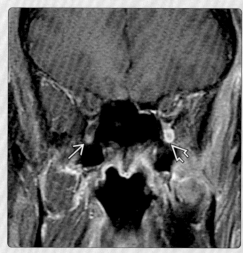

(Left) Sagittal graphic illustrates the classic appearance of perineural tumor (PNT) spread from cheek malignancy. Tumor gains access to infraorbital nerve ➔ and spreads retrograde to pterygopalatine fossa (PPF) ➔, foramen rotundum, and into Meckel cave, involving gasserian ganglion ➔. (Right) Coronal T1WI C+ FS MR in patient with left maxillary SCCa shows dramatic enlargement and enhancement of left CNV2 within the foramen rotundum ➔. Normal right CNV2 is shown for comparison ➔.

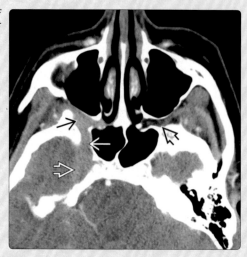 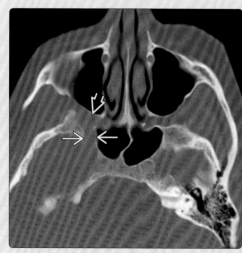

(Left) Axial CECT shows loss of normal fat density in right PPF ➔ as compared to the normal contralateral PPF containing fat and vessels ➔. Soft tissue density fills the right PPF, and there is widening of the right foramen rotundum ➔ and fullness of the right cavernous sinus and Meckel cave ➔ as tumor spreads retrograde. (Right) Axial bone CT in the same patient demonstrates smooth widening of the right foramen rotundum ➔ and PPF ➔. Findings are typical for extracranial and intracranial PNT along CNV2.

Perineural Tumor Spread

TERMINOLOGY

Abbreviations

- Perineural tumor spread (PNT)

Definitions

- Malignant tumor spread along sheath of large nerves distant from 1° site
  - Epineurium & perineurium involved more than endoneurium

IMAGING

General Features

- Best diagnostic clue
  - Abnormal enlargement & enhancement of nerves
  - Widening of associated neural foramen or canal
  - Muscular denervation atrophy
    - Masticator muscles (CNV3) > muscles of facial expression (CNVII)
- Location
  - Intracranial and extracranial
  - CNV and CNVII most frequently involved
    - Maxillary (CNV2) > mandibular (CNV3) > > ophthalmic (CNV1)
- Morphology
  - Tubular enlargement of affected nerve
    - Radiographic **skip areas** possible

CT Findings

- CECT
  - CT shows extracranial > > intracranial PNT
    - Enlarged nerve, ± mild enhancement
    - Abnormal soft tissue density at foramina, canals
    - Effacement of fat within pterygopalatine fossa (PPF), below skull base or in premaxillary region
    - Denervation of supplied musculature ranging from acute swelling/enhancement to chronic fatty atrophy
    - Convex, enhancing cavernous sinus
- Bone CT
  - Smoothly widened foramina or canals

MR Findings

- T1WI
  - **Enlarged nerve** replaces high-signal fat
    - Within canals and foramina
    - Along extracranial course of CN with obliteration of fat pads
      - Beneath foramen ovale or medial to mandibular foramen (CNV3)
      - PPF or premaxillary fat (CNV2)
      - Superomedial orbit (CNV1)
      - Beneath stylomastoid foramen (CNVII)
  - High T1WI in chronically denervated muscles, most obvious in masticator space (CNV3)
- T2WI
  - Tumor replaces normal high signal CSF in Meckel cave (CNV)
  - High T2WI in acute/subacute muscular denervation
- T1WI C+ FS
  - Abnormal enlargement & enhancement of involved nerve
  - Denervated muscles: Enhance in acute/subacute phase

Nuclear Medicine Findings

- PET/CT
  - Rarely detects PNT
    - Small volume of tumor along nerve not classically FDG avid [e.g., adenoid cystic carcinoma (ACCa)]

Imaging Recommendations

- Best imaging tool
  - MR more sensitive than CECT for PNT
  - If only CECT available, carefully evaluate foramina, fat planes, muscles, & cavernous sinus
- Protocol advice
  - T1WI without fat saturation is mainstay of diagnosis
    - T1WI C+ FS helpful for extracranial tumor
      - Susceptibility artifact can obscure PNT at skull base foramen: CNV2, CNV3, & vidian nerve
    - T1WI C+ important for intracranial PNT
  - Scan must include entire nerve from nucleus → end organ

DIFFERENTIAL DIAGNOSIS

Schwannoma

- Tubular, fusiform, lobular mass following nerve
- T2 hyperintense; heterogeneously T1 C+ enhancing
- Larger dimension than perineural tumor

Neurofibroma

- Tubular mass along nerve or plexiform morphology
- T2 shows central target sign
- Homogeneously enhancing

Invasive Fungal Sinusitis

- Infiltrating diffuse disease in face, not exclusively along nerves
- Immunocompromised patients, including diabetics

Skull Base Meningioma

- Homogeneously enhancing dural-based mass ± dural tail
- May extend into neural &/or jugular foramen

Lymphoma

- No cutaneous or mucosal primary lesion as source of PNT

Sarcoidosis

- Dural-based inflammation; may involve cranial nerves
- Typically starts in sinus, mimics PNT

PATHOLOGY

General Features

- Etiology
  - Many H&N cancers have PNT tendency: Mucosal, skin, salivary origin
  - **Neurotropic tumors**
    - ACCa: Minor or major salivary gland
    - Squamous cell carcinoma (SCCa): Mucosal or skin
    - Desmoplastic melanoma
    - Non-Hodgkin lymphoma
  - Primary sites most at risk for PNT
    - Skin: CNV

- Parotid: CNVII
- Hard palate (HP): CNV2
- Nasopharynx: CNV-XII
  - Spread direction: **Retrograde** (toward CNS: Nerve main trunk/brainstem) > > **antegrade** (away from CNS)
  - Most common pathways of PNT spread include
    - **CNV2: Maxillary division** → PPF
      - □ **Infraorbital nerve**: Cheek or maxillary sinus tumors
      - □ **Greater & lesser palatine nerves**: HP minor salivary cancer
    - **CNV3: Mandibular division** → foramen ovale → Meckel cave
      - □ **Mental nerve**: Lip or cutaneous SCCa
      - □ **Inferior alveolar nerve**: Mucosal oral cavity SCCa
      - □ **Auriculotemporal nerve (ATN)**: Branch of CNV3: Enters parotid, & its anterior & posterior communicating rami interface with CNVII
      - □ **Mandibular main trunk**: Masticator space 1° or 2° malignancy
    - **CNV1: Ophthalmic division** → cavernous sinus
      - □ Rare; most often forehead SCCa, melanoma
    - **CNVII: Facial nerve**
      - □ **Intraparotid branches** → intratemporal CNVII → internal auditory canal
      - □ **Greater superficial petrosal nerve (GSPN)**: From geniculate ganglion, joins deep petrosal nerve at foramen lacerum → vidian nerve → PPF
    - **Direct through sphenopalatine foramen** → PPF
      - □ Nasopharynx cancer, nasal malignancies
    - **From PPF, tumor may access multiple sites**
      - □ Through inferior orbital fissure to orbital apex
      - □ Along vidian canal to CNVII geniculate ganglion
      - □ Foramen rotundum → cavernous sinus or to Meckel cave
- Associated features
  - GSPN & ATN = central & peripheral connections between CNV & CNVII: Providing important conduits for PNT between nerves
  - CNV3 supplies muscles of mastication + anterior belly of digastric & mylohyoid muscles
  - CNVII supplies muscles of facial expression + posterior belly of digastric muscle

Gross Pathologic & Surgical Features

- PNT first grows along nerve sheath then invades nerve
- ACCa: Highest propensity for PNT; SCCa most common source since most common H&N tumor

Microscopic Features

- Extension of tumor along nerve via epineurium/perineurium distant from primary site
- Perineural invasion (PNI) not = PNT
  - PNI is microscopic finding of direct nerve invasion at 1° site
- Immunohistochemical markers associated with PNT
  - Presence of growth factor receptor p75
    - Abundant in desmoplastic melanoma, maybe ACCa
- Nerve microenvironment (Schwann cells & macrophages): "Crosstalk" with tumor

CLINICAL ISSUES

Presentation

- Most common signs/symptoms
  - Commonly asymptomatic but with imaging findings
  - CNV: Pain, paresthesia
    - CNV3: Weakness from denervation atrophy of muscles of mastication
    - ATN: Preauricular pain & otalgia
  - CNVII: Facial weakness or paralysis
  - May be confused with "trigeminal neuralgia" & "Bell palsy"
    - High index of suspicion if primary cancer history

Natural History & Prognosis

- PNT = poor prognostic sign indicating increased incidence of local recurrence
  - ACCa has tendency for late recurrence, so long-term follow-up recommended

Treatment

- Surgery combined with postoperative RT ± chemo
- With PNT, entire course of nerve must be radiated
- Presence of PNT may preclude primary surgical therapy
  - 1° RT with neutron or proton beam may be indicated for surgically unresectable salivary tumors

DIAGNOSTIC CHECKLIST

Consider

- Always assess for PNT spread in H&N cancer
  - Findings are subtle; if you don't look, you will not see it
- Even if no history of primary tumor, beware diagnosis of "trigeminal neuralgia"
  - ACCa: Can present as small HP primary with extensive PNT

Image Interpretation Pearls

- Deep face PNT often best seen on precontrast T1 MR without fat saturation
- Denervated muscles disclose affected nerve
- If CECT: Check normal fat planes; evaluate for asymmetry

Reporting Tips

- Examine nerve at risk from end organ to nucleus
  - Knowledge of motor/sensory supply = most effective use of clinical information
- Remember key facts of tumor spread
  - PNT may spread both anterograde & retrograde
  - Beware possibility of radiographic skip lesions
  - Nerves interconnect (e.g., CNV & CNVII)

SELECTED REFERENCES

1. Brown IS: Pathology of perineural spread. J Neurol Surg B Skull Base. 77(2):124-30, 2016
2. Stambuk HE: Perineural tumor spread involving the central skull base region. Semin Ultrasound CT MR. 34(5):445-58, 2013
3. Gandhi MR et al: Detecting and defining the anatomic extent of large nerve perineural spread of malignancy: comparing "targeted" MRI with the histologic findings following surgery. Head Neck. 33(4):469-75, 2011
4. Curtin HD: Detection of perineural spread: fat suppression versus no fat suppression. AJNR Am J Neuroradiol. 25(1):1-3, 2004
5. Ginsberg LE: MR imaging of perineural tumor spread. Magn Reson Imaging Clin N Am. 10(3):511-25, vi, 2002

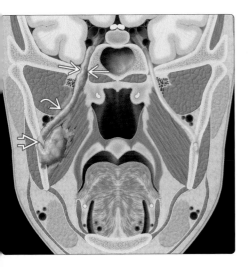

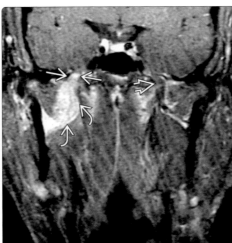

(Left) *Coronal graphic depicts PNT extending from the masticator space into the mandible and along the inferior alveolar nerve ➡. Tumor extends along the nerve ➡ through the foramen ovale ➡ to Meckel cave.* **(Right)** *Coronal T1WI C+ FS MR shows markedly enlarged and enhancing mandibular nerve ➡ coursing through the right masticator space to foramen ovale ➡. Note normal appearance of contralateral mandibular nerve ➡ with normal linear enhancement at foramen ovale from veins traversing the foramen.*

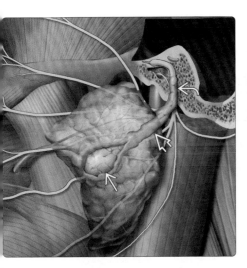

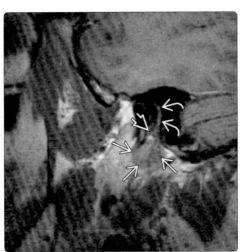

(Left) *Sagittal graphic depicts parotid malignancy ➡ engulfing branches of CNVII. PNT extends along the intraparotid CNVII ➡, through the stylomastoid foramen, to the mastoid segment ➡. Any parotid tumor may spread along CNVII, although adenoid cystic carcinoma is mostly neurotropic.* **(Right)** *Sagittal T1 MR without fat saturation in a patient with facial palsy shows a small parotid mass ➡ immediately beneath the stylomastoid foramen ➡. PNT is evident extending along the mastoid segment of CNVII ➡, which appears enlarged.*

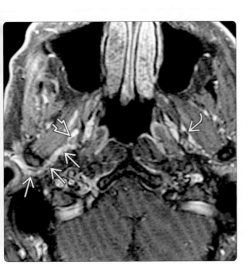

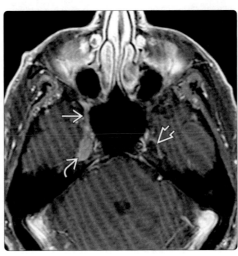

(Left) *Axial MR in a patient with multiple prior SCCa skin reveals linear enhancing right auriculotemporal nerve PNT ➡ posterior to right condyle & medial to the lateral pterygoid muscle, joining enhancing V3 ➡ below the foramen ovale. Note normal left V3 ➡.* **(Right)** *Axial MR shows a PNT from the auriculotemporal nerve tumor filling the right Meckel cave ➡ & extending antegrade along the V2 in the cavernous sinus ➡ through the foramen rotundum into the right PPF. Note the normal CSF-filled left Meckel cave ➡. Biopsy proved SCCa.*

Nodal Squamous Cell Carcinoma

TERMINOLOGY

- Metastatic spread of primary H&N SCCa to nodes

IMAGING

- Change in morphology key to detecting nodal metastasis
- "Malignant nodal criteria" best used in combination
  - Nodal enlargement, typically > 10-mm long axis
  - Round node shape rather than oval
  - Clustered nodes: ≥ 3 nodes 8-9 mm
  - Focal nodal defect/necrosis
  - Extranodal extension
- Ultrasound can help
  - Shows loss of hilar echogenicity & normal hilar flow with ↑ peripheral vascularity

TOP DIFFERENTIAL DIAGNOSES

- Reactive lymph nodes
- 2nd branchial cleft cyst
- Suppurative lymph nodes

- Differentiated thyroid carcinoma nodes
- Non-Hodgkin lymphoma nodes
- Non-head & neck malignancy nodes

PATHOLOGY

- Lymphatic spread of H&N SCCa follows expected pattern

CLINICAL ISSUES

- Nodal metastasis is **most important prognostic factor** for H&N SCCa
  - Unilateral node ↓ prognosis 50%
  - Bilateral nodes ↓ prognosis 75%
- Patient presenting with neck mass from metastatic SCCa + normal clinical & radiographic exam = "**unknown primary**"

DIAGNOSTIC CHECKLIST

- New solid or cystic neck mass in adult is malignant until proven otherwise
- Detection & treatment of metastatic adenopathy is critical for patient survival with primary SCCa

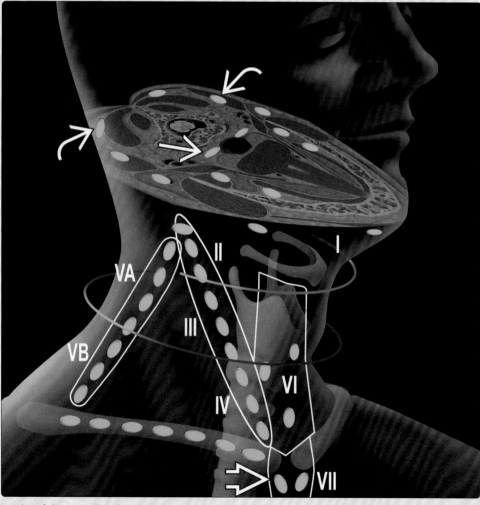

Lateral oblique graphic of the cervical neck depicts the extensive nodal network to which SCCa may metastasize. Superiorly, an axial slice through the suprahyoid neck shows the retropharyngeal nodes ⮕ behind the pharynx and shows multiple superficial nodal groups ⮕. The hyoid bone (blue arc) and cricoid cartilage (orange circle) planes subdivide the internal jugular and spinal accessory nodal group levels. Level II is the most common site of SCCa nodal metastasis, while level VI and level VII are the least common sites. SCCa metastases in level VII ⮕ are considered regional metastases, while nodes more inferiorly in the mediastinum are considered M1 disease.

Nodal Squamous Cell Carcinoma

TERMINOLOGY

Abbreviations

- Nodal squamous cell carcinoma (SCCa)

IMAGING

General Features

- Best diagnostic clue
  - Round, enlarged, &/or heterogeneous node in expected nodal drainage level(s) of H&N SCCa
  - New neck mass in adult, including cystic mass
- Location
  - Level IIA (jugulodigastric) most often involved
- Size
  - Different nodal size criteria used depending on location
  - Nodes > 3 cm are usually confluent nodal masses
- Morphology
  - Change in morphology is key to detecting nodal metastasis
  - **"Malignant nodal criteria" best used in combination rather than individually**
    - Nodal enlargement; several different limits
      - □ Levels I & IIA ≥ 15 mm; levels IIB-VI ≥ 10 mm; retropharyngeal ≥ 8 mm
      - □ Long axis most often used for diameter
      - □ Overall error rate by size criteria alone = 10-20%
    - Round node shape rather than oval
      - □ Ratio of long axis:short axis < 2
    - Clustered nodes: ≥ 3 nodes 8-9 mm
      - □ IIA: 9-10 mm
    - Focal nodal defect/necrosis
      - □ Results in inhomogeneous nodal texture
      - □ May result in diffuse cystic change
      - □ Differentiate from fatty hilum
    - Extranodal extension (ENE)
      - □ Indistinct nodal margins, infiltration of fat ± adjacent soft tissues
      - □ Most sensitive & specific feature of malignancy
      - □ Early ENE may be difficult to detect
- Features of surgical unresectability
  - Carotid encasement ≥ 270°
  - Invasion prevertebral mm, high skull base extension &/or dermal lymphatics

CT Findings

- CECT
  - Variable imaging appearance reflecting 5 malignant nodal criteria
  - Nodal enhancement variable: Increased nodal enhancement may be inflammatory or neoplastic
- CT perfusion: Largely, research for treatment response
  - SCCa: High blood volume & capillary permeability

MR Findings

- DWI
  - Benign nodes have highest ADC values, SCCa have lowest, lymphoma has intermediate
- MR perfusion: Dynamic contrast enhancement
  - Transfer constant (Ktrans) increased, treatment responders show early decrease

Ultrasonographic Findings

- Grayscale ultrasound
  - Round node with loss of hilar echogenicity
- Power Doppler
  - Loss of normal hilar flow, ↑ peripheral vascularity

Nuclear Medicine Findings

- PET
  - SCCa is reliably FDG avid
    - Accuracy ~ 75% for detection of positive nodes
    - Accuracy improves as nodes increase in size
    - False-negative may occur with cystic nodes
    - False-positive reactive nodes in ulcerative tumor
    - Useful for nodal SCCa & unknown primary site
    - High negative predictive value for posttreatment evaluation

Imaging Recommendations

- Best imaging tool
  - Either CECT or MR
    - Stage primary tumor & nodes simultaneously
    - CT performs slightly better than MR for nodal detection
    - MR better for retropharyngeal node detection
  - US helpful for evaluation of suspicious nodes & guidance for fine-needle aspiration

DIFFERENTIAL DIAGNOSIS

Reactive Lymph Nodes

- Tend to retain nodal ovoid contour; not round
- Typically not high FDG avidity; may be moderate

2nd Branchial Cleft Cyst

- Young patient with recurrent angle of mandible mass
- Thin-walled cystic mass posterior to submandibular gland
- May exactly mimic cystic level II nodal metastasis
- FDG uptake may be present if inflammation present
- Diagnosis of exclusion

Suppurative Lymph Nodes

- Clustered cystic or necrotic-appearing nodes with surrounding inflammatory changes
- Often clinically obvious: Hot, tender, febrile patient

Differentiated Thyroid Carcinoma Nodes

- More likely to be heterogeneous than SCCa
- May have calcifications, cystic, high CT density
- MR may have high T1 and high T2 intensity
- ↑ FDG uptake as tumor dedifferentiates
- Most often levels VI, III, IV, & superior mediastinum

Non-Hodgkin Lymphoma Nodes

- Multiple bilateral nonnecrotic nodal masses
- Waldeyer ring involvement or aggressive necrotic nodal non-Hodgkin lymphoma (NHL) mimics SCCa
- Posterior triangle location alone favors nasopharynx, NHL, or scalp SCCa metastases

Nonhead & Neck Malignancy Nodes

- May metastasize to supraclavicular nodes
  - Chest, breast, or abdominal primary tumor
  - Virchow node or Troisier sign on left side

AJCC Nodal Staging in Head and Neck (2010)

Regional Lymph Nodes (N), Most Head and Neck Squamous Cell Carcinoma	Regional Lymph Nodes (N), Nasopharyngeal Carcinoma
NX: Nodes cannot be assessed	**NX**: Nodes cannot be assessed
N0: No regional nodal metastases	**N0**: No regional nodal metastases
N1: Single ipsilateral node ≤ 3 cm	**N1**: Unilateral nodal metastasis ≤ 6 cm **or** any retropharyngeal node
N2a: Single ipsilateral node > 3 cm, ≤ 6 cm	**N2**: Bilateral nodal metastasis ≤ 6 cm
N2b: Multiple ipsilateral nodes, each ≤ 6 cm	**N3a**: Any nodal metastasis > 6 cm
N2c: Bilateral or contralateral nodes, each ≤ 6 cm	**N3b**: Nodal metastasis to supraclavicular fossa
N3: Nodal metastasis > 6 cm	

Adapted from 7th edition AJCC Staging Forms.

PATHOLOGY

General Features

- Etiology
  - Lymphatic spread of primary SCCa generally follows expected pattern in H&N
  - Skip metastasis: Nodes "miss" level
    - Well described with anterior tongue SCCa

Staging, Grading, & Classification

- Level system also useful, as SCCa sites have expected drainage patterns
  - **Nasopharynx**: Retropharyngeal (RPN) > level II, vertebral artery
  - **Oropharynx**: Level IIA > IIB, III; also consider RPN if posterior wall or tonsil
  - **Oral cavity**: Level I & II > III
  - **Hypopharynx**: Level II, III > IV; also consider RPN if pyriform sinus or posterior wall
  - **Larynx**: Level II, III > IV
  - **Scalp skin tumors**: Parotid, suboccipital, level II ± V
- AJCC cervical node classification is used when staging most H&N SCCa
  - Nasopharyngeal carcinoma (NPC) has own nodal staging
  - Thyroid carcinoma has own nodal staging

Gross Pathologic & Surgical Features

- Extranodal extension = tumor infiltration → perinodal fat, adherent to vessels or invading muscles

Microscopic Features

- Metastases 1st lodge in subcapsular sinus then spread through whole node

CLINICAL ISSUES

Presentation

- Most common signs/symptoms
  - Cystic level II metastasis often confused with branchial cleft cyst
  - Painless firm neck mass, may be fixed to adjacent tissues
  - Metastatic node & no obvious primary = "**unknown primary**"
  - Detection of metastatic nodes
    - Clinical exam ~ 75% accuracy, sensitivity 65%
    - Imaging is ~ 80-85% accurate

Demographics

- Epidemiology
  - Presence of nodes varies by primary tumor site
    - Most often: NPC (~ 85%)
    - Least often: Glottic laryngeal SCCa (< 10%)

Natural History & Prognosis

- **Nodal metastasis is most important prognostic factor for H&N SCCa**
  - **Single** ipsilateral node = N1 = **stage III**
  - **Multiple** or **bilateral** nodes = N2 = **stage IVA**
- Unilateral node ↓ prognosis 50%; bilateral nodes ↓ prognosis 75%
- ENE ↓ prognosis further 50% & ↑ recurrence risk by 10
  - Carotid artery encasement, prevertebral mm &/or skull base invasion = surgically unresectable

Treatment

- Resection ± XRT, primary XRT, or chemoXRT

DIAGNOSTIC CHECKLIST

Consider

- New neck mass in adult is malignant until proven otherwise
  - May be solid or cystic node; most often level IIA
  - If calcification, consider thyroid carcinoma
  - If isolated low neck metastasis, consider thyroid or infraclavicular 1°
  - If posterior triangle nodes, consider NPC, NHL, or scalp SCCa

Reporting Tips

- Look carefully at expected nodal drainage site
- Evaluate contralateral neck (upstages to N2c)
- Describe extent for surgical resectability
- Consider skip metastasis, especially in anterior tongue cancer
- Review retropharyngeal nodes as not clinically detectable

SELECTED REFERENCES

1. Gaddikeri S et al: Dynamic contrast-enhanced MR imaging in head and neck cancer: techniques and clinical applications. AJNR Am J Neuroradiol. 37(4):588-95, 2016
2. Gor DM et al: Imaging of cervical lymph nodes in head and neck cancer: the basics. Radiol Clin North Am. 44(1):101-10, viii, 2006

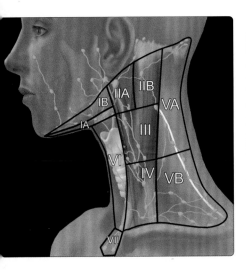

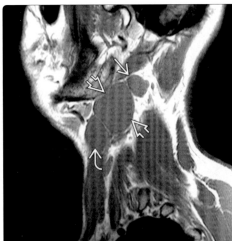

(Left) *Graphic of neck node scheme shows submental (IA) and submandibular (IB) nodes below the jaw. The sternocleidomastoid muscle separates jugular chain (II, III, IV) from spinal accessory chain (VA, VB). Midline anterior nodes are level VI.* (Right) *Sagittal T1WI MR shows 3 solid enlarged metastatic nodes from primary tonsillar SCCa. The largest node is level IIA ➡, beneath the angle of the mandible. Note the smaller adjacent IIB ➡ and adjacent inferior level III node ➡. More than 1 ipsilateral node stages this as N2b.*

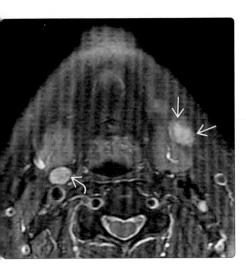

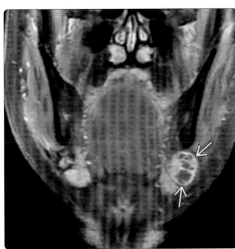

(Left) *Axial T2WI FS MR in a 64-year-old woman with large left oral tongue SCCa demonstrates a clearly enlarged heterogeneous, hyperintense left IB node ➡, which is an expected drainage site for tongue SCCa. Contralateral right IIA node ➡ is rounded, heterogeneously enhancing & very suspicious for tumor.* (Right) *Coronal T1WI C+ FS MR in a patient with large left oral cavity SCCa reveals a left IB node ➡ with cystic necrotic changes & a suspicious right IIA node. Both nodes were positive at resection: T3N2c.*

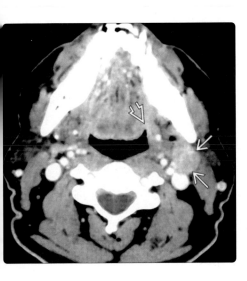

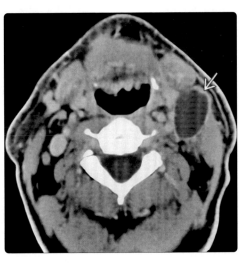

(Left) *Axial CECT in a 49-year-old man shows a unilateral, enlarged, heterogeneous level IIA node ➡. Fine-needle aspiration revealed SCCa. Panendoscopy was negative, but directed biopsies of left glossotonsillar sulcus ➡ revealed SCCa.* (Right) *CECT shows a malignant level II cystic, peripherally enhancing SCCa ➡ node with a clinically occult lingual tonsil SCCa. Cystic level II mass in an adult is tumor until proven otherwise; do not confuse with a branchial cleft cyst, which is diagnosis of exclusion & rarely presents in adults.*

(Left) *Axial T1WI C+ FS MR in a 41-year-old woman smoker with an enlarging neck mass shows a cystic mass ➔ at the right level 2 with a peripheral enhancing rim. Fine-needle aspiration revealed SCCa cells. Asymmetric fullness of the right tongue base ➔ is evident on MR.* (Right) *Sagittal fused PET/CT shows FDG uptake in the rim ➔ with SUV of 2.4 & no uptake in central necrotic portion of node. Uptake may not be evident in cystic nodes. New neck mass is deemed neoplastic until proven otherwise. Patient had a base of tongue primary.*

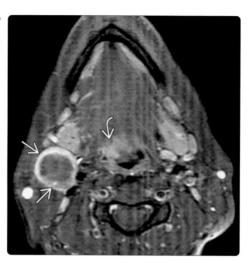
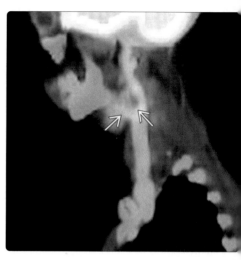

(Left) *Axial CECT in 54-year-old man presenting with neck masses shows multiple pathologic left nodes ➔ secondary to well-defined base of tongue primary SCCa ➔. Notice ill-defined contours of left IIB node ➔, indicating extranodal extension (ENE).* (Right) *Axial T2WI FS MR in 49-year-old patient with lateral tongue SCCa ➔ shows a large heterogeneous nodal mass at level II ➔. Ill-defined margins with infiltration of soft tissues suggest ENE, which involves the carotid sheath ➔.*

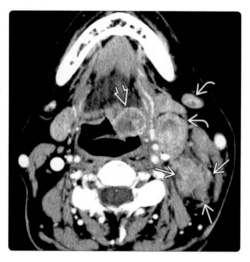
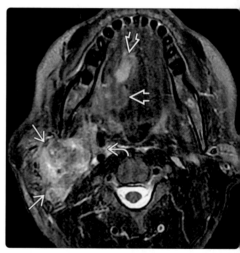

(Left) *Axial CECT shows a left common carotid artery ➔ surrounded by extensive extranodal tumor ➔ that extend to thicken overlying skin ➔. Air pockets throughout left neck within the necrotic tumor are from skin fistulization. The jugular vein is occluded.* (Right) *CTA reformation in a patient with extensive extranodal tumor ➔ reveals multiple outpouchings ➔ along medial carotid wall, indicating significant carotid wall weakening & imminent arterial rupture. Endovascular carotid occlusion was performed.*

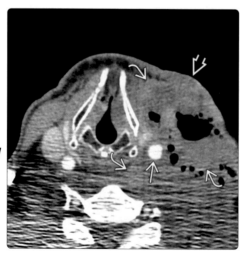
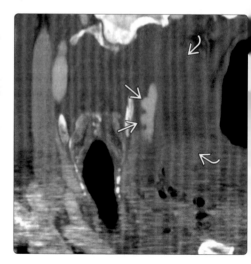

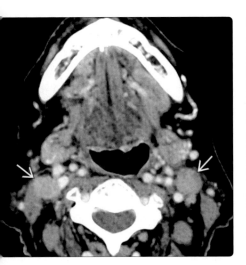
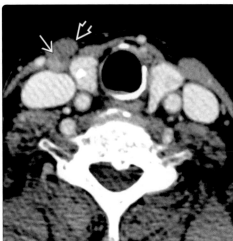

(Left) *Axial CECT in an 83-year-old woman with primary SCCa of anterolateral right tongue demonstrates bilateral level 2 adenopathy* ➡. *While only slightly enlarged, both appear very round in contour and heterogeneous in density. Bilateral adenopathy denotes N2c disease, stage IVA.* (Right) *Axial CECT in a patient with right oral tongue SCCa & IIA nodes shows heterogeneous metastatic level IV node* ➡ *beneath sternocleidomastoid* ⇒, *confirmed with PET and at excision. No nodes are evident at level III. This is known as "skip metastasis."*

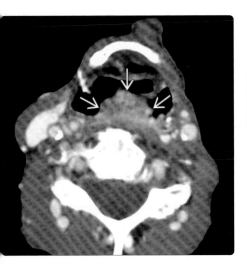
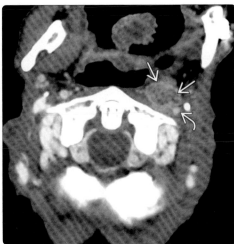

(Left) *Axial CECT demonstrates exophytic heterogeneous SCCa* ➡ *arising from the posterior wall of the pharynx at the level of the hyoid. In all pyriform sinus & posterior pharyngeal wall tumors, always scrutinize retropharyngeal nodes, which are not palpable.* (Right) *Axial CECT in a patient with posterior wall hypopharynx SCCa shows enlarged heterogeneously enhancing node* ➡ *medial to the left internal carotid artery* ⇗, *representing metastatic retropharyngeal node.*

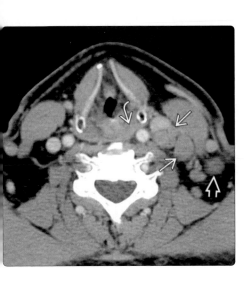
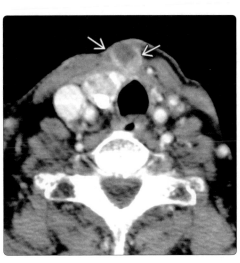

(Left) *Axial CECT in a patient shows cluster of nonnecrotic, large rounded nodes in level III* ➡. *Level VA node* ⇘ *also proved to be metastatic SCCa from subtle postcricoid SCCa* ⇗, *which was apparent on FDG-PET exam.* (Right) *Axial CECT scan shows a rounded, low-density and rim-enhancing mass in the anterior midline of low neck* ➡. *This is location of the Delphian, or prelaryngeal node, and SCCa does not often spread here. Ill-defined margins of this metastasis suggest extracapsular spread.*

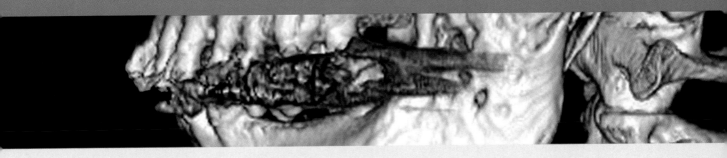

KEY FACTS

TERMINOLOGY

- Neck dissection (ND) performed to treat or accurately stage H&N cancer
- Nodal dissection definitions
  - **Selective ND (SND)**: Resection of known or potential nodal levels while preserving nonlymphatic structures
  - **SND (I-III)**: Resection of nodes in levels I, II, III
  - **SND (II-IV)**: Resection of nodes in levels II-IV
  - **SND (II-V)**: Resection of nodes in levels II-V
  - **SND (VI)**: Resection of nodes in level VI only
- **Modified (radical) ND (MND)**: Nodal resection levels I-V + preservation ≥ 1 nonlymphatic structure (IJV, SCM, or CNXI)
- **Radical ND (RND)**: Nodal resection levels I-V + IJV, SCM, & CNXI; SMG resected with level I nodes
- **Extended neck dissection**: RND + removal of additional structures

IMAGING

- Fibroadipose tissue resected with all NDs

- Imaging findings reflect different tissues resected
  - SND: Loss of fat around CS and beneath SCM; SCM "draped" over CS; IJV & SCM remain
  - MND: Loss of fat around CS; IJV or SCM resected
  - RND: Fibroadipose tissue removed around CS; IJV & SCM resected
- Atrophy of trapezius muscle seen in RND; may be present in MND or SND
- Levator scapulae hypertrophy in RND may mimic tumor
- If level I resected during any nodal dissection, SMG will be absent

CLINICAL ISSUES

- ND may be surgical standard of care even if staging CECT, PET/CECT, or MR do not show nodal metastases
- Physical exam for recurrent adenopathy after ND difficult due to scarring
- Imaging often only way to detect nodal recurrence after ND; PET/CECT has role in difficult cases

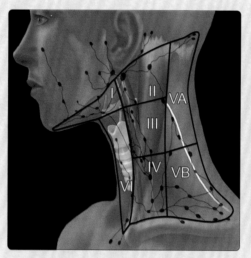
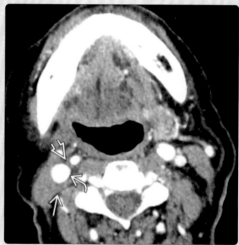

(Left) Graphic illustrates nodal levels that may be removed in different combinations as part of neck nodal dissections. For example, radical neck dissection (RND) involves removal of all groups; selective neck dissection (SND) is removal of levels I through III only. (Right) Axial CECT shows typical selective neck dissection findings at level II on right. Note the loss of fat beneath SCM ➡ and around carotid space ⇒ (compared to normal left side). Right SMG has been resected. Normal flow is present in the right IJV ➡.

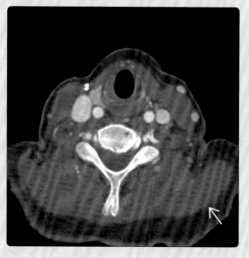
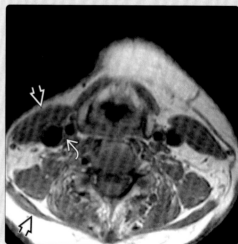

(Left) Axial CECT shows subtle but definite loss of fat around right CS structures, typical appearance following SND. Note the hypertrophy of contralateral trapezius muscle ➡, a common finding after neck dissection. (Right) Axial T1 MR in a different patient shows subtle pericarotid changes ➡ of right SND as compared to left. Note also loss of fat beneath SCM. Right IJV, SCM ➡, and trapezius muscle ⇒ appear normal, as expected with SND.

TERMINOLOGY

Abbreviations

- Neck dissection (ND)
  - Selective neck dissection (SND)
  - Modified (radical) neck dissection (MND)
  - Radical neck dissection (RND)

Synonyms

- Cervical lymph node dissection

Definitions

- SND
  - Most common surgical dissection performed for H&N cancer
  - Resection of known or potential nodal levels while preserving functional, nonlymphatic structures
    - **SND (I-III)**: Resection of nodes in levels I, II, III (supraomohyoid SND)
      - □ Performed in patients with oral cavity squamous cell carcinoma (SCCa)
      - □ Submandibular gland (SMG) usually resected with level IB nodes
    - **SND (II-IV)**: Resection of nodes in levels II-IV (lateral SND)
      - □ Performed in patients with laryngeal and pharyngeal cancer
    - **SND (II-V)**: Resection of nodes in levels II-V (posterolateral SND)
    - **SND (VI)**: Resection of nodes in level VI only (central ND)
      - □ Performed in patients with thyroid carcinoma
- MND
  - Resection of all nodes in levels I or II-V **and** preservation ≥ 1 nonlymphatic structure [internal jugular vein (IJV), sternocleidomastoid muscle (SCM), or CNXI]
- RND
  - Resection of nodal levels I or II-V **and** IJV, SCM, & CNXI
    - SMG resected with level I nodes

IMAGING

General Features

- Best diagnostic clue
  - SND: Loss of fibroadipose tissue of carotid space and beneath SCM
  - MND: SND + absence of IJV or SCM or CNXI
  - RND: SND + absence of IJV and SCM
- Morphology
  - Contour change of neck from fibroadipose tissue resection
  - Imaging findings may be subtle after SND

Imaging Recommendations

- Best imaging tool
  - CECT or PET/CECT
  - MR usually 1st-line study for thyroid carcinoma
    - MR used to avoid patient exposure to iodinated contrast
      - □ Iodinated contrast may delay I-131 therapy by 6 weeks
- Protocol advice
  - CECT from skull base or through primary tumor to thoracic inlet
  - Adequate venous opacification essential to assess for IJV patency, if preserved with SND/MND

CT Findings

- CECT
  - CECT findings depend on type of ND completed
  - **Loss of fat planes around CS and beneath SCM** present in all ND types
    - Fat plane loss secondary to removal of nodes embedded in fibroadipose tissue
  - **SND**: Findings may be **extremely subtle** on imaging
    - Loss of fat around CS and beneath SCM
    - SCM "draped" over CS
    - IJV and SCM remain, but CNXI denervation may be present (atrophy in SCM & trapezius)
    - SMG resected when level IB nodes involved
  - **MND**: IJV **or** SCM removed &/or CNXI
    - CS fibroadipose tissue gone
    - CNXI denervation may be present
  - **RND**: IJV, SCM, & CS fibroadipose tissue all removed
    - Atrophy of trapezius muscle secondary to resection of CNXI
    - Compensatory levator scapulae muscle hypertrophy after 3-6 months

MR Findings

- Like CECT, MR findings reflect type of ND employed
  - Loss of fibroadipose tissue around CS best appreciated on T1WI
- Denervation atrophy of trapezius + SCM may be present with MND and even SND
  - Subacute denervation: Trapezius may enlarge and enhance
  - Chronic denervation: Trapezius loses volume, infiltrated with fat

Ultrasonographic Findings

- Grayscale ultrasound
  - Very high accuracy for detecting recurrent nodal disease when performed by experienced sonographer
  - US not as affected by fatty tissue absence as CECT
    - US better able to detect superficial nodal recurrence
  - Retropharyngeal nodes + level VII not imaged

Nuclear Medicine Findings

- PET/CT
  - Hypermetabolic tissue on PET may diagnose post-ND recurrence
  - Pitfall: Asymmetric muscle uptake after ND

DIFFERENTIAL DIAGNOSIS

Denervation Atrophy CNXI

- Presence of fibroadipose tissue, IJV, and normal nodes & no history of prior surgery
- Check jugular foramen for mass causing CNXI injury
  - Jugular foramen syndrome [vocal cord palsy (CNX), swallowing difficulties (CNIX), CNXI]

PATHOLOGY

General Features

- Etiology
  - ND performed as treatment or staging for H&N cancer
    - Usually SCCa or differentiated thyroid carcinoma
  - SND may remove nodes in en bloc manner or piecemeal
  - RND and MND remove nodes in en bloc manner
- Associated abnormalities
  - Resection of level I nodes also includes removal of ipsilateral SMG
    - Newer surgical techniques aim to preserve SMG to avoid xerostomia

Gross Pathologic & Surgical Features

- Fibroadipose tissue with nodes embedded within fat

Microscopic Features

- Nodes are bisected to determine presence of tumor
- Pathologist determines presence of central nodal necrosis, extranodal tumor extension through nodal capsule, arterial invasion

CLINICAL ISSUES

Presentation

- Most common signs/symptoms
  - Neck is scarred with loss of soft tissue volume
    - Physical exam to detect recurrent adenopathy difficult
    - Posttreatment imaging critical to detect recurrent adenopathy

Demographics

- Epidemiology
  - ND often surgical standard of care even if staging CECT or MR do not show nodal metastases
    - When tongue cancer presents with > 3-mm invasion, SND (I-III) routinely performed as nodal metastases increase in frequency
    - Oropharynx, supraglottic larynx, hypopharynx SCCa are subsites frequently associated with nodal metastases
      - ND or chemo/radiation are standard therapy
  - ND performed in more advanced stage SCCa, either because of malignant nodes on staging CECT/MR or advanced stage

Natural History & Prognosis

- SND by experienced surgeon removes most nodes at risk with less shoulder pain or cosmetic deformity
  - Preservation of IJV important in case nodes recur in contralateral neck, & IJV resection is required because of extracapsular disease
  - Loss of both IJVs undesirable → leads to venous collateral development, neck & face edema, and swelling

Treatment

- Options, risks, complications
  - SND
    - SND is 1st-line surgery for uncomplicated nodal disease

- Removes fewer nodes, but preservation of functional structures reduces morbidity
- Reported as "SND (levels resected)"
- **SND (I-III)**: Resection of levels I, II, III + SMG
  - For oral cavity SCCa
  - Previously called "supraomohyoid ND"
- **SND (II-IV)**: Resection of levels II, III, IV only
  - Performed for all other subsites of SCCa that require treatment or accurate staging of neck disease
  - Previously called "lateral ND"
- **SND (VI)**: Resection of all level VI nodes
  - Nodes between carotids: Hyoid to sternal notch
  - Performed primarily for thyroid malignancy
  - Previously called "central compartment ND"
  - MND
    - Used when extracapsular extension involves SCM or IJV on CECT or MR
    - Attempt to reduce morbidity of RND by preserving functional structures
  - RND
    - Used when extensive extranodal tumor involves IJV or SCM
    - Rarely performed for uncomplicated nodal metastases
    - Marked chronic shoulder pain from CNXI loss main disadvantage

DIAGNOSTIC CHECKLIST

Consider

- Previous ND if fibroadipose tissue, SCM, or IJV not present in patient with history of H&N cancer, especially SCCa

Image Interpretation Pearls

- Post-ND findings evident on CECT or MR but SND findings often subtle
  - History of type of ND helpful for accurate reporting
- Important to detect recurrent nodes ipsilateral or contralateral to side of ND, **so look carefully**
  - After SND, recurrent nodes have ↓ conspicuity, as they may be isodense to SCM with no surrounding fat
    - Consider using PET/CECT or US in difficult cases
  - Recurrent ipsilateral metastatic adenopathy may occur in level IIB or high submuscular recess

Reporting Tips

- Report should include whether IJV, SCM, SMG, or fibroadipose tissue is present
- After SND, comment on opacification of IJV, as IJV thrombosis is undesired outcome of surgery

SELECTED REFERENCES

1. Kito S et al: Alterations in 18F-FDG accumulation into neck-related muscles after neck dissection for patients with oral cancers. Med Oral Patol Oral Cir Bucal. 21(3):e341-8, 2016
2. Mehanna H et al: PET-CT surveillance versus neck dissection in advanced head and neck cancer. N Engl J Med. 374(15):1444-54, 2016
3. Wang K et al: Impact of post-chemoradiotherapy superselective/selective neck dissection on patient reported quality of life. Oral Oncol. 58:21-6, 2016
4. Givi B et al: Selective neck dissection in node-positive squamous cell carcinoma of the head and neck. Otolaryngol Head Neck Surg. 147(4)707-15, 2012

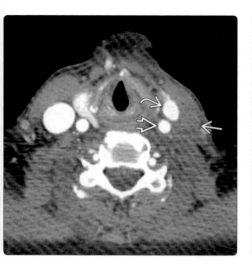

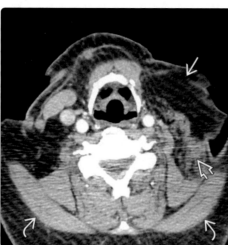

(Left) *Axial CECT shows typical SND findings on left at level III: SCM ➡ draped over carotid artery ➡ and IJV ➡ with no fatty tissue beneath SCM. On right, fat planes around the carotid space are preserved. Note the contour defect with flattening of left neck.* (Right) *Axial CECT shows left modified neck dissection with pectoralis flap reconstruction to fill neck defect. Flap has fat ➡ and muscular components ➡. IJV and SCM were resected, but CNXI was preserved, resulting in symmetric trapezius muscles ➡.*

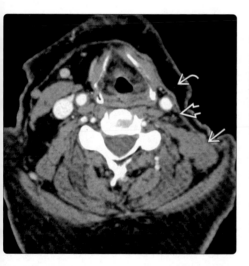

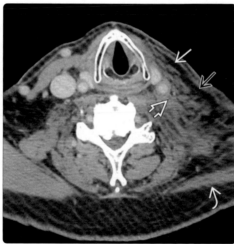

(Left) *Axial CECT in a patient 8 months following left RND reveals absence of left SCM ➡ and IJV ➡ with compensatory levator scapulae muscle hypertrophy ➡ from CNXI surgical resection. Beware of mistaking hypertrophic levator scapulae as recurrent tumor.* (Right) *Axial CECT shows left RND with absence of SCM ➡, IJV ➡ and atrophied trapezius ➡ from CNXI resection. Pectoralis major flap ➡ covers soft tissue defect.*

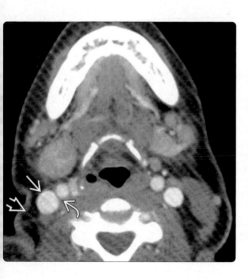

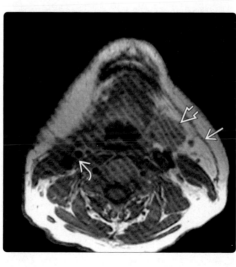

(Left) *Axial CECT at the level of the hyoid bone reveals modified radical neck dissection on right at level II, with surgical resection of SCM ➡ but preservation of normal IJV ➡. Subtle loss of fat planes around carotid space is visible ➡.* (Right) *Axial T1 MR in a patient with SND reveals subtle changes of loss of fat around the carotid space ➡ after resection of nodal groups I through III. The right platysma muscle and submandibular gland are absent, as compared to normal left platysma ➡ and submandibular gland ➡.*

TERMINOLOGY

- Soft tissue or autologous bone used to reconstruct postoperative resection defect in H&N
- Fasciocutaneous flap
  - Deep muscle fascia, arterial perforators, & overlying skin
  - Used for smaller surgical reconstructions
  - Donor site is radial forearm or anterolateral thigh
- Myocutaneous flap
  - Muscle, soft tissue, & skin
  - Used when large surgical defect requires greater tissue volume to fill
  - Donor site is usually pectoralis major muscle
- Osteocutaneous flap
  - Bone, soft tissue, and overlying skin ± muscle
  - Used when surgical reconstruction requires bone replacement (mandible, maxilla, face)
  - Donor site usually fibula or scapula

IMAGING

- CECT/MR
  - Fasciocutaneous, small myocutaneous flaps: May look like normal soft tissue at surgical defect
  - Myocutaneous flap: Denervated at time of transfer to surgical defect; muscle in flap variable depending on time of imaging
  - Osteocutaneous flap: Bone contoured to approximate shape of excised bone

DIAGNOSTIC CHECKLIST

- Essential that history of flap reconstruction available when interpreting complex follow-up scans
  - Flap may be misinterpreted as recurrent tumor
- Look for new enhancing mass (CECT/MR) or hypermetabolic focus (PET) at deep aspect of flap
- Look for splayed/displaced surgical clips

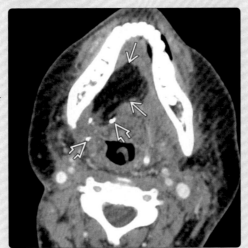
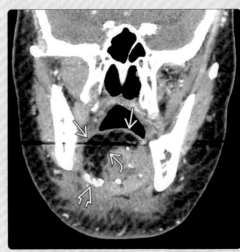

(Left) Axial CECT of the fasciocutaneous radial forearm free flap shows a well-defined, rounded fatty component of the flap ➡ that provides volume to fill the surgical defect. Multiple surgical clips ⮞ in the floor of mouth provide additional evidence that the flap has been placed. (Right) Coronal CECT in the same patient reveals a fatty flap ➡ filling the oral cavity surgical defect, providing soft tissue to reform a smooth contour to the tongue surface ➡. Surgical clips ⮞ are again visible.

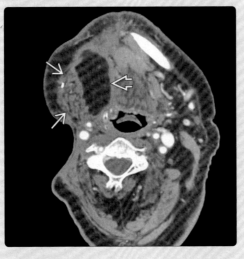
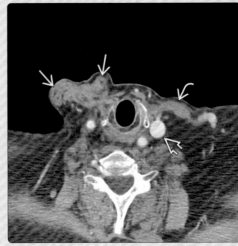

(Left) Axial CECT in a patient with a pectoralis rotational myocutaneous flap following resection of a large retromolar trigone SCCa shows medial hypodense fat component of the flap ⮞ and a lateral striated pectoralis muscle component of flap ➡. (Right) Axial CECT in the low neck (same patient) shows the flap ➡ coming up from the chest. The normal left internal jugular vein ➡ and sternocleidomastoid muscle ⮞ are not seen on the right, as the right radical neck dissection was performed as part of the surgical procedure.

TERMINOLOGY

Definitions

- **Flap**: Soft tissue ± muscle ± bone surgical site reconstruction
  - Also known as **microvascular reconstruction**
- Soft tissue or autologous bone used to reconstruct postoperative resection defect in H&N
  - **Fasciocutaneous flap**
    - Flap constructed of deep muscle **fascia** with its overlying skin
    - Used for smaller surgical reconstructions in H&N
    - Allows harvesting of fasciocutaneous arterial perforators that pass along fascial septa between adjacent muscles
      - □ Results in larger flap size survival at reconstruction site as needed
    - Sensory cutaneous nerves also harvested when sensory reinnervation desired
    - Donor sites primarily radial forearm, lateral arm, temporoparietal, rectus, latissimus dorsi, or anterolateral thigh
  - **Myocutaneous flap**
    - Flap constructed of **muscle**, soft tissue, and overlying skin
    - Used when larger reconstruction site needs more volume (provided by muscle) to adequately fill surgical defect
    - Donor sites include pectoralis major, rectus abdominis, or latissimus dorsi muscles
  - **Osteocutaneous flap**
    - Flap constructed with **bone**, soft tissue, and overlying skin ± muscle
      - □ Also known as **composite** flap
    - Used when reconstruction requires bone replacement
      - □ Primarily employed in oral cavity squamous cell carcinoma (SCCa) reconstructions
      - □ Portion of mandible or maxilla removed during tumor treatment surgery
      - □ Muscle added to osteocutaneous flap if more volume needed for larger surgical defects
    - Donor site usually fibula or scapula
- Flaps most commonly used to reconstruct tumor resection cavity
  - Also used to repair posttraumatic defects in extracranial head and neck
  - Osteocutaneous flap may be used to repair mandibular or maxillary osteonecrosis

IMAGING

General Features

- Best diagnostic clue
  - Soft tissue or bone present in reconstruction site with **nonanatomic** appearance
- Location
  - Fasciocutaneous or myocutaneous flaps
    - Used for large oral cavity > oropharynx > other neck reconstructions
  - Osteocutaneous flaps
    - Used in sinus, orbital, maxillary, or mandibular resection cavities
    - Sites where bone replacement needed
- Size
  - Depends on source of flap
  - Fasciocutaneous flaps smaller
  - Myocutaneous and osteocutaneous flaps larger
- Morphology
  - Depends on donor source: Fascial, muscle, bone density, or combination

Imaging Recommendations

- Best imaging tool
  - PET combined with CECT best imaging study for assessing SCCa flap recurrence
    - PET offers physiologic function
      - □ New nodal recurrence or distant metastases have increased FDG update
      - □ Beware: Surgically denervated muscle can have increased uptake initially
    - CECT best shows new mass or bone destruction at primary site
    - MR affected by motion of ill patients with secretion handling issues
  - CECT may be best imaging study for routine surveillance of reconstruction flaps
    - Physical examination and symptom interpretation clinically challenging
    - Detection of early recurrence key to salvage therapy
- Protocol advice
  - CECT post processed to include complete set of bone algorithm images
    - When osteocutaneous flap present (contains bone), bone component must be viewed at bone windows with bone algorithm
    - Coronal, sagittal, oblique reformations essential to assess all borders of flap/primary site

CT Findings

- CECT
  - Fasciocutaneous or small myocutaneous flaps
    - May look like normal soft tissue at surgical defect
  - Larger fasciocutaneous, myocutaneous, or osteocutaneous
    - Have **nonanatomic** appearance at surgical defect
    - Muscle portion of myocutaneous flaps denervated at time of transfer to surgical defect
      - □ < 6 weeks: May swell and enhance
      - □ > 6 weeks: Shrinkage and fatty infiltrate
    - Osteocutaneous flaps with bone used for mandible, maxilla, orbital wall reconstruction
      - □ Contoured to approximate normal shape of jaw or orbital wall
  - When looking for recurrence in patient with flap
    - Carefully inspect interface between surgical defect and flap at anastomotic site
      - □ Most common site of SCCa recurrence
    - Focal mass-like enhancement suspicious for recurrent tumor
    - Check for change in osseous component or new erosion

– Carefully assess bilateral cervical nodal chains for new nodal mets
- Bone CT
  - Bony portion of flap often contoured to approximate resection site
  - Oral cavity mandible & maxilla are most common sites where osteocutaneous flap is used
  - Interface between native bone and flap = common site of recurrent tumor

MR Findings
- T1WI
  - Signal intensity of flap depends on type of flap used
    – Soft tissue fat (high signal)
    – Muscle (intermediate signal)
    – Bone (low signal cortex, high signal marrow)
- T2WI
  - Muscle portion of flap
    – < 6 weeks: Slightly hyperintense as denervated at time of surgery
    – > 6 weeks: Intermediate to low signal as muscles scar and fat atrophies
  - Postoperative fibrosis usually low signal
    – Fibrosis retracts over time
- T1WI C+
  - Muscle portion of flap
    – < 6 weeks: Muscle may swell and enhance
    – After 6 weeks: Chronic changes are seen
  - Focal area of mass-like enhancement suspicious for recurrent tumor

DIFFERENTIAL DIAGNOSIS

Recurrent SCCa in Reconstruction Flap
- Usually presents with pain or new mass at surgical site months after surgery
  - Neurogenic pain usually implies perineural tumor spread
- Occur at anastomotic site between surgical bed & flap; interface between native bone & flap
- Enhancing irregular mass within or at margin of flap

Postoperative Infection or Abscess
- Presents after surgery with fever, pain, & surgical site induration days to weeks after surgery
- When rim-enhancing lesion seen immediately after surgery, abscess more likely than tumor recurrence
- Found at surgical site with marked homogeneous (phlegmon) or rim (abscess) enhancement

PATHOLOGY

General Features
- Etiology
  - Soft tissue, muscle, or bone from donor site transferred to surgical cavity for reconstruction, cosmesis, and preservation of function
- Associated abnormalities
  - Surgical defect may be extensive, but only part of cavity may require flap

Staging, Grading, & Classification
- Flaps classified based on components

- **Fasciocutaneous flap**: Skin, **fascia**, arterial perforators
- **Myocutaneous flap**: Skin, fascia, **muscle**, arterial perforators
- **Osteocutaneous flap**: Skin, fascia, **bone**, arterial perforators ± muscle (as needed for additional flap volume)

CLINICAL ISSUES

Presentation
- Most common signs/symptoms
  - Known history of H&N SCCa resection with surgical site flap repair
  - Follow-up imaging for recurrence triggered by **pain** or **mass** at surgical site
  - Deep pain without clinical mass suggests recurrence is deep to flap or perineural tumor

Demographics
- Age: Most commonly adults with H&N SCCa

Natural History & Prognosis
- Depends on reason for flap transfer
- Expected survival from tumor determines prognosis
- Overall survival rates poor, as flap reconstructions undertaken in late-stage SCCa
  - ~ 50% 2-year, 30% 5-year survival reported in large series

DIAGNOSTIC CHECKLIST

Consider
- Reconstruction flap has nonanatomic appearance (fat, muscle, or bone in defect)
- Initial **baseline PET/CECT** after treatment changes resolve
  - Best acquired 8-10 weeks after surgery/end of radiation treatment
- Surveillance CECT in postflap patients

Image Interpretation Pearls
- Essential that flap reconstruction history is available when interpreting complex follow-up CECT
  - Anatomic distortion makes scan interpretation challenging
  - Flap may be misinterpreted as recurrent tumor
- Recurrent tumor often occurs at recipient bed where flap placed in surgical defect
  - Look for **new enhancing mass** on CECT in fatty portion of flap
    – Also look for metastatic cervical adenopathy!
  - PET/CT shows recurrent tumor and metastatic cervical adenopathy as high-intensity foci

Reporting Tips
- First describe surgical defect
- Then describe flap composition: Soft tissue and fat ± muscle &/or bone
- Finally, report surgical site or nodal recurrence if present

SELECTED REFERENCES

1. Patel SA et al: Principles and practice of reconstructive surgery for head and neck cancer. Surg Oncol Clin N Am. 24(3):473-489, 2015

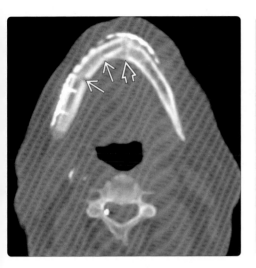

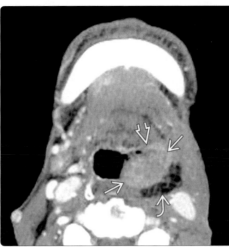

(Left) *Axial bone CT shows an osteocutaneous fibular flap used to reconstruct the mandible following partial mandibulectomy. Note that the osteotomy defects ➡️ allow bone contouring. The donor bone-mandible interface ➡️ is present in the midline.* (Right) *Axial CECT shows recurrent tumor ➡️ at the anastomotic site between the normal tongue base ➡️ and the myocutaneous flap. Recurrence is discrete, homogeneously enhancing, and on the mucosal side of the flap. The fatty portion of flap is seen posterolaterally ➡️.*

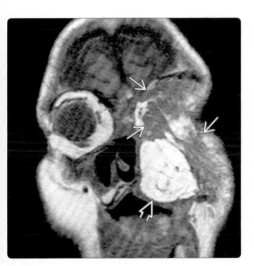

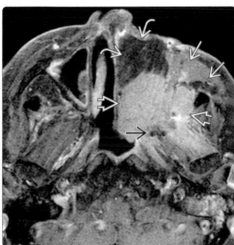

(Left) *Coronal T1WI MR shows a typical rectus abdominis myocutaneous flap ➡️. Striated denervated muscular component of free flap fills orbital exenteration defect. Note the fat component ➡️, providing further volume to fill maxillary & left nasal cavity defect.* (Right) *Axial T1 C+ FS MR (same patient) 18 months later, now with face pain, shows a large enhancing mass ➡️ adjacent to surgical clips ➡️. Mass is deep to fatty ➡️ and muscular ➡️ flap components. This is recurrent SCCa, which typically occurs at deep aspect of flap.*

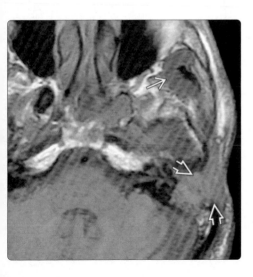

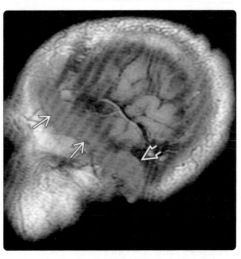

(Left) *Axial T1WI MR shows a patient with a temporalis muscle flap. Part of the temporalis muscle ➡️ remains at the coronoid process of the mandible. The remainder is rotated posteriorly and placed within the mastoid surgical bed ➡️.* (Right) *Sagittal T1WI MR demonstrates a temporalis muscle flap ➡️, which has been rotated posteroinferiorly to cover the mastoid surgical cavity ➡️. Note the value of precontrast T1 images, without fat saturation, in head and neck imaging.*

KEY FACTS

IMAGING

- **Early (1-4 months)**: Diffuse edema of all tissues
  - Reticulation of subcutaneous and deep fat planes
  - Thickening and enhancement of mucosa
  - Swollen, ill-defined enhancing parotid and submandibular glands
  - Subtly swollen muscles, especially pterygoids
- **Late (≥ 12 months)**: Diffuse fibrosis of all tissues
  - Edema and reticulation of fat resolves
  - Mucosal thickening and enhancement may resolve
  - Glandular tissues atrophy; often maintain increased enhancement
  - Lymph nodes and lymphoid tissues atrophy
- **MR**: T2 & T1 C+ accentuate changes seen on CECT
  - Marked T2 intensity & enhancement
- **PET/CT**: No focal uptake unless complication or residual/recurrent tumor

TOP DIFFERENTIAL DIAGNOSES

- Retropharyngeal space edema
- Retropharyngeal space abscess
- Acute parotitis
- Submandibular gland sialadenitis

PATHOLOGY

- XRT destroys endothelial cells lining small vessels
  - **Early**: Results in ischemia, edema, inflammation
  - **Late**: Results in tissue fibrosis

DIAGNOSTIC CHECKLIST

- 1st post-XRT imaging should be 10-12 weeks after end of treatment
- Careful, systematic imaging evaluation is key
- Radiation changes are generally readily identifible
- Severe XRT changes make evaluating scan difficult
  - Residual or recurrent tumor may be easily missed
  - Focal tissue thickening/mass suggests tumor

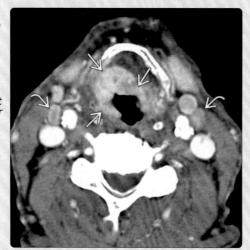
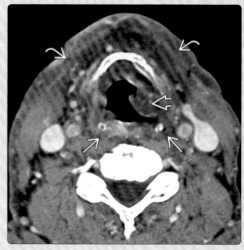

(Left) CECT demonstrates T3 N2c supraglottic SCCa with an enhancing mass ➡ at the base of the epiglottis, aryepiglottic (AE) fold, & pre- & paraglottic fat. Note bilateral nodes ➡. (Right) Axial CECT in the same patient 3 months following chemoXRT shows no residual enhancing tumor or nodes. All fat planes & submucosal tissues, including left AE fold ➡, are edematous with hazy density. Note retropharyngeal ➡ edema as well as thickened skin & platysma muscles ➡. These are expected posttreatment changes.

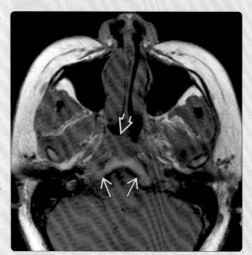
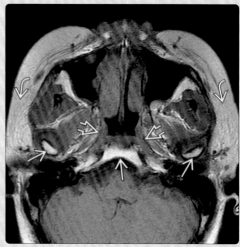

(Left) Axial T1WI MR demonstrates small T1 primary nasopharyngeal carcinoma ➡, which was confined to nasopharynx. There is normal signal intensity in the clivus ➡ suggesting no infiltration by tumor. (Right) Axial T1WI MR after chemoXRT shows resolution of the small nasopharyngeal mass but symmetric, smooth, mild mucosal thickening ➡. Note new marked hyperintensity of the skull base & mandibular condylar marrow ➡. Only minimal facial fat reticulation is evident ➡.

Expected Changes of Neck Radiation Therapy

TERMINOLOGY

Abbreviations

- Radiation therapy (XRT)
- Intensity-modulated radiation therapy (IMRT)
  - Reduces radiation dose to uninvolved surrounding tissues and organs

Definitions

- Expected changes in imaging appearances of neck following XRT

IMAGING

General Features

- Best diagnostic clue
  - **Early**: Diffuse edema of all soft tissues of superficial and deep face & neck
    - Tissues appear diffusely "angry"
  - **Late**: Generalized atrophy of all radiated soft tissues & glands

Imaging Recommendations

- Best imaging tool
  - Post-XRT appearance readily identifiable on either CT or MR
- Protocol advice
  - CECT: ≥ 90-second imaging after contrast to allow mucosal enhancement and increase conspicuity of residual/recurrent mass
  - MR: Fat saturation added to T2 and T1 C+ aids delineation of changes
    - DWI may detect highly cellular tumor recurrence
  - PET/CECT: Complimentary to add specificity for differentiating nonneoplastic change from residual/recurrent tumor
    - PET/MR soon will be available and improve imaging of skull base/sinus/suprahyoid neck XRT-treated tumor beds

CT Findings

- CECT
  - **Early (1-4 months)**: Diffuse edema of all tissues of neck
    - Thickened skin and platysma
    - Reticulation of subcutaneous and deep fat planes
      - □ Edema along fascial planes, such as carotid sheath and retropharyngeal space (RPS)
      - □ Edema of preepiglottic, paraglottic, & parapharyngeal fat
    - Diffuse thickening & enhancement of mucosa, prominent submucosal edema
      - □ Thickened posterior pharyngeal wall
    - Swollen, ill-defined parotid and submandibular glands (SMGs)
      - □ Glands usually enhance robustly after XRT
    - Subtly swollen muscles, especially pterygoids
  - **Late (≥ 12 months)**: Diffuse fibrosis of all tissues of neck
    - Edema and reticulation of fat resolves
    - Concave contour of external neck
    - Thinning of subcutaneous & deep fat planes
    - Mucosal thickening and enhancement may resolve
      - □ Subglottic thickening to 2 mm is common
    - Aryepiglottic (AE) fold and paralaryngeal fat edema remains in ~ 2/3 of patients
    - Retropharyngeal edema resolves by 12 months in 1/3 of patients
    - Glandular tissues (submandibular, parotid, thyroid) atrophy; often maintain increased enhancement
    - Lymph nodes and lymphoid tissues atrophy

MR Findings

- T2 & T1 C+ accentuate changes seen on CECT
  - MR has greater sensitivity to soft tissue inflammation and to contrast enhancement
- Early: Extensive T2 hyperintensity and enhancement of most tissues
  - Neck appears "watery" and diffusely inflamed
    - Symmetric T2 hyperintensity and thickening of platysma, reticulation of subcutaneous and deep fat
    - Linear, hyperintense retropharyngeal edema
  - Muscles may show T2 hyperintensity
  - Symmetric diffuse enhancement of mucosa
  - Increased enhancement of salivary glands
- Late: Most soft tissues return to near-normal signal but appear atrophic
  - Timeline for tissue normalization not defined but likely takes longer than CECT
  - Decrease in enhancement of mucosal and glandular tissues
- T1-hyperintense fatty marrow of cervical vertebrae and skull base
- DWI: Benign post-XRT changes should have mean ACD > 1.3×10^{-3}
  - Always use morphologic imaging with physiologic DWI/ADC maps, as overlap exists between benign tissue & recurrent tumor

Nuclear Medicine Findings

- PET/CT
  - May show asymmetric increased muscular uptake
    - Often compounded by prior surgical resection
    - Increased uptake especially marked in fasciculating residual muscles after oral cavity/tongue resection

DIFFERENTIAL DIAGNOSIS

Retropharyngeal Space Edema

- RPS edema including radiation, jugular vein thrombosis, and pharyngeal infection
- No enhancement of fluid or rim

Retropharyngeal Space Abscess

- Defined pus collection in RPS with local mass effect
- Typically lenticular and rim enhancing
- May be associated with narrowing of internal carotid artery

Acute Parotitis

- Inflammation of gland often with extensive facial cellulitis
- Typically unilateral; ± calculus

Submandibular Gland Sialadenitis

- Inflammation of SMG often associated with calculi
- Typically unilateral with dilated SMG duct

PATHOLOGY

General Features

- Etiology
  - XRT destroys endothelial cells lining small blood vessels
    - **Early**: Results in ischemia, edema, inflammation
    - **Late**: Results in tissue fibrosis
    - Tissues ill-equipped to deal with extreme stressors → XRT complications
    - IMRT goal: Reduce XRT complications in normal tissue surrounding tumor bed
- Associated abnormalities
  - Chemotherapy may be given concurrently to sensitize tissues to XRT
    - Increases severity of acute side effects
    - Probably increases frequency of late effects
    - Improves overall treatment outcome

Microscopic Features

- Histological changes in neck & larynx have been defined
- **Connective tissues (CTs)**
  - Within 2-12 days: Acute inflammatory reaction
    - Leukocyte infiltration, histiocyte formation, necrosis, and occasionally hemorrhage in radiated CTs
    - Small arteries, veins, & lymphatics show detachment of endothelial cells
      □ Increased vessel permeability → interstitial edema
  - Within 1-4 months: Inflammatory CT thickening
    - Deposition of collagenous fibers, sclerosis, hyalinosis
    - Obstruction of vessels by endothelial cell proliferation
      □ Fluid accumulation → interstitial edema
  - At 8 months: CT fibrosis
    - Advanced sclerosis, hyalinosis, fragmentation of collagen fibers
    - Progressive obliterative endarteritis
    - Collateral vessel formation may reduce interstitial edema
- **Muscles**
  - Only minimal abnormalities evident at 1-4 months
  - At 8 months: Waxy degeneration and atrophy
    - Muscle fibers replaced by scar tissue and fat
- **Epithelium**
  - Damage to respiratory epithelium evident at 2-12 days
  - At 8 months: Squamous metaplasia of columnar cells
- **Laryngeal cartilages**
  - 2-12 days: Little response as largely hypocellular
  - 1-4 months: Mild loss of chondrocytes & giant cells
  - At 8 months: Variable thickening and fibrosis of perichondrium
    - Perichondrium is nutrient source to cartilage
  - Resolution of sclerosis of cartilage abutting tumor correlates with local control
    - Converse is not true; ongoing sclerosis may be evident with no evidence of disease

CLINICAL ISSUES

Presentation

- Most common signs/symptoms
  - Oral pain from mucosal inflammation
    - Reduced saliva flow compounds this

- Myositis of masticator space → trismus
  - May occur early with myositis or late with fibrosis
- Glandular atrophy
  - Parotid and SMG atrophy → xerostomia
  - Thyroid atrophy → hypothyroidism; may be subclinical
    □ Seen in 26-48% of H&N squamous cell carcinoma (SCCa) patients

Demographics

- Age
  - Any age, although squamous cell carcinoma, for which most radiation is given, is primarily disease of adults > 45 years

DIAGNOSTIC CHECKLIST

Consider

- Imaging changes are dependent on XRT dose and rate, irradiated tissue volume, & time interval from completion of treatment
  - Edema and inflammation most pronounced 1st few months
  - Many clinical and imaging changes diminish/resolve
  - Tissue atrophy does not resolve

Image Interpretation Pearls

- 1st post-XRT imaging should be 10-12 weeks after end of treatment
- Radiation changes are generally readily recognizable
  - Symmetric diffuse edema → symmetric diffuse fibrosis
- Be aware of asymmetric changes from unilateral XRT
- Severe XRT changes make evaluating scan difficult
  - Residual or recurrent tumor may be easily missed

Reporting Tips

- Image review requires careful, systematic evaluation
  - Important to start with history of tumor site/type
  - Determine whether any structures/tissues resected
  - Review extent of XRT changes in neck
  - Look for focal thickening of mucosa or solid neck mass to suggest residual or recurrent tumor/nodes
    - Evaluate specifically along jugular chains, submandibular space, and posterior triangle
  - More focal inflammatory changes suggest secondary infection or other complication

SELECTED REFERENCES

1. Gutiontov SI et al: Intensity-modulated radiotherapy for head and neck surgeons. Head Neck. 38 Suppl 1:E2368-73, 2016
2. Tol JP et al: A longitudinal evaluation of improvements in radiotherapy treatment plan quality for head and neck cancer patients. Radiother Oncol. 119(2):337-43, 2016
3. Kraaijenga SA et al: Evaluation of long term (10-years+) dysphagia and trismus in patients treated with concurrent chemo-radiotherapy for advanced head and neck cancer. Oral Oncol. 51(8):787-94, 2015
4. Varoquaux A et al: Diffusion-weighted and PET/MR Imaging after Radiation Therapy for Malignant Head and Neck Tumors. Radiographics. 35(5):1502-27, 2015
5. Gunn GB et al: Advances in radiation oncology for the management of oropharyngeal tumors. Otolaryngol Clin North Am. 46(4):629-43, 2013
6. Glastonbury CM et al: The postradiation neck: evaluating response to treatment and recognizing complications. AJR Am J Roentgenol. 195(2):W164-71, 2010
7. Hermans R: Posttreatment imaging in head and neck cancer. Eur J Radiol. 66(3):501-11, 2008

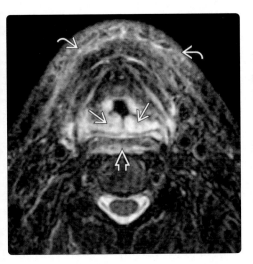

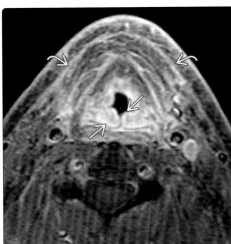

(Left) Axial T2WI FS MR 8 weeks after chemoXRT shows expected changes with hazy hyperintense edema of subcutaneous ➡ and deep fat. Note retropharyngeal edema ➡. Both AE folds ➡ are swollen and diffusely hyperintense from edema. (Right) Axial T1WI C+ FS MR in the same patient shows extensive enhancement of edematous tissues, particularly thickened skin and platysma muscles ➡ but also smooth linear enhancement of AE fold mucosa ➡. MR shows enhancing submucosa not seen on CECT.

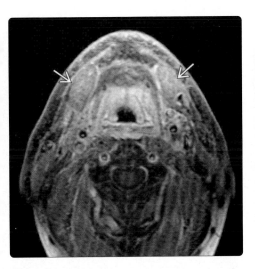

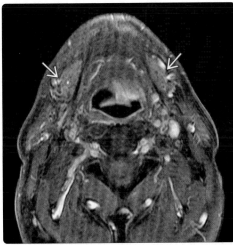

(Left) Axial T1WI C+ FS MR 8 weeks after chemoXRT reveals marked enhancement and thickening of the pharynx and enhancement of deep and subcutaneous fat. Submandibular glands (SMGs) are swollen and enhancing heterogeneously ➡. (Right) Axial T1WI C+ FS MR in the same patient 18 months later shows resolution of the diffuse neck XRT changes with a decrease in the enhancement and size of SMGs ➡ due to chronic radiation-induced sialadenitis. Patients often report xerostomia.

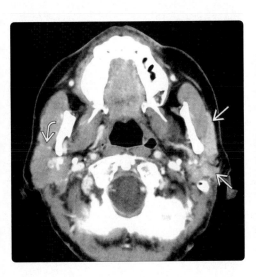

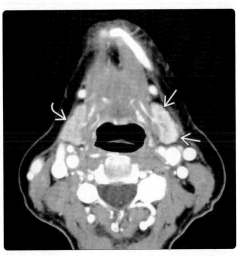

(Left) Axial CECT demonstrates a subtle asymmetric appearance from the prior left XRT. The left parotid gland ➡ appears smaller and hyperdense as compared to the right ➡. (Right) Axial CECT shows a left SMG ➡ robustly enhancing and smaller than the right SMG ➡. Eighteen months prior, subtle asymmetry was secondary to left neck radiation, demonstrating changes of chronic radiation-induced sialadenitis.

TERMINOLOGY

- Uncommon, unintended side effects from radiation therapy (XRT) seen in small proportion of patients

IMAGING

- Potentially involves any radiated neck tissue
  - Excessive inflammation, tissue necrosis, or tumor induction
- CT or MR may be complementary for detection and characterization of abnormality
- CECT typically 1st-order examination; evaluates soft tissues and bones
  - Mucosal ulceration and fistulae, myositis, osteoradionecrosis, chondronecrosis
- MR best for nervous system complications
  - Cerebral radionecrosis, myelopathy, brachial plexitis, cranial neuropathy
- PET may be misleading; intense focal FDG uptake common

TOP DIFFERENTIAL DIAGNOSES

- Recurrent tumor
- Skull base or mandible-maxilla osteomyelitis

PATHOLOGY

- XRT results in obstructive arteriopathy
- Tissues less able to withstand additional stress
- Infection, tumor recurrence, or biopsy may precipitate necrosis

CLINICAL ISSUES

- Uncommon; ~ 1% of patients receiving neck XRT
- Most complications occur ≤ 2 years after XRT
- May occur up to 5-8 years post XRT
- Treatment is largely conservative

DIAGNOSTIC CHECKLIST

- Key differential is always residual/recurrent tumor
- Look for solid enhancing mass

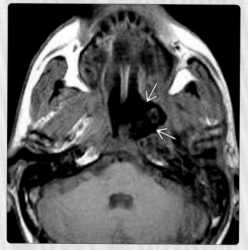 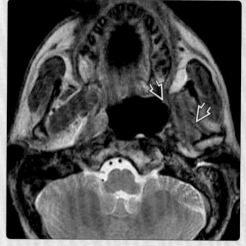

(Left) *Axial T1 MR in a patient treated decade prior for nasopharyngeal carcinoma (NPC) with chemoXRT demonstrates enlarged nasopharyngeal airway following necrosis of the left lateral nasopharyngeal wall tissues* ➡. *(Right) Axial T2 MR in the same patient, slightly more inferiorly at the oropharynx, shows the left medial pterygoid muscle* ➡ *slightly hyperintense & smaller than the contralateral side, suggesting radiation-induced myositis and fibrosis. There are no mass or other imaging features of tumor recurrence.*

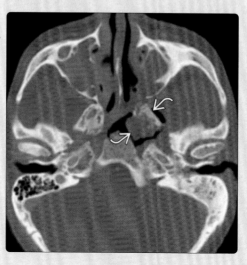 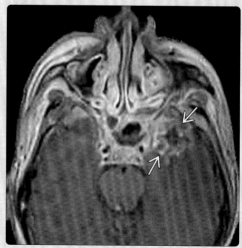

(Left) *Axial bone CT in the same patient shows frank destruction and "crumbling" of the lateral aspect of sphenoid body, creating a sequestrum* ➡. *This is osteoradionecrosis (ORN) of sphenoid bone. (Right) Axial T1 C+ FS MR in the same patient reveals abnormal irregular enhancement of anteromedial left temporal lobe* ➡, *indicating cerebral radionecrosis. This case illustrates potential for radiation-induced complications involving multiple tissues in same field.*

TERMINOLOGY

Definitions

- Uncommon, unintended side effects from radiation therapy (XRT) seen in small proportion of patients

IMAGING

General Features

- Best diagnostic clue
  - No single diagnostic feature, as this potentially involves **any radiated tissue** in neck and may have marked inflammation, tissue necrosis, or tumor induction
    - **Tissue necrosis**: Soft tissue, muscle, cartilage, bone, and brain parenchyma
    - **Marked inflammation**: Brachial plexus, cervical cord, and cranial nerves including optic nerve, muscles
    - **Radiation arteriopathy**: Carotid vessels
    - **Tumor induction**: Radiation-induced neoplasm

Imaging Recommendations

- Best imaging tool
  - CT or MR may be used for detection and characterization of abnormality
    - Solid, enhancing mass raises concern for tumor recurrence
  - MR best for evaluation of nervous system complications
  - **PET/CT often misleading in neck**
    - Focally intense FDG uptake may be seen with necrosis
    - Probably due to accompanying infection/inflammatory response

CT Findings

- CECT
  - Findings vary with site of complication
  - **Mucosa & submucosa**: Necrosis and ulceration → fibrosis
    - Early: Mucosal ulceration common; if solid enhancement, concern for tumor
      - Rarely, severe edema results in airway narrowing
      - Deep ulceration may lead to fistula
    - Late: May result in fibrotic, stenotic pharynx
      - Smooth, minimally enhancing wall
    - Absence of enhancing mass favors necrosis and ulceration over residual/recurrent tumor
  - **Muscles**: Myositis (acute) to fibrosis (late)
    - Early: Marked swelling and decrease in density
    - Late: Marked volume loss of muscles
  - **Cartilage**: Chondronecrosis
    - Fragmentation of cartilage associated with soft tissue swelling
      - ± gas bubbles adjacent to cartilage
  - **Bones**: Osteoradionecrosis (ORN)
    - Bony cortical disruption, loss of trabeculae
    - Often see sequestrum, fragmentation, fracture, gas
  - **Brain parenchyma**: Cerebral radionecrosis
    - Most often anteromedial temporal lobe(s)
    - Vasogenic edema with mass effect
    - Enhancement may be difficult to detect on CECT
  - **Vessels**: Arteriopathy
    - Calcified, atheromatous plaque

  - Carotid most commonly affected; may be asymmetric and unusual segment

MR Findings

- MR findings also vary with site of complication
- Preferred modality for evaluation of CNS/neural complications
- **Brain parenchyma**: Cerebral radionecrosis
  - Cerebral white matter edema & mass effect with focal feathery enhancement
  - Anteromedial temporal lobe: Status post nasopharyngeal or sella radiation
  - Inferior frontal lobes: Sinonasal XRT
  - Key differential is radiation-induced glial tumor
    - Consider if many years (> 10 years) post XRT
  - MR perfusion shows reduced cerebral blood volume relative to normal white matter
  - MR spectroscopy shows reduced metabolites overall
- **Spinal cord**: Myelitis → myelopathy → necrosis
  - Early: Acute cord injury shows edema ± enhancement
  - Late: Delayed XRT myelopathy has expansion, T2 hyperintensity & enhancement
- **Brachial plexus**: XRT-induced plexitis
  - T2 hyperintensity, enhancement, smooth enlargement of nerve roots
- **Cranial nerves**: XRT-induced neuropathy
  - CNXII most often involved: Tongue atrophy with hemitongue T2 hyperintensity
- **Muscles**: Myositis → fibrosis
  - Acute: ↑ T2 SI & enhancement
  - Chronic: ↓ ↓ T2 SI
- **Bone**: ORN
  - Low T1, high T2, enhancing marrow
  - Diffuse inflammation but no mass
- **Cartilage**: Chondronecrosis
  - Loss of T1 signal; cartilage enhances
  - Focal swelling of surrounding soft tissues

DIFFERENTIAL DIAGNOSIS

Recurrent Tumor

- Key differential: Look for solid, enhancing mass

Skull Base or Mandible-Maxilla Osteomyelitis

- Infection often coincident with ORN
- Fragmentation more suggestive of ORN

PATHOLOGY

General Features

- Etiology
  - XRT destroys endothelial cells lining small blood vessels, resulting in obstructive arteriopathy
  - **Tissues less able to withstand additional stress**
    - Infection, tumor recurrence, or biopsy may precipitate necrosis
  - Predisposing factors: Short treatment time, large field, chronic infections, atherosclerosis
    - Many complications seen only with doses **≥ 60 Gy**
    - Ongoing alcohol & tobacco use contribute to mucosal necrosis
  - **Bones**: ORN

Timeline for Radiation-Induced Complications

Radiation Complication	Peak Time of Onset
Early delayed cerebral radiation necrosis	1-6 months
Mucosal deep ulceration	1-9 months
Extreme soft tissue swelling	3-6 months
Chondronecrosis	3-12 months
Osteoradionecrosis	6-12 months
TMJ & pterygoid fibrosis	12-15 months
Late delayed cerebral radiation necrosis	12-15 months
Delayed radiation myelopathy	12-24 months
Accelerated atherosclerosis	1-3 years
Cranial neuropathy	≥ 2 years
Radiation plexopathy	2-4 years
Radiation-induced 2nd neoplasm	> 10 years

- Most often affects mandible
  - Often precipitated by dental infection or extraction
  - Diseased teeth must be extracted prior to XRT
- May affect hyoid, sphenoid, temporal, or frontal bone
- **Cartilage**: Chondronecrosis
  - Perichondrial injury allows infection or tumor to involve cartilage → necrosis
  - Associated with infection &/or recurrent tumor
  - Laryngeal necrosis uncommon, occurs in ~ 1%
    - Peaks in 1st 12 months; may occur years later
- **Spinal cord**: Radiation myelopathy
  - Extensive demyelination, coagulation necrosis
- **Radiation-induced neoplasm**
  - Possibly due to imperfect repair of XRT-induced DNA strand breakage in tumor suppressor genes
  - By definition: > 5 years after XRT, most occur > 15 years
  - Long latency makes necrosis or recurrence less likely than new tumor
  - Meningioma
    - Often multiple, more likely higher grade
  - Sarcoma
    - Rhabdomyosarcoma most common
    - Retinoblastoma patients with *RB* gene especially at risk for sarcoma
  - Parotid malignancy
    - Mucoepidermoid carcinoma most common
  - Glial neoplasm
    - Glioblastoma predominates
    - Same sites as cerebral radionecrosis but much longer latency period

CLINICAL ISSUES

Presentation

- Most common signs/symptoms
  - Symptoms vary by complication site
  - **Pain** is common
    - Odynophagia, otalgia
    - Otalgia and otorrhea if temporal bone
  - Fetor, sputum with cartilage &/or bone fragments

- Masticator muscle fibrosis → trismus
- Pharyngeal muscle fibrosis → dysphagia, aspiration
- Radiation myelitis → paresthesia &/or paralysis

Natural History & Prognosis

- Most complications occur in **1st 2 years** after XRT; this is peak period for squamous cell carcinoma recurrence also
  - May occur up to 5-8 years post XRT

Treatment

- Largely conservative
  - Antibiotics if potentiated or complicated by infection
  - Hyperbaric oxygen therapy if recurrent tumor absolutely excluded
  - Soft tissue healing may take ≥ 6 months
- If extensive/fulminant, may require surgical resection

DIAGNOSTIC CHECKLIST

Image Interpretation Pearls

- Most complications of radiation occur in 1st 2 years but may still occur as long as 5 years post XRT
- Key differential is always residual/recurrent tumor
  - Recurrent tumor or infection may precipitate necrosis
  - Biopsy may also precipitate necrosis
- Look for solid, enhancing mass to favor tumor over radiation necrosis

Reporting Tips

- By being familiar with **expected** XRT changes, it is easier to recognize complications and residual/recurrent tumor
- All tissues in field at risk for complications
  - Not uncommon to see multiple complications

SELECTED REFERENCES

1. Ahmad S et al: Incidence of intracranial radiation necrosis following postoperative radiation therapy for sinonasal malignancies. Laryngoscope. ePub, 2016
2. Horky LL et al: Dual phase FDG-PET imaging of brain metastases provides superior assessment of recurrence versus post-treatment necrosis. J Neurooncol. 103(1):137-46, 2011
3. Glastonbury CM et al: The postradiation neck: evaluating response to treatment and recognizing complications. AJR Am J Roentgenol. 195(2):W164-71, 2010

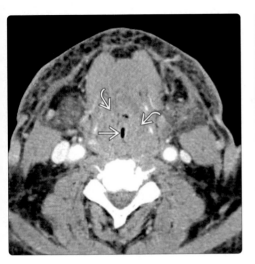
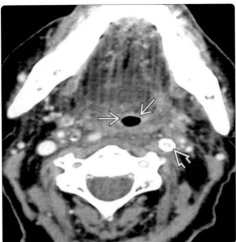

(Left) *Axial CECT was performed 8 weeks after chemoXRT for supraglottic SCCa. Symmetric expected XRT changes are seen throughout neck, but note marked airway narrowing ➡ due to extensive supraglottic edema ➡. Airway edema is common, but airway symptoms are not common after XRT.* (Right) *Axial CECT in a different case shows XRT-induced fibrosis producing narrowed oropharynx ➡ & dysphagia. Mucosal contour is smooth, & there is no mass. Note marked carotid calcification ➡.*

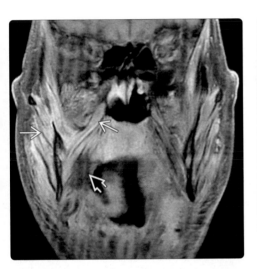
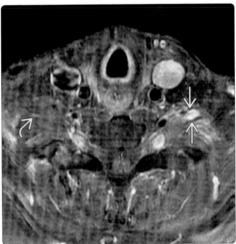

(Left) *Coronal T1 C+ FS MR shows marked enhancement of muscles of mastication, particularly on the right ➡. There is marked pharyngeal mucosa enhancement but a nonenhancing ulcer at the lateral oropharyngeal wall ➡. Absence of mass and enhancement favors ulceration from tissue necrosis.* (Right) *Axial T1 C+ FS MR in a patient with left arm weakness shows enlarged, enhancing left nerve roots ➡ compared to the right ➡. Patient has brachial plexitis 3 years after chemoXRT for tongue base SCCa.*

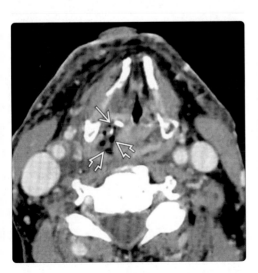
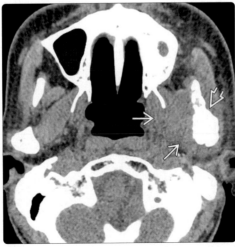

(Left) *Axial CECT 4 months after XRT for hypopharynx SCCa shows air and necrotic debris ➡ posterior to the right cricoarytenoid joint. Arytenoid cartilage ➡ appears fragmented from chondronecrosis.* (Right) *Axial NECT in a patient treated 14 years prior for NPC demonstrates swelling of masticator space tissues ➡ and irregular sclerotic expanded mandible ➡. ORN is less likely in this time frame and more commonly occurs in relation to dental infection. This is radiation-induced osteosarcoma.*

KEY FACTS

TERMINOLOGY

- Osteoradionecrosis
- Complication of radiation therapy (XRT) with necrosis of bone and failure to heal

IMAGING

- Mandible > > maxilla or skull base
- Associated soft tissue edema & induration common
- Difficult to exclude superinfection
- CT: Mixed lytic/sclerotic bone with sequestra
- MR: Diffuse low T1, high T2 signal from edema
- Diffuse enhancement common

TOP DIFFERENTIAL DIAGNOSES

- Osteomyelitis
- Bisphosphonate osteonecrosis
- Alveolar ridge squamous cell carcinoma (SCCa)
- Radiation-induced 2nd primary tumor

PATHOLOGY

- Radiation results in damage to small blood vessels resulting in hypovascular marrow
- Impairs ability of bone to cope with stressors, such as infection or trauma
- May be precipitated by biopsy or tooth extraction
- Pathologic fracture through bone common

CLINICAL ISSUES

- Most often follows XRT for oral cavity SCCa
- Exposed bone from ulcerated mucosa usually present
- Incidence peaks 1st 6-12 months post XRT
- May occur years after XRT

DIAGNOSTIC CHECKLIST

- Jaw pain, nonhealing mucosal ulceration, lytic/sclerotic CT changes
- Must exclude recurrent SCCa as source of changes

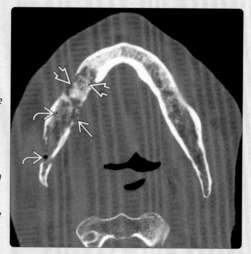
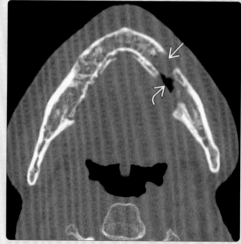

(Left) Axial bone CT demonstrates typical mixed lytic/sclerotic changes and cortical bone interruption ➡ in the right hemimandible following XRT. Note intraosseous gas bubbles ➡ and evolving bone within bone appearance ➡ due to intraosseous bone sequestra. (Right) Axial bone CT in a different patient shows a primarily lytic pattern of osteoradionecrosis (ORN) with interrupted cortex ➡ and intraosseous gas ➡. There is also pathologic fracture of the left mandibular body with off-setting of bone.

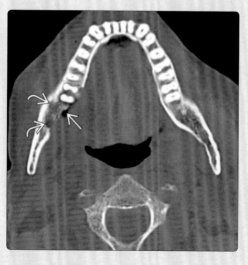
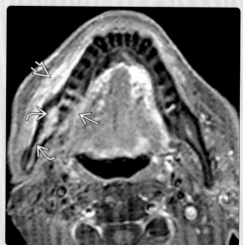

(Left) Axial bone CT shows mandibular extraction socket with small bubble of gas ➡ indicating mucosal erosion, with hazy lucency of adjacent bone ➡. Patient had exposed bone on the physical exam. (Right) Axial T1WI C+ MR in the same patient shows enhancement in the mandible ➡ and diffusely in the lingual ➡ and buccal ➡ soft tissues around the mandible. With a history of prior XRT and now a swollen right face with an exposed bone around socket, imaging is most consistent with early ORN.

Osteoradionecrosis

TERMINOLOGY

Abbreviations

- Osteoradionecrosis (ORN)

Definitions

- Complication of radiation therapy (XRT) with necrosis of bone and failure to heal

IMAGING

General Features

- Best diagnostic clue
  - Mixed lytic/sclerotic bone in patient previously treated with XRT
    - Exposed bone through ulcerated skin or mucosa usually present
    - Often complicated by fracture; may have infection as well
    - Lack of discrete soft tissue mass helps differentiate from recurrent tumor
- Location
  - In H&N, most often seen in jaw and skull base
    - Mandible > > maxilla or other facial bones
    - Temporal or sphenoid bone of skull base
    - Also described in frontal and hyoid bones
- Size
  - May be focal or extensive

Imaging Recommendations

- Best imaging tool
  - Bone CT is best diagnostic modality
  - Soft tissue imaging shows diffuse inflammation but no mass
- Protocol advice
  - Thin bone algorithm CT slices with coronal and sagittal reformations
    - Multiplanar images help plan surgery and potential reconstruction
  - CECT if superimposed infection or recurrent tumor suspected clinically

Radiographic Findings

- Extraoral plain film
  - Mixed lytic/sclerotic bone
  - Extent of involvement & destruction often underestimated by radiography

CT Findings

- CECT
  - Soft tissue edema & induration common, even when no superinfection
  - Focal abnormal enhancement or small abscesses may be evident when infected
  - Fistulization to skin can occur
- Bone CT
  - Cortical bone disruption on background of mixed lysis & sclerosis
    - Loss of trabeculation results in lytic appearance with superimposed sclerosis
  - Sequestered spicules of bone and fragmentation often present
  - Bubbles of air often present within abnormal mandible or in adjacent necrotic tissues
  - Pathological fractures may be evident, may precipitate patient presentation
- PET/CT
  - Marked FDG uptake typically seen with ORN
    - Probably due to inflammatory component
  - CECT important to interpret with PET study to detect recurrent tumor

MR Findings

- T1WI
  - Diffuse low signal intensity of marrow space
  - Disrupted cortex may be evident
- T2WI
  - Diffuse high signal of marrow space
  - Adjacent tissues may appear edematous also
- T1WI C+ FS
  - Diffuse enhancement of marrow common
  - No adjacent solid mass

DIFFERENTIAL DIAGNOSIS

Osteomyelitis

- Mixed lytic/sclerotic bone in patient with infected tooth or extraction site & no history of XRT
- Osteomyelitis may be found with ORN; frequently difficult to differentiate

Bisphosphonate Osteonecrosis

- Mixed lytic/sclerotic bone in patient treated with intravenous bisphosphonates
- Patient has no radiation history

Alveolar Ridge Squamous Cell Carcinoma

- Primarily destructive bone changes with mucosal ulceration
- Solid soft tissue enhancing lesion
- Recurrent squamous cell carcinoma (SCCa) is main imaging differential when ORN is present

Radiation-Induced 2nd Primary Tumor

- Occurs many years after XRT; typically ≥ 8 years
- Sarcoma is most frequent; often associated with soft tissue mass

PATHOLOGY

General Features

- Etiology
  - Radiation results in damage to small blood vessels
    - Endothelial cells lining blood vessels are destroyed, resulting in obstructive arteriopathy
    - Impairs ability of bone to respond to stressors
  - ORN often precipitated by infection or trauma including tooth extraction or **tissue biopsy**
- Associated abnormalities
  - Bacterial infection in necrotic bone often present
    - Current theory suggests osteomyelitis not primary event

Staging, Grading, & Classification

- Various staging or clinical grading systems used
- **Store and Boysen staging for jaw**

- o Stage 0: Mucosal defects only
- o Stage I: Radiologic evidence of ORN + intact mucosa
- o Stage II: Radiologic evidence of ORN + denuded bone
- o Stage III: Exposed radionecrotic bone + orocutaneous fistulae

Gross Pathologic & Surgical Features

- Necrotic fragmented bone with sequestra & spicules
- Fragile, ulcerated mucosa with exposed bone

Microscopic Features

- **Bone necrosis primarily due to hypoxia**
  - o XRT results in obliteration of arteries, including inferior alveolar artery
- Bone is hypocellular and periosteum nonviable
- Biopsy specimen may be complicated with osteonecrosis, osteomyelitis, and recurrent/residual tumor

CLINICAL ISSUES

Presentation

- Most common signs/symptoms
  - o Ulcerated skin or mucosa with exposed necrotic bone in patient with prior history of H&N XRT
    - – Mandible is most common facial bone involved
    - – May be exposed through oral ulceration
- Other signs/symptoms
  - o Fistulization to skin
  - o Oral pain, trismus, dysesthesia, foul breath
  - o Masticator space infection with small abscesses

Demographics

- Epidemiology
  - o Multiple factors influence incidence of ORN
    - – Tumor: Risk increased with stage III/IV primary tumor
    - – XRT plan: Risk increased with higher dose, large field size, short treatment time
      - □ Intensity modulated XRT (IMRT) with lower bone exposure has lower incidence of ORN
    - – Treatment: Risk increased if surgery (mandibulectomy or other osteotomy) in addition to XRT
    - – Patient factors: Risk increased with poor oral hygiene, ongoing alcohol & tobacco exposure

Natural History & Prognosis

- Incidence of ORN is ≤ 6%
- Incidence peaks: 1st 6-12 months post XRT

Treatment

- **Prevention** most important **prior** to XRT
  - o Dental extractions and periodontal care prior to XRT
  - o Improved nutritional status prior and during XRT
  - o Cessation of tobacco & alcohol use
- Conservative treatment includes antibiotics and local irrigation
- Hyperbaric oxygen therapy to promote angiogenesis and aid in treating associated infection
  - o Essential to exclude residual/recurrent tumor prior to hyperbaric oxygen treatment
- Sequestrectomy and primary wound closure for early disease
- Bone resection and reconstruction for severe progressive disease

DIAGNOSTIC CHECKLIST

Consider

- ORN in any patient treated with XRT and new pain, nonhealing mucosal ulceration, lytic/sclerotic CT changes
- Essential to exclude **recurrent SCCa** as source of pain and cortical disruption
  - o Tumor favored when solid soft tissue mass present
- While ORN may occur several years after treatment, if ≥ 8 years, consider **XRT-induced sarcoma,** especially if soft tissue mass associated

Image Interpretation Pearls

- Check for local infection or pathologic fracture

Reporting Tips

- Describe the extent of disease, cortical bone disruption, exposed bone spicules, and sequestrations

SELECTED REFERENCES

1. Deshpande SS et al: Osteoradionecrosis of the mandible: through a radiologist's eyes. Clin Radiol. 70(2):197-205, 2015
2. Mitsimponas KT et al: Osteo-radio-necrosis (ORN) and bisphosphonate-related osteonecrosis of the jaws (BRONJ): the histopathological differences under the clinical similarities. Int J Clin Exp Pathol. 7(2):496-508, 2014
3. Gevorgyan A et al: Osteoradionecrosis of the mandible: a case series at a single institution. J Otolaryngol Head Neck Surg. 42:46, 2013
4. Armin BB et al: Brachytherapy-mediated bone damage in a rat model investigating maxillary osteoradionecrosis. Arch Otolaryngol Head Neck Surg. 138(2):167-71, 2012
5. Dholam KP et al: Dental implants in irradiated jaws: a literature review. J Cancer Res Ther. 8 Suppl 1:S85-93, 2012
6. Hamilton JD et al: Superimposed infection in mandibular osteoradionecrosis: diagnosis and outcomes. J Comput Assist Tomogr. 36(6):725-31, 2012
7. Tchanque-Fossuo CN et al: Amifostine remediates the degenerative effects of radiation on the mineralization capacity of the murine mandible. Plast Reconstr Surg. 129(4):646e-55e, 2012
8. Cannady SB et al: Free flap reconstruction for osteoradionecrosis of the jaws—outcomes and predictive factors for success. Head Neck. 33(3):424-8, 2011
9. Nabil S et al: Incidence and prevention of osteoradionecrosis after dental extraction in irradiated patients: a systematic review. Int J Oral Maxillofac Surg. 40(3):229-43, 2011
10. O'Dell K et al: Osteoradionecrosis. Oral Maxillofac Surg Clin North Am. 23(3):455-64, 2011
11. Tamplen M et al: Standardized analysis of mandibular osteoradionecrosis in a rat model. Otolaryngol Head Neck Surg. 145(3):404-10, 2011
12. Thariat J et al: [Revisiting the dose-effect correlations in irradiated head and neck cancer using automatic segmentation tools of the dental structures, mandible and maxilla.] Cancer Radiother. 15(8):683-90, 2011
13. Bak M et al: Contemporary reconstruction of the mandible. Oral Oncol. 46(2):71-6, 2010
14. Chrcanovic BR et al: Osteoradionecrosis of the jaws–a current overview–part 1: Physiopathology and risk and predisposing factors. Oral Maxillofac Surg. 14(1):3-16, 2010
15. Jacobson AS et al: Reconstruction of bilateral osteoradionecrosis of the mandible using a single fibular free flap. Laryngoscope. 120(2):273-5, 2010
16. Jegoux F et al: Radiation effects on bone healing and reconstruction: interpretation of the literature. Oral Surg Oral Med Oral Pathol Oral Radiol Endod. 109(2):173-84, 2010
17. Scully C et al: Hot topics in special care dentistry. 10. Osteoradionecrosis/radiotherapy. Dent Update. 37(2):127, 2010
18. Spiegelberg L et al: Hyperbaric oxygen therapy in the management of radiation-induced injury in the head and neck region: a review of the literature. J Oral Maxillofac Surg. 68(8):1732-9, 2010
19. Almazrooa SA et al: Bisphosphonate and nonbisphosphonate-associated osteonecrosis of the jaw: a review. J Am Dent Assoc. 140(7):864-75, 2009
20. Bagan JV et al: Osteonecrosis of the jaws by intravenous bisphosphonates and osteoradionecrosis: a comparative study. Med Oral Patol Oral Cir Bucal. 14(12):e616-9, 2009

Osteoradionecrosis

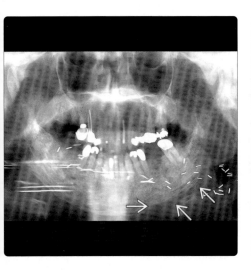

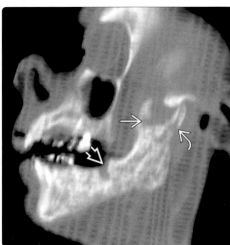

(Left) AP panorex from a patient with prior surgery and XRT to oral cavity reveals diffuse thickening & sclerosis of the mandible with coarsened trabeculae and loss of definition of the cortical bone along the inferior left hemimandibular margin ➡. (Right) Sagittal oblique reconstruction shows heterogeneous multifocal lucency, cortical interruption, and trabecular and cortical thickening and sclerosis. Note deep molar extraction socket ➡. There is fragmentation of the coronoid process ➡ and condylar neck ➡.

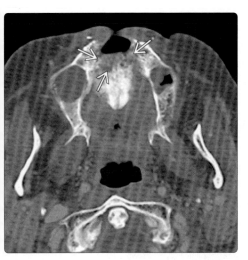

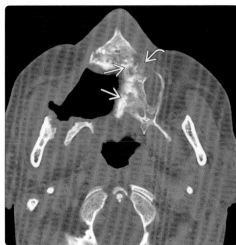

(Left) Axial bone CT in a patient treated with XRT for nasal septal squamous cell carcinoma shows lytic process of the anterior maxilla with a discrete wedge of destroyed and missing bone ➡. (Right) Axial bone CT in a different patient shows right surgical palatectomy but mixed sclerotic ➡ and lytic ➡ changes in the left maxilla, which was included in XRT field. Maxilla is relatively radioresistant, and ORN is rare. Imaging findings are identical as seen in the mandible and other facial and skull base bones.

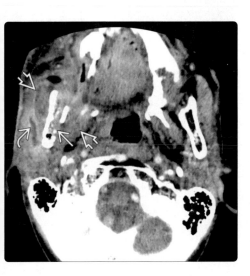

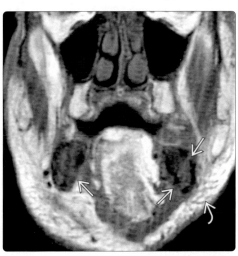

(Left) Axial CECT shows ORN of the right mandible complicated by infection of the masticator space. There is cortical interruption ➡ and diffuse severe edema of the parotid gland and muscles of mastication ➡ and a dilated parotid duct ➡ filled with inflammatory debris. (Right) Coronal T1WI MR shows diffuse replacement of normal mandibular fatty marrow signal. There are multiple focal areas of interrupted cortical bone ➡. Induration and edema of subcutaneous tissues ➡ are common findings in ORN mandible.

Post Laryngectomy

TERMINOLOGY

- Imaging findings following resection of whole larynx or part of larynx
- Most often performed for neoplasm
- **Total laryngectomy (TL)**: Larynx completely resected and neopharynx created
  - Neopharynx connects oropharynx to esophagus
  - Trachea no longer communicates with pharynx
  - Need tracheostomy to breathe, prosthesis to speak
- **Partial laryngectomy (PL)**: Conservative surgery
  - Aim is to preserve voice and breathing, swallowing without aspiration
  - Cordectomy → vertical or horizontal partial laryngectomy → near-total laryngectomy
  - Imaging varies from near-normal to complex reconstruction and deformity
  - Permanent tracheostomy required only with near total laryngectomy

TOP DIFFERENTIAL DIAGNOSES

- Larynx trauma
- Radiated larynx

CLINICAL ISSUES

- **Declining use of both PL and TL** with ↑ use of organ preservation chemoradiation
- Declining use of open surgery in favor of endoscopic transoral laser surgery
- Laryngectomy also used for cartilaginous laryngeal tumors, invasive thyroid tumors, salvage after failed chemoradiation, chondronecrosis, nonfunctioning larynx posttreatment

DIAGNOSTIC CHECKLIST

- Imaging confusion occurs most often with complex appearance of partial laryngectomy
- First determine type of procedure
- Look for recurrent mass and lymphadenopathy

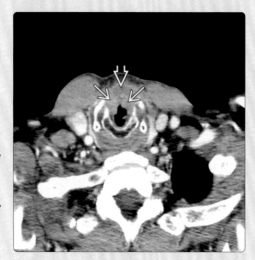
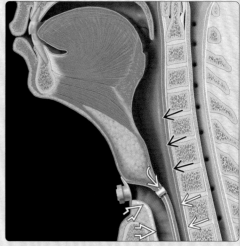

(Left) Axial CECT in a patient with T4N0M0 carcinoma of the larynx shows subglottic extension ➡ and anterior extension to prelaryngeal tissues ➡. (Right) Sagittal graphic depicts expected appearance after total laryngectomy with laryngeal cartilages and hyoid resected. Neopharynx ➡ connects oral cavity to esophagus ➡, while trachea ➡ is brought to skin surface as tracheostomy. Tracheoesophageal voice prosthesis ➡ is a 1-way valve that allows speech when patient manually occludes stoma.

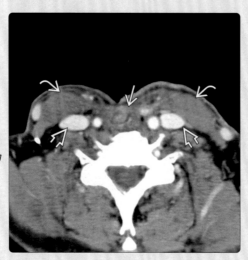
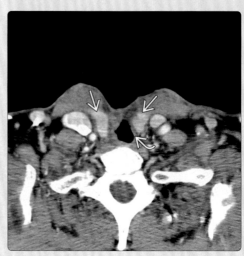

(Left) Axial CECT in the same patient following total laryngectomy, right modified neck dissection, & gastric pull-up demonstrates neopharynx as a multilayered midline tubular structure ➡. Both sternocleidomastoid muscles ➡ and jugular veins ➡ are preserved. (Right) Axial CECT shows new contour of thyroid lobes ➡ after midline splitting of thyroid capsule. If 1 lobe is resected, remaining lobe may be mistaken for node, recurrent mass, or even pseudoaneurysm. Distal anastomosis ➡ often has slightly irregular contour.

TERMINOLOGY

Definitions

- Imaging findings following resection of whole or part of larynx, typically for neoplasm
  - Total laryngectomy (TL): Larynx resected, neopharynx created, permanent tracheal stoma
  - Partial laryngectomy (PL): Preserves voice & breathing without permanent tracheostomy
    - Cordectomy, vertical partial laryngectomy (VPL), horizontal supraglottic laryngectomy (SGL), supracricoid laryngectomy (SCL) with cricohyoidopexy (CHP) or cricohyoidoepiglottopexy (CHEP)
      - "Pexy" indicates surgical fixation of structure
    - Now more often performed as endoscopic **transoral laser surgery (TLS)** rather than open surgery

IMAGING

General Features

- Best diagnostic clue
  - Abnormal contour of pharyngeal airway (vestibule), absence of soft tissue ± part or whole of 1 or more cartilages

CT Findings

- CECT
  - Vestibule of neolarynx appears deformed
  - Soft tissue structures &/or cartilages absent
  - Arytenoid soft tissue thickening common with PL
  - **Pseudocord** scar tissue develops between resected true vocal cord (TVC) and anterior portion of contralateral partially resected cord
    - Usually seen with VPL
  - Not uncommon to see patchy sclerosis or partial resection of cartilages
    - Not often helpful or indicative of recurrence
  - Open resection frequently accompanied by nodal dissection

Imaging Recommendations

- Best imaging tool
  - CECT allows more consistently good-quality larynx imaging
    - MR fraught with motion artifacts
  - PET/CECT: Extremely helpful after TL or PL & radiation, as edematous mucosa makes detecting recurrent squamous cell carcinoma difficult
    - Determine systemic disease prior to salvage TL

DIFFERENTIAL DIAGNOSIS

Larynx Trauma

- Deformity of cartilages following open or closed injury
- Cartilage should not be absent

Radiated Larynx

- Mucosal and deep fat space edema
- Cartilages present unless chondronecrosis

PATHOLOGY

Staging, Grading, & Classification

- Surgeries defined as radical (total laryngectomy) or conservative (cordectomy or partial laryngectomy)
- **Use of chemoradiation and TLS resulted in marked decline of TL and open PL**
- Multiple different forms of PL but goal always preservation of laryngeal function (breathing, voice, swallowing)
  - Defined by plane of resection and form of reconstruction
- Cordectomy
  - Use: Tumor isolated to 1 TVC without fixation
  - Resected: TVC, vocalis muscle, and tendon
    - Typically performed endoscopically (TLS)
  - Imaging: Very subtle; may appear normal
- Vertical partial laryngectomy
  - Use: Early stage glottic to anterior commissure (AC) ± arytenoid, **without** cord fixation
  - **Frontolateral laryngectomy**
    - Use: Tumors to AC without TVC fixation
    - Resected: Vertical midline segment of thyroid cartilage, TVC (± arytenoid) with ventricle and false cord, AC & small part of contralateral anterior cord
    - Reconstruction: Contralateral cord mucosa sutured to perichondrium; ipsilateral side may be left to granulate
    - Imaging: Defect in midline thyroid cartilage, missing aryepiglottic (AE) fold ± ipsilateral arytenoid, dense scar at site of resected cords = **pseudocord**
  - **Hemilaryngectomy**
    - Use: When more posterior extension of tumor to arytenoid cartilage
    - Resected: As with frontolateral **plus** ipsilateral arytenoid, mucosa of AE fold, and thyroid lamina
    - Reconstruction: Grafts, flap, muscle may be used
- **Horizontal laryngectomy**
  - **Supraglottic laryngectomy**
    - Use: Supraglottic tumor not involving ventricle, normal cord mobility
    - Resected: Epiglottis, false cords, AE folds, ventricle, upper 1/3 thyroid cartilage, thyrohyoid membrane
    - Remaining: TVC, arytenoids, lower thyroid cartilage, cricoid
    - Reconstruction: Thyroid sutured to hyoid (thyrohyoidopexy)
    - Imaging: Hyoid & thyroid on same plane, redundant mucosa over arytenoids
  - **Extended SGL**: SGL **plus** 1 arytenoid cartilage, tongue base, or pyriform sinus resected
  - **3/4 laryngectomy**: SGL **plus** ipsilateral TVC & arytenoid cartilage resected
    - Remaining: Hyoid, unilateral glottis, cricoid
  - **Supracricoid laryngectomy**
    - Use: More extensive tumor, no cord fixation
    - Resected: Thyroid cartilage, paraglottic space, TVC, ventricle, false cords, anterior commissure
    - Remaining: Hyoid, 1 or both arytenoids, cricoid
    - Reconstruction: 2 alternative pexy procedures
      - **CHP** if involvement of preepiglottic or paraglottic space, or thyroid cartilage

- □ Imaging: Hyoid sutured to cricoid, no thyroid cartilage, 1 or both cricoarytenoid joints present
- □ **CHEP** if epiglottis and preepiglottic fat can be spared
- □ Imaging: As above but hyoid, cricoid, and epiglottis attached to each other
- **Near total laryngectomy**
  - ○ Use: Advanced unilateral tumor
  - ○ Resected: 1/2 of larynx and anterior part of contralateral TVC **plus** hyoid, epiglottis, preepiglottic space, valleculae
  - ○ Remaining: 1 arytenoid, part of thyroarytenoid muscle, part of thyroid and cricoid cartilages, recurrent laryngeal nerve
  - ○ Reconstruction: Permanent tracheostomy needed for breathing
  - ○ Imaging: Only portion of 1 side of thyroid and cricoid cartilages plus arytenoid present, tracheostomy
- **Total laryngectomy**
  - ○ Use: T4 primary tumor, subglottic extension of tumor to cricoid, salvage for recurrent disease post treatment, nonfunctioning larynx posttreatment, chondronecrosis, thyroid tumors invading larynx, cartilaginous laryngeal tumors
  - ○ Resected: Entire cartilage framework plus endolaryngeal structures, variable thyroid gland
  - ○ Reconstruction: Constrictor muscles or jejunum to create neopharynx
  - ○ Imaging: No larynx, thyroid remnant, tubular neopharynx, ± tracheoesophageal (TE) valve (speech prosthesis)

CLINICAL ISSUES

Presentation

- Most common signs/symptoms
  - ○ Typically performed to maximize local control of laryngeal or hypopharyngeal carcinoma
  - ○ Chemoradiation often results in better speech preservation than PL
  - ○ TL separates trachea from neopharynx and esophagus
    - Speech best with TE valve
    - Breathing occurs through suprasternal stoma
    - Food/liquids swallowed orally then pass through neopharynx to esophagus
  - ○ Partial laryngectomy aims to preserve **voice & breathing** without permanent tracheostomy
    - Also to allow swallowing without aspiration

Demographics

- Epidemiology
  - ○ **Declining use of PL with increasing use of chemoradiation for laryngeal carcinoma**
    - Organ preservation protocols
  - ○ **Declining use of open PL in favor of TLS**
    - Less morbidity, better postoperative function

Treatment

- Laryngeal carcinoma most often treated by **radiation, chemoradiation, and endoscopic surgery**, alone or in combination
  - ○ Increasing use of radiation ± chemo for T1-T3
  - ○ TLS favored over open procedures

- **Glottic carcinoma**
  - ○ With early stage, XRT has better voice preservation
  - ○ Endoscopic laser resection & cordectomy, VPL, SCL with cricohyoidoepiglottopexy
  - ○ TL for T4 tumor
- **Supraglottic carcinoma**
  - ○ With early stage, XRT has better voice preservation
  - ○ Horizontal SGL, SCL with cricohyoidopexy, near total or 3/4 laryngectomy
  - ○ TL for large volume T3 and for T4 tumor
- **Subglottic**
  - ○ TL often; usually advanced presentation
- New directions of surgical management are transoral robotic surgery (TORS) and photodynamic therapy
- Laryngectomies may also be used for **chondronecrosis, invasive thyroid tumors, cartilaginous tumors, caustic destruction of larynx**

DIAGNOSTIC CHECKLIST

Image Interpretation Pearls

- TL typically has straightforward appearance
  - ○ Pitfalls: Misinterpretation of residual thyroid as recurrence; failure to identify residual or new nodes
  - ○ Recurrence tends to occur at proximal &/or distal anastomosis
- Confusion most often occurs when imaging complex PL
  - ○ **Best method to minimize interpretation error is to read surgical notes (if possible)**
  - ○ Have systematic method of evaluating postoperative neck

Reporting Tips

- **Determine which type of procedure was performed**
  - ○ Type of resection: Complete or partial cartilage absence, vertical or horizontal resection plane
  - ○ Type of reconstruction: Relationship of remaining cartilages to hyoid
  - ○ Additional soft tissue flaps placed
- Look for asymmetric neolaryngeal wall thickening or luminal mass
- Look for **abnormal masses** in remaining tissues, particularly at anastomoses
- Check for neck **adenopathy**, apical lung **metastases**

SELECTED REFERENCES

1. Takes RP et al: Current trends in initial management of hypopharyngeal cancer: the declining use of open surgery. Head Neck. 34(2):270-81, 2012
2. Ferreiro-Argüelles C et al: CT findings after laryngectomy. Radiographics. 28(3):869-82; quiz 914, 2008
3. Kelsch TA et al: Partial laryngectomy imaging. Semin Ultrasound CT MR. 24(3):147-56, 2003
4. Mukherji SK et al: Imaging of the post-treatment larynx. Eur J Radiol. 44(2):108-19, 2002
5. Bely-Toueg N et al: Normal laryngeal CT findings after supracricoid partial laryngectomy. AJNR Am J Neuroradiol. 22(10):1872-80, 2001

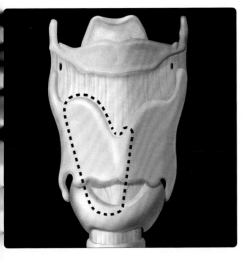

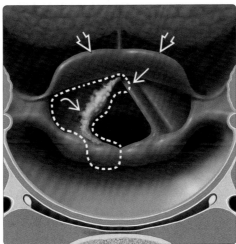

(Left) *Coronal graphic shows cartilaginous components resected with right hemilaryngectomy. Frontolateral vertical partial laryngectomy involves resection of only midline portion of thyroid cartilage.* (Right) *Endoscopic graphic of glottic tumor ➡ with dotted white line shows expected resection plan for right hemilaryngectomy vertical partial laryngectomy (VPL). Resection includes anterior portion of contralateral uninvolved cord ➡ but spares epiglottis ➡.*

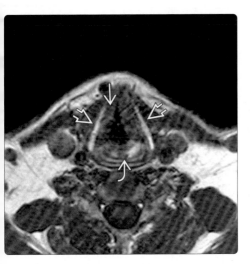

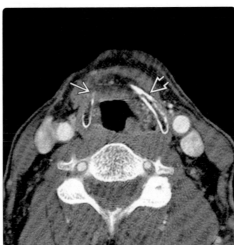

(Left) *Axial T1 MR shows subtle changes to glottis from right endoscopic cordectomy. Note the right true vocal cord is ➡ subtly smaller and deformed compared to normal left cord. Thyroid laminae ➡ and cricoid cartilage ➡ are still present after cordectomy.* (Right) *Axial CECT following open right hemilaryngectomy (VPL) is shown. Hyoid and epiglottis were present on more superior slices. Immediately below hyoid is the superior left thyroid lamina ➡. The anterior aspect of right thyroid cartilage ➡ has been resected.*

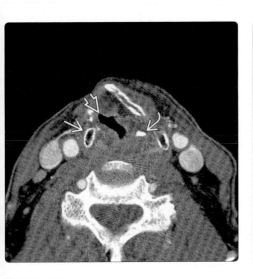

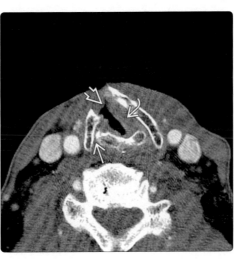

(Left) *Axial CECT shows the same patient with right true and false cords, ventricle, arytenoid, aryepiglottic fold, anterior commissure, and anterior part of left true vocal cord resected, along with most of right anterior thyroid lamina ➡. Left arytenoid ➡ is still present. Note the significant deformity of airway ➡.* (Right) *Axial CECT more inferiorly in the same patient shows left vocal cord ➡ and marked deformity of right glottis from right hemilaryngectomy ➡. Right cricothyroid joint is intact ➡.*

(Left) Axial CECT in a patient with endoscopic resection similar to left frontolateral VPL shows left true vocal cord, ventricle, and thyroarytenoid muscle resected. Anterior commissure and anterior 1/3 of right vocal cord are also removed, but the arytenoids are present ➡. (Right) Axial CECT more inferiorly shows nodular soft tissue pseudocord ➡ that was biopsy-proven scar tissue. Focal defect of right thyroid lamina was thought to be injury at prior anterior right cord resection ➡.

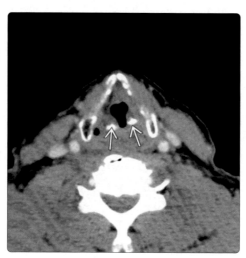
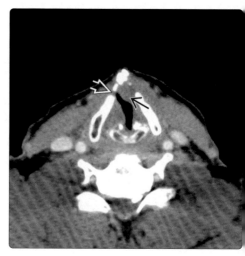

(Left) Sagittal graphic with dotted black line depicts expected resection plane with supraglottic partial laryngectomy (SGL), which is a horizontal hemilaryngectomy. True cord, hyoid ➡, and lower portion of thyroid cartilage are typically retained. (Right) Axial CECT following open SGL shows resection of anterior midportion of hyoid and partial resection of right aryepiglottic fold ➡. Right modified neck dissection was also performed ➡.

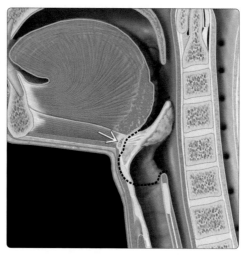
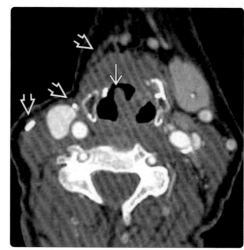

(Left) Sagittal CECT reformat in the same patient shows absence of epiglottis, which should extend up to oropharyngeal airway ➡. Note elevated location of remaining larynx ➡. (Right) Sagittal CECT reformat further laterally in the same patient shows new relationship of hyoid ➡ to remaining lower 1/2 of thyroid lamina ➡ following thyrohyoidopexy. This is routine with open SGL. The glottis, arytenoid, cricoid, and lower 1/3 of thyroid cartilages are typically preserved with this surgery.

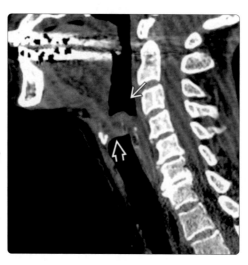
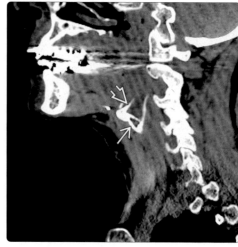

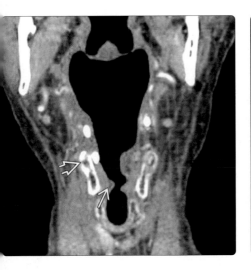
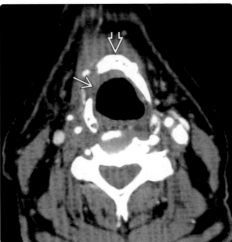

(Left) Coronal CECT reformat following endoscopic right SGL shows resection of entire epiglottis, right false cord, & supraglottic laryngeal mucosa down to right laryngeal ventricle. There is preservation of right true cord ➡ and cartilages. Surgical clip lies medial to thyroid lamina ➡.
(Right) Axial CECT in the same patient after endoscopic SGL shows smooth mucosal scar ➡ and demonstrates absence of superior portion of epiglottis, which should extend above preserved hyoid ➡.

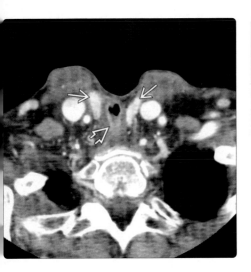
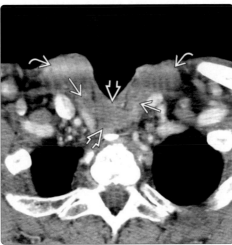

(Left) Baseline axial CECT just above tracheal stoma after total laryngectomy shows distal anastomosis ➡ of neopharynx to esophagus and both thyroid lobes ➡. (Right) Axial CECT in the same patient 9 months later shows new abnormal soft tissue at distal anastomosis ➡. Tumor is infiltrating thyroid lobes ➡, which are now difficult to define from sternocleidomastoid muscles ➡. Recurrent tumor tends to be at proximal or distal anastomosis or is nodal or metastatic.

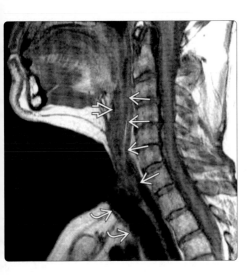
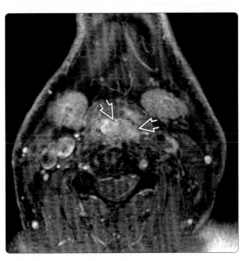

(Left) Sagittal T1 MR after total laryngectomy shows resection of laryngeal cartilages and creation of neopharynx ➡ with cervical trachea ➡ ending at stoma. Proximal anastomosis appears fuller than expected ➡, though this is subtle. (Right) Axial T1 C+ FS MR in the same patient at level of "fullness" seen on sagittal T1 reveals enhancing solid tissue at proximal anastomosis of neopharynx ➡, suggestive of recurrence. This was confirmed at biopsy.

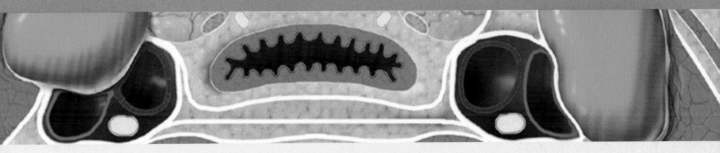

SECTION 19
Pediatric Lesions

Summary Thoughts: Congenital Lesions of Head and Neck

Neck masses are a common indication for imaging the pediatric H&N. The majority of neck masses in children are either congenital or inflammatory in origin, with only 5% of childhood neoplasms occurring in the H&N. The most common extrathyroid, nonneoplastic solid neck masses in children are related to inflammatory disease and do not require imaging unless there is concern for deep neck infection or abscess. The most common cystic masses in the pediatric H&N are congenital lesions secondary to abnormal embryogenesis involving the thyroglossal duct (TGD), branchial apparatus, or vascular endothelium. **Thyroglossal duct cysts** (TGDCs) account for 70-90% of all congenital neck abnormalities in children. The most common **branchial apparatus lesion** is the 2nd branchial cleft cyst (BCC), and **lymphatic malformations** are the most common vascular malformations in the H&N.

Whenever a cystic neck mass in a child is encountered on an imaging study, a very reasonable differential diagnosis can be made based on location (midline, paramidline, or lateral, as well as location relative to carotid sheath), imaging appearance (simple cyst, complicated cyst, enhancement, ± solid component), and clinical presentation (present since birth or acute onset, ± clinical evidence of infection).

Terminology

TGDC or tract is an anomalous remnant of the TGD, which, during normal development, completely involutes. Cysts are located anywhere from the midline posterior tongue at the foramen cecum to the thyroid bed in the lower neck.

Branchial apparatus anomalies may be in the form of cysts, sinus tracts, or fistulae. **Cysts** are fluid-filled with well-defined walls secondary to the failure of obliteration of a branchial cleft or pouch. **Sinus tracts** are congenital tracts with 1 opening, either externally to the skin surface (or external auditory canal) or internally to the pharynx (2nd branchial cleft), superolateral hypopharynx (3rd branchial cleft), or pyriform sinus (4th or 3rd branchial pouch). **Fistulae** are congenital tracts with 2 openings, 1 internally and 1 externally, secondary to failure of obliteration of the branchial cleft and pouch.

Imaging Techniques & Indications

US, CT, and MR are all reasonable options for initial imaging of neck masses in children. Modality choice depends on the clinical presentation, the referring clinical service, and the imaging modalities available at the time of imaging. For instance, if there is concern that a child with cellulitis and cervical adenitis has a drainable abscess deep to a palpable neck mass, US may be very helpful in determining the presence of underlying suppurative adenitis or frank abscess. Likewise, if a child is thought to have a TGDC, US is the imaging modality of choice to evaluate the suspected TGDC and prove the presence of a normal-appearing thyroid gland in the lower neck. Furthermore, US is the imaging modality of choice in patients with suspected infantile hemangioma, and color Doppler findings can be quite characteristic. However, CT is the initial imaging modality of choice to evaluate the total extent of disease in children with suspected deep neck infection and to assess for possible underlying pyriform sinus tract in children with left-sided neck abscesses that involve the left thyroid lobe.

In children who are not presenting with signs and symptoms of infection, CT or MR may be used as the initial imaging modality. The choice of which modality to use may depend on the need for sedation/anesthesia, which is usually required for MR in children under the age of 5 or 6 years. MR is the preferred imaging modality in children with suspected vascular malformations.

Embryology

The thyroid gland migrates from the foramen cecum at the midline posterior tongue to the paramidline location in the lower neck via the path of the **TGD**. The TGD normally involutes during the 5th or 6th week of gestation. However, remnant epithelium anywhere along the tract may persist and form a **TGDC**. As the TGD diverticulum descends caudally, it passes along the anterior surface of the developing hyoid bone, and therefore, remnants may be found anterior to the preepiglottic space of the larynx.

Branchial apparatus structures develop between the 4th and 6th week of gestation and consist of 6 pairs of mesodermal arches separated by 5 paired endodermal pouches internally and 5 paired ectodermal clefts externally. During the 6th week of gestation, the 2nd branchial arch overgrows the 3rd and 4th branchial arches, resulting in a combined 2nd, 3rd, and 4th branchial cleft, termed the "cervical sinus of His." Anomalies of the branchial apparatus include **cysts, sinus tracts, and fistulae**. The most common lesions for which imaging is indicated are **branchial apparatus cysts**, and most of these are related to anomalous development of a branchial cleft. However, a few are related to anomalous development of a branchial pouch.

Location of the lesion is the single most important determinant of the origin of a branchial apparatus anomaly. The **1st BCCs** account for ~ 8% of all branchial anomalies and are located in or around the external auditory canal, ear lobe, or parotid gland and may extend inferiorly to the angle of the mandible. The **2nd BCCs** account for up to 95% of all branchial apparatus anomalies and are subclassified by location using the Bailey classification: Type 1 cysts are located deep to the platysma muscle/anterior to the sternocleidomastoid muscle (SCM), type 2 cysts are posterior to the submandibular gland/anterior to the SCM and are the most common, type 3 cysts protrude between the external and internal carotid arteries, and type 4 cysts are directly adjacent to the pharyngeal wall (thought to be remnant of the 2nd pouch). Fistulas are rare; however, a 2nd branchial apparatus fistula is occasionally identified with an internal opening at the level of the pharynx and an external skin opening anterior to the lower aspect of the SCM.

Third BCCs are rare, located in the posterior compartment of the upper neck or anterior compartment of the lower neck. The 3rd pharyngeal pouch remnants are more common than cleft remnants and are related to descent of the thymic primordium from the lateral margins of the pharynx to the upper anterior mediastinum (via the thymopharyngeal duct) during the 6th to 9th week of gestation. If the duct does not undergo normal involution, a cervical thymic cyst may form that is usually in close association with the anterior margin of the carotid sheath. Formation is from interactions between the endodermal primordia and neural crest cells during normal thymic development and migration. Histologically, Hassall corpuscles will be identifiable within the cyst wall.

Differential Diagnosis of Congenital Lesions

Thyroglossal duct lesions

Thyroglossal duct cyst (TGDC): Tongue base to thyroid bed; embedded in strap muscles when infrahyoid

Ectopic thyroid tissue: Lingual location most common

Branchial apparatus lesions

1st branchial cleft cyst (type 1): Located anterior, inferior, or posterior to EAC

1st branchial cleft cyst (type 2): Located in or adjacent to parotid gland; may extend inferiorly to angle of mandible

2nd branchial cleft cyst: Most common location posterior to submandibular gland, lateral to carotid space, & anteromedial to sternocleidomastoid muscle

3rd branchial cleft cyst: Posterior cervical space upper neck, anterior to SCM lower neck

3rd branchial pouch remnant → thymopharyngeal duct cyst or ectopic thymus: Along course from pharynx to upper mediastinum

4th branchial pouch remnant → pyriform sinus tract: Patients present with left-sided abscess involving thyroid gland

Vascular malformations

Venous malformation: Slow-flow enhancing lesion, phleboliths common

Lymphatic malformation: Nonenhancing unilocular or multilocular ± fluid-fluid levels

Venolymphatic malformation: Mixed enhancing venous and nonenhancing lymphatic components

---

Ectopic foci of solid thymic tissue may also be deposited along the remnant duct.

Pyriform sinus tracts, or, rarely, fistulae represent a unique congenital anomaly of the 4th (or 3rd) pharyngeal pouch. This lesion should be suspected in any child presenting with neck infection involving the left thyroid lobe. The inflammation can frequently be traced superiorly to an asymmetric pyriform sinus apex. Post barium swallow CT study is frequently helpful to define the barium-filled tract extending from the pyriform sinus to the anterior lower neck.

Vascular malformations are congenital malformations of endothelial development that can be divided into capillary, lymphatic, venous, venolymphatic, and arteriovenous malformations based on the predominant endothelial characteristics of the lesion. The most common vascular malformations identified in the H&N are lymphatic malformations, venous malformations, and combined venolymphatic lesions.

Imaging Anatomy

Recognizing the defined location of a congenital abnormality, particularly congenital cysts, is key to arriving at the correct diagnosis or differential diagnosis. **Thyroglossal duct remnants** may be in the form of cysts or solid ectopic thyroid tissue anywhere from the midline tongue base to infrahyoid paramidline thyroid bed. The **1st BCCs** are in or around the EAC or parotid gland. The **2nd BCCs** are most commonly posteromedial to the submandibular gland and anteromedial to the SCM. Cysts in the posterior triangle of the upper neck may be **3rd BCCs or lymphatic malformations**. Cysts along the lower anterior margin of the SCM may be from the 2nd or 3rd branchial cleft or be lymphatic malformations. Cysts or solid masses in close association with the carotid sheath along the tract of the thymopharyngeal duct, from the angle of the mandible to the upper mediastinum, should raise the question of **cervical thymic cyst or ectopic thymus**.

Differential Diagnosis

Thyroglossal Duct Lesions
- Thyroglossal duct lesions are seen anywhere from the tongue base to the thyroid bed.

- The lingual thyroid is the most common ectopic thyroid lesion.

Branchial Apparatus Lesions
- First BCCs include type I and type II cysts. Type 1 cysts are located anterior, inferior, or posterior to the EAC. Type II cysts occur in the superficial, parotid, or parapharyngeal space, and may extend as low as the posterior submandibular space.
- Second BCCs most commonly occur posterolateral to the submandibular gland, lateral to the carotid space, and anteromedial to the SCM.
- Third BCCs are seen in the posterior cervical space of the upper neck or along the anterior border of the SCM in the mid and lower neck.
- Third branchial pouch remnants present as thymopharyngeal duct cysts or ectopic thymus.
- Fourth branchial pouch remnants present as a pyriform sinus tract with recurrent thyroiditis or thyroid abscess, usually left-sided. More recent literature suggests that this may be a 3rd branchial pouch remnant.

Vascular Malformations
- Venous malformations are slow-flow lesions with moderate postcontrast enhancement and phleboliths.
- Lymphatic malformations may be uni- or multilocular, may involve a single or multiple spaces, and most often present as nonenhancing multiseptated cystic masses with fluid-fluid levels.
- Mixed venolymphatic malformations have nonenhancing lymphatic and enhancing venous elements. Characteristic phleboliths may be present.

Selected References

1. Stern JS et al: Imaging of pediatric head and neck masses. Otolaryngol Clin North Am. 48(1):225-46, 2015
2. Wassef M et al: Vascular anomalies classification: recommendations from the international society for the study of vascular anomalies. Pediatrics. 136(1):e203-14, 2015
3. Friedman ER et al: Imaging of pediatric neck masses. Radiol Clin North Am. 49(4):617-32, v, 2011
4. Ibrahim M et al: Congenital cystic lesions of the head and neck. Neuroimaging Clin N Am. 21(3):621-39, viii, 2011

(Left) *Anteroposterior graphic of a 6-week fetus shows the 2nd branchial arch ➡ growing inferiorly over the 3rd & 4th arches, resulting in the cervical sinus of His ➡ that combines the 2nd, 3rd, and 4th branchial clefts (BCs). Notice the thymopharyngeal duct is a remnant of the 3rd branchial pouch ➡.* **(Right)** *Oblique graphic shows tract of type 1, 1st BC anomaly ➡, from medial bony EAC toward the retroauricular area. Tract of type 2, 1st BC anomaly ➡, connects the EAC to the angle of the mandible.*

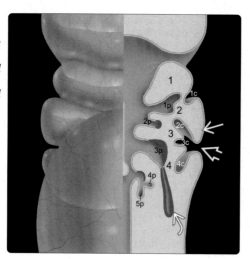
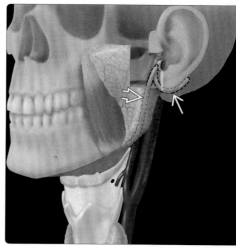

(Left) *Oblique graphic of tract of a 2nd BC cleft fistula ➡ shows a proximal opening ➡ in the faucial tonsil & a distal opening in the anterior supraclavicular neck ➡.* **(Right)** *Oblique graphic of neck illustrates tract of 3rd BC anomaly ➡ extending from the cephalad aspect of the lateral hypopharynx ➡ to the supraclavicular anterior neck skin ➡.*

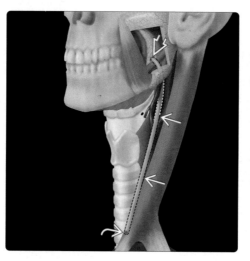
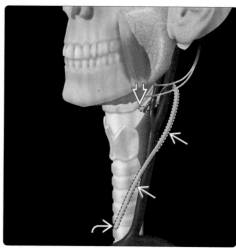

(Left) *Anteroposterior graphic shows both thymopharyngeal duct tracts ➡ extending from the lateral hypopharyngeal area ➡ to the location of the normal lobes of the thymus ➡ in the superior mediastinum.* **(Right)** *Oblique graphic of the neck shows tract of 4th BC anomaly ➡ extending from the hypopharynx ➡ to the location of the left thyroid lobe ➡. This explains why this lesion often presents with thyroiditis.*

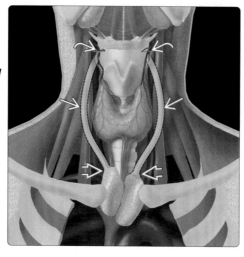
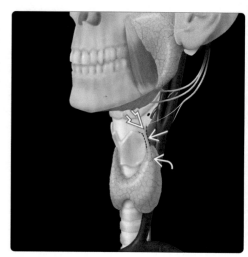

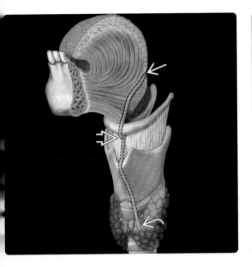

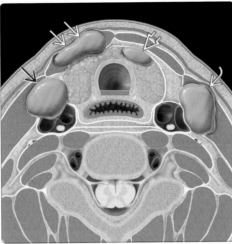

(Left) *Oblique graphic illustrates the tract of the thyroglossal duct descending from the foramen cecum ➡ at the tongue base, under the midline hyoid bone ➡, then tracking off midline to the thyroid lobe ➡.* (Right) *Axial graphic demonstrates the locations of 4 major congenital cystic lesions of the H&N. Shown here are the infrahyoid 2nd & 3rd BC cysts ➡, infrahyoid thyroglossal duct cyst ➡, cervical thymic cysts ➡, and 4th branchial apparatus sinus tracts ➡.*

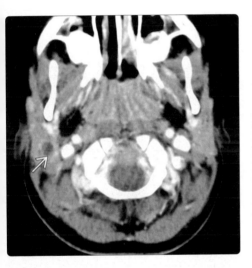

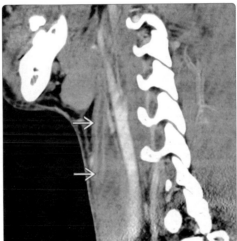

(Left) *Axial CECT in a 2-year-old boy shows intraparotid 1st BC cyst ➡ with mild peripheral enhancement and associated mild enlargement of the ipsilateral parotid gland consistent with parotitis.* (Right) *Sagittal reformatted CECT shows the typical location of a 2nd branchial apparatus fistula ➡ extending from the anterior lower neck skin opening (not included) toward the pharynx in a teenager with intermittent purulent drainage from the skin opening.*

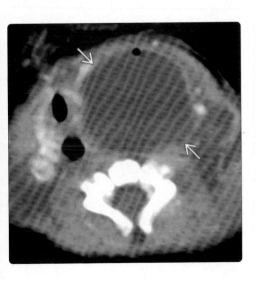

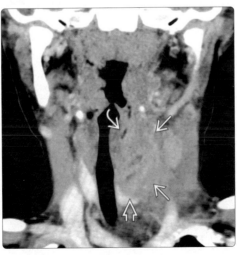

(Left) *Axial CECT in an infant shows a large, well-defined cystic mass ➡ in the left neck that extends into the mediastinum, typical of a cervical thymic cyst. Bubble of gas is concerning for infection.* (Right) *Coronal CECT in a 4-year-old boy shows a phlegmonous mass ➡ in the left neck involving the left thyroid lobe ➡ and a tract of inflammation ➡ coursing toward the left pyriform sinus, consistent with inflamed pyriform sinus tract (remnant of 4th or 3rd branchial pouch).*

TERMINOLOGY

- Subtype of congenital slow-/low-flow vascular malformation due to error in lymphatic vessel formation
- Results in well-defined, cyst-like (macrocystic), ± infiltrative, solid-appearing (microcystic) mass of abnormal lymphatic channels
  - Individual cyst size: Macrocyst > 1 cm, microcyst < 1 cm

IMAGING

- Macrocystic lymphatic malformation (LM): Lobulated, well-defined, **cystic** lesion with numerous thin **internal septations**
  - ± multiple **fluid-fluid levels**, typically due to hemorrhage
  - Soft and compressible by US with internal swirling debris
  - Protein, blood products, chyle/fat may cause bright T1 signal intensity on MR
  - Enhancement limited to rim, septations
- Microcystic LM: More poorly defined and solid-appearing
  - ± diffuse enhancement

- Locations: **Face, neck, chest, axilla** > > abdomen, pelvis, extremities
  - Frequently extend across tissue planes/compartments

TOP DIFFERENTIAL DIAGNOSES

- Infantile hemangioma
- Venous malformation
- Arteriovenous malformation
- Soft tissue sarcoma
- Soft tissue infection

CLINICAL ISSUES

- Soft and pliable mass, often apparent at birth
  - Can compress airway or other vital structures
  - May present later with pain and rapid enlargement due to hemorrhage, inflammation, or hormonal stimulation
- Primary treatment: Surgical resection ± percutaneous sclerotherapy
  - Reports of successful medical therapy with sirolimus

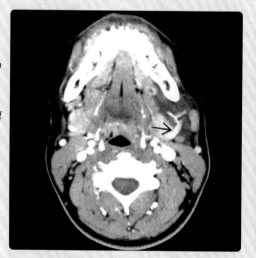
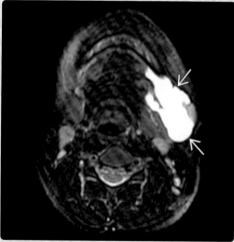

(Left) Axial CECT in a 22-year-old woman with an angle of a mandible mass reveals a low-density submandibular space (SMS) lymphatic malformation (LM) ➡ with venous structures passing through it. The mass conforms to the shape of the SMS. (Right) Axial T2 FS MR in the same patient shows the high fluid signal ➡ of the LM with its lobular margins. In this case, no fluid-fluid levels are seen.

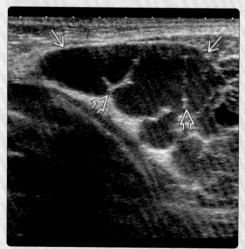
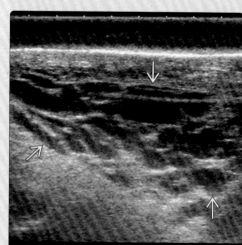

(Left) Ultrasound in a 2-year-old patient with a soft, pliable mass shows a well-defined, lobulated, multicystic lesion ➡ with thin internal septations ➡, typical of a macrocystic LM. (Right) Ultrasound of an LM in a 2 day old with a clinically apparent capillary-venous LM shows a predominantly anechoic mass with thin septations in the subcutaneous soft tissues ➡, typical of a macrocystic LM.

Lymphatic Malformation

TERMINOLOGY

Abbreviations

- Lymphatic malformation (LM)

Synonyms

- Common (cystic) LM, lymphatic anomaly
- Avoid incorrect and confusing terminology
  - Cystic hygroma reserved for abnormal midline posterior nuchal translucency on early fetal ultrasound
    - Different than anterolateral neck LM, which does not implicate chromosomal anomalies
  - Lymphangioma implies neoplasm
    - LM not neoplastic

Definitions

- Subtype of congenital, slow-/low-flow vascular malformation due to error in lymphatic vessel formation
  - Results in well-defined, cyst-like (macrocystic), ± infiltrative, solid-appearing (microcystic) mass of abnormal lymphatic channels
    - Individual cyst size: Macrocyst > 1 cm, microcyst < 1 cm
  - Mass lacks communication with normal lymphatics

IMAGING

General Features

- Location
  - **Face, neck, chest, axilla** > > abdomen, pelvis, extremities
  - Focal > > multifocal
  - Soft tissue > > bone
  - Frequently extend across tissue planes/compartments
- Size
  - Highly variable
  - May enlarge rapidly with hemorrhage, infection, or hormonal stimulation (puberty, pregnancy)
- Morphology
  - Macrocystic: Lobulated, well-defined, cystic lesion with numerous thin internal septations
  - Microcystic: More poorly defined, infiltrative, and solid appearing
  - Components of both may be present

CT Findings

- Multilocular, fluid-attenuation mass
  - Typically uniform but may contain foci of ↑ attenuation (hemorrhage/protein) or ↓ attenuation (fat/chyle)
    - Subtle fluid-fluid levels of blood products
- ± enhancement of septations with contrast
- **Venous structures** in area may pass through LM

MR Findings

- **T2 FS/STIR**: Largely bright fluid signal intensity mass
  - Intervening hypointense septa
  - **Fluid-fluid levels** due to hemorrhage within some cysts
    - Less frequently seen on other sequences
- **T1**: Hemorrhage, protein, fat/chyle within cysts may cause bright signal intensity
- **T1 C+ FS**
  - Macrocystic LM: Thin rim/septal enhancement of cysts
    - Septations may be thicker from prior inflammation or hemorrhage
  - Microcystic LM: ± confluent enhancement of infiltrating tissue
- **MRA/MRV**: No high-flow vessels intrinsic to lesion
  - Nearby normal vessels may be encased by infiltrating LM

Ultrasonographic Findings

- Grayscale ultrasound
  - Macrocystic LM: Anechoic, cystic mass, usually with thin internal septations
    - ± ↑ echogenicity related to hemorrhage or proteinaceous fluid
    - Soft, compressible with swirling debris internally
  - Microcystic LM: Poorly defined region of subcutaneous soft tissue thickening
    - Mildly hypo- or hyperechoic
- Color Doppler
  - No vascular flow identified in cysts
  - Flow may be identified in septations, typically from encased normal vessels

Imaging Recommendations

- Best imaging tool
  - Ultrasound often diagnostic for macrocystic LM, though deep extent and relationship to vital structures may be unclear
  - MR will typically confirm diagnosis and extent of disease
- Protocol advice
  - Ultrasound: For any soft tissue mass, include
    - Compression cine to evaluate internal contents
    - Doppler assessment for presence and types of vascularity
  - MR: For any soft tissue mass, include
    - Subtracted (pre- from post-) contrast-enhanced FS T1
      - □ Particularly relevant in LM, as intrinsic T1 shortening from hemorrhage/protein may confound postcontrast images
  - CECT: Avoid use in children
    - Soft tissue neck CT multiplanar reformations

DIFFERENTIAL DIAGNOSIS

Infantile Hemangioma

- True vascular neoplasm (benign)
- Characteristic life cycle: Small or absent at birth, rapid growth during early infancy, gradual involution over years
- Solid ovoid or lobular, elongated soft tissue mass, typically in cutaneous/subcutaneous tissues
- Variable sonographic echogenicity due to mix of proliferating and involuting components
- Highly vascular by Doppler US
- Bright (but not fluid) T2 signal intensity with diffuse, early enhancement on MR

Venous Malformation

- Focal mass vs. conglomeration of abnormal tubular, slow-flow channels
- Bright (fluid) T2 signal intensity ± fluid-fluid levels on MR
- May have prominent fat along margins or septa
- Phleboliths in soft tissue mass essentially pathognomonic

Arteriovenous Malformation

- Tangle of enlarged tortuous arteries and veins with variable soft tissue components
- High flow with shunting by ultrasound, MRA/MRV

Soft Tissue Sarcoma

- Typically firm, well-defined, round or ovoid hypovascular solid soft tissue mass with variable enhancement
- May have cystic components, but solid components usually visible

Soft Tissue Infection

- Cellulitis: Poorly defined soft tissue thickening with irregular serpentine pockets of fluid
- Abscess: Well-defined hypoechoic collection with mobile debris, thick wall

PATHOLOGY

General Features

- Associated abnormalities
  - Klippel-Trenaunay syndrome
    - Capillary-lymphatic-venous malformation of extremity (usually lower) + lipomatous and osseous overgrowth
    - Port-wine capillary stain on lateral extremity with lymphatic vesicles
    - Varicosities of superficial veins
      - Marginal venous system may dominate over diminutive or absent deep venous system
  - Congenital lipomatous overgrowth with vascular malformations, epidermal nevi, and skeletal anomalies
    - Truncal lipomatous masses ± LM
  - LM not associated with trisomies 13, 18, 21, or Turner syndrome
    - Aneuploidy association occurs with abnormal midline posterior nuchal translucency (cystic hygroma) on early fetal sonography

Staging, Grading, & Classification

- 2014 revised classification by International Society for Study of Vascular Anomalies
  - Common (cystic) LM: Macrocystic, microcystic, mixed
  - Generalized lymphatic anomaly (GLA)
    - Multifocal lesions commonly involving pleura, spleen, bones (axial and appendicular skeleton)
      - Progressive cortical destruction not seen in GLA
    - Macrocystic LM often present
  - Channel-type (or "central conducting-type") LM
    - May see dilated central lymphatics &/or secondary manifestations
      - Intestinal lymphangiectasia with bowel wall thickening and abnormal mesentery causing protein-losing enteropathy
      - Chylous pleural effusions and ascites
      - Extremity edema
  - Primary lymphedema

Microscopic Features

- Variably sized channels lined by flattened endothelium
- Larger channel walls show variable amount of fibrous tissue and smooth muscle
- May be mixed with venous &/or capillary components

Immunohistochemical Features

- Endothelium stains positive for lymphatic markers
  - Prox-1 and VEGFR-3 most sensitive, specific
  - D2-40 and LYVE-1 less sensitive in large channel LM

CLINICAL ISSUES

Presentation

- Most common signs/symptoms
  - Soft and pliable mass without pain
- Other signs/symptoms
  - Pain &/or rapid enlargement due to hemorrhage, inflammation, or hormonal stimulation
  - Cutaneous vesicles suggest LM; skin usually normal
  - Compression of airway or other vital structures

Demographics

- Age
  - Identified at birth or prenatally in majority of cases

Natural History & Prognosis

- LM generally grow commensurate with patient
  - May enlarge rapidly due to hemorrhage, inflammation, or hormonal stimulation
- Prognosis better for small focal lesions
  - Difficult to treat entirety of large infiltrating lesion with surgery or sclerotherapy, leading to recurrence

Treatment

- Surgical resection ± percutaneous sclerotherapy
  - Combination often required for larger infiltrating lesions
  - Sclerotherapy primarily utilized for macrocystic disease
    - Direct injection of sclerosing agent into LM under sonographic/fluoroscopic guidance
      - Doxycycline, bleomycin, OK-432, ethanol
      - Utility of bleomycin also reported in microcystic LM
    - Major complications (skin necrosis, nerve damage, extremity swelling, muscle atrophy, disseminated intravascular coagulation) uncommon
    - Full results of sclerosis can take months to manifest
      - May take multiple staged procedures to treat lesion
- Medical therapy with sirolimus gaining favor
- Compression garments

DIAGNOSTIC CHECKLIST

Image Interpretation Pearls

- **Multicystic** pediatric soft tissue mass with **fluid-fluid** levels strongly suggests slow-/low-flow vascular malformation

SELECTED REFERENCES

1. Koo HJ et al: Ethanol and/or radiofrequency ablation to treat venolymphatic malformations that manifest as a bulging mass in the head and neck. Clin Radiol. pii: S0009-9260(16)00131-8, 2016
2. Wassef M et al: Vascular anomalies classification: recommendations from the International Society for the Study of Vascular Anomalies. Pediatrics. 136(1):e203-14, 2015
3. Elluru RG et al: Lymphatic malformations: diagnosis and management. Semin Pediatr Surg. 23(4):178-85, 2014
4. Trenor CC 3rd et al: Complex lymphatic anomalies. Semin Pediatr Surg. 23(4):186-90, 2014
5. Mulliken JB et al: Mulliken and Young's Vascular Anomalies: Hemangiomas and Malformations. Oxford: Oxford University Press, 2013

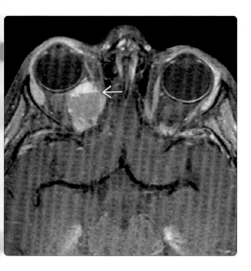
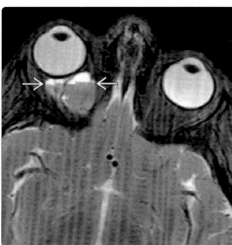

(Left) *Axial T1 C+ FS MR in an older child with acute worsening of longstanding right proptosis with a hemorrhagic orbital LM demonstrates that signal of contents manifests as fluid-fluid levels* ➡, *indicating proteinaceous and hemorrhagic products.* (Right) *Axial T2 FS MR in the same patient shows a large, retrobulbar mass with characteristic fluid-fluid levels* ➡. *The differing heights of the levels are indicative of the multilocular nature of the orbital LM.*

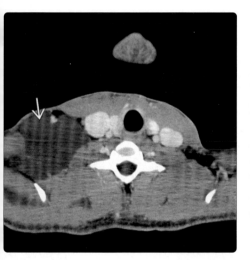
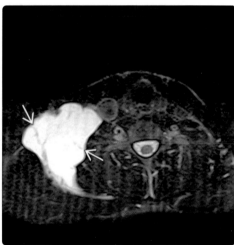

(Left) *Axial CECT in a 25-year-old man shows a ballotable supraclavicular mass* ➡. (Right) *Axial T2 FS MR in the same patient shows the fluid intensity LM conforming to the shape of the posterior cervical space. Note the internal septations* ➡ *seen on MR that are not visible on CECT.*

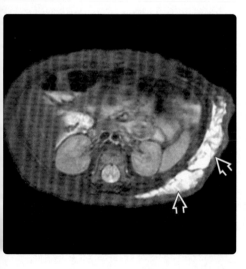
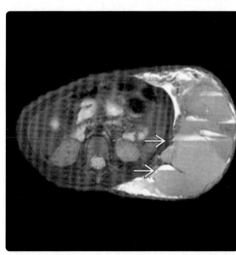

(Left) *Axial T2 FS MR in a child with a flank mass shows an elongated, septated fluid signal intensity lesion* ➡, *typical of an LM.* (Right) *Axial T2 FS MR obtained 1 month later in the same patient shows marked interval enlargement of the mass. Numerous fluid-fluid levels* ➡ *are now seen in the mass, typical of layering blood products due to interval hemorrhage.*

Venous Malformation

TERMINOLOGY

- Venous malformation (VM)

IMAGING

- In child, use MR & US as possible
- General imaging findings
  - Lobulated soft tissue "mass" with **phleboliths**
  - **Solitary or multiple**
  - May be **circumscribed** or **transspatial**, infiltrating adjacent soft tissue compartments
  - ± combined lymphatic malformation (LM), i.e., mixed venolymphatic malformation (VLM)
- CT findings
  - **Rounded calcifications (phleboliths)**
  - Osseous remodeling in adjacent bone
  - Fat hypertrophy in adjacent soft tissues
- Enhancement features
  - **Variable enhancement** pattern reflects sluggish vascular flow to & through lesion

- Patchy & delayed or homogeneous & intense enhancement

TOP DIFFERENTIAL DIAGNOSES

- Lymphatic malformation
- Infantile hemangioma
- Dermoid & epidermoid
- Arteriovenous malformation

PATHOLOGY

- Congenital venous vascular rest
- 70% of patients with periorbital LM or VLM have intracranial vascular & parenchymal anomalies
  - DVA, cerebral cavernous malformation, dural arteriovenous malformation (AVM), pial AVM, sinus pericranii

CLINICAL ISSUES

- Presents as spongy head & neck mass that grows proportionately with patient

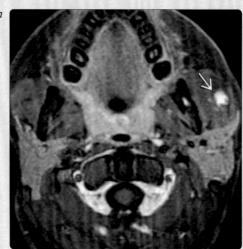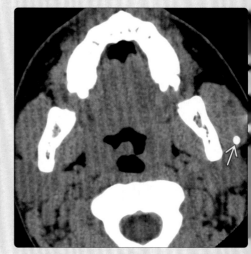

(Left) Axial T1WI C+ FS MR in a 14-year-old boy demonstrates a small focal area of enhancement ➡ in an otherwise nonspecific lesion within the left masseter muscle within the masticator space. (Right) Axial NECT in the same patient shows an ill-defined intramuscular mass with small phlebolith ➡ consistent with venous malformation (VM).

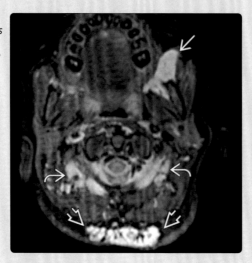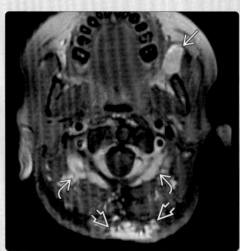

(Left) Axial STIR MR in a 10-year-old girl with multiple VMs demonstrates hyperintense lesions in the left buccal space ➡, the midline posterior subcutaneous neck ➡, and the bilateral paraspinal soft tissues ➡. (Right) Axial T1WI C+ FS MR in the same patient shows variable enhancement of the VM in the left buccal space ➡, the midline posterior subcutaneous neck ➡, and the bilateral paraspinal soft tissues ➡.

Venous Malformation

TERMINOLOGY

Abbreviations
- Venous malformation (VM) = preferred term

Synonyms
- Cavernous malformation, cavernous hemangioma (terms to be avoided)

Definitions
- VM: **Congenital** slow- or low-flow postcapillary lesion composed of endothelial-lined vascular sinusoids

IMAGING

General Features
- Best diagnostic clue
  - Lobulated soft tissue "mass" with **phleboliths**
- Location
  - May be in any space(s) in head and neck
  - Most commonly in buccal region
  - Masticator space, sublingual space, tongue, orbit, & dorsal neck are other common locations
  - Superficial or deep, diffuse or localized
  - Head & neck (40%), extremities (40%), trunk (20%)
- Size
  - Variable, may be very large
- Morphology
  - Multilobulated, **solitary** or **multiple**
  - May be **circumscribed** or **transspatial** (multiple contiguous spaces)
  - ± combined lymphatic malformation (LM), i.e., mixed venolymphatic malformation (VLM)

Radiographic Findings
- Radiography
  - Limited utility, may show phleboliths or trophic changes in adjacent bone

CT Findings
- NECT
  - Lobulated soft tissue mass, isodense to muscle
  - Rounded calcifications (**phleboliths**)
- CECT
  - Flow rate through lesion is variable
    - Influences individual lesion clinical behavior & enhancement pattern
  - **Variable enhancement** pattern reflects sluggish vascular flow to & through lesion
  - Enhancement usually evident but variable
    - Patchy & delayed **or** homogeneous & intense
  - Lymphatic component of VLM does not enhance
  - Osseous remodeling in adjacent bone
  - Fat hypertrophy in adjacent soft tissues
- CTA
  - **No enlarged feeding arteries**
  - Lesion often drained by enlarged veins

MR Findings
- T1WI
  - Multilobulated with **variable signal** intensity
    - Isointense to hypointense relative to muscle

- **Regional fat hypertrophy**
- T2WI
  - Vascular channel size influences appearance
    - Lesions with large vascular channels appear cyst-like, **hyperintense**, septated
    - Lesions with smaller vascular channels appear more solid & intermediate in signal intensity
  - Phleboliths appear as rounded or oval signal voids
  - Vascular signal voids are **atypical**
    - If present = enlarged dysplastic draining veins
- T1WI C+
  - Enhancement variable, may be delayed, heterogeneous or homogeneous, & mild to intense
  - Lymphatic component of VLM will not enhance
- MRV
  - May show enlarged veins associated with lesion
  - May show associated intracranial venous anomalies

Ultrasonographic Findings
- Spongy, compressible
- Lesions with small vascular channels are more echogenic & less compressible than lesions with large vascular lumens
- No arterial flow on Color Doppler
- Venous flow may be observed and augmented by compression with transducer
- Phleboliths = **hyperechoic foci** with acoustic shadowing

Other Modality Findings
- Anatomy & venous drainage best mapped via direct percutaneous injection of venous sinusoids
- Even with direct injection, components of malformation may not freely intercommunicate
- Large channels resemble cluster of grapes; smaller channels have more cotton-wool blush appearance

Imaging Recommendations
- Best imaging tool
  - In adult, CT best identifies phleboliths
  - MR best to map full extent of lesion & identify lymphatic component if VLM
  - Ultrasound if lesion is superficial
- Protocol advice
  - Avoid CT if lesion in child
    - Use US ± MR for imaging evaluation
  - MR with contrast & fat suppression
    - STIR or fat-suppressed T2 images to define full extent of lesion
    - Gradient echo imaging helpful to assure lack of high flow vessels

DIFFERENTIAL DIAGNOSIS

Lymphatic Malformation
- Another common slow- or low-flow lesion
- Compressible fluid-filled macrocystic soft tissue mass
  - Thin enhancing **internal septations**, internal debris, **blood-fluid levels**
- **No phleboliths**; no enhancement unless mixed VLM
- Solitary or multiple; single space or transspatial

Pediatric Lesions

Infantile Hemangioma

- Characteristic life cycle: Small at birth, rapid growth during infancy, gradual involution over years
- Benign, vascular neoplasm of capillaries
  - Endothelial proliferation & GLUT1(+) marker
- Prominent vascular **flow voids** on Doppler US
- Rapid, homogeneous, **intense enhancement**
- No phleboliths

Dermoid and Epidermoid

- Rounded calcifications possible (dermoid)
  - If present, found lying within fat-containing lesion
- Lesion contents very echogenic on ultrasound (dermoid)

Arteriovenous Malformation

- Tangle of **high-flow** vascular flow voids on MR & US
- T2 hyperintense (cystic-appearing) areas unusual
- Phleboliths rare

PATHOLOGY

General Features

- Etiology
  - Congenital venous vascular rest
- Genetics
  - *TEK* mutation in many VM (50% of sporadic VM)
- Associated abnormalities
  - 70% of patients with periorbital LM or VLM have intracranial vascular & parenchymal anomalies
    - Developmental venous anomaly (DVA), cerebral cavernous malformation, dural arteriovenous malformation (AVM), pial AVM, sinus pericranii
- Staging, grading, & classification
  - 2014 revised classification of VM by International Society for Study of Vascular Anomalies
    - Common VM (94%)
    - Familial cutaneomucosal VM: Mutation involving coding for endothelial receptor *TEK*
      - □ Multifocal lesions of lips, tongue
      - □ Dilated neck, upper extremity veins
    - Blue rubber bleb nevus syndrome
      - □ Multifocal cutaneous, muscular, gastrointestinal VM
    - Glomuvenous malformation: Gene mutation involving chromosome 1p
      - □ Glomus cells in VM
    - Cerebral cavernous malformation

Gross Pathologic & Surgical Features

- Poorly circumscribed vascular malformation consisting of irregular venous channels

Microscopic Features

- Venous channels with variable luminal diameter & wall thickness
- Channels lined by flat, mitotically inactive endothelium & scant mural smooth muscle
- Absent internal elastic lamina
- Luminal thrombi, phleboliths

CLINICAL ISSUES

Presentation

- Most common signs/symptoms
  - Spongy soft tissue mass without thrill
    - Bluish skin discoloration when superficial
  - Grows proportionately with patient
  - ↑ ↑ in size with Valsalva, bending over, crying
  - May enlarge rapidly after trauma or infection; or under hormonal influences (puberty, pregnancy)

Demographics

- Age
  - Present at birth
  - Present clinically at any age, usually in children, adolescents, or young adults
- Epidemiology
  - Most common vascular malformation of H&N

Natural History & Prognosis

- Prognosis depends on extent & location
- Larger, extensive VM can cause lifelong morbidity

Treatment

- Conservative therapy
  - Compression garments
  - Antiinflammatory medications
  - Low molecular weight heparin if thrombosis risk ↑
- Percutaneous procedures
  - Direct injection with sclerosing agent under fluoroscopic/ultrasonic guidance
    - Multiple procedures may be required
  - Laser ablation of superficial VM
  - Endovascular ablation of varicosities
    - Radiofrequency vs. laser
- Surgical resection of focal lesions
  - May be used in combination with percutaneous sclerotherapy

DIAGNOSTIC CHECKLIST

Consider

- Does lesion enlarge with Valsalva maneuver, crying, or when head is dependent
  - All these clinical signs suggest VM

Image Interpretation Pearls

- Presence of phleboliths on CT or T2 hyperintense facial mass is most specific imaging finding for VM

SELECTED REFERENCES

1. Wassef M et al: Vascular anomalies classification: recommendations from the International Society for the Study of Vascular Anomalies. Pediatrics. 136(1):e203-14, 2015
2. Kollipara R et al: Current classification and terminology of pediatric vascular anomalies. AJR Am J Roentgenol. 201(5):1124-35, 2013
3. Scolozzi P et al: Intraoral venous malformation presenting with multiple phleboliths. Oral Surg Oral Med Oral Pathol Oral Radiol Endod. 96(2): 197-200, 2003
4. Boukobza M et al: Cerebral developmental venous anomalies associated with head and neck venous malformations. AJNR Am J Neuroradiol. 17(5): 987-94, 1996
5. Baker LL et al: Hemangiomas and vascular malformations of the head and neck: MR characterization. AJNR Am J Neuroradiol. 14(2):307-14, 1993

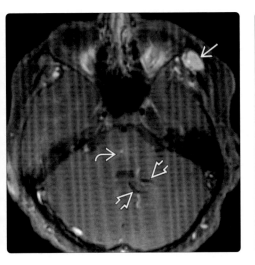
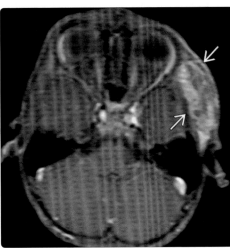

(Left) *Axial T1WI C+ FS MR demonstrates a moderately enhancing VM involving the left temporalis muscle ➡, left cerebellar hemisphere developmental venous anomaly (DVA) ➡, and probable smaller DVA or telangiectasia in the pons ➡.* (Right) *Axial T1WI C+ FS MR shows heterogeneous contrast enhancement within a VM ➡ in the left suprazygomatic masticator space (temporal fossa).*

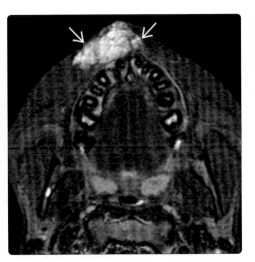
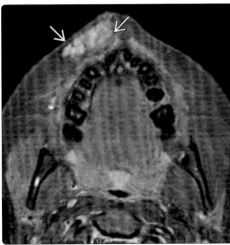

(Left) *Axial STIR MR reveals a well-defined lobulated VM involving the subcutaneous tissues of the upper lip ➡, without underlying osseous or dental abnormality.* (Right) *Axial T1WI C+ FS MR in the same patient shows moderate heterogeneous contrast within the abnormal venous lakes ➡.*

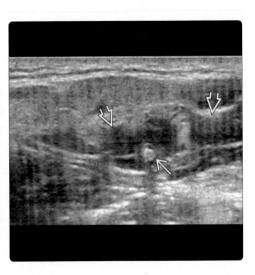
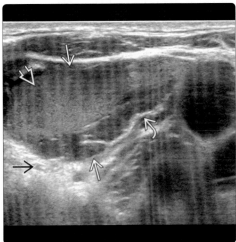

(Left) *Transverse US in upper neck shows a mixed cystic lesion with sinusoidal spaces ➡ & echogenic phlebolith ➡, suggesting diagnosis of VM. While US is able to suggest diagnosis of VM, it cannot define deep extent of larger lesions or confirm multiplicity. (From DI: Ultrasound.)* (Right) *Transverse US in a child with a painless low neck mass shows a well-defined cystic lesion ➡ with large sinusoidal space & fine internal debris ➡ & septa ➡. Note the posterior enhancement ➡ signaling the cystic nature of the lesion. (From DI: Ultrasound.)*

Congenital Vallecular Cyst

TERMINOLOGY

- Epiglottic cyst, base of tongue cyst, ductal cyst, saccular cyst
- Congenital cyst arising in vallecula

IMAGING

- Cystic mass in vallecula of child with stridor
- Most diagnosed with direct laryngoscopy

TOP DIFFERENTIAL DIAGNOSES

- **Thyroglossal duct cyst**
  - When midline tongue base cyst (near foramen cecum), may be indistinguishable from congenital vallecular cyst
- **Retention cyst in pharyngeal mucosal space**
  - Benign postinflammatory retention cyst in nasopharynx or oropharynx
- **Lingual thyroid**
  - Midline, solid mass near foramen cecum
  - Increased attenuation on CT
  - Variable signal intensity on MR

- **Lingual hamartoma**
  - Midline posterior tongue mass near foramen cecum
- **Lymphatic malformation**
  - Cystic, usually transspatial congenital lesion
  - Rarely involves vallecula

CLINICAL ISSUES

- Most common signs/symptoms
  - **Inspiratory stridor**
  - Airway obstruction: May lead to life-threatening airway obstruction if left untreated
  - Apnea
- Other signs/symptoms
  - Laryngomalacia
  - Feeding difficulties
  - Failure to thrive
- Treatment
  - Surgical excision, laser-assisted resection, marsupialization, radiofrequency ablation

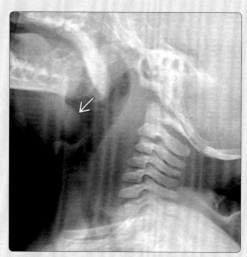
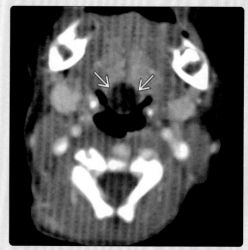

(Left) Lateral radiograph in an infant with stridor shows a well-defined soft tissue mass ➡ at the base of the tongue protruding into the vallecula. (Right) Axial CECT shows a well-defined, low-attenuation, nonenhancing cyst in the midline base of the tongue ➡. Based on CECT findings alone, this lesion cannot be distinguished from thyroglossal duct cyst in the location of the foramen cecum.

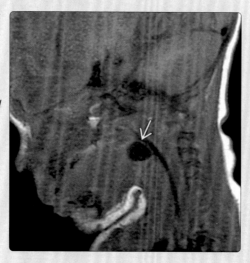
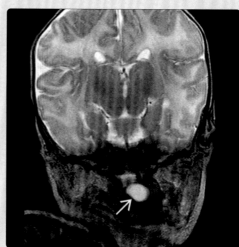

(Left) Sagittal T1WI MR shows an incidentally noted, well-defined, fluid signal intensity congenital vallecular cyst at the base of the tongue ➡ in the anterior oropharynx. (Right) Coronal T2WI MR in the same patient shows a fluid signal intensity vallecular cyst to be somewhat lobulated in contour ➡ and located in the ventral aspect of the oropharynx.

Congenital Vallecular Cyst

TERMINOLOGY

Synonyms

- Epiglottic cyst, base of tongue cyst, ductal cyst, saccular cyst

Definitions

- Congenital cyst arising in vallecula
  - **Proposed theories of origin**
    - Secondary to obstruction of submucosal glands
    - Secondary to congenital cystic distension of laryngeal saccule

IMAGING

General Features

- Best diagnostic clue
  - **Cystic mass in vallecula of child with stridor**
  - Most diagnosed with direct laryngoscopy
- Location
  - Within vallecula
  - Arises from lingual surface of epiglottis
- Size
  - Variable
- Morphology
  - **Round or lobulated**

CT Findings

- Well-defined, low-attenuation, **nonenhancing** mass in vallecula

MR Findings

- Well-defined fluid signal intensity mass in vallecula

Ultrasonographic Findings

- Well-defined, anechoic cyst

DIFFERENTIAL DIAGNOSIS

Thyroglossal Duct Cyst

- When midline tongue base cyst (near foramen cecum), may be indistinguishable from congenital vallecular cyst

Pharyngeal Mucosal Space Retention Cyst

- Benign retention cyst in nasopharynx or oropharynx
- More common in older children and adults

Lingual Thyroid

- Midline, solid mass near foramen cecum
- Increased attenuation on CT
- Variable signal intensity on MR

Lingual Hamartoma

- Midline posterior tongue mass near foramen cecum

Lymphatic Malformation

- Cystic, congenital, usually transspatial lesion
- Rarely involves vallecula

PATHOLOGY

General Features

- Cyst wall contains respiratory &/or squamous epithelium with mucous glands

CLINICAL ISSUES

Presentation

- Most common signs/symptoms
  - Inspiratory stridor
  - Airway obstruction
- Other signs/symptoms
  - Apnea
  - Coexistent laryngomalacia not uncommon, may complicate clinical picture
  - Feeding difficulties
  - Failure to thrive

Natural History & Prognosis

- May lead to life-threatening airway obstruction if left untreated

Treatment

- Surgical excision
- Laser-assisted resection
- Marsupialization
- Radiofrequency ablation

DIAGNOSTIC CHECKLIST

Image Interpretation Pearls

- If well-defined nonenhancing cystic mass discovered in midline vallecula in infant with stridor, suspect vallecular cyst
- May be difficult to differentiate congenital vallecular cyst from thyroglossal duct cyst in foramen cecum of tongue base

SELECTED REFERENCES

1. Cheng J et al: Endoscopic surgical management of inspiratory stridor in newborns and infants. Am J Otolaryngol. 36(5):697-700, 2015
2. Lee DH et al: Clinical characteristics and surgical treatment outcomes of vallecular cysts in adults. Acta Otolaryngol. 1-4, 2015
3. Hsieh LC et al: The outcomes of infantile vallecular cyst post CO_2 laser treatment. Int J Pediatr Otorhinolaryngol. 77(5):655-7, 2013
4. Tsai YT et al: Treatment of vallecular cysts in infants with and without coexisting laryngomalacia using endoscopic laser marsupialization: fifteen-year experience at a single-center. Int J Pediatr Otorhinolaryngol. 77(3):424-8, 2013
5. Gonik N et al: Radiofrequency ablation of pediatric vallecular cysts. Int J Pediatr Otorhinolaryngol. 76(12):1819-22, 2012
6. Chen EY et al: Transoral approach for direct and complete excision of vallecular cysts in children. Int J Pediatr Otorhinolaryngol. 75(9):1147-51, 2011
7. Suzuki J et al: Congenital vallecular cyst in an infant: case report and review of 52 recent cases. J Laryngol Otol. 125(11):1199-203, 2011
8. Breysem L et al: Vallecular cyst as a cause of congenital stridor: report of five patients. Pediatr Radiol. 39(8):828-31, 2009
9. Sands NB et al: Series of congenital vallecular cysts: a rare yet potentially fatal cause of upper airway obstruction and failure to thrive in the newborn. J Otolaryngol Head Neck Surg. 38(1):6-10, 2009
10. Busuttil M et al: Congenital laryngeal cyst: benefits of prenatal diagnosis and multidisciplinary perinatal management. Fetal Diagn Ther. 19(4):373-6, 2004
11. Yao TC et al: Failure to thrive caused by the coexistence of vallecular cyst, laryngomalacia and gastroesophageal reflux in an infant. Int J Pediatr Otorhinolaryngol. 68(11):1459-64, 2004
12. Tibesar RJ et al: Apnea spells in an infant with vallecular cyst. Ann Otol Rhinol Laryngol. 112(9 Pt 1):821-4, 2003
13. Cheng KS et al: Vallecular cyst and laryngomalacia in infants: report of six cases and airway management. Anesth Analg. 95(5):1248-50, table of contents, 2002
14. Ku AS: Vallecular cyst: report of four cases—one with co-existing laryngomalacia. J Laryngol Otol. 114(3):224-6, 2000
15. Myer CM: Vallecular cyst in the newborn. Ear Nose Throat J. 67(2):122-4, 1988

Thyroglossal Duct Cyst

TERMINOLOGY

- Thyroglossal duct cyst (TGDC): Remnant of thyroglossal duct (TDG)
  - Between foramen cecum at tongue base → thyroid bed in infrahyoid neck

IMAGING

- Best diagnostic clue: Midline suprahyoid or midline/paramidline infrahyoid cystic neck mass
- 20-25% in suprahyoid neck
- Almost 50% at hyoid bone
- ~ 25% in infrahyoid neck
  - Embedded in strap muscles = claw sign
- Wall may enhance if infected

TOP DIFFERENTIAL DIAGNOSES

- Lymphatic malformation
- Dermoid or epidermoid in oral cavity
- Lingual thyroid

- Submandibular or sublingual space abscess
- Mixed laryngocele
- Delphian chain necrotic node

PATHOLOGY

- Failure of involution of TGD & persistent secretion of epithelial cells lining duct → TGDC
- Anywhere along route of descent of TGD

CLINICAL ISSUES

- Most common congenital neck lesion
- Treatment: Excision cyst + midline hyoid bone

DIAGNOSTIC CHECKLIST

- Relationship to hyoid bone important to note: Suprahyoid, hyoid, or infrahyoid in location
- Any associated nodularity or chunky calcification suggests associated thyroid carcinoma
- Image thyroid bed with ultrasound: Confirm thyroid gland present

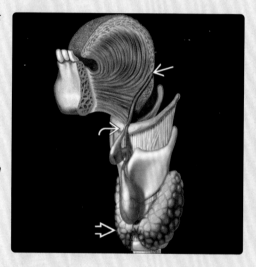 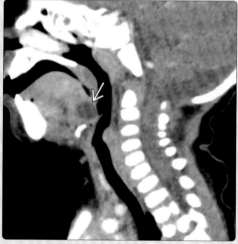

(Left) Sagittal oblique graphic shows course of thyroglossal duct cyst (TGDC), from foramen cecum ➡ to thyroid bed ➡. Note the close relationship to midportion of hyoid bone ➡. A cyst can occur anywhere along the tract. (Right) Sagittal CECT shows a well-defined cystic-appearing mass ➡ at the midline base of the tongue. This was incidentally found on a CT performed to evaluate the extent of deep neck infection (not shown) and subsequently proven to be TGDC.

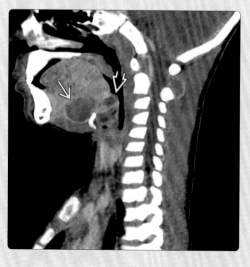 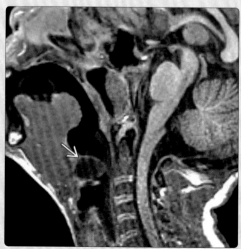

(Left) Sagittal CECT in a child with sore throat and difficulty swallowing shows a lobulated low-attenuation mass in the midline sublingual space ➡, with small posterior extension towards the base of tongue/region of vallecula ➡. This was histologically proved to be inflamed TGDC. (Right) Sagittal T1WI in a child with recurrent TGDC demonstrates a cystic-appearing mass at the midline base of the tongue ➡. Note distortion of the tongue and superior aspect of the mass by the laryngeal mask airway used during anesthesia during image acquisition.

TERMINOLOGY

Synonyms

- Thyroglossal duct cyst (TGDC)
- Thyroglossal duct (TGD) remnant

Definitions

- Remnant of TGD found **between foramen cecum at tongue base & thyroid bed in infrahyoid neck**

IMAGING

General Features

- Best diagnostic clue
  - **Midline suprahyoid or midline/paramidline infrahyoid cystic neck mass**
- Location
  - 20-25% in suprahyoid neck
  - Almost 50% at hyoid bone
  - ~ 25% in infrahyoid neck
  - Suprahyoid neck: Midline; infrahyoid neck midline or paramidline embedded in strap muscles
- Size
  - Variable, usually 2-4 cm
- Morphology
  - Round or ovoid cyst

CT Findings

- CECT
  - Low-attenuation **cystic midline neck mass with thin rim of peripheral enhancement**
    - Wall may enhance if infected
    - Occasional septations
  - Suprahyoid TGDC
    - Base of tongue or within posterior floor of mouth
  - At level of hyoid bone
    - Midline, usually abutting anterior hyoid bone
    - May project into preepiglottic space
  - **Infrahyoid** TGDC
    - **Embedded in strap muscles = claw sign**
    - More inferior TGDC is usually more paramedian location
  - **< 1% contain associated thyroid carcinoma** (usually papillary carcinoma)
    - Solid eccentric mass, often with calcification, within cyst
    - May only be microscopic and therefore not identified prospectively with imaging
    - Majority adults but may occur in teenagers; youngest reported 10 years old

MR Findings

- T1WI
  - Usually hypointense
    - Hyperintense if proteinaceous fluid
- T2WI
  - Homogeneously hyperintense
- T1WI C+
  - **Nonenhancing** cyst
    - Rim enhancement if infected

Ultrasonographic Findings

- **Anechoic or hypoechoic** midline neck mass
  - ± internal echoes (± hemorrhage or infection)
  - Presence of internal echoes does not correlate with histologic evidence of hemorrhage or infection
- Be sure to image lower neck, prove presence of normal-appearing, bilobed thyroid

Imaging Recommendations

- Children: TGDCs have classic clinical presentation
  - Sonography only to confirm normal thyroid gland
  - CT or MR if infected or diagnosis uncertain
- Adults: CT or MR if cyst suprahyoid or infected
- Nuclear scintigraphy if suspect ectopic thyroid

DIFFERENTIAL DIAGNOSIS

Oral Cavity Dermoid and Epidermoid

- Dermoid: **Fat, fluid, or mixed**
- Epidermoid: **Fluid**
- Submandibular space, sublingual space, or root of tongue
- Neither directly involves hyoid bone

Lymphatic Malformation

- **Unilocular or multilocular**
- Focal or transspatial
- **Nonenhancing** unless infected or part of combined venolymphatic vascular malformation
- Fluid-fluid levels common; secondary to hemorrhage

Lingual Thyroid

- **Solid** mass enhances; hyperattenuating on NECT

Submandibular or Sublingual Space Abscess

- Origin: Odontogenic or salivary gland infection
- Not embedded within strap muscles
- Thick, enhancing wall around collections of pus

Mixed Laryngocele

- Traces back to laryngeal origin
- Not embedded within strap muscles

Delphian Chain Necrotic Node

- **May be difficult to differentiate from infected TGDC**
  - Rare in children

PATHOLOGY

General Features

- Genetics
  - Familial cases occur (rare)
    - Usually female
    - Autosomal dominant
  - Thyroid developmental anomalies often occur in same family
- Etiology
  - **Failure of involution of TGD & persistent secretion of epithelial cells lining duct →TGDC**
    - TGDC or ectopic thyroid tissue may occur anywhere along route of descent of TGD
- Associated abnormalities
  - Thyroid agenesis, ectopia, pyramidal lobe
  - Occasionally associated with carcinoma

- – Most commonly papillary carcinoma of TGD
- Embryology/anatomy
  - TGD originates near foramen cecum, at posterior 3rd of tongue
  - Thyroid anlage arises at base of tongue & descends to final location (thyroid bed) along TGD
  - Descends through base of tongue floor of mouth → around or through hyoid bone → anterior to strap muscles → final position in thyroid bed, anterior to thyroid or cricoid cartilage
  - At 5-6 gestational weeks, TGD usually involutes, with foramen cecum & pyramidal thyroid lobe as normal remnants
  - Failure of involution, with persistent secretory activity → TGDC

Gross Pathologic & Surgical Features

- Smooth, benign-appearing cyst, with tract to hyoid bone ± foramen cecum

Microscopic Features

- Cyst lined by respiratory or squamous epithelium
- Small deposits of thyroid tissue with colloid commonly associated
- ± thyroid carcinoma (papillary carcinoma most common)

CLINICAL ISSUES

Presentation

- Most common signs/symptoms
  - Midline or paramedian, doughy, **compressible, painless neck mass** in child or young adult
  - Other signs/symptoms
    - Recurrent midline neck mass with upper respiratory tract infections or trauma
    - ± multiple prior incision & drainage procedures for "neck abscess"
    - **Rarely, lingual TGDC may → airway obstruction in infants**
    - Small lesions may be recognized as incidental finding on brain MR, especially at base of tongue
  - Physical examination
    - If TGDC around hyoid bone, cyst elevates when tongue is protruded

Demographics

- Age
  - < 10 years (up to 90%) at presentation
- Gender
  - M < F in hereditary form
- Epidemiology
  - **Most common congenital neck lesion**
    - 90% of nonodontogenic congenital cysts
    - 3x as common as branchial cleft cysts
  - At autopsy > 7% of population will have TGD remnant somewhere along course of tract

Natural History & Prognosis

- Recurrent, intermittent swelling of mass, usually following minor upper respiratory infection
- Rapidly enlarging mass suggests either infection or associated differentiated thyroid carcinoma
  - Carcinoma is associated with TGDC (< 1%)

- Differentiated thyroid carcinoma (85% papillary carcinoma)

Treatment

- Complete surgical resection = Sistrunk procedure
  - Tract to foramen cecum dissected free
  - Entire cyst & midline portion of hyoid bone resected
    - Even if imaging shows no obvious connection to hyoid bone
    - Exception: Low infrahyoid neck TGDC
  - Decreases recurrence rate from 50% to < 4%
- Isolated lingual TGDC may be treated endoscopically
- Prognosis excellent with complete surgical resection
- Recurrences (incomplete resection) often complicated & lateral
  - Increase risk of recurrence in patients with postoperative infection

DIAGNOSTIC CHECKLIST

Consider

- Relationship to hyoid bone important to note: Suprahyoid, hyoid, or infrahyoid in location
- Any associated nodularity or chunky calcification suggests associated thyroid carcinoma
- Image thyroid bed with ultrasound: Confirm thyroid gland present

SELECTED REFERENCES

1. Oyewumi M et al: Ultrasound to differentiate thyroglossal duct cysts and dermoid cysts in children. Laryngoscope. 125(4):998-1003, 2015
2. Rohof D et al: Recurrences after thyroglossal duct cyst surgery: results in 207 consecutive cases and review of the literature. Head Neck. 37(12):1699-704, 2015
3. Tahir A et al: Thyroglossal duct cyst carcinoma in child†. J Surg Case Rep. 2015(4), 2015
4. Geller KA et al: Thyroglossal duct cyst and sinuses: a 20-year Los Angeles experience and lessons learned. Int J Pediatr Otorhinolaryngol. 78(2):264-7, 2014
5. Zander DA et al: Imaging of ectopic thyroid tissue and thyroglossal duct cysts. Radiographics. 34(1):37-50, 2014
6. Sameer KS et al: Lingual thyroglossal duct cysts—a review. Int J Pediatr Otorhinolaryngol. 76(2):165-8, 2012
7. Burkart CM et al: Update on endoscopic management of lingual thyroglossal duct cysts. Laryngoscope. 119(10):2055-60, 2009
8. Hirshoren N et al: The imperative of the Sistrunk operation: review of 160 thyroglossal tract remnant operations. Otolaryngol Head Neck Surg. 140(3):338-42, 2009
9. Lin ST et al: Thyroglossal duct cyst: a comparison between children and adults. Am J Otolaryngol. 29(2):83-7, 2008
10. Falvo L et al: Papillary thyroid carcinoma in thyroglossal duct cyst: case reports and literature review. Int Surg. 91(3):141-6, 2006
11. Diaz MC et al: A thyroglossal duct cyst causing apnea and cyanosis in a neonate. Pediatr Emerg Care. 21(1):35-7, 2005
12. Koch BL: Cystic malformations of the neck in children. Pediatr Radiol. 35(5):463-77, 2005
13. Marianowski R et al: Risk factors for thyroglossal duct remnants after Sistrunk procedure in a pediatric population. Int J Pediatr Otorhinolaryngol. 67(1):19-23, 2003
14. Glastonbury CM et al: The CT and MR imaging features of carcinoma arising in thyroglossal duct remnants. AJNR Am J Neuroradiol. 21(4):770-4, 2000
15. Ewing CA et al: Presentations of thyroglossal duct cysts in adults. Eur Arch Otorhinolaryngol. 256(3):136-8, 1999
16. Wadsworth DT et al: Thyroglossal duct cysts: variability of sonographic findings. AJR Am J Roentgenol. 163(6):1475-7, 1994
17. Pelausa ME et al: Sistrunk revisited: a 10-year review of revision thyroglossal duct surgery at Toronto's Hospital for Sick Children. J Otolaryngol. 18(7):325-33, 1989
18. Reede DL et al: CT of thyroglossal duct cysts. Radiology. 157(1):121-5, 1985

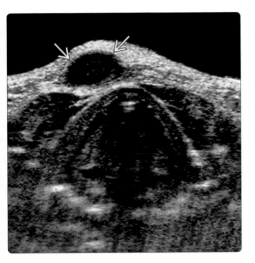

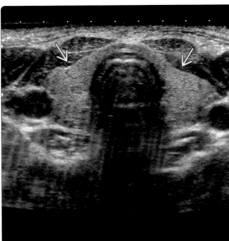

(Left) *Transverse ultrasound shows a well-defined, subcutaneous, right paramidline, hypoechoic mass ➡ ventral to the strap muscles. This was surgically removed and proved to be a TGDC.* (Right) *Transverse ultrasound in child with suspected TGDC demonstrates a normal-appearing, bilobed thyroid ➡ at the expected location in the lower anterior neck. It is important to document this in all patients imaged for work up of TGDC.*

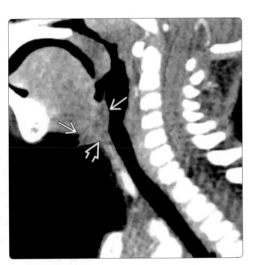

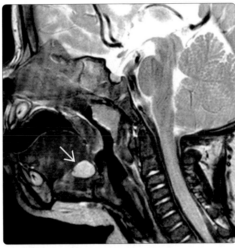

(Left) *Sagittal CECT in a child with recurrent TGDC demonstrates a lobulated, heterogeneous mass ➡ in the midline suprahyoid neck consistent with inflamed recurrent TGD remnant. Notice the absence of the midline hyoid bone ➡ consistent with prior Sistrunk procedure.* (Right) *Sagittal T2WI in a child undergoing brain MR for work-up of seizures shows an incidental, well-defined hyperintense mass at the midline base of the tongue ➡, subsequently proven to be TGDC.*

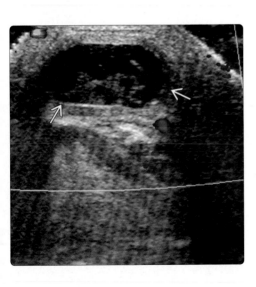

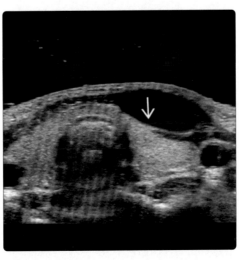

(Left) *Transverse ultrasound in a child with new-onset paramidline anterior left neck mass demonstrates a heterogeneous mass ➡, without internal flow on color Doppler but with significant internal echoes concerning for dermoid or carcinoma within TGDC. Histologically the lesion proved to be TGDC without hemorrhage, infection, or carcinoma.* (Right) *Transverse US in an 8 year old shows a typical infrahyoid TGDC as an anechoic, paramidline mass ➡ causing mild compression of the otherwise normal-appearing thyroid lobe.*

Cervical Thymic Cyst

TERMINOLOGY

- Cervical thymic cyst
- Cystic remnant of **thymopharyngeal duct**
  - Derivative of 3rd pharyngeal pouch

IMAGING

- Cystic mass closely associated with carotid sheath
- Anywhere along thymopharyngeal duct from pyriform sinus to anterior mediastinum
- **Usually lateral infrahyoid neck**
- **Left > right side of neck**
- May splay carotid artery and jugular vein
- Cystic component nonenhancing
- Cyst wall or solid nodules may enhance slightly

TOP DIFFERENTIAL DIAGNOSES

- 2nd branchial cleft cyst
  - Most common: Lateral to carotid sheath, anteromedial to SCM) muscle, posterior to submandibular gland

- 4th branchial anomaly
  - Primary location: Cyst or abscess anterior to left thyroid lobe
- Lymphatic malformation
  - Unilocular or multilocular, focal or infiltrative
  - Fluid-fluid levels common
- Abscess
  - Irregular, thick enhancing wall with low-attenuation center
  - Presents with signs and symptoms of infection
  - If associated with thyroid gland, think 4th branchial pouch anomaly

PATHOLOGY

- **Hassall corpuscles** in cyst wall confirm diagnosis

CLINICAL ISSUES

- Most present between **2-15 years** of age
- Only 33% present after 1st decade

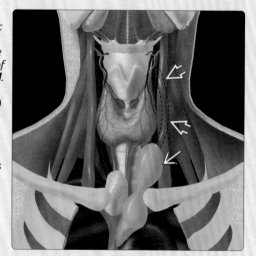
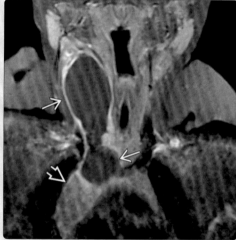

(Left) *Coronal graphic shows typical bilobed cervical thymic cyst ➡ extending from the anterior mediastinum into the lower neck along the course of the thymopharyngeal duct ➡. Notice the close association with the carotid space.* **(Right)** *Coronal T1 C+ FS MR in a 16 month old shows a cystic-appearing right neck mass ➡ causing mild airway compression. The cyst extends to the otherwise normal-appearing thymus ➡. Mild diffuse wall enhancement is consistent with chronic inflammation identified histologically.*

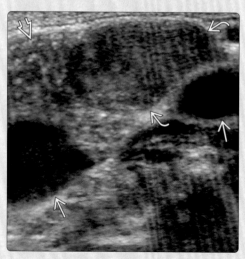
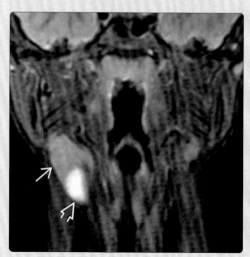

(Left) *Transverse ultrasound in a 7 year old demonstrates a mixed cystic and solid right thymic remnant splaying the carotid sheath vessels ➡. The lateral component demonstrates echogenicity typical of thymus ➡, and the medial component is cystic with mobile intraluminal echoes ➡ on real-time imaging.* **(Right)** *Coronal T2 MR in the same patient shows a mixed solid ➡ and cystic ➡ thymic remnant, the solid portion of which was isointense to intrathoracic thymus on all sequences.*

TERMINOLOGY

Abbreviations

- Cervical thymic cyst (CTC)

Synonyms

- Thymopharyngeal duct cyst; congenital thymic cyst

Definitions

- Cystic remnant of **thymopharyngeal duct**
  - Derivative of **3rd pharyngeal pouch**
- Hassall corpuscles in cyst wall confirm diagnosis

IMAGING

General Features

- Best diagnostic clue
  - Cystic mass in left > right lateral infrahyoid neck, in **lateral visceral space or adjacent to carotid space**
    - **Closely associated with carotid sheath**
      - In lower neck: Medial to carotid sheath, posterior to thyroid
      - In upper neck, or extending from upper neck to mediastinum: Splay carotid artery and jugular vein
- Location
  - Anywhere along thymopharyngeal duct from pyriform sinus to anterior mediastinum
  - **Most common site: Lateral infrahyoid neck**, at level of thyroid gland
    - Left > right
  - May parallel sternocleidomastoid muscle, close to carotid sheath
  - Cervical neck component ± extension to mediastinum
- Size
  - Variable, from several centimeters to very long, along course of thymopharyngeal duct
- Morphology
  - Usually large dominant cyst
  - May be multiloculated
  - May splay carotid artery and jugular vein, especially in upper neck
  - Larger CTC may present as dumbbell-shaped cervicothoracic mass, projecting from lower lateral cervical neck into superior mediastinum

CT Findings

- CECT
  - **Nonenhancing** low-attenuation lateral neck cyst
    - Close association with carotid sheath common
    - Solid components rare = aberrant thymic tissue, lymphoid aggregates, or parathyroid tissue
    - May be connected to mediastinal thymus directly or by fibrous cord

MR Findings

- T1WI
  - Homogeneous hypointense cyst most common
  - May be iso- to hyperintense if filled with blood products, proteinaceous fluid, or cholesterol
  - Thin wall
  - Solid nodules usually isointense to muscle
- T2WI
  - Homogeneously hyperintense fluid contents
- T1WI C+
  - Cystic component nonenhancing
  - Cyst wall or solid nodules may enhance slightly
  - If infected, cyst wall may be thickened and enhancing; surrounding soft tissue may be inflamed

Ultrasonographic Findings

- Thin-walled anechoic or hypoechoic lateral neck mass
- Rarely has solid nodules in wall

Imaging Recommendations

- Best imaging tool
  - CECT or MR preferable to ultrasound to demonstrate total extent of cyst
  - Ultrasound helpful if solid component has typical thymus echotexture
- Protocol advice
  - **Include upper mediastinum** to demonstrate mediastinal extension

DIFFERENTIAL DIAGNOSIS

2nd Branchial Cleft Cyst

- Most common branchial apparatus cyst
- When infrahyoid, anterior to carotid space
- **May mimic CTC when found in lower neck**

4th Branchial Anomaly

- Primary location: Cyst or **abscess anterior to left thyroid lobe**
- Often presents with suppurative thyroiditis
- Inflammation frequently extends to surround apex of pyriform sinus

Lymphatic Malformation

- May affect any space in H&N
- When in posterior cervical space, abuts carotid space posteriorly
- Unilocular or multilocular
- Focal or infiltrative and transspatial
- **Fluid-fluid levels common, secondary to intralesional hemorrhage**

Abscess

- Presents with signs and symptoms of infection
- **Irregular, thick enhancing wall** with low-attenuation center
- If associated with thyroid gland, think 4th branchial pouch anomaly

Thyroid Cyst

- Primary location: Intrathyroidal, left or right
- Large or hemorrhagic colloid cyst
- Usually more medial than CTC

PATHOLOGY

General Features

- Etiology
  - Remnants of thymopharyngeal duct → CTC
  - Ectopic thymus may also occur along thymopharyngeal duct

- Embryology
  - Failure of obliteration of **thymopharyngeal duct, remnant of 3rd pharyngeal pouch**
  - Thymopharyngeal duct arises from pyriform sinus, descends into mediastinum
  - **Persistent sequestered remnants may occur from mandible to thoracic inlet**
  - Thymus and parathyroid glands arise from 3rd and 4th pharyngeal pouches, respectively
  - Embryologic migration follows caudal course along thymopharyngeal duct during 1st trimester
- No malignant association

Gross Pathologic & Surgical Features

- Smooth, thin-walled cervical cyst, often with caudal fibrous strand extending to mediastinal thymus
- Filled with brownish fluid
- Cyst wall may be nodular
- Associated with lymphoid tissue or parathyroid or thymic remnants
- Rarely may extend through thyrohyoid membrane into pyriform sinus

Microscopic Features

- **Hassall corpuscles** in cyst wall confirm diagnosis
  - May not always be identifiable if prior hemorrhage or infection
- Cyst wall may contain
  - Lymphoid tissue
  - Parathyroid tissue
  - Thyroid or thymic tissue
  - Cholesterol crystals and granulomas, probably from prior hemorrhage

CLINICAL ISSUES

Presentation

- Most common signs/symptoms
  - **Often asymptomatic**
  - Gradually enlarging, soft, compressible mid- to lower cervical neck mass
  - When **large, may cause dysphagia, respiratory distress**, or vocal cord paralysis
- Other presentations
  - Large, infantile, cervicothoracic thymic cyst may present with respiratory compromise
  - Rarely may be associated with disordered calcium metabolism if parathyroid component is functioning

Demographics

- Age
  - Most present between **2-15 years** of age
  - Only 33% present after 1st decade
  - Rare reports of primary presentation in adulthood
- Gender
  - Slightly more common in male patients
- Epidemiology
  - Rare compared with other congenital neck masses
  - **Left > right side of neck**

Natural History & Prognosis

- Excellent prognosis if completely resected

- Recurrence common if incompletely resected

Treatment

- Complete surgical resection
- Large cervicothoracic thymic cyst may require H&N and thoracic surgery

DIAGNOSTIC CHECKLIST

Consider

- If cystic mass is intimately associated with anterior carotid sheath, think CTC
- If cystic mass extends from anterior neck to upper mediastinum, think CTC

Image Interpretation Pearls

- Dumbbell-shaped **cervicothoracic cystic mass** highly suggestive of either thymic cyst (vs. lymphatic malformation)
- If unilocular ovoid lesion with discrete margins, may be thymic cyst or unilocular lymphatic malformation

SELECTED REFERENCES

1. Goff CJ et al: Current management of congenital branchial cleft cysts, sinuses, and fistulae. Curr Opin Otolaryngol Head Neck Surg. 20(6):533-9, 2012
2. Pahlavan S et al: Microbiology of third and fourth branchial pouch cysts. Laryngoscope. 120(3):458-62, 2010
3. Thomas B et al: Revisiting imaging features and the embryologic basis of third and fourth branchial anomalies. AJNR Am J Neuroradiol. 31(4):755-60, 2010
4. Sturm-O'Brien AK et al: Cervical thymic anomalies--the Texas Children's Hospital experience. Laryngoscope. 119(10):1988-93, 2009
5. Statham MM et al: Cervical thymic remnants in children. Int J Pediatr Otorhinolaryngol. 72(12):1807-13, 2008
6. Mehrzad H et al: A combined third and fourth branchial arch anomaly: clinical and embryological implications. Eur Arch Otorhinolaryngol. 264(8):913-6, 2007
7. Charous DD et al: A third branchial pouch cyst presenting as a lateral neck mass in an adult. Ear Nose Throat J. 85(11):754-7, 2006
8. Koch BL: Cystic malformations of the neck in children. Pediatr Radiol. 35(5):463-77, 2005
9. Khariwala SS et al: Cervical presentations of thymic anomalies in children. Int J Pediatr Otorhinolaryngol. 68(7):909-14, 2004
10. Pereira KD et al: Management of anomalies of the third and fourth branchial pouches. Int J Pediatr Otorhinolaryngol. 68(1):43-50, 2004
11. Liberman M et al: Ten years of experience with third and fourth branchial remnants. J Pediatr Surg. 37(5):685-90, 2002
12. Ozturk H et al: Multilocular cervical thymic cyst: an unusual neck mass in children. Int J Pediatr Otorhinolaryngol. 61(3): 249-52, 2001
13. Koeller KK et al: Congenital cystic masses of the neck: radiologic-pathologic correlation. Radiographics. 19(1): 121-46; quiz 152-3, 1999
14. Millman B et al: Cervical thymic anomalies. Int J Pediatr Otorhinolaryngol. 47(1): 29-39, 1999
15. Hendrickson M et al: Congenital thymic cysts in children--mostly misdiagnosed. J Pediatr Surg. 33(6): 821-5, 1998
16. Hadi U et al: Valsalva-induced cervical thymic cyst. Otolaryngol Head Neck Surg. 117(6): S70-2, 1997
17. Nguyen Q et al: Cervical thymic cyst: case reports and review of the literature. Laryngoscope. 106(3 Pt 1):247-52, 1996
18. Marra S et al: Cervical thymic cyst. Otolaryngol Head Neck Surg. 112(2): 338-40, 1995
19. Miller MB et al: Cervical thymic cyst. Otolaryngol Head Neck Surg. 112(4): 586-8, 1995
20. Benson MT et al: Congenital anomalies of the branchial apparatus: embryology and pathologic anatomy. Radiographics. 12(5):943-60, 1992

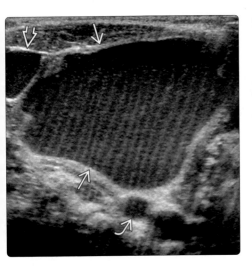

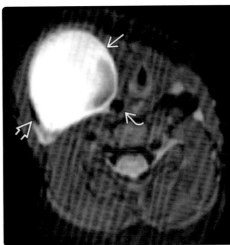

(Left) Transverse ultrasound in a 16 month old shows a large, unilocular cystic mass ➡ with significant internal echoes that were mobile at real-time scanning. The lesion splays the jugular vein ⮞ and carotid artery ⮞ typical of a thymic cyst. However, macrocystic lymphatic malformation would have a similar appearance. (Right) Axial FSE IR image in the same patient demonstrates hyperintense signal within the mass ➡ that displays the right jugular vein ⮞ and carotid artery ⮞, typical of thymic cysts.

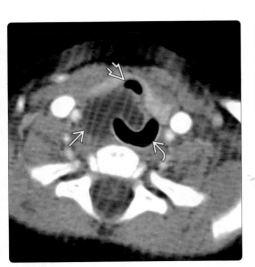

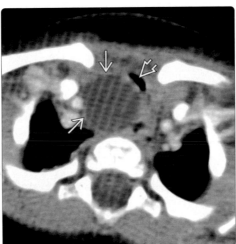

(Left) Axial CECT in a 6 month old with recurrent stridor shows a right-sided cystic neck mass ➡ deep to the right thyroid lobe and trachea ⮞. The cyst is compressible, indented along the posterior margin by the laryngeal mask airway ⮞. Atypical right-sided thymic cyst was found at surgery. (Right) Axial CECT in the same patient shows inferior extension of this thymic cyst ➡ into the upper mediastinum, resulting in leftward deviation of the trachea ⮞.

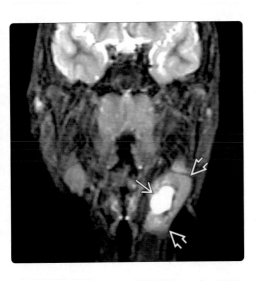

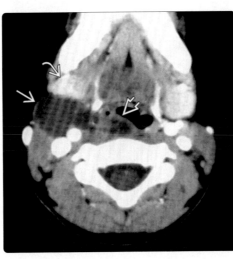

(Left) Coronal T2WI MR shows a rare association of both cystic ➡ and solid ⮞ remnants of thymus in the left neck. (Right) Axial CECT shows a rare appearance of thymic cyst located in the right neck posterior submandibular space ➡ displacing the submandibular gland ⮞ anteromedially. The lesion extends into the retropharyngeal space ⮞.

KEY FACTS

TERMINOLOGY

- Most common 1st branchial cleft (BC) anomalies are cysts (BCCs) or sinus tracts

IMAGING

- Best diagnostic clue: **Cystic mass near pinna & EAC or extending from EAC to angle of mandible**
- CECT: Well-circumscribed, nonenhancing, or rim-enhancing, low-density mass
  - If infected, may have thickened, enhancing rim

TOP DIFFERENTIAL DIAGNOSES

- Cholesteatoma, EAC
  - Submucosal mass with bone erosion
- Granulomatous infection (nontuberculous *Mycobacterium*)
  - Conglomerate parotid space necrotic nodal mass
  - Necrotic material extrudes into subcutaneous fat
- Parotitis complicated by abscess (rare)

- Parotitis with thick-walled, ring-enhancing cystic mass within or adjacent to parotid gland
  - Cellulitis extends to EAC and angle of mandible
- Lymphatic malformation
  - No contrast enhancement, ± fluid-fluid levels
- Venous malformation, EAC
  - Variably enhancing mass, ± phleboliths

PATHOLOGY

- **Remnant of 1st branchial apparatus**
  - Cysts > > sinus or fistula
- Most common location for 1st BCC to terminate is in EAC, between cartilaginous & bony portions

DIAGNOSTIC CHECKLIST

- Think 1st BCC in patient with chronic, unexplained otorrhea or recurrent parotid space abscess
  - Look for cyst in or adjacent to EAC, pinna, parotid gland, or, rarely, parapharyngeal space

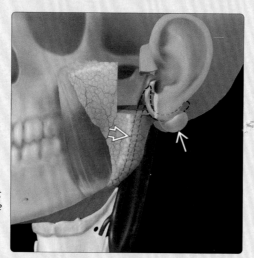
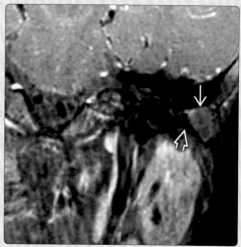

(Left) Oblique graphic of the ear and cheek reveals a Work type I 1st branchial cleft cyst (BCC) ➡ along the tract from the bony-cartilaginous junction of the external auditory canal (EAC) situated just posteroinferior to auricle. The tract of the Work type II BCC ➡ would project inferiorly to the angle of the mandible. (Right) Coronal T1WI C+ FS MR shows an intermediate signal intensity, nonenhancing, Work type I 1st BCC ➡ causing near complete obstruction of the left membranous EAC ➡.

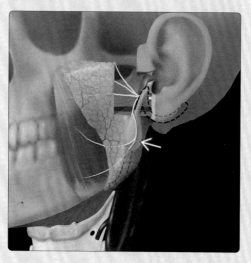
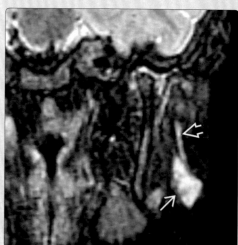

(Left) Oblique graphic of the ear and cheek shows an example of a Work type II 1st BCC ➡ along the course of the tract from the bony-cartilaginous EAC to the angle of the mandible. Note the intimate relationship of the BCC to the facial nerve branches. (Right) Coronal T2WI FS MR demonstrates the cystic inferior component of a type II 1st branchial apparatus cyst ➡ and the sinus tract ➡ extending superiorly toward the EAC.

TERMINOLOGY

Abbreviations

- Branchial cleft cyst (BCC)

Synonyms

- Pharyngeal cleft anomaly = branchial cleft anomaly (BCA)
- Pharyngeal apparatus = branchial apparatus (cleft, arch, or pouch)

Definitions

- **1st branchial cleft anomaly**: Most are **cysts or sinuses**; fistula from skin to external auditory canal (EAC) or middle ear is rare
- 1st BCC: Benign, congenital cyst in or adjacent to parotid gland, EAC, or pinna
  - Remnant of 1st branchial apparatus: Most commonly used classification
    - **Work type I**: Duplication of membranous EAC; ectodermal (cleft) origin
    - **Work type II**: Duplication of membranous EAC & cartilaginous pinna
      - Skin (ectodermal cleft) & cartilage (mesodermal arch) origin
      - May also have contribution from 2nd arch
  - Less commonly used classification
    - Arnot type I: Derived from buried rests of 1st branchial cleft (BC); intraparotid cyst or sinus
    - Arnot type II: Secondary to incomplete closure of 1st BC
      - Cyst or sinus in anterior triangle of neck ± communication with EAC
- **1st BC sinus tract opens near parotid gland**, EAC, parapharyngeal space, or anterior triangle of neck

IMAGING

General Features

- Best diagnostic clue
  - Cystic mass near pinna & EAC (Work type I) or extends from EAC to angle of mandible (Work type II)
- Location
  - Type I: **Periauricular** cyst or sinus tract
    - Anterior, inferior, or posterior to pinna & concha
  - Type II: **Periparotid** cyst or sinus tract
    - More intimately associated with parotid gland, medial or lateral to CNVII
    - Superficial, parotid space, or parapharyngeal space (PPS)
- Size
  - Variable but usually < 3 cm
- Morphology
  - Well-circumscribed cyst

CT Findings

- NECT
  - Low-density cyst
  - If previously infected, can be isodense
- CECT
  - Well-circumscribed, nonenhancing or rim-enhancing, low-density mass
  - If infected, may have thickened, enhancing rim

  - Surrounding fat stranding suggests infection
  - 1st BCC, Work type I
    - Cyst anterior, inferior, or posterior to EAC
    - Lesion may "beak" toward bony-cartilaginous junction of EAC
    - Often runs parallel to EAC
  - 1st BCC, Work type II
    - Cyst superficial, parotid space, or PPS
    - May be as low as posterior submandibular space
    - Deep projection may "beak" to bony-cartilaginous junction of EAC
  - 1st branchial cleft sinus tract (BCST): Linear density courses through subcutaneous fat in vicinity of parotid, EAC, or PPS

MR Findings

- T1WI
  - Low signal intensity unilocular cyst
- T2WI
  - High signal intensity unilocular cyst
  - May see sinus tract to skin, EAC, or, rarely, PPS
  - Edema in surrounding soft tissues when superinfected
- T1WI C+
  - Cyst wall normally does not enhance
  - Previous or concurrent infection may → thickened, enhancing rim

Ultrasonographic Findings

- Anechoic mass in periauricular or periparotid area

Imaging Recommendations

- Best imaging tool
  - CECT or MR for evaluation of cyst
  - MR (T2WI) for small lesions & associated sinus tract
- Protocol advice
  - Coronal reformatted images helpful to evaluate relationship to EAC

DIFFERENTIAL DIAGNOSIS

Congenital Cholesteatoma of EAC

- Nonenhancing submucosal mass with bone erosion
- Lesion matrix may show bone fragments
- Hole in tympanic plate
- Known association with 1st BCC ± fistula to EAC and stenotic or duplicated EAC

Non-TB *Mycobacterium*, Lymph Nodes

- 4- to 6-week history of minimally tender mass with violaceous skin discoloration
- Conglomerate parotid space necrotic nodal mass
- Necrotic tissue may extrude into subcutaneous fat
- Minimal stranding of subcutaneous fat

Parotitis, Acute

- Presents with marked tenderness and fever
- Enlarged/inflamed enhancing parotid
- Cellulitis extends to EAC and angle of mandible
- Complicating abscess is rare: Thick-walled, ring-enhancing cystic mass within/adjacent to parotid gland

Lymphatic Malformation, Periauricular

- Congenital vascular malformation; embryonic lymphatic sacs
- Unilocular or multilocular; microcystic or macrocystic
- Single space or transspatial
- Characteristic fluid-fluid levels are common
- No contrast enhancement or phleboliths unless mixed venous component

Venous Malformation, Periauricular

- Congenital vascular malformation: Endothelial-lined vascular sinusoids
- Single or multiple, lobulated mass ± phleboliths
- Variable enhancement pattern reflects sluggish vascular flow to & through lesion
- ± nonenhancing lymphatic component if mixed venolymphatic malformation

PATHOLOGY

General Features

- Associated abnormalities
  - May be seen in association with other 1st branchial apparatus anomalies
  - May occasionally have associated but separate EAC congenital cholesteatoma
    - Small mass in medial EAC with bony remodeling/erosion EAC and hole in tympanic plate
    - May transgress tympanic membrane (TM) or extend from tympanic plate under TM into middle ear cavity
- Embryology/anatomy
  - Remnant of 1st branchial apparatus
    - **Cleft (ectoderm)** of 1st apparatus → EAC
    - **Arch (mesoderm)** → mandible, muscles of mastication, CNV, incus body, malleus head
    - **Pouch (endoderm)** → eustachian tube, middle ear cavity, & mastoid air cells
  - Branchial remnant occurs with incomplete obliteration of 1st branchial apparatus
  - Isolated BCC has no internal (pharyngeal) or external (cutaneous) communication
  - Branchial cleft fistula has both internal & external connections, from EAC lumen to skin
  - BCST opens externally or (rarely) internally; closed portion ends as blind pouch
  - 2/3 of 1st BC remnants are isolated cysts

Gross Pathologic & Surgical Features

- Cystic neck mass
  - Easily dissected unless repeated infection
- Contents of cyst usually thick mucus
- Cystic remnant may split facial nerve (CNVII) trunk
- CNVII may be medial or lateral to 1st BCC
- Close proximity to CNVII makes surgery more difficult
- Most common location for 1st BCC to terminate is in EAC between cartilaginous & bony portions

Microscopic Features

- Thin outer layer: Fibrous pseudocapsule
- Inner layer: Flat squamoid epithelium
- ± germinal centers & lymphocytes in cyst wall

CLINICAL ISSUES

Presentation

- Most common signs/symptoms
  - Soft, painless, compressible mass: EAC, periauricular, intraparotid or periparotid suprahyoid neck
- Other signs/symptoms
  - Recurrent EAC, preauricular or periparotid swelling
  - Tender mass ± fever if infected
  - EAC or skin sinus tract rare
  - Chronic purulent ear drainage if EAC sinus tract

Demographics

- Age
  - Majority present **< 10 years old**
  - Sinus tracts present earlier
  - When cyst only, may present later, even as adult
- Epidemiology
  - Accounts for 8% of all branchial apparatus remnants
  - Type II > > type I 1st BCC

Natural History & Prognosis

- May enlarge with upper respiratory tract infection
  - Lymph follicles in wall react, wall secretes
- Often incised and drained as "abscess" only to recur
- Prognosis excellent if completely resected
- May recur if residual cyst wall remains

Treatment

- Complete surgical resection
- Proximity to CNVII puts nerve at risk during surgery
  - Work type I: Proximal CNVII
  - Work type II: More distal CNVII branches

DIAGNOSTIC CHECKLIST

Consider

- Think of 1st BCC in patient with chronic, unexplained otorrhea or recurrent parotid gland abscess
  - Look for cyst in or adjacent to parotid gland, EAC, pinna, or, rarely, parapharyngeal space
- Think syndromic etiology for multiple BCA and craniofacial anomaly, e.g., branchiootorenal syndrome

SELECTED REFERENCES

1. Schmidt R et al: Management of first branchial cleft anomalies via a cartilage-splitting technique. Otolaryngol Head Neck Surg. 152(6):1149-51, 2015
2. Shinn JR et al: First branchial cleft anomalies: otologic manifestations and treatment outcomes. Otolaryngol Head Neck Surg. 152(3):506-12, 2015
3. Gonzalez-Perez LM et al: Bilateral first branchial cleft anomaly with evidence of a genetic aetiology. Int J Oral Maxillofac Surg. 43(3):296-300, 2014
4. Bajaj Y et al: Branchial anomalies in children. Int J Pediatr Otorhinolaryngol. 75(8):1020-3, 2011
5. Johnson JM et al: Syndromes of the first and second branchial arches, part 1: embryology and characteristic defects. AJNR Am J Neuroradiol. 32(1):14-9, 2011
6. Johnson JM et al: Syndromes of the first and second branchial arches, part 2: syndromes. AJNR Am J Neuroradiol. 32(2):230-7, 2011
7. Martinez Del Pero M et al: Presentation of first branchial cleft anomalies: the Sheffield experience. J Laryngol Otol. 121(5):455-9, 2007
8. Nicollas R et al: Unusual association of congenital middle ear cholesteatoma and first branchial cleft anomaly: management and embryological concepts. Int J Pediatr Otorhinolaryngol. 69(2):279-82, 2005
9. Mukherji SK et al: Evaluation of first branchial anomalies by CT and MR. J Comput Assist Tomogr. 17(4):576-81, 1993

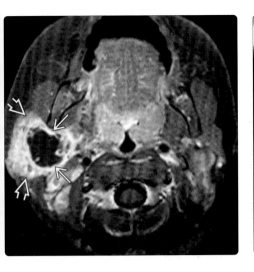

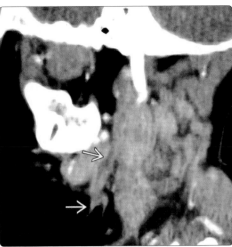

(Left) *Axial T1WI C+ FS MR demonstrates an irregularly shaped, infected 1st BCC ➜ within the right parotid gland, with a thick enhancing wall & diffuse abnormal enhancement of surrounding parotid gland ➜.* **(Right)** *Sagittal CECT in a patient with intermittent drainage at anterior neck and EAC demonstrates a fluid-filled fistula ➜ extending to the skin surface in the left anterior neck that also extended to the EAC at surgery (not shown).*

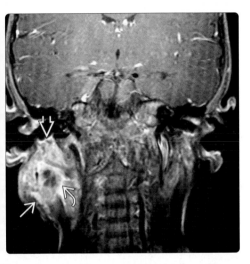

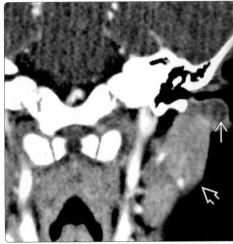

(Left) *Coronal T1WI C+ FS MR demonstrates heterogeneously enhancing inflammatory process ➜ involving the right parotid gland, abutting the inferior aspect of the cartilaginous right EAC ➜. The central area of decreased enhancement represents the infected underlying 1st BCC ➜.* **(Right)** *Coronal CECT in a 3 year old with a left EAC mass shows a well-defined, low-attenuation lesion ➜ superficial to the parotid gland ➜ and abutting the inferior border of the EAC, a typical location for a 1st BCC.*

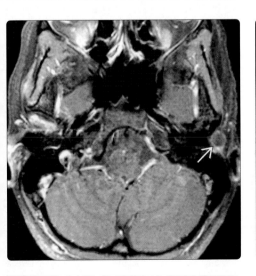

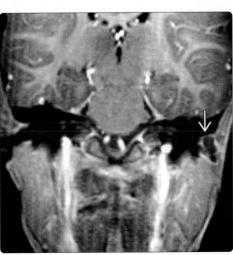

(Left) *Axial T1WI C+ FS MR in a 9 year old with a left EAC mass shows a low signal intensity preauricular 1st BCC with minimal rim enhancement ➜.* **(Right)** *Coronal T1WI C+ FS MR in the same patient clearly shows obstruction of the left EAC by the Work type I BCC ➜.*

2nd Branchial Cleft Cyst

TERMINOLOGY

- Cervical sinus of His cystic remnant: 2nd, 3rd, & 4th branchial clefts & 2nd branchial arch derivative
- Synonyms
  - 2nd branchial cleft cyst (BCC) or anomaly
  - 2nd branchial apparatus cyst or anomaly

IMAGING

- Best diagnostic clue: Cystic neck mass posterolateral to submandibular gland, lateral to carotid space, anterior (or anteromedial) to sternocleidomastoid muscle
- If infected, wall is thicker & enhances with surrounding soft tissue cellulitis

TOP DIFFERENTIAL DIAGNOSES

- Lymphatic malformation
  - Frequently transspatial
- Cervical thymic cyst
  - Remnant of 3rd pharyngeal pouch

- Lymphadenopathy/abscess
  - Presents with signs and symptoms of infection
- Cystic metastatic nodes
  - Squamous cell carcinoma (SCCa) nodal metastasis
  - Differentiated thyroid carcinoma nodal metastasis
- Carotid space schwannoma
  - Occasional large intramural cysts
  - Thick, enhancing wall
  - Rare in children

PATHOLOGY

- 2nd branchial apparatus cyst, sinus or fistulae
- Epidemiology: 2nd branchial apparatus anomalies (BAA) account for up to 95% of all BAA

DIAGNOSTIC CHECKLIST

- Beware of adult with 1st presentation of "2nd BCC"
  - May be necrotic metastasis from head & neck SCCa primary tumor

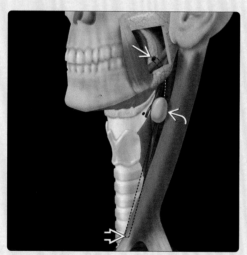
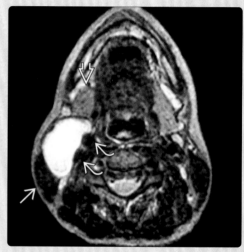

(Left) Sagittal oblique graphic shows 2nd branchial cleft cyst ➡ in its most common location, anterior to the sternomastoid muscle (SCM) & anterolateral to the carotid space. The full tract may extend from the faucial tonsil ➡ to low anterior neck ➡.
(Right) Axial T2WI MR shows a well-defined hyperintense mass anterior to the right SCM ➡, posterolateral to the right submandibular gland ➡, and anterolateral to the right carotid sheath vessels ➡. This is the most common location of 2nd branchial apparatus cysts.

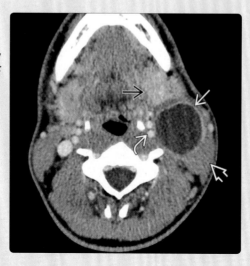
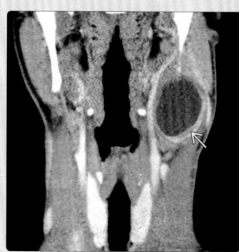

(Left) Axial CECT in a 17-year-old boy shows a well-defined, low-attenuation mass ➡ in the typical location of a Bailey type II 2nd branchial cleft cyst: Anterior to the SCM ➡, lateral to the carotid sheath vessels ➡, and posterior to the submandibular gland ➡.
(Right) Coronal CECT in the same patient demonstrates a thicker wall inferiorly ➡, which histologically represented lymphoid follicles in the wall of the cyst.

TERMINOLOGY

Abbreviations

- 2nd branchial cleft cyst (BCC)

Synonyms

- 2nd branchial apparatus cyst (BAC)
- 2nd branchial apparatus anomaly (BAA)

Definitions

- 2nd BCC: **Most common** branchial apparatus cyst
  - **Cystic remnant of cervical sinus of His**: Derivative of 2nd, 3rd, & 4th branchial clefts
- Sinus: Usually communicates externally along anterior margin of sternocleidomastoid muscle (SCM)
  - Rarely communicates internally to tonsillar fossa
- Fistula: Communicates externally and internally
  - Secondary to persistence of both branchial cleft and pharyngeal pouch remnant
- Combinations
  - Cyst + sinus &/or fistula

IMAGING

General Features

- Best diagnostic clue
  - Cystic neck mass **posterolateral to submandibulargland, lateral to carotid space, anterior to SCM**
  - Most are at or immediately caudal to angle of mandible
- Location
  - Bailey classification of 2nd BACs
    - Type I: Deep to platysma muscle, anterior to SCM
    - **Type II**: Anterior to SCM, posterior to submandibular gland, lateral to carotid sheath
      - □ **Most common**
    - Type III: Protrudes between ICA & ECA, may extend to lateral pharyngeal wall or superiorly to skull base
    - Type IV: Adjacent to lateral pharyngeal wall, probably remnant of 2nd pharyngeal pouch
  - 2nd branchial apparatus fistula extends from anterior to SCM, through carotid artery bifurcation, & terminates in tonsillar fossa
- Size
  - Variable; may range from several cm to > 5 cm
- Morphology
  - Ovoid or rounded, well-circumscribed cyst
  - Focal rim of cyst may extend to carotid bifurcation

CT Findings

- CECT
  - **Low-density cyst with nonenhancing wall**
  - If infected, wall is thicker & enhances with surrounding soft tissue cellulitis

MR Findings

- T1WI
  - Cyst is usually isointense to CSF
  - Infection → increased signal intensity/protein content
- T2WI
  - Hyperintense cyst, no discernible wall
- FLAIR
  - Cyst is iso- or slightly hyperintense to CSF
- T1WI C+
  - No intrinsic contrast enhancement
  - Peripheral wall enhancement if infected

Ultrasonographic Findings

- Anechoic or hypoechoic, thin-walled cyst
  - **May give pseudosolid US appearance**
    - Real time will demonstrate mobile internal echoes to differentiate from solid lesion
- Thickened cyst wall if infected

Imaging Recommendations

- CT, US, or MR clearly demonstrate location of type I, II, and III cysts
- May be difficult to visualize type IV cysts with US
- CT or MR best demonstrate associated findings of infection and rare type IV cysts

DIFFERENTIAL DIAGNOSIS

Lymphatic Malformation

- Unilocular or multilocular
- Frequently transspatial
- Fluid-fluid levels if intralesional hemorrhage
- Isolation to same location as 2nd branchial apparatus anomalies is uncommon

Thymic Cyst

- Remnant of thymopharyngeal duct, derivative of 3rd pharyngeal pouch
- Left side more common than right
- Up to 50% extend into superior mediastinum

Lymphadenopathy/Abscess

- Present with signs and symptoms of infection
- Irregular, thick, enhancing wall with nonenhancing central cavity
- Surrounding soft tissue induration except with *Mycobacterium*
- Associated ipsilateral nonsuppurative adenopathy

Cystic Metastatic Nodes

- Necrotic mass with thick, enhancing wall
- Rare in children, occasional in teenagers
- Cystic squamous cell carcinoma (SCCa) nodal metastasis
- Cystic differentiated thyroid carcinoma nodal metastasis

Carotid Space Schwannoma

- Occasional large intramural cysts
- Thick, enhancing wall
- Centered in posterior carotid space

PATHOLOGY

General Features

- Embryology
  - 2nd branchial arch overgrows 2nd, 3rd, & 4th branchial clefts, forming ectodermally lined cervical sinus of His
  - Remnant of 2nd, 3rd, & 4th branchial clefts opens into cervical sinus of His via cervical vesicles
  - Normally developing cervical sinus of His & vesicles involute

Pediatric Lesions

- Etiology
  - Remnants of 2nd branchial apparatus may form cyst, sinus, or fistula
- Associated abnormalities
  - **Usually isolated lesion**
  - May be part of branchiootorenal (BOR) syndrome
    - Autosomal dominant inheritance
    - Bilateral branchial fistulas or cysts & preauricular tag or pit
    - Profound mixed hearing loss: Cochlear & semicircular canal malformations, stapes fixation
    - Renal anomalies: Cysts, dysplasia, agenesis
    - Patulous eustachian tubes
  - Branchiootic syndrome similar to BOR, without renal involvement

Gross Pathologic & Surgical Features

- Well-defined cyst in locations described by Bailey
- Filled with cheesy material or serous, mucoid, or purulent fluid

Microscopic Features

- Squamous epithelial-lined cyst
- Lymphoid infiltrate in wall, in form of germinal centers
  - Lymphoid tissue suggests epithelial rests may be entrapped within cervical lymph nodes during embryogenesis

CLINICAL ISSUES

Presentation

- Most common signs/symptoms
  - Painless, compressible lateral neck mass in child or young adult
  - **May enlarge during upper respiratory tract infection**
    - Probably due to response of lymphoid tissue
  - Fever, tenderness, and erythema if infected

Demographics

- Age
  - Majority < 5 years; 2nd peak in 2nd or 3rd decade
- Epidemiology
  - 2nd branchial apparatus anomalies account for up to 95% of all branchial apparatus anomalies

Natural History & Prognosis

- Untreated, may become repeatedly infected
- Recurrent inflammation makes surgical resection more difficult
- Excellent prognosis if lesion is completely resected

Treatment

- Complete surgical resection is treatment of choice
- Surgeon must dissect around cyst bed to exclude possibility of associated fistula or sinus
  - If fistula present, usually identified at birth
    - Mucoid secretions are emitted from skin opening
  - If tract proceeds superomedially, it passes through carotid bifurcation into palatine tonsil crypts
  - If tract courses inferiorly, it passes along anterior carotid space, reaching supraclavicular skin
- Endoscope-assisted resection via retroauricular approach feasible alternative to conventional resection

DIAGNOSTIC CHECKLIST

Consider

- Infection if cyst wall enhances or cellulitis
- Does cyst appear adherent to internal jugular vein or carotid sheath?

Image Interpretation Pearls

- Beware of adult with 1st presentation of "2nd BCC"
  - Mass may be metastatic node from head & neck SCCa primary tumor
  - If patient over 30 years of age, first consider cystic nodal metastasis

SELECTED REFERENCES

1. Thottam PJ et al: Complete second branchial cleft anomaly presenting as a fistula and a tonsillar cyst: an interesting congenital anomaly. Ear Nose Throat J. 93(10-11):466-8, 2014
2. Chen LS et al: Endoscope-assisted versus conventional second branchial cleft cyst resection. Surg Endosc. 26(5):1397-402, 2012
3. Goff CJ et al: Current management of congenital branchial cleft cysts, sinuses, and fistulae. Curr Opin Otolaryngol Head Neck Surg. 20(6):533-9, 2012
4. Bajaj Y et al: Branchial anomalies in children. Int J Pediatr Otorhinolaryngol. 75(8):1020-3, 2011
5. Buchanan MA et al: Cystic schwannoma of the cervical plexus masquerading as a type II second branchial cleft cyst. Eur Arch Otorhinolaryngol. 266(3):459-62, 2009
6. Hudgins PA, Gillison M. Second branchial cleft cyst: not!! AJNR Am J Neuroradiol. 30(9):1628-9, 2009
7. Koch BL: Cystic malformations of the neck in children. Pediatr Radiol. 35(5):463-77, 2005
8. Lanham PD et al: Second branchial cleft cyst mimic: case report. AJNR Am J Neuroradiol. 26(7):1862-4, 2005
9. Kemperman MH et al: Evidence of progression and fluctuation of hearing impairment in branchio-oto-renal syndrome. Int J Audiol. 43(9):523-32, 2004
10. Ceruti S et al: Temporal bone anomalies in the branchio-oto-renal syndrome: detailed computed tomographic and magnetic resonance imaging findings. Otol Neurotol. 23(2):200-7, 2002
11. Kemperman MH et al: Inner ear anomalies are frequent but nonobligatory features of the branchio-oto-renal syndrome. Arch Otolaryngol Head Neck Surg. 128(9):1033-8, 2002
12. Shin JH et al: Parapharyngeal second branchial cyst manifesting as cranial nerve palsies: MR findings. AJNR Am J Neuroradiol. 22(3):510-2, 2001
13. Nusbaum AO et al: Recurrence of a deep neck infection: a clinical indication of an underlying congenital lesion. Arch Otolaryngol Head Neck Surg. 125(12):1379-82, 1999
14. Ahuja A et al: Solitary cystic nodal metastasis from occult papillary carcinoma of the thyroid mimicking a branchial cyst: a potential pitfall. Clin Radiol. 53(1):61-3, 1998
15. Choi SS et al: Branchial anomalies: a review of 52 cases. Laryngoscope. 105(9 Pt 1):909-13, 1995
16. Benson MT et al: Congenital anomalies of the branchial apparatus: embryology and pathologic anatomy. Radiographics. 12(5):943-60, 1992
17. Doi O et al: Branchial remnants: a review of 58 cases. J Pediatr Surg. 23(9):789-92, 1988
18. Salazar JE et al: Second branchial cleft cyst: unusual location and a new CT diagnostic sign. AJR Am J Roentgenol. 145(5):965-6, 1985
19. Harnsberger HR et al: Branchial cleft anomalies and their mimics: computed tomographic evaluation. Radiology. 152(3):739-48, 1984
20. Gold BM: Second branchial cleft cyst and fistula. AJR Am J Roentgenol. 134(5):1067-9, 1980

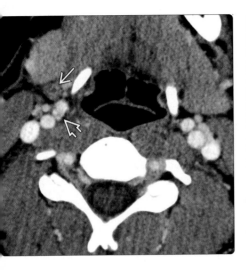
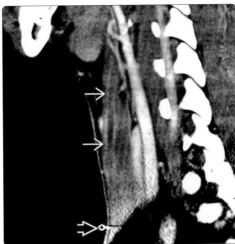

(Left) *Axial CECT in a 15-year-old boy with a pit in the lower anterior neck since birth, now draining purulent fluid, demonstrates a well-defined small lesion ➡ with thick wall anterior to the carotid vessels ➡ and posterior to the submandibular gland.* (Right) *Sagittal CT reconstruction in the same patient demonstrates the course of the infected 2nd branchial cleft sinus tract ➡, extending from the level of the pit (marked with radiodense marker ➡) toward the faucial tonsil.*

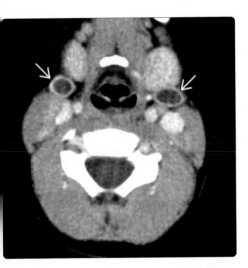
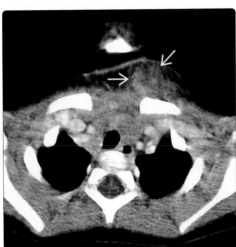

(Left) *Axial CECT in a 2-year-old boy with branchiootorenal syndrome shows bilateral, well-defined, nonenhancing cysts ➡ in the typical location of Bailey type II 2nd branchial cleft cysts.* (Right) *Axial CECT demonstrates a supraclavicular phlegmonous inflammatory mass ➡ deep to a skin dimple in an infant with an infected 2nd branchial apparatus sinus tract. This is the classic location of the lowermost aspect of a remnant sinus tract or fistula.*

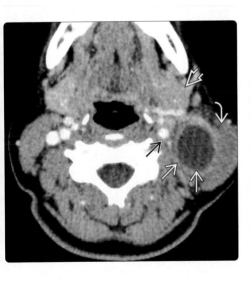
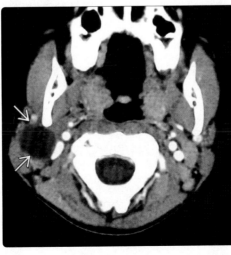

(Left) *Axial CECT shows a well-defined, low-attenuation mass ➡ posterior to the left submandibular gland ➡, deviating the left SCM ➡ posterolaterally and the carotid sheath vessels medially ➡. The thin rim of enhancement was secondary to chronic inflammation and lymphoid hyperplasia in the wall of the cyst.* (Right) *Axial CECT demonstrates a nonenhancing, cystic-appearing mass ➡ at the angle of the right mandible, the most common location of a 2nd branchial cleft cyst.*

TERMINOLOGY

- 3rd branchial cleft cyst (BCC)
  - Epithelial-lined **remnant 3rd branchial cleft**

IMAGING

- CT/MR/US
  - Unilocular thin-walled cyst in **upper posterior cervical space or lower anterior neck**
  - If infected, cyst wall thickens and enhances
  - ± adjacent cellulitis or myositis
- Barium or water-soluble contrast swallow may outline **associated sinus or fistula**

TOP DIFFERENTIAL DIAGNOSES

- 2nd branchial cleft cyst: Most common BCC
- Lymphatic malformation: Uni- or multilocular
- Abscess: Signs and symptoms of infection
- Cervical thymic cyst: 3rd pouch remnant

- 4th branchial apparatus anomaly: Pyriform sinus sinus tract and left neck abscess
- Infrahyoid thyroglossal duct cyst: Embedded in strap muscles when infrahyoid
- Cystic-necrotic metastatic lymph node: Usually known primary H&N squamous cell carcinoma or systemic NHL
- External laryngocele: Communicates with laryngeal ventricle through thyrohyoid membrane

CLINICAL ISSUES

- Fluctuant mass in posterolateral upper neck
- Frequently presents in **adulthood**
- Purulent drainage from skin ostium if associated fistula

DIAGNOSTIC CHECKLIST

- Cyst in posterior triangle of upper neck
  - Think 3rd BCC
- Abscess in posterior triangle of upper neck
  - Think infected preexisting underlying 3rd BCC

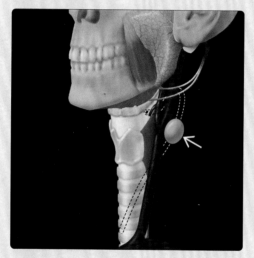
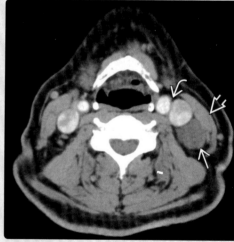

(Left) Lateral graphic illustrates the course of a 3rd branchial anomaly (dashes), along which 3rd branchial cleft cysts arise, most commonly in the upper posterior triangle ➡. (Right) Axial CECT in this adult male patient with a posterior left neck mass demonstrates a well-defined, thin-walled, unilocular cyst ➡ in the posterior cervical space, deep to the sternocleidomastoid muscle ➡ and posterolateral to the carotid space ➡. Note that the cyst wall is imperceptible, indicating the lesion has not been infected.

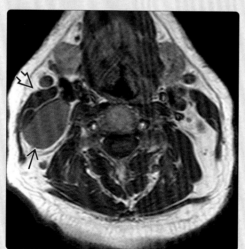
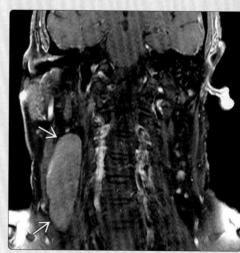

(Left) Axial T1 MR in a 60-year-old man (imaged for other reasons) shows an incidental 3rd branchial cleft cyst in the right posterior triangle ➡ deep to the sternocleidomastoid muscle ➡. (Right) Coronal T1 C+ FS MR in the same patient shows the cyst ➡ deep to the sternocleidomastoid muscle, without significant internal or perilesional enhancement; this is typical of an uncomplicated 3rd branchial cleft cyst.

3rd Branchial Cleft Cyst

TERMINOLOGY

Abbreviations
- 3rd branchial cleft cyst (BCC)

Synonyms
- 3rd branchial apparatus cyst (BAC)

Definitions
- Epithelial-lined cystic remnant of 3rd branchial cleft

IMAGING

General Features
- Best diagnostic clue
  o **Unilocular thin-walled cyst** in upper **posterior cervical space** or lower anterior neck
- Location
  o Anywhere along course of 3rd branchial cleft or pouch
    – Upper neck: Posterior cervical space
    – Lower neck: Anterior border sternocleidomastoid muscle
    – Rarely in submandibular space, lateral to cephalad hypopharynx
  o Classically 3rd branchial fistula would exit base of pyriform sinus, course superior to superior laryngeal and hypoglossal nerves, and inferior to glossopharyngeal nerve
- Size
  o Variable, usually 2-3 cm at presentation
- Morphology
  o Typically ovoid or round cyst

Fluoroscopic Findings
- Barium or water-soluble contrast swallow
  o May outline **associated sinus or fistula**
  o Point of exit from hypopharynx
    – **High lateral margin of pyriform sinus**

CT Findings
- CECT
  o Round or ovoid sharply marginated lesions with central fluid attenuation
  o Cyst wall thin, no calcifications
  o If infected, cyst wall thickens and enhances
    – ± adjacent cellulitis &/or myositis
  o Sternocleidomastoid muscle displaced laterally when cyst in high posterior neck
  o Sternocleidomastoid muscle displaced posterolaterally when cyst in low anterior neck

MR Findings
- T1WI
  o Homogeneous T1 hypointense fluid contents
  o Cyst wall thin or imperceptible
- T2WI
  o Homogeneous T2 hyperintense fluid contents
  o + edema in surrounding tissues if infected
- T1WI C+
  o Thin, uniform minimally enhancing cyst wall
  o If infected
    – Cyst wall thickened and enhancing

- – Fluid contents hyperintense relative to CSF
- – Strand-like enhancement in soft tissues surrounding 3rd BCC

Ultrasonographic Findings
- Thin-walled hypoechoic mass

Imaging Recommendations
- Best imaging tool
  o CECT or MR best to evaluate complete extent
- Protocol advice
  o Barium (or water-soluble contrast) swallow may outline **associated sinus or fistula**
  o **Fistula** may be outlined by direct injection of cutaneous ostium

DIFFERENTIAL DIAGNOSIS

2nd Branchial Cleft Cyst
- Most common branchial apparatus anomaly
- Most common angle of mandible mass in young adult
- Usually lateral to carotid space, posterior to submandibular gland, and anteromedial to sternocleidomastoid muscle

Lymphatic Malformation
- Majority diagnosed before 2 years of age
- Unilocular or multilocular
- Focal or infiltrative
- Fluid-fluid levels if intralesional hemorrhage

Abscess
- Presents with signs and symptoms of infection
- Irregular thick enhancing wall, low-attenuation center
- Surrounding cellulitis
- If associated with thyroid gland, think 4th branchial pouch anomaly
- If in posterior cervical space of upper neck, think infected underlying 3rd BCC

Cervical Thymic Cyst
- 3rd branchial pouch remnant
- Along course of thymopharyngeal duct
- Left > > right
- Closely associated with carotid sheath
- ± extension to anterior mediastinum

4th Branchial Apparatus Anomaly
- Present with suppurative thyroiditis in children
- Abscess closely associated with anterior left thyroid lobe, thyroiditis
- Sinus tract from pyriform sinus apex to anterior lower left neck
- Remnant of 4th (or 3rd) branchial pouch

Infrahyoid Thyroglossal Duct Cyst
- Midline or paramidline anterior neck cyst in child or young adult
- Off midline in strap muscles or anterior to thyroid gland when infrahyoid

Metastases, Cystic-Necrotic Lymph Node
- Spinal accessory malignant necrotic adenopathy in posterior cervical space

- Usually known primary H&N squamous cell carcinoma or systemic non-Hodgkin lymphoma

External Laryngocele

- Adult glassblower or trumpet player with enlarging neck mass
- Communicates with laryngeal ventricle through thyrohyoid membrane

PATHOLOGY

General Features

- Etiology
  - Controversial
    - Failure of obliteration of 3rd branchial cleft, portion of cervical sinus of His or 3rd pharyngeal pouch
- Associated abnormalities
  - 3rd branchial sinus
    - Single opening
      □ Endopharyngeal in high lateral hypopharynx or cutaneous opening in supraclavicular area anterior to carotid artery
  - 3rd branchial fistula
    - 2 openings
      □ Endopharyngeal in high lateral hypopharynx and cutaneous opening in supraclavicular area anterior to carotid artery
      □ Skin opening may be pseudofistula secondary to repeated infection or surgical incision rather than true fistula

Gross Pathologic & Surgical Features

- Smooth thin-walled cysts
- May contain clear, watery to mucinous material
  - ± desquamated cellular debris

Microscopic Features

- Lined by squamous epithelium (occasionally by columnar epithelium)
- Lymphoid tissue in walls of cyst with reactive lymphoid follicles

CLINICAL ISSUES

Presentation

- Most common signs/symptoms
  - Fluctuant mass in posterolateral neck
  - May enlarge rapidly following upper respiratory tract infection
- Other signs/symptoms
  - Recurrent lateral neck or retropharyngeal abscesses
  - Draining fistula along anterior margin of sternocleidomastoid muscle

Demographics

- Age
  - Frequently presents in **adulthood**
  - Presentation of cysts in neonates and infants unusual
  - When sinus or fistula present, early presentation more common
- Epidemiology
  - 3rd branchial cleft anomalies account for only **3%** of all branchial anomalies

- 2nd BCC > 1st BCC > 3rd BCC

Natural History & Prognosis

- Good prognosis if completely resected
- May become infected and present with neck abscess

Treatment

- Surgical resection
  - If infected, treat with antibiotics prior to surgical resection
  - Surgery includes resection of cyst and any associated sinus or fistula

DIAGNOSTIC CHECKLIST

Consider

- When cyst in posterior triangle (posterior cervical space) of upper neck
  - Think 3rd BCC
- Abscess in posterior triangle of upper neck
  - Think infected preexisting underlying 3rd BCC

SELECTED REFERENCES

1. Goff CJ et al: Current management of congenital branchial cleft cysts, sinuses, and fistulae. Curr Opin Otolaryngol Head Neck Surg. 20(6):533-9, 2012
2. Pahlavan S et al: Microbiology of third and fourth branchial pouch cysts. Laryngoscope. 120(3):458-62, 2010
3. Thomas B et al: Revisiting imaging features and the embryologic basis of third and fourth branchial anomalies. AJNR Am J Neuroradiol. 31(4):755-60, 2010
4. Joshi MJ et al: The rare third branchial cleft cyst. AJNR Am J Neuroradiol. 30(9):1804-6, 2009
5. Koch BL: Cystic malformations of the neck in children. Pediatr Radiol. 35(5):463-77, 2005
6. Khariwala SS et al: Cervical presentations of thymic anomalies in children. Int J Pediatr Otorhinolaryngol. 68(7):909-14, 2004
7. Pereira KD et al: Management of anomalies of the third and fourth branchial pouches. Int J Pediatr Otorhinolaryngol. 68(1):43-50, 2004
8. Tsai CC et al: Branchial-cleft sinus presenting with a retropharyngeal abscess for a newborn: a case report. Am J Perinatol. 20(5):227-31, 2003
9. Liberman M et al: Ten years of experience with third and fourth branchial remnants. J Pediatr Surg. 37(5):685-90, 2002
10. Huang RY et al: Third branchial cleft anomaly presenting as a retropharyngeal abscess. Int J Pediatr Otorhinolaryngol. 54(2-3):167-72, 2000
11. Mandell DL: Head and neck anomalies related to the branchial apparatus. Otolaryngol Clin North Am. 33(6):1309-32, 2000
12. Mukherji SK et al: Imaging of congenital anomalies of the branchial apparatus. Neuroimaging Clin N Am. 10(1):75-93, viii, 2000
13. Nicollas R et al: Congenital cysts and fistulas of the neck. Int J Pediatr Otorhinolaryngol. 55(2):117-24, 2000
14. Koeller KK et al: Congenital cystic masses of the neck: radiologic-pathologic correlation. Radiographics. 19(1):121-46; quiz 152-3, 1999
15. Mouri N et al: Reappraisal of lateral cervical cysts in neonates: pyriform sinus cysts as an anatomy-based nomenclature. J Pediatr Surg. 33(7):1141-4, 1998
16. Edmonds JL et al: Third branchial anomalies. Avoiding recurrences. Arch Otolaryngol Head Neck Surg. 123(4):438-41, 1997
17. Kelley DJ et al: Cervicomediastinal thymic cysts. Int J Pediatr Otorhinolaryngol. 39(2):139-46, 1997
18. Nguyen Q et al: Cervical thymic cyst: case reports and review of the literature. Laryngoscope. 106(3 Pt 1):247-52, 1996
19. Benson MT et al: Congenital anomalies of the branchial apparatus: embryology and pathologic anatomy. Radiographics. 12(5):943-60, 1992
20. Zarbo RJ et al: Thymopharyngeal duct cyst: a form of cervical thymus. Ann Otol Rhinol Laryngol. 92(3 Pt 1):284-9, 1983

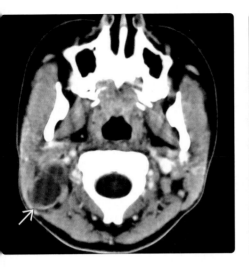
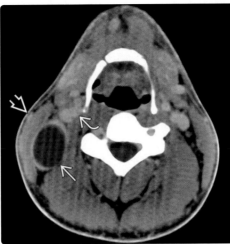

(Left) *Axial CECT demonstrates a 3rd branchial cleft cyst* ➡ *in the posterior triangle of the upper neck. Mild enhancement and internal septation are consistent with superimposed infection.* (Right) *Axial CECT demonstrates a mildly thick-walled, infected 3rd branchial cleft cyst* ➡ *deep to the sternocleidomastoid muscle* ➡ *and posterolateral to the carotid sheath* ➡.

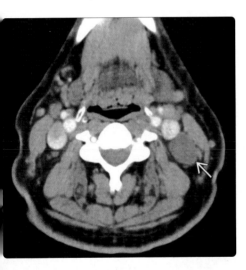
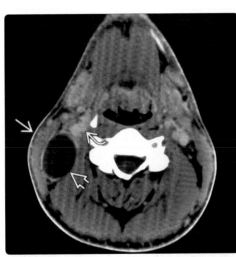

(Left) *Axial CECT shows a 3rd branchial cleft cyst* ➡ *posterolateral to the left carotid sheath.* (Right) *Axial CECT shows well-defined, thin-walled 3rd branchial cleft cyst* ➡ *in the right posterior cervical space, deep to the sternocleidomastoid muscle* ➡ *and posterolateral to the carotid sheath* ➡.

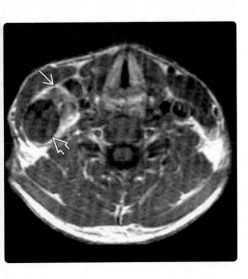
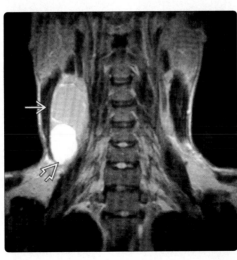

(Left) *Axial T1WI C+ MR demonstrates a variant multiloculated 3rd branchial cleft cyst in the right posterior cervical space. The anterior portion* ➡ *is hyperintense relative to the posterior portion* ➡, *indicating higher protein content secondary to prior infection or hemorrhage.* (Right) *Coronal T2WI MR in the same patient shows superior portion* ➡ *to be hypointense relative to the inferior portion* ➡. *Lymphatic malformation should be included in the preoperative differential diagnosis.*

KEY FACTS

TERMINOLOGY

- Pyriform sinus "fistula" or 4th branchial apparatus anomaly
  - **Most** anomalies are actually **sinus tracts (not cysts) from 4th pharyngeal pouch remnant**
  - Course from apex of pyriform sinus to upper aspect of **left** thyroid lobe

IMAGING

- Sinus tract extending from **apex of pyriform sinus to lower anterior neck** after barium swallow
- CECT best demonstrates phlegmon or abscess
  - Abscess in or adjacent to anterior **left** thyroid lobe
  - CT after barium swallow best identifies sinus tract
- Direct injection of fistula best demonstrates course of fistulous tract

TOP DIFFERENTIAL DIAGNOSES

- Cervical thymic cyst
- Lymphatic malformation

- Thyroglossal duct cyst
- Thyroid colloid cyst
- 3rd branchial cleft cyst

CLINICAL ISSUES

- **Recurrent neck abscesses**
- **Recurrent suppurative thyroiditis**
- Treatment options
  - Initial treatment is antibiotics ± incision and drainage of abscess
  - Complete resection of sinus tract or fistula
  - Thyroid lobectomy for lesions in thyroid lobe

DIAGNOSTIC CHECKLIST

- Suspect sinus tract from pyriform sinus in any child with abscess in or anterior to left thyroid lobe

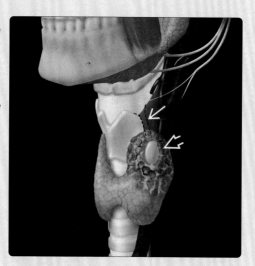
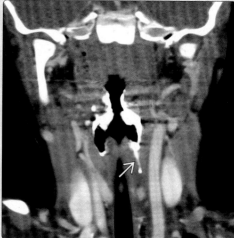

(Left) Sagittal (oblique) graphic shows a sinus tract ⇨ from the pyriform sinus to the left thyroid lobe with associated abscess ⇨ and thyroiditis secondary to a 4th pharyngeal pouch remnant. (Right) Coronal CECT obtained after barium swallow defines a tract ⇨ extending from the apex of the left pyriform sinus to the lower anterior left neck in a patient with prior history of left-sided thyroiditis.

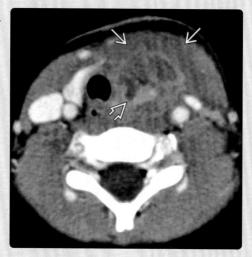
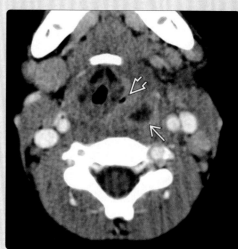

(Left) Axial CECT in a child presenting with acute signs of infection demonstrates a phlegmonous mass ⇨ in the anterior left neck, involving the left thyroid lobe ⇨ and causing deviation of the airway to the right of midline. (Right) Axial CECT in the same patient shows rim-enhancing early abscess ⇨ deviating an air-filled sinus tract ⇨ forward. This constellation of findings should alert the clinician to search for an opening at the apex of the pyriform sinus.

TERMINOLOGY

Synonyms

- Pyriform sinus "fistula"
  - Most 4th branchial anomalies are actually **sinus tracts**, not fistulas or cysts

Definitions

- 4th branchial apparatus sinus tract
  - Course from **apex of pyriform sinus** to upper aspect of left thyroid lobe
- Branchial sinus tract: 1 opening-to-skin surface, external auditory canal, pharynx or hypopharynx
- Branchial fistula: 2 openings; skin and lumen of foregut
  - Arises as epithelial-lined tract left behind when there is persistence of both branchial cleft and its corresponding pharyngeal pouch

IMAGING

General Features

- Best diagnostic clue
  - Sinus tract extending from apex of pyriform sinus to lower anterior neck after barium swallow
  - **Abscess** in or adjacent to anterior **left** thyroid lobe
- Location
  - May occur anywhere from left pyriform sinus apex to thyroid lobe
    - Commonly against or within superior aspect of left thyroid lobe or attached to thyroid cartilage
    - Upper end may communicate with or be adherent to pyriform sinus
- Size
  - Variable
- Morphology
  - Thick-walled sinus tract ± abscess in or adjacent to left thyroid lobe

Fluoroscopic Findings

- Barium swallow
  - Barium-filled sinus tract extending from apex of pyriform sinus to anterior lower neck
  - If performed during acute infection, may not fill portions of sinus tract
  - Scarring secondary to infection may prohibit filling of sinus tract

CT Findings

- CECT
  - Phlegmonous mass or frank abscess in or adjacent to left thyroid lobe with cellulitis extending around and collapsing ipsilateral pyriform sinus
- NECT after barium swallow
  - Barium-filled tract extending from apex of pyriform sinus to lower anterior neck
  - If performed during acute infection, may not fill portions of sinus tract
  - Scarring secondary to infection may prohibit filling of sinus tract

MR Findings

- Phlegmon or abscess in left anterior neck with deep neck inflammation extending to pyriform sinus

Ultrasonographic Findings

- Heterogeneous phlegmonous mass or thick-walled abscess with hyperemic wall anterior to or within left thyroid lobe

Nuclear Medicine Findings

- Cold nodule on thyroid scan

Imaging Recommendations

- Best imaging tool
  - CECT best demonstrates phlegmon or abscess
  - CT after barium swallow best identifies sinus tract
  - Direct injection of fistula best demonstrates course of fistula
- Protocol advice
  - Thin-section postcontrast helical CT with multiplanar reconstructions very helpful

DIFFERENTIAL DIAGNOSIS

Cervical Thymic Cyst

- Congenital cyst: Remnant of **thymopharyngeal duct**, derivative of 3rd pharyngeal pouch
- Left side more common than right
- If confined to visceral space, may mimic 4th branchial apparatus cyst
- Up to 50% extend into superior mediastinum

Lymphatic Malformation

- Uni- or multilocular, focal or infiltrative
- Isolated or transspatial
- **Fluid-fluid levels** if intralesional hemorrhage
- ± enhancing venous malformation if combined velolymphatic malformation

Thyroglossal Duct Cyst

- Anywhere along thyroglossal duct from **base of tongue (foramen cecum) to lower anterior neck** thyroid bed
- Infrahyoid thyroglossal duct cyst
  - Off-midline, anterior to thyroid lobe
  - Closely related to thyroid cartilage or strap muscles

Colloid Cyst Thyroid

- Uncommon in young children, most occur in older children and adults
- True thyroid cysts are rare
- Most "thyroid cysts" = **degenerating adenomas**
- May appear bright on T1 MR due to hemorrhage, colloid, or high protein content

3rd Branchial Cleft Cyst

- Most arise in upper **posterior cervical space**
- Rarely along lower anterior margin of sternocleidomastoid muscle

PATHOLOGY

General Features

- Etiology
  - Controversial
    - Failure of obliteration of 4th branchial **pouch** or distal cervical sinus of His

    – Recent literature suggests course of sinus tract does not follow theoretical tract for 3rd or 4th branchial cleft remnant
        □ Sinus tract may actually be remnant of 3rd branchial pouch
- Associated abnormalities
  - 4th branchial sinus
    – When sinus connection with apex of pyriform sinus is maintained, infection is likely
    – Thyroiditis ± thyroid abscess possible in such circumstances
  - 4th branchial fistula
    – Term fistula denotes 2 openings: 1 in low anterior neck, another into pyriform sinus apex

Gross Pathologic & Surgical Features

- Anterolateral neck cellulitis, phlegmon or abscess
- Direct probing of pyriform apex frequently demonstrates fistula or sinus tract

CLINICAL ISSUES

Presentation

- Most common signs/symptoms
  - Recurrent neck abscesses
  - Recurrent suppurative thyroiditis
  - Fluctuant mass in lower 1/3 of neck anteromedial to sternocleidomastoid muscle
    – Tender if infected
  - Throat pain, dysphagia, stridor

Demographics

- Age
  - Most branchial sinuses & fistulae (all types) present in childhood
  - Most 4th branchial apparatus anomalies are diagnosed in infants and young children
- Gender
  - More common in female patients
- Epidemiology
  - Rarest of all forms of branchial apparatus anomalies (1-2% of all branchial anomalies)
  - Most cases arise on **left**

Natural History & Prognosis

- If sinus tract connection to pyriform sinus unrecognized & untreated, recurrent suppurative thyroiditis ensues
- Recurrence likely if tract contains secretory epithelium, which is not resected

Treatment

- If infected, initial treatment is antibiotics ± incision and drainage of abscess
- Complete resection of sinus tract or fistula, obliterate opening in pyriform sinus
- Thyroid lobectomy is required for lesions in thyroid lobe to prevent recurrence

DIAGNOSTIC CHECKLIST

Consider

- Suspect sinus tract from pyriform sinus in child with phlegmon or abscess in or anterior to left thyroid lobe

SELECTED REFERENCES

1. Goff CJ et al: Current management of congenital branchial cleft cysts, sinuses, and fistulae. Curr Opin Otolaryngol Head Neck Surg. 20(6):533-9, 2012
2. Bajaj Y et al: Branchial anomalies in children. Int J Pediatr Otorhinolaryngol. 75(8):1020-3, 2011
3. Pahlavan S et al: Microbiology of third and fourth branchial pouch cysts. Laryngoscope. 120(3):458-62, 2010
4. Thomas B et al: Revisiting imaging features and the embryologic basis of third and fourth branchial anomalies. AJNR Am J Neuroradiol. 31(4):755-60, 2010
5. Nicoucar K et al: Management of congenital fourth branchial arch anomalies: a review and analysis of published cases. J Pediatr Surg. 44(7):1432-9, 2009
6. Mantle BA et al: Fourth branchial cleft sinus: relationship to superior and recurrent laryngeal nerves. Am J Otolaryngol. 29(3):198-200, 2008
7. James A et al: Branchial sinus of the piriform fossa: reappraisal of third and fourth branchial anomalies. Laryngoscope. 117(11):1920-4, 2007
8. Garrel R et al: Fourth branchial pouch sinus: from diagnosis to treatment. Otolaryngol Head Neck Surg. 134(1):157-63, 2006
9. Koch BL: Cystic malformations of the neck in children. Pediatr Radiol. 35(5):463-77, 2005
10. Jeyakumar A et al: Various presentations of fourth branchial pouch anomalies. Ear Nose Throat J. 83(9):640-2, 644, 2004
11. Pereira KD et al: Management of anomalies of the third and fourth branchial pouches. Int J Pediatr Otorhinolaryngol. 68(1): 43-50, 2004
12. Chaudhary N et al: Fistula of the fourth branchial pouch. Am J Otolaryngol. 24(4): 250-2, 2003
13. Wang HK et al: Imaging studies of pyriform sinus fistula. Pediatr Radiol. 33(5):328-33, 2003
14. Liberman M et al: Ten years of experience with third and fourth branchial remnants. J Pediatr Surg. 37(5): 685-90, 2002
15. Link TD et al: Fourth branchial pouch sinus: a diagnostic challenge. Plast Reconstr Surg. 108(3): 695-701, 2001
16. Minhas SS et al: Fourth branchial arch fistula and suppurative thyroiditis: a life-threatening infection. J Laryngol Otol. 115(12): 1029-31, 2001
17. Cases JA et al: Recurrent acute suppurative thyroiditis in an adult due to a fourth branchial pouch fistula. J Clin Endocrinol Metab. 85(3): 953-6, 2000
18. Mandell DL: Head and neck anomalies related to the branchial apparatus. Otolaryngol Clin North Am. 33(6): 1309-32, 2000
19. Nicollas R et al: Congenital cysts and fistulas of the neck. Int J Pediatr Otorhinolaryngol. 55(2): 117-24, 2000
20. Park SW et al: Neck infection associated with pyriform sinus fistula: imaging findings. AJNR Am J Neuroradiol. 21(5):817-22, 2000
21. Stone ME et al: A new role for computed tomography in the diagnosis and treatment of pyriform sinus fistula. Am J Otolaryngol. 21(5):323-5, 2000
22. Yang C et al: Fourth branchial arch sinus: clinical presentation, diagnostic workup, and surgical treatment. Laryngoscope. 109(3): 442-6, 1999
23. Nicollas R et al: Fourth branchial pouch anomalies: a study of six cases and review of the literature. Int J Pediatr Otorhinolaryngol. 44(1): 5-10, 1998
24. Cote DN et al: Fourth branchial cleft cysts. Otolaryngol Head Neck Surg. 114(1): 95-7, 1996
25. Choi SS et al: Branchial anomalies: a review of 52 cases. Laryngoscope. 105(9 Pt 1): 909-13, 1995
26. Benson MT et al: Congenital anomalies of the branchial apparatus: embryology and pathologic anatomy. Radiographics. 12(5):943-60, 1992
27. Rosenfeld RM et al: Fourth branchial pouch sinus: diagnosis and treatment. Otolaryngol Head Neck Surg. 105(1): 44-50, 1991
28. Godin MS et al: Fourth branchial pouch sinus: principles of diagnosis and management. Laryngoscope. 100(2 Pt 1): 174-8, 1990
29. Lucaya J et al: Congenital pyriform sinus fistula: a cause of acute left-sided suppurative thyroiditis and neck abscess in children. Pediatr Radiol. 21(1):27-9, 1990
30. Taylor WE Jr et al: Acute suppurative thyroiditis in children. Laryngoscope. 92(11):1269-73, 1982

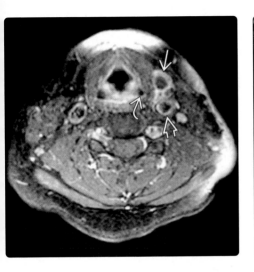

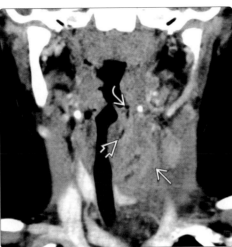

(Left) *Axial T1WI C+ FS MR demonstrates a small, multiloculated, rim-enhancing cystic mass ➡ anterior to the patent left carotid artery ➡ and lateral to the left pyriform sinus apex ➡.* (Right) *Coronal CECT shows the classic appearance of an inflammatory mass ➡ deviating the left thyroid lobe inferiorly, with inflammation surrounding the sinus tract ➡ extending from the pyriform sinus apex ➡.*

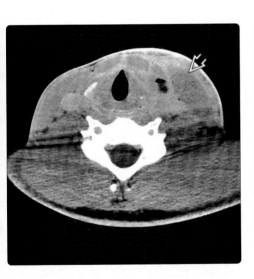

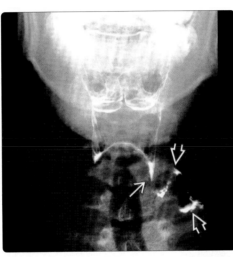

(Left) *Axial CECT demonstrates fluid and gas within a heterogeneously enhancing, multiloculated inflammatory process in the left neck. There is diffuse inflammation and ill definition of the adjacent fat planes and subcutaneous fat. The left sternocleidomastoid muscle is enlarged, consistent with myositis ➡.* (Right) *AP radiograph during barium swallow study in the same patient confirms the sinus tract ➡ with barium extending from apex of left pyriform sinus ➡ to the soft tissues of the lower left neck.*

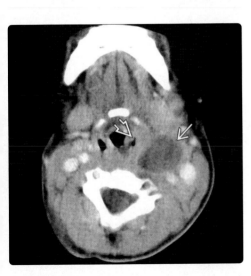

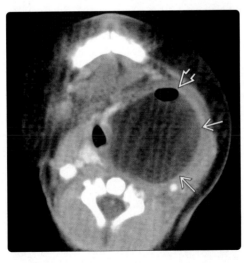

(Left) *Axial radiograph demonstrates a low-attenuation left anterior neck mass ➡ posterior to the left pyriform sinus ➡. Demonstration of extension to the left thyroid lobe should be reason to search for a pyriform apex sinus tract.* (Right) *Axial CECT shows a large, left-sided cystic mass ➡ at the level of the left thyroid lobe, with a small focus of intralesional air ➡, which should suggest connection to the aerodigestive tract.*

TERMINOLOGY

- Definition: Cystic mass resulting from **congenital** epithelial inclusion or rest
  - Epidermoid: Epithelial elements only
  - Dermoid: Epithelial elements + dermal substructure, including dermal appendages

IMAGING

- Epidermoid: Cystic, well-demarcated mass with **fluid contents** only
- Dermoid: Cystic, well-demarcated mass with **fatty, fluid, or mixed contents**
- Location
  - Oral cavity: Submandibular space, sublingual space, or root of tongue
  - Anterior neck, usually midline
  - Orbit: Adjacent to frontozygomatic suture > frontolacrimal suture

- Nasal cyst in association with nasal dermal sinus (NDS) ± intracranial extension
- Scalloping or remodeling of bone common
- Subtle rim enhancement of wall sometimes seen
- Dermoid & epidermoid cysts may see **restricted diffusion**
- Protocol advice
  - Routine CECT of cervical soft tissues
  - MR: T1 precontrast & use fat saturation postcontrast for orbit, neck, & oral cavity lesions
  - High-resolution anterior skull base MR in NDS; image from tip of nose to posterior to crista galli
  - Sagittal to define tract: Nose → anterior skull base

DIAGNOSTIC CHECKLIST

- Complex lesion with fat, consider dermoid cyst
- Simple lesion (may be proteinaceous fluid) = epidermoid or dermoid cyst

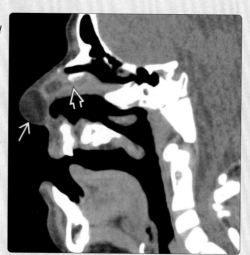
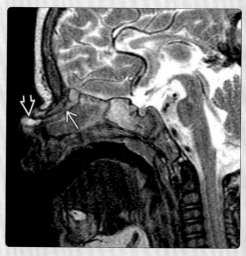

(Left) Sagittal CT reconstruction in a 10-year-old child following cleft palate repair showsh a large nasal dermoid ➡ with nasal dermal sinus tract ⬈ extending toward the cribriform plate. (Right) Sagittal T2WI MR in an 8-month-old girl shows a hyperintense sinus tract ➡ extending from the dermoid at the tip of the nose ⬈ toward the cribriform plate. Notice there is no evidence for intracranial dermoid or epidermoid.

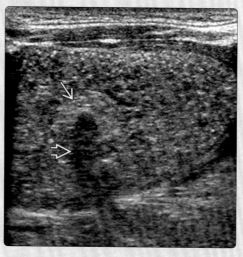
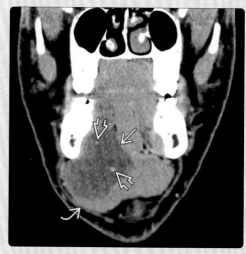

(Left) Longitudinal ultrasound in a 14-year-old boy shows a submental mass with heterogeneous echotexture and minimal increase through transmission. One hyperechoic focus ➡ has posterior acoustical shadowing ⬈, consistent with calcification in a dermoid. (Right) Coronal CECT in the same patient shows a low-density mass ➡ with a few calcifications ⬈ within the oral cavity. Inferior displacement of the mylohyoid muscle ⬈ indicates this dermoid is in the sublingual space.

Dermoid and Epidermoid

TERMINOLOGY

Synonyms
- Developmental cyst, ectodermal inclusion cyst, dermoid cyst

Definitions
- **Congenital** epithelial inclusion or rest → cystic mass
  - **Epidermoid**: Epithelial elements only
  - **Dermoid**: Epithelial elements + dermal substructure, including dermal appendages

IMAGING

General Features
- Best diagnostic clue
  - Epidermoid: Cystic, well-demarcated mass with **fluid contents** only
  - Dermoid: Cystic, well-demarcated mass with **fatty, fluid, or mixed contents**
- Location
  - Epidermoid & dermoid lesions
    - Oral cavity (OC): Submandibular space (SMS), sublingual space (SLS), or root of tongue
    - Anterior neck, usually midline
    - Orbit: Adjacent to frontozygomatic suture > frontolacrimal suture
    - Nasal cyst + nasal dermal sinus (NDS) ± intracranial extension
      - □ Tract or cyst nasal bridge to crista galli
      - □ Large foramen cecum with **bifid or deformed crista galli** or cribriform plate clue to intracranial extension
- Morphology
  - Ovoid or tubular

CT Findings
- NECT
  - Low-density, well-circumscribed cystic mass
    - Epidermoid: Fluid density material inside lesion without complex features
    - Dermoid: Fatty internal material, mixed density fluid, calcification (< 50%) all possible
      - □ When fluid density without complex features, indistinguishable from epidermoid
  - Scalloping or remodeling of bone common
- CECT
  - Lesion wall may be imperceptible
  - Subtle rim enhancement of wall sometimes seen

MR Findings
- T1WI
  - Epidermoid: Well-circumscribed mass with homogeneous fluid signal
    - **Diffuse ↑ signal** if **high protein** fluid
  - Dermoid: Well-circumscribed mass with complex fluid signal
    - If **fatty** elements, **focal or diffuse ↑ signal**
- T2WI
  - Epidermoid: Homogeneous high signal
  - Dermoid: Heterogeneous high signal
    - Intermediate signal if fat

- Focal areas of low signal if calcifications
- DWI
  - Dermoid & epidermoid cysts ± **restricted diffusion**
- T1WI C+
  - Thin rim enhancement or none
  - If fat saturation used, fat will be low signal in dermoid

Ultrasonographic Findings
- Epidermoid: **Pseudosolid** appearance with uniform internal echoes
  - Cellular material in cyst → pseudosolid appearance
  - Posterior wall echo enhancement = cystic lesion
- Dermoid: Mixed internal echoes from fat with echogenic foci & dense shadowing if calcifications

Imaging Recommendations
- Best imaging tool
  - CECT is best imaging tool for OC lesions (unless obscured by dental amalgam, then MR best)
  - CECT or MR for neck lesions
  - MR for orbit lesions
  - MR for NDS to better evaluate intracranial extent
    - CT to evaluate skull base & crista galli deformity
- Protocol advice
  - Routine CECT of cervical soft tissues
  - MR: Include T1 precontrast, & use fat saturation techniques postcontrast for orbit, neck, & OC lesions
  - High-resolution anterior skull base MR in NDS; image from **tip of nose to posterior to crista galli**
    - Sagittal to define tract: Nose → anterior skull base
    - DWI hyperintensity may diagnose epidermoid

DIFFERENTIAL DIAGNOSIS

Pediatric SLS, SMS, or Neck Lesions
- Thyroglossal duct cyst
  - Midline unilocular cystic mass between hyoid bone & foramen cecum
  - No fat or calcifications
- Lymphatic malformation
  - Unilocular or multilocular, transspatial common
  - Fluid-fluid levels common
- Ranula
  - Simple: Unilateral low-density/signal mass in SLS with thin, nonenhancing wall
  - Diving: Comet-shaped unilocular mass with tail in collapsed SLS (tail sign) & head in posterior SMS
- Abscess
  - Clinical: Fever, erythema, elevated white blood cell count
  - Imaging: Rim-enhancing cyst often with soft tissue cellulitis, edema, & adenopathy

Pediatric Orbital Lesions
- Orbital Langerhans cell histiocytosis
  - Enhancing soft tissue mass with smoothly marginated lytic bone lesion
- Rhabdomyosarcoma
  - Moderately enhancing mass frequently inseparable from extraocular muscle
  - Frequently without bone erosion when in orbit
- Orbital infantile hemangioma

- o Significant contrast enhancement, no bone erosion, & presents in infancy
- Orbital lymphatic malformation
  - o Nonenhancing, fluid-fluid levels common
- Orbital venous malformation
  - o Moderate enhancement
  - o Calcifications/phleboliths common
- Orbital idiopathic inflammatory pseudotumor
  - o Painful proptosis common
  - o Moderately enhancing mass, any area of orbit

Pediatric Nasal Lesions

- Normal fatty marrow in crista galli
  - o No mass or pit on nose
- Nonossified foramen cecum
  - o Ossifies postnatally in 1st 5 years of life
- Frontoethmoidal cephalocele
- Nasal glioma (nasal glial heterotopia)
  - o Most commonly projects extranasally onto paramedian bridge of nose

PATHOLOGY

General Features

- Etiology
  - o Congenital inclusion of dermal elements at site of embryonic fusion
    - − Sequestration of trapped surface ectoderm

Staging, Grading, & Classification

- Meyer classification dysontogenetic cysts floor of mouth
  - o **Epidermoid cyst**: Lined with simple squamous epithelium & surrounding connective tissue
  - o **Dermoid cyst**: Epithelium-lined cyst that contains skin appendages
  - o **Teratoid cyst**: Epithelium-lined cyst that contains mesodermal or endodermal elements, such as muscle, bones, teeth, & mucous membranes

Gross Pathologic & Surgical Features

- Oily or cheesy material, tan, yellow, or white
- Cyst wall = fibrous capsule; 2-6 mm in thickness

Microscopic Features

- Epidermoid
  - o Simple squamous cell epithelium with fibrous wall
- Dermoid
  - o Contains dermal structures, including sebaceous glands, hair follicles, blood vessels, fat ± collagen
    - − Lined by keratinizing squamous epithelium
- Teratoid cysts (rare lesion)
  - o Contain elements from all 3 germ cell layers

CLINICAL ISSUES

Presentation

- Most common signs/symptoms
  - o Painless mass in floor of mouth, anterior neck, orbit, or nasoglabellar region
- Other signs/symptoms
  - o OC lesions: Dysphagia, globus oral sensation, airway encroachment when large

- o Orbit lesions: Proptosis, diplopia
- o Nasal lesions: Pit on skin of nasal bridge ± protruding hair, recurrent meningitis, intermittent sebaceous material discharged from pit

Demographics

- Age
  - o OC lesions: Mean age in late teens to 20s
    - − Most dermoid cysts of floor of mouth present at 5-50 years
    - − Average age = 30 years
  - o Orbit lesions: Children or early adulthood
  - o Nasal lesions: Newborn to 5 years
    - − Mean age: 32 months
- Epidemiology
  - o Present from birth; spontaneous occurrence
  - o Dermoid/epidermoid are least common of all congenital neck lesions
  - o Orbit most common dermoid of H&N
  - o OC dermoids account for < 25% of all H&N dermoids

Natural History & Prognosis

- Benign lesion, very slow growth
  - o Present during childhood but small & dormant
  - o Symptomatic during rapid growth phase in young adult
- Sudden growth or change following rupture
  - o Significant inflammation & increased size (rare complication)

Treatment

- Surgical resection is curative
  - o Entire cyst must be removed to prevent recurrence
  - o OC lesions: Surgical approach may be decided by lesion position relative to mylohyoid muscle
    - − SLS: Intraoral approach
    - − SMS: Submandibular approach

DIAGNOSTIC CHECKLIST

Image Interpretation Pearls

- Complex lesion with fat density or signal intensity, consider dermoid cyst
- Simple lesion (may be proteinaceous fluid) = epidermoid or dermoid cyst
- If dermal sinus tract reaches dura anterior cranial fossa, crista galli may be bifid & foramen cecum large

SELECTED REFERENCES

1. Moses MA et al: The management of midline frontonasal dermoids: a review of 55 cases at a tertiary referral center and a protocol for treatment. Plast Reconstr Surg. 135(1):187-96, 2015
2. Paradis J et al: Pediatric teratoma and dermoid cysts. Otolaryngol Clin North Am. 48(1):121-36, 2015
3. Papadogeorgakis N et al: Surgical management of a large median dermoid cyst of the neck causing airway obstruction. A case report. Oral Maxillofac Surg. 13(3):181-4, 2009
4. Lee SS et al: Refinement in technique for pediatric dermoid cyst excision: technical note. Plast Reconstr Surg. 122(4):1059-61, 2008
5. Suzuki C et al: Apparent diffusion coefficient of subcutaneous epidermal cysts in the head and neck comparison with intracranial epidermoid cysts. Acad Radiol. 14(9):1020-8, 2007
6. Hedlund G: Congenital frontonasal masses: developmental anatomy, malformations, and MR imaging. Pediatr Radiol. 36(7):647-62; quiz 726-7, 2006
7. Charrier JB et al: Craniofacial dermoids: an embryological theory unifying nasal dermoid sinus cysts. Cleft Palate Craniofac J. 42(1):51-7, 2005

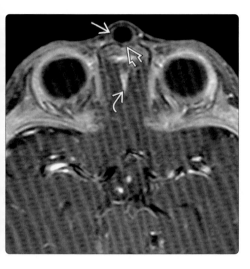

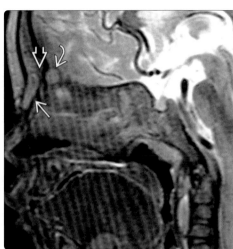

(Left) Axial T1 C+ FS MR in a 6-month-old infant shows a typical nasal glabella dermoid ➡, well defined and nonenhancing, with adjacent osseous remodeling ➡. Notice the normal appearance of the crista galli ➡. (Right) Sagittal T2 MR in an 18-month-old infant shows oblong midline dermoid ➡ remodeling the underlying frontal bone ➡. Deep to the thin but intact frontal bone is a noncontiguous intracranial dermoid at the foramen cecum ➡.

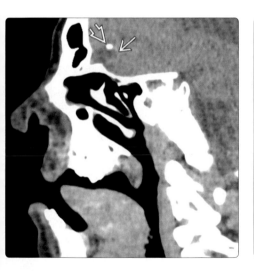

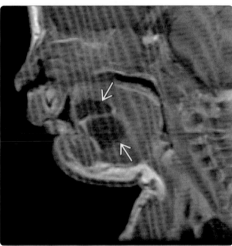

(Left) Sagittal CT reconstruction shows intracranial extension of a dermoid cyst ➡ in a 10-year-old child with nasal dermal sinus. Note the calcification ➡ in the superior margin of the dermoid cyst. (Right) Sagittal T1 C+ FS MR in a 4-day-old infant with floor of mouth mass demonstrates a multiloculated midline mass ➡, histologically proven to be a dermoid cyst. Differential diagnosis would include epidermoid cyst and lymphatic malformation.

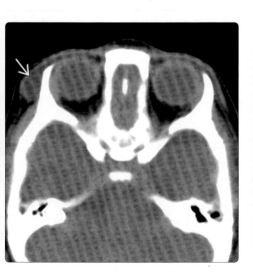

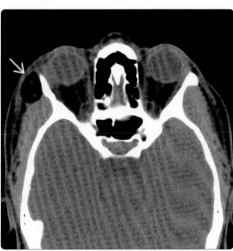

(Left) Axial NECT in a 4-year-old girl shows a well-defined, low-attenuation mass ➡ lateral to the right lateral orbital wall, without fat or calcific attenuation; therefore, differential diagnosis would include epidermoid and dermoid cysts. Histologically, this lesion contained skin appendages and therefore represents a dermoid cyst. (Right) Axial NECT in a child with longstanding history of palpable periorbital mass demonstrates a well-defined fat-containing dermoid ➡ with flattening of the adjacent lateral orbital wall.

TERMINOLOGY

- **Sternocleidomastoid (SCM) tumor of infancy**
- Nonneoplastic SCM muscle enlargement in early infancy

IMAGING

- **Nontender** SCM muscle **enlargement** in infant
- No adjacent inflammation or significant adenopathy
- Location: Right > left; rarely bilateral
- US: Modality of choice when imaging required
  - Variable echogenicity
- CT: Enlarged muscle has similar attenuation to normal muscle pre- and postcontrast
- MR: Variable signal, diffuse enhancement

TOP DIFFERENTIAL DIAGNOSES

- Myositis related to neck infection
  - Tenderness, cellulitis evident clinically
  - Adenopathy conspicuous
- Systemic nodal metastases

- Nodes deep to normal SCM muscle
- Primary cervical neuroblastoma
  - Close association with carotid sheath
- Rhabdomyosarcoma
  - More discrete mass with "aggressive" margins
- Teratoma
  - Often with fat, calcifications

CLINICAL ISSUES

- **Unilateral** longitudinal cervical neck mass
- Torticollis in up to 30%
- Mass appears within 2 weeks of delivery
- Usually **regresses by 8 months** of age
- ↑ in breech presentation & forceps delivery
- Occasionally with developmental dysplasia of hip
- Treatment: Physical therapy/stretching exercises to ↑ range of motion

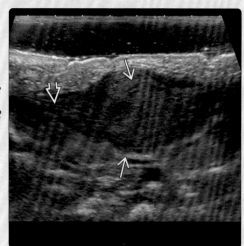

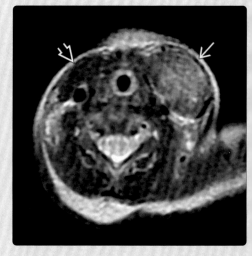

(Left) Longitudinal ultrasound in a 2-week-old infant shows typical fusiform enlargement of the left sternocleidomastoid (SCM) muscle, with mildly increased echogenicity ➡ relative to the uninvolved portion of the muscle ⬦. (Right) Axial T2 MR in the same child shows heterogeneous hyperintensity in the enlarged left SCM muscle ➡, relative to the contralateral normal right SCM muscle ⬦.

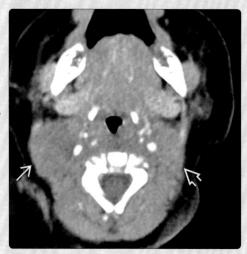

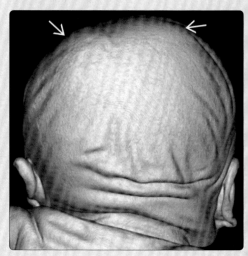

(Left) Axial CECT demonstrates diffuse enlargement of the right SCM muscle ➡, isodense to the normal contralateral SCM muscle ⬦, in a 1-month-old girl with fibromatosis colli. (Right) Posterior 3D surface-rendered soft tissue image in a child evaluated for bilateral cephalohematomas ➡ demonstrates incidental torticollis secondary to left SCM tumor of infancy (large left SCM not included).

TERMINOLOGY

Synonyms
- **Sternocleidomastoid (SCM) tumor of infancy**
- **Congenital muscular torticollis**

Definitions
- Nonneoplastic SCM muscle enlargement in early infancy

IMAGING

General Features
- Best diagnostic clue
  - **Nontender** SCM muscle enlargement in infant
- Location
  - Mid to lower 1/3 of SCM muscle
  - **Right > left; rarely bilateral**

Ultrasonographic Findings
- Grayscale ultrasound
  - Modality of choice when imaging required
  - **Oval or fusiform SCM muscle enlargement**
  - Variable echogenicity
  - **No** discrete extramuscular mass or adenopathy
- Color Doppler
  - Variable hyperemia in acute phase, ↓ blood flow in fibrotic phase

CT Findings
- CECT
  - **Focal or fusiform enlargement of SCM muscle**
  - Similar attenuation compared with normal contralateral muscle
  - No inflammatory "stranding" in adjacent fat
  - No adenopathy or calcifications

MR Findings
- T1WI
  - **Focal or diffuse fusiform enlargement of affected SCM**
  - Variable signal intensity: Iso- to hypointense to normal muscle
- T2WI
  - Variable signal intensity
    - Zones of hypointensity at maximal enlargement, probably due to evolving fibrosis
    - Hyper- to isointense to other muscles
  - Adjacent soft tissues normal
    - Be aware that incidental "reactive" nodal enlargement in infants is common
- T1WI C+
  - Affected muscle **enhances** heterogeneously

Imaging Recommendations
- Best imaging tool
  - Diagnosis usually on clinical exam alone, without imaging
  - Ultrasound confirms clinical suspicion
  - MR recommended for atypical cases

DIFFERENTIAL DIAGNOSIS

Myositis Related to Neck Infection
- + inflammatory changes and adenopathy

Systemic Nodal Metastases
- Adenopathy deep to normal SCM muscle

Primary Cervical Neuroblastoma
- Close association with carotid sheath

Rhabdomyosarcoma
- More discrete mass with "aggressive" margins

Teratoma
- Often with fat, calcifications

Pseudomass From Contralateral SCM Denervation
- CNXI injury → SCM & trapezius muscle atrophy
  - Contralateral normal SCM may appear large

PATHOLOGY

General Features
- Etiology
  - Unknown, several trauma theories → degeneration of fibers & fibrosis
  - ↑ in breech presentation & forceps delivery

CLINICAL ISSUES

Presentation
- Most common signs/symptoms
  - Unilateral longitudinal cervical neck mass
  - Torticollis in up to 30%
- Other signs/symptoms
  - ↓ range of neck motion, facial asymmetry, plagiocephaly

Demographics
- Age
  - 70% present by 2 months of age

Natural History & Prognosis
- Mass appears within 2 weeks of delivery
- Mass may ↑ in size for days to weeks
  - Usually regresses by 8 months of age

Treatment
- Physical therapy/stretching exercises to ↑ range of motion

DIAGNOSTIC CHECKLIST

Consider
- History of traumatic birth?
- Mass confined to SCM muscle?
  - If answer yes to both, dx = fibromatosis colli

Image Interpretation Pearls
- Fusiform mass conforming to shape of SCM muscle = fibromatosis colli

SELECTED REFERENCES

1. Lowry KC et al: The presentation and management of fibromatosis colli. Ear Nose Throat J. 89(9):E4-8, 2010
2. Ablin DS et al: Ultrasound and MR imaging of fibromatosis colli (sternomastoid tumor of infancy). Pediatr Radiol. 28(4):230-3, 1998

KEY FACTS

TERMINOLOGY

- Infantile hemangioma (IH): Benign **vascular neoplasm**; **not** vascular malformation

IMAGING

- Doppler will document characteristic flow
- Well-defined mass with **diffuse enhancement**
- **High-flow vessels** in/adjacent to mass during proliferative phase
- Decrease size with **fatty replacement** during **involuting phase**

TOP DIFFERENTIAL DIAGNOSES

- **Congenital hemangioma**
  - Present at birth or on prenatal imaging
  - GLUT1(-)
- **Venous malformation**
  - Congenital vascular malformation, venous lakes
  - ↑ T2, ↓ T1, diffuse enhancement ± phleboliths

- **Soft tissue sarcoma**
  - Rhabdomyosarcoma, extraosseous Ewing sarcoma, undifferentiated sarcoma
- **Plexiform neurofibroma**
  - Ill-defined margins, transspatial involvement
- **Arteriovenous malformation**
  - Congenital vascular malformation
  - High-flow feeding arteries, arteriovenous shunting, & large draining veins

PATHOLOGY

- **GLUT1** immunohistochemical marker **positive** in all phases of growth & regression

CLINICAL ISSUES

- Typically **inapparent at birth**, appears in 1st few weeks of life
- If age, clinical/imaging appearance, or growth history are atypical for IH, biopsy recommended

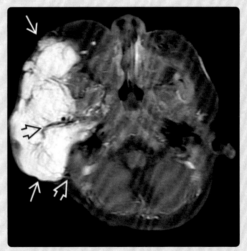
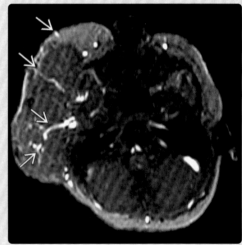

(Left) *Axial T1 C+ FS MR in a 5 month old shows a large, lobulated, intensely enhancing mass ➡ infiltrating the massively enlarged right parotid gland. Notice the prominent intralesional ⇒ and perilesional ⇒ flow voids typical of infantile hemangioma (IH).* (Right) *Axial SPGR flow-sensitive sequence in the same patient shows to better advantage the high-flow nature of the lesion typical of IH. Multiple high-flow vessels are noted within and adjacent to the primary parotid IH ➡.*

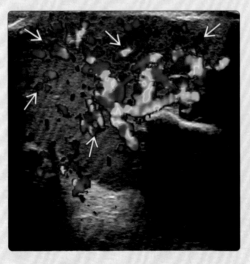
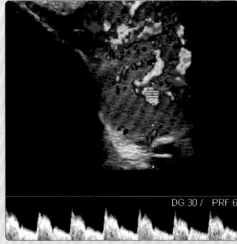

(Left) *Transverse color Doppler ultrasound in a 1-month-old child shows a lobular lesion replacing the parotid gland, with high vessel density ➡ typical of proliferating IH.* (Right) *Transverse color Doppler spectral tracing through the lesion in the same patient demonstrates low-resistance arterial waveforms, typical of IH.*

TERMINOLOGY

Abbreviations

- Infantile hemangioma (IH)

Synonyms

- Older, inappropriate terms: Hemangioma of infancy, capillary hemangioma
  - Widespread misuse of term "hemangioma" in literature
    - Cavernous hemangioma, vertebral body hemangioma, & synovial hemangioma = venous malformations
    - Hemangioendothelioma = higher grade vascular tumor

Definitions

- Benign **vascular neoplasm** of proliferating endothelial cells; most common soft tissue tumor of infancy
- **Not** vascular malformation
- 2014 revised classification by International Society for the Study of Vascular Anomalies (ISSVA) retains 2 main categories
  - Vascular tumors (true neoplasms with cellular proliferation; generally grow out of proportion to patient)
  - Vascular malformations (congenital errors of vessel development; generally grow commensurate with patient)

IMAGING

General Features

- Best diagnostic clue
  - Lobular, well-defined mass with intense, **diffuse contrast enhancement**
  - **High-flow vessels** in/adjacent to mass during proliferative phase (PP)
  - ↓ size with **fatty replacement** during **involuting phase** (IP)
- Location
  - **60% occur in head & neck**
    - Any space: Parotid space, orbit, nasal cavity, subglottic airway, face, neck, rarely intracranial (when intracranial &/or multiple think PHACES association)
- Size
  - Depends on phase of growth & regression
    - Proliferative phase begins few weeks after birth & continues 1-2 years
    - Involuting phase shows gradual regression over next several years
    - Involuted phase usually complete by late childhood; **90% resolve by 9 years**
- Morphology
  - Majority are single lesions in subcutaneous tissues; occasionally multiple, transspatial or deep
  - Associated abnormalities in **PHACES association**
    - **P**osterior fossa & supratentorial brain malformations (Dandy-Walker malformation/variant, migrational anomaly)
    - **H**emangioma of face & neck
    - **A**rterial stenosis, occlusion, aneurysm, hypoplasia, agenesis, aberrant origin
    - **C**ardiovascular defects (aortic coarctation/aneurysm/dysplasia, aberrant subclavian artery ± vascular ring, VSD)
    - **E**ye abnormalities (persistent hyperplasia primary vitreous, coloboma, morning glory disc anomaly, optic nerve hypoplasia, peripapillary staphyloma, microphthalmia, cataract, sclerocornea)
    - **S**upraumbilical raphe & sternal clefts/defects
    - Recent reports of associated endocrine abnormalities (hypopituitarism, ectopic thyroid)
- CECT findings
  - Diffuse & **prominent contrast enhancement**
  - Prominent vessels in/adjacent to mass in PP
  - Fatty infiltration during IP
- MR findings
  - T1: PP isointense to muscle; **IP hyperintense** from **fatty replacement**
  - T2: Mildly hyperintense relative to muscle
  - T1 C+ FS: **Intense contrast enhancement**
    - Best appreciated on fat-saturation T1WI; **serpiginous flow voids** in/adjacent to mass
  - **MR GRE: High-flow vessels** in/adjacent to mass
  - MRA: Stenosis, occlusion, agenesis, aneurysm (PHACES association)
- Sonographic findings
  - Soft tissue mass with variable echogenicity, few macroscopic vessels
  - Proliferative phase: High vessel density on color Doppler (> 5 vessels/cm²), high systolic Doppler shift (> 2 kHz) & low resistive index in arterial vessels, without arterialized veins to suggest shunting
  - Mean venous peak velocities **not** elevated (elevated in true arteriovenous malformation)
  - Involuting phase: ↓ vessel density, ↑ resistive index

Imaging Recommendations

- Best imaging tool
  - No imaging necessary in majority of patients
  - Imaging indications
    - Atypical history, appearance, clinical behavior of lesion
    - Suspect deep extension (e.g., orbit & airway)
    - Pretreatment if considering medical or surgical/laser treatment
    - Assess response to treatment
    - Suspect PHACES association, e.g., large segmental facial IH
  - MR C+ to show diffuse enhancement
  - GRE sequence to identify intralesional/perilesional high-flow vessels
  - MRA to identify associated vascular abnormalities
- Protocol advice
  - Doppler US will document characteristic flow
  - MR imaging should include flow-sensitive, fluid-sensitive, & T1 C+ FS sequences
    - MRA to identify associated vascular anomalies: Stenosis, occlusions, moyamoya, aneurysms
    - Parotid hemangiomas: Evaluate location of CNVII

DIFFERENTIAL DIAGNOSIS

Congenital Hemangioma (RICH/NICH)

- **Present at birth** or on prenatal imaging
  - Rapidly involuting congenital hemangioma (RICH): Involutes by 8-14 months; noninvoluting congenital hemangioma (NICH)
- Solid, heterogeneous, less well-defined mass ± calcification, hemorrhage, necrosis
- Glucose transporter 1 (GLUT1) negative
- Recent reports of partially involuting congenital hemangiomas (initial involution followed by persistent NICH-like lesions)

Venous Malformation

- Congenital **vascular malformation** composed of large venous lakes
- ↑ T2, ↓ T1, **diffuse enhancement**
- Phleboliths

Soft Tissue Sarcoma

- Rhabdomyosarcoma, extraosseous Ewing sarcoma, undifferentiated sarcoma
  - Mild to moderate enhancement ± osseous erosion

Plexiform Neurofibroma

- Infiltrative, swirls, ill-defined margins frequently with **transspatial involvement**
- Associated with additional stigmata of **NF1**

Arteriovenous Malformation

- Congenital vascular malformation
- High-flow feeding arteries, **arteriovenous shunting**, & large draining veins
- ± other soft tissue components

PATHOLOGY

General Features

- Etiology
  - Proposed theory = clonal expansion of angioblasts with high expression of basic fibroblast growth factors & other angiogenesis markers
- Genetics
  - Majority sporadic

Microscopic Features

- Prominent endothelial cells forming small vascular channels (PP), flat endothelial cells + fibrofatty replacement (IP)

Immunohistochemical Features

- GLUT1(+) during all phases of proliferation & regression

CLINICAL ISSUES

Presentation

- Most common signs/symptoms
  - Growing soft tissue mass, typically with warm, reddish or strawberry-like cutaneous discoloration in infant (proliferating phase)
  - Occasionally deeper lesions: Bluish skin coloration secondary to prominent draining veins
- Other signs/symptoms
  - Ulceration of overlying skin
  - Airway obstruction from airway involvement
  - Proptosis from orbital lesion
  - Associated abnormalities in PHACES association

Demographics

- Age
  - Median at presentation 2 weeks, majority present by 1-3 months
    - Typically **inapparent at birth**
    - Up to 1/3 nascent at birth, i.e., pale or erythematous macule, telangiectasia, pseudoecchymotic patch or red spot
- Gender
  - F > M (1.5-4:1)
- Epidemiology
  - Most common H&N tumor in infants
  - Incidence is 1-2% of neonates, 12% by age 1 year
  - ↑ in **preterm infants & low birth weight infants** (up to 30% of infants weighing < 1 kg)
- Ethnicity
  - Most frequent in Caucasians

Natural History & Prognosis

- Majority undergo proliferative phase followed by spontaneous regression by age 9 years
- Large & segmental facial hemangiomas have higher incidence of complications if not treated

Treatment

- Majority do not require treatment; expectant waiting
- Treatment indications: Compromise vital structures, such as optic nerve compression or airway obstruction; significant skin ulceration
- Treatment options
  - Propranolol (β-blocker) has replaced oral steroids as primary therapy due to low side effect profile
  - Intralesional steroids, laser, rarely surgical excision or embolization

DIAGNOSTIC CHECKLIST

Consider

- Phleboliths suggest venous malformation
- Older child, atypical appearance or osseous destruction: Consider sarcoma
- Transspatial mass with café au lait skin lesions suggests plexiform neurofibroma
- Large vessels with ill-defined parenchymal mass suggest arteriovenous malformation

SELECTED REFERENCES

1. Laken PA: Infantile hemangiomas: pathogenesis and review of propranolol use. Adv Neonatal Care. 16(2):135-42, 2016
2. Wassef M et al: Vascular anomalies classification: recommendations from the International Society for the Study of Vascular Anomalies. Pediatrics. 136(1):e203-14, 2015
3. Restrepo R et al: Hemangiomas revisited: the useful, the unusual and the new. Part 1: overview and clinical and imaging characteristics. Pediatr Radiol. 41(7):895-904, 2011
4. Restrepo R et al: Hemangiomas revisited: the useful, the unusual and the new. Part 2: endangering hemangiomas and treatment. Pediatr Radiol. 41(7):905-15, 2011
5. Mulliken JB et al: Hemangiomas and vascular malformations in infants and children: a classification based on endothelial characteristics. Plast Reconstr Surg. 69(3):412-22, 1982

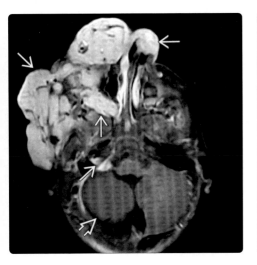
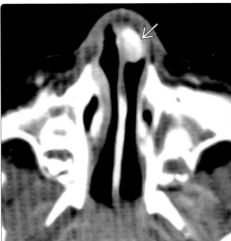

(Left) Axial T1 C+ FS MR in a 4-month-old girl with PHACES syndrome demonstrates multiple enhancing hemangiomas ➡ in the right parotid space, right posterior-inferior orbit, right cheek, nose, and right IAC/CPA. Also notice ipsilateral right cerebellar hemisphere hypoplasia ➡. (Right) Axial CECT in a 7 month old with a nasal mass demonstrates an intensely enhancing mass occluding the left nasal vestibule ➡, characteristics and location typical of IH.

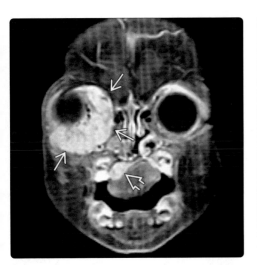
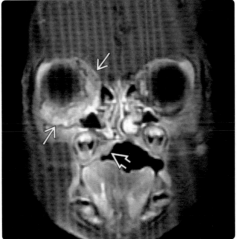

(Left) Coronal T1 C+ FS MR in a 2 month old shows a large, intensely enhancing IH involving the right intraconal and extraconal orbit ➡ and a 2nd lesion involving the right palate ➡. (Right) Coronal T1 C+ FS MR in the same patient after 6 months of Propranolol therapy, instituted to prevent orbital complications, shows significant interval regression of the orbital ➡ and palatal lesions ➡.

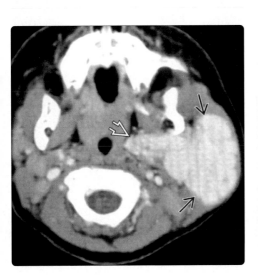
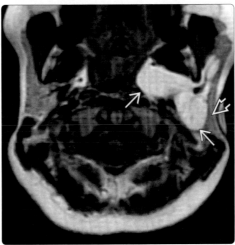

(Left) Axial CECT in a 1-year-old girl demonstrates intense homogeneous enhancement of a very large IH replacing the entire left superficial ➡ and deep lobes ➡ of the parotid gland. (Right) Axial T1 MR in the same child 8 years later shows interval decrease in size and diffuse fatty replacement ➡ of the original IH. Notice the thin sliver of overlying normal-appearing superficial parotid gland tissue ➡.

TERMINOLOGY

- Rhabdomyosarcoma (**RMSa**)
  - Most common childhood soft tissue sarcoma

IMAGING

- Soft tissue mass with variable contrast enhancement
- **Bone destruction** or **remodeling** possible
- Up to **40%** occur in H&N
  - Orbit, parameningeal sites, & all other H&N sites
- Bone CT best to evaluate osseous erosion
- Enhanced MR best to evaluate intracranial spread
- Include neck to rule out cervical metastatic adenopathy

TOP DIFFERENTIAL DIAGNOSES

- Juvenile angiofibroma
- Langerhans cell histiocytosis
- Plexiform neurofibroma
- Nasopharyngeal carcinoma
- Non-Hodgkin & Hodgkin lymphoma

- Leukemia

PATHOLOGY

- Originates from primitive mesenchymal cells (rhabdomyoblasts) committed to skeletal muscle differentiation
- 3 histologic subtypes
  - **Embryonal RMSa**: Most common; younger children
  - **Alveolar RMSa**: 2nd most common; patients 15-25 years of age
  - **Pleomorphic RMSa**: Least common; adults 40-60 years of age

CLINICAL ISSUES

- Age at presentation
  - 70% under 12 years, 40% under 5 years of age
- Treatment: Surgical debulking, chemotherapy ± radiation therapy

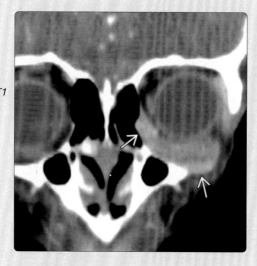
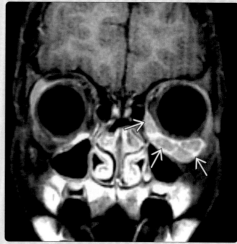

(Left) Coronal CECT in an 8 year old shows a nonspecific, mildly heterogeneous extraconal mass ➡ in the inferior and inferomedial left orbit, without bone destruction. (Right) Coronal T1 C+ FS MR in the same child shows a heterogeneously enhancing mass ➡, atypical appearance for hematoma, hemangioma, and vascular malformation, histologically proven to be embryonal rhabdomyosarcoma (RMSa). The absence of bone destruction does not exclude RMSa.

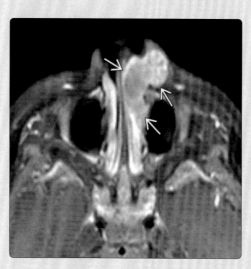
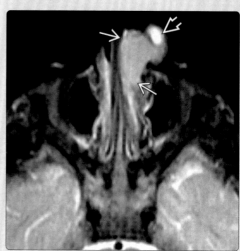

(Left) Axial T1 C+ FS MR in a 15-month-old boy with intermittent nose bleed and swelling of left nasal ala demonstrates a heterogeneously enhancing left nasal/nasal ala mass ➡ obstructing the left nasal cavity. (Right) Axial T2 MR in the same patient demonstrates primarily intermediate signal intensity throughout the mass ➡, with the exception of a small cystic/necrotic region anteriorly ➡, subsequently biopsy proven to represent alveolar RMS.

Primary Cervical Neuroblastoma

TERMINOLOGY

Neuroblastoma (**NBL**): Malignant tumor of primitive neural crest cells

Primary cervical in **1-5%** of cases

o Most cases of NBL arise in adrenal gland (35%), extraadrenal retroperitoneum (30-35%), or posterior mediastinum (20%)

IMAGING

CECT or MR: Well-defined, mild to moderately enhancing soft tissue mass in **posterior carotid space**

o ± adjacent metastatic lymphadenopathy

o Frequently with calcifications

o Unlike primary NBL in abdomen, primary cervical NBL often **displaces carotid sheath vessels** rather than engulfing vessels

I-123 MIBG most specific method of staging and evaluating response to therapy in NBL

TOP DIFFERENTIAL DIAGNOSES

- Reactive lymph nodes
  - o Most common neck mass in child
  - o ± cellulitis, myositis, abscess
- Neurofibroma
  - o Carotid space or brachial plexus common
  - o Plexiform "tangle of worms"
- Lymphoma lymph nodes
  - o Hodgkin or non-Hodgkin lymphoma
- Metastatic NBL
  - o Metastatic H&N disease more common than primary cervical NBL

CLINICAL ISSUES

- **Horner syndrome**
- Palpable mass
- Stridor or feeding difficulties

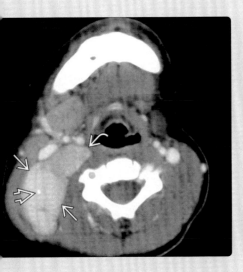
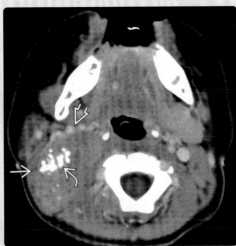

(Left) Axial CECT demonstrates a moderately enhancing right posterior carotid space neck mass ➡ deviating the carotid artery and jugular vein anteriorly. Tiny calcification is present ➡ in a large adherent lymph node ➡, which was positive for neuroblastoma (NBL). (Right) Axial CECT shows a partially calcified right neck mass ➡, deviating the carotid sheath vessels ➡ anteriorly. Course calcifications ➡ are present. Final pathology revealed the lesion to be ganglioneuroblastoma.

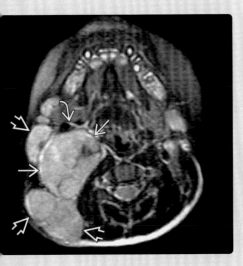
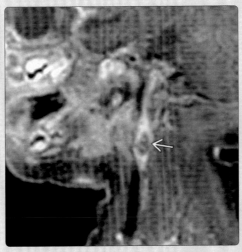

(Left) Axial T2WI FS MR shows a large cervical NBL ➡ situated in the posterior aspect of the carotid sheath. There are multiple large adjacent metastatic lymph nodes ➡. The mass deviates the carotid sheath vessels ➡ anteriorly and deforms the upper airway, both common findings in primary cervical NBL. (Right) Sagittal T1WI C+ FS MR in a 9 month old with Horner syndrome reveals a small rim-enhancing NBL ➡ in the oropharyngeal carotid space.

KEY FACTS

TERMINOLOGY

- Malignant tumor of sympathetic nervous system arising from embryonal neural crest cell derivatives

IMAGING

- Classic imaging appearance
  - "Hair on end" spiculated periostitis of orbits and skull ± bone destruction
- Cranial metastases
  - Nearly always extradural, calvarial-based mass
- Brain metastases rare
  - ↑ prevalence with improved treatment protocols, stage IV metastatic disease
  - Most parenchymal NB mets supratentorial, hemorrhagic

TOP DIFFERENTIAL DIAGNOSES

- Leukemia
- Langerhans cell histiocytosis
- Extraaxial hematoma
- Ewing sarcoma

PATHOLOGY

- Calvarial metastases indicate stage IV disease
  - 60-75% < 1-year survival
  - 15% > 1-year survival despite aggressive treatment

CLINICAL ISSUES

- Most common solid extracranial tumor in children < 5 years of age
  - 8-10% of all childhood cancers
- Most common tumor in neonates/infants < 1 month of age (congenital)
  - Median age at diagnosis: 22 months
  - Ophthalmic manifestation in 20-55%
    - Proptosis and "raccoon eyes"
- Metastasis to bone most common, 2/3 of patients at diagnosis
  - Stage IV disease

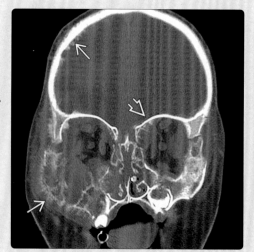
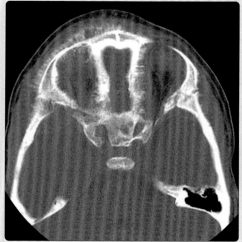

(Left) Coronal NECT of a child with an abdominal mass reveals orbital, facial bone, and calvarial spiculated periostitis giving rise to a hair on end appearance ➡ with associated large soft tissue masses. Note bilateral disease ⇒. Metastatic stage IV neuroblastoma typically involves the skull and bony orbits. (Right) Axial NECT in the same patient shows the "hair on end" appearance. Involvement of the orbits often gives rise to proptosis and ecchymosis "raccoon eyes," which may be mistaken for abuse.

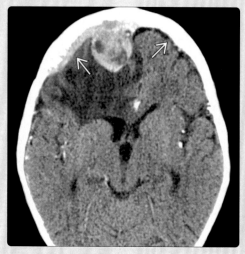
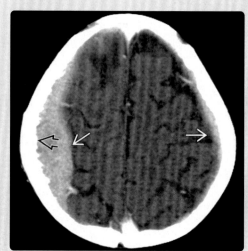

(Left) Axial CECT in a 2-year-old boy with neuroblastoma shows strong, heterogeneously enhancing epidural masses ➡ with mass effect and edema in a frontal lobe. (Right) Cephalad CECT in the same case shows strongly enhancing epidural masses ➡. Irregularity of overlying skull ⇒ indicates calvarial involvement. Intracranial involvement in neuroblastoma is typically from adjacent calvarial metastases with dural invasion. Brain parenchymal metastases are rare.

TERMINOLOGY

Abbreviations

- Neuroblastoma (NB), neuroblastic tumors (NBT)

Definitions

- Malignant tumor of sympathetic nervous system arising from embryonal neural crest cell derivatives

IMAGING

General Features

- Best diagnostic clue
  - Spiculated periorbital bone mass causing proptosis in child with "raccoon eyes"
- Location
  - Cranial metastases nearly always extradural, calvarial-based masses
    - Calvarium, orbit, skull base
  - Brain metastases rare but ↑ with improved treatment protocols, stage IV metastatic disease
    - CNS NB is sole site of disease recurrence in 64% of high-risk patients
    - CNS may represent "sanctuary site" for NB
    - Most parenchymal NB mets supratentorial, hemorrhagic
    - Leptomeningeal, intraventricular lesions also occur
- Morphology
  - Crescentic or lenticular, following contour of bone
  - Typically poorly defined
- Classic imaging appearance: "Hair on end" spiculated periostitis of orbits and skull, ± bony destruction

Radiographic Findings

- Coronal suture widening and periosteal new bone

CT Findings

- NECT
  - Best for showing fine spicules of periosteal bone projecting off skull or sphenoid wings
  - Soft tissue mass typically iso- to hyperdense to brain
    - May mimic epidural or subdural hematoma
  - Mass projects into orbit (extraconal), with extension to surrounding spaces, not preseptal space
  - May project through inner and outer tables of skull
  - May be bilateral
- CECT
  - Enhancing dural metastasis if intracranial
  - Rare ring-enhancing brain parenchymal metastasis

MR Findings

- T1WI
  - Slightly heterogeneous
  - Hypointense to muscle
- T2WI
  - Heterogeneous
  - Hypointense to brain
  - Slightly hyperintense to muscle
- FLAIR: Heterogeneous; hyperintense to muscle
- T2* GRE: Hypointense
- T1WI C+: Vigorously enhances, may be heterogeneous
- MRV: May narrow or invade adjacent dural sinuses

Nuclear Medicine Findings

- Bone scan
  - MIBG (metaiodobenzylguanidine)
    - Catecholamine analog
    - Labeled with I-131 or I-123
    - Avid uptake by neural crest tumors
      - NB, ganglioneuroblastoma, ganglioneuroma, carcinoid, medullary thyroid carcinoma
    - 99% specific for NBT
    - Caveat: Up to 30% of NB not MIBG(+)
      - Misses 50% of recurrent tumors
    - Cannot distinguish marrow disease from bone disease
  - Tc-99m-MDP (methylene diphosphonate)
    - Increased uptake from calcium metabolism of tumor not specific to neural crest tissue
    - 74% sensitivity for bony metastases
    - May distinguish marrow from bone disease
    - Bone scan essential for differentiating stage IV disease from stage IV-S in children < 1 year
  - In-111 pentetreotide
    - Somatostatin analog
    - Not specific to NBT; not superior to MIBG
- PET
  - FDG PET has shown high sensitivity and specificity for recurrent tumor in small numbers of cases, and may identify recurrence when MIBG negative due to dedifferentiation

Imaging Recommendations

- Best imaging tool
  - CT/MR to evaluate primary tumor
  - Nuclear medicine MIBG & Tc-99m MDP bone scan
  - Brain/orbit CT if scintigraphy indicates metastases
- Protocol advice
  - MR C+ and FS complementary to CT

DIFFERENTIAL DIAGNOSIS

Leukemia

- Dural- or calvarial-based masses
- More frequent parenchymal masses
- Less heterogeneous on MR

Langerhans Cell Histiocytosis

- Lytic bone lesions without periosteal new bone
- Often associated with diabetes insipidus

Extraaxial Hematoma

- Subdural or epidural hematoma
- Bleeding disorder or child abuse to be considered

Ewing Sarcoma

- < 1% of cases involve skull
- Aggressive bone destruction
- Spiculated periosteal reaction

Osteosarcoma

- Rarely primary in calvarium

Rhabdomyosarcoma

- Most common soft tissue malignancy of pediatric orbit
- Less likely bilateral; may invade preseptal space

Beta Thalassemia Major

- Classic "hair on end" calvarial expansion
- Not focal or destructive like neuroblastoma

PATHOLOGY

General Features

- Etiology
  - Arises from pathologically maturing neural crest progenitor cells
  - Primary tumors arise at sites of sympathetic ganglia
  - No known causative factor
- Genetics
  - Multiple gene loci associated with NB 1p, 4p, 2p, 12p, 16p, 17q
    - *MYCN* oncogene (chromosome 2) important marker
    - 35% have chromosome 1 short arm deletion
  - 1-2% of cases inherited
- Associated abnormalities
  - Rarely associated with Beckwith-Wiedemann syndrome, neurofibromatosis type 1
  - Some association with neurocristopathy syndromes
    - Hirschsprung disease, congenital central hypoventilation, DiGeorge syndrome

Staging, Grading, & Classification

- Calvarial metastases indicate stage IV disease
- International Neuroblastoma Staging System
  - Stage I: Confined to primary organ
  - Stage IIA: Unilateral tumor, no positive lymph nodes (LN)
  - Stage IIB: Unilateral tumor, unilateral positive LN
  - Stage III: Contralateral involvement
  - Stage IV: Distal metastases
  - Stage IV-S: < 1 year at diagnosis, stage I or II + metastatic disease confined to skin, liver, or bone marrow

Gross Pathologic & Surgical Features

- Grayish-tan soft nodules
- Infiltrating or circumscribed without capsule
- Necrosis, hemorrhage, and calcifications variable

Microscopic Features

- Undifferentiated round blue cells with scant cytoplasm, hyperchromatic nuclei
- May form Homer Wright rosettes
- Ganglioneuroblastoma has interspersed mature ganglion cells
  - Different regions of same tumor may have ganglioneuroblastoma or NB

CLINICAL ISSUES

Presentation

- Most common signs/symptoms
  - "Raccoon eyes" (periorbital ecchymosis)
  - Palpable calvarial masses
- Other signs/symptoms
  - Palpable abdominal or paraspinal mass
  - Cranial metastatic disease rarely occurs in isolation
- Clinical profile
  - Ophthalmic manifestation in 20-55% at presentation
    - Proptosis and "raccoon eyes," 50% bilateral

- Horner syndrome
- Opsoclonus, myoclonus, and ataxia
  - Myoclonic encephalopathy of infancy
  - Paraneoplastic syndrome (not metastatic)
  - Up to 2-4% of NB patients; more favorable prognosis
- Elevated vasoactive intestinal peptides
  - Up to 7% of NBT patients
  - Diarrhea, hypokalemia, achlorhydria
- Elevated homovanillic acid and vanillylmandelic acid in urine (> 90%)

Demographics

- Age
  - Median at diagnosis: 22 months
  - 40% diagnosed by 1 year
  - 35% between 1-2 years
  - 25% > 2 years
  - 89% by 5 years
- Gender
  - M:F = 1.2:1
- Epidemiology
  - Most common solid extracranial tumor in patients < 5 years
  - 8-10% of all childhood cancers
  - Most common tumor in patients < 1 month (congenital)
  - Bony metastasis most common, 2/3 of patients at diagnosis
  - 1-2% spontaneously regress in 6-12 months, mostly stage IV-S
  - NB is most common and aggressive of NBT

Natural History & Prognosis

- Stage I, II, and IV-S have 3-year event-free survival (EFS) of 75-90%
- Stage III: < 1 year old (80-90%) 1-year EFS; > 1 year old (50%) 3-year EFS
- Stage IV: < 1 year old (60-75%) 1-year EFS; > 1 year old (15%) 3-year EFS
- Poor prognostic indicators: Deletion of 1p, translocation of 17q, *MYCN* amplification
- Good prognostic indicators: Localized disease, stage IV-S, decreased *MYCN* amplification

Treatment

- Surgical resection + chemotherapy, radiation
- Bone marrow transplant
- Stage IV-S may spontaneously regress

DIAGNOSTIC CHECKLIST

Consider

- Abdominal imaging to identify primary tumor site

Image Interpretation Pearls

- CT without contrast can help identify bone spicules, eliminating LCH from differential

SELECTED REFERENCES

1. Nabavizadeh SA et al: Imaging findings of patients with metastatic neuroblastoma to the brain. Acad Radiol. 21(3):329-37, 2014
2. Wiens AL et al: The pathological spectrum of solid CNS metastases in the pediatric population. J Neurosurg Pediatr. 14(2):129-35, 2014

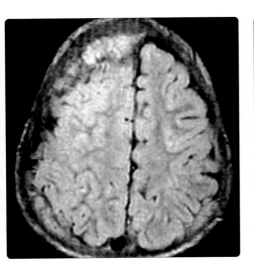 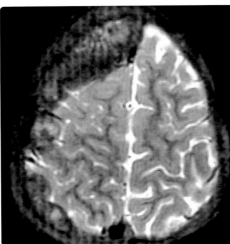

(Left) Axial FLAIR MR shows heterogeneous signal in a patient with extradural metastatic neuroblastoma. Little reactive change is seen in the underlying brain parenchyma despite significant mass effect. (Right) Axial T2WI MR in the same case shows heterogeneous and hypointense signal in this metastatic neuroblastoma. T2 hypointensity is characteristic of densely cellular masses with high nuclear:cytoplasmic ratio.

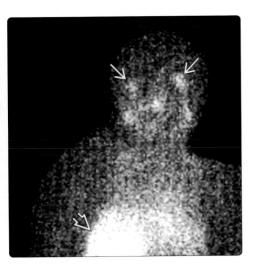 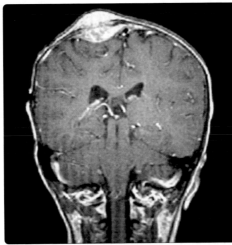

(Left) Coronal I-123-labeled MIBG scan shows areas of increased uptake in the orbits ➡ related to neuroblastoma metastases. Note the large area of uptake in the right abdomen from the primary tumor ➡. Although MIBG scanning is highly specific for neuroblastic tumors, up to 30% of primary and 50% of recurrent neuroblastomas do not take up MIBG. (Right) Coronal T1WI C+ MR shows an enhancing convexity mass centered at the diploic space with subperiosteal and epidural components in a child with neuroblastoma.

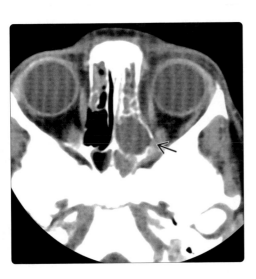 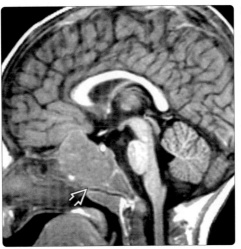

(Left) Axial NECT in a child with neuroblastoma shows an ethmoid mass. There is a small focus of bony erosion ➡ suggesting the correct diagnosis of neuroblastoma metastasis. (Right) Sagittal T1WI MR shows a mildly heterogeneous, large, central skull base mass ➡ with marked expansion of the clivus in this 2 year old with stage IV neuroblastoma. Imaging mimics other malignancies. Neuroblastoma metastases most commonly involve the calvarium or orbital region.

SECTION 20
Syndromic Diseases

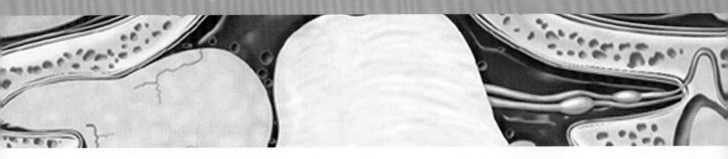

KEY FACTS

TERMINOLOGY

- Neurofibromatosis 1 (**NF1**)
- **Neurofibromas**: Multiple localized neurofibromas & plexiform neurofibromas (PNF) in NF1

IMAGING

- Hyperintense T2 signal
  - **Target** = ↓ signal center, ↑ signal periphery PNF
- Postcontrast CT or MR
  - Localized NF: Homogeneous or patchy enhancement, well-circumscribed fusiform mass
  - PNF: Heterogeneously enhancing, lobulated mass along course of peripheral nerve
- Most conspicuous on STIR & FS T2WI
- Other extracranial H&N manifestations of NF1
  - Orbit: **Optic pathway glioma (OPG)**, optic nerve sheath ectasia, Lisch nodules, buphthalmos, large foramina with PNFs

- Skull & skull base: **Sphenoid dysplasia**, smooth bony foramina with PNF infiltration of cranial nerves, lambdoid suture defect
- Vascular dysplasia: Internal carotid artery stenosis/occlusion & moyamoya; aneurysms & arteriovenous fistula rare

TOP DIFFERENTIAL DIAGNOSES

- Lymphatic malformation
- Venous malformation
- Rhabdomyosarcoma

DIAGNOSTIC CHECKLIST

- Patient with PNF or multiple localized neurofibromas, consider NF1
  - Look for additional findings of brain lesions, OPG, sphenoid wing dysplasia
- Transspatial neurofibroma may be hypodense on CT & mimic lymphatic malformation

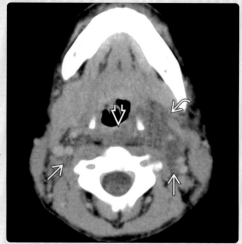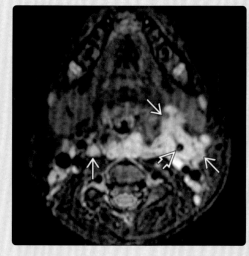

(Left) Axial CECT in a child with neurofibromatosis type 1 (NF1) shows an ill-defined infiltrative transspatial plexiform neurofibroma (PNF) involving the bilateral carotid ➡, retropharyngeal ➡, and left submandibular ➡ spaces. (Right) Axial STIR MR in the same child better defines the margins of the PNF ➡. Notice the infiltrative pattern, with circumferential involvement of the left carotid artery ➡, typical of plexiform lesions.

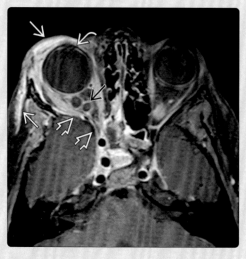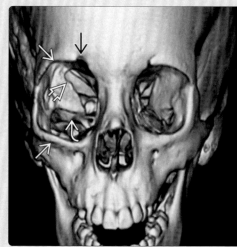

(Left) Axial T1WI C+ FS MR shows diffusely enhancing neurofibroma ➡ involving the right pre- and postseptal orbit and temporalis scalp. There is also sphenoid wing hypoplasia ➡, buphthalmos ➡, and a tortuous optic nerve ➡. (Right) Frontal 3D reformation in the same patient shows diffuse right orbital expansion ➡. There is also enlargement of the superior ➡ and inferior ➡ orbital fissures and supraorbital foramen ➡ related to sphenoid dysplasia and adjacent PNF.

TERMINOLOGY

Abbreviations

- Neurofibromatosis 1 (**NF1**)

Synonyms

- von Recklinghausen disease, autosomal dominant neurofibromatosis

Definitions

- Autosomal dominant neurocutaneous disorder (**phakomatosis**)
- Diagnostic NF1 criteria: If ≥ 2 of following present
  - ○ > 6 café au lait spots measuring ≥ 5 mm in prepubertal & ≥ 15 mm in postpubertal patients
  - ○ ≥ 2 neurofibromas or 1 plexiform neurofibroma (PNF)
  - ○ Axillary/inguinal freckling
  - ○ Visual pathway glioma
  - ○ ≥ Lisch nodules (optic hamartomas)
  - ○ Distinctive bony lesion
    - – Sphenoid wing dysplasia
    - – Thinning of long bones
      - □ ± pseudoarthrosis
  - ○ 1st-degree relative with NF1
- Peripheral nerve sheath tumor (PNST) = schwannoma, neurofibroma, & PNF
- **Neurofibromas**: Localized, plexiform, & diffuse variants

IMAGING

General Features

- Best diagnostic clue
  - ○ **PNF**
    - – Characteristic & diagnostic feature of NF1
  - ○ **Multiple localized neurofibromas**
- Location
  - ○ Neurofibromas may involve **any space in H&N**
    - – Most common: Carotid space, brachial plexus, oral cavity, cheek, retropharyngeal space, posterior cervical space
  - ○ PNST
    - – Usually involves major nerve trunks, including brachial plexus
- Size
  - ○ Localized neurofibroma: Millimeters to multiple centimeters
  - ○ PNF: May reach large size
- Morphology
  - ○ **Localized** neurofibroma
    - – Multiple, well-circumscribed, smooth, fusiform, variably enhancing masses along course of nerves
    - – Paraspinal neurofibroma may be dumbbell-shaped ± smooth enlargement of bony neural foramina
    - – Schwannoma may be indistinguishable from neurofibroma
  - ○ **Diffuse** neurofibroma
    - – Plaque-like or infiltrative, poorly defined, reticulated lesion in skin & subcutaneous fat
  - ○ **PNF**
    - – Transspatial, lobulated, tortuous, rope-like expansion within major nerve distribution
    - – Resembles tangle of worms

CT Findings

- CECT
  - ○ Localized neurofibroma & PNF
    - – Frequently have low attenuation (5–25 HU) on pre- & postcontrast images, mimic lymphatic malformation
    - – Paraspinal neurofibroma may be dumbbell-shaped
      - □ ± enlarged neural foramina

MR Findings

- T2WI
  - ○ Hyperintense
  - ○ Target sign: ↓ signal center, ↑ signal periphery PNF
    - – Fascicular sign: Multiple, small irregular hypointense foci (~ fascicular bundles)
- T1WI C+
  - ○ Localized neurofibroma: Homogeneous or patchy heterogeneous enhancement, well-circumscribed fusiform mass
  - ○ PNF: Heterogeneously enhancing, lobulated mass along course of peripheral nerve
  - ○ Malignant PNST
    - – Differentiation of benign from malignant PNST difficult on imaging alone
    - – If large size (> 5 cm), heterogeneous with central necrosis, infiltrative margins, & rapid growth, consider malignant PNST
  - ○ Diffuse neurofibroma: Plaque-like or infiltrative intense enhancement in skin & subcutaneous fat

Imaging Recommendations

- Best imaging tool
  - ○ MR best to characterize & define total extent
    - – Most conspicuous on STIR & FS T2WI
  - ○ Bone CT delineates associated bone changes
    - – Particularly helpful in patients with sphenoid wing dysplasia & PNF

DIFFERENTIAL DIAGNOSIS

Lymphatic Malformation

- Low attenuation
- Unilocular or multilocular, focal or infiltrative
- No enhancement unless infected or mixed venolymphatic malformation

Venous Malformation

- Phleboliths common

Rhabdomyosarcoma

- Invasive transspatial mass
- Frequently with aggressive bone destruction

PATHOLOGY

General Features

- Etiology
  - ○ *NF1* gene (tumor suppressor gene) normally encodes production of "neurofibromin" that influences cell growth regulation
  - ○ *NF1* gene "turned off" in NF1
    - – Results in cell proliferation & tumor development

- Genetics
  - **Autosomal dominant; 50% new mutations**
  - Gene locus = **chromosome 17q11.2**
    - Nonsense mutation of this gene leads to NF1
- Associated abnormalities
  - Other extracranial H&N manifestations of NF1
    - Orbit: Optic pathway glioma (OPG), optic nerve sheath ectasia, Lisch nodules, **buphthalmos**, **large foramina** with PNFs
    - Skull: Lambdoid suture defect
    - Skull base findings
      - Sphenoid dysplasia with PNF, probably sequelae of PNF interaction with developing underlying bone
      - Smooth, corticated enlargement of skull base bony foramina with PNF infiltration of cranial nerves
    - Vascular dysplasia: Internal carotid artery stenosis/occlusion & moyamoya; aneurysms & arteriovenous fistula rare
    - Neural crest tumors
      - **Pheochromocytoma** 10x ↑ in NF1 patients
      - **Parathyroid adenomas** ↑ incidence
  - Other imaging manifestations of NF1
    - CNS findings
      - Cerebral gliomas, hydrocephalus, cranial nerve schwannomas
      - Dynamic reactive lesions, white matter, dentate nucleus, globus pallidus, brainstem, thalamus, hippocampus
      - Spinal cord astrocytomas

Staging, Grading, & Classification

- Neurofibromas are WHO grade I
- Malignant PNST are WHO grade III/IV

Gross Pathologic & Surgical Features

- **Localized neurofibroma**
  - Fusiform, firm, gray-white mass intermixed with nerve of origin
- **PNF**
  - Diffuse, tortuous, rope-like expansion of nerves resembling tangle of worms
  - Involves adjacent skin, fascia, & deeper tissues
- **Malignant PNST**
  - Fusiform, fleshy, tan-white mass with areas of necrosis & hemorrhage
  - Nerve proximally & distally thickened due to spread of tumor along epineurium & perineurium

Microscopic Features

- Localized neurofibroma
  - Schwann cells, fibroblasts, mast cells in matrix of collagen fibers, & mucoid substance
  - Axons usually embedded within tumor
- PNF
  - Schwann cells & perineural fibroblasts grow along nerve fascicles
- Malignant PNST
  - Fibrosarcoma-like growth of spindle cells
  - Considered high-grade sarcomas
  - PNF: 5% risk of malignant transformation

CLINICAL ISSUES

Presentation

- Most common signs/symptoms
  - Majority of neurofibroma & PNF asymptomatic
  - Cutaneous stigmata of NF1
  - Sudden, painful ↑ size of stable neurofibroma suggests malignant transformation
- Other signs/symptoms
  - Decreased vision with OPG
  - Pulsatile buphthalmos with sphenoid wing dysplasia & PNF

Demographics

- Age
  - Any age, most common presentation in late childhood to early adulthood; new lesions may develop at any time
  - Malignant PNST: Usually in adults, rare in children
- Epidemiology
  - NF1
    - Most common autosomal dominant disorder
      - 1 in 3,000
    - **Most common neurocutaneous syndrome**
    - Most common inherited tumor syndrome
  - Localized neurofibroma
    - **90%** are solitary & not associated with NF1
    - **10%** associated with NF1 → more frequently large, multiple, & involve large deep nerves (e.g., brachial plexus)
  - Malignant PNST
    - **50% associated with NF1**
    - **5%** of patients with NF1 develop malignant PNST
  - Diffuse neurofibroma
    - Majority are in patients **without NF1**

Natural History & Prognosis

- Usually slow growing unless malignant transformation
  - Occasionally massive enlargement in young kids

Treatment

- Resection of neurofibromas that press on vital structures
- Solitary neurofibroma resectable; PNF generally unresectable
- Radiofrequency treatment in PNF may offer new hope

DIAGNOSTIC CHECKLIST

Consider

- If patient has PNF or multiple localized neurofibromas, consider NF1
  - Look for additional findings of brain lesions, OPG, sphenoid wing dysplasia

Image Interpretation Pearls

- Beware: Transspatial neurofibroma may be hypodense on CT & mimic lymphatic malformation

SELECTED REFERENCES

1. McCarville MB: What MRI can tell us about neurogenic tumors and rhabdomyosarcoma. Pediatr Radiol. 46(6):881-90, 2016
2. Rad E et al: Neurofibromatosis type 1: fundamental insights into cell signalling and cancer. Semin Cell Dev Biol. 52:39-46, 2016

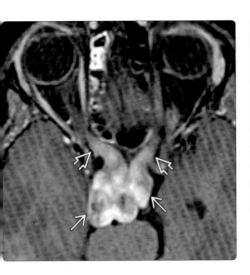
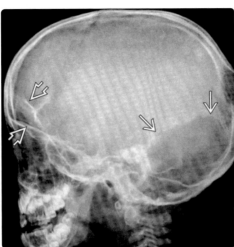

(Left) *Axial T1WI C+ MR shows a large optic pathway glioma involving the chiasm ⮕ and prechiasmatic optic nerves ⮕ in a child with NF1.* (Right) *Lateral radiograph in a child with skull base PNF shows a large lambdoid defect ⮕, a typical but rare lesion in children with NF1. Notice also asymmetry in the orbital roofs ⮕, secondary to unilateral orbital enlargement, typical of patients with sphenoid wing dysplasia and adjacent PNF.*

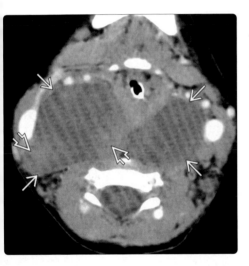
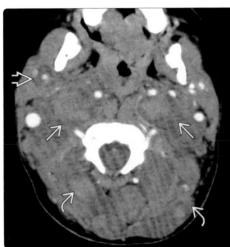

(Left) *Axial CECT in a child with NF1 shows the typical appearance of large carotid space neurofibromas ⮕, low in attenuation with only mild patchy contrast enhancement ⮕.* (Right) *Axial CECT in a child with NF1 shows massive tumor burden, with numerous neurofibromas involving the bilateral carotid spaces ⮕, right parotid space ⮕, and posterior cervical spaces ⮕. Patchy central enhancement with peripheral rim of less enhancement is not uncommon.*

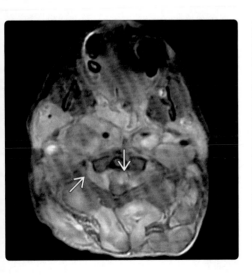
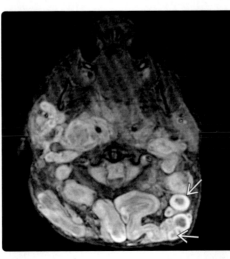

(Left) *Axial T1WI C+ FS MR in the same patient shows a similar pattern of contrast enhancement with patchy central enhancement and peripheral decreased enhancement. Notice also neural foraminal extension into the spinal canal ⮕, compressing the upper cervical cord.* (Right) *All lesions are more conspicuous on axial STIR MR. Notice the typical target appearance to several lesions ⮕ and a more tram track appearance to others, imaged along the long axis rather than a cross section through the neurofibroma.*

IMAGING

- Multiple circumscribed, encapsulated masses following course of cranial or peripheral nerves **without** involvement of CNVIII
- Rare meningiomas (< 5%)
- MR C+ is mainstay of schwannomatosis imaging

TOP DIFFERENTIAL DIAGNOSES

- Neurofibromatosis type 2 (NF2)
- Sporadic schwannoma
- Neurofibromatosis type 1 (NF1)
- Sporadic neurofibroma

PATHOLOGY

- Typically, germline mutation of *SMARCB1* gene
  - *SMARCB1* mutation is **not** found in sporadic (nonsyndromic) schwannomas
  - *SMARCB1* mutation is **not** found in NF2
- Less commonly, germline mutations of *LZTR1* gene

CLINICAL ISSUES

- Incidence thought to be similar to NF2 (~ 1/40,000)
- Typically presents with pain, which may be disabling
  - In contradistinction to NF2, which more frequently presents with neurologic deficits
- Peak incidence between ages 30-60
  - Contrast with NF1 (typically diagnosed in 1st decade)
  - Contrast with NF2 (typically diagnosed in 2nd decade)
- **Normal** life expectancy
  - Contrast with NF2 (↓ life expectancy)

DIAGNOSTIC CHECKLIST

- In patient > 30 years of age with **multiple nonvestibular schwannomas**
  - Consider diagnosis of schwannomatosis
  - Recommend high-resolution MR of temporal bones to screen for NF2
- If multiple schwannomas **and** involvement of CNVIII, alternative NF2 diagnosis should be favored

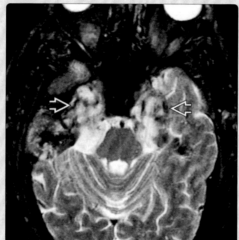 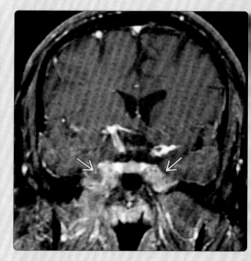

(Left) *Axial T2WI MR of a 47-year-old man with schwannomatosis reveals bulky, fusiform enlargement of the bilateral trigeminal nerves ➡, which demonstrate heterogeneous increased T2 signal and exert mass effect on the pons without associated signal abnormality.* **(Right)** *Coronal T1WI C+ FS MR in the same patient reveals enhancing, globular masses ➡ involving the bilateral trigeminal ganglia, which extend into the infrazygomatic masticator spaces via widened foramina ovale. IACs (not shown) were normal.*

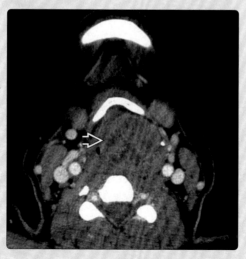 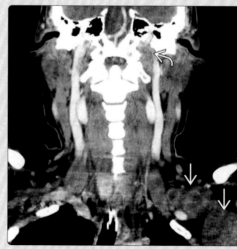

(Left) *Axial CECT of the neck in a 31-year-old woman with schwannomatosis shows a circumscribed, encapsulated, heterogeneously enhancing, submucosal mass ➡ in the supraglottic larynx, which near completely effaces the laryngeal airway.* **(Right)** *Coronal reconstruction reveals additional heterogeneous density masses involving the left brachial plexus ➡ and jugular foramen ➡, compatible with numerous schwannomas in this patient with schwannomatosis.*

TERMINOLOGY

Definitions

- Schwannomatosis: Multiple schwannomas of peripheral nervous system **without** involvement of vestibular nerves

IMAGING

General Features

- Best diagnostic clue
  - Multiple circumscribed, encapsulated masses following course of cranial or peripheral nerves **without** involvement of CNVIII
  - Rarely (< 5%) associated with meningiomas
    - Predilection for falx

CT Findings

- NECT
  - Iso- to slightly hyperdense compared to brain
  - Look for effect on adjacent bone, foramina
    - Smooth enlargement
    - Thin, sclerotic, surgical-appearing margins
- CECT
  - Variable, often heterogenous enhancement

MR Findings

- Variable signal intensity on all sequences due to varying amounts of Antoni A and Antoni B regions
- Hyperintense on T2WI, PD, FLAIR, and STIR
- Intense, typically heterogeneous enhancement on T1WI C+

Imaging Recommendations

- Best imaging tool
  - MR C+ is mainstay of schwannomatosis imaging

PATHOLOGY

General Features

- Genetics
  - Complex, incompletely understood genetics involving germline involvement of *SMARCB1* gene, which is **not** found in sporadic, nonsyndromic schwannomas
    - Tumor supressor gene found on chromosome 22
    - Likely involves multihit mutation phenomenon involving *SMARCB1* and *NF2* genes in affected tissues
  - Germline mutations in *LZTR1* gene found in 80% of schwannomatosis patients **without** *SMARCB1* mutation

Staging, Grading, & Classification

- **Baseline criteria** (all must be met)
  - No germline *NF2* gene mutation
  - Must not meet diagnostic criteria for neurofibromatosis 2 (NF2)
  - No 1st-degree relative with NF2
  - No evidence of vestibular schwannoma on MR
  - Schwannomas cannot be in prior radiation field
- **Definite** diagnosis
  - 2 or more nonintradermal schwannomas (1 histologically proven); **or** 1 pathologically confirmed schwannoma or intracranial meningioma **and** 1st-degree relative meeting diagnostic criteria
- **Possible** diagnosis

  - 2 or more nonintradermal tumors without histopathology proven schwannoma; chronic pain associated with tumor increases likelihood of diagnosis
- **Segmental** schwannomatosis
  - Meets criteria for definite or possible schwannomatosis, but confined to 1 limb or 5 or fewer contiguous spinal elements

CLINICAL ISSUES

Presentation

- Most common signs/symptoms
  - Pain, typically neuropathic in quality; may be disabling
    - In contradistinction to NF2, which more frequently presents with neurologic deficits
  - Symptom onset typically in 2nd or 3rd decade of life
    - Compared to neurofibromatosis 1 (1st decade) and NF2 (2nd decade)

Demographics

- Epidemiology
  - Reported incidence ranges from 1/40,000 to 1/1.7 million, probably closer to 1/40,000 (similar to NF2)

Natural History & Prognosis

- **Normal** life expectancy, unlike NF2 patients who have reduced life expectancy

Treatment

- Symptom control with pain management
- Surgical intervention only if spinal cord compression or symptoms clearly due to schwannoma
- No role for radiation therapy; evolving role of chemotherapy

DIAGNOSTIC CHECKLIST

Consider

- Patient may have schwannomatosis if
  - Age > 30
  - > 1 schwannoma
  - No vestibular schwannoma

Image Interpretation Pearls

- **Caution** favoring diagnosis of schwannomatosis in patient younger than age 30, as vestibular schwannomas may not yet have developed
  - As patient age at time of diagnosis ↑, likelihood of schwannomatosis ↑ and likelihood of NF2 ↓

Reporting Tips

- In patient > 30 years of age, presence of multiple nonvestibular schwannomas should prompt radiologist to
  - Suggest diagnosis of schwannomatosis
  - Recommend high-resolution MR of temporal bones to screen for NF2

SELECTED REFERENCES

1. Blakeley JO et al: Therapeutic advances for the tumors associated with neurofibromatosis type 1, type 2, and schwannomatosis. Neuro Oncol. 18(5):624-38, 2016
2. Ioannidis P et al: Expanding schwannomatosis phenotype. J Neurooncol. 122(3):607-9, 2015
3. Koontz NA et al: Schwannomatosis: the overlooked neurofibromatosis? AJR Am J Roentgenol. 200(6):W646-53, 2013

TERMINOLOGY

- Neurofibromatosis type 2 (**NF2**) = inherited syndrome with multiple **schwannomas, meningiomas, & ependymomas**

IMAGING

- Bilateral **enhancing CPA-IAC masses**
  - Ovoid when small; "ice cream on cone" when large enough to fill IAC & CPA
- CNS
  - Calcifications: Choroid plexus, cerebellar hemispheres, & cerebral cortex
  - Other meningiomas & schwannoma (CNIII-XII)
  - Ependymomas > > gliomas
- Spine
  - Meningiomas, schwannomas, & ependymomas

TOP DIFFERENTIAL DIAGNOSES

- CPA-IAC metastases
  - Bilateral IAC enhancing masses in older patient

- Facial nerve schwannoma, CPA-IAC
  - CPA-IAC mass with labyrinthine canal tail of enhancement
- Meningioma, CPA-IAC
  - Dural-based, eccentric CPA mass with dural tail of enhancement projecting into IAC

PATHOLOGY

- Autosomal dominant disorder
  - Mutation of *NF2* gene chromosome 22
  - **50%** result from **new** dominant gene **mutation**

CLINICAL ISSUES

- Unilateral **sensorineural hearing loss**
- Other symptoms: Tinnitus, vertigo, CNVII paralysis
- Mean age at diagnosis ~ 25 years

DIAGNOSTIC CHECKLIST

- If diagnosis of NF2 made in adult, consider alternative diagnosis of metastases to CPA-IAC

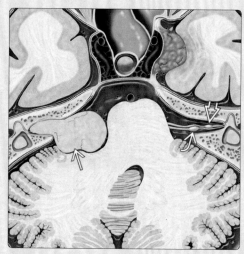
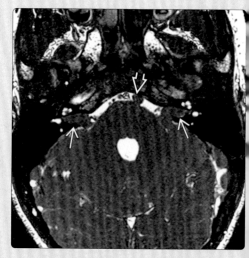

(Left) Axial graphic depicts bilateral cerebellopontine angle-internal auditory canal (CPA-IAC) masses in neurofibromatosis type 2 (NF2). Note large right vestibular schwannoma ➡. On left there is a facial nerve schwannoma ➡ and a vestibular schwannoma ➡. Differentiating facial from vestibular schwannoma is important to assess therapy options. (Right) Axial FIESTA in a 12-year-old boy with NF2 shows bilateral hypointense vestibular schwannomas ➡. Note nodular enlargement of the left CNVI ➡.

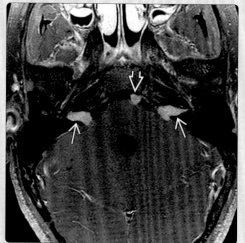
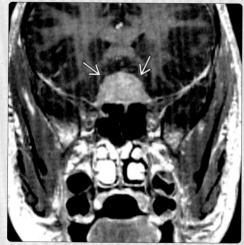

(Left) Axial T1 C+ FS MR in the same child demonstrates typical diffuse postcontrast enhancement of the bilateral vestibular schwannomas ➡ and the left CNVI schwannoma ➡. (Right) Coronal T1 C+ MR in the same patient demonstrates a broad-based, extraaxial planum sphenoidale mass ➡, proven to represent meningioma. This patient had a very high tumor burden at a young age, including multiple other intracranial and extracranial cranial nerve schwannomas as well as spinal lesions (not shown).

TERMINOLOGY

Abbreviations
- Neurofibromatosis type 2 (**NF2**)

Synonyms
- Central neurofibromatosis, bilateral acoustic neurofibromatosis, schwannomatosis
  - Schwannomatosis now considered distinct form of neurofibromatosis, separate from NF1 & NF2

Definitions
- NF2 = inherited syndrome with multiple **schwannomas, meningiomas, & ependymomas**

IMAGING

General Features
- Best diagnostic clue
  - Bilateral enhancing cerebellopontine angle-internal auditory canal (CPA-IAC) vestibular schwannomas
- Location
  - Schwannomas: CPA-IAC, other cranial or spinal nerves
  - Meningiomas: Dural based
  - Extraaxial tumors: Spinal cord & brainstem
- Size
  - Range from millimeters to centimeters
- Morphology
  - Ovoid when small; "ice cream on cone" when large enough to fill IAC & CPA
- Associated imaging findings
  - CNS
    - Calcifications: Choroid plexus, cerebellar hemispheres, & cerebral cortex
    - Other meningiomas & schwannoma (CNIII-XII)
    - Ependymomas > > gliomas
  - Spine
    - Meningiomas, schwannomas, & ependymomas

CT Findings
- Bone CT
  - May show IAC flaring

MR Findings
- T1WI FS C+: Focal, enhancing mass of CPA-IAC cistern centered on porus acusticus
  - Small: Ovoid-enhancing masses in IAC
  - Large: "Ice cream on cone" shape in CPA & IAC
- High-resolution T2 space, CISS, or FIESTA: "Filling defect" in hyperintense CSF of CPA-IAC cistern
  - Helps distinguish vestibular from facial schwannoma

Imaging Recommendations
- NF2 screening MR: T1 C+ MR of brain & spine
- High-resolution T2 of CPA used to follow CPA tumors

DIFFERENTIAL DIAGNOSIS

Metastases, CPA-IAC
- Bilateral IAC enhancing masses in older patient

Facial Nerve Schwannoma, CPA-IAC
- CPA-IAC mass with labyrinthine canal tail of enhancement

Meningioma, CPA-IAC
- Dural-based, eccentric CPA enhancing mass with dural tail projecting into IAC

Sarcoidosis, CPA-IAC
- Multiple focal enhancing meningeal masses

PATHOLOGY

General Features
- Etiology
  - Mutation of *NF2* gene (tumor suppressor) creates environment for multiple tumor growth
    - *NF2* gene encodes for merlin protein
- Genetics
  - **Autosomal dominant** disorder
  - Mutation of *NF2* gene located on long arm of **chromosome 22**
  - 50% result from new dominant gene mutation
- Associated abnormalities
  - Meningiomas & ependymomas

Staging, Grading, & Classification
- Diagnostic criteria
  - Bilateral vestibular schwannomas, or
  - 1st-degree relative with NF2 & 1 vestibular schwannoma, or
  - 1st-degree relative with NF2 & 2 of following: Neurofibroma, meningioma, glioma, schwannoma, juvenile posterior subcapsular lenticular opacity

CLINICAL ISSUES

Presentation
- Most common signs/symptoms
  - Unilateral sensorineural hearing loss (SNHL)
  - Other symptoms: Tinnitus, vertigo, CNVII paralysis

Demographics
- Age
  - Mean age at diagnosis ~ 25 years
- Epidemiology
  - 1 per ~ 35,000; much less frequent than NF1

Natural History & Prognosis
- CPA tumor growth results in profound SNHL
- Significant morbidity & ↓ lifespan associated with NF2

Treatment
- Resection with hearing preservation is possible
- Genetic counseling essential

DIAGNOSTIC CHECKLIST

Image Interpretation Pearls
- If diagnosis of NF2 made in adult, consider alternative diagnosis of metastases to CPA-IAC

SELECTED REFERENCES

1. Slattery WH: Neurofibromatosis type 2. Otolaryngol Clin North Am. 48(3):443-60, 2015
2. Maniakas A et al: Neurofibromatosis type 2 vestibular schwannoma treatment: a review of the literature, trends, and outcomes. Otol Neurotol. 35(5):889-94, 2014

Syndromic Diseases

TERMINOLOGY

- Abbreviation: Basal cell nevus syndrome (**BCNS**)
- Synonyms: Gorlin syndrome, **Gorlin-Goltz syndrome**, nevoid basal cell syndrome, nevoid basal cell carcinoma syndrome
- **Autosomal dominant** disorder with multiple keratocystic odontogenic tumors, basal cell carcinoma (BCCa), **medulloblastoma**, **intracranial dural calcifications**, bifid ribs

IMAGING

- Multiple expansile, lucent lesions of **mandible and maxilla**
- May **displace developing teeth** ± **resorption of roots** of erupted teeth and tooth extrusion
- Variable attenuation/signal intensity depends on protein content &/or hemorrhage

TOP DIFFERENTIAL DIAGNOSES

- Periapical (radicular) cyst

- Dentigerous (follicular) cyst
- Keratocystic odontogenic tumor (nonsyndromic)
- Ameloblastoma

PATHOLOGY

- Etiology: Arise from dental lamina remnants
- Autosomal dominant
  - 1/3 of cases are new mutations
- Associated abnormalities
  - High incidence of **medulloblastomas**
  - Marked calcification of falx (80%), dura
  - Multiple skin **BCCas**
  - Bifid ribs and scoliosis

CLINICAL ISSUES

- Syndrome apparent by **5-10 years**
- Patients present by 3rd decade, with multiple nevoid BCCa; mean age = 19 years

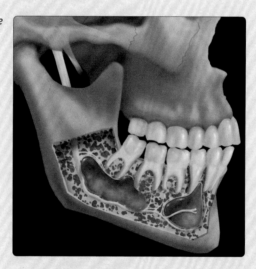
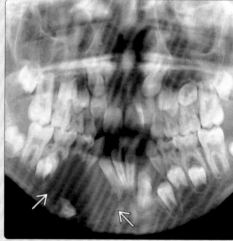

(Left) Lateral graphic with the mandibular cortex removed shows the classic appearance of multiple keratocystic odontogenic tumors in the basal cell nevus syndrome; lesions tend to splay tooth roots and displace nerves. (Right) Anteroposterior panorex radiograph shows a large, expansile radiolucent lesion ➡ in the left paramidline mandible with severe crowding and displacement of involved teeth.

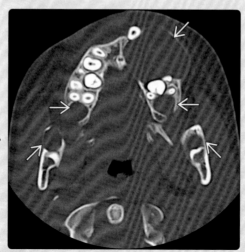
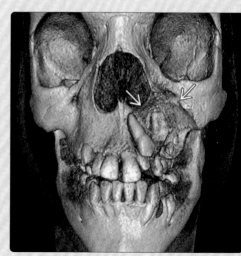

(Left) Axial bone CT demonstrates multiple bilateral lytic lesions ➡ in the maxilla and mandible typical of keratocystic odontogenic tumors in a 9-year-old boy with basal cell nevus syndrome. (Right) Anteroposterior 3D reformation in the same child shows to better advantage the effect of the largest lesion ➡ on the adjacent teeth.

TERMINOLOGY

Abbreviations
- Basal cell nevus syndrome (**BCNS**)

Synonyms
- Gorlin syndrome, **Gorlin-Goltz syndrome**, nevoid basal cell syndrome, nevoid basal cell carcinoma syndrome

Definitions
- **Autosomal dominant** disorder with multiple keratocystic odontogenic tumors (KOT), basal cell carcinoma (BCCa), medulloblastoma, intracranial dural calcifications, bifid ribs

IMAGING

General Features
- Best diagnostic clue
  - Multiple **expansile**, lucent lesions of mandible and maxilla
- Location
  - Mandible and maxilla
- Size
  - 1-9 cm in size, average = 3 cm
- Morphology
  - Unilocular or multilocular

Radiographic Findings
- Radiography
  - Expansile cysts, may have "cloudy" lumen
  - May displace developing teeth ± resorption of roots of erupted teeth and tooth extrusion

CT Findings
- Distinctly corticated expansile cyst, often with scalloped border, extending along mandible length
- High-attenuation precontrast (hemorrhage ± protein)
- Low-attenuation precontrast due to low protein concentration
- No enhancement of wall or matrix

MR Findings
- Low to intermediate T1, high T2 signal

Imaging Recommendations
- Best imaging tool
  - Bone algorithm CT
- Protocol advice
  - Noncontrast thin-section bone CT, axial and coronal

DIFFERENTIAL DIAGNOSIS

Periapical (Radicular) Cyst
- Unilocular cyst associated with tooth root
- Associated with dental caries and infection

Dentigerous (Follicular) Cyst
- Single unilocular cyst surrounds crown of unerupted tooth

Keratocystic Odontogenic Tumor
- Single multilocular cyst with high attenuation

Ameloblastoma
- Can mimic KOT unless enhancing nodule present

PATHOLOGY

General Features
- Etiology
  - Cysts arise from remnants of dental lamina
- Genetics
  - **Autosomal dominant**
  - Mutations of *PTCH1* gene on chromosome arm 9q
  - 1/3 of cases are new mutations
- Associated abnormalities
  - High incidence of **medulloblastomas**
  - Marked **calcification of falx** (80%), dura
  - Multiple skin **BCCas**
  - **Bifid ribs and scoliosis**

CLINICAL ISSUES

Presentation
- Most common signs/symptoms
  - Multiple enlarging jaw masses, may be asymptomatic or present with pain
    - Multiple KOT seen in 80% of cases of BCNS

Demographics
- Age
  - Syndrome apparent by **5-10 years**
  - Patients present by 3rd decade, with multiple nevoid BCCa; mean age = 19 years
    - Aggressive lesions after puberty, may metastasize
- Epidemiology
  - 1 case per 56,000-164,000
    - Prevalence likely higher in patients < 20 years old presenting with BCCas

Natural History & Prognosis
- Morbidity and mortality related to occurrence of neoplasms associated with BCNS
- High recurrence rate of KOT

Treatment
- Surgical methods: Marsupialization, decompression, enucleation, curettage, en block resection

DIAGNOSTIC CHECKLIST

Consider
- Long-term follow-up for possible recurrences

Image Interpretation Pearls
- Can be difficult to differentiate new cyst formation vs. recurrence of treated lesions

SELECTED REFERENCES

1. John AM et al: Basal cell naevus syndrome: an update on genetics and treatment. Br J Dermatol. 174(1):68-76, 2016
2. Ally MS et al: The use of vismodegib to shrink keratocystic odontogenic tumors in patients with basal cell nevus syndrome. JAMA Dermatol. 150(5):542-5, 2014
3. Sartip K et al: Neuroimaging of nevoid basal cell carcinoma syndrome (NBCCS) in children. Pediatr Radiol. 43(5):620-7, 2013
4. Lam EW et al: The occurrence of keratocystic odontogenic tumours in nevoid basal cell carcinoma syndrome. Dentomaxillofac Radiol. 38(7):475-9, 2009
5. Efron PA et al: Pediatric basal cell carcinoma: case reports and literature review. J Pediatr Surg. 43(12):2277-80, 2008

Syndromic Diseases

TERMINOLOGY

- Branchiootorenal syndrome (BOR)
- Autosomal dominant syndrome
  - Deafness and ear anomalies
  - Branchial anomalies/preauricular pits
  - Renal abnormalities

IMAGING

- Neck: Branchial cleft cyst/fistula
- Temporal bone CT findings
  - Dilated eustachian tubes
  - External ear: Variable stenosis/atresia
  - Middle ear: Dysmorphic; fused, malformed ossicles
  - Cochlea: Tapered basal turn, hypoplastic and offset middle/apical turns
  - Semicircular canal anomaly
  - Dilated, bulbous vestibular aqueduct
  - Flared IAC; anomalous CNVII canal
- Abdominal CT findings: Renal cysts, dysplasia, agenesis

- Variable, asymmetric micrognathia

TOP DIFFERENTIAL DIAGNOSES

- Branchiootic syndrome
  - Normal kidneys; BOR genetic overlap
- Otofaciocervical syndrome: BOR genetic overlap
- Congenital nonsyndromic external ear and middle ear malformation

PATHOLOGY

- BOR 1: 8q13.3 locus, *EYA1* gene mutation
- BOR 2: 19q13.3 locus, *SIX5* mutation

CLINICAL ISSUES

- Clinical presentation
  - Hearing loss (sensorineural hearing loss, conductive hearing loss, mixed) (~ 98%)
  - Preauricular tag, pit (~ 84%)
  - Branchial anomalies (~ 70%)
  - Renal anomalies (~ 40%)

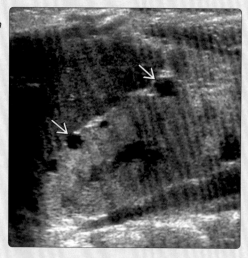
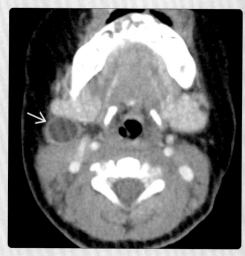

(Left) *Ultrasound of a 4-month-old boy presenting with Potter syndrome is shown. Longitudinal section reveals a solitary echogenic left kidney with numerous peripheral cysts ➡. The patient also had a branchial cleft cyst and microtia.* (Right) *Axial CECT in a 5-month-old boy with preauricular pits and a family history of pits and renal and ear anomalies shows a hypodense lesion ➡ consistent with a 2nd branchial cleft cyst. The patient also had characteristic ear anomalies.*

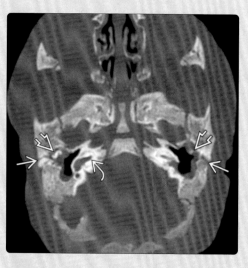
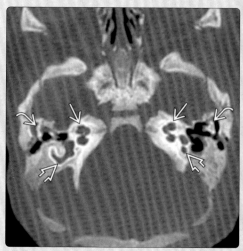

(Left) *Axial bone CT (same patient) imaged at 10 days of age to evaluate microtia, shows bilateral EAC atresia ➡. Ossicles are malformed, fused, and laterally located ➡. Note tapered basal turn of right cochlea ➡.* (Right) *Axial bone CT (same patient) shows "unwound" or offset, hypoplastic middle and apical cochlear turns ➡ and deficiency of the right cochlear modiolus. The posterior semicircular canals ➡ and ossicles ➡ are malformed. CT findings are characteristic of branchiootorenal syndrome.*

TERMINOLOGY

Abbreviations
- Branchiootorenal syndrome (BOR)

Synonyms
- Melnick-Fraser syndrome

Definitions
- Autosomal dominant syndrome
  o Deafness
  o Branchial anomalies/preauricular pits
  o Ear anomalies
  o Renal abnormalities

IMAGING

General Features
- Best diagnostic clue
  o Characteristic cochlear anomaly
    – Tapered basal turn, offset hypoplastic middle and apical turns of cochlea

CT Findings
- CECT
  o Preauricular tags, branchial cysts, sinus tracts and fistulae
- Bone CT
  o Temporal bones findings: Congenital external and middle ear malformation (CEMEM) and inner ear anomalies
    – EAC: Asymmetric angulated and stenotic or atretic
    – Middle ear space: ± underdeveloped and misshapen
    – Ossicles: Dysmorphic, broad incus short process, horizontal orientation long/lenticular process, fusion malleus and incus, ± ossicular fixation
    – Cochlea: **Tapered basal turn, hypoplastic, offset middle/apical turns** → unwound appearance
    – Semicircular canals (SCC): ± globular horizontal SCC, ± absent/hypoplastic posterior SCC
    – Vestibular aqueduct: Dilated, bulbous
    – Internal auditory canal: Flared, widened
    – CNVII canal: Anomalous course labyrinthine segment, obtuse angle anterior genu
  o Skull base
    – Dilated and anomalous eustachian tubes
    – Petrous bone angulation
  o Mandible: Variable asymmetric micrognathia

Ultrasonographic Findings
- Branchial cleft cyst
- Renal abnormalities: Cysts, dysplasia, agenesis

Imaging Recommendations
- Best imaging tool
  o Temporal bone CT
  o US neck and kidneys

DIFFERENTIAL DIAGNOSIS

Branchiootic Syndrome
- Same as BOR except normal kidneys

Bilateral Facial Microsomia
- Bilateral, asymmetric mandibular hypoplasia
- Variable CEMEM

Otofaciocervical Syndrome
- BOR genetic overlap

Congenital External and Middle Ear Malformation
- CEMEM without syndromic features
- Normal mandible, inner ears, eustachian tubes
- No branchial cleft cyst or renal abnormalities

PATHOLOGY

General Features
- Genetics
  o BOR 1: 8q13.3 locus, *EYA1* gene mutation
  o BOR 2: 19q13.3 locus, *SIX5* mutation

CLINICAL ISSUES

Presentation
- Most common signs/symptoms
  o Hearing loss (sensorineural hearing loss, conductive hearing loss, mixed) (~ 98%)
  o Preauricular tag, pit (~ 84%)
  o Branchial anomalies (~ 70%)
  o Renal anomalies (~ 40%)
  o Pinna/EAC anomaly (~ 30%)
- Other signs/symptoms
  o Lacrimal stenosis/aplasia, abnormal palate/mandible

Demographics
- Epidemiology
  o 1:40,000; 2% of profoundly deaf children

Natural History & Prognosis
- High penetrance, variable expression: Mild → lethal

Treatment
- Branchial anomalies: Surgical excision
- Ear anomalies: Hearing augmentation, reconstructive surgery as required for microtia, bilateral EAC atresia
- Renal failure: Dialysis, renal transplant

DIAGNOSTIC CHECKLIST

Consider
- Branchiootic syndrome if normal kidneys

Image Interpretation Pearls
- Characteristic inner ear anomaly: **Unwound cochlea**
- Look for branchial and renal anomalies

Reporting Tips
- Posterior SCC anomaly often overlooked
- Coronal: Differentiate bulbous VA from jugular vein

SELECTED REFERENCES

1. Song MH et al: Mutational analysis of EYA1, SIX1 and SIX5 genes and strategies for management of hearing loss in patients with BOR/BO syndrome. PLoS One. 8(6):e67236, 2013
2. Amin S et al: Incudomalleal joint formation: the roles of apoptosis, migration and downregulation. BMC Dev Biol. 7:134, 2007

(Left) *Axial bone CT in a 4-year-old boy with BOR shows dilatation of an anomalous eustachian tube ➡ terminating in the sphenoid bone. Some mastoid air cells are opacified ➡.* (Right) *Coronal bone CT in a 12-year-old boy with BOR shows angulation of the right EAC ➡ and petrous bones. The right ossicles are malformed and malpositioned in the partially opacified attic ➡. The left EAC is atretic ➡, and the left middle ear cavity is partially opacified.*

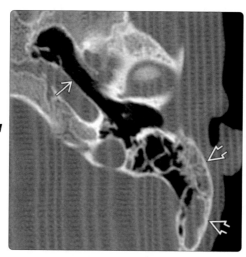
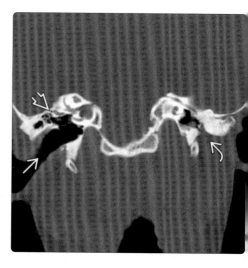

(Left) *Axial bone CT in a 5-year-old girl with BOR shows anterior ligament ossification ➡ fusing the malleus to the attic. Note the hypoplastic middle turn of the cochlea ➡ with an absent modiolus. The vestibular aqueduct is dilated and funnel-shaped ➡.* (Right) *Coronal bone CT in a 10-year-old boy with preauricular pits and mixed hearing loss shows fusion of malleus to incus and fusion of ossicles to the scutum ➡. Note the horizontal orientation of the cochlear basal turn ➡.*

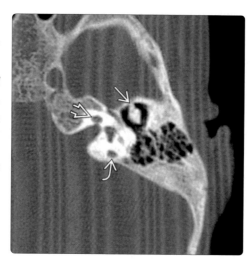
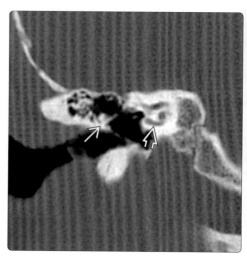

(Left) *Axial HRCT in the same 10-year-old boy demonstrates mild tapering of the cochlear basal turn ➡. Only a small segment of the inferior limb of the posterior SCC is present ➡. The superior limb is absent (not shown).* (Right) *Axial bone CT in a 19-month-old boy with the EYA1 mutation shows hypoplasia of the middle and apical turns of the cochlea ➡, which lack internal septation and appear offset anteriorly from the basal turn ➡.*

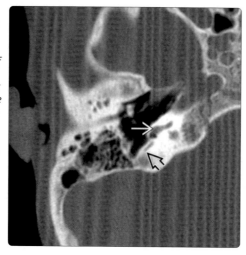
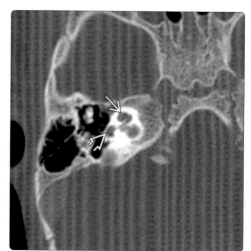

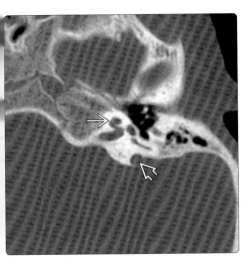

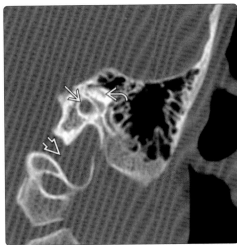

(Left) *Axial bone CT in a 5-year-old girl with hearing loss and BOR reveals characteristic hypoplastic middle and apical cochlear turns ➡, which are offset anteriorly. Bulbous enlargement of the vestibular aqueduct is also seen ➡.* (Right) *Coronal bone CT in a 5-year-old boy shows the utility of the coronal image in distinguishing the dilated vestibular aqueduct ➡ above from the jugular fossa below ➡. Note the hypoplastic posterior SCC ➡.*

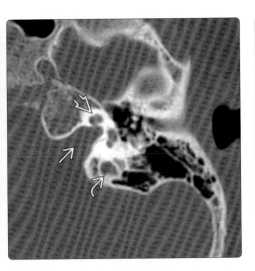

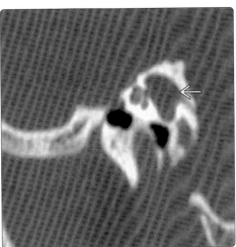

(Left) *Axial bone CT in the same patient demonstrates the broad and funnel-shaped internal auditory meatus ➡. Note also the typical hypoplastic middle and apical turns of the cochlea ➡ and rounded enlargement of the vestibular aqueduct ➡.* (Right) *Sagittal reformatted CT in a 14-year-old boy with BOR demonstrates the bulbous morphology of the IAC ➡.*

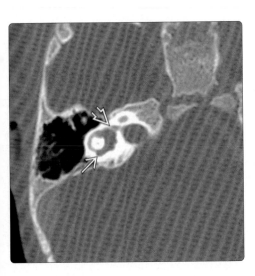

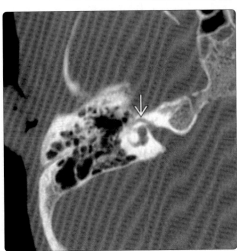

(Left) *Axial bone CT in a 19-month-old patient with hearing loss and preauricular pits demonstrates an anomalous posterior semicircular canal ➡. The canal for the superior vestibular nerve is identified ➡. However, the labyrinthine segment of CNVII is not seen on this image, as it would be in a normal exam.* (Right) *Axial bone CT in the same patient, more cephalad image, shows the anomalous labyrinthine segment of the facial nerve and obtuse angle of the anterior genu ➡.*

KEY FACTS

TERMINOLOGY

- **CHARGE**
  - **C**oloboma
  - **H**eart anomaly
  - **A**tresia choanae
  - **R**etardation: Mental & somatic development
  - **G**enital hypoplasia
  - **E**ar abnormalities
- Major signs: Coloboma, choanal atresia, semicircular canal (SCC) hypoplasia/aplasia, cranial nerve (CN) involvement
- Minor signs: Hindbrain, external/middle ear, cardiac/esophageal malformations, hypothalamo-hypophyseal dysfunction, intellectual disability

IMAGING

- Choanal atresia, coloboma (variable), cleft lip/palate
- Hypoplastic vestibule & hypoplastic/absent SCC
- Mildly flattened apical ± middle turns + thickened modiolus or single cochlear turn/hypoplasia
- Stenotic/atretic cochlear nerve canal
- Stenotic/atretic oval window & overlying anomalous tympanic segment of CNVII
- Large emissary veins, hypoplasia basiocciput, basilar invagination, & vertebral anomalies
- Hypoplastic pons, uplifted vermis ± cerebellar malformation
- CN hypoplasia/aplasia (mainly CNI, VII, & VIII)

TOP DIFFERENTIAL DIAGNOSES

- Kallmann syndrome: Allelic, less severe
- VACTERL association
- Branchiootorenal syndrome

PATHOLOGY

- *CHD7* mutation 60%; *SEMA3E* mutation
- Highly predictive of CHARGE: Cup-shaped pinna, agenesis/hypoplasia SCC, arrhinencephaly

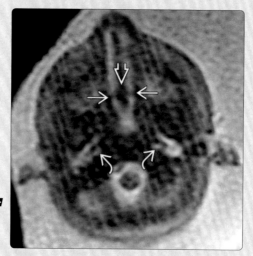
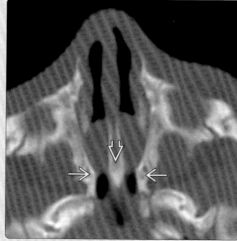

(Left) *Axial FSE T2-weighted fetal MR at 32-weeks gestation shows bilateral choanal atresia with linear hypointensity ➡ extending from the thickened vomer ➡ to the lateral nasal walls, outlined by amniotic fluid. A single cochlear turn is seen bilaterally ➡, and the cochleae appeared isolated from the internal auditory canals (IACs). (Right) Axial bone CT in the same infant at 6 days of age shows lateral nasal wall medial deviation ➡ and a thickened vomer ➡ with bilateral bony and membranous choanal atresia.*

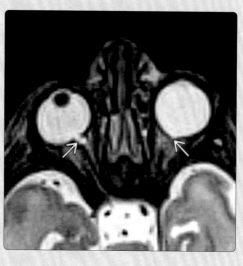
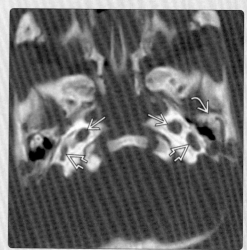

(Left) *Axial FSE T2-weighted MR in the same baby boy (age: 4 days) reveals right microphthalmia and bilateral colobomas ➡. A CHD7 mutation was found, confirming CHARGE syndrome. (Right) Axial bone CT in the same child confirms incomplete cochlear partitioning ➡, hypoplastic vestibules ➡, and absent semicircular canals (SCCs). The ossicles are dysmorphic, and the left malleus is fused to the attic ➡. It is unusual to see the ocular, ear, and nasal findings of CHARGE all in the same patient.*

TERMINOLOGY

Synonyms

- CHARGE association, Hall-Hittner syndrome

Definitions

- **CHARGE** acronym
  - **C**oloboma
  - **H**eart anomaly
  - **A**tresia choanae
  - **R**etardation: Mental & somatic development
  - **G**enital hypoplasia
  - **E**ar abnormalities

IMAGING

General Features

- Best diagnostic clue
  - Inner ear: Hypoplastic vestibules & hypoplastic/absent semicircular canals (SCCs)

CT Findings

- Bone CT
  - Nose: **Choanal atresia**
  - Eyes: **Coloboma**
  - Face & oral cavity: **Cleft lip/palate**
  - Temporal bones
    - **Vestibule: Hypoplastic**
    - **SCC: Hypoplastic/absent**
    - Cochlea: Flattened apical ± middle turns + thickened modiolus or single cochlear turn/hypoplasia
    - Cochlear nerve canal: Stenotic/atretic
    - Vestibular aqueduct: Normal or bulbous endolymphatic duct
    - Oval window: Stenotic/atretic
    - Cranial nerve (CN)VII : Anomalous, hypoplastic, ± dehiscent tympanic segment
    - Ossicles: Dysmorphic, fused
  - Skull base & spine
    - Jugular foraminal stenosis & large emissary veins
    - Hypoplasia basiocciput & spinal anomalies

MR Findings

- Hypoplastic pons (common), uplifted vermis ± cerebellar malformation
- Hypoplasia/aplasia of CN: Primarily CNI, CNVII, & CNVIII
- Hypoplasia basiocciput & vertebral anomalies

Imaging Recommendations

- Best imaging tool
  - MR: Brain, clivus, eyes, inner ears, CNs, & spine
- Protocol advice
  - MR: Brain & 3D T2 (e.g., SPACE, FIESTA) inner ears & CN

DIFFERENTIAL DIAGNOSIS

Kallmann Syndrome

- Allelic, less severe

VACTERL Association

- **V**ertebral/vascular, **a**nal/auricular, **c**ardiac, **t**racheoesophageal fistula, **e**sophageal atresia, **r**enal/radial/rib, **l**imb anomalies

PATHOLOGY

General Features

- Genetics
  - Gene map locus 8q12.1, 7q21.11
  - *CHD7* mutation 60%; *SEMA3E* mutation

Staging, Grading, & Classification

- Major diagnostic characteristics
  - Coloboma, choanal atresia, CN aplasia/hypoplasia (CNI, CNVII, CNVIII, CNIX-X), temporal bone anomalies (90%)
- Minor diagnostic characteristics
  - Genital hypoplasia, developmental delay, cardiac, growth deficiency, orofacial cleft, tracheoesophageal fistula, abnormal faces
- **Definite CHARGE syndrome**: Child with all 4 major characteristics or 3 major & 3 minor characteristics

Gross Pathologic & Surgical Features

- Highly predictive of CHARGE
  - External ear anomalies & agenesis/hypoplasia SCC

CLINICAL ISSUES

Presentation

- Most common signs/symptoms
  - Airway obstruction, feeding difficulty, GE reflux
  - Facial dysmorphism, cleft lip/palate
  - Low-set, cup-shaped ears & deafness
  - Cardiac symptoms (e.g., TOF)
  - Growth retardation
  - Genital hypoplasia (central hypogonadism)
  - Coloboma, microphthalmia, anosmia
  - Developmental delay/autism

Demographics

- Epidemiology
  - Birth incidence: 1 in 12,000; phenotypic variability

DIAGNOSTIC CHECKLIST

Consider

- CHARGE inner ear anomaly highly characteristic
- Consider alternative diagnosis for bilateral choanal atresia & normal inner ears

Image Interpretation Pearls

- Oval window atresia + aberrant/dehiscent CNVII canal on coronal CT
- MR for absent CNs, abnormal pons, & clivus

SELECTED REFERENCES

1. Green GE et al: CHD7 mutations and CHARGE syndrome in semicircular canal dysplasia. Otol Neurotol. 35(8):1466-70, 2014
2. Holcomb MA et al: Cochlear nerve deficiency in children with CHARGE syndrome. Laryngoscope. 123(3):793-6, 2013
3. Legendre M et al: Antenatal spectrum of CHARGE syndrome in 40 fetuses with CHD7 mutations. J Med Genet. 49(11):698-707, 2012
4. Fujita K et al: Abnormal basiocciput development in CHARGE syndrome. AJNR Am J Neuroradiol. 30(3):629-34, 2009
5. Morimoto AK et al: Absent semicircular canals in CHARGE syndrome: radiologic spectrum of findings. AJNR Am J Neuroradiol. 27(8):1663-71, 2006
6. Verloes A: Updated diagnostic criteria for CHARGE syndrome: a proposal. Am J Med Genet A. 133A(3):306-8, 2005

(Left) Axial bone CT in a 1-year-old boy with CHARGE syndrome shows a prominent modiolus ⊒, cochlear nerve canal stenosis ➯, small vestibule ➱, absent SCCs, abnormal course of vestibular aqueduct ➯, and opacified middle ear cavity and mastoid air cells. (Right) Axial bone CT in a 13-month-old boy with a CHD7 mutation shows a thick modiolus ⊒, small vestibule ➯, absent SCCs, narrow malleoincudal joint ➱, middle ear and mastoid air cell opacification, and a large emissary vein ➯.

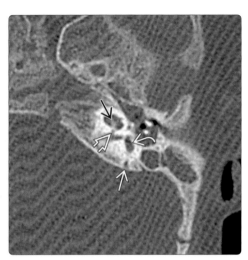
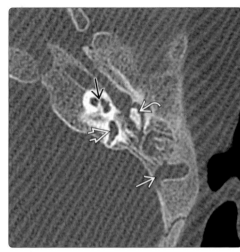

(Left) Axial bone CT in a 16-month-old boy with CHARGE syndrome and a CHD7 mutation shows a single amorphous, unsegmented cochlear turn ➱. The incus and stapes form a single solid bar that is inferiorly angulated ➯. (Right) Axial bone CT in the same patient demonstrates the cephalad aspect of the cochlea ➯, essentially isolated from the IAC ➯. The vestibule is hypoplastic ➱, and the SCCs are absent. The middle ear cavity and mastoid air cells are opacified.

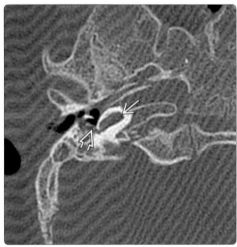
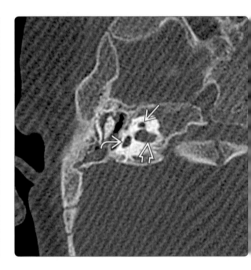

(Left) Coronal bone CT in a 1.5-year-old boy with a CHD7 mutation shows the tympanic segment of CNVII ➱ overlying oval window atresia, hypoplastic vestibule ➯, and absent SCCs. (Right) Coronal bone CT in a 7-year-old girl with CHARGE shows cervical spine anomaly ➯, petrous angulation, hypoplastic vestibule, and absent SCCs. The facial nerve canal is dehiscent and overlies the atretic oval window ➯. The ossicles contact the facial nerve. A large emissary vein indents the tegmen tympani ➱.

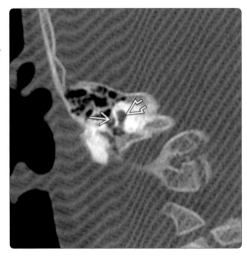
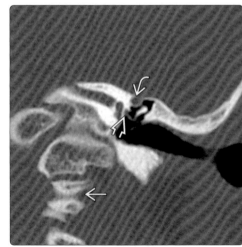

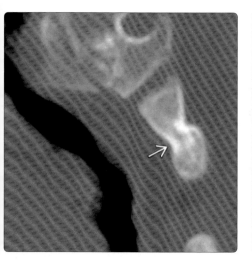
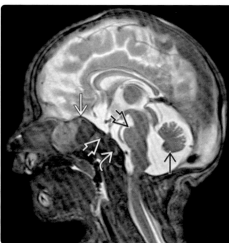

(Left) *Reformatted sagittal CT in a 7-month-old boy with CHARGE shows deformity & constriction of the basiocciput ➡. (Right) Sagittal T2-weighted MR in a 4-day-old boy with a CHD7 mutation shows convexity of the planum sphenoidale ➡, inferior placement of the sella ➡, and a hypoplastic basiocciput ➡. There is uplifting of the vermis with mild inferior vermian hypoplasia ➡ and a mildly prominent 4th ventricle. The pons appears shortened ➡.*

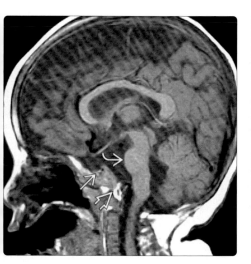
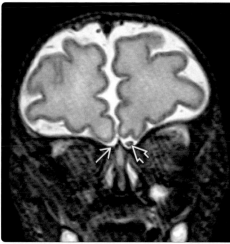

(Left) *Sagittal T1-weighted MR in a 16-month-old boy with a CHD7 mutation demonstrates a partially empty sella ➡, and the infundibulum is not seen. Note the severe hypoplasia of the basiocciput ➡ and basilar invagination. The pons is hypoplastic ➡. (Right) Coronal T2 STIR in the 4-day-old boy with a CHD7 mutation reveals absence of the right olfactory bulb ➡. Note the prominent left olfactory bulb ➡.*

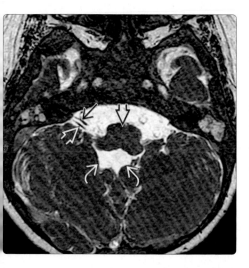
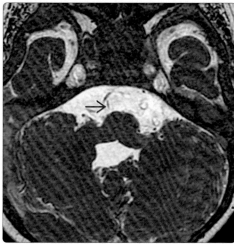

(Left) *Axial 3D FIESTA MR in a 16-month-old patient with CHARGE syndrome shows the right CNVII ➡ and CNVIII ➡. The left CNVII and CNVIII are absent. The pons is hypoplastic and rotated ➡, and the 4th ventricle is asymmetric ➡. (Right) Axial 3D FIESTA MR more cephalad in the same patient shows the right CNVI ➡. The left CNVI is absent.*

Syndromic Diseases

KEY FACTS

TERMINOLOGY

- Oculoauriculovertebral spectrum, Goldenhar syndrome, facioauriculovertebral sequence
- Defect of 1st & 2nd pharyngeal arch derivatives ± neural crest cells

IMAGING

- Mandibular hypoplasia
  - Unilateral; rarely bilateral & asymmetric
- Zygomatic arch hypoplasia
- Hypoplasia muscles of mastication, facial muscles, & parotid gland
- EAC atresia/stenosis
- Middle ear hypoplasia & ossicular malformation/fusion
- Oval window atresia & CNVII anomaly/hypoplasia
- Cervical spine fusion/segmentation anomalies (Klippel-Feil anomaly)
- CNS (variable): Ventriculomegaly, brainstem cleft, cerebellar hypoplasia, cephalocele

TOP DIFFERENTIAL DIAGNOSES

- Teratogenic embryopathy (e.g., diabetes)
- Townes-Brocks syndrome
- Branchiootorenal syndrome
- Treacher Collins syndrome

CLINICAL ISSUES

- Common disorder, prevalence ~ 1 in 3,500 births
- Microtia/anotia, preauricular skin tags
- Hearing loss (~ 85%; CHL > > SNHL)
- Facial asymmetry; unilateral micrognathia
- Facial nerve weakness (~ 50%)
- Variable facial clefts
- Epibulbar lipodermoid, coloboma
- TEF, cardiac, genitourinary, pulmonary abnormalities

DIAGNOSTIC CHECKLIST

- HFM as cause of facial asymmetry & external ear anomalies
- Facial weakness due to CNVII anomaly/hypoplasia

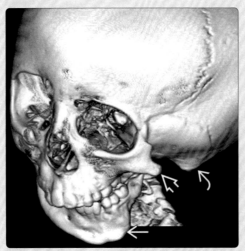
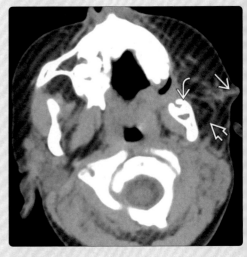

(Left) *3D CT in a 7-year-old girl with hemifacial microsomia (HFM) reveals a smaller left hemimandible ➡, hypoplasia of the zygomatic arch ➡, underdevelopment of the mastoid process ➡, and external auditory canal atresia.* (Right) *Axial NECT in a 4-year-old girl with HFM demonstrates a smaller left mandibular ramus ➡, a preauricular sinus tract, and skin tag ➡. The left muscles of mastication are underdeveloped, and the masticator muscle and parotid tissue are not seen in their expected location ➡.*

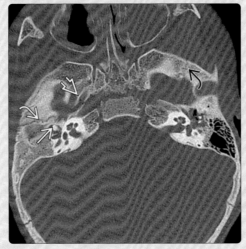
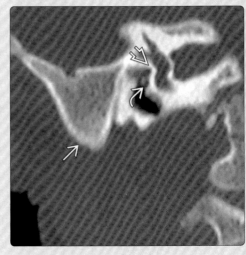

(Left) *Axial bone CT in a 23-month-old boy with HFM shows that the right middle ear cavity is hypoplastic and opacified. The ossicles ➡ are dysmorphic. The right eustachian tube is dilated and anomalous ➡. The right sphenosquamosal suture ➡ is rotated laterally compared with the left ➡.* (Right) *Reformatted coronal bone CT in the same patient shows absent mastoid pneumatization ➡, oval window atresia ➡, and an anomalous inferior course of CNVII tympanic segment ➡, running over the promontory.*

TERMINOLOGY

Abbreviations

- Hemifacial microsomia (HFM)

Synonyms

- Oculoauriculovertebral spectrum, Goldenhar syndrome, facioauriculovertebral sequence

Definitions

- Defect of 1st & 2nd pharyngeal arch derivatives ± neural crest cells
  - **External & middle ear** anomalies
  - Typically unilateral mandibular & TMJ hypoplasia

IMAGING

General Features

- Best diagnostic clue
  - **Unilateral** mandibular hypoplasia, deficient zygomatic arch, & EAC atresia/stenosis

CT Findings

- Bone CT
  - **Micrognathia**
    - Typically unilateral, less commonly bilateral and asymmetric; TMJ hypoplasia or aplasia
  - **Hypoplastic/deficient zygomatic arch**
  - Hypoplasia muscles of mastication & facial muscles
  - Parotid hypoplasia/aplasia ± prominent accessory parotid
  - Temporal bone: **Congenital external & middle ear anomaly (CEMEM)**
    - EAC: Stenosis/atresia, small/absent tympanic plate
    - Mastoid: ± variable decreased pneumatization
    - Middle ear space: Variable hypoplasia
    - Ossicles: Malformed, rotated, fused
    - Oval window: ± stenosis or atresia
    - CNVII canal (FNC): Normal or hypoplastic FNC
      - ☐ Tympanic FNC ± dehiscent/aberrant
      - ☐ Mastoid FNC exits ventrally, sometimes into TMJ
    - Inner ear: Occasional malformation
  - Face: ± facial cleft; ± other structures involved e.g., orbit
  - Spine: ± fusion/segmentation anomalies

MR Findings

- **Mandibular hypoplasia & small muscles of mastication**
- Spine: ± **vertebral anomalies**
- CNS: ± ventriculomegaly, occasional brainstem cleft, cerebellar hypoplasia, cephalocele
- **CNVII: Normal, hypoplasia, or aplasia**

DIFFERENTIAL DIAGNOSIS

Teratogenic Embryopathy (e.g., Diabetes)

- Mandibular & temporal bone anomalies depend on etiology

Townes-Brocks Syndrome

- Simulates Goldenhar phenotype; CEMEM; hand, renal, & anal anomalies

Branchiootorenal Syndrome

- Variable asymmetric micrognathia
- CEMEM, large eustachian tubes

- Tapered cochlear basal turn; small, offset middle/apical turns

Treacher Collins Syndrome

- Bilateral, usually symmetric micrognathia, hypoplastic zygomatic arches, CEMEM

PATHOLOGY

General Features

- Etiology
  - Common disorder, prevalence ~ 1 in 3,500 births
  - Genetic & environmental factors implicated
  - Sporadic, rarely familial (usually autosomal dominant; reduced penetrance)

Staging, Grading, & Classification

- **OMENS** clinical classification (for severity score)
  - **O**rbital asymmetry
  - **M**andibular hypoplasia
  - **E**ar deformity
  - **N**erve dysfunction
  - **S**oft tissue deficiency

CLINICAL ISSUES

Presentation

- Most common signs/symptoms
  - Facial asymmetry (~ 100%): Unilateral micrognathia ± maxillary hypoplasia, clefting, ± CNVII weakness
  - Ear (~ 100%): Microtia/anotia, preauricular skin tags, EAC stenosis/atresia, hearing loss [~ 85%; conductive hearing loss (CHL) > sensorineural hearing loss (SNHL)]
  - Eye (72%): Epibulbar lipodermoid, coloboma, microphthalmia, visual impairment (28%)
  - Cervical spine deformity
  - CNS: Hydrocephalus, cephalocele, mental retardation
- Other signs/symptoms
  - Tracheoesophageal fistula (TEF)/esophageal atresia
  - Cardiac, pulmonary, & genitourinary anomalies

Natural History & Prognosis

- Variable severity, phenotypic heterogeneity

Treatment

- Mandibular reconstruction, hearing aids/ear surgery

DIAGNOSTIC CHECKLIST

Consider

- HFM as cause of facial asymmetry & external ear anomalies
- CNVII anomaly/hypoplasia as cause of facial weakness

SELECTED REFERENCES

1. Beleza-Meireles A et al: Oculo-auriculo-vertebral spectrum: a review of the literature and genetic update. J Med Genet. 51(10):635-45, 2014
2. Gougoutas AJ et al: Hemifacial microsomia: clinical features and pictographic representations of the OMENS classification system. Plast Reconstr Surg. 120(7):112e-120e, 2007
3. Kosaki R et al: Wide phenotypic variations within a family with SALL1 mutations: Isolated external ear abnormalities to Goldenhar syndrome. Am J Med Genet A. 143A(10):1087-90, 2007
4. Rahbar R et al: Craniofacial, temporal bone, and audiologic abnormalities in the spectrum of hemifacial microsomia. Arch Otolaryngol Head Neck Surg. 127(3):265-71, 2001

Treacher Collins Syndrome

TERMINOLOGY

- Treacher Collins syndrome (TCS)
- Nager syndrome: TCS + limb anomalies
- Craniofacial malformation: Down-slanting palpebral fissures, micrognathia, zygomatic and malar hypoplasia, microtia/anotia, ± limb defects

IMAGING

- Temporal bone findings
  - EAC: Stenosis/atresia
  - Decreased/absent mastoid pneumatization
  - Hypoplastic/atretic middle ear space
  - Malformed or absent ossicles ± fixation
  - Oval window stenosis/atresia
  - Facial nerve canal anomalies/dehiscence
  - Normal or malformed cochlea (flattened turns)
  - Normal or malformed lateral semicircular canal ± vestibule

- Relatively symmetric micrognathia, zygomatic/malar hypoplasia
- Coloboma

TOP DIFFERENTIAL DIAGNOSES

- Bilateral facial microsomia
- Nonsyndromic congenital external and middle ear malformation
- Branchiootorenal syndrome

PATHOLOGY

- Autosomal dominant > > recessive, phenotypic variability and genetic heterogeneity, "ribosomopathy"
- TCS: *TCOF1*, *POLR1D*, and *POLR1C* gene mutations
- Nager syndrome: *SF3B4* gene mutation

CLINICAL ISSUES

- Airway obstruction, deafness
- Treatment: Airway support, reconstructive surgery, hearing aids, developmental support

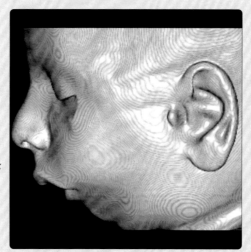
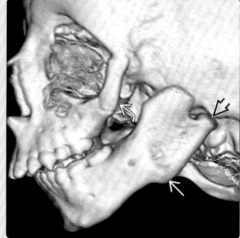

(Left) *Lateral 3D soft tissue surface-rendered reformation CT in an infant with Nager syndrome shows micrognathia, malar flattening, mildly low-set ears, and external auditory meatus atresia.* (Right) *Lateral 3D bone CT in the same infant with Nager syndrome shows micrognathia with an obtuse mandibular angle* ➡ *and marked hypoplasia of the neck and condyle of the mandible* ➡. *There is hypoplasia of the midface and zygomatic complex* ➡ *with absence of the zygomatic arch. There is EAC atresia.*

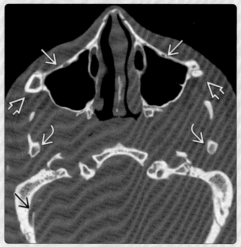
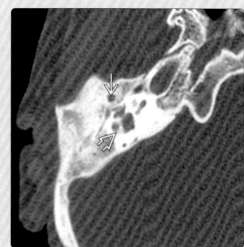

(Left) *Axial bone CT in a 13-year-old girl with Treacher Collins syndrome shows zygomatic complex hypoplasia with posteriorly slanted maxillae* ➡, *absent zygomatic arches* ➡, *& hypoplastic mandibular condyles* ➡. *Note EAC atresia, absent mastoid pneumatization, & an enlarged mastoid emissary vein* ➡. (Right) *Axial bone CT in a 16-year-old girl with TCS shows EAC atresia, absent middle ear space and ossicles, ventrally placed descending facial nerve canal* ➡, *and malformed lateral semicircular canal* ➡ *with small bone island.*

Pierre Robin Sequence

KEY FACTS

TERMINOLOGY

- Pierre Robin sequence (PRS)
- PRS triad: Micrognathia, glossoptosis, respiratory distress

IMAGING

- Bilateral, usually symmetric **micrognathia**
- **Glossoptosis**: Elevated, posteriorly displaced tongue
- Posterior **U-shaped cleft palate**
- Additional features depend on syndromic etiology
- Temporal bone
  - EAC: Normal, stenotic, or atretic [e.g., Treacher Collins syndrome (TCS)]
  - Middle ear & mastoid: Normal or hypoplastic ± opacification
  - Ossicles: Normal, mildly malformed [e.g., stapes in velocardiofacial syndrome (VCFS)], or severely malformed ± fixation (e.g., TCS)
  - Inner ear: Normal or malformed (e.g., small semicircular canal bone island/anlage anomaly in VCFS & TCS)

TOP DIFFERENTIAL DIAGNOSES

- Stickler & related syndromes (18% of PRS)
- VCFS (~ 7% of PRS)
- TCS (~ 5% of PRS)

PATHOLOGY

- Primary micrognathia → glossoptosis → failure of palatal shelf elevation & fusion
- Collagen (*COL*) gene mutations: Stickler syndromes
- 22q11.2 deletion: Velocardiofacial syndrome

CLINICAL ISSUES

- Feeding & breathing difficulties, failure to thrive
- Stickler: Progressive myopia, joint degeneration
- VCFS: Cardiac anomalies, adenoidal hypoplasia, velopharyngeal insufficiency, medial deviation of cervical internal carotid arteries, learning difficulties
- TCS: Malar flattening, downslanting palpebral fissures, coloboma

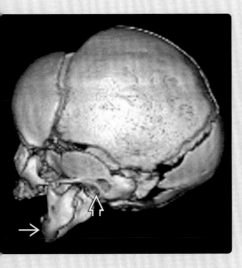

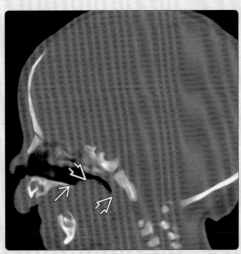

(Left) *Lateral 3D reformation of a 3-week-old girl with Pierre Robin sequence shows moderate, symmetric micrognathia ➡. Note that the zygomatic arch & external auditory canal ➡ are present.* (Right) *Sagittal CT reconstruction (same patient) reveals a shortened hard palate ➡ and glossoptosis (abnormal downward or backward displacement of the tongue) ➡. The tongue, which protrudes above and behind the palate, obstructs the oropharynx, resulting in difficulty with breathing and feeding.*

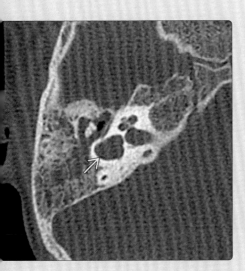

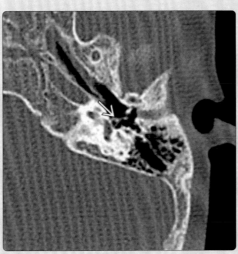

(Left) *Axial bone CT in a 5-year-old boy with velocardiofacial syndrome (VCFS) shows anlage anomaly where lateral semicircular canal (SCC) & vestibule form a single globular space without a bone island ➡. There is diffuse opacification of the middle ear space & mastoid air cells.* (Right) *Axial bone CT in a 7-year-old girl with VCFS & hearing loss shows mild thickening of anterior crus of the stapes ➡ & mildly reduced mastoid pneumatization. More cephalad image (not shown) demonstrated slightly small lateral SCC bone island.*

X-Linked Stapes Gusher (DFNX2)

TERMINOLOGY

- **X-linked mixed hearing loss**
- Conductive hearing loss (CHL) with stapes fixation (DFN3)
- Mixed deafness with **perilymph gusher**
- Profound SNHL ± CHL + bilateral unique inner ear anomaly

IMAGING

- Cochlea: Deficient interscalar septa & osseous spiral lamina, absent modiolus → **corkscrew** appearance
- IAC: Bulbous dilatation laterally + deficient lamina cribrosa
- Vestibule & semicircular canals: ± slightly dilated, ± superior bulge protruding from vestibule ± SCC ossification
- Vestibular aqueduct: ± large
- CNVII canal: Wide labyrinthine & proximal tympanic segments

TOP DIFFERENTIAL DIAGNOSES

- Cochlear incomplete partition type I (IP-I)

- Large vestibular aqueduct + cochlear incomplete partition type II (IP-II)

PATHOLOGY

- X-linked recessive: **Males** affected, female carriers
- Molecular cause: *POU3F4* gene mutation
- Absent lamina cribrosa → communication between CSF & cochlear perilymph → perilymph hydrops

CLINICAL ISSUES

- Bilateral profound SNHL (may be progressive) ± CHL secondary to stapes fixation
  - CHL may be masked by severe SNHL
- Surgical perilymph fistula + perilymph/CSF gusher (e.g., during stapedectomy or cochleostomy)
- Most common cause of X-linked hearing loss

DIAGNOSTIC CHECKLIST

- Essential imaging feature: Widened IAC, deficient lamina cribrosa, cochlear IP-III anomaly (corkscrew cochlea)

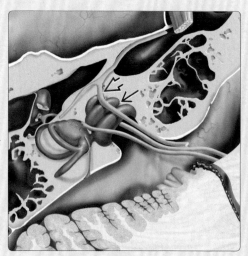
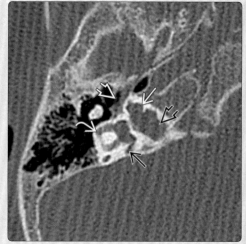

(Left) *Axial graphic of X-linked stapes gusher reveals the corkscrew cochlea ➡ with no modiolus. The internal auditory canal (IAC) is foreshortened & widened. The labyrinthine CNVII segment is enlarged ➡. (Right) Axial bone CT in a 2-year-old boy with profound SNHL shows the internal osseous structures of the cochlea are essentially absent ➡. IAC is widened ➡ and merges with cochlea. The lateral SCC is mildly dilated ➡. The vestibular aqueduct is slightly large ➡, and the proximal tympanic CNVII canal is slightly widened ➡.*

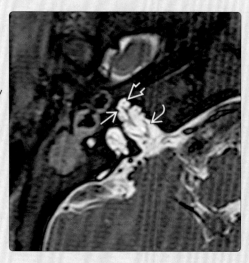
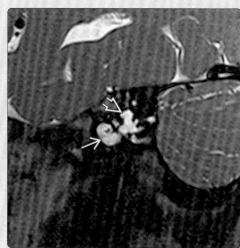

(Left) *Axial T2 SPACE MR in a 1-year-old boy with profound hearing loss shows a corkscrew morphology of the cochlea with deficiency of the interscalar septum ➡ and osseous spiral lamina (partially visualized) ➡ and absence of the modiolus. The IAC is widened and merges with the cochlear turns ➡. (Right) Sagittal oblique T2 SPACE MR in a 2-year-old boy with DFNX2 demonstrates the deficient internal structure of the cochlea ➡, which is dilated. There is a globular protrusion off the superior aspect of the vestibule ➡.*

TERMINOLOGY

Abbreviations

- Deafness X-linked 2 (DFNX2)
- X-linked mixed hearing loss (XLMHL)

Synonyms

- Deafness 3, conductive, with **stapes fixation** (DFN3)
- X-linked deafness with stapes gusher
- **Deafness, mixed, with perilymph gusher**
- Nance deafness
- Cochlear incomplete partition type III (IP-III)

Definitions

- Profound sensorineural hearing loss (SNHL) ± CHL + bilateral unique inner ear anomaly

IMAGING

General Features

- Best diagnostic clue
  - Deficient cochlear partition & absent modiolus → corkscrew appearance + bulbous lateral aspect internal auditory canal (IAC); bilateral and symmetric

CT Findings

- Bone CT
  - **Cochlea**: Deficient interscalar septa & osseous spiral lamina; absent modiolus → **corkscrew** appearance
  - Cochlear nerve canal: Widened
  - **IAC**: **Bulbous dilatation laterally**, absent lamina cribrosa
  - Vestibule & semicircular canals (SCC): Normal or dilated, ± superior bulge protruding from vestibule ± SCC ossification
  - Vestibular aqueduct: ± large
  - Facial nerve canal: Wide labyrinthine & proximal tympanic segments
  - Oval window-stapes: Usually normal
    - May be small with stapes footplate thickening

MR Findings

- T2WI
  - Cochlea: **Deficient interscalar septa & osseous spiral lamina; absent modiolus**
  - Vestibule & SCC: Variable dilatation
  - Endolymphatic sac & duct: ± large
  - IAC: **Bulbous dilatation laterally**
  - CNVII: Normal branches

DIFFERENTIAL DIAGNOSIS

Cochlear Incomplete Partition Type I (IP-I)

- Absent internal cochlear structure without corkscrew morphology

Large Vestibular Aqueduct (IP-II)

- LVA ± absent apical septation & deficient modiolus

PATHOLOGY

General Features

- Genetics
  - Inheritance: **X-linked recessive**
  - Chromosomal locus: **Xq21**; *POU3F4* gene mutation
  - Mutation affects ability of POU3F4 protein to bind DNA, abolishes transcriptional activity

Gross Pathologic & Surgical Features

- Absent lamina cribrosa → communication between subarachnoid space & cochlear perilymph space → perilymphatic hydrops
- Stapes fixation → perilymph/CSF gusher on attempted stapedectomy

CLINICAL ISSUES

Presentation

- Most common signs/symptoms
  - Affected males
    - **Bilateral profound SNHL** (may be progressive)
      - ± CHL from stapes fixation
      - CHL may be masked by severe SNHL
    - Impaired vestibular function
    - Surgical **perilymph fistula + perilymph/CSF gusher** at attempted stapedectomy/cochleostomy
  - Female carriers
    - Normal (most) or mild/delayed-onset hearing loss
    - Normal imaging ± bulbous IACs
- Other signs/symptoms
  - Risk of **meningitis & labyrinthitis ossificans**

Demographics

- Gender
  - Female carriers, affected males
- Epidemiology
  - Most common cause of X-linked hearing loss

Treatment

- Profound SNHL: Cochlear implantation with risk of CSF gusher & meningitis

DIAGNOSTIC CHECKLIST

Image Interpretation Pearls

- Key features: **Bulbous lateral end IAC + deficient lamina cribrosa + cochlear IP-III anomaly**
- Risk of perilymph gusher at stapedectomy/cochleostomy

SELECTED REFERENCES

1. Choi BY et al: Clinical observations and molecular variables of patients with hearing loss and incomplete partition type III. Laryngoscope. 126(3):E123-8, 2016
2. Gong WX et al: HRCT and MRI findings in X-linked non-syndromic deafness patients with a POU3F4 mutation. Int J Pediatr Otorhinolaryngol. 78(10):1756-62, 2014
3. Sennaroglu L: Cochlear implantation in inner ear malformations--a review article. Cochlear Implants Int. 11(1):4-41, 2010
4. Lee HK et al: Clinical and molecular characterizations of novel POU3F4 mutations reveal that DFN3 is due to null function of POU3F4 protein. Physiol Genomics. 39(3):195-201, 2009
5. Friedman RA et al: Molecular analysis of the POU3F4 gene in patients with clinical and radiographic evidence of X-linked mixed deafness with perilymphatic gusher. Ann Otol Rhinol Laryngol. 106(4):320-5, 1997
6. de Kok YJ et al: Association between X-linked mixed deafness and mutations in the POU domain gene POU3F4. Science. 267(5198):685-8, 1995
7. Phelps PD et al: X-linked deafness, stapes gushers and a distinctive defect of the inner ear. Neuroradiology. 33(4):326-30, 1991
8. Nance WE et al: X-linked mixed deafness with congenital fixation of the stapedial footplate and perilymphatic gusher. Birth Defects Orig Artic Ser. 07(4):64-9, 1971

Syndromic Diseases

KEY FACTS

TERMINOLOGY

- McCune-Albright syndrome (MAS)
  - Subtype of **polyostotic fibrous dysplasia (FD)**
- **Classic triad**: Polyostotic FD, endocrine dysfunction, and cutaneous hyperpigmentation

IMAGING

- Best diagnostic clues: Expanded ground-glass bone in child with precocious puberty and skin lesions
- Locations in H&N: Skull, skull base, or facial bones
  - Bilateral and asymmetric common
- CT: Imaging appearance depends on degree of fibrous vs. osseous components
  - **Ground glass**: sclerotic
  - **Mixed** (pagetoid): Radiodensity and radiolucency
  - **Cystic**: Central lucency with thin sclerotic margins
  - Variable enhancement of fibrous component
- MR: Majority ↓ T1, intermediate or ↓ signal T2
  - Rim ↓ signal T2 and central ↑ T2 in cystic lesions

- Fibrous component may enhance intensely

TOP DIFFERENTIAL DIAGNOSES

- Monostotic FD
- Polyostotic FD without MAS
- Jaffe-Campanacci syndrome
  - Nonossifying fibromas, axillary freckling, and café au lait skin lesions, without neurofibromas
- Caffey disease: Usually < 5 months of age
  - Acute onset fever + hot, tender swelling of bones
- Cherubism
  - Familial, symmetric, bilateral fibroosseous lesions of jaw
- Garré sclerosing osteomyelitis
  - Bony expansion, heterogeneous sclerotic pattern
- Intraosseous meningioma
  - Hyperostosis
- Paget disease
  - Cotton wool CT appearance

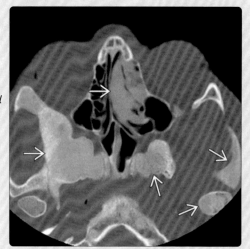 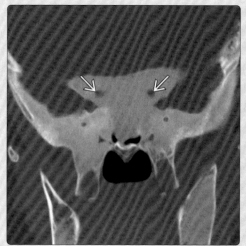

(Left) *Axial bone CT in a 7-year-old girl with McCune-Albright syndrome shows multiple areas of fibrous dysplasia* ➡ *with the typical expanded ground-glass appearance of lesions in the sclerotic stage.* (Right) *Coronal bone CT in the same child shows more extensive involvement of the skull base and typical narrowing of skull base foramina. Despite significant narrowing of both optic canals* ➡, *the child had only mild left-sided optic neuropathy with decreased vision and intermittent diplopia.*

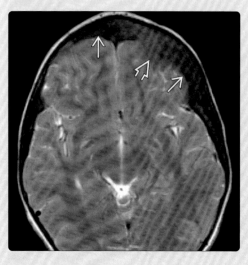 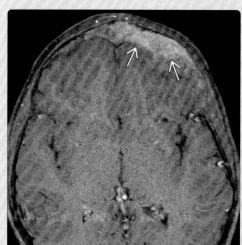

(Left) *Axial T2WI MR in a teenager with a frontal bone fibrous dysplasia lesion shows marked hypointensity within the majority of the expansile, sclerotic frontal bones* ➡, *with patchy hyperintensity typical of a small area of more active fibrous matrix* ➡. (Right) *Axial T1WI C+ FS MR in the same patient shows heterogeneous enhancement* ➡ *in the more active, fibrous component of fibrous dysplasia. This area was more lucent on CT (not shown).*

Cherubism

TERMINOLOGY

- Familial, bilateral fibroosseous jaw lesions
  - Genetically distinct from fibrous dysplasia (FD)

IMAGING

- **Bilateral** multilocular, **expansile** lucent lesions in **mandible**, displacing teeth
- ± submandibular lymph node enlargement

TOP DIFFERENTIAL DIAGNOSES

- FD
  - Ground-glass, mixed cystic and sclerotic, or cystic
- Central giant cell granuloma
  - Expansile lesion with variable septations
  - Anterior midline mandible or ramus > maxilla
- McCune-Albright syndrome
  - Subtype of **polyostotic** FD
  - Classic triad of polyostotic FD, precocious puberty, and cutaneous hyperpigmentation

PATHOLOGY

- Autosomal dominant
  - Heterozygous mutation in *SH3BP2* gene, gene map locus 4p16.3
- Cherubism also reported in patients with Ramon syndrome, Noonan syndrome, and neurofibromatosis type 1

CLINICAL ISSUES

- **Painless** symmetric, swelling of lower face
- Round face and lower eyelid retraction → eyes raised to heaven or cherub-like appearance
- Begins 14 months to 4 years of age
  - Progresses through puberty, then stabilizes
  - May regress in adulthood
  - Clinical swelling usually abates by 3rd decade
  - Radiographic changes seen until 4th decade
- Treatment: Conservative in most, curettage may improve chances of normal dentition and aesthetics

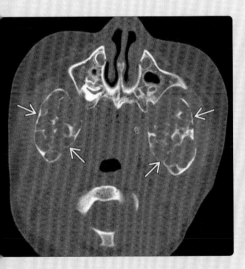
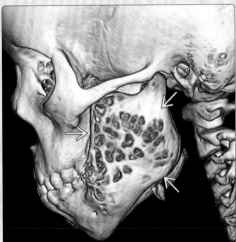

(Left) Axial bone CT in a 17-year-old boy shows bilateral bubbly, expansile lesions ➡ confined to the mandible, a typical appearance of cherubism. Notice there are areas where the cortex appears to disappear without aggressive bone destruction or periosteal reaction. (Right) Lateral 3D reconstruction shows the diffuse expansion of the left mandible ➡ secondary to the multiple bone cysts. (Courtesy J. Cure, MD.)

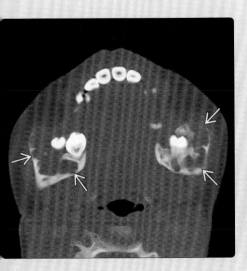
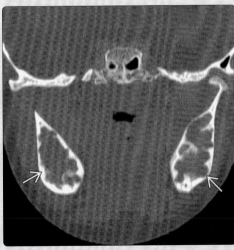

(Left) Axial bone CT in a 4-year-old boy who presented with gradual increase in facial swelling shows bilateral cystic lesions in the mandible ➡ with several areas of diffuse cortical thinning, without aggressive bone destruction or periosteal reaction, typical of cherubism. (Right) Coronal bone CT in the same patient shows the multiloculated cystic, symmetric bilateral mandible lesions ➡ causing expansion of both sides of the mandible.

TERMINOLOGY

- Heterogeneous group of hereditary lysosomal storage diseases due to deficiency of enzymes that degrade glycosaminoglycans (GAGs) or mucopolysaccharides
  - Accumulation of partially degraded GAGs → interference with cell, tissue, & organ function

IMAGING

- Skull & face findings
  - Macrocrania
  - Thickened skull base
  - **Large, J-shaped sella**
  - **Macroglossia**
  - **Stylohyoid ligament** thick Ca⁺⁺/ossification
  - Underpneumatized mastoid air cells
  - Flat or concave mandibular condyle, TMJ ankylosis
- Craniocervical junction: Dens hypoplasia (95%), atlantoaxial instability, cranioverterbal junction stenosis
- Brain findings: Hydrocephalus, large perivascular spaces

TOP DIFFERENTIAL DIAGNOSES

- Down syndrome
  - ± dens hypoplasia without soft tissue dens mass or marrow deposition features
- Achondroplasia
  - Autosomal dominant, abnormal enchondral bone formation
  - Short broad pedicle & thick laminae → spinal stenosis
- Spondyloepiphyseal dysplasia
  - Flattened vertebral bodies, dens hypoplasia, scoliosis may be present at birth
- GM1 gangliosidosis
  - Shares features of vertebral beaking, upper lumbar gibbus, & dens hypoplasia

CLINICAL ISSUES

- Most common signs/symptoms
  - Course facies at 3-6 months
  - Developmental delay in most

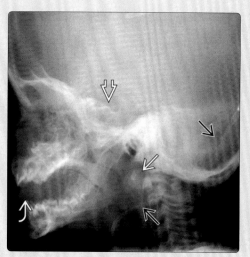
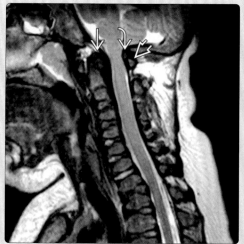

(Left) *Lateral radiograph in a 2-year-old boy with Hurler syndrome shows increased predental space ➡, hypoplastic dens, J-shaped sella ➡, macroglossia ➡, and shunt catheter for treatment of hydrocephalus ➡.* (Right) *Sagittal T2WI MR in a 7-year-old girl with Hurler syndrome shows typical soft tissue "mass" ➡ at tip of hypoplastic dens, hypoplastic posterior ring C1 ➡, and dural thickening ➡ causing minimal cord compression. Notice also the typical bullet-shaped vertebrae.*

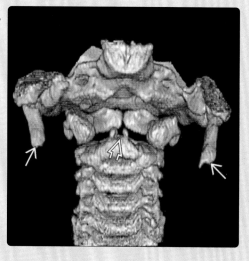
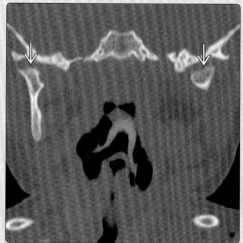

(Left) *Anteroposterior 3D reformation in a 4-year-old girl with Hurler syndrome shows thick bilateral stylohyoid ligament ossification ➡ and a hypoplastic dens ➡.* (Right) *Coronal bone CT in a 3-year-old boy with Morquio syndrome shows bilateral mandibular condyle flattening and cortical irregularity ➡.*

TERMINOLOGY

Abbreviations

- Mucopolysaccharidoses (MPS)

Definitions

- Heterogeneous group of hereditary lysosomal storage diseases due to deficiency of enzymes that degrade glycosaminoglycans (GAGs) or mucopolysaccharides

IMAGING

General Features

- Best diagnostic clue
  - J-shaped sella in child with macrocrania, cervical stenosis, hypoplastic dens, & enlarged perivascular spaces in brain, associated with thoracolumbar gibbus

CT Findings

- Skull & face
  - Macrocrania
  - Thickened skull base
  - Large **J-shaped sella**
  - **Macroglossia**
  - **Stylohyoid ligament calcification**
    - Earlier & thicker than in normal children
  - Underpneumatized mastoid air cells
  - Flat or concave mandibular condyle, TMJ ankylosis
- Craniovertebral junction (CVJ)
  - **Dens hypoplasia** (95%)
  - CVJ stenosis
  - Ligamentous laxity, atlantoaxial instability

MR Findings

- Dens hypoplasia, CVJ stenosis, AO instability
- Thickened dural ring at foramen magnum & C2
- Large J-shaped sella
- CSF signal intensity in large perivascular spaces in cerebral white matter, basal ganglia, & brainstem
  - Accumulation of GAGs within foam cells in Virchow-Robin spaces

Imaging Recommendations

- Best imaging tool
  - Skeletal series to assess associated skeletal abnormalities
  - MR brain & CVJ

DIFFERENTIAL DIAGNOSIS

Down Syndrome (Trisomy 21)

- ± dens hypoplasia without soft tissue dens mass or marrow deposition features

Achondroplasia

- Autosomal dominant, abnormal enchondral bone formation
- Short broad pedicle & thick laminae → spinal stenosis

Spondyloepiphyseal Dysplasia

- Flattened vertebral bodies, dens hypoplasia, scoliosis may be present at birth

PATHOLOGY

General Features

- Etiology
  - Accumulation of GAGs in most organs/ligaments
    - Upper airway obstruction (38%) → difficult intubation
      - □ Macroglossia
      - □ Hypertrophy palatine & adenoid tonsils
      - □ ± thick vocal cords, epiglottis, & aryepiglottic folds
    - Dural thickening foramen magnum → cord compression
    - Submucosal deposition → small, abnormally shaped trachea & bronchi
- Genetics
  - Autosomal recessive (except MPS 2 Hunter X-linked)
- Associated abnormalities
  - Skeletal dysostosis multiplex, joint contractures
  - Lumbar gibbus deformity 2° to beaking vertebrae
  - Dental: Dentigerous cysts, pointed cusps, spade-shaped incisors, thin enamel + pitted buccal surfaces, "rosette" formation of multiple impacted teeth in single follicle

Staging, Grading, & Classification

- MPS subdivisions based on enzyme deficiency
- MPS I-H (Hurler), I-S (Scheie), I-HS (Hurler-Scheie): α-L-iduronidase (4p16.3)
- MPS II (Hunter): Iduronate 2-sulfatase (Xq28)
- MPS III (Sanfilippo): Heparin N-sulfatase (17q25.3)
- MPS IV (Morquio): Galactose 6-sulfatase (16q24.3)
- MPS VI (Maroteaux-Lamy): Arylsulfatase B (5q11-q13)
- MPS VII (Sly): β-glucuronidase
- MPS IX: Hyaluronidase

CLINICAL ISSUES

Presentation

- Most common signs/symptoms
  - Coarse facies at 3-6 months (mild in MPS 3, 6, 7)
  - Developmental delay (not in MPS IV & VI)
  - Macrocrania with frontal bossing

Demographics

- Age
  - Diagnosed in childhood (rare mild form diagnosed in adult); MPS 1H (Hurler) presents in infancy

Natural History & Prognosis

- Prognosis varies with enzyme deficiency
- High spinal cord compression major cause of spinal complications & death

Treatment

- Surgery for more severe symptoms
- Stem cell transplantation replacing conventional bone marrow transplant
  - Using unrelated donor umbilical cord blood

SELECTED REFERENCES

1. Zafeiriou DI et al: Brain and spinal MR imaging findings in mucopolysaccharidoses: a review. AJNR Am J Neuroradiol. 34(1):5-13, 2013
2. Mundada V et al: Lumbar gibbus: early presentation of dysostosis multiplex. Arch Dis Child. 2009 Dec;94(12):930-1. Erratum in: Arch Dis Child. 95(5):401, 2010

SECTION 21
Nose and Sinus

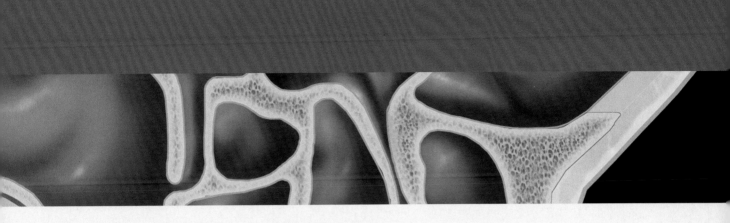

Malignant Tumors

Summary Thoughts: Sinus and Nose

Conditions related to the nose, nasal cavities (NC), and paranasal sinuses (PS) are some of the most common cases encountered by clinicians, prompting 25 million medical visits and costing $2 billion annually. Imaging is required when patients fail 1st-line treatments for inflammatory conditions, invasive disease or neoplasm is suspected, or presurgical planning becomes necessary. Given the complex bony architecture and the intervening air filled spaces, **CT is the most common modality** for evaluating the sinonasal (SN) region. CT determines the extent of disease and is also helpful for surgical planning and intraoperative guidance. MR can be complementary in the evaluation of advanced infectious or inflammatory disease, and in the evaluation of neoplasms. As in all regions of the H&N, information such as patient demographics, presenting symptoms, and clinical exam findings are critical for interpreting imaging studies of this area.

The NC is centrally located and is surrounded by the PS. It is important to understand the drainage pathways of the PS as one can then predict **patterns of disease** based upon the site of an obstructing lesion. However, this can be challenging due to limitless anatomic variation. Infectious/inflammatory diseases are by far the most common pathologies. Neoplasms, both benign and malignant, are relatively rare. They tend to present at an advanced stage and encroach upon vital structures (orbit, skull base, and cranial nerves). These tumors are difficult to completely resect and are associated with high surgical morbidity. Presurgical tumor mapping in such cases is best accomplished with multiplanar MR.

Imaging Approaches and Indications

CT is the preferred modality to evaluate inflammatory disease, depicting mucosal thickening, opacification, air-fluid levels, and soft tissue masses. CT easily depicts osseous changes such as remodeling, scalloping, hyperostosis, or erosion, and is sensitive for detecting Ca^{++} or bone in lesions such as osteomas, chronic fungal disease, fibroosseous lesions, chondrosarcoma, or inverted papilloma. **Coronal images** best demonstrate the anatomy of the **ostiomeatal unit** (OMU). CECT is usually reserved for complicated cases in which soft tissue abscess, neoplasm, or vascular complication (cavernous sinus thrombosis) is suspected.

MR is indicated for evaluation of **complex inflammatory disease and neoplasms**. It is optimal for assessing extension or invasion of disease beyond the SN cavities, evaluating perineural tumor spread, and differentiating tumor from postobstructive secretions.

Imaging Protocols

Historically, direct coronal images were obtained with patient in prone position and ≤ 3-mm slices angled perpendicular to the palate. With multidetector CT, coronal reformatted images can be generated from a thin-slice axial data set acquired in the supine position. This is preferred as images are less degraded by motion artifact and dental amalgam can be avoided. Axial source images can be used in image-guidance systems, obviating additional radiation for "treatment planning" CT prior to surgery. **Sagittal reformatted** images are helpful for delineating **frontal recess** (FR) and the sphenoethmoid region anatomy.

MR imaging protocols generally include axial and coronal T1, STIR, and T1 C+ images, typically with fat suppression.

Imaging Anatomy

The sinonasal region is comprised of the NC and the surrounding PS. There are important anatomic relationships with adjacent structures including orbit, oral cavity, pterygopalatine fossa, and both the anterior and central skull base.

The SN cavities are pneumatized spaces within the maxillary, frontal, sphenoid, and ethmoid bones. Superiorly, the frontal sinuses border the anterior margin of the anterior cranial fossa. The cribriform plate (CP) and fovea ethmoidalis form the roof of the superior NC and ethmoid sinuses, respectively. The hard palate separates the NC from the oral cavity. The NC communicates posteriorly with the nasopharynx via the choanae. The orbits are separated from the ethmoid sinuses by the thin lamina papyracea and are separated from the maxillary sinuses by the orbital floors. Posterior to the maxillary sinuses are the pterygopalatine fossae, which communicate superiorly with the orbital apices, laterally with the masticator space, and posteriorly with central skull base.

The **NC is centrally located** and is divided in the midline by the nasal septum. The posterior septum is bony and formed by the perpendicular plate of the ethmoid superiorly and vomer bone inferiorly. Anteriorly the septum is cartilaginous. The bony superior, middle, and inferior turbinates project into the NC and divide the NC into inferior, middle, and superior meatuses. The middle turbinate is attached superiorly to the CP via the vertical lamella and posterolaterally to the lamina papyracea via the basal (ground) lamella.

The frontal sinuses are divided in the midline by an intersinus septum. Inferomedially, the frontal sinus narrows toward its ostium, which drains into its FR. The **FR is formed by the walls of surrounding structures**, best visualized on **sagittal reformations**. The drainage of the FR is determined by the insertion of the uncinate process. Most often the uncinate inserts laterally onto the lamina papyracea and secretions drain into the middle meatus (MM). Less frequently, the uncinate inserts onto the anterior skull base or middle turbinate.

Paired groups of 13-18 air cells form the ethmoid sinuses. These cells are divided into anterior and posterior groups by the **basal lamella**. The anterior air cells drain into the anterior recess of the hiatus semilunaris and middle meatus via the ethmoid bulla. The posterior air cells drain into the superior meatus and sphenoethmoidal recess (SER).

The maxillary sinuses lie lateral to the NC and inferior to the orbits. Each drains via its maxillary ostium into the infundibulum, then via the hiatus semilunaris into the MM.

The sphenoid sinuses are asymmetric air cells in the body of the sphenoid bone. Important surrounding structures include the maxillary division of CNV in the foramen rotundum laterally, the vidian nerve and artery in the vidian canal inferiorly, the optic nerves and sella superiorly, and the cavernous sinuses laterally. The sphenoid sinuses drain via their ostia into the SER.

The **OMU is a critical intersection** for drainage of the sinuses most affected by inflammatory disease (anterior ethmoid, maxillary, and frontal). Important components of the OMU include the ethmoid infundibulum, uncinate process, hiatus semilunaris, ethmoid bulla, and MM.

Differential Diagnosis of Sinonasal Lesion

Congenital	Benign tumors and tumor-like lesions	Anatomic variations
Nasolacrimal duct mucocele	Osteoma	Sinus hypo- or hyperpneumatization
Choanal atresia	Fibrous dysplasia	Nasal septal deviation and spurs
Nasal glioma	Ossifying fibroma	Frontal cells (types I-IV)
Nasal dermal sinus	Juvenile angiofibroma	**Ethmoid region**
Frontoethmoidal cephalocele	Inverted papilloma	Agger nasi cell
Pyriform aperture stenosis	Hemangioma	Infraorbital (Haller) cell
Infectious and inflammatory	Nerve sheath tumor	Supraorbital ethmoid cell
Acute rhinosinusitis	Benign mixed tumor	Large ethmoid bulla
Chronic rhinosinusitis	**Malignant tumors**	Sphenoethmoidal (Onodi) cell
Complications of rhinosinusitis	Squamous cell carcinoma	Asymmetric fovea ethmoidalis
Allergic fungal sinusitis	Esthesioneuroblastoma	Medial or dehiscent lamina papyracea
Mycetoma (fungal ball)	Adenocarcinoma	**Middle turbinate**
Invasive fungal sinusitis	Melanoma	Concha bullosa
Sinonasal polyposis	Non-Hodgkin lymphoma	Paradoxical curvature
Solitary sinonasal polyp	Sinonasal undifferentiated sarcoma	Hypoplasia
Mucocele	Adenoid cystic carcinoma	**Uncinate process**
Silent sinus syndrome	Chondrosarcoma	Pneumatized
Wegener granulomatosis	Osteosarcoma	Deviated
Sarcoidosis	Rhabdomyosarcoma	Fusion to middle turbinate or skull base
Nasal cocaine necrosis	Metastasis	Atelectatic (approximates orbital floor)

Approaches to Imaging Issues of Sinus and Nose

Congenital lesions can be classified as those presenting with **nasal obstruction vs. nasal mass**. Pyriform aperture stenosis and choanal atresia, for example, cause nasal obstruction without a mass. Frontonasal cephaloceles, dermoids, and extranasal gliomas present as extranasal masses. Frontoethmoidal cephaloceles, intranasal gliomas, and nasolacrimal duct mucoceles present with an intranasal mass. MR imaging can be very helpful for evaluating any connection to the intracranial space.

Rhinosinusitis (RS) is the **most common pathology** of the SN region. Acute RS is usually diagnosed clinically and may not require imaging. Because of the anatomy of the PS drainage pathways, predictable patterns of inflammatory disease exist based upon the point of obstruction. For example, obstruction of the MM would lead to disease in the ipsilateral frontal, anterior ethmoid, and maxillary sinuses. SER obstruction might lead to ipsilateral posterior ethmoid and sphenoid disease. Although uncommon, there are several forms of SN fungal disease. Mycetoma and allergic fungal sinusitis occur in immunocompetent patients and invasive fungal sinusitis (IFS) occurs in the immunocompromised or poorly controlled diabetics. It is important to note that **IFS may appear mass-like** or as **subtle infiltration of fat planes** adjacent to the PS at imaging. Granulomatous disease has a predilection for involving the nasal septum and turbinates.

There are a wide variety of SN neoplasms. Well marginated tumors that cause bony remodeling suggest benign tumors, while infiltrative masses with osseous destruction suggest malignant lesions. The site of origin may also be predictive of histology. For instance, osteomas most often arise in the frontal and ethmoid sinuses, juvenile angiofibromas (JAF) arise in the posterior NC at the sphenopalatine foramen, inverted papillomas often arise along the lateral nasal wall, and esthesioneuroblastoma (ENB) typically arises near the CP. Squamous cell carcinoma is by far the **most common SN malignancy** and most often arises in the maxillary antrum. The imaging features of adenocarcinomas can be nonspecific, but they have a predilection for the ethmoid region. Three malignant neoplasms with a **predilection for the NC** include ENB, lymphoma, and melanoma.

Clinical Implications

It is important to note that studies have shown a poor correlation between symptoms of RS and CT findings. The diagnosis of RS is ultimately a clinical one. Lesions located within the NC can be evaluated with endoscopy. Lesions involving the PS are difficult to evaluate with scopes, so imaging is important for full evaluation.

Disease of the SN cavities often presents with nonspecific symptoms, such as nasal obstruction, discharge, and craniofacial pain. Additional symptoms, such as epistaxis, may be indicative of a vascular lesion (JAF or ENB). Pain may also be caused by mucoceles or neoplasms, while paresthesias can be linked to malignancies such as adenoid cystic carcinoma.

Selected References

1. Amine MA et al: Anatomy and complications: safe sinus. Otolaryngol Clin North Am. 48(5):739-48, 2015
2. Charles Burke M et al: A practical approach to the imaging interpretation of sphenoid sinus pathology. Curr Probl Diagn Radiol. 44(4):360-70, 2015
3. Vaid S et al: An imaging checklist for pre-FESS CT: framing a surgically relevant report. Clin Radiol. 66(5):459-70, 2011
4. Hoang JK et al: Multiplanar sinus CT: a systematic approach to imaging before functional endoscopic sinus surgery. AJR Am J Roentgenol. 194(6):W527-36, 2010

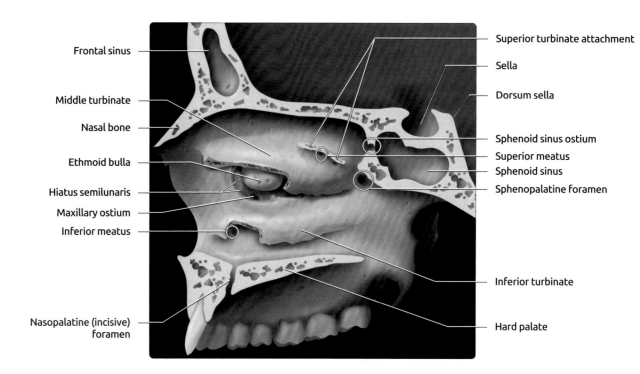

Frontal sinus

Middle turbinate

Nasal bone

Ethmoid bulla

Hiatus semilunaris

Maxillary ostium

Inferior meatus

Nasopalatine (incisive) foramen

Superior turbinate attachment

Sella

Dorsum sella

Sphenoid sinus ostium

Superior meatus

Sphenoid sinus

Sphenopalatine foramen

Inferior turbinate

Hard palate

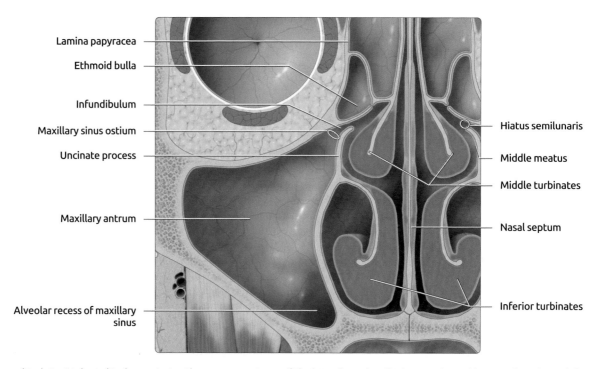

Lamina papyracea

Ethmoid bulla

Infundibulum

Maxillary sinus ostium

Uncinate process

Maxillary antrum

Alveolar recess of maxillary sinus

Hiatus semilunaris

Middle meatus

Middle turbinates

Nasal septum

Inferior turbinates

(Top) *Sagittal graphic demonstrates the osseous anatomy of the lateral nasal wall. The superior turbinate and portions of the middle and inferior turbinates have been resected. The superior, middle, and inferior meatuses drain inferior to their respective turbinates. The ipsilateral frontal, anterior ethmoid, and maxillary sinuses ultimately drain into the middle meatus. The nasolacrimal duct drains into the inferior meatus. The sphenoid ostium is located along the anterior sphenoid sinus wall and drains into the sphenoethmoidal recess.* **(Bottom)** *Coronal graphic of magnified right sinonasal region shows the important structures around the ostiomeatal unit. The vertically oriented uncinate process is bounded laterally by the ethmoid infundibulum, superiorly by the hiatus semilunaris, and medially by the middle meatus. The ethmoid bulla is the dominant anterior ethmoid cell located superior to the uncinate. The middle meatus drains beneath the middle turbinate.*

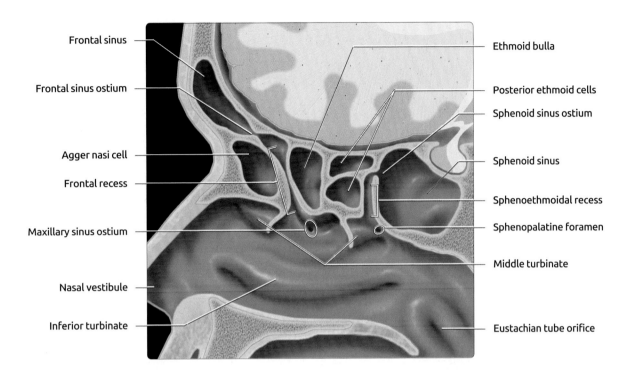

Frontal sinus

Frontal sinus ostium

Agger nasi cell

Frontal recess

Maxillary sinus ostium

Nasal vestibule

Inferior turbinate

Ethmoid bulla

Posterior ethmoid cells

Sphenoid sinus ostium

Sphenoid sinus

Sphenoethmoidal recess

Sphenopalatine foramen

Middle turbinate

Eustachian tube orifice

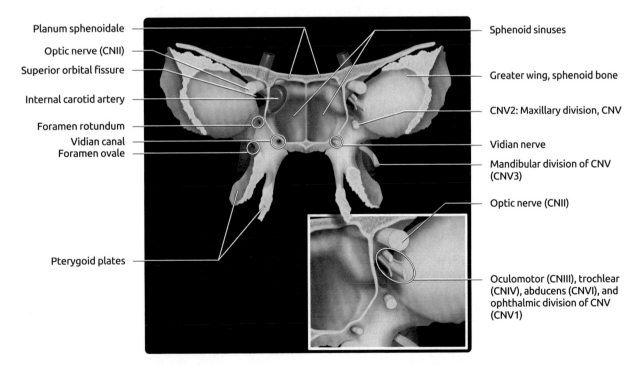

Planum sphenoidale

Optic nerve (CNII)

Superior orbital fissure

Internal carotid artery

Foramen rotundum

Vidian canal
Foramen ovale

Pterygoid plates

Sphenoid sinuses

Greater wing, sphenoid bone

CNV2: Maxillary division, CNV

Vidian nerve

Mandibular division of CNV
(CNV3)

Optic nerve (CNII)

Oculomotor (CNIII), trochlear
(CNIV), abducens (CNVI), and
ophthalmic division of CNV
(CNV1)

(Top) *Sagittal graphic shows the frontal sinus drainage pathway. The frontal sinus narrows inferiorly to its ostium. Secretions drain through the ostium into the frontal recess (FR). The FR is not a true duct in that its walls are comprised of adjacent anatomy. In the graphic, the FR is bounded anteriorly by an agger nasi cell & posteriorly by the ethmoid bulla. Note that FR drainage may vary based upon the point of insertion of the uncinate process.* **(Bottom)** *Coronal graphic shows the important anatomy surrounding the sphenoid sinuses. The cavernous portions of the internal carotid arteries lie lateral and posterior to the sinuses. At the orbital apex, the optic nerve can be seen traversing the optic canal. The maxillary division of CNV in the foramen rotundum and the vidian nerve are positioned lateral and inferior to the sinus, respectively. Multiple cranial nerves pass through the superior orbital fissure (see inset) into the orbit, including CNs III, IV, and VI as well as the ophthalmic division on CNV.*

(Left) *Coronal bone CT shows the paired frontal sinuses ➡ separated by the intersinus septum ➡. The most anterior ethmoid-type cells, the agger nasi, can be seen ➡. Notice the air-filled lacrimal sac on the left ➡.* **(Right)** *Coronal bone CT shows the medial ➡ and lateral ➡ lamellae of the cribriform plate forming the roof of the nasal cavity. The fovea ethmoidalis ➡ forms the ethmoid sinus roof. Note the patent frontal recesses ➡ leading to the middle meatuses.*

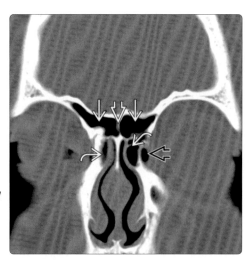
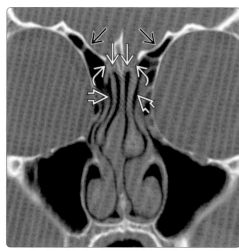

(Left) *Sagittal CT reconstruction shows the frontal sinus drainage pathway. The sinus ➡ drains inferiorly into the frontal recess ➡. A frontal cell ➡ is anterior to the recess and the ethmoid bulla is posterior ➡. Note the middle ➡ and inferior ➡ turbinates.* **(Right)** *Axial T1 MR shows the paired maxillary sinuses ➡ lateral to the nasal cavity. Note the inferior turbinates ➡, midline nasal septum ➡, and air-filled nasolacrimal ducts ➡ above the inferior meatuses.*

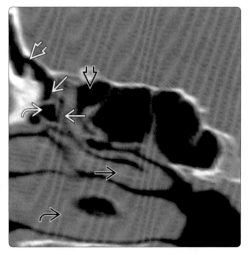
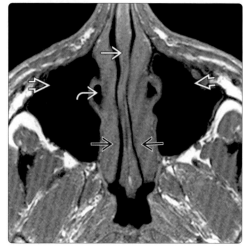

(Left) *Sagittal CT reconstruction shows the nasolacrimal duct ➡ draining into the inferior meatus ➡. Note the pterygopalatine fossa posterior to the maxillary sinus ➡.* **(Right)** *Coronal bone CT at the level of the ostiomeatal units shows the uncinate processes ➡, ethmoid bullae ➡, and middle turbinates ➡. They are pneumatized as is the right inferior turbinate. The middle meatus lies between the uncinate and middle turbinate. A retention cyst blocks the left maxillary ostium.*

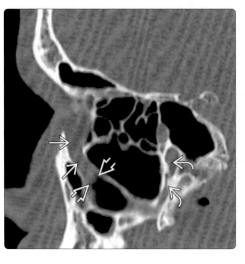
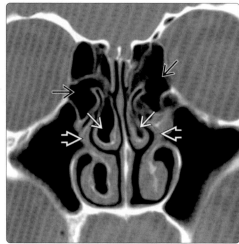

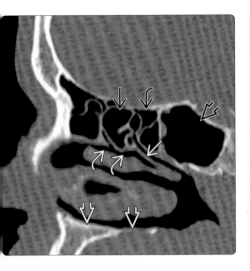

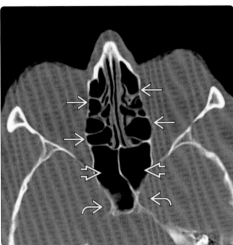

(Left) *Sagittal CT reconstruction shows anterior ➡ and posterior ➡ ethmoid cells and the sphenoid sinus ➡. The lateral attachment of the middle turbinate (basal lamella) is seen ➡. Note the hiatus semilunaris ➡. The palate is noted inferiorly ➡.* (Right) *Axial bone CT shows the thin lamina papyracea ➡ separating the ethmoid air cells from the orbits. The sphenoid sinuses ➡ are separated by an intersinus septum. The internal carotid arteries ➡ are immediately adjacent to the sinuses.*

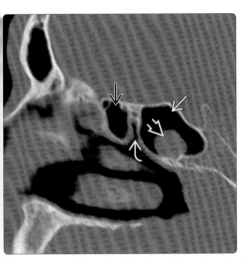

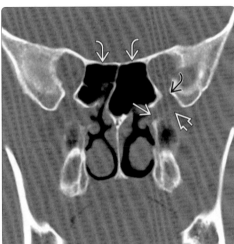

(Left) *Sagittal CT reconstruction shows the sphenoethmoidal recess ➡ bounded anteriorly by the most posterior ethmoid air cell ➡ and posteriorly by the sphenoid sinus ➡. A retention cyst is seen in the sphenoid sinus ➡.* (Right) *Coronal bone CT shows the sphenopalatine foramen ➡ connecting the nasal cavity to the pterygopalatine fossa (PPF) ➡. The inferior orbital fissure ➡ extends from the PPF to the orbital apex. Note the planum sphenoidale above the sphenoid sinuses ➡.*

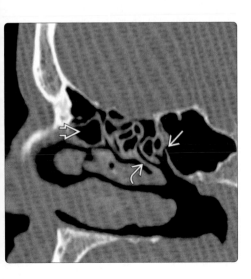

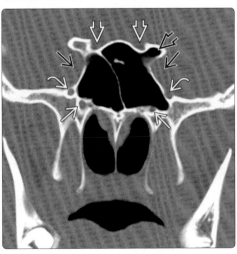

(Left) *Sagittal CT reconstruction shows the sphenoid sinus ostium ➡ along the anterior wall of the sphenoid sinus. An agger nasi cell ➡ & the basal lamella ➡ are also seen.* (Right) *Coronal bone CT shows the important structures around the sphenoid sinuses. The vidian canals ➡ are noted along the sphenoid sinus floors and the foramen rotundum ➡ is located laterally. The optic nerves lie medial to the anterior clinoids ➡ and the cavernous sinuses lie laterally ➡. Pneumatization of the clinoid ➡ is variant anatomy.*

Nasolacrimal Duct Mucocele

TERMINOLOGY

- Synonym: Congenital dacryocystocele

IMAGING

- Well-defined, cystic medial canthal mass in contiguity with enlarged nasolacrimal duct (NLD) in newborn
  - Unilateral or bilateral
- Absent or minimal wall enhancement (unless infected)
- Coronal/sagittal reformatted images show contiguity of cyst at lacrimal sac with NLD and inferior meatus cyst

TOP DIFFERENTIAL DIAGNOSES

- Orbital dermoid and epidermoid
  - Lateral > medial canthus
- Dacryocystocele, acquired lacrimal sac cyst
  - If dacryocystitis: Inflammatory changes in surrounding soft tissues & enhancing cyst rim around cyst

PATHOLOGY

- Tears & mucus accumulate in nasolacrimal duct with imperforate Hasner membrane (distal duct obstruction)

CLINICAL ISSUES

- Proximal lesion: Small, round, bluish, medial canthal mass identified at birth or shortly thereafter
- Distal lesion: Nasal airway obstruction with respiratory distress if bilateral
- Most common abnormality of infant lacrimal apparatus

DIAGNOSTIC CHECKLIST

- Cross-sectional imaging evaluates extent of lesion along lacrimal apparatus & excludes other sinonasal causes of respiratory distress in newborn
- Comment on full extent of lesion from medial canthus to inferior meatus
- Exclude contralateral lesion

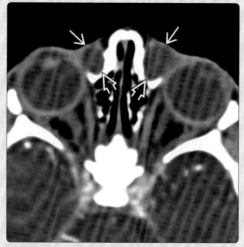
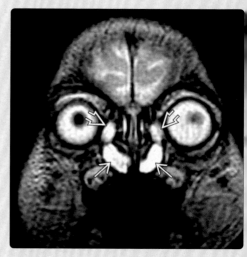

(Left) Axial CECT in a 4 day old with bilateral lacrimal sac enlargement, bluish in color and left side draining purulent material demonstrates bilateral lacrimal sac enlargement ➡. Notice the bilateral enlargement of the lacrimal sac fossa ➡ on both sides. (Right) Coronal T2WI MR in an infant shows hyperintense signal in the mucoceles, not only at the inferior nasolacrimal ducts ➡, but also at the level of the lacrimal sacs ➡. Nasal obstruction results in difficulty breathing, as infants are obligate nose breathers.

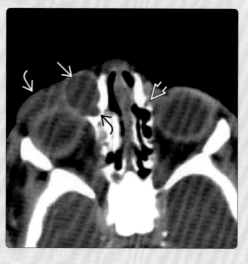
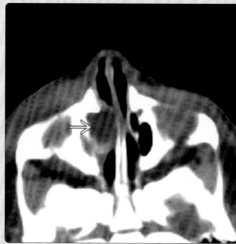

(Left) Axial CECT in an infant demonstrates a cystic mass ➡ with an enhancing rim in the medial right orbit consistent with a mucocele. There is also enlargement of the right lacrimal sac fossa ➡. Note the normal left lacrimal sac fossa ➡. There is a mild amount of right preseptal periorbital soft tissue swelling ➡ consistent with secondary cellulitis. (Right) Axial CECT in the same patient shows extension of the mucocele inferiorly to the level of the inferior meatus ➡. The lesion obstructs the right nasal cavity at that level.

TERMINOLOGY

Abbreviations

- Nasolacrimal duct (NLD) mucocele

Synonyms

- Congenital dacryocystocele

Definitions

- Cystic dilatation of nasolacrimal apparatus secondary to proximal ± distal obstruction of NLD

IMAGING

General Features

- Best diagnostic clue
  - Well-defined, cystic, medial canthal mass in contiguity with enlarged NLD in newborn
- Location
  - Lacrimal sac to inferior aspect of NLD at inferior meatus
  - Unilateral or bilateral

CT Findings

- Hypodense, thin-walled cyst at medial canthus ± inferior meatus extension
- Cyst(s) communicate with enlarged NLD
- Minimal wall enhancement (unless infected)
- Thick rim enhancement ± fluid/debris level if infected

MR Findings

- T1 hypointense/T2 hyperintense, well-circumscribed mass
- Signal intensity varies with protein content &/or infection
- No or minimal wall enhancement (unless infected)
- Thick rim of enhancement with surrounding strandy soft tissue enhancement if inflamed or infected

Imaging Recommendations

- Best imaging tool
  - Thin-section axial bone CT (fast and ↓ need for sedation)

DIFFERENTIAL DIAGNOSIS

Orbital Dermoid and Epidermoid

- Lateral > medial canthus
- 50% fat density/intensity with thin rim enhancement

Dacryocystocele

- Acquired lacrimal sac cyst
- If dacryocystitis: Inflammatory changes in surrounding soft tissues & enhancing cyst rim around cyst

PATHOLOGY

General Features

- Etiology
  - Tears & mucus accumulate in nasolacrimal duct with **imperforate Hasner membrane** (distal duct obstruction)
    - Most membranes perforate during normal breathing and crying at birth
  - Nasolacrimal sac distension &/or anatomic variation compresses canalicular system → trapdoor nasolacrimal sac obstruction
  - If bacteria enter distended sac → dacryocystitis ± cellulitis

CLINICAL ISSUES

Presentation

- Most common signs/symptoms
  - Small, round, bluish, medial canthal mass identified at or shortly after birth = distended lacrimal sac
  - Nasal airway obstruction with respiratory distress if nasal component and bilateral, as infants are obligate nose breathers
    - Submucosal nasal cavity mass at inferior meatus
- Other signs/symptoms
  - Tearing, crusting at medial canthus
  - Preseptal cellulitis
- Clinical profile
  - Infant with medial canthal mass ± nasal cavity mass

Demographics

- Age
  - Infancy; 4 days to 10 weeks typically
- Gender
  - M < F = 1:3
- Epidemiology
  - Most common abnormality of infant lacrimal apparatus
  - Unilateral > bilateral

Natural History & Prognosis

- 90% simple distal obstructions (congenital dacryostenosis) resolve spontaneously by age 1
- Only 50% of patients recognized on prenatal MR ultimately have postnatal symptoms
- Intervention recommended before infection occurs to prevent nasal airway obstruction, dacryocystitis, & permanent sequelae

Treatment

- Daily **manual massage** ± prophylactic systemic/topical antibiotics
  - 10% require probing with irrigation ± Silastic stent placement
  - If endonasal component & no response to above → endoscopic resection with marsupialization
  - Manual massage inappropriate if infected or airway obstruction

DIAGNOSTIC CHECKLIST

Consider

- Cross-sectional imaging evaluates extent of lesion along lacrimal apparatus & excludes other sinonasal causes of respiratory distress in newborn

Image Interpretation Pearls

- Comment on full extent of lesion from medial canthus to inferior meatus, & bilateral or unilateral
- Evaluate for presence of infection, especially abscess

SELECTED REFERENCES

1. Dagi LR et al: Associated signs, demographic characteristics, and management of dacryocystocele in 64 infants. J AAPOS. 16(3):255-60, 2012
2. Takahashi Y et al: Management of congenital nasolacrimal duct obstruction. Acta Ophthalmol. 88(5):506-13, 2010
3. Rand PK et al: Congenital nasolacrimal mucoceles: CT evaluation. Radiology. 173(3):691-4, 1989

TERMINOLOGY

- Congenital obstruction of posterior nasal apertures

IMAGING

- Unilateral or bilateral osseous narrowing of posterior nasal cavity with membranous or osseous obstruction of choana
- Thickening of vomer
- Medial bowing of posterior maxilla
- Unilateral in up to 75%
  - Right > left
- Bilateral in up to 25%
  - 75% of bilateral have other anomalies

TOP DIFFERENTIAL DIAGNOSES

- Choanal stenosis
  - More common than true choanal atresia
- Pyriform aperture stenosis
  - Narrowed anterior nasal passage
- Nasolacrimal duct mucocele

- Bilobed cystic masses in nasolacrimal fossae and inferior meatus
- Nasal foreign body

PATHOLOGY

- Choanal atresia types
  - Mixed bony and membranous atresia in up to 70%
  - Purely bony atresia in up to 30%

CLINICAL ISSUES

- Bilateral choanal atresia → significant respiratory distress in newborn
- Unilateral choanal atresia: Chronic, purulent unilateral rhinorrhea with mild airway obstruction
- Choanal atresia is most common congenital abnormality of nasal cavity

DIAGNOSTIC CHECKLIST

- Respiratory distress and nasal obstruction in newborn should be evaluated with thin-section bone CT

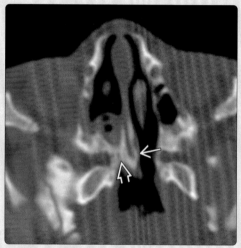
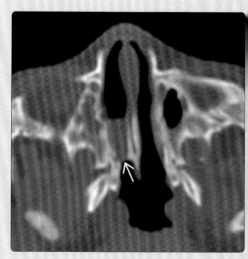

(Left) Axial bone CT through the upper choana in a child with mixed bony/osseous choanal atresia shows osseous choanal obstruction secondary to an enlarged vomer ⇒ fused to the thickened, medially positioned posterior maxilla ⇒. (Right) Axial bone CT through the mid choana in the same patient shows membranous atresia ⇒ bridging the narrowed inferior aspect of the choana. Notice also the retained nasal secretions on the right, secondary to obstruction of the choana.

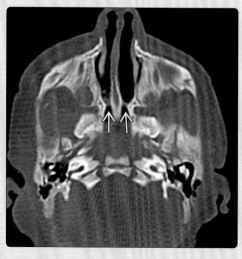
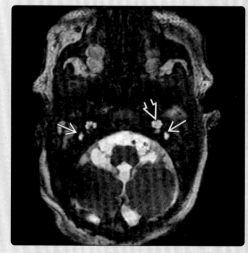

(Left) Axial bone CT in a child with CHARGE syndrome demonstrates bilateral choanal obstruction secondary to linear membranes ⇒ and mildly thickened and medially positioned posterior maxilla, typical of mixed choanal atresia. (Right) Axial volume 3D highly T2-weighted image in the same child shows typical inner ear anomalies of children with CHARGE syndrome, including small/dysplastic vestibules ⇒, absent semicircular canals, and left cochlear dysplasia ⇒.

TERMINOLOGY

Definitions

- Congenital obstruction of posterior nasal apertures
  - Choanae: Junction of posterior nasal cavity and nasopharynx
  - Results in lack of communication between nasal cavity and nasopharynx

IMAGING

General Features

- Best diagnostic clue
  - Bony narrowing of posterior nasal cavity with membranous &/or osseous obstruction of choana
- Location
  - Unilateral in up to 75%
    - Right > left
  - Bilateral in up to 25%
- Size
  - Choanal opening in newborn abnormal if < 0.34 cm; vomer abnormal if > 0.23 cm
- Morphology
  - Medial bowing of posterior maxilla (lateral nasal walls) and pterygoid plate
  - Large/thickened vomer
  - Bony narrowing ± soft tissue membrane/plug obstructs choana
  - Mixed bony and membranous atresia in up to 70%
  - Purely bony atresia in up to 30%

CT Findings

- Bone CT
  - Bony plate narrows or occludes choanal opening(s) ± membranous connection
    - Soft tissue in membranous atresia may be thin/strand-like or thick/plug-like
  - Thickening of vomer, may be fused to maxilla
  - Medial bowing of posterior maxilla and pterygoid plate
  - Nasal cavity filled with air, soft tissue, fluid, hypertrophied inferior turbinates

Imaging Recommendations

- Best imaging tool
  - High-resolution unenhanced bone CT
- Protocol advice
  - Suction secretions from nasal cavity prior to scanning
  - Perform supine with gantry angled 5° cephalad to palate
    - If angle too great → choana at level of skull base → overdiagnosis of choanal atresia
  - High-resolution, edge enhancement bone filters helpful in delineating bone margins in partially ossified skull base
  - Multiplanar reformations as needed
    - Sagittal usually best plane for this
  - 3D reconstructions may be helpful for clinical decision making and surgical planning

DIFFERENTIAL DIAGNOSIS

Choanal Stenosis

- More common than true choanal atresia
- Axial bone CT: Posterior nasal airway narrowed but not completely occluded

Pyriform Aperture Stenosis

- Narrowed anterior nasal passage
- Axial bone CT appearance
  - Narrowing of anterior and inferior nasal passage
  - Thickened anteromedial maxilla
  - Anterior nasal septum may be thinned
  - Single central megaincisor may be present
- Brain evaluation for holoprosencephaly important

Nasolacrimal Duct Mucocele

- Bilobed cystic masses in nasolacrimal fossae and inferior meatus

Nasal Foreign Body

- Older patient with choanal stenosis or unilateral unrecognized choanal atresia

PATHOLOGY

General Features

- Etiology
  - Pathogenesis remains elusive and unproven
    - Failure of perforation of oronasal membrane (normally perforates by 7th week of gestation)
      - Bony choanal atresia: Incomplete canalization of choanae
      - Membranous choanal atresia: Incomplete resorption of epithelial plugs
    - Molecular mechanisms in retinoic acid receptor development recently described in pathogenesis
- Genetics
  - Chromosomal abnormalities, single gene defects, deformations, and teratogens implicated
    - Associated with trisomy 13, 18, 21
    - Familial form exists
    - In patients with CHARGE syndrome, 60% have *CHD7* gene mutation
- Associated abnormalities
  - Syndromic associations common in bilateral atresia
    - **CHARGE syndrome**
      - **C**oloboma, **H**eart defect, **C**hoanal atresia, **R**etarded growth and development, **G**enitourinary abnormalities, **E**ar defects
      - Major diagnostic characteristics: Coloboma, choanal atresia, CN aplasia/hypoplasias (CN I, VII, VIII, IX-X)
      - Minor characteristics: Genital hypoplasia, developmental delay, cardiac anomalies, growth deficiency, orofacial cleft, tracheoesophageal fistula, abnormal faces
      - Definite Dx CHARGE syndrome = all 4 major or 4 major + 3 minor characteristics
    - Acrocephalosyndactyly
    - Amniotic band syndrome
    - Apert syndrome
    - Craniosynostosis
    - Gut malrotations
    - Crouzon syndrome
    - Cornelia de Lange syndrome
    - Fetal alcohol syndrome

- DiGeorge syndrome
- Treacher Collins syndrome

Staging, Grading, & Classification

- Choanal atresia types
  - Mixed bony and membranous atresia in up to 70%
  - Purely bony atresia in up to 30%

Gross Pathologic & Surgical Features

- Membranous soft tissue or bony plate occludes choanal opening

CLINICAL ISSUES

Presentation

- Most common signs/symptoms
  - **Bilateral** choanal atresia: Respiratory distress in newborn
    - Infants are obligate nasal breathers up to 6 months of age
    - Aggravated by feeding
    - Relieved by crying
  - **Unilateral** choanal atresia or stenosis: Chronic, purulent unilateral rhinorrhea &/or mild respiratory distress
- Other signs/symptoms
  - Inability to pass nasogastric tube through nasal cavity beyond 3-4 cm despite aerated lungs on plain film
  - Nasal stuffiness
  - Grunting, snorting, low-pitched stridor
- Clinical profile
  - Bilateral: Infant with respiratory distress
  - Unilateral: Child/young adult with unilateral purulent rhinorrhea

Demographics

- Age
  - Bilateral atresia presents at birth
  - Unilateral choanal atresia/stenosis may present in child/young adult
- Gender
  - F:M = 2:1
- Epidemiology
  - Most common congenital abnormality of nasal cavity
    - 1:5,000-8,000 live births
  - Unilateral choanal atresia more likely to be isolated
  - 75% of bilateral choanal atresia are associated with other anomalies

Natural History & Prognosis

- Bilateral choanal atresia
  - Diagnosed and treated in newborn period
- Unilateral choanal atresia
  - Not life-threatening
  - May present later in childhood
  - Prognosis excellent after surgical therapy
- Some patients prone to restenosis

Treatment

- Establish oral airway immediately to ensure proper breathing
- Membranous atresias may be perforated upon passage of nasogastric tube

- Surgical treatment believed to be effective for alleviating respiratory symptoms
  - Best surgical approaches
    - Endoscopic/laser-assisted techniques
      - ± adjuvant use of stents
    - Use of antiproliferative agents debated
  - Endoscopic approaches frequently used for simple membranous and bony atresias
    - Minimizes traumatic injury leading to ↓ scarring and ↓ restenosis
  - Bilateral bony atresias require transpalatal resection of vomer with choanal reconstruction
- Postoperative scar and incomplete resection of atresia plate best evaluated with bone CT

DIAGNOSTIC CHECKLIST

Consider

- Once airway is established, respiratory distress and nasal obstruction in newborn should be evaluated with thin-section bone CT

Image Interpretation Pearls

- Determine whether unilateral or bilateral choanal atresia
- Look for associated anomalies in H&N

Reporting Tips

- Describe choanal atresia as mixed membranous/bony or purely bony and unilateral or bilateral
  - Comment on thickness of bony atresia plate

SELECTED REFERENCES

1. Strychowsky JE et al: To stent or not to stent? A meta-analysis of endonasal congenital bilateral choanal atresia repair. Laryngoscope. 126(1):218-27, 2016
2. National Organization for Rare Disorders: CHARGE Syndrome. http://rarediseases.org/rare-diseases/charge-syndrome. Published 1988. Updated 2015. Accessed May 16, 2016
3. Gangar M et al: The use of mitomycin C in pediatric airway surgery: does it work? Curr Opin Otolaryngol Head Neck Surg. 22(6):521-4, 2014
4. Aslan S et al: Comparison of nasal region dimensions in bilateral choanal atresia patients and normal controls: a computed tomographic analysis with clinical implications. Int J Pediatr Otorhinolaryngol. 73(2):329-35, 2009
5. Burrow TA et al: Characterization of congenital anomalies in individuals with choanal atresia. Arch Otolaryngol Head Neck Surg. 135(6):543-7, 2009
6. Corrales CE et al: Choanal atresia: current concepts and controversies. Curr Opin Otolaryngol Head Neck Surg. 17(6):466-70, 2009
7. Ramsden JD et al: Choanal atresia and choanal stenosis. Otolaryngol Clin North Am. 42(2):339-52, x, 2009
8. Hengerer AS et al: Choanal atresia: embryologic analysis and evolution of treatment, a 30-year experience. Laryngoscope. 118(5):862-6, 2008
9. Samadi DS et al: Choanal atresia: a twenty-year review of medical comorbidities and surgical outcomes. Laryngoscope. 113(2):254-8, 2003
10. Triglia JM et al: [Choanal atresia: therapeutic management and results in a series of 58 children] Rev Laryngol Otol Rhinol (Bord). 124(3):139-43, 2003
11. Vanzieleghem BD et al: Imaging studies in the diagnostic workup of neonatal nasal obstruction. J Comput Assist Tomogr. 25(4):540-9, 2001
12. Behar PM et al: Paranasal sinus development and choanal atresia. Arch Otolaryngol Head Neck Surg. 126(2):155-7, 2000
13. Keller JL et al: Choanal atresia, CHARGE association, and congenital nasal stenosis. Otolaryngol Clin North Am. 33(6):1343-51, viii, 2000
14. Black CM et al: Potential pitfalls in the work-up and diagnosis of choanal atresia. AJNR Am J Neuroradiol. 19(2):326-9, 1998
15. Harris J et al: Epidemiology of choanal atresia with special reference to the CHARGE association. Pediatrics. 99(3):363-7, 1997
16. Slovis TL et al: Choanal atresia: precise CT evaluation. Radiology. 155(2):345-8, 1985

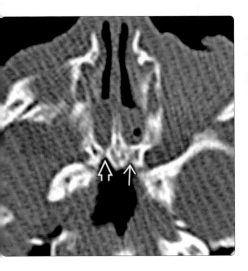

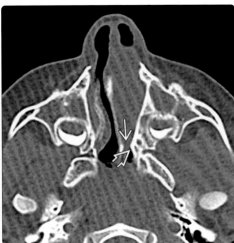

(Left) *Axial bone CT in a neonate with severe respiratory distress demonstrates bilateral choanal atresia, with thick bony atresia on the left* ➡ *and near-complete bony bridge on the right* ➡. *Note retained bilateral nasal cavity secretions secondary to noncommunication between the nasal cavities and nasopharynx.* (Right) *Axial bone CT in a 4 year old with CHARGE syndrome demonstrates left-sided choanal stenosis* ➡ *and thickened, medialized posterior maxilla* ➡.

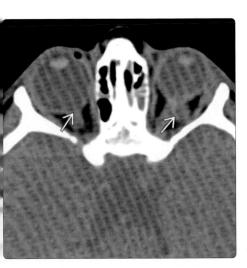

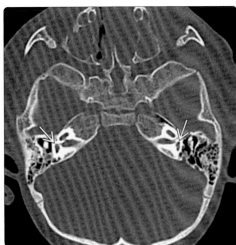

(Left) *Axial NECT in the same child with CHARGE syndrome shows bilateral colobomata* ➡ *and left microphthalmia.* (Right) *Axial bone CT in the same child with CHARGE syndrome shows typical bilateral labyrinthine anomalies with small, diminutive vestibules* ➡ *and absent semicircular canals.*

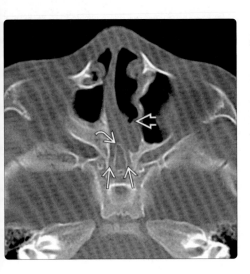

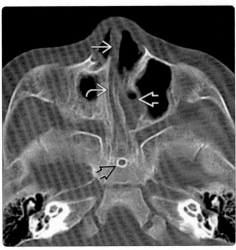

(Left) *Axial bone CT in a newborn with complex nasal anomalies shows bilateral choanal atresia* ➡, *aplasia of the right nasal cavity, fluid layer in the left nasal cavity* ➡, *and thickened vomer* ➡. (Right) *Axial bone CT in the same child shows fluid layering in the left nasal cavity* ➡ *anterior to the absent choanal opening. Note the absent right nasal cavity with the septum* ➡ *apposed to the lateral nasal wall* ➡. *Incidental persistent craniopharyngeal canal* ➡ *is noted.*

Nasal Glioma

TERMINOLOGY

- Developmental mass of dysplastic neurogenic tissue sequestered & isolated from subarachnoid space
  - "**Glioma**" is **misnomer** as this is nonneoplastic tissue
  - Extranasal glioma (ENG), intranasal glioma (ING)

IMAGING

- Well-circumscribed soft tissue mass at superior nasal dorsum (ENG) or within nasal cavity (ING) with no connection to brain
- Multiplanar MR
  - May show pedicle of fibrous tissue (not brain parenchyma) between ING & intracranial cavity
  - Better than CT for differentiating NG from cephalocele or dermoid
  - Gyral structure of gray matter rarely visible
  - Commonly shows hyperintensity related to gliosis

TOP DIFFERENTIAL DIAGNOSES

- Frontoethmoidal cephalocele
- Nasal dermal sinus
- Sinonasal solitary polyp

PATHOLOGY

- Similar spectrum of congenital anomalies as frontoethmoidal cephaloceles
  - Does **not** contain CSF contiguous with subarachnoid or intraventricular spaces
- Rarely associated with other brain or systemic anomalies

CLINICAL ISSUES

- Usually identified at birth
- **ENG: 60%; ING: 30%**; other sites: 10%
- Treatment of choice is complete surgical resection

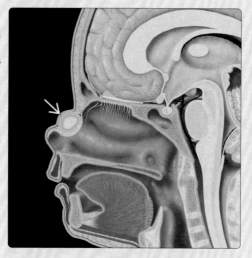
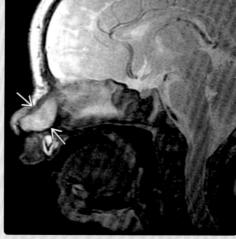

(Left) Sagittal graphic of a nasal glioma shows a mass of dysplastic glial tissue ➡ along the nasal dorsum. Notice the absence of a connection to the intracranial contents. (Right) Sagittal T2 MR in a 3 day old with nasal mass demonstrates an intermediate signal intensity intranasal glioma ➡ without intracranial extension.

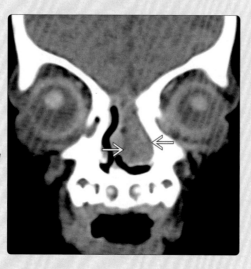
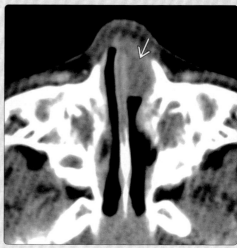

(Left) Coronal NECT shows a well-defined, somewhat polypoid soft tissue mass ➡, consistent with an intranasal glioma, within the left nasal cavity. The nasal septum is slightly deviated toward the right. No definite connection to the frontal lobe parenchyma is appreciated. (Right) Axial CECT shows a left-sided intranasal glioma ➡ widening the anterior nasal vault.

TERMINOLOGY

Abbreviations

- Nasal glioma (NG)
  - Extranasal glioma (ENG), intranasal glioma (ING)

Synonyms

- Nasal cerebral heterotopia, glial heterotopia

Definitions

- Developmental mass of **dysplastic neurogenic tissue** sequestered & isolated from subarachnoid space
  - "**Glioma**" is **misnomer** as this is nonneoplastic tissue
  - Best thought of as cephalocele without intracranial connection to brain

IMAGING

General Features

- Best diagnostic clue
  - Well-circumscribed soft tissue mass at superior nasal dorsum (ENG) or within nasal cavity (ING)
    - **No** connection to brain
- Location
  - Most occur at bridge of nose or in & around nasal cavity
  - Usually off midline; right > left side
  - ENG: Mass along nasal dorsum
    - Glabella most frequent location
    - ENG may also be found at medial canthus
    - May be found in nasopharynx, mouth, pterygopalatine fossa (very rare)
  - ING: Nasal cavity mass
    - May be attached to concha of middle turbinate, nasal septum, or lateral nasal wall
  - Other sites
    - Ethmoid sinus, palate, middle ear, tonsil, & pharynx
- Size
  - 1-3 cm in diameter
- Morphology
  - Well-circumscribed round, ovoid, or polypoid mass

CT Findings

- NECT
  - ENG: Well-circumscribed soft tissue attenuation mass at glabella
    - Isodense to brain
    - Superficial to point of fusion of frontal and nasal bones (fonticulus frontalis)
    - Nasal bones may be thinned
  - ING: Soft tissue attenuation mass within nasal cavity
    - Typically high in nasal vault
    - Fibrous pedicle may extend toward skull base but not intracranially
    - Defect in cribriform plate (10-30%)
  - Calcification rare
- CECT
  - Typically no significant enhancement
  - If intrathecal contrast used
    - Fails to document connection of lesion to subarachnoid space

MR Findings

- T1WI
  - Predominantly mixed to low signal intensity mass
  - Gyral structure of gray matter rarely visible
- T2WI
  - Commonly shows hyperintensity related to gliosis
  - No CSF around lesion connecting to subarachnoid space
- T1WI C+
  - Dysplastic tissue typically does not enhance
    - "Perceived" enhancement at periphery of intranasal lesions may actually represent adjacent nasal mucosa

Imaging Recommendations

- Best imaging tool
  - Multiplanar MR
    - May show pedicle of fibrous tissue (not brain parenchyma) between ING & intracranial cavity
    - MR better than CT for differentiating NG from cephalocele or dermoid
    - Avoids radiation to radiosensitive eye lenses in young patients
- Protocol advice
  - Thin-section sagittal T1 and T2 MR are important sequences
  - Preoperative thin-section axial bone CT with coronal reformatted images may also help in surgical planning
    - Bone only without enhancement

DIFFERENTIAL DIAGNOSIS

Frontoethmoidal Cephalocele

- Frontonasal (FN) & nasoethmoidal (NE) cephaloceles
- Clinical: Congenital mass on or around bridge of nose (FN) or within nasal cavity (NE)
- Imaging: MR shows connection to intracranial brain parenchyma or CSF

Nasal Dermal Sinus

- Clinical: Pit on tip or bridge of nose
- Imaging
  - Associated dermoid or epidermoid along course from tip of nose to foramen cecum, anterior to crista galli
    - Single or multiple
  - Possible intracranial connection via sinus tract

Sinonasal Solitary Polyps

- Clinical: Polyp is less firm, more translucent that ING
  - Unusual < 5 years
- Imaging
  - Typically inferolateral to middle turbinate (ING medial)
  - Homogeneous ↑ T2 MR signal with thin enhancement of peripheral mucosa

Orbital Dermoid and Epidermoid

- Clinical: Focal mass in medial orbit near nasolacrimal suture
- Imaging
  - Dermoid: Fluid or fat density/signal intensity
  - Epidermoid: Fluid density/signal

PATHOLOGY

General Features

- Etiology
  - Dysplastic, heterotopic neuroglial & fibrous tissue separated from brain during development of anterior skull or anterior skull base
  - Similar spectrum of congenital anomalies as frontoethmoidal cephaloceles but does not contain CSF and is not contiguous with subarachnoid or intraventricular spaces
    - ENG: **Fonticulus frontalis** (potential space prior to fusion of frontal & nasal bones) fuses prior to regression of dural diverticulum
      □ Dysplastic parenchyma sequestered over nasal bones/nasofrontal suture
    - ING: **Prenasal space** (potential space prior to fusion of nasal bones with cartilaginous nasal capsule) fuses prior to regression of dural diverticulum
      □ Dysplastic parenchyma sequestered in nasal cavity
- Associated abnormalities
  - Rarely associated with other brain or systemic anomalies

Gross Pathologic & Surgical Features

- Firm, smooth mass
- Rarely recognized as brain tissue at surgery
- 10-30% attached to brain by stalk of fibrous tissue through defect in or near cribriform plate
- Mixed extraintranasal lesions connect through defect in nasal bone

Microscopic Features

- Fibrous or gemistocytic astrocytes & neuroglial fibers
- Fibrous, vascularized connective tissue & sparse neurons
- Glial fibrillary acidic protein (GFAP) & S100 protein positive
- No mitotic features or bizarre nuclear forms

CLINICAL ISSUES

Presentation

- Most common signs/symptoms
  - Extranasal glioma
    - Congenital subcutaneous blue or red mass along nasal dorsum (glabella)
    - Usually nonprogressive midfacial swelling
  - Intranasal glioma
    - Firm, polypoid submucosal nasal cavity mass
    - Nasal obstruction & septal deviation may be present
    - May be confused clinically with nasal polyp
- Other signs/symptoms
  - No change in size with crying, Valsalva, or pressure on jugular vein (vs. frontoethmoidal cephalocele)
  - ENG: Capillary telangiectasia may cover
  - ING: Respiratory distress; epiphora; may protrude through nostril
- Clinical profile
  - Firm mass at glabella (ENG) or within nasal cavity (ING) in newborn

Demographics

- Age
  - Identified at birth or within 1st few years of life

- Epidemiology
  - Very rare lesion
  - **ENG: 60%; ING: 30%**; other sites: 10%

Natural History & Prognosis

- Grows slowly in proportion to adjacent tissue or brain if attached by pedicle
  - May deform nasal skeleton, maxilla, or orbit
- May become infected, resulting in meningitis
- Complete resection is curative
  - 10% recurrence rate with incomplete resection

Treatment

- Treatment of choice is complete surgical resection
  - ENG without intracranial connection removed via external incision with stalk dissection
  - ING without intracranial connection may be removed endoscopically
    - Less postoperative deformity than with craniotomy
  - Rare mixed gliomas (extranasal & intranasal components) best treated with combined intranasal and extracranial approach

DIAGNOSTIC CHECKLIST

Consider

- Most important to **differentiate NG from cephalocele**
- Document lack of connecting brain tissue &/or contiguous CSF space

Image Interpretation Pearls

- Must evaluate images for connection to intracranial cavity through skull base defect (cephalocele)
- Combined use of thin-section MR & bone CT accomplishes this task
  - Focus imaging to frontoethmoid area

SELECTED REFERENCES

1. Gnagi SH et al: Nasal obstruction in newborns. Pediatr Clin North Am. 60(4):903-22, 2013
2. Husein OF et al: Neuroglial heterotopia causing neonatal airway obstruction: presentation, management, and literature review. Eur J Pediatr. 167(12):1351-5, 2008
3. Riffaud L et al: Glial heterotopia of the face. J Pediatr Surg. 43(12):e1-3, 2008
4. De Biasio P et al: Prenatal diagnosis of a nasal glioma in the mid trimester. Ultrasound Obstet Gynecol. 27(5):571-3, 2006
5. Hedlund G: Congenital frontonasal masses: developmental anatomy, malformations, and MR imaging. Pediatr Radiol. 36(7):647-62; quiz 726-7, 2006
6. Huisman TA et al: Developmental nasal midline masses in children: neuroradiological evaluation. Eur Radiol. 14(2):243-9, 2004
7. Penner CR et al: Nasal glial heterotopia. Ear Nose Throat J. 83(2):92-3, 2004
8. Hoeger PH et al: Nasal glioma presenting as capillary haemangioma. Eur J Pediatr. 160(2):84-7, 2001
9. Shah J et al: Pedunculated nasal glioma: MRI features and review of the literature. J Postgrad Med. 45(1):15-7, 1999
10. Belden CJ et al: The developing anterior skull base: CT appearance from birth to 2 years of age. AJNR Am J Neuroradiol. 18(5):811-8, 1997
11. Barkovich AJ et al: Congenital nasal masses: CT and MR imaging features in 16 cases. AJNR Am J Neuroradiol. 12(1):105-16, 1991
12. Kennard CD et al: Congenital midline nasal masses: diagnosis and management. J Dermatol Surg Oncol. 16(11):1025-36, 1990
13. Morgan DW et al: Developmental nasal anomalies. J Laryngol Otol. 104(5):394-403, 1990
14. Younus M et al: Nasal glioma and encephalocele: two separate entities. Report of two cases. J Neurosurg. 64(3):516-9, 1986
15. Whitaker SR et al: Nasal glioma. Arch Otolaryngol. 107(9):550-4, 1981

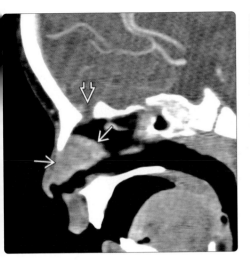

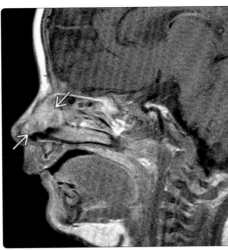

(Left) *Sagittal CECT demonstrates a mildly enhancing soft tissue lesion in the nasal cavity consistent with intranasal glioma ➡. No connection is identified with what appears to be normal foramen cecum ➡ in a child of this age.* (Right) *Sagittal T1 C+ MR in the same patient shows diffuse, slightly heterogeneous enhancement throughout the glioma ➡.*

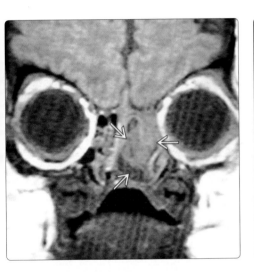

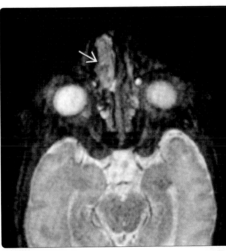

(Left) *Coronal FLAIR MR shows mixed signal intensity within an intranasal glioma ➡. There is no connection to the left frontal lobe to suggest that a cephalocele is present.* (Right) *Axial T2 MR shows a well-circumscribed intranasal glioma ➡. It is slightly heterogeneous but similar in signal intensity to the brain parenchyma. No surrounding CSF can be seen around this glioma, a finding that is more indicative of an cephalocele.*

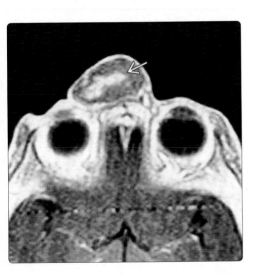

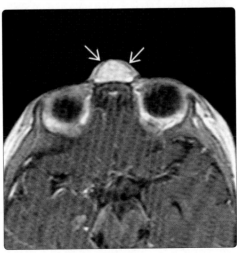

(Left) *Axial T1 C+ MR shows central enhancement ➡ within a large extranasal glioma. The lesion is located slightly off the midline. Enhancement is uncommon in these lesions.* (Right) *Axial T1 C+ MR shows a well-defined extranasal glioma ➡ along the dorsum of the nose in the midline, with diffuse enhancement throughout the lesion. This degree of enhancement is a rare feature of nasal gliomas.*

Nose and Sinus

TERMINOLOGY

- Defective embryogenesis of anterior neuropore resulting in any mixture of dermoid cyst, epidermoid cyst, &/or sinus tract in frontonasal region

IMAGING

- Midline location anywhere from nasal tip to anterior skull base at foramen cecum
- CT
  - Bifid crista galli with large foramen cecum
  - Fluid attenuation tract (sinus)/cyst or fat-containing mass (dermoid) from nasal dorsum to skull base within nasal septum
- MR
  - Fluid signal tract in septum from nasal dorsum to skull base (sinus)
  - Focal low-signal (epidermoid) or high-signal (dermoid) mass found between tip of nose and apex of crista galli

TOP DIFFERENTIAL DIAGNOSES

- Fatty marrow in crista galli
- Nonossified foramen cecum
- Frontoethmoidal cephalocele
- Nasal glioma (nasal glial heterotopia)

PATHOLOGY

- Intracranial extension of nasal dermal sinus (NDS) in 20%
- Associated craniofacial anomalies in 15%

CLINICAL ISSUES

- Nasoglabellar mass (30%)
- Pit on skin of nasal bridge at osteocartilaginous nasal junction ± protruding hair

DIAGNOSTIC CHECKLIST

- Nasoglabellar mass or pit on nose sends clinician in search of NDS with intracranial extension

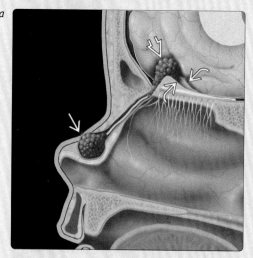

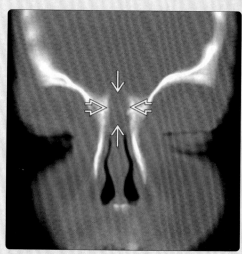

(Left) Lateral graphic depicts a nasal dermal sinus with 2 dermoids. An extracranial dermoid is present just below a cutaneous nasal pit ➡. An intracranial dermoid ⊟ splits a bifid crista galli ➤. (Right) Coronal bone CT demonstrates a nasal dermoid/epidermoid at the skull base. The low-attenuation midline mass ➡ causes remodeling of the adjacent bone ⊟ at the margins of the foramen cecum.

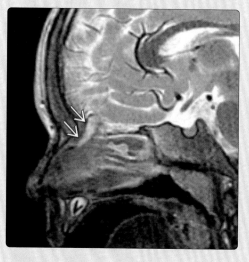

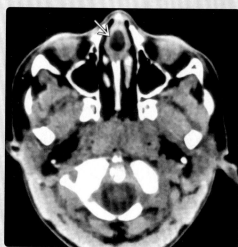

(Left) Sagittal T2WI MR in a 3-year-old boy with a bump on the tip of the nose shows a hyperintense sinus tract ➡ extending from the anterior skull base into the nasal septum. The features are characteristic of a dermal sinus. (Right) Axial NECT demonstrates a low-attenuation dermoid ➡ centered in the cartilaginous portion of the nasal septum. The mass is slightly higher in attenuation than adjacent fat.

TERMINOLOGY

Abbreviations

- Nasal dermal sinus (NDS)

Synonyms

- Nasal dermoid, nasal dermal cyst, anterior neuropore anomaly

Definitions

- Defective embryogenesis of anterior neuropore resulting in any mixture of dermoid cyst, epidermoid cyst, &/or sinus tract in frontonasal region

IMAGING

General Features

- Best diagnostic clue
  - CT
    - Bifid crista galli with large foramen cecum
    - Fluid attenuation tract (sinus)/cyst or fat-containing mass (dermoid)
      - From nasal dorsum to skull base within nasal septum
  - MR
    - Fluid signal tract in septum from nasal dorsum to skull base (sinus)
    - Focal T1 low-signal (epidermoid) or high-signal (dermoid) mass found between tip of nose and apex of crista galli
- Location
  - Midline lesion anywhere from nasal tip to anterior skull base at foramen cecum
- Size
  - 5 mm to 2 cm dermoid/epidermoid
- Morphology
  - Ovoid mass ± tubular sinus tract

CT Findings

- Bone CT
  - Focal tract (sinus) or mass (dermoid or epidermoid) anywhere from nasal bridge to crista galli
    - Fluid-density tract = sinus
    - Fluid-density mass = epidermoid
    - Fat-density mass = dermoid
  - Signs of intracranial extension
    - Large foramen cecum with **bifid or deformed crista galli** or cribriform plate

MR Findings

- T1WI
  - ↓ signal tract = sinus
  - ↑ signal mass = dermoid
  - ↓ signal mass = epidermoid
- T2WI
  - ↑ signal in sinus, epidermoid, or dermoid
  - Coronal plane shows septal lesions to best advantage
- DWI
  - **↑ signal = epidermoid**
  - Susceptibility artifacts at skull base may obscure signal from epidermoid

Imaging Recommendations

- Best imaging tool
  - MR more sensitive for delineating sinus tract and characterizing epidermoid/dermoid lesions and intracranial extension
  - Bone CT optimal for identifying skull base defect and crista galli deformity
- Protocol advice
  - Imaging "sweet spot" is small and anterior
    - **Focus imaging from tip of nose to back of crista galli**
    - Inferior end of axial imaging is hard palate
    - Contrast does not help with diagnosis
  - CT
    - Thin-section (1-2 mm) bone and soft tissue axial and coronal CT
  - MR
    - Sagittal plane displays course of sinus tract from nasal dorsum to skull base
    - Fat-suppressed images confirm fat presence in dermoids
    - **DWI** important additional sequence

DIFFERENTIAL DIAGNOSIS

Fatty Marrow in Crista Galli

- No nasoglabellar mass or pit on nose
- CT and MR otherwise normal

Nonossified Foramen Cecum

- Closes postnatally in 1st 5 years of life
- Crista galli not deformed or bifid

Frontoethmoidal Cephalocele

- Bone dehiscence is larger, involving broader area of midline cribriform plate or frontal bone
- Direct extension of meninges, subarachnoid space ± brain can be seen projecting into cephalocele on sagittal MR

Nasal Glioma

- Solid mass of dysplastic glial tissue separated from brain by subarachnoid space and meninges
- Preferred term = nasal glial heterotopia
- Most commonly projects extranasally onto paramedian bridge of nose
- Less commonly intranasal and along anterior nasal septum, off midline

PATHOLOGY

General Features

- Etiology
  - Anterior neuropore anomaly = general term for anomalous anterior neuropore regression; 3 main types
    - **NDS**
    - **Nasal glioma**
    - **Anterior cephalocele**
  - Embryology-anatomy: Development of anterior neuropore in 4th gestational week
    - Dural stalk passes from area of future foramen cecum to area of osteocartilaginous nasal junction and then normally regresses completely

– Failure of involution may leave neuroectodermal remnants along tract of dural stalk
– Dermoid or epidermoid alone or in association with NDS tract results
- Genetics
  ○ Familial clustering
- Associated abnormalities
  ○ Intracranial extension of NDS seen in **20%**
  ○ Craniofacial anomalies (15%)

Gross Pathologic & Surgical Features

- Sinus = tube of tissue can be followed through bones
- Epidermoid = well-defined cyst; dermoid = lobular, well-defined mass

Microscopic Features

- Sinus = midline epithelial-lined tract
- Epidermoid cyst contains desquamated epithelium
- Dermoid cyst contains epithelium, keratin debris, skin adnexa

CLINICAL ISSUES

Presentation

- Most common signs/symptoms
  ○ Nasoglabellar mass (30%)
  ○ **Pit** on skin of nasal bridge at osteocartilaginous nasal junction ± protruding hair
- Other signs/symptoms
  ○ Intermittent sebaceous material discharge from pit
  ○ < 50% have broadening nasal root & bridge
  ○ If nasal sinus tract present, recurrent meningitis may occur (rare)
- Clinical profile
  ○ Child (mean age = 32 months) with nasal pit ± nasoglabellar mass
  ○ Rarely presents in adult population
    – Episode of meningitis may be 1st problem leading to diagnosis

Demographics

- Age
  ○ Newborn to 5 years old
- Gender
  ○ Male patients with dermal sinus more likely to have intracranial extension
- Epidemiology
  ○ Congenital midline nasal lesions are rare (1 in 20,000-40,000 births)
    – Nasal dermoids are most common

Natural History & Prognosis

- 1-time problem when surgical correction is successful
- Untreated patients have nasal bridge broadening ± recurrent meningitis

Treatment

- 80% require extracranial excision only
  ○ Local procedure to remove pit
  ○ Any associated dermoid or epidermoid also simultaneously removed from nasal bridge
    – Open rhinoplasty vs. transnasal endoscopic excision

- 20% undergo combined extracranial & intracranial resection
  ○ Biorbitofrontal nasal craniotomy approach
    – Dermoid or epidermoid along with involved dura crista galli removed
    – Primary closure of surgical margins of dura completed

DIAGNOSTIC CHECKLIST

Consider

- Nasoglabellar mass or pit on nose sends clinician in search of NDS with intracranial extension
- Focused thin-section MR key to radiologic diagnosis
  ○ Axial coverage from cephalad margin of crista galli to hard palate
  ○ Coronal coverage from tip of nose to crista galli
- Add bone CT if NDS with intracranial extension found on MR

Image Interpretation Pearls

- If dermal sinus tract reaches dura of anterior cranial fossa, crista galli will be bifid and foramen cecum large
- If foramen cecum large but crista galli is not bifid and tract is not seen, foramen cecum is normal and not yet closed
  ○ Beware: Foramen cecum closes postnatally in 1st 5 years of life
  ○ Do not overcall "large foramen cecum," or unnecessary craniotomy may result
  ○ Repeat imaging in 6-12 months to confirm foramen cecum closure good approach in difficult cases

SELECTED REFERENCES

1. Gnagi SH et al: Nasal obstruction in newborns. Pediatr Clin North Am. 60(4):903-22, 2013
2. Holzmann D et al: Surgical approaches for nasal dermal sinus cysts. Rhinology. 45(1):31-5, 2007
3. Hedlund G: Congenital frontonasal masses: developmental anatomy, malformations, and MR imaging. Pediatr Radiol. 36(7):647-62; quiz 726-7, 2006
4. Zapata S et al: Nasal dermoids. Curr Opin Otolaryngol Head Neck Surg. 14(6):406-11, 2006
5. Huisman TA et al: Developmental nasal midline masses in children: neuroradiological evaluation. Eur Radiol. 14(2):243-9, 2004
6. Vaghela HM et al: Nasal dermoid sinus cysts in adults. J Laryngol Otol. 118(12):955-62, 2004
7. Rahbar R et al: The presentation and management of nasal dermoid: a 30-year experience. Arch Otolaryngol Head Neck Surg. 129(4):464-71, 2003
8. Bloom DC et al: Imaging and surgical approach of nasal dermoids. Int J Pediatr Otorhinolaryngol. 62(2):111-22, 2002
9. Lowe LH et al: Midface anomalies in children. Radiographics. 20(4):907-22; quiz 1106-7, 1112, 2000
10. Belden CJ et al: The developing anterior skull base: CT appearance from birth to 2 years of age. AJNR Am J Neuroradiol. 18(5):811-8, 1997
11. Castillo M: Congenital abnormalities of the nose: CT and MR findings. AJR Am J Roentgenol. 162(5):1211-7, 1994
12. Posnick JC et al: Nasal dermoid sinus cysts: an unusual presentation, computed tomographic scan findings, and surgical results. Ann Plast Surg. 32(5):519-23, 1994
13. MacGregor FB et al: Nasal dermoids: the significance of a midline punctum. Arch Dis Child. 68(3):418-9, 1993
14. Barkovich AJ et al: Congenital nasal masses: CT and MR imaging features in 16 cases. AJNR Am J Neuroradiol. 12(1):105-16, 1991
15. Paller AS et al: Nasal midline masses in infants and children. Dermoids, encephaloceles, and gliomas. Arch Dermatol. 127(3):362-6, 1991
16. Wardinsky TD et al: Nasal dermoid sinus cysts: association with intracranial extension and multiple malformations. Cleft Palate Craniofac J. 28(1):87-95, 1991

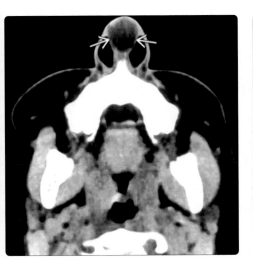

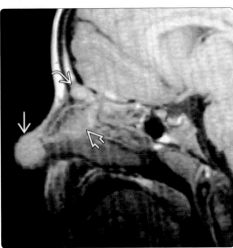

(Left) *Axial NECT shows a well-circumscribed mass ➡️ consistent with a dermoid at the nasal tip. The mass is slightly higher in attenuation than adjacent fat. Dermoids were also seen in the septum and at the foramen cecum in this patient.* (Right) *Sagittal T1WI MR in the same patient again shows the dermoid at the nasal tip ➡️. Additional dermoids are noted in the nasal septum ➡️ and at the skull base ➡️.*

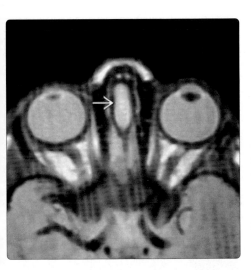

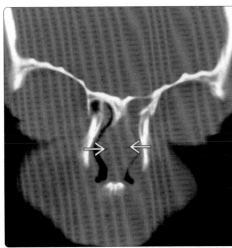

(Left) *Axial PD FSE MR shows the typical features of a nasal dermal sinus tract ➡️ within the nasal septum. The sinus in this infant extended from the skull base to the nasal tip.* (Right) *Coronal bone CT demonstrates the typical appearance of a dermoid lesion within the nasal septum ➡️. The lesion is well defined and low in attenuation.*

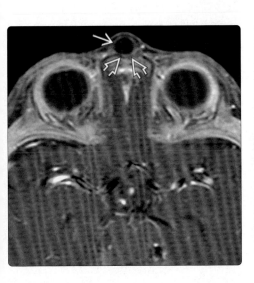

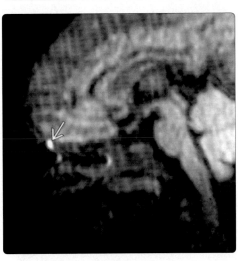

(Left) *Axial T1 C+ FS MR in a 4-month-old infant with glabella mass demonstrates a nonenhancing fluid signal intensity dermoid cyst ➡️ with mild remodeling of the underlying nasal bones ➡️.* (Right) *Sagittal DWI MR reveals an epidermoid in the region of the foramen cecum as a high signal focus of restricted diffusion ➡️. A 2nd (extracranial) lesion is not visible due to air-bone susceptibility artifact.*

TERMINOLOGY

- Congenital herniation of meninges, CSF ± brain tissue through mesodermal defect in anterior skull/skull base
- Synonym: Sincipital cephalocele

IMAGING

- Heterogeneous, mixed-density mass (variable amounts CSF & parenchyma) extending through bony defect
  - Midline frontal: **Frontonasal** type (FNCeph)
  - Intranasal: **Nasoethmoidal** type (NECeph)
  - Inferomedial orbital: **Nasoorbital** type (NOCeph)

TOP DIFFERENTIAL DIAGNOSES

- Nasal glioma
- Orbital dermoid and epidermoid
- Nasal dermal sinus
- Nasolacrimal duct mucocele

PATHOLOGY

- **Frontonasal**
  - Protrudes through unobliterated **fonticulus frontalis**
- **Nasoethmoidal**
  - Protrudes through foramen cecum into **prenasal space**
- **Nasoorbital**
  - Protrudes into inferomedial orbit through defect in lacrimal/frontal process of maxillary bones

CLINICAL ISSUES

- Intracranial abnormalities in **~ 80%**
- F = 67%, M = 33%
- Most common in Southeast Asians

DIAGNOSTIC CHECKLIST

- Sagittal & coronal T1 & T2 MR images optimal for showing contiguity of mass with intracranial contents

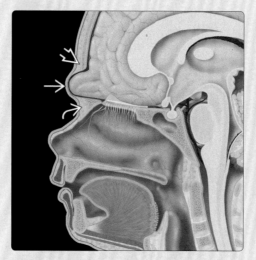
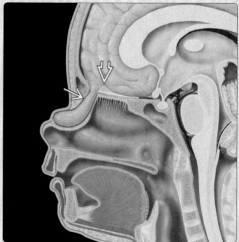

(Left) Sagittal graphic of a frontonasal cephalocele shows herniation of brain through a patent fonticulus frontalis ➡ between the frontal bones above ➡ and nasal bones below ➡. (Right) Nasoethmoidal cephalocele is depicted in this sagittal graphic. Notice the herniation of brain tissue ➡ into the nasal cavity through a patent foramen cecum. Also note the crista galli is positioned posterior to the skull base defect ➡.

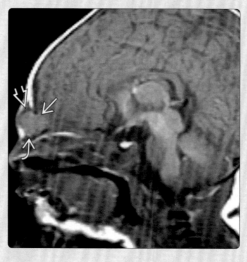
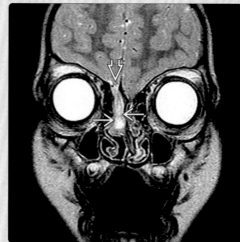

(Left) Sagittal T1 MR in a 1 week old shows a frontonasal cephalocele ➡ with protrusion of the dysplastic-appearing inferior left frontal lobe through a patent ponticulus frontalis. Frontal bone ➡ is above and nasal bone ➡ is below the cephalocele. (Right) Coronal T2 MR shows the typical appearance of a nasoethmoidal cephalocele. The gliotic brain parenchyma ➡ herniating into the nasal cavity is hyperintense. The cephalocele herniates through a skull base defect ➡ to the right of midline.

TERMINOLOGY

Abbreviations

- Frontoethmoidal cephalocele (FECeph)
  - Frontonasal cephalocele (FNCeph)
  - Nasoethmoidal cephalocele (NECeph)
  - Nasoorbital cephalocele (NOCeph)

Synonyms

- Sincipital cephalocele

Definitions

- Congenital herniation of meninges, CSF ± brain tissue through mesodermal defect in anterior skull/skull base presenting as extranasal, intranasal, or medial orbital mass

IMAGING

General Features

- Best diagnostic clue
  - Midline frontal (FNCeph), intranasal (NECeph), or medial orbital (NOCeph) soft tissue mass contiguous with intracranial brain parenchyma extending through bony defect
- Location
  - FNCeph: Anterior forehead at glabella-dorsum of nose
  - NECeph: Superomedial nasal cavity
    - 90% terminate intracranially at single midline defect at foramen cecum
    - 10% terminate intracranially at paired openings at anterior cribriform plates separated by midline bony bridge
  - NOCeph: Inferomedial orbit
- Size
  - Variable
  - 1-2 cm to larger than infant head
- Morphology
  - Well circumscribed, round, globular

CT Findings

- NECT
  - Heterogeneous, mixed-density mass (variable amounts CSF & parenchyma) extending through bony defect
- Bone CT
  - FNCeph: Frontal bones displaced superiorly while nasal bones, frontal processes of maxillae pushed inferiorly
  - NECeph: Nasal bone bowed anteriorly with tract through anterior ethmoid area
    - Crista galli may be bifid or absent
    - Deficient or absent cribriform plate
- CT myelogram
  - Intrathecal contrast: Fills subarachnoid space & surrounds soft tissue extending through bony defect

MR Findings

- T1WI
  - Soft tissue mass with isointense signal to gray matter showing contiguity with intracranial parenchyma extending through bony defect
- T2WI
  - Hyperintense CSF surrounds herniated soft tissue parenchyma
  - Tissue may show ↑ signal due to gliosis
- T1WI C+
  - No abnormal enhancement noted within soft tissue
  - Meninges may enhance if infection/inflammation of meninges present

Ultrasonographic Findings

- OB US: Frontal (FNCeph) or intranasal (NECeph) soft tissue mass
  - FNCeph: Widened interorbital distance

Imaging Recommendations

- Best imaging tool
  - MR superior to CT for cephalocele evaluation
    - Differentiates CSF-filled meningocele and parenchymal components
    - Superior for showing other associated brain anomalies
- Protocol advice
  - Thin, (3 mm) multiplanar T1 & T2 MR
    - Sagittal & coronal planes optimal for visualizing parenchymal herniation through defects
  - Bone CT can provide important information about skull defects for surgical planning
    - CT with intrathecal contrast used only when full MR & bone CT still leave unanswered questions

DIFFERENTIAL DIAGNOSIS

Nasal Glioma

- Clinical: Soft tissue mass along dorsum of nose (extranasal type) or under nasal bones (intranasal type)
- Imaging: MR shows no connection between mass in intracranial contents

Orbital Dermoid and Epidermoid

- Clinical: Focal mass in medial orbit without associated tract
- Imaging: Fat density/intensity if dermoid; fluid density/intensity if epidermoid

Nasal Dermal Sinus

- Clinical: Pit on tip or bridge of nose
- Imaging: Midline sinus from tip of nose to skull base
  - Dermoid or epidermoid may be seen anywhere along tract
  - Possible intracranial connection via sinus tract; does not contain brain parenchyma

Nasolacrimal Duct Mucocele

- Clinical: Small, round, bluish, medial canthal mass identified at birth with submucosal nasal cavity mass at inferior meatus
- Imaging: Nasolacrimal duct dilatation may be present to inferior meatus
  - No connection to skull base or brain parenchyma

PATHOLOGY

General Features

- Etiology
  - Prior to 8th week of gestation, 2 potential spaces present
    - **Fonticulus frontalis**: Between frontal, nasal bones

- **Prenasal space**: Between nasal bones, developing cartilaginous nasal septum
  - Anterior neuropore runs in prenasal space, communicating with anterior cranial fossa via foramen cecum
  - **Dural diverticulum** protruding through defects may fail to regress
    - FNCeph: Protrudes through unobliterated fonticulus frontalis
    - NECeph: Protrudes through foramen cecum into prenasal space
    - NOCeph: Protrudes into inferomedial orbit through defect in lacrimal/frontal process of maxillary bones
- Genetics
  - Sporadic occurrence
  - Not linked to neural tube defects like occipital cephaloceles
  - Siblings have 6% incidence of congenital CNS abnormalities
- Associated abnormalities
  - **Intracranial abnormalities (~ 80%)**
    - Callosal hypogenesis & interhemispheric lipomas
    - Neuronal migration anomalies
    - Microcephaly
    - Aqueductal stenosis & hydrocephalus
    - Colloid or arachnoid cysts
  - Midline craniofacial dysraphisms & hypertelorism
  - Microphthalmos

Staging, Grading, & Classification

- 3 types of sincipital cephaloceles
  - FNCeph
  - NECeph
  - NOCeph

Gross Pathologic & Surgical Features

- Well-defined, meningeal-lined mass containing CSF ± brain tissue

Microscopic Features

- **Meningoencephalocele**: CSF, brain tissue & meninges
- **Meningocele**: Meninges & CSF only
- **Atretic cephalocele**: Forme fruste of cephalocele with dura, fibrous tissue, & degenerated brain tissue
- **Gliocele**: Glial-lined CSF-filled cyst

CLINICAL ISSUES

Presentation

- Most common signs/symptoms
  - Externally visible, firm midline forehead (FNCeph), intranasal (NECeph), or medial orbital (NOCeph) mass
- Other signs/symptoms
  - Hypertelorism & orbital dystopia
  - Hyperpigmentation of overlying skin
  - Change in size with crying, Valsalva, jugular compression
  - Seizures & mental retardation < 50%
- Clinical profile
  - Newborn with mass on forehead, within nasal cavity, or along medial orbital margin

Demographics

- Age
  - Congenital lesion detected on prenatal ultrasound or presenting at birth
- Gender
  - F = 67%, M = 33%
- Ethnicity
  - FECeph most common in Southeast Asians
- Epidemiology
  - Cephaloceles are uncommon in Western countries
  - 1 in 4,000-5,000 live births in Southeast Asia
  - FECeph account for 15% of all cephaloceles
  - FNCeph (50-61%), NECeph (30-33%), NOCeph (6-10%)

Natural History & Prognosis

- Present at birth; require surgical repair
- If untreated, may grow with child
- If thin skin covering or no skin, prone to rupture, CSF leak, & infection
- When CSF filled, may increase rapidly in size
- Hydrocephalus and presence of intracranial abnormalities are predictors of developmental delay/poor outcome

Treatment

- Biopsy contraindicated: CSF leak, seizures, meningitis
- Complete surgical resection
  - Combined plastic surgery & neurosurgery
  - Herniated brain tissue is dysfunctional (no neuro deficits result)
- Meningeal & skull base defect repaired or CSF leak, meningitis, or recurrent herniation may result

DIAGNOSTIC CHECKLIST

Consider

- Sagittal & coronal T1 & T2 MR optimal for showing contiguity of mass with intracranial contents
- Bone CT used to evaluate size & location of bony defect prior to surgical repair

Image Interpretation Pearls

- Determine location of lesion relative to nasal bones
  - Above is FNCeph
  - Below is NECeph
- Evaluate brain for presence of associated intracranial anomalies

SELECTED REFERENCES

1. Keshri AK et al: Transnasal endoscopic repair of pediatric meningoencephalocele. J Pediatr Neurosci. 11(1):42-5, 2016
2. Castelnuovo P et al: Endoscopic endonasal management of encephaloceles in children: an eight-year experience. Int J Pediatr Otorhinolaryngol. 73(8):1132-6, 2009
3. Arshad AR et al: Frontoethmoidal encephalocele: treatment and outcome. J Craniofac Surg. 19(1):175-83, 2008
4. Hedlund G: Congenital frontonasal masses: developmental anatomy, malformations, and MR imaging. Pediatr Radiol. 36(7):647-62; quiz 726-7, 2006
5. Rojvachiranonda N et al: Frontoethmoidal encephalomeningocele: new morphological findings and a new classification. J Craniofac Surg. 14(6):847-58, 2003
6. Naidich TP et al: Cephaloceles and related malformations. AJNR Am J Neuroradiol. 13(2):655-90, 1992
7. David DJ et al: Cephaloceles: classification, pathology, and management. World J Surg. 13(4):349-57, 1989

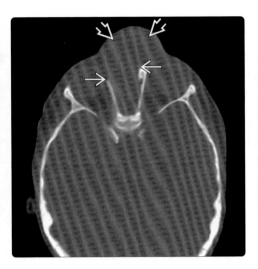

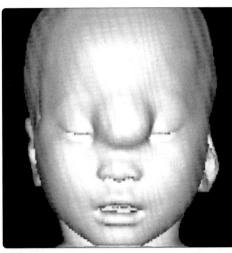

(Left) *Axial bone CT in a newborn with a soft tissue mass in the midline of the forehead shows a large anterior skull defect* ➡ *through which a large frontonasal cephalocele protrudes* ➡. (Right) *Frontal projection 3D surface-rendered CT in the same patient shows the clinical appearance of the large cephalocele between the eyes. This frontonasal cephalocele protrudes through a patent fonticulus frontalis.*

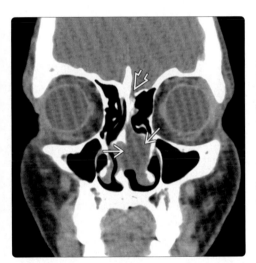

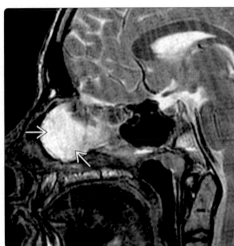

(Left) *Coronal NECT shows a low-density mass* ➡ *in the left nasal cavity in a patient with a nasoethmoidal cephalocele. The small defect in the skull base* ➡ *is somewhat difficult to appreciate on this soft tissue window image.* (Right) *Sagittal T2 FS MR in the same patient shows predominantly CSF signal intensity within the lesion* ➡. *No definite brain parenchyma is seen within the cephalocele on this image.*

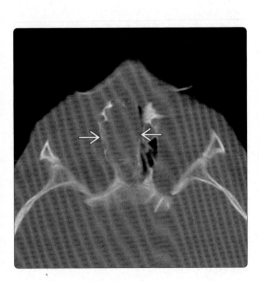

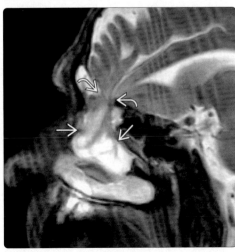

(Left) *Axial bone CT in a 17 month old shows an expansile lesion in the superior nasal cavity and ethmoid region* ➡, *consistent with a nasoethmoidal-type cephalocele. A large skull base defect was noted on coronal images (not shown).* (Right) *Sagittal T2 FS MR in the same patient shows herniation of brain parenchyma and meninges* ➡ *through the defect in the anterior skull base* ➡ *in this case of a nasoethmoidal cephalocele.*

TERMINOLOGY

- Congenital nasal pyriform aperture stenosis (CNPAS): Congenital narrowing of anterior bony nasal passageway

IMAGING

- Best tool: Bone CT in axial & coronal planes
  - Medial deviation of anterior maxillae ± thickening of nasal processes
  - Abnormal maxillary dentition: **Solitary median maxillary central incisor (SMMCI)** (75%)
  - Triangle-shaped palate

TOP DIFFERENTIAL DIAGNOSES

- Nasolacrimal duct mucoceles
  - Intranasal component narrows anterior nasal cavity
- Nasal choanal stenosis/atresia
  - Narrow posterior nasal passage by membrane or bone

PATHOLOGY

- CNPAS without SMMCI almost always isolated anomaly
- Solitary maxillary central incisor in 75% of cases
  - Associated with **holoprosencephaly**

CLINICAL ISSUES

- Respiratory distress in newborn/infant
  - Can mimic choanal atresia/stenosis
  - Breathing problems may be triggered by URI
  - Symptoms may be more pronounced with feeding
- Narrow nasal inlet on clinical exam
- CNPAS 1/5 to 1/3 as common as choanal atresia

DIAGNOSTIC CHECKLIST

- Bone CT recommended for diagnosis or bony narrowing & dental abnormalities
- Brain MR recommended in cases of SMMCI to exclude midline brain anomalies

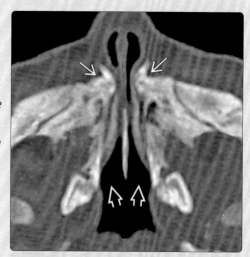
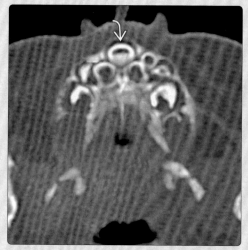

(Left) Axial bone CT in a newborn shows the typical features of congenital nasal pyriform aperture stenosis. There is overgrowth of the anterior maxillae ➡ with marked narrowing of the anterior nasal passages. There is no associated choanal atresia ➡. (Right) Axial bone CT at the level of the palate in the same patient shows a classic associated finding in patients with pyriform aperture stenosis, a solitary median maxillary central incisor or megaincisor ➡.

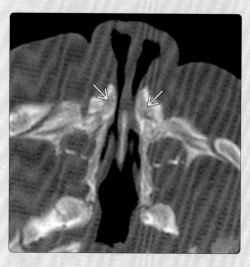
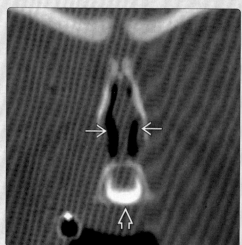

(Left) Axial bone CT in a newborn with respiratory distress demonstrates bilateral congenital nasal pyriform aperture stenosis. The anterior and medial aspects of the maxillae are thickened ➡, causing the narrowing of the anterior nasal airway. (Right) Coronal bone CT in the same patient demonstrates the narrowing of the anterior nasal airway ➡ bilaterally and the associated solitary maxillary central incisor ➡.

TERMINOLOGY

Abbreviations

- Congenital nasal pyriform aperture stenosis (CNPAS)

Definitions

- Congenital narrowing of anterior bony nasal passageway/nasal aperture

IMAGING

General Features

- Best diagnostic clue
  - Medialization and thickening of anterior maxillae with narrowing of nasal airway
- Location
  - Most often **bilateral**
- Size
  - Pyriform aperture (PA) size in CNPAS
    - PA width < 11 mm in term infant diagnostic (normal = 13.4-15.6 mm)
    - PA area = 0.2-0.4 cm² (0.7-1.1 cm² is normal)

Imaging Recommendations

- Best imaging tool
  - Bone CT in axial & coronal planes

CT Findings

- Bone CT
  - **Narrowed bony nasal inlet**
    - Medial deviation of lateral wall of PA (anterior maxillae) ± thickening of nasal processes
  - **Triangle-shaped hard palate**
    - Bony ridge along oral surface of hard palate on coronal images
  - **Abnormal maxillary dentition** may occur
    - Fused or malaligned central & lateral incisors
    - Solitary median maxillary central incisor (SMMCI) syndrome (75%)
  - Posterior choanae normal in caliber

DIFFERENTIAL DIAGNOSIS

Nasolacrimal Duct Mucocele

- Obstruction of distal nasolacrimal ducts results in cysts at inferior meatuses that narrow anterior nasal cavity
- Bony aperture is normal

Nasal Choanal Stenosis/Atresia

- Narrow or occluded posterior nasal passage: Membranous, osseous or mixed
- Anterior nasal passage normal in caliber

PATHOLOGY

General Features

- Etiology
  - 2 theories of pathogenesis
    - **Deficiency of primary palate** derived from midline mesodermal tissue
      - Embryologically, medial maxillary swelling forms structures of primary palate, including 4 incisors
      - Mesoderm thought to have inductive effect on forebrain, hence association of SMMCI syndrome with holoprosencephaly
    - Overgrowth or dysplasia of nasal processes of maxilla
  - CNPAS without SMMCI is almost always isolated anomaly
- Associated abnormalities
  - Upper teeth anomalies
    - **SMMCI syndrome** (75% of CNPAS cases)
  - Semilobar or alobar **holoprosencephaly**
  - Endocrine dysfunction: Pituitary-adrenal axis

CLINICAL ISSUES

Presentation

- Most common signs/symptoms
  - Respiratory distress, especially with feeding, as infants are obligate nasal breathers
    - Can mimic choanal atresia/stenosis
    - Breathing problems may be triggered by upper respiratory infection further compromising narrowed airway
  - Cyanosis
- Other signs/symptoms
  - Symptoms may be more pronounced with feeding
  - Nasogastric tube difficult to pass

Demographics

- Age
  - Newborns or infants in 1st few months of life
- Epidemiology
  - Congenital airway obstruction affects 1 in 5,000 infants
    - Majority are choanal atresia
    - CNPAS 1/5 to 1/3 as common as choanal atresia
      - 1 in 25,000 live births

Treatment

- May be treated conservatively with special feeding techniques
- Surgical intervention in patients with persistent respiratory difficulty & poor weight gain
  - Resection of anteromedial maxilla ± anterior aspect of inferior turbinates & reconstruction of anterior nasal orifice
  - PA width less than 5.7 mm in neonate may correlate with need for surgical intervention

DIAGNOSTIC CHECKLIST

Image Interpretation Pearls

- Brain MR recommended in cases of solitary maxillary central incisor to exclude midline brain anomalies

SELECTED REFERENCES

1. Ginat DT et al: CT and MRI of congenital nasal lesions in syndromic conditions. Pediatr Radiol. ePub, 2015
2. Wormald R et al: Congenital nasal pyriform aperture stenosis 5.7 mm or less is associated with surgical intervention: a pooled case series. Int J Pediatr Otorhinolaryngol. 79(11):1802-5, 2015
3. Osovsky M et al: Congenital pyriform aperture stenosis. Pediatr Radiol. 37(1):97-9, 2007
4. Belden CJ et al: CT features of congenital nasal piriform aperture stenosis: initial experience. Radiology. 213(2):495-501, 1999

KEY FACTS

TERMINOLOGY

- Acute inflammatory sinonasal process lasting ≤ 4 weeks
- Acute bacterial or rhinosinusitis (ABRS or ARS), viral rhinosinusitis (VRS)

IMAGING

- ARS is clinical diagnosis & imaging rarely necessary
- Radiography: Inaccurate and should be supplanted by CT
- NECT: Confirms diagnosis, evaluates when medical therapy has failed, delineates anatomic variants, especially presurgical
  - Axial < 1-mm slice thickness with coronal and sagittal reconstructions
  - Best sign = air-fluid level ± aerosolized secretions with mucosal thickening
  - Most common in ethmoid and maxillary sinuses
  - Often asymmetric sinus involvement
- MR: Indicated for suspected complications

- Consider dictating: "Imaging findings support clinical diagnosis of VRS or ABRS"

TOP DIFFERENTIAL DIAGNOSES

- Pseudo fluid level from large maxillary polyp/cyst
- Posttraumatic blood level
- Postobstructive noninfected secretions

PATHOLOGY

- Most cases follow viral upper respiratory infection

CLINICAL ISSUES

- **Signs/symptoms of ARS**: ≤ 4 weeks of **purulent** nasal drainage, nasal obstruction, and facial pain, pressure, fullness
- VRS usually self-limited
- ARS complications rare
  - Orbital cellulitis, subperiosteal abscess, meningitis, subdural empyema, brain abscess, venous sinus thrombosis

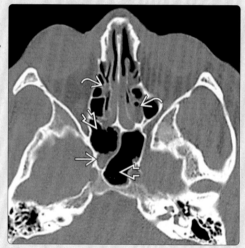
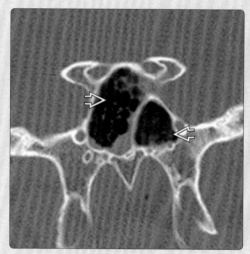

(Left) *Axial NECT in patient with purulent nasal discharge and headache shows patchy bilateral ethmoid sinus disease ⇗, an air-fluid level ⇒ in the right sphenoid sinus, and frothy secretions ⇒ in the bilateral sphenoid sinuses, corroborating the clinical history of acute bacterial rhinosinusitis (ABRS).* (Right) *Coronal reconstruction NECT demonstrates bubbly, frothy secretions in sphenoid sinuses ⇒ in a patient with clinical diagnosis of ABRS.*

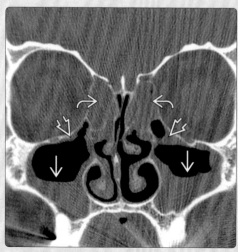
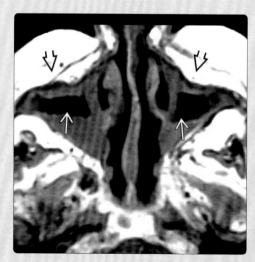

(Left) *Coronal bone CT shows acute bilateral maxillary and ethmoid sinusitis. Note air-fluid levels ⇒ and mucosal thickening ⇒ in maxillary sinuses and complete opacification of ethmoid sinuses ⇗.* (Right) *Axial T1WI MR shows bilateral maxillary air-fluid levels ⇒ and mucosal thickening ⇒ on nondependent anterior sinus walls. The fluid is isointense to soft tissue on this T1 MR image. Note normal surrounding facial fat, with no induration to suggest complicated sinusitis.*

Acute Rhinosinusitis

TERMINOLOGY

Abbreviations

- Acute rhinosinusitis (ARS)
- Acute bacterial rhinosinusitis (ABRS)
- Viral rhinosinusitis (VRS)

Definitions

- Acute inflammatory process of sinonasal mucosa lasting ≤ 4 weeks
  - Classified into VRS vs. ABRS based on clinical presentation
- Generally clinical diagnosis, imaging only needed if complications suspected

IMAGING

General Features

- Best diagnostic clue
  - Air-fluid level ± bubbly/frothy secretions within sinus with mucosal thickening
  - Opacification or mucosal thickening of multiple anterior ethmoid cells ± frontal recess
- Location
  - Most common in ethmoid and maxillary sinuses, typically asymmetric
- Size
  - Normal sinus volume
    - No sinus expansion (mucocele) or reduced volume (chronic rhinosinusitis)

Radiographic Findings

- Radiography
  - **Inaccurate and should be supplanted by CT**
  - Mucosal thickening or sinus opacification ± air-fluid level

CT Findings

- NECT
  - **Air-fluid level**, bubbly or frothy-appearing secretions
  - Moderate mucosal thickening, generally > 1 cm in sinus cavity, ostium, or nasal cavity
  - May see polypoid inflammatory tissue obstructing drainage pathways
- CECT
  - Indicated when orbital or intracranial complications suspected clinically
  - Inflamed sinus mucosa enhances, but thin linear soft tissue deep to mucosa does not
  - Central secretions do not enhance
- Bone CT
  - Bone destruction not typical for acute infection
    - If present, suspect aggressive invasive sinus infection or neoplasm
  - Osteoneogenesis, sinus wall sclerosis and thickening, usually indicates chronic inflammation

MR Findings

- T1WI
  - Mucosal thickening isointense to other soft tissue
  - Air/fluid level
  - Hyperintense secretions when chronic sinusitis present
- T2WI
  - Thickened edematous mucosa especially in maxillary and ethmoids
  - May have air/fluid level in maxillary, frontal, sphenoid sinus
    - Anterior ethmoid cells generally too small for discrete fluid level
  - Secretions ↓ SI when proteinaceous or chronic
- T1WI C+
  - Enhancing mucosa lining sinus cavity
  - Central secretions do not enhance

Imaging Recommendations

- Best imaging tool
  - **ARS is clinical diagnosis**
  - Radiographs inaccurate, and with widespread CT availability, have no role in clinical practice
  - CT: Consider only if evaluating for complications, failed medical therapy, alternative diagnoses, or surgical candidate
    - NECT delineates anatomic variants prior to functional endoscopic sinus surgery
    - CECT indicated if symptoms suggest complicated ABRS
  - MR indicated for orbital or intracranial complications, invasive fungal disease, neoplasm
- Protocol advice
  - Bone CT
    - Axial ≤ 1-mm slice thickness with coronal, sagittal reconstructions to evaluate drainage pathways
  - MR
    - Multiplanar T1 and T2 sequences necessary
    - C+ T1 with fat suppression best for intracranial/orbital complications

DIFFERENTIAL DIAGNOSIS

Pseudofluid Level

- Mucus retention cyst mimics air-fluid level
- Rounded contour with incomplete fluid level

Posttraumatic Blood Level

- Clinical history of recent facial injury
- Increased attenuation of layering fluid (blood)
- Associated sinus wall fractures

Postobstructive Secretions

- Lesion obstructs sinus drainage pathway, resulting in noninfected trapped sinus cavity fluid
- MR differentiates tumor from obstructed secretions
  - Neoplasm generally decreased SI on T2 compared to hyperintense secretions

PATHOLOGY

General Features

- Etiology
  - ABRS uncommonly follows VRS (0.5-2.0% of cases)
    - Upper respiratory infection (URI) → mucosal swelling → sinus outflow obstruction → static secretions in sinus → infection
    - Viral symptoms usually improve in 7-10 days

- Symptoms > 10 days or worsening after 5-7 days suggest bacterial superinfection
  - □ Common organisms: *Streptococcus pneumonia, Haemophilus influenzae, Moraxella catarrhalis*
  - **Odontogenic sinusitis**: Apical periodontitis with dehiscence or transosseous infection extension into maxillary sinus
- Genetics
  - Cystic fibrosis (autosomal recessive disorder) predisposes to rhinosinusitis and polyps
- Associated abnormalities
  - Structural abnormalities may narrow drainage pathways
    - Anatomic variants of septum, uncinate process, middle turbinate, frontal recess, ethmoid sinuses
    - Polyps, either isolated or associated with allergic sinusitis with diffuse polyposis
    - Benign or malignant neoplasms
  - Predisposing systemic disorders: Allergies, immunoglobulin deficiency, immotile cilia syndrome, cystic fibrosis, vitamin D deficiency

Staging, Grading, & Classification

- Can be classified according to etiology: Viral, bacterial, vasomotor

Gross Pathologic & Surgical Features

- Edematous, erythematous mucosa with ostial obstruction, purulent secretions

Microscopic Features

- Tissue-invasive bacteria
- Luminal exudate of neutrophils, eosinophils

CLINICAL ISSUES

Presentation

- Most common signs/symptoms
  - **Cardinal signs/symptoms of ARS**: ≤ 4 weeks of **purulent** nasal drainage & obstruction, facial pain, or pressure
    - VRS: Signs/symptoms last < 10 days, does not progress
    - ABRS: Signs/symptoms fail to improve within 10 days **or** worsen within 10 days after initial improvement
- Other signs/symptoms
  - Fever, cough, malaise, hyposmia, anosmia, dental pain, ear pressure/fullness
    - Facial/dental pain predicts ABRS, but location correlates poorly with site of involvement
- Clinical profile
  - Pediatric or adult patient with nasal discharge and obstruction following viral URI lasting ≤ 4 weeks
  - Laboratory results
    - Nasal/nasopharynx cultures poorly correlate with sinus cultures, do not differentiate ABRS from VRS
      - □ Often contaminated with *Staphylococcus aureus*
    - Endoscopic middle meatus aspiration more specific, but generally not necessary in uncomplicated ARS

Demographics

- Age
  - Generally adult disease but can be seen in children
    - Typically follows viral URI in children

- Epidemiology
  - Sinonasal inflammatory disease is ubiquitous
  - Rhinosinusitis affects nearly 31 million patients in USA annually
    - 12% (1 in 8 adults) of USA population annually
    - > 1 billion physician visits and > $3 billion in ARS healthcare expenditures/year
  - Both VRS and ARS often follow or coexist with common cold

Natural History & Prognosis

- VRS usually self-limited
- ABRS may resolve without antibiotics
- ABRS course may be shortened by medical therapy, surgical drainage, and possibly saline irrigation
- If ABRS untreated, rarely **complications** may ensue
  - Orbital cellulitis, subperiosteal abscess, meningitis, subdural empyema, brain abscess, venous sinus thrombosis

Treatment

- Medical therapy
  - Saline nasal sprays and irrigants, mucolytics to thin secretions
  - Decongestants, antihistamines, antibiotics
  - Nasal steroids
- Surgical therapy
  - More often performed for chronic rhinosinusitis
  - Drainage procedures performed in acute disease (frontal and sphenoid) to prevent development of complications

DIAGNOSTIC CHECKLIST

Consider

- Bone CT if suspect alternative diagnoses, failed therapy, complications, or surgical candidate
  - Acquire ≤ 1-mm axial slices with coronal and sagittal reformations
- CT limitations
  - Cannot differentiate viral from bacterial disease
  - High incidence of sinus mucosal abnormalities in asymptomatic patients

Image Interpretation Pearls

- Air-fluid levels not always present, but most specific indicator
- In correct clinical setting even severe mucosal thickening can indicate ABRS
- Normal nasal mucosal cycle may be impossible to distinguish from ARS mucosal thickening
- Look for signs of invasive fungal sinusitis if immunocompromised patient
- **Consider dictation stating**, "In correct clinical setting, CT findings consistent with ARS or ABRS"

SELECTED REFERENCES

1. Joshi VM et al: Imaging in sinonasal inflammatory disease. Neuroimaging Clin N Am. 25(4):549-68, 2015
2. Rosenfeld RM et al: Clinical practice guideline (update): adult sinusitis. Otolaryngol Head Neck Surg. 152(2 Suppl):S1-S39, 2015
3. Cornelius RS et al: ACR appropriateness criteria sinonasal disease. J Am Coll Radiol. 10(4):241-6, 2013

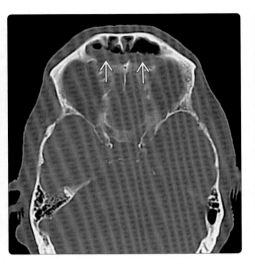

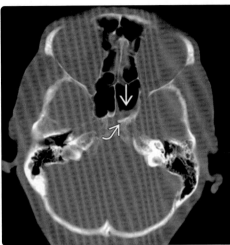

(Left) *Axial NECT performed for headache and fever reveals frothy air-fluid levels ➡ in both frontal sinuses. Although acute rhinosinusitis (ARS) is a clinical diagnosis, imaging may be performed to rule out suspected complications.* (Right) *Axial NECT in patient with clinical diagnosis of ABRS demonstrates an air-fluid level ➡ in left sphenoid sinus. Note osteoneogenesis ➚, or sclerotic sinus wall, suggesting chronic sinus inflammatory disease as well as acute ABRS.*

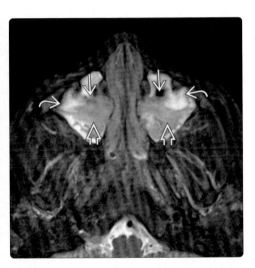

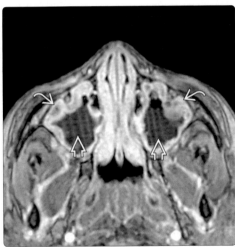

(Left) *Axial T2 FS MR in a pediatric patient with ABRS shows near complete opacification of maxillary sinuses with discrete air-fluid levels ➡. Note circumferential hyperintense edematous mucosa ➚. Fluid relatively hypointense ➡ secondary to increased protein content.* (Right) *Axial T1 C+ SPGR MR in the same patient shows avid enhancement of inflamed sinus mucosa ➚ relative to nonenhancing central secretions ➡. This patient had clinical diagnosis of ABRS.*

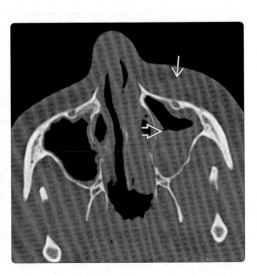

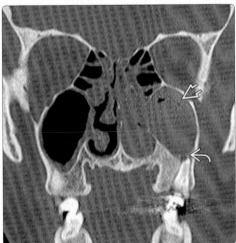

(Left) *Axial NECT in a patient with ABRS shows left maxillary sinus opacification with an air-fluid level ➡. Premaxillary fat soft tissue edema ➡ heralds complicated ABRS with soft tissue infection and facial cellulitis. Note edematous mucosa in left nasal cavity, with near complete obstruction.* (Right) *Coronal NECT shows opacification ➡ of the left maxillary sinus. Apical periodontitis with osseous dehiscence ➡ may contribute an odontogenic component to the ARS.*

KEY FACTS

TERMINOLOGY

- Group of disorders characterized by inflammation of nose & sinuses ≥ 12 consecutive weeks' duration
- This broad definition is based on signs and symptoms and does not restrict to specific etiology

IMAGING

- Nonenhanced bone CT is gold standard for evaluation
  - Sinus mucosal thickening and opacification with thickening & sclerosis of bony walls
  - Involved sinus normal or decreased volume
  - Intrasinus hyperdensity or calcifications common
  - Mucus retention cysts and polyps are common
  - May show established pattern of obstructive sinus disease

TOP DIFFERENTIAL DIAGNOSES

- Wegener granulomatosis, allergic fungal sinusitis, sinonasal polyposis, fungal mycetoma, sarcoidosis

PATHOLOGY

- Causes of CRS are numerous, disparate, & frequently overlapping
- Many factors & processes play role in etiology of chronic rhinosinusitis (CRS)

CLINICAL ISSUES

- Affects 12-14% of USA adult population
- Often associated conditions, such as allergy, underlying anatomic variations

DIAGNOSTIC CHECKLIST

- Coronal sinus CT is study of choice for evaluating changes in bone & identifying anatomic variants that may predispose to recurrent disease
- There is lack of correlation between symptomatology & imaging findings

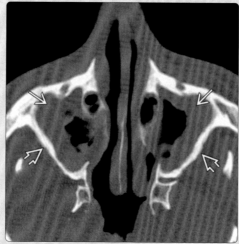
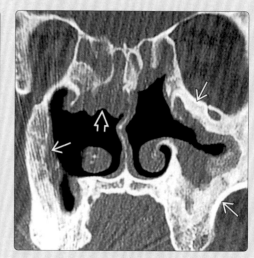

(Left) Axial bone CT in a cystic fibrosis patient shows bilateral maxillary sinus mucosal thickening ➡ and thickening of the bony sinus walls (osteitis) ➡ consistent with chronic inflammatory disease. (Right) Coronal bone CT shows marked diffuse chronic osteitis of the sinus walls ➡ in a patient with chronic rhinosinusitis (CRS) and sinonasal polyposis ➡. Extensive changes from prior endoscopic surgery are present.

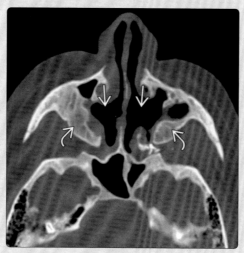
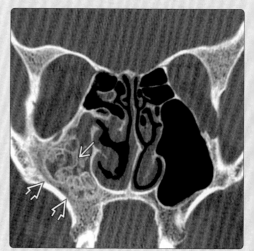

(Left) Axial bone CT demonstrates marked chronic osteitis ➡ of the walls of both maxillary sinuses. The volume of the sinuses is diminished, and there is patchy mucosal thickening. Changes are noted from prior surgery with bilateral antrostomy defects ➡. (Right) Coronal bone CT in a patient with longstanding right maxillary inflammation shows prominent calcifications ➡ within the inspissated right maxillary sinus secretions. Osteitis of the walls of the sinus is also present ➡.

TERMINOLOGY

Abbreviations

- Chronic rhinosinusitis (CRS)

Definitions

- Group of disorders characterized by inflammation of nose & sinuses ≥ 12 consecutive weeks duration
- This broad definition is based on signs and symptoms and does not restrict to specific etiology

IMAGING

General Features

- Best diagnostic clue
  - Sinus cavity opacification or mucosal thickening with hyperostosis/sclerosis of bony walls
- Location
  - Ethmoid sinus > maxillary sinus > frontal & sphenoid sinuses
- Size
  - Involved sinus normal or decreased volume
    - No sinus expansion in uncomplicated cases
- Morphology
  - Disease can be localized or diffuse and may occur in particular pattern (i.e., ostiomeatal unit) in cases caused by obstruction

Radiographic Findings

- Radiography
  - Can demonstrate opacification, mucosal thickening, bony sclerosis and air-fluid levels
  - Lower sensitivity and specificity than CT

CT Findings

- CECT
  - Enhancement of inflamed mucosa may be seen
  - Contrast **not** necessary in uncomplicated cases
- Bone CT
  - Mucosal thickening or opacification of sinus without expansion of sinus
  - Air fluid levels occur with superimposed acute sinusitis
  - Variable density of secretions
    - Isodense to hyperdense depending on protein, water, fungal content
    - Hyperdense secretions may be secondary to inspissated mucus or fungal sinusitis
  - Occasional calcification may be present
  - Bony walls of sinus thickened & sclerotic (osteitis)
  - Mucus retention cysts and polyps are common

MR Findings

- T1WI
  - Thickened mucosa isointense to other soft tissue
  - Variable signal of retained secretions depending on variable water & protein content
    - Higher protein content causes higher T1 signal
- T2WI
  - Mucosa typically hyperintense
  - Retained secretions range from hyperintense (↑ water content) to hypointense (↓ water, desiccated)
  - Thickened sinus walls evident on T2 MR

- T1WI C+
  - Mucosal enhancement typical
  - Contrast not necessary in uncomplicated cases

Imaging Recommendations

- Best imaging tool
  - Thin-section axial bone CT with coronal reformatted images
  - Mucosal thickening, opacification and osseous changes are well depicted
- Protocol advice
  - 0.625- to 1.25-mm thick axial CT in bone algorithm with coronal ± sagittal reformatted images

DIFFERENTIAL DIAGNOSIS

Fungal Sinusitis, Mycetoma

- Sinus opacified; hyperdensity/calcifications common
- Often seen in clinical setting of CRS
  - Bony changes may mimic CRS

Allergic Fungal Sinusitis

- Form of CRS in patients with asthma, allergy
- Involved sinuses opacified and expanded with central high-attenuation material

Sinonasal Polyposis

- Multiple, variable density polypoid soft tissue masses in nasal cavity & sinuses
- Expansion, remodeling of bony walls may be present
- Generally occurs in setting of CRS, with background of chronic mucosal thickening and opacification

Acute Rhinosinusitis

- Clinical course of shorter duration often following viral URI
- Air-fluid levels & bubbly secretions in addition to mucosal thickening
- No bone changes

Sinonasal Wegener Granulomatosis

- Nodular soft tissue thickening ± bone erosion
- Tends to affect nasal cavity > sinuses
  - Involves septum and turbinates

Sinonasal Sarcoidosis

- Nodular soft tissue thickening ± bone erosion
- Sinonasal involvement less common than Wegener
- Predilection for nasal cavity with septal involvement

PATHOLOGY

General Features

- Etiology
  - Definition of CRS is symptom based and does not include specific etiology
  - Causes of CRS are numerous, disparate, & frequently overlapping
    - Inflammation plays greater role than infection
    - Biofilms (antibiotic-resistant bacterial colonies) decrease antibiotic efficacy and release inflammatory mediators
  - Many factors & processes play role in etiology of CRS

- Systemic host factors: Allergic, immunodeficiency, genetic/congenital, mucociliary dysfunction, endocrine, neuromechanism
- Local host factors: Anatomic variants, neoplastic, acquired mucociliary dysfunction
- Environmental: Microorganisms, noxious chemicals, medications, trauma, surgery
- Genetics
  - Sporadic disease in most cases
  - Genetics play role when underlying systemic disorder present
    - Cystic fibrosis, primary ciliary dysmotility, immunodeficiency
- Associated abnormalities
  - Asthma, allergy (> 50% of CRS patients)
  - Dental disease (maxillary)
  - Sinonasal polyposis

Staging, Grading, & Classification

- Rhinosinusitis: 5 clinical categories
  - Acute, subacute, chronic, recurrent acute, acute exacerbation of CRS
- CRS may be bacterial, allergic, or fungal in nature
  - **Bacterial CRS**
    - Bacteria may initiate CRS, cause disease persistence, or exacerbate noninfectious inflammation
    - Common organisms: *Staphylococcus aureus*, coagulase negative *Staphylococcus*, anaerobic & gram-negative bacteria
  - **Allergic CRS**
    - Cytokines & allergic mediators → nasal allergic inflammation → mucosal swelling → obstruction of ostia
  - **Allergic fungal sinusitis**
    - Eosinophilic response to presence of noninvasive fungal elements

Gross Pathologic & Surgical Features

- Mucosal swelling, purulent discharge, polypoid changes, erythema

Microscopic Features

- Mixed inflammatory infiltrate of lymphocytes, plasma cells, eosinophils, interleukin-8, and interferon-γ
- Changes in adjacent bone similar to osteomyelitis

CLINICAL ISSUES

Presentation

- Most common signs/symptoms
  - Nasal obstruction, nasal discharge, hyposmia, anosmia
- Other signs/symptoms
  - Facial pain & pressure, headache
- CRS definition: Sinonasal infection/inflammation **> 12 weeks duration**
- Nasal endoscopy & CT performed to quantify mucosal disease and target culturing

Demographics

- Age
  - All ages affected
- Epidemiology

- CRS results in 18-22 million office visits in USA annually
- Prevalence of CRS difficult to determine due to heterogeneity of disease & diagnostic imprecision

Natural History & Prognosis

- Persistent, recurrent sinusitis often refractory to medical therapy
- Often associated conditions, such as allergy, underlying anatomic variations
  - Patients with mucosal eosinophilia have poorer outcomes
- Nasal endoscopy best objective indicator of early recurrent disease

Treatment

- **Pharmacologic therapy**: Antibiotics, antifungals, decongestants, antihistamines, topical steroids (allergic cases)
- Treatment of comorbid conditions (inhalant sensitivities, polyps, infections, immune deficiencies) critical for treatment success of CRS
- Surgery reserved for cases recalcitrant to medical therapy
  - **Functional endoscopic sinus surgery** current surgical treatment of choice

DIAGNOSTIC CHECKLIST

Consider

- CT study of choice in CRS
  - Evaluates changes in bone & identifies anatomic variants that may predispose to recurrent disease

Image Interpretation Pearls

- Mucosal thickening or opacification in nonexpanded sinus with associated bone thickening/sclerosis most consistent with CRS
- CT yields little information about etiology of mucosal changes
- **Note**: There is lack of correlation between symptomatology & imaging findings

SELECTED REFERENCES

1. Hamilos DL: Pediatric chronic rhinosinusitis. Am J Rhinol Allergy. 29(6):414-20, 2015
2. Huang BY et al: Current trends in sinonasal imaging. Neuroimaging Clin N Am. 25(4):507-25, 2015
3. Joshi VM et al: Imaging in sinonasal inflammatory disease. Neuroimaging Clin N Am. 25(4):549-68, 2015
4. Reddy CE et al: Imaging of granulomatous and chronic invasive fungal sinusitis: comparison with allergic fungal sinusitis. Otolaryngol Head Neck Surg. 143(2):294-300, 2010
5. Nair S: Correlation between symptoms and radiological findings in patients of chronic rhinosinusitis: a modified radiological typing system. Rhinology. 47(2):181-6, 2009
6. Chan Y et al: An update on the classifications, diagnosis, and treatment of rhinosinusitis. Curr Opin Otolaryngol Head Neck Surg. 17(3):204-8, 2009
7. Mafee MF et al: Imaging of rhinosinusitis and its complications: plain film, CT, and MRI. Clin Rev Allergy Immunol. 30(3):165-86, 2006
8. Benninger MS et al: Adult chronic rhinosinusitis: definitions, diagnosis, epidemiology, and pathophysiology. Otolaryngol Head Neck Surg. 129(3 Suppl):S1-32, 2003
9. Emanuel IA et al: Chronic rhinosinusitis: allergy and sinus computed tomography relationships. Otolaryngol Head Neck Surg. 123(6):687-91, 2000
10. Krouse JH: Computed tomography stage, allergy testing, and quality of life in patients with sinusitis. Otolaryngol Head Neck Surg. 123(4):389-92, 2000

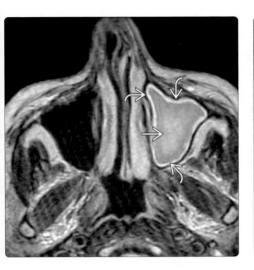

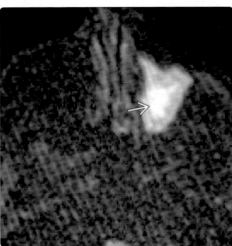

(Left) *Axial T2WI MR in a patient with CRS shows opacification of the left maxillary sinus. The central secretions are somewhat hypointense due to low water and high protein content* ➡. *Hyperintense inflamed mucosa is noted at the periphery* ➡. (Right) *Axial DWI MR in the same patient shows increased signal throughout the left maxillary sinus secretions suggesting restricted diffusion. The restricted diffusion is greatest centrally* ➡.

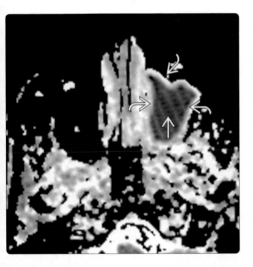

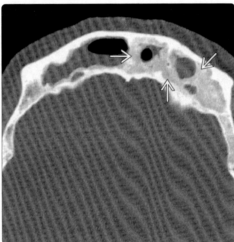

(Left) *Axial ADC map in the same patient confirms that restricted diffusion was the cause of the high signal on the DWI MR. Diminished signal on the ADC is noted in the secretions* ➡ *with high signal in the peripheral mucosa* ➡. (Right) *Axial bone CT in a patient with chronic frontal sinusitis shows mucosal thickening in both frontal sinuses. There is marked thickening of the sinus walls, particularly on the left* ➡. *The changes on the left mimic fibrous dysplasia.*

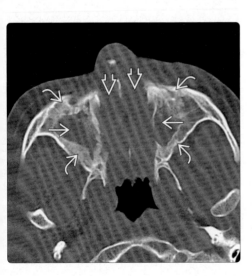

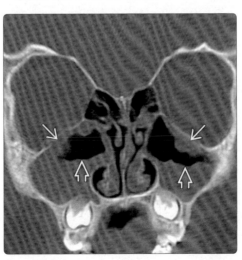

(Left) *Axial bone CT in a Wegener granulomatosis patient shows typical changes of CRS involving maxillary sinuses. Soft tissue opacifies the sinuses* ➡ *& nasal cavity* ➡. *There is prominent osteitis involving the sinus walls* ➡. (Right) *Coronal bone CT in a child with cystic fibrosis shows lobular mucosal thickening in both maxillary sinuses* ➡. *Fluid levels are present* ➡, *suggesting acute infection superimposed on chronic inflammation. Osteitis has not yet developed in this young patient.*

Complications of Rhinosinusitis

TERMINOLOGY

- Superficial complications: Osteomyelitis, subgaleal abscess (Pott puffy tumor), septic thrombophlebitis
- Orbital complications: Preseptal cellulitis/abscess, subperiosteal postseptal abscess (SPA), myositis of extraocular muscles, optic neuritis, septic thrombophlebitis
- Intracranial complications: Meningitis, epidural abscess, subdural empyema (SDE), cerebritis, brain abscess, cavernous sinus thrombosis (CST)

IMAGING

- CECT for SPA
- Contrast-enhanced MR with diffusion-weighted imaging for intracranial complications

TOP DIFFERENTIAL DIAGNOSES

- SPA: Orbital pseudotumor, extraconal neoplasm
- CST: Pseudotumor of cavernous sinus (Tolosa-Hunt), cavernous sinus neoplasm

- SDE: Subdural hygroma/hematoma
- Cerebritis or cerebral abscess: Tumefactive MS, glioblastoma, solitary metastasis, radiation necrosis

PATHOLOGY

- Intraorbital & intracranial complications more likely in acute rhinosinusitis
- Superficial complications more common in chronic rhinosinusitis
- Orbital complication most often from ethmoiditis
- Intracranial complications most often from frontal sinusitis

CLINICAL ISSUES

- Orbital complications more common in children
- Intracranial complications more common from adolescence to 2nd & 3rd decades
- Intracranial complications more common in males
- Intracranial complications → 50-80% mortality if not diagnosed and treated early

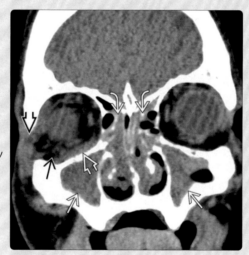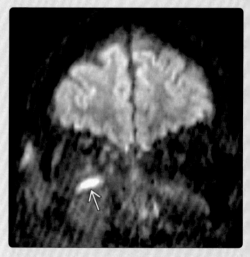

(Left) Coronal NECT in a man with acute sinusitis complicated by orbital cellulitis and subperiosteal abscess shows extensive opacification of maxillary sinuses ➡ and ethmoid air cells ↗, plus retrobulbar, extraconal subperiosteal fluid collection ➡, retrobulbar edema/stranding ➡, and preseptal edema ➡. (Courtesy M. Sturgill, MD.) (Right) Coronal DTI trace in same patient shows reduced diffusivity ➡, confirming subperiosteal abscess complicating acute sinusitis. (Courtesy M. Sturgill, MD.)

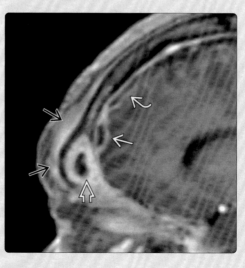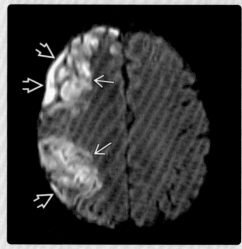

(Left) Sagittal SPGR C+ in frontal sinusitis complicated by subdural empyema, meningitis, cerebritis, and subgaleal abscess shows frontal sinus mucosal thickening and opacification ➡ with rim-enhancing subdural collection ➡ and leptomeningeal enhancement ➡. Note overlying enhancing subgaleal collection ➡. (Right) Axial DTI trace shows reduced diffusivity within a subdural empyema ➡, as well as diffuse cortical reduced diffusivity ➡ from cerebritis and associated acute infarcts complicating frontal sinusitis.

TERMINOLOGY

Abbreviations

- Rhinosinusitis (RS), acute rhinosinusitis (ARS), chronic rhinosinusitis (CRS)
- Subperiosteal postseptal abscess (SPA), cavernous sinus thrombosis (CST), epidural abscess (EDA), subdural empyema (SDE)

Definitions

- Complications of ARS or CRS may affect bone & overlying soft tissues, orbit, or intracranial cavity
  - **Superficial complications**: Osteomyelitis, subgaleal abscess (Pott puffy tumor), septic thrombophlebitis
  - **Orbital complications**: Preseptal cellulitis/abscess, SPA, myositis of extraocular muscles, optic neuritis, septic thrombophlebitis
  - **Intracranial complications**: Meningitis, EDA, SDE, cerebritis, brain abscess, CST

IMAGING

General Features

- Best diagnostic clue
  - SPA: Peripherally enhancing, central low-density mass in extraconal space with surrounding infiltration of fat
  - CST: Heterogeneously enhancing, enlarged cavernous sinus with enlarged or thrombosed superior ophthalmic vein (SOV)
  - EDA & SDE: Extraaxial fluid collection in epidural or subdural space, respectively, with reduced diffusivity & enhancing adjacent meninges
  - Cerebral abscess: Ring-enhancing mass in parenchyma with uniformly thick walls, central reduced diffusivity, & surrounding vasogenic edema
- Location
  - SPA: Superior (frontal sinusitis), medial (ethmoid sinusitis), or inferior (maxillary sinusitis) extraconal space near superior, medial, or inferior rectus muscles, respectively
  - EDA & SDE: Subfrontal when related to frontal or ethmoid sinusitis; above planum sphenoidale from sphenoiditis
  - Cerebral abscess: Most often in frontal lobes related to frontal sinusitis
  - Subgaleal abscess: Soft tissues anterior to frontal sinuses
- Morphology
  - SPA: Lentiform with base along orbital roof, lamina papyracea, or orbital floor
  - CST: Convex lateral margin of affected cavernous sinus
  - EDA: Lenticular pus collection adjacent to infected sinus
  - SDE: Crescentic pus collection conforming to shape of adjacent cerebrum
  - Cerebritis: Ill-defined edema within brain
  - Cerebral abscess: Round or ovoid parenchymal collection

CT Findings

- CECT
  - SPA
    - Peripherally enhancing, central low-attenuation collection in extraconal space

---

  - Infiltration of surrounding fat with swelling of affected extraocular muscle(s) ± dehiscence of sinus wall
  - CST
    - Heterogeneous or ↓ enhancement in sinus compared to contralateral side
    - Convex lateral margins (swollen) cavernous sinus
    - Enlargement of SOV
  - SDE
    - Extraaxial subdural collection with low attenuation centrally & adjacent enhancing dura
  - Cerebral abscess
    - Ring-enhancing lesion with uniform wall & surrounding low-density vasogenic edema
  - Skull osteomyelitis/subgaleal abscess
    - Focal bone lysis, sequestrum formation, reactive bone sclerosis
    - Focal rim-enhancing fluid collection with subgaleal abscess

MR Findings

- SPA
  - Peripherally enhancing extraconal collection with central reduced diffusivity, low to intermediate T1 signal, & ↑ T2 signal
- CST
  - Enlarged, heterogeneous enhancing cavernous sinus
  - Enlarged or thrombosed SOV (absence of flow void)
  - Extraocular muscles may be enlarged from venous engorgement
  - Cavernous carotid may be narrowed
- SDE
  - Crescentic, rim-enhancing extraaxial subdural collection with central reduced diffusivity, low T1 signal, & ↑ T2 signal
  - Adjacent enhancing dura
- EDA
  - Lenticular, rim-enhancing extraaxial epidural collection with central reduced diffusivity, low T1 signal, & ↑ T2 signal
  - Typically subjacent to affected sinus
- Cerebritis
  - Amorphous high signal area of brain on T2 or FLAIR
  - No ring enhancement on T1 C+ sequences
- Cerebral abscess
  - Ring-enhancing lesion with uniform wall thickness
  - Central reduced diffusivity, ↓ T1, & ↑ T2 signal
  - Rim may be ↓ T2 signal surrounded by ↑ T2 signal vasogenic edema

Imaging Recommendations

- Best imaging tool
  - CECT for SPA; contrast-enhanced MR with diffusion-weighted imaging for intracranial complications
- Protocol advice
  - SPA: Thin-section (1 mm) axial CT through sinuses/orbits post contrast with coronal reformats
  - CST: Multiplanar gadolinium-enhanced MR; post contrast with fat suppression; thin-slice axial and coronal through cavernous sinuses/orbits; SPGR +C to assess CST

o SDE/EDA/cerebritis/cerebral abscess: Multiplanar MR with gadolinium; diffusion-weighted imaging imperative

DIFFERENTIAL DIAGNOSIS

Subperiosteal Postseptal Abscess

- Orbital idiopathic inflammatory pseudotumor
- Extraconal neoplasm
  o Orbital lymphoproliferative lesions
  o Rhabdomyosarcoma

Cavernous Sinus Thrombosis

- Skull base idiopathic inflammatory pseudotumor
- Cavernous sinus neoplasm
  o Meningioma
  o Sinonasal non-Hodgkin lymphoma
  o Masticator space CNV3 perineural tumor

Subdural Empyema

- Subdural hygroma
- Chronic subdural hematoma

Cerebritis or Cerebral Abscess

- Cerebral contusion
- Multiple sclerosis
- Glioblastoma
- Radiation & chemotherapy effects on brain

PATHOLOGY

General Features

- Etiology
  o Intraorbital & intracranial complications more likely in ARS; osseous complications more common in CRS
    - Most complications result from bacterial infections; less likely fungal sources
    - Sinocutaneous fistulae reported with CRS of frontal sinus
  o SPA: Valveless ethmoidal veins allow access of ethmoid infection into orbit through thin lamina papyracea
    - Due to ethmoid > sphenoid > frontal > maxillary sinusitis
  o CST: Septic thrombophlebitis of ophthalmic veins
    - Can spread from maxillary sinus via inferior ophthalmic vein or sphenoid sinus via pterygoid plexus
  o Subgaleal abscess (Pott puffy tumor): Osteothrombophlebitis from frontal sinusitis
  o Intracranial complications: Most often from frontal sinusitis because of emissary vein network (Behçet plexus) connecting sinus mucosa with meninges
    - Frontal > > sphenoid > ethmoid > maxillary
- Associated abnormalities
  o Meningitis/meningoencephalitis, ± infarct

CLINICAL ISSUES

Presentation

- Most common signs/symptoms
  o SPA: Proptosis, chemosis, decreased visual acuity, limited ocular motility
  o Subgaleal abscess: Forehead swelling

o CST: Extremely ill patients with retroorbital pain, cranial nerve palsies, & signs of meningitis
o SDE/EDA: Headache, fever, signs of mass effect
o Cerebral abscess: Headache, seizure, focal deficits depending on location

Demographics

- Age
  o Orbital complications of RS more common in children
  o Intracranial complications more common from adolescence to 2nd & 3rd decades
- Gender
  o Intracranial complications more common in males
- Epidemiology
  o 3% of sinusitis patients experience preseptal or orbital inflammation
    - Permanent ocular sequelae in 4.5% of sinogenic orbital infections
    - 15-20% of optic neuritis due to posterior ethmoid & sphenoid sinusitis (rhinogenic optic neuritis)
  o 3% of headaches related to sinusitis
  o 3% of intracranial abscesses secondary to sinusitis

Natural History & Prognosis

- Potential progression of orbital complications if untreated
  o Periorbital cellulitis → SPA → CST → meningitis → SDE → cerebral abscess
  o Prognosis excellent with appropriate antibiotic therapy & surgical drainage
- Intracranial complications → 50-80% mortality if not diagnosed and treated early

Treatment

- Appropriate antibiotic therapy in all cases
- Surgical intervention for SPA (functional endoscopic sinus surgery), some SDE, and cerebral abscesses

DIAGNOSTIC CHECKLIST

Consider

- Imaging valuable in patients with uncertain diagnosis, deteriorating condition despite treatment
- Multiplanar contrast-enhanced MR with diffusion-weighted imaging advantageous for evaluating intracranial complications

Image Interpretation Pearls

- Can be difficult to distinguish SPA from phlegmon
- Compare size & shape of affected cavernous sinus to contralateral side to diagnose CST

SELECTED REFERENCES

1. Marchiano E et al: Characteristics of patients treated for orbital cellulitis: an analysis of inpatient data. Laryngoscope. 126(3):554-9, 2016
2. Cotes C et al: Facial vein thrombophlebitis: an uncommon complication of sinusitis. Pediatr Radiol. 45(8):1244-8, 2015
3. Dankbaar JW et al: Imaging findings of the orbital and intracranial complications of acute bacterial rhinosinusitis. Insights Imaging. 6(5):509-18, 2015
4. Fang A et al: Pediatric acute bacterial sinusitis: diagnostic and treatment dilemmas. Pediatr Emerg Care. 31(11):789-94; quiz 795-7, 2015
5. Cornelius RS et al: ACR appropriateness criteria sinonasal disease. J Am Coll Radiol. 10(4):241-6, 2013

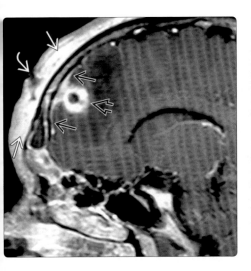

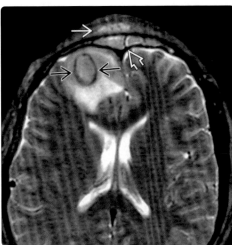

(Left) *Sagittal T1WI C+ MR shows frontal scalp thickening and enhancement* ➡️ *consistent with the diagnosis of Pott puffy tumor (subgaleal abscess) from frontal sinusitis. A draining sinus tract* ➡️ *is noted. Additional intracranial complications, including meningitis* ➡️ *and frontal lobe cerebral abscess* ➡️ *are present.* (Right) *Axial T2WI FS MR shows frontal scalp soft tissue swelling* ➡️ *and frontal sinus opacification* ➡️. *Cerebral abscess has a low T2 signal intensity rim* ➡️ *and extensive surrounding vasogenic edema.*

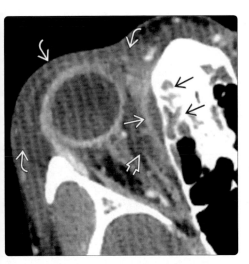

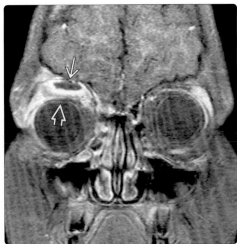

(Left) *Axial CECT shows a rim-enhancing subperiosteal abscess* ➡️ *overlying the orbital lamina with subjacent ethmoid sinus opacification* ➡️. *Note extensive intraconal stranding/edema* ➡️, *proptosis, and diffuse preseptal edema* ➡️ *in this patient with orbital & preseptal cellulitis complicating sinusitis.* (Right) *Coronal T1WI C+ FS MR shows a patient with frontal and ethmoid sinusitis complicated by an abscess* ➡️ *in the extraconal space with mass effect upon the globe, which is displaced* ➡️.

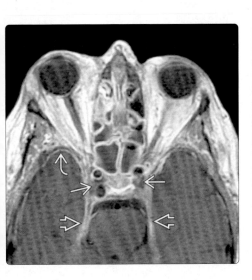

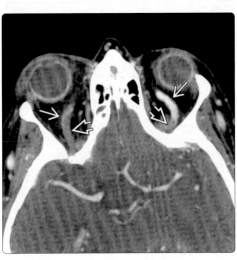

(Left) *Axial T1WI C+ MR in a patient with bilateral cavernous sinus thrombosis secondary to pansinusitis shows foci of nonenhancing thrombus* ➡️ *in both cavernous sinuses. Dural thickening is noted along the tentorium* ➡️ *and along the left greater sphenoid wing* ➡️. (Right) *Axial CECT in the same patient shows enlargement of both superior ophthalmic veins* ➡️ *with filling defects* ➡️ *in the entire vein on the right and posterior portion of the left vein.*

Allergic Fungal Sinusitis

TERMINOLOGY

- Severe form of chronic rhinosinusitis (CRS) with polyposis
- Allergic response to fungi characterized by eosinophilic mucin with noninvasive fungal hyphae

IMAGING

- Opacification and expansion of multiple sinuses with inspissated material
- Centrally hyperdense & peripherally hypodense on CT
- Expansion of sinus with bony remodeling and erosion
- Hypointense on MR (T2WI); may mimic air

TOP DIFFERENTIAL DIAGNOSES

- Sinonasal polyposis
- Eosinophilic mucin rhinosinusitis
- Sinus fungal mycetoma
- Sinonasal solitary polyp
- Sinonasal mucocele
- Sinonasal non-Hodgkin lymphoma

PATHOLOGY

- **Type 1**, IgE-mediated hypersensitivity
- Immune response to fungal antigens
- Viscous, eosinophilic mucin with fungal hyphae
- **Absence** of tissue invasion

CLINICAL ISSUES

- Symptoms: Nasal obstruction, rhinorrhea
- Immunocompetent patient with longstanding CRS
- Serum eosinophilia, elevated IgE
- Cutaneous sensitivity to fungal antigens
- Topical steroids 1st-line medical therapy
- Surgical debridement + perioperative systemic steroids
- Topical & systemic antifungal agents controversial

DIAGNOSTIC CHECKLIST

- Consider AFS in polyposis patient with increased density and expansion involving multiple sinuses
- Hypointense on T2WI, may mimic air

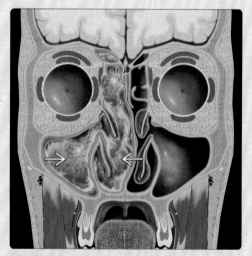
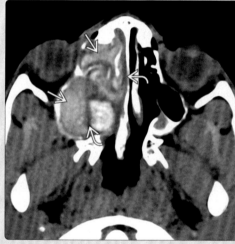

(Left) Coronal graphic shows classic features of allergic fungal sinusitis (AFS), including opacification and expansion of multiple paranasal sinuses and the nasal cavity. Centrally inspissated material is present ➡, surrounded by peripheral edematous mucosa. (Right) Axial NECT shows unilateral involvement of allergic fungal sinusitis. The involved sinuses are expanded, with centrally dense inspissated material ➡, and a peripheral rim of low attenuation ➡. Sinus involvement with AFS may be unilateral, or bilateral.

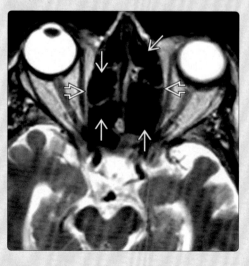
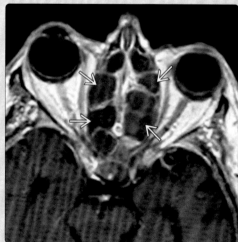

(Left) Axial T2WI MR in a patient with bilateral AFS shows diffuse hypointense signal within the involved ethmoid air cells ➡. There is mild sinus expansion with lateral bowing of the lamina papyracea ➡. Note that the very low signal mimics normal sinus aeration. (Right) Axial T1WI C+ MR in the same patient confirms that the ethmoid sinuses are not aerated, but are in fact completely opacified ➡. The surrounding mucosa shows peripheral linear enhancement.

TERMINOLOGY

Abbreviations

- Allergic fungal sinusitis (AFS) or rhinosinusitis (AFRS)

Definitions

- Severe form of chronic rhinosinusitis (CRS) with polyposis
  - Allergic response to fungi in susceptible individuals
- Characterized by production of eosinophilic mucin containing **noninvasive fungal hyphae**

IMAGING

General Features

- Best diagnostic clue
  - **Opacification** and **expansion** of multiple sinuses with inspissated material
  - Centrally **hyperdense** & peripherally **hypodense** on CT
  - Hypointense on MR (T2WI); may **mimic air**
- Location
  - Involves **multiple sinuses**
  - Unilateral or bilateral (50/50); R > L

CT Findings

- NECT
  - Hyperdense material **centrally** within opacified sinuses
  - Hypodense **rim of mucosa**
  - **Expansion** of sinus with bony remodeling and erosion

MR Findings

- T1WI
  - Signal **variable** (water, protein, & fungal content)
- T2WI
  - **Hypointense** signal **centrally** due to dense fungal concretions & heavy metals; may mimic air
- T1WI C+
  - Peripheral inflamed mucosa enhances

DIFFERENTIAL DIAGNOSIS

Sinonasal Polyposis

- Common form of CRS with polyposis
- Absence of specific antigenic or atopic etiology

Eosinophilic Mucin Rhinosinusitis

- Similar to AFS but without identifiable hyphae
- Systemic immune dysregulation; more often bilateral

Sinus Fungal Mycetoma

- Noninvasive fungal colonization without hyperimmunity
- Isolated, esp. maxillary; hyperdense with fine calcifications

Sinonasal Solitary Polyp

- Low-density mass with rim enhancement
- Classic antrochoanal polyp (ACP)

Sinonasal Mucocele

- Isolated postobstructive lesion
- Chronic expansile features with bony remodeling

Sinonasal Non-Hodgkin Lymphoma

- Sinonasal mass with bone destruction or remodeling

PATHOLOGY

General Features

- Etiology
  - **Type 1**, IgE-mediated hypersensitivity
    - Immune response to **fungal antigens**

Gross Pathologic & Surgical Features

- Viscous brown or greenish-black mucus with peanut butter/cottage cheese consistency

Microscopic Features

- Viscous, eosinophilic mucin with fungal hyphae
- Organisms: *Aspergillus*, *Curvularia*, *Bipolaris*, *Pseudallescheria*, and *Fusarium*
- **Absence** of tissue invasion

CLINICAL ISSUES

Presentation

- Most common signs/symptoms
  - Nasal obstruction, rhinorrhea
- Clinical profile
  - **Immunocompetent** patient with longstanding CRS
  - Polyposis history
  - Serum eosinophilia, elevated IgE
  - Cutaneous sensitivity to fungal antigens

Demographics

- Age
  - Primarily young adults (mean: ~ 30 years)
- Gender
  - Male predominance
- Epidemiology
  - Asthma history in 40%
  - Higher incidence in patients of African descent
  - Predilection for warm, humid climates

Natural History & Prognosis

- Slow, indolent course in face of CRS and allergy

Treatment

- Topical steroids 1st-line medical therapy
- Surgical debridement + perioperative systemic steroids
- Topical & systemic antifungal agents may be beneficial
  - Controversial effectiveness and risks

DIAGNOSTIC CHECKLIST

Consider

- AFS in polyposis patient with increased density and expansion involving multiple sinuses

Image Interpretation Pearls

- Hypointense on T2WI, may **mimic air**

SELECTED REFERENCES

1. Uri N et al: Allergic fungal sinusitis and eosinophilic mucin rhinosinusitis: diagnostic criteria. J Laryngol Otol. 127(9):867-71, 2013
2. Schubert MS: Allergic fungal sinusitis: pathophysiology, diagnosis and management. Med Mycol. 47 Suppl 1:S324-30, 2009

Sinus Mycetoma

TERMINOLOGY

- Fungus ball, aspergilloma
- Chronic, noninvasive form of fungal sinus infection
- Fungal colonization of material within sinus cavity

IMAGING

- Single paranasal sinus containing high-density material
  - Fine, round-to-linear matrix calcifications
- Maxillary > sphenoid > > frontal > ethmoid sinuses
  - Sinus often normal size and nonexpanded
  - May conform to sinus shape or be ball-shaped
- Hypointense T1 signal in solid, mycetomatous mass
- Hypointense T2 signal may be mistaken for air

TOP DIFFERENTIAL DIAGNOSES

- Chronic rhinosinusitis
- Allergic fungal sinusitis
- Sinonasal mucocele
- Invasive fungal sinusitis

PATHOLOGY

- Saprophytic fungal growth within paranasal sinus
  - Usually *Aspergillus fumigatus*
- No tissue invasion (mucosa, blood vessel, bone)
- Tightly packed fungal hyphae without allergic mucin

CLINICAL ISSUES

- Asymptomatic or mild pressure sensation overlying sinuses
- Immunocompetent, nonatopic, otherwise healthy patient
  - Most common in older female patients
  - Indolent course for up to years
- Surgical curettage is treatment of choice and is curative
- Antifungal therapy not effective

DIAGNOSTIC CHECKLIST

- Do not mistake low T2 signal for air
- Check for any signs of invasive disease
- May coexist with other forms of chronic rhinosinusitis

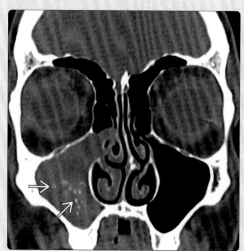
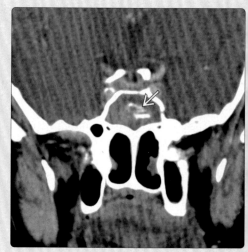

(Left) Coronal bone CT shows the classic features of a mycetoma within the right maxillary sinus. The sinus is opacified but not expanded. Mixed density material consistent with fungal elements and calcium deposits ➡ are present in the sinus. (Right) Coronal CECT in a patient with a sphenoid sinus mycetoma demonstrates multiple foci of calcification ➡ within the fungus ball. The sinus is opacified, and there is mild periosteal thickening but does not show expansion.

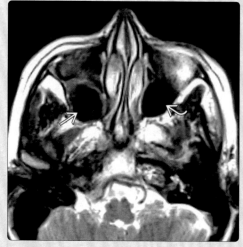
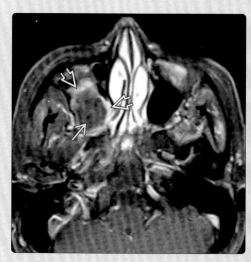

(Left) T2-weighted image in a middle-aged woman with a mild facial pressure sensation shows a normally aerated left maxillary sinus ➡ and opacification of the right maxillary sinus ➡ with material that is nearly as dark in signal as air. (Right) Axial enhanced T1-weighted image with fat suppression shows intermediate signal within the right maxillary sinus ➡, confirming that the cavity is opacified and not air-filled. The material within the sinus is nonenhancing, with rim enhancement evident in the surrounding mucosa ➡.

TERMINOLOGY

Synonyms

- Fungus ball, aspergilloma

Definitions

- Chronic, **noninvasive** form of fungal sinus infection
- Fungal **colonization** of material within sinus cavity

IMAGING

General Features

- Best diagnostic clue
  - Single paranasal sinus containing **high-density** material
    - Fine, round-to-linear matrix calcifications
- Location
  - Usually affects a **single sinus**
  - **Maxillary** > sphenoid > > frontal > ethmoid sinuses
- Size
  - Sinus often normal size and **nonexpanded**
- Morphology
  - May conform to sinus shape or be ovoid (ball-shaped) within sinus lumen

CT Findings

- CECT
  - Thickened mucosa at periphery of sinus may enhance
- Bone CT
  - Opacification or focal mass within sinus lumen
  - Central areas of **high density** ± calcification
  - Chronic mucoperiosteal change may be minor

MR Findings

- T1WI
  - Variable signal material in affected sinus
  - Hypointense **T1 signal** due to absence of free water in thick, solid, mycetomatous mass
- T2WI
  - **Hypointense** signal due to macromolecular protein binding may be mistaken for air
- T1WI C+
  - Inflamed peripheral mucosa may enhance

Imaging Recommendations

- Best imaging tool
  - NECT features diagnostic in typical cases; better for detecting Ca++

DIFFERENTIAL DIAGNOSIS

Chronic Rhinosinusitis

- Less likely to appear mass-like
- Ca++ less likely

Allergic Fungal Sinusitis

- Atopic patient with chronic polypoid rhinosinusitis
- Multiple sinus involvement with expansion & erosion
- High-density (CT) & low T1/T2 (MR) inspissated contents

Sinonasal Mucocele

- Sinus opacified and expanded
- Frontal & ethmoid > > maxillary & sphenoid

Invasive Fungal Sinusitis

- Immunocompromised patient
- Bone destruction & soft tissue invasion

Sinonasal Inverted Papilloma

- Mass in nasal cavity centered at middle meatus
- Convoluted, "cerebriform" architecture

PATHOLOGY

General Features

- Etiology
  - Saprophytic fungal growth within paranasal sinus
  - Usually *Aspergillus fumigatus*

Gross Pathologic & Surgical Features

- Thick, cheesy, gray-green, semisolid material

Microscopic Features

- Tightly packed fungal hyphae without allergic mucin
- No tissue invasion (mucosa, blood vessel, bone) compared to acute invasive fungal sinusitis

CLINICAL ISSUES

Presentation

- Most common signs/symptoms
  - Asymptomatic or mild pressure sensation overlying sinuses
- Clinical profile
  - Immunocompetent, nonatopic, otherwise healthy patient with no or minimal symptoms

Demographics

- Age
  - Most common in older patients but may occur in all ages
- Gender
  - Female predilection

Natural History & Prognosis

- Indolent course for up to years

Treatment

- Surgical curettage is treatment of choice and is curative
- Antifungal therapy not effective

DIAGNOSTIC CHECKLIST

Consider

- Typical patient is only mildly symptomatic & immunocompetent with single sinus involved
- May coexist with other forms of chronic rhinosinusitis

SELECTED REFERENCES

1. Robey AB et al: The changing face of paranasal sinus fungus balls. Ann Otol Rhinol Laryngol. 118(7):500-5, 2009
2. Daudia A et al: Advances in management of paranasal sinus aspergillosis. J Laryngol Otol. 122(4):331-5, 2008
3. Palacios E et al: Sinonasal mycetoma. Ear Nose Throat J. 87(11):606-8, 2008
4. Som PM et al: Hypointense paranasal sinus foci: differential diagnosis with MR imaging and relation to CT findings. Radiology. 176(3):777-81, 1990
5. Zinreich SJ et al: Fungal sinusitis: diagnosis with CT and MR imaging. Radiology. 169(2):439-44, 1988

Invasive Fungal Sinusitis

TERMINOLOGY

- Acute invasive fungal rhinosinusitis (AIFRS): Rapidly progressive (hours to days), transmucosal fungal sinus infection in immunocompromised patients with vascular, bone, soft tissues, orbit, & intracranial invasion resulting in "dry gangrene"

IMAGING

- AIFRS: Commonly starts at middle turbinate, spreads to maxillary & ethmoid sinuses > sphenoid sinus
- Sinus opacification with focal bone erosion, adjacent soft tissue infiltration, & nonenhancing mucosa
- CT: Sinus opacification with focal bone erosion, adjacent soft tissue infiltration
- MR: Superior for evaluating intraorbital & intracranial extension; best defines foci of nonenhancing tissue

TOP DIFFERENTIAL DIAGNOSES

- Acute rhinosinusitis with complication

- Sinonasal granulomatosis with polyangiitis
- Sinonasal squamous cell carcinoma
- Sinonasal non-Hodgkin lymphoma

PATHOLOGY

- 3 distinct clinical/pathologic subgroups of IFRS
  - **Acute (fulminant) invasive** FRS
  - **Chronic** IFRS (CIFRS)
  - **Granulomatous** IFRS (GIFRS)

CLINICAL ISSUES

- AIFRS: Facial swelling (65%), fever (63%), nasal congestion (52%), orbital symptoms (50%), headache (46%), cranial nerve palsy (42%)
  - **Mortality 50-80%**
  - Treatment: Radical debridement until histopathologically normal tissue reached
- CIFRS: Sinus pain, nasal discharge, epistaxis, fever, polyposis
- GIFRS: Enlarging cheek, orbit, or sinonasal mass

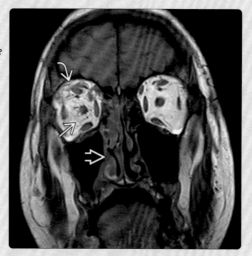
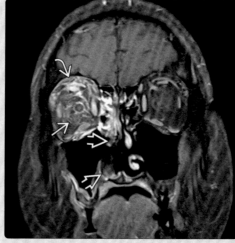

(Left) Coronal T1WI MR in patient with chronic myelogenous leukemia complicated by Rhizopus acute invasive fungal rhinosinusitis (AIFRS) shows subtle asymmetric soft tissue along lateral right nasal cavity & inferior turbinate ➡, & ill-defined soft tissue in intra- ➡ & extraconal ➡ retrobulbar right orbit. (Right) Coronal T1 C+ FS shows mucosal nonenhancement of right inferior & middle turbinates ➡ (black turbinate sign), & enhancing retroorbital intra- ➡ & extraconal ➡ soft tissue in this patient with AIFRS.

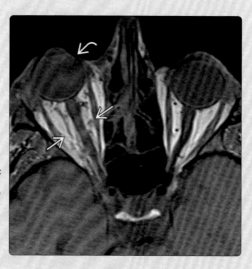
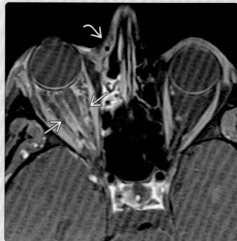

(Left) Axial T1WI MR in a patient with chronic myelogenous leukemia complicated by Rhizopus AIFRS shows ill-defined soft-tissue infiltration ➡ of the retrobulbar fat with associated proptosis ➡. (Right) Axial T1 C+ FS MR better defines the extent of infiltrating retrobulbar soft tissue ➡, as well as early involvement of the soft tissues overlying the nasal bridge ➡ in this patient who succumbed to disease.

TERMINOLOGY

Abbreviations

- Invasive fungal sinusitis
- Acute invasive fungal rhinosinusitis (AIFRS)
- Chronic invasive fungal rhinosinusitis (CIFRS)
- Granulomatous invasive fungal rhinosinusitis (GIFRS)

Definitions

- AIFRS: Rapidly progressive (hours to days), transmucosal fungal sinus infection in immunocompromised patients with vascular, bone, soft tissues, orbit, & intracranial invasion resulting in "dry gangrene"
- CIFRS: Indolent (weeks to months) infection with dematiaceous > hyaline molds or mucormycoses; associated with less severe immunocompromise than AIFRS
- GIFRS: Primarily found in Sudan, India, Pakistan, & Saudi Arabia; gradual onset fungal invasion of orbit, nose, paranasal sinuses, or maxilla with characteristic noncaseating granulomas

IMAGING

General Features

- Best diagnostic clue
  - Sinus opacification with focal bone erosion, adjacent soft tissue infiltration, & nonenhancing mucosa
  - 7-variable model with ≥ 2 positive variables yields 100% specificity & 100% PPV
    - Periantral fat, orbit, pterygopalatine fossa, nasolacrimal duct, lacrimal sac invasion, nasal septal ulceration, bone dehiscence
- Location
  - AIFRS: Commonly starts at middle turbinate, spreads to maxillary & ethmoid sinuses > sphenoid sinus
    - Spread from sinuses can extend in any direction & invade contiguous structures
  - CIFRS: Most common in ethmoid & sphenoid sinuses
- Morphology
  - Ill-defined or mass-like soft tissue lesion

CT Findings

- NECT
  - Earliest finding = unilateral nasal soft tissue thickening
  - Complete or partial soft tissue opacification of affected sinus; mucosal thickening
  - Hyperattenuation of secretions suggests fungal infection; more typical of chronic than acute
  - Focal areas of sinus wall erosion
    - **Subtle bone erosion** as fungi extend along vessels
  - Infiltration of adjacent fat & soft tissues
    - Maxillary sinus: **Perimaxillary fat infiltration** (anterior, premaxillary, or retroantral fat)
    - Can be present without bone destruction due to spread via perivascular channels
    - May be due to edema from vascular congestion, tissue infiltration by fungal elements
- CECT
  - Periantral soft tissues, adjacent musculature may enhance
- CTA

- Arterial narrowing/occlusion; defines extent of territorial ischemia; identifies pseudoaneurysm
- CTV: Better for identifying cavernous sinus thrombosis

MR Findings

- T1WI
  - Variable signal of material within involved sinus
    - Depends on protein/water content, presence of fungal elements
  - ↓ signal (similar to soft tissue) within periantral fat
    - **Key sequence** for identifying infiltration of fat planes
- T2WI
  - Variable signal of sinus secretions
    - Fungal elements may cause hypointense T2 signal
  - High signal edema with fat suppression
- T1WI C+
  - Loss of contrast enhancement lesions
    - **Nonenhancing, hypointense mucosa** (black turbinate sign) corresponds with **necrotic eschar**
  - Enhancement of involved soft tissues
  - Leptomeningeal enhancement
- MRA
  - Vascular involvement (narrowing, dissection, thrombosis)

Angiographic Findings

- Narrowing, dissection, thrombosis, or pseudoaneurysm

Imaging Recommendations

- Best imaging tool
  - CECT with soft tissue & bone windows to evaluate soft tissue infiltration & bone erosion
  - MR superior for evaluating intraorbital & intracranial extension, defining extent of nonenhancing lesions

DIFFERENTIAL DIAGNOSIS

Complicated Rhinosinusitis

- Patient may not be immunocompromised
- Bone erosion less likely
- Homogeneous air-fluid level, peripheral mucosal thickening in sinus
- Complications of subperiosteal postseptal abscess, cavernous sinus thrombosis, meningitis & cerebral abscess may appear similar to AIFRS

Sinonasal Granulomatosis With Polyangiitis

- Usually involves nasal cavity (septum & turbinates)
- Less mass-like soft tissue, prominent bone erosion
- Orbit & skull base involvement possible

Sinonasal Squamous Cell Carcinoma

- Typically immunocompetent patient
- Maxillary antrum most common site
- Solid mass with bone destruction

Sinonasal Non-Hodgkin Lymphoma

- Solid, homogeneous mass in nasal cavity
- ↓ T2 signal due to ↑ N:C ratio could mimic fungus

PATHOLOGY

General Features

- Etiology

○ Vascular & soft tissue invasion by fungi in high-risk patients with **neutropenia/dysfunctional neutrophils**
   – Poorly controlled diabetes mellitus (48%), half present with diabetic ketoacidosis
   – Hematologic malignancy (39%)
   – Corticosteroid use (28%)
   – Renal or liver failure (7%)
   – Solid organ transplant (6%)
   – HIV/AIDS (2%)
   – Autoimmune disease (1%)
○ Rare in patients with normal immune function
○ Spread from sinuses via vascular invasion

Staging, Grading, & Classification

- 3 distinct clinical/pathologic subgroups of IFRS
   ○ **Acute (fulminant) invasive** FRS
   ○ **Chronic invasive** FRS
   ○ **Granulomatous invasive** FRS
- Diagnosis requires identification of invasive fungi from biopsy samples of mucosa, submucosa, bone

Gross Pathologic & Surgical Features

- AIFRS: Necrotic, discolored tissue due to fungus

Microscopic Features

- AIFRS
   ○ Hyphal invasion of mucosa, submucosa, & blood vessels
   ○ Prominent tissue infarction & neutrophilic infiltrates
- CIFRS
   ○ Dense accumulation of hyphae with occasional vascular invasion
   ○ Sparse inflammatory reaction
   ○ > 50% *Aspergillus fumigatus*
- GIFRS
   ○ Noncaseating granulomatous response with considerable fibrosis & scant hyphae
   ○ Vasculitis, vascular proliferation, perivascular fibrosis
   ○ *Aspergillus flavus* most common

CLINICAL ISSUES

Presentation

- Most common signs/symptoms
   ○ AIFRS: Facial swelling (65%), fever (63%), nasal congestion (52%), orbital symptoms (50%), headache (46%), cranial nerve palsy (42%)
   ○ CIFRS: Pain, nasal discharge, epistaxis, fever, polyposis
   ○ GIFRS: Enlarging cheek, orbit, or sinonasal mass
- Clinical profile
   ○ AIFRS: Rapidly progressive (hours to days) invasive fungal infection in immunocompromised patient
   ○ CIFRS: Slowly destructive process (> 12 weeks) seen in patients with AIDS, DM, or those on corticosteroids
      – Can be seen in immunocompetent patient
      – May take months/years to develop, persist, recur
   ○ GIFRS: Immunocompetent host with > 12-week course of enlarging cheek, orbit, or sinonasal mass

Demographics

- Age
   ○ Typically in adults, mean age = 42 years
- Gender
   ○ Male 57%, female 43%
- Epidemiology
   ○ **Diabetic** or **immunocompromised** patients with predisposing conditions
   ○ GIFRS: Geographic predilection, primarily in Sudan, India, Pakistan, & Saudi Arabia

Natural History & Prognosis

- AIFRS: Can be rapidly progressive & fatal in hours to days without appropriate surgical-medical therapy
   ○ **Mortality 50-80%**
   ○ Best prognosis: Limited to sinus & proximal tissues, diabetes, & lack of extrasinonasal nonenhancing lesions
   ○ Poor prognosis: Orbital & intracranial involvement, persistent nonenhancing lesions after debridement, active hematologic disease
   ○ AIFRS of sphenoid sinus can lead to cavernous sinus thrombosis, carotid occlusion, mycotic aneurysm formation, cranial nerve dysfunction, cerebral infarction

Treatment

- Radical debridement until histopathologically normal tissue reached
   ○ Use preoperative identification of nonenhancing lesions as general prediction of surgical margins
- Antifungal therapy with amphotericin B
   ○ *Mucor* species not sensitive to "azole" antifungal
- Treat underlying condition responsible for immunocompromised state

DIAGNOSTIC CHECKLIST

Consider

- AIFRS in diabetic/immunocompromised patient with maxillary sinus disease & "dirty" periantral fat, even if no bone erosion present

Image Interpretation Pearls

- Do not confuse normal variability in volume of periantral fat or normal musculature with fat infiltration
- Evaluate orbit, intracranial cavities for involvement
- Closely examine cavernous sinus, internal carotid & basilar arteries in sphenoid AIFRS
- Identify nonenhancing foci on pre- & postoperative scans

SELECTED REFERENCES

1. Fu KA et al: Basilar artery territory stroke secondary to invasive fungal sphenoid sinusitis: a case report and review of the literature. Case Rep Neurol. 7(1):51-8, 2015
2. Gupta R et al: Allergic fungal rhino sinusitis with granulomas: a new entity? Med Mycol. 53(6):569-75, 2015
3. Kim JH et al: The prognostic value of gadolinium-enhanced magnetic resonance imaging in acute invasive fungal rhinosinusitis. J Infect. 70(1):88-95, 2015
4. Middlebrooks EH et al: Acute invasive fungal rhinosinusitis: a comprehensive update of CT findings and design of an effective diagnostic imaging model. AJNR Am J Neuroradiol. 36(8):1529-35, 2015
5. Rupa V et al: Current therapeutic protocols for chronic granulomatous fungal sinusitis. Rhinology. 53(2):181-7, 2015
6. Lee DH et al: Invasive fungal sinusitis of the sphenoid sinus. Clin Exp Otorhinolaryngol. 7(3):181-7, 2014
7. Aribandi M et al: Imaging features of invasive and noninvasive fungal sinusitis: a review. Radiographics. 27(5):1283-96, 2007
8. Silverman CS et al: Periantral soft-tissue infiltration and its relevance to the early detection of invasive fungal sinusitis: CT and MR findings. AJNR Am J Neuroradiol. 19(2): 321-5, 1998

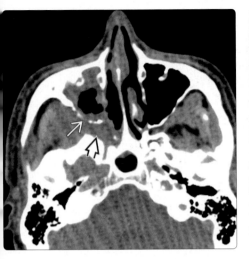
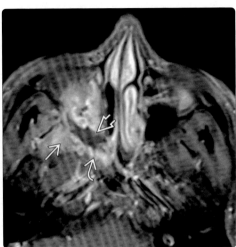

(Left) Axial NECT in a diabetic patient with mucormycosis AIFRS shows circumferential disease in the right maxillary sinus with extensive erosion of the posterior sinus wall ➤ & replacement of the retroantral and pterygopalatine fossa fat with soft tissue ⇨. (Right) Axial T1 C+ FS MR shows focal areas of nonenhancement ⇨ of the maxillary sinus mucosa corresponding to a necrotic eschar, as well as enhancing soft tissue replacement of the retroantral fat ➤ & pterygopalatine fossa ⟶.

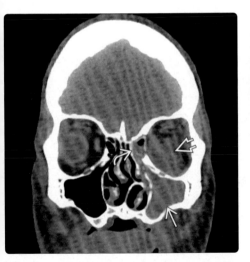
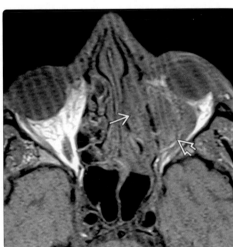

(Left) Coronal NECT in a patient with diabetes, renal failure, & orbital pain shows opacification of the left maxillary sinus ➤ & ethmoid air cells ➤ with extensive extra- & intraconal retroorbital soft tissue ⇨ encasing & displacing the medial & inferior rectus muscles. (Right) Axial T1 MR shows transosseous extension of ethmoid sinus disease ➤ into the retroorbital soft tissues ⇨. Orbital exenteration, maxillectomy, & ethmoidectomy revealed Mucor AIFRS.

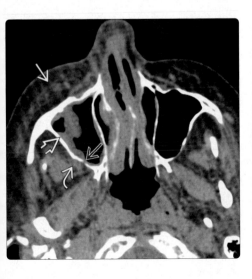
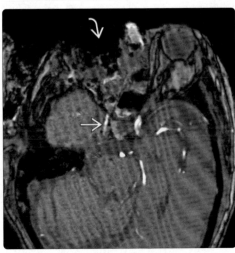

(Left) Axial NECT in a diabetic patient shows relatively unimpressive right maxillary sinus mucosal disease ⇨, but alarming replacement of the premaxillary ➡ & retroantral fat ⟶ by infiltrating soft tissue that proved to be Mucor AIFRS. Note the subtle bony dehiscence ⇨ of posterior wall of maxillary sinus. (Right) Axial TOF MRA following right orbital exenteration ⟶ demonstrates segmental narrowing & luminal irregularity ➤ of the right cavernous internal carotid artery due to Mucor AIFRS.

KEY FACTS

TERMINOLOGY

- Nonneoplastic, inflammatory swelling of sinonasal mucosa that buckles to form "polyps"

IMAGING

- Involves nasal cavity and paranasal sinuses (vs. retention cysts mainly within sinuses)
  - Predominantly along lateral nasal wall and roof of nasal cavity
  - Commonly involves middle turbinate, sparing inferior turbinate
  - Anterior > posterior
  - Primarily mucoid or soft tissue density
  - Remodeling of sinonasal bones common in severe cases
- MR complimentary to CT for assessing intraorbital and intracranial extension, differentiation of sinonasal polyposis (SNP) from neoplasm

TOP DIFFERENTIAL DIAGNOSES

- Allergic fungal sinusitis
- Cystic fibrosis
- Mucous retention cyst
- Solitary polyp
- Granulomatosis with polyangiitis

PATHOLOGY

- Formal pathogenesis of SNP has not been clarified
  - Chronic inflammation is major factor
  - Associated with allergy, asthma, primary ciliary dyskinesia, aspirin sensitivity, and cystic fibrosis

CLINICAL ISSUES

- Although not life threatening, chronic SNP unresponsive to therapy can be chronic, debilitating disease
- Medical therapy = treatment of choice
- Surgery reserved for symptomatic relief and correction of cosmetic deformities, orbital and intracranial involvement

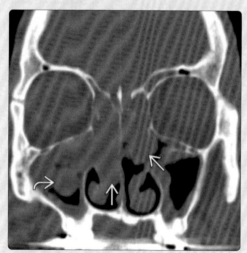
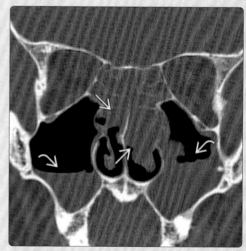

(Left) Coronal bone CT shows the classic appearance of sinonasal polyposis (SNP) with multiple lobular soft tissue masses involving the nasal cavity ➡ and paranasal sinuses ➡. In this case, the involvement is diffuse and bilateral, without expansion. (Right) Coronal bone CT in a patient with polyposis and new onset of acute sinusitis symptoms shows polyps ➡ in the nasal cavity occluding the middle meatuses. Fluid levels ➡ consistent with acute inflammation are present in the maxillary sinuses.

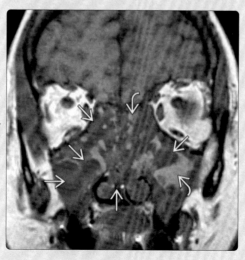
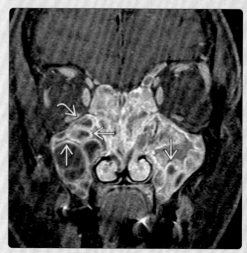

(Left) Coronal T1WI MR shows multiple intermediate signal intensity polyps ➡ filling the nasal cavity maxillary, and ethmoid sinuses. Trapped secretions with high protein content ➡ (T1 shortening) are also noted. (Right) Coronal T1WI C+ FS MR in the same patient shows enhancement of the inflamed mucosa ➡ at the periphery of the polyps. There is slight expansion of the right maxillary sinus with elevation of the orbital floor ➡.

TERMINOLOGY

Abbreviations

- Sinonasal polyposis (SNP)

Synonyms

- Chronic rhinosinusitis with polyposis (CRSwP)
- Polyposis nasi; hypertrophic polypoid rhinosinusitis

Definitions

- Nonneoplastic, inflammatory swelling of sinonasal mucosa that buckles to form "polyps"
- SNP is general term for nonspecific majority of cases
- Specific minority forms of CRSwP are classified separately

IMAGING

General Features

- Best diagnostic clue
  - Polypoid masses involving nasal cavity and paranasal sinuses mixed with chronic inflammatory secretions
- Location
  - Predominantly along lateral nasal wall (near middle meatus), roof of nasal cavity, and ethmoids
  - Commonly involves middle turbinate, sparing inferior turbinate
    - May reflect differences in VCAM1 and CysLT1R protein receptor expression in turbinates
  - Anterior sinonasal cavities > posterior
  - Involves nasal cavity and paranasal sinuses (vs. retention cysts mainly within sinuses)
  - Usually **multiple and bilateral**; may be unilateral
- Size
  - Variable; up to several centimeters
- Morphology
  - Polypoid, lobular

CT Findings

- NECT
  - Primarily mucoid or soft tissue density
    - May be hyperdense with ↑ protein, ↓ water content, or colonization with fungal elements
- CECT
  - Mucosal enhancement at periphery of polyps
    - **No central enhancement** (as seen with neoplasms)
- Bone CT
  - Multiple, polypoid, soft tissue masses within nasal cavity and paranasal sinuses
  - **Remodeling** of sinonasal **bones** common in severe cases
    - May have areas of **bone erosion**
  - Other findings
    - Ethmoid sinus remodeling with trabecular loss and convex lateral walls bulging into orbits
    - **Air-fluid levels** nonspecific and may signal superinfection or trapped fluid
    - Truncation of bulbous, bony, inferior portion of middle turbinates

MR Findings

- T1WI
  - Fresh mucus (high water content) is hypointense
  - Bizarre mixture of layered signals seen in sinuses and nose
    - Results from polyps mixed with various ages of mucus
- T2WI
  - Fresh mucus is hyperintense
  - Chronic, inspissated mucus can appear **low signal** (mimics air)
- T1WI C+
  - Thin mucosal enhancement between polypoid soft tissue lesions without central enhancement

Imaging Recommendations

- Best imaging tool
  - NECT in coronal plane is adequate for most cases
- Protocol advice
  - MR complimentary to CT for assessing intraorbital and intracranial extension, differentiation of SNP from neoplasm

DIFFERENTIAL DIAGNOSIS

Allergic Fungal Sinusitis

- Severe chronic rhinosinusitis with allergic response to fungi
- Eosinophilic mucin containing noninvasive fungal hyphae
- Associated with sinonasal polyps; considered to be specific minority subtype of SNP
- Multiple unilateral or pansinus involvement
- CT shows high-density central material with low-density rim in expanded sinuses
- MR shows low signal particularly on T2WI

Cystic Fibrosis

- Marked paranasal sinus hypoplasia
  - Frontal sinus aplasia and sphenoid hypoplasia useful predictors
- SNP

Sinonasal Retention Cyst

- Clinically asymptomatic or sinusitis history
- Lesions within sinuses with relative sparing of nasal cavity
- Difficult to distinguish from polyps based on density/signal intensity alone
  - Fluid density/signal on CT/MR; no central enhancement

Sinonasal Solitary Polyps

- Unilateral, solitary lesion
- Extends from antrum through widened infundibulum into nasal cavity

Granulomatosis With Polyangiitis

- Multisystem granulomatous disease involving lung and kidney
- Nodular soft tissue most often involving septum, inferior turbinates, and lateral nasal wall
- Bony destruction (septal perforation) rather than remodeling
- Orbital invasion relatively common

PATHOLOGY

General Features

- Etiology
  - Inflammatory swelling of unstable respiratory mucosa

- o Formal pathogenesis of SNP has not been clarified; chronic persistent inflammation is major factor
  - – Principal hypothesis: Allergy and inflammation cause unstable mucosa with epithelial cell proliferation and morphologic changes
  - – Others factors implicated
    - □ Cytokines (*IL-5*, *IL-10*, HLA-G, granulocyte-macrophage colony-stimulating factor, tumor necrosis factor)
    - □ Mechanical forces in areas of contact between opposing mucosal membranes
    - □ Potential role of bacterial biofilms
- Genetics
  - o No causative chromosomal aberrations identified
  - o ↑ in cystic fibrosis patients (autosomal recessive)
- Associated abnormalities
  - o Associated with CRS, allergy, asthma, primary ciliary dyskinesia, aspirin sensitivity, and cystic fibrosis
  - o Polyposis and allergic fungal sinusitis (AFS) are **frequently** seen in association (~ 66% of cases)

Gross Pathologic & Surgical Features

- Pinkish, fleshy, pedunculated polypoid sinonasal masses with glistening mucoid surface

Microscopic Features

- Intact surface respiratory epithelium
- Underlying stroma is edematous with inflammatory cellular infiltrate and variable vascularity, glands, and goblet cells
- Seromucinous glands usually absent
- Eosinophil-dominated inflammation with component of neutrophils and mast cells
- May show squamous, cartilaginous, or osseous metaplasia ± surface ulceration and granuloma formation
  - o Superinfecting bacteria include *Pseudomonas aeruginosa*, *Bacteroides fragilis*, *Staphylococcus aureus*

CLINICAL ISSUES

Presentation

- Most common signs/symptoms
  - o Progressive nasal stuffiness and obstruction
  - o Sensation of secretions that cannot be expelled
- Other signs/symptoms
  - o Rhinorrhea, facial pain, headaches, and anosmia
  - o Cosmetic deformity, hypertelorism in cases of "polypoid mucocele"
- Clinical profile
  - o Allergic patient with progressive nasal stuffiness
  - o Polyps identified with nasal endoscopy

Demographics

- Age
  - o Most common in adults > 20 years
  - o Rare in children < 5 years
- Epidemiology
  - o Frequency of polyps
    - – 1-2% of normal population
    - – 5% of extrinsic asthma patients
    - – 13% of intrinsic bronchial asthma patients
    - – 16% of "dental" sinusitis patients
    - – 20% of cystic fibrosis patients

- – > 50% of aspirin-intolerant patients

Natural History & Prognosis

- Often waxing and waning; chronic, relentless disease
- Eosinophilic-type CRSwP more likely to have postoperative recurrence, shorter disease-free interval
- If left unattended, may become highly deforming in central facial region
- Although not life threatening, chronic SNP unresponsive to therapy can be chronic, debilitating disease

Treatment

- Medical therapy = treatment of choice
- Topical and oral corticosteroids to reduce rhinitis symptoms, ↓ polyp size, and reduce recurrence
- Antibiotics when superinfected
- Surgery reserved for symptomatic relief and correction of cosmetic deformities, orbital and intracranial involvement
  - o Endoscopic polypectomy, functional endoscopic sinus surgery, or sphenoethmoidectomy
  - o Usually only temporary relief

DIAGNOSTIC CHECKLIST

Consider

- If density of expansile polyps is increased ± signal heterogeneous on MR, AFS in setting of polyposis is likely

Image Interpretation Pearls

- Polyps occur in sinuses **and** nasal cavity
  - o Mucous retention cysts typically located in sinuses only
- Individual polyps cannot be differentiated from mucous retention cysts based on density or signal characteristics alone
- Do not be alarmed if areas of **bone erosion** are present in addition to remodeling
  - o If predominant pattern is aggressive-appearing bone destruction, must rule out malignancy or granulomatous disease

SELECTED REFERENCES

1. Brescia G et al: A prospective investigation of predictive parameters for post-surgical recurrences in sinonasal polyposis. Eur Arch Otorhinolaryngol. 273(3):655-60, 2016
2. White LC et al: Why sinonasal disease spares the inferior turbinate: An immunohistochemical analysis. Laryngoscope. 126(5):E179-83, 2015
3. Brescia G et al: Can a panel of clinical, laboratory, and pathological variables pinpoint patients with sinonasal polyposis at higher risk of recurrence after surgery? Am J Otolaryngol. 36(4):554-8, 2015
4. Malagutti N et al: Analysis of Il-10 gene sequence in patients with sinonasal polyposis. Int J Immunopathol Pharmacol. 28(3):434-9, 2015
5. Avelino MA et al: The human leukocyte antigen G molecule (HLA-G) expression in patients with nasal polyposis. Braz J Otorhinolaryngol. 80(3):208-12, 2014
6. Rizzo R et al: Infection and HLA-G molecules in nasal polyposis. J Immunol Res. 2014:407430, 2014
7. Siddiqui J et al: Sinonasal bony changes in nasal polyposis: prevalence and relationship to disease severity. J Laryngol Otol. 127(8):755-9, 2013
8. Blomqvist EH et al: A randomized prospective study comparing medical and medical-surgical treatment of nasal polyposis by CT. Acta Otolaryngol. 129(5):545-9, 2009
9. Bonfils P et al: Evaluation of combined medical and surgical treatment in nasal polyposis - III. Correlation between symptoms and CT scores before and after surgery for nasal polyposis. Acta Otolaryngol. 128(3):318-23, 2008
10. Eggesbø HB et al: Hypoplasia of the sphenoid sinuses as a diagnostic tool in cystic fibrosis. Acta Radiol. 40(5):479-85, 1999
11. Drutman J et al: Sinonasal polyposis: investigation by direct coronal CT. Neuroradiology. 36(6):469-72, 1994

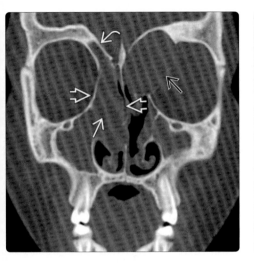

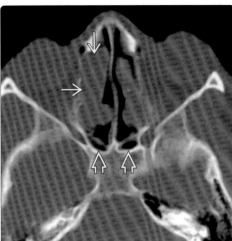

(Left) Coronal bone CT in a 14-year-old girl with cystic fibrosis (CF) shows typical features of SNP, including polypoid material opacifying the right ethmoid air cells and extending into the nasal cavity ➡ with benign osseous remodeling ➡. Note a large left ethmoid mucocele ➡ with dehiscence into the orbit and a hypoplastic right frontal sinus ➡. (Right) Axial bone CT in a CF patient shows a large polyp ➡ in right nasal cavity associated with the middle turbinate. Marked hypoplasia of the sphenoid sinuses ➡ is commonly seen with CF.

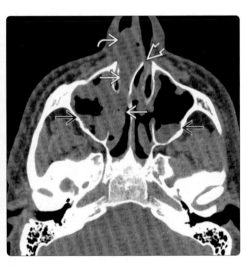

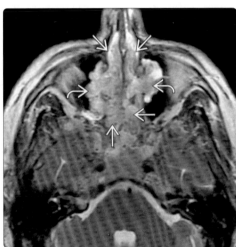

(Left) Axial NECT demonstrates a large polyp filling the right nasal cavity ➡ and extending out the right nare ➡. Note the benign osseous remodeling with leftward deviation of the bony nasal septum ➡. Bubbly air-fluid levels ➡ in the maxillary sinuses are nonspecific but may indicate an acute inflammatory component of the sinusitis. (Right) Axial T2WI MR in a severe case of polyposis shows multiple hyperintense polyps filling the nasal cavity ➡ and involving the medial portions of the maxillary sinuses ➡.

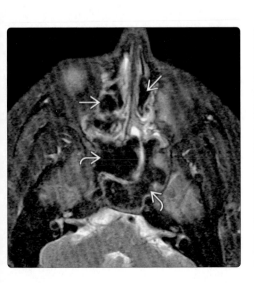

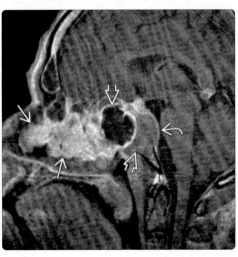

(Left) Axial T2WI FS MR demonstrates hypointense polyps filling and expanding the ethmoid ➡ and sphenoid sinuses ➡. On this sequence, the polyps mimic the hypointense signal of air-filled sinuses. (Right) Sagittal T1WI C+ MR in the same patient shows enhancement in multiple nasal cavity polyps ➡. The sphenoid polyps show mixed signal intensity ➡. Note the marked thinning of the clival cortex ➡.

KEY FACTS

IMAGING

- Most common type is **antrochoanal**
  - Polypoid mass extends from maxillary antrum → enlarged maxillary ostium or accessory ostium → nasal cavity
- Peripheral enhancement with **no** central enhancement
- Bone surrounding infundibulum/accessory ostium smoothly remodeled, not destroyed
- Large lesions extend into nasopharyngeal airway

TOP DIFFERENTIAL DIAGNOSES

- Intranasal glioma
- Nasoethmoidal cephalocele
- Juvenile angiofibroma
- Inverted papilloma
- Esthesioneuroblastoma
- Mucocele, sinonasal

PATHOLOGY

- **Inflammatory polyp** resulting from edematous hypertrophy of respiratory epithelium
- Postobstructive inflammatory disease is often present
  - Greater when antrochoanal polyp exits antrum via natural ostium vs. accessory ostium

CLINICAL ISSUES

- 4-6% of all sinonasal polyps
- Most common in **teenagers** & young adults
- Typical symptoms: Unilateral nasal obstruction, worse on expiration
- Complete surgical removal of nasal & antral components is treatment of choice

DIAGNOSTIC CHECKLIST

- Begin imaging evaluation with coronal bone CT
- If bone CT or endoscopy appearance is atypical, consider MR with contrast to rule out neoplasm

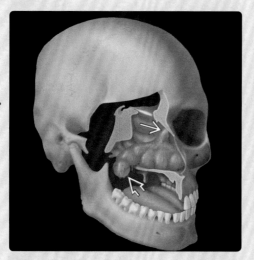
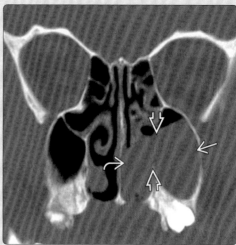

(Left) Longitudinal oblique graphic shows an antrochoanal polyp (ACP) extending from maxillary antrum through a posterior fontanelle ➡ into the nasal cavity. Note the posterior extension of the polyp into the nasopharynx ➡. (Right) Coronal bone CT shows a typical ACP extending from the left maxillary antrum ➡ into the nasal cavity ➡ via a secondary ostium ➡ located posterior to the ostiomeatal complex.

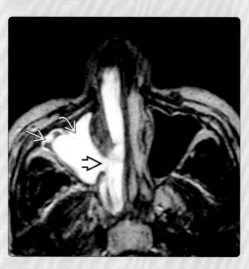
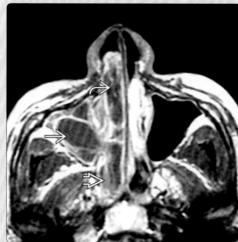

(Left) Axial T2 MR shows diffuse, homogeneous, hyperintense signal ➡ within an ACP. The polyp extends into the nasal cavity via a secondary ostium ➡. A small amount of trapped secretions ➡ are noted lateral to the lesion. (Right) Axial T1 C+ MR shows the antral ➡, nasal ➡, and nasopharyngeal ➡ components of this ACP. Note that there is thin peripheral, but no central or nodular enhancement of the lesion, which helps to distinguish it from a neoplasm.

TERMINOLOGY

Abbreviations

- Antrochoanal polyp (ACP)

Synonyms

- Killian polyp

Definitions

- ACP: Inflammatory polyp arising from maxillary sinus antrum, herniating through major or accessory ostium into nasal cavity ± prolapsing into nasopharynx
  - Other solitary polyps named based upon site of origin → site of termination

IMAGING

General Features

- Best diagnostic clue
  - **Dumbbell-shaped lesion** with maxillary antral origin connected by narrow stalk from maxillary infundibulum/accessory ostium → nasal cavity
- Location
  - Most common type: Antrochoanal polyp
    - Solitary polypoid mass fills maxillary antrum, spills through enlarged maxillary ostium & infundibulum or accessory ostium into nasal cavity
      □ Large lesions extend through choana into nasopharyngeal airway
  - Nasochoanal, sphenochoanal, frontochoanal, & ethmochoanal polyps are less common
- Size
  - Typically large
    - May reach > 5 cm in size
- Morphology
  - Dumbbell-shaped polypoid mass
  - Bulbous nasopharyngeal component in larger lesions

Radiographic Findings

- Lateral radiography: Polypoid soft tissue density resting on nasal surface of soft palate surrounded by air

CT Findings

- CECT
  - Peripheral enhancement of surrounding mucosa with **no central enhancement**
- Bone CT
  - Well-defined, dumbbell-shaped, low mucoid density mass
    - Arises from maxillary antrum, extends through widened maxillary ostium or accessory ostium into ipsilateral nasal cavity
      □ Bone surrounding infundibulum/accessory ostium smoothly remodeled, not destroyed
      □ Stalk or midportion of dumbbell may be difficult to see on coronal sinus CT
    - Large lesions extend into nasopharyngeal airway
    - May have ↑ density centrally depending on chronicity ± fungal colonization
    - Metaplastic ossification rarely occurs with polyps

MR Findings

- T1WI

- Low signal most common due to ↑ water content
  - Variable signal intensity with chronicity
- T2WI
  - High-intensity polyp (near water signal intensity)
- T1WI C+
  - No enhancement of central portion of lesion
  - Thin, peripheral enhancement of mucosa

Imaging Recommendations

- Best imaging tool
  - If endoscopic examination clearly reveals ACP, unenhanced coronal bone CT alone may be sufficient
- Protocol advice
  - Thin-slice axial bone CT with coronal & sagittal reformats
  - MR with contrast may be used in some cases to confirm polyp vs. neoplasm

DIFFERENTIAL DIAGNOSIS

Nasal Glioma

- Intranasal type: Soft tissue mass in nasal cavity
  - Maxillary antrum uninvolved except via secondary obstruction
- Tract through septum to skull base; rare in nasopharynx

Frontoethmoid Cephalocele

- Nasoethmoidal type: Polypoid mass in nose
- Intracranial origin with connection to brain parenchyma
- Defect in cribriform plate

Juvenile Angiofibroma

- Adolescent boys with **enhancing mass** centered in posterior nasal cavity near sphenopalatine foramen
- Often extends into pterygopalatine fossa
- May obstruct maxillary sinus but only extends into this sinus when very large

Sinonasal Inverted Papilloma

- Adult men with **enhancing mass** along lateral nasal wall near middle meatus
- Often herniates into maxillary sinus causing ostiomeatal unit pattern of obstructive sinus opacification
- Convoluted, cerebriform architecture

Esthesioneuroblastoma

- Diffusely **enhancing mass** in superior nasal cavity
- Aggressive, destructive lesion passes through cribriform plate into anterior cranial fossa
- Maxillary involvement unusual

Mucocele, Sinonasal

- Expanded sinus

PATHOLOGY

General Features

- Etiology
  - Inflammatory polyp (retention cyst) of maxillary sinus resulting from edematous hypertrophy of respiratory epithelium
    - Fluid accumulates in lamina propria with polypoid distention, rather than glandular distention

- – Allergy & repeated bouts of sinusitis thought to play role in etiology
- – ↓ lipoxygenase pathway products might be involved in pathogenesis
- – Urokinase-type plasminogen activator and plasminogen activator 1 may also have role
  - o Passage of antral polyp into nose can occur via 2 different routes
    - – Through maxillary infundibulum
    - – Through **accessory ostium** of maxillary sinus
  - o Sphenochoanal polyps route
    - – Sphenoid sinus → sphenoid ostium → sphenoethmoidal recess → choana → nasopharynx
- Associated abnormalities
  - o Postobstructive inflammatory disease
    - – Greater when ACP exits antrum via natural ostium vs. accessory ostium

Gross Pathologic & Surgical Features

- Glistening, pale, mucosa-covered, grape-like mass
- Superficially looks like any other nasal polyp
  - o Careful inspection reveals **stalk** leading laterally through maxillary sinus primary or accessory ostium

Microscopic Features

- Edematous hypertrophy of respiratory epithelium of maxillary antrum
  - o No distention of mucous glands of sinus
- Loose mucoid stroma and mucous glands covered by respiratory epithelium
  - o Reactive atypical stromal cells or cysts may be seen
- Few inflammatory cells with no eosinophils

CLINICAL ISSUES

Presentation

- Most common signs/symptoms
  - o Unilateral nasal obstruction, worse on expiration
    - – When large, protrudes into nasopharyngeal airway
    - – May mimic nasopharyngeal tumor
- Other signs/symptoms
  - o Nasal discharge
  - o Mouth breathing, snoring with sleep apnea
  - o Cheek pain, sore throat, headache
- Clinical profile
  - o Teenager with unilateral nasal obstruction due to unilateral nasal polyp
  - o Rhinoscopic examination: Polyp occludes nasal airway
    - – Obstruction of nasopharynx may be clinically confused with primary nasopharyngeal tumor

Demographics

- Age
  - o Most common in teenagers & young adults
    - – **Mean: ~ 10 years**
    - – 2nd smaller group presents in 3rd-5th decades
- Gender
  - o M > F
- Epidemiology
  - o 4-6% of all sinonasal polyps
  - o Antrochoanal > > sphenochoanal > ethmochoanal polyp
  - o Much more prevalent in pediatric population

- o 40% of patients have allergies but no etiologic link to allergies

Natural History & Prognosis

- Herniation of ACP into nasal cavity may take years to occur
- Surgical removal of both components creates surgical cure
  - o If surgical removal of nasal portion of ACP is completed without removal of antral base, recurrence can be expected
    - – Mean time to recurrence: 45 months

Treatment

- Complete surgical removal of nasal & antral components is treatment of choice
  - o Surgical procedures
    - – Intranasal avulsion, Caldwell-Luc antrostomy, & endoscopic removal through middle meatus
- Corticosteroids are ineffective

DIAGNOSTIC CHECKLIST

Consider

- Begin imaging evaluation with coronal bone CT
- If bone CT or endoscopy appearance is atypical, consider MR with contrast to rule out central enhancement (neoplasm)

Image Interpretation Pearls

- Mucoid density/signal antrochoanal mass with thin rim of peripheral enhancement **only** is highly characteristic of ACP
- Do not mistake nasopharyngeal component for nasopharyngeal neoplasm
  - o Look for ipsilateral opacification of maxillary antrum even if stalk is difficult to see
- Differential diagnosis of ACP in atypical location on coronal sinus CT should include inverting papilloma

SELECTED REFERENCES

1.   Lee DH et al: Difference of antrochoanal polyp between children and adults. Int J Pediatr Otorhinolaryngol. 84:143-6, 2016
2.   Thompson LD et al: Update on select benign mesenchymal and meningothelial sinonasal tract lesions. Head Neck Pathol. 10(1):95-108, 2016
3.   Choudhury N et al: Endoscopic management of antrochoanal polyps: a single UK centre's experience. Eur Arch Otorhinolaryngol. 272(9):2305-11, 2015
4.   Kizil Y et al: Choanal polyps: 98 Cases. J Craniofac Surg. 2014
5.   Frosini P et al: Antrochoanal polyp: analysis of 200 cases. Acta Otorhinolaryngol Ital. 29(1):21-6, 2009
6.   Yuca K et al: Evaluation and treatment of antrochoanal polyps. J Otolaryngol. 35(6):420-3, 2006
7.   Maldonado M et al: The antrochoanal polyp. Rhinology. 42(4):178-82, 2004
8.   Chung SK et al: Surgical, radiologic, and histologic findings of the antrochoanal polyp. Am J Rhinol. 16(2):71-6, 2002
9.   Ozdek A et al: Antrochoanal polyps in children. Int J Pediatr Otorhinolaryngol. 65(3): 213-8, 2002
10. Skladzien J et al: Morphological and clinical characteristics of antrochoanal polyps: comparison with chronic inflammation-associated polyps of the maxillary sinus. Auris Nasus Larynx. 28(2): 137-41, 2001
11. Pruna X et al: Antrochoanal polyps in children: CT findings and differential diagnosis. Eur Radiol. 10(5):849-51, 2000
12. Weissman JL et al: Sphenochoanal polyps: evaluation with CT and MR imaging. Radiology. 178(1):145-8, 1991
13. Towbin R et al: Antrochoanal polyps. AJR Am J Roentgenol. 132(1):27-31, 1979

Solitary Sinonasal Polyp

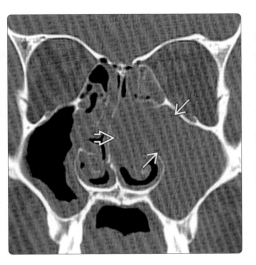

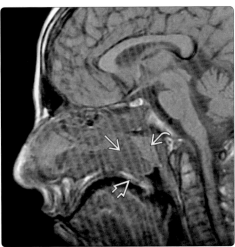

(Left) Coronal bone CT shows an opacified left maxillary sinus. The maxillary ostium is widened ➡, and a large solitary polyp ➡ extends through the ostium into the nasal cavity. The polyp obstructs the middle meatus. (Right) Sagittal T1 MR shows a large, intermediate-signal polyp ➡ extending from the nasal cavity into the nasopharynx. Note normal high signal intensity in the palate ➡ below the polyp. The adenoidal tissue ➡ is slightly hyperintense compared to the polyp.

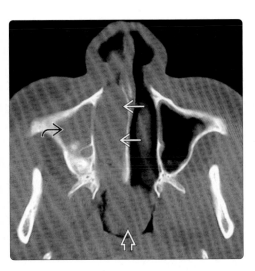

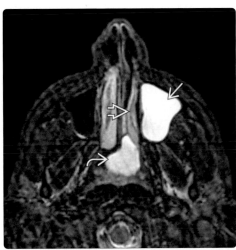

(Left) Axial bone CT shows the typical features of an ACP. The right maxillary antrum is opacified ➡, and there is a polypoid soft tissue mass extending into the nasal cavity ➡. Posteriorly the polyp protrudes through the choana into the nasopharynx ➡. (Right) Axial T2 FS MR in a child shows a hyperintense ACP on the left. The antral ➡ and nasopharyngeal ➡ components of the lesion are shown. The ACP is hyperintense compared to the inferior turbinate ➡.

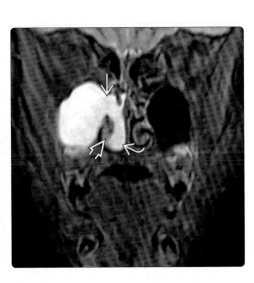

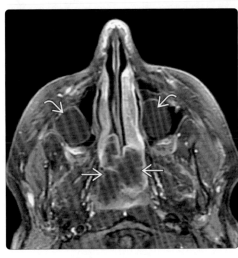

(Left) Coronal STIR MR demonstrates a typical ACP extending through the ostium ➡ between the maxillary sinus into the nasal cavity. The intranasal component ➡ is seen medial to the lower signal intensity inferior turbinate ➡. (Right) Axial T1 C+ FS MR shows a dumbbell-shaped nasochoanal polyp ➡ occluding the choanal openings and filling the nasopharynx. Only peripheral enhancement is seen around the lesion. Note the retention cysts ➡ in the maxillary antra.

IMAGING

- Opacified, **expanded** sinus with **smooth remodeling** of walls
  - May occur in septated sinuses & pneumatized anatomic variant air cells
  - **Frontal (60-65%)** > **ethmoid (25%)** > maxillary (5-10%) > sphenoid (2-5%)
- CT: Thin-section CT with coronal & sagittal reformat helpful for surgical planning and delineation of adjacent normal anatomy
  - Low-density or soft tissue density opacification of sinus with expansion
  - Bony sinus walls remodeled
  - No central enhancement; ± minimal peripheral enhancement
- MR: Enhanced MR recommended for detection of intracranial involvement & identifying potential obstructing neoplasm as underlying cause

- High water content mucus typically shows ↓ T1 signal, ↑ T2 signal, but signal varies with protein content

TOP DIFFERENTIAL DIAGNOSES

- Allergic fungal sinusitis
- Sinonasal polyposis
- Sinonasal solitary polyps

PATHOLOGY

- Cause is obstructed drainage pathway of affected sinus or air cell

CLINICAL ISSUES

- Most common expansile lesion of paranasal sinuses
- Slowly progressive symptoms that vary depending upon lesion location without signs of acute infection
  - > 90% have ophthalmic symptoms & signs
- Surgical cure is goal & expected result when mucocele is present

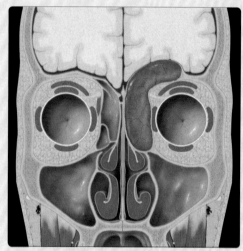
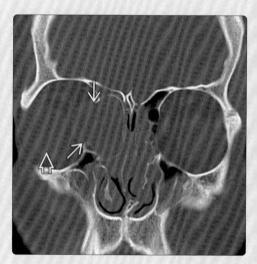

(Left) Coronal graphic shows a large left anterior ethmoid mucocele extending into the left frontal sinus. The affected sinuses are expanded without evidence of aggressive bone destruction. (Right) Coronal bone CT shows the typical features of a right ethmoid mucocele. The sinus is opacified, and there is remodeling of the surrounding bony walls with erosion of the lamina papyracea ➡. Note the mass effect upon the orbit with lateralization of the globe ➡.

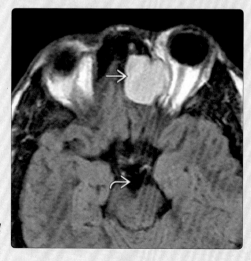
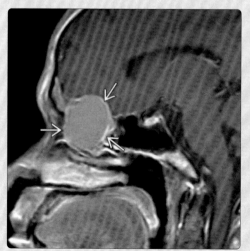

(Left) Axial FLAIR MR in a patient with proptosis and diplopia shows a homogeneous, expansile left ethmoid mucocele. Note that the material within the mucocele ➡ is hyperintense compared to CSF ➡. This likely reflects the high protein content within the mucocele. (Right) Sagittal T1 C+ MR demonstrates increased T1 signal in the mucocele, likely related to elevated protein content. There is no central enhancement within the mucocele (unenhanced T1 MR not shown), with only minimal peripheral enhancement ➡.

TERMINOLOGY

Definitions

- Expanded, chronically obstructed sinus, lined by normal respiratory epithelium and completely filled with mucus

IMAGING

General Features

- Best diagnostic clue
  - **Opacified, expanded sinus** with smooth remodeling of walls
- Location
  - > 90% in frontal & ethmoid sinuses
    - **Frontal (60-65%)** > ethmoid (25%) > maxillary (5-10%) > sphenoid (2-5%)
  - May occur in septated sinuses & pneumatized anatomic variant air cells
  - Ethmoid mucoceles have greatest potential for intraorbital extension
  - Sphenoid mucoceles have greatest potential for intracranial extension
- Morphology
  - Frontal mucocele: Expands anteriorly into skin of forehead or posteriorly into anterior cranial fossa
  - Ethmoid mucocele: Thins & remodels lamina papyracea (lateral ethmoid air cell wall), bowing it into orbit
  - Maxillary mucocele: Expands into ipsilateral nasal cavity, usually in area of secondary ostium of maxillary sinus or into premaxillary soft tissues
  - Sphenoid sinus mucocele: Expands anterolaterally into posterior ethmoids & orbital apex

Radiographic Findings

- Radiography
  - Frontal & maxillary sinus mucocele can be suggested from plain film findings
    - "Clouding" of expanded sinus with loss of normal mucoperiosteal line of sinus wall
  - Ethmoid & sphenoid mucocele may be missed

CT Findings

- CECT
  - No central enhancement; ± minimal peripheral enhancement
    - Thick peripheral enhancement raises suspicion of superinfection (mucopyocele)
- Bone CT
  - Low-density or soft tissue density opacification of sinus with **expansion**
    - High-density areas related to desiccation of secretions or fungal colonization
  - Bony sinus walls remodeled
    - May be thinned, focally absent, or normal thickness
    - Lacks aggressive osseous destruction

MR Findings

- T1WI
  - High water content of mucus interior yields ↓ T1 signal
    - When protein content high, ↑ T1 signal
- T2WI
  - High water content of mucus interior yields ↑ T2 signal

- When areas of inspissated mucus exist, may be ↓ T2 signal
- T1WI C+
  - No central enhancement; ± minimal peripheral enhancement
    - Thickened peripheral mucosa suggests infected mucocele (mucopyocele)
    - Consider tumor obstruction of sinus with secondary mucocele if associated nodular enhancement

Imaging Recommendations

- Best imaging tool
  - Small mucocele may require only unenhanced bone CT
  - Larger mucocele with significant regional compression may benefit from enhanced MR & multiplanar bone CT
- Protocol advice
  - Thin-section CT with coronal & sagittal reformats aid surgical planning & delineation of adjacent normal anatomy
  - Enhanced MR recommended for detection of intracranial involvement & identifying obstructing neoplasm as cause of mucocele

DIFFERENTIAL DIAGNOSIS

Allergic Fungal Sinusitis

- Involves multiple sinuses (key distinguishing feature)
- Typically expansile, especially if seen with polyps
- High central density on CT; mixed MR signal

Sinonasal Polyposis

- Involves multiple sinuses **and** nasal cavity
- May have multiple small mucoceles associated

Sinonasal Solitary Polyps

- "Dumbbell" cystic mass fills maxillary antrum, herniates through sinus ostium into adjacent nasal cavity

Slow-Growing Benign or Malignant Tumor

- May mimic mucocele when seen on bone/unenhanced CT
- Central, nodular enhancement on CT/MR differentiates from mucocele

PATHOLOGY

General Features

- Etiology
  - Results from **obstruction of primary ostium** of affected sinus
    - Obstruction from inflammation, trauma, functional endoscopic sinus surgery, or any space-occupying, sinonasal mass
    - Secretion of mucus into obstructed sinus creates mucocele
    - Sinus expansion from pressure necrosis with slow erosion of inner surface of bony sinus wall matched by new bone formation on outer periosteal surface
- Associated abnormalities
  - Obstructing mass at ostium may cause secondary mucocele

Gross Pathologic & Surgical Features
- Mucocele lumen filled with thick mucoid or gelatinous secretions

Microscopic Features
- Histologically indistinguishable from polyps & retention cysts
- Flattened, pseudostratified, ciliated columnar epithelium = mucus-secreting respiratory epithelium
  - Squamous metaplasia can be seen in longstanding cases
- Retained mucous secretions are sterile
  - Purulent exudate present in cases of mucopyocele
- Reactive bone formation or bony remodeling of adjacent sinus walls may be present

CLINICAL ISSUES

Presentation
- Most common signs/symptoms
  - > 90% have ophthalmic signs & symptoms
  - Principal presenting symptoms depend on site of involvement
    - Frontal mucocele: Forehead bossing, proptosis, diplopia, and mass in superomedial orbit
    - Ethmoid mucocele: Proptosis, blurred vision ± visual loss, periorbital swelling
    - Maxillary mucocele: Nasal obstruction from medial projection with cheek pressure, rhinorrhea
    - Sphenoid mucocele: Visual loss, oculomotor palsy, headache
- Other signs/symptoms
  - Epiphora, decreased color vision, hypoglobus (downward displaced eye)
  - If pain present, consider mucopyocele
- Clinical profile
  - Slowly progressive symptoms that vary depending upon lesion location without signs of acute infection
  - Diagnosis requires correlation between clinical, radiographic, and pathologic findings as diagnosis on histopathology alone can be difficult

Demographics
- Age
  - Most common in adults
    - Occurs in all age groups
  - In children, look for obstructing mass or underlying disorder (cystic fibrosis, immotile cilia syndrome)
- Epidemiology
  - Most common expansile lesion of paranasal sinuses
  - Although rare, sphenoid mucocele has highest complication rate due to proximity of vital structures

Natural History & Prognosis
- Gradual, clinically silent enlargement over months to years
- Cranial neuropathy (CNII-CNVI) may not recover following surgery if chronic at time of presentation
- Complications in untreated cases
  - Include superimposed infection (mucopyocele), meningitis ± brain abscess

Treatment
- Surgical cure is goal & expected result when mucocele is present
  - Endoscopic sinus surgery
    - Reserved for uncomplicated maxillary or ethmoid mucocele
  - Most frontal mucoceles treated with osteoplastic flap ± obliteration
  - Transfacial surgical approaches
    - Reserved for deeper posterior ethmoid or sphenoid mucocele
  - Transcranial surgical approach
    - Reserved for mucoceles with intracranial extension or causing compression of bone structures with optic pathway neurological symptoms

DIAGNOSTIC CHECKLIST

Consider
- Extensive peripheral enhancement may suggest **mucopyocele**
- If central enhancement present, consider neoplasm

Image Interpretation Pearls
- Look for thin peripheral rim of expanded bone
- No central enhancement on postcontrast CT or MR

SELECTED REFERENCES
1. Al-Qudah M: Image-guided sinus surgery in sinonasal pathologies with skull base/orbital erosion. J Craniofac Surg. 26(5):1606-8, 2015
2. Lee JT et al: Intracranial mucocele formation in the context of longstanding chronic rhinosinusitis: A clinicopathologic series and literature review. Allergy Rhinol (Providence). 4(3):e166-75, 2013
3. Scangas GA et al: The natural history and clinical characteristics of paranasal sinus mucoceles: a clinical review. Int Forum Allergy Rhinol. 3(9):712-7, 2013
4. Soon SR et al: Sphenoid sinus mucocele: 10 cases and literature review. J Laryngol Otol. 124(1):44-7, 2010
5. Lee TJ et al: Extensive paranasal sinus mucoceles: a 15-year review of 82 cases. Am J Otolaryngol. 30(4):234-8, 2009
6. Sadiq SA et al: Ophthalmic manifestations of paranasal sinus mucocoeles. Int Ophthalmol. 29(2):75-9, 2009
7. Eggesbø HB: Radiological imaging of inflammatory lesions in the nasal cavity and paranasal sinuses. Eur Radiol. 16(4):872-88, 2006
8. Nicollas R et al: Pediatric paranasal sinus mucoceles: etiologic factors, management and outcome. Int J Pediatr Otorhinolaryngol. 70(5):905-8, 2006
9. Khong JJ et al: Endoscopic sinus surgery for paranasal sinus mucocoele with orbital involvement. Eye. 18(9):877-81, 2004
10. Kosling S et al: Mucoceles of the sphenoid sinus. Eur J Radiol. 51(1):1-5, 2004
11. Landsberg R et al: Magnetic resonance imaging–aided navigation in endoscopic sinus surgery of a bone-destructive sphenoclinoid mucocele. Ann Otol Rhinol Laryngol. 112(8):740-4, 2003
12. Har-El G: Endoscopic management of 108 sinus mucoceles. Laryngoscope. 111(12): 2131-4, 2001
13. Lloyd G et al: Optimum imaging for mucoceles. J Laryngol Otol. 114(3): 233-6, 2000
14. Rombaux P et al: Endoscopic endonasal surgery for paranasal sinus mucoceles. Acta Otorhinolaryngol Belg. 54(2): 115-22, 2000
15. Busaba NY et al: Maxillary sinus mucoceles: clinical presentation and long-term results of endoscopic surgical treatment. Laryngoscope. 109(9): 1446-9, 1999
16. Van Tassel P et al: Mucoceles of the paranasal sinuses: MR imaging with CT correlation. AJR Am J Roentgenol. 153(2):407-12, 1989
17. Hesselink JR et al: Evaluation of mucoceles of the paranasal sinuses with computed tomography. Radiology. 133(2):397-400, 1979

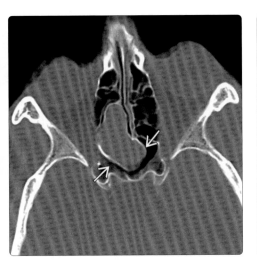

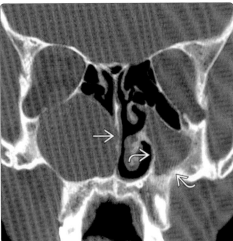

(Left) Axial bone CT demonstrates a posterior ethmoid mucocele that extends into the sphenoid sinuses ➡ rather than into the orbit. The bone surrounding the lesion is thinned and remodeled. (Right) Coronal bone CT shows a large mucocele arising within the right maxillary sinus, an unusual location for a mucocele. The lesion occludes the nasal airway ➡. Note the changes of chronic sinusitis of the left maxillary sinus with decreased volume and thickening of the walls ➡.

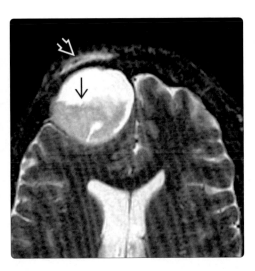

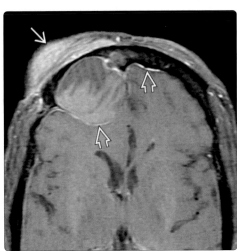

(Left) Axial T2 FS MR shows a large right frontal mucocele containing dependent material with varying signal intensities ➡. This mucocele extended into the superficial soft tissues ➡, causing scalp swelling and edema. (Right) Axial T1 C+ FS MR in a patient with right frontal mucocele shows superficial soft tissue swelling and enhancement ➡ over the ruptured mucocele. There is also enhancement of the dura ➡ in the anterior cranial fossa consistent with early meningeal inflammation.

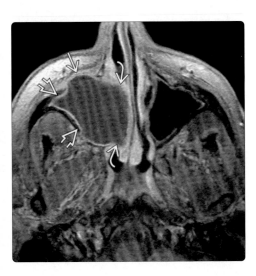

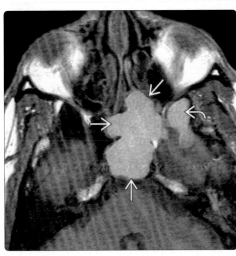

(Left) Axial T1 C+ FS MR shows a mucocele of the right maxillary sinus with erosion of the anterior wall ➡ and extension medially ➡ into the nasal cavity. There is peripheral mucosal enhancement ➡ but no central enhancement. This helps distinguish a mucocele from a neoplasm. (Right) Axial T1 MR demonstrates a large mucocele ➡ of the left sphenoid sinus. The lesion is homogeneously hyperintense, consistent with proteinaceous contents. Note the involvement of the lateral recess ➡.

TERMINOLOGY

- Sinonasal organized hematoma (SOH)
- **Rare**, nonneoplastic, expansile process from recurring hemorrhage within obstructed paranasal sinus provokes proliferative fibrotic response with neovascularization
- Synonyms: Blood boil, hematoma, hematoma-like mass, hematocele, hemorrhagic pseudotumor

IMAGING

- Maxillary sinus location accounts for nearly all cases
  - Medial extension to nasal cavity & ethmoid sinus
- Bone CT
  - Expansile mass in unilateral maxillary sinus
  - Nasal cavity with smooth scalloping and erosion
- MR imaging
  - Mixed T1 and T2 signal
  - Signal compatible with subacute & chronic hemorrhage
- Heterogeneous areas of irregular or nodular **enhancement** seen on both CT and MR can **mimic neoplasm**

TOP DIFFERENTIAL DIAGNOSES

- Solitary sinonasal polyp
- Mucocele
- Inverted papilloma
- Maxillary sinus carcinoma

CLINICAL ISSUES

- Middle-aged patient presents with epistaxis and nasal obstruction

DIAGNOSTIC CHECKLIST

- Subacute and chronic hemorrhage can result in mixed hyperdensity on CT and mixed signal on T2 MR
- Consider SOH when heterogeneous central enhancement occurs in what otherwise appears to represent benign mucocele or polyp
- Consider SOH as **rare** alternative to sinonasal neoplasm in radiologic differential

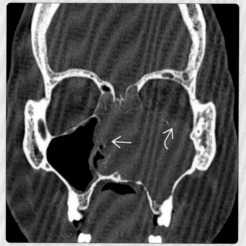
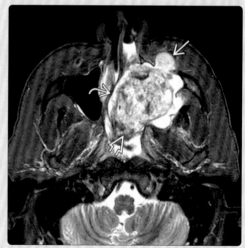

(Left) Coronal sinus CT in a 31 year old with epistaxis and SOH shows soft tissue opacification of left maxillary sinus with expansion. There is resorption of the left orbital floor ➔ with subtle extension into the orbit and complete erosion of the medial wall and septum ➔. (Right) Axial T2 FS MR in the same patient demonstrates a heterogeneous lesion in the left maxillary sinus with focal dehiscence of the anterior wall ➔ and complete erosion of the medial wall as lesion extends to nasal cavity ➔ and nasopharynx ➔.

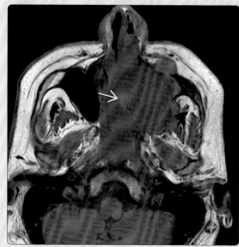
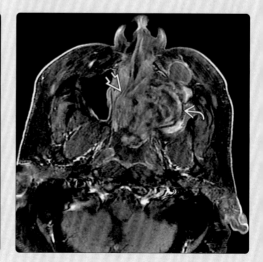

(Left) Axial T1 MR in the same patient reveals an isointense mass expanding the left maxillary sinus. There are scattered areas of T1 hyperintensity suggesting recent hemorrhage ➔. (Right) Axial T1 C+ FS MR in the same patient demonstrates heterogeneous enhancement of the large, expansile, SOH of the left maxillary sinus ➔ and nasal cavity ➔.

TERMINOLOGY

Abbreviations

- Sinonasal organized hematoma (SOH)

Synonyms

- Blood boil, hematoma, hematoma-like mass, hematocele, hemorrhagic pseudotumor

Definitions

- **Rare**, nonneoplastic, expansile process by which recurring hemorrhage within obstructed paranasal sinus provokes proliferative fibrotic response with neovascularization

IMAGING

General Features

- Best diagnostic clue
  - Solitary enhancing, expansile mass in maxillary sinus demonstrates smooth expansion and erosion of bony walls in patient with epistaxis and nasal obstruction
- Location
  - Maxillary sinus location accounts for nearly all cases, with medial extension to nasal cavity and ethmoid sinus
  - Isolated reports of nasal cavity, ethmoid, frontal and sphenoid sinus origins
- Size
  - Usually large (4-5 cm)

CT Findings

- NECT
  - Isodense to hyperdense soft tissue opacification of maxillary sinus
  - Bony margins: Smooth scalloping and erosion indicative of underlying expansile process or mass
  - Bone erosion of medial wall of maxillary sinus and uncinate process common
- CECT
  - Heterogeneous areas of irregular and nodular enhancement

MR Findings

- T1WI
  - Soft tissue is predominantly isointense to normal mucosa with scattered areas of T1 hyperintensity
  - May be mostly **hyperintense** if recent hemorrhage
- T2WI
  - Heterogeneous signal including areas of **marked hypointensity** and **hyperintensity**
  - T2-hypointense rim may be present
- T2* GRE
  - Areas of hemorrhage demonstrate hypointensity due to susceptibility artifact
- T1WI C+
  - Areas of moderate to marked irregular or nodular enhancement

Imaging Recommendations

- Best imaging tool
  - Unenhanced sinus CT in combination with focused enhanced MR of skull base & sinuses
    - CT best demonstrates bony changes related to underlying expanding mass
    - MR best differentiates enhancing portions of lesion and distinguishes SOH from adjacent obstructed secretions

DIFFERENTIAL DIAGNOSIS

Solitary Sinonasal Polyp

- Polypoid or dumbbell-shaped cystic mass extends from maxillary antrum to nasal cavity through enlarged ostium

Mucocele

- Opacified, expanded sinus with smooth remodeling of walls and no central enhancement

Inverted Papilloma

- Most commonly occur along lateral nasal cavity wall, involve middle turbinate and maxillary ostium, and can extend to maxillary antrum with smooth bony remodeling

Maxillary Sinus Carcinoma

- Malignant epithelial tumor occurs most often in maxillary antrum, with aggressive bone destruction

PATHOLOGY

General Features

- Lobulated mass with mixed areas of organized subacute and chronic hemorrhage, fibrin clots, fibrosis, inflammation, and neovascularization

CLINICAL ISSUES

Presentation

- Middle-aged patient presents with epistaxis and nasal obstruction

Demographics

- M > F (2:1)

Treatment

- Complete excision of lesion is curative

DIAGNOSTIC CHECKLIST

Consider

- Consider SOH when heterogeneous central enhancement occurs in what otherwise appears to represent benign mucocele or polyp
- Consider SOH as **rare** alternative to sinonasal neoplasm in radiologic differential

SELECTED REFERENCES

1. Kim JS et al: The increasing incidence of paranasal organizing hematoma: a 20-year experience of 23 cases at a single center. Rhinology. 54(2):176-82, 2016
2. Choi SJ et al: Sinonasal organized hematoma: Clinical features of seventeen cases and a systematic review. Laryngoscope. 125(9):2027-33, 2015
3. Hur J et al: Imaging characteristics of sinonasal organized hematoma. Acta Radiol. 56(8):955-9, 2015
4. Ohta N et al: Clinical and pathological characteristics of organized hematoma. Int J Otolaryngol. 2013:539642, 2013
5. Kim EY et al: Sinonasal organized hematoma: CT and MR imaging findings. AJNR Am J Neuroradiol. 29(6):1204-8, 2008
6. Nishiguchi T et al: Expansile organized maxillary sinus hematoma: MR and CT findings and review of literature. AJNR Am J Neuroradiol. 28(7):1375-7, 2007

TERMINOLOGY

- Acquired asymptomatic process by which walls of maxillary sinus retract, causing reduced volume of sinus, depression of ipsilateral orbital floor, enophthalmos, and hypoglobus

IMAGING

- Diminished volume of maxillary antrum with retraction (concavity) of all walls
- Increase in ipsilateral orbital volume with inferior position ("depression") of orbital floor
- Lateralized uncinate and expanded middle meatus
- Opacification of affected sinus

TOP DIFFERENTIAL DIAGNOSES

- Maxillary sinus hypoplasia
- Posttraumatic or postsurgical change

PATHOLOGY

- Occult chronic obstruction of maxillary ostium → negative pressure within sinus → stagnant mucus fills sinus → osteolysis thins/remodels bony walls → retraction of sinus walls including orbital floor

CLINICAL ISSUES

- Process is typically painless, usually asymptomatic ("silent")
- Adult with **unilateral** enophthalmos or hypoglobus in absence of trauma
- Diplopia is most common visual symptom

DIAGNOSTIC CHECKLIST

- Evaluate extent of pneumatization into malar eminence and superior alveolus to differentiate silent sinus syndrome (SSS) from hypoplasia
  - SSS: Antrum fully pneumatized
  - Sinus hypoplasia: Not fully pneumatized

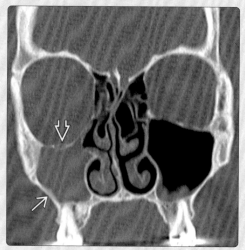
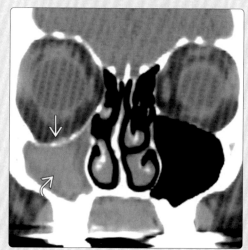

(Left) *Coronal bone CT in SSS shows opacification of the right maxillary sinus with slight thickening of the lateral wall ➡. The orbital floor is bowed inferiorly ➡ with increased orbital volume, which is characteristic of SSS. Enophthalmos is indicated by relative posterior position of globe.* **(Right)** *Coronal NECT shows typical features of SSS with decreased volume of right maxillary sinus, inferior position of the orbital floor ➡, and posterior position of ipsilateral globe. Increased density and chronic secretions ➡ are noted in the sinus.*

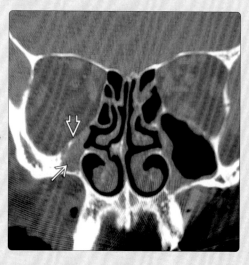
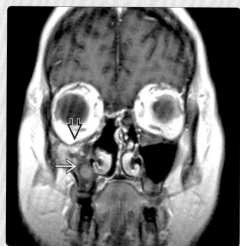

(Left) *Coronal bone CT shows the characteristic features of SSS. The volume of the opacified right maxillary antrum ➡ is diminished. The orbital floor is inferiorly positioned ➡ with increase in overall orbital volume.* **(Right)** *Coronal T1WI C+ MR in a patient with enophthalmos on the right side shows decreased volume of the maxillary sinus ➡, which is opacified with inspissated material. The ipsilateral orbital floor is depressed ➡.*

TERMINOLOGY

Abbreviations

- Silent sinus syndrome (SSS)

Definitions

- Painless, asymptomatic retraction of maxillary sinus walls, causing ↓ volume of involved maxillary sinus, depression of ipsilateral orbital floor, ipsilateral enopthalmus, and hypoglobus

IMAGING

General Features

- Best diagnostic clue
  - Retraction of maxillary sinus walls with diminished sinus volume
- Location
  - Maxillary sinus, typically unilateral
- Size
  - Diminished volume of maxillary antrum
- Morphology
  - Inward bowing of all or most antral walls

CT Findings

- Bone CT
  - Diminished volume of maxillary antrum with retraction (concavity) of all walls
    - Compensatory increase in ipsilateral orbital volume with inferior position of orbital floor
  - Near to complete opacification of affected sinus
  - Lateralized uncinate and expanded middle meatus with variable retraction of middle turbinate and nasal septal deviation
  - Demineralization of sinus walls

MR Findings

- T1WI
  - Opacified sinus with mixed-signal contents and diminished volume
  - Prominence of inferior extraconal orbital fat
- T2WI
  - Mixed signal central secretions with ↑ signal peripheral mucosa
  - Enophthalmos measured in axial plane typically measures 2-6 mm

Imaging Recommendations

- Best imaging tool
  - Axial bone CT with coronal reformats

DIFFERENTIAL DIAGNOSIS

Maxillary Sinus Hypoplasia

- Incomplete pneumatization into malar eminence and maxillary alveolar ridge
- Sinus may be aerated

Posttraumatic or Postsurgical Change

- Look for surgical changes or fractures
- Sinus may not have mucosal disease

PATHOLOGY

General Features

- Etiology
  - Occult chronic obstruction of maxillary ostium → negative pressure within sinus → stagnant mucus fills sinus → osteolysis thins and remodels bony walls → retraction of sinus walls including orbital floor
- Associated abnormalities
  - Ipsilateral enophthalmos

Gross Pathologic & Surgical Features

- Thin or absent orbital floor bone, mucoid material in maxillary sinus, edematous sinus mucosa

Microscopic Features

- Similar to chronic sinusitis with inflammatory debris, but cultures typically negative

CLINICAL ISSUES

Presentation

- Most common signs/symptoms
  - Eye asymmetry or "sagging," diplopia, enophthalmos
  - Symptoms of chronic rhinosinusitis (CRS) typically absent (i.e., "silent")
- Other signs/symptoms
  - Hypoglobus, malar depression, upper lid retraction, vague dental or facial pain
  - Widened middle meatus with retracted uncinate process on nasal endoscopy
- Clinical profile
  - Adult with painless enophthalmos or facial asymmetry ± diplopia with no history of prior trauma

Demographics

- Age
  - Adults: 25-75 years

Treatment

- Functional endoscopic sinus surgery and transconjunctival reconstruction of orbital floor

DIAGNOSTIC CHECKLIST

Image Interpretation Pearls

- Evaluate extent of pneumatization into malar eminence and superior alveolus to differentiate SSS from hypoplasia
  - SSS: Antrum fully pneumatized
  - Sinus hypoplasia: Not fully pneumatized

SELECTED REFERENCES

1. Mangussi-Gomes J et al: Stage II chronic maxillary atelectasis associated with subclinical visual field defect. Int Arch Otorhinolaryngol. 17(4):409-12, 2013
2. Brandt MG et al: The silent sinus syndrome is a form of chronic maxillary atelectasis: a systematic review of all reported cases. Am J Rhinol. 22(1):68-73, 2008
3. Numa WA et al: Silent sinus syndrome: a case presentation and comprehensive review of all 84 reported cases. Ann Otol Rhinol Laryngol. 114(9):688-94, 2005
4. Rose GE et al: Clinical and radiologic characteristics of the imploding antrum, or "silent sinus," syndrome. Ophthalmology. 110(4):811-8, 2003
5. Illner A et al: The silent sinus syndrome: clinical and radiographic findings. AJR Am J Roentgenol. 178(2):503-6, 2002

Granulomatosis With Polyangiitis (Wegener)

TERMINOLOGY

- Idiopathic, autoimmune **necrotizing granulomatous vasculitis** that preferentially involves upper and lower respiratory tracts, kidneys, skin, and joints

IMAGING

- Nodular soft tissue in nose with **septal and nonseptal cartilaginous and bone destruction**
  - **Orbital invasion** most common extrasinonasal H&N site
  - When severe, dura may be involved
- Multiplanar bone CT is best tool for initial evaluation
- Add enhanced MR best if orbital or intracranial involvement suspected

TOP DIFFERENTIAL DIAGNOSES

- Sinonasal sarcoidosis
- Nasal cocaine necrosis
- Chronic rhinosinusitis
- Invasive fungal sinusitis

- Sinonasal non-Hodgkin lymphoma

CLINICAL ISSUES

- H&N involvement in 72-100% of granulomatosis with polyangiitis (GPA) patients
  - Rhinologic symptoms in > 80%
- Symptoms mimic chronic rhinosinusitis
  - Diagnosis often delayed because symptoms mistaken for chronic rhinosinusitis
- Typically 40-60 years
  - Males more commonly affected than females
- Generally indolent disease
  - May transition to fulminating disease

DIAGNOSTIC CHECKLIST

- Consult with clinician for history of other organ system involvement (GPA vs. sarcoidosis) or cocaine abuse
- Can be impossible to differentiate from sinonasal sarcoidosis or lymphoma on imaging

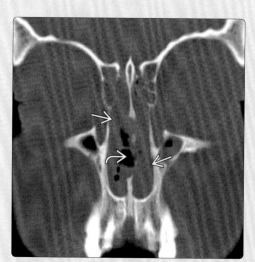
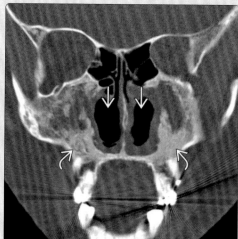

(Left) Coronal bone CT shows the classic features of sinonasal involvement by granulomatosis with polyangiitis (GPA). Nodular soft tissue ➡ is seen in the nasal cavity with an associated septal perforation ⮫. (Right) Coronal bone CT shows sequelae of a severe chronic sinonasal inflammation in GPA with combination of hyperostosis ➡ of sinus walls and bony destruction of turbinates ➡.

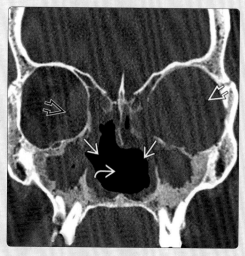
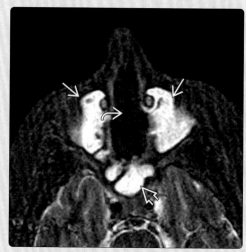

(Left) Coronal bone CT in severe GPA shows extensive soft tissue thickening in the maxillary and ethmoid sinuses and nasal cavity. There is destruction of the nasal septum ➡ and bilateral inferior and middle turbinates ➡. Note: Diffuse soft tissue infiltration of left orbit ➡ and milder disease right orbit ➡. (Right) Axial STIR MR shows hyperintense soft tissue filling the maxillary ➡ and sphenoid sinuses ➡. There is complete destruction of the nasal septum ➡. Thickening of the sinus walls is difficult to appreciate on the MR.

TERMINOLOGY

Abbreviations

- Granulomatosis with polyangiitis (GPA)

Synonyms

- Wegener granulomatosis

Definitions

- Idiopathic, autoimmune **necrotizing granulomatous vasculitis**
- Preferentially affects upper and lower respiratory tracts, kidneys, skin, and joints

IMAGING

General Features

- Best diagnostic clue
  - Severe chronic rhinosinusitis (mucosal thickening and hyperostosis) with additional features of soft tissue mass/nodularity and septal/nonseptal cartilaginous and osseous destruction
- Location
  - Nasal cavity (septum > turbinates) > sinuses (maxillary > ethmoid > frontal > sphenoid)
  - Other H&N sites
    - Orbital invasion most common extrasinonasal site
    - Nasopharynx, subglottic larynx, oral cavity, temporal bone, and salivary glands
- Morphology
  - Ulcerative ± nodular disease

CT Findings

- NECT
  - Chronic rhinosinusitis with localized mucosal nodularity and masses centered in nasal cavity
  - Periantral soft tissue infiltration
  - Orbital extension often 1st extrasinonasal site of invasion
  - Less commonly involves skull base, pterygopalatine fossa, retromaxillary region, and nasopharynx
- CECT
  - Enhancing nodular and mass-like mucosal thickening
- Bone CT
  - Chronic obstruction and inflammation of adjacent sinuses may result in nonspecific hyperostosis of sinus walls
  - **Osseous/cartilaginous erosion** often affects nasal septum primarily, causing **perforation**
  - Destruction then involves turbinates and lateral nasal wall (uncinate process and medial wall maxillary sinus)
  - May affect hard palate leading to sinonasal-oral fistula

MR Findings

- T1WI
  - Low to intermediate signal nodular masses
- T2WI
  - ↓ signal nodular masses (compared to inflamed mucosa = ↑ T2 signal)
  - ↑ signal edema of soft tissues during acute exacerbations with extension into adjacent soft tissues
- T1WI C+

  - Nodular and mass-like enhancing tissue along mucosa
  - **Orbital involvement** presents with enhancing infiltrating mass within orbit, often with contiguous sinonasal disease
  - **Meningeal thickening** with enhancement < 5% (late finding in those with skull base invasion)

Imaging Recommendations

- Best imaging tool
  - Bone-only coronal sinus CT is best tool for initial evaluation
    - Axial MDCT with reformats also very helpful for identifying bone erosion
- Protocol advice
  - If orbital, deep facial, skull base, or meningeal involvement suspected from CT or clinical symptoms → enhanced, fat-saturated MR

DIFFERENTIAL DIAGNOSIS

Sinonasal Sarcoidosis

- Systemic granulomatous disease
  - Sinonasal involvement less common than GPA
  - More common in African Americans
- May be indistinguishable from GPA on imaging

Nasal Cocaine Necrosis

- Septal perforation with nasal inflammatory changes
- May be less nodular than GPA

Chronic Rhinosinusitis

- Symptoms of GPA mimic chronic sinusitis
- Bone thickening and sclerosis **not** destruction
- No systemic disease

Invasive Fungal Sinusitis

- Rapidly progressive sinonasal destructive process in immunocompromised patient
- Sinus > nasal cavity is site of origin; destroys any adjacent bone

Sinonasal Non-Hodgkin Lymphoma

- Midline soft tissue mass with septal and nonseptal bone destruction or remodeling
  - NK/T cell type lymphoma (a.k.a. lethal midline granuloma)
- May exactly mimic GPA on imaging

PATHOLOGY

General Features

- Etiology
  - Autoimmune disease in which antineutrophil cytoplasmic antibodies (ANCA) target proteinase 3, primarily expressed in neutrophils
    - Initiates inflammatory reaction leading to endothelial damage and necrotizing granulomatous vasculitis
- Associated abnormalities
  - Secondary sinus bacterial infections common (e.g., *Staphylococcus aureus*)
  - Other organ system involvement
    - **Lungs (95%), kidneys (85%)**, joints (65%)

– Intracranial abnormalities include **pachymeningitis** and brain infarcts

Gross Pathologic & Surgical Features

- Initial appearance: Diffuse mucosal ulcerations with crusting
- Advanced disease: Cartilaginous and osseous septal destruction leads eventually to saddle nose deformity

Microscopic Features

- Noncaseating, necrotizing, multinucleated, and giant cell granulomas
- Acute ± chronic inflammatory cell infiltrate
- Fibrinoid necrosis of small- to medium-sized vessels

CLINICAL ISSUES

Presentation

- Most common signs/symptoms
  - Nasal obstruction and epistaxis
- Other signs/symptoms
  - Pain, anosmia, purulent rhinorrhea
  - Septal ulcerations and perforation can lead to saddle nose deformity
  - Hoarseness (larynx), stridor (trachea), hearing loss and ear pain (T bone)
  - Constitutional symptoms: Fatigue, night sweats, weight loss
- Clinical profile
  - Classic clinical triad
    - Necrotizing granulomas of upper and lower respiratory tracts
    - Necrotizing vasculitis of both arteries and veins
    - Glomerulonephritis
  - Diagnosis made by biopsy of affected area (nose, sinus, lung, kidney)
    - Multiple biopsies may be inconclusive
      □ Nasal biopsies positive in ~ 40%
  - Laboratory findings
    - ↑ **c-ANCA** (85-98% specificity for GPA)
      □ c-ANCA titers followed for disease response to therapy
    - ↑ ESR
    - ↑ serum creatinine signals presence of renal GPA

Demographics

- Age
  - Typically 40-60 years
- Gender
  - M > F [except laryngeal form (M < F)]
    - May be slightly more prevalent in women when presenting at younger age
- Epidemiology
  - Rare disease
  - H&N involvement in 72-100%
  - Rhinologic symptoms in > 80%

Natural History & Prognosis

- 3-year lag in diagnosis common because initially mistaken for chronic sinusitis
  - Better prognosis if diagnosed at younger age
- Generally indolent disease

- "Limited disease," localized to nose or orbit
  - Treated appropriately, associated with good to excellent prognosis
- May transition to fulminating fatal disease
  - Fulminant sinonasal disease may result in complete nasal destruction (autorhinectomy)
  - Untreated, aggressive disease can be fatal secondary to renal failure or sepsis (major cause of morbidity and mortality)
- Long-term remissions have been achieved
  - Length of remission difficult to predict
  - Spontaneous remissions have been reported

Treatment

- Medical treatments include immunosuppressive agents, cyclophosphamide, and other cytotoxic drugs
  - Fulminant disease treated with high-dose prednisone followed by cyclophosphamide
- Surgery reserved for selected H&N manifestations, such as saddle nose deformity and subglottic stenosis
  - Surgical manipulation may exacerbate neoosteogenesis in sinonasal cavities

DIAGNOSTIC CHECKLIST

Consider

- GPA should be considered when **destructive process** centered **in nasal cavity**, particularly when septal perforation is present
- Consult with clinician for history of other organ system involvement (GPA vs. sarcoidosis) or cocaine abuse

Image Interpretation Pearls

- Can be impossible to differentiate from nongranulomatous rhinosinusitis, sinonasal malignancy, or sarcoid

SELECTED REFERENCES

1. Nwawka OK et al: Granulomatous disease in the head and neck: developing a differential diagnosis. Radiographics. 34(5):1240-56, 2014
2. Cannady SB et al: Sinonasal Wegener granulomatosis: a single-institution experience with 120 cases. Laryngoscope. 119(4):757-61, 2009
3. Fuchs HA et al: Granulomatous disorders of the nose and paranasal sinuses. Curr Opin Otolaryngol Head Neck Surg. 17(1):23-7, 2009
4. Grindler D et al: Computed tomography findings in sinonasal Wegener's granulomatosis. Am J Rhinol Allergy. 23(5):497-501, 2009
5. Erickson VR et al: Wegener's granulomatosis: current trends in diagnosis and management. Curr Opin Otolaryngol Head Neck Surg. 15(3):170-6, 2007
6. Srouji IA et al: Patterns of presentation and diagnosis of patients with Wegener's granulomatosis: ENT aspects. J Laryngol Otol. 121(7):653-8, 2007
7. Lohrmann C et al: Sinonasal computed tomography in patients with Wegener's granulomatosis. J Comput Assist Tomogr. 30(1):122-5, 2006
8. Benoudiba F et al: Sinonasal Wegener's granulomatosis: CT characteristics. Neuroradiology. 45(2): 95-9, 2003
9. Gubbels SP et al: Head and neck manifestations of Wegener's granulomatosis. Otolaryngol Clin North Am. 36(4): 685-705, 2003
10. Langford CA: Wegener's granulomatosis: current and upcoming therapies. Arthritis Res Ther. 5(4): 180-91, 2003
11. Takwoingi YM et al: Wegener's granulomatosis: an analysis of 33 patients seen over a 10-year period. Clin Otolaryngol. 28(3): 187-94, 2003
12. Abdou NI et al: Wegener's granulomatosis: survey of 701 patients in North America. Changes in outcome in the 1990s. J Rheumatol. 29(2): 309-16, 2002
13. Borges A et al: Midline destructive lesions of the sinonasal tract: simplified terminology based on histopathologic criteria. AJNR Am J Neuroradiol. 21(2): 331-6, 2000

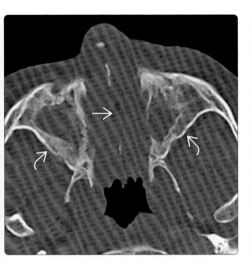

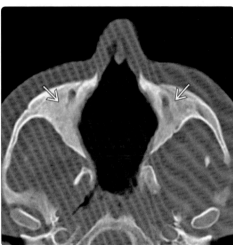

(Left) *Axial bone CT reveals extensive nodular soft tissue filling the nasal cavity with opacification of the maxillary sinuses. A septal perforation ➡ is present, and there is thickening and sclerosis of the sinus walls ➡, all findings consistent with GPA.* (Right) *Axial bone CT in advanced case of GPA demonstrates complete central destruction of the osseous architecture of nasal cavities, including septum, turbinates, and lateral walls. The maxillary sinuses are obliterated by thickened bone ➡.*

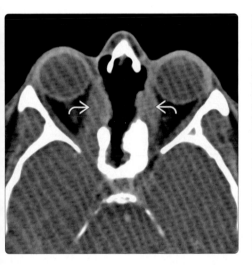

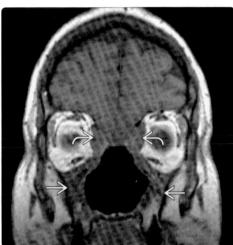

(Left) *Axial NECT shows destruction of the superior nasal septum, ethmoid septations, and the lamina papyracea bilaterally ➡. In this case, there is bilateral orbital extension of the granulomatous disease.* (Right) *Coronal T1WI MR in the same patient again shows the loss of normal nasal anatomy and thickening of the maxillary walls ➡. The fat planes between the abnormal soft tissue and the medial rectus and superior oblique muscles are obscured ➡.*

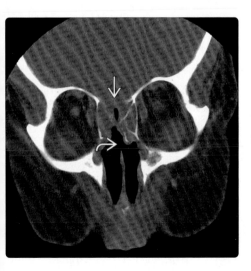

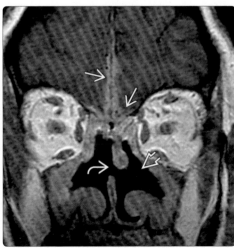

(Left) *Coronal CT shows GPA patient with chronic rhinosinusitis and headache. Perforation of the septum is noted ➡. There is confluent opacification of the ethmoid sinuses bilaterally associated with destruction of the cribriform plate ➡.* (Right) *Coronal MR in same patient demonstrates diffuse mucosal thickening in maxillary and ethmoid sinuses, perforation of the septum ➡, and bilateral destruction of the turbinates and lateral nasal cavity walls ➡. Note the contiguous pachymeningitis in the anterior cranial fossa ➡.*

TERMINOLOGY

- Destruction of osteocartilaginous structures of nose, sinuses, and palate induced by chronic inhalation of cocaine

IMAGING

- Perforation of osteocartilaginous nasal septum ± turbinates/palate **without** soft tissue mass
  - 75% occur in quadrangular cartilage; 25% involve vomer-perpendicular ethmoidal lamina
- Thin-section CT with multiplanar reformat recommended to fully delineate extent of bone destruction

TOP DIFFERENTIAL DIAGNOSES

- Traumatic nasal septal perforation
- Granulomatosis with polyangiitis
- Sinonasal sarcoidosis
- Sinonasal non-Hodgkin lymphoma
- Other drug-related septal perforation

PATHOLOGY

- Nasal septal destruction results from combined effects of chemical irritation, ischemic necrosis from vasoconstriction, and direct trauma from autoinstrumentation
- Chemical agents (i.e., levamisole) added to cocaine to enhance its appearance, add weight, and produce additional psychoactive effects may contribute to necrosis

CLINICAL ISSUES

- Nasal obstruction and discharge are most common symptoms of acquired septal lesions
  - Extension to inferior (68%), middle (44%), and superior (16%) turbinates in 1 large study
- ~ 1.75 million Americans ≥ 12 years old are regular (at least once per month) cocaine users
  - Prevalence of cocaine-induced sinonasal complications ~ 5%
  - Septal perforation most common complication occurring in 4.8% of abusers

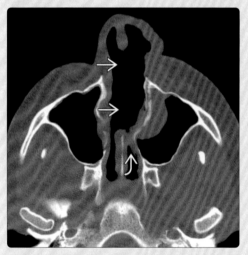

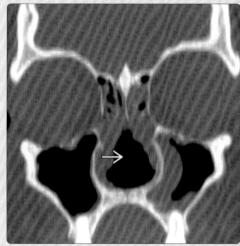

(Left) *Axial bone CT in a patient with a history of chronic cocaine inhalation shows a very large nasal septal perforation ➡. Scarring with adhesion formation ➡ is noted between the lateral nasal wall and septum posteriorly on the left.* (Right) *Coronal CT reconstruction demonstrates a large defect in the nasal septum ➡ related to cocaine necrosis. Note that the concha of the middle and inferior turbinates have been eroded and are absent.*

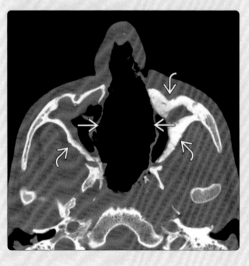

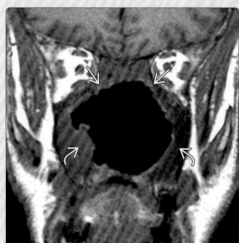

(Left) *Axial bone CT in a severe case of nasal cocaine necrosis shows complete erosion of the nasal septum. The lateral nasal walls ➡ are also involved. Extensive osteitis ➡ of the remaining antral walls is seen from chronic maxillary inflammation.* (Right) *Coronal T1WI MR demonstrates a large nasal septal perforation as well as ethmoid involvement ➡. Inflamed, thickened mucosa ➡ lines the walls of the sinuses.*

TERMINOLOGY

Abbreviations

- Nasal cocaine necrosis (NCN)

Synonyms

- Cocaine-induced midline destructive lesions

Definitions

- Destruction of osteocartilaginous structures of nose, sinuses, and palate induced by chronic inhalation of cocaine

IMAGING

General Features

- Best diagnostic clue
  - Perforation of osteocartilaginous nasal septum ± turbinates/palate **without** soft tissue mass
- Location
  - Nasal septal mucosa and cartilage

Imaging Recommendations

- Best imaging tool
  - Bone CT optimal for evaluating extent of bone destruction

CT Findings

- Bone CT
  - **Nasal septum erosion**
  - Erosion of portions of 1 or both inferior turbinates in > 50%
  - Bone destruction may extend to lateral nasal wall, palate, or orbit

DIFFERENTIAL DIAGNOSIS

Traumatic Nasal Septal Perforation

- Septal necrosis secondary to hematoma in cartilaginous septum leading to ischemia
- Rhinotillexomania (chronic nose picking) causes septal injury due to repetitive trauma/inflammation
  - Imaging findings include septal perforation, absence of anterior/inferior septum

Granulomatosis With Polyangiitis (GPA), Sinonasal

- Necrotizing granulomatous vasculitis
- Nodular soft tissue lesions
- Predilection for nasal septum and turbinates

Sarcoidosis, Sinonasal

- Systemic granulomatous disease (less frequent sinonasal involvement than GPA)
- Predilection for nasal septal and inferior turbinate involvement

Non-Hodgkin Lymphoma, Sinonasal

- Predilection for nasal cavity site of origin with frequent destruction of septum
- Large soft tissue mass in nasal cavity

Fungal Sinusitis, Invasive

- Occurs in immunocompromised population
- Maxillary and sphenoid sinuses more common location of origin than nasal cavity

Other Drug-Related Septal Perforation

- Intranasal opioid/acetaminophen or corticosteroids, bevacizumab

PATHOLOGY

General Features

- Etiology
  - Nasal septal destruction results from combined effects of chemical irritation, ischemic necrosis from vasoconstriction, and direct trauma from autoinstrumentation
  - Perforation results with chronic (> 3 months) intranasal use

Staging, Grading, & Classification

- Diagnosis can be made by identifying cocaine metabolites in urine

Gross Pathologic & Surgical Features

- Atrophic, irritated mucosa with necrosis

Microscopic Features

- Ranges from fibrosis with mild inflammation & necrosis to dense inflammatory infiltrate with extensive necrosis

CLINICAL ISSUES

Presentation

- Most common signs/symptoms
  - Nasal obstruction and discharge are most common symptoms of acquired septal lesions

Demographics

- Age
  - Adolescent to adult age groups
- Gender
  - M > F
- Epidemiology
  - ~ 1.75 million Americans ≥ 12 years old are regular (at least once per month) cocaine users
  - Prevalence of cocaine-induced sinonasal complications ~ 5%

Natural History & Prognosis

- Continued intranasal cocaine use may result in disintegration of nasal cartilage and loss of structural integrity

DIAGNOSTIC CHECKLIST

Consider

- Clinical history of cocaine use is key to diagnosis

SELECTED REFERENCES

1. Laudien M: Orphan diseases of the nose and paranasal sinuses: Pathogenesis - clinic - therapy. GMS Curr Top Otorhinolaryngol Head Neck Surg. 14:Doc 04, 2015
2. Valencia MP et al: Congenital and acquired lesions of the nasal septum: a practical guide for differential diagnosis. Radiographics. 28(1):205-24; quiz 326, 2008
3. Westreich RW et al: Midline necrotizing nasal lesions: analysis of 18 cases emphasizing radiological and serological findings with algorithms for diagnosis and management. Am J Rhinol. 18(4):209-19, 2004

Sinonasal Fibrous Dysplasia

TERMINOLOGY

- Fibroosseous lesion in which normal medullary bone is replaced by weak osseous & fibrous tissue

IMAGING

- Classic appearance: **Ground-glass** density on NECT
  - Density varies with amount of fibrous tissue
  - Variable enhancement of fibrous component
  - Variable presence of lucent/lytic foci
- MR signal & enhancement are highly variable
  - **Expansion of diploic space** key feature of FD
  - **Low T2 signal** characteristic but often not present
  - When T2 hyperintense & enhancing: Neoplasm mimic
- Best imaging tool: Thin-section **bone algorithm NECT**

TOP DIFFERENTIAL DIAGNOSES

- Ossifying fibroma
- Osteoma
- Neo-osteogenesis

PATHOLOGY

- Etiology: Defective gene in bone-forming cells in early fetal life: ↑ osteogenesis in bone marrow
- Can obstruct sinus → recurrent infection, mucocele formation
- 3 forms of FD: Monostotic, polyostotic, & McCune-Albright syndrome

CLINICAL ISSUES

- Headache, pain, sinonasal obstruction & recurrent sinusitis
- Monostotic form most common, 25% in H&N
- Highest incidence: 3-15 years
  - Disease quiescent after cessation of skeletal growth

DIAGNOSTIC CHECKLIST

- MR appearance can be somewhat confusing: Fibrous component **enhances intensely**
  - **Mimics aggressive neoplasm** without comparison CT
  - **NECT critical** to establish correct diagnosis

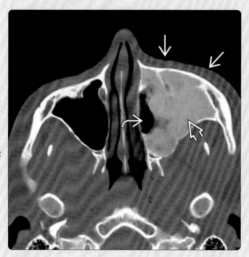
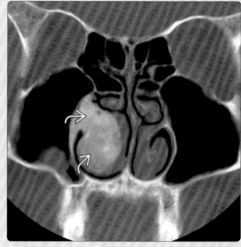

(Left) Axial bone CT demonstrates the classic features of fibrous dysplasia. There is marked expansion of the left maxillary sinus walls with asymmetry of projection of the left cheek ➡. This case shows the typical ground-glass appearance ➡ of this entity. Note the markedly decreased antral volume ➡. (Right) Coronal bone CT shows fibrous dysplasia involving the concha of the right inferior turbinate ➡ and lateral nasal wall. The concha is markedly expanded with ground-glass density.

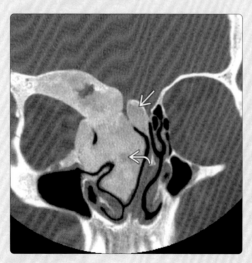
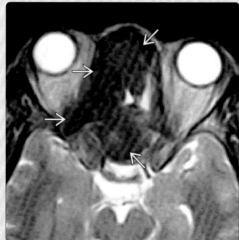

(Left) Coronal bone CT shows extensive fibrous dysplasia involving the orbit, crista galli ➡, ethmoids, and middle turbinate ➡ on the right. The nasal septum is deviated toward the left. (Right) Axial T2 MR shows characteristic marked hypointense signal in fibrous dysplasia ➡. These findings are typical when seen in conjunction with a ground-glass appearance on CT, and are more diagnostic than when T2-hyperintense signal foci are present.

TERMINOLOGY

Abbreviations

- Fibrous dysplasia (FD)

Synonyms

- Lichtenstein-Jaffe disease, cherubism (craniofacial FD)

Definitions

- Normal medullary bone replaced by fibroosseous tissue with varying degree of osseous metaplasia

IMAGING

General Features

- Best diagnostic clue
  o Ill-defined, expansile, ground-glass diploic space
- Location
  o Maxilla > mandible > frontal > ethmoid & sphenoid
- Morphology
  o Generally ill defined, **expansile**, unilateral or asymmetric

CT Findings

- CECT
  o Variable enhancement of fibrous component
- Bone CT
  o **Ground-glass**, expansile lesion with rim of intact cortex
    – Density varies with amount of fibrous tissue
    – Variable lucent/lytic foci

MR Findings

- T1WI
  o **Expanded diploic space with** intermediate to ↓ signal
  o Hypointense peripheral cortical bone
- T2WI
  o Variable: Hyperintense, intermediate, or hypointense
- T1WI C+
  o Homogeneous or heterogeneous
  o Fibrous component **may enhance intensely**
    – **Mimics aggressive neoplasm** without comparison CT

Nuclear Medicine Findings

- PET
  o Can be variably **hot** on FDG PET

Imaging Recommendations

- Best imaging tool
  o Thin-section bone algorithm NECT

DIFFERENTIAL DIAGNOSIS

Sinonasal Ossifying Fibroma

- Solitary, well defined, expansile
- Mixed bone & soft tissue density

Sinonasal Osteoma

- Solitary, well defined; projects into sinus lumen
- Densely ossified

Neo-Osteogenesis

- Slightly thickened, sclerotic sinus walls
- Near site of surgery or chronic inflammation

Meningioma, Skull Base

- Hyperostosis may mimic FD, but enhancing intracranial dural tail distinguishes from FD

PATHOLOGY

General Features

- Genetics
  o Cherubism: Autosomal dominant
- Associated abnormalities
  o Can cause sinus obstruction → recurrent infection, mucocele formation, nasal airway obstruction

Microscopic Features

- Immature (woven), poorly organized osseous component arises metaplastically from fibrous stroma

CLINICAL ISSUES

Presentation

- Most common signs/symptoms
  o Painless swelling, sinus or nasal obstruction

Demographics

- Age
  o 75% < 30 years
- Gender
  o M < F in polyostotic form (1:3)
- Epidemiology
  o Monostotic (70-80%): H&N involved in 25%
  o Polyostotic (20-30%): Bones of H&N involved in ≥ 50%
  o McCune-Albright syndrome (3-10% of FD)

Natural History & Prognosis

- Becomes quiescent with cessation of skeletal growth
- Progression after age 13 years is uncommon and minimal
- Malignant transformation (< 1%)
  o More common if polyostotic or McCune-Albright

Treatment

- Clinical & imaging follow-up if minimally symptomatic
- Surgical excision if functional compromise

DIAGNOSTIC CHECKLIST

Consider

- Consider FD if **expansile enhancing intraosseous lesion on MR**, particularly if **T2 hypointense**, & perform NECT

Image Interpretation Pearls

- MR appearance (signal & enhancement pattern) highly variable & can mimic aggressive neoplasm
  o NECT critical to problem solve

SELECTED REFERENCES

1. Belsuzarri TA et al: McCune-Albright syndrome with craniofacial dysplasia: Clinical review and surgical management. Surg Neurol Int. 7(Suppl 6):S165-9, 2016
2. DeKlotz TR et al: Sinonasal disease in polyostotic fibrous dysplasia and McCune-Albright Syndrome. Laryngoscope. 123(4):823-8, 2013
3. Amit M et al: Surgery versus watchful waiting in patients with craniofacial fibrous dysplasia–a meta-analysis. PLoS One. 6(9):e25179, 2011

KEY FACTS

TERMINOLOGY

- Benign, well-defined, slow-growing, bone-forming tumor

IMAGING

- Well-marginated bone density lesion that arises from wall of paranasal sinus & protrudes into sinus lumen
- Location: Frontal & ethmoid > > > maxillary & sphenoid
- Larger osteomas may be associated with following findings
  - Sinus opacification or mucocele formation from ostial obstruction
  - Orbital mass effect from extraconal extension
  - Pneumocephalus or intraparenchymal tension pneumatocele
  - Brain abscess ± subdural empyema
- CT density depends on "ivory" vs. "mature" components

TOP DIFFERENTIAL DIAGNOSES

- Sinonasal fibrous dysplasia
- Sinonasal ossifying fibroma

- Sinonasal osteosarcoma

PATHOLOGY

- If multiple osteomas are discovered, consider Gardner syndrome
- Etiology not well established; theories include developmental, traumatic, and infectious causes
- Microscopic classifications in literature tend to distinguish between ivory, mature, and mixed types

CLINICAL ISSUES

- Most common benign tumor of paranasal sinuses
- Usually asymptomatic, incidental finding
  - Found in 1% of patients on radiographs & 3% on CT done for sinonasal symptoms
  - < 5% of all osteomas are symptomatic
- M:F ~ 1.5-2.6:1.0
- Symptomatic lesions typically treated surgically

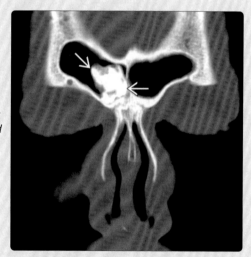
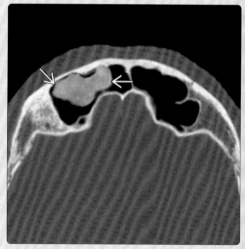

(Left) Coronal bone CT demonstrates the classic appearance of an ivory osteoma ➡ of the right frontal sinus. The lesion is located medially but did not obstruct the frontal recess. The sinus is otherwise well aerated. (Right) Axial bone CT shows a well-defined, calcified mass within the right frontal sinus ➡ consistent with an osteoma. The ground-glass density is suggestive of a mature or mixed-type osteoma, rather than ivory type.

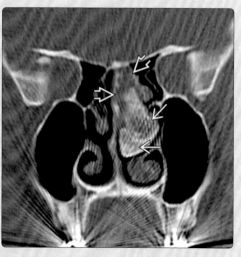
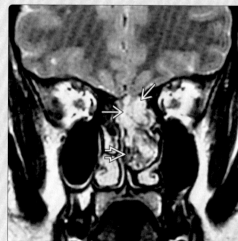

(Left) Coronal bone CT shows a mixed calcified ➡ and soft tissue density ➡ mass involving the left ethmoid sinus and nasal cavity. Using imaging alone, it would be difficult to distinguish this osteoma from other fibroosseous lesions. (Right) Coronal T2WI MR shows high signal intensity ➡ in the superior component of an osteoma that appeared nonossified on CT, and low signal intensity ➡ in the inferior component that appeared densely ossified on CT.

TERMINOLOGY

Synonyms

- Hamartoma of bone

Definitions

- Benign, well-defined, slow-growing, bone-forming tumor

IMAGING

General Features

- Best diagnostic clue
  - Well-marginated bone density lesion that arises from wall of paranasal sinus & protrudes into sinus lumen
- Location
  - Almost exclusively in craniofacial skeleton; paranasal sinuses most common
    - Frontal & ethmoid > > > maxillary & sphenoid
    - Extensive 2009 study concluded: 55.0% ethmoid, 37.5% frontal, 6.0% maxillary, 1.5% sphenoid
  - Traditionally named for sinus lumen invaded by osteoma, not bone of origin (unlike cranial osteomas)
  - May extend intracranially or into orbit
  - Other areas of reported involvement
    - Skull, maxilla, mandible, and T-bone (especially bony external auditory canal)
- Size
  - Range from few mm to several cm (typically 1.5-40.0 mm)
    - Majority < 10 mm
    - > 30 mm = "giant" osteoma
- Morphology
  - Sessile or pedunculated, projecting off wall of sinus

Radiographic Findings

- Radiography
  - Well-defined bone density lesion within sinus lumen ± associated inflammatory mucosal disease

CT Findings

- CECT
  - No appreciable enhancement due to high density of lesion
- Bone CT
  - Ivory type have homogeneous, well-defined, **bone-based, high-density mass**
  - Nonivory-type osteomas may contain areas of soft tissue density
  - Larger osteoma may be associated with following findings
    - Sinus opacification or mucocele formation from ostial obstruction
    - Orbital mass effect from extraconal extension
    - **Pneumocephalus** or intraparenchymal tension pneumatocele
    - Brain abscess ± subdural empyema

MR Findings

- T1WI
  - Low signal on all sequences; often not seen
  - Can be confused with air
  - Central yellow marrow may be high signal

- T2WI
  - Hypointense or follows marrow signal
  - May have hypointense cortical rim
  - Fibrous portions ↑ signal
- T1WI C+
  - No appreciable enhancement (except in fibrous areas)
  - Intracranial complications (e.g., mucocele, abscess) better evaluated with contrast

Imaging Recommendations

- Best imaging tool
  - Thin slice bone CT without contrast

DIFFERENTIAL DIAGNOSIS

Sinonasal Fibrous Dysplasia

- Expansile lesion of bone typically with ground-glass matrix
- Small, old foci may mimic osteoma

Sinonasal Ossifying Fibroma

- Thick, mature bony wall transitioning to immature woven bone centrally
- Most of center of lesion is low density on CT (fibroosseous)

Sinonasal Osteosarcoma

- Bone-forming, invasive, malignant tumor of bone
- Periosteal elevation, permeative margins present
- Soft tissue component often present

Osteoblastoma

- Uncommon in craniofacial skeleton
- Benign but can have more aggressive imaging features (surrounding bone edema & periosteal reaction)

PATHOLOGY

General Features

- Etiology
  - Remains controversial
    - Linked to trauma, infection, or abnormal embryologic development
      - Occurs often at embryologic junction of cartilaginous ethmoid & membranous frontal bones supporting developmental source
    - Some experts believe that osteoma is actually end-stage of fibroosseous lesion not true benign neoplasm
- Genetics
  - Usually sporadic, solitary lesions
  - If multiple osteomas are discovered, consider **Gardner syndrome** (GS): Rare, autosomal dominant transmitted disorder
    - Multiple craniofacial osteomas
    - Intestinal colorectal polyposis progresses to adenocarcinoma
    - Lesions of soft tissues: Fibromatosis, cutaneous epidermoid cysts, lipomas, & leiomyomas
    - Clinically evident osteomas develop ~ 17 years before GS diagnosis
- Associated abnormalities
  - ~ 37% accompanied by pathologic sinonasal findings
    - Focal obstruction & inflammation, generalized inflammation, polyposis

Staging, Grading, & Classification

- Osteomas composed of dense, mature bone without fibrous stroma
  - Ivory
  - Compact
  - Eburnated osteomas
- Osteomas composed of trabeculae of mature bone separated by fibrous stroma
  - Mature
  - Cancellous
  - Spongy
  - Spongious
- Mixed

Gross Pathologic & Surgical Features

- Hard, pale, ossified mass within sinus lumen
- Rock hard, lobulated mass with ivory-like appearance protruding into sinus lumen

Microscopic Features

- Ivory osteomas composed of dense, mature lamellar bone & little fibrous stroma
- Mature osteomas composed of large trabeculae of mature lamellar bone & more abundant fibrous stroma
  - ± osteoblastic rimming
- Those with osteoblastoma-like features more aggressive

CLINICAL ISSUES

Presentation

- Most common signs/symptoms
  - Usually asymptomatic, incidental finding
    - Found incidentally in 1% of patients on radiographs and 3% on CT performed for sinonasal symptoms
    - < 5% of all osteomas are symptomatic
- Other signs/symptoms
  - Sinusitis related to obstruction of sinus ostium
  - Headache, facial pain, swelling, or asymmetry
  - Proptosis & diplopia from intraorbital extension
  - Loss of visual acuity from sphenoethmoidal lesions compressing optic nerve
  - Rarely, dizziness, meningitis, or seizure from pneumocephalus, intracranial mucocele or abscess
- Clinical profile
  - Asymptomatic adult with incidental finding of osteoma on CT performed for other sinonasal complaints

Demographics

- Age
  - Reported in all ages > 20 years
    - > 50% between 50-70 years
    - Rare under age 10
- Gender
  - M:F ~ 1.5-2.6:1.0
- Epidemiology
  - Very common lesion in general population (3% prevalence)
  - Most common primary bone tumor of craniofacial skeleton
    - Almost all osteomas occur in craniofacial skeleton
  - Most common benign tumor of paranasal sinuses

Natural History & Prognosis

- Benign tumor, slowly increases in size by continuous bone formation (0.4-6.0 mm/year)
  - Growth rate greatest at puberty with maximal skeletal growth
- Becomes symptomatic when large, obstructs sinus drainage, or extends intracranially or into orbit
- Degeneration into osteosarcoma has not been reported
- Prognosis is excellent
  - Cure with complete resection, if necessary

Treatment

- If asymptomatic, can treat with watchful waiting
- Complete surgical removal for following indications
  - Unrelenting symptoms
  - Located near frontal sinus ostium
  - > 50% of volume of frontal sinus filled by osteoma
  - Extends intraorbitally or intracranially
  - CT evidence of significant enlargement
- Traditionally removed with open surgical procedures
- Endonasal endoscopic resection possible
  - Small size
  - Frontoethmoidal or orbitoethmoidal in location

DIAGNOSTIC CHECKLIST

Consider

- Other fibroosseous lesions if soft tissue density is major component of lesion
- Be sure to evaluate for affect of osteoma on adjacent structures
  - Patency of sinus drainage pathways; mass effect on orbit, meninges, & brain

Image Interpretation Pearls

- Dense, ossified sinus mass should be considered osteoma until proven otherwise
- If multiple craniofacial osteomas, consider possibility of GS

SELECTED REFERENCES

1. Lee DH et al: Characteristics of paranasal sinus osteoma and treatment outcomes. Acta Otolaryngol. 1-6, 2015
2. Georgalas C et al: Osteoma of the skull base and sinuses. Otolaryngol Clin North Am. 44(4):875-90, vii, 2011
3. Erdogan N et al: A prospective study of paranasal sinus osteomas in 1,889 cases: Changing patterns of localization. Laryngoscope. 119(12):2355-9, 2009
4. McHugh JB et al: Sino-orbital osteoma: a clinicopathologic study of 45 surgically treated cases with emphasis on tumors with osteoblastoma-like features. Arch Pathol Lab Med. 133(10):1587-93, 2009
5. Alexander AA et al: Paranasal sinus osteomas and Gardner's syndrome. Ann Otol Rhinol Laryngol. 116(9):658-62, 2007
6. Eller R et al: Common fibro-osseous lesions of the paranasal sinuses. Otolaryngol Clin North Am. 39(3):585-600, x, 2006
7. Das S et al: Imaging of lumps and bumps in the nose: a review of sinonasal tumours. Cancer Imaging. 5:167-77, 2005
8. de Chalain T et al: Ivory osteoma of the craniofacial skeleton. J Craniofac Surg. 14(5): 729-35, 2003
9. Rao VM et al: Imaging of frontal sinus disease: concepts, interpretation, and technology. Otolaryngol Clin North Am. 34(1): 23-39, 2001
10. Earwaker J: Paranasal sinus osteomas: a review of 46 cases. Skeletal Radiol. 22(6):417-23, 1993

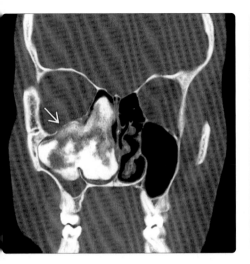

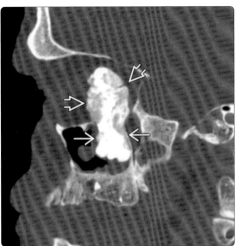

(Left) Coronal bone CT shows a very large, mixed density osteoma involving the right maxillary sinus, ethmoid sinuses, and nasal cavity. There is thinning ➡ of the orbital floor. The turbinates on the right are not visible.
(Right) Sagittal CT reconstruction shows a large, lobulated ivory osteoma involving the posterior aspect of the right maxillary sinus ➡. The mass extends superiorly into the posterior aspect of the orbit ➡ and caused proptosis in this patient.

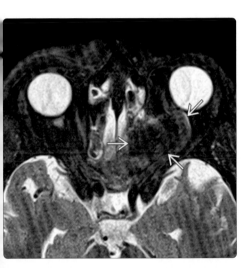

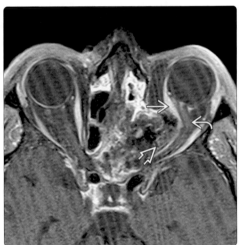

(Left) Axial STIR MR demonstrates a large left ethmoid osteoma ➡ protruding into the left orbit and causing diplopia. The hypointense signal in this lesion is typical for lesions that are densely calcified with low water content. (Right) Axial T1WI C+ FS MR shows lateral displacement of the left medial rectus muscle ➡ and optic nerve ➡. Patchy enhancement is seen in portions of the osteoma ➡ that are less ossified.

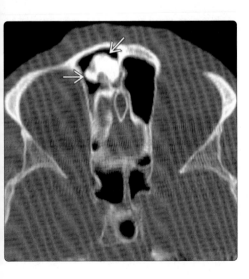

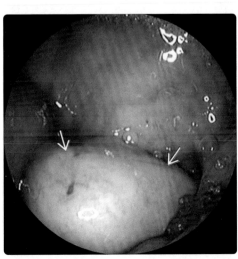

(Left) Axial CT reconstruction shows the classic appearance of an ivory compact osteoma ➡ arising within the right frontal sinus. This mass did not occlude the frontal recess, and there is no associated mucosal disease or mucocele formation. (Right) Intraoperative photograph of the frontal sinus shows a smooth, mucosa-covered pale osteoma ➡ along the floor of the sinus. The osteoma was encroaching upon the frontal sinus ostium.

TERMINOLOGY

- Benign fibroosseous lesion composed of fibrous tissue & mature bone

IMAGING

- Imaging appearance depends on age (↑ ossified portions with age)
  - Classic appearance: Thick, bony peripheral rim surrounding fibrous center
- CT
  - **Expansile mass** with **soft tissue density** (fibrous) **central** area surrounded by **ossified rim**
  - May be indistinguishable from fibrous dysplasia & osteoma
- MR
  - T1: Intermediate to low signal throughout tumor
  - T2: Mixed low-signal (ossified) & high-signal (fibrous) areas
  - Inhomogeneous enhancement of fibrous components

TOP DIFFERENTIAL DIAGNOSES

- Sinonasal fibrous dysplasia
- Sinonasal osteoma
- Sinonasal osteosarcoma

PATHOLOGY

- Thought to arise from mesenchyme of periodontal ligament

CLINICAL ISSUES

- Generally asymptomatic & found incidentally
- Age: 20-40 years most common
- Gender: M:F = 1:5
- Benign, but locally aggressive
  - May obstruct sinus drainage, cause cosmetic deformity & ocular dysfunction
- Complete surgical excision is treatment of choice
- High rate of recurrence with incomplete resection

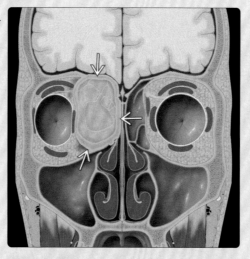
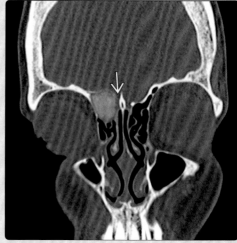

(Left) Coronal graphic shows an ossifying fibroma (OsFib) of the ethmoid region with dense osseous material peripherally ➡ and a fibrous center. The margins are well defined. There is mass effect on the orbital contents. (Right) Coronal bone CT demonstrates a well-circumscribed, expansile, sinonasal OsFib in the right anterior ethmoid sinus with narrowing of the right olfactory groove ➡. The mass is completely ossified and difficult to distinguish from fibrous dysplasia or osteoma.

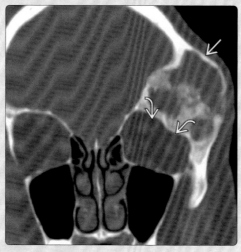
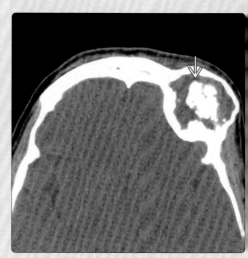

(Left) Coronal bone CT shows a large OsFib of the orbital plate of the frontal bone. This OsFib shows a mixed ossified and fibrous density. It is expansile, and the patient presented with cosmetic deformity from forehead swelling ➡ and proptosis from orbital mass effect ➡. (Right) Axial NECT in the same patient shows that the dominant focus of ossification in this case is central ➡ with surrounding soft tissue density rather than the classic pattern with peripheral ossification.

TERMINOLOGY

Abbreviations

- Ossifying fibroma (OsFib)

Synonyms

- Cementoossifying fibroma, psammomatoid ossifying fibroma, juvenile-aggressive ossifying fibroma

Definitions

- Benign fibroosseous lesion composed of encapsulated mixture of fibrous tissue & mature bone

IMAGING

General Features

- Best diagnostic clue
  - Well-demarcated, expansile mass with soft tissue density (fibrous) central area surrounded by ossified rim
- Location
  - 10-20% of craniofacial OsFib arise from maxilla
    - Most common craniofacial site is mandible (75%)
  - Characteristically **monostotic**
- Size
  - 0.5-10 cm
- Morphology
  - Well circumscribed, expansile

CT Findings

- NECT
  - Well-circumscribed, expansile mass with mixed soft tissue & bone density
  - Most often unilobular
- CECT
  - Fibrous areas may show subtle to more avid enhancement
- Bone CT
  - Imaging appearance depends on age of OsFib (↑ ossified portions with age)
  - Classic appearance
    - **Thick, bony peripheral rim** surrounding **low-attenuation fibrous center**
  - Other appearance
    - Scattered foci of soft tissue density among ossified areas
    - Thin, eggshell appearance of peripheral bone
  - CT appearance may be indistinguishable from fibrous dysplasia & osteoma
  - May absorb maxillary tooth roots

MR Findings

- T1WI
  - Intermediate to low signal throughout tumor
    - Fibrous areas intermediate signal (classically central)
    - Ossified areas hypointense (classically peripheral)
- T2WI
  - Mixed low- & high-signal areas
    - Fibrous areas hyperintense (usually lesion center)
    - Ossified areas hypointense (usually lesion periphery)
  - Obstructed secretions behind lesion & associated mucocele are hyperintense
  - Fluid-fluid levels in portions of these tumors have been reported
- T1WI C+
  - Inhomogeneous enhancement of fibrous portions of tumor matrix
  - Enhancement of outer shell & septa may be seen

Imaging Recommendations

- Best imaging tool
  - Fibroosseous lesions of craniofacial area best studied with bone algorithm CT
- Protocol advice
  - Thin-slice bone CT in axial plane with coronal ± sagittal reformatted images
  - Enhanced T1 fat-saturated MR provides complete presurgical roadmap of surrounding soft tissues at risk

DIFFERENTIAL DIAGNOSIS

Sinonasal Fibrous Dysplasia

- Poorly defined expansion of maxillofacial bones
- Classic ground-glass appearance
- Mixed pattern of less active ground-glass and more active fibrous areas
- May be monostotic (70%) or polyostotic (30%)
- Encompasses rather than absorbs healthy tooth roots

Sinonasal Osteoma

- Mass composed of mostly solid lamellar bone
- Frontal sinus common location

Sinonasal Osteosarcoma

- Destructive, aggressive lesion of craniofacial bones
- Tumor "new bone" in mass matrix
- "Sunburst" periosteal reaction
- Most common in adolescent boys or long-term complication of XRT

Cementoblastoma

- Benign tumor of cementum in young males
- Dense mass associated with tooth root
- Not located in frontal, ethmoid, sphenoid sinuses

PATHOLOGY

General Features

- Etiology
  - Thought to arise from **mesenchyme of periodontal ligament** (related to cementifying fibroma, cementoossifying fibroma)
    - Presumed to originate from mesenchymal blast cells
    - Closely related to fibrous dysplasia & ameloblastoma
  - Densely cellular, well-defined fibrous tumor with ossification progressing from periphery toward center
    - Early stage: Primarily fibrous
    - Late stage: Fills in with mature bone
- Associated abnormalities
  - Large lesions may result in cosmetic deformity, ocular dysfunction
  - May obstruct sinus drainage pathways and lead to mucocele formation
  - Intracranial extension complicated by tension pneumocephalus has been reported

Staging, Grading, & Classification

- Subtypes described
  - Juvenile
  - Active
  - Aggressive
  - Psammomatoid

Gross Pathologic & Surgical Features

- Gritty, gray to white, hard lesion

Microscopic Features

- Islands of osteoid rimmed by osteoblast-forming lamellar bone
- Central OsFib contains immature (woven) bone while periphery has more mature (lamellar) bone
- Fibrous stroma shows parallel & whorl arrangement of collagen & fibroblasts
  - May be densely cellular with hemorrhage, inflammation, & giant cells
- OsFib may be histologically indistinguishable from active form of fibrous dysplasia

CLINICAL ISSUES

Presentation

- Most common signs/symptoms
  - Generally **asymptomatic** & found incidentally
- Other signs/symptoms
  - Chronic sinusitis symptoms: Rhinorrhea, pain, cheek swelling, nasal obstruction
  - Displaced teeth
  - Exophthalmos, diplopia, visual acuity loss due to orbital mass effect
- Clinical profile
  - **20- to 40-year-old woman** with mixed soft tissue-ossified sinus lesion incidentally detected on CT performed for other reasons
  - Appearance mimics other fibroosseous lesions & diagnosis not made of basis of imaging alone
    - Based on combination of clinical, radiological, & pathological criteria

Demographics

- Age
  - 1st appears in young adult
    - 20-40 years most common
  - Wide range reported
- Gender
  - M:F = 1:5
- Epidemiology
  - 10-20% of craniofacial OsFib arise in maxilla
  - < 0.5% risk of malignant degeneration

Natural History & Prognosis

- Slow growing but may be locally aggressive
  - OsFib of paranasal sinuses are more aggressive than OsFib of mandible
  - Juvenile variant (active ossifying fibroma) may have aggressive, locally destructive behavior
- Prognosis excellent after complete resection
- High rate of recurrence if incompletely resected

Treatment

- Complete surgical excision is treatment of choice as permitted by OsFib location
- Lesions with benign behavior that do not produce deformity may be treated with curettage and ostectomy
  - Recurrence rates higher with this approach

DIAGNOSTIC CHECKLIST

Consider

- May not have classic appearance of bony rim with fibrous center
  - Densities may be patchy & randomly distributed

Image Interpretation Pearls

- MR appearance of OsFib highly variable, & lesion may appear more aggressive
  - Careful correlation with CT important
- May be **indistinguishable from fibrous dysplasia** in imaging
  - Refer to more generically as "fibroosseous lesion"
  - If polyostotic process, fibrous dysplasia more likely

Reporting Tips

- Be sure to describe position in relation to sinus drainage pathways
- Be sure to describe mass effect upon adjacent structures, such as orbit, neural foramina, & intracranial cavity

SELECTED REFERENCES

1. Ciniglio Appiani M et al: Ossifying fibromas of the paranasal sinuses: diagnosis and management. Acta Otorhinolaryngol Ital. 35(5):355-61, 2015
2. MacDonald DS: Maxillofacial fibro-osseous lesions. Clin Radiol. 70(1):25-36, 2015
3. McCarthy EF: Fibro-osseous lesions of the maxillofacial bones. Head Neck Pathol. 7(1):5-10, 2013
4. MacDonald-Jankowski DS: Ossifying fibroma: a systematic review. Dentomaxillofac Radiol. 38(8):495-513, 2009
5. Boudewyns AN et al: Sinonasal fibro-osseous hamartoma: case presentation and differential diagnosis with other fibro-osseous lesions involving the paranasal sinuses. Eur Arch Otorhinolaryngol. 263(3):276-81, 2006
6. Eller R et al: Common fibro-osseous lesions of the paranasal sinuses. Otolaryngol Clin North Am. 39(3):585-600, x, 2006
7. Mehta D et al: Paediatric fibro-osseous lesions of the nose and paranasal sinuses. Int J Pediatr Otorhinolaryngol. 70(2):193-9, 2006
8. Kendi AT et al: Sinonasal ossifying fibroma with fluid-fluid levels on MR images. AJNR Am J Neuroradiol. 24(8):1639-41, 2003
9. Alawi F: Benign fibro-osseous diseases of the maxillofacial bones. A review and differential diagnosis. Am J Clin Pathol. 118 Suppl:S50-70, 2002
10. Khoury NJ et al: Juvenile ossifying fibroma: CT and MR findings. Eur Radiol. 12 Suppl 3:S109-13, 2002
11. Williams HK et al: Juvenile ossifying fibroma. An analysis of eight cases and a comparison with other fibro-osseous lesions. J Oral Pathol Med. 29(1):13-8, 2000
12. Engelbrecht V et al: CT and MRI of congenital sinonasal ossifying fibroma. Neuroradiology. 41(7):526-9, 1999
13. Shand JM et al: Juvenile ossifying fibroma of the midface. J Craniofac Surg. 10(5):442-6, 1999
14. Commins DJ et al: Fibrous dysplasia and ossifying fibroma of the paranasal sinuses. J Laryngol Otol. 112(10):964-8, 1998
15. Lawton MT et al: Juvenile active ossifying fibroma. Report of four cases. J Neurosurg. 86(2):279-85, 1997
16. Slootweg PJ: Maxillofacial fibro-osseous lesions: classification and differential diagnosis. Semin Diagn Pathol. 13(2):104-12, 1996
17. Thompson J et al: Nasopharyngeal nonossifying variant of ossifying fibromyxoid tumor: CT and MR findings. AJNR Am J Neuroradiol. 16(5):1132-4, 1995
18. Han MH et al: Sinonasal psammomatoid ossifying fibromas: CT and MR manifestations. AJNR Am J Neuroradiol. 12(1):25-30, 1991

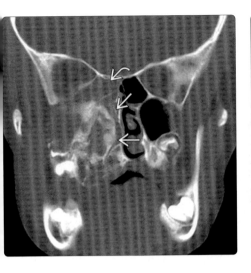
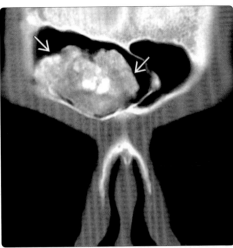

(Left) *Coronal bone CT shows a large maxillary OsFib that nearly fills the entire right maxillary antrum. The right nasal airway is obstructed ➡, and there are postobstructive secretions in the right ethmoid sinuses ➡.* (Right) *Coronal bone CT shows an atypical appearance of an OsFib. This frontal sinus lesion ➡ demonstrates diffuse, slightly heterogeneous ossification with little fibrous component. This OsFib mimics the appearance of an osteoma.*

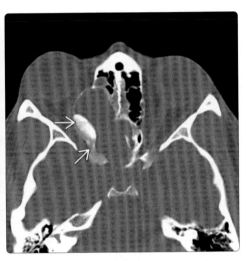
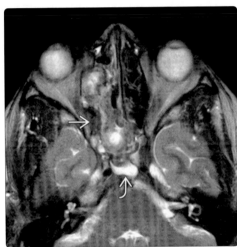

(Left) *Axial bone CT demonstrates an expansile, predominantly soft tissue density mass within the posterior ethmoid region. A focus of peripheral ossification ➡ along the lateral margin suggests that this is a fibroosseous lesion, in this case, an OsFib.* (Right) *Axial T2WI MR in the same patient shows hypointense signal in the ossified portion ➡ of the lesion. Note the hyperintense obstructed secretions ➡ in the sphenoid sinus posterior to the lesion.*

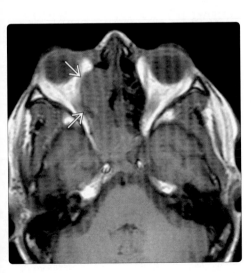
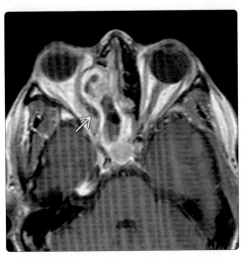

(Left) *Axial T1WI MR in the same patient shows signal intensity similar to that of muscle within the majority of the OsFib. The margins are well defined. Note the mass effect upon the right orbital contents ➡ causing diplopia in this patient.* (Right) *Axial T1WI C+ MR in the same patient reveals heterogeneous enhancement throughout the lesion. The fibrous portions of OsFib typically enhance, and there is little or no enhancement in the ossified ➡ portions.*

TERMINOLOGY

- Benign, vascular, nonencapsulated, locally invasive nasal cavity mass

IMAGING

- Location: Centered in posterior nasal cavity near sphenopalatine foramen
  - Extends into nasopharynx, pterygopalatine fossa, infratemporal fossa
- CT findings in juvenile angiofibroma (JAF)
  - Mass shows diffuse, avid enhancement
  - Posterior wall of maxillary sinus bowed anteriorly
  - Bone remodeling ± destruction
- MR findings in JAF
  - Signal voids represent flow in enlarged vessels
  - Intense enhancement ± flow voids
- Angiography typically performed at time of preoperative embolization shows tumor blush

- Internal maxillary branch of external carotid artery most common feeding vessel

TOP DIFFERENTIAL DIAGNOSES

- Hypervascular polyp
- Rhabdomyosarcoma
- Antrochoanal polyp
- Esthesioneuroblastoma

CLINICAL ISSUES

- Symptoms
  - Unilateral nasal obstruction (90%); epistaxis (60%)
- Almost exclusively occurs in male patients
- Preferred treatment: Complete surgical resection
  - Radiation therapy may be used as adjuvant therapy after surgery or as primary treatment in some cases

DIAGNOSTIC CHECKLIST

- Consider other diagnoses in female patient
- Look for JAF extension into surrounding structures

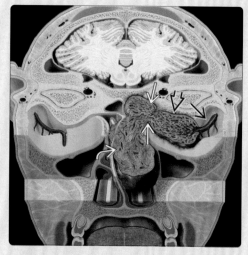
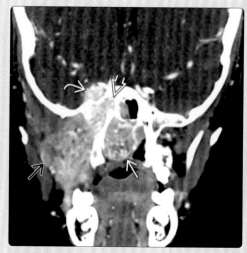

(Left) Transverse oblique graphic shows classic features and location of a juvenile angiofibroma (JAF). Site of origin is in the sphenopalatine foramen ➡ with extension into the pterygopalatine fossa (PPF) ➡ and nasal cavity ➡. The internal maxillary artery ➡ is the dominant feeding vessel of this vascular mass. (Right) Coronal CECT in a 13 year old shows typical growth pattern of a large, hypervascular angiofibroma occluding the nasopharynx ➡, extending into right sphenoid ➡, middle cranial fossa ➡, and masticator space ➡.

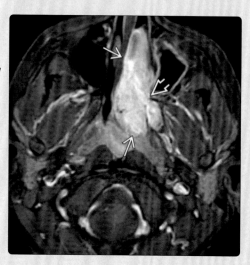
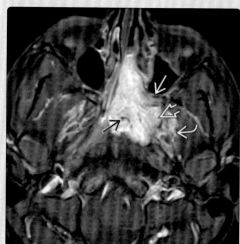

(Left) Axial T1 C+ FS MR in a 15 year old with nasal obstruction shows enhancing angiofibroma ➡ filling the left nasal cavity and extending into the nasopharynx. Presumed site of origin is nasopalatine foramen ➡. (Right) Axial T1 C+ FS MR in the same patient shows a few intralesional high-flow vessels ➡ and extension of angiofibroma into the widened PPF ➡, destruction of the left pterygoid ➡, and extension into the masticator space ➡.

TERMINOLOGY

Abbreviations

- Juvenile angiofibroma (JAF)

Synonyms

- Juvenile nasopharyngeal angiofibroma (JNA); fibromatous or angiofibromatous hamartoma
  - JAF of nasal cavity is more correct terminology
  - JNA is commonly used term, but tumor begins in nose, not in nasopharynx

Definitions

- Benign, vascular, nonencapsulated, locally invasive nasal cavity mass

IMAGING

General Features

- Best diagnostic clue
  - Intensely enhancing mass **originating at sphenopalatine foramen** (SPF) in **adolescent male patient**
- Location
  - Centered in posterior wall of nasal cavity off midline, at margin of SPF
    - Extends from posterior nasal cavity into nasal cavity, nasopharynx, & pterygopalatine fossa (PPF)
      - □ **Penetrates PPF early (90%)** with involvement of upper medial pterygoid lamina
    - Sphenoid sinus extension (60%)
    - May extend into maxillary (43%) & ethmoid sinuses (35%), masticator space (infratemporal fossa), inferior orbital fissure
    - 5-20% extend into middle cranial fossa via vidian canal or foramen rotundum
- Size
  - Usually 2-6 cm but may become massive
- Morphology
  - Lobular, usually well-circumscribed mass
    - Large lesions have infiltrating margins

Radiographic Findings

- Radiography
  - Lateral facial plain film shows **anterior displacement of posterior wall of maxillary antrum** (bow sign)
  - Associated with nasal cavity opacification
  - ± nasal cavity/nasopharyngeal soft tissue mass

CT Findings

- CECT
  - Avidly enhancing soft tissue mass originating near SPF with extension into adjacent nasopharynx & PPF
  - ± opacified sphenoid sinus (obstructed secretions vs. tumor infiltration)
- Bone CT
  - Bone remodeling ± destruction
  - Posterior wall maxillary sinus bowed anteriorly
  - Ipsilateral nasal cavity & PPF enlarged
- CTA
  - Enlarged ipsilateral external carotid artery (ECA) & internal maxillary (IMAX) artery

MR Findings

- T1WI
  - Heterogeneous, intermediate signal
  - **Signal voids** represent flow in enlarged vessels
- T2WI
  - Heterogeneous, intermediate-to-high signal mass
  - Punctate & serpentine flow voids within tumor
- T1WI C+
  - **Intense enhancement** ± flow voids
- T1WI C+ FS
  - Coronal plane shows cavernous sinus, sphenoid sinus, or skull base extension
- MRA
  - Enlarged ipsilateral ECA & IMAX artery
  - Lesional vessels may be too small to evaluate with MRA

Angiographic Findings

- Conventional angiography typically performed at time of preoperative embolization
- **Intense capillary tumor blush** is fed by enlarged feeding vessels from ECA
  - **IMAX** & ascending pharyngeal arteries from ECA are **most common feeding vessels**
  - If skull base or cavernous sinus extension, internal carotid artery (ICA) supply is common
  - Supply may also be from contralateral ECA branches

Imaging Recommendations

- Best imaging tool
  - Maxillofacial bone-only unenhanced CT in axial & coronal planes for evaluating bone remodeling vs. destruction
  - Gadolinium-enhanced MR optimal for mapping lesion extent and determining vascularity
  - Catheter angiography of both ECA & ICA
    - Often in conjunction with embolization therapy
    - Helps plan surgery & ↓ intraoperative blood loss
- Protocol advice
  - Maxillofacial MR with T1 C+ in axial & coronal planes **with fat saturation**
    - Multiplanar imaging optimal for evaluating extension into sphenoid sinus, orbit, skull base
  - CECT may be helpful for evaluating residual disease in postoperative period

DIFFERENTIAL DIAGNOSIS

Hypervascular Polyp

- Nasopharyngeal polyp that becomes hypervascular due to repeated injury
- Does not involve SPF or PPF
- Less hypervascular than JAF

Rhabdomyosarcoma

- Homogeneous mass ± bone destruction
- Not necessarily centered in posterolateral nasal cavity
- Rarely penetrates SPF into PPF

Antrochoanal Polyp

- Maxillary antrum is opacified
- Lesion herniates into anterior nasal cavity, then nasopharynx; PPF not involved
- **Peripheral enhancement** only

Encephalocele

- Nasoethmoidal type presents as intranasal mass
- **Connection to intracranial cavity** seen on imaging
- **No enhancement**
- Usually more anterior in position

Esthesioneuroblastoma

- 1st incidence peaks in 2nd decade; **F > M**
- Presenting symptoms same as JAF
- Nasal cavity mass **near cribriform plate**
- Avidly enhancing

Sinonasal Nerve Sheath Tumor

- Schwannoma or neurofibroma
- Well-defined, enhancing mass with adjacent bone remodeling

PATHOLOGY

General Features

- Etiology
  - Source of fibrovascular tissue of JAF is not known
  - Best current hypothesis: Primitive mesenchyme of SPF is source of JAF

Staging, Grading, & Classification

- Staging systems based on tumor size (< or > 6 cm), invasion to PPF anterior &/or posterior to pterygoid plates, and skull base & intracranial invasion

Gross Pathologic & Surgical Features

- Reddish-purple, compressible, mucosa-covered mass
- Cut surface has spongy appearance

Microscopic Features

- **Unencapsulated, highly vascular polypoid mass** of vascular angiomatous tissue in fibrous stroma
- Myofibroblast is thought to be cell of origin
- Estrogen, testosterone, or progesterone receptors may be present

CLINICAL ISSUES

Presentation

- Most common signs/symptoms
  - Unilateral **nasal obstruction** (90%)
  - **Epistaxis** (60%)
- Other signs/symptoms
  - Nasal voice, nasal discharge
  - Anosmia
  - Pain or swelling in cheek
  - Proptosis
  - Serous otitis media
- Clinical profile
  - **Adolescent male patient with nasal obstruction & epistaxis**
  - Nasal endoscopy: Vascular-appearing nasal cavity mass
    - Biopsy in outpatient setting should be avoided due to risk of hemorrhage

Demographics

- Age
  - 10-25 years reported
    - Average age at onset = 15 years
- Gender
  - Almost **exclusively occurs in male patients**
    - If found in female patient, genetic testing may reveal mosaicism
- Epidemiology
  - 0.5% of all head & neck neoplasms
  - 5-20% of JAF extends to skull base and may have skull base erosion

Natural History & Prognosis

- May rarely spontaneously regress
- Local recurrence rate with surgery: 6-24%
  - Local recurrence more common with large lesions (> 6 cm), intracranial spread, previous treatment

Treatment

- Preferred: **Complete surgical resection** using **preoperative embolization** to ↓ blood loss
- Multiple surgical approaches
  - Open resection (midface degloving) vs. endoscopic removal ± laser assistance
  - Endoscopic resection associated with ↓ bleeding & shorter hospital stay
- Radiation therapy (RT)
  - Adjuvant to surgery for unresectable intracranial disease & cavernous sinus involvement (78% control rates reported)
  - RT alone for cure used in some institutions
  - Used with caution in young patients due to potential to induce malignancies
- Hormonal therapy (estrogen) is controversial

DIAGNOSTIC CHECKLIST

Consider

- JAF in adolescent male patient with epistaxis & enhancing posterior nasal cavity mass

Image Interpretation Pearls

- Be sure to **look for JAF extension** into surrounding structures

SELECTED REFERENCES

1. Schmalbach CE et al: Managing vascular tumors—open approaches. Otolaryngol Clin North Am. 49(3):777-90, 2016
2. Snyderman CH et al: Endoscopic management of vascular sinonasal tumors, including angiofibroma. Otolaryngol Clin North Am. 49(3):791-807, 2016
3. Alshaikh NA et al: Juvenile nasopharyngeal angiofibroma staging: an overview. Ear Nose Throat J. 94(6):E12-22, 2015
4. Huang Y et al: Surgical management of juvenile nasopharyngeal angiofibroma: analysis of 162 cases 1995-2012. Laryngoscope. 124(8):1942-6, 2014
5. Boghani Z et al: Juvenile nasopharyngeal angiofibroma: a systematic review and comparison of endoscopic, endoscopic-assisted, and open resection in 1047 cases. Laryngoscope. 123(4):859-69, 2013
6. Leong SC: A systematic review of surgical outcomes for advanced juvenile nasopharyngeal angiofibroma with intracranial involvement. Laryngoscope. 123(5):1125-31, 2013
7. Yi Z et al: Nasopharyngeal angiofibroma: a concise classification system and appropriate treatment options. Am J Otolaryngol. 34(2):133-41, 2013

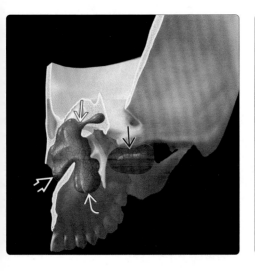

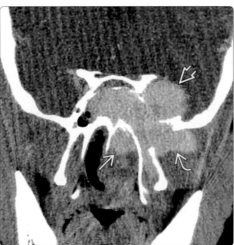

(Left) *Sagittal oblique graphic shows the spread patterns of JAF. The lesion originates at the sphenopalatine foramen ➡ and extends into the nasal cavity ➡, nasopharynx ➡, and infratemporal fossa ➡.* (Right) *Coronal CECT shows a large JAF extending into the nasopharynx ➡, infratemporal fossa ➡, and middle cranial fossa ➡. The sphenoid sinus is replaced by the tumor. Avid enhancement is characteristic of this vascular lesion.*

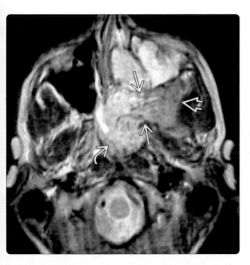

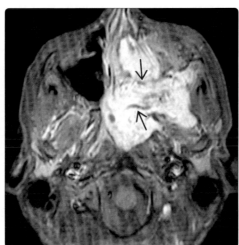

(Left) *Axial T2 MR in a young male patient shows a large, infiltrating JAF in the classic location. The mass is centered at the sphenopalatine foramen ➡ and extends laterally into the masticator space ➡ and medially into the nasopharynx ➡.* (Right) *Axial T1 C+ FS MR in the same patient shows avid enhancement throughout the lesion. Several serpiginous signal voids are noted in the mass ➡, consistent with enlarged feeding vessels, as seen on this sequence.*

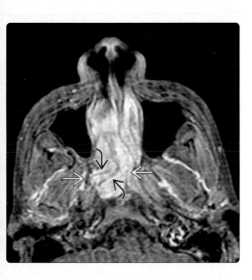

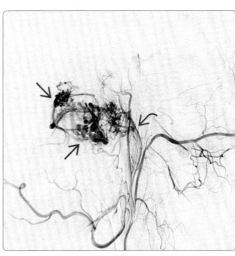

(Left) *Axial T1 C+ FS MR demonstrates a lobular, diffusely enhancing mass filling the right nasal cavity and protruding into the nasopharynx ➡. Flow voids ➡ are also seen in this JAF, consistent with its vascular nature.* (Right) *Lateral catheter angiography shows areas of dense tumor blush ➡ within a JAF prior to embolization. This external carotid artery injection shows that the main arterial feeding vessel is the internal maxillary artery ➡.*

IMAGING

- Typical location: Along lateral nasal wall **centered at middle meatus** ± extension into antrum
- CT findings
  - 40% show entrapped bone
  - Focal bony hyperostosis suggests point of tumor origin
- MR findings
  - T2: Predominantly hyperintense to skeletal muscle
  - T2 & T1 C+ FS: Curvilinear striations or convoluted, cerebriform pattern is characteristic
  - If portion of tumor appears invasive or necrosis present → consider synchronous SCCa
  - Multiplanar MR optimal for tumor mapping & differentiating tumor from obstructed secretions
- PET cannot reliably distinguish benign IPap & SCCa
- Best imaging tool: Multiplanar MR best maps tumor & differentiates tumor from obstructed secretions
- T2 FS & T1 C+ FS MR best show internal architecture

TOP DIFFERENTIAL DIAGNOSES

- Solitary sinonasal (antrochoanal) polyp
- Sinonasal SCCa
- Sinonasal polyposis

PATHOLOGY

- Hyperplastic squamous epithelium replaces seromucinous ducts & glands in stroma with endophytic growth pattern
- **10%** either degenerate into or **coexist with SCCa**
  - SCCa may be synchronous (7%) or metachronous (4%)

CLINICAL ISSUES

- Typically 40-70 years
- M > F (4-5:1)
- High rate of local recurrence if incompletely resected

DIAGNOSTIC CHECKLIST

- Deeply invasive disease may alter surgical approach
- Look for additional masses: 4% are multifocal

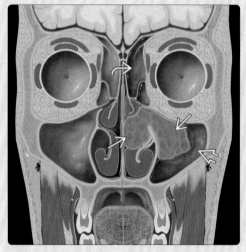
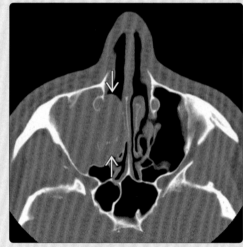

(Left) Coronal graphic shows an inverted papilloma ➡ originating near the middle meatus and extending into the maxillary sinus. Blocked secretions are noted in the ethmoid ➡ and maxillary ➡ sinuses. (Right) Axial bone CT shows a mass in the nasal cavity ➡ along the lateral wall near the middle meatus. The maxillary sinus is opacified, but it is difficult to differentiate obstructed secretions from papilloma on the CT. MR in such a case would be helpful to delineate the margins of the mass.

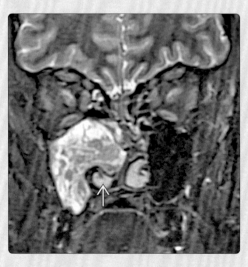
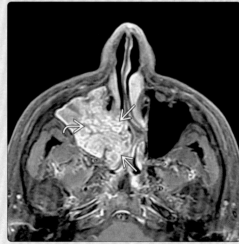

(Left) Coronal T2 FS MR shows characteristic features on an inverted papilloma that involves the right maxillary sinus and nasal cavity. The lesion has a convoluted, cerebriform architecture. Note the inferior displacement of the inferior turbinate ➡. (Right) Axial T1 C+ FS MR shows classic features of an inverted papilloma. The lesion is centered at the middle meatus with nasal cavity ➡ and antral ➡ components. This lesion shows characteristic convoluted, cerebriform architecture.

TERMINOLOGY

Abbreviations

- Inverted papilloma (IPap)

Synonyms

- Endophytic papilloma, schneiderian papilloma, squamous cell papilloma, transitional cell papilloma, cylindrical epithelioma

Definitions

- Benign epithelial tumor of nasal mucosa with histology showing epithelium proliferating into underlying stroma

IMAGING

General Features

- Best diagnostic clue
  - Mass along lateral nasal wall **centered at middle meatus** ± extension into antrum with local bone remodeling & obstructive sinus disease
- Location
  - Most commonly originates along lateral nasal wall near middle meatus
  - Spreads into adjacent sinuses
    - Maxillary (69%), ethmoid (50-90%), sphenoid (10-20%), frontal (10-15%), orbit & CNS (~ 30%)
  - Uncommonly originates in maxillary antrum, sphenoid, frontal, or ethmoid sinuses
- Size
  - Small IPap: < 3-cm mass centered in middle meatal region of lateral wall of nose
  - Large IPap: > 3-cm mass that remodels nasal cavity, invades or obstructs ipsilateral sinuses

CT Findings

- NECT
  - Soft tissue mass along lateral nasal wall at middle meatus ± extension into maxillary sinus
    - 40% show entrapped bone
    - 10% show tumorous calcification
    - Focal hyperostosis of adjacent bone (plaque or cone-shaped) may indicate point of tumor origin
  - Unilateral obstruction yields ostiomeatal unit pattern of inflammatory sinus disease
  - Small IPap may show no bone changes, making identification of tumor difficult
  - Larger IPap shows bone remodeling & mass effect in middle meatal region
    - Consider synchronous squamous cell carcinoma (SCCa) if bony destruction ± focal loss of cerebriform morphology
- CECT
  - IPap enhances while obstructed sinus secretions do not
    - Variable enhancement pattern from diffuse to heterogeneous
    - **Convoluted, cerebriform appearance** evident with contrast

MR Findings

- T1WI
  - Isointense to slightly hyperintense to soft tissue & muscle
- T2WI
  - Heterogeneous, predominantly hyperintense to skeletal muscle
    - Curvilinear striations or convoluted, cerebriform pattern is distinctive
  - Areas of necrosis & postobstructive secretions are high signal on T2
- T1WI C+
  - Enhancement may have convoluted, cerebriform appearance
  - If portion of tumor appears invasive or necrosis present → consider synchronous SCCa

Imaging Recommendations

- Best imaging tool
  - Tumor usually 1st detected on sinus CT performed for evaluation of "sinusitis" symptoms
  - When mass is found on CT, MR completed for preoperative tumor mapping
- Protocol advice
  - Multiplanar MR optimal for tumor mapping & differentiating tumor from obstructed secretions
  - T2 FS & T1 C+ FS sequences best show internal architecture

Nuclear Medicine Findings

- PET/CT
  - High FDG uptake with SUV max > 3.0 typical in IPap with higher SUV in associated SCCa
    - PET cannot be reliably distinguish benign IPap & SCCa

DIFFERENTIAL DIAGNOSIS

Sinonasal Solitary Polyps

- Antrochoanal polyp: Dumbbell-shaped lesion involving maxillary antrum & ipsilateral nasal cavity
- Peripheral, **not central**, enhancing lesion with mucus or fluid density (CT) or intensity (MR) contents

Sinonasal SCCa

- Destroys rather than remodels bones in most cases
- Typically originates within maxillary antrum > nasal cavity

Sinonasal Polyposis

- Polypoid lesions in nasal cavity & paranasal sinuses
- Bone remodeling & sinus expansion

Juvenile Angiofibroma

- Adolescent boys with nose bleeds
- Mass centered at margin of sphenopalatine foramen in posterior nasal cavity
- Intense enhancement of this highly vascular mass is typical

Esthesioneuroblastoma

- Typically centered in superior nasal cavity near cribriform plate
- Intense enhancement; more likely to invade orbit/anterior skull base

PATHOLOGY

General Features

- Etiology

- o Maturation of sinonasal mucosa into ciliated columnar epithelium & mucous glands gives rise to papillomas
- o Neither etiology nor factors responsible for malignant transformation are fully elucidated
  - − Viral origin has been postulated (e.g., human papilloma virus)
- Associated abnormalities
  - o **10%** either degenerate into or **coexist with SCCa**
    - − SCCa may be either synchronous (7%) or metachronous (4%)

Staging, Grading, & Classification

- 3 schneiderian papilloma types arise from nasal mucosa
  - o Inverted papilloma (47%)
  - o Fungiform papilloma (50%): Occurs on nasal septum in young males; rarely imaged prior to surgical treatment
  - o Cylindric cell papilloma (3%)
- No widely accepted, clinically relevant staging system

Gross Pathologic & Surgical Features

- Endoscopic or surgical observations
  - o Bulky, opaque, polypoid mucosal mass with red-gray color characteristic of lobulated tumor surface

Microscopic Features

- Hyperplastic squamous epithelium replacing seromucinous ducts & glands in underlying stroma
  - o Mucosal infoldings into stroma without interrupting basement membrane
- Surrounding nasal mucosa often shows squamous metaplasia

CLINICAL ISSUES

Presentation

- Most common signs/symptoms
  - o Similar to recurrent sinusitis with nasal obstruction & discharge
- Other signs/symptoms
  - o Epistaxis, anosmia, headache, pain
- Clinical profile
  - o Adult **male** patient with symptoms similar to chronic rhinosinusitis

Demographics

- Age
  - o Typically 40-70 years
- Gender
  - o M > F (4-5:1)
- Epidemiology
  - o 0.5-7% of all tumors of nasal cavity
  - o Involves at least 1 paranasal sinus 82% of time
  - o Typically unifocal; causes unilateral "sinusitis"
    - − Multifocal in 4% of cases
  - o Bilateral in up to 13% due to transseptal extension

Natural History & Prognosis

- Benign, but locally aggressive tumor
  - o Strong potential for local recurrence if incompletely resected
  - o When SCCa is associated, prognosis changes to survival rates associated with nasal SCCa

Treatment

- Type of surgery depends on location and size of lesion as well as involvement of critical structures
  - o Surgical resection using variety of methods
    - − Endoscopic resection is effective for most smaller tumors
    - − Midfacial degloving & sublabial approaches for larger lesions
    - − Medial maxillectomy through lateral rhinotomy + wide en bloc excision in more extensive IPap

DIAGNOSTIC CHECKLIST

Consider

- T1 C+ FS MR used to search for convoluted, cerebriform appearance
- MR used to evaluate for extension beyond sinonasal cavities & differentiate tumor from secretions

Image Interpretation Pearls

- Identify invasion of deeper areas (ethmoid sinuses, pterygopalatine fossa, orbit) at imaging as this may alter surgical approach
- Areas of necrosis or frank bony destruction should raise suspicion for coexistent SCCa
- Look for additional masses as 4% multifocal

SELECTED REFERENCES

1. Adriaensen GF et al: Challenges in the management of inverted papilloma: a review of 72 revision cases. Laryngoscope. 126(2):322-8, 2016
2. Zhao RW et al: Human papillomavirus infection and the malignant transformation of sinonasal inverted papilloma: a meta-analysis. J Clin Virol. 79:36-43, 2016
3. Jeon TY et al: 18F-FDG PET/CT findings of sinonasal inverted papilloma with or without coexistent malignancy: comparison with MR imaging findings in eight patients. Neuroradiology. 51(4):265-71, 2009
4. Karkos PD et al: Computed tomography and/or magnetic resonance imaging for pre-operative planning for inverted nasal papilloma: review of evidence. J Laryngol Otol. 123(7):705-9, 2009
5. Jeon TY et al: Sinonasal inverted papilloma: value of convoluted cerebriform pattern on MR imaging. AJNR Am J Neuroradiol. 29(8):1556-60, 2008
6. Sham CL et al: The roles and limitations of computed tomography in the preoperative assessment of sinonasal inverted papillomas. Am J Rhinol. 22(2):144-50, 2008
7. Cannady SB et al: New staging system for sinonasal inverted papilloma in the endoscopic era. Laryngoscope. 117(7):1283-7, 2007
8. Head CS et al: Radiographic assessment of inverted papilloma. Acta Otolaryngol. 127(5):515-20, 2007
9. Lee DK et al: Focal hyperostosis on CT of sinonasal inverted papilloma as a predictor of tumor origin. AJNR Am J Neuroradiol. 28(4):618-21, 2007
10. Shojaku H et al: Positron emission tomography for predicting malignancy of sinonasal inverted papilloma. Clin Nucl Med. 32(4):275-8, 2007
11. Yousuf K et al: Site of attachment of inverted papilloma predicted by CT findings of osteitis. Am J Rhinol. 21(1):32-6, 2007
12. Chiu AG et al: Radiographic and histologic analysis of the bone underlying inverted papillomas. Laryngoscope. 116(9):1617-20, 2006
13. Maroldi R et al: Magnetic resonance imaging findings of inverted papilloma: differential diagnosis with malignant sinonasal tumors. Am J Rhinol. 18(5):305-10, 2004
14. Klimek T et al: Inverted papilloma of the nasal cavity and paranasal sinuses: clinical data, surgical strategy and recurrence rates. Acta Otolaryngol. 120(2):267-72, 2000
15. Ojiri H et al: Potentially distinctive features of sinonasal inverted papilloma on MR imaging. AJR Am J Roentgenol. 175(2):465-8, 2000
16. Phillips PP et al: The clinical behavior of inverting papilloma of the nose and paranasal sinuses: report of 112 cases and review of the literature. Laryngoscope. 100(5):463-9, 1990

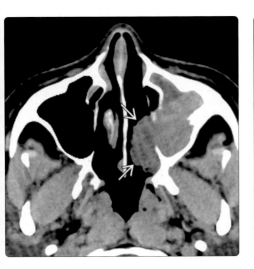

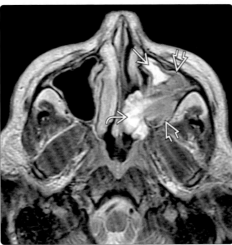

(Left) *Axial NECT shows a slightly lobular soft tissue mass within the left nasal cavity* ⮕ *with extension into the left maxillary sinus. The location is typical of a papilloma. It is difficult to differentiate the mass from obstructed secretions on the CT.* (Right) *Axial T2 MR shows a heterogeneous inverted papilloma* ⮕ *that occupies most of the maxillary antrum. The mass is hypointense compared to secretions* ⮕ *trapped anteromedially. The nasal component of this papilloma* ⮕ *is hyperintense.*

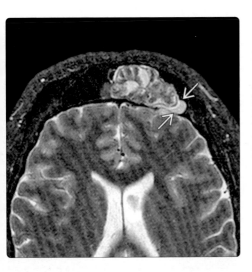

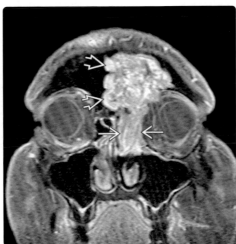

(Left) *Axial STIR MR shows the classic architecture of inverted papilloma. The lesion shows a convoluted, cerebriform appearance. Trapped secretions laterally* ⮕ *are hyperintense compared to the mass. The frontal sinus is an unusual location for this lesion.* (Right) *Coronal T1 C+ FS MR shows inverted papilloma involving the ethmoid sinuses* ⮕ *in addition to the frontal sinus. Trapped secretions* ⮕ *along the margin of frontal tumor component are proteinaceous with intrinsic T1 shortening.*

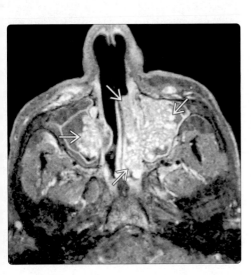

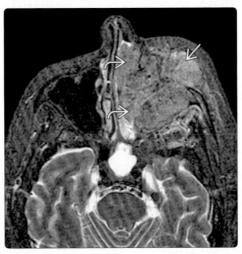

(Left) *Axial T1 C+ MR shows an unusual case of bilateral inverted papillomas* ⮕ *due to transseptal extension involving the maxillary sinuses. The larger lesion on the left nearly fills the nasal cavity. Both lesions demonstrate the typical convoluted morphology.* (Right) *Axial STIR MR demonstrates a squamous carcinoma arising within an inverted papilloma. Papilloma involves the left nasal cavity* ⮕ *and maxillary sinus. The carcinoma has destroyed the anterior maxillary wall and extends into the premaxillary soft tissues* ⮕.

Sinonasal Hemangioma

TERMINOLOGY

- Lobular capillary hemangioma (LCH): Benign capillary proliferation with distinct lobular architecture
  - Old term: Pyogenic granuloma

IMAGING

- Location: LCH: Nasal septum (55%), particularly anteriorly (17%)
- Typically ≤ 2 cm
- CT
  - Central areas of lobular enhancement surrounded by iso- to hypodense "cap" of variable thickness
  - May cause bone erosion or remodeling
- MR
  - Usually **T2 hyperintense**
  - Homogeneous, **avid enhancement ± flow voids**
- Lobular areas of capillary blush on angiography
  - Preoperative embolization ↓ intraoperative bleeding

TOP DIFFERENTIAL DIAGNOSES

- Venous malformation (old term: Cavernous hemangioma)
  - No central avid enhancement or flow voids
  - Centripetal pattern of enhancement with delayed filling
  - Variable T2 signal
- Sinonasal melanoma
- Juvenile angiofibroma
- Angiomatous polyp
- Hemangiopericytoma

PATHOLOGY

- Predisposing factors include trauma & hormonal influences

CLINICAL ISSUES

- Symptoms: Epistaxis & nasal obstruction
- Peak incidence in 5th decade with slight F > M

DIAGNOSTIC CHECKLIST

- Multiplanar MR if lesion near skull base

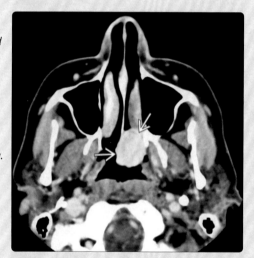
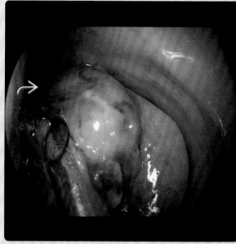

(Left) *Axial CECT demonstrates an avidly enhancing, well-circumscribed soft tissue mass ➡ in the posterior nasal cavity and protruding into the nasopharynx. No bony destructive changes were seen. This lobular hemangioma arose from the inferior turbinate; the patient presented with nasal bleeding.* (Right) *Endoscopic view of a lobular capillary hemangioma shows a lobulated, epithelial lined, red hypervascular mass ➡.*

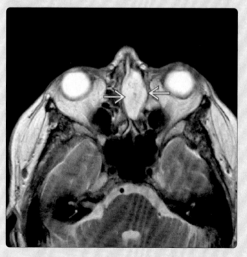
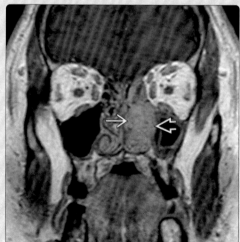

(Left) *Axial T2 MR demonstrates a well-defined, ovoid soft tissue mass ➡ in the superior aspect of the left nasal cavity in an adult patient with intermittent epistaxis. The lesion is homogeneously hyperintense on this sequence, typical of hemangioma. No orbital invasion is appreciated.* (Right) *Coronal T1 C+ MR shows homogeneous enhancement with a left nasal cavity hemangioma ➡. Note the mild expansion of the lateral nasal wall ➡ but no overtly invasive features.*

TERMINOLOGY

Synonyms

- Lobular capillary hemangioma (LCH) (old term: Pyogenic granuloma)
  - Misnomer: No evidence for infectious origin & granulation tissue not present histologically
- Other archaic terms: Telangiectatic granuloma, granuloma pedunculatum, human botryomycosis

Definitions

- LCH: Benign capillary proliferation with microscopically distinct lobular architecture affecting skin and mucous membranes of oral cavity & nasal region

IMAGING

General Features

- Best diagnostic clue
  - Well-defined, enhancing nasal cavity mass arising from **anterior septum or turbinates**
- Location
  - LCH: Nasal septum most common (55%), particularly anterior nasal vestibule (17%)
- Size
  - Typically ≤ 2 cm (CH is generally larger than LCH)
- Morphology
  - Well defined, lobulated

CT Findings

- CECT
  - **Avid enhancement**
  - Central areas of lobular enhancement surrounded by iso- to hypodense "cap" of variable thickness

MR Findings

- T1WI
  - Low- to intermediate-signal mass (compared to muscle)
- T2WI
  - Most often **hyperintense**
  - Larger lesions may show signal voids (**flow voids**)
- T1WI C+
  - Intense homogeneous enhancement

Angiographic Findings

- Lobular areas of capillary blush
- Preoperative embolization ↓ intraoperative bleeding

Imaging Recommendations

- Best imaging tool
  - Multiplanar enhanced MR
  - If large, bone CT for bone changes

DIFFERENTIAL DIAGNOSIS

Venous Malformation

- Old term is cavernous hemangioma; historical misnomer applies to nonneoplastic **venous malformation**
- May mimic LCH clinically & even pathologically, but imaging differs
- Lateral nasal wall typical location
- Centripetal-lobular & mild contrast enhancement or multifocal nodular

- Fills in centrally on delayed imaging
- Heterogeneous & variable T2 signal: Mixed hypo & hyperintensity
- May cause bone erosive changes

Juvenile Angiofibroma

- Occurs exclusively in males, usually adolescent
- Posteriorly nasal cavity near sphenopalatine foramen

Sinonasal Melanoma

- Clinical: Middle-aged patient
- ↑ precontrast T1 signal, ↓ T2 signal

Hemangiopericytoma

- More likely within sinus
- May contain bone or cartilage

PATHOLOGY

General Features

- Etiology
  - Predisposing factors include **trauma** (nose picking, nasal packing) & **hormonal factors** (pregnancy, oral contraceptives)

Gross Pathologic & Surgical Features

- Solitary, red-to-purple hypervascularized nasal mass ± superficial ulceration

Microscopic Features

- Lobular growth pattern of capillary proliferation

CLINICAL ISSUES

Presentation

- Most common signs/symptoms
  - **Epistaxis** & nasal obstruction

Demographics

- Age
  - Peak incidence in 5th decade
- Gender
  - Slight female predominance

Natural History & Prognosis

- "Pregnancy tumor" may regress after parturition

Treatment

- Local surgical excision

DIAGNOSTIC CHECKLIST

Consider

- Multiplanar MR for tumor mapping if lesion extends superiorly toward skull base

SELECTED REFERENCES

1. Kim JH et al: Computed tomography and magnetic resonance imaging findings of nasal cavity hemangiomas according to histological type. Korean J Radiol. 16(3):566-74, 2015
2. Iwata N et al: Hemangioma of the nasal cavity: a clinicopathologic study. Auris Nasus Larynx. 29(4):335-9, 2002
3. Dillon WP et al: Hemangioma of the nasal vault: MR and CT features. Radiology. 180(3):761-5, 1991

Sinonasal Nerve Sheath Tumor

KEY FACTS

TERMINOLOGY

- Slow-growing, benign tumors arising from nerve sheath (schwannoma) or peripheral nerve tissue (neurofibroma)
- Peripheral nerve sheath tumor (PNST)

IMAGING

- Well-defined, **expansile** soft tissue mass arising in nasoethmoid region with adjacent bone remodeling
- MR shows extent & differentiates obstructed secretions
  - Hypo- to hyperintense ± **intramural cysts**
  - Schwannoma: **Whorled** pattern of enhancement
- NECT best shows **benign osseous remodeling**

TOP DIFFERENTIAL DIAGNOSES

- Inverted papilloma
- Sinonasal benign mixed tumor (pleomorphic adenoma)
- Sinonasal solitary polyp
- Sinonasal lymphoma
- Sinonasal melanoma

PATHOLOGY

- Several PNST types: Schwannoma, neurofibroma, perineurioma (rare in sinonasal region), & malignant PNST
- ↑ incidence of sinonasal neurofibromas in *NF1*
- ↑ incidence of sinonasal schwannomas in *NF2*
- FNA may confuse schwannoma with spindle cell sarcoma

CLINICAL ISSUES

- Rare sinonasal benign tumor
- Nonspecific symptoms may mimic inflammatory disease
  - Nasal obstruction, epistaxis, anosmia
- < 4% of H&N schwannomas arise in sinonasal cavities
- Treatment: Surgical excision is curative

DIAGNOSTIC CHECKLIST

- Imaging role: Direct biopsy, accurately map extent of lesion, & look for orbital/intracranial extension
- Imaging features usually not specific enough to make histologic diagnosis

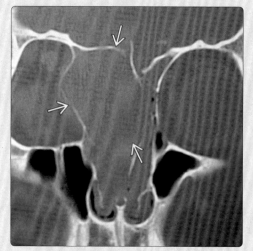
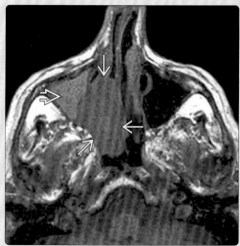

(Left) *Coronal bone CT demonstrates an expansile mass involving the right nasal cavity and ethmoid region ➡. Note the smooth remodeling of the bone surrounding the lesion suggestive of a benign mass. This schwannoma could be confused with a mucocele on CT alone.* (Right) *Axial T1 MR shows a schwannoma in the right nasal cavity ➡ deviating the septum to the left. Trapped secretions with high T1 signal are noted lateral to the mass in the maxillary sinus ➡.*

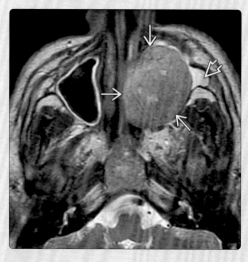
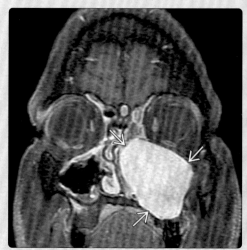

(Left) *Axial T2 MR in a young male patient with facial swelling and nasal obstruction shows a well-defined, low-signal mass centered in the left maxillary sinus ➡ with trapped secretions lateral to the lesion ➡.* (Right) *Coronal T1 C+ FS MR shows diffuse enhancement throughout neurofibroma ➡, easily distinguishing this solid enhancing tumor from mucocele, a more common expansile paranasal sinus lesion.*

TERMINOLOGY

Synonyms

- Peripheral nerve sheath tumor (PNST)
  - Schwannoma = neurilemoma

Definitions

- Slow-growing, benign tumors of nerve sheath (schwannoma) or peripheral nerve tissue (neurofibroma)

IMAGING

General Features

- Best diagnostic clue
  - Well-defined, expansile soft tissue mass arising in nasoethmoid region with adjacent bone remodeling
- Location
  - Schwannomas most common in nasal cavity & ethmoids
  - Rare cases extend into orbit or intracranially
- Size
  - Can reach large size
- Morphology
  - Usually ovoid-round, smooth margin

Imaging Recommendations

- Best imaging tool
  - MR for extent & differentiate from obstructed secretions
  - Bone CT best shows benign pattern of bone remodeling
- Protocol advice
  - Multiplanar MR with T1, STIR/T2 FS, & T1 C+ FS

CT Findings

- NECT
  - Schwannoma: Isodense to other soft tissue
  - Neurofibroma: May show homogeneous ↓ attenuation
- CECT
  - Variable enhancement, but usually mild
- Bone CT
  - **Expansile** mass with **bone remodeling**, not destruction

MR Findings

- T1WI
  - Intermediate signal typical
- T2WI
  - Hypo- to hyperintense ± **intramural cysts**
- T1WI C+ FS
  - Schwannoma: **Whorled** pattern of enhancement

DIFFERENTIAL DIAGNOSIS

Sinonasal Inverted Papilloma

- Convoluted or "cerebriform" architecture

Sinonasal Benign Mixed Tumor

- Imaging looks benign, but is nonspecific

Sinonasal Mucocele

- Peripheral **(no central) enhancement** with contrast

Solitary Sinonasal Polyps

- Homogeneous ↓ T1 & ↑ T2 MR signal
- Peripheral **(no central) enhancement**

Juvenile Angiofibroma

- Adolescent boys with nasal obstruction & epistaxis
- Highly vascular with avid enhancement & flow voids on MR

Sinonasal Non-Hodgkin Lymphoma

- Malignant lymphoid neoplasm with nasal cavity predilection

Sinonasal Melanoma

- Malignancy typically arising in septum/turbinates
- ↑ T1 & ↓ T2 MR signal typical of highly melanotic lesions

PATHOLOGY

General Features

- Etiology
  - Schwannomas arise from Schwann cells of CNV (V1 & V2) & autonomic nerves to septal vessels & mucosa
- Genetics
  - ↑ incidence of sinonasal neurofibromas in *NF1*
  - ↑ incidence of sinonasal schwannomas in *NF2*

Microscopic Features

- Schwannoma: Compact spindle cell proliferations of hypercellular (Antoni A) and myxoid (Antoni B) areas

CLINICAL ISSUES

Presentation

- Most common signs/symptoms
  - Symptoms often nonspecific, mimics inflammation
  - Nasal obstruction, epistaxis, anosmia

Demographics

- Age
  - Children to elderly
  - Most schwannomas present in 4th-6th decades
- Epidemiology
  - 45% of PNST arise in H&N
  - < 4% of H&N schwannomas are sinonasal

Natural History & Prognosis

- Prognosis excellent for benign nerve sheath tumors
- Malignant transformation: Neurofibroma > schwannoma

Treatment

- Surgical excision is curative
- Adjuvant radiotherapy reserved for malignant lesions

DIAGNOSTIC CHECKLIST

Image Interpretation Pearls

- Role of imaging is to direct biopsy, accurately map extent of lesion, evaluate for orbital/intracranial extension

SELECTED REFERENCES

1. Yang B et al: Magnetic Resonance imaging features of schwannoma of the sinonasal tract. J Comput Assist Tomogr. 39(6):860-5, 2015
2. Fang WS et al: An unusual sinonasal tumor: soft tissue perineurioma. AJNR Am J Neuroradiol. 30(2):437-9, 2009
3. Yu E et al: CT and MR imaging findings in sinonasal schwannoma. AJNR Am J Neuroradiol. 27(4):929-30, 2006

KEY FACTS

TERMINOLOGY

- Synonym: Pleomorphic adenoma
- Benign, histologically heterogeneous tumor with epithelial, myoepithelial, & stromal components

IMAGING

- Originates in nasal cavity (septum > lateral nasal) > paranasal sinuses
- CT findings
  - Well-demarcated soft tissue mass in anterior nasal cavity often arising from septum
  - Bone remodeled rather than destroyed
- MR findings
  - Typically **very high T2 signal** and low T1 signal
  - Variable enhancement; heterogeneous in larger lesions

TOP DIFFERENTIAL DIAGNOSES

- Sinonasal solitary polyp
- Sinonasal inverted papilloma

- Juvenile angiofibroma
- Sinonasal nerve sheath tumor

PATHOLOGY

- Thought to arise from minor salivary rests
  - Nasal septal BMT tends to be highly cellular with little stromal component (compared to salivary gland tumors)

CLINICAL ISSUES

- Presentation
  - Nasal obstruction ± epistaxis
  - Most present at 30-60 years
  - More common in women
- Slow growing with excellent prognosis
- Treatment is local surgical excision
- Consider BMT in adult patient with benign-appearing anterior nasal mass
- Consider dermoid cysts, intranasal gliomas, & nasoethmoidal encephalocele in children

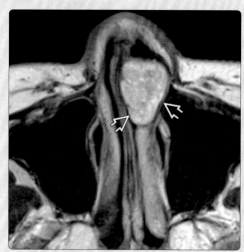

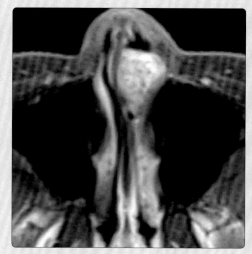

(Left) *Axial T2 MR shows a well-circumscribed, heterogeneous, hyperintense benign mixed tumor (BMT) in the left anterior nasal cavity* ➡ *arising from the anterior nasal septum.* (Right) *Axial T1 C+ FS MR shows an avidly enhancing BMT in the anterior nasal cavity. Central enhancement excludes nasal polyp, but imaging is not specific and other neoplastic processes are in the differential diagnosis for this appearance.*

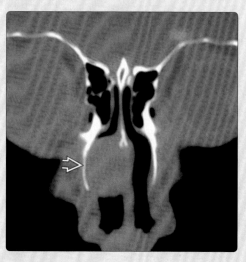

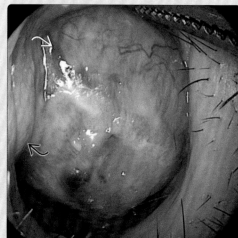

(Left) *Coronal bone CT demonstrates a circumscribed BMT in the right nasal cavity adjacent to the nasal septum. There is lateral displacement and remodeling, but not destruction, of the lateral nasal wall* ➡, *which is typical of a benign lesion.* (Right) *Nasal endoscopic view demonstrates a well-circumscribed, round BMT* ➡ *in the anterior nasal cavity originating from the anterior nasal septum* ➡.

TERMINOLOGY

Abbreviations

- Benign mixed tumor (BMT)

Synonyms

- Pleomorphic adenoma

Definitions

- Benign, histologically heterogeneous tumor with epithelial, myoepithelial, & stromal components

IMAGING

General Features

- Best diagnostic clue
  - Sharply marginated, round-ovoid soft tissue mass ± adjacent bone remodeling
- Location
  - Nasal cavity (septum > lateral nasal) > paranasal sinuses
    - Maxillary sinus & nasopharynx less common
- Size
  - Most < 2 cm
- Morphology
  - Round or ovoid with well-defined margins
  - Larger lesions may have lobular margins

Imaging Recommendations

- Best imaging tool
  - CECT vs. multiplanar enhanced MR
- Protocol advice
  - Bone window images helpful for evaluating bone remodeling

CT Findings

- NECT
  - Well-demarcated soft tissue mass in anterior nasal cavity often arising from septum
- CECT
  - Variable enhancement; heterogeneous in larger lesions
- Bone CT
  - Bone **remodeled** rather than destroyed

MR Findings

- T1WI
  - Well-circumscribed, low-signal mass
- T2WI
  - Typically **very high T2** signal
    - Heterogeneous signal in larger lesions
- T1WI C+ FS
  - Small lesions enhance homogeneously
  - Heterogeneous enhancement in larger BMT

DIFFERENTIAL DIAGNOSIS

Sinonasal Solitary Polyp

- Low attenuation with peripheral enhancement only
- Usually arises in maxillary antrum & extends into nasal cavity

Sinonasal Inverted Papilloma

- Arises along lateral nasal wall near middle meatus
- Convoluted, cerebriform architecture ± Ca++

Juvenile Angiofibroma

- Adolescent male patient with nasal obstruction & epistaxis
- Arises in posterior nasal cavity near sphenopalatine foramen
- Vascular lesion with avid enhancement & flow voids

Sinonasal Nerve Sheath Tumor

- Rare, benign mass
- Usually arises in superior nasal cavity

Sinonasal Osteoma

- Most common in frontal & ethmoid sinuses > nasal cavity
- Dense bony lesion or mixed soft tissue & bone density

PATHOLOGY

General Features

- Etiology
  - Thought to arise from **minor salivary rests**

Microscopic Features

- Lobular architecture of loose chondromyxoid stroma and cellular component of rounded epithelial & spindle-shaped myoepithelial cells

CLINICAL ISSUES

Presentation

- Most common signs/symptoms
  - Nasal obstruction
- Other signs/symptoms
  - Intermittent epistaxis
  - Swelling or mass of nose

Demographics

- Age
  - Most present at 30-60 years but can occur at any age
    - Consider dermoid cysts, intranasal gliomas, & nasoethmoidal encephalocele in children
- Gender
  - F > M
- Epidemiology
  - 8% of BMTs arise outside of major salivary glands (mainly in minor salivary rests in oral cavity)

Natural History & Prognosis

- Slow growing with excellent prognosis
- Tendency to recur if incompletely resected
  - Lower recurrence rate compared to parotid & intraoral BMT
- Carcinoma may arise rarely in BMT

Treatment

- Local surgical excision with clear margins generally curative

DIAGNOSTIC CHECKLIST

Consider

- Imaging features are nonspecific, but consider BMT in adult patient with benign-appearing anterior nasal mass

SELECTED REFERENCES

1. Kuan EC et al: Sinonasal and skull base pleomorphic adenoma: a case series and literature review. Int Forum Allergy Rhinol. 5(5):460-8, 2015

Sinonasal Squamous Cell Carcinoma

TERMINOLOGY

- Malignant epithelial tumor with squamous cell or epidermoid differentiation

IMAGING

- Location: Maxillary antrum involved in > 80%
- CT findings
  ○ Soft tissue density mass with irregular margins
  ○ Aggressive **bone destruction**
- MR findings
  ○ ↓ T2 signal due to ↑ nuclear:cytoplasmic ratio
  ○ Enhances to lesser degree than other sinonasal malignancies
- Multiplanar enhanced MR optimal for tumor mapping, detection of perineural tumor spread & nodes

TOP DIFFERENTIAL DIAGNOSES

- Sinonasal adenocarcinoma
- Sinonasal undifferentiated carcinoma
- Invasive fungal sinusitis
- Sinonasal non-Hodgkin lymphoma
- Wegener granulomatosis
- Adenoid cystic carcinoma

PATHOLOGY

- Risk factors: Inhaled wood dust, metallic particles (nickel & chromium), chemicals, HPV, inverted papilloma
  ○ Formaldehyde, arsenic & asbestos exposure may ↑ risk
  ○ HPV, pre- or coexisting inverted papilloma ↑ risk

CLINICAL ISSUES

- Symptoms mimic chronic sinusitis & delay diagnosis
- Age at presentation: 50-70 years old
- Most common malignancy of sinonasal area
- 15% maxillary sinus squamous cell carcinomas have malignant adenopathy
- Overall **5-year survival: 60%**
- Combined surgery & XRT most common treatment

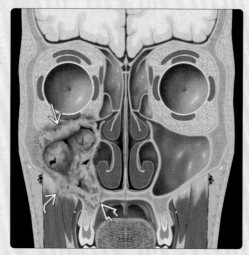
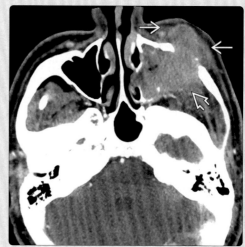

(Left) Coronal graphic shows the typical features of an aggressive right maxillary squamous cell carcinoma (SCCa) with destruction of the maxillary sinus walls. Extension into the orbit ➡, maxillary alveolus ➡, and buccal space ➡ is noted. (Right) Axial CECT shows the typical location and appearance of an antral SCCa. There is extension into the premaxillary soft tissues anteriorly ➡ and through the posterior maxillary wall into the infratemporal fossa ➡.

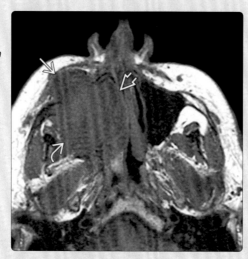
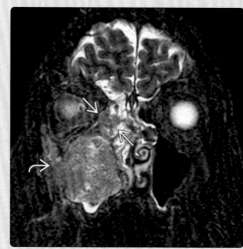

(Left) Axial T1 MR shows a large antral SCCa. The signal of the mass is similar to other soft tissues. There is extension anteriorly into the premaxillary soft tissues ➡, medially into the nasal cavity ➡, and posteriorly into the masticator space ➡. (Right) Coronal T2 FS MR of SCCa demonstrates ethmoid sinus involvement ➡ and masticator space extension ➡. The low T2 signal of this mass is consistent with high cellularity and N:C ratio.

Sinonasal Squamous Cell Carcinoma

TERMINOLOGY

Abbreviations
- Squamous cell carcinoma (SCCa)

Synonyms
- Epidermoid carcinoma, transitional carcinoma, nonkeratinizing carcinoma, respiratory mucosal carcinoma

Definitions
- Malignant epithelial tumor growing from sinus surface epithelium into sinus lumen with squamous cell or epidermoid differentiation

IMAGING

General Features
- Best diagnostic clue
  - Aggressive antral soft tissue mass with invasion & destruction of sinus walls
- Location
  - 75% arise in sinuses; ~ 30% arise primarily in nose
    - **Maxillary antrum (85%)**, ethmoid (10%), frontal/sphenoid (< 5%)
  - Radiologist creates presurgical tumor map of spread
    - Medial: Nasal cavity → ethmoid sinuses
    - Anterior: Premaxillary soft tissues of cheek
    - Posterior: Retroantral fat pad, pterygopalatine fossa (PPF) & masticator space
    - Lateral: Malar eminence & subcutaneous tissues
    - Superior: Through orbital floor into orbit proper or via PPF → inferior orbital fissure → orbit
    - Inferior: Maxillary alveolar ridge, buccal space, & hard palate
    - Perineural tumor spread (PNTS): Inferior orbital nerve or PPF → V2 (foramen rotundum) → cavernous sinus
- Size
  - Usually fills maxillary antrum
- Morphology
  - Well defined to poorly defined with irregular, **spiculated margins**

CT Findings
- CECT
  - Solid, moderately enhancing mass with aggressive bone destruction
  - Enhancement tends to be heterogeneous
  - Nonenhancing areas may represent necrosis
- Bone CT
  - **Bone destruction** is characteristic
  - Soft tissue density mass with irregular margins

MR Findings
- T1WI
  - Intermediate-signal mass, similar to muscle signal
  - Areas of intratumoral hemorrhage may show ↑ T1 signal
- T2WI
  - Intermediate to high signal compared to musculature, but lower than other sinonasal malignancies
    - **↓ T2 signal** due to ↑ cellularity & ↑ nuclear:cytoplasmic (N:C) ratio

- T2 differentiates high-signal obstructed sinus secretions from tumor
- DWI
  - Mildly restricted diffusion due to ↑ N:C ratio
- T1WI C+
  - Enhancement typically mild to moderate; diffuse, but heterogeneous
    - **Enhances to lesser degree** than adenocarcinoma, esthesioneuroblastoma, melanoma
  - Areas of necrosis do not enhance
  - T1 C+ FS images optimal for detecting PNTS

Nuclear Medicine Findings
- PET
  - Avid uptake of F-18 FDG due to hypermetabolism
    - Useful in staging to identify metastatic disease
  - If SCCa arose in inverted papilloma, both may show avid FDG uptake

Imaging Recommendations
- Best imaging tool
  - Most are initially diagnosed on routine NECT for evaluation of "sinusitis" symptoms
  - Multiplanar enhanced MR optimal for tumor mapping, detection of PNTS, & retropharyngeal nodes
- Protocol advice
  - Precontrast T1 & postcontrast T1 MR with fat suppression from sellar floor to hyoid bone

DIFFERENTIAL DIAGNOSIS

Sinonasal Adenocarcinoma
- Imaging features can be similar to SCCa
- Predilection for ethmoid sinus
- Tends to enhance more than SCCa

Sinonasal Undifferentiated Carcinoma
- Can be impossible to distinguish from SCCa
- Rapidly growing

Invasive Fungal Sinusitis
- Immunocompromised patient
- Rapidly progressive destructive lesion
- ICA invasion and thrombosis may be associated

Sinonasal Non-Hodgkin Lymphoma
- Bulky homogeneous sinonasal mass (B-cell type)
- Tendency to cause nasal septum destruction (NKTL type)
- May exactly mimic Wegener granulomatosis

Wegener Granulomatosis
- Septal and nonseptal bone destruction in nose
- Chronic sinusitis associated
- Sinonasal disease associated with tracheobronchial and renal disease

PATHOLOGY

General Features
- Etiology
  - Risk factors: Inhaled wood dust, metallic particles (nickel, chromium), & chemicals used in leather & textile industries; Thorotrast exposure

- Formaldehyde & asbestos exposure may ↑ risk
- HPV, pre- or coexisting inverted papilloma ↑ risk
- No direct link to alcohol or tobacco use

Staging, Grading, & Classification

- Staging taken from AJCC staging tables (7th edition)
- **Maxillary sinus** primary tumor (T) staging criteria
  - **T1**: Maxillary antrum only; **no bone destruction**
  - **T2**: Bone invasion (hard palate, nasal wall); **not** involving posterior wall maxillary sinus or pterygoid plates
  - **T3**: Invades bone of posterior wall ± subcutaneous tissues ± floor of medial orbital wall ± pterygoid fossa ± ethmoid sinuses
  - **T4a** (resectable): Invades anterior orbit, skin, infratemporal fossa, pterygoid plates, cribriform plate, frontal or sphenoid sinuses
  - **T4b** (unresectable): Involves orbital apex, dura, brain, middle fossa, clivus, nasopharynx, cranial nerves (other than V2)

Gross Pathologic & Surgical Features

- Friable, polypoid, papillary, or fungating soft tissue mass
- Aggressive spread into adjacent structures

Microscopic Features

- 2 main subtypes: Keratinizing (80%) & nonkeratinizing (20%)
  - Keratinizing: Papillary or inverted architectural patterns; dyskeratosis, poorly to well differentiated
  - Nonkeratinizing: Exophytic pattern; interconnecting ribbon-like growth, hypercellular, pleomorphism, used to be called transitional cell carcinoma
- Papillary variant of SCCa uncommon

CLINICAL ISSUES

Presentation

- Most common signs/symptoms
  - **Symptoms mimic chronic sinusitis** & delay diagnosis
  - Nasal cavity primaries present earlier with nasal obstruction, bleeding
- Other signs/symptoms
  - Larger maxillary tumors: Unilateral nasal obstruction, epistaxis, & cheek numbness
  - Tooth pain or loosening, proptosis & diplopia, trismus, facial asymmetry
- Clinical profile
  - Older male patient presenting with unilateral sinusitis refractory to medical therapy

Demographics

- Age
  - 50-70 years old
- Gender
  - M > F
- Epidemiology
  - 3% of H&N neoplasms
  - **Most common malignancy** of sinonasal area
    - SCCa accounts for 80% of malignant tumors of sinonasal area
  - 15% of maxillary sinus SCCa have malignant adenopathy
    - Retropharyngeal or level II jugular chain nodes

- ↑ incidence if history of radiation therapy to H&N
- ↑ incidence in immunosuppressed patients

Natural History & Prognosis

- Overall **5-year survival: 60%**
- Survival statistics heavily influenced by tumor stage
  - T1 SCCa treated aggressively have 100% survival (rarely diagnosed at T1 primary stage)
  - 5-year survival rates for T4a primary SCCa drop to 34%
- Better prognosis: Nasal cavity SCCa, low tumor stage, HPV-positive tumor & history of inverted papilloma
- Worse prognosis: Extension beyond sinus walls, regional nodal disease, PNTS, large primary size
- Relapse occurs at primary site > regional lymph nodes
  - If tumor recurs, 90% < 1-year survival

Treatment

- Combined treatment with surgery & XRT
  - En bloc resection vs. endoscopic resection depending on tumor size & structures involved
  - XRT may be conventional, 3D conformal, or IMRT
- Chemotherapy gaining popularity as genetics of SCCa better understood

DIAGNOSTIC CHECKLIST

Consider

- SCCa primary diagnosis in adult male with aggressive soft tissue mass in maxillary antrum

Image Interpretation Pearls

- ↓ T2 signal & tendency to enhance less than other sinonasal malignancies

Reporting Tips

- Evaluate for extension into orbit, masticator space, palate
  - Check PPF & foramen rotundum for V2 PNTS

SELECTED REFERENCES

1. Dubal PM et al: Squamous cell carcinoma of the maxillary sinus: a population-based analysis. Laryngoscope. 126(2):399-404, 2016
2. Roh JL et al: 18F fluorodeoxyglucose PET/CT in head and neck squamous cell carcinoma with negative neck palpation findings: a prospective study. Radiology. 271(1):153-61, 2014
3. Sanghvi S et al: Epidemiology of sinonasal squamous cell carcinoma: a comprehensive analysis of 4994 patients. Laryngoscope. 124(1):76-83, 2014
4. Ansa B et al: Paranasal sinus squamous cell carcinoma incidence and survival based on Surveillance, Epidemiology, and End Results data, 1973 to 2009. Cancer. 119(14):2602-10, 2013
5. Alos L et al: Human papillomaviruses are identified in a subgroup of sinonasal squamous cell carcinomas with favorable outcome. Cancer. 115(12):2701-9, 2009
6. Cohen EG et al: 18F-FDG PET evaluation of sinonasal papilloma. AJR Am J Roentgenol. 193(1):214-7, 2009
7. Jeon TY et al: 18F-FDG PET/CT findings of sinonasal inverted papilloma with or without coexistent malignancy: comparison with MR imaging findings in eight patients. Neuroradiology. 51(4):265-71, 2009
8. Jo VY et al: Papillary squamous cell carcinoma of the head and neck: frequent association with human papillomavirus infection and invasive carcinoma. Am J Surg Pathol. 33(11):1720-4, 2009
9. Raghavan P et al: Magnetic resonance imaging of sinonasal malignancies. Top Magn Reson Imaging. 18(4):259-67, 2007
10. El-Mofty SK et al: Prevalence of high-risk human papillomavirus DNA in nonkeratinizing (cylindrical cell) carcinoma of the sinonasal tract: a distinct clinicopathologic and molecular disease entity. Am J Surg Pathol. 29(10):1367-72, 2005
11. Loevner LA et al: Imaging of neoplasms of the paranasal sinuses. Magn Reson Imaging Clin N Am. 10(3): 467-93, 2002

Sinonasal Squamous Cell Carcinoma

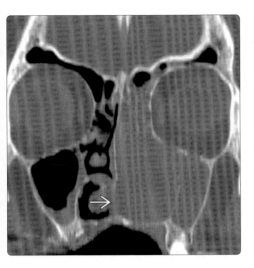
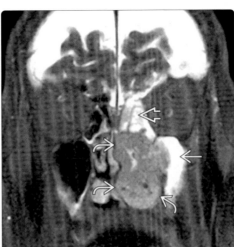

(Left) Coronal CT reconstruction shows a large mass filling the left nasal cavity with erosion of ipsilateral turbinates. This SCCa eroded the inferior nasal septum ➡. The margins of the mass are difficult to delineate here. (Right) Coronal STIR MR defines hypointense signal intensity tumor margins ➡. Obstructed secretions within the maxillary ➡ & ethmoid sinuses ➡ are hyperintense compared to the tumor. The low T2 tumor signal may be related to its high N:C ratio.

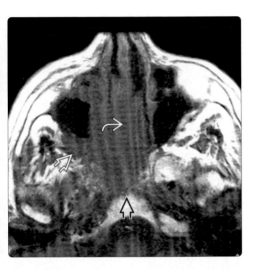
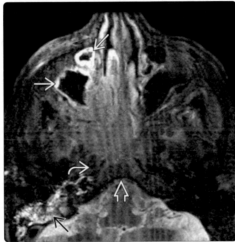

(Left) Axial T1 MR shows an SCCa of the nasal cavity with involvement of the nasal septum ➡, lateral spread into the pterygopalatine fossa ➡, and posterior extension into the nasopharynx ➡ toward the skull base. (Right) Axial T2 FS MR delineates tumor margins compared to mucosal thickening in the maxillary antrum ➡, prevertebral muscles ➡, and suppressed clival marrow ➡. Mastoid mucosal thickening ➡ is present due to eustachian tube obstruction.

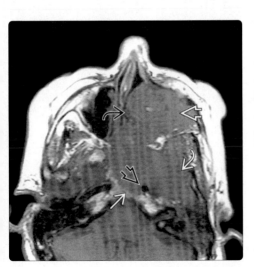
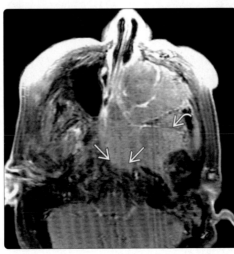

(Left) Axial T1 MR shows a very large antral SCCa ➡ with extension into the nasal cavity ➡, infratemporal fossa ➡, and clivus ➡. The mass encases the left internal carotid artery ➡, but the flow void is preserved. (Right) Axial T1 C+ FS MR shows homogeneous enhancement of a maxillary sinus carcinoma with no definite areas of necrosis. Note invasion of the clivus ➡ and diffuse infiltration of the muscles of mastication ➡.

Esthesioneuroblastoma

TERMINOLOGY

- Malignant neuroectodermal tumor arising from **olfactory neuroepithelium** in superior nasal cavity

IMAGING

- Enhanced MR & bone CT best delineate ENB for en bloc craniofacial surgery
- **Dumbbell-shaped** mass with "waist" at cribriform plate
- Bone CT: Bone remodeling mixed with bone destruction, especially of cribriform plate
- CECT/T1 C+ MR: Homogeneously enhancing mass
  - **Cysts** at intracranial tumor-brain margin
- Mildly restricted diffusion: Small round blue cell tumor
- T2 MR sequences best differentiate tumor from sinus secretions

TOP DIFFERENTIAL DIAGNOSES

- Sinonasal squamous cell carcinoma
- Sinonasal adenocarcinoma
- Sinonasal non-Hodgkin lymphoma
- Sinonasal undifferentiated carcinoma

PATHOLOGY

- No etiologic, genetic, or risk factors elucidated
- Staging: **Kadish classification**; good predictor of outcome
- Histologic grading: Hyams system

CLINICAL ISSUES

- **Adolescent or middle-aged** patient with unilateral nasal obstruction & mild epistaxis
  - Bimodal distribution in 2nd & 6th decades
  - Slight male predilection
- Combined surgical resection & radiotherapy is treatment of choice
- Excellent prognosis vs. other sinonasal malignancies
  - 5-year survival rates: 75-77% overall
  - Recurrence in ~ 30%
  - Metastases in 10-30% of patients

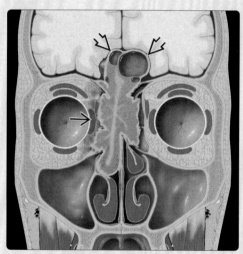
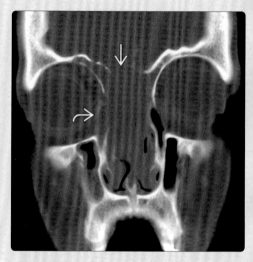

(Left) Coronal graphic shows the classic features of esthesioneuroblastoma (ENB) centered below the cribriform plate and extending into the anterior cranial fossa and right orbit ➡. Cyst formation ⇗ is noted at the tumor-brain interface. (Right) Coronal bone CT shows an ENB filling the upper nasal cavity and ethmoid sinuses. The lesion extends through the anterior skull base ➡. The lamina papyracea on the right is thinned and laterally displaced ➡.

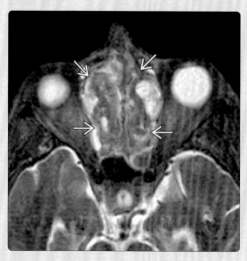
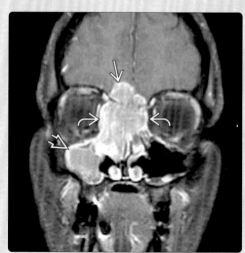

(Left) Axial STIR MR demonstrates a large, heterogeneous ENB ➡ centered in the midline below the skull base and occupying the nasal cavity and ethmoid sinuses. The mass is predominantly hypointense in this case and causes hypertelorism. (Right) Coronal T1 C+ FS MR shows an avidly enhancing ENB with extension into anterior cranial fossa ➡ and both orbits ➡. Avid enhancement is characteristic of this highly vascular neoplasm. Note the trapped maxillary secretions ➡.

TERMINOLOGY

Abbreviations
- Esthesioneuroblastoma (ENB)

Synonyms
- Olfactory neuroblastoma, pleomorphic olfactory neuroblastoma

Definitions
- Rare, malignant, neuroectodermal sinonasal (SN) tumor

IMAGING

General Features
- Best diagnostic clue
  - Dumbbell-shaped mass with upper portion in anterior cranial fossa, lower portion in upper nasal cavity, & "waist" at level of cribriform plate
  - **Peripheral tumor cysts** at intracranial tumor-brain margin is highly suggestive of diagnosis of ENB
- Location
  - Superior nasal cavity **at cribriform plate**
    - Smaller ENB: Unilateral nasal mass centered on superior nasal wall; local spread in nose & sinuses
    - Large ENB: Tumor in anterior cranial fossa with parenchymal & dural infiltration, extension into orbits
  - Cervical nodal metastases may occur at initial presentation or as later recurrence, especially upper cervical levels (I-III) & retropharyngeal
    - Important to report; impacts treatment planning
- Size
  - Range from < 1-cm nodule to mass filling entire nasal cavity & lower anterior cranial fossa
- Morphology
  - Polypoid mass when small; dumbbell-shaped when large

CT Findings
- NECT
  - Bone CT
    - Bone remodeling causing enlargement of nasal cavity mixed with bone destruction, especially of cribriform plate area
    - Speckled pattern of calcification within tumor matrix unusual
- CECT
  - Homogeneously enhancing mass
  - When large, may see nonenhancing areas of necrosis

MR Findings
- T1WI
  - Hypointense to intermediate signal intensity mass compared to brain
  - Areas of hemorrhage can be hyperintense
- T2WI
  - Tumor is intermediate to hyperintense to brain with areas of cystic degeneration
    - Obstructed secretions in adjacent sinuses often hyperintense (provide inherent contrast to tumor)
  - Hemorrhagic foci are hypo- to hyperintense depending on age of blood
  - Intracranial cysts at tumor-brain interface are hyperintense
- DWI
  - Mildly restricted diffusion as ENB is small round blue cell tumor
- T1WI C+
  - **Avid homogeneous tumor enhancement**
  - Enhancement heterogeneous in areas of necrosis

Nuclear Medicine Findings
- FDG PET positive, higher sensitivity of detecting nodal and distant metastases

Imaging Recommendations
- Best imaging tool
  - Enhanced MR with bone CT best delineates ENB for en bloc craniofacial surgery
- Protocol advice
  - Bone CT shows precise extent of bone destruction & may alter extent of craniofacial resection
  - T2 MR best differentiates tumor from sinus secretions
  - Multiplanar T1 C+ FS MR for evaluating tumor extension beyond SN cavities

DIFFERENTIAL DIAGNOSIS

Sinonasal Squamous Cell Carcinoma
- More common in **maxillary antrum** than nasal cavity
- Does not enhance to same degree as ENB

Sinonasal Adenocarcinoma
- **Wood dust & occupational exposures** are risk factors
- Predilection for ethmoid origin with nasal cavity involvement
- Enhances less avidly & more heterogeneously than ENB

Anterior Skull Base Meningioma
- May cause hyperostosis in adjacent skull base
- Not associated with cyst formation at tumor-brain interface

Non-Hodgkin Lymphoma
- Dense on NECT, restricted diffusion
- Does not enhance to same degree as ENB
- Rarely breaches skull base

Sinonasal Melanoma
- Favors **lower nasal cavity as site** of origin (septum & turbinates)
- ↑ T1 & ↓ T2 signal classic

Sinonasal Undifferentiated Carcinoma
- Difficult to distinguish from ENB on imaging
- Not confined to cribriform plate/superior nasal cavity
- Usually in older patients

PATHOLOGY

General Features
- Etiology
  - No etiologic basis or risk factors elucidated
  - Tumor of neural crest origin & **begins in olfactory neuroepithelium** in superior nasal cavity at cribriform plate
- Associated abnormalities

- ○ ENB patients occasionally present with paraneoplastic symptoms
  - – Cushing syndrome → adrenocorticotrophic hormone secretion
  - – Hyponatremia → antidiuretic hormone secretion

Staging, Grading, & Classification

- Staging criteria: Modified **Kadish classification**; good predictor of outcome; stage C is most common
  - ○ Stage A: Localized to nasal cavity
  - ○ Stage B: Localized to nasal cavity & sinuses
  - ○ Stage C: Orbital and intracranial extension
  - ○ Stage D: Cervical and distant metastases
- Histologic grading: Hyams system; stronger prediction of prognosis
  - ○ Grades 1-4 based upon architectural pleomorphism, neurofibrillary matrix, rosette formation, mitoses, necrosis, presence of gland formation, & calcifications

Gross Pathologic & Surgical Features

- Clinically appears as firm, nonpulsatile mass covered by intact respiratory mucosa
  - ○ Tumor may bleed profusely on biopsy
- Broad-based, pedunculated, lobulated, mucosal-covered mass at cribriform plate; soft, glistening
  - ○ May show engorged, red appearance due to rich, vascular stroma

Microscopic Features

- Submucosal lesion with prominent nested appearance
  - ○ Neurofibrillary intercellular matrix & rosette formations
  - ○ Mild nuclear pleomorphism with low mitotic activity most common
- Frequently contains areas of necrosis & calcification
- Electron microscopy
  - ○ Shows neurosecretory granules
  - ○ May help make correct diagnosis when light microscopy is inconclusive
- ENB is type of small round blue cell tumors (SRBCT); difficult to differentiate from other SRBCT
  - ○ Lymphoma, Ewing sarcoma, melanoma, rhabdomyosarcoma, Merkel cell carcinoma

CLINICAL ISSUES

Presentation

- Most common signs/symptoms
  - ○ Nasal obstruction & **epistaxis**
    - – Symptoms usually predate diagnosis by 6-12 months
- Other signs/symptoms
  - ○ Anosmia, rhinorrhea
  - ○ Hypertelorism, proptosis, diplopia, & epiphora
  - ○ Headache
  - ○ Cranial neuropathies suggest skull base/cavernous sinus involvement
- Clinical profile
  - ○ **Adolescent or middle-aged patient** with unilateral nasal obstruction & mild epistaxis

Demographics

- Age
  - ○ **Bimodal distribution** in 2nd & 6th decades

- Gender
  - ○ Slight male predominance
- Epidemiology
  - ○ 2-3% of all intranasal neoplasms

Natural History & Prognosis

- **5-year survival rates: 75-77% overall**
  - ○ Staging & tumor grade are significant prognostic indicators
    - – 5-year disease-free survival
      - □ Kadish stage A: > 90%; stage B: 70-90%; stage C: 35-70%; stage D: < 35%
- Negative prognostic indicators
  - ○ Female sex, age < 20 or > 50 years at presentation
  - ○ Higher tumor histology grade, higher staging (Kadish C and D)
- Recurrence in ~ 30% up to 15 years after primary diagnosis
- Metastases in 10-30% of patients
  - ○ Nodal &/or distant metastases to lung, bone, liver

Treatment

- Combined therapy using craniofacial resection & radiotherapy is treatment of choice
  - ○ Radiotherapy offers better local control since negative resection margins often difficult to achieve
  - ○ Low-stage resectable tumors may be approached endoscopically in selected patients
- Chemotherapy reserved for larger, high-grade ENB & disseminated disease

DIAGNOSTIC CHECKLIST

Consider

- Using both preoperative CT & MR imaging
  - ○ CT for detection of extent of bone destruction
  - ○ MR for precise mapping of tumor soft tissue extent

Image Interpretation Pearls

- Dumbbell-shaped mass with waist at cribriform plate + intracranial marginal cysts are characteristic of ENB

SELECTED REFERENCES

1. Saade RE et al: Prognosis and biology in esthesioneuroblastoma: the emerging role of Hyams grading system. Curr Oncol Rep. 17(1):423, 2015
2. Kaur G et al: The prognostic implications of Hyam's subtype for patients with Kadish stage C esthesioneuroblastoma. J Clin Neurosci. 20(2):281-6, 2013
3. Papacharalampous GX et al: Olfactory neuroblastoma (esthesioneuroblastoma): towards minimally invasive surgery and multi-modality treatment strategies - an updated critical review of the current literature. J BUON. 18(3):557-63, 2013
4. Broski SM et al: The added value of 18F-FDG PET/CT for evaluation of patients with esthesioneuroblastoma. J Nucl Med. 53(8):1200-6, 2012
5. Howell MC et al: Patterns of regional spread for esthesioneuroblastoma. AJNR Am J Neuroradiol. 32(5):929-33, 2011
6. Devaiah AK et al: Treatment of esthesioneuroblastoma: a 16-year meta-analysis of 361 patients. Laryngoscope. 119(7):1412-6, 2009
7. Tseng J et al: Peripheral cysts: a distinguishing feature of esthesioneuroblastoma with intracranial extension. Ear Nose Throat J. 88(6):E14, 2009
8. Yu T et al: Esthesioneuroblastoma methods of intracranial extension: CT and MR imaging findings. Neuroradiology. 51(12):841-50, 2009
9. Zollinger LV et al: Retropharyngeal lymph node metastasis from esthesioneuroblastoma: a review of the therapeutic and prognostic implications. AJNR Am J Neuroradiol. 29(8):1561-3, 2008

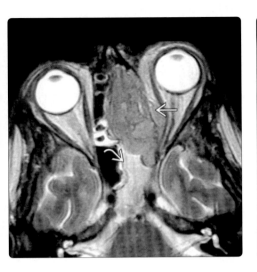

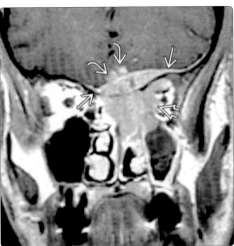

(Left) *Axial T2 FS MR shows diffuse intermediate to low signal within an ENB centered in the left nasal cavity. Extension into the left orbit ➡ is seen. Trapped secretions ➡ are noted in the left sphenoid sinus.* (Right) *Coronal T1 C+ MR shows intracranial extension of a left nasal cavity ENB. The tumor avidly enhances and invades dura causing a dural tail ➡. Invasion of left frontal lobe ➡ and left orbit ➡ was present in this case.*

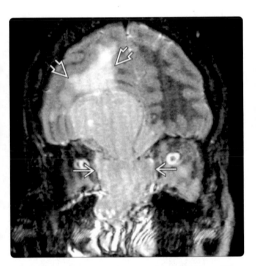

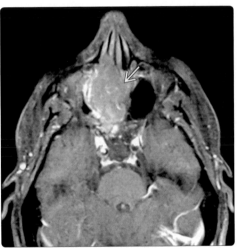

(Left) *Coronal T2 MR demonstrates a very large ENB with extension into both orbits ➡ and into the anterior cranial fossa. Despite the large intracranial component, only brain edema ➡ and not parenchymal invasion was seen in this case.* (Right) *Axial T1 C+ MR shows diffuse, homogeneous enhancement throughout an ENB centered in the right nasal cavity. This ENB crossed the midline ➡ through the nasal septum.*

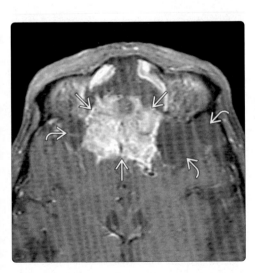

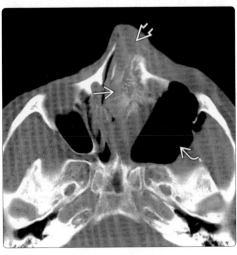

(Left) *Axial T1 C+ FS MR in an elderly man shows the intracranial component of a large, avidly enhancing ENB ➡. Multiple cysts ➡ are noted at the tumor-brain interface, a characteristic feature of this tumor.* (Right) *Axial bone CT shows a somewhat unusual calcified tumor matrix ➡ within a recurrent left-sided ENB. Invasion of anterior nasal soft tissues ➡ is present. Note air-filled cavity ➡ resulting from prior maxillectomy.*

Sinonasal Melanoma

TERMINOLOGY

- Arises from melanocytes migrated from **neural crest origin** to sinonasal epithelium

IMAGING

- Soft tissue mass in nasal cavity > paranasal sinuses with bone destruction ± remodeling
  - Predilection for nasal septum, lateral nasal wall, and inferior turbinate
- MR (melanotic melanoma)
  - ↑ **T1** & ↓ **T2 signal** results from melanin, free radicals, metal ions, and hemorrhage
  - T2* GRE may show **blooming** when hemorrhage present in sinonasal melanoma (SNM)
  - Avidly enhances due to vascularity in SNM; enhancement may be difficult to appreciate if high precontrast T1 signal present

TOP DIFFERENTIAL DIAGNOSES

- Squamous cell carcinoma
- Non-Hodgkin lymphoma
- Esthesioneuroblastoma

CLINICAL ISSUES

- Adult with nasal stuffiness, epistaxis, and pigmented mass identified at nasal endoscopy
  - 5th-8th decades most common
  - > 90% occurs in whites, M > F
- Poor prognosis with 6-17% chance of 5-year survival
  - Mean survival ~ 24 months
  - Systemic metastatic disease typically precedes death

DIAGNOSTIC CHECKLIST

- Look for hemorrhagic mass arising in lower nasal cavity with ↑ T1 and ↓ T2 signal

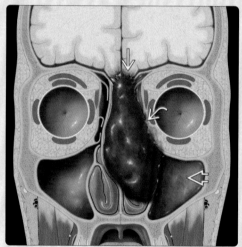
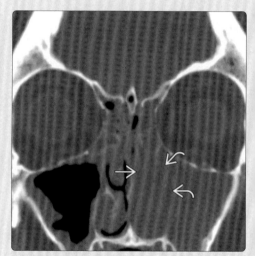

(Left) Coronal graphic shows a darkly pigmented (highly melanotic) mass centered in the nasal cavity. Invasion of the skull base ➡, orbit ➡, and lateral nasal wall is seen, but the septum is deviated rather than invaded. Trapped secretions ➡ are noted in the left maxillary sinus. (Right) Coronal bone CT in a patient with left nasal obstruction and epistaxis shows a mass in the left nasal cavity with erosion of the left middle turbinate ➡ and portions of the lateral nasal wall ➡.

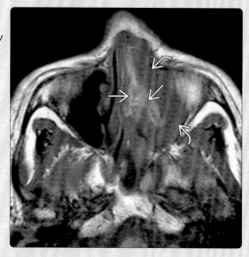
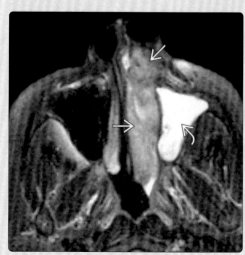

(Left) Axial T1 MR demonstrates a mass in the left nasal cavity with maxillary sinus extension. The lesion is heterogeneous with areas of T1 shortening ➡ and intermediate signal ➡. T1 shortening on unenhanced images may indicate the presence of melanin or hemorrhage. (Right) Axial T2 FS MR shows a lobular melanoma ➡ within the left nasal cavity. It is somewhat hypointense and is readily distinguishable from the hyperintense obstructed secretions ➡ in the maxillary sinus.

TERMINOLOGY

Abbreviations

- Sinonasal melanoma (SNM)

Definitions

- Malignant transformation of melanocytes migrating from neural crest in sinonasal cavity

IMAGING

General Features

- Best diagnostic clue
  - ↑ T1 MR signal mass in nasal cavity
- Location
  - **Nasal cavity** > sinuses
    - Nasal septum, lateral wall, and inferior turbinate
- Size
  - Large polypoid sinonasal mass

CT Findings

- Bone CT
  - Lobular soft tissue mass in nasal cavity
  - Bone destruction ± remodeling

MR Findings

- T1WI
  - **Melanotic** melanoma: **↑ signal** due to melanin, free radicals, metal ions, hemorrhage
  - **Amelanotic** melanoma: Intermediate (soft tissue) signal
- T2WI
  - **Melanotic** melanoma: **↓ signal**
  - Amelanotic melanoma: Variable signal
- T2* GRE
  - Areas of hemorrhage may show blooming
- T1WI C+
  - Avid enhancement

Imaging Recommendations

- Best imaging tool
  - Multiplanar MR imaging with contrast

DIFFERENTIAL DIAGNOSIS

Sinonasal Squamous Cell Carcinoma

- Arises in maxillary antrum > nasal cavity
- Aggressive bone destruction; heterogeneous with variable enhancement

Sinonasal Non-Hodgkin Lymphoma

- Nasal cavity mass with bone destruction ± remodeling
- Homogeneous; ↓ T2 signal; ↓ ADC

Esthesioneuroblastoma

- Mass near cribriform plate with bone destruction

Juvenile Angiofibroma

- Young male patient
- Posterior nasal cavity near sphenopalatine foramen

PATHOLOGY

General Features

- Etiology

  - Arises from melanocytes of **neural crest origin** migrated to sinonasal epithelium

Gross Pathologic & Surgical Features

- Pink to dark colored, soft vascular nasal mass, arise from septum and lateral nasal wall

Microscopic Features

- Epithelioid, spindle, and mixed cell types
- Melanin heavily deposited, limited, or absent

CLINICAL ISSUES

Presentation

- Most common signs/symptoms
  - Nasal obstruction, epistaxis, pain, hyposmia
- Physical exam
  - Bulky, brownish black, friable vascular nasal mass

Demographics

- Age
  - 5th-8th decades most common (range: 30-85 years)
- Gender
  - M > F
- Epidemiology
  - SNM < 2% of melanomas and 4-12% of sinonasal malignancies
  - > 90% occur in whites

Natural History & Prognosis

- Poor prognosis with 6-17% chance of 5-year survival
- Metastasis to lungs, lymph nodes, and brain typically precedes death

Treatment

- Radical surgery with adjuvant radiotherapy

DIAGNOSTIC CHECKLIST

Consider

- Can appear similar to nasal polyp on CT if low melanin content
- Consider SNM for pigmented appearance on nasal endoscopy

Image Interpretation Pearls

- Look for mass arising in lower nasal cavity with ↑ T1 and ↓ T2 signal

SELECTED REFERENCES

1. Gras-Cabrerizo JR et al: Management of sinonasal mucosal melanomas and comparison of classification staging systems. Am J Rhinol Allergy. 29(1):e37-40, 2015
2. Gilain L et al: Mucosal melanoma of the nasal cavity and paranasal sinuses. Eur Ann Otorhinolaryngol Head Neck Dis. 131(6):365-9, 2014
3. Michel J et al: Sinonasal mucosal melanomas: the prognostic value of tumor classifications. Head Neck. 36(3):311-6, 2014
4. Moreno MA et al: Mucosal melanoma of the nose and paranasal sinuses, a contemporary experience from the M. D. Anderson Cancer Center. Cancer. 116(9):2215-23, 2010
5. Dauer EH et al: Sinonasal melanoma: a clinicopathologic review of 61 cases. Otolaryngol Head Neck Surg. 138(3):347-52, 2008
6. Chang PC et al: Perineural spread of malignant melanoma of the head and neck: clinical and imaging features. AJNR Am J Neuroradiol. 25(1):5-11, 2004
7. Loevner LA et al: Imaging of neoplasms of the paranasal sinuses. Magn Reson Imaging Clin N Am. 10(3):467-93, 2002

Sinonasal Adenocarcinoma

TERMINOLOGY

- Malignant neoplasm with glandular differentiation arising from surface epithelium or minor salivary rests

IMAGING

- Predilection for nasal cavity & ethmoid sinuses
- May reach large size due to delay in diagnosis
  - 75% with involvement of > 1 SN region at diagnosis
- CT
  - Well- to poorly defined mass with bone destruction or remodeling
- MR
  - Typically intermediate to hyperintense T2 signal
  - Diffuse, heterogeneous enhancement
- Goals of imaging: Determine malignant characteristics & orbital or intracranial extension

TOP DIFFERENTIAL DIAGNOSES

- Sinonasal squamous cell carcinoma

- Esthesioneuroblastoma
- Sinonasal undifferentiated carcinoma
- Sinonasal non-Hodgkin lymphoma

PATHOLOGY

- 2 major subtypes
  - Intestinal (related to wood dust exposure): Most frequent form colonic > solid > papillary > mucinous & mixed type
  - Nonintestinal: Unrelated to wood dust exposure
- Accounts for 15% of all SN cancers

CLINICAL ISSUES

- 6th decade most common
- M > F (~ 3:1)
- Poor prognosis with higher grades, incomplete resection, & intracranial involvement
- 5-year survival rates generally poor (~ 50%)
- Complete surgical excision for cure

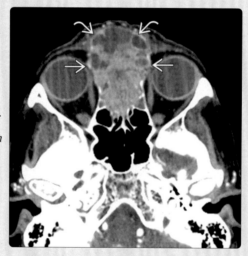
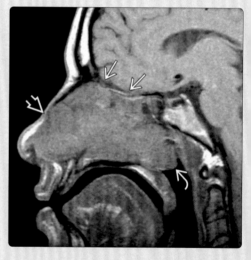

(Left) Axial CECT shows a large, heterogeneously enhancing adenocarcinoma filling the upper nasal cavity and ethmoid sinuses. There is anterior extension into the soft tissues of the nasal dorsum ⮕ and destruction of bilateral lamina papyracea ➡. (Right) Sagittal T1WI MR shows a large adenocarcinoma filling the nasal cavity and extending into the nasopharynx ⮕. No extension through the skull base ➡ is seen. The lesion invades subcutaneous fat ⮕ of the dorsum of the nose.

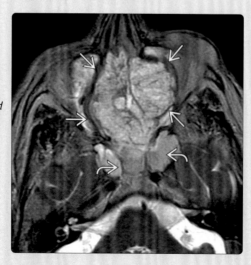
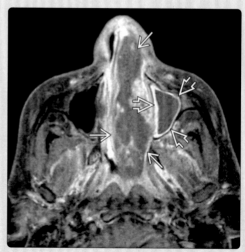

(Left) Axial T2WI FS MR demonstrates a large, hyperintense, heterogeneous adenocarcinoma of ethmoids ➡ filling the nasal cavity and causing mass effect on both orbits. Obstructed secretions ⮕ are present in the sphenoid sinuses. (Right) Axial T1WI C+ FS MR shows a left nasal cavity adenocarcinoma ➡, with heterogeneous enhancement. Note the left maxillary sinus is obstructed with peripheral (but no central) enhancement of retained secretions ⮕.

TERMINOLOGY

Abbreviations

- Sinonasal adenocarcinoma (SN AdenoCa)

Definitions

- Malignant neoplasm with glandular differentiation arising from surface epithelium or minor salivary rests

IMAGING

General Features

- Best diagnostic clue
  - Poorly defined, enhancing sinonasal mass with ethmoid sinus, nasal cavity, & skull base involvement
- Location
  - Predilection for **nasal cavity & ethmoid sinuses**
- Size
  - May reach large size due to **delay in diagnosis**

CT Findings

- CECT
  - Diffuse, often heterogeneous enhancement
- Bone CT
  - Bone destruction > remodeling

MR Findings

- T1WI
  - Intermediate signal; ↑ signal in foci of hemorrhage
- T2WI
  - Variable; typically intermediate to hyperintense
- T1WI C+
  - Diffuse, heterogeneous enhancement

Imaging Recommendations

- Best imaging tool
  - Multiplanar enhanced MR
- Protocol advice
  - C+ FS MR to map tumor extension & detect perineural spread

DIFFERENTIAL DIAGNOSIS

Sinonasal Squamous Cell Carcinoma

- Usually in maxillary antrum; more ill defined

Esthesioneuroblastoma

- Adolescent or middle-aged
- Near cribriform plate; intense enhancement

Sinonasal Undifferentiated Carcinoma

- Can look very similar to SN AdenoCa
- Aggressive with rapid growth

Sinonasal Non-Hodgkin Lymphoma

- Predilection for nasal cavity
- Homogeneous, ↓ T2 signal

PATHOLOGY

General Features

- Etiology
  - **Wood dust exposure** has strong link to intestinal-type AdenoCa
  - Other exposure: Inhaled metal dust, leather & textile industry chemicals

Staging, Grading, & Classification

- AJCC TNM staging system most frequently used for lesions originating in nasal cavity & ethmoids
- Subtypes include
  - Intestinal: Most frequent form colonic (40%) followed by solid (20%), papillary (18%), and mucinous and mixed type (together 22%)
  - Nonintestinal: Unrelated to wood dust exposure

Gross Pathologic & Surgical Features

- Tan-white-pink; flat, exophytic, or papillary; friable to firm

Microscopic Features

- Well differentiated
  - Unencapsulated tumor, uniform glands with cystic spaces, no stroma
- Poorly differentiated
  - Invasive, solid growth pattern, pleomorphism, ↑ mitoses
- Colonic (intestinal) type: Invasive with various growth patterns (papillary-tubular, alveolar-mucoid, alveolar-goblet/signet ring, & mixed)

CLINICAL ISSUES

Presentation

- Most common signs/symptoms
  - Nasal stuffiness & obstruction
  - Epistaxis

Demographics

- Age
  - **6th decade most common** (mean: 64 years)
- Gender
  - **M > F** (~ 3:1)
- Epidemiology
  - 15% of all SN cancers

Natural History & Prognosis

- Prognosis excellent for low grade, poor for high grade
- 5-year survival rates generally poor (~ 50%)

Treatment

- Complete surgical excision for cure
- Radiation therapy & chemotherapy used alone or in conjunction with surgery

DIAGNOSTIC CHECKLIST

Consider

- AdenoCa if history of occupational exposure & involvement of nasal cavity & ethmoid sinuses

SELECTED REFERENCES

1. Hoeben A et al: Intestinal-type sinonasal adenocarcinomas: The road to molecular diagnosis and personalized treatment. Head Neck. ePub, 2016
2. Leivo I: Sinonasal adenocarcinoma: update on classification, immunophenotype and molecular features. Head Neck Pathol. 10(1):68-74, 2016
3. Rawal RB et al: Endoscopic resection of sinonasal malignancy: a systematic review and meta-analysis. Otolaryngol Head Neck Surg. ePub, 2016
4. Sklar EM et al: Sinonasal intestinal-type adenocarcinoma involvement of the paranasal sinuses. AJNR Am J Neuroradiol. 24(6):1152-5, 2003

Sinonasal Non-Hodgkin Lymphoma

TERMINOLOGY

- Sinonasal non-Hodgkin lymphoma: Extranodal lymphoproliferative malignancy

IMAGING

- Appearance can mimic variety of neoplasms & aggressive inflammatory disorders
- Predilection for nasal cavity > sinuses
- CT: Homogeneous mass ± bone remodeling or destruction
  - May be hyperdense due to high N:C ratio
- Imaging modality of choice: Multiplanar MR with T1 C+ FS
- MR: ↓ T2 signal
- Restricted diffusion due to high cellularity
- PET for initial staging & treatment response

TOP DIFFERENTIAL DIAGNOSES

- Sinonasal granulomatosis with polyangiitis; (Wegener granulomatosis)
- Sinonasal adenocarcinoma

- Esthesioneuroblastoma
- Sinonasal squamous cell carcinoma

PATHOLOGY

- 3 pathologic subgroups
  - B-cell (Western) phenotype most common
  - T-cell (Asian) phenotype
  - Natural killer/T-cell lymphoma (Asian): Subtype of T cell

CLINICAL ISSUES

- Male patient in 6th decade with nonspecific symptoms of nasal obstruction & discharge
- Local radiotherapy (XRT) is primary treatment ± combination chemotherapy

DIAGNOSTIC CHECKLIST

- NHL could be included in DDx for almost any aggressive adult nasal soft tissue mass
- Imaging clue to diagnosis: Presence of enlarged cervical nodes & Waldeyer ring lymphatic mass

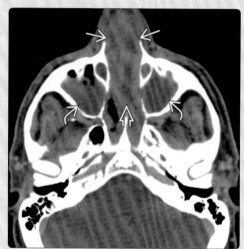
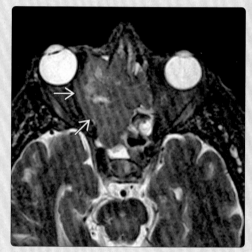

(Left) *Axial CECT shows a large non-Hodgkin lymphoma (NHL)* ➡ *centered in the nasal cavity with slightly heterogeneous enhancement. There is gross destruction of the nasal septum* ⇨. *Obstructed secretions* ➡ *are noted in both maxillary sinuses.* (Right) *Axial STIR MR shows a large lymphoma involving the nasal cavity and ethmoid sinuses. Relatively hypointense signal is characteristic of this tumor with high nuclear:cytoplasmic ratio. Note the involvement of the right orbit* ➡ *with resulting proptosis.*

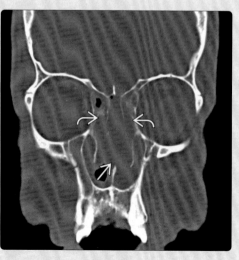
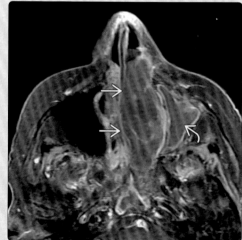

(Left) *Coronal bone CT shows the classic location of sinonasal non-Hodgkin lymphoma (NHL-SN). The mass is centered around the nasal septum, and there is destruction of the septum* ➡ *as well as multiple ethmoid septations* ➡. (Right) *Axial T1 C+ FS MR demonstrates a large lymphoma filling the left nasal cavity. The septum is displaced* ➡ *but not eroded. Homogeneous mild enhancement is present. Trapped secretions* ➡ *are present in the left maxillary antrum.*

TERMINOLOGY

Abbreviations
- Sinonasal non-Hodgkin lymphoma (NHL-SN)
- Natural killer/T-cell lymphoma (NKTL)

Definitions
- NHL-SN: Extranodal lymphoproliferative malignancy, most often of B-cell, T-cell, or NK-/T-cell origin
  o NKTL: Subtype of peripheral T-cell lymphoma
    – Previously called lethal midline granuloma, polymorphic reticulosis, angiocentric T-cell lymphoma

IMAGING

General Features
- Best diagnostic clue
  o **Homogeneous soft tissue mass** with predilection for nasal cavity ± bone destruction
  o Very nonspecific imaging features
    – NHL-SN **can mimic** variety of neoplasms & aggressive inflammatory disorders
- Location
  o **Nasal cavity** > maxillary > ethmoid > frontal sinuses
    – NKTL may have simultaneous involvement of nasopharynx & oropharynx in addition to sinonasal cavities
- Size
  o Usually 2-5 cm
- Morphology
  o Variable: Diffusely infiltrative & ill-defined, nodular, or bulky mass

CT Findings
- NECT
  o Bulky, lobular, soft tissue mass in nasal cavity ± sinuses
  o May be **hyperdense** compared to soft tissue due to high N:C ratio
  o NKTL: Infiltrative > polypoid soft tissue mass in nasal cavity ± ulceration/necrosis/bone destruction
- CECT
  o Moderate **homogeneous enhancement**
- Bone CT
  o Tends to remodel &/or erode bone
  o B-cell (Western) type: Soft tissue & osseous destruction
    – More likely to invade orbit
  o T-cell (Asian) type: Nasal septal destruction & perforation more common

MR Findings
- T1WI
  o Intermediate, homogeneous signal similar to or slightly higher than muscle
- T2WI
  o **Low to intermediate** homogeneous signal
    – Due to highly cellular nature & ↑ N:C ratio
- DWI
  o Restricted diffusion, significantly lower ADC values as compared with squamous cell carcinomas
- T1WI C+
  o Variable but diffuse & homogeneous enhancement
    – Typically > muscle but < mucosa

---

  o Nonenhancing areas of necrosis more common in NKTL than in other NHL-SN

Nuclear Medicine Findings
- PET
  o May show moderate to avid uptake
  o Valuable for initial staging and treatment response evaluation

Imaging Recommendations
- Best imaging tool
  o Multiplanar MR with T1 C+ FS
    – MR better delineates tumor margins & differentiates tumor from mucosal thickening & secretions
- Protocol advice
  o Begin with thin-section axial & coronal T1 & T2 sequences without FS
  o Follow with T1 C+ FS MR in same planes through sinonasal area

DIFFERENTIAL DIAGNOSIS

Sinonasal Wegener Granulomatosis
- **Can be indistinguishable** from NHL-SN on imaging
- Favors nasal cavity (septum & turbinates)
- Requires laboratory/biopsy confirmation

Sinonasal Adenocarcinoma
- More likely to originate in sinuses, particularly ethmoids
- May be related to occupational exposure (wood dust)

Esthesioneuroblastoma
- Adolescent or middle-aged adult
- Superior nasal cavity near cribriform plate
- Typically higher T2 signal, more prominent enhancement

Sinonasal Squamous Cell Carcinoma
- Most common in maxillary sinus
- More heterogeneous with frank bone destruction

Sinonasal Melanoma
- Originates in nasal cavity
- ↑ T1 & ↓ T2 signal with avid enhancement
- Tendency for bony remodeling > destruction

PATHOLOGY

General Features
- Etiology
  o Malignant lymphoproliferative disorder arising from variety of immune cell types
  o 3 subgroups
    – **B-cell (Western) phenotype**: Most frequent type in paranasal sinuses; less aggressive
    – **T-cell (Asian) phenotype**: More common in nasal cavity; more aggressive
    – **NKTL**: Subtype of T-cell lymphoma; more common in nasal cavity; more aggressive
      □ Epstein-Barr virus (EBV) likely has role in pathogenesis of NKTL
- Associated abnormalities
  o Lymph nodes **infrequently** involved

- o Distant metastases seen in stage IV: Liver, spleen, brain, & bone marrow

Staging, Grading, & Classification

- Multiple staging systems: Ann Arbor staging system (IE to IVE), Murphy staging system
- Histologic classification: WHO system for lymphoid neoplasms (1999)
  - o Multiple additional classification systems: Rappaport, Luke-Collins, Revised European American Lymphoma (REAL)
- Large tumors & those with extranasal extension represent higher tumor stage

Gross Pathologic & Surgical Features

- Polypoid, soft to rubbery mass with homogeneous pink-tan or bluish color
- Locally destructive & ulcerative

Microscopic Features

- Monomorphous malignant cellular infiltrate of various types
- Various types are characterized immunophenotypically
- NKTL: Polymorphous cellular infiltrate of mononuclear cells growing in angiocentric, angiodestructive growth pattern
  - o Mucosal ulceration, pseudoepitheliomatous hyperplasia, & inflammatory infiltrate may be seen
  - o EBV(+) in nearly all cases

CLINICAL ISSUES

Presentation

- Most common signs/symptoms
  - o Nasal obstruction & discharge
    - **Symptoms mimic sinusitis**, which leads to delay in diagnosis
  - o Bleeding more common in NKTL due to ulceration & necrosis
- Other signs/symptoms
  - o Unilateral facial swelling, otitis media, cervical adenopathy, headache
  - o NKTL: Septal cartilage destruction leads to "saddle-nose" deformity
- Clinical profile
  - o Male patient in 6th decade with nonspecific symptoms of nasal obstruction & discharge

Demographics

- Age
  - o B-cell (Western) type: 6th decade
  - o T-cell (Asian) type: 7th decade
- Gender
  - o Western form: M = F
  - o Asian form: M > F
- Ethnicity
  - o B-cell type more common in USA & Europe
    - Accounts for 55-85% of SN lymphomas in Western populations
  - o T-cell type more common in **East Asia & Latin America**
    - NKTL type more common in Asians & South Americans
- Epidemiology
  - o < 1% of all H&N malignancies

- 0.2-2% of all lymphomas arise in SN cavities
- Malignant lymphoma is **2nd most common SN malignancy** after squamous cell carcinoma
  - o < 50% of NHL occurs in H&N
    - 60% of H&N NHL is extranodal (sinonasal, oral cavity, laryngopharynx, salivary glands)
    - **44%** of H&N extranodal lymphomas occur **in sinonasal cavities**

Natural History & Prognosis

- B-cell type can have slow, indolent course if left untreated
  - o Prognosis generally good with > 50% 5-year survival
- Asian (T-cell) type has much worse prognosis; can be rapidly fatal
  - o NKTL: Worse prognosis than B-cell lymphoma even though usually manifests as local disease in nasal cavity
  - o 42% 5-year survival in stages I & II; 0% in stages III & IV

Treatment

- Primary treatment: Local radiotherapy (XRT)
- Intermediate or more aggressive NHL-SN usually treated with combination chemotherapy or combination of radiation & chemotherapy
- NKTL: XRT for local disease; XRT & chemotherapy for multifocal or disseminated disease

DIAGNOSTIC CHECKLIST

Consider

- Sinonasal NHL can be **difficult to distinguish** from other neoplasms, chronic sinusitis, & granulomatous disorders
  - o NHL could be included in DDx for almost any aggressive adult nasal soft tissue mass
- Differentiation from granulomatous disease requires biopsy & laboratory studies

Image Interpretation Pearls

- Presence of enlarged homogeneous cervical nodes may be clue to diagnosis
  - o Simultaneous involvement of nasopharynx & oropharynx in addition to sinonasal cavities is suggestive of NKTL, particularly in Asian patients

SELECTED REFERENCES

1. Wang X et al: Effectiveness of 3 T PROPELLER DUO diffusion-weighted MRI in differentiating sinonasal lymphomas and carcinomas. Clin Radiol. 69(11):1149-56, 2014
2. Sandner A et al: Primary extranodal Non-Hodgkin lymphoma of the orbital and paranasal region-a retrospective study. Eur J Radiol. 82(2):302-8, 2013
3. Kim J et al: Extranodal nasal-type NK/T-cell lymphoma: computed tomography findings of head and neck involvement. Acta Radiol. 51(2):164-9, 2010
4. Tempescul A et al: 18F-FDG PET/CT in primary non-Hodgkin's lymphoma of the sinonasal tract. Ann Hematol. 89(6):635-7, 2010
5. Sands NB et al: Extranodal T-cell lymphoma of the sinonasal tract presenting as severe rhinitis: case series. J Otolaryngol Head Neck Surg. 37(4):528-33, 2008
6. Hatta C et al: Non-Hodgkin's malignant lymphoma of the sinonasal tract–treatment outcome for 53 patients according to REAL classification. Auris Nasus Larynx. 28(1):55-60, 2001
7. Borges A et al: Midline destructive lesions of the sinonasal tract: simplified terminology based on histopathologic criteria. AJNR Am J Neuroradiol. 21(2):331-6, 2000
8. Gaal K et al: Sinonasal NK/T-cell lymphomas in the United States. Am J Surg Pathol. 24(11):1511-7, 2000
9. Harnsberger HR et al: Non-Hodgkin's lymphoma of the head and neck: CT evaluation of nodal and extranodal sites. AJR Am J Roentgenol. 149(4):785-91, 1987

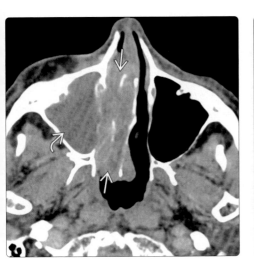

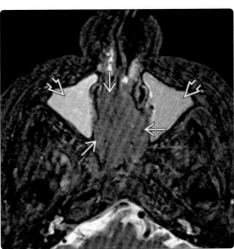

(Left) *Axial CECT shows a homogeneous soft tissue mass ➡ filling the right nasal cavity. This NHL did not destroy the nasal septum. The lesion obstructs the right middle meatus, and trapped secretions ➡ are present in the right maxillary antrum.* (Right) *Axial STIR MR shows the typical hypointense appearance of NHL on long TR images. The highly cellular tumor ➡ is homogeneously low in signal compared to the obstructed secretions ➡ in the adjacent maxillary sinuses.*

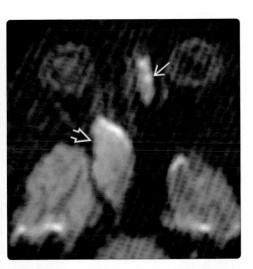

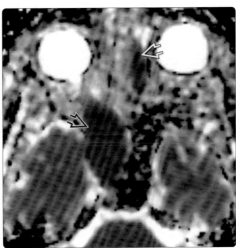

(Left) *Axial DWI MR of NHL-SN shows restricted diffusion corresponding to a right posterior ethmoid and sphenoid mass ➡. In addition, there is a smaller lesion in the left anterior ethmoid sinus, which also shows high signal ➡, corresponding to additional focus of NHL.* (Right) *Axial ADC map of a patient with NHL-SN shows marked restricted diffusion within a large mass in the right posterior ethmoid and sphenoid sinuses ➡ and within a small lesion in the left anterior ethmoid sinus ➡.*

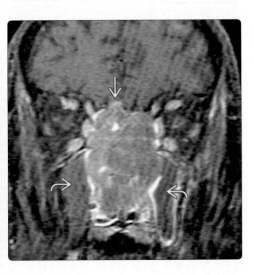

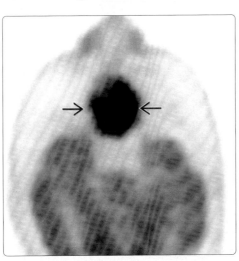

(Left) *Coronal T1 C+ FS MR shows diffuse enhancement throughout this sinonasal lymphoma. There is extension through the skull base ➡ into the anterior cranial fossa. On this sequence, there is good differentiation of the tumor from trapped secretions in the maxillary sinuses ➡.* (Right) *Axial PET performed at the time of sinonasal lymphoma diagnosis shows diffuse, avid uptake of FDG ➡ within the primary mass. No other areas of uptake were noted in the neck.*

Sinonasal Neuroendocrine Carcinoma

TERMINOLOGY

- Rare malignancy of epithelial origin expressing neuroendocrine markers
- Pathologically distinguishable from other sinonasal neuroectodermal tumors: ENB, SNUC, SCUNC

IMAGING

- SN neuroectodermal tumors **cannot** reliably be distinguished with radiologic criteria
- Predilection for superior **nasal cavity** & **ethmoid sinuses**
- Variably enhancing, ill-defined mass; bone destruction & invasion of adjacent compartments

TOP DIFFERENTIAL DIAGNOSES

- Esthesioneuroblastoma (ENB)
- Sinonasal undifferentiated carcinoma (SNUC)
- Sinonasal squamous cell carcinoma
- Sinonasal adenocarcinoma

PATHOLOGY

- Sinonasal neuroendocrine neoplasms range from more differentiated (ENB) to less differentiated (SNEC) to poorly differentiated (SCUNC)
- 2/3 positive for epithelial markers (low molecular weight cytokeratins & epithelial membrane antigen)
- Immunoreactive for neuroendocrine markers (chromogranin, synaptophysin, S100, CD57)

CLINICAL ISSUES

- Wide age range; average: ~ 50 years
- Usually present with locally advanced disease
  - **70%** present as **stage IV disease**
- Management of these rare neoplasms often based on analogous treatment principles for NEC of other anatomic sites (lung & larynx) & treatment of SNUC
- Overall 5-year survival: ~ 64%

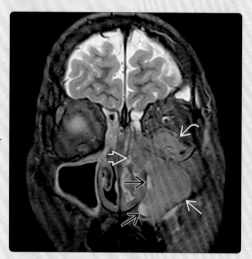

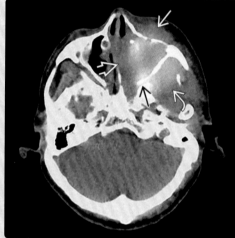

(Left) Coronal T2 FS MR demonstrates a hypointense soft tissue mass filling the left maxillary sinus ➡ with extension into the left nasal cavity ➡ and orbit ➡. Note hyperintense trapped secretion in medial left maxillary sinus ➡. (Right) Axial Indium-111 pentetreotide-fused SPECT/CT in the same patient shows increased radiotracer uptake of the left maxillary sinus SNEC. There is extension into the left premaxillary soft tissues ➡, nasal cavity ➡, retromaxillary fat ➡, and pterygopalatine fossa ➡.

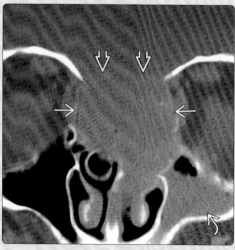

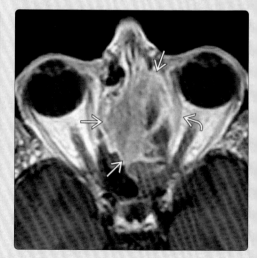

(Left) Coronal bone CT shows a large mass centered in the superior nasal cavity bilaterally with involvement of both ethmoid labyrinths ➡. There is aggressive bone destruction with erosion of ethmoid septations and the anterior skull base ➡. Obstructed secretions ➡ are seen in the left maxillary sinus. (Right) Axial T1WI C+ MR in the same patient shows diffuse, heterogeneous enhancement throughout this SNEC ➡. There is mass effect on the left orbital contents ➡ with lateral bowing of medial rectus muscle.

TERMINOLOGY

Abbreviations

- Sinonasal neuroendocrine carcinoma (SNEC)
- Esthesioneuroblastoma (ENB)
- Sinonasal undifferentiated carcinoma (SNUC)
- Small cell undifferentiated neuroendocrine carcinoma (SCUNC)
- Neuroendocrine carcinoma (NEC)

Definitions

- Rare malignancy of epithelial origin expressing neuroendocrine markers
  - Pathologically distinguishable from other sinonasal neuroectodermal tumors: ENB, SNUC, SCUNC

IMAGING

General Features

- Best diagnostic clue
  - SN neuroectodermal tumors cannot generally be distinguished by clinical or radiologic criteria
- Location
  - Predilection for superior **nasal cavity** & **ethmoid sinuses**
  - In H&N, more common in larynx

CT Findings

- CECT
  - Variably enhancing soft tissue mass with ill-defined borders & invasion of adjacent compartments
- Bone CT
  - Aggressive bone destruction

MR Findings

- T1WI
  - Ill-defined soft tissue mass; isointense to musculature
- STIR
  - Heterogeneous, low to intermediate long TR signal
- T1WI C+ FS
  - Variable, typically diffuse enhancement

Nuclear Medicine Findings

- Indium-111 pentetreotide scintigraphy
  - ↑ uptake in well & moderately differentiated SNEC

Imaging Recommendations

- Best imaging tool
  - Multiplanar gadolinium-enhanced MR imaging with fat suppression best delineates tumor extent

DIFFERENTIAL DIAGNOSIS

Esthesioneuroblastoma

- Arises near cribriform plate; highly vascular with avid enhancement ± flow voids

Sinonasal Undifferentiated Carcinoma

- Aggressive, ill-defined mass; often with necrosis
- Least differentiated of neuroectodermal tumors with tenuous neuroendocrine differentiation

Sinonasal Adenocarcinoma

- Nonspecific imaging features; ethmoid predilection; rare < 40-50 years

Sinonasal Squamous Cell Carcinoma

- Most common sinonasal malignancy; commonly arises in maxillary antrum (~ 70%)

Small Cell Undifferentiated Neuroendocrine Carcinoma

- Rare; nonspecific features; cannot distinguish from SNEC or SNUC on imaging

PATHOLOGY

General Features

- Etiology
  - Cell of origin not clearly known
    - Derived from endocrine cells of dispersed neuroendocrine system vs. basal progenitor cells in olfactory mucosa

Staging, Grading, & Classification

- SNEC is **part of spectrum of neuroendocrine tumors**
  - ENB (most differentiated) → SNEC → SCUNC → SNUC
- SNEC is morphologically distinct from SCUNC and immunohistochemically distinct from SNUC

Microscopic Features

- 2/3(+) for epithelial markers (low molecular weight cytokeratins & epithelial membrane antigen)
- Neurosecretory granules
  - Immunoreactive for neuroendocrine markers (chromogranin, synaptophysin, S100, CD57)

CLINICAL ISSUES

Presentation

- Most common signs/symptoms
  - Nasal obstruction, discharge, & epistaxis

Demographics

- Age
  - Wide range (20-70 years); average: ~ 50 years

Natural History & Prognosis

- Usually present with locally advanced disease
  - **70%** present as **stage IV disease**

Treatment

- Management of these rare neoplasms often based on analogous treatment principles for NEC of other anatomic sites (lung & larynx) & treatment of SNUC
  - Multimodality approach utilized at most institutions (surgery + chemo & XRT)

SELECTED REFERENCES

1. Subedi N et al: Neuroendocrine tumours of the head and neck: anatomical, functional and molecular imaging and contemporary management. Cancer Imaging. 13(3):407-22, 2013
2. Mitchell EH et al: Multimodality treatment for sinonasal neuroendocrine carcinoma. Head Neck. Nov 2. 34(10):1372-6, 2011
3. Likhacheva A et al: Sinonasal neuroendocrine carcinoma: impact of differentiation status on response and outcome. Head Neck Oncol. 3:32, 2011
4. Rischin D et al: Sinonasal malignancies of neuroendocrine origin. Hematol Oncol Clin North Am. 22(6):1297-316, xi, 2008
5. Rosenthal DI et al: Sinonasal malignancies with neuroendocrine differentiation: patterns of failure according to histologic phenotype. Cancer. 101(11):2567-73, 2004

KEY FACTS

TERMINOLOGY

- Sinonasal undifferentiated carcinoma (**SNUC**)
- Rare, aggressive, sinonasal nonsquamous cell epithelial or nonepithelial malignant neoplasm of varying histogenesis

IMAGING

- Aggressive sinonasal mass with bone destruction & rapid growth
- Large, typically > 4 cm at presentation
- Origin most common in nasal cavity with extension into paranasal sinuses; ethmoid origin more common than maxillary
- Bone CT: Poorly defined, soft tissue sinonasal mass with aggressive bone destruction
- MR: Isointense to muscle on T1
  - Low to intermediate T2 signal
  - Heterogeneous enhancement with necrosis

TOP DIFFERENTIAL DIAGNOSES

- Sinonasal squamous cell carcinoma
- Esthesioneuroblastoma
- Sinonasal non-Hodgkin lymphoma
- Sinonasal adenocarcinoma

CLINICAL ISSUES

- Higher propensity for distant metastases to bone, brain & dura, liver, & cervical nodes than other sinonasal malignancies

DIAGNOSTIC CHECKLIST

- Imaging features are nonspecific
- Tumor growth rate & presence of nodes/distant metastases helpful for suggesting SNUC
- Consider extending coverage to evaluate for intracranial (particularly dural) & cervical nodal disease

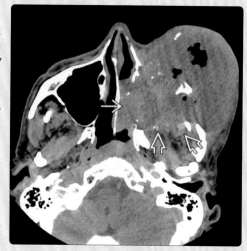
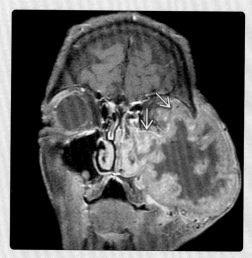

(Left) *Axial NECT demonstrates a large mass in the left maxillary antrum with marked bone destruction and extension into the nasal cavity ➡, masticator space ➡, and soft tissues of the cheek. Foci of air are seen within the necrotic portion of this rapidly growing lesion.* **(Right)** *Coronal T1WI C+ FS MR in the same patient shows a thick, nodular, enhancing rim at the periphery of the mass with central necrosis. There is aggressive invasion of the orbit ➡.*

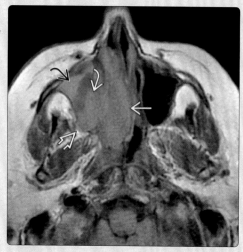
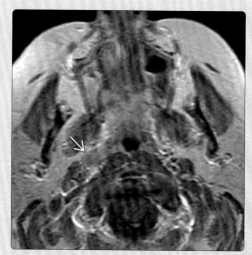

(Left) *Axial FLAIR MR demonstrates a large mass filling the right nasal cavity ➡ and extending into the right maxillary antrum ➡. There is extension into the retroantral fat ➡. Note the trapped secretions in the lateral aspect of the maxillary sinus ➡.* **(Right)** *Axial T1WI C+ MR in the same patient at the level of the nasopharynx shows a pathologic lateral retropharyngeal nodal metastasis ➡ from the patient's sinonasal undifferentiated carcinoma.*

KEY FACTS

TERMINOLOGY

- Malignant salivary type of adenocarcinoma

IMAGING

- Location: **Maxillary** > nasal cavity
- Low grade: Solidly enhancing, well-defined soft tissue mass
- High grade: Poorly defined, heterogeneous + bone destruction ± perineural tumor spread (PNTS)
- Multiplanar, **gadolinium-enhanced MR with fat suppression** recommended
  - Improves detection of PNTS

TOP DIFFERENTIAL DIAGNOSES

- Sinonasal squamous cell carcinoma
- Sinonasal adenocarcinoma (intestinal type)
- Esthesioneuroblastoma
- Sinonasal undifferentiated carcinoma

PATHOLOGY

- Not associated with inhalation exposures
- 3 histologic types
  - Cribriform (52%)
  - Tubular (20%)
  - Solid (29%); worst outcome; higher tendency for PNTS
- Most patients present with **T4 disease (65%)**

CLINICAL ISSUES

- Sinonasal adenoid cystic carcinoma (ACCa) accounts for 10-25% of H&N ACCa
  - Most common sinonasal salivary tumor
- Symptoms mimic sinusitis
  - **Facial pain ± numbness** (CNV2) → PNTS
- More common in Caucasians
- Overall 5-year survival rate: 50-86%
  - Late recurrences are not uncommon even > 15 years after initial therapy

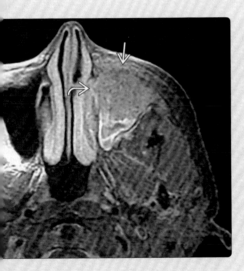
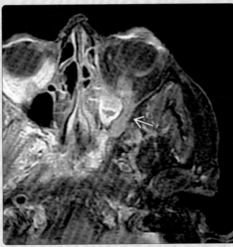

(Left) Axial T1WI C+ FS MR demonstrates diffuse enhancement of a left maxillary sinus adenoid cystic carcinoma (ACCa). There is osseous destruction and extension through the anterior ➡ and medial ➡ maxillary sinus walls. (Right) Axial T1WI C+ FS MR in the same patient demonstrates linear enhancing soft tissue along CNV2 ➡ involving the left inferior orbital fissure extending toward foramen rotundum, compatible with perineural tumor spread.

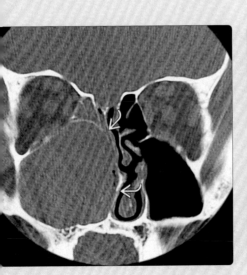
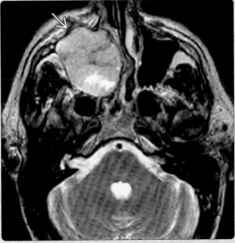

(Left) Coronal bone CT shows opacification of the right maxillary sinus by a large, expansile ACCa. The medial maxillary wall is eroded, and the mass extends into the nasal cavity. Note the leftward deviation of the nasal septum ➡. (Right) Axial T2WI MR in the same patient shows slightly heterogeneous, high signal throughout the mass. Slight extension into the premaxillary soft tissues is noted ➡. The relatively well-defined appearance of the ACCa may suggest a lower grade histology.

IMAGING

- Arises from maxilla, nasal septum, and skull base
  - Nasal septum location: Posterosuperior vomer
- Bone CT: **Chondroid matrix calcification** and narrow bony transition zone
  - 50% with chondroid matrix
- MR: Increased (high) signal on T2 images and heterogeneous enhancement

TOP DIFFERENTIAL DIAGNOSES

- Sinonasal osteosarcoma
- Skull base meningioma
- Sinonasal ossifying fibroma
- Sinonasal fibrous dysplasia
- Esthesioneuroblastoma

PATHOLOGY

- Malignant neoplasm arising from chondrocytes, embryonal rests, or mesenchymal cells

- May complicate Ollier and Maffucci syndromes

CLINICAL ISSUES

- Presents in 5th-7th decades
  - Duration from symptom onset to diagnosis: 3 months to 1 year
- Accounts for only 0.1% of H&N cancers
- Surgical resection is primary treatment modality
  - Difficult to achieve oncologic resection due to proximity of vital structures
  - Late recurrences after long disease-free periods are reported; long-term follow-up advised
- Overall 5-year survival: 54-81%

DIAGNOSTIC CHECKLIST

- **Arc-whorl** or **ring-like calcified matrix** on CT in lesion with ↑ T2 signal on MR may suggest diagnosis of chondrosarcoma

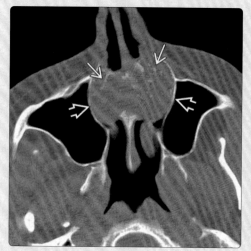
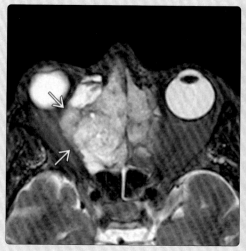

(Left) Axial bone CT shows a bilobed chondrosarcoma centered around the nasal septum at the bone-cartilage junction. Note involvement of bilateral nasal cavities. Multiple chondroid calcifications ➡ are characteristic. The lateral nasal walls ⇨ are remodeled but not destroyed. (Right) Axial STIR MR demonstrates a large chondrosarcoma involving the ethmoid sinuses bilaterally. There is extension into the right orbit ➡. High signal on T2-weighted images is a common feature of this histology.

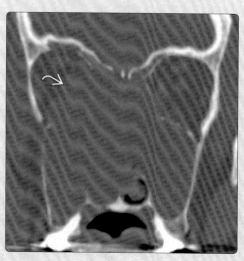
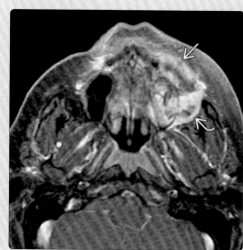

(Left) Coronal CT reconstruction shows a large, aggressive mass filling ethmoid sinuses and nasal cavity with bone destruction and extension into right orbit ➡. No classic chondroid matrix, but malignant features are present. (Right) Axial T1WI C+ FS MR shows a chondrosarcoma of the left maxilla with involvement of maxillary antrum. Lesion enhances heterogeneously and extends into premaxillary ➡ and retromaxillary ➡ soft tissues.

Sinonasal Osteosarcoma

KEY FACTS

TERMINOLOGY

- Rare malignant bone tumor arising from **primitive bone-forming mesenchyma**

IMAGING

- > 50% of craniofacial sinonasal osteosarcoma (OSa) arise in jaw
  - Mandible > maxilla
  - < 50% involve extragnathic bones (skull, orbit, sphenoid & ethmoid bones, or zygoma)
- CT best for delineating osteoid matrix & cortical involvement
  - **Hyperdense mass** with osteoid matrix & periosteal reaction
- MR optimal for evaluating extent within marrow & adjacent structures

TOP DIFFERENTIAL DIAGNOSES

- Chondrosarcoma, ossifying fibroma, osteoma, fibrous dysplasia, metastasis

PATHOLOGY

- Up to 25% are secondary malignancy in **prior radiation field**
- Increased incidence in hereditary retinoblastoma
- May arise in bone affected by Paget disease, fibrous dysplasia, multiple exostoses, enchondromatosis

CLINICAL ISSUES

- Most present in 3rd-4th decades
  - Older than classical OSa of long bones
- No strong gender predilection
- Craniofacial OSa accounts for 6-13% of all OSa
- Surgical resection is mainstay of treatment
  - Neoadjuvant chemotherapy has significantly improved cure rates

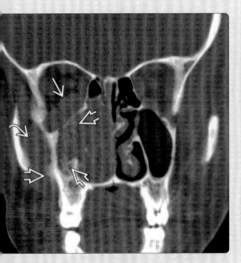
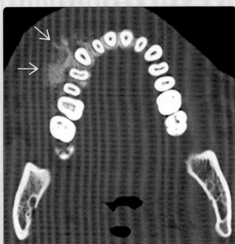

(Left) Coronal bone CT shows an aggressive mass involving the maxilla with soft tissue filling the maxillary antrum and nasal cavity. There is extension into the orbit ➡ and infratemporal fossa ➡. Note the sunburst periosteal reaction ➡ consistent with osteosarcoma. (Right) Axial NECT bone algorithm demonstrates an osteosarcoma projecting exophytically from the right maxillary alveolar ridge with aggressive sunburst periosteal reaction ➡.

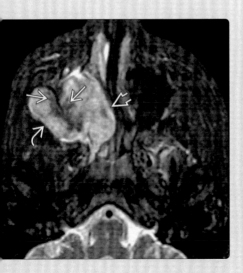
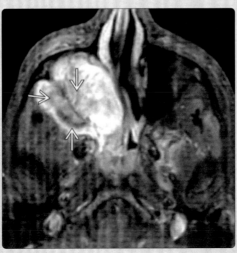

(Left) Axial T2WI FS MR demonstrates a large osteosarcoma centered around the lateral wall of the right maxillary sinus. There is medial extension into the nasal cavity ➡ and lateral extension into the masticator space ➡. Linear hypointense radiating periosteal reaction ➡ is noted along the bone of origin. (Right) Axial T1WI C+ FS MR in the same patient shows diffuse, avid enhancement throughout the soft tissue component of the mass. The hypointense periosteal reaction ➡ is noted.

SECTION 22
Orbit

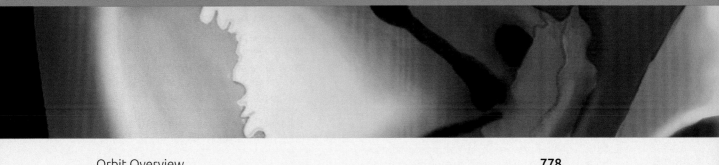

Imaging Approach & Indications

General Approach

Imaging of the orbit encompasses 2 clinically distinct areas of ophthalmology.

- The eye (or globe)
- The bony orbit, soft tissues, & periorbita

Lesions in these 2 areas result in specific clinical profiles. When a patient is referred for imaging, it is usually clear to the clinician whether the problem involves the globe versus some other structure of the orbit.

The term "orbital" refers to those bony structures and soft tissues that are extrinsic to the eye, as opposed to the term "ocular," which refers to the globe itself.

Most imaging referrals come from ophthalmologists, oculoplastic surgeons, neuro-ophthalmologists, neurosurgeons, and otolaryngologists. Imaging of the orbit and globe provides complementary information to the physical and ophthalmoscopic examination.

Ultrasound

Ultrasound of the eye is a readily available complement to funduscopic examination and is traditionally performed in the ophthalmology clinic. In addition to providing imaging of the globe, transocular ultrasound provides a limited, high-resolution assessment of other intraorbital soft tissues.

CT

Because of its superior bony characterization, CT has advantages over MR for orbital lesions that arise from or directly affect the bones, such as epithelial inclusions, osteocartilaginous tumors with matrix, osteodystrophic processes, benign masses that cause bony scalloping, and aggressive malignancies that cause bony destruction.

The presence of calcification is a specific differentiating feature in some lesions, and CT can provide essential diagnostic information, even after an MR has been obtained. For example, an indeterminate diagnosis of perioptic nerve meningioma on MR might be confirmed with identification of calcification on CT.

In some instances, CT can provide enough information to allow for a definitive diagnosis and guide therapy without the need for MR. Examples include thyroid ophthalmopathy, clinically benign lacrimal mass, orbital cavernous malformation, and orbital disease that is secondary to a sinonasal process.

MR

For evaluating complex orbital disease, MR is the preferred modality. Superior soft tissue differentiation and enhancement make MR ideal for characterizing the extent of complicated lesions, including extraocular tumors, vascular malformations, and complex infectious or inflammatory processes.

In particular, MR is the optimal modality for delineating the extent of malignant orbital disease. Important features visible on MR include optic nerve invasion, perineural extension of tumor to the orbit, intracranial extension of disease, and hematogeneous or CSF disseminated metastases.

Although ultrasound is usually the 1st line for imaging the globe, MR can provide a more accurate visualization of retrobulbar extension of intraocular malignancy, including retinoblastoma, ocular melanoma, and ocular metastases.

Additionally, MR provides exquisite characterization of the globe itself, which is particularly useful in circumstances where funduscopic evaluation is obscured, such as swollen or injured eye, retinal detachment, large intraocular mass, vitreal hemorrhage, or opaque media from any cause.

Imaging Anatomy

Bony Orbit

Major components of the bony orbital walls are the frontal bone superiorly, zygomatic bone laterally and inferiorly, maxillary bone inferiorly and medially, and ethmoid bone medially. Smaller contributions medially include the lacrimal bone, nasal bone, and a tiny portion of the palatine bone. The sphenoid bone makes up a large portion of the orbit posteriorly and laterally, forming the complex foramina at the orbital apex.

Globe

The aqueous-filled anterior segment includes anterior and posterior chambers, both anterior to the lens. The vitreous-filled posterior segment occupies the bulk of the globe posteriorly. The layers, or tunica, of the eye include the inner retina, vascular choroid, and outer structural sclera. The anterior refractive constructs include the iris and ciliary body, which are specialized portions of the uvea, as well as the lens.

Orbital Septum

The orbital septum is comprised of fascia arising from the orbital periosteum that inserts onto the aponeurosis of the tarsal plates of the lids, providing a barrier between the anterior periorbita and the intraorbital contents. Although the septum itself is often not discernible as a discrete structure on routine imaging, its presence is readily evident when a disease process, especially preseptal infection, is contained on 1 side of the barrier.

Lacrimal Apparatus

The lacrimal gland lies in a bony fossa at the anterior aspect of the superolateral orbit. Lacrimal drainage is via canaliculi and sac at the inferomedial orbit, and from there it passes through the nasolacrimal duct, which drains via the inferior meatus.

Extraocular Muscles

The 4 rectus muscles originate from the annulus of Zinn at the apex and insert on the corneoscleral surface. The superior oblique has similar origin and insertion but courses through the trochlea ("pulley") at the superomedial orbital rim. The inferior oblique has a short, more direct course originating from the anteroinferior orbital rim. The levator palpebrae superioris originates at the annulus, coursing just above the superior rectus, forming the superior muscle complex, and inserts at the upper eyelid.

Optic Nerve-Sheath Complex

The optic nerve (CNII) is actually a central nervous tract that traverses the optic canal and orbit to insert at the optic nerve head. The surrounding dural sheath is contiguous with the intracranial dura posteriorly and with the sclera anteriorly. A thin rim of CSF surrounding the nerve is typically visible on MR and is contiguous with CSF in the intracranial cisterns.

Peripheral Cranial Nerves

CNIII, CNIV, & CNVI supply motor innervation to the extraocular muscles (EOMs), as well as parasympathetics to the iris via CNIII. The individual branches of these nerves are not reliably distinguished within the orbit. However, knowledge of their course through the cavernous sinus and

Differential Diagnosis: Orbit

Congenital lesions (globe)	Infectious lesions (globe)	Benign tumors
Coloboma	Ocular toxocariasis	Lacrimal benign mixed tumor
Persistent hyperplastic primary vitreous	Acute endophthalmitis	Optic pathway glioma
Coats disease		Optic nerve sheath meningioma
Congenital lesions (orbit)	**Infectious lesions (orbit)**	**Malignant tumors (globe)**
Orbital dermoid and epidermoid	Orbital subperiosteal abscess	Retinoblastoma
Orbital neurofibromatosis, type 1	Orbital cellulitis	Uveal melanoma
Vascular malformations	**Inflammatory lesions**	**Malignant tumors (orbit)**
Orbital lymphatic malformation	Orbital idiopathic pseudotumor	Lacrimal epithelial carcinoma
Orbital varix	Orbital sarcoidosis	Lymphoproliferative lesions
Orbital cavernous malformation	Thyroid ophthalmopathy	Orbital Langerhans histiocytosis
Vascular neoplasms	Optic neuritis	Metastases
Orbital infantile hemangioma		

superior orbital fissure (SOF) allows localization of pathology that involves these nerves.

Two of the branches of CNV course through the orbit. V1 passes with other nerves through the SOF and exits the orbit through the supraorbital foramen. V2 passes through foramen rotundum and inferior orbital fissure and exits the orbit through the infraorbital foramen.

Vascular Structures
The ophthalmic artery enters the orbit alongside the optic nerve within the optic canal; it is frequently visible in the orbit, as it diverges from the nerve near the apex. High-resolution angiography, CT, and MR show the artery originating as the 1st intradural branch of the internal carotid artery. The superior ophthalmic vein is variable but typically found coursing between the superior rectus muscle and the optic nerve.

Orbital Fat
In addition to acting as a volume "filler" for the orbital cavity, orbital fat provides intrinsic imaging contrast, making other structures and disease processes more conspicuous.

Anatomy-based Imaging Issues

In approaching orbital lesions, it is useful to localize the process to a subregion of the orbit and ascertain the relationship of the lesion to critical structures.

- **Globe**: Is the lesion entirely intraocular, or is there transscleral extension, particularly with regard to the optic nerve head?
- **Optic nerve**: Does the lesion arise within the nerve proper or involve primarily the dural sheath?
- **EOM**: Is the lesion intraconal or extraconal, or does it arise from the muscles themselves? Is muscle involvement symmetric or otherwise characteristic?
- **Lacrimal gland**: Is the lesion unilateral, or is it bilateral, indicating a systemic process?
- **Bone**: Does the lesion arise from the bone itself? If the lesion is adjacent to bone, does the bone show benign scalloped remodeling or aggressive destruction?
- **Focality**: Is the lesion isolated or multiple, focal or diffuse and poorly defined? Does the lesion extend beyond the orbit?

Imaging Protocols
CT
Routine imaging of the orbit with CT does not require special discussion, except for 1 clinical circumstance: Intermittent proptosis due to orbital varix. This dynamic lesion enlarges with increases in venous pressures and is best demonstrated with provocation. After performing routine enhanced CT, the scan is repeated with the breath held in Valsalva maneuver, increasing venous pressures and dynamically enlarging the varix.

MR
Routine imaging of the orbit with MR is usually adequate for the majority of ophthalmologic indications. The protocol includes 3 sequence types, each of these performed in axial and coronal planes, at 3-mm slice thickness and 18-cm field of view. Whole-brain imaging is added when indicated.
- Precontrast T1WI (without fat suppression)
- T2WI with fat suppression (alternatively STIR)
- Postcontrast T1WI with fat suppression

Pathologic Issues: Vascular Malformations

Vascular malformations are congenital, nonneoplastic lesions, with classification that reflects their histologic and hemodynamic features.

Orbital cavernous malformation: This common mass is unique to the orbit. It is encapsulated with low-flow venous channels. The term hemangioma is commonly used to refer to this lesion but is actually a misnomer.

Venolymphatic malformation: Lesions may have no flow (type 1), venous flow (type 2), or may be mixed. There may be a distensible component, resulting in varix. Outdated terminology to be avoided includes "lymphangioma" and "cystic hygroma."

Arteriovenous malformations (AVM): True orbital AVMs are rare lesions, with high-flow arterial (type 3) hemodynamics.

Selected References
1. Yanoff M, Duker J: Ophthalmology. Expert Consult (4th ed.). Saunders: Philadelphia, PA, 2013
2. Rootman J. Diseases of the Orbit: A Multidisciplinary Approach. Philadelphia, PA: Lippincott, 2003

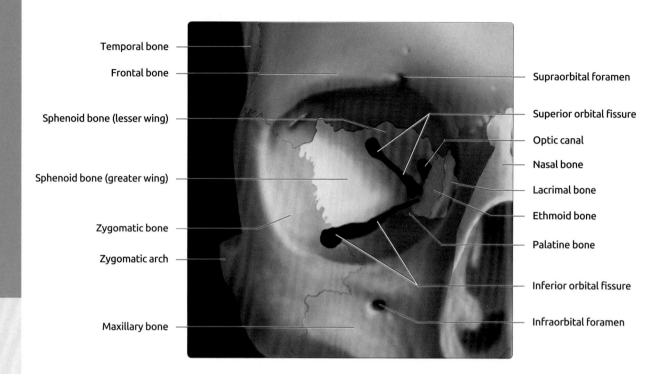

Temporal bone
Frontal bone
Sphenoid bone (lesser wing)
Sphenoid bone (greater wing)
Zygomatic bone
Zygomatic arch
Maxillary bone

Supraorbital foramen
Superior orbital fissure
Optic canal
Nasal bone
Lacrimal bone
Ethmoid bone
Palatine bone
Inferior orbital fissure
Infraorbital foramen

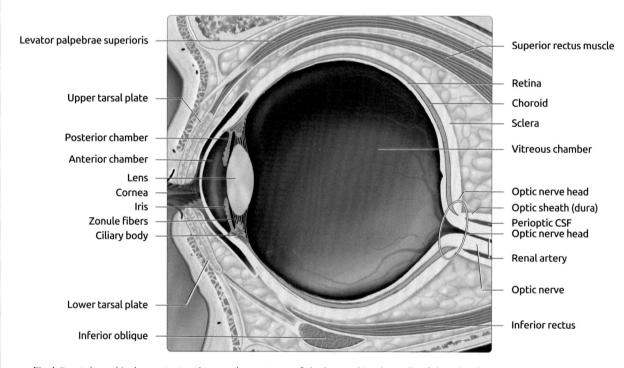

Levator palpebrae superioris
Upper tarsal plate
Posterior chamber
Anterior chamber
Lens
Cornea
Iris
Zonule fibers
Ciliary body
Lower tarsal plate
Inferior oblique

Superior rectus muscle
Retina
Choroid
Sclera
Vitreous chamber
Optic nerve head
Optic sheath (dura)
Perioptic CSF
Optic nerve head
Renal artery
Optic nerve
Inferior rectus

(Top) *Frontal graphic demonstrates the complex anatomy of the bony orbit. The walls of the orbital cavity receive contributions from 8 different bones of the skull. The complex foramina and fissures at the apex are located primarily within the greater & lesser wings of the sphenoid bone and its junctions with adjacent bones.* **(Bottom)** *Sagittal graphic demonstrates the anterior and posterior segments of the globe. The aqueous anterior segment is comprised of the anterior chamber and very small posterior chamber. The much larger posterior segment is filled by the vitreous chamber. The layered tunicae of the retina, choroid, and sclera are demonstrated as well as the components of the optic nerve at its insertion. Some of the extraocular muscles and eyelid structures are also demonstrated.*

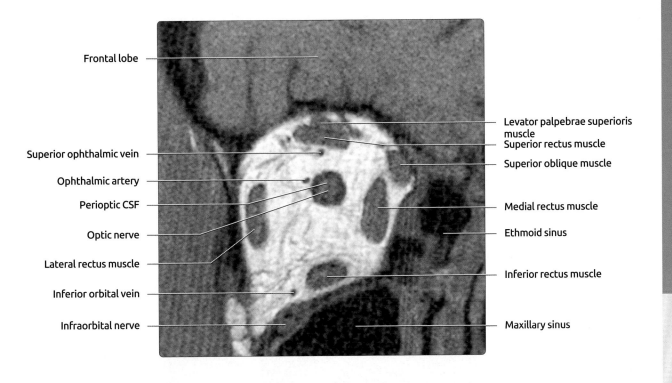

Frontal lobe

Levator palpebrae superioris muscle

Superior rectus muscle

Superior oblique muscle

Superior ophthalmic vein

Ophthalmic artery

Medial rectus muscle

Perioptic CSF

Ethmoid sinus

Optic nerve

Lateral rectus muscle

Inferior rectus muscle

Inferior orbital vein

Infraorbital nerve

Maxillary sinus

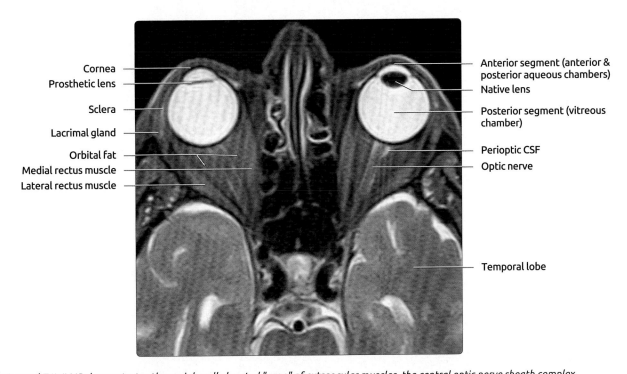

Cornea

Anterior segment (anterior & posterior aqueous chambers)

Prosthetic lens

Native lens

Sclera

Posterior segment (vitreous chamber)

Lacrimal gland

Orbital fat

Perioptic CSF

Medial rectus muscle

Optic nerve

Lateral rectus muscle

Temporal lobe

(Top) *Coronal T1WI MR demonstrates the peripherally located "cone" of extraocular muscles, the central optic nerve sheath complex, and the vascular structures of the orbit. The intrinsic T1 signal of the orbital fat provides excellent contrast for visualizing the intraorbital contents.* **(Bottom)** *Axial T2WI MR with fat suppression nearly eliminates signal from orbital fat, allowing for conspicuity of fluid signal structures. A small amount of CSF surrounding the optic nerve is usually visible on T2WI. The normal extraocular muscles show intermediate to low signal. A small portion of the lacrimal gland is seen, but the majority of the gland is located further superiorly. The anterior segment of the eye shows water signal, primarily representing the anterior chamber; the posterior chamber is not separately discernible on routine MR. The posterior segment also shows water signal, comprised of the vitreous chamber. Note that this patient has a prosthetic lens on the right.*

Coloboma

TERMINOLOGY

- Coloboma = gap or defect of ocular tissue
- May involve any or all structures of embryonic cleft
- Types of posterior coloboma
  - Optic disc coloboma
  - Choroidoretinal coloboma
- Related but distinct anomalies
  - Morning glory disc anomaly
  - Peripapillary staphyloma

IMAGING

- Focal defect at posterior pole of globe
- Outpouching contiguous with vitreous
- Oriented posteriorly with long axis of globe
- Microphthalmos and retrobulbar cysts often present
- Isodense to vitreous on CT
- Isointense to vitreous on MR
- Bulging of posterior globe on prenatal MR

TOP DIFFERENTIAL DIAGNOSES

- Congenital microphthalmos
- Congenital glaucoma
- Neurofibromatosis type 1
- Degrenative staphyloma
- Axial myopia

PATHOLOGY

- Failure of embryonic fissure fusion
- Isolated, sporadic, and syndromic genetic etiologies
- Bilateral when syndromic

CLINICAL ISSUES

- Decreased visual acuity; leukocoria
- Treatment to address refractive errors, strabismus, amblyopia, retinal detachment

DIAGNOSTIC CHECKLIST

- Look for syndromic and systemic associations

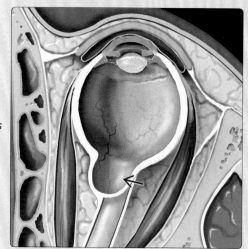
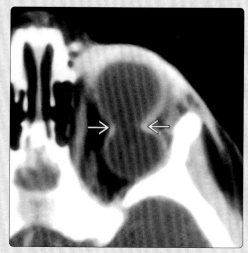

(Left) Axial graphic of classic optic disc coloboma shows a focal defect in the posterior globe at the site of the optic nerve head insertion ➡. (Right) Axial CECT demonstrates a broad colobomatous defect ➡ centered on the upper margin of the optic disc. Note vitreous appears contiguous to retrobulbar outpouching. Apart from the retrobulbar outpouching, the globe is small.

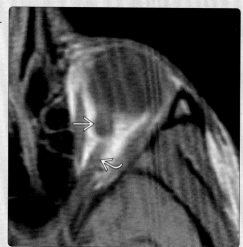
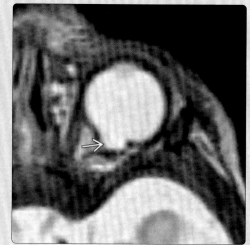

(Left) Axial T1 MR of the orbit demonstrates a focal posterior pole outpouching of the globe ➡, located just above and medial to optic nerve head. Note posterior intraorbital optic nerve ➡. (Right) Axial T2 MR in the same patient demonstrates a focal globe defect near the optic nerve insertion ➡. Note fluid signal within the outpouching is identical to the intraocular vitreous.

TERMINOLOGY

Abbreviations

- Optic disc coloboma (ODC)
- Choroidoretinal coloboma (CRC)

Definitions

- Coloboma = **gap** or defect of ocular tissue
- Types of **posterior** coloboma
  - **ODC**: Excavation confined to **optic disc**
  - **CRC**: Defect separate from or extends **beyond disc**
- Related anomalies
  - Morning glory disc anomaly (**MGDA**): Defect with glial tissue & pigmented rim
  - Peripapillary staphyloma (**PPS**): Congenital scleral defect at optic nerve head
- Other colobomatous lesions
  - May involve any or all structures of **embryonic cleft**
    - Iris, ciliary body, lens, or eyelid
  - Fuchs coloboma
    - Inferiorly tilted disc with crescent-shaped defect along inferonasal margin

IMAGING

General Features

- Best diagnostic clue
  - Focal defect with outpouching at posterior pole of globe; vitreous contiguous with defect
  - **Microphthalmos** and retrobulbar **cysts** often present
- Location
  - Posterior globe at optic **nerve head** insertion
- Size
  - Usually small (few to several mm)
  - MGDA & PPS larger than simple coloboma
- Morphology
  - **Crater-shaped** excavation, contiguous with vitreous
  - Oriented posteriorly with **long axis** of globe
  - MGDA defect funnel-shaped with central glial tissue
  - PPS defect encircles optic disc
- Laterality
  - Unilateral when sporadic, bilateral when syndromic
  - MGDA almost always unilateral, R > L
  - PPS usually unilateral

CT Findings

- NECT
  - Fluid in defect ± retrobulbar cyst **isodense to vitreous**
  - Subretinal hyperdensity if hemorrhage
- Bone CT
  - Ca++ may develop at margins of chronic defects

MR Findings

- T1WI and T2WI
  - **Isointense to vitreous**
  - Complex signal if retinal detachment, including hemorrhagic or proteinaceous fluid (T1 hyperintense)
  - Glial tuft of MGDA isointense to white matter
- Enhancement
  - Sclera enhances; glial tuft in MGDA may enhance
  - Otherwise no abnormal enhancement within defect

- Prenatal MR
  - Bulging of posterior globe profile

Ultrasonographic Findings

- Outpouching of posterior globe at optic nerve head
- Hypoechoic retrobulbar mass if cyst present

Imaging Recommendations

- Best imaging tool
  - MR or CT show globe and extraocular features, especially if defects prevent direct visualization
  - CT provides reasonable depiction without sedation
  - MR of brain helpful if **syndromic** to evaluate for associated **intracranial abnormalities**

DIFFERENTIAL DIAGNOSIS

Congenital Microphthalmos

- Congenital severe ocular derangement
- Deformed small globe with adjacent cyst

Congenital Glaucoma

- Present at birth, usually bilateral
- Enlarged globe

Neurofibromatosis Type 1

- Globe enlargement = "buphthalmos"
- May have associated optic glioma, sphenoid wing dysplasia, plexiform neurofibroma

Degenerative Staphyloma

- Degenerative ectasia of globe
- Thinning of posterior sclera-uveal rim
- Enlarged globe, associated with myopia

Axial Myopia

- Elongated anteroposterior dimension

PATHOLOGY

General Features

- Etiology
  - Embryological considerations
    - Embryonic fissure extends along **inferonasal** aspect of optic cup and stalk
    - Fissure fusion (**5th-7th week**) required for normal globe and nerve formation
  - Coloboma (ODC/CRC)
    - Failure of embryonic fissure fusion superiorly
  - MGDA
    - Faulty scleral closure (4th week)
    - Mesoectodermal dysgenesis of optic nerve head
  - PPS
    - Incomplete differentiation of sclera
    - Diminished peripapillary structural support
- Genetics
  - **Sporadic** coloboma
    - Noninherited
    - Unilateral; especially isolated ODC
    - Possible maternal environmental factors
  - **Nonsyndromic** coloboma
    - Typically **autosomal dominant**
    - Identified with many specific mutations

- ○ **Syndromic** coloboma
  - – Usually **autosomal recessive**
  - – Typically bilateral, especially CRC
  - – Associated with trisomies
  - – Dozens of syndromes (CHARGE, Aicardi, papillorenal, COACH, Meckel, Warburg, Lenz)
- ○ **MGDA**
  - – Typically sporadic; rare familial cases
  - – Unilateral, except when familial
- ○ **PPS**
  - – Typically sporadic
  - – Unilateral, usually isolated anomaly
- Associated abnormalities
  - ○ Triad of major congenital globe anomalies
    - – Microphthalmos, anophthalmos, and coloboma (**MAC**)
  - ○ Orbital
    - – Microphthalmia; optic tract & chiasm atrophy
    - – Retrobulbar colobomatous cyst
    - – Retinal detachment (25-40%) (ODC, MGDA)
    - – Congenital optic pit (ODC, MGDA)
    - – Cataract; hyaloid artery (ODC, MGDA)
    - – Iris coloboma (ODC)
    - – Persistent hyperplasic primary vitreous, aniridia (MGDA)
  - ○ Systemic
    - – Renal, CNS, and many other systemic associations, particularly when bilateral

Staging, Grading, & Classification

- Simple coloboma (normal globe and cornea): ~ 15%
  - ○ Best prognosis for vision
- Coloboma with microcornea (< 30 mm): ~ 40%
  - ○ Better prognosis
- Coloboma with microcornea & microphthalmos: ~ 40%
  - ○ Worse prognosis
- Coloboma with microphthalmos and cyst: ~ 5%
  - ○ Worst prognosis for vision

Gross Pathologic & Surgical Features

- Coloboma (ODC/CRC)
  - ○ Funnel-shaped depression at fundus
- MGDA
  - ○ Tuft of whitish tissue overlying enlarged disc
- PPS
  - ○ Excavation that incorporates sunken optic disc

Microscopic Features

- Coloboma (ODC/CRC)
  - ○ Invagination of gliotic retina into defect
- MGDA
  - ○ Central core of vascular connective and glial tissue
- PPS
  - ○ Large peripapillary defect, thinned sclera

CLINICAL ISSUES

Presentation

- Most common signs/symptoms
  - ○ Decreased **visual acuity** (VA)
- Other signs/symptoms
  - ○ **Leukocoria**

- ○ Iris involvement causes typical "keyhole" defect
- ○ Microphthalmia or anophthalmia in severe cases
- ○ Associated **syndromic** features
- Clinical profile
  - ○ Vision depends on extent of optic disc involvement and retinal detachment
    - – Strabismus and nystagmus secondary to poor VA
    - – Reduced visual evoked potentials
- Funduscopic examination
  - ○ ODC
    - – Enlarged disc with excavation
    - – May resemble glaucomatous cupping
  - ○ CRC
    - – White with pigmented margins
    - – Extends inferiorly from or inferior to disc
  - ○ MGDA
    - – Enlarged, excavated disc; central core of tissue
    - – Central tuft of tissue with surrounding ring of pigment; resembles morning glory blossom
  - ○ PPS
    - – Central crater with recessed optic nerve
    - – Optic disc sunken, otherwise normal; atrophy of surrounding pigment epithelium

Demographics

- Gender
  - ○ No predilection
    - – Except MGDA: M < F (1:2)
- Epidemiology
  - ○ Coloboma (nonsyndromic): 1:12,000
  - ○ MGDA and PPS: Rare

Natural History & Prognosis

- Visual acuity correlates with retinal status
  - ○ Detachment leads to precipitous vision loss
  - ○ Nerve atrophy and cataracts may lead to more insidious vision loss

Treatment

- Address refractive errors, strabismus, amblyopia
- Retinal detachment management

DIAGNOSTIC CHECKLIST

Consider

- Coloboma is ophthalmoscopic diagnosis
- Imaging confirms ocular features, identifies retrobulbar findings such as cyst, and evaluates coexistent anomalies

Image Interpretation Pearls

- Look for **syndromic** and systemic associations

SELECTED REFERENCES

1. Dar SA et al: Prenatal diagnosis of colobomatous microphthalmos. J Pediatr Ophthalmol Strabismus. 52 Online:e22-5, 2015
2. Williamson KA et al: The genetic architecture of microphthalmia, anophthalmia and coloboma. Eur J Med Genet. 57(8):369-80, 2014
3. Righini A et al: Prenatal magnetic resonance imaging of optic nerve head coloboma. Prenat Diagn. 28(3):242-6, 2008
4. Altun E et al: Anterior coloboma with macrophthalmos and cyst: MR findings. Clin Imaging. 29(6):430-3, 2005
5. Vogt G et al: A population-based case-control study of isolated ocular coloboma. Ophthalmic Epidemiol. 12(3):191-7, 2005
6. Chan RT et al: Morning glory syndrome. Clin Exp Optom. 85(6):383-8, 2002

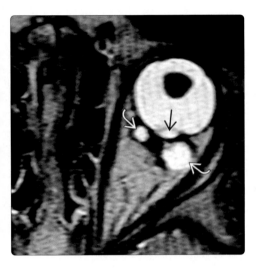

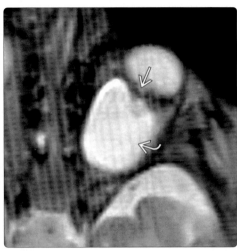

(Left) Axial T2 FS MR shows a small left globe with a broad posterior coloboma ➡. Two associated distinct colobomatous cysts ➡ are present in retrobulbar fat immediately posterior to the globe. (Right) Axial T2 FS MR in an infant with multiple congenital anomalies demonstrates a small colobomatous defect at the posterior pole of ➡ small, irregular left globe. An associated large retrobulbar cyst ➡ is present.

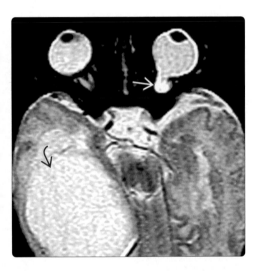

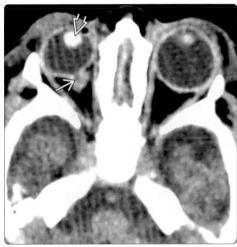

(Left) Axial STIR MR in a patient with Aicardi syndrome demonstrates a moderate-sized left coloboma ➡ at the optic nerve insertion. A large choroid plexus cyst is present ➡, a common finding in patients with this X-linked syndrome. (Right) Axial CECT in a patient with CHARGE syndrome shows small defect at posterior pole of right eye with focal vitreal herniation ➡. The right eye is microphthalmic, with abnormal appearance of the lens ➡.

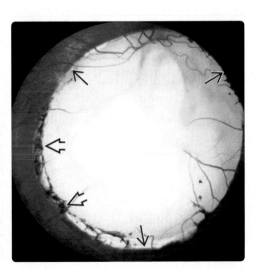

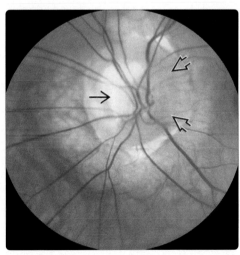

(Left) Funduscopy shows a large posterior coloboma centered at the optic nerve head ➡. Associated marginal pigmentation ➡ suggests chorioretinal involvement. (Right) Funduscopy shows an enlarged, funnel-shaped optic disc ➡ with central glial tissue as well as annular pigmentation ➡, resulting in an appearance that resembles a morning glory flower.

Persistent Hyperplastic Primary Vitreous

TERMINOLOGY

- Congenital lesion due to incomplete regression of embryonic ocular blood supply
- Persistent fetal vasculature = new term in recent literature

IMAGING

- **Martini glass shape** of enhancing soft tissue
  - Triangular retrolental vascular tuft of tissue
  - Central tissue stalk of hyaloid remnant
- Retinal detachment common
- Small globe, hyperdense vitreous
- Calcification rare
- Hyperintense blood with layering debris

TOP DIFFERENTIAL DIAGNOSES

- Retinoblastoma
- Congenital cataract
- Coats disease
- Retinopathy of prematurity

PATHOLOGY

- Normal fetal primary vitreous involutes by birth
- **Failure of hyaloid regression** causes remnant to persist in Cloquet canal

CLINICAL ISSUES

- **Leukocoria** with poor vision and small eye
- Anterior type has better prognosis for vision
- Surgical options include lensectomy, vitrectomy
- Long-term management
  - Amblyopia therapy and refractive correction
  - Management of glaucoma and detachments

DIAGNOSTIC CHECKLIST

- Primary vitreous may be incompletely regressed and normally visible in premature infant
- Persistent hyperplastic primary vitreous is most common intraocular abnormality to be confused with retinoblastoma

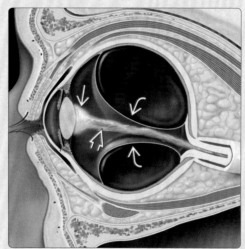
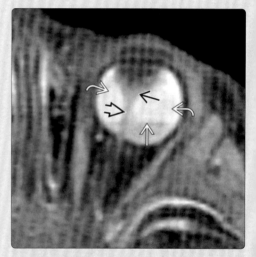

(Left) Sagittal graphic depicts persistent hyperplastic primary vitreous. A triangular retrolental soft tissue mass is present ➡, with stalk-like hyaloid remnant ➡. Note the large V-shaped retinal detachment ➡. (Right) Axial T1WI C+ FS MR shows the martini glass appearance of retrolental tuft of tissue ➡ with linear stalk ➡ extending to the optic nerve head. A large hyperintense detachment is present ➡, with associated hemorrhage and fluid level ➡.

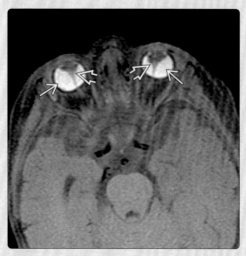
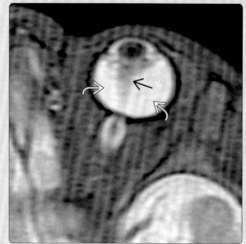

(Left) Axial T1 FS MR shows bilateral microphthalmia and abnormal hyperintense, hemorrhagic retinal detachments within the bilateral posterior globes ➡. The hypointense signal intensity extending from the lens to the optic disc represents the hyaloid remnant ➡. (Right) Axial T2 FS MR shows the hyaloid remnant in the right eye ➡ extending from the lens to the posterior pole at the nerve insertion. A large hyperintense retinal detachment ➡ is relatively inconspicuous compared to vitreous on T2WI.

TERMINOLOGY

Abbreviations

- Persistent hyperplastic primary vitreous (**PHPV**)

Definitions

- Congenital lesion due to **incomplete regression of embryonic ocular blood supply**
- Persistent fetal vasculature = new term in recent literature

IMAGING

General Features

- Best diagnostic clue
  - **Retrolental soft tissue** and **stalk**
  - **Hyperdense or hyperintense small globe**
- Location
  - Isolated posterior form (15-25%)
  - Isolated anterior form (5-25%)
  - Both anterior and posterior (50-80%)
  - **Unilateral > bilateral** (3:1)
- Morphology
  - **Martini glass shape** of enhancing soft tissue
    - Triangular retrolental vascular tuft of tissue
    - Central tissue stalk of hyaloid remnant
  - **Retinal detachment** common
- Enhancement
  - Retrolental tissue enhances, as does vitreous depending on degree of persistent vascularity

CT Findings

- NECT
  - Small globe, hyperdense vitreous
  - Layering blood or debris may be present
  - Calcification rare

MR Findings

- Spin-echo MR
  - Small globe, vitreous abnormally hyperintense on both T1WI and T2WI
  - Hemorrhage and layering debris in vitreous
    - Signal varies with age of blood

Ultrasonographic Findings

- Lens displacement, hyperechoic retrolental stalk

Imaging Recommendations

- Best imaging tool
  - CT differentiates from retinoblastoma (Ca^{2+})
  - **MR superior for differentiating noncalcified retinoblastoma from other causes of leukocoria**
- Protocol advice
  - Contrast enhancement is essential

DIFFERENTIAL DIAGNOSIS

Retinoblastoma

- Calcification differentiates from PHPV

Congenital Cataract

- Malformed lens due to prenatal insult

Coats Disease

- Exudative retinopathy with detachments

Retinopathy of Prematurity

- Retrolental fibroplasia; small, dense globe

PATHOLOGY

General Features

- Etiology
  - Primary vitreous = embryonic hyaloid vasculature of developing globe
  - Normal fetal primary vitreous involutes by 8th month of gestation
  - Failure of hyaloid regression causes remnant to persist in Cloquet canal
- Associated abnormalities
  - PHPV usually isolated and unilateral
  - Bilateral lesions associated with systemic or syndromic conditions including Norrie, Warburg

Microscopic Features

- Fibrovascular loose connective tissue
- Hyaloid artery remnant

CLINICAL ISSUES

Presentation

- Most common signs/symptoms
  - Leukocoria with poor vision and small globe
- Other signs/symptoms
  - Cataract, strabismus, nystagmus, uveitis

Natural History & Prognosis

- Anterior: Best prognosis for vision
- Posterior: May have light/motion perception only
- Risk of secondary glaucoma

Treatment

- Goals: Salvage vision, avoid glaucoma, pupil cosmesis
- Surgical options
  - Anterior: Lensectomy, intraocular prosthetic lens
  - Posterior: Vitrectomy, removal of hyaloid stalk
- Long-term management
  - Amblyopia therapy and refractive correction
  - Management of glaucoma and detachments

DIAGNOSTIC CHECKLIST

Consider

- Primary vitreous may be incompletely regressed and normally visible in premature infant

Image Interpretation Pearls

- PHPV is most common intraocular abnormality to be confused with retinoblastoma

SELECTED REFERENCES

1. Burns NS et al: Diagnostic imaging of fetal and pediatric orbital abnormalities. AJR Am J Roentgenol. 201(6):W797-808, 2013
2. Brennan RC et al: US and MRI of pediatric ocular masses with histopathological correlation. Pediatr Radiol. 42(6):738-49, 2012

Coats Disease

TERMINOLOGY

- Retinal telangiectasias, exudative retinopathy
- Abnormal retinal capillary development leading to subretinal accumulation of exudate

IMAGING

- Subretinal exudate with retinal detachment
- Unilateral in 90%; bilateral when syndromic
- Affected eye slightly smaller than normal eye
- Typical V-shaped contour of retinal detachment
- CT
  - Hyperdense exudate, calcification very uncommon
- MR
  - Hyperintense proteinaceous, hemorrhagic exudate
  - Nerve enhancement in advanced disease
- Ultrasound
  - Linear detached retina and tiny cholesterol crystals

TOP DIFFERENTIAL DIAGNOSES

- Retinoblastoma
- Persistent hyperplastic primary vitreous
- Retinopathy of prematurity

PATHOLOGY

- Breakdown of blood-retinal endothelial barrier
- Cholesterol crystals and hemosiderin in exudate

CLINICAL ISSUES

- Presents with leukocoria, vision loss
- Tortuous and dilated capillaries with tiny aneurysms
- Male predominance; onset within 1st decade
- Laser photocoagulation and cryotherapy

DIAGNOSTIC CHECKLIST

- Retinoblastoma is most important differential consideration

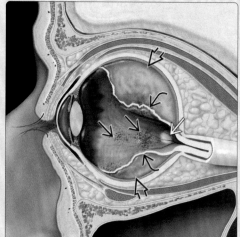

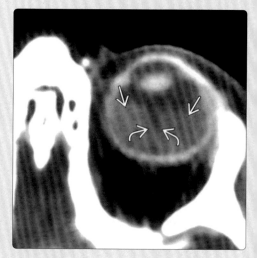

(Left) Sagittal graphic depicts both dilatation and tiny aneurysms of retinal capillaries ➡ with associated large subretinal exudates ➡ and retinal detachments ➡. A subfoveal nodule ➡ is also demonstrated. (Right) Axial NECT shows left globe posterior segment hyperdensity ➡ representing subretinal exudate composed of proteinaceous fluid and blood products. The classic "V" shape of the detached retina is faintly visible ➡.

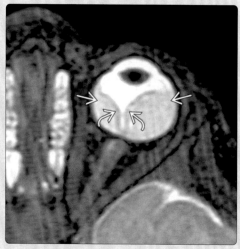

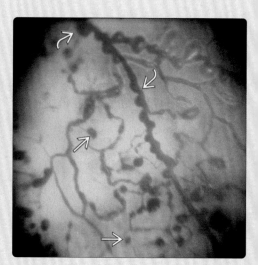

(Left) Axial STIR MR demonstrates subretinal fluid ➡ that is less hyperintense than normal vitreous. The detached retina shows a characteristic "V" shape ➡ extending from the optic nerve head. (Right) This slit-lamp photograph shows characteristic telangiectasias ➡ and aneurysms ➡ atypical of Coats disease.

TERMINOLOGY

Synonyms
- **Retinal telangiectasias**
- Exudative retinitis, **exudative retinopathy**

Definitions
- Abnormal retinal capillary development leading to subretinal accumulation of exudate

IMAGING

General Features
- Best diagnostic clue
  o **Subretinal exudate** with retinal detachment
- Location
  o **Unilateral** in 90%; bilateral when syndromic
- Size
  o Affected eye **slightly smaller** than normal eye
- Morphology
  o Typical **V-shaped** contour of **retinal detachment**

Imaging Recommendations
- Protocol advice
  o Correlate with CT to assess for calcification
  o Always include contrast enhancement

CT Findings
- NECT
  o Hyperdense exudate, calcification very **uncommon**

MR Findings
- T1WI
  o Hyperintense proteinaceous, hemorrhagic exudate
- T2WI
  o Hyperintense proteinaceous, hemorrhagic exudate
- T1WI C+ FS
  o Nerve enhancement in advanced disease
- MRS
  o Large peak at 1-1.6 ppm (lipids/proteolipids)

Ultrasonographic Findings
- Grayscale ultrasound
  o Linear detached retina and tiny cholesterol crystals

DIFFERENTIAL DIAGNOSIS

Retinoblastoma
- Most common ocular tumor in children
- **Calcification** present in vast majority

Persistent Hyperplastic Primary Vitreous
- Normal fetal hyaloid fails to regress
- **Retrolental tissue** and stalk in small eye

Retinopathy of Prematurity
- Altered development of retinal vasculature in premature newborns related to supplemental oxygen therapy
- **Small globe**, hyperdense, bilateral

Ocular Toxocariasis
- **Uveoscleral** enhancement

PATHOLOGY

General Features
- Etiology
  o Leakage of exudate into subretinal space
  o Cause unknown, possible genetic component
- Associated abnormalities
  o Usually isolated, but some syndromic associations
  o Norrie disease
    – X-linked recessive, mutation of *NDP* gene
    – Bilateral, infantile onset, more severe

Gross Pathologic & Surgical Features
- Retinal detachment with yellowish subretinal exudate
- May demonstrate fibrous nodule

CLINICAL ISSUES

Presentation
- Most common signs/symptoms
  o **Leukocoria**, vision loss
- Other signs/symptoms
  o Tortuous and dilated capillaries with tiny aneurysms on funduscopy

Demographics
- Age
  o Onset within 1st decade of life
  o Uncommon variation presents in adults
- Gender
  o Male predominance

Natural History & Prognosis
- Vision spared in early stages
- Increasing exudate leads to retinal detachment
- Secondary glaucoma and blindness in late stages
- Adult variation shows limited involvement, slower progression, and tendency to hemorrhage

Treatment
- Laser photocoagulation and cryotherapy
- Vitrectomy and retinal reattachment when advanced
- Bevacizumab (Avastin) to inhibit angiogenesis

DIAGNOSTIC CHECKLIST

Consider
- Retinoblastoma is most important differential consideration

Image Interpretation Pearls
- Lack of calcification and enhancement distinguish Coats disease from retinoblastoma
- Smaller size of affected globe may help distinguish Coats disease from noncalcifying retinoblastoma

SELECTED REFERENCES
1. Sigler EJ et al: Current management of Coats disease. Surv Ophthalmol. 59(1):30-46, 2014

Orbital Dermoid and Epidermoid

TERMINOLOGY

- Congenital orbital ectodermal inclusion lesion resulting in choristomatous cyst
- Dermoid: Includes dermal appendages
- Epidermoid: Dermal adnexal structures absent

IMAGING

- Cystic, well-demarcated, extraconal mass with lipid, fluid, or mixed contents
- Adjacent to orbital periosteum, near suture lines
- Superolateral at frontozygomatic suture most common
- May contain debris or fluid levels
- Osseous remodeling in majority of lesions, with smooth scalloped margins and thinning or dehiscence
- Distinguishing features
  - Dermoid: Typically but not exclusively contains fat; more heterogeneous, with complex signal on MR
  - Epidermoid: Density and intensity similar to fluid; more homogeneous; diffusion restriction on MR

TOP DIFFERENTIAL DIAGNOSES

- Dermolipoma
- Frontal or ethmoid sinus mucocele
- Lacrimal gland cyst

PATHOLOGY

- Congenital inclusion of trapped ectoderm at suture site
- Fibrous capsule lined by squamous epithelium

CLINICAL ISSUES

- Firm, nontender mass, fixed to underling bone
- Slowly progressive; may rupture with acute inflammation
- Presentation typically in childhood; deeper lesions in adults
- Surgical resection is curative

DIAGNOSTIC CHECKLIST

- Features are distinctive, but deep or inflamed lesions may present diagnostic challenge
- Presence of fat is essentially pathognomonic

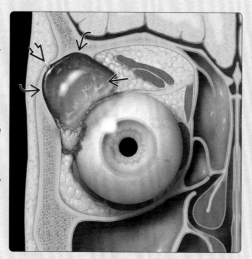
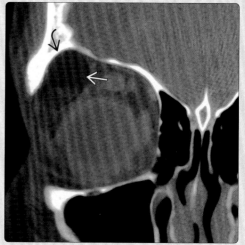

(Left) Coronal graphic depicts a superotemporal dermoid cyst ⊡ located adjacent to the frontozygomatic suture of the right orbit ⊡. There is resultant mass effect on the globe with remodeling of the bony orbit ⊡. (Right) Coronal CT demonstrates an ovoid, well-marginated cystic mass in the superotemporal quadrant of the right orbit ⊡. Even on bone windows, the lipid density within the mass can be readily appreciated. Smooth remodeling of the adjacent bony orbit is evident ⊡.

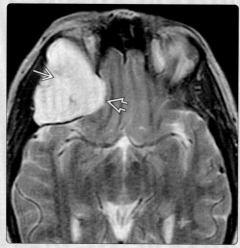
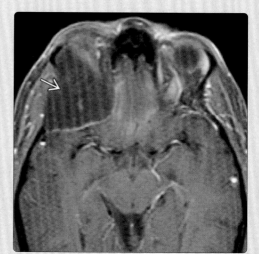

(Left) Axial T2-weighted MR shows a very large, lobulated mass centered at the deep right orbit and sphenoid ⊡. This epidermoid cyst shows fluid signal with some internal heterogeneity. Marked thinning of the adjacent bony orbit and skull base is evident ⊡. (Right) Axial T1-weighted postcontrast MR in the same patient shows low signal with mild irregularity in the epidermoid cyst ⊡ but no appreciable enhancement. The lesion showed no evidence of lipid signal on precontrast images.

TERMINOLOGY

Synonyms

- Congenital orbital **ectodermal inclusion cyst**
- Dermoid = epidermal dermoid cyst
- Epidermoid = epidermal or epithelial cyst

Definitions

- Cystic, **choristomatous** mass lesion of orbit resulting from congenital epithelial **inclusion**
- Dermoid lesions
  - Epithelial elements plus dermal substructure, including **dermal appendages**
- Epidermoid lesions
  - Epithelial elements **without adnexal structures**

IMAGING

General Features

- Best diagnostic clue
  - Cystic, well-demarcated, anterosuperior extraconal mass with **lipid, fluid,** or **mixed contents**
- Location
  - Adjacent to orbital periosteum, near **suture lines**
  - Majority extraconal in **superolateral** aspect of anterior orbit, at **frontozygomatic** suture (65-75%)
  - Remainder mostly in **superonasal** aspect, at frontolacrimal suture, but can occur anywhere
- Size
  - Typically < 1-2 cm in superficial lesions
  - Larger in deep, complicated lesions
- Morphology
  - Ovoid, **well-demarcated** cystic mass
  - Most show thin definable wall (75%)
  - No nodular soft tissue outside cyst (80%)
- Subtypes
  - **Superficial** (simple, exophytic)
    - Typically smaller, discrete, rounded
    - Present in early childhood
  - **Deep** (complicated, endophytic)
    - More insidious, extensive bony changes
- Contents
  - Lipid components evident in 40-50% of lesions
  - May contain mixed **fluid** or **debris**
  - **Fluid-fluid levels** in 5-10% of lesions
- Distinguishing features
  - Dermoid: Typically but not exclusively contain **fat**; more heterogeneous
  - Epidermoid: Density and intensity similar to **fluid**; more homogeneous

Radiographic Findings

- Radiography
  - Scalloped bony lucency with sclerotic margins

CT Findings

- NECT
  - **Hypodense fat** in about half
    - Density -30 to -80 HU
  - **Calcification** in 15%
    - Fine or punctate, in cyst wall

- CECT
  - Mild, thin rim enhancement
  - Irregular margins and enhancement indicate rupture with inflammatory reaction
- Bone CT
  - **Osseous remodeling** in majority of lesions (85%)
    - Pressure excavation; smooth, **scalloped** margins
    - **Thinning** of bone, may cause focal dehiscence
    - Bony tunnel, cleft, or pit in up to 1/3, leading to dumbbell appearance

MR Findings

- T1WI
  - Strongly **hyperintense** if **fatty** contents
  - Isointense or slightly hyperintense otherwise
- T2WI
  - Isointense or mildly hypointense
  - Heterogeneous **debris**
  - May show fluid-fluid levels
- DWI
  - Epidermoid shows diffusion restriction
- T1WI C+
  - Thin **rim enhancement**
  - More extensive **inflammation if ruptured**
- Fat-saturation techniques
  - Dermoid shows **suppression** of lipid signal

Ultrasonographic Findings

- Grayscale ultrasound
  - Adequate for evaluation of simple superficial lesions without posterior extension
  - High internal **reflectivity**, variable attenuation
  - Debris may impair determination of cystic nature

Imaging Recommendations

- Best imaging tool
  - CT without contrast often adequate for diagnosis
- Protocol advice
  - Pursue MR with contrast if features not characteristic, particularly with lesion growth

DIFFERENTIAL DIAGNOSIS

Orbital Dermolipoma

- Clinical: Soft solid lateral canthus mass
- Imaging: Homogeneous episcleral fat

Frontal or Ethmoid Sinus Mucocele

- Clinical: Chronic obstructive sinusitis
- Imaging: Expansile obstructed sinus space

Lacrimal Gland Cyst

- Clinical: Lacrimal swelling and inflammation
- Imaging: Fluid density and intensity within gland

Orbital Cellulitis

- Clinical: May mimic ruptured dermoid
- Imaging: Preseptal or intraorbital infiltration

Orbital Rhabdomyosarcoma

- Clinical: Enlarging orbital mass in child
- Imaging: Variably enhancing aggressive orbital mass

PATHOLOGY

General Features

- Etiology
  - **Congenital inclusion** of dermal elements
  - Sequestration of trapped surface **ectoderm**
  - Typically at site of embryonic **suture** closure
  - Acquired epidermoid may occur after remote surgery or trauma (**implantation** cyst)

Gross Pathologic & Surgical Features

- Whitish or yellowish, well-delineated mass
- Tethered to orbital **periosteum** by fibrovascular tissue
- Oily or cheesy material that is tan, yellow, or white

Microscopic Features

- Fibrous **capsule** lined by keratinizing stratified squamous epithelium
- Granulomatous reaction, particularly in deep or complicated lesions
- May show evidence of **rupture**, particularly dermoid
  - Disruption of lining, acute or remote
  - Chronic inflammatory changes in 40%
- Dermoid
  - **Sebaceous** glands and hair **follicles**, blood vessels, **fat**, and collagen; sweat glands in minority (20%)
  - Contains keratin, sebaceous secretions, lipid metabolites, and hair
- Epidermoid
  - **No adnexal** structures
  - Filled with **keratinaceous** debris and cholesterol

CLINICAL ISSUES

Presentation

- Most common signs/symptoms
  - Firm, rounded mass at **lateral eyebrow**
  - **Nontender**, slowly progressive
- Other signs/symptoms
  - Painless in 90% but **inflamed if ruptured**
  - Relatively **fixed** to underlying bone
- Clinical profile
  - Childhood presentation
    - More common than adult
    - **Subcutaneous** nodule near orbital rim
    - Smaller, little globe displacement
  - Adult presentation
    - Often arises **deep** to orbital rim
    - Typically in superolateral extraconal orbit, near lacrimal gland
    - Less easily palpated; **larger**, globe displacement
    - Less well-defined borders, more likely to erode into adjacent structures
  - May present with **rupture** (10-15%)
    - Secondary to **trauma** or **spontaneously**
    - Acute inflammation **mimics cellulitis** or inflammatory tumor
    - Can result in entrapment, neuropathy
  - Mass effect if very large
    - Diplopia due to restricted movement
    - Compromise of globe or optic nerve

Demographics

- Age
  - Usually presents in **childhood** and teenage years
  - Simple, superficial lesions often present in infancy
  - May present or **grow at any age**
  - Occasionally will appear in adult and grow significantly over several months
- Gender
  - Equal or slight male predominance
- Epidemiology
  - Most common noninflammatory nonneoplastic space-occupying lesion of orbit
    - Half of childhood orbital lesions
    - 90% of cystic orbital lesions
  - 10% of head and neck dermoid and epidermoid cysts are periorbital in location

Natural History & Prognosis

- Benign lesion, usually cosmetic considerations
- Very **slow growth**, usually dormant for years
  - Present during childhood but small and dormant
  - May become symptomatic during **rapid growth** phase in **young adult**
- Sudden growth or change following **rupture**
  - Significant **inflammation** and increased size

Treatment

- **Surgical resection** is curative
  - Entire cyst must be removed to prevent recurrence
    - Including growth center at periosteal interface
  - **Brow** or **eyelid crease** incision most common
    - Approach depends on location in orbit
  - Lesions evident in early childhood should be removed to avoid traumatic rupture
- Steroids or nonsteroidal drugs to calm inflammation in ruptured lesions
- Asymptomatic small lesions may be observed expectantly
  - Particularly small epidermoid, with less inflammatory response in event of rupture

DIAGNOSTIC CHECKLIST

Consider

- Features of typical lesions are distinctive, but deep or inflamed lesions may present diagnostic challenge
- Dermoid cyst is distinct from dermolipoma

Image Interpretation Pearls

- Presence of fat is essentially **pathognomonic**
- Posterior extent of **complex lesions** may not be clinically apparent; therefore, imaging is warranted

SELECTED REFERENCES

1. Burnham JM et al: Intracranial extension of an orbital epidermoid cyst. Ophthal Plast Reconstr Surg. 2014
2. Golden RP et al: Percutaneous drainage and ablation of orbital dermoid cysts. J AAPOS. 11(5):438-42, 2007
3. Yen KG et al: Current trends in the surgical management of orbital dermoid cysts among pediatric ophthalmologists. J Pediatr Ophthalmol Strabismus. 43(6):337-40; quiz 363-4, 2006
4. Shields JA et al: Orbital cysts of childhood--classification, clinical features, and management. Surv Ophthalmol. 49(3):281-99, 2004
5. Nugent RA et al: Orbital dermoids: features on CT. Radiology. 165(2):475-8, 1987

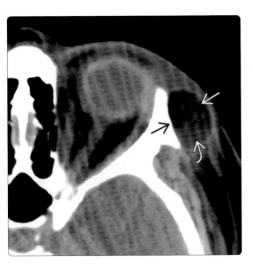
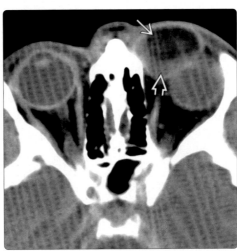

(Left) *Axial NECT shows an ovoid mass in the temporal fossa adjacent to the lateral orbit ➡. This dermoid cyst shows fat density, with slightly more dense debris layering dependently ➡. Note the broad scalloped remodeling of the adjacent bone ➡.* (Right) *Axial NECT shows a dermoid cyst ➡ located medially in the orbit, near the location of the frontolacrimal suture. The cyst has fat density contents, as well as dependent soft tissue density debris ➡.*

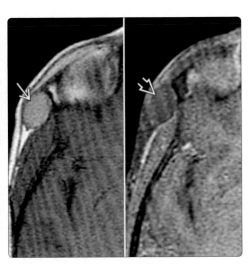
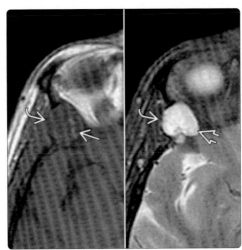

(Left) *Axial MRs show a dermoid cyst located lateral to orbit in region of temporal fossa, demonstrated on T1 noncontrast ➡ and T1 fat-saturated postcontrast ➡ images. Signal suppression with fat saturation indicates lipid contents.* (Right) *Axial MRs in an adult show an example of a deep epidermoid cyst, which is demonstrated on T1 ➡ and T2 ➡ images. The lesion shows near fluid signal without indication of fatty contents. The lateral orbital wall shows benign scalloped thinning ➡.*

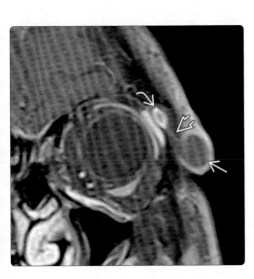
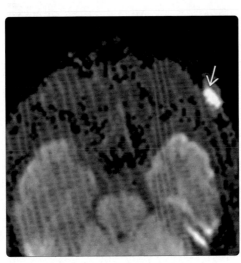

(Left) *Coronal T1-weighted postcontrast MR shows an epidermoid cyst with thin marginal enhancement ➡ lateral to the left orbital rim. A smaller intraorbital component is seen along the inner margin of the orbital wall ➡, with scalloping of the bone at the lacrimal fossa. A small connecting stalk is visible in the region of the frontozygomatic suture ➡.* (Right) *Axial diffusion MR in the same patient shows diffusion restriction within the lesion at the left lateral orbital rim ➡ consistent with epidermoid cyst.*

TERMINOLOGY

- Neurocutaneous disorder (inherited tumor syndrome) with distinct orbitocranial manifestations

IMAGING

- Constellation of features is pathognomonic of NF1
  - Plexiform neurofibroma (PNF)
  - Optic nerve glioma (ONG)
  - Sphenoid dysplasia (SD)
  - Buphthalmos
  - Optic nerve sheath ectasia
- Orbitofacial NF1 typically unilateral

TOP DIFFERENTIAL DIAGNOSES

- **PNF**
  - Rhabdomyosarcoma, infantile hemangioma, Langerhans cell, venolymphatic malformation
- **ONG**
  - Glioma without NF1, nerve sheath meningioma

- **SD**
  - Congenital cephalocele, traumatic cephalocele
- **Buphthalmos**
  - Congenital glaucoma, coloboma
- **Optic nerve sheath ectasia**
  - Normal variant, intracranial hypertension

PATHOLOGY

- Autosomal dominant, 50% new mutations

CLINICAL ISSUES

- Presentation: Periorbital masses, proptosis, & ptosis
- Natural history: Progressive orbitofacial deformity and progressive visual and ophthalmologic dysfunction

DIAGNOSTIC CHECKLIST

- Although NF1 is inherited disorder, orbital manifestations are progressive and develop over time
- Rapid change in PNF concerning for malignant sarcomatous degeneration

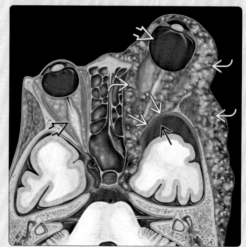
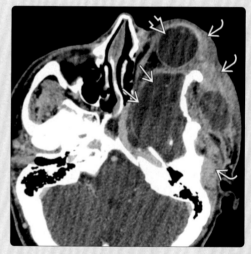

(Left) Axial graphic depicts features of orbital NF1, including sphenoid wing dysplasia ➡, with arachnoid cyst protruding through the bony defect ➡. Extensive plexiform neurofibromas are demonstrated ➡ as well buphthalmos ➡. An optic nerve glioma is evident on the right ➡. (Right) Axial CECT shows a large defect in the left greater sphenoid wing ➡, with middle fossa contents protruding into the orbit and causing marked proptosis ➡. Extensive orbitotemporal plexiform neurofibromas are evident ➡.

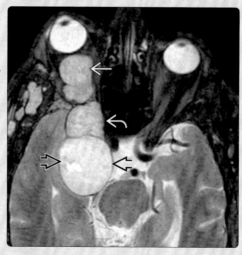
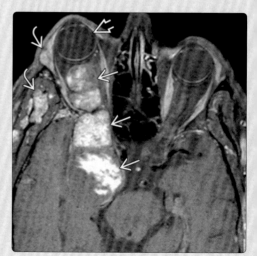

(Left) Axial STIR MR shows hyperintense multilobulated plexiform masses in the orbit ➡ extending through an enlarged superior orbital fissure and dysplastic sphenoid wing ➡ into the middle fossa and cavernous sinus ➡. (Right) Axial T1-weighted postcontrast MR in the same patient shows patchy enhancement of the massive orbital and skull base neurofibromas ➡. The right globe is severely proptotic ➡. Extracranial plexiform tumors in the orbitotemporal regions are also evident ➡.

TERMINOLOGY

Abbreviations

- Neurofibromatosis type 1 (NF1)

Synonyms

- von Recklinghausen disease

Definitions

- **Neurocutaneous disorder** (inherited tumor syndrome) with distinct orbitofacial and cranial manifestations

IMAGING

General Features

- Best diagnostic clue
  - Constellation of orbital, skull base, and intracranial features is **pathognomonic** of NF1
- Location
  - Orbitofacial NF1 typically **unilateral**
- Morphology
  - **Plexiform neurofibroma** (PNF)
    - Serpentine, unencapsulated infiltrative masses
    - May involve cranial nerves, intraorbital branches, muscles, optic nerve sheath, and sclera
    - Associated enlargement of skull base foramina
  - **Optic nerve glioma** (ONG)
    - Tubular or lobular enlargement of optic nerve
    - May involve any segment of nerve
    - May extend posterior to chiasm and brainstem
  - **Sphenoid dysplasia** (SD)
    - Bony defects, decalcification, or remodeling of greater sphenoid wing & lateral orbital wall
    - Enlargement of middle fossa with herniation of intracranial contents into orbit
    - Associated middle fossa arachnoid cyst common
  - **Buphthalmos**
    - Increased axial and AP globe diameter
    - Remodeling & enlargement of anterior orbital rim
    - Thickening of uveal/scleral layer
  - **Optic nerve sheath ectasia**
    - Nontumorous enlargement of dural sheath
    - Increased CSF surrounding optic nerve

Radiographic Findings

- Radiography
  - Defect of greater sphenoid wing
  - Enlarged egg-shaped anterior orbital rim
  - Harlequin eye appearance

CT Findings

- NECT
  - **PNF**: Hypodense **infiltrative** soft tissue masses
  - **ONG** or **dural ectasia**: Enlarged nerve/sheath contour
  - **SD**: Bony **defect** with **herniation** of middle fossa into orbit; proptosis may be marked

MR Findings

- T1WI
  - **PNF**: Hypointense **ill-defined** soft tissue masses
  - **ONG**: Isointense ON mass ± **cystic** hypointensity
- T2WI
  - **PNF**: Hyperintense nodular masses with central low-signal **target sign**
  - **ONG**: Hyperintense **fusiform** optic nerve mass
  - **Buphthalmos**: Enlarged globe, thickened sclera
  - **Nerve sheath ectasia**: Increased **perioptic fluid**
- T1WI C+
  - **PNF**: Irregular infiltrative **serpentine** masses; variable enhancement, may be intense
  - **ONG**: Variably enhancing optic nerve mass

Ultrasonographic Findings

- **PNF**: Irregular, compressible, **highly** reflective
- **ONG**: Smooth nerve enlargement, **minimally** reflective
- **SD**: Defect of posterior bony orbital wall
- **Buphthalmos**: Increased eye diameter

Imaging Recommendations

- Best imaging tool
  - MR ideal for assessment of orbital, extracranial, and intracranial lesions
  - CT to assess skull base defects and surgical planning
- Protocol advice
  - Dedicated brain and orbit examinations indicated for extensive abnormalities

DIFFERENTIAL DIAGNOSIS

DDx of Plexiform Neurofibroma

- Rhabdomyosarcoma
- Infantile hemangioma
- Langerhans cell histiocytosis
- Leukemia
- Venolymphatic malformation

DDx of Optic Nerve Glioma

- Optic pathway glioma (isolated)
- Optic nerve sheath meningioma

DDx of Sphenoid Dysplasia

- Congenital sphenorbital cephalocele
- Posttraumatic sphenoid cephalocele

DDx of Buphthalmos

- Congenital glaucoma
- Coloboma

DDx of Optic Nerve Sheath Ectasia

- Normal variant
- Idiopathic intracranial hypertension
- Optic nerve sheath meningioma

PATHOLOGY

General Features

- Etiology
  - Disorder of histogenesis, classified as neurocutaneous inherited tumor syndrome
  - **Constellation** of orbital NF1 findings is characteristic
- Genetics
  - **Autosomal dominant**; variable expression
  - 50% **new mutations**; gene locus = 17q11.2
  - Loss of NF1 **tumor suppressor** gene function
- Associated abnormalities

- o **CNS tumors** on brain imaging
- o Characteristic nonneoplastic focal areas of signal intensity
- o Diffuse soft tissue neurofibromas; skeletal deformities

Staging, Grading, & Classification

- Diagnostic criteria for NF1 established by NIH consensus statement on neurofibromatosis
- Treatment-based classification of orbital disease
  - o Orbital soft tissue with seeing eye
  - o Soft tissue & bone, with seeing eye
  - o Soft tissue & bone, with blind malpositioned eye

Gross Pathologic & Surgical Features

- **PNF**
  - o Worm-like infiltrating tortuous masses
  - o May involve eyelid, anterior periorbita, scalp, orbit, temporal fossa, and skull base
- **ONG**
  - o Diffuse nerve enlargement; tan-white tumor
  - o Cystic component with mucinous changes
- **SD**
  - o Bony defect of posterior lateral orbit
  - o Middle cranial fossa expansion with arachnoid cyst
- **Buphthalmos**
  - o Associated with PNF in anterior orbit

Microscopic Features

- **PNF**
  - o Myxoid endoneural accumulation early
  - o Schwann cell proliferation, collagen accumulation
- **ONG**
  - o Spindle-shaped astrocytes with hyperplasia of fibroblasts and meningothelial cells
- **SD**
  - o Bone decalcification; premature suture closure
- **Buphthalmos**
  - o Periscleral infiltration by plexiform tumors

CLINICAL ISSUES

Presentation

- Most common signs/symptoms
  - o Infiltrative periorbital masses, proptosis, and ptosis
- Other signs/symptoms
  - o **PNF**
    - – Bulky soft tissue masses; **bag-of-worms** texture
    - – PNF anywhere is indicative of NF1
  - o **ONG**
    - – Visual deficit, often relatively **mild**
    - – Proptosis associated with poor vision
  - o **SD**
    - – Pulsatile **exophthalmos** due to orbital encroachment by middle fossa contents
  - o **Buphthalmos**
    - – Enlarged eye; impaired vision
    - – May present with **glaucoma**
- Clinical profile
  - o Child with progressive proptosis, visual impairment, soft tissue masses, & cosmetic deformities

Demographics

- Age
  - o Findings may not be evident at birth
  - o Cutaneous signs present at birth or 1st year
  - o Tumors begin to appear in childhood
- Gender
  - o No significant gender predilection
- Epidemiology
  - o NF1 is **most common** inherited tumor syndrome
  - o Prevalence 1:2,500-5,000
  - o Orbital involvement in up to 1/3 of NF1

Natural History & Prognosis

- Orbital features of NF1 are **progressive** developmental lesions rather than simply congenital defects
- **Progressive worsening** of complications over time
  - o Orbitofacial deformity
  - o Glaucoma, optic nerve compromise, blindness
  - o Proptosis, corneal exposure
  - o Muscle impairment, amblyopia
- PNF may undergo **sarcomatous degeneration** to malignant peripheral nerve sheath tumor (2-16%)
- Decreased life expectancy
  - o Malignancy most common cause of death

Treatment

- **PNF**
  - o Generally not surgically curable due to infiltrative nature
  - o Anterior orbit and eyelid procedures most common
  - o Debulking may be required for vision or cosmesis
  - o Radiation therapy not effective
- **ONG**
  - o Observation unless vision threatened
  - o Radiation therapy or surgery for bulky tumors
- **SD**
  - o Transcranial reconstruction with bone grafts for severe posterior defects
  - o Management of resultant proptosis; may ultimately require enucleation
  - o Debulking of associated PNF

DIAGNOSTIC CHECKLIST

Consider

- Although NF1 is inherited disorder, orbital manifestations are progressive and develop over time

Image Interpretation Pearls

- Rapid change in appearance of PNF tumors worrisome for malignant sarcomatous degeneration

SELECTED REFERENCES

1. Pessis R et al: Surgical care burden in orbito-temporal neurofibromatosis: Multiple procedures and surgical care duration analysis in 47 consecutive adult patients. J Craniomaxillofac Surg. 43(8):1684-93, 2015
2. Chaudhry IA et al: Orbitofacial neurofibromatosis: clinical characteristics and treatment outcome. Eye (Lond). 26(4):583-92, 2012
3. Erb MH et al: Orbitotemporal neurofibromatosis: classification and treatment. Orbit. 26(4):223-8, 2007
4. Zeid JL et al: Orbital optic nerve gliomas in children with neurofibromatosis type 1. J AAPOS. 10(6):534-9, 2006
5. Jacquemin C et al: Orbit deformities in craniofacial neurofibromatosis type 1. AJNR Am J Neuroradiol. 24(8):1678-82, 2003

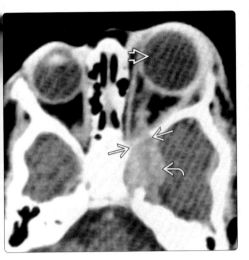

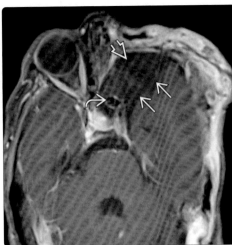

(Left) *Axial CECT in a young girl shows mild sphenoid dysplasia with widening of the superior orbital fissure ⮕ and a neurofibroma extending into the central skull base ⮕. The left globe shows buphthalmos ⮕. (Right) Axial T1-weighted postcontrast MR in the same patient 2 decades later shows a massive sphenoid defect ⮕ demonstrating the progressive nature of this process. There is herniation of a large associated arachnoid cyst ⮕ into the orbit. An internal carotid artery aneurysm is noted incidentally ⮕.*

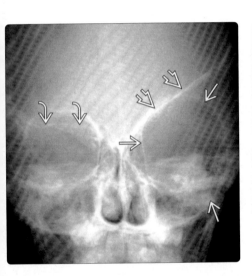

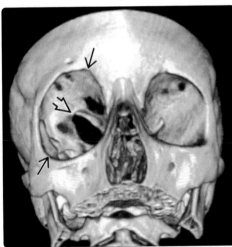

(Left) *Anteroposterior radiograph in a child with NF1 and sphenoid wing dysplasia shows enlargement of the left orbital rim ⮕. The normal contour of the greater wing of the sphenoid is distorted and displaced ⮕, in contrast to the normal appearance on the right ⮕. (Right) 3D CT surface rendering in a patient with NF1 shows an enlarged, egg-shaped contour of the right orbital rim ⮕. A defect is evident in the sphenoid bone at the orbital apex ⮕ in the region of the superior orbital fissure.*

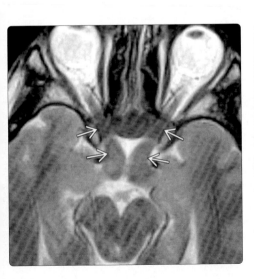

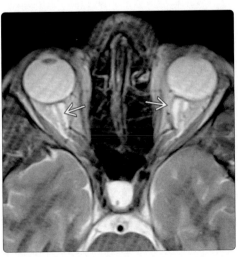

(Left) *Axial T2-weighted MR in a patient with NF1 shows diffuse enlargement of the optic nerves bilaterally ⮕, consistent with optic pathway gliomas. The lesions extend posteriorly to involve the chiasm and optic tracts. (Right) Axial T2-weighted MR in a patient with NF1 but no orbital masses shows ectasia of the optic dural sheaths, which manifest as increased CSF signal surrounding the intraorbital segments of the optic nerves bilaterally ⮕.*

Orbital Lymphatic Malformation

TERMINOLOGY

- Congenital vascular malformation with variable lymphatic and venous vascular elements

IMAGING

- Poorly marginated, lobulated, transspatial mass
- Multiloculated cystic features with fluid-fluid levels, blood products, and variable irregular enhancement
- Variants: Superficial vs. deep, macrocystic vs. microcystic
- CT: Irregular cystic hypodense mass with mixed hyperdense blood products
- MR: Variable signal resulting from mixed age hemorrhagic, lymphatic, or proteinaceous fluid
- Variable enhancement, typically at margins, more pronounced if prominent venous components
- US: Hypoechoic with heterogeneous internal echoes
- Best imaging tool
  - Dedicated enhanced orbital MR with fat suppression

TOP DIFFERENTIAL DIAGNOSES

- Orbital varix
- Orbital cavernous malformation
- Infantile hemangioma
- Plexiform neurofibroma

PATHOLOGY

- Congenital nonneoplastic vascular malformation
- Dilated dysplastic lymphatic ± venous channels

CLINICAL ISSUES

- Mass effect with proptosis in pediatric patient
- May rapidly ↑ in size due to acute hemorrhage
- Conservative therapy preferred due to surgical risk
- Percutaneous sclerotherapy for suitable lesions
- Surgical resection difficult, recurrence common

DIAGNOSTIC CHECKLIST

- Blood products & fluid-fluid levels highly suggestive

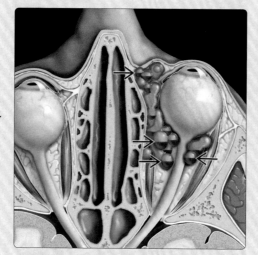
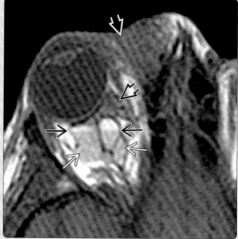

(Left) *Axial graphic depicts typical features of orbital lymphatic malformation, including transspatial extension, and characteristic fluid-fluid levels within loculations ➡. (Right) Axial T1-weighted MR shows an infiltrative, transspatial mass. The posterior intraconal component ➡ demonstrates fluid-blood levels ➡ within macrocystic loculations. The preseptal ➡ and anterior intraorbital ➡ components appear more homogeneously hypointense, suggesting microcystic or venous elements.*

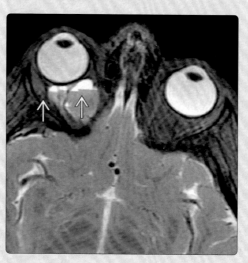
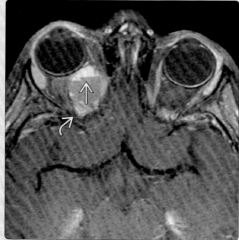

(Left) *Axial T2-weighted MR in an older child with acute worsening of longstanding right proptosis shows a large lobulated retrobulbar mass with characteristic fluid-fluid levels ➡. The differing heights of levels are indicative of the multilocular nature of the lesion. (Right) Axial T1-weighted postcontrast MR in the same patient demonstrates the variable signal of contents again manifest as fluid-fluid levels ➡ indicating proteinaceous and hemorrhagic products. Mild venous enhancement is evident posteriorly ➡.*

TERMINOLOGY

Abbreviations

- Orbital lymphatic malformation (LM or OLM)
- Orbital venolymphatic malformation (VLM or OLVM)

Synonyms

- Outdated terms: Lymphangioma, cystic hygroma

Definitions

- Congenital vascular malformation with variable **lymphatic** and **venous** vascular elements

IMAGING

General Features

- Best diagnostic clue
  - **Poorly marginated**, lobulated, **transspatial** mass
  - Multiloculated cystic features with **fluid-fluid levels**, **blood products**, and variable **irregular enhancement**
- Location
  - **Superficial**: Often confined to conjunctiva
    - Relatively common type of VLM
  - **Deep**: Extending into orbit
    - Extraconal > intraconal but often transspatial
- Morphology
  - **Irregular** margins, **multilocular cysts** with fluid levels
  - Macrocystic (> 1 cm), microcystic (< 1 cm), or mixed
  - Posterior venous lesions with more well-defined margins may mimic orbital cavernous malformation

CT Findings

- NECT
  - Irregular multicystic **hypodense** mass
  - Hemorrhage with mixed hyperdense **blood products**
  - Punctate calcification or phleboliths uncommon
- CECT
  - Cystic structures with mild **rim enhancement**
  - More diffuse enhancement of **venous components**
- Bone CT
  - **Remodeling** of bony orbit with large lesions

MR Findings

- T1WI
  - **Lobulated**, poorly circumscribed mass
  - **Fluid-fluid levels** with variable signal due to mixed age hemorrhagic, lymphatic, or proteinaceous fluid in multilocular cystic spaces
  - Different ages of **blood products**; subacute blood characteristically **hyperintense**
- T2WI FS
  - Lobulated, **very hyperintense** fluid signal
  - **Fluid-fluid levels** show signal corresponding to age of blood products
  - No flow voids (unlike infantile hemangioma)
- T1WI C+ FS
  - **Variable enhancement**, typically rim pattern at margins of cysts
  - More pronounced irregular enhancement if prominent venous components present
  - Nonenhancing **thrombus** may be visible with acute exacerbation

Ultrasonographic Findings

- Grayscale ultrasound
  - **Hypoechoic** blood and lymph-filled cystic spaces
  - **Heterogeneous** internal echoes
  - Echoic spikes at endothelial walls

Imaging Recommendations

- Best imaging tool
  - Dedicated enhanced orbital MR with fat suppression

DIFFERENTIAL DIAGNOSIS

Orbital Varix

- Clinical: **Intermittent** pain and **proptosis**
- Imaging: Similar to VLM, but **dynamic expansion** demonstrated with **Valsalva**
- Pathology: Often considered part of **VLM spectrum** but with **distensible** venous component

Orbital Cavernous Malformation

- Clinical: Slowly growing, **painless** mass, most **common** benign orbital mass in **adults**
- Imaging: Circumscribed ovoid **intraconal** solid mass with **dynamic** fill-in enhancement
- Pathology: **Pseudoencapsulated** venous malformation, unique to eye

Infantile Hemangioma

- Clinical: Highly vascular tumor of **infancy**; frequently **regresses** spontaneously
- Imaging: Poorly marginated, intensely enhancing orbitofacial mass with **flow voids**
- Pathology: True vascular **neoplasm**

Plexiform Neurofibroma

- Clinical: Associated with **neurofibromatosis** type 1
- Imaging: Infiltrative, transspatial masses, associated with **sphenoid dysplasia** and orbitofacial deformity
- Pathology: Nerve sheath tumor of neurocutaneous syndrome

Rhabdomyosarcoma

- Clinical: **Most common primary** orbital malignancy in children
- Imaging: Infiltrative, **destructive** orbital mass
- Pathology: **Embryonal** and **alveolar** subtypes most common

Lymphoproliferative Lesions

- Clinical: Lymphoid **proliferation** with mass primary to orbit, may be associated with systemic disease
- Imaging: Pliable mass, commonly involving **lacrimal** gland, or **multifocal** or diffuse in orbit
- Pathology: **Spectrum** ranging from benign reactive hyperplasia to malignant Non-Hodgkin lymphoma

Idiopathic Inflammatory Pseudotumor

- Clinical: Inflammatory changes with **painful** proptosis and ophthalmoplegia
- Imaging: Asymmetric **mass-like inflammation** of muscles, lacrimal gland, and other orbital structures
- Pathology: **Unknown**; some cases associated with **IgG4**

PATHOLOGY

General Features

- Etiology
  - Congenital **nonneoplastic vascular malformation** with low or no venous flow
  - Arise from pluripotent venous anlage
  - Lymphatic tissue not normally found in orbit
- Associated abnormalities
  - Malformations in other regions of head and neck
  - Generalized lymphangiomatosis
  - Noncontiguous **intracranial** vascular malformations

Staging, Grading, & Classification

- General classification of orbital vascular malformations
  - **Type 1**: No flow (lymphatic malformation)
  - **Type 2**: Venous flow (venolymphatic malformation)
    - Nondistensible vs. distensible (associated with varix)
  - **Type 3**: Arterial flow (high flow, AVM)

Gross Pathologic & Surgical Features

- Thin-walled **multilocular** mass
- **Cystic** structures containing clear or chocolate-colored fluid
- Poorly marginated with **insinuation** along tissue planes; difficult to dissect

Microscopic Features

- **Unencapsulated** mass of irregularly shaped sinuses; infiltrates into adjacent stroma
- Dilated **dysplastic** venous ± lymphatic channels lined with flattened endothelial cells
- **Cystic** spaces with lymphatic fluid or chronic blood products
- **Lymphoid follicles** and lymphocyte infiltration
- Positive **lymphatic** immunohistochemical **markers** confirms lymphatic origin

CLINICAL ISSUES

Presentation

- Most common signs/symptoms
  - Progressive **proptosis** with **sudden episodic worsening**
- Other signs/symptoms
  - Mass effect; compressive optic neuropathy
  - Diplopia, restricted extraocular muscles, ptosis
  - Periorbital ecchymosis associated with hemorrhage
- Clinical profile
  - Lesions may **rapidly ↑** in size due to **acute hemorrhage**
    - Recurrent hemorrhages in 50%
    - Associated with lesion **recurrence** after surgery
    - **Thrombosis** may precipitate hemorrhage; related to stasis, congestion, and inflammation
  - Lesions may intermittently ↑ and ↓ in size in conjunction with upper respiratory infection
    - Related to presence of **lymphatic tissue**

Demographics

- Age
  - Younger patients: **Infants to young adults**
  - 40% present by age 6; 60% present by age 16
- Gender
  - Slight female predominance

- Epidemiology
  - Incidence 3:100,000
  - 5% of childhood orbital masses

Natural History & Prognosis

- **Progressive slow growth** during childhood, through puberty and into early adulthood, with **episodic acute enlargement** due to **hemorrhage**
- Infiltrating nature results in frequent **recurrence**
- Refractory visual problems & disfigurement common
- Poor visual acuity associated with multiple surgical resections
- Optic nerve compromise with recurrent large lesions

Treatment

- Options, risks, complications
  - Conservative therapy
    - **Observation** preferred if vision is not threatened due to hazards of surgery
    - Systemic **steroids** may decrease pain, swelling, and proptosis; especially in younger patients
    - 45% of smaller lesions show **regression**
  - Image-guided sclerotherapy
    - Percutaneous **intralesional** injection of sclerosing agent, particularly for macrocystic lesions
  - Surgery
    - Difficult resection due to complex **insinuation** with normal orbital structures
    - **Recurrence** after surgery common (~ 50%)
    - Acute mass effect due to hemorrhage may require emergent **decompression**
    - Indications include optic nerve dysfunction, corneal compromise, & intractable amblyopia

DIAGNOSTIC CHECKLIST

Consider

- Deep circumscribed lesions in adults may mimic orbital cavernous hemangioma
- VLM and orbital varix are related lesions
  - VLM is hemodynamically isolated
  - Varix has systemic drainage, which accounts for pressure-dependent distensibility

Image Interpretation Pearls

- Presence of blood products with **fluid-fluid levels** is highly suggestive of VLM

SELECTED REFERENCES

1. Lally SE: Update on orbital lymphatic malformations. Curr Opin Ophthalmol. ePub, 2016
2. Balakrishnan K et al: Standardized outcome and reporting measures in pediatric head and neck lymphatic malformations. Otolaryngol Head Neck Surg. 152(5):948-53, 2015
3. Hill RH 3rd et al: Percutaneous drainage and ablation as first line therapy for macrocystic and microcystic orbital lymphatic malformations. Ophthal Plast Reconstr Surg. 28(2):119-25, 2012
4. Chadha V et al: Orbital venous-lymphatic malformation. Eye (Lond). 23(12):2265-6, 2009
5. Smoker WR et al: Vascular lesions of the orbit: more than meets the eye. Radiographics. 28(1):185-204; quiz 325, 2008
6. Lewin JS: Low-flow vascular malformations of the orbit: a new approach to a therapeutic dilemma. AJNR Am J Neuroradiol. 25(10):1633-4, 2004
7. Graeb DA et al: Orbital lymphangiomas: clinical, radiologic, and pathologic characteristics. Radiology. 175(2):417-21, 1990

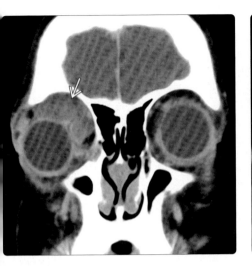
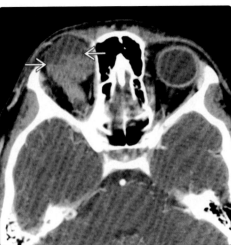

(Left) *Coronal CECT in a child with intermittently progressive proptosis shows a lobulated intermediate- to low-density mass in the superomedial anterior orbit ➡️, which causes displacement of the globe.* (Right) *Axial CECT in the same patient shows multiple loculations within the mass and demonstrates fluids of varying density with discrete levels ➡️. The more dense chronic hemorrhagic products are seen layering dependently.*

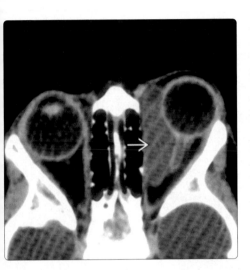
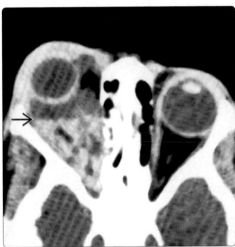

(Left) *Axial CECT shows a cystic, well-defined, nonenhancing mass with imperceptible wall in the medial left orbit ➡️. The mass has a simple, unilocular appearance but is transspatial with intraconal, extraconal, and preseptal components.* (Right) *Axial NECT in a 4-year-old child reveals an irregular, multilocular, transspatial orbital lymphatic malformation. Layering hyperdense fluid-fluid levels ➡️ represent blood products from spontaneous hemorrhage.*

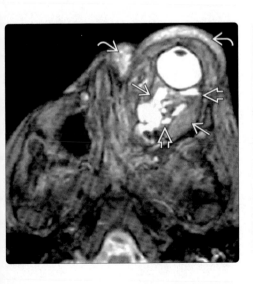
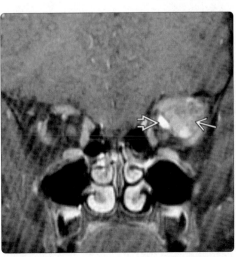

(Left) *Axial T2-weighted MR shows a massive, complex lymphatic malformation ➡️ with proptosis. Variable signal with fluid-fluid levels ➡️ represents sequelae of multiple bouts of hemorrhage. Additional preseptal component is also evident ➡️.* (Right) *Coronal T1WI C+ FS MR demonstrates a large complex mass in the left orbit, which mostly contains nonenhancing material with differing amounts in intrinsic T1 signal ➡️. Enhancing structure medially represents a venous component ➡️, possibly a small varix.*

Orbital Venous Varix

TERMINOLOGY

- Low-flow venous malformation with systemic venous connection and dynamically distensible varix

IMAGING

- Intensely enhancing orbital mass that distends with increased venous pressure
- Nonenhancing foci of flow, hemorrhage, thrombosis, or cystic lymphatic spaces
- Best imaging tool: Dynamic CT without and with provocation maneuver

TOP DIFFERENTIAL DIAGNOSES

- Orbital venolymphatic malformation
  - Multiloculated with fluid levels; may coexist with varix
- Orbital cavernous malformation
  - Common adult orbital mass, "hemangioma"
- Orbital infantile hemangioma
  - Benign neoplasm of infancy that typically regresses

PATHOLOGY

- Congenital venous malformation with slow flow, distensible component, and systemic venous connection
- May coexist with venolymphatic malformation
- Dilated venous channels with fibrotic walls ± phleboliths

CLINICAL ISSUES

- Intermittent reversible proptosis
- Proptosis elicited by change in head position or Valsalva
- Variable pain and ophthalmoplegia
- Sudden worsening due to thrombosis or hemorrhage
- **Treatment options**
  - Observation if symptoms mild and stable
  - Transcatheter embolization or sclerosis
  - Surgery for intractable pain or threatened vision

DIAGNOSTIC CHECKLIST

- Routine imaging may be negative unless provocative test performed (e.g., Valsalva)

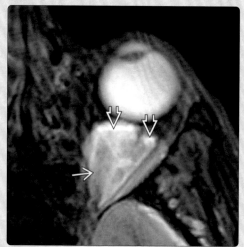
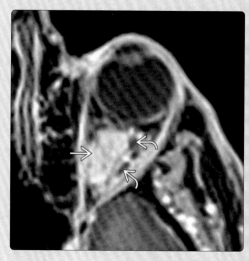

(Left) Axial MR in a patient with intermittent left proptosis shows a heterogeneously T2-hyperintense mass ➡ with multiple internal fluid levels ⮕. (Right) Axial T1 C+ FS MR in the same patient shows intense, somewhat heterogeneous enhancement of the retrobulbar mass ➡. Nonenhancing regions ➡ may reflect cystic noncommunicating or lymphatic vascular spaces or may reflect relatively rapid or turbulent venous flow artifact.

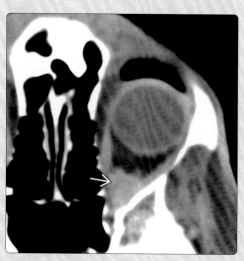
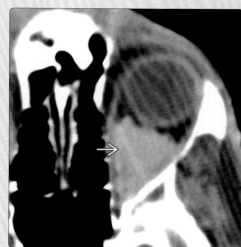

(Left) Dynamic enhanced CT at quiet breathing shows a relatively small, enhancing retrobulbar mass ➡. The mass appears smaller than on comparison MR, as patient was lying down for only a short time prior to CECT scan. (Right) Dynamic CT performed immediately following 15 seconds of Valsalva shows marked enlargement of the retrobulbar mass ➡, indicating a varix with systemic venous connection.

TERMINOLOGY

Synonyms

- **Distensible** orbital venous malformation

Definitions

- **Low-flow** venous malformation with **systemic venous connection** and dynamically distensible varix

IMAGING

General Features

- Best diagnostic clue
  - Intensely enhancing orbital mass that **distends** with increased **venous pressure**
- Location
  - May occur anywhere in orbit
  - Usually retrobulbar and extraconal, often superolateral
- Size
  - Changes **dynamically** with venous pressure
    - Increases in size with prone position or Valsalva maneuver
  - May be undetectable unless elicited
- Morphology
  - Well-defined margins but may have irregular or lobulated contours; often **tubular** or **tortuous**

CT Findings

- NECT
  - Well-defined, tubular or tortuous soft tissue density lesion in retrobulbar space
- CECT
  - Intense enhancement; **increases in size on Valsalva**
- Bone CT
  - May contain **phleboliths**

MR Findings

- T1WI
  - Complex signal, blood products, fluid levels
- T2WI
  - Complex signal, blood products, fluid levels
- T1WI C+
  - **Intense enhancement**
  - Variable areas of nonenhancement
    - Heterogeneous fast or turbulent **flow void**
    - Cystic or **lymphatic** spaces
    - Areas of **thrombosis** or acute **hemorrhage**

Ultrasonographic Findings

- Grayscale ultrasound
  - **Hypoechoic**; slow flow on Doppler

Angiographic Findings

- Filling of dilated structure on late venous phase

Imaging Recommendations

- Best imaging tool
  - **Dynamic** CECT with **provocation** maneuver
  - MR indicated if thrombosis or hemorrhage suspected
- Protocol advice
  - CECT without and with provocation maneuver
    - Valsalva for 10-15 seconds
    - Varix will distend when venous pressure raised
  - US useful for bedside provocative challenge

DIFFERENTIAL DIAGNOSIS

Orbital Venolymphatic Malformation

- May present with sudden proptosis due to hemorrhage
- Multiloculated spaces, fluid levels, variable enhancement

Orbital Cavernous Malformation

- Most common isolated orbital mass in adults
- Well-defined, intense dynamic "fill-in" enhancement

Orbital Infantile Hemangioma

- Infant lesion, frequently regresses spontaneously
- Irregular, intense enhancement and flow voids

PATHOLOGY

General Features

- Etiology
  - **Congenital** venous malformation with slow flow, **distensible** component, and **systemic** venous connection
- Associated abnormalities
  - May **coexist** with **venolymphatic malformation**

Gross Pathologic & Surgical Features

- Single or multiple dilated valveless vessels
- Acute hemorrhage or thrombosis may be present

Microscopic Features

- Dilated venous channels with fibrotic walls ± **phleboliths**

CLINICAL ISSUES

Presentation

- Most common signs/symptoms
  - Intermittent **reversible proptosis**
- Other signs/symptoms
  - Variable pain and ophthalmoplegia
- Clinical profile
  - Proptosis elicited by change in head position or Valsalva

Natural History & Prognosis

- **Congenital** nonprogressive lesion
- Sudden worsening due to **thrombosis** or **hemorrhage** often prompts attention or intervention

Treatment

- Observation if symptoms mild and stable
- Transcatheter **embolization** or **sclerosis rarely needed**
- Surgery for intractable pain or threatened vision

DIAGNOSTIC CHECKLIST

Image Interpretation Pearls

- Routine imaging may be negative unless provocative test performed (e.g., Valsalva)

SELECTED REFERENCES

1. Kiang L et al: Images in clinical medicine. Orbital varix. N Engl J Med. 372(7):e9, 2015
2. Smoker WR et al: Vascular lesions of the orbit: more than meets the eye. Radiographics. 28(1):185-204, 2008

Orbital Cavernous Venous Malformation (Hemangioma)

TERMINOLOGY

- Venous vascular malformation of orbit characterized by endothelial-lined cavernous spaces
- Pseudo-encapsulated morphology distinguishes orbital cavernous venous malformation from venous malformations elsewhere in the head & neck
- Synonymous with cavernous "hemangioma" (misnomer)

IMAGING

- Solid enhancing intraorbital mass
  - Most intraconal, usually lateral
  - Ovoid or round, sharply marginated
  - Pseudocapsule of compressed surrounding tissue
- CT
  - Benign remodeling of bone in larger lesions
- MR
  - T2 hyperintense; internal septations may be visible
  - Characteristic dynamic enhancement
    - Heterogeneous early patchy central enhancement

- Fills in homogeneously on delayed images

PATHOLOGY

- Slowly growing vascular malformation
- ISSVA classification as slow-flow venous lesion
- Dilated vascular channels of thin-walled sinusoidal spaces, flattened endothelial cells, scant fibrous connective stroma
- Pseudocapsule with surrounding compressed tissue
- No evidence of cellular proliferation

CLINICAL ISSUES

- Slowly progressive painless proptosis
- Most common isolated orbital mass in adults
- Female predominance; faster growth during pregnancy
- Excellent prognosis; rare recurrence after surgery

DIAGNOSTIC CHECKLIST

- Often discovered incidentally during brain MR
- "Hemangioma" is common term but misnomer
- Patchy dynamic enhancement is characteristic

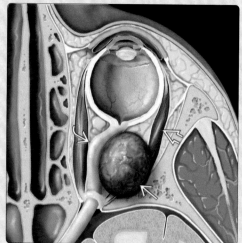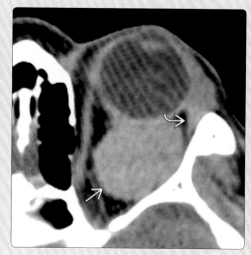

(Left) Axial graphic through the orbit shows an ovoid, well-demarcated, intraconal mass ➡ that displaces the optic nerve ➡ and adjacent lateral rectus muscle ➡. Note the lack of adjacent structure invasion. (Right) Axial NECT shows a well-demarcated, ovoid, slightly hyperdense mass centered in the lateral aspect of the left orbit ➡. The lateral rectus muscle is seen draping around the lateral margin of this intraconal mass ➡.

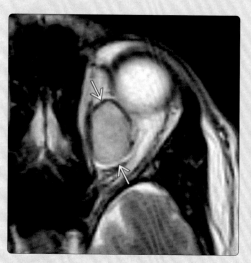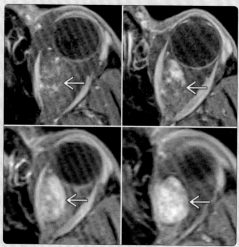

(Left) Axial T2WI MR reveals a sharply marginated, ovoid, hyperintense intraconal mass. A thin rim of signal ➡ represents the pseudocapsule, accentuated by a chemical shift artifact. (Right) Axial T1 C+ FS MR demonstrates progressive enhancement of a vascular mass in the medial left orbit ➡. Serial scans were obtained over the course of several minutes, from earliest (top left) to latest (bottom right) following contrast injection.

Orbital Cavernous Venous Malformation (Hemangioma)

TERMINOLOGY

Abbreviations

- Orbital cavernous venous malformation (**OCVM**)

Synonyms

- Cavernous hemangioma (misnomer)
- **Encapsulated** cavernous lesion of orbit

Definitions

- Venous vascular **malformation** of orbit characterized by endothelial-lined **cavernous** spaces

IMAGING

General Features

- Best diagnostic clue
  - Well-demarcated, ovoid, enhancing **intraconal** mass
  - Avid **dynamic** enhancement
    - Initially patchy, homogeneously on delayed images
- Location
  - Most (> 75%) **intraconal**, usually lateral
  - Involves orbital fissures or optic canal in 10-20%
- Size
  - Ranging from few millimeters (incidental) to very large (with mass effect)
- Morphology
  - **Ovoid** or round, sharply **marginated**
  - **Pseudocapsule** of compressed surrounding tissue
  - Indents rather than conforms to globe
  - Does not expand with Valsalva

CT Findings

- NECT
  - Homogeneously isodense
  - Benign remodeling of bone in large lesions
- CECT
  - Avid enhancement

MR Findings

- T1WI
  - Homogeneous and isointense to muscle
  - Pseudocapsule may be visible as hypointense rim
- T2WI
  - Hyperintense; internal septations may be visible, particularly in larger lesions
  - Chemical shift artifact visible in frequency encoded direction
- T1WI C+
  - Characteristic fill-in pattern on dynamic enhancement
    - Heterogeneous early patchy central enhancement
    - Diffuse enhancement in venous phase
    - Homogeneous on delayed post-contrast images
- MRA
  - Does not show high flow characteristics
  - Not visible on routine MRA

Ultrasonographic Findings

- Grayscale ultrasound
  - Well-demarcated hyperechoic retrobulbar mass
  - Highly reflective borders representing pseudocapsule

Imaging Recommendations

- Best imaging tool
  - Enhanced thin-section dedicated orbital MR
    - Specific MR features include patchy dynamic enhancement, septations, and pseudocapsule
- Protocol advice
  - CT usually diagnostic in appropriate clinical setting
  - MR appearance is characteristic
    - Use fat-suppressed FSE or STIR for T2WI
    - Use fat-suppressed T1WI post contrast
    - Include dynamic enhanced scan to show characteristic enhancement pattern

DIFFERENTIAL DIAGNOSIS

Lymphoproliferative Lesion

- Spectrum from polyclonal reactive to lymphoma (MALT)
- Infiltrative or "plastic" homogeneously enhancing mass

Orbital Metastasis

- Muscles and globe more common
- May involve any area of orbit or extend from bone

Optic Nerve Sheath Meningioma

- Fusiform enhancing mass surrounding optic nerve
- Tram-track calcification and enhancement

Optic Nerve Glioma

- Minor association with neurofibromatosis type 1 (NF1)
- Tubular mass indistinguishable from optic nerve

Orbital Varix

- Uniformly enhancing vascular mass
- Distensible, enlarges with Valsalva maneuver

Orbital Lymphatic Malformation

- Prone to hemorrhage with sudden proptosis
- Multilocular mass, transspatial, fluid levels

Hemangiopericytoma

- Uncommon; may mimic OCVM
- Intense enhancement; margins less well defined

Schwannoma

- Uncommon in orbit
- Ovoid to fusiform, homogeneously enhancing mass

Neurofibroma

- Diagnostic feature of NF1
- Irregular, lobulated, or serpentine masses

PATHOLOGY

General Features

- Etiology
  - Slowly growing vascular malformation
  - Slow-flow venous lesion with dilated vascular spaces
  - Nonneoplastic; not a true hemangioma
- Associated abnormalities
  - Multiple lesions associated with systemic disorders
    - e.g., blue rubber bleb nevus syndrome

Staging, Grading, & Classification

- International Society for the Society of Vascular Anomalies classification of vascular malformations
  - OCVM classified as slow-flow venous lesion
  - Some arterial imaging features have been observed; however, no arterial elements present histologically, and OCVM is considered essentially venous lesion

Gross Pathologic & Surgical Features

- Round, well-defined, reddish mass; vascular channels
- Fibrous pseudocapsule, distinct from surrounding compressed tissue
- Apical vascular tag frequently present

Microscopic Features

- Network of dilated vascular channels, larger than capillaries, filled with red blood cells
- Thin-walled sinusoidal spaces lined with mature flattened endothelial cells, surrounded by few layers of smooth muscle, separated by scant fibrous connective stroma
- No evidence of cellular proliferation
  - Lack of GLUT-1, desmin, and Ki-67 immunohistochemical markers supports malformative rather than neoplastic pathophysiology
  - Apparent proliferative endothelial features noted in early descriptions may relate to reactive effects of in situ thrombosis within cavernous channels

CLINICAL ISSUES

Presentation

- Most common signs/symptoms
  - Slowly progressive painless proptosis
- Other signs/symptoms
  - Headache or retrobulbar pain
  - Vision loss due to compressive optic neuropathy
- Clinical profile
  - Diplopia, visual impairment, increased intraocular pressure with large lesions
- Funduscopic examination
  - Choroidal striae, optic nerve elevation, and posterior indentation with large lesions

Demographics

- Age
  - Range = 10-60 years; mean = 40 years
- Gender
  - Female predominance, approximately 2:1
- Ethnicity
  - No known predilection
- Epidemiology
  - Most common isolated orbital mass in adults
    - 5% of orbital masses

Natural History & Prognosis

- Slow, progressive enlargement over years
  - On average 10-15% volume growth per year
- Faster growth during pregnancy
- Eventually compress and displace orbital structures
- Excellent prognosis; very low recurrence rate

Treatment

- Surgical resection indicated for visual disturbance, cosmesis, or other significant mass effect
  - Lateral orbitotomy is conventional surgical approach
  - Transconjunctival techniques may be option
  - More extensive surgery for apex lesions
    - Higher complication rate
- Pseudocapsule promotes easy extraction
- Observation alone for stable lesions, lesions without significant symptoms, or poor surgical candidates

DIAGNOSTIC CHECKLIST

Consider

- Most common adult orbital mass lesion
  - Often discovered incidentally during brain MR
- "Hemangioma" is common term but misnomer
  - OCVM is malformation, not neoplasm
- Hemangiopericytoma is rare but has similar imaging appearance
- Distinct lesion from infantile ("capillary") hemangioma, neoplastic tumor of infancy

Image Interpretation Pearls

- Patchy dynamic enhancement is characteristic feature reminiscent of cavernous malformations seen elsewhere
- Macroscopic calcifications or phleboliths are not typical, unlike venous malformations elsewhere

Reporting Tips

- Radiologist should be confident diagnosing this common benign adult lesion with characteristic appearance

SELECTED REFERENCES

1. McNab AA et al: The natural history of orbital cavernous hemangiomas. Ophthal Plast Reconstr Surg. 31(2): 89-93, 2015
2. Rootman DB et al: Comparative histology of orbital, hepatic and subcutaneous cavernous venous malformations. Br J Ophthalmol. 99(1):138-40, 2015
3. Wassef M et al: Vascular anomalies classification: recommendations from The International Society for the Study of Vascular Anomalies. 136(1):e203-14, 2015
4. Rootman DB et al: Cavernous venous malformations of the orbit (so-called cavernous haemangioma): a comprehensive evaluation of their clinical, imaging and histologic nature. Br J Ophthalmol. 98(7):880-8, 2014
5. Rootman J et al: Vascular malformations of the orbit: classification and the role of imaging in diagnosis and treatment strategies. Ophthal Plast Reconstr Surg. 30(2):91-104, 2014
6. Bonavolontà G et al: An analysis of 2,480 space-occupying lesions of the orbit from 1976 to 2011. Ophthal Plast Reconstr Surg. 29(2):79-86, 2013
7. Osaki TH et al: Immunohistochemical investigations of orbital infantile hemangiomas and adult encapsulated cavernous venous lesions (malformation versus hemangioma). Ophthal Plast Reconstr Surg. 29(3):183-95, 2013
8. Gupta A et al: Orbital cavernous haemangiomas: immunohistochemical study of proliferative capacity, vascular differentiation and hormonal receptor status. Orbit. 31(6):386-9, 2012
9. Tian YM et al: Adhesion of cavernous hemangioma in the orbit revealed by CT and MRI: analysis of 97 cases. Int J Ophthalmol. 4(2):195-8, 2011
10. Jinhu Y et al: Dynamic enhancement features of cavernous sinus cavernous hemangiomas on conventional contrast-enhanced MR imaging. AJNR Am J Neuroradiol. 29(3):577-81, 2008
11. Smoker WR et al: Vascular lesions of the orbit: more than meets the eye. Radiographics. 28(1):185-204; quiz 325, 2008
12. Rootman J: Vascular malformations of the orbit: hemodynamic concepts. Orbit. 22(2):103-20, 2003
13. Harris GJ: Orbital vascular malformations: a consensus statement on terminology and its clinical implications. Orbital Society. Am J Ophthalmol. 127(4):453-5, 1999

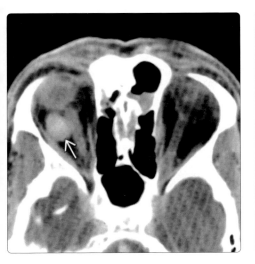

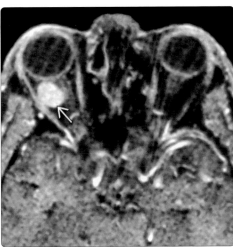

(Left) *Axial CECT shows an ovoid, well-circumscribed, enhancing mass ➡ within the intraconal fat of the right orbit, abutting the optic nerve and lateral rectus muscle.* (Right) *Axial T1WI C+ FS MR demonstrates avid enhancement of an intraconal mass ➡. The mass is relatively small, with little mass effect, and no aggressive features. Such lesions are frequently asymptomatic or have gradual changes that may go unnoticed by the patient.*

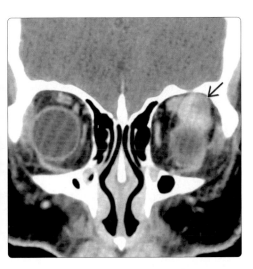

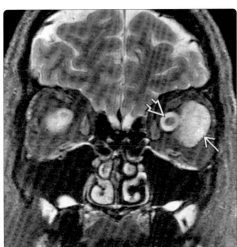

(Left) *Coronal CECT shows an intraconal mass ➡ with a patchy early enhancement pattern, highly suggestive of orbital cavernous malformation. Although the lesion extends to the periphery of the orbit, its center is intraconal.* (Right) *Coronal STIR MR shows a large intraconal cavernous malformation ➡. The mass shows high signal similar to the CSF that surrounds the displaced optic nerve ➡.*

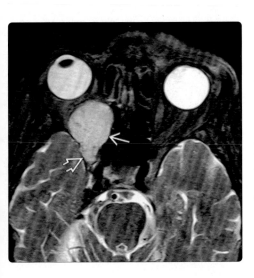

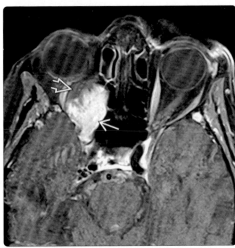

(Left) *Axial T2WI FS MR shows a large, hyperintense, slightly lobulated mass extending the apex of the right orbit ➡. There is enlargement of the superior orbital fissure from this slowly growing mass ➡.* (Right) *Axial T1WI FS MR shows incomplete but intense enhancement of the large orbital cavernous malformation that involves the apex ➡. The nonenhancing portions ➡ would be expected to fill in on delayed images.*

Ocular Toxocariasis

TERMINOLOGY

- Ocular larva migrans (OLM)
- Sclerosing endophthalmitis
- Granulomatous retinal nematode infection

IMAGING

- Enhancing granulomatous nodule posteriorly in eye with inflammatory features
- Posterior pole of eye; almost always unilateral
- CT
  - Nodular mass without calcification
  - Vitreal hyperdensity due to retinal detachment
- MR
  - Intravitreal membranes, retinal detachments
  - Enhancing retinal nodule
- US
  - Echogenic nodular granuloma

TOP DIFFERENTIAL DIAGNOSES

- Retinoblastoma
- Coats disease
- Persistent hyperplastic primary vitreous
- Retinopathy of prematurity
- Acute endophthalmitis

PATHOLOGY

- *Toxocara* species of roundworm parasites
- Humans are paratenic (accidental) hosts

CLINICAL ISSUES

- Progressive forms of disease
  - Chronic endophthalmitis
  - Posterior granuloma
  - Peripheral granuloma

DIAGNOSTIC CHECKLIST

- May closely mimic retinoblastoma

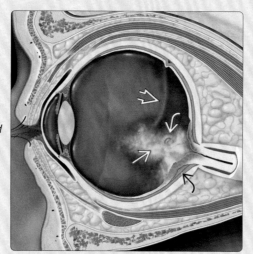
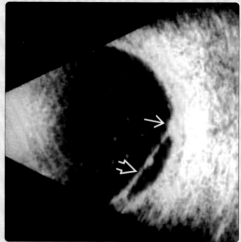

(Left) Sagittal graphic demonstrates a granulomatous reaction ➡ secondary to a dead Toxocara larva ➡. A retinal fold is present ➡ due to postinflammatory changes and traction, as well a small subretinal fluid collection ➡. (Right) Transocular ultrasound shows an echoic nodule at the posterior pole of the globe ➡ corresponding to a Toxocara granuloma. An intravitreal membrane ➡ is seen extending from the nodule.

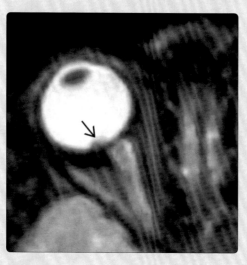
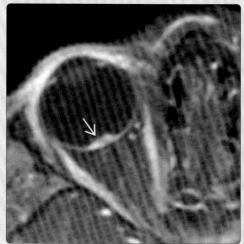

(Left) Axial T2 FS MR shows a small, retinal-based mass at the posterior pole of the globe ➡, representing granulomatous reaction at the site of the expired nematode larva. There was no Ca++ on CT. No other retinal complications are evident. (Right) Axial T1 C+ FS MR shows moderate enhancement of a retinal-based nodule at the posterior pole of the right globe ➡, representing granulomatous reaction at the site of the expired nematode larva.

TERMINOLOGY

Synonyms

- Ocular larva migrans (OLM)
- Sclerosing **endophthalmitis**

Definitions

- Granulomatous retinal nematode infection

IMAGING

General Features

- Best diagnostic clue
  - Enhancing granulomatous **nodule** posteriorly in eye with **inflammatory** and postinflammatory features
- Location
  - **Posterior pole** of eye; almost always **unilateral**
- Morphology
  - Retinal-based **nodular mass**

Imaging Recommendations

- Best imaging tool
  - CT & MR adjuncts to ultrasound & funduscopy

CT Findings

- NECT
  - Posterior nodular mass **without calcification**
  - Vitreal hyperdensity due to **retinal detachment**

MR Findings

- T2WI
  - Isointense or hypointense to vitreous
  - Intravitreal **membranes** and retinal **detachments**
  - Variable signal subretinal fluid
- T1WI C+
  - Moderately **enhancing retinal nodule**

Ultrasonographic Findings

- Grayscale ultrasound
  - Echogenic **nodular** granuloma
  - Vitreous membranes and **retinal folds**

DIFFERENTIAL DIAGNOSIS

Retinoblastoma

- Most **common** ocular tumor in children
- **Calcification** present in vast majority

Coats Disease

- More common in **males**
- Retinal **detachments** with large complex exudates

Persistent Hyperplastic Primary Vitreous

- Normal fetal hyaloid **fails to regress**
- **Retrolental tissue** and stalk in small eye

Retinopathy of Prematurity

- **Retrolental fibroplasia** related to excess **oxygen**
- Small globe, hyperdense, **bilateral**

Acute Endophthalmitis

- **Bacterial** or **fungal** infection of eye
- **Uveoscleral** enhancement

PATHOLOGY

General Features

- Etiology
  - Ingestion of **contaminated** food or geophagia
  - Disease due to **immunoallergic** reaction to antigens following larval death

Parasitology

- *Toxocara* species of **roundworm parasites**
  - *Toxocara canis* (dog host) and *Toxocara cati* (cat host)
- Humans are paratenic (accidental) hosts
  - Ingestion of eggs from ova-laden **pet feces**
  - Larvae migrate from intestine to eye

Laboratory Tests

- Serum ELISA for anti-*Toxocara* antibodies
  - **Low titers** in ocular compared to visceral disease

CLINICAL ISSUES

Presentation

- Most common signs/symptoms
  - Loss of visual acuity, **leukocoria**
- Other signs/symptoms
  - Squinting, perceived light flashes
  - Chorioretinitis, optic papillitis, endophthalmitis

Demographics

- Age
  - Mean: 8 years (may occur in young adults)
- Gender
  - 60% male, 40% female
- Epidemiology
  - Ocular infection rare in developed world
  - Majority of **pets** are infested (33-100%)

Natural History & Prognosis

- Ocular disease **months to years** after initial infection
- Chronic endophthalmitis
- Posterior granuloma
- Peripheral granuloma

Treatment

- Pharmaceutical
  - Antihelmintic (mebendazole, albendazole)
  - Corticosteroids
- Surgical
  - Vitrectomy and subretinal surgery
  - Photocoagulation

DIAGNOSTIC CHECKLIST

Image Interpretation Pearls

- May closely mimic retinoblastoma
- Lack of Ca^{++} on CT helps differentiate

SELECTED REFERENCES

1. Despreaux R et al: Ocular toxocariasis: clinical features and long-term visual outcomes in adult patients. Am J Ophthalmol. 166:162-8, 2016
2. Arevalo JF et al: Ocular toxocariasis. J Pediatr Ophthalmol Strabismus. 50(2):76-86, 2013

Orbital Subperiosteal Abscess

TERMINOLOGY

- **Purulent** accumulation between bony **orbital wall** and orbital **periosteum**

IMAGING

- Lentiform, rim-enhancing collection along orbital wall
  - Loculated fluid density/signal on CT/MR
  - Adjacent sinusitis
- Demineralization &/or dehiscence of orbital wall
- Diffusion restriction within abscess on MR
- **Imaging recommendations**
  - CT with contrast for diagnosis and monitoring
  - MR with contrast for complications or to avoid radiation

TOP DIFFERENTIAL DIAGNOSES

- Orbital cellulitis
- Idiopathic orbital inflammation
- Sinonasal mucocele
- Nasolacrimal duct mucocele

PATHOLOGY

- Secondary to adjacent sinusitis
- Upper respiratory microbes: Simple and aerobic in children; polymicrobial and anaerobic in adults

CLINICAL ISSUES

- Presentation and natural history
  - Eye swelling, erythema, gaze restriction
  - Rapidly progressive, potentially blinding disease
  - Venous thrombosis, intracranial extension complications
- Treatment
  - Targeted IV antibiotics
  - Surgical drainage for larger abscesses and older patients
  - Factors that may indicate surgical drainage
    - > 10 years, mass effect, or visual compromise
    - Large volume abscess or frontal sinus origin

DIAGNOSTIC CHECKLIST

- Risk of blindness, which requires immediate attention

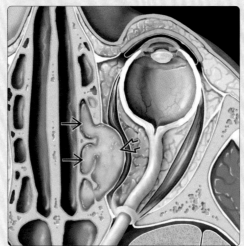
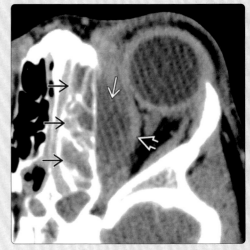

(Left) Axial graphic depicts spread of infection from the left ethmoid sinuses ➡ through the lamina papyracea into the medial orbit. Resultant subperiosteal abscess ⇨ causes mass effect, displacing the adjacent muscle cone and putting the optic nerve at risk. (Right) Axial CECT shows asymmetric opacification of the left ethmoid sinuses ➡ with a large subperiosteal abscess extending into the medial extraconal orbit ➡. Displacement of the medial rectus ⇨ is a typical finding.

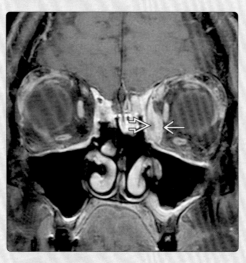
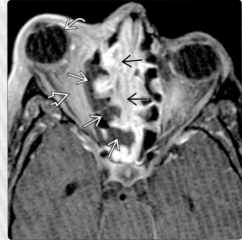

(Left) Coronal T1WI C+ FS MR in a patient status post endoscopic sinus surgery shows phlegmonous enhancement in the medial right extraconal fat ➡ with a small abscess pocket forming centrally ⇨. (Right) Axial T1WI C+ FS MR shows a large subperiosteal abscess ➡ extending through the lamina papyracea with findings of acute sinusitis ➡ and extensive right orbital cellulitis ⇒. Marked proptosis is evident ➚. Posterior extension of the abscess implies higher risk of vision loss.

TERMINOLOGY

Abbreviations

- Orbital subperiosteal abscess (SPA)

Definitions

- Purulent accumulation between bony orbital wall and orbital periosteum

IMAGING

General Features

- Best diagnostic clue
  - **Lentiform**, **rim-enhancing** collection along orbital wall
    - Adjacent **sinusitis**, particularly ethmoid
- Location
  - **Medial extraconal** orbit, along lamina papyracea
    - More common; associated ethmoid/maxillary sinusitis
  - **Superior and lateral** location less common
    - Associated ethmoid/frontal sinusitis
- Size
  - Surgery indicated for larger volume
  - SPA may appear relatively small relative to degree of orbital **edema** and **proptosis**
- Morphology
  - Flat or **lenticular** collection bowing into extraconal space
  - **Displacement** of adjacent **rectus** muscle

CT Findings

- NECT
  - Confluent density in **medial** &/or superior orbit
  - Opacified ethmoid, maxillary, &/or frontal sinuses
  - Inflammatory stranding of orbital fat ("**dirty fat**")
- CECT
  - **Rim-enhancing** hypodense **fluid** collection
  - Prominently enhancing paranasal sinus mucosa
  - Displaced, enlarged, irregular rectus muscle
- Bone CT
  - **Demineralization** &/or **dehiscence** of orbital wall, particularly lamina papyracea

MR Findings

- T1WI
  - Hypointense **fluid** signal within abscess
  - Infiltrative inflammatory hypointensity in orbital fat
- T2WI FS
  - Hyperintense **fluid** signal within abscess
  - Infiltrative inflammatory hyperintensity in orbital fat
  - Opacified ethmoid, maxillary, &/or frontal sinuses
- DWI
  - Diffusion **restriction** within abscess, due to viscosity and dense cellular material within pus
- T1WI C+
  - **Rim-enhancing** fluid collection in medial orbit
  - Prominently enhancing paranasal sinus mucosa
  - Irregular infiltrative enhancement of orbital fat

Ultrasonographic Findings

- Grayscale ultrasound
  - Fusiform collection between bone and highly reflective **periosteum**, adjacent to muscle

Imaging Recommendations

- Best imaging tool
  - CT with contrast for diagnosis and monitoring
    - Abscess volume measurements aid surgical decision
- Protocol advice
  - Serial CTs helpful for monitoring response
  - MR with contrast for problem solving
    - Evaluate for potential intracranial complications
    - More sensitive than CT and should be pursued when strong clinical suspicion
  - Use low-dose CT technique, or consider using MR in pediatric patients

DIFFERENTIAL DIAGNOSIS

Orbital Cellulitis

- Infiltration and enhancement without discrete collection
- Trauma or sinusitis; may be preseptal or intraorbital

Idiopathic Orbital Inflammation

- Inflammatory pseudotumor, without fever/leukocytosis

Sinonasal Mucocele

- Chronic obstruction with expansion and osseous remodeling

Nasolacrimal Duct Mucocele

- Cystic mass in enlarged lacrimal sac, with enlarged and opacified nasolacrimal duct

Subperiosteal Hematoma

- Extraconal collection, hyperdense on NECT if acute

Dermoid/Epidermoid

- Developmental epithelial inclusion
- May show localized inflammation if ruptured

PATHOLOGY

General Features

- Etiology
  - Secondary to adjacent **sinusitis**
    - Hematogenous transmission of bacteria through valveless **orbital veins**
    - Direct extension through congenital or acquired **dehiscence**, particularly in lamina papyracea
    - Orbital **cellulitis** precedes SPA
  - Microbiology
    - **Upper respiratory** flora, varies by age group
      - □ Children: Commonly single **aerobes**
      - □ Adolescents: Mixed, mostly aerobes
      - □ Adults: **Mixed aerobes** and **anaerobes**
    - Emergence of more aggressive aerobes, including methicillin-resistant *Staphylococcus aureus* (**MRSA**), over recent decades
  - Abscess formation
    - Sinusitis leads to orbital **periostitis**
    - Relatively **avascular** subperiosteal space promotes accumulation of pus
- Associated abnormalities
  - Underlying sinus disease
    - Polyposis, mechanical sinonasal obstruction
    - Cystic fibrosis, ciliary dyskinesia

Staging, Grading, & Classification

- Chandler grouping of sinus-related orbital disease (does not necessarily imply order of disease progression)
  - **I**: Preseptal cellulitis
  - **II**: Orbital (postseptal) cellulitis
  - **III**: Subperiosteal abscess
  - **IV**: Large intraorbital abscess
  - **V**: Extraorbital complications
    - Cavernous sinus thrombosis, intracranial extension

Gross Pathologic & Surgical Features

- Pocket of yellow-green fluid in expanded space between bone and periosteum

Microscopic Features

- Necrotic debris with inflammatory cell and microorganisms

CLINICAL ISSUES

Presentation

- Most common signs/symptoms
  - Orbital **edema** and painful **proptosis** with **fever**
- Other signs/symptoms
  - Eye swelling, erythema, gaze restriction
  - Visual disturbance in 15-30%
    - Optic neuritis due to intraconal extension
    - Retinal ischemia from central artery occlusion
- Clinical profile
  - Associated with acute or chronic sinusitis
  - Preceded by upper respiratory infection in children

Demographics

- Age
  - Most common in children
  - More severe in adults
- Gender
  - Male patients more likely to require surgical drainage

Natural History & Prognosis

- Rapidly progressive, **potentially blinding** disease
- IV antibiotics with surgical drainage when indicated results in **excellent prognosis** in most cases
- Progression of SPA leads to frank intraorbital abscess
  - Increased proptosis, increased pressure
  - Worsening vision, ophthalmoplegia
- Other complications
  - **Superior ophthalmic vein** thrombosis
  - **Cavernous sinus thrombosis**, rare but devastating
  - **Intracranial** extension
    - Meningitis, empyema, cerebritis, brain abscess

Treatment

- Medical therapy (IV antibiotics)
  - Manageable with antibiotics alone in 25-50%
    - Children under 10 years
      - □ Majority of small SPA manageable without surgery
      - □ Simple aerobic microbes responsive to antibiotics
    - Absence of visual signs or surgical indications
    - Phlegmon with small or no abscess
  - Antibiotic regimen
    - Broad polymicrobial coverage, targeted with cultures
    - Add anaerobe coverage when indicated

- Surgical indications
  - **Emergent** (immediate drainage)
    - Optic nerve or retinal compromise
    - Intracranial involvement
  - **Urgent** (antibiotics alone inadequate)
    - Age 10 years or older or immunocompromised
    - Visual compromise or disproportionate pain
    - Proptosis, muscle restriction, elevated pressure
    - Frontal sinus origin
    - Superior or inferior extension of abscess
    - Larger volume (> 3.8 mL or > 1.25 mL if superior)
    - Gas in collection (suggests anaerobic infection)
    - Bone destruction
  - **Expectant** (after failed medical therapy)
    - Visual changes at any time
    - Persistent fever after 36 hours
    - Clinical deterioration after 24-48 hours
    - No improvement after 72 hours
- Surgical options
  - Endoscopic drainage
    - Generally preferred for small SPA
  - External drainage
    - Larger abscesses, abscesses extending along roof or floor of orbit or originating from frontal sinus

DIAGNOSTIC CHECKLIST

Consider

- Orbital disease may be **1st sign** of sinusitis

Image Interpretation Pearls

- Superior location and larger abscess volume increase likelihood of surgical drainage
- Presence of diffusion restriction on MR increases diagnostic confidence when contrast cannot be administered

Reporting Tips

- Requires immediate attention (may cause blindness)

SELECTED REFERENCES

1. Marchiano E et al: Characteristics of patients treated for orbital cellulitis: an analysis of inpatient data. Laryngoscope. 126(3):554-9, 2016
2. Quintanilla-Dieck L et al: Characteristics of superior orbital subperiosteal abscesses in children. Laryngoscope. ePub, 2016
3. Erickson BP et al: Orbital cellulitis and subperiosteal abscess: a 5-year outcomes analysis. Orbit. 34(3):115-20, 2015
4. Liao JC et al: Subperiosteal abscess of the orbit: evolving pathogens and the therapeutic protocol. Ophthalmology. 122(3):639-47, 2015
5. Le TD et al: The effect of adding orbital computed tomography findings to the Chandler criteria for classifying pediatric orbital cellulitis in predicting which patients will require surgical intervention. J AAPOS. 18(3):271-7, 2014
6. Smith JM et al: Predicting the need for surgical intervention in pediatric orbital cellulitis. Am J Ophthalmol. 158(2):387-394.e1, 2014
7. Todman MS et al: Medical management versus surgical intervention of pediatric orbital cellulitis: the importance of subperiosteal abscess volume as a new criterion. Ophthal Plast Reconstr Surg. 27(4):255-9, 2011
8. Migirov L et al: Endoscopic sinus surgery for medial orbital subperiosteal abscess in children. J Otolaryngol Head Neck Surg. 38(4):504-8, 2009
9. Sepahdari AR et al: MRI of orbital cellulitis and orbital abscess: the role of diffusion-weighted imaging. AJR Am J Roentgenol. 193(3):W244-50, 2009
10. McIntosh D et al: Failure of contrast enhanced computed tomography scans to identify an orbital abscess. The benefit of magnetic resonance imaging. J Laryngol Otol. 122(6):639-40, 2008
11. Tanna N et al: Surgical treatment of subperiosteal orbital abscess. Arch Otolaryngol Head Neck Surg. 134(7):764-7, 2008
12. Chandler JR et al: The pathogenesis of orbital complications in acute sinusitis. Laryngoscope. 80(9):1414-28, 1970

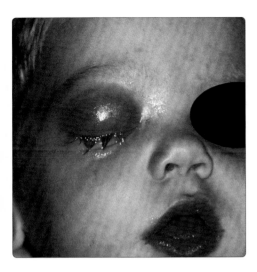

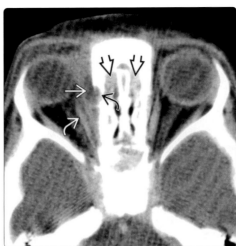

(Left) *Clinical photograph in a young child with sinusitis and cystic fibrosis shows a swollen eyelid but relatively minor periorbital edema, indicating postseptal disease.* (Right) *Axial CECT in the same child shows opacification of the ethmoid sinuses ➡, with dehiscence of the right lamina papyracea ➡. A small subperiosteal abscess is present ➡ with displacement of the adjacent medial rectus ➡. The patient responded well to IV antibiotics without surgery.*

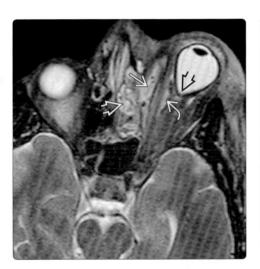

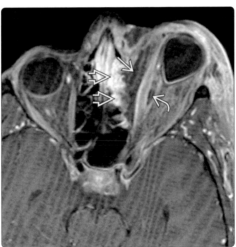

(Left) *Axial T2WI FS MR in a patient who failed antibiotic therapy for cellulitis shows marked intraorbital edema with proptosis and tenting of the globe ➡. An abscess is present with subperiosteal extraconal ➡ and intraconal ➡ components. Adjacent sinusitis is evident ➡.* (Right) *Axial T1WI C+ FS MR in the same patient demonstrates low-intensity extraconal ➡ and intraconal ➡ pus with rim enhancement. Ethmoid sinusitis with mucosal enhancement is evident ➡. This patient suffered total vision loss in the left eye.*

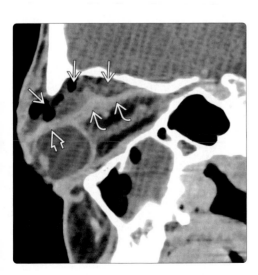

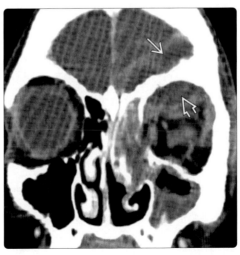

(Left) *Sagittal CT reconstruction in a patient with acute frontal sinusitis shows a complex abscess in the superior extraconal orbit ➡ containing fluid and gas. Mass effect is evident on the globe ➡ and muscle cone ➡. The location of this abscess would preclude the use of endoscopic drainage.* (Right) *Coronal CECT reformation shows unilateral left sinusitis with superiorly located subperiosteal abscess ➡. Intracranial spread is present, manifest as epidural empyema ➡.*

TERMINOLOGY

- Preseptal cellulitis
  - Infection limited to superficial periorbita
- Intraorbital (postseptal) cellulitis
  - Infection posterior to orbital septum
- Orbital septum
  - Connective tissue plane that acts as diaphragm

IMAGING

- Superficial periorbital or deep intraorbital soft tissue infiltration with mass effect & enhancement
- Enhanced CT adequate for uncomplicated cases
- MR shows diffusion restriction if abscess is present

TOP DIFFERENTIAL DIAGNOSES

- Orbital subperiosteal abscess
- Invasive fungal infection
- Idiopathic orbital inflammatory disease
- Orbital sarcoidosis

PATHOLOGY

- Etiology
  - Preseptal cellulitis: Trauma, insect bites common
  - Intraorbital cellulitis: Sinusitis most common
- Microbiology
  - Related to traumatic & sinogenic etiologies
  - Adults more likely polymicrobial & less responsive

CLINICAL ISSUES

- Presentation
  - Preseptal cellulitis
    - Periorbital edema & erythema
  - Intraorbital cellulitis
    - Axial (forward) displacement of globe
- Treatment
  - Targeted antimicrobials with cultures
  - Concomitant corticosteroids to reduce inflammation
  - Surgical drainage may be required if abscess develops

(Left) *Axial CECT in a patient with facial impetigo shows edema and enhancement of the preseptal soft tissues* ➡️ *with normal appearance of the intraorbital fat* ➡️. *Note that the adjacent sinuses are clear.* (Right) *Axial STIR MR in a teenage girl shows infiltrating signal representing both preseptal* ➡️ *and postseptal* ➡️ *cellulitis secondary to ethmoid sinusitis* ➡️. *Although no abscess is present, there is significant proptosis with tenting of the posterior globe* ➡️.

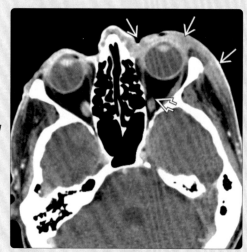
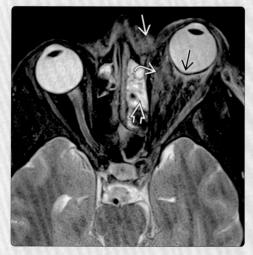

(Left) *Axial T1-weighted postcontrast MR in a patient with recent penetrating facial trauma shows extensive preseptal* ➡️ *and intraorbital* ➡️ *infiltration and enhancement. A rim-enhancing collection is seen extending along the trajectory of injury* ➡️. (Right) *Diffusion-weighted image in the same patient shows restriction within the collection* ➡️, *indicating acute abscess. The abscess crosses the plane of the orbital septum, which was violated due to the trauma.*

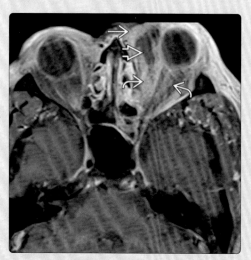
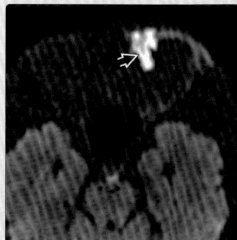

TERMINOLOGY

Synonyms

- **Preseptal cellulitis**
  - Infection limited to superficial periorbita
- **Intraorbital (postseptal) cellulitis**
  - Infection posterior to orbital septum
  - Extraconal &/or intraconal

Definitions

- **Orbital septum**
  - Connective tissue plane that acts as **diaphragm** at anterior boundary of orbit
- **Phlegmon**
  - Infectious infiltrate **without** discrete **abscess**
- **Subperiosteal abscess**
  - Complication of cellulitis

IMAGING

General Features

- Best diagnostic clue
  - Superficial periorbital or deep intraorbital **soft tissue infiltration & inflammation** with **mass effect** & **enhancement**
- Location
  - **Preseptal**: Anterior periorbital soft tissues
  - **Intraorbital**: Extraconal &/or intraconal
- Morphology
  - **Infiltrative** & ill defined with **mass effect**

Imaging Recommendations

- Best imaging tool
  - CECT adequate for uncomplicated cases
  - MR with contrast for difficult or aggressive cases
- Protocol advice
  - Serial CECT useful if treatment response indeterminate

CT Findings

- CECT
  - **Infiltration** of periorbital &/or intraorbital fat; diffuse heterogeneous **enhancement**

MR Findings

- T1WI
  - Hypointense infiltration of normal fat
- T2WI FS
  - Heterogeneous hyperintensity
- DWI
  - Restriction demonstrated if abscess is present
- T1WI C+ FS
  - Diffuse heterogeneous enhancement

DIFFERENTIAL DIAGNOSIS

Orbital Subperiosteal Abscess

- Progressive complication of sinogenic orbital cellulitis

Invasive Fungal Infection

- Opportunistic sinus infection with orbital extension

Idiopathic Orbital Inflammatory Pseudotumor

- Mass-like features, multifocal involvement

Orbital Sarcoidosis

- Multifocal involvement, especially lacrimal

PATHOLOGY

General Features

- Etiology
  - **Preseptal** cellulitis
    - Trauma most common cause; insect bites also common, particularly in children
  - **Intraorbital** cellulitis
    - Sinusitis most common cause
    - May be secondary to foreign bodies
- Associated abnormalities
  - Underlying **sinus disease**
    - Sinonasal polyposis or obstructive lesion

Microbiology

- Bacterial
  - **Preseptal**: *Staphylococcus*, *Streptococcus*, & *Haemophilus influenzae*
  - **Intraorbital**: Polymicrobial including anaerobes

CLINICAL ISSUES

Presentation

- Most common signs/symptoms
  - **Preseptal** cellulitis
    - Periorbital edema & erythema
  - **Intraorbital** cellulitis
    - Axial (forward) displacement of globe
- Other signs/symptoms
  - **Fever**, pain, chemosis, malaise
  - **Loss of vision** & movement are ominous signs

Natural History & Prognosis

- **Preseptal** cellulitis
  - Responds well to antibiotics
  - Postseptal extension uncommon
- **Intraorbital** cellulitis
  - May progress to abscess if inadequately treated

Treatment

- Targeted **antimicrobials** with cultures
  - Intravenous therapy when fulminant or aggressive
- Concomitant **corticosteroids** to reduce inflammation
- Surgical drainage may be required if abscess develops
  - Younger children usually respond without surgery

DIAGNOSTIC CHECKLIST

Image Interpretation Pearls

- Serial imaging may play role in assessing treatment response

SELECTED REFERENCES

1. Marchiano E et al: Characteristics of patients treated for orbital cellulitis: an analysis of inpatient data. Laryngoscope. 126(3):554-9, 2016
2. Erickson BP et al: Orbital cellulitis and subperiosteal abscess: a 5-year outcomes analysis. Orbit. 34(3):115-20, 2015
3. Kapur R et al: MR imaging of orbital inflammatory syndrome, orbital cellulitis, & orbital lymphoid lesions: role of diffusion-weighted imaging. AJNR Am J Neuroradiol. 30(1):64-70, 2009

Idiopathic Orbital Inflammation (Pseudotumor)

TERMINOLOGY

- Nonspecific orbital inflammation, not due to any known etiology or systemic illness

IMAGING

- Poorly marginated, mass-like, or infiltrative enhancing inflammatory tissue involving any area of orbit
  - **Myositic** (extraocular muscles)
  - **Lacrimal** (lacrimal gland)
  - **Anterior** (globe, retrobulbar orbit)
  - **Diffuse** (multifocal intraconal ± extraconal)
  - **Apical** (orbital apex, intracranial extension)
- Diffuse irregularity, muscle enlargement, and enhancement
- T2/STIR hypointense due to cellular infiltrate and fibrosis
- Best imaging tool: Contrast-enhanced MR with fat suppression
- Disease variants
  - Tolosa-Hunt: Through fissures into cavernous sinus
  - Sclerosing: More often bilateral, may extend into sinuses

- IgG4: Predilection for lacrimal gland and nerves

TOP DIFFERENTIAL DIAGNOSES

- Lymphoproliferative lesions, especially lymphoma
- Thyroid ophthalmopathy
- Sarcoidosis
- Granulomatosis with polyangiitis (Wegener)
- Orbital cellulitis

PATHOLOGY

- Polymorphous chronic inflammation and fibrosis

CLINICAL ISSUES

- Acute to subacute orbital pain, swelling, restricted motion, diplopia, proptosis, and impaired vision
- Steroid treatment effective in most patients

DIAGNOSTIC CHECKLIST

- Idiopathic orbital inflammation (pseudotumor) is diagnosis of exclusion

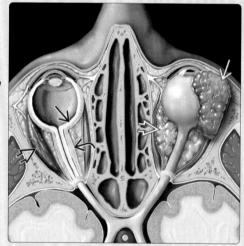
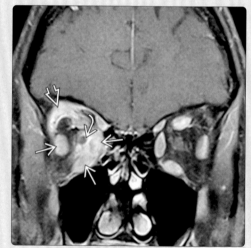

(Left) Axial graphic depicts multifocal idiopathic orbital inflammation, including involvement of the extraocular muscles ➡, orbital fat ➡, lacrimal gland ➡, sclera ➡, and optic sheath ➡. (Right) Coronal T1WI C+ FS MR demonstrates extensive orbital inflammation, with ill-defined enlargement and enhancement of the rectus muscles ➡, extraconal infiltration extending to the lacrimal gland ➡, and intraconal enhancement partially surrounding the optic nerve ➡.

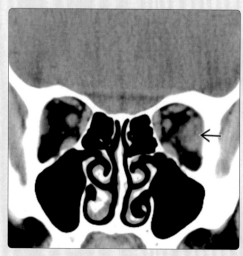
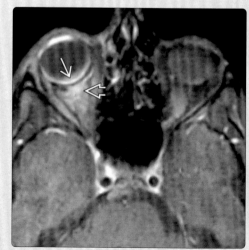

(Left) Coronal NECT in a middle-aged woman with left eye pain and diplopia shows enlargement and hypodensity of the left lateral rectus muscle ➡. Isolated lateral rectus myositis is a typical manifestation of idiopathic orbital inflammatory disease, rare in thyroid orbitopathy. (Right) Axial T1WI C+ FS MR in a patient with uveitis shows inflammatory changes of the anterior right orbit. Marked uveoscleral "shaggy" enhancement is evident ➡, as well as ill-defined enhancement of retrobulbar fat ➡.

Idiopathic Orbital Inflammation (Pseudotumor)

TERMINOLOGY

Abbreviations

- Idiopathic orbital inflammation (IOI)

Synonyms

- Orbital pseudotumor (or simply "**pseudotumor**")

Definitions

- **Tolosa-Hunt**
  - Variant **apical** form extending into cavernous sinus
- **Sclerosing** orbital inflammatory pseudotumor
  - Variant form with chronic progressive **fibrosis**
- **IgG4**-related disease (IgG4-RD)
  - Variant form, recently identified, with **plasma cell**-mediated inflammation
  - Accounts for minority of IOI

IMAGING

General Features

- Best diagnostic clue
  - Poorly marginated, mass-like, **enhancing inflammatory** soft tissue involving any area of orbit
- Location
  - Typically unilateral, bilateral in 25% of cases
  - Categorized by area(s) of involvement
    - **Myositic** [extraocular muscles (EOM)]
      - □ Most common pattern
      - □ Any muscle affected; lateral rectus, medial rectus, and superior complex most frequent
      - □ Involves tendinous insertions (unlike thyroid disease), tubular configuration, shaggy margins
    - **Lacrimal** (lacrimal gland)
      - □ 2nd most common pattern
      - □ Diffuse enlargement of gland in AP dimension
      - □ Cannot differentiate from lymphoproliferative lesions or sarcoidosis by imaging alone
    - **Anterior** (globe, retrobulbar orbit)
      - □ 3rd most common pattern
      - □ Uveal-scleral (episcleritis or sclerotenonitis): Thickened sclera with shaggy enhancement
      - □ Variable involvement of retrobulbar fat, optic nerve and sheath
    - **Diffuse** (multifocal intraconal ± extraconal)
      - □ Overlaps with other patterns
      - □ Frequently mass-like but tends not to distort globe or erode bone
    - **Apical** (orbital apex, intracranial extension)
      - □ Less common; involves orbital apex with posterior extension through fissures
  - Disease variants
    - **Tolosa-Hunt**: Apical disease that extends through orbital fissures into cavernous sinus
    - **Sclerosing** pseudotumor: More often bilateral, may extend into sinuses
    - **IgG4-RD**: Any part of orbit, predilection for lacrimal gland and infraorbital nerve
- Morphology
  - May be focally mass-like or diffuse
  - Irregular margins, **infiltrative** features

CT Findings

- NECT
  - Lacrimal, EOM, or other orbital mass
  - **Multifocal** or **infiltrative** soft tissue
- CECT
  - Moderate diffuse irregularity and enhancement of involved structures
- Bone CT
  - May rarely remodel or erode bone

MR Findings

- T1WI
  - Hypointense, particularly sclerosing disease
- T2WI FS
  - Isointense or slightly hyperintense to muscle
  - **Hypointense** compared to many orbital lesions due to **cellular infiltrate** and **fibrosis**
    - Portends worse treatment response
    - Characteristic feature of IgG4-RD
- STIR
  - Similar to T2WI FS, less prone to artifact
- T1WI C+
  - Moderate to marked diffuse irregularity, enlargement, and enhancement of involved structures
  - Tolosa-Hunt: Enhancement and fullness of anterior cavernous sinus and orbital fissures

Imaging Recommendations

- Best imaging tool
  - Contrast-enhanced thin-section MR with fat suppression

DIFFERENTIAL DIAGNOSIS

Lymphoproliferative Lesions

- Non-Hodgkin lymphoma, primary to orbit or with systemic disease; MALT variety typical
- Pliable mass, involving lacrimal gland, multifocal or diffusely in orbit; often bilateral

Thyroid Ophthalmopathy

- Thyroid dysfunction clinically; less often painful
- Bilateral, characteristic pattern of EOM involvement; affects muscle bellies, spares tendons

Sarcoidosis

- Orbital involvement in 20% of patients with systemic sarcoidosis
- Granulomatous enhancement of multiple orbital structures, particularly lacrimal gland

Granulomatosis With Polyangiitis (Wegener)

- Necrotizing vasculitis of multiple organs
- Paranasal sinus and orbital involvement with bone destruction; commonly bilateral

Orbital Cellulitis

- Secondary to adjacent sinusitis (ethmoid) or trauma
- Phlegmonous periorbital and intraconal infiltration; may be accompanied by subperiosteal abscess

Carotid-Cavernous Fistula

- Presents with pulsatile exophthalmos, chemosis

- Enlarged arterialized venous structures (signal voids) without discrete orbital mass

PATHOLOGY

General Features

- Etiology
  - Pathogenesis unknown; probably related to underlying **immune-mediated** processes
  - Not due to infection, granulomatous disease, thyroid orbitopathy, lymphoproliferative disease, or other specific systemic illness
- Associated abnormalities
  - Secondary angle-closure glaucoma
  - **Autoimmune** disorders

Gross Pathologic & Surgical Features

- Typically soft, compressible mass
- Occasionally hard, fibrotic; particularly chronic

Microscopic Features

- Polymorphous infiltration of **chronic inflammatory** cells with variable fibrosis
- Proliferating fibroblastic **connective tissue**
- Capillary proliferation with perivasculitis
- Histological variations
  - **Sclerosing**: Disproportionate connective tissue and early fibrosis with sclerosis
  - **Granulomatous**: Histiocytes, multinucleated giant cells, and granuloma formation
  - **Vasculitic**: Small vessel inflammatory infiltrate
  - **Eosinophilic**: Infiltration of eosinophilia without vasculitis; more common in children
  - **IgG4-RD**: Plasma cell infiltrate with fibrosis

CLINICAL ISSUES

Presentation

- Most common signs/symptoms
  - Acute to subacute onset of orbital **pain**, **inflammation**, and **edema**
  - Restricted eye motion, **diplopia**, and **proptosis**
- Other signs/symptoms
  - Impaired vision (perineuritis)
- Clinical profile
  - **Myositic**
    - Diplopia; painful limitation of ocular movement
    - Conjunctival injection at muscle insertions
  - **Lacrimal**
    - Enlarged, tender gland
    - Proptosis and globe displacement
    - More likely to have systemic disorder
  - **Anterior**
    - Proptosis, ptosis, lid swelling, injection
    - Uveitis, sclerotenonitis, retinal detachments
    - Decreased vision and limited movement
  - **Apical**
    - Milder signs of inflammation
    - Decreased vision; optic neuropathy
  - **Tolosa-Hunt**
    - Painful ophthalmoplegia (CNIII, IV, V, VI)
- Diagnosis

- Biopsy for confirmation indicated in patients unresponsive to or relapse after 1st-line therapy
- Serologic studies indicated for IgG and subtypes, including IgG4

Demographics

- Age
  - Any may be affected; mean: **5th decade**
- Gender
  - Overall F = M; myositic form F > M (2:1)
- Epidemiology
  - Most common painful orbital mass in adults
    - 10% of all orbital masses
  - 3rd most common orbital disorder
    - After thyroid and lymphoproliferative lesions

Natural History & Prognosis

- 5-10% **resolve spontaneously**
- Pattern of involvement affects prognosis
  - Recurrence more likely with multifocal disease
  - Poorer visual outcome in apical and diffuse disease
- Intermittent disease more likely in younger patients
- Chronic sclerosing disease not as responsive, but therapy may slow progression
- Rarely severe cases progress to fixed, painless, sightless eye requiring exenteration
- **Risk factors** include low socioeconomic status, elevated BMI, and bisphosphonate therapy

Treatment

- **Systemic steroids** are 1st-line therapy
  - **80-85%** of patients respond
  - Dramatic and rapid improvement typical
  - Recurrence after initial response in **25-40%**
- Second-line therapies for nonresponsive or refractory cases or when steroids contraindicated
  - Low-dose radiotherapy
  - Cytotoxic chemotherapy
  - Other immunosuppressive agents

DIAGNOSTIC CHECKLIST

Consider

- IOI is **diagnosis of exclusion**
- Atypical onset, poor response, or recurrence should prompt biopsy to confirm and exclude lymphoma
- Consider other **systemic causes** with bilateral, multifocal, lacrimal, or apical involvement
- Consider infectious cellulitis and carotid fistula when acute onset

Image Interpretation Pearls

- Isolated **lateral rectus** enlargement most likely IOI

SELECTED REFERENCES

1. McNab AA et al: IgG4-related ophthalmic disease. Part I: background and pathology. Ophthal Plast Reconstr Surg. 31(2):83-8, 2015
2. Bijlsma WR et al: Risk factors for idiopathic orbital inflammation: a case-control study. Br J Ophthalmol. 95(3):360-4, 2011
3. Mendenhall WM et al: Orbital pseudotumor. Am J Clin Oncol. 33(3):304-6, 2010

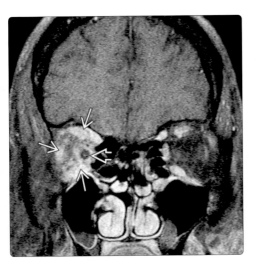

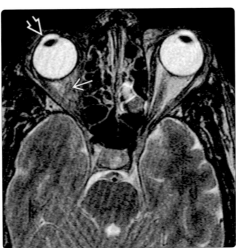

(Left) *Coronal T1WI C+ FS MR in a patient with painful, fixed right eye shows extensive, ill-defined intra- and extraconal enhancement. The extraocular muscles are enlarged, with poorly defined contours ➡. Note infiltration surrounding the optic sheath ➡. (Right) Axial T2WI MR in the same patient shows ill-defined, hypointense infiltration of right orbit ➡. Low T2 signal is indicative of chronic fibrosis due to sclerosing IOI (pseudotumor). Note lateral gaze ➡, which was fixed.*

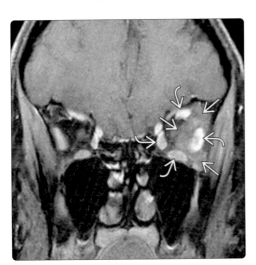

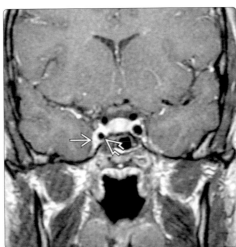

(Left) *Coronal T1WI C+ FS MR in a patient with restricted gaze shows poorly enhancing infiltrative tissue involving the intraconal and extraconal left orbit ➡, with mild enlargement of the extraocular muscles ➡. Patient responded to multimodal drug therapy. (Right) Coronal T1WI C+ FS MR in a patient with facial pain and ophthalmoplegia shows lateral dural wall bulging and enhancement of cavernous sinus ➡ when compared to left. Note decreased caliber of cavernous carotid artery ➡ in this Tolosa-Hunt variant.*

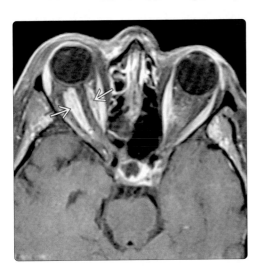

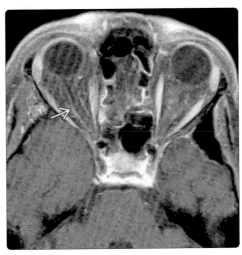

(Left) *Axial T1WI C+ FS MR in an older woman with optic neuropathy shows an intraconal mass encasing the optic nerve sheath ➡. A presumptive diagnosis of meningioma was made based on initial clinical presentation. (Right) Axial T1WI C+ FS MR in the same patient 2 years later shows near-complete spontaneous resolution of the intraconal mass, with thin minimal residual enhancement along the optic nerve sheath ➡. Presumptive diagnosis was idiopathic orbital inflammation.*

TERMINOLOGY

- Noncaseating granulomatous inflammation of orbit

IMAGING

- Multiple sites of orbital involvement
  - Diffuse lacrimal gland infiltration
  - Optic nerve-sheath thickening, enhancement
  - Asymmetric extraocular muscle infiltration
  - Intraorbital enhancing soft tissue masses
  - Eyelid and periorbital preseptal infiltration
  - Uveitis, especially anterior, but also posterior
- Best imaging tool: T2 FS MR and T1 C+ MR
- Ga-67 scintigraphy supportive but nonspecific

TOP DIFFERENTIAL DIAGNOSES

- Idiopathic orbital inflammatory disease
- Lymphoproliferative lesions
- Granulomatosis with polyangiitis
- Thyroid ophthalmopathy

PATHOLOGY

- Unknown etiology
- Noncaseating granulomas are pathologic hallmark
- Elevated ACE levels support diagnosis

CLINICAL ISSUES

- Most common signs/symptoms
  - Uveitis, lacrimal mass, and dacryoadenitis
  - Swelling, ptosis, and globe displacement
- Other signs/symptoms
  - Eye pain, conjunctivitis, vitreous and retinal changes
  - Vision loss, diplopia, perineuritis, papillitis,
- Associated with systemic sarcoidosis
- Female predilection
- Oral corticosteroids are treatment of choice

DIAGNOSTIC CHECKLIST

- Imaging appearance similar to that of idiopathic inflammation and lymphoproliferative lesions

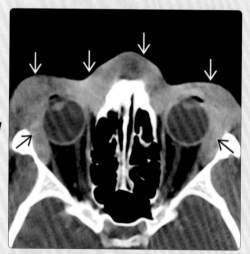
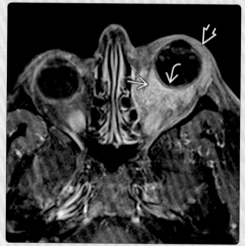

(Left) Axial CECT shows marked bilateral enlargement and enhancement of the lacrimal glands ➡, with medial displacement of the globes. Marked thickening of preseptal periorbital soft tissues is also evident ➡. (Right) Axial T1 FS C+ MR shows mass-like infiltration ➡ of left retrobulbar orbit, with associated proptosis and mild globe tenting ➡. Preseptal thickening and inflammation are also present ➡. Patient had mild systemic sarcoidosis elsewhere, with mediastinal adenopathy.

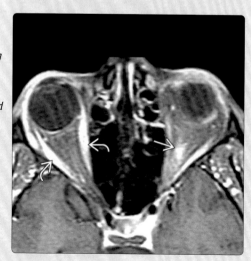
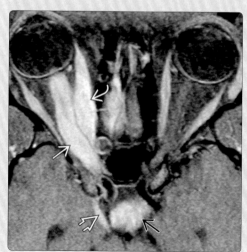

(Left) Axial T1 C+ MR in a patient with sarcoidosis and acute vision loss shows abnormal enhancement along left intraorbital optic nerve ➡. In addition, the right medial and lateral rectus muscles show mildly increased size and enhancement ➡. (Right) Axial T1 C+ FS MR shows numerous ophthalmologic manifestations of sarcoidosis, with thickening and enhancement of right optic nerve ➡, medial rectus ➡, and oculomotor CNIII ➡. Suprasellar granulomatous mass is also present ➡.

TERMINOLOGY

Definitions

- **Noncaseating granulomatous** inflammation of orbit

IMAGING

General Features

- Best diagnostic clue
  - Orbital mass effect or enlargement involving 1 or more typical structure(s)
- Location
  - Diffuse **lacrimal gland** infiltration
    - Most common orbital site of involvement (~ 60%)
  - Optic **nerve-sheath** thickening, enhancement
  - Asymmetric **extraocular muscle** (EOM) infiltration
  - Intraorbital enhancing **soft tissue masses**
  - Eyelid and **periorbital preseptal** infiltration
  - **Uveitis**; especially anterior, but also posterior

CT Findings

- CECT
  - Enhancing orbital structures or masses

MR Findings

- T1WI
  - **Hypointensity** of involved orbital structures or masses
- T2WI
  - Variable **hyperintensity** of involved orbital structures or masses
- T1WI C+
  - Diffuse **enlargement** and homogeneous **enhancement** of involved structures
    - Lacrimal gland, muscles, optic nerve ± sheath
  - Enhancing intraorbital soft tissue **masses**
  - **Intracranial** involvement with enhancement & nodularity

Nuclear Medicine Findings

- Ga-67 scintigraphy
  - Increased uptake; supportive but nonspecific

Imaging Recommendations

- Best imaging tool
  - T2 FS MR and T1 C+ MR

DIFFERENTIAL DIAGNOSIS

Idiopathic Orbital Inflammatory Disease

- Nonspecific inflammation, protean manifestations

Lymphoproliferative Lesions

- Soft, homogeneous orbital masses

Thyroid Ophthalmopathy

- Predictable medial/inferior EOM enlargement pattern

Granulomatosis With Polyangiitis (Wegener)

- Necrotizing vasculitis, sinonasal and orbital disease

PATHOLOGY

General Features

- Etiology
  - Unknown
- Genetics
  - Gene expression profiles are suggestive of diagnosis
- Laboratory
  - Elevated CSF and serum **ACE levels** support diagnosis
  - Serum **lysozyme** is more sensitive but less specific

Microscopic Features

- **Noncaseating** granulomas are pathologic hallmark
  - Central **multinucleated giant cells** and rim of lymphocytes

CLINICAL ISSUES

Presentation

- Most common signs/symptoms
  - Uveitis, lacrimal mass, and dacryoadenitis
  - Swelling, ptosis, and globe displacement
- Other signs/symptoms
  - **Anterior uveitis**: Eye pain, conjunctivitis
  - **Posterior uveitis**: Vitreous and retinal changes
  - **Lacrimal gland**: Palpable, enlarged gland; dry eye
  - **Optic nerve**: Perineuritis, papillitis, vision loss
  - **EOM**: Limited movement, diplopia
- Clinical profile
  - Associated with **systemic** sarcoidosis
    - Orbital disease common **initial presentation**
    - 20-25% of have ophthalmic disease

Demographics

- Age
  - 20-40 years most common
- Gender
  - **Female** predominance (2:1)
- Ethnicity
  - Highest in African & Northern European descent
- Epidemiology
  - Prevalence: 2-60 per 100,000

Natural History & Prognosis

- Remission in 1/2 in 3 years, 2/3 in 10 years

Treatment

- Observation for mild disease, although orbital involvement typically warrants treatment
- Oral **corticosteroids** are treatment of choice
- Other immunosuppressants for recalcitrant disease

DIAGNOSTIC CHECKLIST

Image Interpretation Pearls

- Imaging appearance similar to that of **idiopathic inflammation** and **lymphoproliferative** lesions

SELECTED REFERENCES

1. Rosenbaum JT et al: Parallel gene expression changes in sarcoidosis involving the lacrimal gland, orbital tissue, or blood. JAMA Ophthalmol. 133(7):770-7, 2015
2. Demirci H et al: Orbital and adnexal involvement in sarcoidosis: analysis of clinical features and systemic disease in 30 cases. Am J Ophthalmol. 151(6):1074-1080, 2011
3. Mavrikakis I et al: Diverse clinical presentations of orbital sarcoid. Am J Ophthalmol. 144(5):769-775, 2007

Thyroid-Associated Orbitopathy

TERMINOLOGY

- Graves ophthalmopathy, thyroid eye disease
- Autoimmune orbital inflammation associated with autoimmune thyroid dysfunction

IMAGING

- Bilateral extraocular muscle (EOM) enlargement in typical distribution
  - Nonuniform, symmetric involvement
  - I'M SLO mnemonic for sites of predilection
  - Enlargement of muscle bellies; typically spares tendons
- Heterogeneous areas of internal lower density
- Exophthalmos and increased orbital fat
- T2/STIR signal correlates with disease activity
  - Increase in acute disease due to edema and inflammation
  - Decrease in chronic disease due to involutional changes with fibrosis
- Decreased EOM enhancement compared to normal

TOP DIFFERENTIAL DIAGNOSES

- Idiopathic orbital inflammation
- Orbital sarcoidosis
- Orbital cellulitis
- Lymphoproliferative disease

PATHOLOGY

- Autoimmune inflammation due to thyrotropin receptor autoantigens present in both thyroid gland and orbit
- Orbital fibroblasts and adipocytes involved in T-cell lymphocyte cytokine-mediated inflammation
- Associated with other autoimmune diseases

CLINICAL ISSUES

- Typical patient is middle-aged woman with lid retraction, periorbital edema, proptosis, and restricted gaze
- Orbital disease may not be concordant with thyroid disease
- Corticosteroids 1st line of therapy in acute disease
- Surgery for decompression in severe cases

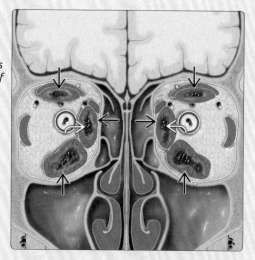
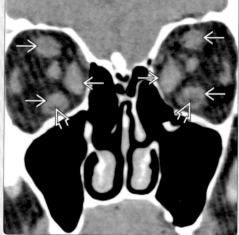

(Left) Coronal graphic shows bilateral symmetric enlargement of extraocular muscles (EOMs) ➡. Irregularity within the muscles ➡ represents accumulation of lymphocytes and mucopolysaccharide deposition. (Right) Coronal NECT shows enlargement of the bilateral inferior, medial, and superior rectus muscles ➡ in a patient with thyroid eye disease. Mucopolysaccharide deposition manifests as areas of low density ➡ within the muscles, particularly inferior recti.

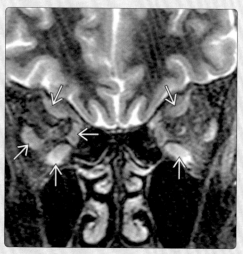
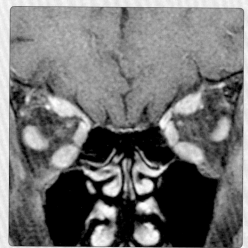

(Left) Coronal STIR MR demonstrates bilateral diffuse enlargement of multiple rectus muscles ➡. Hyperintensity on STIR imaging correlates with acuity of disease, as well as responsiveness to glucocorticoid therapy. (Right) Axial enhanced MR in the same patient with acute thyroid eye disease shows diffuse enlargement of essentially all of the rectus muscles. EOMs affected by acute thyroid orbitopathy typically enhance less intensely than normal muscles.

TERMINOLOGY

Synonyms

- **Graves** ophthalmopathy, thyroid eye disease

Definitions

- **Autoimmune** orbital inflammatory condition associated with autoimmune thyroid dysfunction

IMAGING

General Features

- Best diagnostic clue
  - Bilateral **extraocular muscle** (EOM) enlargement in typical distribution
- Location
  - Nonuniform, symmetric EOM involvement
    - Bilateral in 90%; symmetrical in 70%
    - **I'M SLO** mnemonic for sites of predilection
    - Inferior ≥ medial ≥ superior > lateral ≥ oblique
    - Isolated muscle involvement in 5%
- Size
  - EOM enlargement varies with disease severity
  - Thickness > 5 mm considered abnormal
    - Midbelly thickness correlates with muscle volume
  - Normative EOM thickness (mm) at midbelly (CT data)
    - Inferior: 4.8; medial: 4.2; superior: 4.6; lateral: 3.3
- Morphology
  - Enlargement of **muscle bellies**; typically **spares tendons**, but may be involved in acute phase
  - Increased **orbital fat**, especially in patients < 40 years

CT Findings

- NECT
  - Enlargement of EOM bellies
  - Heterogeneous areas of internal lower density
    - Due to glycosaminoglycan deposition
  - Exophthalmos
    - Line drawn between lateral orbital rims demonstrates degree of exophthalmos
  - Other features
    - Straightened ("stretched") optic nerve
    - Lacrimal gland enlargement

MR Findings

- T1WI
  - Isointense enlargement of EOM bellies
- T2WI FS
  - Increased EOM signal in acute disease
    - Increased water due to edema and inflammation
  - Decreased EOM signal in chronic disease
    - Involutional changes with fibrosis
  - Decreased optic nerve diameter posteriorly
- STIR
  - Signal intensity ratio correlates with clinical activity
    - Correlates with increased muscle volume
- T1WI C+
  - Decreased EOM enhancement compared to normal
    - Impaired microcirculation, decreased perfusion
    - Secondary to intraorbital mass effect

Ultrasonographic Findings

- Grayscale ultrasound
  - Enlarged EOM bellies, spares tendons
  - Internal reflectivity lower in acute disease
    - Edema and inflammation
  - Internal reflectivity higher in chronic disease
    - End-stage changes and fibrosis

Imaging Recommendations

- Best imaging tool
  - CT to assess uncomplicated disease and plan surgical decompression
  - MR to assess disease activity in deciding therapy and to assess optic nerve compromise
  - MR in atypical cases to exclude other pathology
- Protocol advice
  - Imaging not routinely necessary in patients with mild disease if diagnosis is established clinically
  - Volumetric analysis (EOM)
    - Can be used to monitor treatment response
    - Transverse diameter correlates with volume

DIFFERENTIAL DIAGNOSIS

Idiopathic Orbital Inflammation

- Inflammatory changes with painful proptosis and ophthalmoplegia
- Unilateral, often involving lateral rectus; may involve other orbital structures (especially lacrimal gland)

Sarcoidosis

- Orbital disease in 20% of patients with systemic sarcoid
- Granulomatous multifocal orbital enhancement

Orbital Cellulitis

- Proptosis, fever, associated sinus infection (ethmoid)
- Fat infiltration, subperiosteal abscess, myositis

Lymphoproliferative Lesions

- Non-Hodgkin lymphoma, primary to orbit or with systemic disease; MALT variety typical
- Pliable, homogeneously enhancing mass may originate from or infiltrate EOM

Metastasis

- History of known primary
- Isolated or multiple masses within EOM, orbital fat, globe, or bony orbit

PATHOLOGY

General Features

- Etiology
  - Autoimmune inflammation of EOM, periorbital fat, and connective tissues
  - Thyrotropin receptor-like autoantigens present in both thyroid gland and orbital fibroblasts
  - Orbital fibroblasts react to lymphocyte (T-cell) infiltration and cytokine-mediated inflammation
    - Glycosaminoglycan (hyaluron) deposition
    - Fibroblast proliferation, differentiation into adipocytes, and adipogenesis
- Associated abnormalities

- Increased incidence of myasthenia gravis
  - Potential confounding cause of EOM dysfunction
- Associated with other autoimmune diseases

Staging, Grading, & Classification

- Functional classification (clinical severity and risk)
  - Mild: Eyelid lag and retraction with proptosis in setting of active hyperthyroidism
  - Moderate: Soft tissue inflammation, intermittent myopathy, stabilizes without major sequelae
  - Severe: Rapid and fulminant, greater mass effect, severe sequelae including optic nerve compromise
- VISA scheme
  - **Vision**: Specifically, optic neuropathy
  - **Inflammation**: Indicated by pain and swelling
  - **Strabismus**: Limitations in motility
  - **Appearance**: Proptosis, lid function, and exposure

Gross Pathologic & Surgical Features

- Gross enlargement of EOM, increased orbital fat

Microscopic Features

- Mixed cellular infiltration with lymphocytes, plasma cells, macrophages, and eosinophils
- Glycosaminoglycan (hyaluron) deposition
- Enlargement of fibroblasts, increased collagen
- Fibrosis and muscle degeneration in chronic phase

CLINICAL ISSUES

Presentation

- Most common signs/symptoms
  - Eyelid retraction, periorbital edema, proptosis, pain, restricted gaze
- Other signs/symptoms
  - Eyelid lag on downgaze, incomplete closure
  - Dry eyes, chemosis, and corneal ulceration
  - Diplopia, restricted EOM movement, strabismus
  - Dysthyroid optic neuropathy in severe cases
    - Vision loss due to optic nerve compression at apex
- Clinical profile
  - Orbitopathy common in systemic Graves disease
    - 30-50% have clinically evident orbital symptoms
    - 70-90% have orbital involvement if subclinical disease included
    - 5% have severe orbital disease
  - Associated with systemic thyroid disease
    - 80-90% hyperthyroid
    - 10-20% hypothyroid or euthyroid
    - Orbit symptoms precede systemic disease in 20%; coincident in 40%; afterwards in 40%

Demographics

- Age
  - Young and middle-aged adults (30-50 years)
  - Orbitopathy more severe in older patients
  - Graves disease uncommon in children
- Gender
  - F >> M (3-6x more common)
  - More severe and later onset in males
- Ethnicity

- More common and more severe in patients of European descent
- Epidemiology
  - Incidence 1:2,000 to 1:5,000
  - Most common cause of exophthalmos in adults
  - 40% and 25% of Graves patients, with & without eyelid signs, respectively

Natural History & Prognosis

- Orbitopathy often self-limited, favorable outcome
- Significant chronic disease in 10-15%; severe in 5%
- Treatment of systemic thyroid disease may worsen orbitopathy, particularly radioiodine treatment
- Smoking exacerbates orbital disease
  - 15-20% higher recurrence rate

Treatment

- Supportive therapy for early and mild cases
  - Corneal care; observation for vision impairment
- More aggressive therapy for patients with severe inflammation or optic nerve compromise
- Medical therapy
  - Corticosteroids 1st-line therapy in acute disease
    - 85% stabilization and 40% reduction of disease
- Radiation therapy
  - Rapid palliation with 60-70% response
- Surgical therapy
  - Decompression for uncontrolled mass effect
    - Chronic disease, failed medical therapy
    - Resection of lateral orbital walls/orbital floors
    - Muscle volumes may increase following decompression, unrelated to disease reactivation
  - Restoration of eyelid position and function
  - Correction of strabismus

DIAGNOSTIC CHECKLIST

Consider

- Most common cause of exophthalmos in adult
- Typical patient is middle-aged woman

Image Interpretation Pearls

- Fluid-sensitive MR sequence can help differentiate acute edema from late change fibrosis
- MR shows optic nerve compression better than CT

Reporting Tips

- Consider other diagnoses if isolated to lateral rectus

SELECTED REFERENCES

1. Shan SJ et al: The pathophysiology of thyroid eye disease. J Neuroophthalmol. 34(2):177-85, 2014
2. Borumandi F et al: Classification of orbital morphology for decompression surgery in Graves' orbitopathy: two-dimensional versus three-dimensional orbital parameters. Br J Ophthalmol. 97(5):659-62, 2013
3. Dolman PJ et al: Orbital radiotherapy for thyroid eye disease. Curr Opin Ophthalmol. 23(5):427-32, 2012
4. Bahn RS: Graves' ophthalmopathy. N Engl J Med. 362(8):726-38, 2010
5. Dodds NI et al: Use of high-resolution MRI of the optic nerve in Graves' ophthalmopathy. Br J Radiol. 82(979):541-4, 2009
6. Kirsch E et al: Imaging in Graves' orbitopathy. Orbit. 28(4):219-25, 2009

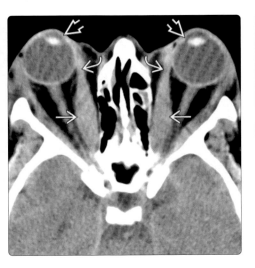
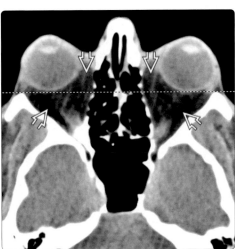

(Left) Axial CECT shows marked thickening of the medial rectus bellies ➡, with relative sparing of the tendinous insertions ➡. The disconjugate orientation of the lenses ➡ is evidence of impaired muscle movement. (Right) Axial NECT in a patient with clinical exophthalmos shows prominent intraorbital fat ➡. The degree of proptosis is made evident by a line drawn between the lateral orbital rims (dotted line).

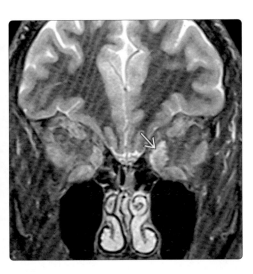
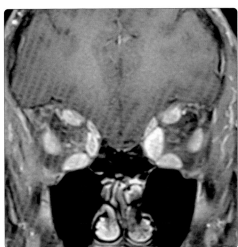

(Left) Coronal STIR MR in a patient with acute thyroid eye disease shows enlargement of multiple EOMs. Regions of more intense signal, such as the left medial rectus ➡, correlate with more active disease and can be used for assessment of treatment response. (Right) Coronal enhanced MR in the same patient demonstrates mild asymmetry of EOM enlargement with otherwise typical distribution. Of note, lateral rectus thickness may be overestimated on coronal images due to oblique course relative to the imaging plane.

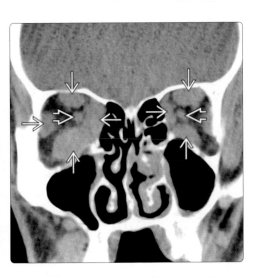
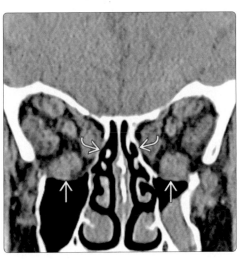

(Left) Coronal NECT in a patient with advanced thyroid eye disease shows marked enlargement of the rectus muscle bellies ➡, worse on the right. This results in crowding at the orbital apex, with the potential for compression of the optic nerves ➡. (Right) Coronal NECT shows diffuse marked enlargement of rectus muscles. In this patient, decompression of the medial ➡ and inferior ➡ orbital walls has been performed to decrease the degree of mass effect on the optic nerves.

Optic Neuritis

IMAGING

- Focal or segmental T2 hyperintensity of optic nerve
- Central or diffuse optic nerve enhancement
- Optic nerve diffusely & mildly enlarged
- Increased diffusivity due to disruption of myelinated axons

TOP DIFFERENTIAL DIAGNOSES

- Ischemic optic neuropathy
- Infectious optic neuritis
- Idiopathic perineuritis (pseudotumor)
- Granulomatous optic neuropathy (sarcoid)
- Optic nerve sheath meningioma
- Optic nerve glioma

PATHOLOGY

- Autoimmune demyelination in susceptible patients
- Triggered by infection, systemic disease, or other stressor
- Nerve edema acutely, atrophy chronically

CLINICAL ISSUES

- Symptoms
  - Acute loss of visual acuity & color vision; eye pain
- Distinct clinical profiles
  - Acute multiple sclerosis-associated optic neuritis (ON)
  - Neuromyelitis optica (Devic syndrome)
  - Acute demyelinating encephalomyelitis (ADEM)
  - Pediatric ON
- Spontaneous recovery of vision is characteristic
- 2x or more as common in female patients

DIAGNOSTIC CHECKLIST

- Identification of demyelinating lesions in CNS is critical neuroimaging task in setting of ON
  - High incidence of MS in patients with ON
  - Findings on MR strongly predictive of MS
- Recommend brain & spinal cord imaging

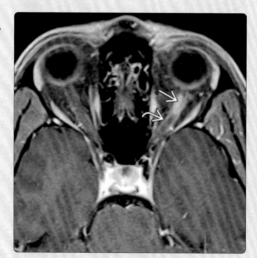

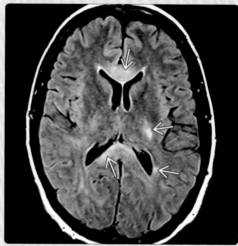

(Left) *Axial T1WI C+ FS MR in an adult woman with left eye pain and decreased color vision shows intense segmental enhancement of the left intraorbital optic nerve ➡. A component of peripheral nerve sheath enhancement is seen extending posteriorly ➡.* (Right) *Axial FLAIR MR of the brain in the same patient shows multiple periatrial, capsular, and callosal white matter lesions ➡. CSF analysis yielded oligoclonal bands, and the patient was diagnosed with multiple sclerosis.*

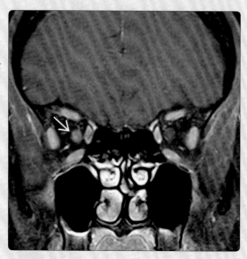

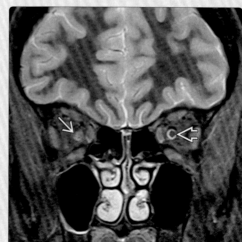

(Left) *Coronal T1WI C+ FS MR in a young adult woman with right eye vision loss, pain, & afferent pupillary defect shows moderate enhancement of the intraorbital optic nerve ➡. There are no other inflammatory changes in the orbit.* (Right) *Coronal STIR MR in the same patient shows increased signal in the right optic nerve ➡. Note that the hyperintense signal of the right nerve is similar to CSF in the optic nerve sheath, whereas the normal left nerve is distinct from the surrounding CSF ➡.*

TERMINOLOGY

Abbreviations

- Optic neuritis (ON)

IMAGING

General Features

- Best diagnostic clue
  - **Enhancement** & mild **enlargement** of optic nerve
- Location
  - **Unilateral** in 70%
    - More commonly bilateral in children
  - Segment(s) of nerve involvement
    - Anterior intraorbital: 45%
    - Mid intraorbital: 60%
    - Intracanalicular: 35%
    - Prechiasmatic & chiasm: 10%
- Size
  - Optic nerve diffusely mildly **enlarged**

CT Findings

- CECT
  - Often normal, may show mild optic nerve enlargement or enhancement

MR Findings

- T1WI
  - Optic nerve diffusely & mildly **enlarged**
- T2WI
  - Focal or segmental **hyperintensity** of optic nerve
  - ± coexistent brain & spinal cord lesions
- STIR
  - Hyperintensity of optic nerves similar to T2WI
- FLAIR
  - ± coexistent **white matter** lesions in brain
    - Presence is **predictor** for **multiple sclerosis** (MS)
    - Especially if increased on early follow-up brain scan
- DWI
  - **Increased diffusivity** in demyelinating plaques
    - Related to disruption of myelinated axons
    - Differentiates acute ON from ischemic optic neuropathy
  - Decreased fractional anisotropy
- T1WI C+
  - **Nerve enhancement** centrally or diffusely > 90%
    - Consistent with active demyelination
  - Variant peripheral sheath enhancement pattern
    - May simulate nerve sheath meningioma
    - Less likely to be associated with MS
- Functional MR
  - Reduced visual cortex activation

Ultrasonographic Findings

- Grayscale ultrasound
  - Mild enlargement of optic nerve

Other Modalities

- Optical coherence tomography (OCT)
  - Decreased retinal nerve fiber layer thickness

Imaging Recommendations

- Best imaging tool
  - Enhanced MR is imaging tool of choice
    - Caveat: Optic nerves, brain, & spinal cord may appear **normal** in early MS
- Protocol advice
  - Thin-section axial & coronal sequences
  - **Fat-suppressed** T2 FSE or STIR & T1 C+
  - Include **whole brain** sagittal & axial FLAIR

DIFFERENTIAL DIAGNOSIS

Ischemic Optic Neuropathy

- Restricted diffusion at nerve head, otherwise often normal
- More likely in **male**, advanced age
- Visual acuity does **not** improve, unlike acute ON

Infectious Optic Neuritis

- Nerve enlargement more pronounced
- May be indistinguishable from ON on imaging

Idiopathic Perineuritis (Pseudotumor)

- Enlarged, enhancing optic nerve-sheath complex
- Inflammation may involve any orbital structure
- **Painful proptosis**; mobility restriction & diplopia

Granulomatous Optic Neuropathy (Sarcoid)

- Enlarged, enhancing optic nerve similar to ON
- EOM & lacrimal gland involvement
- **Intracranial disease** with meningeal enhancement

Optic Nerve Sheath Meningioma

- Thickened, enhancing optic nerve sheath
- "Tram-track" **calcifications** are diagnostic
- Progressive vision loss, **lack of pain**

Optic Nerve Glioma

- **Tubular enlarged, variably enhancing** optic nerve
- NF1 often present but not majority
- Rare malignant optic glioma in adults

Radiation-Induced Optic Neuropathy

- Bilateral optic nerve enhancement
- 1-3 years following radiation
- Pituitary, parasellar, & skull base tumors

Toxic Optic Neuropathy

- Methanol, carbon monoxide, many pharmaceuticals

Other Systemic or Inflammatory Conditions

- SLE, Sjögren syndrome, rheumatoid arthritis, antiphospholipid antibody, paraneoplastic syndrome

PATHOLOGY

General Features

- Etiology
  - Presumed **autoimmune** process
    - T cells & autoreactive antibodies cross blood brain barrier resulting in demyelinating inflammation
    - Infection, systemic disease, or other stressor may be inciting event that triggers autoimmune response
- Genetics

○ HLA alleles associated with risk of developing ON & MS

Staging, Grading, & Classification

- Subtypes of optic neuritis
  - ○ Neuroretinitis
  - ○ Papillitis
    - – Less likely to lead to MS
  - ○ Retrobulbar neuritis
  - ○ Perineuritis
- McDonald criteria
  - ○ Based on clinical, imaging, & CSF findings

Gross Pathologic & Surgical Features

- Nerve edema acutely, atrophy chronically

Microscopic Features

- Acute: Macrophages, lymphocytes, & plasma cells
  - ○ Myelin loss, axonal damage, cholesterol droplets
  - ○ Oligodendrocyte precursors & remyelination attempts suggest potential for intervention
- Chronic: Atrophy, gliosis, astrocytic scar
  - ○ Axonal loss, little remyelination, may cavitate

CLINICAL ISSUES

Presentation

- Most common signs/symptoms
  - ○ Acute loss of visual acuity & eye pain
- Other signs/symptoms
  - ○ Dyschromatopsia (impaired color vision)
  - ○ Vision worse in bright light
  - ○ Phosgenes (light flashes)
  - ○ Eye tenderness or pain with movement
  - ○ Uhthoff symptom: Exertion-induced vision loss
  - ○ Relative afferent pupillary defect
  - ○ Swollen optic disc (papillitis) in 33%
  - ○ Delayed visual evoked potential (VEP) latency
- Clinical profile
  - ○ Typical acute ON
    - – May present as clinically isolated syndrome (CIS)
    - – High risk of developing clinical definite MS (CDMS)
  - ○ Neuromyelitis optica (NMO) = Devic syndrome
    - – Acute ON, typically bilateral, with myelitis
    - – ON more likely to relapse
    - – Seropositive autoantibody marker, NMO-IgG (antibody to aquaporin-4 water channels)
  - ○ Acute demyelinating encephalomyelitis (ADEM)
    - – Clinically isolated syndrome without overt MS
    - – May involve optic nerves primarily or exclusively
  - ○ Pediatric ON
    - – Rare, ≤ 5% of cases
    - – More frequently bilateral (40-60%)
    - – Less likely to develop MS (15-35%)
    - – May follow viral illness or vaccination
    - – More frequently attributable to ADEM
  - ○ Isolated ON
    - – May be solitary, recurrent, or chronic relapsing

Demographics

- Age
  - ○ Presentation 15-50 years, average early 30s

- Gender
  - ○ M:F = 1:2
- Ethnicity
  - ○ Highest prevalence among Northern European ancestry
  - ○ Moderately high with Mediterranean ancestry
  - ○ Low with African or Asian ancestry
- Epidemiology
  - ○ Incidence: 4-6 per 100,000 in USA & Europe
  - ○ 40-60% of ON patients ultimately develop MS
    - – Up 75% of women, 35% of men
  - ○ MR findings highly correlated with subsequent MS
    - – Up to 75% of patients with brain lesions
    - – 25% of patients with normal brain MR
  - ○ 70-90% of MS patients develop ON at some point

Natural History & Prognosis

- Acute symptom onset over hours to days
- Spontaneous **recovery of vision** is characteristic
  - ○ Begins in 2 weeks, continues for months to years
  - ○ Acuity: 70% ≥ 20/25; 80% ≥ 20/30; 90% ≥ 20/40
- ON frequently **initial demyelinating event** in MS
- Recurrent ON is common
  - ○ Overall 35%, more frequent in MS & NMO
  - ○ Recurs in same eye in 20-30%

Treatment

- Corticosteroid treatment (IV with PO taper)
  - ○ Accelerates short-term recovery
  - ○ Does not alter long-term vision outcome
- Optic Neuritis Treatment Trial
  - ○ National Eye Institute sponsored investigation

DIAGNOSTIC CHECKLIST

Consider

- Spontaneous **recovery** of vision is typical
  - ○ Consider other diagnosis if vision remains poor
  - ○ Ischemic neuropathy more likely in older patients

Image Interpretation Pearls

- Identification of demyelinating lesions in CNS is critical neuroimaging task in setting of ON
  - ○ High incidence of MS in patients with ON
  - ○ Findings on MR strongly predictive of MS

Reporting Tips

- Recommend brain & spinal cord imaging

SELECTED REFERENCES

1. Toosy AT et al: Optic neuritis. Lancet Neurol. 13(1):83-99, 2014
2. Swanton JK et al: Early MRI in optic neuritis: the risk for clinically definite multiple sclerosis. Mult Scler. 16(2):156-65, 2010
3. Volpe NJ: The optic neuritis treatment trial: a definitive answer and profound impact with unexpected results. Arch Ophthalmol. 126(7):996-9, 2008
4. Hickman SJ et al: Optic nerve diffusion measurement from diffusion-weighted imaging in optic neuritis. AJNR Am J Neuroradiol. 26(4):951-6, 2005

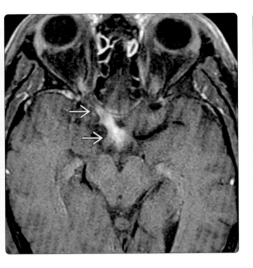

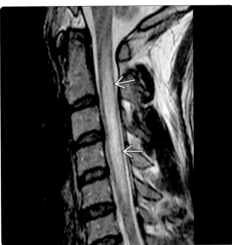

(Left) *Axial T1WI C+ FS MR in a patient with severe acute vision loss shows marked enhancement of the right optic nerve, involving the cisternal segment and extending from the optic canal to the chiasm* ➡. **(Right)** *Sagittal T2WI MR in the same patient also with acute myelopathy shows a long segment of cervical cord enlargement with T2 hyperintensity* ➡. *MR of the brain was normal, and CSF did not show oligoclonal bands. Serum antibody testing confirmed neuromyelitis optica.*

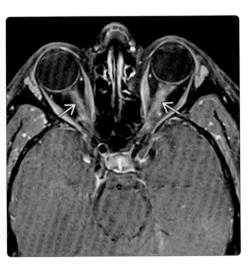

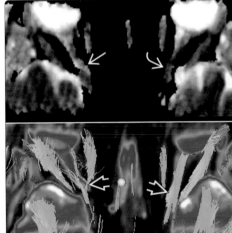

(Left) *Axial T1WI C+ FS MR in a young male patient with blurry vision and eye pain shows patchy enhancement and mild enlargement of the optic nerves* ➡, *worse on the left. CSF and clinical course were consistent with ADEM.* **(Right)** *Axial diffusivity image (above) in a patient with optic neuritis shows increased mean diffusivity in the right optic nerve* ➡ *compared to the left* ➡. *Tractography (below) shows corresponding loss of fiber bundle distinction of the right compared to left optic nerves* ➡.

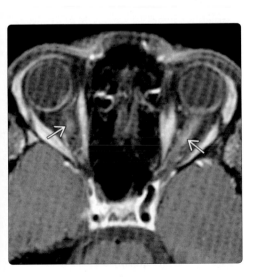

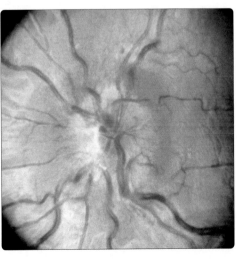

(Left) *Axial T1WI C+ FS MR in a 7-year-old girl with acute vision loss following a viral illness shows bilateral irregular enhancement of the optic nerves* ➡, *worse on the left. CSF analysis was unremarkable, and the patient had an uneventful recovery.* **(Right)** *Funduscopic image in a child with postviral optic neuritis shows the typical appearance of papillitis. The fundus returned to normal after corticosteroid therapy, and the patient did not go on to develop multiple sclerosis.*

Orbital Langerhans Cell Histiocytosis

TERMINOLOGY

- Spectrum of diseases with Langerhans-type histiocytes
- Eosinophilic granuloma: Unifocal, single system
- Hand-Schüller-Christian: Multifocal, single system
- Letterer-Siwe: Multifocal, multisystem

IMAGING

- Orbital disease typically unifocal but may occur in conjunction with multifocal/multisystem disease
- Anterior or lateral orbitofrontal skull most common; greater sphenoid wing common in multifocal disease
- "Punched out" or geographic lytic bone lesion
- Associated soft tissue mass with heterogeneous enhancement
- CT adequate in young patients with localized disease
- MR to assess extensive or intracranial involvement

TOP DIFFERENTIAL DIAGNOSES

- Rhabdomyosarcoma

- Metastasis
- Leukemia

PATHOLOGY

- Unknown etiology (immunoreactive vs. neoplastic)
- Staging
  - Unifocal, unisystem: Bone; older children & adults
  - Multifocal, unisystem: Bone, skin, viscera; young children
  - Multifocal, multisystem: Disseminated, fulminant; infants
- Birbeck granules on electron microscopy

CLINICAL ISSUES

- Periorbital pain and swelling, proptosis
- Local curettage and intralesional corticosteroid injection
  - Excellent prognosis for localized lesions
- Systemic chemotherapy for extensive disease
  - High mortality with disseminated disease

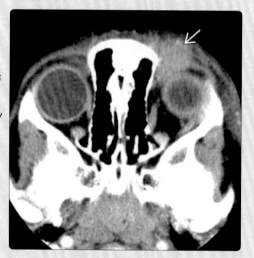
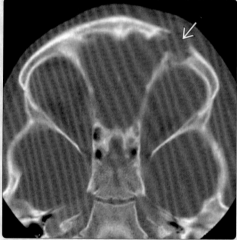

(Left) Axial CECT in a child with focal swelling over left medial eye shows a homogeneously enhancing soft tissue mass ➡ that extends into the subcutaneous soft tissues and medial extraconal orbit. Imaging features on soft tissue window CT are nonspecific. (Right) Axial bone CT in the same patient shows a focal lytic lesion in the frontal bone at the superior orbital rim ➡ with irregular geographic margins. Note the absence of periosteal reaction or calcification.

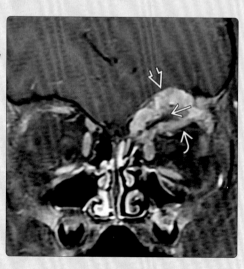
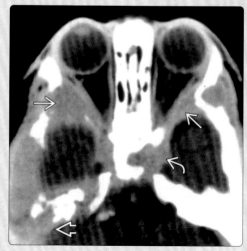

(Left) Coronal T1 C+ FS MR demonstrates a destructive enhancing mass at the left orbital roof ➡. Intraorbital ➡ and intracranial ➡ tumors are present. Intracranial mass has a smooth dural interface, suggesting extradural in location. (Right) Axial CECT in a young child with disseminated Langerhans cell histiocytosis shows bulky soft tissue masses involving the lateral orbits and sphenoid triangle bilaterally ➡, as well as the central skull base ➡ and right temporal bone ➡.

TERMINOLOGY

Synonyms

- Eosinophilic granuloma (EG)
  - Unifocal disease involving single location
- Hand-Schüller-Christian (HSC)
  - Multifocal disease in single organ
- Letterer-Siwe (LS)
  - Multifocal disease involving multiple organs

Definitions

- Spectrum of diseases characterized by proliferation of pathological Langerhans-type **histiocytes**

IMAGING

General Features

- Best diagnostic clue
  - Geographic, **lytic** lesion of skull/orbit with associated enhancing **soft tissue mass**
- Location
  - Orbital disease typically **unifocal** but may occur in conjunction with multifocal/multisystem disease
  - **Anterior** or **lateral** orbitofrontal skull most common
  - Lateral orbital wall and greater sphenoid wing also common, particularly multifocal disease
- Size
  - Ranges from small discrete lesion to diffuse bony involvement
- Morphology
  - **Destructive** bony changes with soft tissue mass

CT Findings

- CECT
  - **Homogeneous** soft tissue mass with diffuse, moderate enhancement
- Bone CT
  - Destructive osteolytic changes
    - Classic "**punched out**" bone lesion with beveled margins
    - May be irregular and **geographic**

MR Findings

- T1WI
  - Isointense to hypointense soft tissue mass
- T2WI
  - Isointense to hyperintense soft tissue mass
- T1WI C+ FS
  - **Diffusely enhancing** soft tissue mass
  - Frequently mildly heterogeneous
  - Intracranial extension with dural involvement

Imaging Recommendations

- Best imaging tool
  - CT adequate in young patients with localized disease
  - MR to assess extensive or intracranial involvement

DIFFERENTIAL DIAGNOSIS

Rhabdomyosarcoma

- Aggressive, destructive primary orbital malignancy

Metastasis

- Particularly neuroblastoma in young children

Leukemia

- Acute myeloid leukemia, chronic lymphotic leukemia, or granulocytic sarcoma

PATHOLOGY

General Features

- Etiology
  - Unknown etiology (**immunoreactive** vs. **neoplastic**)

Staging, Grading, & Classification

- **Unifocal, single system**
  - Bony lesions; older patient population; best prognosis
- **Multifocal, single system**
  - Bone, skin, viscera; younger patient population
- **Multifocal, multisystem involvement**
  - Disseminated, fulminant; infants; worst prognosis

Microscopic Features

- Proliferation of Langerhans cells mixed with **eosinophils**
- Positive **CD1a** and **S100** immunostaining
- Characteristic **Birbeck granules** (electron microscopy)

CLINICAL ISSUES

Presentation

- Most common signs/symptoms
  - Periorbital pain and swelling, proptosis
- Other signs/symptoms
  - Diplopia or nerve palsies due to mass effect
  - Effects on visual acuity may lead to amblyopia in younger patients.

Demographics

- Age
  - EG: 5-20+ years; HSC: 1-4 years; LS: < 2 years
- Gender
  - M:F = **2:1**

Natural History & Prognosis

- Excellent prognosis for localized lesions
- High mortality with disseminated disease

Treatment

- Local **curettage** and **intralesional corticosteroid** injection extremely effective in unifocal lesions
- Systemic **chemotherapy** for extensive disease

DIAGNOSTIC CHECKLIST

Reporting Tips

- Recommend skeletal survey or radionuclide bone scan to exclude multifocal disease

SELECTED REFERENCES

1. Bhanage AB et al: Langerhans cell histiocytosis with presentation as orbital disease. J Pediatr Neurosci. 10(2):162-5, 2015

Orbital Infantile Hemangioma

TERMINOLOGY

- Synonyms: Orbital capillary hemangioma, infantile periocular hemangioma
- Definition: **Benign vascular tumor** of infancy
- Distinct lesion from vascular malformation

IMAGING

- Location: Preseptal &/or postseptal orbit
  - Exclusively retrobulbar in 10%
- CT findings
  - Lobular, slightly hyperdense, homogeneous
  - Intense enhancement
- MR findings
  - T1 intermediate; prominent internal **flow voids**
  - Moderate T2 hyperintensity (high cellularity)
- US: High vessel density, absent arteriovenous shunting, high peak arterial Doppler shift
  - When superficial, US confirms clinical diagnosis
- MR best for mapping larger, deeper lesions

TOP DIFFERENTIAL DIAGNOSES

- Rhabdomyosarcoma
- Metastatic neuroblastoma
- Orbital cellulitis
- Orbital Langerhans cell histiocytosis
- Orbital venous malformation
- Plexiform neurofibroma
- Orbital non-Hodgkin lymphoma

CLINICAL ISSUES

- Distinguish from vascular malformations
  - Present at birth; grow in monophasic fashion
- 3 distinct phases
  - **Proliferative phase**: Appears few weeks after birth and grows rapidly for 1st year or 2
  - **Involuting phase**: Regression over 3-5 years
  - **Involuted phase**: Usually complete regression by late childhood

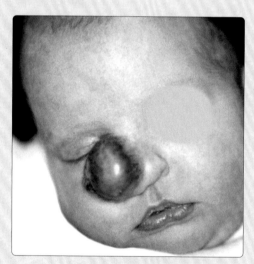
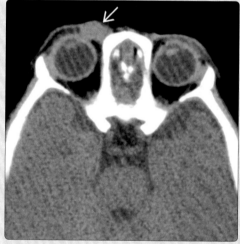

(Left) *Clinical photograph shows a superficial vascular mass centered at the medial orbit and nose, with typical violaceous discoloration seen in infantile hemangioma.* (Right) *Axial CT without contrast demonstrates the most common location for orbital infantile hemangioma, within the superior medial preseptal soft tissues ➡. There is no evidence of postseptal extension.*

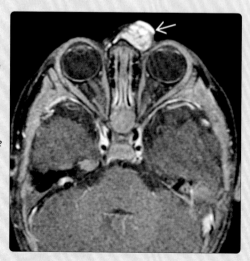
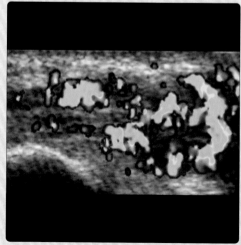

(Left) *Axial enhanced T1WI depicts a well-delineated intensely enhancing infantile hemangioma ➡ with internal septations &/or flow voids in a typical periorbital location. Once again, postseptal extension is absent.* (Right) *Doppler ultrasound in the same patient shows striking internal flow, typical for phase I (proliferating) infantile hemangioma.*

Orbital Infantile Hemangioma

TERMINOLOGY

Synonyms
- Orbital capillary hemangioma, infantile periocular hemangioma

Definitions
- **Benign vascular tumor** of infancy
- Distinct lesion from vascular malformation

IMAGING

General Features
- Best diagnostic clue
  - Lobular or infiltrative, **hypervascular, intensely enhancing** mass in infant
- Location
  - May involve multiple contiguous areas
  - Predilection for eyelids, supranasal periorbita
  - Sites of orbital involvement
    - Most commonly superficial superomedial extraconal location
    - May extend postseptal, into superior orbital fissure or into intraconal space
    - Exclusively retrobulbar in 10%
- Size
  - Variable, small superficial lesions rarely imaged
- Morphology
  - Ranges from lobular to infiltrative
    - Infiltrative pattern typical in postseptal component

CT Findings
- CECT
  - Intense enhancement, usually homogeneous
    - Decreases with involution
  - Prominent vessels during proliferative phase
  - Increasing fat content & septations with involution
  - No calcifications

MR Findings
- T1WI
  - Slightly hyperintense to muscle
  - Internal flow voids
- T2WI
  - Moderate hyperintensity reflects high cellularity
  - **Flow voids** frequently visible
- T1WI C+
  - Diffuse, **intense enhancement**
  - Enhancement may appear heterogeneous, particularly in involuting phase
- MRA
  - Generally not necessary for diagnosis but helpful in assessing associated arterial abnormalities in **PHACES** syndrome (**p**osterior fossa anomalies, **h**emangioma, **a**rterial, **c**ardiac, **e**ye & **s**ternal anomalies)
- MPGR
  - Intralesional high-flow vessels

Ultrasonographic Findings
- Lobular soft tissue mass with high vessel density, high peak arterial Doppler shift, absent arteriovenous (AV) shunting

Angiographic Findings
- Enlarged feeding branches from external carotid, ophthalmic arteries
- Dense parenchymal stain, no AV shunting

Imaging Recommendations
- Best imaging tool
  - When small and superficial, ultrasound may be sufficient to confirm clinical diagnosis
  - MR best for mapping larger, deeper, and more complex lesions
- Protocol advice
  - Enhanced MR in multiple planes with fat suppression best for tumor mapping

DIFFERENTIAL DIAGNOSIS

Rhabdomyosarcoma
- Rapidly progressive invasive orbital mass
- Bone destruction present when large

Metastatic Neuroblastoma
- Rapidly progressive osseous metastatic mass
- Predilection for greater sphenoid wing

Orbital Cellulitis
- Inflammatory changes ± abscess formation

Orbital Langerhans Cell Histiocytosis
- Well-defined, lytic bone lesion with enhancing soft tissue mass in children

Orbital Venous Malformation
- Hypointense T1, hyperintense T2, diffuse contrast enhancement, ± phleboliths

Plexiform Neurofibroma
- Infiltrative + sphenoid dysplasia
- + other stigmata of neurofibromatosis type 1

Orbital Non-Hodgkin Lymphoma
- Multicompartmental infiltrating mass

Orbital Leukemia
- Homogeneous masses that mold to 1 or more orbital walls ± periosteal reaction, usually without frank bone destruction

PATHOLOGY

General Features
- Etiology
  - **Proliferation** of vascular endothelium
    - Grows by endothelial cellular hyperplasia
    - Distinguish from vascular malformation: Localized defect of vascular morphogenesis with quiescent endothelium
- Genetics
  - Most cases sporadic
  - Some associated with pleiotropic genetic syndromes
  - Small percent autosomal dominant
    - Gene map locus 5q35.3, 5q31-q33
- Associated abnormalities

- Large lesions may involve ectodermal structures of face, neck, and airway
  - Parotid involvement common
- PHACES syndrome

Staging, Grading, & Classification

- Classification by location
  - Deep: Within deep tissues of lid and anterior orbit, or entirely retrobulbar
  - Superficial: Confined to dermis
  - Combined: Both dermal and deep components

Gross Pathologic & Surgical Features

- Bluish hue of overlying skin
- May have external or internal carotid arterial supply
- Capable of profuse bleeding

Microscopic Features

- Unencapsulated lobulated **cellular neoplasm**
- Thin-walled, capillary-sized vascular spaces in lobules with thin fibrous septa
  - Venous malformation has larger vascular spaces
- Increased numbers of endothelial and mast cells during proliferative phase
- Decreased cellularity during involutional phase
- Immunohistochemical marker **Glut1-positive in all phases**

CLINICAL ISSUES

Presentation

- Most common signs/symptoms
  - Unilateral eyelid, brow, or nasal vascular lesion
  - Ophthalmologic symptoms common: Amblyopia, astigmatism, proptosis, and decreased visual acuity
    - Risk of amblyopia highest when diffuse, > 1 cm in size, and associated with PHACES syndrome
- Clinical profile
  - Rubbery, soft mass
  - **Bluish discoloration of skin** or conjunctiva (80%)
    - Blanche with pressure, unlike port-wine stain
  - Enlarge with Valsalva or crying in 50%
  - Occasional periorbital fat excess following involution

Demographics

- Age
  - Typically not present at birth; most **appear within 1st few weeks**
    - Vascular malformations present at birth, deep lesions may not become apparent until later in life
- Gender
  - M:F 1:2-3
  - Even higher female predominance in genetic syndromes
- Epidemiology
  - Affects about 1% of neonates

Natural History & Prognosis

- 3 distinct phases
  - **Proliferative phase**: Appears few weeks after birth and grows rapidly for 1st year or 2
  - **Involuting phase**: Regression over 3-5 years
  - **Involuted phase**: Usually complete regression by late childhood

- Distinguish from vascular malformations: Present at birth & grow in monophasic fashion with age
- Variants: Noninvoluting congenital hemangioma (**NICH**) and rapidly involuting congenital hemangioma (**RICH**)
  - Present at or before birth, Glut1-negative

Treatment

- Expectant observation unless complications
- Indications for treatment
  - Ophthalmologic: Visual disturbance, nerve compromise, proptosis
  - Dermatologic: Ulceration, infection, cosmesis
- Propanolol now recognized as very effective treatment
- Corticosteroids: Intralesional, systemic, or topical administration
- Intratumoral laser therapy in larger lesions
- Interferon, vincristine, surgical resection, or laser ablation for recalcitrant lesions
- Intravascular embolization contraindicated for intraorbital lesions

DIAGNOSTIC CHECKLIST

Consider

- Remember differential diagnosis for rapidly growing mass in infant includes malignancy

Image Interpretation Pearls

- US can provide easy bedside evaluation
- In appropriate age group, cellular enhancing mass with prominent flow voids nearly diagnostic

Reporting Tips

- Map lesion with particular reference to critical structures in orbit & intracranial compartment

SELECTED REFERENCES

1. Stass-Isern M: Periorbital and orbital infantile hemangiomas. Int Ophthalmol Clin. 54(3):73-82, 2014
2. Xu S et al: Treatment of periorbital infantile haemangiomas: a systematic literature review on propranolol or steroids. J Paediatr Child Health. 50(4):271-9, 2014
3. Drolet BA et al: Initiation and use of propranolol for infantile hemangioma: report of a consensus conference. Pediatrics. 131(1):128-40, 2013
4. Frank RC et al: Visual development in infants: visual complications of periocular haemangiomas. J Plast Reconstr Aesthet Surg. 63(1):1-8, 2010
5. Nguyen J et al: Pharmacologic therapy for periocular infantile hemangiomas: a review of the literature. Semin Ophthalmol. 24(3):178-84, 2009
6. Chan LK et al: The management of periorbital fat excess in haemangioma involution. J Plast Reconstr Aesthet Surg. 61(2):133-7, 2008
7. Léauté-Labrèze C et al: Propranolol for severe hemangiomas of infancy. N Engl J Med. 358(24):2649-51, 2008
8. Tronina SA et al: Combined surgical method of orbital and periorbital hemangioma treatment in infants. Orbit. 27(4):249-57, 2008
9. Weiss AH et al: Reappraisal of astigmatism induced by periocular capillary hemangioma and treatment with intralesional corticosteroid injection. Ophthalmology. 115(2):390-397, 2008
10. Chung EM et al: From the archives of the AFIP: pediatric orbit tumors and tumorlike lesions: nonosseous lesions of the extraocular orbit. Radiographics. 27(6):1777-99, 2007
11. Judd CD et al: Intracranial infantile hemangiomas associated with PHACE syndrome. AJNR Am J Neuroradiol. 28(1):25-9, 2007
12. Levi M et al: Surgical treatment of capillary hemangiomas causing amblyopia. J AAPOS. 11(3):230-4, 2007
13. Reddy AR et al: Is this really a capillary haemangioma? Orbit. 26(4):327-9, 2007

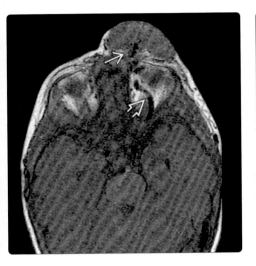
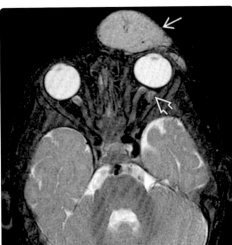

(Left) *Axial T1WI MR in a large supraorbital infantile hemangioma reveals prominent internal flow voids* ➡ *and enlargement of the superior ophthalmic vein* ⇉, *which serves as the primary venous drainage pathway.* (Right) *Axial T2WI MR of a large infantile hemangioma in a similar location* ➡ *demonstrates a small lobular retrobulbar component* ⇶. *Careful inspection of the postseptal soft tissues is critical when reviewing imaging studies in periorbital hemangioma.*

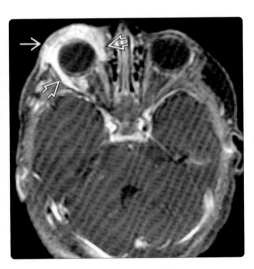
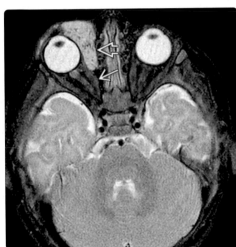

(Left) *Pre-* ➡ *and postseptal* ⇶ *components are present in this child with right orbital hemangioma demonstrating typical intense enhancement. While some lesions are lobular and well demarcated, others show a more infiltrative pattern.* (Right) *The medial rectus muscle* ➡ *is displaced medially by this infantile hemangioma with postseptal component* ⇶, *confirming extraconal location. Though the lesion appears "soft" and is deformed by the globe, subtle globe deviation and distortion are present.*

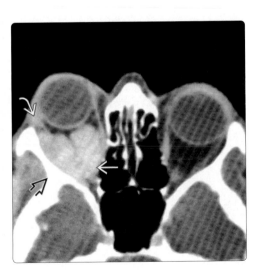
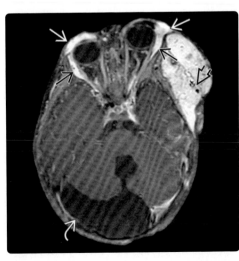

(Left) *Axial CECT demonstrates an intensely enhancing, lobular, primarily retrobulbar hemangioma. The mass is multicompartmental, with intraconal* ➡ *and extraconal* ⇶ *components, as well as a small superficial preseptal component laterally* ⬈. *The globe is markedly proptotic.* (Right) *Axial T1 C+ FS MR shows a child with PHACES syndrome. Bilateral orbital hemangiomas have preseptal* ➡ *and postseptal* ⇨ *components. The component in the masticator space has flow voids* ⇶. *Note cerebellar asymmetry* ⬈.

TERMINOLOGY

- Optic pathway glioma (OPG)
- Primary neuroglial tumor of optic pathway
- 3 broad subtypes
  - Childhood syndromic [neurofibromatosis type 1 (NF1)], childhood sporadic, adult

IMAGING

- Fusiform optic nerve (ON) mass with variable posterior pathway involvement
  - Sporadic lesions tend to be larger and cause more distortion of normal morphology than syndromic lesions
- MR is preferred imaging modality
  - Isointense to mildly hypointense on T1WI
  - Variably hyperintense on T2WI
  - Enhancement varies from minimal to intense
- Associated neuroimaging findings in NF1
  - ↑ T2 foci in brain, other central nervous system tumors, sphenoid dysplasia, buphthalmos

TOP DIFFERENTIAL DIAGNOSES

- Optic neuritis
- ON sheath meningioma
- Idiopathic orbital inflammatory pseudotumor
- Sarcoidosis

PATHOLOGY

- Childhood OPG: Low-grade glioma
- Adult OPG: Anaplastic astrocytoma or glioblastoma multiforme

CLINICAL ISSUES

- Decreased vision, proptosis; often asymptomatic
- Childhood OPG: Onset 0.5-15.0 years
- 30-40% of patients with OPG have NF1
- 11-30% of patients with NF1 have OPG
- Natural history highly variable, but generally indolent in childhood OPG

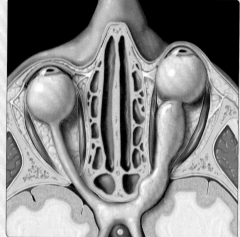
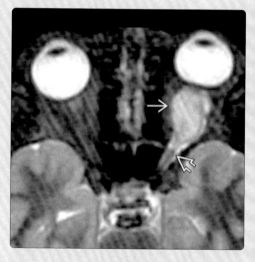

(Left) Axial graphic depicts a left optic pathway glioma (OPG) extending along the length of the intraorbital nerve, through the enlarged optic canal, and into the prechiasmatic segment. The fusiform pattern of enlargement is typical. (Right) Axial T2WI FS MR shows fusiform enlargement and buckling of the left intraorbital optic nerve (ON) resulting in mild proptosis. The tumor ➡ is hyperintense on T2WI, as is typical for OPG. Note normal cerebrospinal fluid ➡ in the sheath posterior to the tumor.

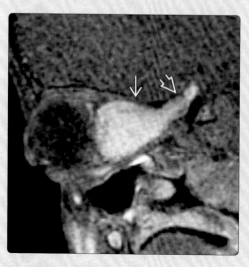
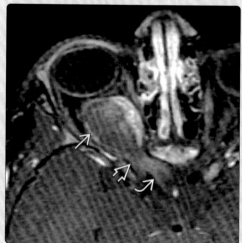

(Left) Oblique sagittal T1WI C+ FS MR reveals globular enlargement and intense homogeneous enhancement of intraorbital ON ➡ extending posteriorly into widened optic canal ➡. (Right) Axial T1WI C+ FS MR shows mild, patchy enhancement and marked fusiform enlargement of intraorbital ➡, intracanalicular ➡, and prechiasmatic ➡ segments of right ON. Lesions in children with neurofibromatosis type 1 (NF1) may demonstrate only minimal contrast enhancement.

TERMINOLOGY

Abbreviations

- Optic pathway glioma (OPG)

Synonyms

- Optic nerve glioma; anterior visual pathway glioma

Definitions

- Primary neuroglial tumor of optic pathway
- 3 broad subtypes
  o Childhood benign tumors: **With** neurofibromatosis type 1 (**NF1**), syndromic 30-40%
  o Childhood benign tumors: **Without** NF1 (sporadic)
  o Adult tumors: Typically malignant

IMAGING

General Features

- Best diagnostic clue
  o Fusiform optic nerve (ON) mass with variable posterior pathway involvement
- Location
  o **Childhood lesions with NF1 (syndromic)**
    – Anterior pathways, unilateral or bilateral
    – Bilateral highly associated with NF1
    – 50% extend to chiasm, hypothalamus, and retrochiasmal optic pathways
    – Optic radiation involvement is rare
  o **Childhood lesions without NF1 (sporadic)**
    – Affects chiasm and retrochiasmal segment predominantly
  o **Adult lesions**
    – Unilateral ON with posterior extension
- Size
  o Syndromic (with NF1): 0.5-2.0 cm long
  o Sporadic (without NF1): 1-8 cm long
  o Adult lesions: Varies depending on posterior extent
- Morphology
  o General
    – Diffuse **sausage-shaped or fusiform** enlargement of nerve and chiasm
    – Characteristic kinking or buckling of nerve
  o Syndromic: Smooth, tubular, tortuous ON enlargement
  o Sporadic: Smooth, nodular, with cystic components
  o Adult: Diffuse ON enlargement, invasive features
- Associated neuroimaging findings if NF1 present: ↑ T2 foci in brain, other central nervous system (CNS) tumors, sphenoid dysplasia, buphthalmos, plexiform neurofibromas

CT Findings

- NECT
  o Isodense fusiform nerve enlargement; focal hypodensity if cystic spaces
- Bone CT
  o Ca^{2+} rare (unlike ON sheath meningioma)
  o Enlargement of bony optic canal if intracranial extension

MR Findings

- T1WI
  o Isointense to mildly hypointense compared to brain
  o Focal hypointensity if cystic spaces present
- T2WI
  o Signal is variable, but moderate hyperintensity typical
  o Peripheral hyperintensity due to perineural arachnoid gliomatosis (PAG) in NF1
  o Focally hyperintense cystic spaces of mucinous degeneration in sporadic cases
- DWI
  o Elevated mean ADC values have been demonstrated
- T1WI C+
  o Enhancement varies from minimal to intense
    – Syndromic: Often little enhancement
    – Sporadic: Moderate to intense enhancement
    – Adult: Moderate heterogeneous enhancement
  o DCE MR: Increased mean permeability values demonstrated in clinically aggressive tumors

Imaging Recommendations

- Best imaging tool
  o MR is preferred imaging modality
    – Defines involvement of proximal optic pathways
    – Allows assessment of related intracranial findings in patients with NF1

DIFFERENTIAL DIAGNOSIS

Optic Neuritis

- Acute-onset pain and vision loss
- Enhancing ON with minimal nerve enlargement

ON Sheath Meningioma

- Slow-onset proptosis and ↓ vision in adult
- Perineural mass, may be calcified

Idiopathic Orbital Inflammatory Pseudotumor

- Painful proptosis, mass-like inflammation
- Can involve any structure in orbit
- Variable imaging appearance, including perineural enhancement

Sarcoidosis

- Systemic illness, orbital inflammation
- Predilection for lacrimal gland
- ON, orbital, and intracranial enhancement

PATHOLOGY

General Features

- Genetics
  o NF1 (if present): Autosomal dominant with variable penetrance and variable clinical expressivity
- Associated abnormalities
  o Focal brain T2 hyperintensities in NF1 patients
    – Seen in 80-90% of NF1 patients who have OPG
    – Seen in 50-70% of all NF1 patients
  o Other CNS tumors in NF1 patients (most commonly low-grade astrocytomas)

Staging, Grading, & Classification

- Low-grade gliomas
  o Vast majority of childhood lesions
  o 60% WHO grade I pilocytic astrocytoma
  o 40% WHO grade II fibrillary astrocytoma

- o In NF1, tumor may represent PAG rather than true astrocytoma
- High-grade gliomas
  - o Most adult lesions, occasionally childhood lesions
  - o Anaplastic astrocytoma, glioblastoma multiforme
- Dodge classification defines locoregional extent of tumor
  - o Stage A: Limited to 1 ON
  - o Stage B: Involves chiasm ± ON
  - o Stage C: Extends toward hypothalamus or posterior visual pathways

Gross Pathologic & Surgical Features

- Diffuse ON enlargement; tan-white tumor
- Cystic component related to mucinous degeneration or infarction

Microscopic Features

- Syndromic: Circumferential perineural infiltration with arachnoid gliomatosis
  - o Central nerve sparing (relatively preserved vision)
- Sporadic: Expansile intraneural infiltration

CLINICAL ISSUES

Presentation

- Most common signs/symptoms
  - o Decreased vision
- Other signs/symptoms
  - o Proptosis, optic atrophy
  - o Nystagmus
  - o Intracranial mass effect
- Clinical profile
  - o Childhood OPG
    - – Syndromic: Frequently asymptomatic; lesions detected on routine imaging
    - – Sporadic: Larger, more aggressive
  - o Adult OPG
    - – Aggressive course with rapid deterioration of vision

Demographics

- Age
  - o Childhood: Onset 0.5-15.0 years (mean: 5 years)
  - o Adult: Onset 20-80 years (mean: 50 years)
- Gender
  - o Slight female predominance in childhood OPG
- Epidemiology
  - o Childhood benign lesions
    - – 3% of orbital tumors; 5% of intracranial tumors
    - – 30-40% of patients with OPG have NF1
    - – 11-30% of patients with NF1 have OPG
  - o Adult malignant lesions: Very rare

Natural History & Prognosis

- Natural history highly variable
  - o Ranges from spontaneous regression to progressive visual and neurologic impairment, culminating in death
- Syndromic: Generally indolent course, progression typically stops by age 6, though can continue to age 12
  - o Progression most frequent first 2 years following diagnosis
  - o Spontaneous regression can occur
- Sporadic: Less indolent, more intervention required

- o Shorter time to relapse
- Adult: Poor prognosis, rapidly fatal
- Specific location impacts prognosis
  - o Rate of complications and death
    - – Optic chiasm/retrochiasmal gliomas > ON gliomas

Treatment

- Childhood lesions with NF1
  - o Biopsy generally not required; **presumptive diagnosis**
  - o Observation unless vision threatened
  - o Chemotherapy is first line for tumor progression
  - o Radiation therapy (XRT) and surgery reserved for patients with bulky tumor or older children with progressive disease
    - – XRT complications: Secondary tumors, radiation necrosis, moyamoya disease, impaired growth, cognitive deficits
- Childhood lesions without NF1
  - o Biopsy typically indicated
  - o Surgical debulking for large tumors when there is severe visual loss and proptosis
  - o Adjunctive radiation ± chemotherapy
- Adult OPG
  - o Multimodality therapy

DIAGNOSTIC CHECKLIST

Consider

- Clinical and imaging features vary with specific subtype: Syndromic, sporadic, adult
- Bilateral intraorbital lesions indicate syndromic disease (NF1)

SELECTED REFERENCES

1. Aquilina K et al: Optic pathway glioma in children: does visual deficit correlate with radiology in focal exophytic lesions? Childs Nerv Syst. 31(11):2041-9, 2015
2. Shofty B et al: The effect of chemotherapy on optic pathway gliomas and their sub-components: a volumetric MR analysis study. Pediatr Blood Cancer. 62(8):1353-9, 2015
3. Nicolin G et al: Natural history and outcome of optic pathway gliomas in children. Pediatr Blood Cancer. 53(7):1231-7, 2009
4. Schupper A et al: Optic-pathway glioma: natural history demonstrated by a new empirical score. Pediatr Neurol. 40(6):432-6, 2009
5. Jost SC et al: Diffusion-weighted and dynamic contrast-enhanced imaging as markers of clinical behavior in children with optic pathway glioma. Pediatr Radiol. 38(12):1293-9, 2008
6. Taylor T et al: Radiological classification of optic pathway gliomas: experience of a modified functional classification system. Br J Radiol. 81(970):761-6, 2008
7. Walrath JD et al: Magnetic resonance imaging evidence of optic nerve glioma progression into and beyond the optic chiasm. Ophthal Plast Reconstr Surg. 24(6):473-5, 2008
8. Lee AG: Neuroophthalmological management of optic pathway gliomas. Neurosurg Focus. 23(5):E1, 2007
9. Zeid JL et al: Orbital optic nerve gliomas in children with neurofibromatosis type 1. J AAPOS. 10(6):534-9, 2006
10. Liu GT et al: Optic radiation involvement in optic pathway gliomas in neurofibromatosis. Am J Ophthalmol. 137(3):407-14, 2004
11. Thiagalingam S et al: Neurofibromatosis type 1 and optic pathway gliomas: follow-up of 54 patients. Ophthalmology. 111(3):568-77, 2004
12. Laithier V et al: Progression-free survival in children with optic pathway tumors: dependence on age and the quality of the response to chemotherapy–results of the first French prospective study for the French Society of Pediatric Oncology. J Clin Oncol. 21(24):4572-8, 2003

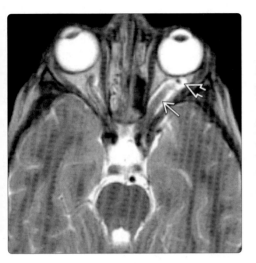

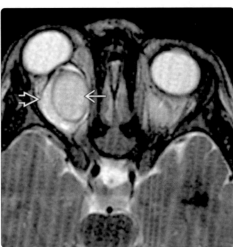

(Left) Axial T2W MR shows abnormal thickness of left intraorbital ON ➡. The optic sheath anterior to the tumor is kinked and dilated ➡. (Right) Axial T2WI MR demonstrates enlargement and moderate T2 hyperintensity of the intraorbital segment of the right ON ➡. A peripheral zone of higher signal intensity ➡ is compatible with associated arachnoid hyperplasia.

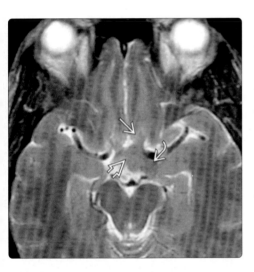

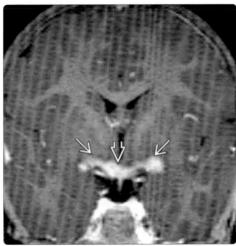

(Left) Axial T2WI MR shows an OPG involving the intracranial prechiasmatic segment ➡, chiasm ➡ and left optic tract ➡. OPGs typically demonstrate higher T2 signal than this isointense lesion. (Right) Coronal T1 C+ MR demonstrates vivid enhancement of the chiasm ➡ and bilateral proximal optic tracts ➡ in a patient with bilateral OPGs. The degree of contrast enhancement is extremely variable in OPGs.

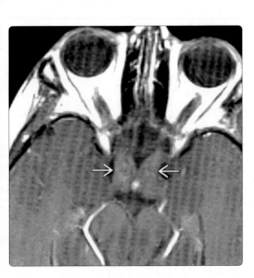

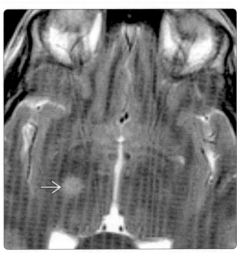

(Left) Axial T1WI C+ MR shows diffuse enlargement of the prechiasmatic and chiasmatic segments of the bilateral ONs ➡, with only minimal patchy enhancement. The presence of bilateral optic gliomas generally heralds the diagnosis of NF1. (Right) Axial T2WI MR of the brain demonstrates a rounded, high signal lesion in the basal ganglia ➡, typical for NF1. These lesions do not demonstrate significant enhancement.

Optic Nerve Sheath Meningioma

TERMINOLOGY

- Optic nerve sheath meningioma
  - Also known as perioptic meningioma
- Benign, slow-growing tumor of optic nerve sheath
- Distinct entity from intracranial (spheno-orbital) meningioma that extends through orbital apex

IMAGING

- Uniformly enhancing mass surrounding intraorbital optic nerve with Ca++ in 1/3 to 1/2 of cases
- Tram-track pattern of enhancement or Ca++ around optic nerve
- Variably hyperintense to hypointense on T2WI

TOP DIFFERENTIAL DIAGNOSES

- Optic nerve glioma
- Orbital pseudotumor
- Orbital sarcoidosis
- Metastasis

- Orbit lymphoproliferative lesions

PATHOLOGY

- Benign tumor arising from arachnoid "cap" cells within optic nerve sheath
- Histologic subtypes and degree of calcification affect signal intensity on T2WI MR

CLINICAL ISSUES

- Classic triad: Visual loss, optic atrophy, optociliary venous shunting
- Fractionated radiotherapy currently 1st-line therapy, radiosurgery also being explored

DIAGNOSTIC CHECKLIST

- MR is preferred imaging modality, but look for Ca++ on CT when diagnosis in doubt
- Look for other findings of neurofibromatosis type 2, especially in pediatric patients

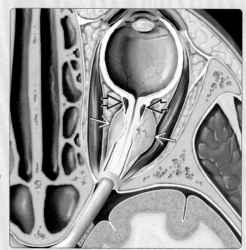
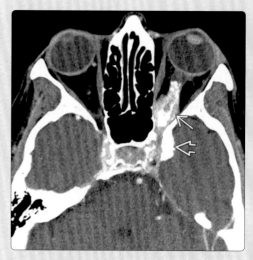

(Left) Axial graphic depicts a fusiform meningioma ➡ arising from the optic nerve sheath. Characteristic "perioptic cyst" ➡ behind the globe represents trapped cerebrospinal fluid (CSF) within nerve sheath. (Right) Axial CECT shows enhancing optic nerve sheath meningioma (ONSM) ➡ with punctate and linear calcification surrounding left optic nerve complex extending through orbital apex. Note adjacent hyperostosis ➡.

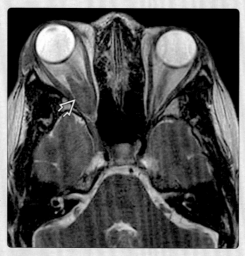
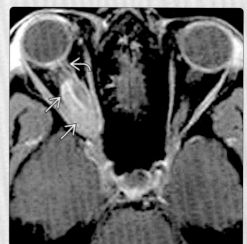

(Left) Axial T2WI FS MR reveals a globular meningioma involving intraorbital segment of right optic nerve ➡. Note T2 signal similar to brain parenchyma. Though SI may be variable, ONSMs, like intracranial lesions, are often relatively hypointense on T2WI. (Right) Axial T1WI FS MR demonstrates globular configuration of avidly enhancing ONSM ➡ eccentrically surrounding orbital segment of right optic nerve. Note tumor spares optic nerve immediately posterior to globe ➡, a common pattern.

TERMINOLOGY

Abbreviations

- Optic nerve sheath meningioma (ONSM)

Synonyms

- Perioptic meningioma

Definitions

- Benign, slow-growing neoplasm of optic nerve (ON) dural sheath
- Distinct entity from intracranial (spheno-orbital) meningioma that extends through orbital apex
  - 90% of meningiomas that involve orbit are secondary lesions rather than primary ONSM

IMAGING

General Features

- Best diagnostic clue
  - Enhancing mass surrounding intraorbital ON with Ca++
- Location
  - Intraconal or orbital apex mass that arises from ON sheath complex
- Size
  - Intraorbital ONSM relatively small at presentation because of early symptoms
  - Spheno-orbital tumors have larger intracranial component
- Morphology
  - Solid, well-defined enlargement of ON complex
  - Encases ON in circumferential pattern but may be eccentric or pedunculated
  - Tubular shape (65%) > pedunculated (25%) > fusiform (10%)
    - Diffuse thickening more common than segmental
    - En plaque variants may occur

CT Findings

- NECT
  - Linear or punctate Ca++ characteristic in 1/3-1/2 cases
    - Typically spares distal segment of ON at nerve head insertion
  - If no Ca++, tumor is isodense to other soft tissue
- CECT
  - Uniform, moderately intense enhancement
  - **Tram-track** appearance: Tumor enhancement or Ca++ around ON
    - Although relatively specific, tram-track enhancement **not** pathognomonic
      - Pseudotumor, lymphoma, or sarcoid have peripheral perioptic enhancement

MR Findings

- T1WI
  - Isointense to other soft tissue
- T2WI
  - Variably hyperintense to hypointense depending on degree of Ca++ and histologic subtype
  - "**Perioptic cysts**" are specific feature
    - Defined as ↑ cerebrospinal fluid within nerve sheath surrounding distal ON between tumor and globe

- STIR
  - Similar to T2 but lesions more conspicuous because of suppression of orbital fat signal
- T1WI C+
  - Uniform moderate to marked enhancement of tumor with central nonenhancing ON
  - Tumor best demonstrated with fat suppression

Imaging Recommendations

- Best imaging tool
  - Contrast-enhanced MR with fat suppression
    - MR better than CT for characterizing tumor relative to adjacent orbital structures
    - MR best shows extent of disease involving orbital apex, optic canal, optic nerve chiasm, and intracranial structures
  - CT may help in indeterminate cases by demonstrating Ca++
- Protocol advice
  - Postcontrast, fat-suppressed T1WI delineates tumor margins best
  - Perioptic cysts best demonstrated on T2WI with fat saturation

DIFFERENTIAL DIAGNOSIS

Optic Nerve Glioma

- Neoplastic enlargement of ON
- No tram-track enhancement, Ca++, or perioptic cysts
- Typically low-grade pediatric tumor (ONSM usually adult tumor)
- May be associated with neurofibromatosis type 1 (NF1); ONSM with NF2

Optic Neuritis

- T2 hyperintense, enhancing ON with minimal nerve enlargement or patchy sheath enhancement
- Often associated with inflammatory and demyelinating processes such as multiple sclerosis

Orbital Idiopathic Inflammatory Pseudotumor

- Ill-defined and usually not isolated to ON sheath
- Presents with painful exophthalmos

Orbital Sarcoidosis

- When no systemic disease, can be indistinguishable from ONSM on enhanced CT and MR
- Predilection for lacrimal glands

Metastasis

- Breast and lung most common primaries
- Often involve choroid and extraocular muscles

Orbit Lymphoproliferative Lesions

- Usually not isolated to nerve sheath
- Typically well-defined, pliable mass
- ↓ T2 signal due to high cellularity

PATHOLOGY

General Features

- Etiology
  - Benign tumor arising from **arachnoid "cap" cells** within ON sheath

- Genetics
  - **NF2** present in 4-12% of patients
    - 28% of juveniles diagnosed with ONSM are concomitantly diagnosed with NF2
- Associated abnormalities
  - Patients with NF2 show characteristic findings, such as bilateral vestibular schwannoma

Staging, Grading, & Classification

- Same WHO classification as for intracranial meningiomas

Gross Pathologic & Surgical Features

- Sharply circumscribed, unencapsulated
- Circumferential to ON
- Tightly adherent to perineural pial microvascular structures
  - Rarely invades ON

Microscopic Features

- Histologic features similar to intracranial meningiomas
- Meningothelial subtype most common in orbit
- Transitional (54%) and meningotheliomatous (38%) subtypes most common in children
- Positive for progesterone receptors in 40-80%, more so in women
- Fibroblastic and transitional subtypes tend to be hypointense to cerebral cortex on T2WI MR

CLINICAL ISSUES

Presentation

- Most common signs/symptoms
  - Slow, usually painless, progressive unilateral vision loss and proptosis
  - Central vision preserved until late in disease
- Other signs/symptoms
  - Diplopia, transient visual obscuration, headache
  - Funduscopic examination
    - Optic disc pallor and swelling typical
    - Optociliary venous shunting in association with optic disc changes very suggestive of ONSM
- Clinical profile
  - Classic triad: Visual loss, optic atrophy, optociliary venous shunting

Demographics

- Age
  - Typically presents in 4th and 5th decades, but broad age range
  - ONSM in juvenile patients has distinct natural history
    - Average age at presentation: 10 years
    - More likely associated with NF2
- Gender
  - F:M ~ 2:1 to 4:1
    - In children, slightly more common in boys
- Epidemiology
  - ~ 5% of primary orbital tumors
  - Only 2% of meningiomas are ONSM
  - Radiation exposure, hereditary predisposition, and hormonal influence are cited risk factors

Natural History & Prognosis

- Progressive but slow vision loss expected in most untreated patients
- More aggressive behavior in juvenile patients
  - Relative increased size, growth, recurrence rates, and incidence of malignant degeneration
- Postoperative visual impairment inevitable as tumor tightly adherent to pia and shares blood supply

Treatment

- **Fractionated stereotactic radiotherapy** (and more recently radiosurgery) used when vision still present but visual loss progressive
- Observation with regular visual testing and MR surveillance recommended if vision normal and stable
- Surgical excision indicated if intracranial extension or if vision preservation impossible
  - Generally poor results with optic canal or ON sheath decompression

DIAGNOSTIC CHECKLIST

Consider

- ON nerve glioma is major differential consideration in young patients
- When imaging appearance characteristic, radiation therapy without biopsy may provide best chance of vision preservation

Image Interpretation Pearls

- MR is preferred imaging modality for tumor assessment
  - CT shows Ca^{++} when diagnosis in doubt

SELECTED REFERENCES

1. Conti A et al: CyberKnife multisession stereotactic radiosurgery and hypofractionated stereotactic radiotherapy for perioptic meningiomas: intermediate-term results and radiobiological considerations. Springerplus. 4:37, 2015
2. Vanikieti K et al: Pediatric primary optic nerve sheath meningioma. Int Med Case Rep J. 8:159-63, 2015
3. Shapey J et al: Diagnosis and management of optic nerve sheath meningiomas. J Clin Neurosci. 20(8):1045-56, 2013
4. Milker-Zabel S et al: Fractionated stereotactic radiation therapy in the management of primary optic nerve sheath meningiomas. J Neurooncol. 94(3):419-24, 2009
5. Wilhelm H: Primary optic nerve tumours. Curr Opin Neurol. 22(1):11-8, 2009
6. Harold Lee HB et al: Primary optic nerve sheath meningioma in children. Surv Ophthalmol. 53(6):543-58, 2008
7. Eddleman CS et al: Optic nerve sheath meningioma: current diagnosis and treatment. Neurosurg Focus. 23(5):E4, 2007
8. Miller NR: New concepts in the diagnosis and management of optic nerve sheath meningioma. J Neuroophthalmol. 26(3):200-8, 2006
9. Miller NR: Primary tumours of the optic nerve and its sheath. Eye. 18(11):1026-37, 2004
10. Jackson A et al: Intracanalicular optic nerve meningioma: a serious diagnostic pitfall. AJNR Am J Neuroradiol. 24(6):1167-70, 2003
11. Narayan S et al: Preliminary visual outcomes after three-dimensional conformal radiation therapy for optic nerve sheath meningioma. Int J Radiat Oncol Biol Phys. 56(2):537-43, 2003
12. Saeed P et al: Optic nerve sheath meningiomas. Ophthalmology. 110(10):2019-30, 2003
13. Turbin RE et al: A long-term visual outcome comparison in patients with optic nerve sheath meningioma managed with observation, surgery, radiotherapy, or surgery and radiotherapy. Ophthalmology. 109(5):890-9; discussion 899-900, 2002
14. Ortiz O et al: Radiologic-pathologic correlation: meningioma of the optic nerve sheath. AJNR Am J Neuroradiol. 17(5):901-6, 1996

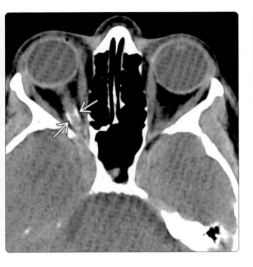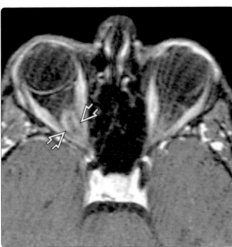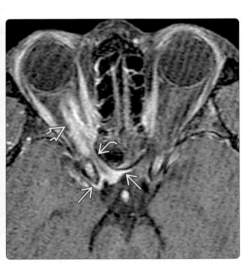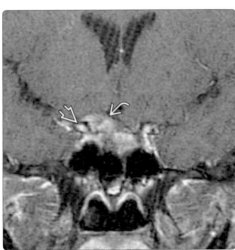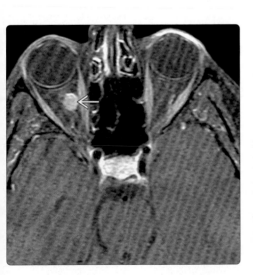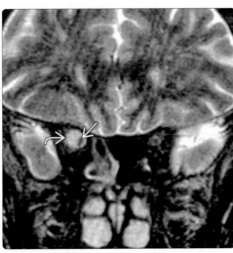

(Left) Axial NECT shows typical tram-track calcifications ➡ of ONSM without obvious soft tissue mass. Occasionally, posttraumatic or idiopathic optic nerve sheath calcification can mimic this appearance. (Right) Axial T1WI C+ FS MR, same patient, shows typical optic nerve encasement by enhancing tumor ➡, the MR equivalent of tram-track sign. Presence of enhancing tumor rules out traumatic or idiopathic etiologies.

(Left) Axial T1WI C+ FS MR demonstrates tumor surrounding the intraorbital ➡ and intracanalicular ➡ segments of right optic nerve. Note dural tail ➡ along sphenoid lesser wing. (Right) Coronal T1WI C+ FS MR, same patient, confirms enhancement of tumor in right optic canal, medial to anterior clinoid process ➡ and diffusely over sphenoid lesser wing ➡. As the bulk of the tumor is intraorbital, ONSM is favored over spheno-orbital-type meningioma.

(Left) Axial T1WI FS MR reveals pedunculated eccentric ONSM ➡. This small lesion resulted in late symptoms, as optic nerve compression was mild. There is considerable variability in imaging appearance of ONSM, though enhancement and sparing of optic nerve are consistent findings. (Right) Coronal T2WI FS MR demonstrates flattened right optic nerve ➡ eccentric within ONSM ➡. Note bulk of tumor located laterally and superiorly. Tumor is hyperintense relative to brain.

Lacrimal Gland Benign Mixed Tumor

TERMINOLOGY

- Benign mixed tumor of lacrimal gland
  - a.k.a. pleomorphic adenoma
- Benign epithelial neoplasm of lacrimal gland

IMAGING

- Unilateral circumscribed lacrimal fossa mass with **scalloped bony remodeling**
- Anterior superotemporal extraconal orbit
  - Majority originate in orbital lobe of lacrimal gland
- CT: Mild heterogeneity; occasional punctate calcifications
- MR: Increased conspicuity of cystic elements
- Moderate to marked enhancement on CECT and T1 MR

TOP DIFFERENTIAL DIAGNOSES

- Lacrimal gland lymphoproliferative lesion
- Lacrimal gland carcinoma
- Orbital dermoid/epidermoid
- Orbital idiopathic inflammatory pseudotumor

- Lacrimal cyst

CLINICAL ISSUES

- Most common lacrimal gland tumor
  - Up to 90% benign tumors of lacrimal gland
  - Up to 50% of primary epithelial tumors of lacrimal gland
- Cumulative low risk of malignant transformation
  - 5% at 10 years; 10% at 20 years; 20% at 30 years
  - Carcinoma ex pleomorphic adenoma accounts for ~ 10% of lacrimal gland carcinoma
- Occurs in 2nd to 5th decades (younger age than malignant neoplasms)
- Presents with slowly progressive painless proptosis
- Complete surgical excision is curative
  - If capsular disruption, need long-term follow-up

DIAGNOSTIC CHECKLIST

- Scalloped bony remodeling on CT is characteristic
- Small cystic elements may be seen on CT or MR

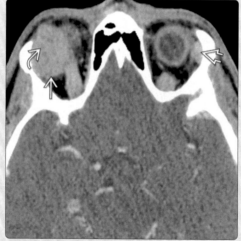
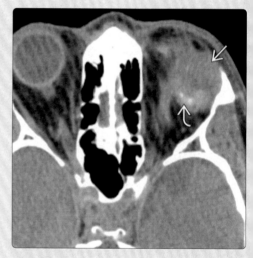

(Left) *Axial CECT demonstrates a slightly heterogeneous, well-circumscribed, enhancing superolateral orbital mass ➡. Small internal cysts ➡ are a common finding. Note opposite normal lacrimal gland ➡. (Right) Axial NECT shows a well-defined lobular mass of the left lacrimal gland ➡ with internal calcifications identified posteriorly ➡.*

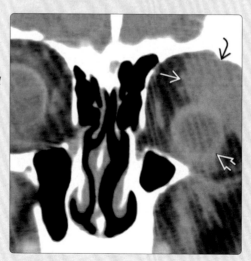
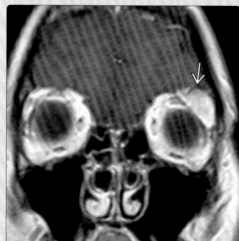

(Left) *Coronal NECT reveals a lobular mass in the superior temporal aspect of the left orbit ➡ associated with scalloped remodeling of the lacrimal fossa ➡. Note typical inferomedial displacement of the globe ➡ associated with tumors of the lacrimal region. (Right) Coronal T1 C+ MR shows a well-circumscribed, enhancing mass in the left superolateral orbit, with smooth scalloped osseous remodeling ➡.*

Lacrimal Gland Benign Mixed Tumor

TERMINOLOGY

Abbreviations
- Benign mixed tumor (BMT) of lacrimal gland

Synonyms
- Pleomorphic adenoma of lacrimal gland

Definitions
- Benign epithelial neoplasm of lacrimal gland

IMAGING

General Features
- Best diagnostic clue
  - Unilateral lacrimal mass with scalloped bony remodeling of lacrimal fossa
- Location
  - Anterior **superotemporal extraconal** orbit
    - Majority originate in orbital lobe of gland
- Morphology
  - Solid, round or oval, circumscribed

CT Findings
- CECT
  - Moderate to marked enhancement
  - Small cystic elements common
- Bone CT
  - Soft tissue mass with **scalloping/remodeling** of **lacrimal fossa**
  - Occasional punctate calcification (33%)

MR Findings
- T1WI
  - Hypointense to isointense; mild heterogeneity
- T2WI
  - Isointense to hyperintense
  - Increased conspicuity of cystic elements
- T1WI C+
  - Moderate to marked enhancement

Imaging Recommendations
- Best imaging tool
  - Enhanced MR to confirm circumscribed nature
  - Coronal bone CT to assess bony remodeling

DIFFERENTIAL DIAGNOSIS

Orbital Lymphoproliferative Lesions
- Homogeneous enlargement of gland; molds to shape of globe
- ↑ density on NECT; ↓ T2 MR signal; homogeneous enhancement

Lacrimal Gland Carcinoma
- Lacrimal mass with ill-defined margins and invasion of adjacent bone/soft tissue
- Imaging features can be nonspecific

Orbital Dermoid and Epidermoid
- Well-circumscribed extraconal mass near frontozygomatic suture

- DWI high signal if epidermoid; presence of fat = dermoid; scalloping of adjacent bone

Orbital Idiopathic Inflammatory Pseudotumor
- Palpably enlarged, tender gland
- Diffuse anterior-posterior enlargement of gland with stranding of fat at margins

Lacrimal Cyst
- Well-defined, fluid density/signal within parenchyma

Dacryoadenitis
- Tender, enlarged gland often with overlying cellulitis
- Infiltration and stranding in surrounding fat

PATHOLOGY

Staging, Grading, & Classification
- Follows WHO classification for salivary neoplasms

Microscopic Features
- "Pleomorphic" refers to diverse epithelial and myoepithelial components

CLINICAL ISSUES

Presentation
- Most common signs/symptoms
  - Slowly progressive painless proptosis
  - Inferomedial globe displacement

Demographics
- Age
  - 2nd to 5th decades
    - Generally younger age than malignant neoplasms
- Epidemiology
  - **2%** of all orbital neoplasms
  - Most common lacrimal gland tumor

Natural History & Prognosis
- Cumulative low risk of malignant transformation
  - 5% at 10 years; 10% at 20 years; 20% at 30 years
  - Carcinoma ex pleomorphic adenoma may be any type, but adenocarcinoma, not otherwise specified and mucoepidermoid most common

Treatment
- Complete surgical excision is curative
  - Lateral orbitotomy for wide exposure
  - Intact removal without rupture or incision
    - Capsular disruption requires long-term follow-up for possible seeding, which may lead to recurrence with risk of malignancy

DIAGNOSTIC CHECKLIST

Image Interpretation Pearls
- Scalloped bony remodeling is characteristic but not pathognomonic

SELECTED REFERENCES

1. von Holstein SL et al: Tumors of the lacrimal gland. Semin Diagn Pathol. 33(3):156-63, 2016

KEY FACTS

TERMINOLOGY

- Retinoblastoma (RB)
- Malignant primary retinal neoplasm
- Trilateral/quadrilateral RB: Bilateral ocular RB plus pineal ± suprasellar tumors

IMAGING

- Unilateral in 60%, bilateral in 40%
- Trilateral or quadrilateral disease rare
- **Extraocular extension** in **< 10%**
  - Indicates poor prognosis
- CT: **Calcification** in **> 90%**
- MR: Assess extent of intraocular tumor and presence of optic nerve, orbital, or intracranial involvement
  - T1: Mild hyperintensity
  - T2: Moderate to marked hypointensity
  - Moderate to marked heterogeneous enhancement

TOP DIFFERENTIAL DIAGNOSES

- Persistent hyperplastic primary vitreous
- Coats disease
- Retinopathy of prematurity
- Orbital toxocariasis

PATHOLOGY

- **Primitive neuroectodermal tumor**
- Inherited (germline): Multilateral > unilateral

CLINICAL ISSUES

- Most common intraocular tumor of childhood
- **Leukocoria** in 50-60%
- 90-95% diagnosed by age 5 years

DIAGNOSTIC CHECKLIST

- Calcified intraocular mass in child is RB until proven otherwise

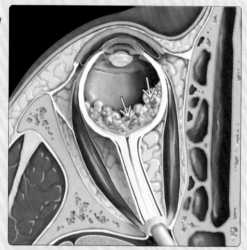
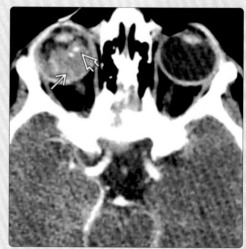

(Left) Axial graphic depicts retinoblastoma with lobulated tumor extending through the limiting membrane into the vitreous. Punctate calcifications ➡ are characteristic. (Right) Axial CECT demonstrates a lobular endophytic retinoblastoma ➡ containing small calcifications ➡ and filling much of the vitreous compartment. A calcified ocular mass in a child represents retinoblastoma until proven otherwise.

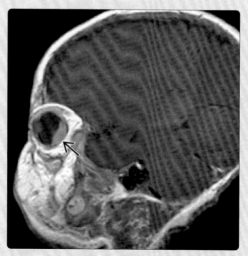
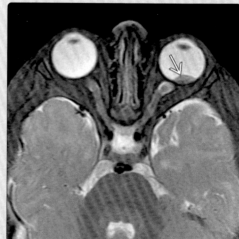

(Left) Sagittal postcontrast T1WI through the orbit shows an enhancing intraocular mass ➡ without visible extraocular extension. (Right) Axial T2WI FS MR shows a mass at the margin of the left optic disc ➡. Virtually all retinoblastomas demonstrate hypointensity relative to vitreous on T2WI; the lenticular shape is typical for early lesions.

TERMINOLOGY

Abbreviations

- Retinoblastoma (RB)

Definitions

- Malignant primary retinal neoplasm
- **Trilateral** RB: Bilateral ocular tumors plus midline intracranial neuroblastic tumor, typically pineal
- **Quadrilateral** (tetralateral) RB: Bilateral disease plus pineal and suprasellar tumors

IMAGING

General Features

- Best diagnostic clue
  - Intraocular **calcified** mass in child
- Location
  - Diagnosis typically with ophthalmoscopy and ultrasound
    - MR for tumor mapping and prognostication
  - Unilateral in 60%, **bilateral in 40%**
  - Trilateral or quadrilateral disease rare
  - Extraocular extension in < 10%
    - Spreads along scleral vessels into orbit and along optic nerve to subarachnoid space
  - Predictors for metastatic disease: Involvement of optic nerve, choroid, anterior chamber or orbit
    - Anterior chamber enhancement reflects neoangiogenesis and is associated with more aggressive tumor behavior
  - Role of MR
    - Exclude pseudoneoplastic lesions
    - Assess intraocular (choroid, sclera, prelaminar optic nerve), extraocular (postlaminar optic nerve, orbital), and intracranial (pineal, parasellar, metastatic) involvement
- Size
  - Decreased ocular size in RB
- Growth patterns
  - **Endophytic** form (45%)
    - Inward protrusion into vitreous
    - Associated with vitreous seeding
  - **Exophytic** form (45%)
    - Outward growth into subretinal space, typically with hemispherical configuration
    - Associated retinal detachment and subretinal exudate
  - **Mixed** endophytic and exophytic (10%)

CT Findings

- NECT
  - Punctate or finely speckled **calcification** (> 90-95%)
- CECT
  - Moderate to marked heterogeneous enhancement

MR Findings

- T1WI
  - Variable, mildly hyperintense (vs. vitreous)
- T2WI
  - Moderate to markedly hypointense (vs. vitreous)
    - Helps distinguish from other congenital lesions (persistent hyperplastic primary vitreous, Coats) that are hyperintense

  - Best for identifying subretinal fluid ± vitreous hemorrhage
- T1WI C+
  - Moderate to marked heterogeneous enhancement
  - Best to assess extent of intraocular disease and presence of optic nerve or extraocular invasion
    - **Choroidal invasion**: Localized thickening and heterogeneous contrast enhancement near tumor
    - **Scleral invasion**: Interruption in thin hypointense zone surrounding enhancing choroid
    - **Optic nerve invasion**: Thickening of optic disc (prelaminar), enhancement of nerve (postlaminar)
      - MR shown to have low sensitivity and specificity in assessing optic nerve invasion

Ultrasonographic Findings

- A scan: Highly reflective spikes at calcifications
- B scan: Echodense, irregular mass with focal shadows

Imaging Recommendations

- Best imaging tool
  - Enhanced MR with fat-saturated T1- and T2-weighted imaging best for tumor mapping
  - Calcification on CT relatively specific
- Protocol advice
  - Include whole brain to assess for trilateral disease

DIFFERENTIAL DIAGNOSIS

Persistent Hyperplastic Primary Vitreous

- Small globe, hyperdense; no Ca^{++}
- Hyperintense on T2WI; retrolental tissue stalk

Coats Disease

- Normal-size globe, hyperdense; no Ca^{++}
- Hyperintense on T1WI and T2WI

Retinopathy of Prematurity

- Retrolental fibroplasia; associated with excess oxygen and premature retinal vessels
- Small globe, hyperdense, bilateral; Ca^{+++} if advanced

Toxocariasis, Orbit

- Uveoscleral enhancement; no Ca^{++} acutely

Other Causes of Leukocoria

- Retinal detachment
  - Subretinal hemorrhage, retinal folds
- Choroidal osteoma
- Choroidal hemangioma (hamartoma)
- Retinal dysplasia

PATHOLOGY

General Features

- Etiology
  - Primitive neuroectodermal tumor
  - **Sporadic** (nongermline): **60%** of RB
    - Majority (85%) of unilateral disease
  - **Inherited** (germline): **40%** of RB
    - Essentially all bilateral and multilateral disease
      - Minority (15%) of unilateral disease
    - Autosomal dominant with 90% penetrance

- – Positive family history in 5-10%
- – New germline mutations in 30-35%
- Genetics
  - ○ *RB1* gene: Chromosome 13, q14 band
  - ○ Somatic mosaicism in 10-20% of RB patients
- Associated abnormalities
  - ○ Risk of 2nd malignancy ↑ in germline disease
    - – Sarcoma, melanoma, CNS tumors, epithelial tumors (lung, bladder, breast)
    - – 20-30% in nonirradiated patients
    - – 50-60% in irradiated patients
    - – Occur within 30 years, average 10-13 years
  - ○ 13q deletion syndrome: RB plus multiple organ system anomalies

Staging, Grading, & Classification

- Reese-Ellsworth classification
  - ○ Groups 1-5
  - ○ Based on size, location, and multifocality
  - ○ More useful in radiation therapy management
- International (Murphree) classification of RB (ICRB); newer
  - ○ Groups A through E
  - ○ Based on size, retinal location, subretinal or vitreous seeding, and several specific prognostic features
  - ○ More useful in chemotherapy management

Gross Pathologic & Surgical Features

- Yellowish-white irregular pedunculated retinal mass

Microscopic Features

- Small round cells, scant cytoplasm, and large nuclei
- Flexner-Wintersteiner rosettes and fleurettes

CLINICAL ISSUES

Presentation

- Most common signs/symptoms
  - ○ **Leukocoria** (50-60%)
- Other signs/symptoms
  - ○ Severe vision loss
  - ○ Strabismus common with macular involvement or retinal detachment
  - ○ Proptosis if significant orbital disease
  - ○ Rubeosis iridis (redness of iris secondary to neovascularization) correlates with anterior chamber enhancement on MR
  - ○ Inflammatory signs in 10%

Demographics

- Age
  - ○ RB is congenital but usually not apparent at birth
  - ○ Average age at diagnosis: 18 months
    - – Unilateral: 24 months, bilateral: 13 months
    - – Earlier with family history and routine screening
  - ○ 90-95% diagnosed by age 5 years
- Epidemiology
  - ○ Most common intraocular tumor of childhood
  - ○ Incidence of 1:17,000 live births
    - – Has increased in past 60 years
  - ○ 3% of cancers in children under 15
  - ○ 1% of cancer deaths; 5% of childhood blindness

Natural History & Prognosis

- Poor prognosis for extraocular disease
  - ○ < 10% 5-year disease-free survival
- Degree of nerve involvement correlates with survival
  - ○ Superficial or no invasion: 90%
  - ○ Invasion to lamina cribrosa (prelaminar): 70%
  - ○ Invasion beyond lamina cribrosa (postlaminar): 60%
  - ○ Involvement at surgical margin: 20%
- Poor prognosis for trilateral disease or cerebrospinal fluid spread
  - ○ < 24-month survival

Treatment

- > 95% of children with RB in USA are cured with modern techniques
  - ○ Challenge is maintaining eye and vision
- Based on tumor volume and localization, intraocular tumor extension, and extraocular stage of disease
- Enucleation
  - ○ Advanced disease with no chance of preserving useful vision
- External beam radiation therapy
  - ○ Indicated for bulky tumors with seeding
  - ○ Unfavorable complications, e.g., arrested bone growth and radiation-induced tumors
- Chemotherapy ("chemoreduction")
  - ○ Currently favored 1st-line therapy for lower grade intraocular tumors
  - ○ Limits need for external radiation and enucleation
  - ○ Combine with other local modalities to achieve cure
  - ○ Intraarterial chemotherapy is recently developed treatment option
- Plaque radiotherapy
  - ○ Locally directed, I-125 or other isotope
  - ○ Selected solitary or small tumors
- Cryotherapy
  - ○ Primary local treatment of small anterior tumors
- Photocoagulation
  - ○ Primary local treatment of small posterior tumors

DIAGNOSTIC CHECKLIST

Consider

- Assess for intraocular and extraocular spread, including optic nerve
  - ○ Check for intracranial trilateral or quadrilateral disease in pineal and suprasellar regions

Image Interpretation Pearls

- Calcified intraocular mass in child is RB until proven otherwise

SELECTED REFERENCES

1. Wyse E et al: A review of the literature for intra-arterial chemotherapy used to treat retinoblastoma. Pediatr Radiol. 46(9):1223-33, 2016
2. Sirin S et al: High-resolution MRI using orbit surface coils for the evaluation of metastatic risk factors in 143 children with retinoblastoma: Part 1: MRI vs. histopathology. Neuroradiology. 57(8):805-14, 2015
3. de Graaf P et al: Contrast-enhancement of the anterior eye segment in patients with retinoblastoma: correlation between clinical, MR imaging, and histopathologic findings. AJNR Am J Neuroradiol. 31(2):237-45, 2010
4. Dunkel IJ et al: Trilateral retinoblastoma: potentially curable with intensive chemotherapy. Pediatr Blood Cancer. 54(3):384-7, 2010

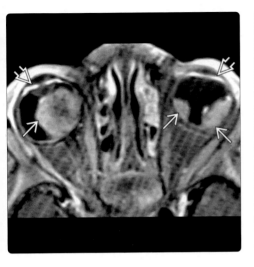

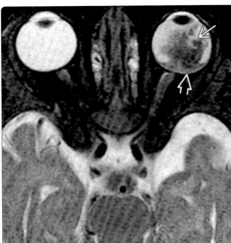

(Left) *Enhanced T1WI MR shows bulky enhancing intraocular masses compatible with bilateral retinoblastomas ➡. Note prominent enhancement of each iris ➡; anterior segment enhancement is associated with more aggressive tumor behavior.* (Right) *Axial T2WI FS MR reveals lobular, hypointense mass filling much of the vitreous compartment of the left globe ➡. Note posterior fluid level indicating associated vitreous hemorrhage ➡.*

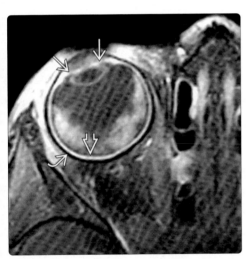

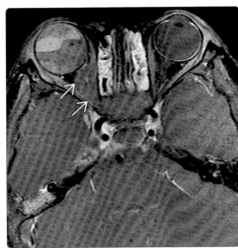

(Left) *Axial T1WI C+ MR shows moderately enhancing retinoblastoma, associated with prominent anterior segment enhancement ➡. Note intact thin lines of enhancing choroid ➡ and hypointense sclera ➡, indicating absence of invasion of these structures.* (Right) *Axial T1WI C+ FS MR demonstrates retinoblastoma virtually filling the right globe. There is subtle thickening and enhancement of the right optic nerve ➡, indicating postlaminar invasion.*

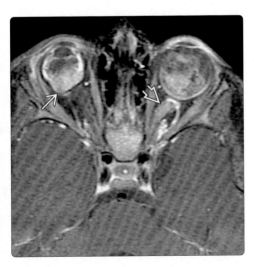

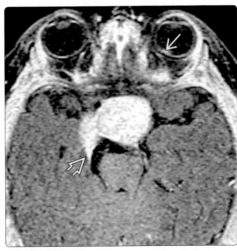

(Left) *On T1WI C+ FS MR, interruption of linear hypodensity with focal contour abnormality indicates scleral invasion of retinoblastoma on the right ➡. The left postlaminar optic nerve demonstrates asymmetric enlargement and enhancement ➡.* (Right) *In this patient with pathologically proven trilateral retinoblastoma, only 1 ocular lesion is identified on this FS enhanced T1WI ➡. There is a bulky enhancing suprasellar and parasellar mass, with extension along dural reflections ➡.*

Ocular Melanoma

TERMINOLOGY

- Synonyms: Uveal melanoma, choroidal melanoma, ocular adnexal melanoma
- Malignancy arising from melanocytes
  - Most often in choroid

IMAGING

- Choroid > ciliary > iris
- Dome- or mushroom-shaped with broad choroidal base
- Often with associated retinal detachment
- **Ultrasound** is primary imaging modality for evaluation of intraocular disease
- **Enhanced MR** with fat suppression to assess extraocular disease
  - Mildly to strongly T1 hyperintense to vitreous
  - T2 hypointense
  - Moderate, diffuse tumor enhancement

TOP DIFFERENTIAL DIAGNOSES

- Choroidal metastasis
- Choroidal hemangioma
- Retinal detachment
- Choroidal osteoma

PATHOLOGY

- Sun exposure, light-colored irides increase risk

CLINICAL ISSUES

- **Painless vision disturbance**
- Blurred vision, scotoma, field loss, floaters
- Most common primary intraocular tumor in adults
- Globe-sparing treatment options for small/medium tumors
- Prognosis worsens with extraocular invasion, extension through Bruch membrane, and ↑ size
- Death from systemic metastases; liver most common

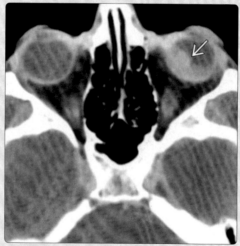
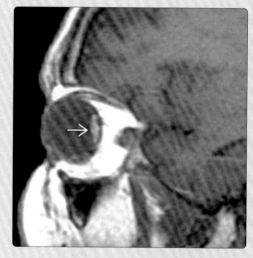

(Left) Axial CECT demonstrates a bilobed left choroidal lesion ➡, homogeneously hyperdense on this enhanced study. Distinction between tumor and retinal detachment is difficult. (Right) Sagittal T1W MR without contrast demonstrates a small mass along the posterior choroid ➡ that is moderately hyperintense relative to vitreous.

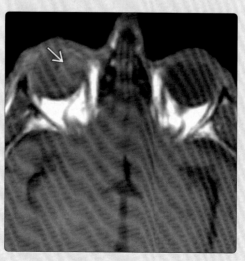
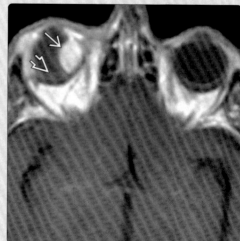

(Left) Axial T1WI MR reveals a tumor along the nasal choroidal surface of the right globe ➡, which is only mildly hyperintense relative to vitreous. Ocular melanomas distant from the macula may be quite large before significant visual defects are apparent. (Right) Axial C+ T1WI MR shows intense enhancement of dome-shaped ocular melanoma ➡. Lenticular-shaped mild hyperintensity ➡ lateral to the enhancing lesion is compatible with associated retinal detachment.

Ocular Melanoma

TERMINOLOGY

Synonyms

- **Uveal melanoma**, ocular adnexal melanoma, choroidal melanoma

Definitions

- Primary malignancy of uveal tract

IMAGING

General Features

- Best diagnostic clue
  - Enhancing intraocular mass with ↑ **T1WI MR signal** in adult
- Location
  - Temporal hemisphere posterior to equator most common site of origin
  - Posterior uvea
    - **Choroidal lesions (85%)**
      - ☐ Posterior segment peripheral mass
      - ☐ Transscleral/optic nerve extension when advanced
    - Ciliary body (10%): Behind posterior chamber
  - Anterior uvea
    - Iris lesions (5%): Within anterior chamber
- Size
  - Criteria for therapeutic decisions
    - Small: 5- to 16-mm diameter, < 3-mm depth
    - Medium: 5- to 16-mm diameter, 3- to 10-mm depth
    - Large: > 16-mm diameter, > 10-mm depth
- Morphology
  - Dome- or mound-shaped, broad choroidal base
  - **Mushroom shape** implies penetration through Bruch membrane (separates choroid from retina)
  - Diffuse, laterally spreading form in 5%
  - Typically solid
    - Cavitary variant appears cystic

CT Findings

- NECT
  - Solid soft tissue density mass
  - Calcification rare; may occur after therapy
- CECT
  - Diffuse moderate enhancement

MR Findings

- T1WI
  - Mildly to strongly **hyperintense** compared with vitreous
    - Signal increases with ↑ melanotic pigmentation
  - **Retinal detachments** with subretinal fluid: Variably hyperintense, due to blood products or protein
- T2WI
  - Strongly **hypointense** compared with vitreous
  - Subretinal fluid: Isointense to hypointense, depending on nature of exudate
- T1WI C+
  - Moderate, diffuse tumor enhancement
  - No enhancement of retinal detachment or subretinal fluid

Ultrasonographic Findings

- A scan
  - Low to medium internal reflectivity
  - Spike at tumor surface; vascular oscillations
- B scan
  - Domed, lobulated, or mushroom-shaped mass
  - Choroidal excavation/scleral bowing indicate invasion

Nuclear Medicine Findings

- PET/CT
  - Limited utility at primary site, sensitive for detection of metastases
  - Higher tumor SUV correlated with chromosome 3 loss and larger tumor size (poor prognostic signs)
- I-123-IMP SPECT
  - May be helpful in diagnosis of atypical or indeterminate lesions

Imaging Recommendations

- Best imaging tool
  - Ultrasound for intraocular tumor evaluation
  - Enhanced MR of orbits with fat suppression to assess extraocular disease

DIFFERENTIAL DIAGNOSIS

Choroidal Metastasis

- Breast and lung primaries most common
  - Located on temporal side of macula

Choroidal Hemangioma (Hamartoma)

- Benign vascular lesion
- Circumscribed form in adults ± retinal detachment
- Diffuse form in infants associated with Sturge-Weber
- > T2 signal and enhancement than melanoma

Retinal Detachment

- Serous, exudative, or hemorrhagic
- Myriad etiologies, including trauma, inflammation, underlying tumor, or systemic disease
- Does not enhance but may obscure underlying mass

Choroidal Osteoma

- Tendency to occur in young women
- Often asymptomatic, found incidentally
- Curvilinear, plaque-like Ca^{++} lesion along posterior globe

Idiopathic Inflammatory Pseudotumor

- May affect any orbital structure
  - Globe/scleral involvement → endophthalmitis
- Painful, inflammatory presentation

Retinoblastoma

- Most common intraocular tumor in children
- Rarely occurs in adults
- Calcification in 95%

PATHOLOGY

General Features

- Etiology
  - Primary malignancy arising from melanocytes within choroid
- Genetics

- o Several mutations and familial melanoma syndromes have been identified
- Associated abnormalities
  - o Ocular melanocytosis, dysplastic nevus syndrome, xeroderma pigmentosum
- Risk factors
  - o Genetic factors have greatest influence on risk
  - o Sun exposure, light-colored irides increase risk

Staging, Grading, & Classification

- Modified Callender classification
  - o Spindle cell nevus: Premalignant
  - o Spindle cell melanoma: A and B cell types
  - o Fascicular: Palisaded B cells (spindle subtype)
  - o Necrotic: Significant necrosis prior to treatment
  - o Mixed: Spindle and epithelioid cells
  - o Epithelioid: Predominantly epithelioid cells

Gross Pathologic & Surgical Features

- Range from heavily pigmented to amelanotic
- Discoloration and atrophy of overlying retina

Microscopic Features

- 3 cell types used for classification
  - o Spindle A: Elongated nuclei, few mitoses
  - o Spindle B: Plump nuclei, more prominent nucleoli
  - o Epithelioid: Ovoid nuclei, anaplastic, poor prognosis

CLINICAL ISSUES

Presentation

- Most common signs/symptoms
  - o **Painless vision disturbance**
  - o Frequent coexisting retinal detachment
- Other signs/symptoms
  - o Blurred vision, scotoma, field loss, floaters
  - o Pain rare (due to ciliary nerve involvement)
- Clinical profile
  - o **Frequently asymptomatic**
    - – Often discovered on routine eye exam
    - – Presentation more advanced when located farther from fovea and nerve head
- Ophthalmoscopy
  - o Dome-shaped mass of variable pigmentation
  - o Orange discoloration of overlying retina; exudative detachment may obscure mass

Demographics

- Age
  - o Peak incidence: **6th decade**
    - – Iris melanoma presents slightly younger
- Ethnicity
  - o **Northern European descent highest risk**
  - o Hispanic, Asian uncommon
  - o African descent rare
- Epidemiology
  - o **Most common primary intraocular tumor in adults**
  - o Incidence 6-8 per 1 million
    - – 5% of all melanomas

Natural History & Prognosis

- Appears to be systemic disease at presentation with treatment of primary disease curative in some patients
- Death from systemic metastases (liver most common)
  - o 5-year cumulative metastasis rate: 25%
  - o 10-year cumulative metastasis rate: 34%
  - o No effective treatment for metastatic disease
- Worse prognosis if any of the following
  - o Large size, anterior location, extension through Bruch membrane, transscleral/nerve invasion
    - – Optic nerve invasion most common in juxtapapillary or diffuse tumors
  - o Amelanotic, epithelioid pattern, highly mitotic

Treatment

- Protocols largely driven by results of Collaborative Ocular Melanoma Study (COMS) Group
  - o Multicenter NIH/National Eye Institute trial
- Observation
  - o Suitable for indeterminate stable small nevi
  - o Sequential ultrasound to document stability
- Transpupillary thermotherapy
  - o Option for small tumors; preserves vision
  - o Tumor heating by infrared radiation
- Surgical block excision (sclerouvectomy)
  - o Option for small tumors < 1/3 of globe circumference
  - o Preserves some vision
- Plaque brachytherapy
  - o Common option for medium-sized tumors
  - o Isotope plaque (I-125) sutured over tumor site
- External beam irradiation
  - o Alternative for medium-sized tumors
  - o Charged particles (protons, helium ions)
  - o Gamma knife radiosurgery
- Surgical enucleation
  - o Standard for large tumors, treatment failures
  - o Radical exenteration for widespread tumor

DIAGNOSTIC CHECKLIST

Consider

- Most common ocular tumor in adults
- Ultrasonography remains most frequently utilized diagnostic modality for intraocular disease
- MR more accurate than US for extraocular spread

Image Interpretation Pearls

- Enhancement reliably distinguishes tumor from associated retinal detachment on MR

SELECTED REFERENCES

1. Luke JJ et al: Biology of advanced uveal melanoma and next steps for clinical therapeutics. Pigment Cell Melanoma Res. 28(2):135-47, 2015
2. Mashayekhi A et al: Primary transpupillary thermotherapy for choroidal melanoma in 391 cases: importance of risk factors in tumor control. Ophthalmology. 122(3):600-9, 2015
3. Matsuo T et al: Clinicopathological correlation for the role of fluorodeoxyglucose positron emission tomography computed tomography in detection of choroidal malignant melanoma. Int J Clin Oncol. 19(2):230-9, 2014
4. McCannel TA et al: Association of positive dual-modality positron emission tomography/computed tomography imaging of primary choroidal melanoma with chromosome 3 loss and tumor size. Retina. 30(1):146-51, 2010

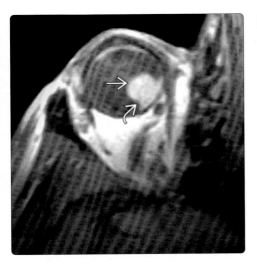

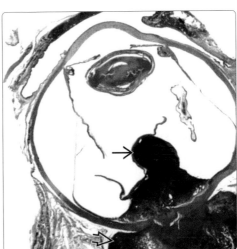

(Left) *Axial T1WI MR obtained with a regional orbit coil demonstrates a well-defined hyperintense mass* ➡ *within the posterior nasal quadrant of the right globe. The mushroom-shaped configuration with waist-like narrowing at the tumor base* ➡ *indicates that invasion of Bruch membrane is likely.* (Right) *Micropathology at low power shows a mushroom-shaped melanoma* ➡ *penetrating through Bruch membrane. Bulky extraocular tumor is seen extending posteriorly through the optic nerve head* ➡.

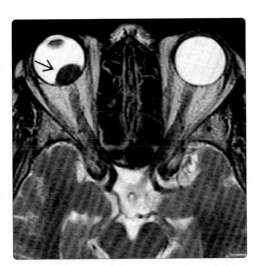

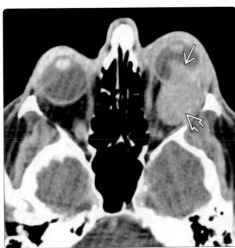

(Left) *Axial T2WI shows marked hypointensity of a choroidal melanoma* ➡. (Right) *Axial CECT shows an enhancing tumor within the posterior aspect of the left globe* ➡ *with an unusually large extraocular (retrobulbar) component* ➡ *resulting in proptosis. The very large size of this melanoma and the presence of extraocular extension are both poor prognostic factors.*

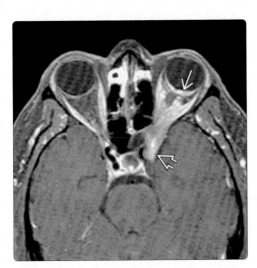

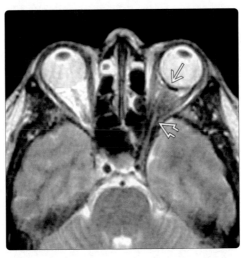

(Left) *Axial T1WI C+ FS MR shows thickening of the posterior choroid of the left globe* ➡ *with extraocular tumor extending through the superior orbital fissure into the cavernous sinus* ➡. *This is a variant case, both because of the large volume of extraocular disease and its highly infiltrative appearance.* (Right) *Axial T2WI MR demonstrates characteristic low T2 signal in both intraocular* ➡ *and extraocular* ➡ *components of infiltrative lesion, supporting the diagnosis of ocular melanoma.*

Orbital Lymphoproliferative Lesions

TERMINOLOGY

- Spectrum of lesions ranging from benign lymphoid hyperplasia to malignant lymphoma

IMAGING

- Solid, pliable, homogeneously enhancing tumor
  - Can involve any part of orbit; lacrimal predilection
- Mass with lobulated margins
  - Molds to adjacent structures in "plastic" fashion
- Mildly T2 hyperintense to muscle (high cellularity)
- Decrease ADC, particularly in true lymphoma
- Moderate to marked homogeneous enhancement

TOP DIFFERENTIAL DIAGNOSES

- IgG4-related disease
- Idiopathic orbital inflammation
- Orbital sarcoidosis
- Orbital Sjögren syndrome
- Lacrimal gland epithelial tumor

PATHOLOGY

- Spectrum of lymphocytic proliferation
  - Benign **lymphoid hyperplasia**
    - Reactive, polyclonal; indeterminate when atypical
  - Non-Hodgkin **lymphoma**
    - Low-grade MALT/ENMZL most common

CLINICAL ISSUES

- Presentation: Insidious anterior orbital/eyelid swelling
- Long-term risk of developing systemic lymphoma
- Lymphoid hyperplasia responsive to steroids
- Lymphoma responsive to radiation therapy

DIAGNOSTIC CHECKLIST

- Benign hyperplasia vs. malignant lymphoma
  - **Hyperplasia**: Well-defined, bilateral, flow void sign, higher enhancement ratio, sinusitis, less elderly
  - **Lymphoma**: Irregular, unilateral, diffusion restriction, lower enhancement ratio, more elderly

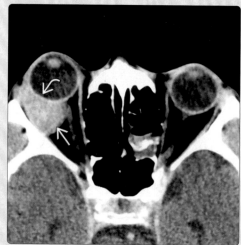
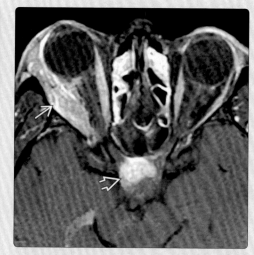

(Left) *Axial CECT shows a lobular retrobulbar mass ➡ conforming to the shape ("molding") of the posterior aspect of the right globe ➡ with minimal flattening of the scleral margin. This MALT lymphoma demonstrates homogeneous density and enhancement.* (Right) *Coronal T1 C+ MR shows a homogeneously enhancing extraconal MALT lymphoma involving the lacrimal gland with posterior extension along the lateral rectus ➡. Note the presence of intracranial suprasellar tumor ➡.*

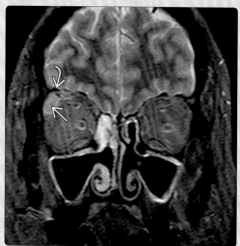
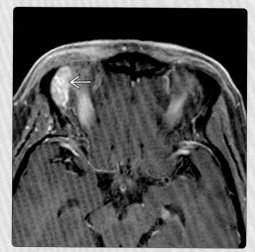

(Left) *Coronal STIR MR in a 50-year-old woman shows a mildly hyperintense, ovoid, well-marginated mass in the right lacrimal gland ➡. Note the presence of an adjacent small flow void ➡.* (Right) *Axial T1 C+ FS MR in the same patient shows homogeneous enhancement of the mass ➡ in the left lacrimal gland. Pathology revealed benign lymphoid hyperplasia. The lesion responded to localized steroid injection.*

Orbital Lymphoproliferative Lesions

TERMINOLOGY

Abbreviations
- Orbital lymphoproliferative lesions (OLPL)

Synonyms
- Mucosa-associated lymphoid tissue (MALT) lymphoma = extranodal marginal zone lymphoma (ENMZL)

Definitions
- OLPL represents **spectrum** of lesions ranging from benign lymphoid hyperplasia (LH) to malignant non-Hodgkin lymphoma (NHL)

IMAGING

General Features
- Best diagnostic clue
  - **Solid, pliable, homogeneously enhancing** tumor that molds to and encases orbital structures
- Location
  - Can involve **any part of orbit**
    - Predilection for **lacrimal gland** & may be only site of involvement
    - Anterior extraconal orbit, often centered in **superotemporal** quadrant
    - **Conjunctival** disease frequent; isolated in 20%
    - May present with primary **extraocular** muscle involvement, simulating thyroid orbitopathy
    - **Diffuse infiltrative** form may occur with intraconal, muscular, or perineural involvement
  - **Unilateral** in most cases of 1° **lymphoma** (60-75%)
  - **Bilateral** in most cases of **benign** OLPL (50-80%)
- Morphology
  - Mass with **lobulated** margins
    - Margins more **well-defined** in **benign** OLPL
    - Margins more **irregular** in true **lymphoma**
  - Often molds to adjacent structures in "**plastic**" fashion
  - May have infiltrative or inflammatory appearance
- Associated findings
  - Concomitant **sinusitis** associated with **benign** OLPL

CT Findings
- NECT
  - Isodense to slightly **hyperdense**, due to highly **cellular** nature and nuclear:cytoplasmic ratio
- CECT
  - Moderate diffuse, **homogeneous** enhancement
  - Dynamic enhancement pattern helps distinguish from inflammatory disease
- Bone CT
  - Bone destruction indicates aggressive histology
    - Molding associated with more indolent disease

MR Findings
- T1WI
  - Mildly hyperintense to muscle; homogeneous
- T2WI
  - Only **mildly hyperintense** to muscle (high **cellularity**)
  - Adjacent vessel flow void associated with benign OLPL
- DWI
  - **Decrease ADC**, particularly in true **lymphoma**

- T1WI C+
  - Moderate to marked **homogeneous enhancement**
  - Enhancement ratio (to muscle) higher with benign OLPL

Imaging Recommendations
- Best imaging tool
  - MR modality of choice for evaluating location and extent of disease
- Protocol advice
  - Axial and coronal MR: T1, T2, diffusion, and C+ FS

DIFFERENTIAL DIAGNOSIS

IgG4-Related Disease
- Infiltrative masses with subacute presentation
- Accounts for significant number of previously diagnosed LH
- Characteristic T2 hypointensity
- Predilection for lacrimal and perineural involvement

Idiopathic Orbital Inflammation (Pseudotumor)
- Presentation typically more acute & painful
- Similar wide range of imaging appearances

Orbital Sarcoidosis
- Painless masses anywhere in orbit
- Predilection for lacrimal glands; may be bilateral

Orbital Sjögren Syndrome
- Lacrimal involvement with keratoconjunctivitis sicca
- Look for bilateral parotid enlargement, cysts, Ca++

Thyroid Ophthalmopathy
- Painless, often bilateral symmetric proptosis
- Characteristic pattern of extraocular muscle enlargement

Orbital Cellulitis
- Pain, erythema, fever; associated with sinusitis
- Discrete orbital masses are less common

Lacrimal Gland Epithelial Tumor
- Unilateral lacrimal mass, painless when benign
- T2 MR signal more hyperintense

Orbital Metastasis
- Can occur anywhere in orbit
- Breast & lung carcinoma are common primaries

PATHOLOGY

General Features
- Etiology
  - **Reactive** or **malignant** lymphocytic proliferation
- Genetics
  - Hyperplasia = **polyclonal**
  - Lymphoma = **monoclonal**
  - ENMZL markers often indeterminate
- Associated abnormalities
  - Systemic conditions: Collagen vascular disease, Sjögren disease, hematologic malignancy
  - Immunocompromised status: AIDS, transplant patients

Staging, Grading, & Classification
- Classification of OLPL spectrum
  - **Benign lymphoid hyperplasia**: 10-40%

- – Reactive hyperplasia, polyclonal
- – Atypical hyperplasia; indeterminate
- o **Non-Hodgkin lymphoma**: 60-90%
  - – Low-grade MALT/ENMZL most common
  - – Other: Follicular, diffuse large B-cell, mantle cell, T-cell & NK/T, Burkitt, and other lymphomas
- Staging of orbital lymphomas
  - o Ann Arbor system: Stages I-IV; (E) if extranodal disease
    - – Subclassification: (A) without, or (B) with systemic symptoms (weight loss, fever, night sweats)
  - o Most MALT/ENMZL stage IE-A or IIE-A at presentation

Microscopic Features

- Common feature of all OLPL subtypes: Cellular lymphocytic infiltration
- Hyperplasia: Polymorphous infiltrate of lymphocytes, follicle formation, endothelial proliferation
- Small B-cell lymphoma: Small round lymphocytes, vaguely nodular, plasma cells
  - o Characteristic **marginal zone** cells in ENMZL

CLINICAL ISSUES

Presentation

- Most common signs/symptoms
  - o **Insidious** anterior orbital/eyelid swelling
    - – Fleshy mass visible if conjunctiva involved
  - o Intraorbital **mass** effect with **proptosis**, **diplopia**
    - – Globe **displacement** (nonaxial, inferior) in 50%
- Other signs/symptoms
  - o Fever, night sweats, weight loss
- Clinical profile
  - o 4 basic clinical syndromes
    - – Indolent painless orbital mass (most common)
    - – Fulminant orbital mass (immunocompromised)
    - – Regional bony mass (secondary orbit extension)
    - – Neuro-ophthalmic (CNS disease)

Demographics

- Age
  - o Older patients (5th to 8th decades)
    - – **Benign** OLPL in **younger** patients
    - – **Lymphoma** in **elderly** patients
- Epidemiology
  - o 5-10% of orbital masses; most common adult neoplasm
  - o Constitutes 1-2% of NHL, 8% of extranodal lymphoma
  - o Orbit involvement develops in 5% of systemic NHL
  - o Systemic lymphoma in up to 50% at presentation

Natural History & Prognosis

- **Indolent** course for primary low-grade and low-stage (IE-A) tumors
- Major long-term **risk** of developing **systemic lymphoma**
  - o Systemic relapse in 25-75%
  - o Typically abdominal, pelvic, or neck lymph nodes
- Histology affects risk of systemic disease
  - o Small B cell (atypical hyperplasia, MALT, etc.): 25-50%
  - o All others (large B cell, mantle cell, T cell, etc.): 50-75%
- Orbital site affects risk of systemic disease
  - o Eyelid: 67%; orbit: 35%; conjunctiva: 20%
  - o Increased risk of systemic disease if bilateral

- **Excellent prognosis** for **MALT/ENMZL** with radiotherapy
  - o Survival: 5 year = 90-100%, 10 year = 70-90%
  - o Local control approaches 100%
  - o Indolent course even after relapse
- Good local control for other types of lymphoma but poorer long-term survival with systemic disease

Treatment

- Lymphoid hyperplasia
  - o Responsive to **steroids**, given systemically or injected locally
- Low-grade small B-cell lymphoma (MALT/ENMZL)
  - o Excellent response to **radiation** therapy alone
- High-grade diffuse B-cell lymphoma
  - o Systemic chemotherapy or immunotherapy
  - o Local radiation treatment may be beneficial in selected areas

DIAGNOSTIC CHECKLIST

Consider

- Whole-body **staging** and **surveillance** are indicated because of risk of development of systemic lymphoma
- Tumor location has significant impact on eventual risk of systemic lymphoma

Image Interpretation Pearls

- **Broad range** of imaging manifestations
  - o Carefully examine anterior compartment structures, including orbital septum, conjunctiva, and lids
  - o May involve any portion of orbit
- Consider OLPL in differential for any orbital mass
- Features that help distinguish benign hyperplasia from true lymphoma
  - o **Benign**: Well-defined, bilateral, flow void sign, higher enhancement ratio, sinusitis, less elderly
  - o **Lymphoma**: Irregular, unilateral, diffusion restriction, lower enhancement ratio, more elderly

SELECTED REFERENCES

1. Xu XQ et al: Benign and malignant orbital lymphoproliferative disorders: Differentiating using multiparametric MRI at 3.0T. J Magn Reson Imaging. ePub, 2016
2. Amin S et al: Diagnostic pitfalls in "low-grade lymphoma" of the orbit and lacrimal gland. Orbit. 34(4):206-11, 2015
3. Andrew NH et al: An analysis of IgG4-related disease (IgG4-RD) among idiopathic orbital inflammations and benign lymphoid hyperplasias using two consensus-based diagnostic criteria for IgG4-RD. Br J Ophthalmol. 99(3):376-81, 2015
4. Kharod SM et al: Radiotherapy in the management of orbital lymphoma: a single institution's experience over 4 decades. Am J Clin Oncol. ePub, 2015
5. Haradome K et al: Orbital lymphoproliferative disorders (OLPDs): value of MR imaging for differentiating orbital lymphoma from benign OPLDs. AJNR Am J Neuroradiol. 35(10):1976-82, 2014
6. Andrew NH et al: Intraorbital corticosteroid injection for orbital reactive lymphoid hyperplasia. Eye (Lond). 27(4):561-3, 2013
7. Demirci H et al: Orbital lymphoproliferative tumors: analysis of clinical features and systemic involvement in 160 cases. Ophthalmology. 115(9):1626-31, 1631, 2008
8. Akansel G et al: MRI patterns in orbital malignant lymphoma and atypical lymphocytic infiltrates. Eur J Radiol. 53(2):175-81, 2005
9. Valvassori GE et al: Imaging of orbital lymphoproliferative disorders. Radiol Clin North Am. 37(1):135-50, x-xi, 1999

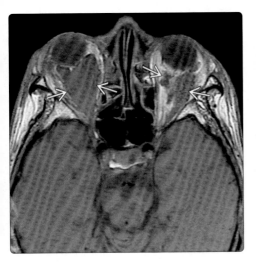

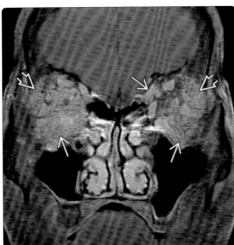

(Left) *Axial T1 MR through the orbits reveals extensive bilateral, lobular, infiltrative soft tissue masses ➡, which involve the intraconal and intraconal spaces.* (Right) *Coronal T1 C+ FS MR in the same patient shows moderate diffuse enhancement of the infiltrating tissue. There are bilateral lacrimal gland lesions ➡ along with intraconal, conal, and extraconal involvement ➡.*

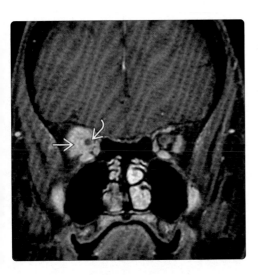

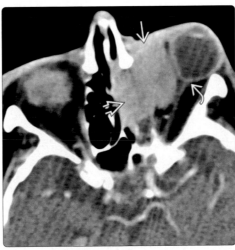

(Left) *Coronal T1 C+ FS MR shows typical features of MALT lymphoma with a homogeneous, enhancing intraconal mass ➡. The tumor surrounds the optic nerve ➡, potentially mimicking meningioma.* (Right) *Axial CECT shows a homogeneously enhancing mass in the medial orbit ➡, with severe left proptosis and tenting of the optic disc ➡. This mantle cell lymphoma is more aggressive than typical orbital MALT lymphoma and has destroyed much of the left ethmoid complex ➡.*

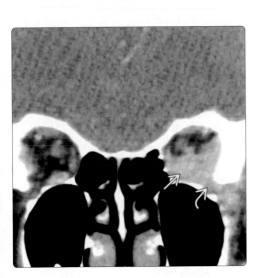

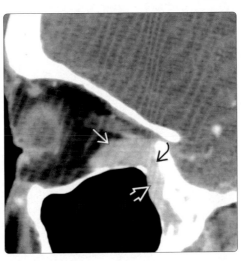

(Left) *Coronal CECT reveals an infiltrative OLPL in the inferior aspect of the left orbit ➡ with extension into the inferior orbital fissure ➡. This typically homogeneous lesion has ill-defined margins.* (Right) *Sagittal CECT in the same patient demonstrates further infiltrative extension from the posterior orbital lesion ➡ through the inferior orbital fissure ➡ and into the pterygopalatine fossa ➡. Ill-defined lesions often demonstrate more aggressive histology.*

Lacrimal Gland Carcinoma

TERMINOLOGY

- Malignant epithelial neoplasm of lacrimal gland
- Subtypes: Adenoid cystic carcinoma (ACCa), adenocarcinoma, squamous cell carcinoma, carcinoma ex pleomorphic adenoma

IMAGING

- Irregular or lobular lacrimal gland mass
  o Bone destruction seen in 70%; best indicator of malignant nature
- CT: Isodense with moderate enhancement
  o Bone algorithm CT to delineate bone erosion
- MR: T1 isointense with moderate to prominent T2 hyperintensity and enhancement
  o C+ FS images best for tumor mapping & identifying perineural spread
- PET/CT: FDG uptake variable

TOP DIFFERENTIAL DIAGNOSES

- Benign mixed tumor
- Lymphoproliferative lesion
- Dacryoadenitis
- Idiopathic inflammatory pseudotumor
- Sarcoidosis
- Sjögren syndrome
- Wegener granulomatosis

PATHOLOGY

- Parallels that of salivary gland neoplasms
- Divided into low and high grade based on WHO classification of salivary tumors

CLINICAL ISSUES

- ~ 2% of orbital neoplasms
- ACCa most common malignant lacrimal tumor
  o Must assess for perineural spread

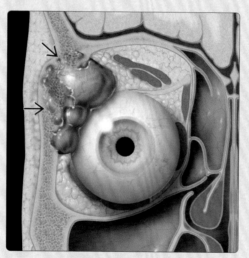
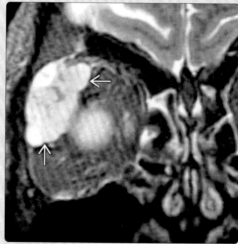

(Left) Coronal graphic depicts an infiltrating mass of the right lacrimal gland. The superolateral bony orbit is invaded ➡ by this lacrimal gland carcinoma, and the globe is displaced inferomedially. (Right) Coronal T2WI FS MR shows a markedly hyperintense, somewhat heterogeneous mass ➡ with lobulated, circumscribed borders centered in the right lacrimal fossa. In the absence of bone destruction, this adenoid cystic carcinoma cannot be distinguished from a benign lacrimal tumor.

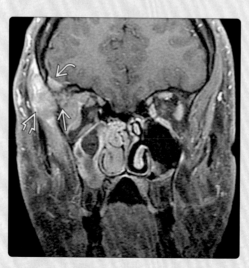
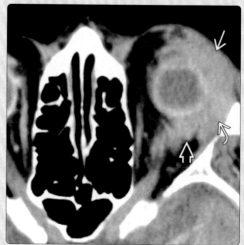

(Left) Coronal T1WI C+ FS MR reveals an irregular mass in the superolateral right orbit with bone destruction ➡ and extension into both the anterior cranial ➡ and temporalis ➡ fossae. Biopsy showed carcinoma ex pleomorphic adenoma. (Right) Axial NECT shows extensive local infiltration of an adenocarcinoma that invades the preseptal tissues ➡, as well as conal ➡ and intraconal ➡ retrobulbar spaces. The mass is closely apposed to the globe with scleral irregularity suspicious for invasion.

TERMINOLOGY

Synonyms

- Subtypes include adenoid cystic carcinoma (ACCa), adenocarcinoma, squamous cell carcinoma, acinic cell carcinoma, carcinoma ex pleomorphic adenoma

Definitions

- Malignant epithelial neoplasm of lacrimal gland

IMAGING

General Features

- Best diagnostic clue
  - Irregular lacrimal fossa mass **with bone erosion**
- Location
  - Superior temporal quadrant of orbit
  - Contiguous or perineural spread to surrounding structures and skull base

CT Findings

- NECT
  - Lobular or infiltrative isodense mass
- CECT
  - Moderate to intense enhancement
- Bone CT
  - Bone destruction in 70%
    - **Best indicator of malignant nature**
    - Bone remodeling typical of benign mixed tumor

MR Findings

- T1WI
  - Isointense to mildly hypointense to muscle
- T2WI
  - Moderate to prominent hyperintensity
- T1WI C+
  - Moderate to intense enhancement

Imaging Recommendations

- Best imaging tool
  - Enhanced MR with fat suppression best for mapping tumor extent & perineural spread
- Protocol advice
  - Bone algorithm CT to identify osseous erosion

DIFFERENTIAL DIAGNOSIS

Lacrimal Benign Mixed Tumor

- Slow-growing mass
- Scalloped, **bone remodeling**

Orbital Lymphoproliferative Lesion

- Typically shows **lower T2 signal** intensity

Dacryoadenitis

- Acute to subacute onset of painful swelling

Orbital Idiopathic Inflammatory Pseudotumor

- Steroid-responsive, noninfectious inflammation
- Painful & may be bilateral

Orbital Sarcoidosis

- Granulomatous process ± concurrent sinusitis

Orbital Sjögren Syndrome

- Autoimmune sialadenitis

Orbital Wegener Granulomatosis

- Granulomatous vasculitis with aggressive sinusitis

PATHOLOGY

Staging, Grading, & Classification

- AJCC 7th edition major changes in lacrimal staging
  - Parallels that of salivary gland neoplasms
  - Divided into low- & high-grade WHO classification
    - **Low-grade tumors** include carcinoma ex pleomorphic adenoma and acinic cell carcinoma
    - **High-grade tumors** include ACCa, squamous cell carcinoma, and adenocarcinoma

CLINICAL ISSUES

Presentation

- Most common signs/symptoms
  - Inferomedial globe displacement (75%)
- Other signs/symptoms
  - Diplopia
  - **Pain → bone/perineural involvement**
  - Sensory loss in distribution of lacrimal nerve

Demographics

- Epidemiology
  - Rare: 2% of orbital neoplasms
  - Epithelial neoplasms = 4% of lacrimal gland lesions
  - ACCa most common lacrimal malignancy (50%)

Natural History & Prognosis

- Low grade: Good prognosis following local resection
- High grade: High incidence local & distant recurrence, esp. ACCa
  - Disease-free survival rate 50% at 10 years for ACCa

Treatment

- Primarily surgical, ranging from local resection to exenteration ± bone removal
- Adjuvant radiation therapy for high-grade lesions

DIAGNOSTIC CHECKLIST

Consider

- Consider lacrimal carcinoma if unilateral mass + bone destruction

Image Interpretation Pearls

- Perineural spread is important feature of ACCa, most common lacrimal carcinoma

SELECTED REFERENCES

1. Sanders JC et al: Adenoid cystic carcinoma of the lacrimal gland. Am J Otolaryngol. 37(2):144-7, 2016
2. von Holstein SL et al: Tumors of the lacrimal gland. Semin Diagn Pathol. 33(3):156-63, 2016
3. Ahmad SM et al: American Joint Committee on Cancer classification predicts outcome of patients with lacrimal gland adenoid cystic carcinoma. Ophthalmology. 116(6):1210-5, 2009
4. Rootman J et al: Changes in the 7th edition of the AJCC TNM classification and recommendations for pathologic analysis of lacrimal gland tumors. Arch Pathol Lab Med. 133(8):1268-71, 2009

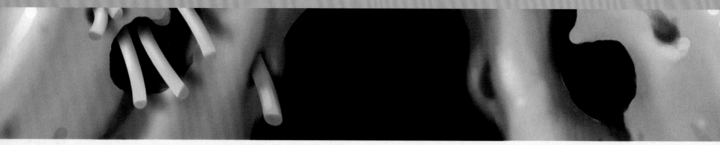

SECTION 23
Skull Base Lesions

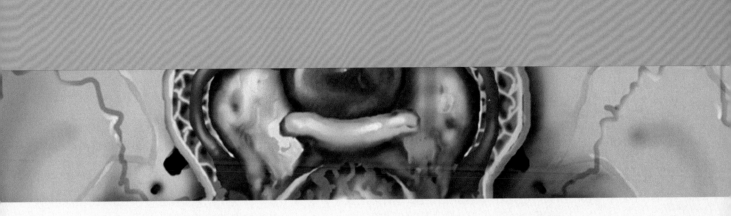

Skull Base Lesions

Imaging Approaches and Indications

CT is the primary imaging tool for evaluating the bony details of the skull base (SB). Multislice CT scanners allow thin slices (≤ 1 mm) and provide excellent multiplanar reformatted images. These function as the mainstay for evaluating bony changes associated with SB diseases as well as providing evidence for calcific or bony matrices of these lesions.

MR is an essential partner to bone CT in evaluating SB lesions as it provides the best understanding of lesion soft tissue extent. T1 precontrast images show lesion margins against the contrast of skull base marrow fat. T1 also reveals high-signal subacute blood and intralesion high-velocity flow voids to best advantage. Enhanced, fat-saturated T1 sequences define enhancement characteristics of the lesion in question. GRE may show blooming if hemorrhage or venous sinus thrombosis is present. DWI hyperintensity in a focal SB lesion suggests the diagnosis of epidermoid. MRA and MRV are important sequences to acquire if internal carotid and vertebral artery or venous sinus involvement is suspected.

Imaging Anatomy

The SB is made up of five bones: The paired frontal and temporal bones and the unpaired ethmoid, sphenoid, and occipital bones. Two major surfaces of the SB can be described: The **endocranial surface**, which faces the brain, cisterns, cranial nerves (CN), and intracranial vessels, and the **exocranial surface**, which faces the extracranial H&N. The exocranial surface anteriorly interfaces with the sinus, nose, and orbits, centrally with the masticator (MS), parotid (PS), parapharyngeal, and anterior pharyngeal mucosal spaces (PMS), and posteriorly with the carotid (CS), retropharyngeal (RPS), perivertebral (PVS), and posterior PMS.

The **endocranial surface** can be further divided into three regions: The anterior, central, and posterior SB.

- **Anterior SB** (ASB): Floor of anterior cranial fossa, comprised of orbital plate of frontal bone, ethmoid bone cribriform plate and ethmoid sinus roof, and planum sphenoidale and lesser wing (LWS) of sphenoid bone; important ASB foramina include **foramen cecum** (FC) and **cribriform plate foramina**
- **Central SB** (CSB): Floor of middle cranial fossa, made up of **basisphenoid**, **greater wing** of sphenoid bone (GWS), and **temporal bone** (T-bone) anterior to petrous ridge; bony landmarks of CSB include sella turcica, tuberculum sellae, and posterior clinoid process; important CSB foramina and fissures are optic canal, superior orbital fissure (SOF), inferior orbital fissure (IOF), foramen rotundum, foramen ovale, foramen spinosum, vidian canal, carotid canal, and foramen lacerum
- **Posterior SB** (PSB): Bony bowl that makes up floor of posterior cranial fossa, made up of **posterior wall** of **T-bone** and **occipital bone**; occipital bone has 3 parts: Basilar part (lower clivus/basiocciput), condylar part lateral to foramen magnum, including occipital condyles, and squamous part (large bony plate posterosuperior to foramen magnum); important PSB foramina and fissures include internal auditory canal (IAC), jugular foramen, hypoglossal canal, stylomastoid foramen, and foramen magnum

Skull Base Foramina/Fissures and Contents

Anterior Skull Base
- **Foramen cecum**: Midline, anterior to crista galli; embryologic remnant of anterior neuropore, which normally involutes in early childhood
- **Cribriform plate foramina**: Roof of nasal cavity; transmits afferent fibers from nasal mucosa to olfactory bulbs of **CNI**

Central Skull Base
- **Optic canal**: Medial LWS; transmits **CNII** to **globe**, dura, arachnoid and pia, CSF, ophthalmic artery
- **SOF**: Between LWS and GWS; transmits **CNIII**, **CNIV**, **CNVI**, **CNV1**, and superior ophthalmic vein
- **IOF**: Cleft between maxilla body and GWS; transmits inferior orbital artery, vein, and nerve
- **Foramen rotundum**: Conduit to pterygopalatine fossa (PPF) within sphenoid bone superolateral to vidian canal; transmits **CNV2** to **PPF**, artery of foramen rotundum, emissary veins from cavernous sinus to pterygoid plexus
- **Foramen ovale**: Within GWS; conduit to masticator space; transmits **CNV3** into **masticator space**, lesser petrosal nerve, and accessory meningeal branch of internal maxillary artery
- **Foramen spinosum**: Within GWS posterolateral to foramen ovale; transmits middle meningeal artery and vein and recurrent branch of CNV3
- **Vidian canal**: Inferolateral to foramen rotundum within GWS; connects foramen lacerum to PPF; transmits vidian nerve and artery
- **Carotid canal**: In T-bone and GWS; transmits petrous (C2) and lacerum (C3) segments of internal carotid artery (ICA) and **sympathetic plexus**
- **Foramen lacerum**: Pseudoforamen; cartilaginous floor of lacerum ICA segment

Posterior Skull Base
- **IAC**: In posterior wall of T-bone; opening called porus acusticus; transmits **CNVII**, **CNVIII**, and labyrinthine artery
- **Jugular foramen** (JF): Cleft between temporal and occipital bones with 2 parts (pars nervosa and vascularis); pars nervosa transmits **CNXI** into **CS**, Jacobsen nerve, inferior petrosal vein; pars vascularis transmits **CNX**, **CNXI**, Arnold nerve, posterior meningeal artery, jugular bulb
- **Hypoglossal canal**: Found with condylar occipital bone inferomedial to JF; transmits **CNXII** into **CS**
- **Stylomastoid foramen**: Exocranial surface of T-bone between medial mastoid tip and styloid process; transmits **CNVII** into **parotid space**
- **Foramen magnum**: Occipital bone inferior ring; transmits medulla oblongata, vertebral arteries, and **CNXI** (ascending spinal component)

Embryology

ASB embryology is key to understanding disease in this area (anterior neuropore anomaly, cephalocele, nasal glioma). The **prenasal space** is a transient prenatal region separating nasal bones and cartilaginous nasal capsule. The anterior neuropore extends from intracranial space to prenasal space and briefly contacts skin at the bridge of the nose but involutes prior to birth. The prenasal space reduces to a small canal anterior to the crista galli called the **foramen cecum**. The newborn FC

Skull Base Differential Diagnosis: Tumors & Tumor-Like Lesions by Site

Skull base, anterior, central, or posterior	Melanoma, N
Meningioma	Lacrimal gland carcinoma, O
Giant cell tumor	**Central skull base**
Hemangiopericytoma	Sella: Pituitary macroadenoma
Metastases	Clivus: Chordoma, ecchordosis physaliphora
Multiple myeloma	Petrooccipital fissure: Chondrosarcoma
Plasmacytoma	Meckel cave: Trigeminal schwannoma
Osteosarcoma	T-bone: Tumor
Rhabdomyosarcoma, parameningeal	Endolymphatic sac tumor
Langerhans cell histiocytosis	T-bone: Tumor-like lesions
Tumor-like lesions	Acquired cholesteatoma
Fibrous dysplasia	Congenital cholesteatoma
Paget disease	Cholesterol granuloma
Idiopathic extraorbital inflammation (pseudotumor)	**Posterior skull base**
Anterior skull base	Clivus (occipital bone): Chordoma
Mucocele, SN	Jugular foramen
Osteoma, SN	Glomus jugulare paraganglioma
Esthesioneuroblastoma, N	Jugular foramen schwannoma
Squamous cell carcinoma, SN	Jugular foramen meningioma
Non-Hodgkin lymphoma, SN or O	Hypoglossal canal: Hypoglossal schwannoma

SN = sinonasal; N = nasal; O = orbit.

diameter is ~ 4 mm. The FC should be completely ossified by 2 years of age.

As the ASB originates largely from cartilaginous precursors, the process of ossification can be confusing on imaging. The ASB ossifies from posterior to anterior and lateral to medial. At birth the ASB is composed of cartilage, which progressively ossifies. Ossification of the crista galli and cribriform plate begins at 2 months and is nearly complete by 24 months. The crista galli contains fat at about 12 months (**do not** call it a dermoid). The area of the FC ossifies last, reaching its adult configuration by 2 years (**do not** overcall an anterior neuropore anomaly).

The CSB forms from ~ 24 ossifications centers. Major centers include the presphenoid (planum sphenoidale), postsphenoid (basisphenoid containing sella, dorsum, sphenoid sinus), alisphenoid (GWS), and orbitosphenoid (LWS). The **sphenooccipital synchondrosis** lies between the basisphenoid and basiocciput. It is the site of most postnatal SB growth and one of the last sutures to fuse (completed by age 20 years). Persistence of the **craniopharyngeal canal** (remnant of Rathke pouch) may occur between the presphenoid and basisphenoid. Persistence of the **median basal canal** may be seen between the basioccipital ossification centers.

Approaches to Skull Base Imaging Issues

Creating skull base lesion DDx can be difficult because some lesions can occur anywhere along the SB. Understanding the DDx list of the lesions that can occur anywhere in the SB is essential. Adding this group to a site-specific DDx can yield a near complete set of possible lesions to be considered. ASB, CSB, and PSB DDx lists can be constructed. The CSB can be further refined into shorter site-specific DDx lists for the sella, clivus, petrooccipital fissure, and Meckel cave. The PSB has one important site-specific DDx for the jugular foramen.

Knowledgeable reports about SB lesions require the radiologist to understand the interface relationships between the SB and the extracranial H&N. The ASB sits atop the frontal and ethmoid sinuses, orbit, and nose. Many of the ASB lesions originate in these structures. The CSB resides superior to the MS, PS, and PMSs. Nasopharyngeal carcinoma directly accesses the intracranial compartment via the foramen lacerum (perivascular spread). MS and PS space malignancies may reach the intracranial compartment via perineural spread along CNV3 and CNVII, respectively. The PSB directly interacts with the CS, RPS, and PVSs. When JF lesions exit the skull base inferiorly, they plunge directly into the nasopharyngeal CS.

Without a clear understanding of perineural tumor (PNT) SB spread, the radiologist may not identify this key imaging finding. PNT from PS malignancy enters the stylomastoid foramen and climbs the CNVII mastoid segment. MS malignancy at CNV3 PNT traverses foramen ovale on its way to Meckel cave. Cheek skin, palate, sinus, or orbit carcinoma can access CNV2 via the infraorbital nerve or PPF, following CNV2 through the foramen rotundum into the middle cranial fossa. PPF malignancy may also show PNT spread via the vidian nerve to the foramen lacerum. PNT also connects between CNV and CNVII along the greater superficial petrosal nerve on the superior ridge of the petrous T-bone.

Selected References

1. Borges A: Skull base tumours part I: imaging technique, anatomy and anterior skull base tumours. Eur J Radiol. 66(3):338-47, 2008
2. Borges A: Skull base tumours Part II. Central skull base tumours and intrinsic tumours of the bony skull base. Eur J Radiol. 66(3):348-62, 2008

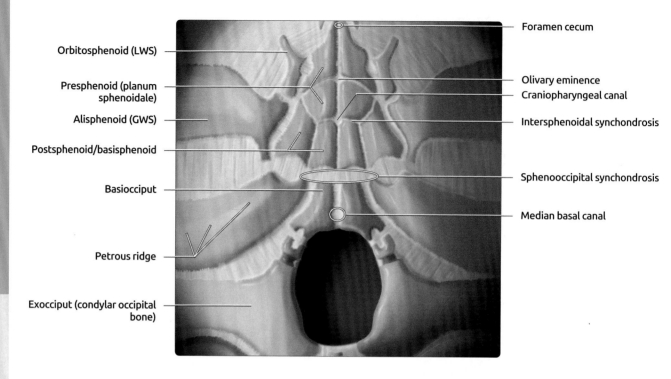

Orbitosphenoid (LWS)

Presphenoid (planum sphenoidale)

Alisphenoid (GWS)

Postsphenoid/basisphenoid

Basiocciput

Petrous ridge

Exocciput (condylar occipital bone)

Foramen cecum

Olivary eminence

Craniopharyngeal canal

Intersphenoidal synchondrosis

Sphenooccipital synchondrosis

Median basal canal

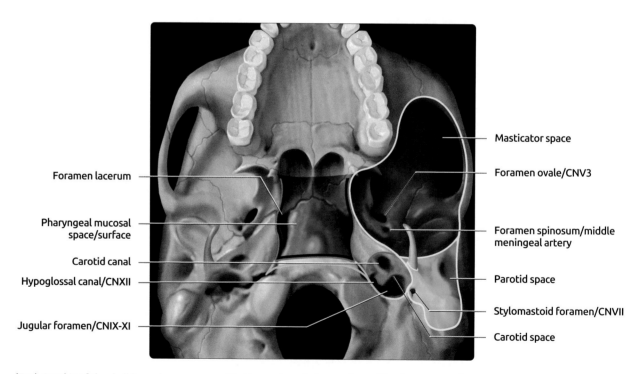

Foramen lacerum

Pharyngeal mucosal space/surface

Carotid canal

Hypoglossal canal/CNXII

Jugular foramen/CNIX-XI

Masticator space

Foramen ovale/CNV3

Foramen spinosum/middle meningeal artery

Parotid space

Stylomastoid foramen/CNVII

Carotid space

(Top) *Graphic of the skull base shows many ossification centers. Between the ossification centers of presphenoid is a cartilaginous gap called the olivary eminence, which is obliterated shortly after birth. In the midline, note the craniopharyngeal canal, sphenooccipital synchondrosis, and median basal canal. The sphenooccipital synchondrosis fuses over the first 20 years of life while the craniopharyngeal and median basal canals are rarely persistent into childhood. When persistent, these two canals can rarely be the source of meningitis.* **(Bottom)** *Graphic of the skull base viewed from below shows the relationship of spaces of the suprahyoid neck to the skull base. Four spaces have key interactions with skull base: Masticator, parotid, carotid, and pharyngeal mucosal spaces. Parotid space (green) malignancy can follow CNVII into the stylomastoid foramen. Masticator space (purple) receives CNV3 while CNIX-XII enter the carotid space (red). The pharyngeal mucosal space abuts the foramen lacerum, which is covered by fibrocartilage in life.*

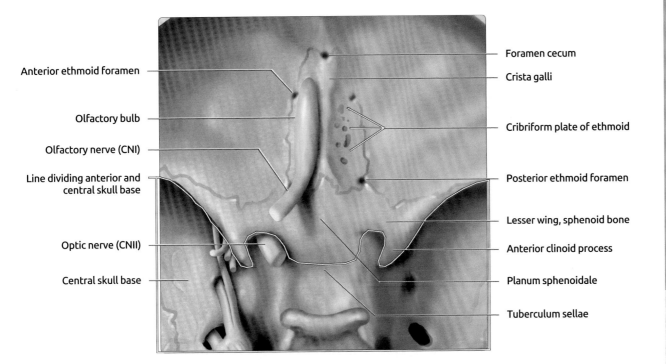

Anterior ethmoid foramen

Olfactory bulb

Olfactory nerve (CNI)

Line dividing anterior and central skull base

Optic nerve (CNII)

Central skull base

Foramen cecum

Crista galli

Cribriform plate of ethmoid

Posterior ethmoid foramen

Lesser wing, sphenoid bone

Anterior clinoid process

Planum sphenoidale

Tuberculum sellae

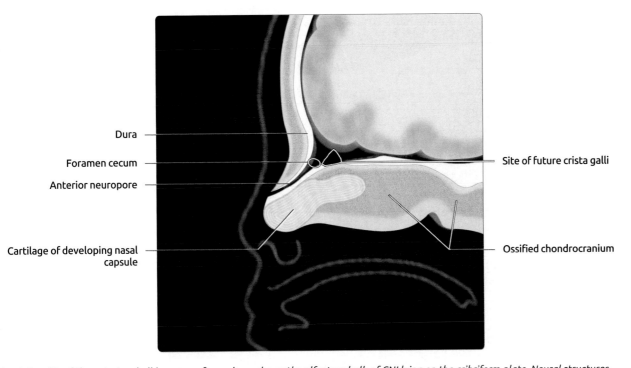

Dura

Foramen cecum

Anterior neuropore

Cartilage of developing nasal capsule

Site of future crista galli

Ossified chondrocranium

(Top) *Graphic of the anterior skull base seen from above shows the olfactory bulb of CNI lying on the cribriform plate. Neural structures have been removed on right, allowing visualization of numerous perforations in the cribriform plate, through which afferent fibers from olfactory mucosa pass to form the olfactory bulb. The posterior margin of the anterior skull base is formed by the lesser wing of sphenoid and planum sphenoidale. Note the foramen cecum, a small pit anterior to the crista galli, bounded anteriorly by frontal bone and posteriorly by ethmoid bone. If the anterior neuropore persists, an enlarged foramen cecum, bifid crista galli, and epidermoid along the neuropore tract are possible. (Bottom) Sagittal graphic of the anterior skull base during development shows ossification of the chondrocranium proceeding from posterior to anterior. The prenasal space is now encased in bone and has become the foramen cecum. A normal stalk of dura extends through the foramen cecum to skin (anterior neuropore).*

Skull Base Overview

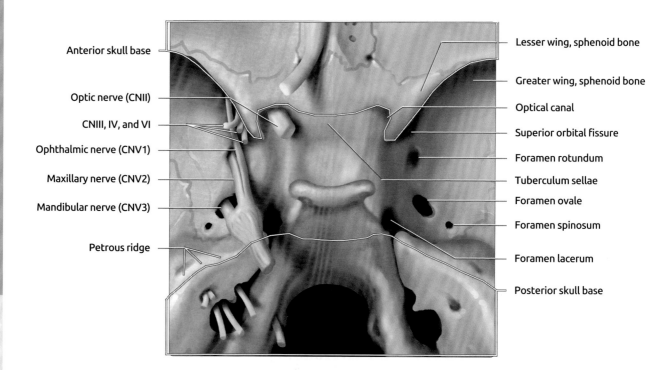

Anterior skull base

Optic nerve (CNII)

CNIII, IV, and VI

Ophthalmic nerve (CNV1)

Maxillary nerve (CNV2)

Mandibular nerve (CNV3)

Petrous ridge

Lesser wing, sphenoid bone

Greater wing, sphenoid bone

Optical canal

Superior orbital fissure

Foramen rotundum

Tuberculum sellae

Foramen ovale

Foramen spinosum

Foramen lacerum

Posterior skull base

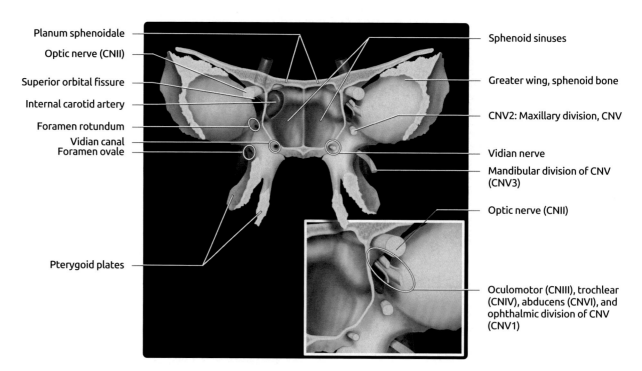

Planum sphenoidale

Optic nerve (CNII)

Superior orbital fissure

Internal carotid artery

Foramen rotundum

Vidian canal
Foramen ovale

Pterygoid plates

Sphenoid sinuses

Greater wing, sphenoid bone

CNV2: Maxillary division, CNV

Vidian nerve

Mandibular division of CNV
(CNV3)

Optic nerve (CNII)

Oculomotor (CNIII), trochlear
(CNIV), abducens (CNVI), and
ophthalmic division of CNV
(CNV1)

(Top) *Graphic of the central skull base seen from above shows the important nerves on the left and the numerous fissures and foramina on the right. The greater wing of the sphenoid bone forms the anterior wall of the middle cranial fossa. The posterior limit of the central skull base is the dorsum sella medially and the petrous ridge laterally.* **(Bottom)** *Coronal graphic shows the important anatomy of the central skull base/sphenoid bone. The cavernous portions of the internal carotid arteries lie lateral and posterior to the sinuses. At the orbital apex, the optic nerve can be seen traversing the optic canal. Multiple cranial nerves pass through the superior orbital fissure into the orbit, including CNs III, IV, and VI as well as the ophthalmic division on CNV. The maxillary division of CNV in foramen rotundum and the vidian nerve are positioned lateral and inferior to the sinus, respectively.*

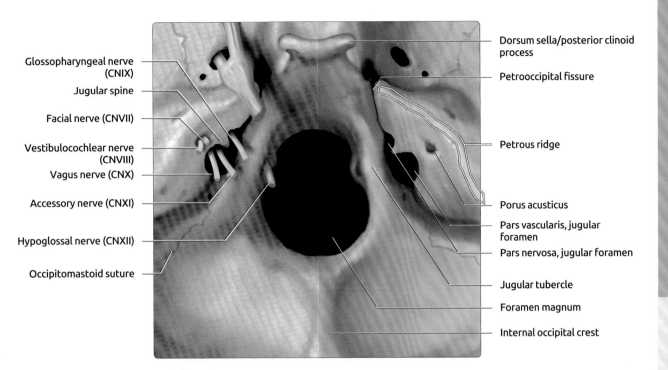

Glossopharyngeal nerve (CNIX)
Jugular spine
Facial nerve (CNVII)
Vestibulocochlear nerve (CNVIII)
Vagus nerve (CNX)
Accessory nerve (CNXI)
Hypoglossal nerve (CNXII)
Occipitomastoid suture

Dorsum sella/posterior clinoid process
Petrooccipital fissure
Petrous ridge
Porus acusticus
Pars vascularis, jugular foramen
Pars nervosa, jugular foramen
Jugular tubercle
Foramen magnum
Internal occipital crest

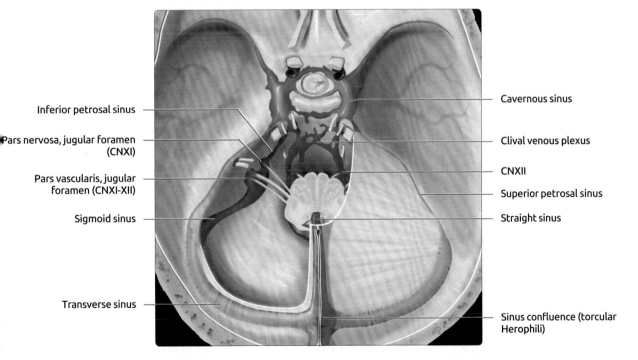

Inferior petrosal sinus
Pars nervosa, jugular foramen (CNXI)
Pars vascularis, jugular foramen (CNXI-XII)
Sigmoid sinus
Transverse sinus

Cavernous sinus
Clival venous plexus
CNXII
Superior petrosal sinus
Straight sinus
Sinus confluence (torcular Herophili)

(Top) *Graphic shows the posterior skull base as seen from above. The neural structures are shown on the left while the bony landmarks are seen on the right. The anterior boundary of posterior skull base is clivus medially and petrous ridge laterally. The major foramina are the foramen magnum, porus acusticus, jugular foramen, and hypoglossal canal. Notice that the jugular foramen connects anteriorly with the petrooccipital fissure.* (Bottom) *Graphic of the posterior skull base shows the major dural venous sinuses and jugular foramen from above. The midbrain and pons as well as the left half of the tentorium cerebelli have been removed. Notice the transverse sinus is in the wall of the occipital bone while the sigmoid sinus is in the medial wall of the temporal bone. The two portions of the jugular foramen are also visible. The anterior pars nervosa receives the glossopharyngeal nerve (CNIX), while the pars vascularis has the vagus (CNX) and accessory (CNXI) nerves passing through it.*

Ecchordosis Physaliphora

TERMINOLOGY

- Benign **cystic mass arising dorsal to clivus with intradural component in prepontine cistern**
  - Considered to be ectopic notochordal remnant

IMAGING

- CT: Prepontine intradural mass connected by osseous stalk or pedicle to clivus
  - May have associated well-marginated, scalloped lesion of clivus with sclerotic margins
- MR: Provides best depiction of lesion, stalk, and intradural component
  - Uniformly T2 hyperintense
  - Clival component hypointense compared to normal marrow
  - Restricted diffusion often noted
  - **Lack of enhancement** differentiates from chordoma

TOP DIFFERENTIAL DIAGNOSES

- Chordoma
- Skull base metastasis
- Dermoid or epidermoid
- Arachnoid cyst

PATHOLOGY

- Few clear cells ("**physaliphorous cells**") surrounded by chondromyxoid stroma

CLINICAL ISSUES

- Asymptomatic & usually found incidentally on head MR
  - Found in 2% of autopsies & 1.6% of MR studies
- Indolent lesion, which does not appear to grow
- Typically not managed surgically unless significant brainstem compression or symptoms are present

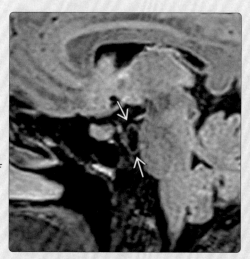
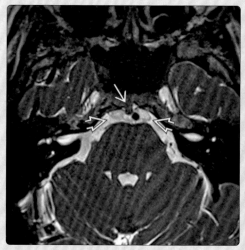

(Left) Sagittal T2 FLAIR demonstrates the intradural component of a classic ecchordosis physaliphora with a notable thin-walled ⊸ cyst, which is otherwise isointense with CSF. Clival portion of lesion is not well seen. (Right) Axial 3D T2 MR SSFSE demonstrates a small bony strut ⊸ of classic ecchordosis physaliphora (EP) and the intradural cystic component of the lesion ⊸, which is surrounding the basilar artery. Cystic lesion within the clivus is not apparent on this section.

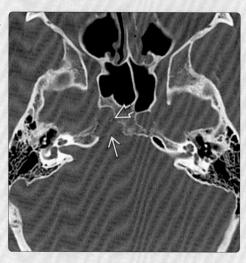
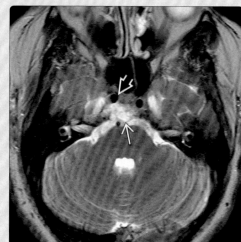

(Left) Axial bone CT shows a well-marginated lytic lesion of the clivus with sclerotic borders ⊸. This lesion extended to the carotid canal ⊸, but the carotid artery was normal. No intradural component is appreciated on this bone window CT. (Right) Axial T2 MR in the same patient shows hyperintense T2 signal with internal septations within the clival portion of the lesion and demonstrates intradural extension into the prepontine cistern ⊸, adjacent to the basilar artery. A normal internal carotid artery flow void is evident ⊸.

TERMINOLOGY

Abbreviations

- Ecchordosis physaliphora (EP)

Definitions

- Benign cystic mass arising from dorsal clivus considered to be **ectopic notochordal remnant**

IMAGING

General Features

- Best diagnostic clue
  - Well-defined lesion of clivus with prepontine intradural cystic mass connected by stalk or pedicle to clival lesion
- Location
  - **Prepontine cistern** along dorsal midline clivus most common; occasionally paramedian
  - Recently proposed classification system depends on EP appearance; clivus alone or clivus and intradural component
- Morphology
  - Well defined, lobular ± stalk

Imaging Recommendations

- Best imaging tool
  - MR provides best depiction of lesion, stalk, and intradural component
- Protocol advice
  - Sagittal images and 3D T2 best for identifying osseous stalk attaching lesion to clivus and cyst

CT Findings

- NECT
  - CT may not identify intradural component (similar density to CSF)
- Bone CT
  - Variable osseous stalk or pedicle connecting basisphenoid portion of clivus to intradural component
  - Well-marginated, scalloped clival component with sclerotic margins

MR Findings

- T1WI
  - Intradural component may be nearly isointense to CSF
  - Intraclival component (if present) hypointense compared to normal clivus marrow
- T2WI
  - Uniformly hyperintense in most cases
- DWI
  - **Restricted diffusion** often noted
- T1WI C+
  - No enhancement noted (differentiates from chordoma)

DIFFERENTIAL DIAGNOSIS

Clivus Chordoma

- Malignant clival mass that typically remains extradural
- Always enhances; destroys bone
- Aggressive & symptomatic

Skull Base Metastasis

- Multiple lesions, enhancement is common

Dermoid and Epidermoid

- Rarely located in clivus but may closely resemble imaging characteristics

Arachnoid Cyst

- Follows CSF density/signal intensity exactly

PATHOLOGY

General Features

- Etiology
  - Benign congenital malformation arising from ectopic notochordal tissue

Gross Pathologic & Surgical Features

- Small cystic or gelatinous mass, which has intradural component and is attached to clivus by stalk

Microscopic Features

- Few clear cells ("physaliphorous cells") surrounded by chondromyxoid stroma

CLINICAL ISSUES

Presentation

- Most common signs/symptoms
  - Asymptomatic lesion may be found incidentally on head MR or CT
- Other signs/symptoms
  - Rare brainstem compressive symptoms, pontine hemorrhage, CSF fistulae with rhinorrhea

Demographics

- Epidemiology
  - Found in 2% of autopsies & 1.6% of MR studies

Natural History & Prognosis

- Indolent lesion, which **does not** appear to **grow**

Treatment

- Typically not managed surgically unless significant brainstem compression or symptoms are present

DIAGNOSTIC CHECKLIST

Image Interpretation Pearls

- Identification of stalk arising from clivus with intradural extension of lesion into prepontine cistern is characteristic

SELECTED REFERENCES

1. Golden LD et al: Benign notochordal lesions of the posterior clivus: retrospective review of prevalence and imaging characteristics. J Neuroimaging. 24(3):245-9, 2014
2. Chihara C et al: Ecchordosis physaliphora and its variants: proposed new classification based on high-resolution fast MR imaging employing steady-state acquisition. Eur Radiol. 23(10):2854-60, 2013
3. Alkan O et al: A case of ecchordosis physaliphora presenting with an intratumoral hemorrhage. Turk Neurosurg. 19(3):293-6, 2009
4. Ciarpaglini R et al: Intradural clival chordoma and ecchordosis physaliphora: a challenging differential diagnosis: case report. Neurosurgery. 64(2):E387-8; discussion E388, 2009
5. Srinivasan A et al: Case 133: ecchordosis physaliphora. Radiology. 247(2):585-8, 2008
6. Roberti F et al: Intradural cranial chordoma: a rare presentation of an uncommon tumor. Surgical experience and review of the literature. J Neurosurg. 106(2):270-4, 2007
7. Mehnert F et al: Retroclival ecchordosis physaliphora: MR imaging and review of the literature. AJNR Am J Neuroradiol. 25(10):1851-5, 2004

TERMINOLOGY

- Fossa navicularis magna (FNM)
  - Congenital defect resulting from minor pharyngeal formation miscue creating boat-shaped defect in ventral surface of midclivus

IMAGING

- Sagittal bone CT
  - FNM appears as **boat-shaped corticated divot** of **midline, ventral, midclivus**
- Sagittal MR
  - Nasopharyngeal **adenoids/mucosa** project into FNM lumen

TOP DIFFERENTIAL DIAGNOSES

- Persistent craniopharyngeal canal (P-CPC)
- Median basal canal (MBC)
- Extraosseous chordoma
- Ecchordosis physaliphora

PATHOLOGY

- Best etiology hypothesis
  - During notochord ascent, focal adhesions form between notochord and foregut endoderm
  - Pharyngeal mucosa is then carried along with notochord toward developing skull base
  - Final result is midline divot (FNM) in ventral midclivus lined with pharyngeal mucosa/adenoidal tissue

CLINICAL ISSUES

- **Asymptomatic, incidental finding**
- Rarely infected ± meningitis

DIAGNOSTIC CHECKLIST

- **Location comparison** of congenital lesions in area
  - P-CPC anterior to sphenoccipital synchondrosis
  - FNM and MBC posterior to sphenoccipital synchondrosis
  - FNM affects ventral cortex of midclivus
  - MBC is most commonly transclival in lower clivus

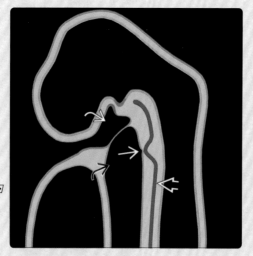
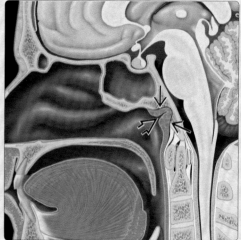

(Left) Sagittal graphic of a 4- to 5-week-old fetus shows that as the notochord ➡ ascends, it forms focal adhesions with the foregut endoderm ➡, & a portion of pharyngeal mucosa is carried along with the notochord to the developing skull base. A diverticulum (FNM) lined with pharyngeal mucosa/adenoids will appear in the midline; see the stomodeum ➡ & foregut ➡. (Right) Sagittal graphic of adult FNM shows the lesion ➡ in the sagittal plane is boat-shaped, midline, in the ventral mid-clivus, & filled with mucosa & adenoidal tissue ➡.

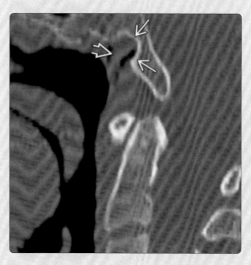
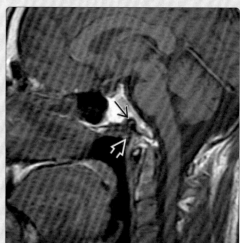

(Left) Sagittal bone CT reformation in a patient scanned for neck pain reveals an incidental boat-shaped FNM ➡ with nasopharyngeal adenoids/mucosa projecting into its lumen ➡. (Right) Sagittal T1 MR in the same patient shows the FNM is in the ventral midclivus ➡. The MR better shows the mucosa/adnoids projecting into the FNM ➡. The low signal areas are due to air trapped in the adenoidal tissues.

TERMINOLOGY

Abbreviations

- Fossa navicularis magna (FNM)

Synonyms

- Pharyngeal bursa or pharyngeal fossa

Definitions

- FNM: Congenital defect resulting from minor pharyngeal formation miscue creating boat-shaped defect in ventral surface of midclivus

IMAGING

General Features

- Best diagnostic clue
  - Sagittal bone CT: **Boat-shaped corticated divot of midline, ventral, midclivus**
  - Sagittal MR: **Nasopharyngeal adenoids/mucosa project into FNM lumen**
- Location
  - Defect found in ventral surface of mid to midclivus
  - FNM posterior to sphenoccipital synchondrosis
- Size
  - Variable: Barely visible to 15 mm
- Morphology
  - Ovoid on axial view; boat-shaped on sagittal view

CT Findings

- Bone CT
  - Axial: Ovoid, corticated lesion of midclivus
  - Sagittal: Boat-shaped lesion; ventral clival surface
  - Air may be trapped in adenoidal tissue within FNM
  - Small fossa navicularis defects may be subtle

MR Findings

- T1WI FS
  - Mucosa/adenoidal tissue project into FNM
- T1WI C+ FS
  - Mild enhancement of adenoidal tissue in FNM
  - If significant enhancement ± adjacent skull base bone abnormalities, consider infection
    - Infected FNM is extremely rare

DIFFERENTIAL DIAGNOSIS

Persistent Craniopharyngeal Canal

- Persistent bony canal between anterior floor of sella and nasopharyngeal roof
- Results from developmental nonobliteration of adenohypophyseal stalk
- If small, incidental
- May be intermediate in size and contain ectopic pituitary
- May be large and contain cephalocele, tumors, or both

Median Basal Canal

- Persistent bony canal spanning lower clivus inner cortex to posterior nasopharynx
- Notochordal track remnant
- Very rare lesion

Extraosseous Chordoma

- Midline nasopharyngeal chordoma with soft tissue and bony components
- May have median basal canal component

Ecchordosis Physaliphora

- Superior dorsal clival cortex scalloping lesion
- Benign congenital malformation arising from ectopic notochordal tissue

PATHOLOGY

General Features

- Best etiology hypothesis
  - During notochord ascent, **focal adhesions** form **between notochord and foregut endoderm**
  - Pharyngeal mucosa will be carried along with notochord as result toward developing skull base
  - Midline divot in ventral midclivus lined with pharyngeal mucosa/lymphoid tissue results (FNM)

CLINICAL ISSUES

Presentation

- Most common signs/symptoms
  - **Asymptomatic; incidental finding**
  - Rarely infected ± meningitis

Demographics

- Age
  - Present at birth; age of discovery based on incidental lesion discovery while imaging for another reason
- Epidemiology
  - ~ 5% if count smaller fossa navicularis and FNM

Natural History & Prognosis

- Incidental finding
- Very rarely may cause skull base osteomyelitis ± meningitis

Treatment

- No treatment required unless infected

DIAGNOSTIC CHECKLIST

Consider

- FNM is **not** associated with Tornwaldt cyst
- **Location comparison** of congenital lesions in area
  - Persistent craniopharyngeal canal anterior to sphenoccipital synchondrosis (SOS)
  - FNM and median basal canal (MBC) posterior to SOS
  - FNM affects ventral cortex of midclivus
  - MBC is most commonly transclival in lower clivus

SELECTED REFERENCES

1. Ginat DT et al: Multi-detector-row computed tomography imaging of variant skull base foramina. J Comput Assist Tomogr. 37(4):481-5, 2013
2. Segal N et al: Intracranial infection caused by spreading through the fossa naviclaris magna - a case report and review of the literature. Int J Pediatr Otorhinolaryngol. 77(12):1919-21, 2013
3. Ben Salem D et al: Fossa navicularis: anatomic variation at the skull base. Clin Anat. 19(4):365, 2006
4. Cankal F et al: Fossa navicularis: anatomic variation at the skull base. Clin Anat. 17(2):118-22, 2004
5. Beltramello A et al: Fossa navicularis magna. AJNR Am J Neuroradiol. 19(9):1796-8, 1998

Invasive Pituitary Macroadenoma

TERMINOLOGY

- Invasive, benign pituitary adenoma with inferior extension into skull base

IMAGING

- Multiplanar gadolinium-enhanced MR is imaging modality of choice
- Mass invading central skull base **contiguous with and inseparable from soft tissue mass in sella**
- Ill-defined soft tissue mass centered in sella with invasion of surrounding bone and soft tissue
- Intense enhancement may be heterogeneous as tumor enlarges
- May **extend into cavernous sinus**

TOP DIFFERENTIAL DIAGNOSES

- Clival chordoma
- Skull base meningioma
- Skull base metastasis

- Petrooccipital chondrosarcoma
- Skull base plasmacytoma

CLINICAL ISSUES

- Mean age at presentation: ~ 40 years
- If hormone secreting, symptoms depend on which hormone secreted
- 25% visual field defect or other cranial nerve palsy
- Treatment: Multimodality therapy required for best outcome
  - Surgery often indicated for decompression of optic apparatus
  - Resection often incomplete and leads to recurrences
  - ↑ morbidity due to proximity to vital structures

DIAGNOSTIC CHECKLIST

- Look at sagittal images for normal pituitary gland, and, if absent, invasive adenoma should be at top of DDx

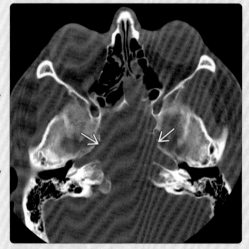
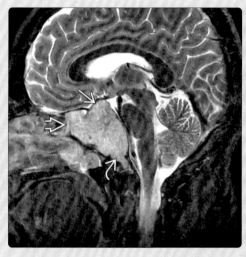

(Left) CT of invasive pituitary macroadenoma shows extensive bone erosion of central skull base and dorsal clivus. Sella and basisphenoid are largely destroyed. Tumor extends to medial aspects of petrous internal carotid artery canals ➡. (Right) Sagittal T2WI MR shows extensive invasive pituitary tumor with suprasellar extension ➡ and invasion anteriorly into basisphenoid ➡ and inferiorly into clivus ➡. Tumor also extends anteroinferiorly into nasopharynx and posterior nasal cavity.

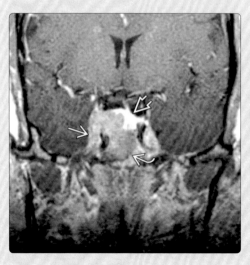
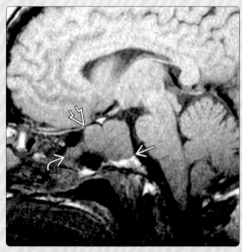

(Left) Coronal T1WI C+ MR demonstrates pituitary adenoma with invasion of right cavernous sinus ➡ and encasement of carotid artery. Tumor extends inferiorly into skull base ➡. Residual normal enhancing pituitary gland is seen superior to invasive adenoma ➡. (Right) Sagittal T1WI MR shows an invasive pituitary adenoma extending inferiorly into the clivus and replacing normal clival fat ➡. The mass also invades sphenoid sinus ➡ and posterior nasal cavity ➡. The normal pituitary gland is not visualized.

TERMINOLOGY

Definitions

- Invasive benign pituitary macroadenoma with inferior extension into skull base

IMAGING

General Features

- Best diagnostic clue
  - Mass invading central skull base **contiguous with and inseparable from soft tissue mass in sella**
- Size
  - Generally > 5 cm

CT Findings

- NECT
  - Ill-defined soft tissue mass centered in sella with invasion of surrounding bone and soft tissue
  - Hemorrhage in 10%; calcification in 2%

MR Findings

- T1WI
  - Sellar and infrasellar mass typically isointense to gray matter
- T2WI
  - Variable signal on long TR images
- T1WI C+
  - Intense enhancement may be heterogeneous as tumor enlarges
    - Dural tail may be seen and mimic meningioma
    - May **extend into cavernous sinus**

Imaging Recommendations

- Best imaging tool
  - Multiplanar gadolinium-enhanced MR

DIFFERENTIAL DIAGNOSIS

Clival Chordoma

- Midline clival mass
- ↑ **T2 signal** characteristic

Skull Base Meningioma

- Centered along lateral margin of cavernous sinus or tentorium
- Avidly enhancing ± dural tail, tumoral Ca^+

Skull Base Metastasis

- Destructive mass that can be anywhere in skull base

Chondrosarcoma (Petrooccipital Fissure)

- Centered along lateral margin of clivus in petrooccipital fissure
- **Chondroid calcifications** (50%)

Skull Base Plasmacytoma

- T2 signal is low to intermediate
- > 50% have concurrent multiple myeloma

PATHOLOGY

General Features

- Etiology

- Hypothesis for pituitary tumor formation
  - Hypophysiotrophic hormone excess, suppressive hormone insufficiency, or growth factor excess → hyperplasia
  - Hyperplasia predisposes to genetic instability → cell transformation → adenoma formation

Staging, Grading, & Classification

- Radioanatomical classification of adenomas
  - Stage I: Microadenoma < 1 cm without sellar expansion
  - Stage II: Macroadenoma ≥ 1 cm and may be suprasellar
  - Stage III: Macroadenoma with enlargement and invasion of floor or suprasellar extension
  - Stage IV: Destruction of sella

Microscopic Features

- Monotonous sheets of uniform cells

CLINICAL ISSUES

Presentation

- Most common signs/symptoms
  - **Pituitary hormonal abnormality** (symptoms depend on which hormone secreted)
- Other signs/symptoms
  - 25% visual field defect or other cranial nerve palsy

Demographics

- Age
  - Mean age at presentation: ~ 40 years
- Epidemiology
  - Pituitary adenoma: 15% of intracranial tumors
  - Invasive adenomas account for 35% of all pituitary neoplasms

Natural History & Prognosis

- Adenomas typically slow growing
- > 1/3 behave in more aggressive manner with high recurrence rate

Treatment

- Multimodality therapy and long-term follow-up required for best outcome
- Surgical resection is treatment of choice if possible
  - Surgery often followed by radiation ± chemotherapy

DIAGNOSTIC CHECKLIST

Image Interpretation Pearls

- **Look at sagittal images for normal pituitary gland**; if absent, invasive adenoma should be at top of DDx

SELECTED REFERENCES

1. Sav A et al: Invasive, atypical and aggressive pituitary adenomas and carcinomas. Endocrinol Metab Clin North Am. 44(1):99-104, 2015
2. Hornyak M et al: Multimodality treatment for invasive pituitary adenomas. Postgrad Med. 121(2):168-76, 2009
3. Gürlek A et al: What are the markers of aggressiveness in prolactinomas? Changes in cell biology, extracellular matrix components, angiogenesis and genetics. Eur J Endocrinol. 156(2):143-53, 2007
4. Nakasu Y et al: Tentorial enhancement on MR images is a sign of cavernous sinus involvement in patients with sellar tumors. AJNR Am J Neuroradiol. 22(8):1528-33, 2001
5. Yokoyama S et al: Are nonfunctioning pituitary adenomas extending into the cavernous sinus aggressive and/or invasive? Neurosurgery. 49(4):857-62; discussion 862-3, 2001

KEY FACTS

TERMINOLOGY

- Rare, locally aggressive tumor of clivus arising from cranial end of primitive notochord remnant

IMAGING

- Location: **Clivus**; sphenooccipital synchondrosis
  - Can occur anywhere along primitive notochord
- CT findings
  - **Midline**, expansile, multilobulated, well-circumscribed mass
  - Lytic bone destruction with intratumoral Ca^{++}
  - Variable enhancement
- MR findings
  - T1: Intermediate to low signal ≈ brain
  - T2: Classically ↑ ↑ signal
  - T1WI C+: Moderate to marked enhancement
  - DWI: Mean ADC value $1474 \pm 117 \times 10^{-6}$ mm²/s, generally less than chondrosarcoma

TOP DIFFERENTIAL DIAGNOSES

- Invasive pituitary macroadenoma
- Ecchordosis physaliphora
- Skull base chondrosarcoma
- Skull base plasmacytoma
- Skull base metastasis
- Skull base meningioma

CLINICAL ISSUES

- **35%** of all chordomas arise in **skull base**
- Common symptoms: Headache & diplopia (CNVI)
- Most common age: 30-50 years
- M:F = 1:1
- Treatment
  - Should be managed by multidisciplinary skull base team
  - Surgical resection (conventional surgery vs. endonasal transclival resection)
  - Proton beam RT: Postop & unresectable tumors
- Brachyury: Molecular marker distinctive for chordoma

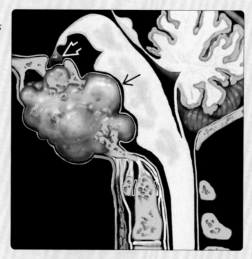
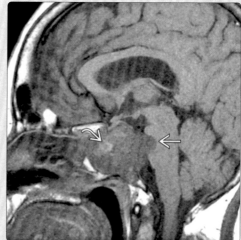

(Left) *Sagittal graphic shows an expansile, destructive mass originating from clivus, "thumbing" pons ➥ & elevating the pituitary gland ➡. Note bone fragments floating in chordoma.* **(Right)** *Sagittal T1 MR shows near-complete involvement of the clivus with expansile low-signal tumor. Note the classic "thumb" ➡ of tumor compressing the pons. Note foci of high signal ➥ from intratumoral hemorrhage, calcificiatio, or mucin.*

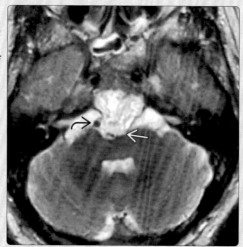
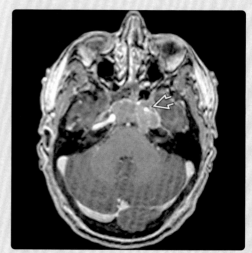

(Left) *Axial T2 MR shows characteristic marked, diffuse hyperintensity with an internal matrix. Notice right posterolateral displacement of the basilar artery ➥ & compression of the pons ➡ without parenchymal edema from this slow-growing tumor.* **(Right)** *Axial T1 C+ MR shows minimal enhancement, but extension into left cavernous sinus encasing the internal carotid artery (ICA) ➡. Angiographic balloon occlusion testing of the left ICA may be warranted should surgery be considered in this patient.*

TERMINOLOGY

Abbreviations

- Clival chordoma (CCh)

Synonyms

- Basicranial chordoma

Definitions

- Rare, locally aggressive tumor of clivus arising from cranial end of primitive notochord remnant

IMAGING

General Features

- Best diagnostic clue
  - **Destructive, expansile, midline clival mass** with ↑ T2 signal
- Location
  - Can occur anywhere along primitive notochord
    - Clivus near sphenooccipital synchondrosis
    - Commonly found in midline from sella to coccyx
  - Other rare locations in head & neck
    - Sellar region, sphenoid sinus, nasopharynx, maxilla, & paranasal sinuses
- Size
  - Usually 2-5 cm at presentation
- Morphology
  - Expansile, multilobulated, well-circumscribed mass
  - Expanding tumor **invades or displaces** local structures

CT Findings

- NECT
  - Centrally located, well-circumscribed, expansile soft tissue mass
  - Hyperdense relative to adjacent neural axis
- CECT
  - Variable enhancement
  - May contain low-attenuation areas representing myxoid/gelatinous material
- Bone CT
  - Mass causes lytic bone destruction
  - **Intratumoral Ca^{++}** = sequestra from destroyed bone > dystrophic Ca++

MR Findings

- T1WI
  - Intermediate to low signal compared to brain
    - ↓ tumor signal easily distinguished from adjacent fatty marrow
  - Small foci ↑ signal: Hemorrhage or mucoid material
  - Tumor "thumb" **indents anterior pons** on sagittal images
- T2WI
  - Classically ↑ **T2 signal**
    - Secondary to high fluid content
  - Foci of ↓ signal from Ca^{++}, hemorrhage, & mucoid
  - ↓ signal septations can separate ↑ signal lobules
- T2* GRE
  - Foci of hemorrhage ↓ signal
- DWI

- Mean ADC value 1474 ± 117 x 10^{-6} mm²/s: Generally less than chondrosarcoma
- T1WI C+
  - Moderate to marked enhancement
  - **Honeycomb enhancement pattern** secondary to intratumoral areas of low signal intensity
  - Subtle or no enhancement reflects necrosis ± ↑ volume mucinous material
- MRA
  - Vessel encasement/displacement frequent
    - Arterial narrowing rare; therefore, MRA less useful than MR

Angiographic Findings

- Avascular mass
- Propensity to displace & encase internal carotid arteries & vertebrobasilar system
- Balloon test occlusion evaluates risk of neurologic impairment with vessel sacrifice

Imaging Recommendations

- Best imaging tool
  - Both CT & MR usually needed for treatment planning
  - MR without & with contrast best confirms diagnosis & extent of tumor
- Protocol advice
  - Focused enhanced MR of skull base
  - Thin-section axial CT imaging of skull base with coronal ± sagittal reformations

DIFFERENTIAL DIAGNOSIS

Invasive Pituitary Macroadenoma

- Originates in sella & involves pituitary gland
- Extends into sphenoid sinus, not prepontine cistern

Ecchordosis Physaliphora

- Rare, benign notochord remnant lesion
- Nonenhancing, T2-hyperintense mass posterior to clivus

Skull Base Chondrosarcoma

- Arises off midline at petrooccipital fissure
- Similar T1 & T2 characteristics to CCh
- Chondroid calcifications more common
- ADC values 2051 ± 261 x 10^{-6} mm²/s, much higher than chordoma

Skull Base Plasmacytoma

- Can be midline destructive mass of clivus
- T2 signal usually intermediate to low

Skull Base Metastasis

- Destructive lesion; extraosseous component < CCh
- Known primary neoplasm

Skull Base Meningioma

- Sclerosis/hyperostosis of adjacent bone
- Homogeneous enhancement with dural tails
- Commonly causes narrowing of encased vessels

PATHOLOGY

General Features

- Etiology

- ○ Arises from remnants of primitive notochord
- Genetics
  - ○ Brachyury gene: Molecular marker distinctive for chordoma

Staging, Grading, & Classification

- Low to intermediate malignancy, slow-growing but locally aggressive
- 2 histopathologic subtypes
  - ○ Typical (classic) chordoma & chondroid chordoma

Gross Pathologic & Surgical Features

- Gross appearance: Multilobulated, gelatinous, gray mass

Microscopic Features

- Classic chordoma: Cords of physaliphorous cells with areas of necrosis, hemorrhage, & entrapped bone
  - ○ **Physaliphorous cells** have bubbly appearance & confirm diagnosis
    - – Large cell containing mucin & glycogen vacuoles
- Chondroid chordoma: Stroma resembles hyaline cartilage with neoplastic cells in lacunae
  - ○ Term "chondroid" in chondroid chordoma is misnomer; refers to histologic mimic
  - ○ Lesion does not contain true cartilage or cells of cartilage origin
- Classic & chondroid chordomas immunopositive for epithelial markers cytokeratin & epithelial membrane antigen
  - ○ Compared to chondrosarcoma, which is negative for those markers
- Transcription factor **brachyury**: Recently described specific for chordoma

CLINICAL ISSUES

Presentation

- Most common signs/symptoms
  - ○ Headaches & diplopia from CNVI involvement
- Other signs/symptoms
  - ○ Ophthalmoplegia results from tumor proximity to cranial nerves
    - – Cranial nerves III, IV, & VI in cavernous sinus
    - – CNVI in Dorello canal
  - ○ Visual loss (optic nerve, chiasm, optic tracts involved)
  - ○ Facial pain (CNV2)
  - ○ Lateral growth can injure CNVII or VIII in CPA-IAC
  - ○ Large chordoma may reach jugular foramen inferolaterally affecting CNIX-XII
  - ○ Headache likely related to stretching of dura
- Clinical profile
  - ○ Adult with gradual onset of ophthalmoplegia & headache

Demographics

- Age
  - ○ 30-50 years old
    - – Can occur at any age
- Gender
  - ○ M:F = 1:1
- Ethnicity
  - ○ Caucasians > African Americans

- Epidemiology
  - ○ **35%** of all chordomas arise in **skull base**
  - ○ 50% are sacrococcygeal
  - ○ 15% arise from vertebral body

Natural History & Prognosis

- Begins as expansile destructive bone lesion
  - ○ Infiltrates/transgresses dura, encases CN & vessels, & compresses brain/brainstem
  - ○ Rarely begins as intradural/intracranial
- Better prognosis if young age at presentation
- Chondroid chordoma has better prognosis than classic chordoma
- Poorer 5-year survival than chondrosarcoma
- Local recurrence is common despite combined therapy
  - ○ Rarely tumor recurrence along surgical tract
- Distant metastasis rare: Lymph nodes, bone, lung, liver
  - ○ Distant metastases more common in recurrent CCh

Treatment

- Should be managed by multidisciplinary skull base team
- Surgical resection (conventional surgery vs. endonasal transclival resection)
  - ○ Complete excision difficult due to close proximity of critical structures
- Proton beam RT: Postop & unresectable tumors

DIAGNOSTIC CHECKLIST

Consider

- Destructive midline mass originating from clivus **hyperintense on T2** is most common presentation

Image Interpretation Pearls

- T1WI C+ MR best for tumor characteristics & extent
- Bone CT can better characterize bony destruction
- Look for encasement of ICA & vertebrobasilar system

Reporting Tips

- Comment on involvement of adjacent vital structures
- ADC values 1474 ± 117 x 10^{-6} mm²/s differentiates from higher ADC values of chondrosarcoma
  - ○ Must exclude hemorrhage/Ca^{++}, cystic areas/necrosis from ROI when measuring ADC

SELECTED REFERENCES

1. Campbell RG et al: Contemporary management of clival chordomas. Curr Opin Otolaryngol Head Neck Surg. 23(2):153-61, 2015
2. Choy W et al: Predictors of recurrence following resection of intracranial chordomas. J Clin Neurosci. 22(11):1792-6, 2015
3. Kanamori H et al: Genetic characterization of skull base chondrosarcomas. J Neurosurg. 123(4):1036-41, 2015
4. Müller U et al: Is there a role for conventional MRI and MR diffusion-weighted imaging for distinction of skull base chordoma and chondrosarcoma? Acta Radiol. ePub, 2015
5. Van Gompel JJ et al: Chordoma and chondrosarcoma. Otolaryngol Clin North Am. 48(3):501-14, 2015
6. Yeom KW et al: Diffusion-weighted MRI: distinction of skull base chordoma from chondrosarcoma. AJNR Am J Neuroradiol. 34(5):1056-61, S1, 2013
7. Pamir MN et al: Analysis of radiological features relative to histopathology in 42 skull-base chordomas and chondrosarcomas. Eur J Radiol. 58(3):461-70, 2006
8. Noël G et al: Chordomas of the base of the skull and upper cervical spine. One hundred patients irradiated by a 3D conformal technique combining photon and proton beams. Acta Oncol. 44(7):700-8, 2005

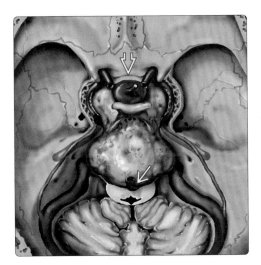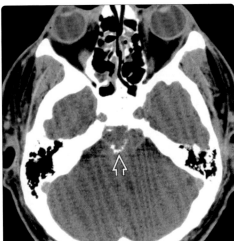

(Left) *Axial graphic illustrates a large clival chordoma pushing posteriorly to indent the low pons & basilar artery ⇨. Basisphenoid invasion ⇨ is also seen lifting pituitary gland in the sella.* **(Right)** *Axial NECT demonstrates a typical midline clival chordoma (CCh) with irregular posterior intratumoral calcifications ⇨ representing associated matrix calcifications &/or bone fragments. This tumor compresses the pons posteriorly.*

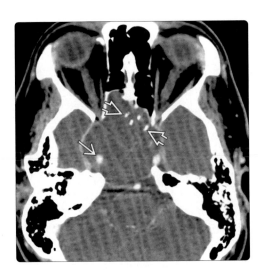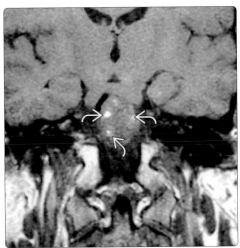

(Left) *Axial CECT shows an unenhancing CCh with significant myxoid content engulfing the right internal carotid artery ⇨ without significant narrowing. Bone fragments ⇨ in anterior tumor margin are typical.* **(Right)** *Coronal T1 MR shows focal areas of T1 shortening within the mass consistent with calcification, hemorrhage, &/or mucoid degeneration ⇨.*

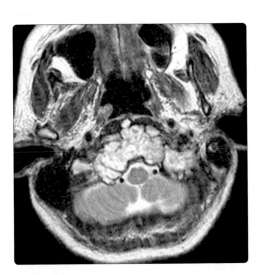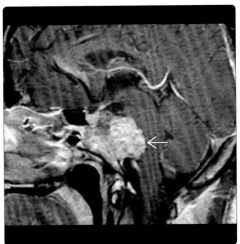

(Left) *Axial T2 MR shows extensive T2-hyperintense clival tumor involving the occipital bone. Marked hyperintense T2 signal is a classic feature of chordoma. Surgical excision would also require stabilization of craniocervical junction.* **(Right)** *Sagittal T1 C+ MR demonstrates heterogeneous enhancement of CCh. Note posterior extension into prepontine cistern, with resulting "thumbing" of pons ⇨.*

KEY FACTS

TERMINOLOGY

- Persistent craniopharyngeal canal (PCPC)
- Synonyms: Transsphenoidal canal, craniopharyngeal duct, hypophyseal canal, basipharyngeal canal, persistent hypophyseal canal
- Developmental anomaly with persistent tract from nasopharynx to pituitary fossa
- Believed by many to be persistent Rathke duct

IMAGING

- Skull base bone CT
  - Midline, well-marginated tract from sella to roof of nasopharynx
  - Anterior to sphenooccipital synchondrosis
  - Typically < 1.5 mm in diameter
- Multiplanar MR
  - Smoothly marginated cylindrical "canal" extending from sella to nasopharynx
  - Variable signal intensity in canal itself

- MR best to evaluate pituitary and suprasellar structures for associated abnormality
- Coronal sections reveal adenohypophysis perched on craniopharyngeal canal like **ball on tee**

TOP DIFFERENTIAL DIAGNOSES

- Skull base cephalocele
- Sphenobasilar synchondrosis
- Persistent medial basal canal

PATHOLOGY

- Associations with pituitary abnormalities, cephaloceles, midline craniofacial anomalies

CLINICAL ISSUES

- Typically incidental finding
- Seen in 0.42% of population
- Usually obliterated by 12th week of gestation
- **"Leave alone" lesion** when isolated finding

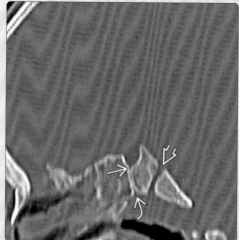
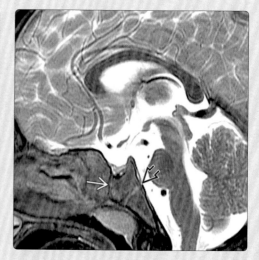

(Left) Sagittal reformatted CT shows bony tract originating in floor of sella turcica ➡ extending to roof of nasopharynx ➡. Note sphenooccipital synchondrosis ➡ posteriorly and unfused in this child. (Right) T2 sagittal MR in same patient shows persistent craniopharyngeal canal ➡ evident as small tract with central intermediate signal and hypointense margins extending from pituitary fossa to nasopharynx. Normal sphenooccipital synchondrosis ➡ is posterior to craniopharyngeal canal.

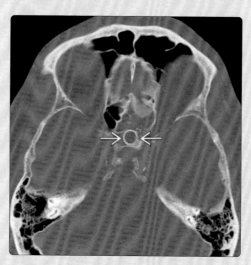
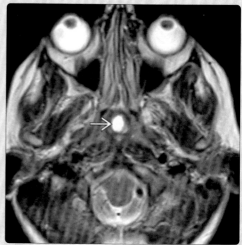

(Left) Axial bone CT demonstrates an incidental well-defined sclerotic ovoid "lesion" in the sphenoid bone ➡, consistent with midsegment of a persistent craniopharyngeal canal. This smooth canal should be demonstrated in contiguity with the sella and nasopharynx. (Right) Axial T2 MR in same patient demonstrates large persistent craniopharyngeal canal ➡. Note CSF-signal intensity smoothly ovoid structure. Fluid-filled canal extended from pituitary fossa to nasopharynx.

TERMINOLOGY

Abbreviations

- Persistent craniopharyngeal canal (PCPC)

Synonyms

- Transsphenoidal canal, craniopharyngeal duct, hypophyseal canal, basipharyngeal canal, persistent hypophyseal canal

Definitions

- Developmental anomaly with **persistent tract from nasopharyngeal roof to pituitary fossa**
  o May represent persistent Rathke duct
    – Alternative hypothesis: Persistent vascular channel unrelated to Rathke duct

IMAGING

General Features

- Best diagnostic clue
  o Midline well-marginated cylindrical to ovoid tract from sella to nasopharyngeal roof
- Location
  o Extends between superior surface of nasopharynx to sella turcica floor in oblique fashion
    – Terminates in nasopharynx near junction of vomer & sphenoid rostrum
  o Lies anatomically between presphenoid and basisphenoid
    – **Anterior to sphenooccipital synchondrosis**
- Size
  o Typically < 1.5 mm in diameter
    – When larger, evaluate carefully for **associated pituitary abnormality**
- Morphology
  o Tubular canal
    – Occasionally ends blindly without communication with sella

Imaging Recommendations

- Best imaging tool
  o High-resolution skull base CT
  o Multiplanar MR to exclude pituitary abnormality or cephalocele
- Protocol advice
  o Sagittal and coronal CT reconstructions

CT Findings

- Bone CT
  o Smoothly marginated cylindrical-to-ovoid **midline bony "canal"** extending from sella to nasopharynx
  o **Oblique orientation** to nasopharynx

MR Findings

- Smoothly marginated tubular canal in sphenoid
- Variable signal intensity in canal
- May demonstrate central enhancement on postcontrast T1W images
- Coronal sections reveal adenohypophysis perched on craniopharyngeal canal like **ball on tee**
- Evaluate pituitary and suprasellar structures for potential associated abnormality

DIFFERENTIAL DIAGNOSIS

Skull Base Cephalocele

- Nasopharyngeal or basioccipital nasopharyngeal cephalocele types in similar location
- Contain variable meningeal-lined CSF/brain parenchyma

Sphenooccipital Synchondrosis

- Linear cleft between basisphenoid & basiocciput
- Conspicuity decreases from childhood to adulthood

Persistent Medial Basal Canal (Basilaris Medianus)

- Developmental variant of lower midline clivus
- Posteroinferior to sphenooccipital synchondrosis

PATHOLOGY

General Features

- Associated abnormalities
  o Pituitary abnormalities, cephaloceles, midline craniofacial anomalies

CLINICAL ISSUES

Presentation

- Most common signs/symptoms
  o Typically **incidental finding**
- Other signs/symptoms
  o Pituitary dysfunction may be presenting symptom

Demographics

- Epidemiology
  o Seen in 0.42% of population

Natural History & Prognosis

- Usually obliterated by 12th week of gestation
- Rarely reported to cause upper airway obstruction (during infancy), CSF leak, meningitis, sinusitis, hydrocephalus

Treatment

- **"Leave alone" lesion** when isolated finding

DIAGNOSTIC CHECKLIST

Image Interpretation Pearls

- Evaluate hypothalamic-pituitary axis for associated abnormality

SELECTED REFERENCES

1. Mohindra S et al: A novel minimally invasive endoscopic repair in a case of spontaneous CSF rhinorrhea with persistent craniopharyngeal canal. Neurol India. 63(3):434-6, 2015
2. Abele TA et al: Craniopharyngeal canal and its spectrum of pathology. AJNR Am J Neuroradiol. 35(4):772-7, 2014
3. Ginat DT et al: Multi-detector-row computed tomography imaging of variant skull base foramina. J Comput Assist Tomogr. 37(4):481-5, 2013
4. Kaushik C et al: Ectopic pituitary adenoma in persistent craniopharyngeal canal: case report and literature review. J Comput Assist Tomogr. 34(4):612-4, 2010
5. Pinilla-Arias D et al: Recurrent meningitis and persistence of craniopharyngeal canal: case report. Neurocirugia (Astur). 20(1):50-3, 2009
6. Marsot-Dupuch K et al: A rare expression of neural crest disorders: an intrasphenoidal development of the anterior pituitary gland. AJNR Am J Neuroradiol. 25(2):285-8, 2004
7. Ekinci G et al: Transsphenoidal (large craniopharyngeal) canal associated with a normally functioning pituitary gland and nasopharyngeal extension, hyperprolactinemia, and hypothalamic hamartoma. AJR Am J Roentgenol. 180(1):76-7, 2003

Sphenoid Benign Fatty Lesion

TERMINOLOGY

- Synonym: Arrested pneumatization of sphenoid
- Definition: Well-corticated, fat-containing lesion of sphenoid bone
  - Occurs in regions where primary or accessory pneumatization known to occur
  - Usually adjacent to posterior sinus wall

IMAGING

- Bone CT findings
  - Thin-section axial images best for depicting uniform cortical bone rim
  - Well-defined, **low-attenuation** (fat density), nonexpansile lesion with **sclerotic rim**
  - May have occasional curvilinear calcification or soft tissue density
- MR
  - Can help delineate smaller lesions

- Central ↑ **T1**, variable T2, & ↓ T1 signal post fat suppression
  - Hypointense rim
  - Minimal if any enhancement

TOP DIFFERENTIAL DIAGNOSES

- Fibrous dysplasia
- Hemangioma
- Chordoma
- Ossifying fibroma

CLINICAL ISSUES

- Common **incidental finding** on CT or MR depicting skull base
- **"Leave alone"** lesion

DIAGNOSTIC CHECKLIST

- Identification of internal fat & sclerotic margin is essentially pathognomonic

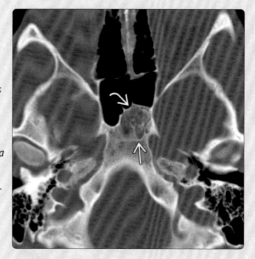
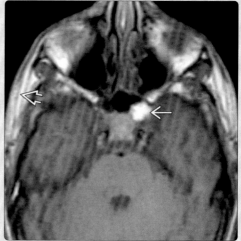

(Left) Axial bone CT shows characteristic features of an incidentally discovered fatty lesion of the sphenoid. The lesion ➡ bulges into left sphenoid sinus ➚ and has well-defined sclerotic margins and predominantly low density (fat) centrally. Note normal trabeculae traverse lesion. (Right) Axial T1WI MR (same patient) demonstrates a homogeneously hyperintense, nonexpansile lesion ➡ in left aspect of basisphenoid similar in signal to subcutaneous fat ➨. MR may be useful to confirm internal fatty contents.

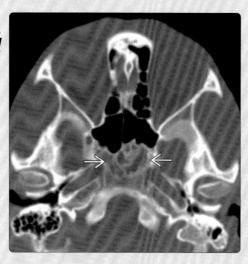
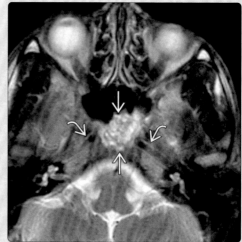

(Left) Axial bone CT demonstrates a typical benign, fatty lesion of the sphenoid ➡ with well-defined margins and a low-density central component, confirmed on MR to represent fat. (Right) Axial T2WI MR in the same patient confirms predominantly hyperintense (paralleling fat) signal with a lobulated contour to the lesion ➡. There is no significant distortion of skull base foramina or normal structures, such as petrous segments of internal carotid arteries ➨.

TERMINOLOGY

- Synonyms: Giant TS, "dumbbell" TS

IMAGING

- Tubular mass along course of trigeminal nerve
  - Can involve preganglionic (cisternal) segment, Meckel cave, CNV1 (superior orbital fissure), CNV2 (foramen rotundum), CNV3 (foramen ovale)
  - May extend extracranially via CNV exit foramina
- Size: Small to giant
- Morphology: "Dumbbell" shape secondary to constriction at porus trigeminus or skull base foramen
- CT: Soft tissue mass with smooth bony erosion of central skull base, ± foraminal widening
- MR: T1 iso- to hypointense, T2 hyperintense, variable enhancement
  - Cyst formation is common

TOP DIFFERENTIAL DIAGNOSES

- Meningioma
- CNV3 perineural tumor
- CNV2 perineural tumor
- Non-Hodgkin lymphoma

PATHOLOGY

- Benign nerve sheath tumor
  - 2nd most common intracranial schwannoma next to vestibular schwannoma
- May occur in setting of neurofibromatosis

DIAGNOSTIC CHECKLIST

- Dumbbell-shaped or tubular mass along course of trigeminal nerve is characteristic
- Enhanced MR best to identify intracranial and extracranial extent of lesion
- Search for additional intracranial schwannomas, which may indicate neurofibromatosis

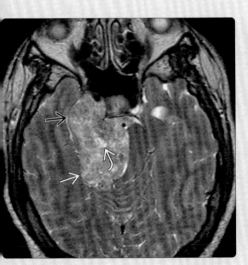
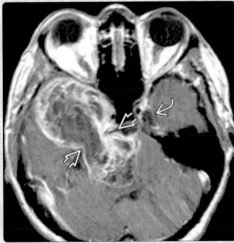

(Left) *Axial T2WI MR shows a mass in both middle* ⊐ *and posterior* ➡ *cranial fossae, consistent with extraaxial location. Internal areas of higher T2 signal intensity* ⇗ *may indicate cystic degeneration.* (Right) *Axial T1WI C+ MR reveals a dumbbell-shaped giant TS with a waist formed at the level of the porus trigeminus* ⇗. *Extensive cystic components are present. Note the normal left Meckel cave containing CSF signal* ➡.

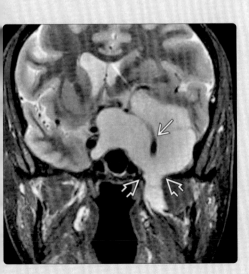
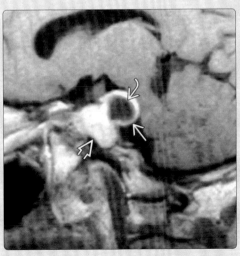

(Left) *Coronal T2WI FS MR demonstrates a well-demarcated, hyperintense, giant TS encasing, but not significantly compressing, the left internal carotid artery* ➡. *In this location, a waist is formed as the mass extends through the enlarged foramen ovale* ⇗. (Right) *Sagittal T1WI C+ MR reveals a "dumbbell" TS affecting the preganglionic* ➡ *and Meckel cave* ⇗ *segments of the trigeminal nerve. Notice the intramural cyst in the preganglionic segment* ➡, *common in schwannomas.*

Hypoglossal Nerve Schwannoma

TERMINOLOGY

- Benign tumor of differentiated Schwann cells surrounding CNXII

IMAGING

- Multiplanar contrast-enhanced MR with bone CT for delineation of bone margins
- CT findings
  - Sharply marginated fusiform mass with enlarged hypoglossal canal (HC)
  - Coronal plane: Remodeling of undersurface of jugular tubercle
  - Tongue muscle atrophy with fatty replacement
- MR: Homogeneous, enhancing mass following course of CNXII
  - Cephalad growth toward preolivary sulcus
  - Caudal growth into nasopharyngeal carotid space
- Distal lesions may present in carotid space, submandibular space, or in tongue

TOP DIFFERENTIAL DIAGNOSES

- Asymmetric HC venous drainage
- Skull base metastasis
- Persistent hypoglossal artery
- Jugular foramen meningioma
- Glomus jugulare paraganglioma

PATHOLOGY

- Smooth, encapsulated mass arising eccentrically from CNXII
- Multiple schwannomas are associated with NF2

CLINICAL ISSUES

- Hypoglossal neuropathy results in unilateral tongue denervation
- Larger lesions may produce multiple lower cranial neuropathies
- Surgical removal in single operation is curative

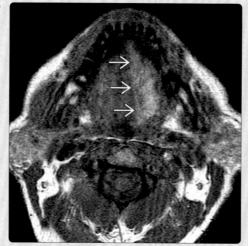
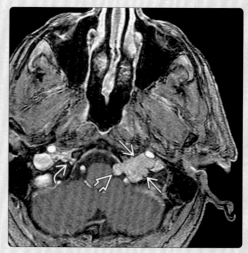

(Left) Axial T1 MR through the tongue demonstrates asymmetric signal of tongue. Right hemitongue is normal; left hemitongue has sharply marginated abnormally ↑ signal ➡. Increased signal signifies fatty infiltration and should direct attention to hypoglossal canal (HC). (Right) Axial T1 C+ MR at HC reveals lobulated mass ➡ on left extending into medullary cistern ➡. Note normal right hypoglossal canal ➡. Mass demonstrates uniform enhancement consistent with schwannoma. Cystic change is common with large tumors.

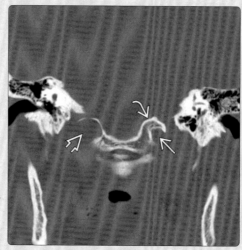
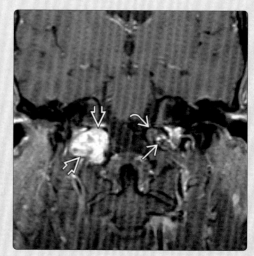

(Left) Coronal bone CT shows a markedly expanded HC on the right ➡, eroding undersurface of "eagle's beak." Contrast this with the normal left HC ➡ and jugular tubercle ➡. (Right) Coronal T1 C+ FS MR in the same patient reveals heterogeneous enhancement of the schwannoma ➡ with marked scalloping of adjacent occipital bone & obliteration of normal "eagle's beak" as seen on CT. The normal hypoglossal canal ➡ & jugular tubercle ➡ are identified on left.

TERMINOLOGY

Abbreviations

- Hypoglossal nerve schwannoma (HNS), hypoglossal canal (HC)

Definitions

- Extremely rare benign tumor of differentiated Schwann cells surrounding CNXII

IMAGING

General Features

- Best diagnostic clue
  o Fusiform, well-defined soft tissue mass along expected course of CNXII
- Location
  o May occur anywhere along course of CNXII
    – Distal lesions may present in carotid space, submandibular space, or in tongue
- Size
  o Usually large at presentation
- Morphology
  o Fusiform lesions that may attain **dumbbell shape**

CT Findings

- NECT
  o Sharply marginated soft tissue density mass along course of CNXII
  o Fatty attenuation in ipsilateral hemitongue secondary to denervation atrophy
- CECT
  o Uniformly enhancing ± intramural cysts
- Bone CT
  o Smooth, sharply marginated and enlarged HC
  o Coronal plane: Enlargement, remodeling of undersurface of jugular tubercle (below "eagle's beak")

MR Findings

- T1WI
  o Typically isointense to gray matter
  o Associated denervation may cause ipsilateral tongue muscle atrophy & fatty replacement with ↑ signal
- T2WI
  o Typically ↑ signal
  o Large HNS may have ↑ T2 signal **intramural cysts**
- T1WI C+
  o Uniform enhancement when small

Imaging Recommendations

- Best imaging tool
  o Enhanced multiplanar MR with bone CT providing detail on bony remodeling of HC

DIFFERENTIAL DIAGNOSIS

Asymmetric HC Venous Drainage (Pseudolesion)

- Nonenlarged HC with normal cortical margins
- Linear transcanalicular venous enhancement surrounding normal nerve

Skull Base Metastasis

- Bony margins of HC are lytic or permeative

- Enhancing, invasive mass

Persistent Hypoglossal Artery

- MR + MRA: Flow void passes through enlarged HC to basilar artery

Jugular Foramen Meningioma

- Dural-based mass with enhancing dural tail; secondarily involves HC
- Permeative-sclerotic bony changes or hyperostosis

Glomus Jugulare Paraganglioma

- Permeative-destructive bone margins of jugular foramen
- Multiple flow voids are characteristic on MR

PATHOLOGY

Gross Pathologic & Surgical Features

- Smooth, tan, ovoid, encapsulated, & lobulated mass
- Arises eccentrically from CNXII nerve sheath

CLINICAL ISSUES

Presentation

- Most common signs/symptoms
  o Hypoglossal neuropathy results in **unilateral tongue denervation**
    – Tongue deviates toward side of lesion on protrusion

Demographics

- Epidemiology
  o Extremely rare schwannoma (much less common than CN V, VII, IX or X)

Natural History & Prognosis

- Slowly growing, benign tumor

Treatment

- Surgical removal of tumor in single operation is optimal
  o Proposed tumor grading system for operative care
    – Type A, intradural; type B, dumbbell; type C, extracranial; type D, peripheral

DIAGNOSTIC CHECKLIST

Consider

- HNS if well-defined fusiform mass identified along expected course of CNXII

Reporting Tips

- Be sure to follow entire craniocaudal extent of lesion

SELECTED REFERENCES

1. Ram H et al: Hypoglossal schwannoma of parapharyngeal space: an unusual case report. J Maxillofac Oral Surg. 14(Suppl 1):73-6, 2015
2. Nonaka Y et al: Microsurgical management of hypoglossal schwannomas over 3 decades: a modified grading scale to guide surgical approach. Neurosurgery. 69(2 Suppl Operative):ons121-40; discussion ons140, 2011
3. Edizer DT et al: Hypoglossal schwannoma presenting only with headache. J Craniofac Surg. 21(1):261-2, 2010
4. Rachinger J et al: Dumbbell-shaped hypoglossal schwannoma. A case report. Magn Reson Imaging. 21(2):155-8, 2003
5. Sarma S et al: Nonvestibular schwannomas of the brain: a 7-year experience. Neurosurgery. 50(3):437-48; discussion 438-9, 2002
6. Ogawa T et al: A multifocal neurinoma of the hypoglossal nerve with motor paralysis confirmed by electromyography. Int J Oral Maxillofac Surg. 30(2):176-8, 2001

Jugular Bulb Pseudolesion

TERMINOLOGY

- Asymmetric, large jugular bulb (JB) flow phenomenon simulates neoplasm or thrombosis on MR sequences

IMAGING

- Best diagnostic clue: Complex MR signal in JB with normal jugular foramen (JF) cortex & jugular spine
  - Complex MR signal does not persist on all MR sequences
  - Normal bony margins of JB on temporal bone CT

TOP DIFFERENTIAL DIAGNOSES

- High JB
- JB diverticulum
- Dehiscent JB
- Sigmoid sinus-JB thrombosis
- Jugular foramen schwannoma
- Jugular foramen meningioma

CLINICAL ISSUES

- Found incidentally on brain MR during work-up for unrelated symptoms
- Surgical exploration must be avoided by radiologist making correct diagnosis
- No treatment or follow-up required

DIAGNOSTIC CHECKLIST

- JB pseudolesion is most common JB "lesion"
- Once abnormality is seen in JF on MR, 1st question to ask is, "Am I looking at JB pseudolesion?"
  - Do not mistake JB pseudolesion for schwannoma or venous sinus thrombosis
- If JB pseudolesion is observed while patient is in imaging center, add MRV to protocol to clarify
- Use bone CT to evaluate bony margins of JF if MR diagnosis uncertain

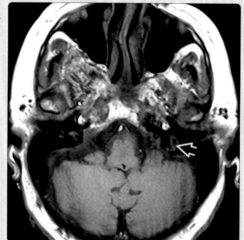
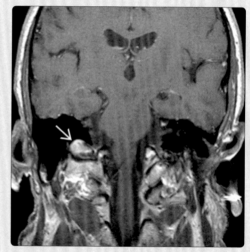

(Left) *Axial T1WI MR shows heterogeneous signal intensity within the left jugular foramen ⮕, concerning for pathology. Other MR sequences proved this to be a jugular bulb pseudolesion, related to an asymmetric, large jugular bulb.* (Right) *Coronal T1WI C+ MR shows a jugular bulb pseudolesion ⮕ related to turbulent flow in a mildly asymmetric right jugular bulb. This pseudolesion may be mistaken for a schwannoma or venous thrombosis. Other MR sequences confirmed this pseudolesion.*

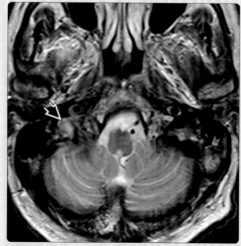
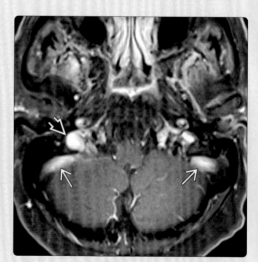

(Left) *Axial T2WI MR shows a hyperintense right jugular foramen "lesion" ⮕, concerning for a jugular foramen schwannoma in this elderly patient with new-onset right-sided numbness.* (Right) *Axial T1WI C+ FS MR in the same patient shows normal enhancement of a mildly prominent right jugular bulb ⮕. The enhancement is similar to the enhancement of the normal sigmoid sinuses ⮕. Other sequences including an MRA/MRV confirmed this as a jugular bulb pseudolesion.*

TERMINOLOGY

Synonyms

- Jugular bulb (JB) pseudomass; "leave alone" lesion of jugular foramen (JF)

Definitions

- Asymmetric, large JB flow phenomenon simulates neoplasm or thrombosis on MR sequences

IMAGING

General Features

- Best diagnostic clue
  o **Complex MR signal** intensity in **JB** with normal JF cortex & jugular spine
- Location
  o JF bulb
    − Prominent JB more commonly **right-sided**
- Size
  o Typical JB measures 1.0-1.5 cm
- Morphology
  o Rounded area of heterogeneous signal intensity centered on JF

CT Findings

- CECT
  o Normal enhancing sigmoid sinus (SS) & JB
    − No filling defect to suggest thrombosis
- Bone CT
  o Asymmetric JB, with **intact cortical margins** & jugular spine
- CTV: Asymmetric JB shows same enhancement as internal jugular vein (IJV) & SS

MR Findings

- T1WI
  o Variable signal; may have soft tissue intensity or heterogeneous signal
- T2WI
  o Heterogeneous signal intensity
    − Usually conspicuous when iso- to hyperintense
- FLAIR
  o Heterogeneous signal intensity, often hyperintense
- T2* GRE
  o No significant blooming
- T1WI C+
  o Avid enhancement of JB
    − Identical enhancement to adjacent IJV & SS
- MRV
  o JB shows asymmetric enlargement without evidence of thrombosis
    − Phase contrast MRV: Shows normal flow in JB & SS

Angiographic Findings

- Catheter venography: Normal, asymmetrically large SS & JB fill with contrast
  o JB often "high-riding"

DIFFERENTIAL DIAGNOSIS

High Jugular Bulb

- Most cephalad portion of JB extends superior to floor of IAC ± basal turn of cochlea
- Bone CT: JB cortical margins intact; no middle ear extension

Jugular Bulb Diverticulum

- Focal polypoid mass extending from cephalad JB into middle ear
- Smooth bone margins, intact sigmoid plate

Dehiscent Jugular Bulb

- Usually present with vascular "mass" behind intact tympanic membrane
- Sigmoid plate dehiscence on CT

Sigmoid Sinus-Jugular Bulb Thrombosis

- NECT: Hyperdense SS/JB, normal bony margins
- CECT/CTA/CTV: Look for intraluminal thrombus
  o Vasa vasorum of vein wall may enhance as thin white rim (empty delta sign)
- MRV: Filling defect or lack of flow

Glomus Jugulare Paraganglioma

- Permeative bony changes along JF
- T1 MR: JF mass with high-velocity flow voids
- Vector of spread: Superolateral from JB to middle ear

Jugular Foramen Schwannoma

- Smoothly scalloped, enlarged JF
- T1 C+ MR: Dumbbell-shaped, enhancing mass in JF
- Vector of spread: Superomedial along CNIX-XI

Jugular Foramen Meningioma

- Permeative-sclerotic or hyperostotic bony change around JF
- T1 C+ MR: Enhancing dural tails along margins
- Vector of spread: Centrifugal along dural surfaces

PATHOLOGY

General Features

- Etiology
  o Normal developmental variant

CLINICAL ISSUES

Presentation

- Most common signs/symptoms
  o **Asymptomatic**
    − Found incidentally on brain MR during work-up for unrelated symptoms

Demographics

- Epidemiology
  o Most common "lesion" of JF found on MR imaging

SELECTED REFERENCES

1. Kizildag B et al: The relationship between tinnitus and vascular anomalies on temporal bone CT scan: a retrospective case control study. Surg Radiol Anat. ePub, 2016
2. Bae SC et al: Single-center 10-year experience in treating patients with vascular tinnitus: diagnostic approaches and treatment outcomes. Clin Exp Otorhinolaryngol. 8(1):7-12, 2015

TERMINOLOGY

- High jugular bulb (JB): Superior aspect of JB extends above floor of IAC with **no** middle ear connection
  - If dehiscence into middle ear present, use "dehiscent JB" not "high JB" to describe

IMAGING

- Most cephalad portion of JB extends superior to **floor of IAC** ± at level of basal turn of cochlea
  - Jugular foramen cortical margins intact
- Axial: JB at level of IAC or cochlea
- Coronal: JB medial ± inferior to semicircular canals
- T1 C+: High JB enhances same as jugular vein
- MRV: Same signal as surrounding venous structures
- High JB occurs most commonly on **right**
- Best imaging tool: T-bone CT

TOP DIFFERENTIAL DIAGNOSES

- Jugular bulb pseudolesion

- Jugular bulb diverticulum
- Dehiscent jugular bulb
- Glomus jugulare paraganglioma
- Jugular foramen schwannoma
- Jugular foramen meningioma

PATHOLOGY

- High JB is more commonly seen with poorly aerated mastoid air cells
- JB diverticulum present in 35% of cases with high JB

CLINICAL ISSUES

- High JB is typically **incidental**
  - May ↑ risk of inadvertently entering JB during mastoidectomy
- Otoscopic exam: Normal
- Conservative management most common treatment
- Rarely reported to be associated with pulsatile tinnitus or Meniere disease; causality uncertain

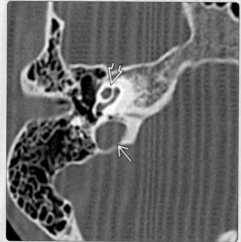
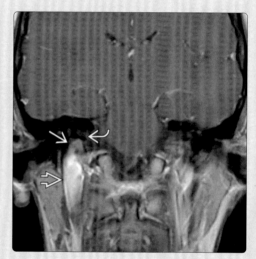

(Left) Axial T-bone CT of the right ear shows a high jugular bulb ➔ at the level of the cochlea ➔ with intact cortical margins. These congenital lesions are typically incidental, but may be associated with pulsatile tinnitus. (Right) Coronal T1WI C+ FS MR shows a high jugular bulb ➔ connected inferiorly to a large internal jugular vein ➔. The top of the high jugular bulb reaches the level of the floor of the internal auditory canal ➔. On axial images, this may mimic an inner ear lesion if the connection to the jugular vein is not appreciated.

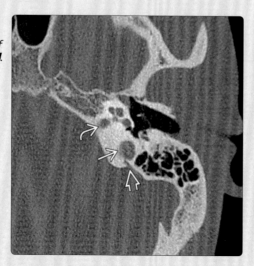
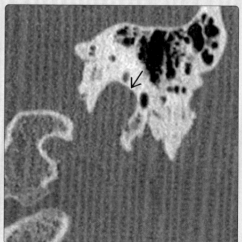

(Left) Axial T-bone CT of the left ear shows a high jugular bulb ➔ present at the level of the internal auditory canal ➔. The high jugular bulb abuts the bony vestibular aqueduct ➔ on its posterior margin. (Right) Coronal T-bone CT in the same patient shows the high jugular bulb ➔ as a cephalad extension of the jugular foramen. A high jugular bulb occurs most commonly on the right side. This congenital lesion can be associated with jugular bulb dehiscence or a jugular bulb diverticulum.

TERMINOLOGY

Abbreviations

- High jugular bulb (JB)

Synonyms

- High-riding jugular bulb

Definitions

- Superior aspect of JB extends above floor of IAC with **no** connection to middle ear
  - If dehiscent JB into middle ear, use "dehiscent JB" not "high JB" to describe

IMAGING

General Features

- Best diagnostic clue
  - Bone CT: Most cephalad portion of JB extends superior to floor of IAC ± at level of basal turn of cochlea
- Location
  - When JB reaches or exceeds floor of IAC
  - Occurs most commonly on right
- Size
  - Variable; JB typically 1.0-1.5 cm
- Morphology
  - Superior extension of JB with smooth bony margins

Imaging Recommendations

- Best imaging tool: T-bone CT

CT Findings

- NECT
  - Axial: JB at level of IAC, often at cochlea basal turn
  - Coronal: JB medial ± inferior to semicircular canals
- Bone CT: Jugular foramen (JF) cortical margins intact, including sigmoid plate

MR Findings

- T1: May be heterogeneous
- T2: Most commonly hypointense (invisible), may be heterogeneous
- T1 C+: High JB enhances same as internal jugular vein (IJV)
  - Coronal: Extends to level of IAC
- MRV: Same signal as surrounding venous structures

DIFFERENTIAL DIAGNOSIS

Jugular Bulb Pseudolesion

- MR shows asymmetric large JB with mass-like signal
- Usually found incidentally in skull base work-up
- Bone CT: Intact jugular spine & JB cortical margins

Jugular Bulb Diverticulum

- Bone CT: Focal projection extending off JB margin superiorly into deep temporal bone just behind IAC
- T1 C+ MR: Enhancing middle ear mass connects to enhancing JB

Dehiscent Jugular Bulb

- Vascular retrotympanic mass
- Protruding mass extends into posteroinferior middle ear cavity

- Bone CT: Sigmoid plate shows focal dehiscence
- T1 C+ MR: Enhancing mass connects to enhancing JB

Glomus Jugulare Paraganglioma

- Enhancing mass in jugular foramen (JF)
- Bone CT: Permeative destructive JF bony changes
- T1 MR: High-velocity flow voids ("pepper")

Jugular Foramen Schwannoma

- Dumbbell-shaped mass along cranial nerves IX-XI
- Bone CT: Smoothly scalloped, enlarged JF
- T1 C+ MR: Fusiform enhancing JF mass

Jugular Foramen Meningioma

- Mass in JF spreading centrifugally along dural planes
- Bone CT: Permeative-sclerotic or hyperostotic margins
- T1 C+ MR: Avidly enhancing mass with dural tails

PATHOLOGY

General Features

- Etiology
  - Congenital abnormality, benign vascular variant
  - High JB is more commonly seen with poorly aerated mastoid & perilymphatic structures

CLINICAL ISSUES

Presentation

- Most common signs/symptoms
  - Most commonly an **incidental** finding
  - Rarely reported to be associated with pulsatile tinnitus or Meniere disease; causality uncertain

Demographics

- Age: May be discovered at any age
- Gender: Slight female predominance
- Epidemiology: **5%** of temporal bone specimens
  - JB diverticulum present in 35% of cases with high JB

Treatment

- Conservative management

DIAGNOSTIC CHECKLIST

Consider

- High JB is typically incidental
- ↑ risk of entering JB during mastoidectomy

Image Interpretation Pearls

- MR: Complex or increased signal of high JB does not persist on all MR sequences

SELECTED REFERENCES

1. Singla A et al: High jugular bulb: different osseous landmarks and their clinical implications. Surg Radiol Anat. ePub, 2016
2. Brook CD et al: The Prevalence of High-Riding Jugular Bulb in Patients with Suspected Endolymphatic Hydrops. J Neurol Surg B Skull Base. 76(6):471-4, 2015
3. Park JJ et al: Jugular bulb abnormalities in patients with Meniere's disease using high-resolution computed tomography. Eur Arch Otorhinolaryngol. 272(8):1879-84, 2015
4. Redfern RE et al: High jugular bulb in a cohort of patients with definite Ménière's disease. J Laryngol Otol. 128(9):759-64, 2014

TERMINOLOGY

- DJB: Normal venous variant with superior & lateral extension of jugular bulb (JB) into middle ear (ME) cavity through dehiscent sigmoid plate

IMAGING

- Soft tissue mass in ME contiguous with JB through **dehiscent sigmoid plate**
  - **Lateral outpouching** from JB best seen on coronal CT
  - Enhances to same degree as adjacent venous structures on C+ CT and MR
  - CTA or MRA may be performed in equivocal cases

TOP DIFFERENTIAL DIAGNOSES

- Asymmetrically large jugular bulb
- High-riding jugular bulb
- Jugular bulb diverticulum
- Glomus tympanicum paraganglioma
- Glomus jugulare paraganglioma

- Jugular foramen schwannoma
- Jugular foramen meningioma

CLINICAL ISSUES

- DJB has been reported as linked to many symptoms, though **causality** is **disputed**
  - Pulsatile tinnitus, hearing loss, Ménière disease
- Otoscopy: **Vascular blue "mass"** behind intact tympanic membrane may prompt imaging
- Otoscopic findings + bone CT findings make correct diagnosis
  - Corrected DJB diagnosis provides warning to surgeons when surgery contemplated for other indications
  - Helps avoid injury to JB

DIAGNOSTIC CHECKLIST

- DJB in differential diagnosis list of any vascular retrotympanic mass
- Coronal temporal bone CT will show direct continuity of middle ear mass with JB

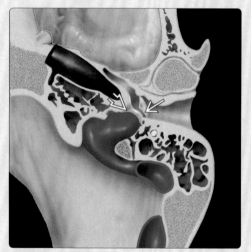
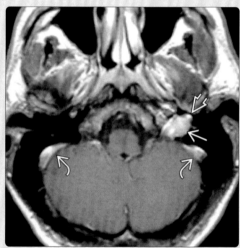

(Left) Axial graphic depicts a dehiscent jugular bulb projecting superolaterally into the middle ear through the dehiscent sigmoid plate ➡. Typically, a blue-colored vascular "mass" is identified behind the posteroinferior quadrant of the intact tympanic membrane ➡. (Right) Axial T1WI C+ MR shows enhancement of the prominent jugular bulb ➡ contiguous with the dehiscent component in the middle ear ➡. Enhancement is identical to the sigmoid sinuses ➡.

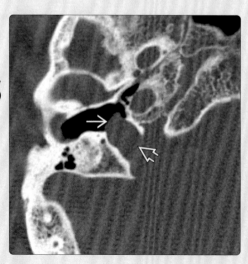
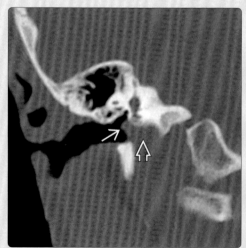

(Left) Axial bone CT demonstrates the jugular bulb ➡ and soft tissue density mass ➡ within the inferior right middle ear cavity contiguous through the widely dehiscent jugular plate. (Right) Coronal bone CT shows a laterally lobulated extension ➡ of the dehiscent jugular bulb ➡ into the right middle ear. Dehiscent jugular bulb is the most common vascular variant of the temporal bone and is more frequent on the right.

TERMINOLOGY

Abbreviations

- Dehiscent jugular bulb (DJB)

Definitions

- Normal venous variant with superior & lateral extension of JB into middle ear (ME) through dehiscent sigmoid plate

IMAGING

CT Findings

- CECT
  - Protruding mass enhances to same degree as JB
- Bone CT
  - Soft tissue mass in posteroinferior ME
    - Sigmoid plate dehiscent
- CTA
  - Enhancement pattern mirrors sigmoid sinus & internal jugular (IJ) vein

MR Findings

- T1WI
  - May have heterogeneous intensity or flow void
- T2WI
  - May have heterogeneous intensity or flow void
- T1WI C+
  - Enhancing ME mass connects to enhancing JB
- MRV
  - Coronal images show **lateral lobulation** best

DIFFERENTIAL DIAGNOSIS

Jugular Foramen Asymmetry

- Common normal variant, right more common
- Bone CT: Intact sigmoid plate

High Jugular Bulb

- Defined by superior portion extending to floor of IAC
- Bone CT: JB cortical margins intact, including sigmoid plate

Jugular Bulb Diverticulum

- Bone CT: Focal polypoid mass extending from superior JB

Glomus Tympanicum Paraganglioma

- Bone CT: Focal mass on cochlear promontory with ME floor intact

Glomus Jugulare Paraganglioma

- Bone CT: Permeative-destructive bony changes along JB superolateral margins
- Unenhanced T1 MR: Jugular foramen (JF) mass with high-velocity flow voids ("pepper")

Jugular Foramen Schwannoma

- Bone CT: Smoothly scalloped, enlarged JF
- T1 C+ MR: Dumbbell-shaped enhancing JF mass

Jugular Foramen Meningioma

- CT: Permeative-sclerotic or hyperostotic bony changes
- T1 C+ MR: May show dural tails
- T2 MR: Intermediate signal intensity, similar to cortex

PATHOLOGY

General Features

- Etiology
  - Congenital lesion
- Associated abnormalities
  - Most often associated with high-riding JB

CLINICAL ISSUES

Presentation

- Most common signs/symptoms
  - **Asymptomatic** incidental finding
- Other signs/symptoms
  - DJB has been reported as linked to many symptoms, though causality disputed
    - Pulsatile tinnitus, hearing loss, Ménière disease
- **Otoscopy**: Blue-colored vascular mass behind intact TM, prompting imaging
  - Seen in **posteroinferior TM quadrant**

Demographics

- Age
  - May be discovered on otoscopic or radiologic exam at any age
- Epidemiology
  - Most common vascular variant of petrous bone
  - More common on right side
    - Dural venous sinuses and jugular vein are larger on right in 75% of individuals

Natural History & Prognosis

- Renders JB vulnerable to trauma
  - Important to warn surgeons of presence of DJB when surgery is contemplated for other indications

DIAGNOSTIC CHECKLIST

Consider

- DJB in differential diagnosis list of any vascular retrotympanic mass

Image Interpretation Pearls

- Coronal TB CT will show direct continuity of middle ear mass with jugular bulb
- Smooth bony margins exclude more aggressive processes, such as tumor or infection

SELECTED REFERENCES

1. Atmaca S et al: High and dehiscent jugular bulb: clear and present danger during middle ear surgery. Surg Radiol Anat. 36(4):369-74, 2014
2. Huang BR et al: Dehiscent high jugular bulb: a pitfall in middle ear surgery. Otol Neurotol. 27(7):923-7, 2006
3. Caldemeyer KS et al: The jugular foramen: a review of anatomy, masses, and imaging characteristics. Radiographics. 17(5):1123-39, 1997
4. Smith B et al: Dehiscent jugular bulb. Ann Otol Rhinol Laryngol. 96(2 Pt 1):232-3, 1987
5. Daniels DL et al: Jugular foramen: anatomic and computed tomographic study. AJR Am J Roentgenol. 142(1):153-8, 1984
6. Lo WW et al: High-resolution CT of the jugular foramen: anatomy and vascular variants and anomalies. Radiology. 150(3):743-7, 1984

TERMINOLOGY

- Congenital vascular anomaly of jugular bulb (JB), with **focal finger-like projection extending from JB** into surrounding skull base

IMAGING

- T-bone CT: Focal projection extending off JB margin **superiorly** into deep T-bone just behind IAC
- Other directions of extension: **Lateral, medial, anterior, or posterior**
- Imaging protocol: Start with thin-section T-bone CT
  - If concern lingers, MR with contrast & MRV

TOP DIFFERENTIAL DIAGNOSES

- JB pseudolesion
- High JB
- Dehiscent JB
- Glomus jugulare paraganglioma
- Jugular foramen schwannoma or meningioma

PATHOLOGY

- JBD thought to represent expansion of high JB into surrounding bone but hindered by dense otic capsule

CLINICAL ISSUES

- **Asymptomatic**, incidental finding commonly
- Many symptoms have been linked to JBD
- JBD present in 35% of cases with high-riding JB

DIAGNOSTIC CHECKLIST

- JB diverticulum (JBD) in differential of medial temporal bone mass with smooth margins on CT
- Turbulent flow makes JB & JBD difficult to evaluate by MR
- Look for smooth bony remodeling on bone CT & continuity with JB
- On axial T1 C+ MR enhancing foci behind IAC may be mistaken for acoustic schwannoma or intralabyrinthine schwannoma

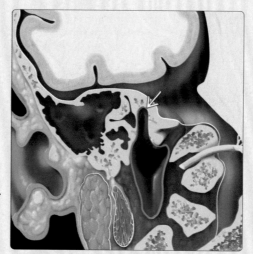
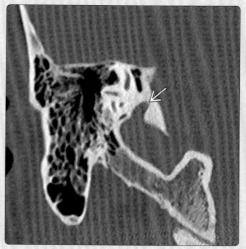

(Left) Coronal graphic depicts a jugular bulb diverticulum (JBD) as a finger-like superior projection off the JB into the petrous temporal bone ➡ without extension into the middle ear. (Right) Coronal right ear CT shows a JBD ➡ as a thumb-like projection arising from the superior JB margin. Continuity with the normal JB and smooth bony margins helps confirm the diagnosis. This JB lesion is more common on the left side. Patients are asymptomatic as a rule.

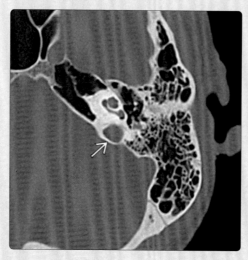
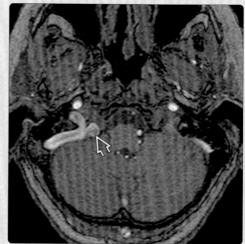

(Left) Axial left T-bone CT shows a JBD ➡ projecting cephalad from the JB into the medial temporal bone. These diverticula are typically located posterior to the internal auditory canal and have smooth bony margins. (Right) Axial MRV source image shows a medially projecting JBD ➡. This polypoid extension from the JB has similar enhancement characteristics as the JB and jugular vein. A JBD may be discovered at any age.

TERMINOLOGY

Abbreviations

- Jugular bulb diverticulum (JBD)

Synonyms

- Jugular diverticulum, petrous jugular malposition

Definitions

- JBD: **Congenital vascular anomaly** of jugular bulb (JB) with focal **finger-like projection** extending from JB into surrounding skull base

IMAGING

General Features

- Best diagnostic clue
  - T-bone CT: **Focal polypoid projection** extending off JB margin superiorly into deep temporal bone just behind IAC
- Location
  - JBD most commonly extends superiorly
  - Other directions of extension
    - Lateral, medial, anterior, or posterior
    - Lateral extension is often through dehiscent sigmoid plate = dehiscent JB
  - JB itself may be **high** or less commonly in normal position
- Size
  - Typical JB measures 1.0-1.5 cm
  - Diverticulum smaller than JB, typically < 1 cm in diameter & length
- Morphology
  - Lobulated outpouching arising from JB
  - May be finger-like or broad-based

CT Findings

- Bone CT: JBD is **well-corticated, smooth polypoid extension** off JB margin
  - Axial: Most commonly seen behind IAC
  - Coronal: Finger-like projection off top of JB
- CECT: Uniform enhancement of JB & JBD
- CTA: Contiguous with JB, similar enhancement

MR Findings

- T1WI: Heterogeneous signal intensity
- T2WI: Low signal from high-velocity flow (invisible)
  - Turbulent flow, heterogeneous high intensity (uncommon)
- T1WI C+: Avid enhancement, similar to JB & IJV
  - May mimic IAC or intralabyrinthine schwannoma
- MRV: Finger-like projection off JB

Imaging Recommendations

- Protocol advice: Start with thin-section T-bone CT
  - If concern lingers, MR with contrast & MRV

DIFFERENTIAL DIAGNOSIS

JB Pseudolesion

- MR shows asymmetric large JB with mass-like signal
- Usually found incidentally in skull base work-up
- Bone CT: Intact jugular spine & JB cortical margins

High JB

- Defined by most as cephalad portion of JB extending superior to floor of IAC ± at level of basal turn of cochlea
- CT: Jugular foramen (JF) cortical margins intact, including sigmoid plate
- MR: Complex or increased signal does not persist on all MR sequences

Dehiscent JB

- Vascular retrotympanic mass
- Protruding mass extends into posteroinferior middle ear cavity
- CT: Sigmoid plate shows focal dehiscence
- T1 C+ MR: Avidly enhancing middle ear mass connects to avidly enhancing JB

Glomus Jugulare Paraganglioma

- Enhancing mass in jugular foramen
- CT: Permeative destructive JF margin bony changes
- T1 MR: High-velocity flow voids ("pepper")

Jugular Foramen Schwannoma

- Dumbbell-shaped mass along cranial nerve IX-XI
- CT: Smoothly scalloped bony margins of enlarged JF
- T1 C+ MR: Fusiform enhancing mass in JF

PATHOLOGY

General Features

- Etiology
  - JBD may be secondary to hemodynamic factors
  - JBD more commonly seen with high-riding JB
  - Thought to represent expansion of high JB into surrounding bone, hindered by dense otic capsule

CLINICAL ISSUES

Presentation

- Most common signs/symptoms
  - **Asymptomatic**, incidental finding
- Many symptoms have been linked to JBD, based on direction of diverticulum extension: Sensorineural hearing loss, tinnitus, vertigo
- Symptoms reported have tenuous link to JBD

Demographics

- Epidemiology
  - Present in 8% of T-bone specimen studies
  - More common on left side

Treatment

- Conservative management of symptoms
- **Caveat**: Include in radiology report to warn surgeon if ear surgery planned

SELECTED REFERENCES

1. Mortimer AM et al: Endovascular treatment of jugular bulb diverticula causing debilitating pulsatile tinnitus. BMJ Case Rep, 2015
2. Park JJ et al: Jugular bulb abnormalities in patients with Meniere's disease using high-resolution computed tomography. Eur Arch Otorhinolaryngol. 272(8):1879-84, 2015
3. Chong VF et al: Radiology of the jugular foramen. Clin Radiol. 53(6):405-16, 1998

TERMINOLOGY

- Benign tumor arising from **neural crest** progenitor crest cells (glomus bodies) located in & around jugular foramen (JF)

IMAGING

- Bone CT: **Permeative-destructive** bone changes along JF margins
  - Jugular spine erosion is common
  - Floor of middle ear cavity dehisced
- MR: Lesions > 2 cm demonstrate characteristic **salt & pepper** appearance
- CTA/angiography: Main arterial supply is from **ascending pharyngeal artery**
- **Paraganglia rests** occur in 3 distinct bodies around JF: Jugular bulb, tympanic branch of CNIX (Jacobsen nerve), & auricular branch of CNX (Arnold nerve)
- Vector of spread: **Superolateral** through floor of middle ear is typical

TOP DIFFERENTIAL DIAGNOSES

- Glomus tympanicum paraganglioma
- Jugular foramen schwannoma
- Jugular foramen meningioma
- Jugular foramen metastasis
- Dehiscent jugular bulb

CLINICAL ISSUES

- Presentation: Objective pulsatile tinnitus most common
  - Other symptoms: CNIX-XI ± CNXII cranial neuropathy
  - CNVII or CNVIII neuropathy less often
- Otoscopic exam: **Red, pulsatile** retrotympanic mass
- M:F = 1:4
- Glomus jugulare paraganglioma (GJP) is most common JF tumor
- GJP & carotid body paraganglioma account for 80% of H&N paragangliomas
- Treatment: Surgical resection ± radiation
  - Radiosurgery may be used as primary therapy

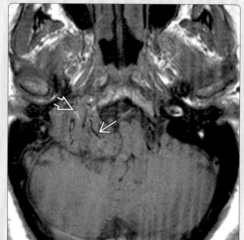
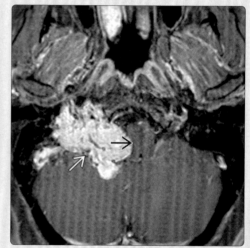

(Left) *Axial T1WI MR shows a large mass arising from the jugular foramen with multiple areas of salt & pepper. The "salt"* ⇒ *represents blood products or slow flow, while the "pepper"* ➡ *represents high-velocity arterial branch flow voids that help differentiate this tumor from other lesions in this location.* (Right) *Axial T1WI C+ FS MR in the same patient shows the classic intense enhancement of this large vascular tumor* ➡. *There is intracranial extension in this patient with mass effect upon the adjacent medulla* ➡.

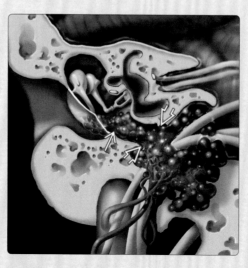
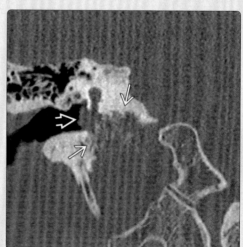

(Left) *Coronal graphic shows a glomus jugulare paraganglioma (GJP) centered in the jugular foramen dehiscing the middle ear floor* ⇒ *to reach the middle ear cavity* ➡. *The main arterial supply for this vascular tumor is the ascending pharyngeal artery.* (Right) *Coronal T-bone CT of the right ear shows the classic permeative-destructive margins* ➡ *of GJP. Note the typical vector of spread superolateral from the jugular foramen to the middle ear* ➡, *seen as a vascular retrotympanic mass at otoscopy.*

Glomus Jugulare Paraganglioma

TERMINOLOGY

Abbreviations
- Glomus jugulare paraganglioma (GJP)

Synonyms
- Glomus jugulotympanicum paraganglioma, jugular foramen (JF) paraganglioma, chemodectoma

Definitions
- Benign tumor arising from neural crest progenitor cells (glomus bodies) located in & around JF

IMAGING

General Features
- Best diagnostic clue
  - Mass in JF with **permeative-destructive** change of adjacent bone on CT
  - Multiple black dots ("**pepper**") in tumor mass indicating high-velocity flow voids from feeding arterial branches on MR
- Location
  - Paraganglia rests occur in 3 distinct bodies around jugular foramen
    - Jugular bulb (JB), tympanic branch of CNIX (Jacobsen nerve), & auricular branch of CNX (Arnold nerve)
  - Vector of spread: **Superolateral** through floor of middle ear (most common)
- Size
  - Large at presentation
    - 2-6 cm most commonly
- Morphology
  - Poorly marginated JF tumor with adjacent bone invasion

CT Findings
- NECT
  - Poorly defined soft tissue mass centered over JF
- CECT
  - Diffuse, intense enhancement
- Bone CT
  - **Permeative-destructive** bone changes along superolateral margin of JF mark extent of tumor
    - Jugular spine erosion is common
    - Vertical segment of petrous ICA posterior wall often dehiscent
    - Mastoid segment of facial nerve may be engulfed
  - Mimics malignancy

MR Findings
- T1WI
  - Lesions > 2 cm demonstrate characteristic **salt & pepper** appearance
    - "Salt" refers to hyperintense foci within tumor related to hemorrhage or slow flow
      - Hyperintense foci relatively rare MR finding
    - "Pepper" refers to numerous hypointense foci within tumor representing high-velocity arterial flow voids
      - Hypointense foci common MR finding
- T2WI
  - Mixed hyperintense mass with hypointense foci ("pepper")

- T1WI C+
  - Intense enhancement is characteristic
  - Delineates tumor extent in skull base & middle ear
  - Tumor may extend intraluminal within internal jugular vein or sigmoid sinus
  - Coronal: May show tongue of tumor curving up from JF, through middle ear floor, terminating on cochlear promontory
- MRV
  - Delineates sigmoid sinus and jugular vein status

Angiographic Findings
- Hypervascular mass with enlarged feeding arteries, rapid, intense tumor blush, & early draining veins
  - Main arterial supply is from **ascending pharyngeal artery** that supplies inferomedial territory
  - Caroticotympanic branches of ICA & meningeal branches of vertebral artery may contribute
  - Anterior tympanic artery from ECA supplies anterior compartment
  - Stylomastoid artery from ECA supplies posterolateral compartment

Nuclear Medicine Findings
- PET
  - Paragangliomas show **avid** F-18 FDG uptake
  - Useful in detecting metastasis or response to therapy

Imaging Recommendations
- Best imaging tool
  - Combination of bone CT and enhanced MR
- Bone CT, MR, & angiography all done before surgery
- Bone CT delineates areas of bone destruction
  - Shows bony landmarks less well seen on MR
- MR reveals exact soft tissue extent of tumor
- Angiography provides vascular road map for surgeon
  - Embolization used for preoperative hemostasis

DIFFERENTIAL DIAGNOSIS

Glomus Tympanicum Paraganglioma
- Bone CT: Globoid mass on cochlear promontory
  - Middle ear floor intact
- T1 C+ MR: Mass enhances
  - May differentiate location of glomus tympanicum paraganglioma (GTP) from obstructed secretions
- Otoscopy: Larger GTP may mimic GJP

Jugular Foramen Schwannoma
- Bone CT: Smooth remodeling, enlargement of JF
- T1 C+ MR: Fusiform enhancing mass ± cysts
- Angiography: Absence of tumor blush or enlarged feeding arteries; "puddling" on venous phase
- Vector of spread: Superomedial along CNIX-XI course

Jugular Foramen Meningioma
- Bone CT: Permeative-sclerotic bony JF margins
- T1 C+ MR: Enhancing mass with dural tails
- Angiography: Prolonged but mild tumor blush
- Vector of spread: Centrifugal spread along dural surfaces

Jugular Foramen Metastasis
- Bone CT: Destructive bone changes on JF margins

- T1 C+ MR: Heterogeneously enhancing invasive mass
- Vector of spread: Irregular centrifugal spread pattern

Dehiscent Jugular Bulb

- Bone CT: Sigmoid plate is focally dehiscent
- Coronal CT or MR: Superolateral extension of jugular bulb into middle ear
- Otoscopy: Blue-black posteroinferior quadrant retrotympanic mass

PATHOLOGY

General Features

- Etiology
  - Benign tumor arising from jugular foramen **paraganglia**
  - Paraganglia (glomus bodies): Chemoreceptors that respond to changes in blood oxygen, carbon dioxide levels
- Genetics
  - Familial prevalence ~ 10% for all paragangliomas
  - Germline *SDHB* and *SDHD* mutations
    - Higher risk of malignant paraganglioma
- Associated abnormalities
  - Increased risk of thyroid malignancy
  - Increased risk of paragangliomas in MEN1, NF1, multiple myocutaneous neuromas

Staging, Grading, & Classification

- **Glasscock-Jackson classification** of GJP: Correlates tumor extent with surgical approach
  - I: Small tumor involving JB, middle ear, mastoid
  - II: Tumor extends under IAC; may have intracranial extension
  - III: Extends into petrous apex (PA); may have intracranial extension
  - IV: Extends beyond PA, into clivus or infratemporal fossa; ± intracranial extension
- **Fisch classification**: Anatomic classification
  - A: Tumor limited to middle ear
  - B: Limited to tympanomastoid area, no infralabyrinthine involvement
  - C: Invades infralabyrinthine compartment & PA
    - C1: Limited involvement of vertical carotid canal
    - C2: Invades vertical carotid canal
    - C3: Invades horizontal carotid canal
  - D1: Intracranial extension < 2 cm
  - D2: Intracranial extension > 2 cm

Gross Pathologic & Surgical Features

- Lobulated, solid mass with fibrous pseudocapsule
- Cut surface shows multiple enlarged feeding arteries

Microscopic Features

- Biphasic cell pattern composed of chief cells & sustentacular cells surrounded by fibromuscular stroma
  - Chief cells arranged in characteristic compact cell nests or balls of cells (zellballen)
- Electromicroscopy: Shows neurosecretory granules

CLINICAL ISSUES

Presentation

- Most common signs/symptoms

  - Objective **pulsatile tinnitus**
  - Otoscopic exam: **Red, pulsatile** retrotympanic mass
  - Other symptoms: CNIX-XI ± CNXII cranial neuropathy; CNVII or CNVIII cranial neuropathy less often
  - Otologic symptoms predominate initially with cranial nerve palsies occurring late
- Clinical profile
  - 50-year-old woman with progressive pulsatile tinnitus & red, pulsatile retrotympanic mass

Demographics

- Age
  - 40-60 years
- Gender
  - M:F = 1:4
- Epidemiology
  - GJP & carotid body paraganglioma account for 80% of H&N paragangliomas
  - GJP is most common JF tumor
    - GJP is 2nd most common temporal bone tumor (glomus tympanicum paraganglioma is 1st)
  - Multicentric 5-10% in sporadic GJPs
  - Multicentric 25-50% in familial GJPs

Natural History & Prognosis

- Slow-growing tumor can be watched in older patients
- 60% have postoperative cranial neuropathy
- Aggressive behavior is seen in 2-13% of cases
  - Increased in patients with familial tumor syndromes
- Mortality rates are estimated at 15%

Treatment

- Surgery: Infratemporal fossa approach (Fisch type A)
- Larger lesions may require surgery & radiation
- Radiation therapy or radiosurgery may be used as primary therapy

DIAGNOSTIC CHECKLIST

Consider

- Look for multicentric lesions when evaluating GJP
- Both GJP & JF metastases will have permeative bone destruction
- Vascular schwannoma may mimic GJP on MR

Image Interpretation Pearls

- GJP diagnosed when mass shows
  - Bone CT: Permeative-destructive bone invasion
  - MR: JF mass with prominent flow voids ("pepper")
  - Vector of spread: Superolateral → JF into middle ear

SELECTED REFERENCES

1. Li D et al: Less-aggressive surgical management and long-term outcomes of jugular foramen paragangliomas: a neurosurgical perspective. J Neurosurg. 1-12, 2016
2. Griauzde J et al: Imaging of vascular lesions of the head and neck. Radiol Clin North Am. 53(1):197-213, 2015
3. Wanna GB et al: Contemporary management of jugular paragangliomas. Otolaryngol Clin North Am. 48(2):331-41, 2015
4. Gilbo P et al: Radiotherapy for benign head and neck paragangliomas: a 45-year experience. Cancer. 120(23):3738-43, 2014
5. Collins N et al: Contiguous bilateral head and neck paragangliomas in a carrier of the SDHB germline mutation. J Vasc Surg. 55(1):216-9, 2012

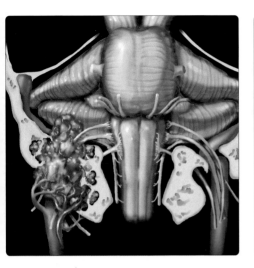

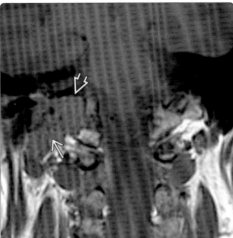

(Left) *Coronal graphic shows a large GJP arising from the jugular foramen engulfing the jugular vein and CNIX-XII and infiltrating the adjacent skull base.* (Right) *Coronal T1WI MR shows a large GJP* ➡ *involving the skull base with extension superiorly and laterally to the external auditory canal. Note the multiple high-velocity flow voids* ➡, *characteristic of paraganglioma. A GJP is the 2nd most common tumor of the temporal bone.*

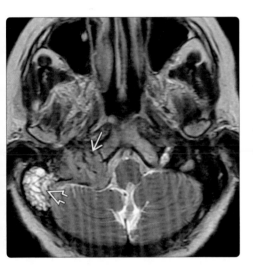

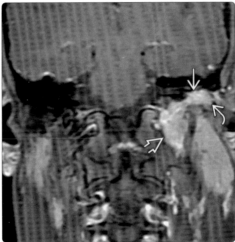

(Left) *Axial T2WI MR shows a large mass arising from the jugular foramen with multiple high-velocity flow voids* ➡ *that help differentiate this tumor from other lesions in this location. There is a mastoid effusion related to eustation tube obstruction* ➡. (Right) *Coronal T1WI C+FS MR shows an enhancing GJP* ➡ *involving the skull base with extension superiorly and laterally to the middle ear* ➡ *and external auditory canal* ➡. *This 15 year old with an SDHB mutation is at risk for a more aggressive paraganglioma.*

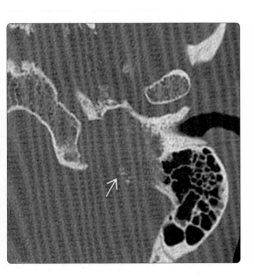

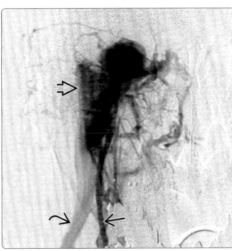

(Left) *Axial T-bone CT of the left ear shows a GJP with typical bony permeative-destructive margins* ➡. *A pulsatile, red retrotympanic mass and pulsatile tinnitus would be expected clinical findings.* (Right) *Anteroposterior selective ascending pharyngeal artery* ➡ *angiogram reveals extensive filling of a GJP* ➡. *Note the early draining vein* ➡ *related to arteriovenous shunting. Endovascular embolization is often done preoperatively for control of blood loss.*

TERMINOLOGY

- Benign tumor of differentiated Schwann cells wrapping around cranial nerves (CNs) IX, X, or XI within jugular foramen (JF)

IMAGING

- Bone CT: Sharply marginated, enlarged JF
- T1WI C+ MR
  - Tubular or dumbbell-shaped, uniformly enhancing
  - No flow voids ("pepper") (vs. paraganglioma)
  - Nonenhancing cystic areas in large lesions
- T2WI hyperintense
- Superomedial vector of tumor growth
  - Follows craniocaudal course of CNs IX-XI
  - Grows cephalad from JF through basal cistern toward retroolivary sulcus of lateral medulla
  - Grows inferiorly from JF into nasopharyngeal carotid space
- MRV: Dural sinus compressed, not occluded

TOP DIFFERENTIAL DIAGNOSES

- JF pseudolesion
- Glomus jugulare paraganglioma
- JF meningioma
- Skull base metastasis

CLINICAL ISSUES

- Mean age: 45 years old
- Sensorineural hearing loss in 90% at presentation
  - May present clinically like vestibular schwannoma
- 2nd most common JF tumor
  - Glossopharyngeal nerve (CNIX) most common nerve of origin
- Complete surgical removal of tumor in single procedure is goal
  - May be complicated by lower cranial neuropathy
- Radiosurgery as primary or adjuvant therapy

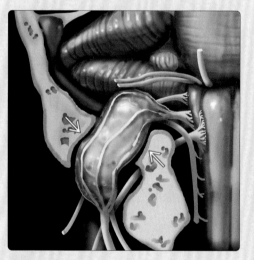
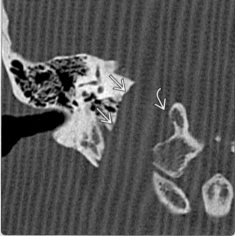

(Left) Coronal graphic depicts a classic jugular foramen (JF) schwannoma as a fusiform mass arising on 1 of the cranial nerves (IX-XI) within the JF. Note the vector of spread is superomedial. The JF ➡ is enlarged with an intact cortex. (Right) Coronal bone CT shows a sharply marginated, enlarged JF with amputation of the lateral jugular tubercle ➡. The smooth enlargement ➡ with sclerotic margins is characteristic of JF schwannoma.

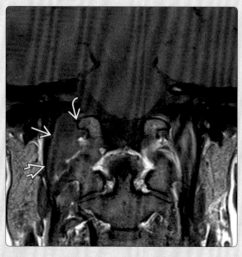
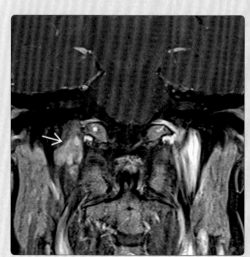

(Left) Coronal T1 MR shows a JF schwannoma ➡ projecting superomedially from the JF toward the brainstem. Inferiorly, the schwannoma extends into the nasopharyngeal carotid space ➡. There is amputation of the lateral aspect of the jugular tubercle ➡. Lack of flow voids helps differentiate this schwannoma from the more common glomus jugulare paraganglioma. (Right) Coronal T1 C+ MR in the same patient shows enhancement of the JF schwannoma ➡.

Jugular Foramen Schwannoma

TERMINOLOGY

Abbreviations

- Jugular foramen schwannoma (JFS)

Synonyms

- Neuroma, neurilemoma, neurinoma

Definitions

- Benign tumor of differentiated Schwann cells wrapping around cranial nerves (CNs) IX, X, or XI within JF

IMAGING

General Features

- Best diagnostic clue
  - Sharply marginated, enlarged JF on bone CT
  - Fusiform, enhancing mass enlarging JF on T1WI C+ MR
- Location
  - JF
    - Vector of tumor growth
      □ Follows general craniocaudal course of CNs IX-XI
      □ Grows cephalad from JF through basal cistern toward retroolivary sulcus of lateral medulla
      □ Grows inferiorly from JF into nasopharyngeal carotid space
- Size
  - Often large at presentation (> 3 cm)
- Morphology
  - Fusiform or "dumbbell" mass
    - Waist is within JF

CT Findings

- NECT
  - Well-defined soft tissue mass isodense to brain, occasionally hypodense
- CECT
  - Dense contrast enhancement is typical
  - Larger JFS often show nonenhancing intramural cysts
- Bone CT
  - **Smooth JF enlargement** with thin, sclerotic margins
  - Coronal plane may show amputation of lateral jugular tubercle ("bird's beak")
  - Multilobular intraosseous extension into adjacent skull base may be marked

MR Findings

- T1WI
  - Tubular or dumbbell-shaped JF mass
  - Typically isointense to brain
  - Internal carotid artery characteristically displaced over anteromedial margin of JFS in nasopharyngeal carotid space
  - **No flow voids** ("pepper") or hyperintensity related to blood products ("salt") even when large
- T2WI
  - High signal relative to white matter
  - ↑ signal **cystic areas** can be seen in large JFS
    - 25% of JFS show intramural cysts
- DWI
  - No diffusion restriction

- May be mildly hyperintense related to T2 "shine-through"
- T1WI C+
  - Uniformly enhancing JF mass
  - Nonenhancing intramural cystic components in larger tumors may be seen
  - When small, may be difficult to differentiate enhancing normal jugular bulb (JB) from small JFS
    - Tissue-intensity mass seen better on unenhanced T1 & T2WI
- MRV
  - Dural sinuses usually compressed, not occluded
    - Occlusion can be evaluated with phase-contrast MRV employing low-velocity encoding setting

Angiographic Findings

- Tumor is moderately vascular
- Feeding vessels are tortuous but not enlarged
- Scattered contrast "puddles" are characteristic in venous phase
- No arteriovenous shunting or vascular encasement

Imaging Recommendations

- Best imaging tool
  - Enhanced brain/skull base MR best delineates internal architecture & soft tissue extent of JFS
  - Bone CT is best for assessing JF cortex for typical smooth, sclerotic margins

DIFFERENTIAL DIAGNOSIS

JF Pseudolesion

- Venous flow phenomenon mimics schwannoma or other lesion
- Asymmetric large JB with complex MR signal
- Asymmetric large JF with normal margins on CT
- T1 C+ MR: Slow flow in JF enhances
- MRV: Normal dural sinuses & jugular bulb

Glomus Jugulare Paraganglioma

- Permeative-destructive JF bone margins on bone CT
- High-velocity flow voids ("pepper") on unenhanced MR sequences
- Rapid tumor blush with early draining veins on angiography
- Growth vector: Superolateral from JF into middle ear

JF Meningioma

- Permeative-sclerotic bone margins of JF on CT
- Intermediate to low signal on T2WI
- Dural-based mass with enhancing dural "tails"
- Prolonged blush into capillary phase on angiography
- Growth vector: Centrifugally along dural surfaces

Skull Base Metastasis

- Bony margins of JF are destructive on CT
- Heterogeneously enhancing, invasive JF mass
- Growth vector: All directions from JF
- Multiple lesions commonly seen

PATHOLOGY

General Features

- Etiology

- o Arises from differentiated neoplastic Schwann cells wrapping around CNs IX, X, or XI
- Genetics
  - o 90% are solitary and sporadic
  - o 4% arise in setting of Neurofibromatosis type 2 (NF2
  - o < 5% associated with schwannomatosis
- Associated abnormalities
  - o Multiple schwannomas are associated with NF2 or schwannomatosis

Staging, Grading, & Classification

- Kaye & Pellet Surgical Classification (from surgical & radiologic findings)
  - o Type A: Extends to cerebellopontine angle (CPA)
  - o Type B: Within JF
  - o Type C: Nasopharyngeal carotid space &/or JF
  - o Type D: Intracranial and extracranial (cisternal & carotid space)
- WHO grade I

Gross Pathologic & Surgical Features

- Smooth, lobulated mass arising from nerve sheath
  - o Arises eccentrically from nerve sheath
- Tan, round/ovoid, encapsulated mass

Microscopic Features

- Differentiated neoplastic Schwann cells
- Spindle cells with elongated nuclei
  - o Antoni A: Areas of compact, elongated cells
  - o Antoni B: Areas of less cellular, loosely arranged tumor, ± clusters of lipid-laden cells
- Immunochemistry: Strong, diffuse immunostaining for S100 protein = neural crest marker antigen present in supporting cells of nervous system
- No necrosis but may have intratumoral cysts ± hemorrhage

CLINICAL ISSUES

Presentation

- Most common signs/symptoms
  - o Sensorineural hearing loss (SNHL) in 90% at presentation
    - May present clinically like vestibular schwannoma
- Other signs/symptoms
  - o CNs IX-XI neuropathy occurs late in disease progression
  - o Hoarseness, aspiration (recurrent laryngeal nerve, branch of CNX)
  - o Dizziness may be related to cerebellar compression
  - o Pulsatile tinnitus may be related to dural sinus thrombosis and dAVF
  - o Hemifacial spasm (mass effect on CNVII in CPA)
- Clinical profile
  - o Middle-aged (~ 45 years old) individual with unilateral SNHL

Demographics

- Age
  - o Mean: 45 years old
- Gender
  - o No gender predilection
- Epidemiology
  - o Schwannomas represent 8% of intracranial tumors
    - 85-90% of CPA tumors are schwannoma

- o 2nd most common JF tumor
  - Glomus jugulare paraganglioma > > schwannoma > meningioma
  - Nonvestibular schwannoma incidence: CNV > > CNIX > CNX > CNVII > CNXI > CNXII > CNIII > CNIV > CNVI
- o Glossopharyngeal nerve (CNIX) most common nerve of origin of JFS

Natural History & Prognosis

- Benign, slow-growing tumor
- Advanced disease or treatment may result in late CNVII-XII neuropathy

Treatment

- Complete surgical removal of tumor in single procedure is goal
- Surgical approach dictated by presence or absence of cisternal or nasopharyngeal carotid space extension
  - o Surgical cure may be complicated by lower cranial neuropathy, often CNIX & CNX
- Stereotactic radiosurgery is being used more frequently as primary or adjuvant therapy

DIAGNOSTIC CHECKLIST

Consider

- JFS most likely when smooth, scalloped margins seen around JF soft tissue mass on CT

Image Interpretation Pearls

- Lack of flow voids help differentiate JFS from more common glomus jugulare paraganglioma

Reporting Tips

- Be sure to describe extension below skull base into carotid space

SELECTED REFERENCES

1. Hasegawa T et al: Gamma knife surgery for patients with jugular foramen schwannomas: a multiinstitutional retrospective study in Japan. J Neurosurg. 1-10, 2016
2. Komune N et al: Surgical approaches to jugular foramen schwannomas: an anatomic study. Head Neck. 38 Suppl 1:E1041-53, 2016
3. Park ES et al: A single-institution retrospective study of jugular foramen schwannoma management: radical resection versus subtotal intracranial resection through a retrosigmoid suboccipital approach followed by radiosurgery. World Neurosurg. 88:552-62, 2016
4. Li W et al: Lesions involving the jugular foramen: clinical characteristics and surgical management. Acta Otolaryngol. 135(6):565-71, 2015
5. Thomas AJ et al: Nonparaganglioma jugular foramen tumors. Otolaryngol Clin North Am. 48(2):343-59, 2015
6. Hasegawa T: Stereotactic radiosurgery for nonvestibular schwannomas. Neurosurg Clin N Am. 24(4):531-42, 2013
7. Sedney CL et al: Microsurgical management of jugular foramen schwannomas. Neurosurgery. 72(1):42-6; discussion 46, 2013
8. Fayad JN et al: Jugular foramen tumors: clinical characteristics and treatment outcomes. Otol Neurotol. 31(2):299-305, 2010
9. Safavi-Abbasi S et al: Nonvestibular schwannomas: an evaluation of functional outcome after radiosurgical and microsurgical management. Acta Neurochir (Wien). 152(1):35-46, 2010
10. Fukuda M et al: Long-term outcomes after surgical treatment of jugular foramen schwannoma. Skull Base. 19(6):401-8, 2009
11. Eldevik OP et al: Imaging findings in schwannomas of the jugular foramen. AJNR Am J Neuroradiol. 21(6):1139-44, 2000
12. Caldemeyer KS et al: The jugular foramen: a review of anatomy, masses, and imaging characteristics. Radiographics. 17(5):1123-39, 1997

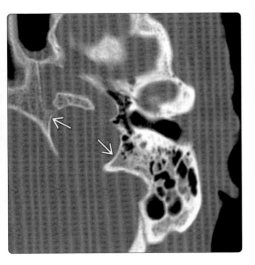

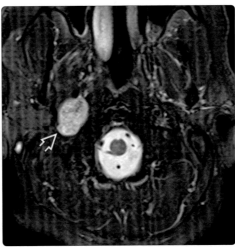

(Left) *Axial bone CT shows the classic smooth enlargement of the JF with thin sclerotic margins ➡ in this patient with a JF foramen schwannoma. These bone changes can help differentiate this lesion from other common lesions of the JF, including glomus jugulare paraganglioma and meningioma.* (Right) *Axial T2 FS MR shows a hyperintense right carotid space mass ➡ related to extension of a JF schwannoma into the carotid space. Note the typical hyperintensity and absence of flow voids.*

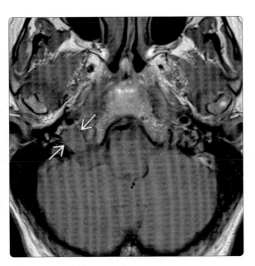

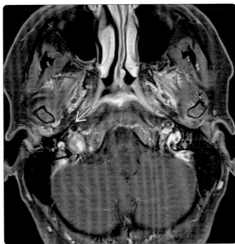

(Left) *Axial T1WI MR shows a small right JF schwannoma ➡. Note the typical lack of high-velocity flow voids, which helps differentiate this lesion from the more common glomus jugulare paraganglioma. Small lesions may be difficult to differentiate from jugular bulb asymmetry.* (Right) *Axial T1 C+ FS MR in the same patient shows heterogeneous enhancement ➡ of the schwannoma. When lesions are large, intramural cystic, nonenhancing components may be present.*

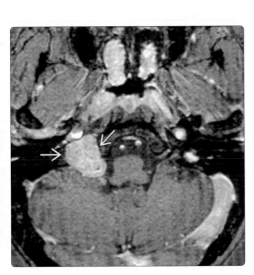

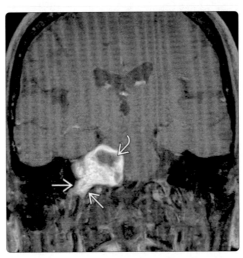

(Left) *Axial T1 C+ FS MR shows a fusiform, homogeneously enhancing right JF schwannoma ➡ with extension into the adjacent cistern. Most of these patients have associated sensorineural hearing loss.* (Right) *Coronal T1WI C+ FS MR shows a heterogeneously enhancing, lobulated mass arising from the JF ➡. Note typical superomedial vector of spread toward brainstem. Large tumors may have nonenhancing components related to intramural cysts ➡.*

TERMINOLOGY

- Benign neoplasm arising from arachnoid cap cells found along cranial nerves within jugular foramen (JF)

IMAGING

- Bone CT: **Permeative-sclerotic** JF margins
- T1WI C+ MR: Enhancing JF mass spreading along dural surfaces
  - Enhancing **dural tails** may be seen
  - No high-velocity flow voids
- **Centrifugal** vector of spread: Extends in all directions from JF along dural surfaces and through surrounding bones
  - May protrude into basal cisterns or nasopharyngeal carotid space

TOP DIFFERENTIAL DIAGNOSES

- Glomus jugulare paraganglioma
- JF schwannoma
- JF metastasis

- JF pseudolesion
- Dehiscent jugular bulb

PATHOLOGY

- Proliferation of arachnoid meningothelial cap cells along CNs IX-XI in JF

CLINICAL ISSUES

- CNs IX-XI neuropathy most common presentation
- Risk factors
  - Prior nasopharynx, skull base, or brain radiation; neurofibromatosis type 2; female sex hormones
- Meningioma is 3rd most common JF mass
  - Paraganglioma > > schwannoma > meningioma
- Treatment: Complete surgical removal is goal
  - Surgical cure often results in multiple lower cranial neuropathies
  - Radiotherapy for elderly patients, poor surgical risk or subtotal resection

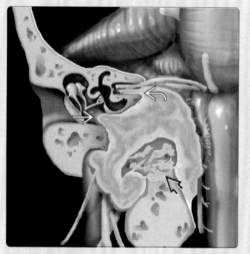
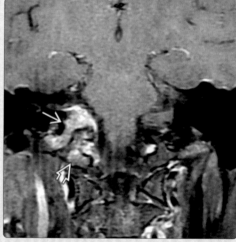

(Left) Coronal graphic shows a large jugular foramen meningioma invading the middle ear ➡, skull base marrow ⊠, and internal auditory canal ➡. Note the cranial nerves of the jugular foramen (CN IX-XI) are engulfed. (Right) Coronal T1WI C+ FS MR shows a large jugular foramen meningioma ➡ with invasion of the skull base marrow ⊠. Jugular foramen meningiomas have a centrifugal vector of spread and often extend along dural surfaces and through the surrounding bones.

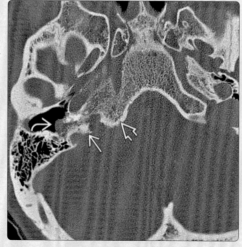
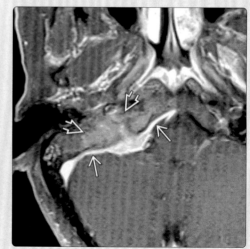

(Left) Axial bone CT shows the characteristic permeative sclerotic changes along the jugular foramen ➡ and lateral clivus ⊠ of this jugular foramen meningioma. The meningioma extends into the middle ear ➡ and may present clinically as a vascular retrotympanic mass on otoscopy. (Right) Axial T1WI C+ FS MR shows a jugular foramen meningioma with en plaque morphology and dural tails ➡. Note the lack of flow voids and the jugular foramen involvement with extensive adjacent skull base infiltration ➡.

TERMINOLOGY

Definitions

- Benign neoplasm arising from arachnoid cap cells found along cranial nerves within jugular foramen (JF)

IMAGING

General Features

- Best diagnostic clue
  - **Permeative-sclerotic** involvement of bone around JF on CT
  - Enhancing JF mass spreading **centrifugally** along dural surfaces on enhanced MR
- Location
  - Centered within JF
  - Vector of spread: Centrifugal pattern (away from center)
    - Extends in all directions from JF along dural surfaces and through surrounding bones
      □ Dural-based spread into basal cistern most common
    - May protrude into nasopharyngeal carotid space below
- Morphology
  - Poorly circumscribed mass

CT Findings

- NECT
  - Hyperdense JF mass
- Bone CT
  - **Permeative-sclerotic** JF margins

MR Findings

- T1WI
  - Hypo- to isointense JF mass compared to brain parenchyma
  - **No** high-velocity flow voids
- T2WI
  - Relative T2 hypointensity suggests dense histology
- T1WI C+
  - Dense, uniform contrast enhancement
  - Enhancing **dural tails** may be visible along adjacent dural surfaces of basal cisterns
- MRV
  - May occlude dural sinuses and jugular bulb
    - Patency of adjacent dural sinuses should be documented prior to surgery

Angiographic Findings

- Supply primarily from dural branches of external carotid artery and vertebral artery
- Angiography provides vascular road map for surgeon
  - Evaluates collateral arterial and venous circulation
  - Embolization used for preoperative hemostasis

DIFFERENTIAL DIAGNOSIS

Glomus Jugulare Paraganglioma

- **Permeative-destructive** JF bony margins on CT
- High-velocity flow voids ("pepper") characteristic on MR
- Vector of spread: Superolateral into middle ear

Jugular Foramen Schwannoma

- **Smooth** enlargement of JF on CT
- Tubular JF mass on MR ± intramural cysts when large
- Vector of spread: Superomedial along CNs IX-XI

Jugular Foramen Metastasis

- **Destructive** bone margins of JF on CT
- Heterogeneously enhancing invasive JF mass on MR

Jugular Foramen Pseudolesion

- Asymmetric JF MR signal suggests lesion
- JF bony margins intact on CT
- Complex JF signal does not persist on all MR sequences

Dehiscent Jugular Bulb

- Superolateral extension of jugular bulb into middle ear
- Sigmoid plate focally dehiscent on CT

PATHOLOGY

General Features

- Etiology
  - Meningioma arises from proliferation of arachnoidal cap cells of meninges
- Genetics
  - Sporadic: Isolated defect on chromosome 22
  - Inherited: Associated with NF2 and systemic chromosome 22 abnormality

Staging, Grading, & Classification

- Typical meningioma (90%): WHO grade I
- Atypical meningioma (7%): WHO grade II
- Anaplastic meningioma (3%): WHO grade III

CLINICAL ISSUES

Presentation

- Most common signs/symptoms
  - CNs IX-XI neuropathy

Demographics

- Age
  - Typically 40-60 years
- Gender
  - F > M = 2:1

DIAGNOSTIC CHECKLIST

Image Interpretation Pearls

- Large JF meningioma may mimic glomus jugulare paraganglioma

SELECTED REFERENCES

1. Samii M et al: Endoscope-assisted retrosigmoid infralabyrinthine approach to jugular foramen tumors. J Neurosurg. 1-7, 2015
2. Guinto G et al: Nonglomic tumors of the jugular foramen: differential diagnosis and prognostic implications. World Neurosurg. 82(6):1283-90, 2014
3. Fayad JN et al: Jugular foramen tumors: clinical characteristics and treatment outcomes. Otol Neurotol. 31(2):299-305, 2010
4. Hamilton BE et al: Imaging and clinical characteristics of temporal bone meningioma. AJNR Am J Neuroradiol. 27(10):2204-9, 2006
5. Macdonald AJ et al: Primary jugular foramen meningioma: imaging appearance and differentiating features. AJR Am J Roentgenol. 182(2):373-7, 2004

TERMINOLOGY

- Arachnoid granulation (AG)
  - Defined as enlarged arachnoid villi projecting into major dural venous sinus lumen
- Aberrant arachnoid granulation (AbAG)
  - Defined as AG that penetrates dura, but fails to reach venous sinus, typically in sphenoid or T-bone

IMAGING

- Intrasinus AG: Well-circumscribed, discrete, filling defect in venous sinus ± inner calvarial table erosion
  - CECT: Nonenhancing; density like CSF
  - MR: T1/T2 intensity follows CSF; FLAIR often hyperintense
- AbAG: Multiple focal outpouches in sphenoid bone or T-bone
  - Sphenoid bone location: Greater wing
  - T-bone location: Posterior wall or tegmen
  - CT: Multiple smooth pits in sphenoid or T-bone

- MR: T1 and T2 intensity follows CSF

TOP DIFFERENTIAL DIAGNOSES

- Dural sinus hypoplasia-aplasia
- Transverse-sigmoid sinus pseudolesion
- Dural sinus thrombosis
- Dural arteriovenous fistula

CLINICAL ISSUES

- Intrasinus AG: Asymptomatic with rare exception
- AbAG: Mostly asymptomatic
  - If large with rupture, **CSF leak** ± meningitis possible
  - Sphenoid bone: CSF leak → sphenoid fluid → rhinorrhea
  - T-bone: CSF leak → middle ear-mastoid fluid → otorrhea
  - Large AG may have associated **cephalocele** (± seizure)
  - **Meningitis** may complicate CSF leak
- Treatment
  - Intrasinus AG: No treatment required
  - AbAG: No treatment unless CSF leak present

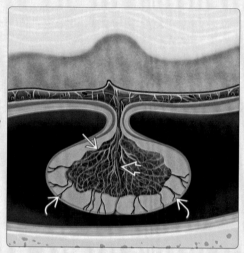
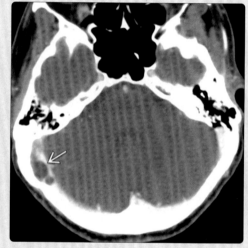

(Left) Graphic shows a giant arachnoid granulation (AG) projecting from subarachnoid space into transverse sinus. CSF core ➡ extends into the AG and is separated by arachnoid cap cells from the venous sinus endothelium ➚. Giant AGs often contain prominent venous channels ➡ and septations. (Right) Axial CECT shows a giant arachnoid granulation cluster at the transverse-sigmoid venous sinus junction ➡. The 1st imaging interpretation of this finding mistakenly suggested venous sinus thrombosis.

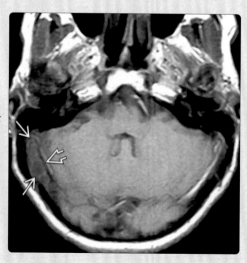
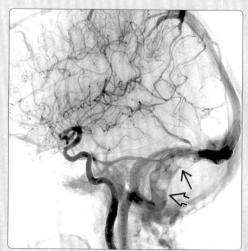

(Left) Axial T1WI MR in the same patient reveals the multiple giant AGs ➡ as low signal within the transverse and proximal sigmoid sinuses. The medial low-signal line ➡ is the dura. (Right) Lateral internal carotid artery angiogram in the same patient clearly depicts multiple giant AGs in the transverse ➡ and proximal sigmoid ➡ venous sinuses. No intrasinus pressure gradient was present across the lesion.

Dural Sinus and Aberrant Arachnoid Granulations

TERMINOLOGY

Abbreviations

- Arachnoid granulation (AG)
- Aberrant arachnoid granulation (AbAG)

Synonyms

- Pacchionian depressions, granulations, or bodies
- When large → "giant" arachnoid granulation
- When in sphenoid bone and temporal bone (T-bone) → AbAG

Definitions

- Arachnoid villi: Term used to describe smaller AG
- AG: Enlarged arachnoid villi projecting into major dural venous sinus lumen
- AbAG: AG that penetrated dura, but fails to reach venous sinus, typically in sphenoid or T-bone
  - Also referred to as arachnoid pits or osteodural defects

IMAGING

General Features

- Best diagnostic clue
  - Intrasinus AG: Discrete filling defect in venous sinus ± inner calvarial table erosion
    - CECT: Nonenhancing; similar density to CSF
    - MR: T1/T2 intensity follows CSF; often hyperintense on FLAIR
  - AbAG: Multiple focal outpouches in sphenoid bone, often greater wing
    - Bone CT: Multiple smooth pits in sphenoid bone
    - MR: T1 and T2 intensity follows CSF
- Location
  - Most common location: Transverse sinus
  - Other locations: Sigmoid, sagittal, or straight sinus
  - AbAG location: Sphenoid bone, often greater wing, or lateral sinus wall
    - T-bone: Posterior wall or tegmen tympani
- Size
  - Range: 5-15 mm
  - If > 15 mm, called "giant" AG
- Morphology
  - Single or multiple ovoid lesions
  - Focal osseous pits in inner table of calvaria

CT Findings

- NECT
  - Intrasinus AG isodense with CSF
  - CSF pulsations may result in erosion or scalloping of inner table
  - AbAG: Focal osseous erosions in sphenoid bone
    - If large, may appear multilocular; mimic cystic bone lesion
- CECT
  - Nonenhancing, ovoid focal filling defect within venous sinus
  - Isodense to CSF
  - AbAG: CSF density with subtle rim (dural) enhancement
- CT venogram
  - Focal filling defect within venous sinus

MR Findings

- T1WI
  - Venous sinus defect isointense to CSF
- T2WI
  - Hyperintense (like CSF)
  - Surrounded by normal flow void of major venous sinus
  - AbAG: High-signal outpouching into sphenoid bone
    - If large, may see arachnoid pouch bulging into sphenoid sinus lumen
      □ Arachnoid strands seen as low signal lines within pouch
    - Larger lesions may have **CSF leak** into sphenoid sinus
      □ Fluid levels seen in sphenoid sinus if leak present
    - Larger lesions may have **cephalocele** associated
- T1WI C+
  - Intrasinus AG: Ovoid without enhancement surrounded by enhancing blood in dural sinus
    - Veins, septa may enhance
  - AbAG: Nonenhancing foci in sphenoid bone
- MRV
  - Intrasinus AG
    - Source images show focal signal loss in location of AG
    - MRV reformation shows focal defect in affected sinus

Imaging Recommendations

- Best imaging tool
  - Intrasinus AG: Enhanced MR with MRV
  - AbAG: Bone CT of skull base
    - Enhanced MR focused to sphenoid bone area

DIFFERENTIAL DIAGNOSIS

Dural Sinus Hypoplasia-Aplasia

- Congenital hypoplastic-aplastic transverse sinus
- "High-splitting" tentorium

Transverse-Sigmoid Sinus Pseudolesion

- Asymmetric complex flow phenomenon in sinus mimics lesions
- Not present on all sequences; MRV sorts out

Dural Sinus Thrombosis

- Long-segment region of ↓ venous sinus flow
- NECT: Hyperdense
- CECT: Nonenhancing clot in venous sinus lumen
- MR: Hyperintense on T1 or lack of flow void on T2
  - T1 C+: Nonenhancing clot in venous sinus lumen

Dural AV Fistula

- MR: Recanalized, irregular transverse-sigmoid sinuses
  - MRA: Enlarged, feeding external carotid artery branches; early venous drainage
- Angio: Enlarged, feeding external carotid artery branches

PATHOLOGY

General Features

- Etiology
  - Intrasinus AG: Normal variant enlarged arachnoid villi
    - Penetrates dura overlying venous sinus
    - Arachnoid cap cells in margin of AG responsible for CSF resorption

○ AbAG: Penetrates dura, but fails to reach venous sinus in sphenoid or T-bone
  – CSF pulsations enlarge AbAG, causing arachnoid pouch bulging
  – Bulging arachnoid pouch penetrates subjacent structures (dura, then underlying bone)
  – If pouch stretches to point of rupture, CSF enters air cells if involved
    □ Sphenoid bone-sphenoid sinus: CSF leak → sphenoid fluid → rhinorrhea
    □ T-bone air cells: CSF leak → middle ear-mastoid fluid → otorrhea
    □ Cephalocele possible in larger AbAG

Gross Pathologic & Surgical Features

- AG: Smooth arachnoid granulation projecting into venous sinus or subarachnoid space
- AbAG: Osteodural defects in lateral sphenoid sinus wall or greater wing of sphenoid

Microscopic Features

- Enlarged arachnoid villi
- Central core of loose connective tissue with CSF
- Peripheral zone of dense connective tissue
- Projects through dura of venous sinus wall

CLINICAL ISSUES

Presentation

- Most common signs/symptoms
  ○ Intrasinus AG: Asymptomatic with rare exception
    – If suspect giant AG in venous sinus causing venous hypertension with headache, angiography with pressure measurements needed
    – In most cases, no pressure gradient across giant AG in dural venous sinus found
  ○ AbAG: Mostly asymptomatic
    – If CSF pulsations enlarge AbAG in sphenoid sinus or T-bone wall, CSF leak ± meningitis possible
      □ Sphenoid sinus wall rupture: Rhinorrhea
      □ T-bone air cell rupture: Otorrhea
    – If significant cephalocele occurs, seizure possible
- Other signs/symptoms
  ○ Benign intracranial hypertension in obese middle-aged females with rhinorrhea
    – Look for AbAG in sphenoid bone adjacent to sphenoid sinus

Demographics

- Age
  ○ ↑ in frequency with ↑ age; ≥ 40 years
- Epidemiology
  ○ Intrasinus AG: 25% CECT or T2WI MR
  ○ AbAG: Rare to see with imaging
    – Sphenoid bone: < 2%
    – T-bone: < 1%

Natural History & Prognosis

- Intrasinus AG: Remains asymptomatic
- AbAG: May remain small
  ○ If enlarge in response to CSF pulsations may penetrate dura, bone and air cells

  – CSF leak, cephalocele, or meningitis may result

Treatment

- Intrasinus AG: No treatment required
- AbAG: No treatment needed unless enlarged with resulting CSF leak
  ○ Can follow large, asymptomatic AbAG
  ○ If CSF leak present into sphenoid sinus or T-bone, surgical dural repair necessary
    – Surgical repair prevents meningitis possibility

DIAGNOSTIC CHECKLIST

Consider

- If **intrasinus giant AG** with history of headache, consider angiogram to look for intrasinus pressure gradient
- If **AbAG** presents in lateral wall **sphenoid bone**, look for fluid in sphenoid sinus as evidence for CSF leak
  ○ Also use MR to evaluate for possible associated cephalocele
- If **AbAG** found in posterior wall of **T-bone**, look for fluid in mastoid air cells as evidence for CSF leak

Image Interpretation Pearls

- Intrasinus AG
  ○ Confirm AG remains CSF density (as seen with CECT or CT angiogram) and intensity (as seen with T1 and T2 MR sequences)
  ○ Make sure proximal and distal venous sinus is normal from imaging perspective
- AbAG in lateral sphenoid sinus wall or posterior wall T-bone
  ○ If large or multiple, look for evidence of CSF leak

SELECTED REFERENCES

1. Battal B et al: Brain herniations into the dural venous sinuses or calvarium: MRI of a recently recognized entity. Neuroradiol J. 27(1):55-62, 2014
2. De Keyzer B et al: Giant arachnoid granulations mimicking pathology. A report of three cases. Neuroradiol J. 27(3):316-21, 2014
3. Settecase F et al: Spontaneous lateral sphenoid cephaloceles: anatomic factors contributing to pathogenesis and proposed classification. AJNR Am J Neuroradiol. 35(4):784-9, 2014
4. La Fata V et al: CSF leaks: correlation of high-resolution CT and multiplanar reformations with intraoperative endoscopic findings. AJNR Am J Neuroradiol. 29(3):536-41, 2008
5. Lloyd KM et al: Imaging of skull base cerebrospinal fluid leaks in adults. Radiology. 248(3):725-36, 2008
6. Schuknecht B et al: Nontraumatic skull base defects with spontaneous CSF rhinorrhea and arachnoid herniation: imaging findings and correlation with endoscopic sinus surgery in 27 patients. AJNR Am J Neuroradiol. 29(3):542-9, 2008
7. Haroun AA et al: Arachnoid granulations in the cerebral dural sinuses as demonstrated by contrast-enhanced 3D magnetic resonance venography. Surg Radiol Anat. 29(4):323-8, 2007
8. Amlashi SF et al: Intracranial hypertension and giant arachnoid granulations. J Neurol Neurosurg Psychiatry. 75(1):172, 2004
9. Liang L et al: Normal structures in the intracranial dural sinuses: delineation with 3D contrast-enhanced magnetization prepared rapid acquisition gradient-echo imaging sequence. AJNR Am J Neuroradiol. 23(10):1739-46, 2002
10. Casey SO et al: Prevalence of arachnoid granulations as detected with CT venography of the dural sinuses. AJNR Am J Neuroradiol. 18(5):993-4, 1997
11. Leach JL et al: Normal appearance of arachnoid granulations on contrast-enhanced CT and MR of the brain: differentiation from dural sinus disease. AJNR Am J Neuroradiol. 17(8):1523-32, 1996
12. Roche J et al: Arachnoid granulations in the transverse and sigmoid sinuses: CT, MR, and MR angiographic appearance of a normal anatomic variation. AJNR Am J Neuroradiol. 17(4):677-83, 1996

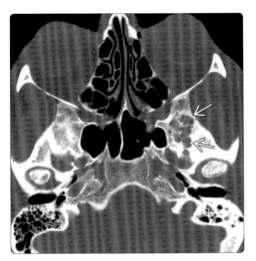

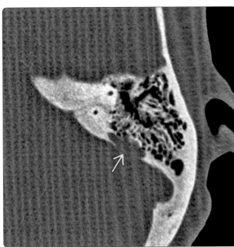

(Left) *Axial bone CT through the midsphenoid sinus shows multiple ovoid bony defects in the greater wing of sphenoid bone* ➡ *representing aberrant AGs (AbAGs) (arachnoid pits). These AGs may enlarge from CSF pulsations.* **(Right)** *Axial left ear temporal bone CT reveals an example of incidental AbAG* ➡ *in posteromedial tegmen mastoideum. No CSF in the mastoid is present.*

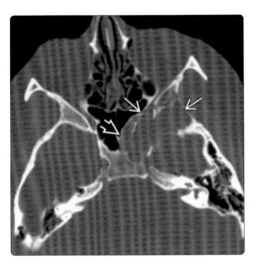

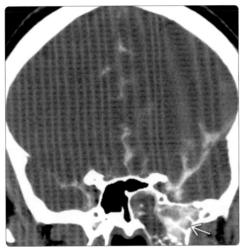

(Left) *Axial bone CT reveals a multilocular lesion in the left greater wing of the sphenoid* ➡ *and basisphenoid* ➡. *The most likely etiology of this lesion is CSF pulsations enlarging AbAGs.* **(Right)** *Coronal CT cisternography in the same patient reveals contrast leaking* ➡ *from the subarachnoid space into the giant AbAGs.*

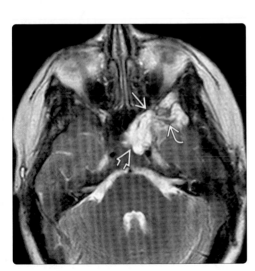

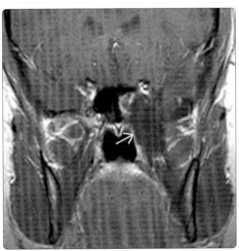

(Left) *Axial T2WI MR in the same patient demonstrates CSF signal within the greater wing of the sphenoid bone* ➡ *and basisphenoid* ➡. *Arachnoid outpouching with arachnoid stranding* ➡ *can be seen within the giant AbAGs.* **(Right)** *Coronal T1WI C+ MR in the same patient shows fluid within the expanded pterygoid wing of sphenoid* ➡. *This represents CSF within an arachnoid pouch filling giant AbAGs.*

Skull Base Dural Sinus Thrombosis

TERMINOLOGY

- Abbreviation: Dural sinus thrombosis (DST)

IMAGING

- MR with MRV is best single imaging exam for DST
- CT findings
  - ↑ **density** thrombus in affected dural sinus
  - Conforms to shape of sinus; fusiform enlargement acutely
  - CECT → enhancing dura surrounding less dense thrombus
- MR findings
  - ↓ **signal** (blooming) on **T2*** sequences in thrombus
  - Restricted diffusion in parenchymal venous infarction in temporal/occipital lobes or cerebellum
  - Parenchymal hemorrhage more common than arterial infarct

TOP DIFFERENTIAL DIAGNOSES

- Arachnoid granulation
- Physiologic sinus flow asymmetry
- Dural sinus hypoplasia-aplasia
- Subdural hematoma

PATHOLOGY

- Wide variety of causes (> 100 identified)
  - Otomastoiditis most common
  - Pregnancy & oral contraceptives
  - Trauma (temporal bone fracture)
  - Metabolic (dehydration, thyrotoxicosis, cirrhosis)

CLINICAL ISSUES

- Headache most common symptom (70-90%)
- Young female most common (autoimmune, oral contraceptives)
- ≤ **50%** of DSTs progress to venous **infarction**

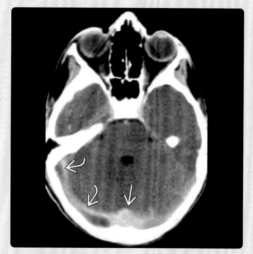
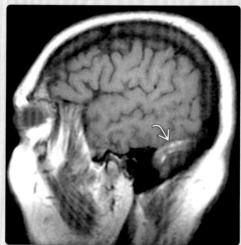

(Left) *Axial CECT shows sinus thrombosis secondary to oral contraceptive use. A tubular filling defect ➡ represents thrombus in the right transverse sinus with enhancement of the anterior dura of the sinus. The torcular enhances normally ➡. (Right) Sagittal T1WI MR demonstrates heterogeneous signal representing acute & subacute blood products within the transverse sinus clot extending into the sigmoid sinus ➡. No evidence of temporal lobe infarction is seen.*

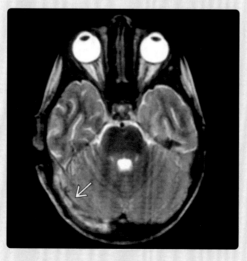
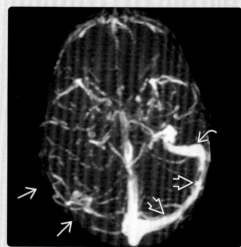

(Left) *Axial T2WI MR shows heterogeneous but largely high signal ➡ representing thrombus in the right transverse & sigmoid sinuses. No abnormal signal is identified in the right cerebellar hemisphere that would suggest venous infarction. (Right) Axial MRV in the same patient confirms the absence of flow-related signal in the thrombosed portions of the right transverse and sigmoid sinuses ➡ and confirms the patency of other dural sinuses and contralateral transverse ➡ and sigmoid ➡ sinuses.*

TERMINOLOGY

Abbreviations

- Dural sinus thrombosis (DST)

Synonyms

- Cerebral venous sinus thrombosis, sinovenous thrombosis

Definitions

- In situ thrombosis of posterior fossa dural venous sinus due to variety of causes

IMAGING

General Features

- Best diagnostic clue
  - Increased density (CT) or abnormal signal intensity (MR) in affected dural sinus of posterior fossa
- Location
  - Thrombophlebitis most commonly starts at transverse-sigmoid confluence
  - DST may involve ≥ 1 of following posterior fossa sinuses: Torcular Herophili, transverse sinus (TS) ± vein of Labbé, sigmoid sinus (SS), jugular bulb
- Size
  - In acute thrombosis, affected sinus may be enlarged
    - **Caveat**: Transverse sinus size typically asymmetric from side to side in individual
- Morphology
  - Conforms to shape of dural sinus affected
    - Fusiform enlargement of venous structure acutely
    - Important for distinguishing DST from arachnoid granulation (focal filling defect)

CT Findings

- NECT
  - ↑ **density** thrombus in affected dural sinus
  - Dense triangle of thrombus, **δ** sign, if sinus seen in cross section
    - Phrase used mainly to describe sagittal sinus thrombosis
    - Sagittal CT reconstruction of TS or coronal reconstruction of SS could show **δ** sign
  - Parenchymal venous infarction may be associated (~ 1/3 of cases)
    - Parenchymal hypodensity (edema ± infarction)
      - ☐ Temporal or occipital lobe location with TS thrombosis
      - ☐ Cerebellar hemisphere location with distal TS & SS thrombosis
      - ☐ Cortical/subcortical hemorrhages (may be petechial)
- CECT
  - Reverse or empty **δ** sign, enhancing dural leaves surrounding less dense thrombus (25% of cases)
  - **Filling defect** in TS ± SS; may extend into jugular bulb or vein
  - Shaggy, dilated, irregular cortical veins (collateral channels)
  - CECT alone unreliable for diagnosis of DST extent (high-density clot may appear like patent enhancing sinus)
- CTA
  - When performed per arterial protocol, enhancement phase too early to evaluate venous sinuses
  - Hyperdense sinus could potentially be confused with venous contrast
- CTV
  - 10-15 second delay beyond CTA image acquisition allowing venous timing for CT venogram
  - Filling defect in dural venous sinus with surrounding dural enhancement

MR Findings

- T1WI
  - Acute DST: Absent flow void with isointense clot (similar to gray matter)
  - **Subacute DST: Hyperintense clot** (methemoglobin)
  - Chronic DST: Isointense clot
- T2WI
  - Acute DST: Hypointense clot (deoxyhemoglobin)
  - **Subacute DST: Hyperintense clot**
  - Chronic DST: Hyperintense clot
  - Additional findings if parenchymal infarction present
    - Gyral swelling, sulcal effacement in temporal lobe
- T2* GRE
  - Profound hypointense signal or **blooming** on T2* sequences with acute or subacute thrombosis
    - May be difficult to discern against bone, air (in adjacent temporal bone)
  - Parenchymal hemorrhage in venous infarct ↓ signal in acute stage
- DWI
  - Acute & subacute clot may demonstrate restricted diffusion
  - Acute parenchymal venous infarct shows restricted diffusion
    - Parenchymal DWI abnormalities are more likely reversible compared to arterial ischemic insults
- T1WI C+
  - Filling defect may nearly completely fill dural sinuses
  - **Peripheral enhancement** may be reactive dura or residual flow around clot
  - Chronic DST may enhance intensely & should be correlated with MRV findings
    - Irregular enhancing venous channels may be seen with incomplete recanalization; enhancement within recanalized clot may mimic normal sinus enhancement
  - Associated parenchymal venous infarction may show patchy enhancement
- MRV
  - Lack of flow-related signal in TS-SS, ± jugular bulb

Angiographic Findings

- Late venous phase images critical
  - Complete lack of flow in affected dural sinuses
  - Central filling defect with surrounding contrast

Imaging Recommendations

- Best imaging tool
  - MR with MRV is best single imaging exam for DST
    - Almost all MR sequences show signal abnormality in dural sinuses

     – Complications (venous infarct, hemorrhage) easily identified

     – Susceptibility weighted imaging (SWI) may prove to be useful technique

- Protocol advice
  - Coronal & sagittal CTV reconstructions ± MRV sequences very helpful for TS & SS thrombosis evaluation
  - Contrast-enhanced MRV decreases false-positive DST in small but patent dural sinus
  - Use MRV with multiple encoding gradients to distinguish physiological flow asymmetry from thrombus

DIFFERENTIAL DIAGNOSIS

Arachnoid Granulation

- Focal ovoid filling defect extending into TS-SS
- CSF density (CT) & intensity (MR)

Physiologic Sinus Flow Asymmetry

- Slow or asymmetric flow creates MR variable signal

Normal Dural Sinus

- Flowing blood in normal, asymmetric dural sinus
- Slightly more dense than brain on NECT

Dural Sinus Hypoplasia-Aplasia

- 33% of normal individuals have unilateral hypoplastic TS
- Congenitally small TS may show no flow or enhancement on MRV
- Sagittal T1 shows no TS structure along posterior tentorium

Subdural Hematoma

- Subdural blood adjacent to TS-SS mimics clot within dural sinus; false reverse (empty) δ sign

PATHOLOGY

General Features

- Etiology
  - Most common cause: **Otomastoiditis ± subdural empyema → dural sinus thrombophlebitis**
    - Wide variety of causes (> 100 identified)
      - ☐ Pregnancy, oral contraceptives
      - ☐ Trauma (temporal, occipital bone fracture adjacent to sinus); variable rate of DST depending on sinus involved
      - ☐ Metabolic (dehydration, thyrotoxicosis, cirrhosis)
      - ☐ Hematologic (coagulopathy)
- Associated abnormalities
  - DST with arterial infarctions in patients with Behçet disease

CLINICAL ISSUES

Presentation

- Most common signs/symptoms
  - Headache (70-90%)
  - May be confused clinically with idiopathic intracranial hypertension (pseudotumor cerebri)
    - No diagnosis of **pseudotumor cerebri** should be made without venous evaluation
- Other signs/symptoms
  - Nausea, vomiting, & papilledema

  - Neurologic deficits & seizures
- Clinical profile
  - Young woman with sudden onset of unrelenting headache & ear infection or history of oral contraceptive use

Demographics

- Age
  - May be seen at any age
  - Young female most common (autoimmune, oral contraceptives)
- Gender
  - F > M
- Epidemiology
  - **1% of acute stokes** arise from **DST**

Natural History & Prognosis

- **≤ 50% of DSTs** progress to venous **infarction**
  - Extension to straight sinus or vein of Labbé dramatically increases complication risk
    - Temporal lobe infarction ± parenchymal hemorrhage

Treatment

- Anticoagulation (heparin) is mainstay of therapy
- Endovascular thrombolysis may be utilized for subacute or chronic thrombosis or if lack of improvement with anticoagulation
- Treat inciting cause of thrombosis

DIAGNOSTIC CHECKLIST

Image Interpretation Pearls

- Use contralateral cortical veins, dural sinuses, or arterial structures for density comparison on NECT
- CECT may be misleading, may mask clot

Reporting Tips

- Identify cause of DST if possible
- Identify which veins are secondarily involved
- Identify complications

SELECTED REFERENCES

1. Bonneville F: Imaging of cerebral venous thrombosis. Diagn Interv Imaging. 95(12):1145-50, 2014
2. Delgado Almandoz JE et al: Prevalence of traumatic dural venous sinus thrombosis in high-risk acute blunt head trauma patients evaluated with multidetector CT venography. Radiology. 255(2):570-7, 2010
3. Leach JL et al: Partially recanalized chronic dural sinus thrombosis: findings on MR imaging, time-of-flight MR venography, and contrast-enhanced MR venography. AJNR Am J Neuroradiol. 28(4):782-9, 2007
4. Leach JL et al: Imaging of cerebral venous thrombosis: current techniques, spectrum of findings, and diagnostic pitfalls. Radiographics. 26 Suppl 1:S19-41; discussion S42-3, 2006
5. Rodallec MH et al: Cerebral venous thrombosis and multidetector CT angiography: tips and tricks. Radiographics. 26 Suppl 1:S5-18; discussion S42-3, 2006
6. Khandelwal S et al: Distinguishing dural sinus thrombosis from benign intracranial hypertension. Emerg Med J. 21(2):245-7, 2004
7. Canhão P et al: Thrombolytics for cerebral sinus thrombosis: a systematic review. Cerebrovasc Dis. 15(3):159-66, 2003
8. Liang L et al: Evaluation of the intracranial dural sinuses with a 3D contrast-enhanced MP-RAGE sequence: prospective comparison with 2D-TOF MR venography and digital subtraction angiography. AJNR Am J Neuroradiol. 22(3):481-92, 2001
9. Provenzale JM et al: Dural sinus thrombosis: findings on CT and MR imaging and diagnostic pitfalls. AJR Am J Roentgenol. 170(3):777-83, 1998

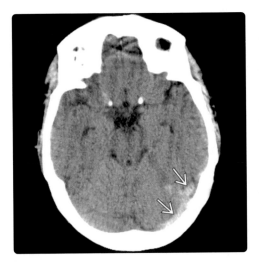

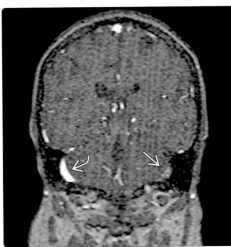

(Left) Axial NECT demonstrates high-attenuation thrombus ➡ in the left transverse sinus. In a case like this, differentiation from subdural hematoma may be difficult. MR imaging or CECT could be helpful for making that distinction. (Right) Coronal MRV source image shows high signal from normal blood flow in the right sigmoid sinus ➡. Absence of flow-related signal in the contralateral sinus ➡ has resulted from dural sinus thrombosis.

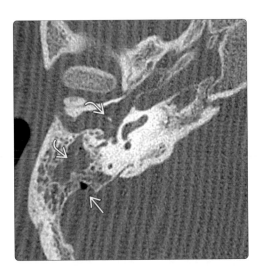

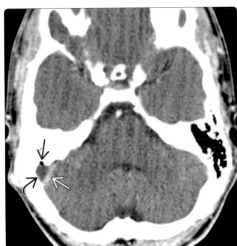

(Left) Axial bone CT in a patient with acute coalescent otomastoiditis ➡ shows thinning of the sigmoid plate and a small focus of air in the expected location of the sigmoid sinus ➡. (Right) Postcontrast head CT in the same patient depicts only compressed sigmoid sinus ➡. Intracranial air ➡ is again noted adjacent to a hypodense epidural abscess ➡ lateral to the compressed sigmoid sinus.

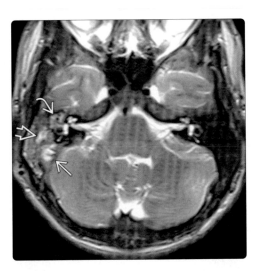

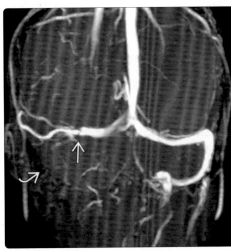

(Left) Axial T2WI MR (same patient) shows inflammatory material in the right mastoid ➡ and middle ear ➡, as well as a high-signal epidural abscess and compressed &/or thrombosed sigmoid sinus ➡. Note the normal appearance of the right temporal lobe and cerebellum. (Right) Anteroposterior MRV (MIP) in the same patient demonstrates abrupt occlusion ➡ of the right transverse sinus and lack of flow-related signal in the right sigmoid sinus ➡ and jugular bulb/vein.

TERMINOLOGY

- Cavernous sinus thrombosis/thrombophlebitis (CST)
- CST: Blood clot in CS ± infection/thrombophlebitis

IMAGING

- Relevant anatomy
  - CS = trabeculated venous cavities
  - Receive blood from multiple valveless veins
  - Blood flows in any direction (depending on pressure gradient)
- CECT or MR
  - CT findings often subtle or negative in CST
  - Enlarged CS with convex margins
  - Filling defects in cavernous sinus
  - Enlarged superior ophthalmic vein ± clot, proptosis
  - Enlarged extraocular muscles
  - Intracavernous carotid artery: Rarely stenosis, thrombosis, or pseudoaneurysm formation

TOP DIFFERENTIAL DIAGNOSES

- Cavernous sinus neoplasm
  - Meningioma, lymphoma, metastasis
- Cavernous carotid aneurysm, fistula
- Infection/inflammation
  - Idiopathic inflammatory orbital pseudotumor, sarcoidosis, Wegener granulomatosis

PATHOLOGY

- Often complication of sinusitis/midface infection
  - *Staphylococcus aureus* most common pathogen

CLINICAL ISSUES

- Headache most common early symptom
- Orbital pain, ophthalmoplegia, visual loss

DIAGNOSTIC CHECKLIST

- Clinical setting + high index of suspicion
- Negative CT → MR/MRV or CTA

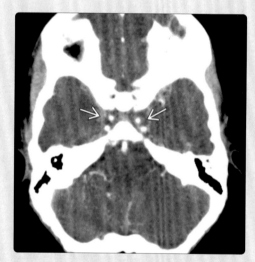
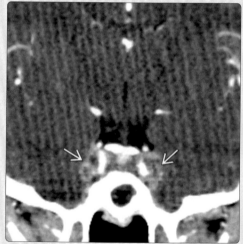

(Left) *Axial CECT of the head in a child with extensive sinusitis (not shown), demonstrates near-complete lack of cavernous sinus enhancement* ➡️. **(Right)** *Coronal CECT shows classic laterally convex margins of the heterogeneously enhancing cavernous sinuses* ➡️.

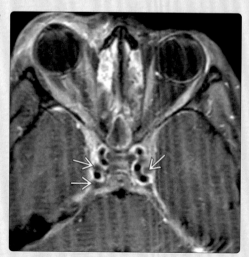
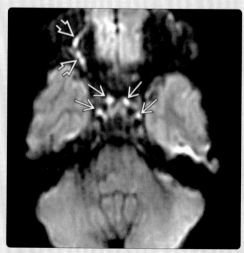

(Left) *Axial T1 C+ FS MR in the same patient demonstrates multiple filling defects in the cavernous sinuses* ➡️*, right preseptal cellulitis, proptosis, lateral rectus muscle enlargement, and extensive sinus disease.* **(Right)** *Axial DWI MR in the same patient shows corresponding hyperintense signal within cavernous sinus clots* ➡️ *and associated right superior ophthalmic vein thrombus* ➡️.

TERMINOLOGY

Abbreviations

- Cavernous sinus thrombosis/thrombophlebitis (CST)

Definitions

- CST: Blood clot in cavernous sinus (CS)
  - ± infection/thrombophlebitis

IMAGING

General Features

- Best diagnostic clue
  - Appropriate clinical setting + high index of suspicion
- Location
  - Relevant anatomy
    - CS = trabeculated venous cavities, not single pool of blood, with multiple venous interconnections
    - Receive blood from multiple valveless veins
      - □ Facial veins via superior ophthalmic vein (SOV) and inferior ophthalmic vein (IOV)
      - □ Sphenoid, deep middle cerebral veins
    - CSs drain into
      - □ Inferior petrosal sinuses → internal jugular veins (IJVs)
      - □ Superior petrosal sinuses → sigmoid sinuses

Imaging Recommendations

- Best imaging tool
  - CTA
    - 1- to 3-mm sections through orbits and CSs
  - MR + contrast, MRA/MRV

CT Findings

- NECT
  - Findings often subtle or negative
- CECT
  - Filling defects in involved CS
    - CS margins convex, not flat/concave
  - Orbits: SOVs ↑ ± clot
    - Proptosis, enlarged extraocular muscles
  - Intracavernous carotid artery: Rarely stenosis, thrombosis, or pseudoaneurysm formation
- CTA/CTV
  - Filling defects in 1 or both CSs

MR Findings

- Enlarged CS with convex lateral margins
- Isointense to gray matter on T1WI, heterogeneous high signal intensity on T2WI
- Variable contrast enhancement, filling defects in CS
- May see hyperintense clot in CS on DWI

DIFFERENTIAL DIAGNOSIS

Cavernous Sinus Neoplasm

- Meningioma, schwannoma
- Metastasis, lymphoma, invasive carcinomas

Cavernous Carotid Aneurysm, Fistula

- Flow voids

Infection/Inflammation

- Idiopathic inflammatory orbital pseudotumor, sarcoidosis, Wegener granulomatosis

PATHOLOGY

General Features

- Etiology
  - Complication of sinusitis or other infection
    - Skin infection, orbital complication of sinusitis, odontogenic disease, or otomastoiditis
  - Other causes
    - Trauma
    - Underlying malignancy

CLINICAL ISSUES

Presentation

- Most common signs/symptoms
  - Headache and fever most common early symptoms
    - Often localized to regions innervated by V1 and V2
  - Orbital pain, periorbital edema, chemosis
  - Proptosis, ophthalmoplegia, visual loss
- Other signs/symptoms
  - Hypoesthesia or hyperesthesia in V1 and V2 dermatomes
  - Decreased pupillary responses
  - Signs/symptoms in contralateral eye diagnostic of CST
  - Meningeal signs
  - Systemic signs indicative of sepsis are late findings

Demographics

- Epidemiology
  - *Staphylococcus aureus* ~ 70% of infections
  - *Streptococcus pneumoniae*, gram-rods, anaerobes
  - Fungi (*Aspergillus*, *Rhizopus*) rare

Natural History & Prognosis

- Without therapy, signs appear in contralateral eye in 24-48 hours
  - Spread via communicating veins to contralateral CS
- Can be fatal (death from sepsis or CNS involvement)
- Incidence/fatality significantly ↓ with early antibiotics
- Complete recovery infrequent
  - Permanent visual impairment (15%)
  - Cranial nerve deficits (50%)

Treatment

- Intravenous antibiotics
- Supportive care, hydration, steroids

DIAGNOSTIC CHECKLIST

Image Interpretation Pearls

- Maintain high clinical suspicion
- Negative CT → MR/MRV or CTA

SELECTED REFERENCES

1. Desa V et al: Cavernous sinus thrombosis: current therapy. J Oral Maxillofac Surg. 70(9):2085-91, 2012
2. Madhusudhan KS et al: Cavernous sinus thrombophlebitis causing reversible narrowing of internal carotid artery. Neurol India. 57(1):102-3, 2009

Dural Arteriovenous Fistula

TERMINOLOGY

- Dural arteriovenous fistula (DAVF)
- Acquired direct shunt between dural artery and dural venous sinus or cortical vein

IMAGING

- Best imaging modality: DSA
- Most common site: Transverse sinus (TS)
- CECT findings in DAVF
  - Tortuous, enhancing dural feeders with enlarged dural sinus
  - Enlarged cortical draining veins → aggressive DAVF
  - ± flow-related aneurysms
- MR findings in DAVF
  - Localized or generalized venous dilatation
  - Focal T2 hyperintensity in adjacent WM (venous congestion)

TOP DIFFERENTIAL DIAGNOSES

- Hypoplastic TS-sigmoid sinus (TS-SS)
- Jugular bulb pseudolesion
- Dural sinus thrombosis
- Pial arteriovenous malformation

CLINICAL ISSUES

- Accounts for 35% of infratentorial vascular malformations
- TS-SS DAVF presents with pulsatile tinnitus
- Usually present in middle-aged, older patients
- Prognosis depends on location, venous drainage pattern

DIAGNOSTIC CHECKLIST

- If patient has objective pulsatile tinnitus and no other vascular lesion on cross-sectional imaging, angiography necessary to completely exclude DAVF
- Single pedicle or small DAVF may not be seen on MR or MRA

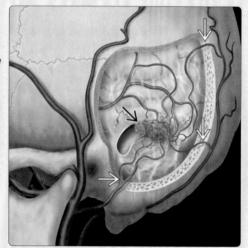
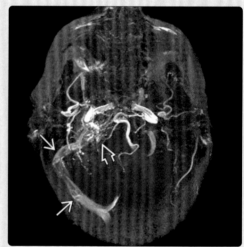

(Left) *Typical dural arteriovenous fistula (DAVF) with short segment of thrombosed transverse sinus (TS) ➾ shows DAVF consisting of multiple dural vessels in wall of thrombosed segment. Multiple dural & transosseous feeders arise from external ➡ (ECA) & internal carotid arteries (ICA).* (Right) *MRA shows extensive prominent vascularity in right skull base ➡ from DAVF. Source images from MRA should be reviewed for correlation with MIP images. Dural sinuses ➡ remain patent in this case. Thrombosis is often seen.*

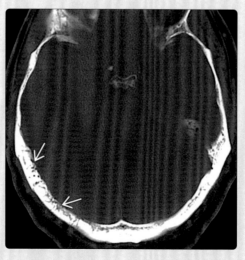
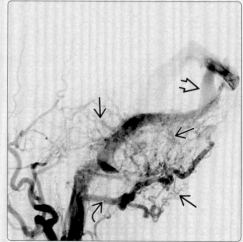

(Left) *Bone CT in a patient with DAVF shows innumerable enlarged transcalvarial vascular channels ➡. These particularly numerous vascular markings are usually noted, but less impressive findings may go overlooked. Clinical suspicion may be helpful information.* (Right) *Selective right ECA angiogram shows a large occipital artery ➾ and auricular artery with prominent transosseous perforating vessels ➡. Venous reflux into a large right TS ➾ is present.*

Dural Arteriovenous Fistula

TERMINOLOGY

Abbreviations
- Dural arteriovenous fistula (DAVF)

Synonyms
- Dural arteriovenous (AV) shunt, dural fistula

Definitions
- Abnormal acquired direct shunt between dural artery and dural venous sinus or cortical vein
  - Heterogeneous group of lesions with common angioarchitecture (AV shunts within dura)
  - Distinct from true AV malformation because most DAVFs are acquired
    - Exception is vein of Galen malformation

IMAGING

General Features
- Best diagnostic clue
  - Network of tiny vessels in wall of thrombosed dural venous sinus
- Location
  - Skull base dural venous sinuses
    - Most common site → transverse sinus (TS)
    - 2nd most common site → cavernous sinus (CS)
- Size
  - Variable size, but actual shunt nidus usually < 2 cm
- Morphology
  - Innumerable serpiginous AV shunts in wall of dural sinus

CT Findings
- NECT
  - Usually normal in cases presenting without hemorrhage
  - Subarachnoid, subdural, or parenchymal hemorrhage may be seen in cases presenting acutely with hemorrhage
    - Parenchymal hemorrhage not in typical location for hypertensive bleed
- CECT
  - If small, CECT normal
  - Larger DAVFs show tortuous dural feeders with enlarged dural sinus ± flow-related aneurysms
  - Dilated vessels in proximity to parenchymal hemorrhage (if present)
  - Enlarged, tortuous cortical draining veins
- Bone CT
  - Transosseous collateral channels may be seen in area of occipitomastoid suture

MR Findings
- T1WI
  - May be normal
  - Isointense thrombosed dural sinus ± flow voids
- T2WI
  - Isointense thrombosed sinus ± flow voids
  - Localized or generalized venous dilatation
  - Focal T2 hyperintensity in adjacent white matter (WM) (venous congestion)
- T2* GRE
  - Usually normal in uncomplicated DAVF
  - May show parenchymal hemorrhage in DAVF with cortical venous drainage
  - Thrombosed dural sinus will bloom
- DWI
  - Normal unless venous infarct or ischemia present
- T1WI C+
  - Chronically thrombosed sinus enhances intensely
  - Rare: Diffuse dural enhancement
- MRA
  - Time-resolved contrast-enhanced MRA useful for depiction of angioarchitecture and dynamics
  - TOF MRA positive in larger DAVF
- MRV
  - Occluded involved sinus, collateral flow
  - 3D-phase contrast MRA with low-velocity encoding can identify fistula, feeding arteries, flow reversal in draining veins

Angiographic Findings
- Conventional
  - Most common site = wall of TS or sigmoid sinus (SS) (35-40%)
    - Multiple arterial feeders are typical with dural/transosseous branches from external carotid artery, most commonly followed by internal carotid artery and vertebral artery tentorial/dural branches
    - Arterial inflow into parallel venous channel ("recipient pouch") common
    - Involved dural sinus often thrombosed
    - Flow reversal in dural sinus/cortical veins correlates with ↑ symptoms, hemorrhage risk
    - Tortuous engorged pial veins with venous congestion/hypertension (clinically aggressive)
    - High flow may result in high-flow vasculopathy with progressive stenoses, outlet occlusion, bizarre vascular appearance

Imaging Recommendations
- Best imaging tool
  - DSA with superselective catheterization of involved dural supply

DIFFERENTIAL DIAGNOSIS

Dural Sinus Hypoplasia-Aplasia
- Congenitally small TS-SS may have low flow on MRV, no enhancement on T1 C+ MR
- Sagittal T1WI shows no or very small sinus in normal anatomic location
- No signal abnormalities on T2, FLAIR, or GRE

Sigmoid Sinus-Jugular Bulb Pseudolesion
- Slow or asymmetric flow creates variable signal on MR sequences
- Use MRV to clarify

Thrombosed Dural Sinus
- Collateral/congested venous drainage can mimic DAVF
- Can be spontaneous, traumatic, infectious (thrombophlebitis)

Pial Arteriovenous Malformation
- Congenital lesion with intraaxial nidus

- Pial arterial supply with possible parasitization of dural supply

PATHOLOGY

General Features

- Etiology
  - Adult DAVFs are usually **acquired**, not congenital
    - May be idiopathic
    - Can occur in response to **trauma**, **craniotomy**, **venous occlusion**, or **venous hypertension**
- Associated abnormalities
  - Cortical drainage may lead to edema, encephalopathy, hemorrhage

Staging, Grading, & Classification

- **Cognard classification** of intracranial DAVFs correlates venous drainage pattern with clinical course
  - Type I: Located in sinus wall; normal antegrade venous drainage; benign clinical course
  - Type IIA: Located in main dural sinus; reflux into sinus but not cortical veins
  - Type IIB: Reflux (retrograde drainage) into cortical veins; 10-20% hemorrhage
  - Type III: Direct cortical drainage; no venous ectasia; 40% hemorrhage
  - Type IV: Direct cortical drainage; venous ectasia; 65% hemorrhage
  - Type V: Spinal perimedullary venous drainage; progressive myelopathy

CLINICAL ISSUES

Presentation

- Most common signs/symptoms
  - 2 major modes of presentation
    - Hemorrhage (parenchymal, subarachnoid, or subdural)
    - Venous hypertension/congestion (pulsatile tinnitus, dementia, seizures, encephalopathy)
  - Symptoms vary with site, type of shunt
    - TS-SS → pulsatile tinnitus
    - CS → pulsatile exophthalmos, chemosis, retroorbital pain
    - Brainstem DAVF → quadriparesis, lower cranial nerve palsies
- Clinical profile
  - Middle-aged patient with pulse-synchronous tinnitus

Demographics

- Age
  - DAVFs usually present in middle-aged or older patients
- Epidemiology
  - Rare, acquired lesions
  - Account for 6% of supratentorial and 35% of infratentorial vascular malformations
  - Account for 10-15% of all cerebrovascular malformations with AV shunting

Natural History & Prognosis

- Prognosis, clinical course depends on location, venous drainage pattern

- 98% of DAVFs without retrograde venous drainage have benign course
  - DAVFs draining into major dural sinus usually follow benign clinical course
  - DAVFs with retrograde cortical venous drainage have aggressive clinical course
- Overall risk of hemorrhage from DAVF = 2% per year (depends on location and hemodynamics)
- Spontaneous closure rare
- Acute deterioration has been reported after lumbar puncture

Treatment

- Observation in selected cases
- Treatment options if hemorrhage risk exists
  - Endovascular → embolization
  - Surgical resection → skeletonization of involved sinus
  - Stereotactic radiosurgery
- Recurrences common

DIAGNOSTIC CHECKLIST

Consider

- DAVFs are rare but treatable, so consider in patient with hemorrhage in atypical location for hypertensive bleed and no other cause
- If patient has objective pulsatile tinnitus and no other vascular lesion on cross-sectional imaging, DSA necessary to completely exclude DAVF

Image Interpretation Pearls

- Single pedicle or small DAVF may not be seen on MR or MRA
- Venous collateral flow in dural sinus thrombosis can become very prominent and mimic DAVF

Reporting Tips

- Evaluate both internal/external carotid and vertebral arteries when performing angiography in patient with spontaneous intracranial hemorrhage
- Identification of associated venous varix is important, as this finding signals ↑ risk of hemorrhage

SELECTED REFERENCES

1. Josephson CB et al: Computed tomography angiography or magnetic resonance angiography for detection of intracranial vascular malformations in patients with intracerebral haemorrhage. Cochrane Database Syst Rev. 9:CD009372, 2014
2. Kobayashi A et al: Prognosis and treatment of intracranial dural arteriovenous fistulae: a systematic review and meta-analysis. Int J Stroke. 9(6):670-7, 2014
3. Lin N et al: Non-galenic arteriovenous fistulas in adults: transarterial embolization and literature review. J Neurointerv Surg. 7(11):835-40, 2014
4. Morales H et al: Documented development of a dural arteriovenous fistula in an infant subsequent to sinus thrombosis: case report and review of the literature. Neuroradiology. 52(3):225-9, 2010
5. Noguchi K et al: Intracranial dural arteriovenous fistulas: evaluation with combined 3D time-of-flight MR angiography and MR digital subtraction angiography. AJR Am J Roentgenol. 182(1):183-90, 2004
6. Kai Y et al: Pre- and post-treatment MR imaging and single photon emission CT in patients with dural arteriovenous fistulas and retrograde leptomeningeal venous drainage. AJNR Am J Neuroradiol. 24(4):619-25, 2003
7. Rucker JC et al: Diffuse dural enhancement in cavernous sinus dural arteriovenous fistula. Neuroradiology. 45(2):88-9, 2003
8. van Dijk JM et al: Venous congestive encephalopathy related to cranial dural arteriovenous fistulas. Neuroimaging Clin N Am. 13(1):55-72, 2003

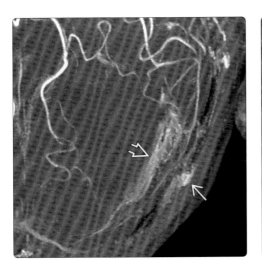

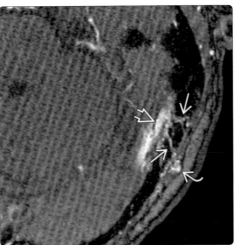

(Left) *Axial MRA MIP reveals irregular flow-related enhancement in partially recanalized TS* ➡ *with compact transosseous* ➡ *DAVF arterial supply.* (Right) *Axial MRA source image in the same patient demonstrates numerous transosseous collateral vessels as linear areas of flow-related signal in temporal bone* ➡. *Note enlarged distal occipital artery* ➡ *and partially recanalized TS* ➡.

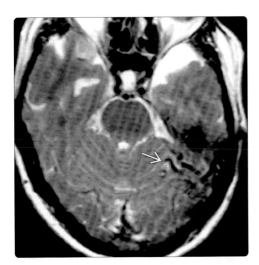

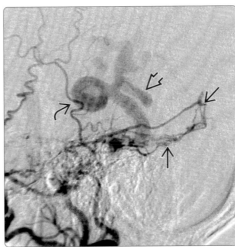

(Left) *Axial T2WI MR in patient with DAVF shows enlargement of multiple prominent cerebellar veins* ➡. *Lesions with enlarged cortical veins have an increased incidence of intracranial hemorrhage. White matter edema from venous congestion may also be evident.* (Right) *Lateral ECA angiography in the same patient shows enlarged dural feeders* ➡ *to DAVF. Deep cortical venous drainage is well seen* ➡, *and venous varix is displayed* ➡. *Tentorial DAVFs may have particularly complex anatomy.*

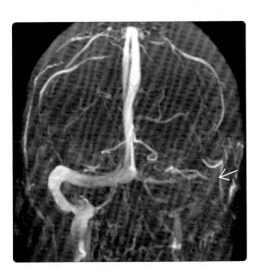

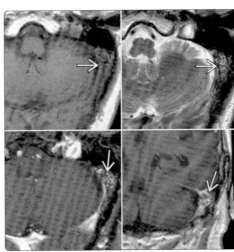

(Left) *AP MRV reveals that the left TS and sigmoid sinus (SS) are smaller than the right with distal TS occlusion* ➡. *The distal TS-proximal SS confluence is the most common site for DAVFs of posterior skull base.* (Right) *Composite MR shows atypical DAVF with innumerable small flow voids* ➡ *in the thrombosed segment of TS-SS junction. MRA may show flow-related enhancement of vessels, but angiography is often necessary to confirm.*

KEY FACTS

TERMINOLOGY

- Basal cephalocele = congenital extracranial herniation of meninges, CSF, ± brain tissue through mesodermal defect in sphenoid, ethmoid, or basiocciput

IMAGING

- Nasopharyngeal
  - Transethmoid: Defect in cribriform plate
  - Sphenoethmoid: Bony defect junction of cribriform plate and planum sphenoidale
  - Sphenonasopharyngeal = transsphenoid: Defect in body of sphenoid bone
    - Most common
  - Basioccipital-nasopharyngeal (transbasioccipital): Bony defect parallel & inferior to sphenooccipital synchondrosis
    - Area of median basal canal
- Sphenoorbital
- Sphenomaxillary

Best imaging tool

- Best imaging tool
  - MR best identifies meninges, CSF, brain, pituitary, and optic nerves/chiasm position
  - Bone CT defines osseous defects prior to surgery

TOP DIFFERENTIAL DIAGNOSES

- Nasal glioma
- Nasal dermal sinus
- Teratoma

CLINICAL ISSUES

- Most common signs/symptoms
  - May be clinically occult
  - Hypertelorism, nasal mass, nasal stuffiness, endocrine dysfunction
  - Recurrent meningitis
- Combined surgical procedure may involve neurosurgery, otolaryngology, &/or plastic surgery

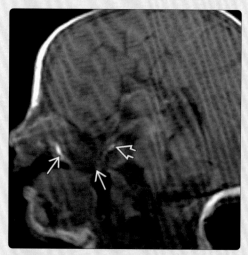
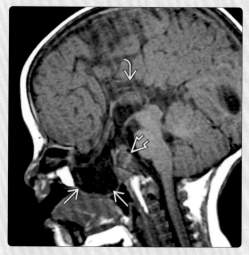

(Left) Sagittal T1WI MR in a 3-day-old boy with a nasal mass shows CSF signal intensity transsphenoidal meningocele ➡ protruding into the nasopharynx via a skull base defect in the floor of the sella. Notice posterior pituitary hyperintensity in the dorsal aspect of the sella ➡. (Right) Sagittal T1WI MR in the same child at 9 months of age demonstrates increase in size of the cephalocele ➡, a defect anterior to the sphenooccipital synchondrosis ➡, and associated callosal agenesis ➡.

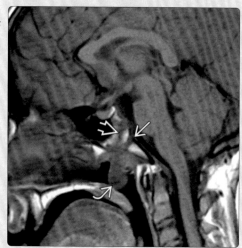
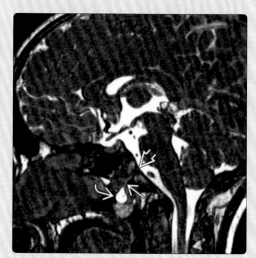

(Left) Sagittal T1 MR in a 13 year old with meningitis shows a median basilar canal ➡ inferior to residual sphenooccipital synchondrosis ➡ and an associated nasopharyngeal mass ➡. (Right) Sagittal FIESTA in the same child shows the nasopharyngeal mass to be mixed signal intensity with a hyperintense linear tract ➡ extending from the median basilar canal ➡ to the cystic-appearing portion of the nasopharyngeal mass ➡. Histologically the mass was thought to be infarcted Thornwaldt cyst.

TERMINOLOGY

Synonyms

- Basal cephaloceles
- "Occult" cephaloceles

Definitions

- Basal cephalocele = congenital extracranial herniation of **meninges, CSF ± brain tissue** through mesodermal defect in **sphenoid, ethmoid,** or **basiocciput**
  - Nasopharyngeal
    - Transethmoid
    - Sphenoethmoid
    - Sphenonasopharyngeal = transsphenoid (large craniopharyngeal canal)
    - Basioccipital-nasopharyngeal (transbasioccipital)
  - Sphenoorbital
  - Sphenomaxillary

IMAGING

General Features

- Best diagnostic clue
  - Midline inferior herniation of CSF ± brain or pituitary gland into nasopharynx through defect in skull base
- Location
  - **Nasopharyngeal**
    - Transethmoid: Bone defect in cribriform plate
    - Sphenoethmoid: Bony defect at junction of cribriform plate & planum sphenoidale
    - Sphenonasopharyngeal = transsphenoid = craniopharyngeal canal
      □ Bony defect in midline body of sphenoid bone
    - Basioccipital-nasopharyngeal (transbasioccipital)
      □ Bony defect parallel and 1.0-1.5 cm inferior to sphenooccipital synchondrosis
      □ In area of persistent median basal canal
      □ May simulate patent sphenooccipital synchondrosis
      □ Communicates with prepontine cistern
  - **Sphenoorbital**
    - Posterior orbital cephaloceles communicate with **middle cranial fossa** through optic foramen, superior orbital fissure, or orbital wall defect
  - **Sphenomaxillary**
    - Extend through **superior orbital fissure** into posterior orbit ± extension through inferior orbital fissure and pterygopalatine fossa
- Size
  - Variable
- Morphology
  - Well circumscribed, round or ovoid

Imaging Recommendations

- Best imaging tool
  - MR best identifies meninges, CSF, brain, pituitary, and optic nerves/chiasm position
  - Bone CT complimentary to define osseous defects prior to surgery
- Protocol advice
  - Thin (3 mm) multiplanar T1 & T2 MR
  - CT with multiplanar reformations for surgical planning

CT Findings

- NECT
  - Variable attenuation mass protruding into nasopharynx (or orbit)
    - Most commonly CSF attenuation
- Bone CT
  - Depicts osseous defect in skull base

MR Findings

- Mass with variable signal intensity protruding into nasopharynx, oropharynx, or orbit
  - Depends on content of cephalocele: CSF, meninges, brain
  - Pituitary gland variable location within cephalocele
    - Frequently lines posterior wall of cephalocele
- No abnormal enhancement
  - Presence of enhancement may suggest infection/inflammation

DIFFERENTIAL DIAGNOSIS

Nasal Glioma

- Well-defined soft tissue mass
- No intracranial extension

Nasal Dermal Sinus

- nasal dorsum skin pit ± cyst tip of nose to foramen cecum
- ± bifid crista galli

Teratoma

- Oropharyngeal location
- Mixed cystic/solid mass with soft tissue, fat, & calcium

PATHOLOGY

General Features

- Etiology
  - Majority **congenital**, rarely posttraumatic/postsurgical
    - Osseous defect secondary to faulty separation of neurectoderm from surface ectoderm during neural tube formation
      □ Prevents mesodermal tissue, which should form bone, from interposing between 2 germ layers
- Genetics
  - Sporadic
  - No well-defined genetic link
- Associated abnormalities
  - Callosal dysgenesis
  - Eye abnormalities: Optic pits or posterior coloboma
  - Midline facial clefts: Lip, nose, palate
  - Rare reports
    - Internal carotid artery (ICA) dysgenesis
    - Epignathus teratoma
    - Hypothalamic hamartoma
    - Thornwaldt cyst & enterogenous cyst reported with median canalis basilaris

Staging, Grading, & Classification

- Cephaloceles classified **by contents** of sac
  - Meningocele: Leptomeninges & CSF
  - Meningoencephalocele (encephalocele): Leptomeninges, CSF, & brain

- ○ Atretic cephalocele is forme fruste of cephaloceles, i.e., small, noncystic, flat nodules in scalp
  - – Parietal are near vertex, occipital are cephalic to external occipital protuberance
- Cephaloceles classified **by site** of osseous defect
  - ○ Calvarium
    - – Occipitocervical, occipital, parietal, lateral, interfrontal, temporal
  - ○ Skull base
    - – Frontoethmoidal = sincipital
      - □ Nasofrontal, nasoethmoidal, and nasoorbital
    - – Basal cephaloceles
      - □ Nasopharyngeal: Transethmoid, sphenoethmoid, sphenonasopharyngeal (transsphenoid or craniopharyngeal canal), basioccipital-nasopharyngeal (transbasioccipital)
      - □ Sphenoorbital
      - □ Sphenomaxillary
- Craniopharyngeal canal classification
  - ○ Type 1: Small, incidental canal
  - ○ Type 2: Medium-sized canals + ectopic pituitary tissue
  - ○ Type 3: Large canals containing cephaloceles &/or tumors
    - – 3A: Contain cephaloceles
    - – 3B: Contain tumors
    - – 3C: Contain cephaloceles & tumors

Gross Pathologic & Surgical Features

- Well-defined, meningeal-lined mass containing CSF ± brain tissue

Microscopic Features

- Meningoceles: Leptomeninges & CSF
- Meningoencephaloceles: Leptomeninges, CSF, & brain
- Atretic cephaloceles: Dura, fibrous tissue, & degenerated brain tissue

CLINICAL ISSUES

Presentation

- Most common signs/symptoms
  - ○ May be clinically **occult**
  - ○ Hypertelorism
  - ○ Nasal mass & nasal stuffiness
  - ○ Endocrine dysfunction
- Other signs/symptoms
  - ○ **Recurrent meningitis**
    - – Highest incidence in patients with basioccipital-nasopharyngeal cephalocele
  - ○ Developmental delay primarily related to associated malformations

Demographics

- Age
  - ○ Congenital lesion
    - – May be recognized on prenatal US/MR or present after birth

Natural History & Prognosis

- Present at birth
  - ○ May not be diagnosed at birth due to occult location
- May increase in size rapidly if CSF-filled

- Prognosis depends in part on associated abnormalities

Treatment

- Combined surgical procedure may involve neurosurgery, otolaryngology, &/or plastic surgery
- Continued increase in success with endoscopic repair

DIAGNOSTIC CHECKLIST

Consider

- Look for cephalocele in patients with recurrent meningitis history
- High-resolution sagittal & coronal T1 & T2 images
  - ○ Optimal evaluation of contents of mass and contiguity with intracranial space
- Bone CT with multiplanar reformations defines osseous defect prior to surgical repair

Reporting Tips

- Identify lesion contents and osseous defect prior to surgical repair
- Recognize associated intracranial and craniofacial abnormalities

SELECTED REFERENCES

1. Keshri AK et al: Transnasal endoscopic repair of pediatric meningoencephalocele. J Pediatr Neurosci. 11(1):42-5, 2016
2. Abele TA et al: Craniopharyngeal canal and its spectrum of pathology. AJNR Am J Neuroradiol. 35(4):772-7, 2014
3. Morabito R et al: Pharyngeal enterogenous cyst associated with canalis basilaris medianus in a newborn. Pediatr Radiol. 43(4):512-5, 2013
4. Lohman BD et al: Not the typical Tornwaldt's cyst this time? A nasopharyngeal cyst associated with canalis basilaris medianus. Br J Radiol. 84(1005):e169-71, 2011
5. Borges A: Imaging of the central skull base. Neuroimaging Clin N Am. 19(4):669-96, 2009
6. Castelnuovo P et al: Endoscopic endonasal management of encephaloceles in children: an eight-year experience. Int J Pediatr Otorhinolaryngol. 73(8):1132-6, 2009
7. Lesavoy MA et al: Nasopharyngeal encephalocele: report of transcranial and transpalatal repair with a 25-year follow-up. J Craniofac Surg. 20(6):2251-6, 2009
8. Lee TJ et al: Endoscopic treatment of traumatic basal encephaloceles: a report of 8 cases. J Neurosurg. 108(4):729-35, 2008
9. Schuknecht B et al: Nontraumatic skull base defects with spontaneous CSF rhinorrhea and arachnoid herniation: imaging findings and correlation with endoscopic sinus surgery in 27 patients. AJNR Am J Neuroradiol. 29(3):542-9, 2008
10. Gupta DK et al: Transethmoidal transpharyngeal nasal encephalocele: neuroimaging. Pediatr Neurosurg. 42(5):335-7, 2006
11. Kizilkilic O et al: Hypothalamic hamartoma associated with a craniopharyngeal canal. AJNR Am J Neuroradiol. 26(1):65-7, 2005
12. Ekinci G et al: Transsphenoidal (large craniopharyngeal) canal associated with a normally functioning pituitary gland and nasopharyngeal extension, hyperprolactinemia, and hypothalamic hamartoma. AJR Am J Roentgenol. 180(1):76-7, 2003
13. Daniilidis J et al: Intrasphenoidal encephalocele and spontaneous CSF rhinorrhoea. Rhinology. 37(4):186-9, 1999
14. Koch BL et al: Congenital malformations causing skull base changes. Neuroimaging Clin N Am. 4(3):479-98, 1994
15. Naidich TP et al: Cephaloceles and related malformations. AJNR Am J Neuroradiol. 13(2):655-90, 1992
16. Cohen R et al: Epignathic teratoma associated with craniopharyngeal canal. AJNR Am J Neuroradiol. 10(3):652, 1989
17. Currarino G: Canalis basilaris medianus and related defects of the basiocciput. AJNR Am J Neuroradiol. 9(1):208-11, 1988
18. Nager GT: Cephaloceles. Laryngoscope. 97(1):77-84, 1987
19. Currarino G et al: Transsphenoidal canal (large craniopharyngeal canal) and its pathologic implications. AJNR Am J Neuroradiol. 6(1):39-43, 1985

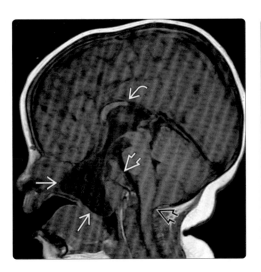

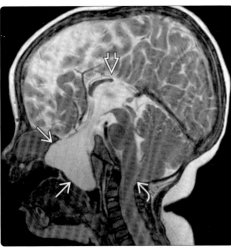

(Left) *Sagittal T1WI MR in an 18-month-old boy shows a large transsphenoidal cephalocele* ➡ *occluding the nasopharynx anterior to the sphenooccipital synchondrosis* ➡. *The pituitary gland is not identifiable; the corpus callosum is dysplastic* ➡. *There is associated Chiari 1 configuration of the cerebellar tonsil* ➡. (Right) *Sagittal T2WI MR in the same child shows similar findings of skull base cephalocele* ➡, *corpus callosum dysgenesis* ➡, *and low-lying cerebellar tonsil* ➡.

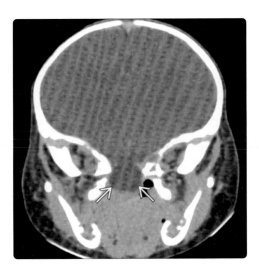

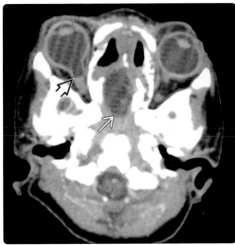

(Left) *Coronal CECT in a 5 day old with a nasal mass shows a transsphenoidal cephalocele* ➡ *extending into the nasopharynx via a large skull base defect. On this image, the contents of the cephalocele appear to be predominantly CSF. MR is better for determining the nature of the contents.* (Right) *Axial CECT in the same child shows hypertelorism secondary to the cephalocele extending through the skull base defect* ➡ *and a well-defined optic nerve coloboma* ➡.

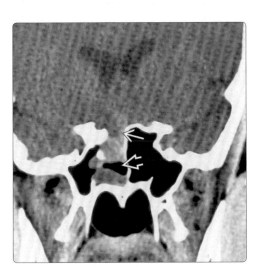

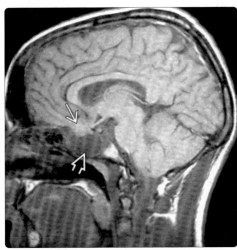

(Left) *Coronal NECT defines a defect* ➡ *in the roof of the partially opacified right sphenoid sinus* ➡ *in a teenager. In this case, the skull defect was related to previous head trauma, and the patient had a posttraumatic CSF leak.* (Right) *Sagittal T1WI MR in the same patient better defines the nature of the cephalocele herniating through a skull base defect into the sphenoid sinus. It contains posterior inferior frontal lobe tissue* ➡ *and a large amount of CSF* ➡.

Skull Base CSF Leak

IMAGING

- Best clue: Anterior or central **skull base (SB) defect** on bone CT with **positive β2-transferrin** test on nasal secretions
- Anterior skull base bone CT findings
  - Bone defect in cribriform plate, lateral lamella of middle turbinate or ethmoid roof
  - Other evidence for fracture, endoscopic sinus surgery, congenital cephalocele
- Central skull base bone CT findings
  - Bone defect in sella floor (transnasal pituitary surgery), lateral wall sphenoid (osseous dural defect)
- Multiple defects often present in obese patient with **idiopathic intracranial hypertension**
- MR used if cephalocele suspected

TOP DIFFERENTIAL DIAGNOSES

- Vasomotor rhinitis
- Skull base defect without CSF leak

PATHOLOGY

- Congenital CSF leak
  - Cribriform defect ± congenital cephalocele, persistent craniopharyngeal canal
- Acquired leak: Spontaneous leak from osseous dural defect
  - Lateral roof of sphenoid sinus
- Posttraumatic leak: Can occur with any facial or SB fx, or even closed head injury
  - Roof or lateral wall of sphenoid sinus, or cribriform plate/ethmoid roof
- Postoperative defect: Can occur after sinonasal or skull base surgery

CLINICAL ISSUES

- Rhinorrhea with Valsalva or head down maneuvers
- **β2-transferrin** is best test to confirm fluid from nose is CSF
- Persistent CSF leaks endoscopically repaired

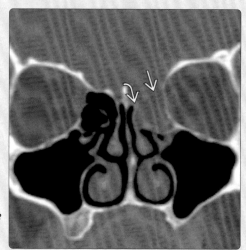
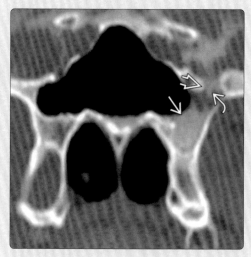

(Left) Coronal bone CT shows large bony defect ➡ in left ethmoid roof, lateral to insertion of middle turbinate ⬈. Because there is complete opacification of the ethmoid cells, an MR was performed that showed meningoencephalocele.
(Right) Coronal bone CT after intrathecal contrast shows CSF ➡ in left sphenoid chamber, bone defect ⬈, and contrast extending through defect ⬈. CT cisternography is rarely necessary when high-resolution bone CT and MR are performed 1st for CSF leak.

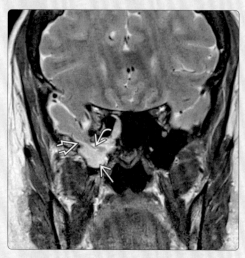
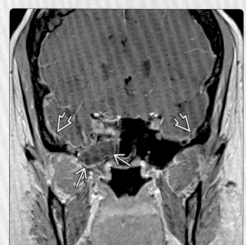

(Left) Coronal T2WI MR reveals lateral sphenoid sinus filled with CSF ➡. Note the osseous defect in lateral sphenoid roof ⬈, and brain herniating through defect ⬈. Patient had a spontaneous CSF leak. Many such leaks are caused by large osseous dural defects. (Right) Coronal T1WI C+ MR in same patient shows peripheral enhancement ➡ of the sphenoid meningoencephalocele. Note diffuse thin dural enhancement ⬈, including at the defect site. Dural enhancement may be present without infection.

TERMINOLOGY

Definitions

- Osseous dural defect (ODD): Focal gap though dura and underlying skull base (SB) bone
  - Acquired; seen commonly with intracranial hypertension
  - May result from underlying bone thinning or aberrant arachnoid granulations

IMAGING

Imaging Recommendations

- Best imaging tool
  - Bone CT with multiplanar reformations
    - Large defects easily visualized on multiplanar CT, obviating need for CT cisternography
    - Small, < 4-mm defects difficult to see, especially if present in bone that is normally thin
      □ May require CT cisternography
  - MR used if cephalocele suspected
  - **CT cisternogram** indicated if > 1 potential site of leak
    - Positive study much more likely if active leak
    - Be sure to scan SB prior to intrathecal contrast as osteoneogenesis can mimic contrast in sinus cavity
    - After LP and intrathecal contrast placed, have patient do maneuvers that ↑ rhinorrhea

General Features

- Best diagnostic clue
  - Anterior or central **SB defect** on bone CT, ± fluid level or opacified sinus with **positive β2-transferrin** test on nasal secretions
- Location
  - Anterior SB: Cribriform plate, lateral lamella, ethmoid roof
  - Central SB: Sella floor, lateral sphenoid sinus wall in pneumatized inferolateral recess
  - Multiple defects common in obese patient

CT Findings

- Bone CT
  - Anterior skull base
    - Bone defect in cribriform plate, lateral lamella of middle turbinate, or ethmoid roof
  - Central skull base
    - Bone defect in sella floor (transnasal pituitary surgery), lateral wall sphenoid near foramen rotundum, especially in obese patient

MR Findings

- T2WI
  - Osseous defect, fluid in sinus cavity
  - Traction encephalomalacia at leak site, especially if cephalocele present
- T1WI C+
  - Dural enhancement at defect site common

DIFFERENTIAL DIAGNOSIS

Vasomotor Rhinitis

- Rhinorrhea from sinuses with negative β2-transferrin

Skull Base Defect Without CSF Leak

- Not all bony defects leak

PATHOLOGY

General Features

- Etiology
  - Congenital CSF leak: Cribriform plate defect, congenital cephalocele, persistent craniopharyngeal canal
  - Acquired leak: Spontaneous leak from ODD
    - Most common at lateral roof of sphenoid sinus near foramen rotundum in obese patient
    - Usually secondary to **idiopathic intracranial hypertension (IIH)** → gradual SB thinning → SB defect
  - Posttraumatic leak: Can occur after facial or SB fracture, or closed head injury
    - Most commonly seen at roof or lateral wall of sphenoid sinus, or cribriform plate/ethmoid roof
  - Postoperative defect: May occur after sinonasal, or anterior or central SB surgery
- Associated abnormalities
  - Cephalocele can be associated with herniation of meninges or brain through osseous dural defect

CLINICAL ISSUES

Presentation

- Most common signs/symptoms
  - Rhinorrhea
  - **β2-transferrin** best 1st test to confirm nasal fluid is CSF

Demographics

- Age
  - Spontaneous leaks most common in **middle-aged, obese women**

Natural History & Prognosis

- Posttraumatic CSF leaks: Usually resolve spontaneously due to scarring at SB defect
- Spontaneous CSF leak: Usually secondary to IIH, gradual SB thinning → frank defect

Treatment

- Persistent CSF leaks endoscopically repaired
- Fascia-bone graft placed on intracranial side of defect
- Treated spontaneous leaks from IIH may recur unless bariatric surgery or medical therapy

DIAGNOSTIC CHECKLIST

Consider

- CSF leak in patient with risk factors, especially obesity or prior surgery, rhinorrhea with sinus opacification

Image Interpretation Pearls

- If β2-transferrin of nasal fluid is positive, carefully assess skull base on bone CT

SELECTED REFERENCES

1. Oakley GM et al: Diagnosis of cerebrospinal fluid rhinorrhea: an evidence-based review with recommendations. Int Forum Allergy Rhinol. 6(1):8-16, 2016
2. Lloyd KM et al: Imaging of skull base cerebrospinal fluid leaks in adults. Radiology. 248(3):725-36, 2008

Skull Base Fibrous Dysplasia

TERMINOLOGY

- Fibrous dysplasia (FD)
- Congenital disorder with defect in osteoblastic differentiation and maturation, resulting in progressive replacement of normal cancellous bone by mixture of fibrous tissue and immature woven bone

IMAGING

- May affect calvarium, skull base, and facial bones
- Density (CT) and signal (MR) appearance highly variable
- CT findings
  - Expansile lesion centered in medullary space with variable attenuation
  - Sclerotic FD: Ground-glass density
  - Pagetoid FD: Mixed lucent and sclerotic areas
  - Cystic FD: Centrally lucent with thin sclerotic borders
- MR findings
  - Low signal in ossified ± fibrous portions of lesion
  - Variable enhancement depending on lesion pattern

- PET findings
  - Can be variably hypermetabolic on FDG PET

TOP DIFFERENTIAL DIAGNOSES

- Paget disease
- Ossifying fibroma
- Meningioma
- Skull base metastasis

PATHOLOGY

- Contains fibrous tissue with interspersed trabeculae of immature woven bone that resemble Chinese letters
- Sporadic mutation of GNAS gene; is not inherited
- Associated abnormalities include aneurysmal bone cyst, multiple endocrine disorders in McCune-Albright syndrome

CLINICAL ISSUES

- 3 presentations: Monostotic, polyostotic, and McCune-Albright syndrome

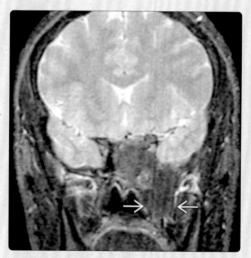
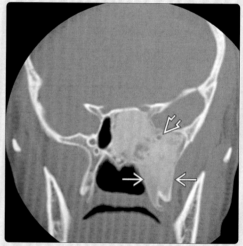

(Left) Coronal T2WI MR in a patient with fibrous dysplasia (FD) of skull base shows expanded bone and marked hypointensity extending into pterygoid processes ➡. (Right) Coronal CT in the same patient demonstrates expansion of body and greater wing of the sphenoid with obliteration of left sphenoid sinus lumen. Left foramen rotundum ➡ is narrowed and laterally displaced. Note the marked expansion of left pterygoid process and medial and lateral pterygoid plates ➡.

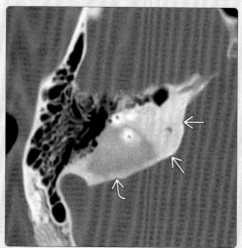
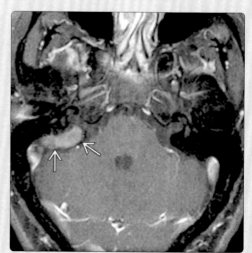

(Left) Axial bone CT shows FD involving temporal bone with smooth, expanded appearance of the bone ➡. Petrous temporal bone is extensively involved with sparing of inner ear structures. More posterior-lateral component ➡ shows the classic ground-glass density. (Right) Axial T1WI C+ FS MR in the same patient demonstrates enhancement of entire extent of involved petrous bone ➡. In this case, enhancement is diffuse and homogeneous.

TERMINOLOGY

Abbreviations

- Fibrous dysplasia (FD)

Synonyms

- Craniofacial FD (CFD), osteitis fibrosa, osteodystrophy fibrosa
- McCune-Albright syndrome

Definitions

- Congenital disorder with **defect in osteoblastic differentiation and maturation** resulting in progressive replacement of normal cancellous bone by mixture of fibrous tissue and immature woven bone

IMAGING

General Features

- Best diagnostic clue
  - **Ground-glass matrix** in **expansile bone** lesion on bone CT
- Location
  - Affects any bone, including skull, skull base, and facial bones
  - Often > 1 bone involved
- Size
  - Polyostotic lesions can be massive
- Morphology
  - Expanded bone

Radiographic Findings

- Radiography
  - Expanded, thickened bone with ground-glass density
  - May be accompanied by areas of sclerosis or lucency

CT Findings

- NECT
  - Appearance varies with relative content of fibrous vs. osseous tissue
  - Expansile lesion with abrupt transition zone between lesion and normal bone typical
- CECT
  - Enhancement often difficult to appreciate except in areas of lucent bone
- Bone CT
  - **Expansile** lesion centered in **medullary space** with variable attenuation
    - **Pagetoid (mixed) pattern** (50%): Mixed radiopacity and radiolucency
    - **Sclerotic FD** (25%): Ground-glass density
    - **Cystic FD** (25%): Centrally lucent lesions with thinned but sclerotic borders

MR Findings

- T1WI
  - Expansile mass with ↓ signal in ossified ± fibrous portions of lesion
- T2WI
  - **Low signal** in ossified ± fibrous portions of lesion
  - In active phase, heterogeneous signal pattern often present
- T1WI C+
  - Variable enhancement depending on lesion pattern
    - None, rim, or diffuse
  - Impressive enhancement may also be seen in fibrous areas
- MRA
  - Vascular narrowing or displacement where affected bone encroaches on arterial vascular canals/foramina
- MRV
  - Vascular narrowing or displacement where affected bone encroaches on venous vascular canals/foramina

Nuclear Medicine Findings

- Bone scan
  - Nonspecific; sensitive to extent of skeletal lesions in polyostotic FD
  - Increased radionuclide accumulation, perfusion, and delayed bone phase
- PET
  - Accumulation of [11C]methyl-L-methionine on PET
  - Can be variably hypermetabolic on FDG PET

Imaging Recommendations

- Best imaging tool
  - Bone CT best for most cases
- Protocol advice
  - T1 C+ FS MR in complicated cases (cranial neuropathy, suspected malignant transformation)

DIFFERENTIAL DIAGNOSIS

Paget Disease

- Typically presents in elderly
- Involves T-bone and calvarium more frequently than craniofacial area
- Cotton-wool CT appearance

Ossifying Fibroma

- May mimic cystic form of FD
- Thick, bony rim and lower density center
- Tends to appear more mass-like and localized than FD

Meningioma

- Intraosseous meningioma may mimic FD
- En plaque soft tissue mass may be evident on enhanced MR

Skull Base Metastasis

- Mixed sclerotic-destructive may mimic FD
- Prostate and breast carcinoma most common primary tumors to metastasize to skull base

Chondrosarcoma

- Centered on petrooccipital fissure
- Arc or ring-like matrix calcifications on bone CT
- Hyperintense on T2WI MR

Giant Cell Tumor

- May mimic sclerotic FD
- Hypointense on T2 MR due to hemosiderin deposition
- More intense enhancement on MR than FD

PATHOLOGY

General Features
- Etiology
  - **Benign tumor-like lesion** of bone with local arrest of normal structural/architectural development
- Genetics
  - Sporadic mutation of *GNAS* gene; is not inherited
  - All cells descended from mutated cell line can manifest features of monostotic or polyostotic FD
- Associated abnormalities
  - Aneurysmal bone cysts
  - Multiple endocrine disorders may be seen in McCune-Albright syndrome

Staging, Grading, & Classification
- **Monostotic vs. polyostotic**
- Specific lesion type relates to disease activity
  - Pagetoid
  - Sclerotic
  - Cystic

Gross Pathologic & Surgical Features
- Tan-yellow to white mass
- Rubbery to gritty consistency depending on fibrous vs. osseous content

Microscopic Features
- Fibrous tissue with interspersed trabeculae of immature woven bone that resemble Chinese letters

CLINICAL ISSUES

Presentation
- Most common signs/symptoms
  - Symptoms depend on lesion location
    - Temporal bone: CHL; EAC stenosis; CNVII weakness
    - Orbital: Proptosis, optic neuropathy
    - Sinonasal: Ostial obstruction → mucocele formation
- Other signs/symptoms
  - Pain, focal swelling, tenderness
  - Leontiasis ossea (lion facies) with extensive facial bone involvement
    - Alters facial and calvarial contours
    - Obstructs sinuses
    - Complex cranial neuropathy possible from foraminal encroachment
- Clinical profile
  - 3 presentations: Monostotic, polyostotic, and McCune-Albright syndrome
  - **Monostotic FD (70%)**
    - Single osseous site affected
    - Older children and young adults (75% present before age 30)
    - Skull base and face involved in 25%; maxilla (especially zygomatic process) and mandible (molar area) > > frontal bone > ethmoid and sphenoid bones > T-bone
    - May be asymptomatic, incidental finding
  - Polyostotic FD (25%)
    - Involves ≥ 2 separate osseous sites
    - Skull base and face involved in 50%
    - Younger patients (mean age at diagnosis 8 years)

- 2/3 have symptoms, including craniofacial asymmetry, by age 10
  - McCune-Albright syndrome (3-5%)
    - Polyostotic FD (usually unilateral)
    - Associated with endocrine dysfunction (precocious puberty) and cutaneous hyperpigmentation (*café au lait* spots)
    - Appears earlier and affects more bones more severely

Demographics
- Age
  - **Most < 30 years**
- Gender
  - M:F = 1:2
  - McCune-Albright syndrome usually female
- Epidemiology
  - One of most common fibroosseous lesions
  - Monostotic FD 6x more common than polyostotic FD
  - Polyostotic form more likely to have calvarial involvement

Natural History & Prognosis
- Monostotic CFD has excellent prognosis
  - Often ceases to progress after puberty
- Polyostotic FD rarely life threatening but has poor prognosis
  - May progress beyond 3rd decade
- Malignant (sarcomatous) transformation of FD is rare (< 0.5% of cases)
  - Osteosarcoma most common

Treatment
- Aggressive surgical management typically not recommended
- Radiation therapy generally avoided (may cause malignant transformation)
- Bisphosphonate therapy may ameliorate course (↓ pain and fractures)

DIAGNOSTIC CHECKLIST

Image Interpretation Pearls
- Classic appearance → **ground-glass on bone CT**; ↓ signal on T2WI MR

SELECTED REFERENCES

1. Lee SE et al: The diagnostic utility of the GNAS mutation in patients with fibrous dysplasia: meta-analysis of 168 sporadic cases. Hum Pathol. 43(8):1234-42, 2012
2. Wei YT et al: Fibrous dysplasia of skull. J Craniofac Surg. 21(2):538-42, 2010
3. Hullar TE et al: Paget's disease and fibrous dysplasia. Otolaryngol Clin North Am. 36(4):707-32, 2003
4. Chong VF et al: Fibrous dysplasia involving the base of the skull. AJR Am J Roentgenol. 178(3):717-20, 2002
5. Itshayek E et al: Fibrous dysplasia in combination with aneurysmal bone cyst of the occipital bone and the clivus: case report and review of the literature. Neurosurgery. 51(3):815-7; discussion 817-8, 2002
6. Sharma RR et al: Symptomatic cranial fibrous dysplasias: clinico-radiological analysis in a series of eight operative cases with follow-up results. J Clin Neurosci. 9(4):381-90, 2002
7. Sirvanci M et al: Monostotic fibrous dysplasia of the clivus: MRI and CT findings. Neuroradiology. 44(10):847-50, 2002
8. Lustig LR et al: Fibrous dysplasia involving the skull base and temporal bone. Arch Otolaryngol Head Neck Surg. 127(10):1239-47, 2001
9. Jee WH et al: Fibrous dysplasia: MR imaging characteristics with radiopathologic correlation. AJR Am J Roentgenol. 167(6):1523-7, 1996

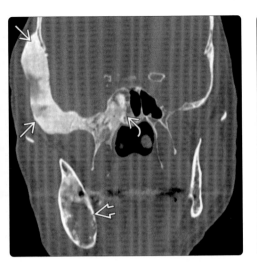

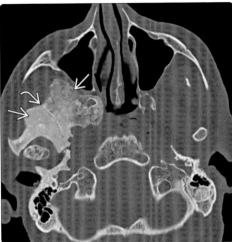

(Left) Coronal bone CT shows expanded mixed density within squamous temporal bone ➡. Mixed density involvement of sphenoid bone is also noted with expansion ➡. A predominantly cystic (fibrous) focus of FD involvement is seen in mandibular body ➡. (Right) Axial bone CT in same patient with polyostotic FD shows mixed lucent and sclerotic pattern of bone involvement ➡. Note abrupt transition of imaging appearance at a suture ➡, characteristic of FD.

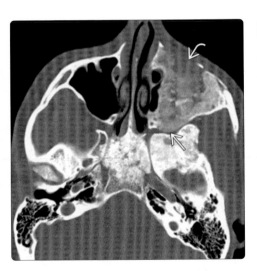

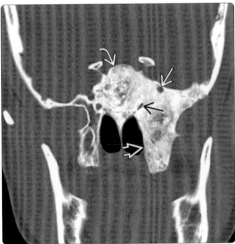

(Left) Axial bone CT demonstrates mixed sclerotic and lucent FD affecting the sphenoid bone and maxilla. Note the narrowing of left pterygomaxillary fissure ➡. A cortical defect along maxilla ➡ represents previous biopsy. (Right) Coronal bone CT shows extensive FD involvement of sphenoid ➡ and pterygoid processes ➡. Significant narrowing of left vidian canal ➡ and displacement and minimal narrowing of left foramen rotundum ➡ are noted.

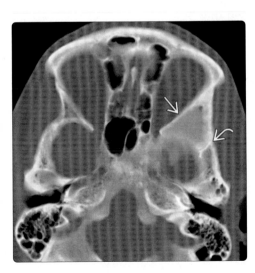

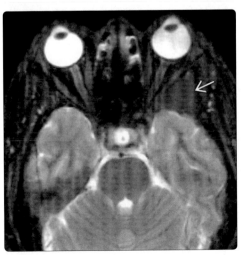

(Left) Axial bone CT shows bony expansion and sclerosis and ground-glass density ➡ in left greater sphenoid wing. Note abrupt change to normal-appearing bone at left sphenotemporal suture ➡, typical of FD. (Right) Axial T2WI FS MR in same patient shows predominantly hypointense signal ➡ in affected bone. MR signal characteristics and enhancement can be highly variable on MR imaging depending on the amount of fibrous vs. sclerotic tissue.

Skull Base Paget Disease

TERMINOLOGY

- Primary metabolic bony disease of unknown etiology

IMAGING

- CT findings
  - Bone CT most demonstrative of mixed sclerosis & lysis
  - Well-defined lytic regions with expansion of bone in early-phase disease
  - Cotton-wool appearance in later lytic-sclerotic phase
- MR findings
  - T1WI: Hypointense signal due to fibrovascular replacement of marrow space
  - Heterogeneous enhancement due to hypervascular nature of new bone
- Basilar invagination from bone softening & expansion

TOP DIFFERENTIAL DIAGNOSES

- Fibrous dysplasia
- Skull base metastasis
- Osteopetrosis
- Osteogenesis imperfecta

PATHOLOGY

- Cases may have autosomal dominant transmission
  - Some consistent mutations identified in familial cases & some sporadic cases
- Both environmental and genetic causes likely
- Histologic mosaic bone pattern in final stage of disease

CLINICAL ISSUES

- Common presentation: Expansile, lytic, & sclerotic bony disease of axial skeleton and skull in elderly male patient
  - Hearing loss if temporal bone involvement
  - May be incidental finding
- Malignant transformation in < 1% of cases
- Pagetic bone pain is uncommon (constant, boring character)
- Treatment: Lasting response to bisphosphonate agents

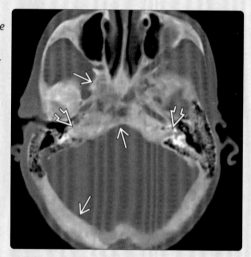

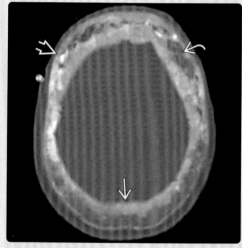

(Left) Axial bone CT of the skull base shows Paget disease with diffuse expansion and hyperdensity of the skull base ➡ and a fluffy appearance of the abnormally thickened bone. This process also involves the temporal bones and otic capsules ➡. (Right) Axial bone CT in the same patient demonstrates the extensive nature of the disease with diffuse irregular calvarial cortical thickening ➡, patchy osteolysis ➡, and islands of sclerotic bone ➡ representing cotton-wool lesions.

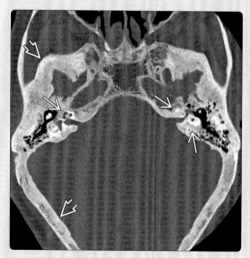

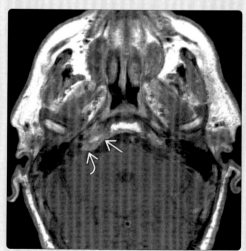

(Left) Axial bone CT demonstrates diffuse skull base sclerosis with mild bony expansion, irregular cortical thickening ➡, and poor corticomedullary differentiation. There is demineralization of the otic capsules ➡ bilaterally. Temporal bone involvement may result in hearing loss. (Right) Axial T1WI C+ MR in the same patient demonstrates avid enhancement of the pagetoid focus ➡, which is mildly expanded and results in stenosis of the internal auditory canal ➡.

TERMINOLOGY

Abbreviations

- Paget disease (PD)

Synonyms

- Osteitis deformans

Definitions

- Primary metabolic bony disease of unknown etiology caused by waves of osteoclastic and osteoblastic activity

IMAGING

General Features

- Best diagnostic clue
  - Mixed **expansile, lytic, & sclerotic** bony disease of axial skeleton and skull in elderly male patient

Imaging Recommendations

- Best imaging tool
  - Bone CT most demonstrative of mixed sclerosis & lysis

CT Findings

- Bone CT
  - Characteristic stages of bone remodeling with progression from bony lysis to sclerosis
    - Well-defined lytic regions with expansion of bone in early phase of disease
    - **Cotton-wool** appearance in later mixed lytic-sclerotic phase
  - Basilar invagination from bone softening & expansion

MR Findings

- T1WI
  - **Hypointense signal** due to fibrovascular replacement of fat in marrow space
  - Patchy ↑ signal possible with hemorrhage, slow flow in vascular channels
- T2WI
  - Heterogeneous, occasional hyperintense signal
- T1WI C+
  - Heterogeneous enhancement due to vascular channels in involved bone

DIFFERENTIAL DIAGNOSIS

Fibrous Dysplasia

- Classic ground-glass appearance and expansion in segments of diseased bone
- Can have more focal areas of soft tissue & sclerosis → mimics Paget disease

Skull Base Metastasis

- Investigate for history of known malignancy
- Associated soft tissue mass more common
- Typically less diffuse & lesions more well defined

Osteopetrosis

- Presents in childhood
- Uniform bony sclerosis, diffuse involvement
- Spiculated periosteal reaction

Osteogenesis Imperfecta

- Age of onset usually much younger

PATHOLOGY

General Features

- Etiology
  - Admixture of environmental and genetic factors seem responsible for PD
- Genetics
  - Some cases have clear autosomal dominant transmission
  - Mutations in *SQSTM1* and *OPTN* locus of chromosome 10p13 have been discovered

Staging, Grading, & Classification

- 1st stage of disease is lysis
- Progresses to mixed lytic & sclerotic disease
- Final stage of disease is dense sclerosis

Microscopic Features

- Histologic mosaic bone pattern in final stage of disease

CLINICAL ISSUES

Presentation

- Most common signs/symptoms
  - Occasional incidental finding
  - Pagetic bone pain is uncommon
    - Constant, boring character
  - Hearing loss with temporal bone involvement
    - **Conductive hearing loss** may result from involvement of ossicles
    - **Sensorineural hearing loss** may result from bony compression of CNVIII or cochlear involvement
- Other signs/symptoms
  - Wide range of other presentations, including
    - Skull deformity & fractures
    - Cranial neuropathies
    - Brainstem and cerebellar dysfunction
    - ↑ alkaline phosphatase levels

Demographics

- Age
  - Typically disease of elderly (uncommon under age 55)
- Gender
  - M:F = 3:2

Natural History & Prognosis

- Generally benign course
- Malignant transformation to osteosarcoma in < 1% of cases

Treatment

- Lasting response to bisphosphonate agents

SELECTED REFERENCES

1. Gruener G et al: Paget's disease of bone. Handb Clin Neurol. 119:529-40, 2014
2. Ralston SH et al: Genetics of Paget's disease of bone. Curr Osteoporos Rep. 12(3):263-71, 2014
3. Theodorou DJ et al: Imaging of Paget disease of bone and its musculoskeletal complications: review. AJR Am J Roentgenol. 196(6 Suppl):S64-75, 2011
4. Swartz JD: The otodystrophies: diagnosis and differential diagnosis. Semin Ultrasound CT MR. 25(4):305-18, 2004

Skull Base Langerhans Cell Histiocytosis

TERMINOLOGY

- Langerhans cell histiocytosis (LCH): Spectrum of disorders caused by neoplastic clonal proliferations of CD1a, CD207, S100 (+) dendritic cells
  - Single system (SS) (unifocal or multifocal) vs. multisystem (MS) disease
  - Bone and skin most frequently involved
  - High-risk organ involvement: Liver, spleen, marrow: Worse prognosis
  - Other organs: Lymph nodes, pituitary, thymus, GI tract, CNS
  - 70% have involvement of H&N: Skull base, temporal bone (T-bone), craniofacial

IMAGING

- CT findings
  - Geographic, lytic lesion of skull base/T-bone
  - Associated with enhancing soft tissue mass
- MR findings
  - Heterogeneous, strongly enhancing soft tissue mass ± intracranial/dural extension

TOP DIFFERENTIAL DIAGNOSES

- Acute coalescent otomastoiditis
- Rhabdomyosarcoma
- Acquired cholesteatoma

CLINICAL ISSUES

- Typical presentation: Young male patient with otalgia, otorrhea, & postauricular mass
  - Usually presents in 1st decade
  - M:F = 1.2-3:1
  - Otologic symptoms may be only initial sign of disease
  - More common among Caucasians
- 90% cure rate for unifocal disease of T-bone
- Usually responds well to medical management
- Surgical curettage or mastoidectomy for localized mastoid-middle ear disease

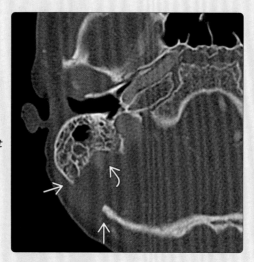
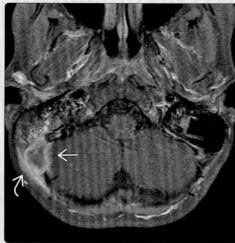

(Left) Axial CECT in Langerhans cell histiocytosis (LCH) demonstrates involvement of the posterior mastoid with well-defined destruction ➡ displacing the adjacent sigmoid sinus ➡. (Right) Axial T1 C+ FS MR of the same case demonstrates heterogeneous enhancement of LCH & depicts extent of soft tissue disease ➡ contiguous with bony lesion & involvement of contiguous dura ➡.

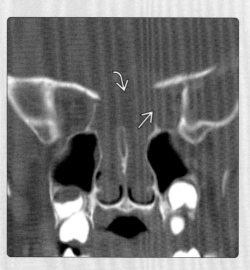
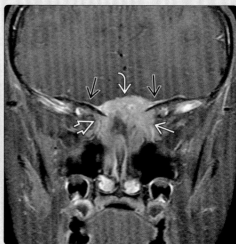

(Left) Coronal bone CT shows LCH lesion centered in the basisphenoid and extending into the left ➡ orbital apex through the medial orbital wall. A large area of bone dehiscence involves planum sphenoidale ➡. (Right) Coronal T1WI C+ MR in the same patient shows involvement of the left orbit near apex ➡, right orbital apex ➡, & anterior cranial fossa ➡. Dural involvement is also noted with abnormal dural enhancement ➡ at the tumor margins.

TERMINOLOGY

Abbreviations

- Langerhans cell histiocytosis (LCH)

Synonyms

- Eosinophilic granuloma, histiocytosis X, Hand-Schüller-Christian disease, Letterer-Siwe disease

Definitions

- LCH: Spectrum of disorders caused by neoplastic clonal proliferations of CD1a, CD207, S100 (+) dendritic cells
- Single system (SS) (unifocal or multifocal) vs. multisystem (MS) disease
  - Bone and skin most frequently involved
  - Worse prognosis: Organs at high risk are liver, spleen, marrow
  - Other organs: Lymph nodes, pituitary, thymus, GI tract, CNS
  - H&N: Skull base, temporal bone (T-bone), craniofacial

IMAGING

General Features

- Best diagnostic clue
  - Well-marginated, **geographic, lytic lesion** of skull base/T-bone + enhancing soft tissue mass
- Location
  - **Mastoid portion** of T-bone common site for H&N disease
    - Petrous apex less common
  - Skull lesions (frontal & parietal bones) more common than skull base
  - Mandible, maxilla, & vertebral body lesions also may occur
  - Unifocal 50-75%; multifocal SS 10-20%; all others multifocal/MS disease
- Size
  - Varies from small, punched-out lesion to total diffuse bony involvement
- Morphology
  - Destructive, marginated lesion most often

Radiographic Findings

- Radiography
  - Lytic bone lesion with punched-out borders
  - "Button sequestrum" occasionally noted in skull lesions

CT Findings

- CECT
  - Variably enhancing soft tissue mass with mastoid destruction
  - May involve contiguous dura
- Bone CT
  - Bony lesions of variable appearance, typically lytic
    - Most have sharply defined punched-out appearance
    - Geographic bone destruction in mastoid T-bone
      □ Ossicular & otic capsule destruction
    - Lytic lesions with beveled margins, ± sclerosis (common appearance in skull)
    - May have more diffuse bone destructive change

MR Findings

- T1WI
  - Iso- to hypointense bone lesion ± soft tissue mass
  - ↑ signal in proliferative LCH lesions due to lipid-laden macrophages
- T2WI
  - Hyper- to isointense mass
  - Rarely blood products in soft tissue mass
- STIR
  - Similar findings to T2WI
  - Whole-body STIR to assess for multifocal disease
    - More sensitive for skeletal & extraskeletal LCH than radiographs or bone scan
    - Limited ability to distinguish active vs. residual disease
- T1WI C+
  - Heterogeneous, strongly enhancing soft tissue mass
  - May show defined or infiltrative borders
  - ± intracranial extension/dural enhancement

Nuclear Medicine Findings

- Bone scan: Most lesions ↑ radiotracer uptake, few ↓ or absent radiotracer uptake
- PET/CT: FDG highly sensitive for active LCH (↑ radiotracer uptake)

Imaging Recommendations

- Best imaging tool
  - Bone CT delineates geographic pattern of T-bone/skull base involvement
  - Gadolinium-enhanced MR best for depicting soft tissue extent & intracranial involvement
  - CECT or MR help differentiate inflammatory mastoid lesions from LCH
- Protocol advice
  - C+ FS MR

DIFFERENTIAL DIAGNOSIS

Acute Coalescent Otomastoiditis

- Acutely ill patient; responsive to antibiotics
- Trabecular loss, cortical dehiscence usually less extensive than in LCH
- No soft tissue component unless abscess present

Rhabdomyosarcoma

- Aggressive unilateral soft tissue mass with bone destruction
- More common in petrous apex & middle ear than mastoid
- Biopsy may be required to differentiate from LCH

Acquired Cholesteatoma

- Tympanic membrane perforation with white mass on otoscopy
- Bone destruction involves scutum & ossicles; usually less extensive than LCH
- Does not enhance; + diffusion restriction

Congenital Cholesteatoma

- White, retrotympanic mass on otoscopy
- Does not enhance; + diffusion restriction

Cholesterol Granuloma

- Preceded by history of chronic ear infections

- More common in petrous apex & middle ear than mastoid
- Hyperintense on T1 MR

Fibrous Dysplasia

- Lytic phase lesions may mimic LCH
- Typically causes bone expansion & areas of ground-glass attenuation

PATHOLOGY

General Features

- Genetics
  - Monoclonality of pathologic Langerhans cell
  - > 50% carry mutations in BRAF

Staging, Grading, & Classification

- Location of LCH lesion & SS vs. MS involvement → treatment decisions & prognosis
  - Young age, multifocal involvement, multiorgan dysfunction, relapse
  - Low-risk organs: Skin, bone, lungs, lymph nodes, GI tract, pituitary gland & CNS
  - High-risk organs: Liver, spleen & bone marrow
- Formerly classified into 1 of 3 overlapping forms
  - Unifocal LCH (eosinophilic granuloma)
  - Hand-Schüller-Christian disease
    - Multifocal bone, skin, viscera, & brain involvement
  - Letterer-Siwe disease
    - Acute, fulminant, disseminated multiorgan disease, including liver, spleen, lymphatic, lung, & bone

Microscopic Features

- Active lesion: Granuloma of dendritic Langerhans cells > inflammatory cells
- Later stages: Macrophages > Langerhans cells + fibrotic & xanthomatous changes
- Birbeck granule: Classic "tennis racquet" organelle found by electron microscopy in up to 40% of Langerhans cells
  - Diagnostic importance diminished due to immunostaining of specific markers now available (CD1a, CD207, S100 protein)

CLINICAL ISSUES

Presentation

- Most common signs/symptoms
  - **Otologic symptoms** may be only initial sign of disease
    - Initial presentation with otologic symptoms in 25%
    - Conductive hearing loss & otorrhea
      - □ Otorrhea from secondary infection with granulation tissue formation
- Other signs/symptoms
  - Otalgia, vertigo
  - Otitis externa/media
  - Postauricular swelling
  - Facial nerve palsy, sensorineural hearing loss
  - Aural polyp from erosion of EAC wall by lesion
  - Proptosis, ptosis with orbital involvement
- Clinical profile
  - Male child or adolescent with otalgia, otorrhea, & postauricular mass

Demographics

- Age
  - 90% of cases < 15 years at presentation
  - SS, unifocal (70% of cases); peak age: 5-15 years
  - SS, multifocal (20% of cases); peak age: 1-5 years
  - MS high-risk organ-positive (10% of cases); peak age: 0-2 years
- Gender
  - **M:F = 2:1**
- Epidemiology
  - Rare (0.2-2.0 cases per 100,00 children)
  - **70% have involvement of H&N**
    - Bilateral disease in up to 45% of cases
  - Bone lesions most common manifestation of disease (80-95% of children with LCH)

Natural History & Prognosis

- 90% cure rate for unifocal disease of T-bone
- Soft tissue component resolves initially, then reossification of lytic bone lesion
- Local recurrence may occur

Treatment

- SS disease
  - Unifocal bone disease: Watchful waiting vs. curettage & local steroid injection
  - Multifocal bone disease or CNS-risk lesion: Chemotherapy & steroids x 6-12 months
- MS disease (± high-risk organ): Multiagent chemotherapy x 12 months

DIAGNOSTIC CHECKLIST

Consider

- Consider LCH when destructive T-bone lesion does not respond to antibiotics & tympanostomy tubes

Reporting Tips

- Differentiation of LCH lesion from rhabdomyosarcoma essential

SELECTED REFERENCES

1. Chevallier KM et al: Differentiating pediatric rhabdomyosarcoma and Langerhans cell histiocytosis of the temporal bone by imaging appearance. AJNR Am J Neuroradiol. 37(6):1185-9, 2016
2. Egeler RM et al: Langerhans cell histiocytosis is a neoplasm and consequently its recurrence is a relapse: In memory of Bob Arceci. Pediatr Blood Cancer. ePub, 2016
3. Modest MC et al: Langerhans cell histiocytosis of the temporal bone: A review of 29 cases at a single center. Laryngoscope. 126(8):1899-904, 2016
4. Collin M et al: Cell(s) of Origin of Langerhans cell histiocytosis. Hematol Oncol Clin North Am. 29(5):825-38, 2015
5. Demellawy DE et al: Langerhans cell histiocytosis: a comprehensive review. Pathology. 47(4):294-301, 2015
6. Rollins BJ: Genomic Alterations in Langerhans cell histiocytosis. Hematol Oncol Clin North Am. 29(5):839-51, 2015
7. Chung EM et al: From the archives of the AFIP. Pediatric orbit tumors and tumorlike lesions: osseous lesions of the orbit. Radiographics. 28(4):1193-214, 2008
8. Krishna H et al: Solitary Langerhans-cell histiocytosis of the clivus and sphenoid sinus with parasellar and petrous extensions: case report and a review of literature. Surg Neurol. 62(5):447-54, 2004
9. Prayer D et al: MR imaging presentation of intracranial disease associated with Langerhans cell histiocytosis. AJNR Am J Neuroradiol. 25(5):880-91, 2004

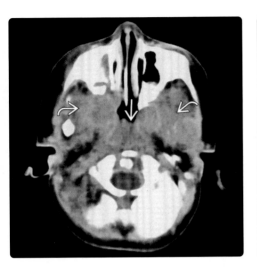

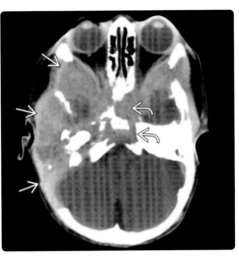

(Left) *Axial CECT demonstrates extensive LCH lesion with considerable soft tissue involvement. LCH extends into nasopharynx ➡ & bilateral nasopharyngeal masticator space ➡.* (Right) *Higher section axial CECT demonstrates a large LCH lesion of central skull base ➡ & temporal bone (T-bone) ➡ with relatively homogeneous enhancement. Mass results in extensive destruction of right T-bone, sphenoid wings, & clivus.*

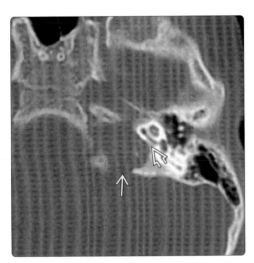

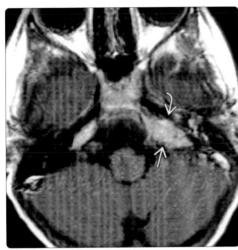

(Left) *Axial CT demonstrates LCH lesion in left petrous apex ➡ with scalloping of otic capsule ➡. Lesion is also contiguous with petrous segment of internal carotid artery (ICA) along anterior margin.* (Right) *Axial T1 C+ MR of the same patient demonstrates uniform enhancement of LCH lesion in petrous apex ➡. Contiguity with petrous ICA ➡ is evident.*

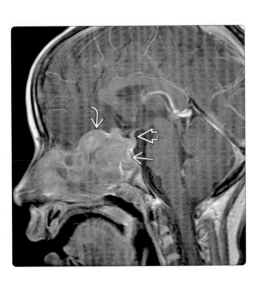

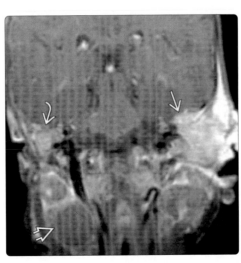

(Left) *Sagittal T1 C+ MR shows a large, heterogeneously enhancing, central skull base LCH lesion extending into sella ➡. Note intracranial extension into anterior fossa through planum sphenoidale ➡ & involvement of infundibulum ➡.* (Right) *Coronal T1 C+ MR demonstrates bilateral T-bone LCH. On left, irregular LCH lesion involves dura ➡, while on right, it extends to dural surface ➡. In right neck, there is associated heterogeneously enhancing cervical adenopathy ➡.*

Skull Base Osteopetrosis

TERMINOLOGY

- Rare heritable metabolic bone disease with defective bone remodeling resulting in overproduction of immature bone
- **Autosomal recessive osteopetrosis** (AROP): Childhood severe form
- **Autosomal dominant osteopetrosis** (ADOP): Adult benign, less severe form

IMAGING

- **AROP**: CT findings seen in **infancy**
  - Diffuse increase in overall bone density
  - Temporal bone: Internal auditory canal (IAC) & internal carotid artery canal stenoses, middle ear encroachment
  - Skull base: Foraminal & dural sinus stenoses
- **ADOP type 1**: Adult CT findings
  - Universal otosclerosis
    - Spares spine
  - Dense sclerosis of calvarium
- **ADOP type 2**: Adult CT findings
  - Dense sclerosis of skull base, spine, pelvis
    - Spares calvarium
  - Generalized ↑ density of entire skull base
  - Endobones (unresorbed primary ossification centers)
  - Sclerotic otic capsule beyond normal bony labyrinth margins
  - IAC short & trumpet-shaped
  - Enlarged subarcuate fossa possible

TOP DIFFERENTIAL DIAGNOSES

- Skull base Paget disease
- Skull base fibrous dysplasia

PATHOLOGY

- Hereditary disorder: *CLCN7* gene mutation

CLINICAL ISSUES

- **AROP** is apparent in **infancy**
- ADOP manifests later in life

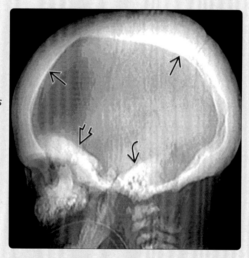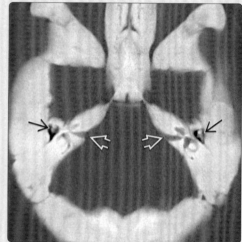

(Left) *Lateral radiograph shows diffuse thickening of calvarium ⊃, cranial base ⊃, and the temporal bone ⊃, characteristic of the more severe form of osteopetrosis (autosomal recessive).* **(Right)** *Axial skull base bone CT shows diffuse sclerosis of entire cranial base. There is narrowing of both middle ears ⊃. Note also compromise of each internal auditory canal ⊃. This child has autosomal recessive osteopetrosis.*

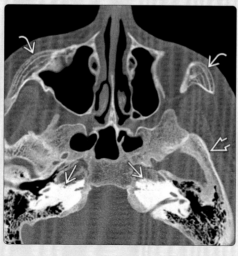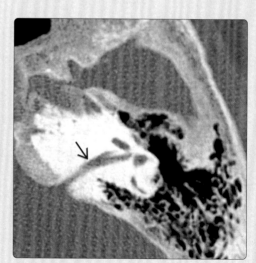

(Left) *Axial bone CT through the skull base in a young adult with type 2 autosomal dominant osteopetrosis shows bilateral dense sclerosis of temporal bone ➡ with thickening of the calvarium ➡ without increased density. Notice the endobone appearance of both malar eminences ➡ from unresorbed primary ossification centers.* **(Right)** *Axial bone CT of the left temporal bone in the same patient reveals encroachment upon the internal auditory canal ⊃ by osteopetrosis of inner ear bone.*

Skull Base Osteopetrosis

TERMINOLOGY

Synonyms
- Marble bone disease

Definitions
- Rare heritable metabolic bone disease with defective bone remodeling resulting in overproduction of immature bone
- **Autosomal recessive osteopetrosis** (AROP)
  - Childhood severe form; malignant infantile osteoporosis
- **Autosomal dominant osteopetrosis** (ADOP), type 2
  - Adult less severe form; Albers-Schönberg disease

IMAGING

General Features
- Best diagnostic clue
  - Dense, sclerotic bones (chalk bones)
- Location
  - Temporal bone (T-bone), calvarium, & skull base

Radiographic Findings
- Radiography
  - Dense bone is easily appreciated in AROP

CT Findings
- NECT
  - **AROP**: Calcifications within basal ganglia, thalami, dentate nuclei, & white matter
    - From renal tubular acidosis secondary to associated carbonic anhydrase II deficiency
- Bone CT
  - **AROP**: CT findings seen in **infancy**
    - Diffuse increase in overall bone density
    - T-bone: Internal auditory canal (IAC) & internal carotid artery (ICA) canal stenoses, middle ear encroachment
    - Skull base: Foraminal & dural sinus stenoses
  - **ADOP**: Adult CT findings
    - **Type 1**: Dense sclerosis of calvarium
      - Universal otosclerosis; spares spine
    - **Type 2**: Dense sclerosis of skull base, spine, pelvis; spares calvarium
      - Generalized ↑ density of entire skull base
      - Endobones (unresorbed primary ossification centers)
      - Sclerotic otic capsule beyond normal bony labyrinth margins
      - IAC short & trumpet shaped
      - Enlarged subarcuate fossa possible

MR Findings
- T1WI
  - AROP: Thickening of calvarium, skull base, & T-bone
- T2* GRE
  - ADOP type 2: Blooming of Ca^{++}
    - Basal ganglia, thalami, dentate nuclei, & white matter
- T1WI C+
  - AROP: C+ in suprahyoid neck = extramedullary hematopoiesis
- MRA: Petrous ICA stenosis (AROP)
- MRV: Dural venous sinus stenosis (AROP)

DIFFERENTIAL DIAGNOSIS

Skull Base Paget Disease
- Clinical: Elderly patients
- Usually seen as diffuse, cotton-wool appearance
- Demineralized otic capsule correlates with SNHL

Skull Base Fibrous Dysplasia
- Clinical: < 30 yr old
- Relative sparing of otic capsule
- Lytic, sclerotic, or mixed
- Increased bone volume is characteristic

PATHOLOGY

General Features
- Etiology
  - Hereditary disorder: *CLCN7* gene mutation
- Genetics
  - Autosomal recessive or dominant
- Overproduction of immature bone
  - Osteoclast function is defective

Microscopic Features
- Persistent primary bony spongiosa

CLINICAL ISSUES

Presentation
- Most common signs/symptoms
  - AROP
    - Cranial neuropathies, poor bone growth, petrous ICA & dural venous sinus stenoses
    - Marrow replaced: Anemia & neutropenia
      - Extramedullary hematopoiesis possible
    - Fragile bones: **Fractures** with minor trauma
  - ADOP
    - Asymptomatic to progressive symptoms
    - Eustachian tube obstruction with otitis media
    - Facial nerve, other cranial nerve deficits
    - External auditory canal stenosis

Demographics
- Age
  - **AROP** is apparent in **infancy**
  - ADOP manifests later in life

Natural History & Prognosis
- Children with AROP rarely survive childhood
- Progressive bilateral hearing loss in ADOP type 2

SELECTED REFERENCES
1. Szymanski M et al: Osteopetrosis of the temporal bone treated with cochlear implant. J Int Adv Otol. 11(2):173-5, 2015
2. Turgut M et al: Autosomal recessive osteopetrosis as an unusual cause of hydrocephalus, extensive calcification of tentorium cerebelli, and calvarial hyperostosis. J Neurosurg Pediatr. 5(4):419-21, 2010
3. Curé JK et al: Cranial MR imaging of osteopetrosis. AJNR Am J Neuroradiol. 21(6):1110-5, 2000
4. Elster AD et al: Autosomal recessive osteopetrosis: bone marrow imaging. Radiology. 182(2):507-14, 1992
5. Elster AD et al: Cranial imaging in autosomal recessive osteopetrosis. Part II. Skull base and brain. Radiology. 183(1):137-44, 1992

TERMINOLOGY

- Definition: Nonspecific, nonneoplastic benign inflammatory lesion without identifiable local or systemic causes characterized by polymorphous lymphoplasmacytic infiltrate
- Idiopathic orbital inflammation (IOI)
  - May involve any part(s) of orbit
- Idiopathic extraorbital inflammation
  - **Intracranial involvement**: Spread through superior orbital fissure (SOF) or optic canal (OC)
    - Cavernous sinus, dura, Meckel cave
  - **Skull base-extracranial involvement**: Spreads from inferior orbital fissure (IOF) or through orbital wall
    - Anterior skull base, sinuses, nasopharyngeal spaces
- IgG4-related disease: Subgroup of idiopathic inflammation with systemic involvement
  - Intracranial noncontiguous sites: Pituitary, infundibulum
  - Extracranial noncontiguous H&N sites: Parotid, submandibular glands, thyroid

IMAGING

- T1WI C+ FS MR: Diffusely enhancing, infiltrating mass
  - Extends from orbit through SOF ± OC to cavernous sinus, dura, Meckel cave
  - Extends through IOF to pterygopalatine fossa, nose, deep nasopharyngeal spaces
- T2: Iso- to **hypointense** lesion; ↑ fibrosis, ↓ intensity

TOP DIFFERENTIAL DIAGNOSES

- En plaque meningioma
- Meningeal non-Hodgkin lymphoma
- Nasopharyngeal carcinoma
- Neurosarcoid

CLINICAL ISSUES

- Symptoms: Painful proptosis ± headaches ± cranial neuropathies
- Diagnosis of exclusion; must be biopsied
- Treatment: High-dose systemic **steroids**

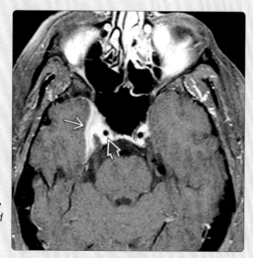
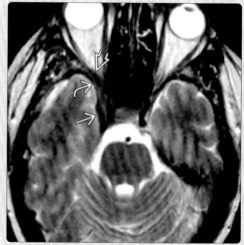

(Left) Axial T1WI C+ FS MR shows a focus of enhancing idiopathic extraorbital inflammation (IEI) involving the right cavernous sinus ➡ with subtle narrowing ➡ of the intracavernous internal carotid artery. (Right) Axial T2WI MR in the same patient reveals an idiopathic orbital inflammation (IOI) lesion ➡ connects to the cavernous sinus IEI ➡ through the superior orbital fissure (SOF) ➡. Both areas of idiopathic inflammation are hypointense due to the fibrosis often found within this lesion.

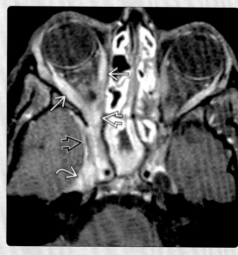
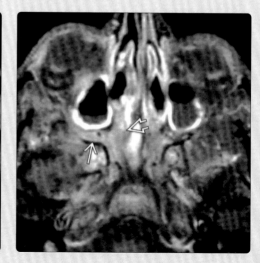

(Left) Axial T1WI C+ FS MR through the orbits shows enlarged, enhancing orbital rectus muscles ➡ connecting through the SOF ➡ with the cavernous sinus ➡ and Meckel cave ➡. The initial impression of adenoid cystic carcinoma gave way to biopsy-proven idiopathic inflammation with both intraorbital and intracranial components. (Right) Axial T1WI C+ FS MR in the same patient shows the lesion invading inferiorly through the inferior orbital fissure into the pterygopalatine fossa ➡ and nose ➡.

TERMINOLOGY

Abbreviations
- Idiopathic extraorbital inflammation (IEI)

Synonyms
- Idiopathic inflammatory disease, Tolosa-Hunt syndrome, hypertrophic cranial pachymeningitis, plasma cell granuloma

Definitions
- Nonspecific, nonneoplastic benign inflammatory lesion without identifiable local or systemic causes characterized by polymorphous lymphoplasmacytic infiltrate
  - IgG4-related disease (IgG4-RD): Subgroup of idiopathic orbital inflammation (IOI) IEI lesions where multisystem manifestation is present with positive cell immunostain showing IgG4-rich plasma cells

IMAGING

General Features
- Best diagnostic clue
  - IOI combined with contiguous extraorbital (intracranial, skull base, or extracranial) idiopathic inflammation
- Location
  - IOI
    - May involve any part(s) of orbit
  - IEI
    - **Intracranial involvement**: Spread through superior orbital fissure (SOF) or optic canal (OC)
      - □ Cavernous sinus
      - □ Dural thickening (previously called "pachymeningitis")
      - □ Meckel cave area
      - □ Noncontiguous IgG4-RD: Pituitary, infundibulum
    - **Skull base-extracranial involvement**: Spreads from inferior orbital fissure (IOF) or through orbital wall
      - □ Pterygopalatine fossa, nose, sinuses
      - □ Anterior skull base, sinuses
      - □ Deep spaces of nasopharynx
      - □ Noncontiguous IgG4-RD: Parotid, submandibular glands, thyroid
- Size
  - Small, subtle to very extensive extraorbital involvement
  - Skull base and extracranial soft tissue masses may be large (many centimeters)
- Morphology
  - Soft tissue infiltrating lesions mimic invasive malignancy

CT Findings
- CECT
  - Orbital enhancing, infiltrating mass with extension through SOF or OC to cavernous sinus, dura, skull base
    - If extension through IOF, lesion reaches pterygopalatine fossa, nose, sinuses, deep spaces
    - If extension through orbital wall, sinuses or anterior skull base affected
- Bone CT
  - Associated bone erosion unusual
- CTA

- If cavernous internal carotid artery (ICA) involved, often narrowed

MR Findings
- T1WI
  - Lesion isointense to gray matter
- T2WI
  - Iso- to **hypointense** infiltrating mass
    - Increased **fibrosis** yields increased hypointensity
- FLAIR
  - No adjacent brain edema
- T1WI C+
  - Orbital enhancing, infiltrating lesion spread to intra- ± extracranial contiguous sites
    - Extends though SOF-OC to cavernous sinus, local dura, Meckel cave
    - Extends through IOF to pterygopalatine fossa, nose, sinuses, deep spaces
    - If extension through orbital wall, sinuses or anterior skull base affected
- MRA
  - If cavernous sinus involved, **ICA narrowing** common

Imaging Recommendations
- Best imaging tool
  - MR: Delineates extraorbital intracranial and extracranial extensions best
- Protocol advice
  - Begin with MR, including full brain FLAIR and T1WI C+ with fat saturation
    - T1 C+ FS best sequence
  - Bone CT may help differentiate this lesion from en plaque meningioma

DIFFERENTIAL DIAGNOSIS

En Plaque Meningioma
- Enhancing meningeal mass with dural tails
- Permeative-sclerotic invasive bone changes typical
- May exactly mimic intracranial IEI

Meningeal Non-Hodgkin Lymphoma
- More diffuse, multifocal with underlying bone involvement
- "Great pretender" (can mimic many intracranial diseases)

Nasopharyngeal Carcinoma
- Arises in nasopharyngeal mucosal space
- Invades cephalad into skull base, sinuses
- Orbit usually spared

Neurosarcoid
- Systemic manifestations abound
- Increased erythrocyte sedimentation rate (ESR) and serum angiotensin converting enzyme (ACE)

Skull and Meningeal Metastases
- Simultaneous orbital metastases unusual
- Nodular meningeal carcinomatosis less common than diffuse carcinomatosis
- Cranial neuropathy occurs early

PATHOLOGY

General Features

- Etiology
  - Benign inflammatory process of unknown origin
  - Immune-autoimmune pathophysiology suspected
  - IgG4-RD is now recognized as subgroup of IOI-IEI

Microscopic Features

- Characteristic histopathologic features of IOI and IEI
  - Diffuse lymphoplasmacytic infiltration
  - Varying degrees of **fibrosis** present

IgG4-Related Disease Subtype Additional Features

- Microscopic features
  - IgG4-RD subgroup: IgG4-rich plasma cells
  - IgG4-RD subgroup: Mild to moderate eosinophil infiltrate
- Immunohistochemical features
  - Semiquantitative analysis of **IgG4 immunostaining** may provide compelling features
    - > 30 IgG4-positive cells per high-power field
    - IgG4:IgG ratio > 50%
    - Lower values of IgG4-positive cells acceptable for diagnosis when characteristic microscopic appearance is present
- Serum IgG4 levels
  - Serum IgG4 is not by itself sufficient to diagnose IgG4-related disease
  - Serum IgG4 is elevated in majority (can reach ≥ 25x normal) but can be seen in 20-40% of normals

CLINICAL ISSUES

Presentation

- Most common signs/symptoms
  - IOI and IEI
    - Orbital lesion: **Painful proptosis**
    - Intracranial lesion only: Chronic headaches
    - Cavernous sinus: Cranial neuropathy (CNIII, IV, V, VI)
    - Extracranial soft tissues: Focal or diffuse mass
      □ Sinonasal, nasopharyngeal space mass
  - IgG-RD subtype: Other sites involved
    - Tumor-like lesion with indolent disease course (develops over months to years)
    - Head and neck: Salivary glands > thyroid gland, lymph nodes, laryngeal disease
      □ Orbit: Bilateral > unilateral proptosis ± CNII symptoms from optic nerve compression
      □ Suprahyoid neck: Chronic sialoadenitis (submandibular = Küttner tumor; parotid = Mikulicz disease)
      □ Infrahyoid neck: Hypothyroidism ± goiter (Hashimoto and Riedel thyroiditis); lymph nodes
    - Involvement outside of head and neck
      □ Brain: Pituitary hypophysitis
      □ Chest: Lung lesions; fibrosing mediastinitis and pleuritis
      □ Abdomen: Type 1 autoimmune pancreatitis, sclerosing cholangitis, cholecystitis, renal lesions, retroperitoneal fibrosis
      □ Vascular: Aortitis, arteritis

- Clinical profile
  - Adult presenting with painful proptosis, headaches, and cranial nerve palsies

Demographics

- Age
  - Extraorbital: Adults (40-65 years of age)

Natural History & Prognosis

- Idiopathic intraorbital and extraorbital inflammation
  - Rapid response to steroid therapy common
  - When extensive extraorbital involvement present, may be resistant to all therapies
    - May cause severe disability or death

Treatment

- Options, risks, complications
  - **Diagnosis of exclusion**
    - Extraorbital disease must be biopsied
    - Biopsy excludes infectious and neoplastic (meningioma, NHL) causes of focal dural thickening
  - **High-dose systemic steroids** with slow taper is principal treatment option
    - 70% success rate
  - Steroid-resistant cases ± cases with extensive skull base involvement
    - Radiotherapy ± chemotherapy
    - Surgical resection as possible

DIAGNOSTIC CHECKLIST

Consider

- IEI is diagnosis of exclusion
  - 1st exclude infection and malignancy with biopsy
  - Realize that intracranial IEI affecting dura and hypertrophic cranial pachymeningitis are same disease

Image Interpretation Pearls

- If infiltrating mass in orbit with contiguous dural and cavernous sinus lesion, consider IEI
- IOI alone > > IOI + IEI > > IEI alone (rare)
- If IOI + IEI with noncontiguous head and neck lesions of salivary glands, thyroid, lymph nodes ± systemic disease, consider subgroup IgG-RD
  - Recommend IgG4 immunostaining of tissue biopsy and serum IgG4 analysis

SELECTED REFERENCES

1. Bhatti RM et al: IgG4-related disease of the head and neck. Adv Anat Pathol. 20(1):10-6, 2013
2. Fujita A et al: IgG4-related disease of the head and neck: CT and MR imaging manifestations. Radiographics. 32(7):1945-58, 2012
3. Toyoda K et al: MR imaging of IgG4-related disease in the head and neck and brain. AJNR Am J Neuroradiol. 33(11):2136-9, 2012
4. Battineni ML et al: Idiopathic hypereosinophilic syndrome with skull base involvement. AJNR Am J Neuroradiol. 28(5):971-3, 2007
5. Mangiardi JR et al: Extraorbital skull base idiopathic pseudotumor. Laryngoscope. 117(4):589-94, 2007
6. Narla LD et al: Inflammatory pseudotumor. Radiographics. 23(3):719-29, 2003
7. Cho YS et al: Inflammatory pseudotumour involving the skull base and cervical spine. J Laryngol Otol. 115(7):580-4, 2001
8. Bencherif B et al: Intracranial extension of an idiopathic orbital inflammatory pseudotumor. AJNR Am J Neuroradiol. 14(1):181-4, 1993

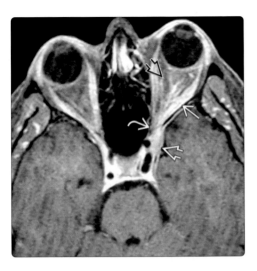
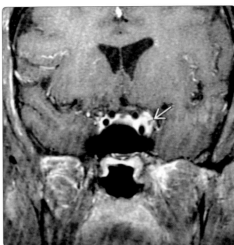

(Left) In this patient with painful proptosis, axial T1WI C+ FS MR shows an intraorbital lateral rectus ➡ and intraconal ⧉ lesion. Note the idiopathic inflammation spreads through the (SOF) ➡ to the anterior cavernous sinus ➡. (Right) Coronal T1WI C+ FS MR in the same patient shows the intracranial extension of the lesion into the left cavernous sinus ➡. Idiopathic orbital inflammation extending into the cavernous sinus is the most common form of extraorbital extension.

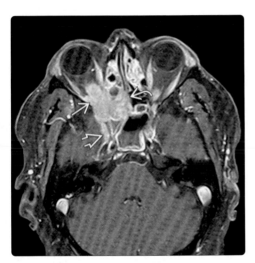
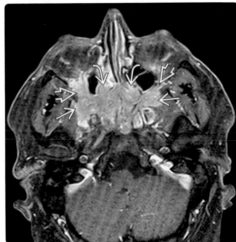

(Left) Axial T1WI C+ FS MR shows extensive orbital apex ➡, ethmoid sinus ➡, and foramen rotundum ➡ infiltrating, enhancing idiopathic inflammation. (Right) On a more inferior slice in the same patient, axial T1WI C+ FS MR reveals bilateral pterygopalatine fossa ➡ involvement with continuous intranasal IEI ➡. Both inferior orbital fissures are also affected ➡. Large IOI-IEI deposits often respond poorly to steroid treatment.

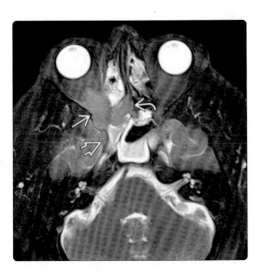
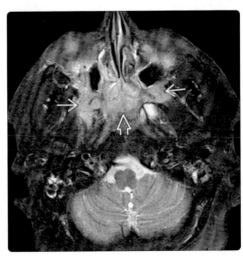

(Left) Axial T2WI FS MR in the same patient shows an infiltrating idiopathic inflammation in the orbital apex ➡, ethmoid sinus ➡, and foramen rotundum ➡. Hyperintense obstructed sinuses are easily differentiated from the IOI-IEI. Hypointensity results from diffuse fibrosis often seen within larger lesions. (Right) Axial T2WI FS MR in the same patient shows extensive IEI involving the pterygopalatine fossae ➡ and posterior nose ➡.

Skull Base Giant Cell Tumor

TERMINOLOGY

- Giant cell tumor (GCT)
- Benign intraosseous neoplasm arising from **multinucleated giant cells**

IMAGING

- CT: **Expansile** intraosseous soft tissue mass with thinned surrounding **cortical shell**
- MR: **Hypointense rim** & prominent internal enhancement
- Sphenoid bone > temporal bone > > frontal bone

TOP DIFFERENTIAL DIAGNOSES

- Aneurysmal bone cyst (ABC)
- Chordoma
- Chondrosarcoma
- Fibrous dysplasia
- Plasmacytoma

PATHOLOGY

- Hemorrhage/hemosiderin deposition common
- Overlap with other giant cell containing tumors, such as giant cell lesion, aneurysmal bone cyst, brown tumor, pigmented villonodular synovitis
- Major neoplastic component of GCT comprised by the stromal cells, not the multinucleated giant cells

CLINICAL ISSUES

- Rare lesion: 2% of all GCT arise in skull base
- Peak incidence: 3rd-4th decade
- Metastases in 2% of cases
- Recurrence rate 40-60% after resection

DIAGNOSTIC CHECKLIST

- If in patient < 30 yr of age, consider fibrous dysplasia
- If lesion centered in sella & normal pituitary not seen, consider invasive adenoma
- If patient has known malignancy, consider metastasis

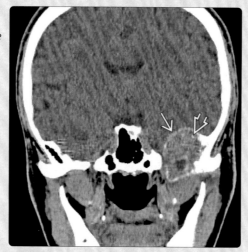
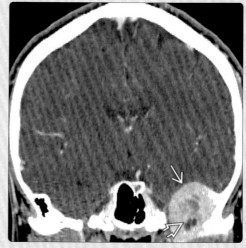

(Left) Coronal NECT image demonstrates expansile mass centered in floor of left middle cranial fossa. There is thin peripheral (egg shell) calcification ➡, as well as specks of internal matrix calcification ➡. (Right) Coronal CECT image of same patient shows the mass enhances intensely ➡, except for areas of cystic change ➡.

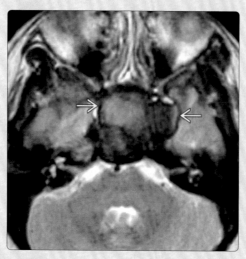
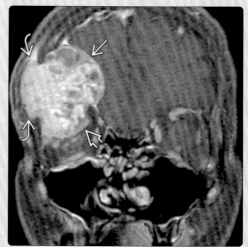

(Left) Axial T2WI MR shows expansile sphenoid giant cell tumor with central heterogeneous hypointensity with a markedly hypointense rim ➡. Fibrous dysplasia may mimic this appearance. (Right) Coronal T1 C+ FS MR demonstrates a giant cell tumor in its least common skull base location, the frontal bone. There is intracranial ➡ and extracranial ➡ extension, including involvement of the superior orbit ➡.

TERMINOLOGY

Abbreviations

- Giant cell tumor (GCT)

Synonyms

- Osteoclastoma

Definitions

- Benign intraosseous neoplasm featuring **multinucleated giant cells**

IMAGING

General Features

- Best diagnostic clue
  - CT: **Expansile** intraosseous soft tissue mass with thin surrounding cortical shell
  - MR: **Hypointense rim** with prominent internal enhancement
- Location
  - Sphenoid bone > temporal bone > > frontal bone
- Size
  - Variable, usually > 3 cm

CT Findings

- NECT
  - Mildly hyperdense soft tissue mass
- CECT
  - Marked enhancement
- Bone CT
  - Overlying **cortical shell** may be focally dehiscent
  - Occasional scant matrix calcification

MR Findings

- T1WI
  - Mixed iso- to hyperintense to gray matter
  - **Hypointense rim** common
- T2WI
  - Mixed iso- to hyperintense to gray matter
    - Occasionally diffusely hypointense (due to hemosiderin, calcification)
  - Markedly hypointense rim
- T1WI C+
  - Marked enhancement

DIFFERENTIAL DIAGNOSIS

Aneurysmal Bone Cyst

- Soap bubble appearance with blood-fluid levels
- May arise secondarily from GCT

Chordoma

- Destructive midline clival mass with bone fragments

Chondrosarcoma

- Eccentric erosive mass, chondroid calcifications

Fibrous Dysplasia

- Diffuse ground-glass density, hypointense on T2WI
- < 30 yr old, rarely progressive

Plasmacytoma

- Homogeneous soft tissue mass
- Solitary or seen in association with multiple myeloma

PATHOLOGY

General Features

- Etiology
  - Unknown
  - Can arise secondarily in pagetoid bone

Microscopic Features

- Multinucleated osteoclastic giant cells, often with hemorrhage/hemosiderin
- Light microscopic findings very similar to other lesions with giant cells
  - Patient demographics, lesion location, and radiographic features often necessary to arrive at specific diagnosis
    - Giant cell lesion (formerly known as giant cell reparative granuloma)
    - Brown tumor
    - Aneurysmal bone cyst and pigmented villonodular synovitis

CLINICAL ISSUES

Presentation

- Most common signs/symptoms
  - Headache & local pain
  - Cranial nerve palsies
- Other signs/symptoms
  - Sphenoid GCT: Diplopia, ophthalmoplegia
  - Temporal bone (TB) GCT: Otalgia, hearing loss, facial palsy, TMJ dysfunction

Demographics

- Age
  - Peak incidence: 3rd-4th decade
- Gender
  - Female predominance
- Epidemiology
  - Only 2% of all GCT in skull base

Natural History & Prognosis

- Rare sarcomatous transformation
  - Usually seen only after radiation therapy
- Metastases in 2% of cases

Treatment

- Preoperative embolization
- Surgical resection/curettage
  - Reported recurrence rate after resection: 40-60%
- Radiation therapy for inoperable lesions

SELECTED REFERENCES

1. Billingsley JT et al: A locally invasive giant cell tumor of the skull base: case report. J Neurol Surg Rep. 75(1):e175-9, 2014
2. Prasad SC et al: Giant cell tumors of the skull base: case series and current concepts. Audiol Neurootol. 19(1):12-21, 2014
3. Chakarun CJ et al: Giant cell tumor of bone: review, mimics, and new developments in treatment. Radiographics. 33(1):197-211, 2013
4. Kim Y et al: Modern interpretation of giant cell tumor of bone: predominantly osteoclastogenic stromal tumor. Clin Orthop Surg. 4(2):107-16, 2012
5. Isaacson B et al: Giant-cell tumors of the temporal bone: management strategies. Skull Base. 19(4):291-301, 2009

TERMINOLOGY

- Benign extraaxial neoplasm arising from arachnoid cap cells

IMAGING

- Anterior skull base: Olfactory groove, tuberculum sella, and sphenoid wing
- Central skull base: Petroclival and pericavernous
- Posterior skull base: Lower clival and foramen magnum
- Morphology: Sessile (en plaque)/lentiform > globose/spherical
- CT findings
  - Hyperdense, homogeneously enhancing mass
  - 25% intramural calcification
  - Hyperostosis > permeative sclerotic
- MR findings
  - Isointense to gray matter with prominent enhancement
  - Enhancing reactive dural tail in 60%
  - Cerebrospinal fluid-vascular cleft between tumor and parenchyma

TOP DIFFERENTIAL DIAGNOSES

- Skull base schwannoma
- Giant pituitary macroadenoma
- Chordoma
- Skull base/dural metastasis
- Sarcoidosis

CLINICAL ISSUES

- 2nd most common primary intracranial tumor
- Middle-aged to elderly patients
- M:F = 1:3

DIAGNOSTIC CHECKLIST

- Assess involvement of critical skull base structures: Optic canal, vessels, cavernous sinus, Meckel cave

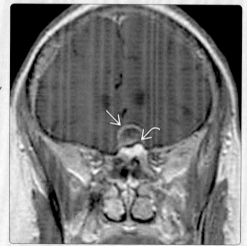
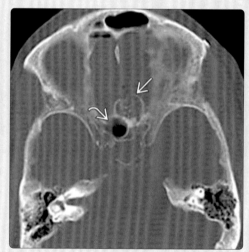

(Left) Coronal T1WI C+ MR demonstrates a peripherally enhancing mass ➡ based along the floor of the anterior fossa. Although the central low signal is atypical (reflecting heavy calcification), the presence of hyperostosis and upward "blistering" ➡ of the planum sphenoidale is highly characteristic of meningioma. (Right) Axial bone CT in the same patient shows the calcified meningioma ➡ along the planum sphenoidale, with accompanying pneumatosis dilatans of the adjacent sphenoid sinus ➡.

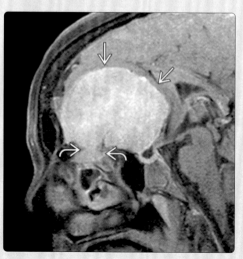
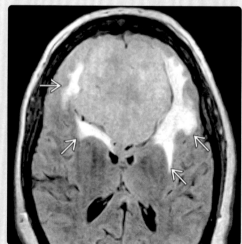

(Left) Sagittal T1WI C+ FS MR shows a large, avidly enhancing anterior cranial fossa meningioma buckling the medial frontal lobe ➡. There is inferior extension through the cribriform plate into the olfactory recess of the nasal cavity ➡. (Right) Axial FLAIR MR in the same patient demonstrates signal intensity similar to gray matter, with only mild heterogeneity. There is extensive peritumoral edema ➡, a finding that increases surgical morbidity and likelihood of recurrence.

TERMINOLOGY

Definitions

- Benign extraaxial neoplasm arising from arachnoid cap cells

IMAGING

General Features

- Best diagnostic clue
  - Avidly enhancing, extraaxial **dural-based mass with enhancing tails**
- Location
  - **Anterior skull base** (40% of intracranial meningiomas)
    - 50% in olfactory groove and tuberculum sella
      - 15% of olfactory groove meningiomas grow into sinonasal cavity
      - Tuberculum sella meningiomas may grow into 1 or both optic canals
    - 50% in sphenoid wing
      - Clinoidal (medial sphenoid wing)
      - Spheno-orbital (lateral sphenoid wing); most frequently symptomatic
  - **Central skull base**
    - Petroclival (upper clivus, cavernous sinus, tentorium, and petrous apex)
  - **Posterior skull base**
    - Lower clival, foramen magnum
      - Foramen magnum lesions may be posterior, anterior, or lateral
  - Additional skull base locations: Cerebellopontine angle/internal auditory canal, temporal bone, jugular foramen
- Morphology
  - Sessile/lentiform > globose/spherical
  - Occasional en plaque configuration
    - Carpet-like tumor overlying hyperostotic bone
    - Common in spheno-orbital lesions (lateral sphenoid wing)

CT Findings

- NECT
  - **75% hyperdense** compared with brain parenchyma
  - **25% intramural calcification**
    - May occasionally be entirely calcified
- CECT
  - 90% show strong, uniform enhancement
- Bone CT
  - Hyperostotic > permeative sclerotic adjacent bone changes
    - **Hyperostotic bone** may or may not be invaded
    - Upward "blistering" may be seen along planum sphenoidale
      - **Pneumosinus dilatans** of adjacent sphenoid sinus may occur

MR Findings

- T1WI
  - Hypo- to isointense to gray matter
    - May be low or absent signal in heavily calcified areas
  - Rare ↑ signal in foci of hemorrhage
- T2WI
  - Hypo- to isointense to gray matter
  - 25% atypical appearance with ↑ signal in necrosis, cysts
  - **Cerebrospinal fluid-vascular cleft** at periphery of large lesions
    - Thin space between tumor and brain containing fluid and vessels
  - Peritumoral brain edema correlates with pial blood supply
    - Increased incidence surgical morbidity and early recurrence
- T2* GRE
  - If significantly calcified, may "bloom"
- T1WI C+
  - **Prominent enhancement in 95%**
    - Enhancing dural tail in 60%
  - Meningioma within cavernous sinus typically enhances to lesser degree than uninvolved sinus

Angiographic Findings

- Dural vessels supply center, pial vessels supply periphery
- Sunburst or spoke-wheel pattern of enlarged dural feeders common
- Prolonged vascular "stain" into venous phase

Imaging Recommendations

- Best imaging tool
  - Enhanced, fat-suppressed MR generally best for precise tumor mapping

DIFFERENTIAL DIAGNOSIS

Trigeminal Schwannoma

- Parasellar mass, often with cystic components
- May extend through trigeminal exit foramina or prepontine cistern

Giant Pituitary Macroadenoma

- Large, invasive mass with skull base invasion
- No identifiable normal pituitary tissue

Clival Chordoma

- Midline destructive mass
- High T2 signal; heterogeneous enhancement

Chondrosarcoma

- Eccentric mass with chondroid matrix
- ↑ T2 signal

Skull Base Metastasis

- Variable appearance depending on histology of primary and whether metastases are to skull base marrow or dura
  - Multiple dural-based, enhancing masses

Plasmacytoma

- Lytic destructive mass of clivus
- May be solitary or multiple in setting of multiple myeloma

Neurosarcoid

- Multifocal, dural-based, enhancing foci
- Look for infundibular stalk enhancement and enlargement

Rosai-Dorfman Disease

- Rare histiocytic disease

- May demonstrate multiple dural-based, T2-hypointense masses

PATHOLOGY

General Features

- Etiology
  - Most are sporadic
  - Multiple inherited schwannomas, meningiomas, and ependymomas (MISME) in neurofibromatosis type 2 (NF2)
  - Increased incidence following radiotherapy
    - More commonly over convexities than skull base
    - Develop 20-35 years following radiation
- Genetics
  - Mutations in *NF2* gene on chromosome 22 are detected in ~ in 60% of sporadic meningiomas

Staging, Grading, & Classification

- WHO classification (2016)
  - Grade I: Benign (90%), e.g., meningothelial
  - Grade II: Atypical (7%), e.g., clear cell
  - Grade III: Anaplastic/malignant (2%), e.g., rhabdoid
- Grade II and III meningiomas are less common at skull base than along convexities
- Poor correlation between histologic grade and imaging features

Gross Pathologic & Surgical Features

- Semilunar or en plaque > round or globose
- Sharply circumscribed
- Adjacent dural thickening (tail)
  - **Not specific for meningioma**; may accompany any dural-based process
  - Usually reactive, not neoplastic

Microscopic Features

- Arise from meningothelial (arachnoid "cap") cells
  - Relatively uniform cells with tendency to form whorls
  - Fibrous content correlates with T2 signal hypointensity
- Psammoma bodies (laminated calcific concretions)
- Highly vascularized

CLINICAL ISSUES

Presentation

- Most common signs/symptoms
  - May be incidental finding
    - 33% of incidental intracranial neoplasms
  - Symptoms often nonspecific
    - Headache
    - Dizziness
    - Syncope
- Other signs/symptoms
  - Anterior skull base: Anosmia, visual loss, proptosis
  - Central skull base: Ophthalmoplegia
  - Posterior skull base: Myelopathy, lower cranial neuropathy

Demographics

- Age
  - Middle-aged to elderly patients
  - Peak age: 60 years
- Gender
  - M:F = 1:3
- Epidemiology
  - 2nd most common primary intracranial tumor
  - Most common extraaxial tumor
  - 15-25% of primary intracranial tumors
  - 10% multiple (NF2; multiple meningiomatosis)

Natural History & Prognosis

- Indolent course is typical
- More aggressive course in WHO grade II/III lesions
- Those with peritumoral brain edema have **higher surgical complication and recurrence rates**

Treatment

- Surgery most likely to achieve cure but often requires complex combined approach with significant morbidity risk
  - Preoperative angiography/embolization may be employed to reduce intraoperative blood loss
  - Simpson grading system used to estimate completeness of resection
    - Grade I (complete removal including dura and underlying bone) → grade IV (subtotal resection)
  - Prognosis for cure more dependent on tumor location than grade
- Radiotherapy/radiosurgery may be used primarily or adjunctive when resection is incomplete

DIAGNOSTIC CHECKLIST

Consider

- Solitary, enhancing, dural-based extraaxial mass = meningioma, particularly in adult patient without known malignancy

Reporting Tips

- Assess caliber of internal carotid, basilar, or vertebral arteries if surrounded by tumor
  - Meningioma often narrows internal carotid artery
    - Other parasellar lesions, such as schwannoma, macroadenoma, and lymphoma, typically will not
- Assess for Meckel cave or optic canal involvement
- Always **search for 2nd meningioma**
  - Multiple meningiomas in 10% of sporadic cases
- Report brain edema, as it increases rate of surgical morbidity and recurrence

SELECTED REFERENCES

1. Louis DN et al: The 2016 World Health Organization Classification of Tumors of the Central Nervous System: a summary. Acta Neuropathol. 131(6):803-20, 2016
2. Lin BJ et al: Correlation between magnetic resonance imaging grading and pathological grading in meningioma. J Neurosurg. 121(5):1201-8, 2014
3. Saraf et al: Update on meningomas. Oncologist. 16(11):1604-1613, 2011
4. Hsu CC et al: Do aggressive imaging features correlate with advanced histopathological grade in meningiomas? J Clin Neurosci. 17(5):584-7, 2010
5. Li Y et al: Sphenoid wing meningioma en plaque: report of 37 cases. Chin Med J (Engl). 122(20):2423-7, 2009
6. Minniti G et al: Radiotherapy and radiosurgery for benign skull base meningiomas. Radiat Oncol. 4:42, 2009
7. Mirone G et al: En plaque sphenoid wing meningiomas: recurrence factors and surgical strategy in a series of 71 patients. Neurosurgery. 65(6 Suppl):100-8; discussion 108-9, 2009

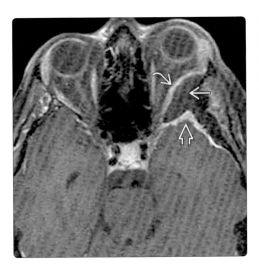

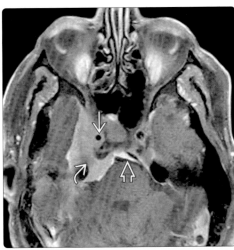

(Left) *Axial T1WI C+ FS MR in a patient with left proptosis reveals an en plaque meningioma of the left sphenoid wing characterized by striking hyperostosis ➡ and only thin intraorbital ➡ and intracranial ➡ rinds of enhancing tumor.* (Right) *Axial T1WI C+ FS MR demonstrates a meningioma of the central skull base encasing and narrowing the right internal carotid artery ➡. The tumor extends through the porus trigeminus ➡ into the prepontine cistern. A dural tail is present medially ➡.*

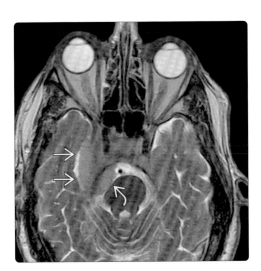

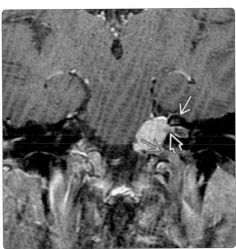

(Left) *Axial T2WI MR in the same patient shows a central skull base meningioma approximately isointense to gray matter with a CSF-vascular cleft between the tumor and the displaced temporal lobe ➡. The small posterior fossa component is associated with deformity of the pons ➡.* (Right) *Coronal T1WI C+ FS MR shows an extraaxial mass based along medial surface of petrous bone with involvement of the internal auditory canal (IAC) ➡ and jugular foramen ➡. There is hyperostosis of the roof of the IAC ➡.*

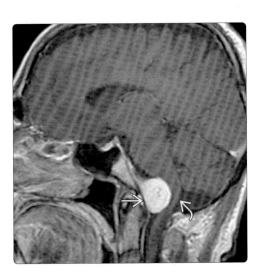

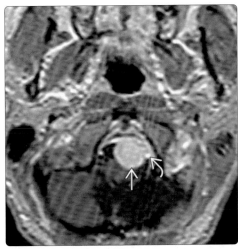

(Left) *Sagittal T1WI C+ MR shows a globose mass at the anterior foramen magnum ➡ buckling the medulla posteriorly ➡. The broad base along the dura favors meningioma over other foramen magnum lesions, such as schwannoma.* (Right) *Axial T1WI C+ MR shows an anterior foramen magnum meningioma ➡ lying medial to the left vertebral artery ➡. Given the plethora of critical vascular and neural structures at the skull base, resection of even small lesions may be difficult.*

Skull Base Plasmacytoma

KEY FACTS

TERMINOLOGY

- Abbreviations: Solitary bone plasmacytoma (SBP), extramedullary plasmacytoma (EMP), multiple myeloma (MM)
- Definition: Isolated intramedullary or extramedullary neoplasm of plasma cells in absence of clinical or radiographic findings of MM

IMAGING

- CT findings
  - SBP: Solitary intraosseous, **lytic mass with nonsclerotic margins**
  - EMP: Sinonasal mass with secondary osseous invasion of skull base
- MR findings
  - Homogeneously enhancing intraosseous/extraosseous skull base mass
  - More sensitive for marrow space involvement and excluding additional small/early lesions

- Bone CT best defines trabecular and cortical destruction
- MR best defines marrow extent & extraosseous soft tissue tumor

TOP DIFFERENTIAL DIAGNOSES

- Multiple myeloma
- Skull base metastasis
- Invasive pituitary macroadenoma
- Chordoma

PATHOLOGY

- Monoclonal proliferation of immunoglobulin-secreting plasma cells

CLINICAL ISSUES

- Symptoms: Local pain, headache, cranial nerve deficits
- M > F in 5th-9th decade
- SBP has higher rate of conversion to MM than EMP
- If skull base plasmacytoma diagnosed, complete clinical and radiologic work-up for MM required

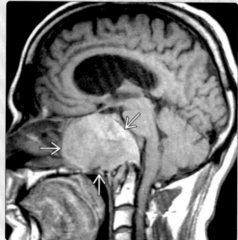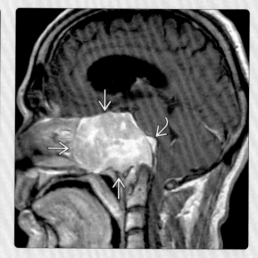

(Left) Sagittal T1WI MR in a 61-year-old man demonstrates a large solitary mass ➡ expanding the clivus, obliterating the sphenoid sinus, and extending into the posterior nasal cavity and nasopharynx. The plasmacytoma is slightly hyperintense to brain parenchyma. (Right) Sagittal T1WI C+ MR shows heterogeneous enhancement of the lesion ➡ without necrosis. Dural thickening ➡ is noted posteriorly as epidural extension begins to compress the medulla.

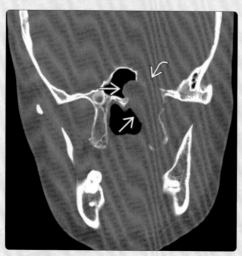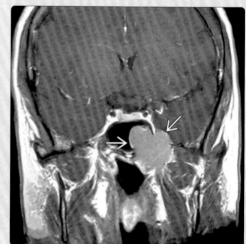

(Left) Coronal bone CT in a 45-year-old woman with sinus pain demonstrates an expansile mass ➡ centered in the left sphenoid bone. The mass expands medially into the sphenoid sinus and erodes medial floor of the middle cranial fossa ➡. The margins of the tumor are relatively sharp, and in some areas there is preservation of thin eggshell margin of cortical bone. (Right) Coronal T1WI C+ MR demonstrates homogeneous enhancement of this skull base plasmacytoma ➡.

TERMINOLOGY

Abbreviations

- Solitary bone plasmacytoma (SBP)
- Extramedullary plasmacytoma (EMP)
- Multiple myeloma (MM)

Definitions

- Solitary bone plasmacytoma
  - Monoclonal plasma cell neoplasm of bone marrow seen in absence of other criteria to fulfill diagnosis of MM
  - Generally presents as single osteolytic lesion
  - Can affect any bone of skull base, but has predilection for sphenoid bone and petrous apex
- Extramedullary plasmacytoma
  - Solitary extraosseous plasma cell proliferation in absence of other criteria to fulfill diagnosis of MM
- Multiple solitary plasmacytoma
  - Multiple sites of extramedullary or osseous lesions in absence of MM criteria
- Malignant plasmacytoma
  - Focal intramedullary or extramedullary tumor in context of MM
  - Once diagnosis of MM is established, most no longer use term plasmacytoma

IMAGING

General Features

- Best diagnostic clue
  - CT shows solitary intraosseous mass causing **lytic destruction** of skull base
- Location
  - SBP: Epicenter is marrow space of sphenoid, temporal (petrous), or occipital bones
    - Soft tissue mass may be isolated to bone
    - Can have significant extraosseous soft tissue component
  - EMP: Involves skull base secondarily when lesion originates in sinonasal cavities, orbit, or nasopharynx
    - Sinonasal region is most common site of origin
    - Predominantly extraosseous with secondary skull base invasion
    - EMPs that occur in nasopharynx or sphenoid sinus can invade clivus and be indistinguishable from SBPs
    - Rarely affects dura or leptomeninges primarily
- Morphology
  - SBP: Intraosseous mass with biconvex expansion of involved bone, ± extraosseous mass
  - EMP: Infiltrative soft tissue mass adjacent to skull base with secondary osseous erosion

CT Findings

- NECT
  - Hyperdense (relative to muscle or brain) soft tissue attenuation
- CECT
  - Mild-moderate homogeneous enhancement
  - Epidural space involvement common
- Bone CT
  - SBP: Lytic lesion with **scalloped, nonsclerotic margins**

- No tumoral calcification, but peripherally displaced osseous fragments may be seen

MR Findings

- T1WI
  - Homogeneous, iso- to hypointense to gray matter (GM)
- T2WI
  - Homogeneous, isointense to GM most often
- STIR
  - Homogeneous, iso- or hyperintense to GM
- FLAIR
  - Homogeneous, iso- or hyperintense to GM
- T1WI C+
  - Moderate, homogeneous enhancement

Nuclear Medicine Findings

- Bone scan
  - No Tc-99m pertechnetate uptake (cold lesion)
- PET/CT
  - Moderate to marked FDG uptake

Imaging Recommendations

- Best imaging tool
  - Bone CT best defines trabecular and cortical destruction
  - MR best defines marrow extent & extraosseous soft tissue tumor
- Protocol advice
  - MR of skull base to include **multiplanar T1, followed by T1 C+ FS** in same planes for direct comparison
  - Follow with bone CT without contrast to assess bony margins & extent of bone destruction
  - **Whole-body work-up** necessary to confirm isolated nature of solitary plasmacytoma & exclude MM

DIFFERENTIAL DIAGNOSIS

Multiple Myeloma

- Key is identifying additional lesions
- Multiple radiolucent lesions on radiographs & CT
- MR shows additional focal bone marrow lesions or diffuse marrow replacement

Skull Base Metastasis

- Known primary tumor
- Multiple lesions common

Invasive Pituitary Macroadenoma

- Expansile mass of clivus indistinguishable from pituitary gland
- Predominant growth vector of macroadenoma is inferior into clivus and sphenoid sinus

Chordoma

- Solitary midline clivus lesion
- May contain calcifications or ossific fragments on CT
- Typically very hyperintense on T2 MR

Non-Hodgkin Lymphoma

- Soft tissue mass with bony destruction of skull base
- Secondary invasion of skull base from nasal cavity site of origin

Skull Base Meningioma

- Dural meningioma can invade bony skull base secondarily
  - Dural component may be inconspicuous compared with invasive osseous component
- Rarely meningioma originates from intraosseous location
- Permeative, sclerotic expansile intraosseous mass on CT
- Avid enhancement on CT & MR

Nasopharyngeal Carcinoma

- Mass originates in nasopharyngeal mucosal space
- Destructive upward invasion of basisphenoid & basiocciput

Giant Cell Tumor

- Expansile intraosseous clival neoplasm arising from multinucleated giant cells

PATHOLOGY

General Features

- SBP: Monoclonal proliferation of immunoglobulin-secreting plasma cells
  - Considered benign in absence of MM criteria and no conversion to MM in 3-yr period

Staging, Grading, & Classification

- 2 types
  - Plasmacytic plasmacytomas
  - Plasmablastic plasmacytomas

Gross Pathologic & Surgical Features

- Bony defects filled with soft, red tumor of gelatinous consistency

Microscopic Features

- Plasma cells in reticular stroma
- Plasmacytic plasmacytomas
  - Mature plasma cells with eccentric round nuclei, condensed clumped chromatin, basophilic cytoplasm, prominent pale Golgi zone
- Plasmablastic plasmacytomas
  - Plasma cells with large vesicular nuclei, prominent nucleoli, amphophilic to basophilic cytoplasm, small often indistinct Golgi zone

CLINICAL ISSUES

Presentation

- Most common signs/symptoms
  - Highly dependent on lesion location
  - Local pain & headache
  - Various cranial neuropathies

Demographics

- Age
  - Most present in 5th-9th decade
- Gender
  - M > F
  - EMP: Occurs predominately in males
- Ethnicity
  - More common in African American patients
- Epidemiology
  - SBP: From all locations, represent only 3% of plasma cell neoplasms

- EMP: **80%** of primary EMPs occur in head & neck

Natural History & Prognosis

- SBP: Progression to MM common with skull base lesions, often within 1 yr of initial presentation
  - Higher rates of progression to MM associated with
    - Tumoral proliferative activity
    - Plasmablastic histology
    - Intraosseous skull base location
- EMP: Conversion to MM is significantly less compared with SBP

Treatment

- Surgical resection
  - Skull base resection highly morbid with cranial nerve dysfunction common postop
- Radiation therapy
  - Plasmablastic variety may require higher radiation doses
- Follow-up critical to monitor for evolution of multiple myeloma

DIAGNOSTIC CHECKLIST

Consider

- When plasmacytoma diagnosed, patient needs complete work-up for MM
- If **no MM** is present, then lesion considered **benign plasmacytoma**
  - Routine follow-up is then employed to watch for possible emergence of MM

Image Interpretation Pearls

- SBP: CT shows solitary intraosseous, osteolytic soft tissue mass with nonsclerotic margins
- Use enhanced MR with fat suppression to exclude additional lesions in commonly overlooked regions
  - Mandibular condyle, greater wing of sphenoid, occipital condyle, calvarium, upper cervical spine

Reporting Tips

- Include broad differential for solitary, expansile clival lesion
- Recommend whole body work-up, including skeletal survey, MR, or PET/CT to exclude additional lesions

SELECTED REFERENCES

1. Kalwani N et al: Plasmacytoma of the clivus presenting as bilateral sixth nerve palsy. J Neurol Surg Rep. 76(1):e156-9, 2015
2. Neelakantan A et al: Benign and malignant diseases of the clivus. Clin Radiol. 69(12):1295-303, 2014
3. Bag AK et al: Neuroimaging: intrinsic lesions of the central skull base region. Semin Ultrasound CT MR. 34(5):412-35, 2013
4. Gagliardi F et al: Solitary clival plasmocytomas: Misleading clinical and radiological features of a rare pathology with a specific biological behaviour. Acta Neurochir (Wien). 155(10):1849-56, 2013
5. Soutar R et al: Guidelines on the diagnosis and management of solitary plasmacytoma of bone and solitary extramedullary plasmacytoma. Br J Haematol. 124(6):717-26, 2004
6. Schwartz TH et al: Association between intracranial plasmacytoma and multiple myeloma: clinicopathological outcome study. Neurosurgery. 49(5):1039-44; discussion 1044-5, 2001
7. Okamoto K et al: Solitary plasmacytomas of the occipital bone: a report of two cases. Eur Radiol. 7(4):503-6, 1997
8. Provenzale JM et al: Craniocerebral plasmacytoma: MR features. AJNR Am J Neuroradiol. 18(2):389-92, 1997
9. Toland J et al: Plasmacytoma of the skull base. Clin Radiol. 22(1):93-6, 1971

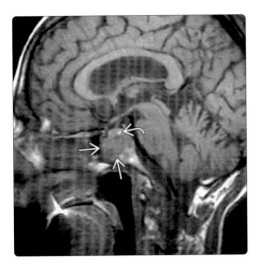
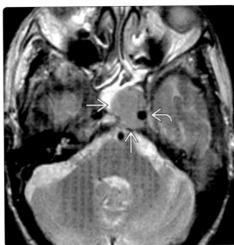

(Left) *Sagittal T1WI MR in an 82-year-old man with headache and abnormal sinus CT reveals a solitary infiltrating plasmacytoma of the basisphenoid ➔ bulging anteriorly into the sphenoid sinus. The lesion is distinct from the inferior margin of the pituitary gland ➔.* (Right) *Axial T2WI MR shows a slightly hyperintense mass relative to brain ➔ that extends into the sphenoid sinus and laterally into the left cavernous sinus, encasing the left internal carotid artery ➔.*

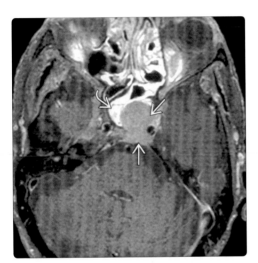
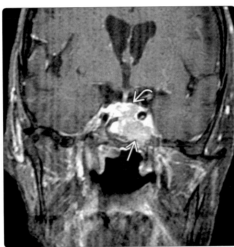

(Left) *Axial T1WI C+ FS MR shows solid homogeneous enhancement ➔ without necrosis or flow voids. Notice the anterior margin of the mass is easily distinguished from the enhancing mucosa of the sphenoid sinus ➔.* (Right) *Coronal T1WI C+ FS MR shows contrast enhancement of this plasmacytoma ➔, that makes it difficult to separate the mass from enhancing pituitary tissue ➔. This plasmacytoma mimics an invasive macroadenoma.*

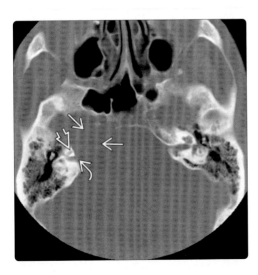
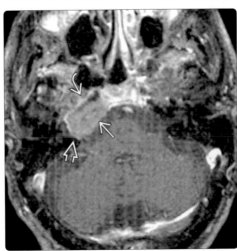

(Left) *Axial bone CT in a 72-year-old man with headaches, diplopia, and multiple myeloma reveals a solitary lytic mass of the right petrous apex ➔. This plasmacytoma invades the cochlea ➔ and internal auditory canal ➔.* (Right) *Axial T1WI C+ FS MR shows moderate enhancement of this malignant plasmacytoma of the petrous apex ➔. There is encasement of petrous internal carotid artery ➔ and erosion into the inner ear and internal auditory canal posteriorly ➔.*

Skull Base Multiple Myeloma

TERMINOLOGY

- Malignant monoclonal plasma cell proliferation

IMAGING

- CT shows osteolytic lesion(s) of skull base with additional skeletal lesions of calvarium, facial bones, cervical spine, etc.
- MR is most sensitive for evaluation of marrow involvement & assessing soft tissue characteristics
  - Homogeneous, isointense to gray matter on T1 & T2WI with moderate, diffuse enhancement

TOP DIFFERENTIAL DIAGNOSES

- Skull base metastases
- Non-Hodgkin lymphoma
- Chordoma
- Chondrosarcoma
- Invasive macroadenoma

CLINICAL ISSUES

- Most patients > 40 yr (average: 62 yr)
- 70% men
- Patients have localized pain and cranial neuropathy depending on lesion location
- Systemic symptoms related to anemia, renal failure, hypercalcemia

DIAGNOSTIC CHECKLIST

- Key to imaging diagnosis is demonstrating multiple marrow replacing, **osteolytic lesions** on CT or plain films
- **Use T1 MR C+ FS** images to evaluate commonly overlooked regions of skull base & face
  - Clivus, petrous apex, occipital condyle, greater wing of sphenoid, mandibular condyle
- Whole-body imaging is recommended to evaluate for extracranial disease

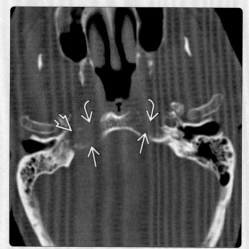
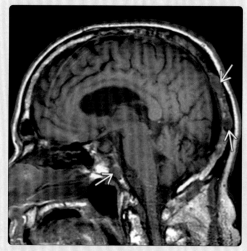

(Left) Axial bone CT demonstrates nearly symmetric bilateral occipital bone lytic lesions ➡ of multiple myeloma. Symmetry can reduce conspicuity; however, loss of the expected outer white cortical line is clearly abnormal ➡. Note erosion into the right carotid canal ➡. (Right) Sagittal T1 MR shows multiple low-signal foci of multiple myeloma ➡. This is a relatively sensitive sequence (without FS) for osseous malignancy, particularly if the whole skull enhances &/or no FS is applied on the postcontrast sequence.

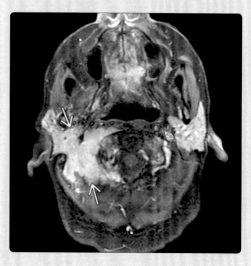
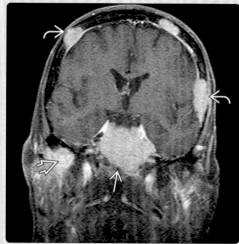

(Left) Axial T1 C+ FS MR in a patient with right facial nerve palsy shows homogeneously enhancing osseous and extraosseous tumor ➡ destroying the mastoid segment of the right temporal bone and obliterating the stylomastoid foramen. T1 C+ FS MR is typically the most sensitive sequence to detect marrow involvement. (Right) Coronal T1 C+ FS MR shows a dominant enhancing mass in the clivus ➡ with additional smaller myelomatous lesions in the calvarium ➡ and right infratemporal fossa ➡.

TERMINOLOGY

Definitions

- Multiple myeloma (MM) is malignant monoclonal plasma cell neoplasm of bone marrow

IMAGING

Imaging Recommendations

- Best imaging tool
  - CT optimally shows **lytic lesions** in osseous skull base and calvarium
  - MR best for detection of marrow-replacing lesions and to evaluate extraosseous soft tissue
- Protocol advice
  - MR of skull base to include multiplanar **T1WI, followed by T1WI C+ FS** in same planes for direct comparison

Radiographic Findings

- Limited value in evaluating skull base
- Classic punched-out lytic lesions of calvaria

CT Findings

- Bone CT
  - Multiple **intraosseous lytic lesions** with nonsclerotic margins

MR Findings

- T1WI
  - Homogeneous, isointense to gray matter (GM)
- T2WI
  - Homogeneous, typically isointense to GM
- DWI
  - Sensitive to marrow malignancy (low ADC)
- T1WI C+ FS
  - Moderate, homogeneous enhancement ± soft tissue extension

Nuclear Medicine Findings

- Bone scan
  - Often little or no uptake of Tc-99m pertechnetate (cold lesion)
- PET
  - Can detect bone marrow lesions and extramedullary lesions with high sensitivity and specificity
  - FDG avidity indicates active disease and can be used to assess treatment response
- PET/CT
  - 90% sensitive & specific for focal MM
- Tc-99m MIBI
  - Radiotracer accumulates inside plasma cells infiltrating bone marrow
  - > 90% sensitivity & specificity for marrow and extramedullary lesions

DIFFERENTIAL DIAGNOSIS

Skull Base Metastases

- Often late stage with known primary extracranial neoplasm

Non-Hodgkin Lymphoma

- Lymphoproliferative neoplasm with focal or multifocal, osseous &/or extraosseous involvement of skull base

Chordoma

- Solitary, expansile clival mass with marked T2 hyperintensity

Chondrosarcoma

- Solitary, expansile, destructive paramidline or midline skull base mass, typically with significant T2 hyperintensity

Invasive Pituitary Macroadenoma

- Benign lesion with invasion inferiorly into clivus

CLINICAL ISSUES

Presentation

- Most common signs/symptoms
  - Pain at site of lesion
  - Site-dependent cranial neuropathy
  - Diplopia, compressive optic neuropathy

Demographics

- Age
  - Majority > 40 yr (average: 62)
- Gender
  - M > F (70% vs. 30%)
- Epidemiology
  - Associated with exposure to radiation & agricultural agents (pesticides)

Treatment

- Oral regimen of melphalan and prednisone has been mainstay of therapy
  - Newer treatments include thalidomide, bortezomib, lenalidomide
- Autologous stem cell transplantation prolongs survival

DIAGNOSTIC CHECKLIST

Image Interpretation Pearls

- Use T1 C+ FS MR to evaluate commonly overlooked regions of skull base & face
  - Petrous apex, mandibular condyle, occipital condyle, greater wing of sphenoid

Reporting Tips

- Can be difficult to differentiate MM from metastatic disease
- If skull base & calvarial lesions identified, whole-body imaging recommended to evaluate for additional lesions

SELECTED REFERENCES

1. Lasocki A et al: Intracranial involvement by multiple myeloma. Clin Radiol. 70(8):890-7, 2015
2. Sachpekidis C et al: Comparison of (18)F-FDG PET/CT and PET/MRI in patients with multiple myeloma. Am J Nucl Med Mol Imaging. 5(5):469-78, 2015
3. Giles SL et al: Whole-body diffusion-weighted MR imaging for assessment of treatment response in myeloma. Radiology. 271(3):785-94, 2014
4. Joshi A et al: Skull base presentation of multiple myeloma. Ear Nose Throat J. 90(1):E6-9, 2011
5. Delorme S et al: Imaging in multiple myeloma. Eur J Radiol. 70(3):401-8, 2009
6. Lütje S et al: Role of radiography, MRI and FDG-PET/CT in diagnosing, staging and therapeutical evaluation of patients with multiple myeloma. Ann Hematol. 88(12):1161-8, 2009
7. Baur-Melnyk A et al: Role of MRI for the diagnosis and prognosis of multiple myeloma. Eur J Radiol. 55(1):56-63, 2005

Skull Base Metastasis

TERMINOLOGY

- Metastatic disease (mets) affecting osseous skull base &/or adjacent dura

IMAGING

- Enhancing, destructive mass of osseous skull base in patient with **known extracranial primary malignancy**
- Often dominant lesion seen in context of multiple additional skeletal lesions affecting skull base, calvarium, spine, etc.
- MR most sensitive modality
  - ○ **Osseous metastasis**: Enhancing marrow space mass ± extraosseous extension
  - ○ **Dural metastasis**: Enhancing, infiltrating, dural-based lesion
- Noncontrast T1 & T1 C+ FS MR best sequences
- CT shows variable pattern of cortical and trabecular bone involvement: Lytic, permeative, sclerotic

TOP DIFFERENTIAL DIAGNOSES

- Multiple myeloma
- Non-Hodgkin lymphoma
- Skull base meningioma
- Solitary central skull base mass
  - ○ Invasive pituitary adenoma, chordoma, chondrosarcoma

PATHOLOGY

- Cancer sources: Breast (40%) > lung (14%) > prostate (12%)

CLINICAL ISSUES

- Skull base mets from extracranial primaries occur in 4% of cancer patients

DIAGNOSTIC CHECKLIST

- Consider metastatic disease if skull base lesion seen in patient with known malignancy who develops craniofacial pain or cranial neuropathy
- Look for additional skeletal/osseous lesions of cervical spine, skull base, calvarium

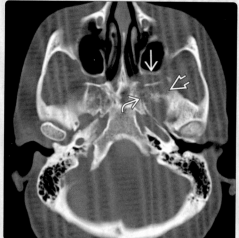
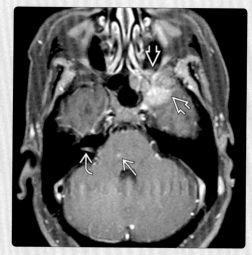

(Left) Axial bone CT in a lung cancer patient with new left facial pain and dizziness shows a lytic lesion of the left sphenoid body ➡. Note erosion of the vidian canal ➡ and cortical irregularity of the margins of pterygopalatine fossa ➡ with associated soft tissue invasion. (Right) Axial T1 C+ FS MR reveals an enhancing mass ➡ of the sphenoid wing with dural invasion. Close inspection shows leptomeningeal tumor in right internal auditory canal ➡ and tiny pontine brain metastasis ➡.

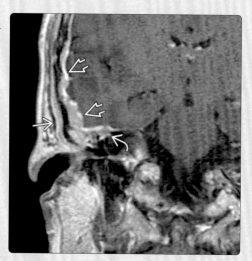
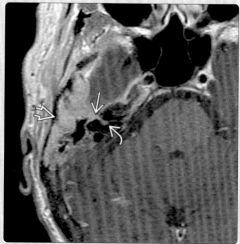

(Left) Coronal T1 C+ MR in a 60 year old with breast cancer and right facial palsy shows a smooth, enhancing dural metastasis ➡ along the squamous temporal bone and petrous ridge. Tumor extends to the geniculate ganglion ➡. Note extracranial tumor lateral to the involved squamous temporal bone ➡. (Right) Axial T1 C+ MR shows thick dural tumor ➡ infiltrating the petrous ridge with perineural extension to CNVII geniculate ganglion ➡ to the fundus of the internal auditory canal ➡.

TERMINOLOGY

Definitions

- Metastatic disease affecting osseous skull base &/or adjacent dura

IMAGING

General Features

- Best diagnostic clue
  - Enhancing, destructive mass of osseous skull base in patient with **known extracranial primary malignancy**
  - Often dominant lesion seen in context of multiple additional skeletal lesions affecting skull base, calvarium, spine, etc.
- Location
  - Osseous
    - Occurs where bone marrow is most abundant: Clivus, nonpneumatized petrous apex, and greater wing of sphenoid
  - Dural
    - Occurs anywhere along dura of anterior, central, or posterior skull base
- Size
  - Often large, dominant, symptomatic lesion with subsequent detection of **additional lesions**
  - Small, "strategically located" lesions can affect cranial nerves and produce neurologic deficit

Imaging Recommendations

- Best imaging tool
  - Enhanced MR best evaluates skull base lesions within bone & delineates invasion into adjacent soft tissues
    - Can miss enhancing lesions without soft tissue invasion without FS or comparison to T1 precontrast
- Protocol advice
  - Axial and coronal **precontrast T1 without FS** identifies low-signal marrow lesions
  - **T1 C+ FS** in identical planes to demonstrate osseous and extraosseous tumor

CT Findings

- CECT
  - Skull base & calvarial metastases: Enhancing mass infiltrating bone marrow
- Bone CT
  - Variable pattern of cortical and trabecular bone involvement: Lytic, permeative, sclerotic
  - Sclerotic lesions may mimic benign enostosis (bone island)
    - Bone scan of enostosis is cold

MR Findings

- T1WI
  - Hypointense marrow lesion **replaces high-signal fat**
- T2WI
  - Variable marrow signal depending on cellularity &/or sclerosis
- T1WI C+ FS
  - Enhancing marrow space mass ± extraosseous extension
  - Pearl: Without FS, ↑ signal of enhancing tumor may be inconspicuous against background of ↑ signal from fat

Nuclear Medicine Findings

- PET/CT
  - Combination of lytic-destructive lesions on CT with moderate to marked FDG uptake

DIFFERENTIAL DIAGNOSIS

Multiple Myeloma

- Plasma cell neoplasm
- Multiple enhancing lytic lesions of skull base & calvarium

Non-Hodgkin Lymphoma

- Lymphoproliferative neoplasm
- Can have multifocal extranodal & extralymphatic lesions of skull base and dura

Skull Base Meningioma

- Primary dural-based enhancing neoplasm(s) with secondary sclerosis or invasion of skull base
- May be multiple & mimic metastatic disease

Solitary Central Skull Base Mass

- Invasive pituitary macroadenoma
- Chordoma
- Chondrosarcoma

Idiopathic Inflammatory Pseudotumor

- Enhancing, nonneoplastic fibroinflammatory process of orbital apex, cavernous sinus, or skull base

PATHOLOGY

General Features

- Etiology
  - Source of mets: Breast cancer (40%) > lung cancer (14%) > prostate cancer (12%)

CLINICAL ISSUES

Presentation

- Most common signs/symptoms
  - Headache, craniofacial pain, & progressive unilateral cranial neuropathy

Demographics

- Epidemiology
  - Skull base metastasis from extracranial primaries occurs in 4% of cancer patients

Treatment

- Radiation therapy is mainstay of treatment for focal/isolated disease

DIAGNOSTIC CHECKLIST

Image Interpretation Pearls

- In metastatic evaluation of brain, remember to include osseous skull base and adjacent dura in search pattern

SELECTED REFERENCES

1. Bag AK et al: Neuroimaging: intrinsic lesions of the central skull base region. Semin Ultrasound CT MR. 34(5):412-35, 2013
2. Mitsuya K et al: Metastatic skull tumors: MRI features and a new conventional classification. J Neurooncol. 104(1):239-45, 2011
3. Nayak L et al: Intracranial dural metastases. Cancer. 115(9):1947-53, 2009

Skull Base Chondrosarcoma

TERMINOLOGY

- Skull base chondrosarcoma (CSa-SB): Chondroid malignancy of skull base

IMAGING

- Typical location **off-midline**, centered on **petrooccipital fissure**
- CT
  - Characteristic **chondroid tumor matrix calcification** in **50%**
  - Arc or ring-like calcifications
  - Sharp, narrow, nonsclerotic transition zone to adjacent normal bone
- MR
  - High T2 signal with scattered hypointense foci (calcifications)
  - Heterogeneously enhancing
  - Whorls of enhancing lines within tumor matrix often seen

TOP DIFFERENTIAL DIAGNOSES

- Chordoma
- Skull base metastasis
- Plasmacytoma
- Nasopharyngeal carcinoma (invasive)
- Meningioma
- Benign petrous apex lesions

CLINICAL ISSUES

- Typically middle-aged patient with insidious onset of headache & cranial nerve palsies (especially CNVI)

DIAGNOSTIC CHECKLIST

- Is lesion **off-midline** (CSa) or in midline (chordoma)?
- Do calcifications represent **arc-whorl intralesional calcifications** (CSa) or fragmented destroyed bone (chordoma)?
- Consider MR angiography or CTA for preoperative characterization of vessel involvement

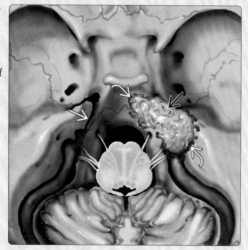
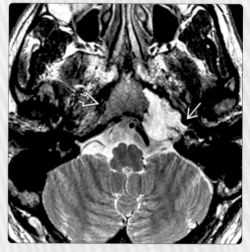

(Left) Axial graphic depicts the classic location of a chondrosarcoma of the skull base centered in the left petrooccipital fissure ➡. Note the normal right petrooccipital fissure ➡. Chondroid calcifications, depicted in yellow, are present within the lesion ➡. (Right) Axial T2 MR reveals a large, high-signal chondrosarcoma of the left petrooccipital fissure. Note that the vertical segment of the petrous internal carotid artery is compressed ➡. Note normal right petrooccipital fissure ➡.

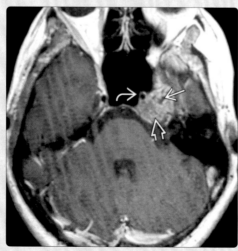
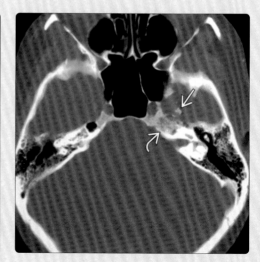

(Left) Axial T1 C+ MR shows mottled enhancement ➡ within a chondrosarcoma centered at the left petrooccipital fissure. Calcified matrix is seen as a focal low signal intensity area ➡ within the otherwise enhancing tumor. The left internal carotid artery is patent ➡. (Right) Axial bone CT demonstrates typical chondroid calcification ➡ in a left petrooccipital fissure chondrosarcoma. In this case, no significant destruction of the adjacent petrous apex ➡ is appreciated.

TERMINOLOGY

Abbreviations

- Chondrosarcoma-skull base (CSa-SB)

Definitions

- CSa-SB: Chondroid malignancy of skull base

IMAGING

General Features

- Best diagnostic clue
  - Solitary enhancing osteolytic soft tissue mass, centered at petrooccipital fissure (POF) ± chondroid matrix
- Location
  - Off midline at **POF** (2/3)
  - Anterior basisphenoid (1/3)
- Size
  - Variable, usually > 3 cm at time of diagnosis
- Morphology
  - Well-circumscribed, lobulated margins

CT Findings

- NECT
  - Soft tissue component is relatively dense
- CECT
  - Variable, heterogeneous enhancement
- Bone CT
  - Expansile mass at POF producing erosive or destructive bone changes in clivus and petrous apex
  - ~ 50% will have radiographically classic chondroid matrix with **"rings and arcs" calcification**
  - Sharp, narrow, nonsclerotic transition zone to adjacent normal bone

MR Findings

- T1WI
  - Low to intermediate signal intensity relative to gray matter
    - ↓ signal foci within tumor may suggest underlying coarse matrix mineralization or fibrocartilaginous elements
- T2WI
  - Variable, usually **high signal**
  - Hypointense foci (calcifications) less conspicuous than on CT
- T1WI C+
  - Heterogeneous enhancement

Angiographic Findings

- Avascular or hypovascular mass
- Internal carotid artery displacement ± encasement

Imaging Recommendations

- Best imaging tool
  - Combination of multiplanar, gadolinium-enhanced MR & high-resolution bone CT
- Protocol advice
  - High-resolution axial bone CT for evaluation of chondroid matrix & pattern of bone destruction
  - MR of skull base to include T2WI and multiplanar T1WI, followed by T1WI C+ FS in same planes for direct comparison
  - MRA & MRV, or CTA helpful to assess vascular involvement preoperatively

DIFFERENTIAL DIAGNOSIS

Chordoma

- Destructive clival lesion; bone fragments within matrix
- Midline > lateral location
- Low T1 & markedly high T2 MR signal; enhancing mass
- Chondroid chordomas more aggressive & worse prognosis

Skull Base Metastasis

- Bone CT: Destructive mass that can be anywhere in skull base
- MR: Often multiple enhancing, invasive lesions
- Typically low to intermediate T2 signal
- Known primary tumor

Plasmacytoma and Multiple Myeloma

- Usually more midline, within clivus
- **T2 signal is low** to intermediate
- > 50% have concurrent multiple myeloma

Nasopharyngeal Carcinoma

- Primary mass in nasopharyngeal mucosal space
- Tumor invades superiorly to clivus, foramen lacerum, and POF

Meningioma

- Calcification in meningioma can mimic chondroid matrix
- Hyperostosis possible; not typically destructive in absence of invasion
- Low to intermediate T2 MR signal; enhancing with dural tails

Non-Hodgkin Lymphoma

- Lymphoproliferative neoplasm with focal or multifocal, osseous &/or extraosseous involvement of skull base
- Low to intermediate T2 MR signal, may restrict on DWI

Nonneoplastic Lesion of Petrous Apex

- Includes benign expansile lesions: Cholesteatoma, mucocele, cholesterol granuloma
  - Should be nonenhancing, smoothly marginated without calcified matrix
- High signal from asymmetric petrous apex marrow can mimic enhancing tumor

Chondromyxoid Fibroma

- Rare, expansile, noninfiltrating skull base mass
- Areas of ground-glass density may be seen
- Appearance may overlap with CSa-SB

PATHOLOGY

General Features

- Etiology
  - Arises from remnants of embryonal cartilage, endochondral bone, or from primitive mesenchymal cells in meninges
    - May arise from metaplasia of meningeal fibroblasts

- Genetics
  - May complicate Ollier disease & Maffucci syndromes

Staging, Grading, & Classification

- Classification
  - Conventional CSa: Hyaline (7%), myxoid (30%), or mixed (63%)
  - Clear cell
  - Mesenchymal
  - Dedifferentiated
- Grading from low to high grade
  - Based on degree of cellularity, pleomorphism, mitoses, & multinucleated cells

Microscopic Features

- Hypercellular tumor composed of chondrocytes with hyperchromatic, pleomorphic nuclei & prominent nucleoli
  - Binucleate or multinucleate cells are rule
- Hyaline matrix may calcify in "ringlets"
  - Intercellular matrix is solid in hyaline type compared to mucinous/gelatinous matrix in myxoid or mixed types
- Histology may overlap with or be confused with that of chordoma
  - Histology particularly confusing in chondroid chordoma, myxoid chondrosarcoma
  - Differentiation facilitated by immunohistochemical staining

CLINICAL ISSUES

Presentation

- Most common signs/symptoms
  - **Abducens (CNVI) palsy** due to proximity of Dorello canal
  - **Headache**
  - Mean duration of symptoms at diagnosis = 27 months
- Other signs/symptoms
  - Other cranial nerve palsies (CNs III, V, VII, VIII)
- Clinical profile
  - Middle-aged patient with insidious onset of headaches & cranial nerve palsies

Demographics

- Age
  - Range: 10-80 years
    - Mean: 40 years
- Epidemiology
  - 6% of all skull base tumors
  - 75% of all cranial CSa occur in skull base

Natural History & Prognosis

- Prognosis depends on extent at diagnosis, histologic grade, & completeness of surgical resection
  - Disease-specific 10-year survival rates of 99% recently reported
  - Most central skull base chondrosarcomas are well to moderately differentiated
  - High-grade CSa metastasizes to bones & lung more frequently
- Conventional CSa: Indolent growth pattern
  - Most are slow growing, locally invasive, but rarely metastasize

- Mesenchymal & dedifferentiated forms: Aggressive behavior; poor prognosis

Treatment

- Aggressive resection associated with significant morbidity and low likelihood of complete resection
- Combined radical resection & postoperative, high-dose, fractionated precision conformal radiation therapy most often utilized
  - Charged particle RT (protons or carbon ions) alone or combined with subtotal resection

DIAGNOSTIC CHECKLIST

Consider

- Is lesion in off-midline (CSa) vs. midline (chordoma)?
- Do calcifications represent arc-whorl intralesional calcifications (CSa) or fragmented destroyed bone (chordoma)?
- Does patient have known primary neoplasm (metastasis), myeloma (plasmacytoma), or nasopharyngeal mass (nasopharyngeal carcinoma)?

Image Interpretation Pearls

- Classic appearance: Heterogeneously enhancing tumor located at **POF** with hyperintense signal on T2 MR
  - CT shows chondroid mineralization & bone destruction
- When no tumor matrix found, difficult to tell from CSa plasmacytoma, focal metastasis, or chondromyxoid fibroma

SELECTED REFERENCES

1. Awad M et al: Skull base chondrosarcoma. J Clin Neurosci. 24:1-5, 2016
2. Bag AK et al: Neuroimaging: intrinsic lesions of the central skull base region. Semin Ultrasound CT MR. 34(5):412-35, 2013
3. Bloch O et al: Skull base chondrosarcoma: evidence-based treatment paradigms. Neurosurg Clin N Am. 24(1):89-96, 2013
4. Gardner PA et al: Carotid artery injury during endoscopic endonasal skull base surgery: incidence and outcomes. Neurosurgery. 73(2 Suppl Operative):ons261-9; discussion ons269-70, 2013
5. Sbaihat A et al: Skull base chondrosarcomas: surgical treatment and results. Ann Otol Rhinol Laryngol. 122(12):763-70, 2013
6. Bloch OG et al: Cranial chondrosarcoma and recurrence. Skull Base. 20(3):149-56, 2010
7. Borges A: Imaging of the central skull base. Neuroimaging Clin N Am. 19(4):669-96, 2009
8. Gallia GL et al: Skull base chondrosarcoma presenting with hemorrhage. Can J Neurol Sci. 36(6):774-5, 2009
9. Hong P et al: Chondrosarcoma of the head and neck: report of 11 cases and literature review. J Otolaryngol Head Neck Surg. 38(2):279-85, 2009
10. Cho YH et al: Chordomas and chondrosarcomas of the skull base: comparative analysis of clinical results in 30 patients. Neurosurg Rev. 31(1):35-43; discussion 43, 2008
11. Almefty K et al: Chordoma and chondrosarcoma: similar, but quite different, skull base tumors. Cancer. 110(11):2457-67, 2007
12. Lustig LR et al: Chondrosarcomas of the skull base and temporal bone. J Laryngol Otol. 121(8):725-35, 2007
13. Schmidinger A et al: Natural history of chondroid skull base lesions--case report and review. Neuroradiology. 44(3):268-71, 2002
14. Richardson MS: Pathology of skull base tumors. Otolaryngol Clin North Am. 34(6):1025-42, vii, 2001
15. Korten AG et al: Intracranial chondrosarcoma: review of the literature and report of 15 cases. J Neurol Neurosurg Psychiatry. 65(1):88-92, 1998
16. Brown E et al: Chondrosarcoma of the skull base. Neuroimaging Clin N Am. 4(3):529-41, 1994
17. Meyers SP et al: Chondrosarcomas of the skull base: MR imaging features. Radiology. 184(1):103-8, 1992

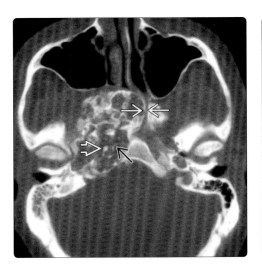
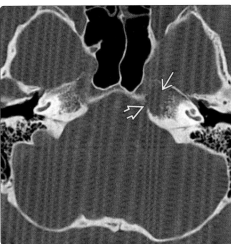

(Left) *Axial bone CT shows rounded ➡ and arc-like ➡ calcified foci in this large chondrosarcoma centered at the petrooccipital fissure. Up to 50% of chondrosarcomas demonstrate matrix calcification. Note slight narrowing of the left vidian canal ➡.* (Right) *Axial bone window CT shows subtle bone destruction ➡ with cortical erosion ➡ in this small left petrous apex chondrosarcoma. No calcified matrix is seen. MR showed a corresponding T2-hyperintense and enhancing mass in this location.*

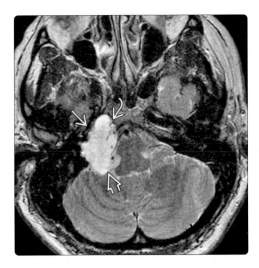
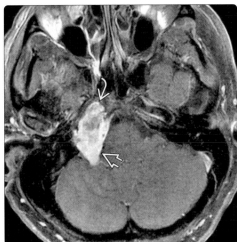

(Left) *Axial T2 MR shows a hyperintense chondrosarcoma involving the right petrous apex ➡ and extending into the right cerebellopontine angle cistern (CPA) ➡. The petrous carotid artery is displaced anteriorly ➡.* (Right) *Axial T1 C+ FS MR demonstrates avid enhancement in this chondrosarcoma. Note petrous apex ➡ and CPA cistern ➡ involvement. Most skull base chondrosarcomas emanate from the petrooccipital fissure. However, when they become large it may be hard to see the point of origin.*

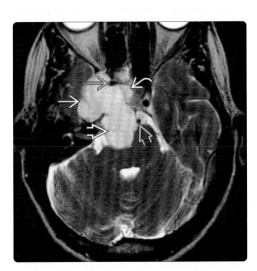
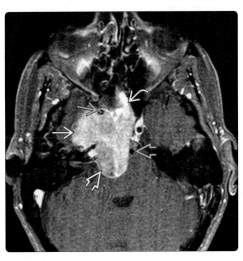

(Left) *Axial T2 MR shows a hyperintense right parasellar chondrosarcoma ➡ that extends into the prepontine cistern ➡ and sphenoid sinus ➡. Note internal carotid ➡ and basilar ➡ arterial displacement by the mass.* (Right) *Axial T1 C+ FS MR shows moderate enhancement within a right parasellar chondrosarcoma ➡. The patient presented with intractable headache, epistaxis, & diplopia. Tumor invades prepontine cistern ➡ & sphenoid sinus ➡, partly encases the right ICA ➡, and displaces the basilar artery ➡.*

Skull Base Osteosarcoma

TERMINOLOGY

- Neoplasm composed of malignant cells producing osteoid matrix, or immature bone

IMAGING

- Very rare in skull base → clivus, parasellar, sphenoid wing, & anterior skull base
- CT findings
  - Often destructive & expansile
  - May be **lytic** or **blastic**
  - May show **tumor bone formation** & periosteal reaction
- MR findings
  - Heterogeneous low to intermediate T1 signal
  - Intermediate to high T2 signal; bone components ↓ T2WI signal
  - Marrow/soft tissue enhancement

TOP DIFFERENTIAL DIAGNOSES

- Chordoma
- Chondrosarcoma
- Metastatic disease
- Plasmacytoma
- Non-Hodgkin lymphoma
- Invasive macroadenoma

PATHOLOGY

- May occur as late effect of previous irradiation
- Associated with Paget disease, fibrous dysplasia, giant cell tumor, Ollier disease, chronic osteomyelitis

CLINICAL ISSUES

- Nonspecific symptoms: Swelling, pain
- Present in 3rd-4th decade; M = F
- Difficult to completely resect due to proximity to critical structures within skull base
- Relatively resistant to XRT

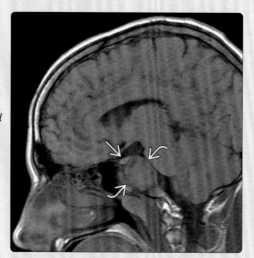
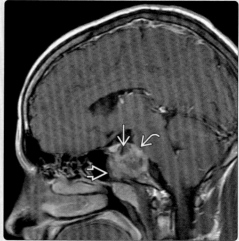

(Left) Sagittal T1WI MR demonstrates an expansile, intermediate-signal clival osteosarcoma ➦. Normal pituitary parenchyma ➡ is seen at the superior aspect of the mass. This finding helps to exclude invasive pituitary adenoma from the differential diagnosis. (Right) Sagittal T1WI C+ MR in the same patient shows heterogeneous enhancement throughout the mass ➦. Note extension into the sphenoid sinus ➡. Nonenhancing foci with hypointense signal ➡ may represent areas of osteoid.

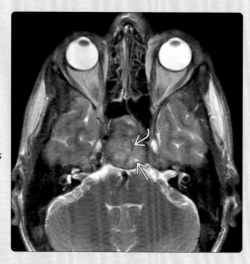
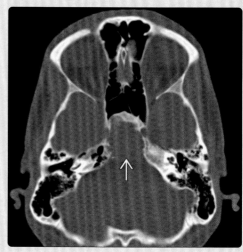

(Left) Axial T2WI MR in the same patient shows heterogeneous, intermediate signal with areas of higher signal ➡, which may be due to focal necrosis. Curvilinear lower signal area may represent an area of internal calcification ➦. (Right) Axial bone CT in the same patient shows that this osteosarcoma is predominantly lytic. There is some expansion of the clivus with a large area of bone destruction posteriorly ➡. This lesion does not show osteoid matrix.

TERMINOLOGY

Abbreviations
- Osteosarcoma of skull base (OSa-SB)

Definitions
- Neoplasm composed of malignant spindle cells producing osteoid or immature bone

IMAGING

General Features
- Best diagnostic clue
  - Aggressive, ill-defined mass arising from bone with soft tissue & **osteoid matrix**
- Location
  - Occurs rarely in skull base: Clivus, sphenoid-sella, greater sphenoid wing, anterior skull base

Imaging Recommendations
- Best imaging tool
  - Multiplanar contrast-enhanced MR best for evaluating marrow space and soft tissue involvement
  - Bone CT shows internal osteoid matrix & periosteal reaction to better advantage

CT Findings
- Bone CT
  - Expansile mass may be **lytic** or **blastic**
  - May show **tumor bone formation** or malignant periosteal reaction

MR Findings
- T1WI
  - Heterogeneous, low to intermediate signal
- T2WI
  - Heterogeneous intermediate to high T2 signal with densely ossified components showing ↓ signal
- T1WI C+ FS
  - Marrow/soft tissue components show enhancement

DIFFERENTIAL DIAGNOSIS

Chordoma
- Midline clival mass
- Hyperintense on T2WI MR

Chondrosarcoma
- Expansile mass at POF producing erosive or destructive bone changes in clivus and petrous apex
- 50% will have radiographically classic chondroid matrix with **rings and arcs** of calcification

Skull Base Metastasis
- Patient has known primary neoplasm
- Lesions often multiple

Plasmacytoma
- Solitary or multiple if in setting of multiple myeloma
- Homogeneous, lytic, & well defined

Invasive Macroadenoma
- Can be significantly or predominantly invasive to clivus
- Cannot distinguish pituitary gland separate from mass

PATHOLOGY

General Features
- Etiology
  - Primary etiology unknown
  - May occur secondary to **prior irradiation**
- Associated abnormalities
  - May be associated with Paget disease, fibrous dysplasia, giant cell tumor, solitary or multiple osteochondroma, enchondroma, Ollier disease

Staging, Grading, & Classification
- Classification based upon histology: Osteoblastic, chondroblastic, fibroblastic, telangiectatic, & juxtacortical types
- Grading (low, intermediate, high) based on degree of cellular atypia and recognizable histologic architecture

Microscopic Features
- Osteoid production by atypical neoplastic osteoblasts

CLINICAL ISSUES

Presentation
- Most common signs/symptoms
  - Swelling, mass, & pain
- Other signs/symptoms
  - Cranial nerve deficits

Demographics
- Age
  - 3rd-4th decade
- Gender
  - M = F
- Epidemiology
  - Most common primary bone malignancy overall but only 6-10% in head & neck

Natural History & Prognosis
- Poor overall survival

Treatment
- Maximal safe surgical resection with adjuvant radiation

SELECTED REFERENCES

1. Ahrari A et al: Primary osteosarcoma of the skull base treated with endoscopic endonasal approach: a case report and literature review. J Neurol Surg Rep. 76(2):e270-4, 2015
2. Hadley C et al: Osteosarcoma of the cranial vault and skull base in pediatric patients. J Neurosurg Pediatr. 13(4):380-7, 2014
3. Mohindra S et al: Primary osteosarcoma of clivus: a short report. Br J Neurosurg. 28(4):531-3, 2014
4. Sun TT et al: Spontaneous osteosarcoma in craniomaxillofacial fibrous dysplasia: clinical and computed tomographic features in 8 cases. Oral Surg Oral Med Oral Pathol Oral Radiol. 118(1):e24-31, 2014
5. O'Neill JP et al: Head and neck sarcomas: epidemiology, pathology, and management. Neurosurg Clin N Am. 24(1):67-78, 2013
6. Ottaviani G et al: The etiology of osteosarcoma. Cancer Treat Res. 152:15-32, 2010
7. Chennupati SK et al: Osteosarcoma of the skull base: case report and review of literature. Int J Pediatr Otorhinolaryngol. 72(1):115-9, 2008
8. Hansen MR et al: Osteosarcoma of the skull base after radiation therapy in a patient with McCune-Albright syndrome: case report. Skull Base. 13(2):79-83, 2003
9. Smith RB et al: National Cancer Data Base report on osteosarcoma of the head and neck. Cancer. 98(8):1670-80, 2003

Skull Base Osteomyelitis

TERMINOLOGY

- Skull base osteomyelitis (SBO)
- Severe infection of temporal, sphenoid, ± occipital bone causing bone destruction
- Typical SBO: Temporal bone involved 1st, most often from necrotizing external otitis (NEO)
- Atypical SBO: Usually secondary to invasive sinusitis or deep face infection; can be idiopathic

IMAGING

- Ill-defined, infiltrative process involving temporal bone &/or central skull base
  - CT demonstrates cortical erosion & destruction
  - MR shows abnormal marrow signal & enhancement
  - Extraosseous inflammation mimics neoplasm

TOP DIFFERENTIAL DIAGNOSES

- Metastatic disease of skull base
- Nasopharyngeal carcinoma
- Non-Hodgkin lymphoma of skull base

PATHOLOGY

- **Pseudomonas** #1 pathogen (in typical SBO/NEO)
- **Bacterial or fungal** (*Mucor* & *Aspergillus*) in atypical SBO

CLINICAL ISSUES

- Most often seen in **immunocompromised** patients, especially **elderly diabetics**
- Elevated erythrocyte sedimentation rate (ESR)
- Indolent course & nonspecific symptoms, difficult to diagnose clinically
- High morbidity & mortality despite intensive antibiotic therapy

DIAGNOSTIC CHECKLIST

- **Bone CT & enhanced MR** best evaluate osseous destruction & marrow involvement
- Consider SBO for any infiltrative skull base process if **biopsies are negative for malignancy**

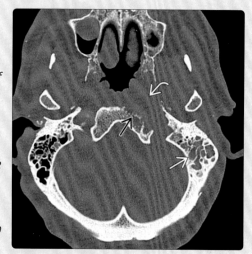
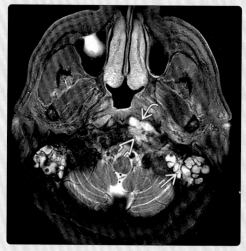

(Left) *CT of a 55-year-old patient with type II diabetes, presenting with low-grade fever, severe pain, and drainage from left ear demonstrates opacification of mastoid air cells ➡, soft tissue fullness left nasopharynx ➡, and cortical erosions of clivus ➡. Pathogen in this case identified as Staphylococcus aureus.* (Right) *Axial T2 FS MR with SBO demonstrates fluid opacification of mastoid air cells ➡, abnormal increased marrow signal in left side of clivus ➡, and small abscess in left longus capitus muscle ➡.*

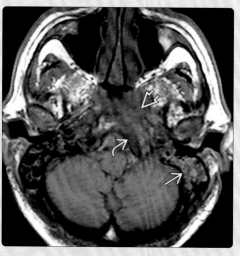
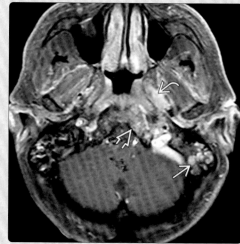

(Left) *Axial T1 MR demonstrates opacification of left mastoid ➡, ill-defined infiltration into the left nasopharynx with loss of normal fat signal and fat planes ➡, and loss of normal marrow fat signal in left side of clivus ➡. (Right) Axial T1 C+ FS MR of SBO shows enhancing inflammatory tissue in left mastoid ➡, abnormal enhancement in the clivus ➡, and ill-defined enhancement in the left nasopharynx and surrounding soft tissues ➡. Pathogen in this case identified as S. aureus.*

TERMINOLOGY

Abbreviations

- Skull base osteomyelitis (SBO)

Definitions

- SBO: Severe infection of temporal, sphenoid, &/or occipital bone that results in osseous destruction &/or marrow space involvement
- **Typical SBO**: Infection involves temporal bone initially, occurs most often as result of **necrotizing external otitis** (NEO)
  - Many authors consider part of spectrum of NEO
  - SBO can occur secondary to other infections related to temporal bone including otomastoiditis or petrous apicitis
  - Can occur secondary to trauma or surgery of temporal bone
  - Pseudomonas aeruginosa is most common pathogen
- **Atypical SBO**: Occurs secondary to **invasive sinusitis** or deep face infections, not temporal bone
  - No recent history of NEO or otomastoiditis
  - Also referred to as central skull base osteomyelitis
  - Less common than typical SBO
  - Can be idiopathic, without specific localized head & neck infection

IMAGING

General Features

- Best diagnostic clue
  - Ill-defined infiltrative process of skull base with osseous erosion & destruction on CT, abnormal marrow signal & enhancement on MR, usually with extraosseous inflammation of intracranial &/or extracranial soft tissues
- Location
  - Temporal bone & central skull base
- Morphology
  - Ill defined and infiltrative with osseous and extraosseous abnormalities

Radiographic Findings

- Opacified mastoid air cells, external auditory canal (EAC) soft tissue fullness, or sphenoid sinus opacification with cortical erosions of skull base

CT Findings

- Typical SBO
  - Early: Swollen EAC soft tissues with localized bone erosion & adjacent cellulitis or abscess
  - Destruction of petrous apex & central skull base occurs with advanced or inadequately treated disease
- Atypical SBO
  - Early findings: Sphenoid sinus opacification
  - Late: Cortical erosion, trabecular demineralization, and late osteolysis of central skull base

MR Findings

- T1WI
  - Soft tissue opacification, thickened EAC, temporal bone, or sphenoid sinus
  - Low signal replaces normal T1-hyperintense marrow fat
- STIR
  - High signal within inflamed EAC, auricle, adjacent soft tissues, & infected marrow
- DWI
  - ADC values tend to be higher with SBO than malignancy
- T1WI C+ FS
  - Abnormal marrow enhancement & infiltrative extraosseous enhancing soft tissue
  - Soft tissue infiltration in nasopharyngeal soft tissues may mimic neoplasm such as nasopharyngeal carcinoma
  - MR may show combination of enhancing soft tissue & nonenhancing areas of devitalized tissue in *Mucor*

Imaging Recommendations

- Best imaging tool
  - Combined bone CT & enhanced MR best evaluate cortical and trabecular integrity, marrow space, & soft tissue cellulitis, phlegmon, or abscess
- Protocol advice
  - CT performed using high-resolution thin-slice technique with bone algorithm
  - MR performed using **multiplanar precontrast T1 (without FS)** & **corresponding T1 C+ FS,** & STIR
    - MR more sensitive than CT for early marrow involvement in nonpneumatized petrous apex, basisphenoid, & basiocciput

DIFFERENTIAL DIAGNOSIS

Metastatic Disease of Skull Base

- Usually known primary tumor
- Multiple lesions common
- SBO may be mistaken for metastatic disease in neutropenic cancer patients

Nasopharyngeal Carcinoma

- Mass originates in nasopharyngeal mucosal space
  - Usually mucosal primary is visible clinically
- Destructive upward invasion of basisphenoid & basiocciput
- May mimic SBO when advanced skull base invasion is present

Non-Hodgkin Lymphoma of Skull Base

- Soft tissue mass with bony destruction of skull base
- Secondary invasion of skull base from nasal cavity site of origin
- Other hematologic malignances (e.g., leukemia) can appear similar

Granulomatosis With Polyangiitis

- Rare mimic of SBO due to destructive changes
- Other granulomatous diseases (e.g., TB, sarcoid) also rarely can mimic SBO

Idiopathic Skull Base Inflammation (Inflammatory Pseudotumor)

- Noninfectious source of inflammation may appear identical
- May primarily involve skull base or extend secondarily from idiopathic orbital inflammation
- Diagnosis of exclusion

Bone Dysplasias

- Fibrous dysplasia, skull base

- o MR mimic of SBO; CT shows ground-glass opacification & bone expansion with variable lytic foci
- Paget disease, skull base
  - o MR mimic of SBO; CT shows osseous expansion with lytic lesion (osteoporosis circumscripta) or mixed lytic-sclerotic foci having cotton-wool appearance

PATHOLOGY

General Features

- **Necrotizing otitis externa = typical SBO**
  - o Infection starts in external ear & surrounding soft tissues, spreads lateral to medial in temporal bone
  - o Occurs most often in **diabetics**
  - o Partially treated NOE may create confusing clinical & imaging picture of relatively normal EAC but persistent SBO (may spread to central skull base)
  - o **Pseudomonas aeruginosa** identified in 98% of cases
- **Atypical SBO** usually due to invasive sinusitis, which spreads to central skull base
  - o Also occurs most often in **immunocompromised** (diabetes, HIV, chronic steroid use)
  - o Typical pathogens: Gram-positive bacteria; fungal: **Zygomycetes** (*Mucor* in ketoacidosis) and *Aspergillus* (neutropenia)
  - o **Angioinvasion** is common in invasive fungal disease, often affecting cavernous sinuses &/or intracranial vessels
    - – May result in intracranial infarcts

Gross Pathologic & Surgical Features

- Specimens contain variable inflammatory changes ranging from edema to frank purulence
- Tissue demonstrates variable necrosis, particularly with fungal etiology
- Specimens may not demonstrate microorganisms at histology
- Cultures important for definitive treatment

CLINICAL ISSUES

Presentation

- Most common signs/symptoms
  - o Typical SBO: Otalgia, otorrhea, & hearing loss in diabetic patient
  - o Atypical SBO: Sinusitis, headache, fever, malaise, cranial neuropathies in immunocompromised patient
- Other signs/symptoms
  - o **Elevated sedimentation rate**
    - – Helps distinguish infection from malignancy
  - o Elevated WBC
  - o Fever and generalized signs of infection
  - o Purulent sinusitis or otorrhea
  - o Cranial nerve deficits

Demographics

- Most commonly seen in elderly patients with diabetes
- Seen in other immunosuppressed patients all ages

Natural History & Prognosis

- Associated with high morbidity & mortality despite intensive antibiotic therapy

Treatment

- Intensive pathogen-specific antibiotic therapy including IV antibiotics
- Surgical approaches
  - o Biopsy & culture for definitive diagnosis & organism identification
  - o Surgical debridement of necrotic bone & soft tissue, especially for fungal disease
  - o Drainage of pneumatized spaces
  - o Drainage of abscesses

DIAGNOSTIC CHECKLIST

Consider

- Radiologic & clinical diagnosis of SBO requires high index of suspicion
  - o SBO is more common than reported
  - o Delay in diagnosis is common
- Consider SBO for any infiltrative skull base process if **biopsies are negative for malignancy**

Image Interpretation Pearls

- High-resolution bone CT of skull base necessary to identify **early cortical erosion**
- Multiplanar MR including **precontrast T1 without FS** & **T1 C+ FS** images required to identify marrow space involvement
  - o High-yield target areas: Nonpneumatized petrous apex, basisphenoid, & basiocciput

Reporting Tips

- Improvement in soft tissue abnormalities best indicator of early radiologic improvement
- Abnormalities of bone & bone marrow may persist for weeks to months despite response to treatment

SELECTED REFERENCES

1. Orioli L et al: Central skull base osteomyelitis: a rare but life-threatening disease. Acta Clin Belg. 70(4):291-4, 2015
2. Johnson AK et al: Central skull base osteomyelitis: an emerging clinical entity. Laryngoscope. 124(5):1083-7, 2014
3. Bag AK et al: Neuroimaging: intrinsic lesions of the central skull base region. Semin Ultrasound CT MR. 34(5):412-35, 2013
4. Adams A et al: Central skull base osteomyelitis as a complication of necrotizing otitis externa: Imaging findings, complications, and challenges of diagnosis. Clin Radiol. 67(10):e7-e16, 2012
5. Ozgen B et al: Diffusion MR imaging features of skull base osteomyelitis compared with skull base malignancy. AJNR Am J Neuroradiol. 32(1):179-84, 2011
6. Borges A: Imaging of the central skull base. Neuroimaging Clin N Am. 19(4):669-96, 2009
7. Clark MP et al: Central or atypical skull base osteomyelitis: diagnosis and treatment. Skull Base. 19(4):247-54, 2009
8. Lin YJ et al: Posterior fossa intracranial inflammatory pseudotumor: a case report and literature review. Surg Neurol. 72(6):712-6; discussion 716, 2009
9. Carfrae MJ et al: Malignant otitis externa. Otolaryngol Clin North Am. 41(3):537-49, viii-ix, 2008
10. Bouccara D et al: [Osteomyelitis of the skull base due to otologic or sinus infections. 5 cases.] Ann Otolaryngol Chir Cervicofac. 124(1):25-32, 2007
11. Lee EJ et al: MR imaging of orbital inflammatory pseudotumors with extraorbital extension. Korean J Radiol. 6(2):82-8, 2005
12. Singh A et al: Skull base osteomyelitis: diagnostic and therapeutic challenges in atypical presentation. Otolaryngol Head Neck Surg. 133(1):121-5, 2005
13. Chang PC et al: Central skull base osteomyelitis in patients without otitis externa: imaging findings. AJNR Am J Neuroradiol. 24(7):1310-6, 2003
14. Chan LL et al: Imaging of mucormycosis skull base osteomyelitis. AJNR Am J Neuroradiol. 21(5): 828-31, 2000

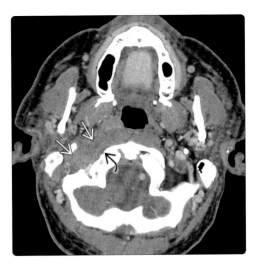
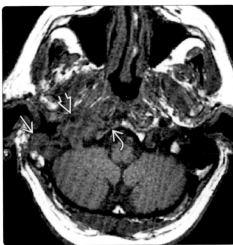

(Left) *Elderly patient with recent mastoidectomy for chronic otitis media developed fever, headache, and 6th-nerve palsy. CT demonstrates abnormal soft tissue thickening involving carotid space and prevertebral space ➡. Note small abscess adjacent to right occipital bone ⮎.* (Right) *Axial T1 MR demonstrates abnormal soft tissue in the right mastoids ➡ and prevertebral soft tissues surrounding the narrowed right ICA ➡. Notice replacement of normal fat signal in the right occipital bone ➡.*

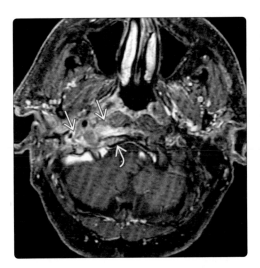
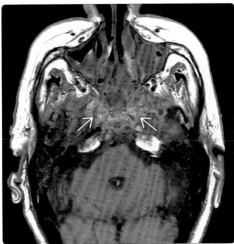

(Left) *Axial T1 C+ FS MR in an elderly patient with postoperative SBO demonstrates marked enhancement of the carotid space and preclival soft tissues ➡. Note abnormal enhancement of marrow in right side of occipital bone ➡.* (Right) *Axial T1 MR in 70-year-old diabetic patient with several months of sinusitis, headache, fever, and visual loss demonstrates patchy, widespread replacement of normal marrow signal in sphenoid bone ➡. Pathogens are Mucor and Pseudomonas.*

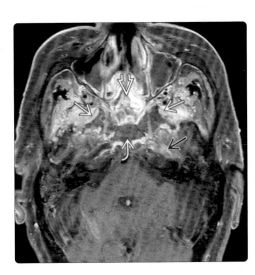
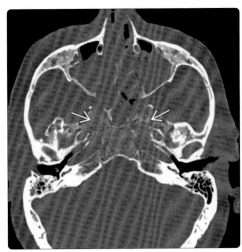

(Left) *Axial T1 C+ FS MR in 70-year-old diabetic patient with polymicrobial SBO secondary to sinusitis demonstrates enhancing sphenoid sinus ➡ and abnormal soft tissue enhancement ➡ surrounding the centrally nonenhancing, devitalized sphenoid bone ➡. Notice loss of flow void in the left ICA, which is occluded ➡.* (Right) *Axial CT in 70-year-old diabetic patient with polymicrobial SBO secondary to sinusitis demonstrates severe, diffuse osteolysis of the central skull base ➡. Pathogens are Mucor and Pseudomonas.*

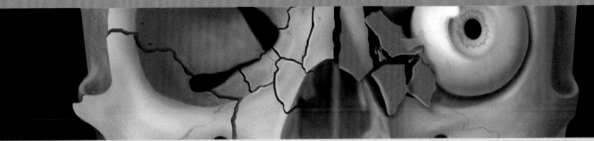

SECTION 24
Skull Base and Facial Trauma

Summary Thoughts: Skull Base & Facial Trauma

Skull base fractures (fxs) require considerable force & are often associated with other craniofacial injuries. Blunt trauma is responsible for over 90% of skull base & facial fxs & are frequently related to vehicular accidents. Injuries may range from a solitary linear fx to complex injuries involving the craniofacial skeleton. Associated intracranial injuries, such as cerebral contusion, intra-/extraaxial hemorrhage, dural tears, & vascular injuries, are common in these cases. The objective of imaging in these trauma patients is to depict the location & extent of fxs & to recognize associated injuries to vital structures. Accurate imaging interpretation also aids in surgical planning & in preventing complications.

Imaging Approaches & Indications

High-resolution bone algorithm CT is the modality of choice for imaging skull base & facial trauma. Thin-slice (0.6-1.0 mm) axial images extend from the skull vertex through the facial bones with coronal & sagittal reformatted images generated from the axial data set. Sagittal reformatted images are helpful for assessing injuries to the anterior & central skull base (ASB & CSB), particularly in patients with CSF leak. **3D-reformatted** images of facial fxs are beneficial for surgical planning as they provide a more anatomic representation of fx malalignment prior to reconstruction.

Patients with **CSF leak** or **recurrent meningitis** usually have visible defects in the ASB & CSB that are demonstrated with high-resolution bone CT. If a defect is not identified on bone CT or there are multiple fxs & it is unclear which is the source of the leak, CT cisternography may better delineate the leak site.

Arterial vascular injuries may be seen with CSB fxs that traverse the carotid canals. CTA can be performed in these patients to assess for **dissection**, traumatic **pseudoaneurysm**, or presence of **carotid-cavernous fistula**. Fxs of the petrous temporal bones & posterior fossa may extend into the major venous sinuses, resulting in posterior fossa epidural hematoma or posttraumatic venous thrombosis. CTV or MRV may be obtained in such cases. Conventional angiography is typically not necessary but used for treating vascular complications.

Cerebral injuries are often seen in high-impact trauma. Although MR is not performed initially, it is more sensitive for assessing the degree of parenchymal injury.

Approaches to Imaging Issues in Skull Base & Facial Trauma

Anterior Skull Base

ASB, or frontobasal, trauma is frequently associated with injury to the sinonasal cavities & orbits. The majority of these patients have facial injuries, including fxs of the frontal bone, orbital roofs, & cribriform plates (CP). Imaging analysis should address the following questions.

- Do fx lines involve CP or traverse anterior or posterior walls of frontal sinuses?
- Do fxs involve orbital apex or optic canals?

Central Skull Base

CSB (lateral basal) trauma may involve the sphenoid sinus walls, cavernous sinuses, & clivus & may present with carotid vascular injury or cranial nerves (CNs) III, IV, VI, or CNVI-III

deficits. Imaging analysis should address the following questions.

- Are walls of sphenoid sinuses, carotid canals, & clivus intact?
- Do cavernous sinuses appear symmetric?

Temporal Bone

Petrous temporal fxs typically have a longitudinal or transverse trajectory. The longitudinal type more often spares the otic capsule traversing the mastoid & middle ear cavities, & squamous portion, & may result in ossicular chain disruption. Transverse fxs more often involve the otic capsule extending into the occipital bone after traversing the inner ear. Imaging analysis should address the following questions.

- Does main fx line involve or spare otic capsule?
- Is ossicular chain intact?
- Does fx traverse inner ear or CNVII canal?
- Does fx traverse tegmen?

Posterior Skull Base

Fxs of the occipital bones may be isolated or associated with transverse petrous ridge fxs. The fx may extend into a dural venous sinus, jugular foramen (CNIX-XI), or CNXII canal. Craniocervical junction injuries should also be suspected in these patients. Imaging analysis should address the following questions.

- Does fx extend into transverse sinus, sigmoid sinus, or jugular foramen?
- Does fx involve internal auditory canal or hypoglossal canal?

Orbital Trauma

Orbital fxs are classified as: (1) Those involving the orbital walls, frequently the inferior orbital rim, & (2) the orbital "blowout" fx. Blowout fxs may involve the orbital floor or medial orbital wall, but the inferior orbital rim remains intact. Imaging analysis should address the following questions.

- Is there **entrapment** of inferior ± medial rectus muscles & fat; how large & displaced are fx fragments?
- Is fx isolated or are other orbital or facial fxs present [zygomaticomaxillary complex fracture (ZMC), nasoorbitalethmoid fracture (NOE), Le Fort]?

Transfacial Fracture (Le Fort)

There are 3 types of Le Fort fxs, & a consistent feature of all 3 types is the presence of bilateral pterygoid plate fxs. Le Fort I is a horizontal fx through the maxilla involving the piriform aperture. Le Fort II is a pyramidal fx involving the nasofrontal junction, infraorbital rims, medial orbital walls & orbital floors, & zygomaticomaxillary suture lines. Le Fort III (craniofacial separation) consists of fxs at the nasofrontal junction extending laterally through the lateral orbital walls & zygomatic arches. Le Fort fxs are rarely pure & are often seen in combination with other fxs. Imaging analysis should address the following questions.

- Which Le Fort types are involved; are fxs same on each side of face?
- Are other facial fx patterns present (ZMC, NOE)?

Zygomaticomaxillary Complex Fracture

The prominent position of the zygomatic arch makes it susceptible to trauma. This fx type was formerly referred to as the tripod fx; however, that is a misnomer as the zygoma has 4 involved articulations, & 5 distinct fxs are evident. Imaging analysis should address the following questions.

- How displaced & comminuted is ZMC fx?

Temporal Bone, Skull Base, & Facial Trauma Complications

Fracture Locations/Type	Potential Complications
Skull base trauma	
Anterior skull base	Posterior wall frontal sinus contaminated fx; cribriform plate fx: CSF leak/cephalocele/meningitis, CNI injury; orbital apex or optic canal fx: CNII injury
Central skull base	Internal carotid artery injury: Thrombosis, dissection, pseudoaneurysm, CCF; sphenoid sinus superior wall fx: CSF leak/cephalocele if dural tear; CNs at risk: CNIII, IV, VI, CNVI-III
Posterior skull base	Transvenous sinus fx: Venous sinus thrombosis, epidural hematoma; CNs at risk: CNVII-VIII (internal auditory canal); CNIX-XI (jugular foramen); CNXII (hypoglossal canal)
Temporal bone	Tegmen mastoideum/tympani fx: CSF leak/cephalocele if dural tear; CNs at risk: CNVII (facial nerve canal fx), CNVIII (transcochlear fx)
Orbital trauma	
Medial blowout	Medial rectus entrapment; diplopia, enophthalmos
Inferior blowout	Inferior rectus entrapment; infraorbital nerve injury, diplopia, enophthalmos
Foreign body	Globe rupture; CNII laceration/transection; infection
Facial trauma	
Transfacial (Le Fort I-III), zygomaticomaxillary complex fx, complex midfacial, nasoorbitalethmoid fxs	Traumatic telecanthus, nasolacrimal apparatus injury, epiphora, inferior orbital nerve injury (CNV2), malocclusion, mucocele
Mandibular fx	Trismus, inferior alveolar nerve injury, infection, loss of teeth

- What is extent of involvement of orbital floor, orbital apex, & lamina papyracea?
- How is lateral orbital wall displaced & is pterygoid plate fractured?

Complex Midfacial Fracture

The complex midfacial fx or "facial smash injury" consists of multiple facial fxs that cannot be classified as one of the named patterns (Le Fort, ZMC, NOE). Imaging analysis should address where the fxs are concentrated & the presence of associated orbital or skull base injuries.

Nasoorbitalethmoid Fracture

High-force trauma to the nasal bones is transmitted to the ethmoid sinuses & orbits in NOE fxs. The **medial canthal tendon** (MCT) may be disrupted in these cases & fxs may extend into the lacrimal apparatus. Imaging analysis should address the following questions.
- Is bone fragment to which MCT attaches displaced or comminuted?
- Is nasal bridge displaced posteriorly into ethmoids or superiorly into anterior fossa?
- Are there injuries to CP, frontal recess, or globes?

Mandible Fracture

Mandible fxs may occur within the alveolus (parasymphysis, body, or angle) or posterior to the teeth (ascending ramus, subcondylar region, condyle, or coronoid process). The mandible is essentially a ring of bone & multiple fxs are common, often bilaterally. Fx fragment displacement is affected by muscular attachments to the bone. Imaging analysis should address the following questions.
- Where are fxs located & what is degree & direction of displacement?
- Is inferior alveolar foramen or canal involved?
- Are condyles subluxed or dislocated?
- Do fxs involve periodontal ligament space (tooth socket)?

Clinical Implications

Understanding the mechanisms & complications of injury is essential for managing skull base trauma. The objective of treatment in patients with facial trauma is to stabilize & restore facial anatomy & to provide skeletal support for the function of mastication. Treatment is also directed toward relief of early & prevention of late complications.

Clinical signs of ASB injury include epistaxis, proptosis, chemosis, rhinorrhea, anosmia, & visual deficits. In addition to CSF leak, patients with fxs of the posterior frontal sinus wall or cribriform plate are at risk for subsequent meningitis. Fxs at the orbital apex & optic canal may cause visual deficits. Signs of temporal bone trauma may include postauricular hematoma (Battle sign), hemotympanum, otorrhea, conductive or sensorineural hearing loss, vertigo, or facial weakness. Clinical signs of posterior skull base trauma include symptoms of mass effect from epidural hematoma related to dural sinus trauma or lower cranial never deficits.

In patients with midfacial trauma, injuries to the palate, maxilla, & mandible should be assessed at imaging, as lack of appropriate repair can result in malocclusion. Depending on the degree, orbital floor involvement in patients with a ZMC fx will likely require surgical reduction. Orbital wall fxs will be treated if there is entrapment of the extraocular muscles, impingement upon the orbital apex or middle cranial fossa, or to prevent globe malposition that is resulting in diplopia or enophthalmos. Traumatic telecanthus & damage to the lacrimal drainage pathway are complications of NOE fxs that require surgical intervention.

Selected References

1. Fraioli RE et al: Facial fractures: beyond Le Fort. Otolaryngol Clin North Am. 41(1):51-76, vi, 2008
2. Samii M et al: Skull base trauma: diagnosis and management. Neurol Res. 24(2):147-56, 2002

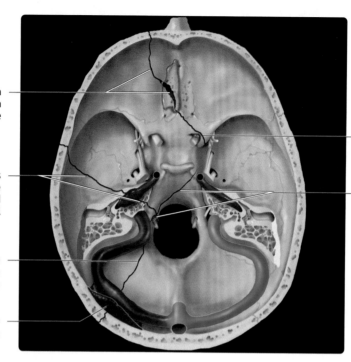

Frontal bone fracture with extension across cribriform plate

T-bone fracture of squamous portion & petrous ridge traversing petrous carotid canal

Occipital bone fracture extending into transverse sinus & jugular foramen

Posterior fossa (venous) epidural hematoma

Fracture extends through lesser sphenoid wing involving optic canal with optic nerve injury

Linear fracture through clivus with posterior extension into hypoglossal canal (CNXII)

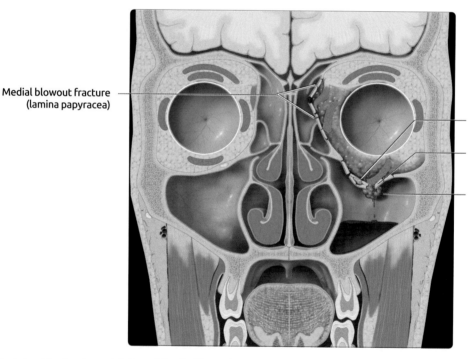

Medial blowout fracture (lamina papyracea)

Injured infraorbital nerve (CNV2)

Entrapped inferior rectus muscle

Orbital fat herniating into maxillary sinus

(Top) *Graphic of endocranial view of the skull base shows multiple fractures with expected complications. An anterior skull base fracture crosses the cribriform plate & extends into the optic canal. A fracture through the right middle fossa extends through the petrous apex involving the petrous carotid canal. An oblique clival fracture extends into the hypoglossal canal. A posterior fossa occipital fracture damages the transverse sinus & causes an extraaxial hemorrhage.* **(Bottom)** *Coronal graphic illustrates a medial & an inferior blowout fracture on the left. The medial blowout fracture displaces the lamina papyracea medially into the ethmoid sinus. An inferior blowout fracture of the floor of the orbit (maxillary sinus roof) with infraorbital nerve injury is depicted. Herniation of the inferior rectus muscle & orbital fat into the maxillary sinus may occur with variably sized floor fractures. A blow to the anterior orbit/globe, such as from a baseball, may cause either both or one of these fractures.*

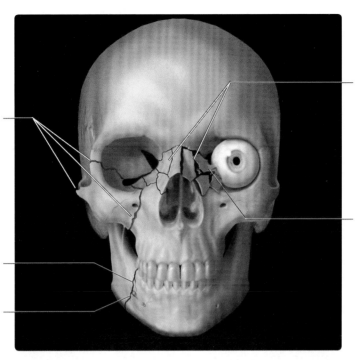

Nasoorbitalethmoid fracture

Zygomaticomaxillary complex fracture shows fracture lines through lateral orbital wall, zygomatic arch, & anterior maxillary wall with orbital floor involvement

Nasoorbitalethmoid fracture with a dominant fracture fragment attached to medial canthal tendon

Mandibular body fracture crosses inferior alveolar canal

Inferior alveolar nerve injury from transmandibular fracture

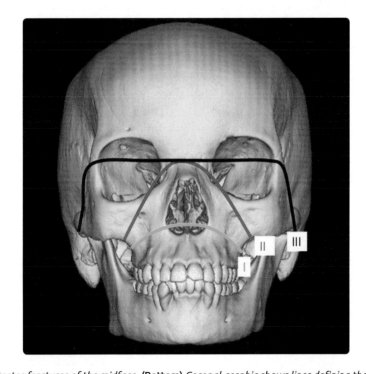

(Top) Frontal graphic demonstrates fractures of the midface. (Bottom) Coronal graphic shows lines defining the 3 types of Le Fort fractures. Le Fort I (green) involves the nasal aperture & essentially separates the maxilla & palate from the remaining midface. Le Fort II (red) traverses the inferior orbital rim & is also known as the pyramidal fracture due to its configuration. The Le Fort III (black), or craniofacial separation, extends through the zygomatic arches. A common feature of all 3 Le Fort fracture types is involvement of the pterygoid plates (not shown).

KEY FACTS

TERMINOLOGY

- Temporal bone (T-bone) fracture

IMAGING

- Bone algorithm MDCT with coronal reconstructions, CTA/MRA for suspected vascular injury
  - Dedicated brain imaging critical to evaluate for intracranial injuries (present in up to 90%)
- **Longitudinal fractures**: Vertical plane parallels long axis of petrous ridge (PR)
  - External auditory canal (EAC), middle ear (ME)/ossicular involvement common; otic capsule (OC) involvement rare
- **Transverse fractures**: Perpendicular to PR long axis
  - OC involvement, facial nerve (CNVII) injury very common; EAC/ME involvement rare
- **Oblique fractures**: Mixed features, typically horizontal and parallel to PR long axis

- OC-violating vs. OC-sparing classification better predicts complications, such as sensorineural hearing loss, CNVII injury, and CSF leak
- **Ossicular injuries**: Dislocations > > fractures, incus most commonly involved
- **CNVII injuries**: Most commonly at **geniculate ganglion**; symptoms often resolve spontaneously
- All varieties: Assess for tegmen fracture (CSF leak), carotid canal injury, extension to central skull base, intracranial, and cervical spine injury

TOP DIFFERENTIAL DIAGNOSES

- Pseudofractures: Sutures, fissures, canaliculi, aqueducts

DIAGNOSTIC CHECKLIST

- Always assess most clinically relevant structures: CNVII canal, otic capsule, tegmen, carotid canal, ossicles
- Do not misdiagnose pseudofracture

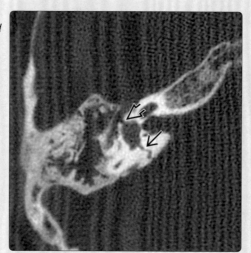
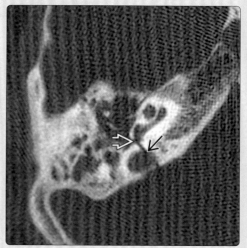

(Left) Axial bone CT in a 14 year old following severe head injury shows a medial transverse, otic capsule-violating fracture ➡ traversing the vestibule, with extension into the medial aspect of the tympanic facial nerve canal ➡. (Right) Axial bone CT more inferiorly in the same patient shows typical inferior extension of the fracture across the jugular foramen ➡, into the round window niche ➡.

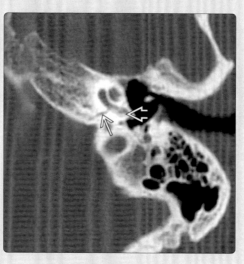
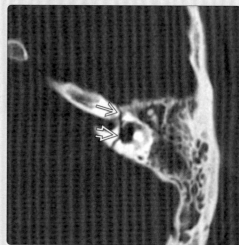

(Left) Axial bone CT shows a chronic transverse fracture line extending through the otic capsule ➡ to the basal turn of the cochlea ➡, where abnormal high density indicates the presence of labyrinthitis ossificans. (Right) Axial bone CT reveals a transverse otic capsule-violating fracture extending through the labyrinthine CNVII canal ➡ and the vestibule ➡. This medial subtype of transverse fracture often results in complete and permanent sensorineural hearing loss and facial palsy.

TERMINOLOGY

Synonyms

- Temporal bone (T-bone) fracture

Definitions

- Traumatic injury of temporal bone ± ossicle injury

IMAGING

General Features

- Best diagnostic clue
  - Bone CT shows fracture line
  - Secondary signs include **hemotympanum**, **pneumolabyrinth**, intracranial (IC) or extracranial air/hemorrhage near mastoid
    - Unexplained **parapharyngeal space air** should prompt search for **mastoid fracture**
- Morphology
  - Longitudinal fracture: Vertical plane parallels long axis of petrous ridge (PR), runs with (not across) petrotympanic fissure
  - Transverse fracture: Perpendicular to PR long axis; foramen magnum or jugular foramen to middle fossa
  - Oblique fracture: Mixed features, horizontal and parallel to PR long axis, crosses petrotympanic fissure
  - Newer classification: **Otic capsule** (OC) **violating** vs. **OC sparing**, more clinically relevant classification
    - **OC violating fractures**: Increased incidence of **sensorineural hearing loss** (SNHL), **CNVII injury**, & **CSF leak**
      □ 5-20% of fractures violate otic capsule

CT Findings

- Bone CT
  - **Longitudinal fractures**
    - Often involve temporal squamosa, external auditory canal (EAC), tympanic membrane (TM), and middle ear (ME); usually spare otic capsule
      □ Hemotympanum & ossicular disruption common
    - CNVII canal involvement most often occurs at geniculate or tympanic segments
      □ CNVII injury less common than with transverse fractures
  - **Transverse fractures**
    - Medial subtype: Posterior petrous surface through IAC to geniculate CNVII canal
    - Lateral subtype: Posterior petrous surface through OC
      □ **Pneumolabyrinth** common
    - Frequent CNVII injury, often at geniculate or IAC
    - EAC, TM, and ME involved less commonly than in longitudinal fractures
  - **Oblique fractures**
    - Involve EAC & ME; usually spare otic capsule
  - **Ossicular injuries**
    - **Dislocations** > > fractures
      □ Incus most commonly fractured ossicle
    - Incudostapedial > incudomalleolar > complete incus dislocation
    - Stapediovestibular disruption: Increasingly diagnosed with high-resolution MDCT

- Malleus dislocation rare (supported by malleal ligaments, TM attachments)
  - **Perilymph fistula (PLF)**: Oval or round window rupture with communication between middle ear & membranous labyrinth
    - Subtle findings include pneumolabyrinth and fluid at oval/round windows
  - All fracture types: Assess for tegmen fractures, carotid canal injuries, propagation to central skull base, and IC and cervical spine injuries
    - Up to 90% of patients with T-bone fractures have concomitant IC injury and up to 9% have cervical spine injury
- CTA
  - Consider CTA if fracture extends to carotid canal
    - Carotid canal fracture only moderately associated with internal carotid artery (ICA) injury
      □ Risk similar to other findings not typically associated with ICA injury (e.g., subdural hematoma)
  - Consider CTV if fracture extends to dural venous sinus or jugular bulb
  - Both carotid and dural venous sinus injuries are rare

MR Findings

- T1WI
  - Hemotympanum, hemolabyrinth (low signal acutely, high signal subacutely)
  - ICA injury: Dissection (fried-egg sign) or occlusion (loss of ICA flow void)
- T2WI
  - ME & mastoid debris appears hyperintense
  - Look for hypointense line of intact dura over tegmen on coronal images if CSF leak suspected
  - Loss of expected high signal in labyrinth may indicate hemolabyrinth, pneumolabyrinth, or posttraumatic labyrinthitis ossificans if subacute imaging
- T1WI C+
  - Most valuable for suspected subacute intracranial complications (meningitis, abscess)
  - CNVII, membranous labyrinth may enhance when involved by fracture
- MRA
  - Internal carotid artery occlusion or dissection, carotid cavernous fistula
- MRV
  - Sigmoid sinus or jugular vein thrombosis

Imaging Recommendations

- Best imaging tool
  - Temporal bone CT
- Protocol advice
  - Bone algorithm MDCT with reconstructed coronal images
    - 3D CT reconstructions helpful for clarifying fracture orientation, ossicular alignment
  - Routine brain CT or MR for intracranial complications
  - Consider CTA/MRA if involves carotid canal, CTV/MRV if involves dural sinus or jugular foramen

DIFFERENTIAL DIAGNOSIS

Pseudofractures

- Sclerotic, well-corticated margins, typically bilateral and symmetric
- Sutures/fissures
  - External: Temporoparietal, petrooccipital, sphenopetrosal (angular), occipitomastoid
  - Internal: Petrotympanic, petrosquamosal, tympanosquamous, tympanomastoid
- Canaliculi
  - Mastoid, inferior tympanic, subarcuate (petromastoid canal), singular canaliculi
- Aqueducts
  - Cochlear, vestibular aqueducts

Incus Interposition Procedure

- Surgical remodeling/realignment of incus, to bridge deficient ossicular chain and correct conductive hearing loss (CHL)
- Mimics chronic incus dislocation

Mastoiditis/Mastoid Effusion

- Preexisting mastoid or middle ear opacification may not reflect hemotympanum or CSF leak

PATHOLOGY

General Features

- Etiology
  - T-bone fracture requires application of great force, typically high-velocity impact
    - Motor vehicle accident (MVA) most common etiology
  - Longitudinal fractures due to lateral impact
  - Transverse fracture due to occipital or frontal impact
  - Tympanic plate fracture due to blow on chin

CLINICAL ISSUES

Presentation

- Most common signs/symptoms
  - Physical findings: Periauricular swelling and ecchymosis (Battle sign), EAC hemorrhage, hemotympanum
  - **Conductive hearing loss**: Initially may reflect hemotympanum ± tympanic membrane injury
    - If persistent, must evaluate for ossicular injury
  - **SNHL**: Injury to OC, IAC, brainstem, or PLF
    - If fracture absent, may reflect labyrinthine concussion
    - Intralabyrinthine hemorrhage may ultimately lead to labyrinthitis ossificans
  - Facial nerve dysfunction: CNVII injuries represent spectrum from stretching/crushing/compression to complete transection
    - Delayed paresis often reflects reversible injury; typically managed conservatively
    - Immediate, complete paralysis: Poor prognosis for recovery; may be managed surgically
  - **CSF leak**: Most resolve spontaneously within 7 days
    - Surgery for persistent leak
    - ≤ 10% develop meningitis
  - **Vertigo**: Common after even minor head trauma

- When severe/persistent, may reflect brain stem injury, labyrinthine concussion, benign paroxysmal positional vertigo, Ménière syndrome (endolymphatic hydrops), PLF
  - **Perilymphatic fistula**: Symptoms often vague; dizziness, vertigo, imbalance, fluctuating SNHL
    - Early detection facilitates surgical repair, hearing preservation
  - Chronic presentations
    - Acquired cephalocele
    - Acquired cholesteatoma
      - Squamous invasion of fracture site
    - EAC stenosis
- Other signs/symptoms
  - Intracranial pathology on CT in up to 90%
    - Extracerebral (epidural, subdural, subarachnoid) or intracerebral (contusion, diffuse axonal injury)
  - CNVI injury
  - Trismus if glenoid fossa is involved

Demographics

- Age
  - All ages; CNVII paralysis less common in pediatric T-bone fractures
- Gender
  - M > F
- Epidemiology
  - Most common fractures of skull base
  - Incidence is increasing, likely reflecting increasing traffic and population

Natural History & Prognosis

- Related to presence or absence of facial nerve injury, ossicular injury, PLF, and associated intracranial complications

Treatment

- Management of severe head injury is priority
- Anticoagulation ± endovascular therapy for carotid injury
- Antibiotics if CSF leak is present
- Management of CNVII injuries remains controversial; most advocate observation ± steroids for paresis
  - Surgical decompression or CNVII repair may be performed in patients with immediate paralysis

DIAGNOSTIC CHECKLIST

Consider

- Systematically assess most clinically relevant structures: CNVII canal, otic capsule, tegmen, carotid canal, ossicles
- Do not forget to evaluate intracranial contents

Image Interpretation Pearls

- Check contralateral side to exclude pseudofracture

Reporting Tips

- Classify fractures with regard to both anatomic (longitudinal/transverse/oblique) and otic capsule violating/sparing criteria

SELECTED REFERENCES

1. Kennedy TA et al: Imaging of temporal bone trauma. Neuroimaging Clin N Am. 24(3):467-86, viii, 2014

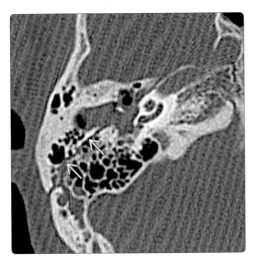
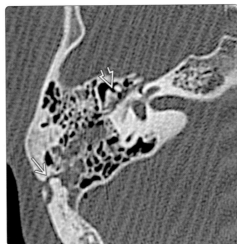

(Left) *Axial bone CT in a 16 year old following a fall from a truck demonstrates a nondepressed otic capsule-sparing longitudinal temporal bone fracture ➡. (Right) Axial bone CT in the same patient shows posterior aspect of the longitudinal fracture ➡ and subtle medial subluxation of the malleus head ⇨ seen as the "ice cream" sliding off of the "cone."*

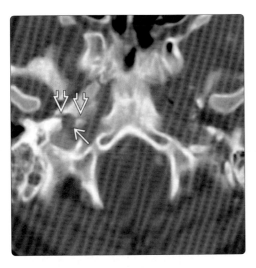
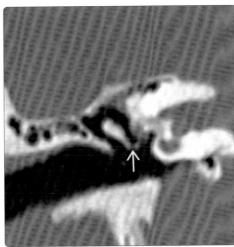

(Left) *Axial CTA demonstrates lack of enhancement in the left distal internal carotid artery ➡ secondary to posttraumatic occlusion in a teenager with bilateral complicated T-bone fractures (not shown) and involvement of the carotid canal ⇨. (Right) Coronal bone CT shows a lucency at the junction of the long and lenticular processes of the incus ➡. Persistent conductive hearing loss should prompt a careful search for ossicular injury; this subtle fracture was confirmed at surgery.*

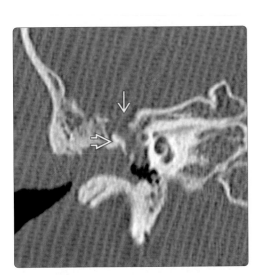
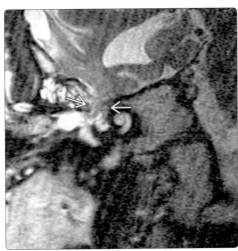

(Left) *Coronal bone CT in a 15 year old who suffered longitudinal otic capsule-sparing temporal bone fracture 8 years ago demonstrates a large tegmen tympani defect ➡ at the site of the original fracture plane and middle ear opacification, concerning for cephalocele. Note the ossicle displacement laterally ⇨. (Right) Coronal T2WI FSE MR in the same patient confirms herniation of the inferior right temporal lobe ➡ through the tegmen tympani defect, consistent with posttraumatic cephalocele.*

KEY FACTS

TERMINOLOGY

- Injury to middle ear ossicles; dislocation or subluxation >> fracture

IMAGING

- **Malalignment or dislocation** of ossicle articulations
- **Incudostapedial** > incudomalleolar > complete incus dislocation > stapediovestibular disruption > malleus dislocation
- **Incudostapedial dislocation**
  - Incus lenticular process anterior or posterior to stapes head
- **Incudomalleolar dislocation/disruption**
  - Axial CT: "Ice cream falling off of cone"
  - Sagittal CT: Disruption of molar tooth
- **Incus dislocation**
  - Disrupted incudomalleolar & incudostapedial joints → incus dissociating from malleus & stapes
- **Stapes dislocation/stapediovestibular disruption**

- Suspect if transverse fracture through oval window
- Actual disruption difficult to see, < 1-mm images may identify stapes fragments or footplate malalignment
- **Malleus dislocation**
  - Rare traumatic ossicle finding

TOP DIFFERENTIAL DIAGNOSES

- **Congenital ossicular anomalies and fixation**
  - Abnormal shape, size, or orientation; fixation of ossicles to wall of ME cavity
- **Ossicular prosthesis**
  - Stapes prosthesis: Missing all or part of stapes superstructure
  - Incus interposition graft: Mimics chronic incus dislocation
- **Chronic otomastoiditis with ossicular erosions**
  - Erosive ossicular changes in absence of cholesteatoma, in patient with history of chronic otitis media
- **Congenital cholesteatoma with ossicular erosions**
- **Acquired cholesteatoma with ossicular erosions**

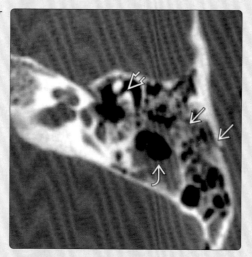
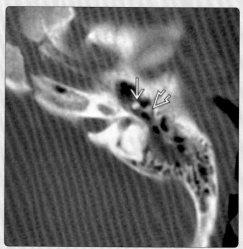

(Left) Axial bone CT in a 7 year old who fell 8 feet shows a longitudinal, otic capsule-sparing temporal bone fracture ➡, mild widening of the incudomalleolar joint ➡, and blood in the antrum ➡. (Right) Axial bone CT in a 12 year old involved in an all-terrain vehicle accident demonstrates medial dislocation of the malleus head ➡ relative to the incus body ➡, resulting in the ice cream falling off of the cone appearance, typical of incudomalleolar dislocation.

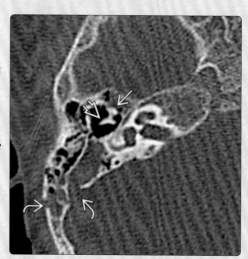
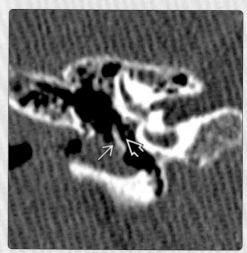

(Left) Axial bone CT in an 18 month old after a TV fell on his head shows malposition and malrotation of the malleus head ➡ and the incus body ➡, as well as a diastatic mastoid fracture ➡. (Right) Coronal reformat bone CT in the same child also shows inferior position of the incus long process ➡ relative to the stapes head ➡, consistent with incus dislocation secondary to incudomalleolar and incudostapedial joint disruption.

TERMINOLOGY

Definitions

- Injury to middle ear ossicles
  - Dislocation or subluxation >> fracture

IMAGING

General Features

- Best diagnostic clue
  - **Malalignment or dislocation** of ossicle articulations
- Location
  - **Incudostapedial** > incudomalleolar > complete incus dislocation > stapediovestibular disruption > malleus dislocation
- Morphology
  - **Incudostapedial** dislocation difficult to diagnose on CT, oblique reconstructions helpful
    - **Incus lenticular process anterior or posterior to stapes head**
  - **Incudomalleolar** dislocation/disruption
    - Axial CT: **Malleus head offset** from incus short process looks like **ice cream falling off of cone**
    - Sagittal CT: **Disruption of molar tooth**
  - **Incus** dislocation
    - **Incudomalleolar & incudostapedial joints disrupted** → incus dissociates from malleus & stapes
  - **Stapes** dislocation/stapediovestibular disruption rare
    - Suspect if **transverse fracture line passing through oval window**
    - Actual disruption difficult to see, < 1-mm images may identify stapes fragments or footplate malalignment
  - **Malleus** dislocation **rare**

Imaging Recommendations

- Best imaging tool
  - High-resolution temporal bone CT
    - 0.50- to 0.75-mm slice thickness
- Protocol advice
  - Bone algorithm MDCT with reconstructed coronal ± oblique &/or sagittal images
    - 3D CT reconstructions helpful for clarifying ossicular alignment

DIFFERENTIAL DIAGNOSIS

Congenital Ossicular Anomalies and Fixation

- Ossicular fixation: **Rigid bar or fibrous band** connects ossicle to wall of middle ear cavity
- Ossicular malformation: Abnormal **shape, size, or orientation**

Ossicular Prosthesis

- Surgical reconstruction of malfunctioned portions of ossicular chain to improve hearing
  - Stapes prosthesis
    - **Missing all or part of stapes superstructure**
  - Incus interposition graft
    - **Mimics chronic incus dislocation**
  - Partial ossicular replacement prosthesis (PORP)
  - Total ossicular replacement prosthesis (TORP)

Chronic Otomastoiditis With Ossicular Erosions

- Erosive ossicular changes in absence of cholesteatoma, in patient with history of chronic otitis media

Congenital Cholesteatoma With Ossicular Erosions

- Smooth, well-circumscribed middle ear mass ± ossicular erosions

Acquired Cholesteatoma With Ossicular Erosions

- Soft tissue mass in Prussak space with scutum, ossicle, &/or lateral epitympanum wall erosion

PATHOLOGY

General Features

- Etiology
  - Disruption of ossicle support: Ligaments and tendons; tetanic contraction of stapedius and tensor tympani muscles contribute to many of injuries
    - Head trauma >> blast injury; rarely secondary to foreign body insertion or lightning strike
    - Incus involved in most posttraumatic ossicular disruptions; weaker ligamentous support compared to malleus and stapes
    - Malleus support: Anterior, lateral, & superior malleolar ligaments; tensor tympani tendon; embedded in tympanic membrane
    - Stapes support: Stapedius tendon (stapes hub); stapediovestibular articulation (stapes footplate & annular ligament)
- Associated abnormalities
  - Temporal bone fractures
    - **Longitudinal, transverse, or mixed**
    - **Otic capsule violating or otic capsule sparing**
  - **Pneumolabyrinth** secondary to posttraumatic perilymph fistula
  - Middle ear/mastoid opacification/**hemotympanum**
  - **Intracranial injury**: Extraaxial hematoma, parenchymal contusion, pneumocephalus, cerebral edema, diffuse axonal injury
  - **Facial nerve canal fracture** with facial nerve injury
  - **CSF leak**
  - **Carotid artery canal &/or jugular foramen fracture**

CLINICAL ISSUES

Presentation

- Most common signs/symptoms
  - Posttraumatic **conductive hearing loss**
    - Secondary to hemotympanum &/or injury to TM, tympanic ring, or ossicles
    - Suspect ossicular injury if persistent hearing loss ≥ 30 decibels lasting ≥ **2 months following trauma**

Treatment

- Ossicular reconstruction with repositioning or interpositioning of various materials: Ossicles, cortical bone grafts, bone cement, PORP, or TORP

SELECTED REFERENCES

1. Kennedy TA et al: Imaging of temporal bone trauma. Neuroimaging Clin N Am. 24(3):467-86, viii, 2014

KEY FACTS

TERMINOLOGY

- Traumatic injury of bony anterior, middle, or posterior cranial fossa

IMAGING

- Noncorticated, noninterdigitating lucency + pneumocephalus or intraorbital emphysema
- Location
  - Anterior fossa: Frontal bone-sinus, cribriform plate
  - Middle fossa: Greater sphenoid wing, sphenoid sinus, clivus
  - Posterior fossa: Petrous temporal bone, occiput
- Protocol advice
  - Bone CT: Skull + facial bones + cervical spine
  - NECT: Brain + neck soft tissues
  - CTA or MRA: Suspected neurovascular injury
  - MR brain: Suspected cerebral injury

TOP DIFFERENTIAL DIAGNOSES

- Pseudofractures
  - Sutures and fissures
  - Canals and foramina
  - Emissary veins and venous sinuses

PATHOLOGY

- Associated abnormalities
  - Intracranial contusion, hematoma
  - Pneumocephalus
  - Neurovascular injury
  - CSF fistula/leak
  - Cranial nerve deficits

CLINICAL ISSUES

- Results from high-velocity impact: Motor vehicle accident, gunshot/missile
- Management triaged according to degree/severity of intracranial injury

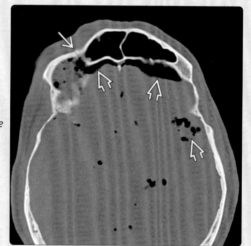
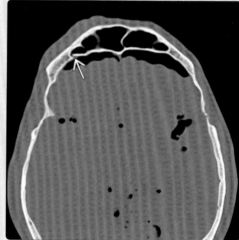

(Left) Axial bone CT shows an anterior skull base or type I/II frontobasal fracture with a fracture line extending through the superomedial orbit ➡ just lateral to the frontal sinus. There is significant associated pneumocephalus ➡. (Right) Axial bone CT shows a fracture through the posterior wall of the right frontal sinus ➡. This fracture, in addition to other small fractures in the cribriform plate (not shown), accounts for the source of pneumocephalus and places the patient at risk for meningitis.

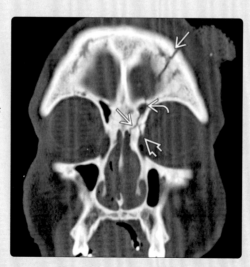
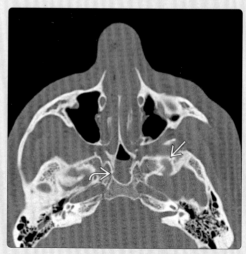

(Left) Coronal bone CT shows an anterior skull base/type III frontobasal fracture with a large fracture ➡ extending through the left frontal bone to the nasoorbitoethmoid complex. The fracture traverses the left frontal sinus ➡ and terminates in the region of the left lacrimal sac ➡. (Right) Axial bone CT shows middle cranial fossa (MCF) fractures through the left greater wing of sphenoid bone ➡ and lateral wall of the right sphenoid sinus ➡. Fractures of the MCF often involve vascular canals or neural foramina.

TERMINOLOGY

Definitions

- Traumatic injury of anterior, middle, or posterior skull base

IMAGING

General Features

- Best diagnostic clue
  - Noncorticated, noninterdigitating lucency in skull base bone ± pneumocephalus or intraorbital emphysema
- Location
  - Anterior cranial fossa (ACF)
    - Frontal bone, ethmoid bone, & anterior sphenoid bone
    - Includes frontal sinus, medial 1/3 superior orbital rim, nasoethmoid, cribriform plate, and planum sphenoidale
  - Middle cranial fossa (MCF): Greater wing of sphenoid (GWS) bone, sphenoid sinus, clivus
    - Includes cavernous sinus, horizontal and vertical petrous carotid canals
  - Posterior cranial fossa (PCF): Petrous temporal bone & occiput
- Size
  - Fractures involving cribriform plate, fovea ethmoidalis, carotid canal **may be subtle**
- Morphology
  - Linear
    - Longitudinal, transverse, or oblique
      - May be vertical or horizontal
      - ACF longitudinal fractures run **parallel to cribriform plate**
      - ACF transverse or oblique fractures usually extend to involve orbit and sphenoid
      - MCF fractures typically **transverse or oblique**
  - Comminuted
    - Often associated skull or midface fractures

Imaging Recommendations

- Best imaging tool
  - Thin-slice axial bone CT with multiplanar reconstruction
- Protocol advice
  - Bone CT: Head + facial bones
    - Multidetector CT (MDCT) higher accuracy for detection of fracture
    - Thin-section axial acquisition with 1-mm coronal and sagittal reformats
    - 3D volumetric reconstruction for assessment of deformity, fracture orientation, & reconstruction planning
  - NECT: Head + facial bones
    - Assess **associated intracranial injury**
    - Assess soft tissue injury of orbit, face, upper neck
  - CTA or MRA: **Suspected carotid/vertebral dissection, thromboembolism, carotid-cavernous fistula (CCF)**
    - Fracture involves carotid canal or extends through clivus
    - Enlarged superior ophthalmic vein, significant air in cavernous sinus
  - MR brain: Suspected **cerebral parenchymal injury**

CT Findings

- NECT
  - Associated intracranial injury
    - Epidural, subdural hematoma, parenchymal contusion, subarachnoid blood, infarct
  - Associated intraorbital soft tissue injury
    - Globe rupture or tenting; intraocular hemorrhage
    - Lens dislocation
    - Retrobulbar or subperiosteal hematoma
  - Paranasal sinus hemorrhage or hematoma
- Bone CT
  - Noncorticated, noninterdigitating lucency
    - May have associated diastasis of sutures
  - Comminution of bone typically mild to moderate
    - Displacement of bone fragments
    - Highly comminuted cribriform or ethmoid fractures usually associated with complex facial fractures
  - Associated pneumocephalus, intraorbital emphysema
  - Air-fluid levels in frontal, ethmoid, sphenoid sinuses
- CTA
  - Arterial occlusion/**dissection**
    - Vessel wall irregularity, luminal narrowing, pseudoaneurysm
    - Lack of contrast opacification
      - Segmental high-grade flame-shaped or tapered narrowing/string sign → dissection
    - 16 slice or greater MDCT: **92% negative predictive value** for carotid/vertebral occlusion, dissection
  - **Carotid-cavernous fistula**
    - Focal bulging, asymmetric distension of involved cavernous sinus
    - Enlargement of ipsilateral superior ophthalmic vein
    - Fistula tract between cavernous carotid and cavernous sinus

MR Findings

- T1WI FS
  - Consider T1 FS without contrast for cervical dissection
- T1/T2/FLAIR/DWI: Hemorrhage, infarction, shear injury
  - Loss of flow void in ICA/vertebral or fried egg/crescent sign → occlusion or dissection
- MRA: Carotid/vertebral occlusion or dissection, CCF

DIFFERENTIAL DIAGNOSIS

Pseudofractures of Skull Base

- Sutures and fissures
  - Sphenofrontal suture and metopic suture
  - Sphenooccipital synchondroses
  - Petrooccipital fissure
  - Sphenopetrosal synchondrosis and sphenosquamosal suture
  - Tympanosquamous suture and petrotympanic fissure
  - Occipitomastoid suture
- Canals and foramina
  - Anterior, posterior ethmoidal artery canal
  - Supraorbital artery foramen
  - Vidian canal
  - Neurovascular channels from foramen rotundum and ovale

- – Inferior and lateral rotundal canals
- – Accessory meningeal artery canal and foramen of Vesalius
- Emissary veins and venous sinuses
  - Mastoid, occipital, petrosquamosal, posterior condylar
  - Superior petrosal sinus

PATHOLOGY

General Features

- Etiology
  - ACF: Results from frontal bone impact
    - **Predominately** secondary to **motor vehicle accident (MVA)**
    - Low-velocity frontal bone injuries → linear fractures of anterior ± central skull base
    - High-velocity lateral or inferior frontal bone/glabella, supraorbital region & zygoma → anterior + central skull base involvement
  - MCF: High-velocity impact to lateral frontal bone, zygoma, temporal or parietal bone
- Associated abnormalities
  - Intracranial contusion, hematoma
  - Pneumocephalus
  - CSF fistula/leak
    - – ↑ probability with linear or comminuted fractures involving ACF, central anterior skull base
  - Carotid or vertebrobasilar dissection, thromboembolism
    - – Fracture involving sphenoid sinus or carotid canal → ↑ probability of neurovascular injury
  - Dural AV fistula
    - – CCF: ↑ **incidence of CCF with sphenoid, carotid canal fracture**
  - Cranial nerve deficits
    - – Frontobasal: CNI, less commonly CNIII, IV, VI
    - – MCF: CNIII-VI
  - Horner syndrome

Staging, Grading, & Classification

- AOCMF classification divides skull base into 9 regions: Left and right frontal, central, middle, and posterior cranial fossa
  - Anterior skull base: Frontal bone and LWS
  - Central skull base
    - – Central anterior: Cribriform plate and planum sphenoidale
    - – Central middle: Sella and parasellar compartments
    - – Central posterior: Clivus
  - Middle: Sphenoid, GWS, and temporal bone
  - Posterior: Parietal and occipital bone
- Other classifications
  - Frontobasal: Type I, type II, and type III
    - – Types I and II are linear fractures involving frontal bone, nasoorbitoethmoid, cribriform plate or planum sphenoidale (type 1) or extend through orbit and squamous temporal bone (type II)
    - – Type III: Combined comminuted type 1 and type II fractures

CLINICAL ISSUES

Presentation

- Most common signs/symptoms

- Frontal or temporal scalp laceration, hematoma
  - – Periorbital hematoma (raccoon eyes)
- Proptosis, other orbital injuries
- Altered mental status, loss of consciousness, & neurological deficit
- Other signs/symptoms
  - Nausea, vomiting, seizure, drowsiness

Demographics

- Age
  - All ages
    - – Less common in pediatric populations
- Gender
  - M > F
- Epidemiology
  - High-velocity impact predominately MVA, gunshot/missile
  - Lower velocity blunt trauma more often following falls, assault/nonaccidental trauma

Natural History & Prognosis

- ACF/Type II and III frontobasal
  - Higher risk for intracranial injuries
  - Higher risk for CSF leak
- MCF fractures
  - Higher risk for intracranial injuries
  - Higher risk for neurovascular injuries
  - Higher risk for cranial nerve deficits

Treatment

- Management triaged according to degree/severity of intracranial injury
- Endovascular treatment for neurovascular injury
- Antibiotic coverage for meningitis/CSF leak
- Management of orbital injuries
- CSF leak repair

SELECTED REFERENCES

1. Di Ieva A et al: The comprehensive AOCMF classification: skull base and cranial vault fractures - level 2 and 3 tutorial. Craniomaxillofac Trauma Reconstr. 7(Suppl 1):S103-13, 2014
2. Maillard AA et al: Trauma to the intracranial internal carotid artery. J Trauma. 68(3):545-7, 2010
3. Bächli H et al: Skull base and maxillofacial fractures: two centre study with correlation of clinical findings with a comprehensive craniofacial classification system. J Craniomaxillofac Surg. 37(6):305-11, 2009
4. Manson PN et al: Frontobasal fractures: anatomical classification and clinical significance. Plast Reconstr Surg. 124(6):2096-106, 2009
5. Mithani SK et al: Predictable patterns of intracranial and cervical spine injury in craniomaxillofacial trauma: analysis of 4786 patients. Plast Reconstr Surg. 123(4):1293-301, 2009
6. Atabaki SM et al: A clinical decision rule for cranial computed tomography in minor pediatric head trauma. Arch Pediatr Adolesc Med. 162(5):439-45, 2008
7. Nakstad PH et al: Correlation of head trauma and traumatic aneurysms. Interv Neuroradiol. 14(1):33-8, 2008
8. Feiz-Erfan I et al: Incidence and pattern of direct blunt neurovascular injury associated with trauma to the skull base. J Neurosurg. 107(2):364-9, 2007
9. Madhusudan G et al: Nomenclature of frontobasal trauma: a new clinicoradiographic classification. Plast Reconstr Surg. 117(7):2382-8, 2006
10. Pretto Flores L et al: Positive predictive values of selected clinical signs associated with skull base fractures. J Neurosurg Sci. 44(2):77-82; discussion 82-3, 2000

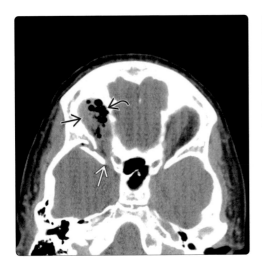

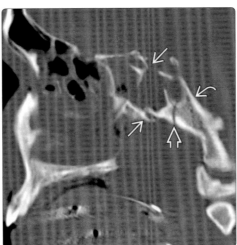

(Left) Axial NECT shows a displaced fracture through the posterior rim of the right lesser wing of the sphenoid bone with orbital emphysema ⮕ & a subperiosteal hematoma ⮕. Note that slight rotation of the sphenoid wing fracture fragment impinges on the superior orbital fissure ⮕. (Right) Sagittal bone CT in a patient following a motor vehicle accident (MVA) shows multiple comminuted sphenoid ⮕ and clival ⮕ fractures. The posterior clivus is intact ⮕, reducing the probability of vertebral artery injury.

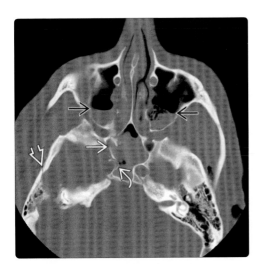

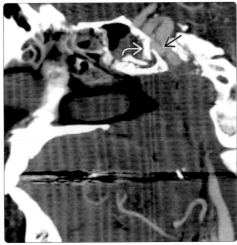

(Left) Axial bone CT shows a comminuted fracture through the lateral wall of the right sphenoid sinus ⮕ and carotid canal. Note the "double wall" ⮕ in the carotid canal. Additional small fractures are seen in the right squamous temporal bone ⮕, and there are air-fluid levels in the maxillary sinuses ⮕. (Right) Sagittal CTA shows a pseudoaneurysm ⮕ in the cavernous (C4) segment of the internal carotid artery adjacent to the sphenoid fracture fragments ⮕.

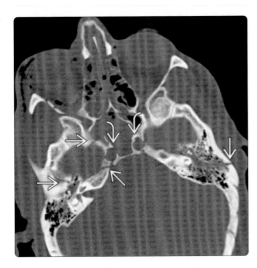

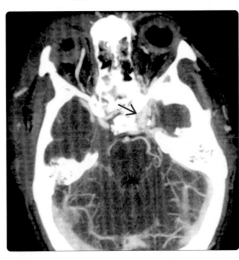

(Left) Axial bone CT in a patient following high-speed MVA shows multiple temporal, petrous temporal bone and sphenoid fractures ⮕. Both carotid canals are fractured ⮕, increasing the probability of carotid injury. (Right) Axial CTA shows asymmetric abnormal venous enhancement in conjunction with arterial enhancement in this traumatic carotid-cavernous fistula (CCF) ⮕ in the left cavernous carotid. The superior ophthalmic vein was also enlarged (not shown). The CCF was confirmed on digital subtraction angiography.

TERMINOLOGY

- Foreign material introduced into orbit via trauma

IMAGING

- CT is sensitive and safe modality for detecting foreign body (FB)
  - Density and shape indicate nature of object
  - **Metal** density > 1,000-2,000 HU, attenuation artifact
    - Firearms, workplace materials
  - **Glass** denser than bone, wide variation
    - Pane shards or safety glass fragments
  - **Wood** typically low density, similar to air when dry
    - Pencils with dense stylus core, tree branches
  - **Miscellaneous** objects of any origin
    - Plastic or sponge very low density, similar to air
    - Sand or gravel dense granular material
- Consider MR for possible FB if CT negative
  - Contraindicated if unknown ferromagneticity
  - Inflammation or granulation suggests organic material

TOP DIFFERENTIAL DIAGNOSES

- Ophthalmic surgical device
- Phthisis bulbi
- Dystrophic calcification

PATHOLOGY

- Most FB occur with high-velocity or projectile injury
  - Hammering, occupational, assault, MVA
  - May occur after apparently trivial trauma

CLINICAL ISSUES

- Organic FB more likely to incite cellulitis and abscess
- All puncture wounds require exploration
- Surgical decision depends on type and location of FB

DIAGNOSTIC CHECKLIST

- CT is study of choice and should be performed 1st
- Occult FB discoveries are surprisingly common
- Assess for globe rupture and optic nerve injury

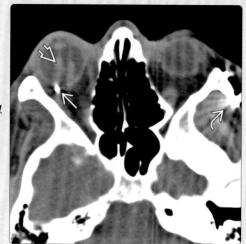
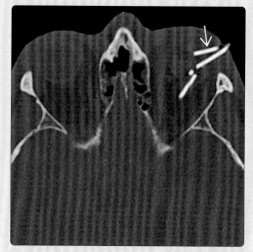

(Left) Axial NECT in a patient who sustained a shotgun injury to the face shows shrapnel ➡ in the sclera posteriorly. The globe was ruptured, and there is intraocular hemorrhage ➡. Additional foreign body artifact is noted on the left ➡. (Right) Axial bone CT shows multiple well-defined hyperdense shards of glass penetrating the left orbit and perforating globe ➡. The patient had fallen face first onto a drinking glass while intoxicated.

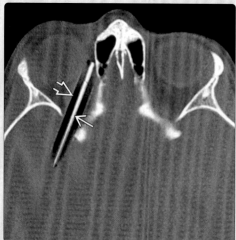
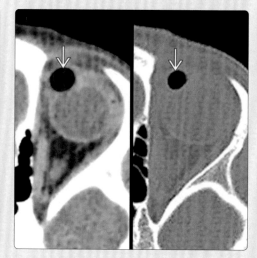

(Left) Axial bone CT shows a piece of a broken pencil within the right orbit. The center dense core represents the pencil stylus ("lead") ➡. The outer casing of wood is low density ➡. (Right) Axial CT demonstrates a foreign body with very low density ➡ displayed at 2 different grayscale levels. Variable grayscale display is useful when assessing the nature of a foreign body, demonstrating in this case that the object is comprised of polystyrene foam, rather than air or a lipoid mass.

TERMINOLOGY

Abbreviations

- Foreign body (FB)

Definitions

- Foreign material introduced into orbit via trauma

IMAGING

General Features

- Size
  - Larger FB easier to detect
    - Glass: > 90% if ≥ 1.5 mm; < 50% if ≤ 0.5 mm

Imaging Recommendations

- Best imaging tool
  - **CT** most sensitive modality for detecting FB
    - Safe in presence of metallic object
  - Consider **MR** to assess for possibility of plastic, wooden, or other organic FB if CT negative
    - Contraindicated if unknown ferromagneticity

CT Findings

- NECT
  - **Metal** FB very high density (> 1,000-2,000 HU)
    - Streak artifact due to **beam-hardening** effect
    - Firearm projectiles, workplace materials
  - **Glass** FB denser than bone, varies with type
    - High-density glass (e.g., crystal) easiest to detect
    - Shape: Shards (panes) or angular fragments (safety)
  - **Wood** FB appears as **air** density with **geographic** margin
    - Dry wood (-600 HU); fresh wood (-20 HU)
    - Pencils (with dense stylus core); tree branches
  - **Miscellaneous** FB range from ordinary to bizarre
    - **Plastic** or **sponge** very low density, similar to air
    - **Sand** or **gravel** appear as dense granular material
    - **Bone** from displaced fracture or animal **tooth**

MR Findings

- STIR
  - Hyperintense inflammatory response surrounding FB, particularly organic material
- T1WI C+ FS
  - Enhancement of inflammatory or granulation tissue suggests organic origin

DIFFERENTIAL DIAGNOSIS

Ophthalmic Surgical Device

- Intraocular lens (refractive correction)
- Scleral band (sponge, rubber, or plastic)
- Intraocular retinopexy tamponade (oil or gas)
- Ocular prosthesis (following enucleation)

Phthisis Bulbi

- Shrunken, disfigured, calcified globe
- Chronic end-stage due to severe eye injury

Dystrophic Calcification

- Drusen (punctate calcification at optic disc)
- Rectus muscle insertion, trochlear sling
- Nonspecific senile scleral calcification

PATHOLOGY

General Features

- Etiology
  - Most FB occur with **high-velocity** or **projectile** injury
    - Hammering is common mechanism (metal on metal)
    - Occupational hazard (nail gun, glass workers)
    - Assault (knives, gunshot, BB pellets)
    - Motor vehicle collision (glass, metallic fragments)
  - May occur after apparently trivial trauma
- Associated abnormalities
  - **Fractures** and **globe injury** in path of introduced object
  - More complications with heavier and posterior FB

Staging, Grading, & Classification

- Metallic, inorganic (steel, lead, copper, etc.)
- Nonmetallic, inorganic (glass, plastic, fiberglass, etc.)
- Nonmetallic, organic (wood, plant material, etc.)

CLINICAL ISSUES

Presentation

- Most common signs/symptoms
  - Sharp, stabbing pain at time of injury
  - Pain on eye movement, ↓ visual acuity
  - Hyphema, vitreal hemorrhage
- Other signs/symptoms
  - Orbital mass, cellulitis, or abscess
  - Optic neuropathy
  - Orbital wall fracture

Demographics

- Epidemiology
  - Penetrating injury is component of 50% of trauma to eye
  - Intraocular FB present in 20-40% of open globe injuries

Natural History & Prognosis

- **Organic** FB more likely to incite **cellulitis and abscess** compared with metallic FB

Treatment

- All puncture wounds require exploration
- Inorganic FB may be treated conservatively
- Decision regarding surgical removal depends on **type** and **location** of FB
  - Anterior metallic FB may be removed to prevent infection, motility impairment, ptosis, or fistula formation
  - FB at orbital apex adjacent to optic nerve may require optic canal decompression

DIAGNOSTIC CHECKLIST

Image Interpretation Pearls

- CT is **study of choice** and should be performed 1st
- **Occult** FB discoveries are surprisingly common

Reporting Tips

- Assess for **globe rupture** and **optic nerve** injury

SELECTED REFERENCES

1. Kubal WS: Imaging of orbital trauma. Radiographics. 28(6):1729-39, 2008

KEY FACTS

TERMINOLOGY

- Traumatic deformity of orbital floor or medial wall resulting from impact of blunt object larger than orbital aperture

IMAGING

- High-resolution axial bone CT with coronal & sagittal reconstructions is modality of choice
- 2 broad categories of blowout fractures
  - Open door: Large, displaced, frequently comminuted
  - Trapdoor: Linear, hinged, minimally displaced
- Associated findings
  - Herniation of orbital contents through bony defect
  - Involvement of infraorbital canal
  - Orbital soft tissue injury
  - May occur in combination with other facial fractures (nasal, transfacial, zygomaticomaxillary complex)

TOP DIFFERENTIAL DIAGNOSES

- Dehiscent lamina papyracea

- Orbital decompression surgery
- Nasoorbitalethmoidal fracture

CLINICAL ISSUES

- Most common symptoms
  - Diplopia: Typically related to entrapment
  - Enophthalmos: Due to prolapse of orbital contents into sinuses
  - Hypesthesia of cheek and upper gum: Due to infraorbital nerve injury

DIAGNOSTIC CHECKLIST

- Entrapment is clinical, not radiographic, diagnosis
  - Note abnormal position & morphology of extraocular muscles
- In children, minimally displaced but highly symptomatic trapdoor fractures are common

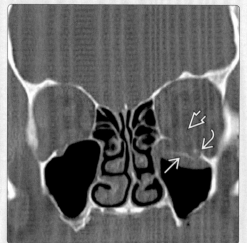
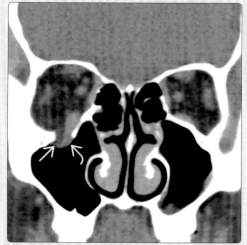

(Left) Coronal bone CT demonstrates a mildly depressed left orbital floor orbital blowout fracture (OBF) ➡ just medial to the infraorbital canal ➡. The inferior rectus muscle ➡ is grossly normal in position and configuration. (Right) Coronal NECT reveals a chronic right orbital floor OBF with herniation of a small volume of fat ➡ and a portion of the inferior rectus muscle ➡ through the fracture defect. The muscle also demonstrates an abnormal vertical orientation.

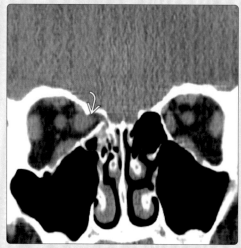
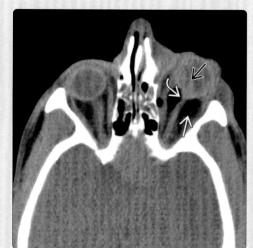

(Left) Coronal soft tissue NECT shows deformity of the right medial rectus muscle, entering the osseous defect of a lamina papyracea fracture ➡. (Right) Axial NECT shows retrobulbar orbital emphysema ➡ with associated proptosis and tenting of the optic nerve insertion ➡. There is also an intraocular hemorrhage ➡.

TERMINOLOGY

Abbreviations

- Orbital blowout fracture (OBF)

Definitions

- Orbital floor or medial wall fracture resulting from impact of blunt object of diameter greater than orbital aperture
  o Pure: Without orbital rim fracture
  o Impure: With orbital rim fracture

IMAGING

General Features

- Best diagnostic clue
  o Deformity of orbital floor/medial wall ± herniation of orbital contents through bony defect
- Location
  o Floor fractures: Middle 1/3, near infraorbital canal
  o Conflicting data exist regarding relative frequency of floor vs. medial wall fractures
- Morphology
  o Open door: Large, displaced, frequently comminuted
  o Trapdoor: Linear, hinged, minimally displaced
    - High frequency of extraocular muscle (EOM) entrapment despite scant external signs of trauma
    - May be difficult to diagnose radiographically because of minimal displacement
    - Most pediatric blowout fractures are trapdoor type

CT Findings

- Bone CT
  o Simple or comminuted fracture of orbital floor/medial wall, ±
    - Herniation of orbital contents (fat, EOMs)
    - Fracture through infraorbital canal
    - Injury to orbital soft tissues (globe rupture, retrobulbar hematoma)
  o Significant orbital emphysema more common in medial wall fractures
  o May occur in combination with other facial fractures, e.g., nasal, transfacial (Le Fort), zygomaticomaxillary complex (ZMC)

Imaging Recommendations

- Best imaging tool
  o Thin-slice bone algorithm MDCT in axial plane with coronal, sagittal reconstructions
    - Involvement of infraorbital canal best seen in coronal plane
    - Involvement/sparing of orbital rim best determined in sagittal plane
- Protocol advice
  o Include soft tissue algorithm reconstructions to evaluate orbital contents

DIFFERENTIAL DIAGNOSIS

Dehiscent Lamina Papyracea

- Medial wall deformity may reflect congenital dehiscence &/or is associated with ethmoid hypoplasia

Orbital Decompression Surgery

- Resection of medial orbital wall performed for thyroid orbitopathy

Nasoorbitalethmoidal Fracture

- Fractures also involve nasal bridge with nasal depression and traumatic telecanthus

Zygomaticomaxillary Complex Fracture

- Fractures also seen in zygomatic arch, lateral orbital wall, maxillary sinus walls

CLINICAL ISSUES

Presentation

- Most common signs/symptoms
  o Diplopia
    - Typically secondary to EOM ± fat entrapment
    - May occur without entrapment, secondary to edema/hemorrhage
  o Enophthalmos
    - Secondary to prolapse of orbital contents into maxillary (or ethmoid) sinus
  o Hypesthesia of cheek and upper gum
    - Secondary to fracture through infraorbital canal
- Other signs/symptoms
  o Visual loss
    - Secondary to globe/optic nerve injury
  o Oculocardiac reflex

Natural History & Prognosis

- Small uncomplicated fractures: No treatment
- Urgent surgery recommended for nonresolving oculocardiac reflex, white-eyed OBF with severe gaze restriction, early enophthalmos
- Timing otherwise controversial
  o Most advocate surgery within 2 weeks for diplopia, herniation of orbital contents on CT, or large orbital floor fractures (> 50% of floor area) that may result in delayed enophthalmos

Treatment

- Orbital floor reconstruction typically performed with alloplast (titanium mesh, porous polyethylene)

DIAGNOSTIC CHECKLIST

Consider

- In children, minimally displaced but highly symptomatic trapdoor fractures are common

Image Interpretation Pearls

- Entrapment is clinical, not radiographic, diagnosis

Reporting Tips

- Assess position, orientation, and configuration of EOMs, as functional entrapment can occur without significant displacement
- Check for mass effect on optic nerve insertion from retrobulbar hematoma or emphysema

SELECTED REFERENCES

1. Layton CJ: Factors associated with significant ocular injury in conservatively treated orbital fractures. J Ophthalmol. 2014:412397, 2014

Transfacial Fractures (Le Fort)

TERMINOLOGY

- Fractures disrupting **pterygomaxillary junction**, disjoining portions of face (maxilla) from skull

IMAGING

- Best diagnostic clue: Pterygoid process and pterygoid plate fractures in patients with clinically mobile facial skeleton
- **Le Fort I**
  - Pyriform rim + medial & lateral walls of maxillary sinus or alveolus + nasal septum
- **Le Fort II**
  - Medial orbital wall, including frontomaxillary suture + nasofrontal junction; inferior orbital wall, including zygomaticomaxillary suture + inferior rim
- **Le Fort III**
  - Medial orbital wall, including frontomaxillary suture + nasofrontal junction; lateral orbital wall, including zygomaticofrontal suture + zygomaticosphenoid suture + zygomatic arch

TOP DIFFERENTIAL DIAGNOSES

- Zygomaticomaxillary complex fracture
- Nasoorbitalethmoidal fracture
- Complex facial fracture
- Pterygoid plate avulsion

PATHOLOGY

- **Type I: "Floating palate"**
  - Inferior portions of medial & lateral maxillary buttresses
- **Type II: "Pyramidal fracture"**
  - Superior portion of medial maxillary buttress + inferior portion of lateral maxillary buttress
- **Type III: "Craniofacial dissociation"**
  - Superior portions of lateral and medial maxillary buttresses + upper transverse maxillary buttress

DIAGNOSTIC CHECKLIST

- Involvement of pterygoid processes/plates is common feature and sine qua non of Le Fort fractures

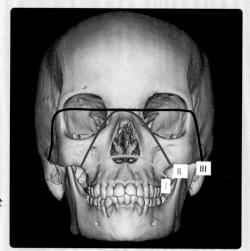
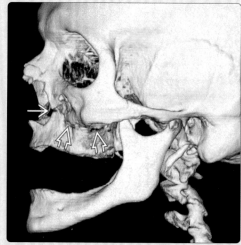

(Left) *Frontal graphic demonstrates the 3 types of Le Fort fractures. Le Fort I (green) involves the nasal aperture and piriform rim; Le Fort II (red) traverses the inferior and medial orbital walls; and Le Fort III (black) extends through the zygomatic arches and lateral and medial orbital walls.* (Right) *3D CT reformation shows a horizontal Le Fort I fracture ⮕ separating the maxillary alveolus from the midface. Note the involvement of the nasal aperture ⮕. The inferior orbital rim and zygomatic arch are intact.*

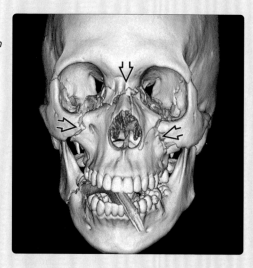
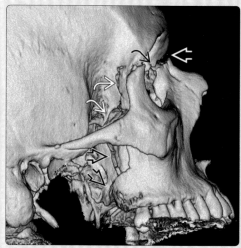

(Left) *AP 3D CT reformation shows a Le Fort II fracture ⮕ with subtle clockwise rotation of the midface and an asymmetric bite. Note the bilateral inferior orbital rim involvement with sparing of the nasal aperture.* (Right) *Lateral bone CT 3D reformation shows a right Le Fort III fracture with nasofrontal diastasis ⮕, medial ⮕ and lateral ⮕ orbital wall fractures, and pterygoid plate fractures ⮕. The inferior orbital rim is spared.*

TERMINOLOGY

Synonyms

- Le Fort fracture

Definitions

- Fractures disrupting **pterygomaxillary junction**, disjoining portions of face (maxilla) from skull

IMAGING

General Features

- Best diagnostic clue
  - **Pterygoid process and pterygoid plate** fractures in patients with clinically mobile facial skeleton

Imaging Recommendations

- Best imaging tool
  - Thin-section bone CT
- Protocol advice
  - Noncontrast helical CT (slice thickness ≤ 1 mm) in bone algorithm, with multiplanar and 3D reformations
  - Shaded surface 3D renderings facilitate Le Fort fracture analysis and assist in surgical planning

CT Findings

- Le Fort I
  - Fracture involving **pyriform rim** + **medial & lateral walls** of maxillary sinus or alveolus + nasal septum
- Le Fort II
  - Fracture involving **medial orbital wall**, including **frontomaxillary suture** + **nasofrontal junction**
  - Fracture involving involving i**nferior orbital wall** including **zygomaticomaxillary suture** + **inferior rim**
- Le Fort III
  - Fracture involving **medial orbital wall**, including **frontomaxillary suture** + **nasofrontal junction**
  - Fracture involving **lateral orbital wall**, including **zygomaticofrontal suture** + **zygomaticosphenoid suture** + **zygomatic arch**

DIFFERENTIAL DIAGNOSIS

Zygomaticomaxillary Complex Fracture

- Spares pterygoid process/plates
- Involves zygomaticofrontal, zygomaticomaxillary, zygomaticosphenoid, and zygomaticotemporal sutures

Nasoorbitalethmoidal Fracture

- Spares pterygoid processes/plates
- Depression of nasal pyramid ± telecanthus due to displacement of medial canthal ligament

Complex Facial Fracture

- Highly comminuted midface fracture
- In pure form, spares pterygoid processes/plates, but frequently coexists with LF patterns

Pterygoid Plate Avulsion

- Associated with violent trauma to mandible
- Lateral pterygoid plate typically involved, pterygoid process proper usually spared

PATHOLOGY

Staging, Grading, & Classification

- **Type I: "Floating palate"**
  - Pterygomaxillary disjunction + fractures of inferior portions of medial and lateral maxillary buttresses
- **Type II: "Pyramidal fracture"**
  - Pterygomaxillary disjunction + fractures of superior portion of medial maxillary buttress + inferior portion of lateral maxillary buttress
- **Type III: "Craniofacial dissociation"**
  - Pterygomaxillary disjunction + fractures of superior portions of lateral and medial maxillary buttresses + upper transverse maxillary buttress
- **Combinations of Le Fort types**
  - Unilateral/asymmetric Le Fort fracture and combinations of Le Fort fracture with other facial fracture types (zygomaticomaxillary complex, nasoorbitoethmoid) are common

CLINICAL ISSUES

Presentation

- Most common signs/symptoms
  - "Mobile face"
    - Maxillary alveolus/hard palate; midface; or entire face
- Other signs/symptoms
  - Enophthalmos, diplopia (Le Fort II)
  - Infraorbital nerve injury with facial sensory loss (Le Fort II)
  - Periorbital ecchymosis (Le Fort II and III)
  - Lacrimal apparatus injury with epiphora (Le Fort II and III)
  - Dental malocclusion

Natural History & Prognosis

- Long-term complications may include
  - Facial deformity, breathing difficulty, and masticatory problems/malocclusion
  - Telecanthus, visual loss, diplopia, and epiphora
  - Anosmia, facial numbness, and headaches

Treatment

- Surgical reduction and fixation of facial fractures
  - Starts with frontal bone "bar"
  - Other facial bones "suspended" from frontal bar
  - Zygomaticofrontal injuries repaired 1st, palatoalveolar complex last
  - Orbital fractures repaired after horizontal and vertical buttresses surgically reconstituted

DIAGNOSTIC CHECKLIST

Image Interpretation Pearls

- Involvement of **pterygoid processes/plates** is common feature and sine qua non of Le Fort fractures

SELECTED REFERENCES

1. Winegar BA et al: Spectrum of critical imaging findings in complex facial skeletal trauma. Radiographics. 33(1):3-19, 2013
2. Kim SH et al: Analysis of 809 facial bone fractures in a pediatric and adolescent population. Arch Plast Surg. 39(6):606-11, 2012
3. Fraioli RE et al: Facial fractures: beyond Le Fort. Otolaryngol Clin North Am. 41(1):51-76, vi, 2008

(Left) *Oblique bone CT 3D reformation shows a right Le Fort I fracture ➡ mobilizing the right hemimaxilla, which is rotated inferiorly ➡. In addition, there are multiple nasal bone fractures ➡ and comminuted left maxillary fractures ➡.* **(Right)** *Sagittal bone CT reformation shows the utility of sagittal reformats for demonstrating the maxillary disjunction of a Le Fort I with fracture, extending from the lateral aspect of the nasal aperture ➡ through the pterygoid process ➡.*

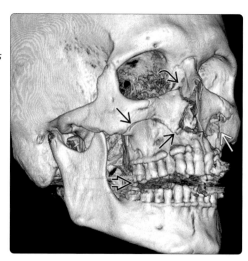
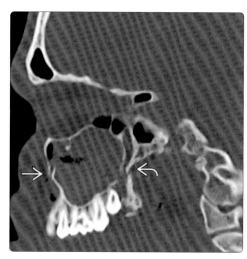

(Left) *Frontal bone CT 3D reformation shows a left Le Fort II fracture extending from the nasal bones ➡ through the ethmoid complex and anteroinferiorly to the inferior orbital rim ➡. Note the associated bilateral Le Fort I fractures ➡. Microplate fixation is evident from an old zygomaticomaxillary repair ➡.* **(Right)** *Lateral bone CT reformation shows a Le Fort II fracture involving the nasal bones ➡ and inferior orbital rim ➡. There is an associated Le Fort I fracture ➡. The fractured pterygoid plate is obscured by the mandible.*

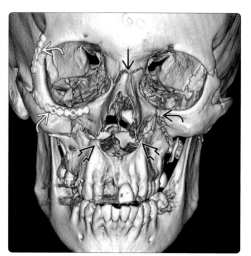
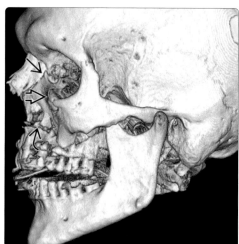

(Left) *Bone CT 3D reformation displays features of a right Le Fort III fracture with craniofacial disjunction, including depressed nasal fracture ➡, zygoma fractures ➡, and depressed zygomatic arch fracture ➡. Note accompanying comminuted orbital and maxillary smash fractures ➡.* **(Right)** *Bone CT of right Le Fort III fracture shows bilateral nasal bone fractures ➡, lateral orbital wall fracture ➡, & right zygomatic arch fracture ➡. A combination of nasoethmoid and zygoma fractures should prompt search for Le Fort III.*

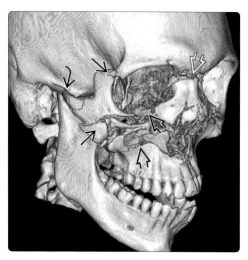
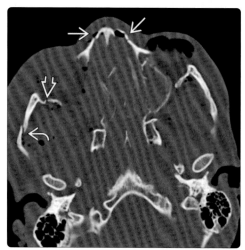

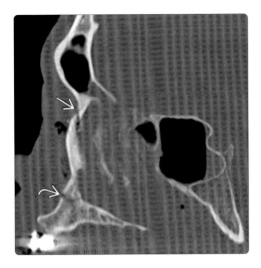

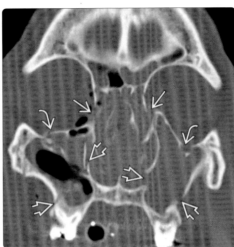

(Left) *Bone CT reformation shows combined Le Fort I & II features with a nasofrontal junction fracture* ➡ *representing Le Fort II pattern & a medial maxillary buttress fracture* ➡ *representing Le Fort I pattern.* (Right) *Coronal bone CT reformation shows fractures involving inferomedial orbital walls* ➡ *extending from nasofrontal junction. Fractures go through the upper transverse maxillary buttresses (orbital rim & floors)* ➡, *as well as inferior medial & lateral maxillary buttresses* ➡. *This constitutes Le Fort I & II patterns.*

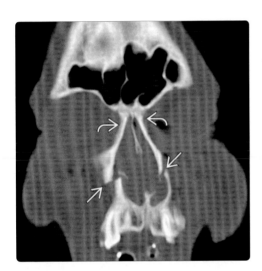

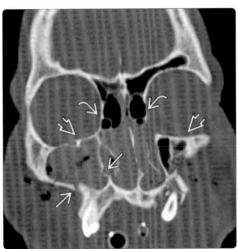

(Left) *Coronal bone CT reformation illustrates the transverse and vertical buttresses. There are fractures through the inferior medial (lower transverse) maxillary buttress* ➡ *representing a component of the Le Fort I pattern. Note that the vertical medial maxillary buttress is preserved* ➡. (Right) *Coronal bone CT reformation shows fractures through the right lower transverse medial and lateral maxillary buttresses* ➡ *in a Le Fort I pattern. The upper transverse* ➡ *and vertical* ➡ *buttresses are intact.*

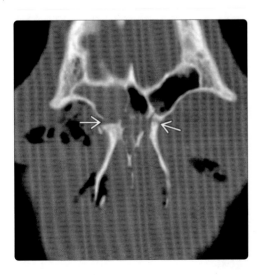

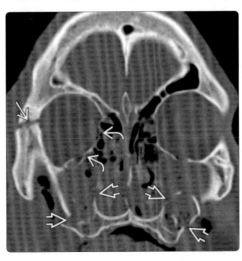

(Left) *Coronal bone CT reformation shows fractures through nasofrontal junction* ➡ *common to Le Fort II & III patterns. This fracture site is at the confluence of the vertical (medial maxillary) & transverse (upper maxillary) buttresses, forming the anterior point of midfacial (craniofacial) disjunction.* (Right) *Coronal bone CT reformation shows fracture of the right upper transverse buttresses* ➡ *and zygomaticofrontal suture* ➡ *representing Le Fort II and III patterns. Also present is a complete Le Fort I fracture* ➡.

Zygomaticomaxillary Complex Fracture

TERMINOLOGY

- ZMC fracture definition: Fracture complex with fracture lines involving zygomatic arch, lateral orbital wall, anterior & lateral walls of maxillary sinus, & orbital floor
  - Previous called **trimalar** or **tripod** fracture, ZMC fracture terminology most accurate as fracture involves lateral orbital wall along zygomaticosphenoid suture

IMAGING

- Fracture lines through or near sutures of zygoma
- Modality of choice: Thin-slice axial bone algorithm CT
  - Can be reformatted in coronal plane
  - 3D reformatted images very helpful for demonstrating degree of fracture displacement & angulation for surgical planning

TOP DIFFERENTIAL DIAGNOSES

- Complex midfacial fracture
- Transfacial (Le Fort) fractures

- Zygomatic arch fracture

PATHOLOGY

- Most common mechanism of injury: Direct blow to cheek (malar eminence)
- Classification systems not often used to plan treatment since advent of miniplates & microplates

CLINICAL ISSUES

- Teenage to young adult males most commonly affected
- Signs & symptoms
  - Loss of cheek projection with increased facial width
  - Impaired sensation or anesthesia of cheek/upper lip
    - Inferior orbital nerve injury
  - Trismus
    - Depressed zygomatic arch impinges on temporalis muscle or coronoid process of mandible
- Excellent prognosis for restored cosmesis after surgical fixation

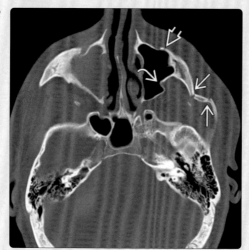
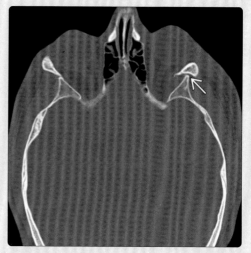

(Left) *Axial bone CT shows the typical fracture patterns of a zygomaticomaxillary complex (ZMC) fracture. There is a comminuted fracture of the left zygomatic arch* ➡ *and a fracture of the lateral maxillary sinus wall that is buckled* ➡. *The anterior wall fracture is subtle* ➡. (Right) *Axial bone CT through the orbits in the same patient shows a displaced lateral orbital wall fracture* ➡. *The bone fragment protrudes into the extraconal fat near the lateral rectus muscle.*

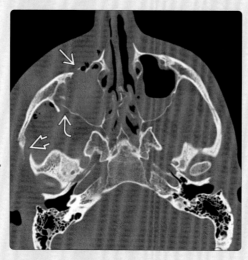
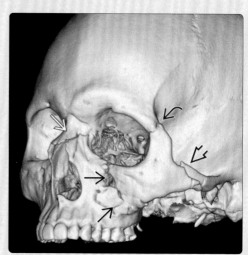

(Left) *Axial bone CT shows a right ZMC fracture. There is premaxillary soft tissue swelling. Fractures of the anterior* ➡ *and lateral* ➡ *right maxillary sinus walls are noted, in addition to a right zygomatic arch fracture* ➡. (Right) *3D reformation demonstrates the classic features of a ZMC fracture. Fractures involve the walls of the left maxillary sinus* ➡, *the left zygomatic arch* ➡, *and the lateral orbital wall* ➡. *This patient also sustained trauma to the nasal dorsum* ➡.

TERMINOLOGY

Abbreviations

- Zygomaticomaxillary complex (ZMC) fracture

Synonyms

- Trimalar fracture; tripod fracture; displaced ZMC fracture = quadripod or quadramalar fracture
- **ZMC fracture terminology most universally accepted**

Definitions

- Fracture complex with fracture lines involving zygomatic arch, lateral orbital wall, anterior & lateral walls of maxillary sinus, & orbital floor

IMAGING

General Features

- Best diagnostic clue
  - Fracture complex with fracture lines involving zygomatic arch, lateral orbital wall, anterior & lateral walls of maxillary sinus, & orbital floor
- Location
  - **Fracture lines through or near sutures of zygoma**

CT Findings

- Bone CT
  - Lucent fracture line locations
    - Along lateral orbital wall (**zygomaticofrontal & zygomaticosphenoid sutures**)
    - From inferior orbital fissure to orbital floor (**near infraorbital canal**)
    - Down anterior maxilla (**near zygomaticomaxillary suture**)
    - Up posterior maxillary wall to inferior orbital fissure
    - Also fracture through **zygomatic arch (near zygomaticotemporal suture)**

Imaging Recommendations

- Best imaging tool
  - Thin-slice (0.6-1.0 mm) axial bone algorithm CT

DIFFERENTIAL DIAGNOSIS

Complex Midfacial Fracture

- Multiple markedly comminuted fractures not fitting into classification
- Bilateral

Transfacial (Le Fort) Fractures

- All 3 Le Fort types involve pterygoid processes
- LeFort III is only type involving zygomatic arch

Zygomatic Arch Fracture

- Isolated zygomatic arch fracture(s) without maxillary wall or lateral orbital wall involvement

Inferior Orbital (Blowout) Fracture

- Fractures involve orbital floor ± inferior orbital rim
- Sparing of zygomatic arch, lateral orbital wall, maxillary sinus walls

PATHOLOGY

General Features

- Etiology
  - Most commonly occurs after **direct blow to cheek (malar eminence) during assault**
  - Zygomas have 2 attachments to cranium & 2 to midface creating portions of inferior & lateral orbital walls
    - **ZMC fracture + ipsilateral nasoorbitoethmoidal fracture**, higher incidence of postop complications/deformities

Staging, Grading, & Classification

- Classification systems not often used to plan treatment with use of miniplates & microplates
- 1 of more complete classification systems based upon type, frequency, & postreduction stability of malar fractures

CLINICAL ISSUES

Presentation

- Most common signs/symptoms
  - Loss of cheek projection with increased facial width
  - **Impaired sensation** or anesthesia of cheek/upper lip
    - Infraorbital nerve injury (**> 90% of cases**)
  - Trismus

Demographics

- Age
  - Teenage to young adults most common
- Gender
  - More common in males
- Epidemiology
  - Zygomatic fractures are **2nd most common facial fractures** after nasal bone trauma

Natural History & Prognosis

- Excellent prognosis for restored cosmesis after surgical fixation
- Surgical results depend somewhat upon degree of comminution, fracture displacement, & angulation

Treatment

- Surgical exposure indicated if angulated or severely comminuted
- Surgery goals
  - Correct 3D position of malar prominence
  - Restore orbital volume by correcting alignment of zygoma & sphenoid

SELECTED REFERENCES

1. Winegar BA et al: Spectrum of critical imaging findings in complex facial skeletal trauma. Radiographics. 33(1):3-19, 2013
2. Buchanan EP et al: Zygomaticomaxillary complex fractures and their association with naso-orbito-ethmoid fractures: a 5-year review. Plast Reconstr Surg. 130(6):1296-304, 2012
3. Fraioli RE et al: Facial fractures: beyond Le Fort. Otolaryngol Clin North Am. 41(1):51-76, vi, 2008
4. Hopper RA et al: Diagnosis of midface fractures with CT: what the surgeon needs to know. Radiographics. 26(3):783-93, 2006
5. Linnau KF et al: Imaging of high-energy midfacial trauma: what the surgeon needs to know. Eur J Radiol. 48(1):17-32, 2003
6. Salvolini U: Traumatic injuries: imaging of facial injuries. Eur Radiol. 12(6):1253-61, 2002

Complex Facial Fracture

TERMINOLOGY

- Synonyms: Facial smash injury, panfacial fracture
- No widely accepted definition
  - Severely comminuted fractures involving multiple facial bones
  - Does not follow pattern described for traditional transfacial (Le Fort) fracture

IMAGING

- Thin-section axial bone CT with multiplanar reconstruction is modality of choice
  - 3D CT reformatted images improve appreciation of disrupted facial architecture for surgical planning
- Fractures may involve frontal, nasoethmoid, midfacial, or craniofacial regions
  - May also involve mandible
- CTA may be necessary to exclude carotid artery injury
- MR helpful for assessing associated intracranial & orbital injuries

TOP DIFFERENTIAL DIAGNOSES

- Transfacial (Le Fort) fracture
- Zygomaticomaxillary complex fracture
- Nasoorbitalethmoidal fracture

PATHOLOGY

- High association with intracranial injuries

CLINICAL ISSUES

- Soft tissue injuries & loss of bone structure may lead to malocclusion, "dish" face deformity, & enophthalmos
- Treatment often delayed because of other life-threatening injuries
- Reconstruction often performed in multiple stages
- Preoperative CT, virtual surgical planning, intraoperative navigation, & 3D reconstructions aid in planning & execution of complex craniofacial fracture reconstruction

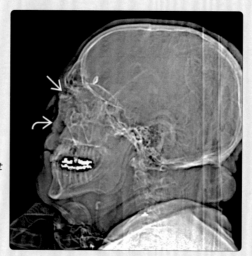
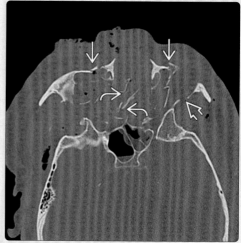

(Left) Lateral CT scout image in a patient status post high-force blunt facial trauma demonstrates flattening of facial projection involving the nasal dorsum ➡ & midface ➡, referred to as "dish" face deformity. (Right) Axial bone CT in same patient demonstrates extensive injuries to the facial soft tissues & underlying facial skeleton. Lacerations with soft tissue emphysema are noted. Severely comminuted fractures involve the maxillae ➡, orbital walls ➡, & nasal septum ➡. The entire face is depressed.

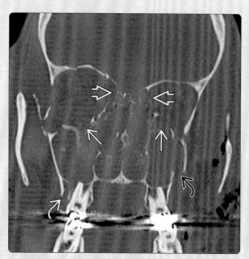
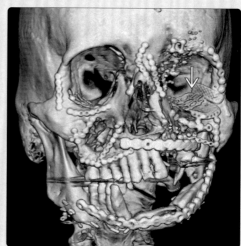

(Left) Coronal bone CT demonstrates extensive fractures of the midface involving the medial orbital walls ➡, orbital floors ➡, right maxillary alveolus ➡, & left lateral maxillary sinus ➡. The fractures do not conform to a classic Le Fort fracture pattern. (Right) Anteroposterior 3D reformation in a patient after reconstruction of panfacial injuries shows numerous malleable screw plates bridging fractures & mesh along the left orbital floor ➡.

TERMINOLOGY

Abbreviations

- Complex facial fracture (CFFx)

Synonyms

- Facial smash injury, panfacial fracture

Definitions

- No widely accepted definition of CFFx or panfacial fracture
- Definitions include
  - Severely comminuted fractures involving multiple facial bones that do not follow pattern described for traditional transfacial (Le Fort) fracture
  - Fractures involving upper, middle, & lower face (nasoorbitalethmoidal, zygomaticomaxillary complex, central midface, & mandible)
  - Fracture patterns involving both midface & mandible

IMAGING

General Features

- Best diagnostic clue
  - Numerous, markedly comminuted fractures from high-energy impact that cannot be classified as traditional transfacial types
- Location
  - May involve frontal, nasoethmoid, midfacial, or craniofacial regions; may also involve mandible

Imaging Recommendations

- Best imaging tool
  - Thin-section axial bone CT with multiplanar & 3D reconstruction
- Protocol advice
  - 3D CT reformatted images improve appreciation of disrupted facial architecture for surgical planning
  - CTA may be necessary to exclude carotid artery injury
  - MR helpful for assessing associated intracranial & orbital injuries

CT Findings

- Bone CT
  - Multiple, severely comminuted fractures
  - Fractures do not conform to classic patterns of facial trauma

DIFFERENTIAL DIAGNOSIS

Transfacial (Le Fort) Fractures

- Fractures occur along 3 lines of weakness in facial skeleton
- Bilateral pterygoid plate fractures required

Zygomaticomaxillary Complex Fracture

- Lateral midface fracture complex from blunt trauma to malar eminence
- Fractures involve anterior & lateral walls of maxillary sinus, zygomatic arch, & lateral orbital wall
- Orbital floor frequently involved

Nasoorbitalethmoidal Fracture

- Comminuted fractures from high-impact force to nasal bridge
- Frequently involve frontal recess, cribriform plate, nasolacrimal duct, & medial canthal tendon

PATHOLOGY

General Features

- Etiology
  - High-energy impact to face causes highly comminuted fractures
- Associated abnormalities
  - High association with intracranial injuries
  - CFFx involving frontal & nasoethmoid regions have ↑ incidence of dural tears
  - CFFx of nasoethmoid region may have associated injuries to lacrimal apparatus, medial canthal tendon, frontal recess, & cribriform plate

Staging, Grading, & Classification

- No widely accepted definition or classification of CFFx
  - Some authors describe them as involving both midface & mandible
  - Others describe them as involving upper, middle, & lower face (nasoorbitoethmoid, zygomaticomaxillary complex, central midface, & mandible)
  - Some authors divide panfacial (smash) fractures into 4 types: Frontal smash, naso-ethmoid smash, central midface smash, craniofacial smash

CLINICAL ISSUES

Presentation

- Most common signs/symptoms
  - Gross facial deformity
- Other signs/symptoms
  - Telecanthus, cerebrospinal fluid leak, visual loss

Demographics

- Age
  - Most common in adolescents & young adults
- Gender
  - Predominantly male patients

Natural History & Prognosis

- Soft tissue injuries & loss of bone structure may lead to malocclusion, "dish" face deformity, & uni- or bilateral enophthalmos
- Difficult to completely repair, & patients often left with cosmetic deformity & functional deficits

Treatment

- Goal of treatment → restore function & preinjury 3D facial contours
  - Multispecialty surgical team often required for best intracranial & extracranial outcome
- Advantages of early treatment include reduced risk of postop infection & maintained soft tissue expansion

SELECTED REFERENCES

1. Uzelac A et al: Orbital and facial fractures. Neuroimaging Clin N Am. 24(3):407-24, vii, 2014
2. Mundinger GS et al: Blunt-mechanism facial fracture patterns associated with internal carotid artery injuries: recommendations for additional screening criteria based on analysis of 4,398 patients. J Oral Maxillofac Surg. 71(12):2092-100, 2013

Nasoorbitalethmoidal Fracture

TERMINOLOGY

- **Central upper midface fracture** complex involving confluence of medial and upper maxillary buttresses and their posterior extensions
  - Disruption of medial canthal regions, ethmoids, and medial orbital walls

IMAGING

- Bone CT: Nasal bone fracture in combination with fractures of medial orbital wall and frontal process of maxilla

TOP DIFFERENTIAL DIAGNOSES

- Complex midfacial fracture
- Nasal bone fracture
- Medial orbital blowout fracture

PATHOLOGY

- Force transmitted through nasal bones and involves ethmoid sinuses and medial orbits

- May involve frontal recess resulting in impaired frontal sinus drainage
- May involve cribriform plate → CSF leak, meningoencephalocele, intracranial infection
- Manson classification
  - Type I: Medial canthal insertion on large fracture fragment
  - Type II: Canthal tendon attached to small bone fragment
  - Type III: Complete avulsion of medial canthal tendon

CLINICAL ISSUES

- Symptoms and signs
  - Loss of nasal projection in profile
  - Increased distance between inner corners of eyes (telecanthus)
- Nasoorbitalethmoidal fractures can be among most difficult facial fracture patterns to accurately repair

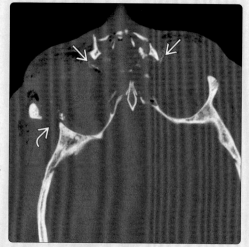
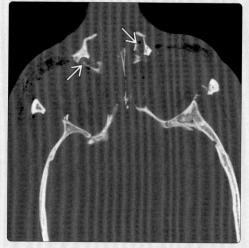

(Left) Axial bone CT shows markedly comminuted fractures involving the naso-orbital-ethmoidal (NOE) complex. Multiple small fracture fragments are noted in the medial canthal regions ➡, and there is a degree of telecanthus. Soft tissue swelling, emphysema, and a lateral orbital fracture ➡ are noted. (Right) Axial bone CT in the same patient inferior to the previous image shows that the fractures involve both nasolacrimal ducts ➡. In such a patient, epiphora would be an expected complication of the injury.

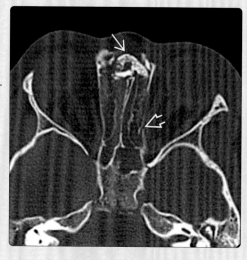
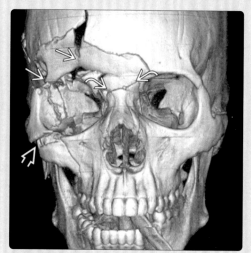

(Left) Axial bone CT demonstrates comminuted fractures involving the NOE complex with retropulsion of the nasal bridge ➡ and fracture of the left lamina papyracea ➡. (Right) Anterior 3D reconstructed bone CT in a 20 year old demonstrates highly comminuted fractures involving the NOE ➡, orbit ➡, and maxilla ➡.

TERMINOLOGY

Abbreviations

- Nasoorbitalethmoidal fracture (NOE fx)

Definitions

- **Central upper midface fracture** complex
  - Involving confluence of medial and upper maxillary buttresses and their posterior extensions along medial orbital wall and floor
  - Distinguished from simple nasal fractures by posterior disruption of medial canthal regions, ethmoids, and medial orbital walls

IMAGING

General Features

- Best diagnostic clue
  - Nasal bone fracture in combination with fractures of medial orbital wall and frontal process of maxilla
- Location
  - Central upper midface; nasal dorsum and medial orbits
  - Includes damage to ethmoid sinus and walls

Imaging Recommendations

- Best imaging tool
  - Thin-section bone algorithm CT + multiplanar reformats

CT Findings

- Bone CT
  - Nasal bone fractures in combination with fractures of medial orbital wall and frontal process of maxilla
  - Frontal recess involvement likely if there is displaced anterior table fracture medial to supraorbital notch involving frontal sinus floor

DIFFERENTIAL DIAGNOSIS

Complex Midfacial Fracture

- Severe injury with fracture pattern not falling into other classifications

Nasal Bone Fracture

- Intact medial orbital walls and frontal process of maxilla

Medial Orbital Blowout Fracture

- Orbital rims spared

PATHOLOGY

General Features

- Etiology
  - NOE = facial unit composed of nasal bones, medial orbital walls, and frontal process of maxillary bones
  - **High-force trauma**
    - Thin nasal bones, ethmoid sinus walls, & medial orbits act as "crumple zone," allow traumatic force to be dissipated
    - Critical structures (brain and optic nerve) lie in stronger bone posteriorly and are relatively protected
- Associated abnormalities
  - Fractures through **frontal recess** with disruption of frontal sinus drainage
  - Associated fractures of **cribriform plate**

- Severe **ocular injuries**
- Orbital hematoma
- Contiguous skull fractures

Staging, Grading, & Classification

- Manson classification system (3 major subsets based on degree of injury to medial canthal attachment)
  - Type I: Fractured piece is large, and medial canthal insertion on it is intact
  - Type II: Comminution of bony buttress and canthus is attached to small bone fragment
  - Type III: Avulsion of medial canthal tendon from its osseous insertion
    - Diagnosis is made clinically, not with imaging

CLINICAL ISSUES

Presentation

- Most common signs/symptoms
  - Loss of nasal projection in profile
  - ↑ distance between inner corners of eyes (telecanthus)
- Other signs/symptoms
  - Epiphora (5-31% of NOE fx patients)
  - Globe malposition
  - Vision loss

Demographics

- Age
  - Most common in teens to young adults

Natural History & Prognosis

- Significant cosmetic and functional deficits may arise from high-force NOE injury
  - Midface retrusion and nasal shortening
    - From telescoping of nasal bones
  - Telecanthus results from disruption of medial canthal tendons
    - From bony insertion or displacement of medial canthal tendon fragment
  - Epiphora from injury to lacrimal puncta, canaliculi, sac, or nasolacrimal duct

DIAGNOSTIC CHECKLIST

Reporting Tips

- Imaging description should include
  - **Degree of comminution** of medial vertical maxillary buttress in region of medial canthal tendon attachment
  - Distance between 2 lacrimal fossae in coronal plane
  - Involvement of frontal sinus drainage pathway and orbit
- Also report degree of comminution of surrounding nasal, maxillary, and orbital walls for surgical planning purposes

SELECTED REFERENCES

1. Pawar SS et al: Frontal sinus and naso-orbital-ethmoid fractures. JAMA Facial Plast Surg. 16(4):284-9, 2014
2. Wolff J et al: Late reconstruction of orbital and naso-orbital deformities. Oral Maxillofac Surg Clin North Am. 25(4):683-95, 2013
3. Chapman VM et al: Facial fractures in children: unique patterns of injury observed by computed tomography. J Comput Assist Tomogr. 33(1):70-2, 2009
4. Papadopoulos H et al: Management of naso-orbital-ethmoidal fractures. Oral Maxillofac Surg Clin North Am. 21(2):221-5, vi, 2009

IMAGING

- Mandible simulates bony ring: **2 breaks** common (50%)
  - Parasymphyseal fracture often associated with contralateral angle/body or subcondylar fracture
  - Bilateral subcondylar fractures after direct impact to symphysis
- CT has largely replaced plain film evaluation of facial trauma
  - Thin-slice axial bone algorithm CT with coronal & 3D reformat
- Bone CT appearance
  - Lucent, noncorticated lines with variable diastasis, angulation, & comminution
  - Fracture tends to follow long axis of teeth
  - In condylar neck fracture, condylar head pulled medially by lateral pterygoid muscle
  - Empty temporomandibular joint (TMJ) sign when TMJ dislocated

TOP DIFFERENTIAL DIAGNOSES

- Pseudofractures: Nutrient canal, Inferior alveolar nerve canal, mental foramen

PATHOLOGY

- Causes of mandibular fracture
  - Motor vehicle accidents: 40%
  - Assault: 40%
  - Fall: 10%
  - Sports-related injury: 5%
- 15% have ≥ 1 other facial bone fracture

CLINICAL ISSUES

- 2nd most commonly fractured facial bone
- Goals of treatment are restoration of normal occlusion & complete bony union
- Wound infection is potential complication of fracture to tooth-bearing portion of mandible

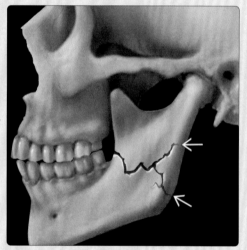
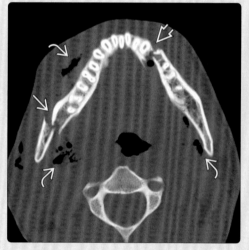

(Left) Sagittal graphic shows a complex mandibular ramus fracture obliquely crossing the posterior margin of the mandible ➡️. Inferior alveolar nerve may be injured in such a fracture, resulting in numb chin. (Right) Axial bone CT shows displaced mandibular fractures of right angle ➡️ and left parasymphysis ➡️. A fracture through the teeth is considered open, requiring antibiotics. Two fractures are often present as the mandible is essentially a fixed ring of bone. Extensive lacerations resulted in associated soft tissue emphysema ➡️.

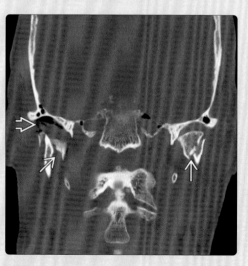
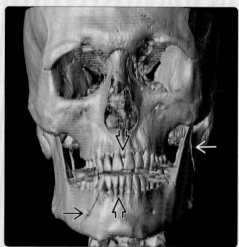

(Left) Coronal bone CT demonstrates bilateral mandibular condyle fractures ➡️ with severe displacement of fracture fragments on the right. Trauma to the right TMJ was significant, and air is noted in the joint ➡️. (Right) 3D reformation shows obliquely oriented fractures through the right mental foramen ➡️ and left mandibular ramus ➡️. There is associated malocclusion ➡️. 3D reformatted images are often helpful for surgical repair of facial fractures.

TERMINOLOGY

Abbreviations

- Fracture of mandible

Definitions

- Traumatic break in mandibular cortex

IMAGING

General Features

- Best diagnostic clue
  - Focal noncorticated lucency in mandibular cortex
- Location
  - Mandible simulates bony ring
    - **2 breaks in ring common** (50%) & bilateral fracture result
      - □ Parasymphyseal fracture on 1 side often associated with contralateral angle/body or subcondylar fracture
      - □ Bilateral subcondylar fractures after direct impact to symphysis
    - Alternatively unilateral mandibular fracture may occur with **contralateral temporomandibular joint (TMJ) dislocation**

CT Findings

- Bone CT
  - Lucent, noncorticated fracture lines with variable diastasis, angulation, & comminution
  - Fracture lines tend to follow long axis of teeth
  - In condylar neck fracture, **condylar head pulled medially** by lateral pterygoid muscle
  - **Empty TMJ sign** may be seen on axial CT images when TMJ dislocated

MR Findings

- T1WI
  - ↓ marrow signal intensity from edema
  - May see discrete, well-defined hypointense fracture line
  - Hypointense joint effusion if TMJ affected
- T2WI
  - ↑ marrow signal due to edema
    - Surrounding edema on MR may be more extensive than fracture length
  - Hypointense fracture line
  - Surrounding ↑ signal soft tissue edema

Imaging Recommendations

- Best imaging tool
  - Thin-slice axial bone algorithm CT through mandible & TMJs

DIFFERENTIAL DIAGNOSIS

Nutrient Canal

- Pseudofracture caused by radiolucent channels extending through osseous structures
- Commonly mistaken for fracture lines

Inferior Alveolar Nerve Canal (V3)

- Normally located inferior & medial within mandibular body running parallel to body

- Corticated, begins at mandibular foramen & ends at mental foramen

Mandibular Lingula

- Small bony projection extending from medial mandible at mandibular foramen for inferior alveolar nerve
- Usually symmetric and triangular in shape

PATHOLOGY

General Features

- Etiology
  - Fracture causes
    - Motor vehicle accidents: 40%
    - Assault: 40%
    - Fall: 10%
    - Sports-related injury: 5%
- Associated abnormalities
  - 15% of cases with mandibular fracture have ≥ 1 other facial bone fracture

CLINICAL ISSUES

Presentation

- Most common signs/symptoms
  - Jaw pain or trismus (normal opening > 40 mm)
  - Abnormal mobility on palpation and mouth opening

Demographics

- Epidemiology
  - Mandible is **2nd most commonly fractured facial bone**
    - Account for ~ 25% of facial fracture
  - Mandibular fracture frequencies
    - Condylar process: 30%
    - Angle: 25%
    - Body: 25%
    - Symphyseal/parasymphyseal: 15%
    - Ramus: 3%
    - Coronoid process: 2%

Treatment

- Goals of treatment are restoration of normal occlusion & complete bony union

DIAGNOSTIC CHECKLIST

Consider

- Mandible is considered ring of bone → look for 2nd fracture, TMJ dislocation (empty TMJ socket), or facial fracture
- Posterior wall of TMJ is anterior wall of external auditory canal (EAC), so check for fracture or EAC opacification

SELECTED REFERENCES

1. Rudderman RH et al: The biophysics of mandibular fractures: an evolution toward understanding. Plast Reconstr Surg. 121(2):596-607, 2008
2. Ellis E 3rd et al: Fractures of the mandible: a technical perspective. Plast Reconstr Surg. 120(7 Suppl 2):76S-89S, 2007
3. Hobbs DL et al: Trauma radiography of the mandible. Radiol Technol. 78(4):265-8, 2007
4. Ceallaigh PO et al: Diagnosis and management of common maxillofacial injuries in the emergency department. Part 2: mandibular fractures. Emerg Med J. 23(12):927-8, 2006
5. Stacey DH et al: Management of mandible fractures. Plast Reconstr Surg. 117(3):48e-60e, 2006

KEY FACTS

TERMINOLOGY

- Internal derangement (ID) of TMJ
- Abnormal positional and functional relationship between articular disc and articulating surfaces

IMAGING

- Best imaging tool: Oblique corrected sagittal PD or T1WI and T2WI MR
- Articular disc most commonly positioned **anterior** to mandibular condyle
- Normal or dysmorphic disc morphology

TOP DIFFERENTIAL DIAGNOSES

- Rheumatoid arthritis
- Synovial chondromatosis
- Calcium pyrophosphate deposition disease
- Pigmented villonodular synovitis

CLINICAL ISSUES

- Very prevalent: 20-30% of population
  - Majority asymptomatic
  - **ID seen in > 80% of symptomatic TMJ patients**
  - Symptoms: Trismus, preauricular pain, limited range of motion
- Most prevalent at 20-40 years
- Symptomatic joints: F:M = 4:1
  - More common in males if 2° to trauma
- Treatment
  - Conservative: Bite splint
  - Surgical: Arthrocentesis & discectomy

DIAGNOSTIC CHECKLIST

- Report anterior disc displacement ± reduction
- Report associated effusion or synovitis

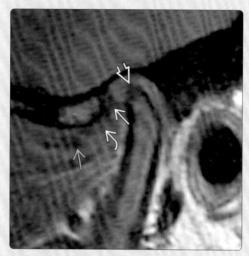
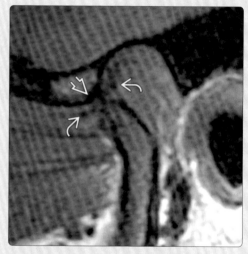

(Left) Sagittal T1 MR shows the articular disc anteriorly displaced with the posterior band ➡ anterior to the condyle, thinned intermediate zone ➡, and dysmorphic anterior band ➡. Note the thinning of cortex and flattening of the articular surface of the condyle ➡. (Right) Sagittal T1 MR in open mouth position shows the condyle translating to the articular eminence ➡ and recapture of the articular disc ➡. This case shows anterior disc displacement with reduction.

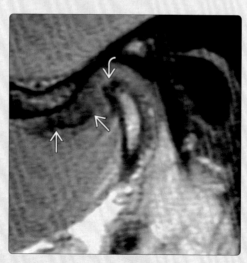
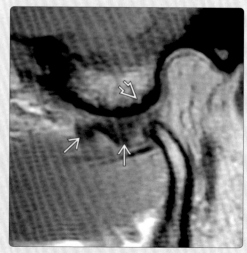

(Left) Sagittal T1 MR shows a dysmorphic articular disc ➡ completely dislocated anteriorly with respect to the mandibular condyle. Note the flattening and beaking of the anterior aspect of the mandibular condyle ➡. (Right) Sagittal T1 MR in open mouth position shows translation of the mandibular condyle to the articular eminence ➡ but with the disc remaining anterior to the condyle ➡. This case shows anterior disc displacement without reduction.

TERMINOLOGY

Synonyms

- Internal derangement (ID) of TMJ

Definitions

- Abnormal positional & functional relationship between articular disc & articulating surfaces

IMAGING

General Features

- Best diagnostic clue
  - Articular disc positioned anterior to mandibular condyle
- Location
  - Usually intracapsular
  - Unilateral or bilateral
- Morphology
  - Normal disc shape or dysmorphic

Imaging Recommendations

- Best imaging tool
  - Thin-section oblique corrected sagittal & coronal MR in **closed** and **open mouth positions**
- Protocol advice
  - MR sequences should include sagittal PD or T1 & T2
  - Cine images provide more accurate functional information

MR Findings

- T1WI
  - Displacement may be anterior, medial, lateral, or combination
    - Posterior band of articular disc **anterior to 12 o'clock position** relative to mandibular condyle
    - Anterior displacement = angle > 10° between posterior band and vertical orientation of condyle
    - Posterior disc displacement is rare
- T2WI
  - May have superior or inferior joint space **effusion** with ↑ **signal**
  - ↑ signal in condyle if associated marrow edema
- T1WI C+
  - Disc nonenhancing
  - Associated acute synovitis will enhance

DIFFERENTIAL DIAGNOSIS

Rheumatoid Arthritis

- Proliferating, inflamed synovial tissue ("pannus")
- Enhancing, enlarged synovium
- Moderate to significant osteoarthritis often present also

Synovial Chondromatosis

- Chondrometaplasia of synovial membrane
- Cartilaginous nodules detach from synovium and calcify
  - These are known as loose bodies

Calcium Pyrophosphate Dihydrate Deposition Disease

- Metabolic disease associated with chondrocalcinosis
- Uncommon in TMJ
- Calcified, enhancing intracapsular mass

Pigmented Villonodular Synovitis

- Rare in TMJ
- Tumefactive proliferation of synovium
- Locally aggressive

Synovial Cyst

- Rare in TMJ
- Cyst arising from synovium

PATHOLOGY

General Features

- Etiology
  - Multifactorial; arises from dysfunctional remodeling
    - ↓ adaptive capacity of articular surface ± functional overloading
    - Ligamentous laxity
  - May occur secondary to trauma (condylar fracture/dislocation)

Gross Pathologic & Surgical Features

- Hyperemic, deformed articular disc

Microscopic Features

- Connective tissue hyalinization, hyperplasia, and vascular reaction

CLINICAL ISSUES

Presentation

- Most common signs/symptoms
  - **Majority asymptomatic**
  - Trismus
  - Preauricular pain
- Other signs/symptoms
  - Limited range of motion on opening
  - "Clicking" or locking

Demographics

- Age
  - Adults: Most prevalent from 20-40 years
- Gender
  - Symptomatic: **F:M = 4:1**
  - More common in **male patients if 2° to trauma**
- Epidemiology
  - 20-30% of population
  - ID seen in > 80% of symptomatic TMJ patients

SELECTED REFERENCES

1. Kakimoto N et al: Comparison of the T2 relaxation time of the temporomandibular joint articular disk between patients with temporomandibular disorders and asymptomatic volunteers. AJNR Am J Neuroradiol. 35(7):1412-7, 2014

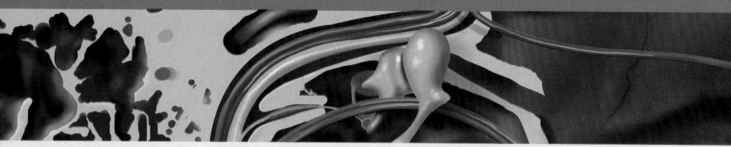

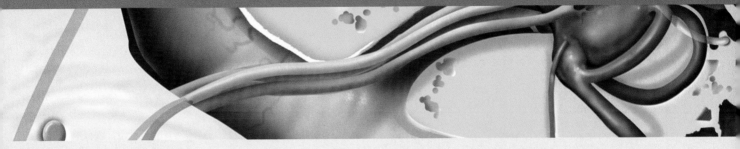

Summary Thoughts: Temporal Bone

The temporal bone (T-bone) is 1 of the most complex and intriguing areas of the head and neck. Understanding normal anatomy is key to accurate T-bone image interpretation. Incorporating the otologic findings of a middle ear mass also helps the radiologist to arrive at a correct preoperative diagnosis. If the clinical question is conductive hearing loss (CHL), an abnormality on CT is almost always present and should be extensively searched for, especially in children.

Cholesteatoma is a very common clinical concern in most ear, nose, throat (ENT) practices. The following questions should be addressed in a patient with a cholesteatoma: (1) Is the tegmen tympani intact? (2) Is there potential for a fistula into the membranous labyrinth? (3) Is the facial nerve canal adjacent to or eroded by the cholesteatoma? (4) Is there tissue in the sinus tympani? (5) What is the relationship of the mass to the ossicles?

Imaging Techniques & Indications

CT is the primary imaging tool for evaluating the fine bony detail of the T-bone. Current multislice CT scanners allow thin slices (≤ 1 mm) and provide excellent multiplanar reformatted images, which have become the mainstay for diagnosis of T-bone disease. Current protocols include direct axial and reformatted coronal views, vestibular oblique or short-axis views (Poschl plane), and cochlear oblique or long-axis views (Stenver plane). A window width of 4,000 HU is ideal.

CT is the imaging study of choice when the clinical question is CHL, external auditory canal (EAC) atresia/stenosis, or possible cholesteatoma.

MR is best for evaluation of inner ear pathology, particularly sensorineural hearing loss (SNHL). High-resolution 3D MR cisternographic sequences provide an excellent screening examination for patients with SNHL. These thin-section (≤ 1 mm) T2-weighted MR sequences (SPACE, FIESTA, etc.) in the axial and coronal planes can help identify mass lesions of the internal auditory canal (IAC), particularly a vestibular schwannoma. Sagittal oblique planes are excellent for evaluation of a child with SNHL to easily identify the 4 nerves within the IAC.

The gold standard for imaging patients with acquired SNHL is enhanced thin-section (≤ 3 mm) axial and coronal images through the T-bone with fat-saturated, postcontrast images. Precontrast T1-weighted images are helpful to evaluate for T1-hyperintense lesions, such as hemorrhage or lipoma.

When the clinical question is SNHL, a petrous apex lesion, or possible IAC or cerebellopontine angle (CPA) lesion, MR is the imaging study of choice.

Embryology

The otocyst buds from the neuroectoderm, migrates to the location of the inner ear, and becomes the membranous labyrinth. The EAC forms from the 1st branchial groove or cleft. The middle ear (tympanic) cavity forms from the 1st branchial (pharyngeal) pouch. The tympanic membrane (TM) forms where the EAC (1st branchial cleft) and middle ear (1st branchial pouch) meet. The middle ear cavity and the eustachian tube form from the same 1st branchial pouch. The middle ear cavity envelops the ossicles.

The **ossicles** form primarily from the 1st and 2nd branchial arches, separately from the inner ear. The endolymphatic system forms from the otocyst. The perilymphatic space and otic capsule form from surrounding mesenchyme.

In nonsyndromic EAC atresia, the inner ear is spared, as it forms from migration of the otocyst, which is independent from the 1st and 2nd branchial groove-pouch-arch interaction. Therefore, inner ear anomalies in most cases form without EAC or ME anomalies. A combination of external, middle, and inner ear anomalies suggests a syndromic etiology or teratogenic insult.

Consider the following questions when evaluating a patient with **EAC atresia**: (1) Is the EAC atresia plate thick, thin, or part membranous in nature? (2) How small is the middle ear cavity? (3) What is the status of the ossicles? (4) Is the facial nerve canal anomalous in its course or dehiscent? (5) What is the status of the oval and round windows? (6) Is there a congenital cholesteatoma? (7) Are the inner ear structures normal?

Imaging Anatomy

The T-bone is located in the middle cranial fossa posterolateral floor. Its boundaries include the sphenoid bone anteriorly, occipital bone posteriorly and medially, and parietal bone superiorly and laterally.

There are **5 bony parts** of the adult T-bone: Squamous, mastoid, petrous, tympanic, and styloid portions. The squamous portion forms the lateral wall of the middle cranial fossa. The mastoid process represents the postnatal development of the posteroinferior mastoid. The petrous portion of the T-bone contains the middle and inner ear, IAC, and petrous apex. The tympanic segment is a U-shaped bone that forms most of the bony external ear. The styloid portion forms the styloid process after birth.

The **petrous portion** of the T-bone includes 2 important structures anteriorly. The tegmen tympani (Latin for "roof of the cavity") serves as the roof of the tympanic cavity. The arcuate eminence is the bony prominence over the superior semicircular canal (SCC) and serves as an important surgical landmark along the middle cranial fossa floor.

There are 5 major anatomic components of the T-bone: EAC, middle ear-mastoid (ME-M), inner ear, petrous apex, and facial nerve. These anatomic components help define the various differential diagnosis lists of the T-bone.

The **EAC** is made up of the tympanic bone medially and fibrocartilage laterally. The medial border of the EAC is formed by the TM, which attaches to the scutum superiorly and the tympanic annulus inferiorly. The nodal drainage of the EAC and the adjacent scalp is to the parotid lymph nodes.

The **middle ear** includes the epitympanum, mesotympanum, and hypotympanum. The **epitympanum** (attic) is defined superiorly by the tegmen tympani, which forms the roof. The inferior margin is defined by a line between the scutum and the tympanic segment of the facial nerve. The tegmen tympani is the thin bony roof between the epitympanum and the middle cranial fossa dura. **Prussak space** represents the lateral epitympanic recess and is a classic location for acquired (pars flaccida) **cholesteatoma**. The malleus head and body and the short process of the incus are present within the epitympanum.

The **mesotympanum** is the middle ear area between the epitympanum above and the hypotympanum below. It is defined superiorly by a line between the scutum and tympanic segment of the facial nerve and inferiorly by a line between the tympanic annulus and the base of the cochlear promontory. The remainder of the ossicles (manubrium of the malleus, long and lenticular process of the incus and stapes) is located in the mesotympanum. The 2 muscles of the middle ear, the tensor tympani and stapedius muscles, are also in the mesotympanum and function to dampen sound. The posterior wall of the mesotympanum has 3 important structures: Facial nerve recess, pyramidal eminence, and sinus tympani. The **facial nerve recess** contains the mastoid facial nerve and may be dehiscent or have a bony covering. The **pyramidal eminence** contains the belly and tendon of the stapedius muscle. The **sinus tympani** is a clinical blind spot during a standard mastoid surgical approach to the T-bone, where cholesteatomas may hide. The medial wall contains the lateral SCC, the tympanic segment of the facial nerve, and the oval and round windows. The **hypotympanum** is a shallow trough on the floor of the middle ear cavity.

The **mastoid** sinus contains 3 important anatomic structures. The **mastoid antrum** (Latin for "cave") is the large, central mastoid air cell. The **aditus ad antrum** (Latin for "entrance to the cave") connects the epitympanum of the middle ear to the mastoid antrum. **Körner septum** is part of the petrosquamosal suture running posterolaterally through the mastoid air cells. This septum functions as an important surgical landmark within the mastoid air cells and also serves as a barrier to the extension of infection from the lateral mastoid air cells to the medial mastoid air cells. The mastoid T-bone continues to develop after birth. As the mastoid eminence protects the facial nerve, this nerve is relatively unprotected until the eminence is formed. This is why the facial nerve is vulnerable to birth trauma.

The **inner ear** contains the **membranous labyrinth**, which is housed within the bony labyrinth (otic capsule). The membranous labyrinth consists of the fluid spaces within the bony labyrinth, including the fluid and soft tissues within the vestibule, SCCs and cochlea, the endolymphatic duct and sac, and cochlear duct. The vestibule houses the largest part of the membranous labyrinth, consisting of the utricle and saccule. The utricle is the more cephalad portion, and the saccule is the more caudal portion of the vestibule. The vestibule is separated laterally from the middle ear by the oval window niche. The SCCs project off the superior, posterior, and lateral aspects of the vestibule. The lateral (or horizontal) SCC is at risk for fistula formation from an epitympanic cholesteatoma as it projects into the epitympanum. The endolymphatic duct and sac contain endolymph, whereas the cochlear duct contains perilymph.

The **bony labyrinth** (otic capsule) forms the cochlea, vestibule, SCCs, and vestibular and cochlear aqueducts. The **cochlea** has approximately 2.5 turns. The entire cochlea encircles a central bony axis, the **modiolus**. The modiolus houses the spiral ganglion, cell bodies of the cochlear nerve. The 3 spiral chambers of the cochlea are the scala tympani (posterior chamber), scala vestibuli (anterior chamber), and scala media (contains organ of Corti = hearing apparatus).

The **SCCs** project off the superior, lateral, and posterior aspects of the vestibule. The superior SCC projects cephalad. The bony ridge over the superior SCC in the roof of the petrous pyramid is the arcuate eminence, an important surgical landmark. The lateral (or horizontal) SCC projects into the middle ear. The tympanic segment of the facial nerve is on the undersurface of the lateral SCC. The posterior SCC projects posteriorly along the petrous ridge. The crus

communis is the common origin of the superior and posterior SCCs.

The **petrous apex** is anteromedial to the inner ear and lateral to the petrooccipital fissure. It is pneumatized in ~ 33% of people. The abducens nerve (CNVI) passes along the medial surface of the petrous apex and through the Dorello canal. The trigeminal nerve (CNV) passes through the porus trigeminus into Meckel cave on the cephalad-medial surface of the petrous apex. In petrous apicitis, CNV and CNVI are commonly affected.

The petrous **internal carotid artery** (ICA) includes the vertical and horizontal segments within the petrous temporal bone. The vertical segment rises to the genu beneath the cochlea. The horizontal segment projects anteromedially to turn cephalad as the cavernous segment.

The **intratemporal facial nerve (CNVII)** is composed of the IAC and labyrinthine, tympanic, and mastoid segments. The IAC segment is located anterosuperiorly within the IAC. The labyrinthine segment extends from the IAC fundus to the geniculate ganglion. The geniculate ganglion is also known as the anterior genu, and the greater superficial petrosal nerve originates here. The tympanic segment leaves the geniculate ganglion and passes under the lateral SCC. The posterior genu is the portion where the tympanic segment bends inferiorly to become the mastoid segment. The mastoid segment leaves the posterior genu to pass inferiorly to the stylomastoid foramen. It first gives off the motor nerve to the stapedius muscle, then the chorda tympani nerve. The facial nerve then exits the skull base through the stylomastoid foramen.

The motor root of CNVII innervates the muscles of facial expression, stapedius, platysma, and posterior belly of the digastric muscles. The sensory-parasympathetic root (nervus intermedius) contains special sensory visceral afferent fibers that convey taste to the anterior 2/3 of the tongue; the parasympathetic portion provides general visceral efferent secretomotor fibers to lacrimal, submandibular, and sublingual glands.

CNVII has 4 major functions that help localize a lesion along its course. Lacrimation is via the greater superficial petrosal nerve. The stapedius nerve provides the stapedius reflex, which creates sound dampening. Taste to the anterior 2/3 of the tongue is via the chorda tympani nerve to the lingual nerve to the oral tongue. Motor branches supply muscles of facial expression.

The 2 muscles of the temporal bone, the **tensor tympani** and **stapedius** muscles, function to dampen sound. When dysfunctional, the patient presents with hyperacusis. The tensor tympani is innervated by a trigeminal nerve (CNV3) branch. It is located in the anteromedial wall of the mesotympanum. The tensor tympani muscle tendon goes through the cochleariform process and turns laterally to attach to the manubrium of the malleus. The stapedius muscle is innervated by CNVII. The stapedius muscle belly is located in the pyramidal eminence. The stapedius tendon attaches to the head of the stapes.

There are 3 ossicles of the middle ear: **Malleus, incus**, and **stapes**. The malleus is the most anterior ossicle and is composed of the umbo, manubrium, and head. The incus is located posteriorly and is composed of the short process, body, long process, and lenticular process. The stapes is

Differential Diagnosis: Location

External auditory canal	Inner ear
External auditory canal atresia/stenosis	Superior semicircular canal dehiscence
Cholesteatoma	Labyrinthitis & labyrinthine ossificans
Squamous cell carcinoma	Large endolymphatic sac anomaly
Exostoses (surfer's ear)	Fenestral & cochlear otosclerosis
Osteoma	Intralabyrinthine schwannoma
Medial canal fibrosis	Endolymphatic sac tumor
Keratosis obturans	Intralabyrinthine hemorrhage
Necrotizing otitis externa	Labyrinthine malformations
Middle ear-mastoid	**Petrous apex**
Acquired cholesteatoma	Trapped fluid
Congenital cholesteatoma	Cholesterol granuloma
Cholesterol granuloma	Congenital cholesteatoma
Acute coalescent mastoiditis	Cephalocele
Chronic otitis media ± tympanosclerosis	Apical petrositis
Dehiscent jugular bulb	Mucocele
Aberrant internal carotid artery	**Intratemporal facial nerve**
Glomus tympanicum paraganglioma	Herpetic facial neuritis (Bell palsy)
Glomus jugulare paraganglioma	Facial nerve venous malformation ("hemangioma")
Meningioma	Facial nerve schwannoma
Rhabdomyosarcoma	Perineural parotid malignancy

located medially and is composed of the head, crura, and footplate.

Approaches to Imaging Issues of the Temporal Bone

When faced with a T-bone study, use a systematic approach through the 5 major functional components (EAC, ME-M, inner ear, petrous apex, and facial nerve). Evaluate and report on the location of the ICA, status of the ossicles, location of CNVII and integrity of the facial nerve canal, presence of the oval window, and integrity of the fissula ante fenestram (anterior margin of the oval window). If a lesion of the T-bone is found, its location as well as clinical findings help refine the differential diagnosis list.

CHL is caused by a disruption of the conductive chain, which may be due to diseases of the EAC, TM, ossicles, or oval window. Typical lesions to consider in a patient with CHL include acquired cholesteatoma, chronic otitis media, EAC atresia/stenosis, fenestral otosclerosis, and cholesterol granuloma. Less common etiologies include oval window atresia, congenital cholesteatoma, ossicular fixation, and medial canal fibrosis.

SNHL involves lesions of the cochlea, modiolus, or cochlear nerve. These lesions may occur in the T-bone, IAC, CPA, or brainstem. Inner ear abnormalities in congenital SNHL may provide clues to a specific syndromic etiology. Positive findings help direct genetic testing and affect patient management. The most common lesion to present with acquired unilateral SNHL is vestibular schwannoma (~ 90% of lesions). Other much less common etiologies include meningioma, otosclerosis, facial nerve schwannoma, metastases, and labyrinthitis.

Whenever the T-bone is imaged, the entire facial nerve canal should be visualized and inspected. If a lesion of CNVII is found, it should be precisely localized to 1 of the CNVII segments: Cisternal segment (brainstem to porus acusticus), IAC (canalicular) segment, labyrinthine segment, tympanic segment, mastoid segment, or parotid segment.

Some lesions of the T-bone may result in **facial nerve paralysis**, including Bell palsy, T-bone fractures, cholesteatoma, schwannoma, venous malformation, glomus jugulare paraganglioma, meningioma, metastases, middle ear rhabdomyosarcoma, and Langerhans histiocytosis.

Clinical Implications

When a middle ear lesion is present, correlation with **otoscopic findings** provides critical clues to precise preoperative diagnosis. If a ruptured TM is present, a cholesteatoma may be seen through the defect. Most retrotympanic lesions have a distinctive hue and location. When the ENT surgeon sees a **white** middle ear lesion behind an intact TM, diagnoses to consider include a congenital cholesteatoma or schwannoma. If there is a **red** hue, the list includes a paraganglioma or aberrant ICA. If there is a **blue** hue, cholesterol granuloma, chronic otitis media with hemorrhage, or a dehiscent jugular bulb should be considered.

Peripheral facial nerve paralysis is defined as unilateral facial nerve injury with involvement of the entire face, including the forehead. This type of CNVII injury includes loss of the 4 facial nerve functions: Lacrimation (parasympathetic), stapedius reflex (sound dampening), taste to the anterior 2/3 of the tongue, and facial expression. Injury to CNVII at any point as it winds through the T-bone results in peripheral facial nerve paralysis.

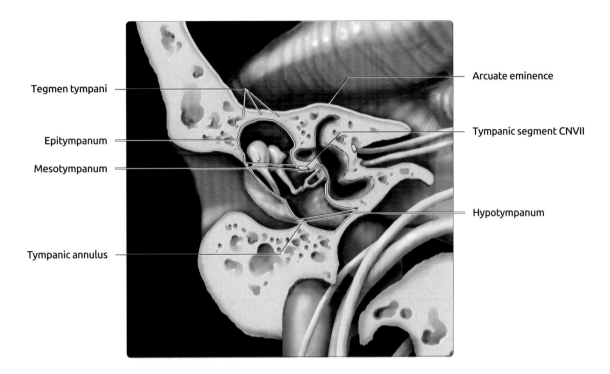

Tegmen tympani

Epitympanum

Mesotympanum

Tympanic annulus

Arcuate eminence

Tympanic segment CNVII

Hypotympanum

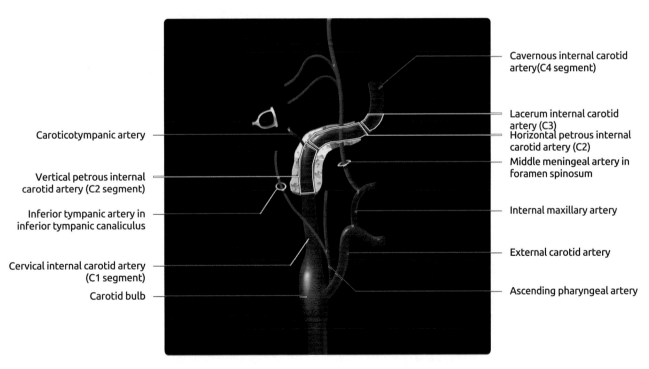

Caroticotympanic artery

Vertical petrous internal carotid artery (C2 segment)

Inferior tympanic artery in inferior tympanic canaliculus

Cervical internal carotid artery (C1 segment)

Carotid bulb

Cavernous internal carotid artery(C4 segment)

Lacerum internal carotid artery (C3)

Horizontal petrous internal carotid artery (C2)

Middle meningeal artery in foramen spinosum

Internal maxillary artery

External carotid artery

Ascending pharyngeal artery

(Top) *Coronal magnified graphic shows the middle ear. The middle ear is divided into 3 portions: Epitympanum, mesotympanum, and hypotympanum. The epitympanum is defined as the middle ear cavity above a line drawn from the tip of the scutum to the tympanic segment of CNVII. The epitympanic roof is called the tegmen tympani. The mesotympanum extends from this line inferiorly to a line connecting the tympanic annulus to the base of the cochlear promontory.* (Bottom) *Sagittal graphic shows the petrous internal carotid artery (ICA). The cervical ICA enters the carotid canal of the skull base to become the vertical petrous ICA (C2 subsegment ICA). It then turns anteromedially to become the horizontal petrous ICA (C2 subsegment ICA). The segment of the intracranial ICA just above the foramen lacerum is called the lacerum segment (C3 ICA segment). Note that the inferior tympanic artery rises through the inferior tympanic canaliculus, and the middle meningeal artery arises off the internal maxillary artery passing through the foramen spinosum.*

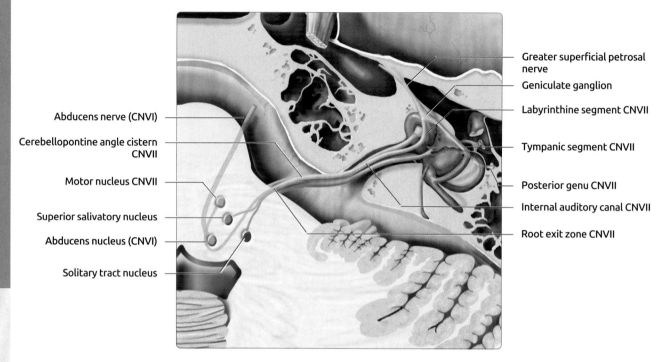

Abducens nerve (CNVI)

Cerebellopontine angle cistern CNVII

Motor nucleus CNVII

Superior salivatory nucleus

Abducens nucleus (CNVI)

Solitary tract nucleus

Greater superficial petrosal nerve

Geniculate ganglion

Labyrinthine segment CNVII

Tympanic segment CNVII

Posterior genu CNVII

Internal auditory canal CNVII

Root exit zone CNVII

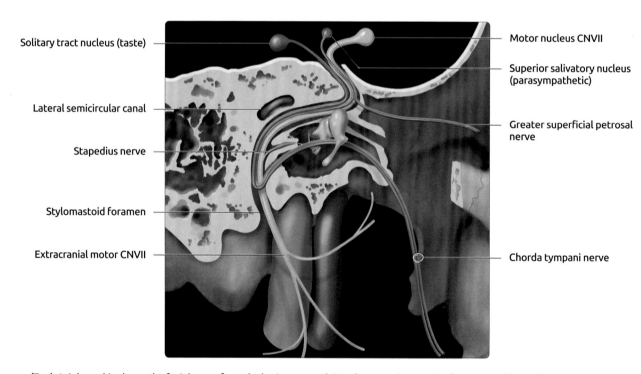

Solitary tract nucleus (taste)

Lateral semicircular canal

Stapedius nerve

Stylomastoid foramen

Extracranial motor CNVII

Motor nucleus CNVII

Superior salivatory nucleus (parasympathetic)

Greater superficial petrosal nerve

Chorda tympani nerve

(Top) *Axial graphic shows the facial nerve from the brainstem nuclei to the posterior genu in the temporal bone. The motor nucleus sends out fibers, which encircle the CNVI nucleus before reaching the root exit zone at the pontomedullary junction. Superior salivatory nucleus sends parasympathetic secretomotor fibers to the lacrimal, submandibular, and sublingual glands. The solitary tract nucleus receives the anterior 2/3 of tongue taste information, via the chorda tympani nerve, to the lingual nerve, to the oral tongue.* (Bottom) *Sagittal graphic depicts CNVII within the temporal bone (T. Motor fibers pass through the T-bone, giving off the stapedius nerve to the stapedius muscle, then exit via the stylomastoid foramen to the extracranial CNVII (entirely motor). Parasympathetic fibers from the superior salivatory nucleus reach the lacrimal gland via the greater superficial petrosal nerve and the submandibular-sublingual glands via the chorda tympanic nerve. The anterior 2/3 of tongue taste fibers come via the chorda tympani nerve.*

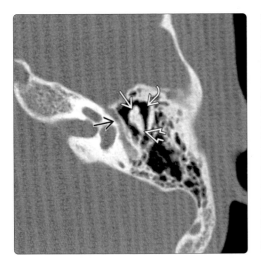

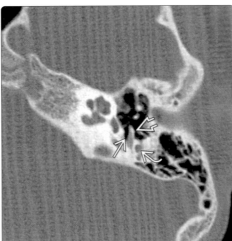

(Left) *Axial T-bone CT through the epitympanum shows the malleus head* ➡️ *anterior to the incus short process* ➡️. *Prussak space is the lateral epitympanic recess* ➡️ *and is a typical location for acquired cholesteatoma. Tympanic segment CNVII is well seen* ➡️. (Right) *Axial T-bone CT through the mesotympanum shows the posterior wall sinus tympani* ➡️ *and pyramidal eminence* ➡️, *which contains the stapedius muscle & mastoid CNVII* ➡️. *The most anterior ossicle is the malleus. The posterior ossicle is the incus.*

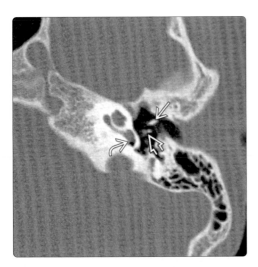

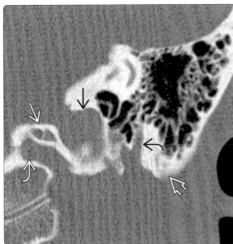

(Left) *Axial T-bone CT through the low mesotympanum shows the normal manubrium of malleus* ➡️ *and the incudostapedial articulation* ➡️. *Basal turn of the cochlea ends at the round window* ➡️. (Right) *Coronal T-bone CT through the posterior mastoid region shows the mastoid segment of CNVII* ➡️, *which then exits at the stylomastoid foramen. The mastoid tip* ➡️ *helps protect this portion of CNVII. The jugular foramen* ➡️ *and the hypoglossal canal* ➡️ *are separated by the jugular tubercle* ➡️.

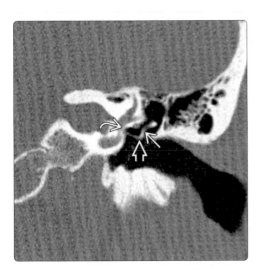

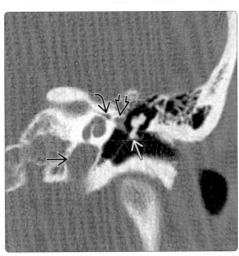

(Left) *Coronal T-bone CT through the semicircular canals demonstrates the long process* ➡️ *and the lenticular process* ➡️ *of the incus. Notice the normal absence of bone evident in the oval window niche* ➡️. *The oval window is best visualized in the coronal plane.* (Right) *Coronal T-bone CT through the anterior middle ear shows the malleus* ➡️, *labyrinthine* ➡️, *and tympanic* ➡️ *facial nerve segments. Notice the horizontal petrous ICA* ➡️ *below the cochlea.*

Foramen Tympanicum

TERMINOLOGY

- Synonyms: Foramen of Huschke; tympanic bone dehiscence
- Definition: Developmental ossification defect in anteroinferior aspect of bony EAC
  - Should be considered normal EAC variant

IMAGING

- Axial temporal bone CT: ~ 4- to 6-mm bony dehiscence in medial, anteroinferior aspect of bony EAC
- Axial diameter: Variable; 2-8 mm (mean: ~ 4 mm)

TOP DIFFERENTIAL DIAGNOSES

- 1st branchial cleft cyst
- EAC cholesteatoma
- EAC squamous cell carcinoma

PATHOLOGY

- Foramen tympanicum is formed in tympanic plate of temporal bone before 1 yr of age

- Usually closes before 5 yr of age
- Persistence seen on bone CT after 5 yr of age in ~ 5% of patients
- Pathology associated with foramen tympanicum
  - **Spontaneous herniation of TMJ soft tissues** into EAC
  - Parotid gland and synovial TMJ fistulas into EAC
  - Foramen tympanicum may facilitate ear injury during TMJ arthroscopy

CLINICAL ISSUES

- **Asymptomatic** normal variant found incidentally during temporal bone CT
- Otorrhea with otalgia possible if dehiscence is large
  - Physical examination reveals polypoid lesion in anteroinferior bony EAC
  - If patient opens mouth, polypoid lesion disappears
- Gustatory otorrhea (occurs with eating)
  - Sialo-aural fistula from parotid gland through foramen tympanicum to EAC

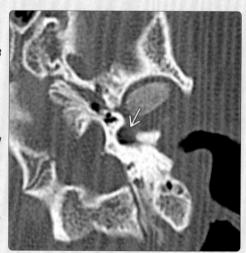
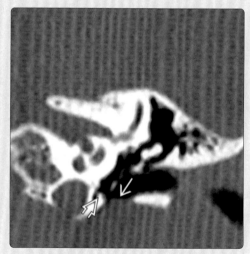

(Left) Axial temporal bone CT of the left ear shows appearance of incidental foramen tympanicum ➡ in a 3 year old. Notice the anteroinferior tympanic bone dehiscence that normally closes by 5 years of age. (Right) Coronal temporal bone CT in the same patient demonstrates the well-defined areas of incomplete ossification in the anterior medial aspect of the osseous external auditory canal ➡. Note the proximal relationship of the foramen tympanicum to the tympanic annulus ➡.

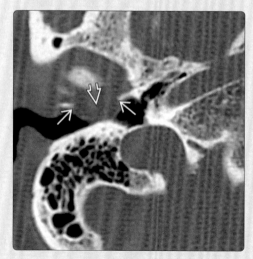
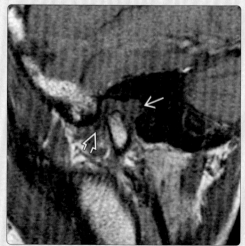

(Left) Axial bone CT through the EAC reveals a large (14 mm) foramen tympanicum in the anteroinferior bony EAC ➡. The posterior TMJ soft tissues have prolapsed through a dehiscence ➡ into the EAC lumen. (Right) Sagittal T1 MR in the closed mouth position shows posterior TMJ soft tissues filling the lumen of the EAC ➡. The meniscus ➡ is in normal position. With mouth open (not shown), the soft tissue in the EAC diminishes considerably, suggesting it is the joint capsule that has prolapsed into the EAC.

TERMINOLOGY

Synonyms

- Foramen of Huschke
- Tympanic bone dehiscence

Definitions

- Foramen tympanicum
  - Developmental ossification defect in anteroinferior aspect of bony EAC

IMAGING

General Features

- Best diagnostic clue
  - Axial temporal bone CT: ~ 4- to 6-mm bony dehiscence in medial, anteroinferior aspect of bony EAC
- Location
  - Located at anteroinferior aspect of EAC, posteromedial to temporomandibular joint (TMJ)
- Size
  - Axial diameter: Variable; 2-8 mm (mean: ~ 4 mm)
  - Mean sagittal diameter: 3.5 mm

CT Findings

- Bone CT
  - Focal dehiscence visible on axial bone CT in medial, anteroinferior aspect of bony EAC
    - In bony wall, shared in common with the TMJ
  - **Dehiscence** found in **~ 5%** of normal temporal bones
    - **Focal thinning** of bone in this location: **35%**
  - More commonly unilateral than bilateral (2:1)
  - Larger lesions have additional findings
    - Polypoid mass in anteroinferior EAC
      - □ From **prolapse of TMJ retrodiscal soft tissues**
      - □ Rarely results from **parotid prolapse**

MR Findings

- Only positive in case of larger dehiscence when TMJ soft tissues or parotid prolapse is present

Imaging Recommendations

- Best imaging tool
  - T-bone CT defines extent of foramen tympanicum
  - When large with prolapsing tissue, TMJ MR is used to define tissue type

DIFFERENTIAL DIAGNOSIS

1st Branchial Cleft Cyst

- Cyst intraparotid or periauricular

EAC Cholesteatoma

- Bony EAC destruction with bone fragments

EAC Squamous Cell Carcinoma

- Begins as obvious auricular squamous cell carcinoma
- After multiple treatments, invades EAC ± focal bony wall destruction

PATHOLOGY

General Features

- Etiology

- Foramen tympanicum is formed in tympanic plate of temporal bone at ~ 1 yr of age
- Usually closes before 5 yr of age
- Persistence after 5 yr of age seen on bone CT in ~ 5% of patients
- Foramen is defined by traversing structure
  - Foramen tympanicum is **not** true foramen
  - More appropriate term than foramen tympanicum is **tympanic bone dehiscence**
  - Considered **normal variant**
- Pathology associated with foramen tympanicum
  - Spontaneous herniation of TMJ soft tissues into EAC
  - Foramen tympanicum may facilitate ear injury during TMJ arthroscopy
  - Parotid gland and synovial TMJ fistulas into EAC
  - Infection spread through foramen tympanicum from EAC outward or from TMJ inward

CLINICAL ISSUES

Presentation

- Most common signs/symptoms
  - **Asymptomatic** bony defect found incidentally during temporal bone CT
- Other signs/symptoms
  - Otorrhea with otalgia possible if dehiscence is large
    - Physical examination reveals polypoid lesion in anteroinferior bony EAC
    - If patient opens mouth, polypoid lesion disappears
  - Salivary fistula formation with **gustatory otorrhea** and otalgia
    - Extremely rare lesion
    - Sialo-aural fistula from parotid gland through foramen tympanicum to EAC
    - Otorrhea fluid tests positive for amylase
    - Gustatory otorrhea occurs when eating
  - Complication during TMJ arthroscopy
    - Inadvertent passage of arthroscope into EAC or middle ear
    - Resultant otologic complications possible
  - TMJ/masticator space infection or EAC infection may spread in either direction

Demographics

- Gender
  - Persistence seen in females > males

Natural History & Prognosis

- Persistent foramen tympanicum at 5 yr of age continues to close with increasing age in some patients

SELECTED REFERENCES

1. Akbulut N et al: Evaluation of foramen tympanicum using cone-beam computed tomography in orthodontic malocclusions. J Craniofac Surg. 25(2):e105-9, 2014
2. Nakasato T et al: Spontaneous temporomandibular joint herniation into the external auditory canal through a persistent foramen tympanicum (Huschke): radiographic features. J Comput Assist Tomogr. 37(1):111-3, 2013
3. Park YH et al: Temporomandibular joint herniation into the external auditory canal. Laryngoscope. 120(11):2284-8, 2010
4. Lacout A et al: Foramen tympanicum, or foramen of Huschke: pathologic cases and anatomic CT study. AJNR Am J Neuroradiol. 26(6):1317-23, 2005

TERMINOLOGY

- Congenital external & middle ear malformation (CEMEM)

IMAGING

- Auricle: Anotia or microtia
- EAC stenosis: Narrow EAC, tympanic plate (TP) hypoplasia
  - Normal or thickened tympanic membrane (TM)
  - Small middle ear cavity
  - Subtle ossicular anomaly
- EAC atresia: Absent EAC, TP, and TM; moderate or severe CEMEM + middle ear findings
- Moderate CEMEM middle ear findings
  - Small middle ear cavity ± low tegmen tympani
  - Fusion, malformation, & rotation of malleus & incus
  - Oval window atresia (35%) ± aberrant CNVII tympanic segment
  - Mastoid CNVII more anterolateral than normal
- Severe CEMEM middle ear findings
  - Tiny or absent middle ear cavity, low tegmen tympani

- Ossicles absent or rudimentary
- Oval window atresia (35%) ± aberrant CNVII tympanic segment
- Aberrant facial nerve canal course
- Erosive opacity in stenotic EAC or MEC suggests congenital cholesteatoma

TOP DIFFERENTIAL DIAGNOSES

- Acquired EAC stenosis (surfer's ear)
- EAC osteoma
- Tympanosclerosis

CLINICAL ISSUES

- Conductive hearing loss = most common symptom
- Severity of microtia approximates severity of CEMEM

DIAGNOSTIC CHECKLIST

- EAC atresia = clinical diagnosis
- CT provides preoperative roadmap

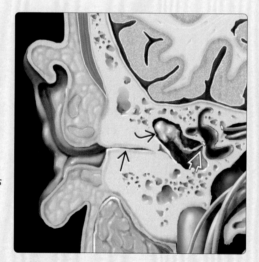
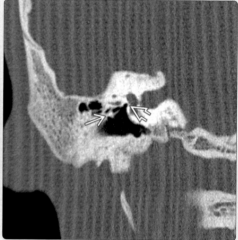

(Left) Coronal graphic of the right ear shows deformed auricle with absent external auditory canal ➡. Ossicular fusion mass ➡ and rotation with oval window atresia ➡ are also present. (Right) Coronal bone CT in this patient with congenital external ear malformation shows the ossicular fusion mass ➡ ankylosed to the lateral wall of the middle ear cavity. Oval window atresia is present, diagnosed by observing the narrowed oval window niche and thin bone covering the oval window itself ➡.

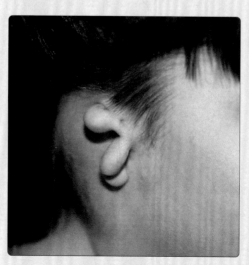
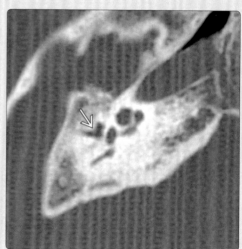

(Left) Clinical photograph reveals small, severely malformed auricle with no identifiable external auditory canal. Severe microtia will be reflected in severe EAC and middle ear malformation on temporal bone CT. (Right) Axial bone CT in a patient with severe microtia reveals a normal-appearing inner ear with a very small middle ear cavity ➡ and no ossicles. The absence of ossicles combined with near absence of the middle ear cavity makes surgical correction extremely difficult.

TERMINOLOGY

Abbreviations

- Congenital external & middle ear malformation (CEMEM)

Synonyms

- Congenital aural atresia or dysplasia

Definitions

- Anotia: Absent auricle
- Microtia: Small, malformed auricle
- External ear malformation [auricle & external auditory canal (EAC)]
  - EAC atresia: Absent EAC, tympanic plate (TP), & tympanic membrane (TM)
  - EAC stenosis: Narrow EAC, TP hypoplasia, TM present
  - EAC duplication: Duplication of part or all of EAC
- Middle ear cavity (MEC) malformation: Aplasia or hypoplasia MEC + ossicular anomaly

IMAGING

General Features

- Best diagnostic clue
  - Microtia or anotia + absent EAC
  - Microtia or normal pinna + narrow EAC
- Location
  - EAC & MEC; unilateral or bilateral
- Morphology
  - Small, malformed auricle (microtia) or anotia
  - Mildest CEMEM has narrowed EAC
  - More severe CEMEM has no identifiable EAC or TP
  - Hypoplastic middle ear cavity
  - Dysmorphic ossicles, especially malleus & incus

CT Findings

- Bone CT
  - Auricle & EAC in CEMEM
    - Dysmorphic auricle: Anotia or microtia
    - EAC stenosis
      - Narrow or "blind-ending" EAC
      - TP present but small; TM thickened ± Ca++
      - Erosive opacity suggests keratosis obturans or EAC cholesteatoma
    - EAC atresia
      - Absent EAC
      - Absent TP & TM
      - Membranous ± (thick or thin) bony "atresia plate"
    - Duplicated EAC
      - Duplication of membranous or entire EAC
  - Middle ear malformation
    - Mild CEMEM: EAC stenosis
      - MEC: Mild hypoplasia, shallow facial recess
      - Oval window: Normal or stenotic ± anomalous course of tympanic segment CNVII
      - Ossicles: Variable malformation, rotation, fusion to lateral MEC, fusion of malleolar-incudal articulation
      - Mastoid segment CNVII: Near normal in location
    - Moderate CEMEM: EAC stenosis or atresia
      - MEC: Moderate hypoplasia ± low tegmen tympani

- Oval window: Atresia (35%) ± anomalous course ± dehiscent tympanic segment CNVII
  - Round window: Atresia (5%)
  - Ossicles: Malformed, rotated, fused (malleus & incus > stapes)
  - Mastoid CNVII: More anterolateral than normal
  - Rounded or erosive opacity = associated congenital cholesteatoma (2%)
    - Severe CEMEM: EAC atresia
      - MEC: Tiny or absent, low tegmen tympani
      - Oval & round windows: Atresia
      - Ossicles: Absent or rudimentary
      - CNVII: ± hypoplasia; anomalous/bizarre course
  - Facial nerve canal findings
    - Aberrant tympanic & mastoid segments common
    - Tympanic segment may be dehiscent, overlying oval or round windows
    - Mastoid segment usually anterolaterally displaced
    - May exit skull base into glenoid fossa, or lateral to styloid process
  - Mastoid pneumatization: Normal to absent
  - Inner ear & IAC: < 30% anomaly = syndromic
  - Mandible: Micrognathia + low-set pinna = syndromic

MR Findings

- Limited utility, e.g., large congenital cholesteatoma

Imaging Recommendations

- Best imaging tool
  - High-resolution CT
- Protocol advice
  - 0.6-mm axial CT with coronal & oblique reformats

DIFFERENTIAL DIAGNOSIS

Acquired EAC Stenosis (Surfer's Ear)

- Bilateral acquired lesions + normal auricle

EAC Osteoma

- Unilateral acquired benign bony growth obliterates EAC

EAC Cholesteatoma

- Erosive opacity in normal or stenotic EAC

Tympanosclerosis

- EAC normal in size
- Inflammatory calcifications of TM, ossicles, MEC

Keratosis Obturans, EAC

- Keratin debris opacifies and erodes stenotic EAC

PATHOLOGY

General Features

- Etiology
  - Variety of causes of CEMEM, often unknown
  - Known syndromic/genetic causes
  - Epithelial cells of 1st branchial groove fail to split & canalize, resulting in CEMEM
- Genetics
  - 14% have positive prior family history
  - May be associated with various syndromes
    - Hemifacial microsomia spectrum

– Branchio-oto-renal syndrome
– Treacher Collins syndrome
- Associated abnormalities
  o Isolated or part of craniofacial syndrome
    – Suggested by micrognathia + low-set pinna
    – Branchial cleft anomalies
  o Inner ear anomaly occurs < 10% (syndromic cases)
    – Inner ear forms earlier from otocyst
- Embryology-anatomy in CEMEM
  o 1st & 2nd branchial arches & 1st pharyngeal pouch develop at same time during embryogenesis
  o Branchial groove & 1st pharyngeal pouch give rise to EAC
    – Initially, solid core of epithelial cells
    – In 3rd trimester, cell core canalizes into EAC
    – Failure of canalization leads to CEMEM
  o 1st branchial arch forms malleus head, incus body & short process, & tensor tympani tendon
  o 2nd branchial arch forms manubrium of malleus, long process of incus, stapes (except footplate), & stapedial muscle and tendon
    – Ossicular fusion mass very common in CEMEM
    – Oval window atresia may be associated with CEMEM
  o Inner ear forms earlier than EAC; anomalies unusual in CEMEM unless syndromic

Staging, Grading, & Classification

- Jahrsdoerfer scale and surgical outcomes
  o Score of ≥ 7 points predicts adequate surgical success
- Scoring system; best possible score = 10 points
  o Stapes present: 2
  o Oval window open: 1
  o Middle ear space present: 1
  o Facial nerve course identified: 1
  o Malleus-incus complex present: 1
  o Incus-stapes connection present: 1
  o Mastoid pneumatization present: 1
  o Round window present: 1
  o External ear present: 1
- Recommendations
  o Operate on unilateral CEMEM score ≥ 7
  o Operate on bilateral CEMEM score ≥ 5-6

Gross Pathologic & Surgical Features

- Malformed auricle; low set if + micrognathia
- Stenosis or absence of EAC
  o Atresia plate membranous &/or bony

CLINICAL ISSUES

Presentation

- Most common signs/symptoms
  o Conductive hearing loss = most common symptom
  o Physical exam
    – Absent, small ± low-set auricle
      □ Severity of microtia approximates severity of CEMEM & MEC malformation
    – EAC is stenotic or absent

Demographics

- Age
  o Present at birth

- Gender
  o Occurs more commonly in males
- Epidemiology
  o 1 in 10,000-20,000 live births
  o Unilateral:bilateral cases = 4:1
    – Nonsyndromic CEMEM usually unilateral
    – Bilateral CEMEM common when syndromic

Natural History & Prognosis

- Static clinical course, unless associated MEC cholesteatoma or syndromic
- Bilateral atresia: Bilateral conductive hearing loss
  o After surgery, hearing is adequate but not normal
- Auricle reconstruction may require 4-5 staged surgeries

Treatment

- Cosmetic reconstruction of auricle usually in adolescence
- CT to assess course of CNVII & oval window & inner ear status prior to surgery
- Bilateral atresia is treated at 5-6 years of age, when head has reached 90% of adult size
  o Auricle reconstruction precedes surgical treatment of MEC & ossicles
  o Surgical reconstruction of ear with mildest EAC atresia
  o Both auricles are repaired for cosmetic reasons
- Normal morphology & location of stapes important for surgical reconstruction & ossicular function

DIAGNOSTIC CHECKLIST

Consider

- EAC atresia = clinical diagnosis
  o CT provides preoperative roadmap
  o CT scoring systems suggest when to operate

Reporting Tips

- Preoperative CT checklist used for surgical planning
  o Atresia plate: Bony vs. membranous; note thickness
  o Report size of MEC as normal or small
  o Status of ossicles: Presence, morphology, & ankylosis
  o Oval window present? Stapes?
    – If no stapes, ossicular reconstruction is difficult
  o Trace course of CNVII; aberrant CNVII at risk during surgery
  o Survey for erosive opacity suggesting cholesteatoma

SELECTED REFERENCES

1. Bartel-Friedrich S: Congenital auricular malformations: description of anomalies and syndromes. Facial Plast Surg. 31(6):567-80, 2015
2. Jacob R et al: High-resolution CT findings in children with a normal pinna or grade I microtia and unilateral mild stenosis of the external auditory canal. AJNR Am J Neuroradiol. 36(1):176-80, 2015
3. Zhao S et al: An imaging study of the facial nerve canal in congenital aural atresia. Ear Nose Throat J. 94(10-11):E6-13, 2015
4. Casale G et al: Acquired ear canal cholesteatoma in congenital aural atresia/stenosis. Otol Neurotol. 35(8):1474-9, 2014
5. Mukherjee S et al: The "boomerang" malleus-incus complex in congenital aural atresia. AJNR Am J Neuroradiol. 35(11):2181-5, 2014
6. Kösling S et al: Congenital malformations of the external and middle ear. Eur J Radiol. 69(2):269-79, 2009
7. Shonka DC Jr et al: The Jahrsdoerfer grading scale in surgery to repair congenital aural atresia. Arch Otolaryngol Head Neck Surg. 134(8):873-7, 2008
8. Selesnick S et al: Surgical treatment of acquired external auditory canal atresia. Am J Otol. 19(2):123-30, 1998

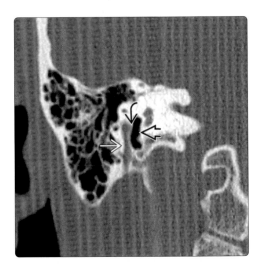

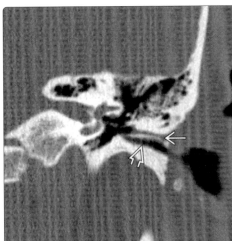

(Left) *Coronal bone CT in a patient with congenital external ear malformation through the pyramidal eminence ➡ demonstrates the mastoid segment of the facial nerve canal ➡ at the same level as the sinus tympani ➡. This is anterior to its normal location.* (Right) *Coronal bone CT in a patient with bilateral EAC malformation shows that the left narrowed EAC canal has 2 channels, 1 aerated ➡ and 1 with a membranous plug ➡. Such a "duplicated EAC" is a rare variant seen in EAC atresia.*

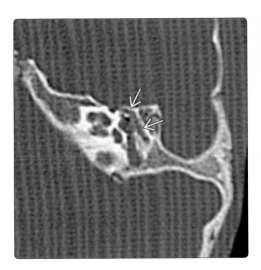

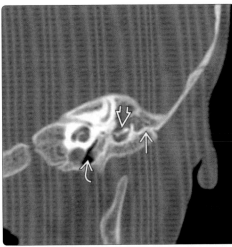

(Left) *Axial bone CT in a patient with severe congenital external ear malformation reveals an ectopic tympanic segment of the facial nerve canal ➡ arching lateral to the opacified middle ear cavity.* (Right) *Coronal bone CT in the same patient shows complete absence of the EAC ➡ associated with bilobed, hypoplastic middle ear cavity partially aerated inferiorly ➡ with the ossicular fusion mass in the superolateral cavity ➡.*

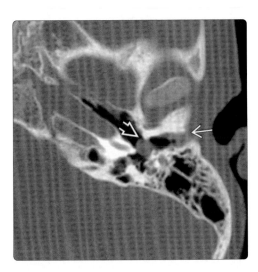

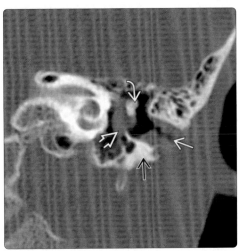

(Left) *Axial bone CT in a 9-year-old boy with left conductive hearing loss reveals EAC stenosis ➡ with partial EAC opacification. There is a rounded opacity ➡ within the mildly hypoplastic MEC, consistent with a congenital cholesteatoma.* (Right) *Coronal bone CT in a 9-year-old boy with EAC stenosis ➡. The congenital cholesteatoma ➡ surrounds and erodes the malleus ➡, which also has an abnormal orientation. Note the small tympanic plate ➡.*

Necrotizing External Otitis

TERMINOLOGY

- Necrotizing external otitis (NEO)
- NEO definition: Severe **invasive infection** of EAC, adjacent soft tissues, and skull base

IMAGING

- Swollen EAC soft tissues with **bony erosion** (bone CT) and adjacent cellulitis or abscess
- MR findings
  - Low T1 signal in bony marrow: Osteomyelitis
  - Tissues of EAC and auricle diffusely enhance
- T1WI C+ MR findings
  - **Phlegmon**: Heterogeneously enhancing tissue
  - **Abscesses**: Rim-enhancing fluid collections
- Nuclear medicine findings
  - Bone and gallium scans often done together
  - If both positive with gallium scan showing larger activity area, high correlation with NEO

TOP DIFFERENTIAL DIAGNOSES

- EAC squamous cell carcinoma
- EAC cholesteatoma
- Postinflammatory medial canal fibrosis
- EAC keratosis obturans

PATHOLOGY

- Diabetic vasculopathy and immune dysfunction
- **Pseudomonas aeruginosa**: 98% NEO infections

CLINICAL ISSUES

- Presentation: Severe otalgia and otorrhea
  - "Silent" disease if **diabetic microangiopathy**
- 95% of adults with NEO have **diabetes**
  - Predisposition equal for types I and II
- Treatment
  - Glucose control, granulation debridement
  - Topical and systemic antibiotic therapy
  - Surgical drainage of any abscess

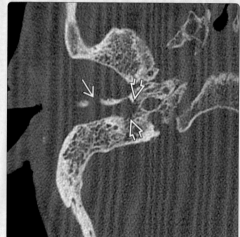
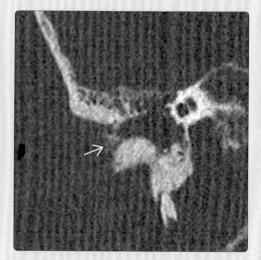

(Left) Axial bone CT shows EAC opacification with focal anterior wall ➡ and floor of middle ear ⮆ erosion in this diabetic patient with painful otorrhea and early necrotizing external otitis. (Right) Coronal bone CT in the same patient demonstrates anterior EAC wall bony destruction ➡ accompanied by complete opacification of the EAC. The middle ear is also opacified. In this case, the Pseudomonas infection involved both the EAC and the middle ear cavity.

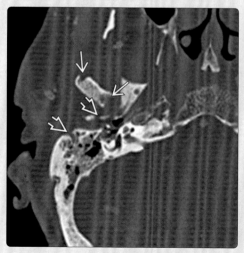
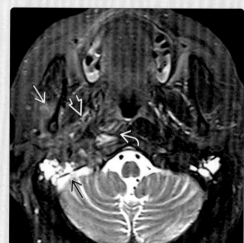

(Left) Axial bone CT reveals EAC opacification associated with multiple areas of erosive bony change ➡. The mandibular condyle is also eroded ➡, indicating that the infection has spread to involve the TMJ. (Right) Axial T2WI FS MR in the same patient shows abnormal high signal in the masticator ➡, parapharyngeal ➡, and prevertebral ➡ spaces secondary to spread of the EAC infection into the subjacent spaces of the suprahyoid neck. Sigmoid sinus high signal is from thrombosis ➡.

TERMINOLOGY

Abbreviations

- Necrotizing external otitis (NEO)

Synonyms

- Malignant external otitis, malignant otitis externa

Definitions

- NEO: Severe **invasive infection** of EAC, adjacent soft tissues, and skull base

IMAGING

General Features

- Best diagnostic clue
  o Swollen EAC soft tissues with bony erosion and adjacent cellulitis or abscess

CT Findings

- Bone CT
  o Early: Thickened mucosa of EAC and auricle
  o Late: Bony EAC **erosion** (especially floor)
    – Adjacent skull base destructive change possible

MR Findings

- T1WI
  o Muscle signal in EAC and adjacent soft tissues
  o Diffuse low signal in normal high-signal fatty marrow seen in infected temporal bone and skull base
- T2WI
  o Diffuse transspatial high signal suggests cellulitis
  o Focal high-signal areas suggest abscess
- STIR
  o Increased signal intensity within inflamed EAC, auricle, adjacent soft tissues, and infected bone
- T1WI C+ FS
  o Tissues of EAC and auricle diffusely enhance
  o Heterogeneous enhancement with cellulitis-phlegmon in adjacent soft tissues
  o Abscesses present as rim-enhancing fluid collections

Nuclear Medicine Findings

- General comments
  o Less commonly used compared to a decade ago

Imaging Recommendations

- Best imaging tool
  o Bone CT may identify subtle cortical erosions signaling early osteomyelitis
  o MR more sensitive for intracranial complications, bone marrow edema, extent of extracranial soft tissue involvement
  o Follow-up treatment
    – Bone changes persist on CT for up to 1 year
    – Resolution of soft tissue and marrow changes on MR may be better marker of treatment response

DIFFERENTIAL DIAGNOSIS

External Auditory Canal Squamous Cell Carcinoma

- Known, often treated auricle squamous cell carcinoma
- CT-MR: Imaging mimics NEO

External Auditory Canal Cholesteatoma

- Submucosal EAC mass
- CT: Unilateral EAC mass with bony erosion (intramural bony "flakes" in 50%)

Postinflammatory Medial Canal Fibrosis

- CT: Fibrous crescent in medial EAC
  o No underlying bony erosion

PATHOLOGY

General Features

- Etiology
  o Diabetic vasculopathy and immune dysfunction
  o **Pseudomonas aeruginosa**: 98% of NEO infections

CLINICAL ISSUES

Presentation

- Most common signs/symptoms
  o Severe otalgia and otorrhea
- Other signs/symptoms
  o Cranial nerve palsies herald skull base osteomyelitis
  o CNVII, CNIX-XII cranial neuropathies
  o WBC normal or mildly ↑, ESR invariably ↑

Demographics

- Age
  o Diabetic patients older (> 60 years)
  o Nondiabetic, immunocompromised patients younger
- Epidemiology
  o **95%** of adults with NEO have **diabetes**

Natural History & Prognosis

- Begins as soft tissue EAC infection
  o Spreads into adjacent osseous and soft tissue structures
  o May progress to skull base osteomyelitis
  o May progress to deep spatial abscess
- 20% recurrence rate

Treatment

- Glucose control, aggressive granulation debridement
- Systemic (ciprofloxacin) and topical antibiotic therapy
- Surgical drainage if deep facial abscess

DIAGNOSTIC CHECKLIST

Consider

- EAC squamous cell carcinoma can mimic NEO on imaging
  o Auricle squamous cell carcinoma clinically obvious

Image Interpretation Pearls

- Early cortical erosions best seen with bone CT

SELECTED REFERENCES

1. Le Clerc N et al: Skull base osteomyelitis: incidence of resistance, morbidity, and treatment strategy. Laryngoscope. 124(9):2013-6, 2014
2. Adams A et al: Central skull base osteomyelitis as a complication of necrotizing otitis externa: Imaging findings, complications, and challenges of diagnosis. Clin Radiol. 67(10):e7-e16, 2012
3. Franco-Vidal V et al: Necrotizing external otitis: a report of 46 cases. Otol Neurotol. 28(6):771-3, 2007
4. Grandis JR et al: Necrotizing (malignant) external otitis: prospective comparison of CT and MR imaging in diagnosis and follow-up. Radiology. 196(2):499-504, 1995

TERMINOLOGY

- Keratosis obturans (KO): Abnormal accumulation & obstruction of bony EAC from desquamated keratin without erosive bony changes

IMAGING

- Temporal bone CT findings
  - Benign-appearing **luminal** soft tissue lesion partially or completely filling EAC
  - May diffusely enlarge EAC
  - **No** bony erosive change (cf. EAC cholesteatoma)
  - Bilateral (50%)
  - Middle ear spared unless KO neglected

TOP DIFFERENTIAL DIAGNOSES

- Benign EAC debris
- EAC cholesteatoma
- Necrotizing external otitis
- EAC squamous cell carcinoma

PATHOLOGY

- Benign keratin "plug" filling EAC without focal bony erosion

CLINICAL ISSUES

- Clinical presentation
  - Acute **severe otalgia**
  - Conductive hearing loss
- KO treatment
  - Excision of keratin "plug"
  - Removal of reaccumulated debris often required

DIAGNOSTIC CHECKLIST

- "KO" & "EAC cholesteatoma" terms often confused
  - KO: EAC luminal lesion **without** bony erosions
    - If large, may involve middle ear through damaged tympanic membrane
  - EAC cholesteatoma: Submucosal lesion with EAC erosions ± bony flecks (50%)
    - If large, may involve mastoid air cells

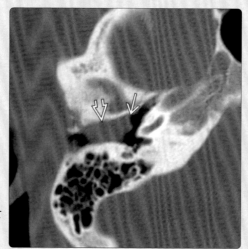
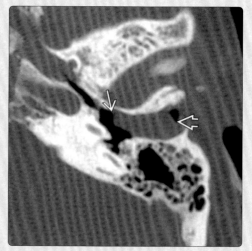

(Left) Axial bone CT in this patient with otoscopic evidence of EAC obstruction shows a soft tissue "plug" ⇨ in the EAC extending laterally from the tympanic membrane ➡. Note absence of underlying bony changes. (Right) Axial bone CT in a patient with conductive hearing loss demonstrates a benign-appearing soft tissue lesion in the left EAC extending from the tympanic membrane ➡ to the lateral bony EAC margin ⇦. The middle ear and underlying EAC bone are not involved.

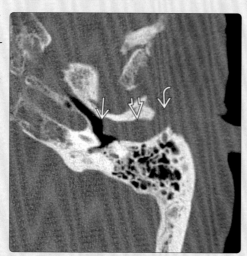
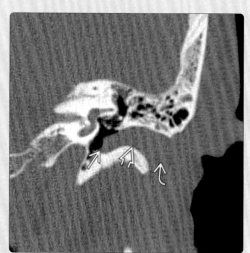

(Left) Axial bone CT of the left ear shows the EAC is filled with soft tissue ➡. This bland-appearing lesion extends from the tympanic membrane ➡ laterally into the cartilaginous EAC ➡. (Right) Coronal bone CT in the same patient reveals benign-appearing soft tissue within the EAC ➡ extending from the tympanic membrane ➡ laterally into the cartilaginous EAC ➡. There is slight flaring of the lateral bony EAC, but no other bony change is apparent.

TERMINOLOGY

Abbreviations

- External auditory canal (EAC)
- Keratosis obturans (KO)

Synonyms

- Laminated epithelial "plug;" keratin "plug"

Definitions

- KO: Abnormal accumulation & obstruction of bony EAC from desquamated keratin without erosive bony changes

IMAGING

General Features

- Best diagnostic clue
  - KO appears as homogeneous soft tissue filling EAC
    - Mild EAC enlargement common
    - Focal bony erosion **not** present
- Morphology
  - Soft tissue conforms to EAC

CT Findings

- Bone CT
  - Benign-appearing soft tissue filling EAC
    - May diffusely enlarge EAC
    - **No** bony erosive change (cf. EAC cholesteatoma)
  - Bilateral (50%)
  - Middle ear spared unless KO neglected

MR Findings

- T1WI
  - Homogeneous low-intermediate signal soft tissue filling EAC
- T2WI
  - Isointense or low signal intensity
- T1WI C+
  - May rim enhance

Imaging Recommendations

- Best imaging tool
  - Temporal bone CT

DIFFERENTIAL DIAGNOSIS

Benign EAC Debris

- CT: Partially filled EAC; no bony erosion
- Clinical: Waxy debris visible

EAC Cholesteatoma

- CT: Unilateral EAC soft tissue with bony erosion
  - Bony intramural flakes (50%)
- Clinical: Mucosal irregularity; submucosal mass

Necrotizing External Otitis

- CT: EAC swelling ± bone erosion ± abscess
- Clinical: Diabetic patient; otorrhea

EAC Squamous Cell Carcinoma

- CT: Irregular mass ± bony erosion
  - Extends from external ear to involve EAC
- Clinical: Known squamous cell carcinoma on auricle

PATHOLOGY

General Features

- Etiology
  - 2 common theories
    - Abnormal epithelial migration with keratinaceous debris build-up
    - Sympathetic reflex stimulation of ceruminous glands in EAC causes hyperemia & epidermal plugging
  - Radiation dermatitis can also produce radiation KO
- Associated abnormalities
  - Chronic sinusitis & bronchiectasis

Gross Pathologic & Surgical Features

- Marked inflammation in subepithelial tissue
- Benign keratin "plug" fills EAC without focal bony erosion

Microscopic Features

- Desquamated keratin tissue
- Keratin tightly organized in lamellar pattern in KO
  - EAC cholesteatoma organized in random keratin pattern

CLINICAL ISSUES

Presentation

- Most common signs/symptoms
  - Acute **severe otalgia**
  - Conductive hearing loss

Demographics

- Age
  - Younger patients (< 40 years old)
- Epidemiology
  - Rare EAC lesion

Treatment

- Excision of keratin "plug"
- Direct treatment of granulations when present
  - Excision, cauterization, topical steroids
- Removal of reaccumulated debris often required

DIAGNOSTIC CHECKLIST

Image Interpretation Pearls

- "KO" & "EAC cholesteatoma" terms often confused
  - KO: EAC luminal lesion **without** bony erosions
  - EAC cholesteatoma: Submucosal lesion with EAC erosions ± bony flecks (50%)
  - Both lesions consist of exfoliated keratin

SELECTED REFERENCES

1. Park SY et al: Clinical characteristics of keratosis obturans and external auditory canal cholesteatoma. Otolaryngol Head Neck Surg. 152(2):326-30, 2015
2. Spielmann PM et al: Surgical management of external auditory canal lesions. J Laryngol Otol. 127(3):246-51, 2013
3. Saunders NC et al: Complications of keratosis obturans. J Laryngol Otol. 120(9):740-4, 2006
4. Kuczkowski J et al: Immunohistochemical and histopathological features of keratosis obturans and cholesteatoma of the external auditory canal. Atypical keratosis obturans. J Laryngol Otol. 118(3):249-50; author reply 250-1, 2004
5. Naiberg J et al: The pathologic features of keratosis obturans and cholesteatoma of the external auditory canal. Arch Otolaryngol. 110(10):690-3, 1984

Temporal Bone

TERMINOLOGY

- Medial canal fibrosis (MCF)
  - Discrete clinicopathological disease characterized by formation of fibrous tissue in medial aspect of bony EAC

IMAGING

- **Early stage MCF**
  - Thickened TM with edematous, mildly thickened medial EAC mucosa
- **Late stage MCF**
  - Thick tissue "crescent" overlying lateral TM surface
  - TM **cannot** be resolved as separate from MCF fibrous mass
  - No underlying bony changes present

TOP DIFFERENTIAL DIAGNOSES

- Benign EAC debris
- EAC keratosis obturans
- EAC cholesteatoma

- EAC exostoses (surfer's ear)
- EAC squamous cell carcinoma
- Necrotizing external otitis

PATHOLOGY

- MCF is final common pathophysiologic pathway for multiple mechanisms of injury to EAC
  - Chronic otitis externa: Most common etiology
  - Secondary to surgical procedure or trauma
  - Suppurative otitis media
  - Radiotherapy to EAC

CLINICAL ISSUES

- Common presentation
  - 50-year-old woman with bilateral otorrhea, conductive hearing loss (CHL), history of chronic otitis
- Treatment options
  - Early: Topical steroids
  - Late phase: Surgery corrects CHL; recurrence frequent

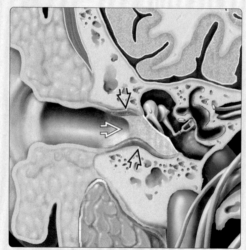
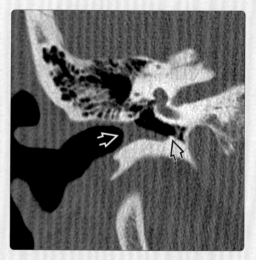

(Left) Coronal graphic of the right ear shows medial canal fibrosis (MCF) as a thick fibrous crescent ⮞ overlying the TM and filling the medial external auditory canal (EAC). Inflammatory changes ⮊ of medial EAC walls are also depicted. (Right) Coronal T-bone CT reveals a band of soft tissue ⮞ filling the medial EAC and abutting the TM. The middle ear is unaffected by MCF. The inferior insertion of the TM is marked by the tympanic annulus ⮞.

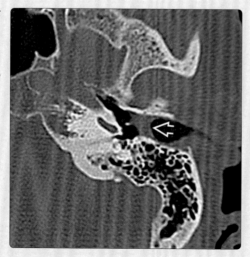
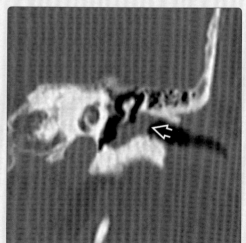

(Left) Axial bone CT of the left ear demonstrates the characteristic appearance of mature MCF as a crescentic area of soft tissue thickening ⮞ on the outer surface of the TM extending laterally into the EAC. (Right) Coronal bone CT in the same patient reveals the fibrous rind ⮞ on the outer surface of the TM. Notice that the middle ear is spared, as is typical for MCF.

TERMINOLOGY

Abbreviations

- Medial canal fibrosis (MCF)

Synonyms

- Idiopathic inflammatory medial meatal fibrotizing otitis (IMFO)
- Postinflammatory MCF, acquired MCF, acquired atresia, chronic stenosing external otitis

Definitions

- Discrete clinicopathological disease characterized by formation of fibrous tissue in medial aspect of bony external auditory canal (EAC)

IMAGING

General Features

- Best diagnostic clue
  - Fibrous crescent overlying lateral surface of TM
- Location
  - Medial EAC, adjacent to TM
  - ~ 50% bilateral
- Size
  - Variable
    - May have mild thickening of TM with edematous EAC walls early
    - More advanced cases show near-complete opacification of EAC
- Morphology
  - Homogeneous soft tissue conforming to medial EAC

CT Findings

- CECT
  - May see slight enhancement of edematous EAC thickened walls
- Bone CT
  - Unilateral or bilateral medial EAC fibrous plug
  - **Early stage MCF**
    - Thickened TM with edematous, mildly thickened medial EAC mucosa
  - **Late stage MCF**
    - Looks like thick crescent of tissue overlying lateral surface of TM
    - TM cannot be resolved as separate from MCF fibrous mass
    - No underlying bony changes present
    - Middle ear mastoid uninvolved

MR Findings

- T1WI
  - Homogeneous low signal soft tissue in medial EAC
- T2WI
  - Intermediate to low signal soft tissue in medial EAC
  - More fibrous tissue present = lower signal
- T1WI C+
  - Enhancement of thickened, inflamed/edematous EAC walls and TM common

Imaging Recommendations

- Best imaging tool
  - Temporal bone CT
- Protocol advice
  - Temporal bone thin section (1 mm or less) nonenhanced, bone algorithm CT
    - Acquire in axial plane; reconstruct coronal plane
    - Be sure to include entire EAC in magnified images

DIFFERENTIAL DIAGNOSIS

Benign EAC Debris

- Clinical: Usually obvious on otoscopic exam
- Temporal bone CT: Luminal soft tissue in EAC without osseous erosion
  - Air often present in clefts and interstices of EAC debris

EAC Keratosis Obturans

- Clinical: Younger patients with sinusitis and bronchiectasis
- Temporal bone CT: Bilateral keratin plugs filling EAC
  - Mild diffuse EAC enlargement seen without focal bony erosions
  - Spares middle ear cavity

EAC Cholesteatoma

- Clinical: Otorrhea and EAC mass in older patient population
- Temporal bone CT: Unilateral EAC soft tissue with underlying bony destruction
  - Bony "flakes" seen within mass in 50% of cases

EAC Exostoses

- Clinical: Younger patients with repetitive exposure to cold water (surfer's ear)
- Temporal bone CT: Bilateral osseous encroachment of EAC canal
  - Diffuse broad-based overgrowth of osseous EAC with normal mucosal surfaces
  - Usually begins at medial osseous EAC

EAC Squamous Cell Carcinoma

- Clinical: Ulcerating lesion affects external ear
  - Spreads to involve EAC mucosal surfaces
- CT: Irregular, ill-defined mass with underlying aggressive bony erosion
  - Can mimic EAC cholesteatoma

Necrotizing External Otitis

- Clinical: Elderly diabetics with *Pseudomonas aeruginosa* EAC infection
- Temporal bone CT: EAC mucosal swelling ± underlying bone erosion ± deep space abscess (extension of disease inferiorly)
  - Diagnosis confirmed with biopsy and culture

PATHOLOGY

General Features

- Etiology
  - Chronic inflammation of medial EAC heals via granulation tissue formation
    - Granulation tissue slowly matures into mature fibrous plug
  - MCF is final common pathophysiologic pathway for multiple mechanisms of injury to EAC
    - Chronic otitis externa

□ Most common underlying etiology
- Secondary to surgical procedure or trauma
- Suppurative otitis media
- Radiotherapy to EAC
- Ectopic apocrine glands in medial canal mucosa
○ Autoimmune mechanism suspected

Staging, Grading, & Classification

- Early (wet) stage
  ○ Chronic otitis media with otorrhea and conductive hearing loss (CHL)
- Late (dry) stage (mature MCF)
  ○ Medial EAC fibrous plug with CHL

Gross Pathologic & Surgical Features

- Inflamed, edematous margins to fibrous plug covering TM

Microscopic Features

- Early stage
  ○ Granulation tissue
  ○ May demonstrate lymphocyte infiltration
- Late stage
  ○ Layered fibrous connective tissue
  ○ May demonstrate focal areas of calcification

CLINICAL ISSUES

Presentation

- Most common signs/symptoms
  ○ CHL
    - Typically 20-40 decibels
  ○ Other signs/symptoms
    - Chronic otitis externa
    - Chronic dermatitis (eczema or psoriasis)
    - Tinnitus
    - Otorrhea
  ○ Early stage
    - Chronic otitis media with otorrhea and CHL (wet)
  ○ Late stage
    - Mature fibrous plug present with CHL (dry)
- Clinical profile
  ○ 50-year-old woman with bilateral otorrhea, CHL, and history of chronic otitis

Demographics

- Age
  ○ Mean age: 50 years old
  ○ Range: 5-80 years old
    - Usually rare in pediatric population
- Gender
  ○ M:F = 1:2
- Epidemiology
  ○ Rare lesion

Natural History & Prognosis

- Surgical complication
  ○ Recurrence of EAC stenosis (< 5%)
  ○ Restenosis may occur years after treatment

Treatment

- Surgical intervention alone corrects CHL
- Early phase

○ Topical steroids
- Late phase
  ○ Surgical intervention required to correct CHL
  ○ Excision of all fibrous tissue and involved skin
    - Wide canaloplasty
    - Meatoplasty followed by reconstruction by split skin graft
  ○ Recurrence frequent
- Squamous epithelium may be needed to repopulate EAC and lateral TM
  ○ Skin grafts may be needed from posterior pinna

DIAGNOSTIC CHECKLIST

Consider

- Differentiate MCF from keratosis obturans and EAC cholesteatoma
  ○ Medial canal fibrosis: Look for medial EAC tissue plug with no EAC bone changes
  ○ Keratosis obturans: Look for complete opacification and subtle EAC bony widening
  ○ EAC cholesteatoma: Look for focal EAC soft tissue mass with underlying bony erosion ± intramural bone flecks

Image Interpretation Pearls

- Crescentic soft tissue plug against TM highly suggestive of MCF
- No role for MR imaging in MCF diagnosis or imaging evaluation
- Long-term follow-up is recommended to evaluate risk of recurrence

SELECTED REFERENCES

1. Moser G et al: Ectopic apocrine glands as a predisposing factor for postinflammatory medial meatal fibrosis: a clinicopathologic study. Otol Neurotol. 36(1):191-7, 2015
2. Ghani A et al: Postinflammatory medial meatal fibrosis: early and late surgical outcomes. J Laryngol Otol. 127(12):1160-8, 2013
3. Hopsu E et al: Idiopathic inflammatory medial meatal fibrotizing otitis presenting in children. Otol Neurotol. 29(3):350-2, 2008
4. Lin VY et al: Medial canal fibrosis: surgical technique, results, and a proposed grading system. Otol Neurotol. 26(5):825-9, 2005
5. Luong A et al: Acquired external auditory canal stenosis: assessment and management. Curr Opin Otolaryngol Head Neck Surg. 13(5):273-6, 2005
6. Hopsu E et al: Idiopathic inflammatory medial meatal fibrotizing otitis. Arch Otolaryngol Head Neck Surg. 128(11):1313-6, 2002
7. Lavy J et al: Chronic stenosing external otitis/postinflammatory acquired atresia: a review. Clin Otolaryngol. 25(6):435-9, 2000
8. el-Sayed Y: Acquired medial canal fibrosis. J Laryngol Otol. 112(2):145-9, 1998
9. Slattery WH 3rd et al: Postinflammatory medial canal fibrosis. Am J Otol. 18(3):294-7, 1997
10. Magliulo G et al: Medial meatal fibrosis: current approach. J Laryngol Otol. 110(5):417-20, 1996
11. Keohane JD et al: Medial meatal fibrosis: the University of Western Ontario experience. Am J Otol. 14(2):172-5, 1993
12. Katzke D et al: Postinflammatory medial meatal fibrosis. A neglected entity? Arch Otolaryngol. 108(12):779-80, 1982

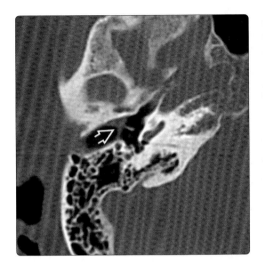
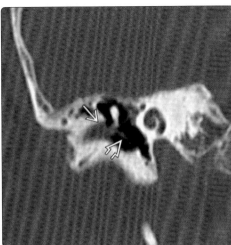

(Left) Axial bone CT of the right ear shows the early findings of MCF as thin crescentic TM thickening ➡. Clinical diagnosis at this stage is necessary as CT will not differentiate this appearance from other causes of TM thickening. (Right) Coronal bone CT in the same patient reveals that the upper TM ➡ is thicker than the lower portion ➡. As the lesion progresses, the fibrous crescent will affect the whole lateral TM surface.

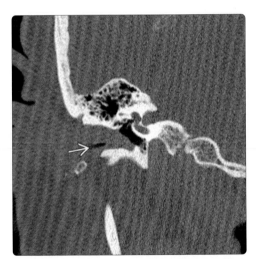
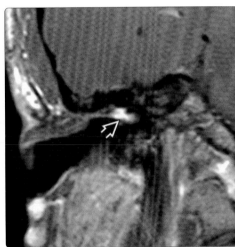

(Left) Coronal bone CT in this patient with a more aggressive case of MCF reveals a sliver of air ➡ remaining as the EAC lumen. The fibrous plug has nearly obliterated the EAC. (Right) Coronal T1 C+ MR in this patient with early phase MCF demonstrates enhancing fibrous tissue ➡ within the medial right EAC. As expected, the middle ear is spared.

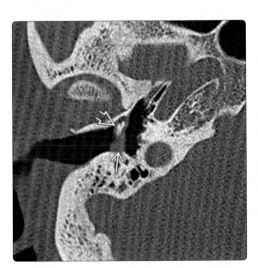
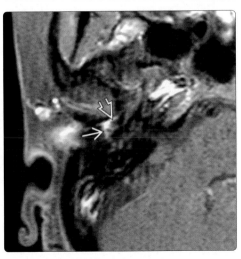

(Left) Axial bone CT of the right ear reveals a thick TM ➡ with foci of calcification ➡. Calcification has been reported in pathologic specimens of MCF. Whether this is a part of the lesion or an associated locus of tympanosclerosis cannot be determined. (Right) Axial T1WI C+ FS MR in the same patient shows that the MCF is enhancing ➡ with the area of calcification ➡ seen as a low signal foci.

EAC-Acquired Cholesteatoma

TERMINOLOGY

- External auditory canal cholesteatoma (EACC)
- EACC: EAC erosive lesion composed of exfoliated keratin within stratified squamous epithelium

IMAGING

- **Unilateral** scalloping soft tissue bony EAC mass
- **Bone fragments** within soft tissue mass (50%)
- May extend locally into subjacent bony structures
- Tympanic membrane intact; middle ear spared

TOP DIFFERENTIAL DIAGNOSES

- Medial canal fibrosis of EAC
- Necrotizing external otitis
- Squamous cell carcinoma of EAC
- Keratosis obturans of EAC

PATHOLOGY

- Spontaneous: Abnormal migration of EAC ectoderm

- Secondary: Postoperative or posttraumatic
- Congenital: Ectodermal rest within EAC wall (rare)
  - May be associated with congenital external ear malformation

CLINICAL ISSUES

- Presentation
  - Primary symptoms: Otorrhea & otalgia
- Demographics
  - Older population: 40-75 years old
- Natural history: Relentless increase in size & erosion of EAC bony wall
  - May show less aggressive behavior in pediatric patients
- Treatment options
  - Surgical excision for larger lesions with bony invasion

DIAGNOSTIC CHECKLIST

- Focal, unilateral EAC mass + EAC bony scalloping ± bony flecks = EACC

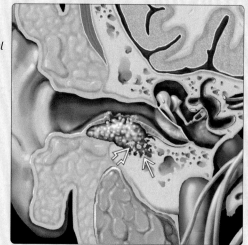

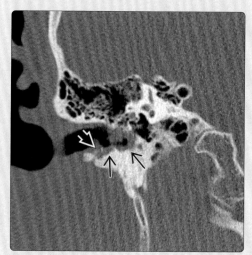

(Left) Coronal graphic shows an external auditory canal cholesteatoma (EACC) as an erosive, scalloping submucosal mass in the inferior bony EAC. Note bone erosion ➡ with bony flecks ➡ within the cholesteatoma matrix. (Right) Coronal bone CT reveals an EACC as a soft tissue mass along the inferior bony canal with underlying osseous erosion ➡ and bony flecks within the cholesteatoma matrix ➡.

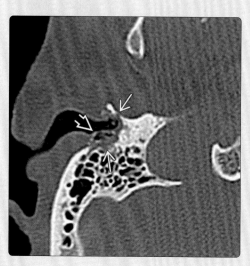

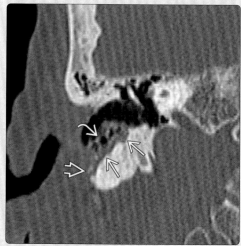

(Left) An elderly woman presented with otorrhea, otalgia, and a heaped-up submucosal lesion in the EAC area. Axial bone CT shows an erosive lesion of the bony EAC ➡ affecting the anterior, posterior, and inferior walls. Note multifocal bony flecks ➡ within the soft tissue component of the lesion. (Right) Coronal bone CT reveals an EACC with bony flecks ➡ and underlying bone erosions ➡. Note air foci ➡ within the lesion.

TERMINOLOGY

Abbreviations

- External auditory canal cholesteatoma (EACC)

Definitions

- EAC erosive lesion composed of exfoliated keratin within stratified squamous epithelium

IMAGING

General Features

- Best diagnostic clue
  - Erosive EAC soft tissue mass ± internal bony flecks

CT Findings

- Bone CT
  - **Unilateral** scalloping soft tissue bony EAC mass
  - **Bone fragments** within soft tissue mass (50%)
  - May extend locally into subjacent bony structures
  - Tympanic membrane intact; middle ear spared

MR Findings

- T1WI
  - Soft tissue intensity mass in EAC
- T2WI
  - Intermediate signal; compared to ↑ signal of inflammatory tissues
- DWI
  - Reduced diffusivity/marked hyperintensity
- T1WI C+
  - Low intensity, rim-enhancing EAC mass

Imaging Recommendations

- Best imaging tool
  - Axial & coronal bone CT of temporal bone

DIFFERENTIAL DIAGNOSIS

Medial Canal Fibrosis of EAC

- CT: Obstructive fibrous tissue within medial EAC
  - **Bilateral**; no bony erosion present

Necrotizing External Otitis

- Elderly diabetic patients with P*seudomonas* infection
- Infectious process of EAC
- **CT**: **Unilateral** inflammatory soft tissue changes
  - Bony osteomyelitis changes

Squamous Cell Carcinoma of EAC

- Elderly patients with known external ear skin squamous cell carcinoma
- **CT**: **Unilateral** invasive soft tissue mass

Keratosis Obturans of EAC

- Younger patients with sinusitis & bronchiectasis
- **CT**: **Bilateral** keratin plugs filling EAC
  - No focal EAC bony changes

PATHOLOGY

General Features

- Etiology
  - Spontaneous: Abnormal migration of EAC ectoderm

- Secondary: Postoperative or posttraumatic
- Congenital: Ectodermal rest within EAC wall (rare)
  - May be associated with congenital external ear malformation

Staging, Grading, & Classification

- Staging criteria (histopathology + clinical stage)
  - Stage I: Superficial; hyperplasia of canal epithelium
  - Stage II: Periosteitis; localized to ear pocket
  - Stage III: Extension into bony canal
  - Stage IV: Extension into adjacent bony structures

Gross Pathologic & Surgical Features

- Different type of cholesteatoma; not pearly white
- Waxy material discolored by inflammatory change
- Intramural bony fragments possible

Microscopic Features

- Similar to epidermoid inclusion cyst
- Stratified squamous epithelium with progressive exfoliation of keratinous material
- Contents may be rich in cholesterol crystals

CLINICAL ISSUES

Presentation

- Most common signs/symptoms
  - Otorrhea & otalgia
- Other signs/symptoms
  - Conductive hearing loss

Demographics

- Age
  - Older population: 40-75 years
- Epidemiology
  - 0.1% incidence in new ENT patients

Natural History & Prognosis

- Relentless increase in size & erosion of EAC bony wall
  - May show less aggressive behavior in pediatric patients
- Typical vector of spread = EAC bony wall into mastoid cavity
  - Transtympanic spread less common
- Recurrences more common with increasing lesion size & invasion of surrounding osseous structures

Treatment

- Most controlled with periodic office debridement
- Surgical excision for larger lesions with bony invasion

DIAGNOSTIC CHECKLIST

Consider

- EAC cholesteatoma **unilateral** lesion
  - Medial canal fibrosis & keratosis obturans bilateral

Image Interpretation Pearls

- Focal, unilateral EAC mass + EAC bony scalloping ± bony flecks = EACC

SELECTED REFERENCES

1. Chawla A et al: Computed tomography features of external auditory canal cholesteatoma: a pictorial review. Curr Probl Diagn Radiol. 44(6):511-6, 2015
2. Baráth K et al: Neuroradiology of cholesteatomas. AJNR Am J Neuroradiol. 32(2):221-9, 2011

TERMINOLOGY

- Osteoma: Rare, benign, focal, pedunculated, bony overgrowth of osseous EAC with normal overlying mucosa

IMAGING

- Most common site: Bony-cartilaginous EAC junction
- Bone CT: Benign-appearing, focal, **pedunculated**, bony overgrowth of osseous EAC
  - Wax, squamous debris, or **secondary cholesteatoma** possible with large, lateral lesions

TOP DIFFERENTIAL DIAGNOSES

- EAC exostoses (surfer's ear)
- EAC cholesteatoma
- Medial canal fibrosis
- Necrotizing external otitis
- Benign EAC debris

PATHOLOGY

- Irregularly oriented **lamellated bone** with surrounding discrete, fibrovascular channels
- Osteoma found in other temporal bone sites
  - Ossicles, mastoid, internal auditory canal

CLINICAL ISSUES

- Asymptomatic, usually incidental finding
- Treatment
  - Permanent cure with adequate surgical excision

DIAGNOSTIC CHECKLIST

- Differentiate from EAC exostoses
  - EAC osteoma: Narrow-based, single lesion, lateral EAC, **unilateral**
  - EAC exostosis: Broad-based, circumferential, multilobular, medial EAC, **bilateral**

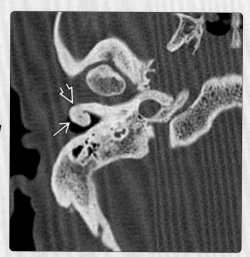
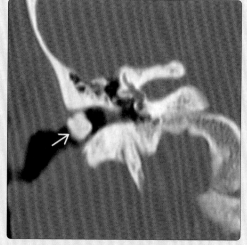

(Left) Patient presents with hard submucosal mass in midexternal auditory canal. Axial bone CT shows an osteoma ➡ pedunculating from the anterolateral aspect ➡ of the bony external auditory canal (EAC). (Right) Coronal bone CT in the same patient shows the osteoma ➡ almost completely plugging the EAC lumen. There is still sufficient room for wax and squamous debris to exit the medial EAC.

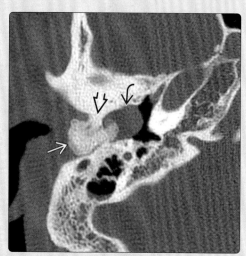
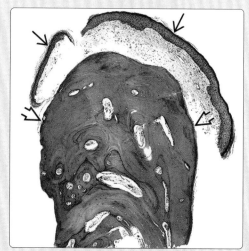

(Left) Clinical exam shows occlusion of the EAC. Axial bone CT shows a pedunculated osteoma ➡ arising from the anterior EAC bony wall ➡. Note the secondary cholesteatoma ➡ within the medial EAC. (Right) H&E micrograph reveals surface squamous epithelium ➡ is uninvolved by the osteoma ➡. There is well-formed, mature compact bone within the osteoma. This osteoma expanded from the adjacent bony EAC cortex, creating an obstructing submucosal mass. (From DP: H&N.)

TERMINOLOGY

Abbreviations

- External auditory canal (EAC) osteoma

Definitions

- Rare, benign, focal, pedunculated, bony overgrowth of osseous EAC with normal overlying soft tissues

IMAGING

General Features

- Best diagnostic clue
  - Unilateral, solitary, **pedunculated**, bony overgrowth of EAC without aggressive features
- Location
  - Unilateral EAC, single lesion typical
  - Most common site: Bony cartilaginous junction EAC
- Size
  - Variable, usually small (< 1 cm)
- Morphology
  - Variable, usually oval

CT Findings

- Bone CT
  - Benign-appearing, focal, **pedunculated**, bony overgrowth of osseous EAC
  - Wax, squamous debris, or secondary cholesteatoma possible with large, lateral lesions

Imaging Recommendations

- Best imaging tool
  - Axial & coronal temporal bone CT
  - MR not useful in this setting

DIFFERENTIAL DIAGNOSIS

EAC Exostoses (Surfer's Ear)

- Most common solid tumor of EAC
- Broad-based, **bilateral** bony EAC overgrowths
- Circumferential, multilobular

EAC Cholesteatoma

- Unilateral EAC destructive mass
- Intramural bony flakes (50%)

Medial Canal Fibrosis

- Fibrous mass in medial EAC without bony erosion
- Follows otitis externa or surgical procedure

Necrotizing External Otitis

- Severe EAC infectious process
- Granulation tissue with possible bony erosion at inferior bony-cartilaginous junction

Benign EAC Debris

- Soft tissue density in EAC without bony changes

PATHOLOGY

General Features

- Etiology
  - Likely spontaneous bony growth
  - Reaction to repeated external insult

- Associated abnormalities
  - Osteomas associated with EAC cholesteatoma
  - Gardener syndrome: Variant of familial adenomatous polyposis; autosomal dominant
- Embryology/anatomy
  - May be attached to tympanosquamous or tympanomastoid suture line

Gross Pathologic & Surgical Features

- Osteoma connected to underlying EAC bone

Microscopic Features

- Pathologically similar to exostoses
- Irregularly oriented **lamellated bone** with surrounding discrete, fibrovascular channels

CLINICAL ISSUES

Presentation

- Most common signs/symptoms
  - Asymptomatic, usually incidental finding
  - Other signs/symptoms
    - If large, conductive hearing loss
    - If associated with cholesteatoma, serous otitis media

Demographics

- Age
  - Broad age range
- Epidemiology
  - Unilateral & solitary
  - EAC osteoma is less common than exostoses
  - 20% prevalence in surfers (possible early exostoses)

Natural History & Prognosis

- Permanent cure with adequate surgical excision
- Possible surgical complications
  - EAC stenosis
  - Temporomandibular joint prolapse

Treatment

- Medical therapy is adequate without surgical excision for symptomatic lesions
- Surgical removal may be performed through EAC under local anesthesia

DIAGNOSTIC CHECKLIST

Image Interpretation Pearls

- Differentiate from EAC exostoses
  - EAC osteoma: Narrow-based, single lesion, lateral EAC, **unilateral**
  - EAC exostosis: Broad-based, circumferential, multilobular, medial EAC, **bilateral**

SELECTED REFERENCES

1. Carbone PN et al: External auditory osteoma. Head Neck Pathol. 6(2):244-6, 2012
2. Viswanatha B: Extracanalicular osteoma of the temporal bone. Ear Nose Throat J. 87(7):381-3, 2008
3. Yuen HW et al: External auditory canal osteoma. Otol Neurotol. 29(6):875-6, 2008
4. Ramirez-Camacho R et al: Fibro-osseous lesions of the external auditory canal. Laryngoscope. 109(3):488-91, 1999
5. Orita Y et al: Osteoma with cholesteatoma in the external auditory canal. Int J Pediatr Otorhinolaryngol. 43(3):289-93, 1998

TERMINOLOGY

- Definition: Benign overgrowth of bony EAC in response to chronic cold water exposure

IMAGING

- Temporal bone CT
  - **Bilateral** lesions in all cases
  - Broad-based or more focal circumferential bony overgrowth of osseous EAC
  - Variable EAC stenosis results

TOP DIFFERENTIAL DIAGNOSES

- EAC osteoma
- EAC cholesteatoma
- EAC medial canal fibrosis
- Necrotizing external otitis

CLINICAL ISSUES

- Most common symptom
  - Conductive hearing loss
- Other signs/symptoms
  - Otitis externa, tinnitus, otalgia
- Patient profile
  - 20-50 yr olds
  - Male predominance
  - 70% prevalence in surfers
    - Increased incidence with increased time of exposure
- Treatment options
  - Often require no treatment
  - May require surgical excision

DIAGNOSTIC CHECKLIST

- Image interpretation pearls
  - Most common differential diagnosis: EAC osteoma
  - EAC osteoma: Unilateral, lateral bony EAC focal osseous protuberance
  - EAC exostoses: Bilateral midbody EAC circumferential, multilobular narrowing

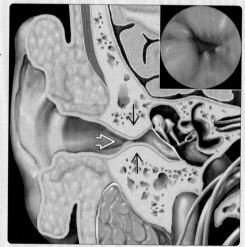
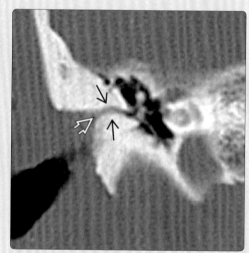

(Left) Coronal graphic shows benign-appearing bony overgrowth of the right EAC ➡ in a case of EAC exostoses. Insert shows otoscopic view of circumferential submucosal EAC narrowing ➡. (Right) Coronal bone CT of the right temporal bone shows severe EAC stenosis ➡ secondary to circumferential exostoses ➡ that developed bilaterally as a result of chronic cold water exposure from surfing.

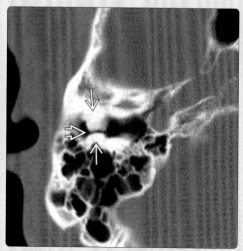
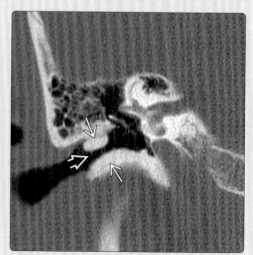

(Left) Axial bone CT reveals bilateral EAC exostoses ➡ with moderate EAC luminal stenosis ➡. (Courtesy C. Schatz, MD.) (Right) Coronal temporal bone CT in the same patient shows EAC exostoses ➡ with moderate EAC luminal stenosis ➡. The bilaterality (not shown) and circumferential bony involvement differentiate this lesion from unilateral, focal EAC osteoma.

TERMINOLOGY

Synonyms

- Surfer ear; cold water ear

Definitions

- Benign overgrowth of bony EAC in response to chronic cold water exposure

IMAGING

General Features

- Best diagnostic clue
  - Benign, overgrowth of osseous EAC with normal overlying soft tissues
- Location
  - Bony EAC; **bilateral**
  - Usually located medial to EAC isthmus
    - EAC osteoma usually located lateral to isthmus
- Size
  - Variable, narrowing of EAC
- Morphology
  - Broad-based or focal; circumferential

CT Findings

- CECT
  - Normal soft tissues overlying stenotic EAC
- Bone CT
  - Broad-based or more focal circumferential bony overgrowth of osseous EAC
  - Bilateral; variable EAC stenosis results

Imaging Recommendations

- Best imaging tool
  - Temporal bone CT
  - MR of no help with this diagnosis

DIFFERENTIAL DIAGNOSIS

EAC Osteoma

- Unilateral focal, pedunculated, bony overgrowth

EAC Cholesteatoma

- Unilateral, bone flakes (50%)
- Underlying bony scalloping

EAC Medial Canal Fibrosis

- Inflammatory fibrous EAC plug

Necrotizing External Otitis

- EAC infection in immunocompromised patient

PATHOLOGY

General Features

- Etiology
  - Bony EAC reaction to cold water exposure
  - Theory: Irritation of EAC results in increased vascular flow
  - Occurs exclusively in humans

Gross Pathologic & Surgical Features

- Benign, bony overgrowth of osseous EAC

Microscopic Features

- Pathologically similar to osteoma
- Parallel, concentric layers of subperiosteal bone
  - Broad-based lamellar bone

CLINICAL ISSUES

Presentation

- Most common signs/symptoms
  - Conductive hearing loss (CHL)
  - Other signs/symptoms
    - Otitis externa, tinnitus, otalgia
  - Although bilateral, 80% present with unilateral symptoms
- Clinical profile
  - CHL in adult male with history of prolonged cold water exposure (swimmers, surfers, divers)

Demographics

- Age
  - 20-50 yr olds
- Gender
  - Male predominance
- Ethnicity
  - Lesion not usually found in African Americans
- Epidemiology
  - 70% prevalence in surfers
  - Increasing incidence with increasing time of exposure

Natural History & Prognosis

- Complete occlusion of EAC is rare
- Normal hearing & normal epithelial migration patterns seen postoperatively
- 5% surgical complication rate
  - Canal stenosis, TMJ prolapse, sensorineural hearing loss, & persistent tempanic membrane (TM) perforation

Treatment

- Often requires no treatment
- May require surgical excision
  - Complications of superior EAC drilling
    - TM perforation
    - TMJ dehiscence
  - Drilling excision along posterior, inferior, & anterior walls performed with less risk of complications
    - Allows preservation of canal skin, leading to permanent cure

DIAGNOSTIC CHECKLIST

Image Interpretation Pearls

- Biggest differential diagnosis: EAC osteoma
  - Osteoma: Unilateral, focal osseous protuberance
  - Exostoses: Bilateral circumferential, multilobular bony EAC narrowing

SELECTED REFERENCES

1. Spielmann PM et al: Surgical management of external auditory canal lesions. J Laryngol Otol. 127(3):246-51, 2013
2. Carbone PN et al: External auditory osteoma. Head Neck Pathol. 6(2):244-6, 2012

EAC Skin Squamous Cell Carcinoma

TERMINOLOGY

- SCCa most common malignancy of EAC

IMAGING

- Bone destruction or soft tissue invasion indicates aggressive malignancy
- Temporal bone CT best predicts osseous invasion
- Enhanced MR superior for intracranial, parotid, and perineural spread
- Either CECT or MR of neck for adenopathy

TOP DIFFERENTIAL DIAGNOSES

- Benign EAC debris
- EAC cholesteatoma
- Necrotizing external otitis
- Osteoradionecrosis

PATHOLOGY

- Disease of elderly (median age: 65 years)
- ↑ incidence in patients with otological diseases

CLINICAL ISSUES

- Biopsy critical as early SCCa appears identical to other Dx on imaging
- Secondary EAC involvement from regional primary skin SCCa more common than primary EAC SCCa
- EAC SCCa 1st destroys bony canal, then invades surrounding anatomic structures
- **5-year survival** for early stage (T1/T2) = 70%; advanced stage (T3) = 41%
- With small tumors, en bloc resection often curative

DIAGNOSTIC CHECKLIST

- Soft tissue extent, bone or parotid invasion, intracranial extension, CNVII perineural spread
- Look for intraparotid nodes, pre- and postauricular nodes, then levels II and Va

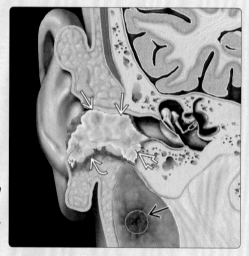
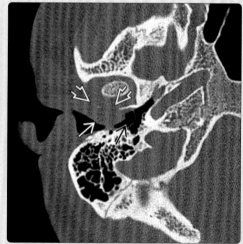

(Left) Coronal graphic illustrates large EAC squamous cell carcinoma (SCCa) presenting as a mass ➡ filling canal. Note the aggressive features with infiltration of the auricle and its cartilages ➡, invasion of temporal bone ➡, and metastatic intraparotid node ➡. (Right) Axial CT of temporal bone reveals a SCCa of right EAC with prominent soft tissue mass ➡ filling the EAC. Osseous invasion through the posterior wall of TMJ condylar fossa ➡ is present. Distal EAC at TM ➡ is clear of tumor.

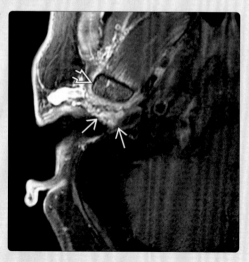
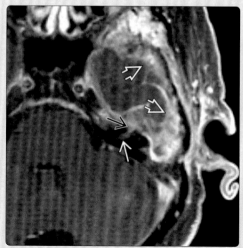

(Left) Axial T1WI C+ MR shows a solidly enhancing EAC SCC ➡ filling the canal and invading anteriorly into the TMJ. Note the soft tissue tumor around the right condylar head ➡. (Right) Axial T1WI C+ FS MR shows more advanced EAC SCCa with gross transdural ➡ extension into left middle cranial fossa. Marked thickening and enhancement along CNVII at the geniculate ganglion ➡ and in the internal auditory canal ➡ represents a perineural tumor.

TERMINOLOGY

Definitions

- Squamous cell carcinoma (SCCa) involving external auditory canal (EAC)

IMAGING

General Features

- Best diagnostic clue
  - EAC mass ± aggressive underlying bony changes
- Relevant anatomy
  - EAC, auricle, and adjacent scalp
  - Nodal drainage to parotid and pre- and postauricular nodes

CT Findings

- CECT
  - Heterogeneously enhancing EAC lesion
  - Intraparotid and periauricular nodes at risk
- Bone CT
  - Early: EAC soft tissue mass without bony destruction
  - EAC nonossified cartilage invasion difficult to diagnose
  - EAC bone destruction early sign of progressing disease

MR Findings

- T2WI
  - Heterogeneous high signal
- T1WI C+
  - Homogeneous or heterogeneous enhancement
  - Rarely, advanced disease spreads to middle ear, CNVII, or intracranial
    - Posterior cranial fossa invasion can involve sigmoid sinus

Nuclear Medicine Findings

- PET
  - Useful for detecting residual/recurrent disease post treatment

DIFFERENTIAL DIAGNOSIS

Benign EAC Debris

- CT: Soft tissue debris in EAC without bony erosion

EAC Cholesteatoma

- Unilateral EAC mass ± bony "flakes" with underlying bony destruction

Necrotizing External Otitis

- Older **diabetic** patients with *Pseudomonas* infection
- CT: Granulation tissue with possible bony erosion at inferior bony-cartilaginous junction

Osteoradionecrosis

- Disruption of mastoid air cells septa superimposed on radiation-induced otomastoiditis

PATHOLOGY

General Features

- Etiology
  - Auricle skin SCCa spreads into EAC > > 1° EAC Ca

Staging, Grading, & Classification

- T1: Tumor limited to EAC without bony erosion or soft tissue invasion
- T2: Tumor with limited EAC bone or soft tissue involvement
- T3: Tumor with osseous EAC erosion and limited soft tissue/middle ear/mastoid involvement
- T4: Tumor erodes inner ear structures/TMJ/extensive soft tissue, or CNVII paresis

CLINICAL ISSUES

Presentation

- Most common signs/symptoms
  - Early small lesions mimic benign processes both clinically and imaging
  - Ulcerating auricle: EAC skin lesion
    - Presentation may **mimic otitis externa** or **EAC cholesteatoma**
  - Otorrhea, otalgia, and conductive hearing loss

Demographics

- Age
  - Disease of elderly (median: 65 years)
- Epidemiology
  - Malignant tumors of EAC are very rare
    - 85% of all EAC malignant tumors are SCCa

Natural History & Prognosis

- EAC SCCa destroys osseous EAC, then invades surrounding anatomic structures
  - Posterior extension into mastoid bone
  - Anterior extension into temporomandibular joint
- Lymph node metastases rare, poor prognostic indicator

Treatment

- En bloc resection nearly always performed
- T1-T2 tumors: Surgery or radiation therapy
- T3-T4 tumors: Surgery and radiation ± chemotherapy

DIAGNOSTIC CHECKLIST

Consider

- Secondary EAC involvement from adjacent skin SCCa much more common than 1° EAC SCCa
- Radiologically interrogate surrounding structures for possible involvement
  - Parotid gland (direct invasion or nodes)
  - Temporomandibular joint
  - Mastoid temporal bone

Image Interpretation Pearls

- Look for osseous destructive changes
- CECT or MR should include parotid gland for 1st-order nodes

Reporting Tips

- Soft tissue extent, bone or parotid invasion, regional nodal disease, intracranial extension, CNVII perineural spread

SELECTED REFERENCES

1. Takenaka Y et al: Chemoradiation therapy for squamous cell carcinoma of the external auditory canal: a meta-analysis. Head Neck. 37(7):1073-80, 2015

Congenital Middle Ear Cholesteatoma

TERMINOLOGY

- Congenital middle ear cholesteatoma (CMEC)
- Definition: Cholesteatoma in middle ear behind intact TM in patient with no history of surgery, otitis media, or otorrhea

IMAGING

- Temporal bone CT findings
  - Small: Well-circumscribed soft tissue middle ear mass medial to ossicles
  - Large: Erodes ossicles, middle ear wall, lateral semicircular canal, or tegmen tympani
  - Long process of incus & stapes superstructure most commonly destroyed ossicles
  - If aditus ad antrum occluded, mastoid air cells opacify with retained secretions
  - Mastoid pneumatization usually normal
- MR findings
  - T1WI C+: Rim-enhancing middle ear mass
  - Non-echo-planar DWI sequences recommended
    - Minimize susceptibility artifacts
    - ↑ sensitivity for detection of smaller lesions (2 mm)
    - Highly specific due to high keratin content

TOP DIFFERENTIAL DIAGNOSES

- Pars flaccida-acquired cholesteatoma
- Pars tensa-acquired cholesteatoma
- Glomus tympanicum paraganglioma
- Facial nerve schwannoma of tympanic segment
- Middle ear cholesterol granuloma

CLINICAL ISSUES

- Younger patient (< 20 years old)
- **Incidental** avascular ME mass behind **intact TM**
- Unilateral conductive hearing loss (30%)
- Complete surgical extirpation = treatment of choice

DIAGNOSTIC CHECKLIST

- Consider CMEC when avascular mass seen behind intact TM in younger patient (< 20 years old)

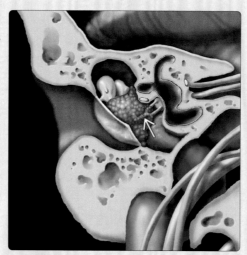
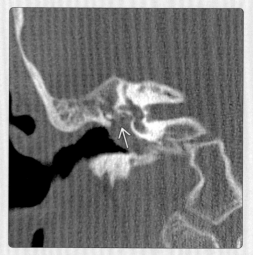

(Left) Coronal graphic shows congenital middle ear cholesteatoma (CMEC). Notice that the lesion surrounds and is medial to the ossicles ➡. The tympanic membrane is intact. (Right) Coronal temporal bone CT of the right ear demonstrates a large congenital cholesteatoma filling the middle ear cavity with subtle long process of incus and stapes hub erosion ➡ and deossification. The tympanic membrane bulges laterally but is intact by otoscopic examination.

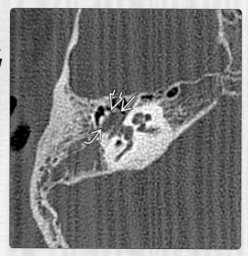
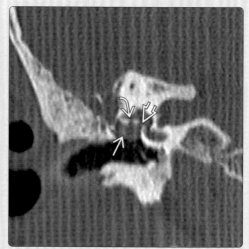

(Left) Axial bone CT of the right ear reveals a medial epitympanic congenital cholesteatoma ➡ eroding the medial head of the malleus ➡ and short process of the incus ➡. Aditus ad antrum block causes mastoid effusion. (Right) Coronal bone CT in the same patient shows CMEC eroding the long process of the incus ➡ and filling the oval window niche ➡. The tympanic segment of CNVII canal enlargement ➡ is secondary to cholesteatoma focal invasion.

TERMINOLOGY

Abbreviations
- Congenital middle ear cholesteatoma (CMEC)

Synonyms
- Primary cholesteatoma, epidermoid

Definitions
- Cholesteatoma in middle ear (ME) behind intact TM in patient with no history of surgery, otitis media, or otorrhea

IMAGING

General Features
- Best diagnostic clue
  - Temporal bone CT shows smooth, well-circumscribed ME mass ± ossicular erosions
- Location
  - Multiple ME locations
    - Anterosuperior quadrant of tympanic cavity near eustachian tube
    - Posterior epitympanum at tympanic isthmi (area between ME cavity & attic)
    - Epitympanum medial to ossicles
- Size
  - Usually small because identified on otoscopic exam
  - Entire ME cavity not involved at presentation
- Morphology
  - Lobular, discrete ME mass

CT Findings
- Bone CT
  - Temporal bone CT appearance depends on size of lesion
  - Small: Detected early, appears as well-circumscribed soft tissue ME mass
  - Large: Larger CMEC may erode ossicles, ME wall, lateral semicircular canal, or tegmen tympani
    - Long process of incus & stapes superstructure most commonly destroyed ossicles
    - Bone erosion less common than in acquired cholesteatoma
    - Labyrinthine extension may occur, but only late in disease process
    - If aditus ad antrum occluded, mastoid air cells opacify with retained secretions
    - Associated inflammatory changes infrequent
      □ Mastoid pneumatization usually normal
  - Common ME locations
    - **Anterosuperior quadrant** of ME, adjacent to eustachian tube & anterior tympanic ring
      □ Inferior but adjacent to tensor tympani muscle
    - Peristapedial region
    - Posterior epitympanum, at tympanic isthmi

MR Findings
- T1WI
  - Iso- to hypointense ME mass
- T2WI
  - Intermediate-intensity ME mass
  - With larger lesions, aditus ad antrum obstruction seen as high signal retained secretions in mastoid
- DWI
  - Non-echo-planar DWI sequences recommended
    - Minimize susceptibility artifacts
    - ↑ sensitivity for detection of smaller lesions (2 mm)
    - Highly specific due to high keratin content
- T1WI C+
  - Peripherally enhancing ME mass
    - CMEC is nonenhancing material with subtle rim enhancement
  - If lesion is longstanding, associated scar may be seen as thickened area of enhancement adjacent to CMEC

Imaging Recommendations
- Best imaging tool
  - Temporal bone CT = exam of choice
  - T1WI C+ MR is complementary exam in certain circumstances
    - Recommended if recurrent or large CMEC
    - Recommended if diagnosis uncertain, with glomus tympanicum or facial nerve schwannoma possible considerations
      □ Glomus tumor & CNVII schwannoma enhance
- Protocol advice
  - If large cholesteatoma, DWI sequence diagnostic

DIFFERENTIAL DIAGNOSIS

Pars Flaccida-Acquired Cholesteatoma
- Otoscopy shows **pars flaccida TM perforation**
- CT findings
  - Scutum erosion with lesion in lateral epitympanum
  - Ossicular chain & lateral semicircular canal erosion
  - Chronic inflammatory changes present
    - Mastoid underpneumatized

Pars Tensa-Acquired Cholesteatoma
- Otoscopy shows **pars tensa TM perforation**
- CT findings
  - Lesion enlarges medial to ossicles
  - Ossicular erosion common

Glomus Tympanicum Paraganglioma
- Otoscopy shows pulsatile, vascular mass behind TM
  - Unusual in pediatric or adolescent patient
- CT findings
  - Sessile mass on cochlear promontory
  - No bony erosions present
- MR findings
  - Focal enhancing mass on T1WI C+ MR

Facial Nerve Schwannoma of Tympanic Segment
- Otoscopy shows avascular mass behind intact TM
  - Appearance can closely mimic congenital cholesteatoma
- CT findings
  - Tubular mass emanating from tympanic CNVII canal
  - Enlarged bony facial nerve canal
  - Enlarged geniculate fossa
- MR findings
  - Tubular enhancing mass on T1WI C+ MR
  - Extends from geniculate ganglion along tympanic segment of facial nerve

Middle Ear Cholesterol Granuloma

- Otoscopy reveals blue TM
  - History of prior surgery or recurrent ME infection
- CT findings
  - ME mass with ossicular erosion common
- MR findings
  - T1 nonenhanced MR shows high signal in ME

PATHOLOGY

General Features

- Etiology
  - 2 principal theories
    - Congenital **ectodermal rest** in ME cavity left behind at time of closure of neural tube (3rd-5th week of fetal life)
    - Lack of regression of epidermoid formation
      - □ Epidermoid formation: Point of epithelial transformation between tympanic cavity & eustachian tube
      - □ When it does not regress, becomes mass-like ME accumulation of stratified epithelial squamous cells
      - □ **Anterosuperior** CMEC results
  - Neither theory is unifying
- Associated abnormalities
  - EAC atresia can present with associated congenital cholesteatoma: In EAC or ME
  - Rarely associated with 1st branchial cleft remnant
- Other locations of congenital cholesteatoma in temporal bone
  - Petrous apex, mastoid, EAC, facial nerve canal

Staging, Grading, & Classification

- CMEC staging system
  - Stage 1: Single quadrant; no ossicular involvement or mastoid extension
  - Stage 2: Multiple quadrants; no ossicular involvement or mastoid extension
  - Stage 3: Ossicular involvement; no mastoid involvement
  - Stage 4: Mastoid extension

Gross Pathologic & Surgical Features

- Circumscribed, pearly white mass with capsular sheen

Microscopic Features

- Identical to epidermoid inclusion cyst
- Stratified squamous epithelium, with progressive exfoliation of keratinous material
- Contents rich in cholesterol crystals

CLINICAL ISSUES

Presentation

- Most common signs/symptoms
  - **Incidental** avascular ME mass behind **intact TM**
- Other signs/symptoms
  - Unilateral conductive hearing loss (30%)
  - Large CMEC can obstruct eustachian tube with resultant ME-mastoid effusion & infection

Demographics

- Age

- Average age of presentation or detection
  - Anterior or anterosuperior: 4 years
  - Posterosuperior & mesotympanum: 12 years
  - Attic & mastoid antrum involvement: 20 years
- Gender
  - M:F = 3:1
- Epidemiology
  - Accounts for 5% of all temporal bone cholesteatomas

Natural History & Prognosis

- Smaller, anterior lesions have better outcome with complete surgical resection
  - Smaller lesions may be encapsulated & easily removed
- If untreated, keratin debris accumulates over time, with resultant larger lesion
  - Enlarging, cyst-like lesion may rupture, extending throughout ME
  - If eustachian tube obstructed, otomastoiditis occurs
  - Larger lesions with infection may be difficult to differentiate from acquired cholesteatoma
- Large lesions or posterior epitympanic cholesteatoma have recurrence rates as high as 20%

Treatment

- Complete surgical extirpation = treatment of choice
  - Tympanoplasty for small, well-encapsulated CMEC
  - Tympanoplasty with canal wall up mastoidectomy for large CMEC
  - Tympanoplasty with canal wall down mastoidectomy for very large CMEC
- Ossicle chain reconstruction often necessary

DIAGNOSTIC CHECKLIST

Consider

- CMEC when avascular mass seen behind **intact TM**
- CMEC when no history of repeat ME infections
- CMEC when ME is opacified with wall erosion in congenital external ear dysplasia

Image Interpretation Pearls

- Younger patient + CT lesion medial to ossicles + normal mastoid pneumatization = CMEC

SELECTED REFERENCES

1. Bacciu A et al: Open vs closed type congenital cholesteatoma of the middle ear: two distinct entities or two aspects of the same phenomenon? Int J Pediatr Otorhinolaryngol. 78(12):2205-9, 2014
2. Más-Estellés F et al: Contemporary non-echo-planar diffusion-weighted imaging of middle ear cholesteatomas. Radiographics. 32(4):1197-213, 2012
3. Ganaha A et al: Efficacy of diffusion-weighted magnetic resonance imaging in the diagnosis of middle ear cholesteatoma. Auris Nasus Larynx. 38(3):329-34, 2011
4. De Foer B et al: The value of single-shot turbo spin-echo diffusion-weighted MR imaging in the detection of middle ear cholesteatoma. Neuroradiology. 49(10):841-8, 2007
5. Kutz JW Jr et al: Congenital middle ear cholesteatoma. Ear Nose Throat J. 86(11):654, 2007
6. Shirazi MA et al: Surgical treatment of pediatric cholesteatomas. Laryngoscope. 116(9):1603-7, 2006
7. Nelson M et al: Congenital cholesteatoma: classification, management, and outcome. Arch Otolaryngol Head Neck Surg. 128(7):810-4, 2002
8. Potsic WP et al: A staging system for congenital cholesteatoma. Arch Otolaryngol Head Neck Surg. 128(9):1009-12, 2002
9. Friedberg J: Congenital cholesteatoma. Laryngoscope. 104(3 Pt 2):1-24, 1994

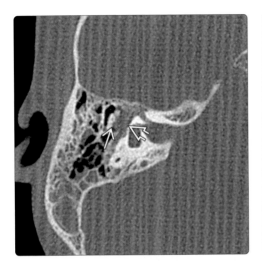

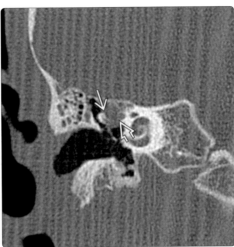

(Left) *Axial bone CT of the right ear in a patient with recurrent otomastoiditis and conductive hearing loss reveals a soft tissue mass in the medial epitympanum eroding the medial surface of the head of the malleus & short process of the incus ➡. The anterior tympanic CNVII canal is also dehiscent ➡.* (Right) *Coronal bone CT in the same patient shows erosion of medial malleus head ➡ and lateral margin of anterior tympanic segment of CNVII canal ➡ by this medial epitympanic CMEC.*

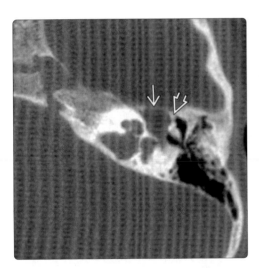

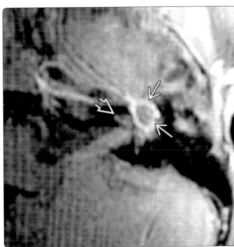

(Left) *Axial bone CT of the left ear reveals a CMEC in the anterior epitympanic recess scalloping the adjacent middle ear wall ➡ and bowing the epitympanic cog posteriorly ➡. The malleus head abuts the posterior margin of the CMEC.* (Right) *Axial T1WI C+ MR in the same patient reveals typical rim enhancement ➡ along the margins of this anterior epitympanic CMEC. The central nonenhancing component is the CMEC. Notice the more medial cochlear signal ➡.*

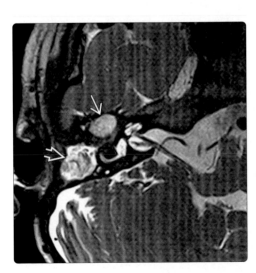

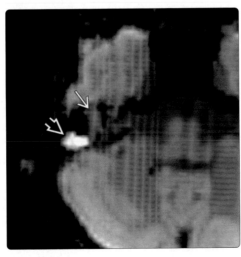

(Left) *Axial T2 MR in a 5-year-old boy previously operated on for CMEC reveals material in middle ear cavity ➡ and mastoid antrum ➡. Differentiating postoperative changes from recurrent cholesteatoma is impossible in this image.* (Right) *Axial DWI in the same patient shows the mastoid collection with reduced diffusivity ➡ indicating recurrent congenital cholesteatoma. Middle ear collection does not restrict ➡ and is not recurrent cholesteatoma.*

TERMINOLOGY

- Definition congenital mastoid cholesteatoma: Cholesteatoma in mastoid secondary to epithelial rest

IMAGING

- Bone CT findings
  - Expansile soft tissue mass
  - Smooth erosion of mastoid bone
- MR findings
  - T1 low, T2 high
  - T1WI C+ nonenhancing; bows sigmoid sinus
  - **DWI hyperintensity** (restricted diffusion)
- Mastoid locations
  - Anywhere in mastoid area
  - Medial mastoid ± IAC ± petrous apex

TOP DIFFERENTIAL DIAGNOSES

- Large pars flaccida-acquired cholesteatoma
- Mastoid cholesterol granuloma

- Temporal bone fibrous dysplasia
- Temporal bone Langerhans cell histiocytosis

PATHOLOGY

- Microscopic: Stratified squamous epithelium with progressive exfoliation of keratinous material

CLINICAL ISSUES

- Presentations
  - Older patient group (20-40 years)
    - Compared to middle ear cholesteatoma
  - Retroauricular swelling and pain; ± headache
  - May be **incidentally found** on head MR
- Treatment
  - Surgical removal is treatment of choice
  - Sigmoid sinus preservation important

DIAGNOSTIC CHECKLIST

- DWI **restricted diffusion** confirms congenital mastoid cholesteatoma diagnosis

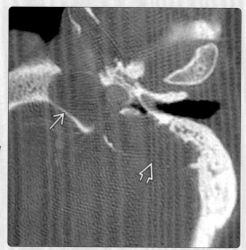
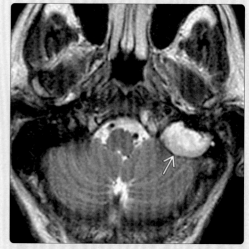

(Left) Axial bone CT shows a multilobular congenital cholesteatoma involving the lateral clivus ➡ and the medial mastoid ⇨. The expansile bony margins are suggestive of this diagnosis. (Right) Axial T2WI MR in the same patient reveals a giant temporal bone congenital mastoid cholesteatoma as a high signal sharply marginated mass ➡.

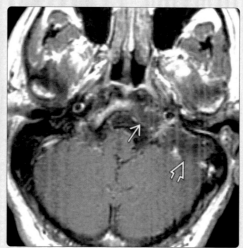
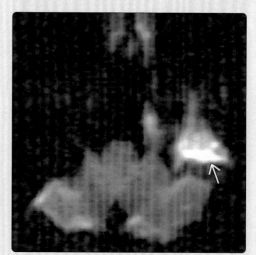

(Left) Axial T1WI C+ MR in the same patient shows both the lateral clival ➡ and mastoid ⇨ components of a large temporal bone congenital cholesteatoma. As in this case, nonenhancement would be expected. (Right) Axial DWI MR in the same patient shows high signal ➡ in the location of the giant temporal bone congenital cholesteatoma. Restricted diffusion within the lesion is highly suggestive of the diagnosis of cholesteatoma.

TERMINOLOGY

Abbreviations

- Congenital mastoid cholesteatoma (CMC)

Synonyms

- Primary mastoid cholesteatoma or epidermoid

Definitions

- Congenital cholesteatoma in mastoid secondary to epithelial rest

IMAGING

General Features

- Best diagnostic clue
  - Bone CT: Smooth erosion of mastoid bone
  - MR: T1 low, T2 high, T1WI C+ nonenhancing, DWI high signal
- Location
  - Anywhere in mastoid area
    - Medial mastoid ± IAC ± petrous apex
    - Occipitomastoid suture
- Size
  - Usually large (> 3 cm) as clinically silent
- Morphology
  - Lobular, ovoid

CT Findings

- Bone CT
  - Lobular soft tissue mastoid mass erodes trabeculae, thins or dehisced cortex
    - May exit mastoid into EAC, parotid space, carotid space

MR Findings

- T1WI
  - Iso- to hyperintense mastoid area mass
- T2WI
  - Intermediate to high intensity
- DWI
  - High signal (restricted diffusion)
- T1WI C+ FS
  - Subtle rim enhancement
  - CMC itself nonenhancing

Imaging Recommendations

- Best imaging tool
  - Temporal bone CT = exam of choice
  - MR helpful in assessing extramastoid spread
    - Transverse-sigmoid sinus status
    - Extracranial spread

DIFFERENTIAL DIAGNOSIS

Large Pars Flaccida Acquired Cholesteatoma

- Middle ear & mastoid affected; erosive
- MR: T1 low, T2 high signal

Mastoid Cholesterol Granuloma

- Middle ear & mastoid affect; erosive
- MR: T1 high, T2 signal high

Temporal Bone Fibrous Dysplasia

- Expansile bony process
- MR: Variable; usually T1 low, T2 low

Temporal Bone Langerhans Histiocytosis

- Destructive bony process
- MR: T1 low, T2 high signal; enhancing

PATHOLOGY

General Features

- Etiology
  - Congenital ectodermal rest in mastoid or occipitomastoid suture

Microscopic Features

- Same as epidermoid inclusion cyst
- Stratified squamous epithelium with progressive exfoliation of keratinous material

CLINICAL ISSUES

Presentation

- Most common signs/symptoms
  - Retroauricular swelling and pain
    - ± headache
  - May be **incidental** head MR finding
- Other signs/symptoms
  - When large, involving medial mastoid, IAC area, may present with meningitis
  - Retroauricular abscess

Demographics

- Age
  - Older patient group compared to middle ear congenital cholesteatoma
    - Presents in 20-40 year olds

Natural History & Prognosis

- If untreated, keratin debris accumulates, lesion grows larger

Treatment

- Surgical removal treatment of choice
- Mastoidectomy

DIAGNOSTIC CHECKLIST

Consider

- Suspect CMC if globular nonenhancing mastoid area mass
  - DWI restricted diffusion confirms diagnosis

Reporting Tips

- In all lesions of mastoid area, comment on status of transverse-sigmoid sinus

SELECTED REFERENCES

1. Cvorović L et al: Congenital cholesteatoma of mastoid origin–a multicenter case series. Vojnosanit Pregl. 71(7):619-22, 2014
2. Más-Estellés F et al: Contemporary non-echo-planar diffusion-weighted imaging of middle ear cholesteatomas. Radiographics. 32(4):1197-213, 2012
3. Giannuzzi AL et al: Congenital mastoid cholesteatoma: case series, definition, surgical key points, and literature review. Ann Otol Rhinol Laryngol. 120(11):700-6, 2011

Oval Window Atresia

TERMINOLOGY

- Oval window atresia (OWA): Absent space between lateral semicircular canal above and cochlear promontory below associated with anomalous stapes and malpositioned CNVII

IMAGING

- Temporal bone CT findings
  - Normal OW replaced by ossific "web" or plate
  - **Inferomedially positioned** tympanic segment **CNVII**
    - May completely overlie OW
    - May reside on superior or inferior OW margin
- Key surgical finding on CT = facial nerve location prevents safe surgical correction
- Best imaging tool: Multiplanar temporal bone CT
  - OW niche best seen in coronal plane
  - CNVII location relative to OW best seen in coronal plane
  - Stapes crura best seen in axial plane
- Bony plate over OW + inferomedially displaced tympanic CNVII = OWA

- If both findings present, no differential diagnosis present

TOP DIFFERENTIAL DIAGNOSES

- Tympanosclerosis
- Fenestral otosclerosis
- Congenital external ear malformation

PATHOLOGY

- Best hypothesis for OW etiology
  - Primitive stapes fails to fuse with primitive vestibule during 7th week of gestation

CLINICAL ISSUES

- Clinical presentation
  - Nonprogressive conductive hearing deficit from birth
  - Lack of history of otomastoiditis; normal EAC
- Best treatment: Vestibulotomy with ossiculoplasty
  - **Facial nerve ectopia** into oval window niche is relative surgical contraindication

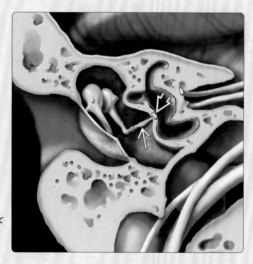 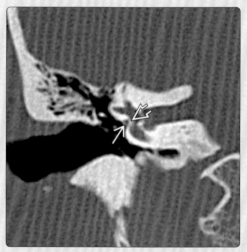

(Left) Coronal graphic illustrates features of oval window atresia, including malformation of the stapes crura and footplate ➡ and tympanic segment of the facial nerve in an abnormal location ➡. (Right) Coronal bone CT through the IAC demonstrates that the oval window is absent with bone density ➡ in its expected location. The tympanic segment of the facial nerve is not in its expected location inferior to the horizontal SCC but instead overlies the atretic window ➡. The stapes is not seen.

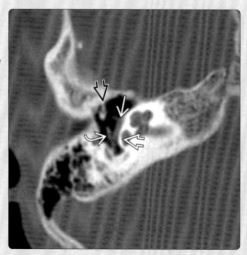 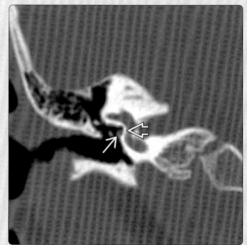

(Left) Axial bone CT in an adolescent patient with conductive hearing loss shows deformed ossicles with angulation of the incus ➡ and anterior malleolar ligament calcification ➡. The oval window is bone covered ➡ with the tympanic segment of CNVII traversing its margin ➡. (Right) Coronal bone CT in the same patient reveals the bony plate within the oval window ➡. Notice that the tympanic segment is present along the inferior margin of the oval window niche ➡.

TERMINOLOGY

Abbreviations

- Oval window atresia (OWA)

Synonyms

- Congenital absence of oval window (OW)

Definitions

- Absent space between lateral semicircular canal above and cochlear promontory below associated with anomalous stapes and malpositioned CNVII

IMAGING

CT Findings

- Bone CT
  - Normal OW replaced by ossific web
  - Malformed stapes superstructure (absence of normal paired crura) and distal incus
  - **Inferomedially positioned** tympanic segment **CNVII**
    - May reside on superior or inferior margin of OW
    - May completely overlie expected location of OW
      - □ **Critical surgical importance**
      - □ OW drill-out may be contraindicated if present
    - Common associated finding (> 60%)
  - Normal EAC

Imaging Recommendations

- Best imaging tool
  - Multiplanar high-resolution temporal bone CT
    - OW niche best seen in coronal plane
    - Stapes crura best seen in axial plane
- Protocol advice
  - Thin-section (< 1 mm) axial and coronal temporal bone CT
    - Additional reformations for oval window, CNVII, and stapes visualization
      - □ Transverse and longitudinal obliques
      - □ Custom oblique views as needed

DIFFERENTIAL DIAGNOSIS

Tympanosclerosis

- Clinical: Chronic otomastoiditis
- Imaging: Stapes may be thickened, including footplate
  - Ossific deposits on ossicle surface may be seen
  - Middle ear debris/sclerotic mastoid = chronic otomastoiditis
  - Stapes and facial nerve are normal

Fenestral Otosclerosis

- Clinical: Rare in childhood
- Imaging: Lucent lesions anterior to OW
  - Obliterative variety (< 10%) results in similar appearance to OWA, but stapes and facial nerve are intrinsically normal

Congenital External Ear Malformation

- Clinical: Microtia, EAC malformation
- Imaging: Variable EAC narrowing or absence
  - Ossicle fusion, rotation; CNVII anomalous course
  - OWA may be associated

PATHOLOGY

General Features

- Etiology
  - Best hypothesis: Primitive stapes fails to fuse with primitive vestibule during 7th week of gestation
  - If stapes forms but annular ligament does not, congenital stapes fixation results (instead of OWA)
    - Caution: This may result in congenital conductive hearing loss in absence of imaging findings

Gross Pathologic & Surgical Features

- Tympanic segment of CNVII abnormal in most cases
  - Inferomedially positioned
- Abnormal incus lenticular process associated
  - Expected since distal incus and stapes superstructure are both formed from 2nd branchial arch

CLINICAL ISSUES

Presentation

- Most common signs/symptoms
  - Profound conductive hearing deficit in child
    - Nonprogressive; air-bone gap of over 40dB

Demographics

- Age
  - Usually discovered in children
- Gender
  - M > F
- Epidemiology
  - OWA **bilateral** in ~ **40%**

Natural History & Prognosis

- Surgical correction results modest over long term

Treatment

- Vestibulotomy with ossiculoplasty
  - Stapes prosthesis or total ossicular replacement prosthesis
- Alternative treatment (round window vibroplasty) under investigation
  - Version of active middle ear implants
- CNVII ectopia into OW niche is relative surgical contraindication

DIAGNOSTIC CHECKLIST

Consider

- Inspect OW in children with congenital conductive deficit

Image Interpretation Pearls

- Thickened bone over OW + inferomedially displaced tympanic CNVII = OWA

SELECTED REFERENCES

1. Su Y et al: Congenital middle ear abnormalities with absence of the oval window: diagnosis, surgery, and audiometric outcomes. Otol Neurotol. 35(7):1191-5, 2014
2. de Alarcon A et al: Congenital absence of the oval window: diagnosis, surgery, and audiometric outcomes. Otol Neurotol. 29(1):23-8, 2008
3. Booth TN et al: Imaging and clinical evaluation of isolated atresia of the oval window. AJNR Am J Neuroradiol. 21(1):171-4, 2000
4. Zeifer B et al: Congenital absence of the oval window: radiologic diagnosis and associated anomalies. AJNR Am J Neuroradiol. 21(2):322-7, 2000

KEY FACTS

TERMINOLOGY

- Lateralized internal carotid artery (Lat-ICA)
- Rare temporal bone vascular variant

IMAGING

- CTA best shows ICA entering anterior middle ear cavity lateral to normal position
- Petrous ICA genu lateral to line drawn perpendicular to midpoint cochlea basal turn on axial images
- Dehiscent lateral ICA often associated
- Coronal bone CT: Tympanic canaliculus not enlarged
- On maximal intensity projection, CTA/MRA vessel contour mimics aberrant ICA
- Source images best for clarifying exact anomalous course of ICA through temporal bone

TOP DIFFERENTIAL DIAGNOSES

- Aberrant internal carotid artery
- Glomus tympanicum paraganglioma
- Glomus jugulare paraganglioma
- ICA aneurysm at petrous apex

PATHOLOGY

- Developmental anomaly
- Not associated with persistent stapedial artery

CLINICAL ISSUES

- Often asymptomatic; incidental on CT or otoscopy
- Patient may present with pulsatile tinnitus
- Important finding to avoid inadvertent surgical injury

DIAGNOSTIC CHECKLIST

- Differentiate from aberrant ICA
  - Aberrant ICA: Inferior tympanic canaliculus enlarged, vertical carotid canal hypoplastic or absent, courses across cochlear promontory
  - Lat-ICA: Inferior tympanic canaliculus and vertical carotid canal normal, courses in anterior middle ear cavity at level of cochlear basal turn

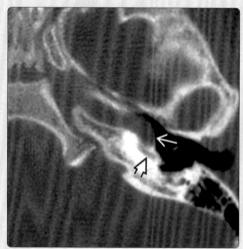
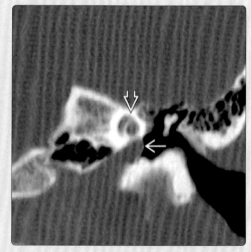

(Left) *Axial left ear temporal bone CT shows a lateralized petrous internal carotid artery (ICA), with its genu ➥ located lateral to a line drawn perpendicular to the midportion of the cochlear basal turn ➦. Position in the anterior middle ear is typical. Inferior tympanic canaliculus was normal (not shown), helping to differentiate from aberrant ICA.* (Right) *Coronal bone CT shows left ICA ➥ extending more lateral to the cochlea ➥ than expected within the anterior hypo- and mesotympanum.*

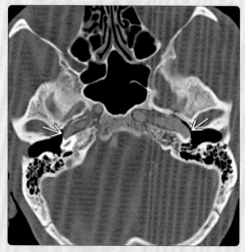
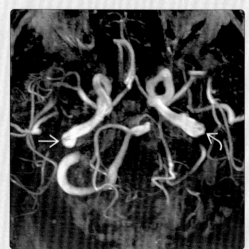

(Left) *CTA bone window images depict bilateral petrous ICA genus projecting laterally into the anterior middle ear cavities. There is associated lateral wall dehiscence ➥, a common finding in lateralized ICA.* (Right) *MRA maximal intensity projection shows asymmetry of contour of ICAs with posterior genu (where ascending carotid turns to become petrous portion) on right side appearing more posterior ➥ and slightly more lateral than on left ➥.*

TERMINOLOGY

Abbreviations

- Lateralized internal carotid artery (Lat-ICA)

Definitions

- Anomalous intratemporal course of ICA
  - Enters anterior mesotympanum
  - Often has dehiscent lateral ICA bony wall

IMAGING

General Features

- Best diagnostic clue
  - Temporal bone CT/CTA shows lateral course of ICA in mesotympanum
- Location
  - ICA lies in anteromedial aspect of middle ear cavity as it turns medially to petrous segment

CT Findings

- Bone CT
  - Bone CT shows protrusion of ICA into anterior aspect of middle ear
    - Dehiscence usually near basal turn of cochlea
  - Coronal temporal bone CT shows laterally displaced ICA at level of cochlear promontory
- CTA
  - Intermediate window/level setting shows course and contour of Lat-ICA projecting into middle ear
  - Bone window shows lateral wall dehiscence

MR Findings

- MRA
  - On maximal intensity projections, mimics aberrant ICA
  - Source images show lateral position of genu of vertical and horizontal portions of petrous ICA
  - Basilar projection reveals bulbous, posterolaterally placed petrous ICA
- Routine MR sequences
  - Lat-ICA may be "invisible" because of low-signal mastoid air and bone

Imaging Recommendations

- Best imaging tool
  - Temporal bone CT/CTA best show course and distinguish from aberrant ICA
  - MRA source images key for clarification of anomalous course
- Protocol advice
  - CTA most readily confirms diagnosis
  - Carefully evaluate coronal and axial planes

DIFFERENTIAL DIAGNOSIS

Aberrant Internal Carotid Artery

- ICA enters hypotympanum through enlarged inferior tympanic canaliculus
- Aberrant ICA then courses through middle ear across cochlear promontory

Glomus Tympanicum Paraganglioma

- Focal mass on cochlear promontory

- No tubular shape; normal ICA on MRA/CTA

Glomus Jugulare Paraganglioma

- Mass arising in jugular foramen and projecting superolaterally into middle ear
- Permeative-destructive bony changes on CT

Internal Carotid Artery Aneurysm at Petrous Apex

- Focal or fusiform expansion of petrous ICA canal
- MRA and CTA show focal vascular mass

PATHOLOGY

General Features

- Etiology
  - Developmental variation
    - No etiology known
- Associated abnormalities
  - Lat-ICA appears to be isolated finding
  - Not associated with persistent stapedial artery

CLINICAL ISSUES

Presentation

- Most common signs/symptoms
  - Often asymptomatic; incidental finding on CT or otoscopy
  - Patient may present for imaging with objective or subjective pulsatile tinnitus

Demographics

- Gender
  - No gender predilection known
- Epidemiology
  - Rare temporal bone vascular lesion

Natural History & Prognosis

- Developmental anomaly
- No long-term sequelae reported

Treatment

- None; probably incidental developmental anomaly
- Important radiologic observation
- **Inadvertent surgical vascular injury can result in significant neurologic deficits**

DIAGNOSTIC CHECKLIST

Consider

- Must differentiate from aberrant ICA
  - Lat-ICA does not enter middle ear through enlarged inferior tympanic canaliculus
  - ICA does not course across cochlear promontory
- Important normal vascular variant to recognize and report to avoid surgical injury to ICA

Image Interpretation Pearls

- Always check course of ICA on temporal bone CT or CTA
- Always check integrity of lateral wall of temporal ICA

SELECTED REFERENCES

1. Glastonbury CM et al: Lateralized petrous internal carotid artery: imaging features and distinction from the aberrant internal carotid artery. Neuroradiology. 54(9):1007-13, 2012

Aberrant Internal Carotid Artery

TERMINOLOGY

- Aberrant internal carotid artery (AbICA): Congenital vascular anomaly resulting from failure of formation of extracranial ICA with arterial collateral pathway

IMAGING

- Appearance of AbICA on thin-section (< 1 mm) temporal bone CT is diagnostic
- AbICA appears as tubular lesion crossing middle ear from posterior to anterior
- Enlarged inferior tympanic canaliculus important observation
- Caution: Do not mistake AbICA for glomus tympanicum paraganglioma

TOP DIFFERENTIAL DIAGNOSES

- Vascular middle ear lesion
  - Glomus tympanicum paraganglioma
  - Dehiscent jugular bulb
  - Lateralized internal carotid artery

PATHOLOGY

- Best explanation: "Alternative blood flow" theory
  - Persistence of pharyngeal artery system means C1 portion of ICA is absent
  - Mature arterial collateral system compensates for absent C1 and vertical petrous ICA segments
  - Ascending pharyngeal artery → inferior tympanic artery → caroticotympanic artery → posterolateral aspect of horizontal petrous ICA
- 30% of AbICA have persistent stapedial artery

CLINICAL ISSUES

- Typically asymptomatic and discovered at time of routine physical exam, during middle ear surgery, or as incidental imaging finding
- Associated symptoms: Pulsatile tinnitus and conductive hearing loss
- No treatment is best treatment

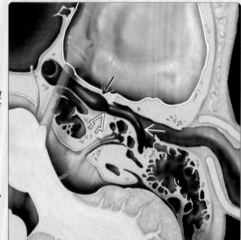
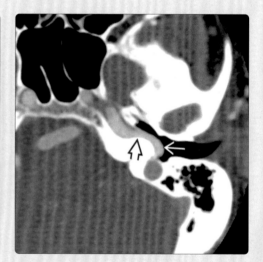

(Left) Axial graphic of the left temporal bone illustrates classic aberrant internal carotid artery (AbICA) ➡ rising along the posterior cochlear promontory, crossing along the medial middle ear wall, & rejoining the horizontal petrous ICA ➡. At the point of reconnection to the horizontal petrous ICA, stenosis ➡ is often present. (Right) Axial CTA through the middle ear shows the looping aberrant internal carotid ➡ on the low cochlear promontory. Note the caliber change ➡ as the AbICA rejoins the normal horizontal segment of the ICA.

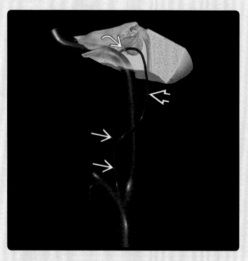
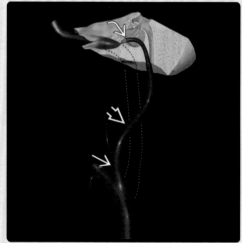

(Left) Lateral graphic of a normal adult cervical & petrous ICA reveals inferior tympanic artery ➡ branching off the ascending pharyngeal artery ➡, passing into the temporal bone to anastomose with the very small caroticotympanic artery ➡ on the cochlear promontory. (Right) Lateral graphic depicts failure of the cervical ICA to develop (dotted lines), with the ascending pharyngeal ➡, inferior tympanic ➡, caroticotympanic ➡ arteries providing an alternative collateral arterial channel resulting in an AbICA.

TERMINOLOGY

Abbreviations
- Aberrant internal carotid artery (AbICA)

Synonyms
- Aberrant carotid artery

Definitions
- Congenital vascular anomaly resulting from failure of formation of extracranial internal carotid artery (ICA) with arterial collateral pathway

IMAGING

General Features
- Best diagnostic clue
  o Tubular structure running horizontally through middle ear cavity from posterior to anterior
- Location
  o Enters posterior middle ear through enlarged inferior tympanic canaliculus
    – Posterior and lateral to expected site of petrous carotid canal
  o Courses anteriorly across cochlear promontory to join horizontal petrous ICA through dehiscent carotid plate
  o Most commonly unilateral
- Size
  o Smaller than horizontal petrous ICA
- Morphology
  o Tubular morphology is key observation

CT Findings
- CECT
  o Enhancement equivalent to other arteries
    – **Caution**: Glomus tympanicum paraganglioma also enhances; use morphology to differentiate tubular AbICA from ovoid paraganglioma
- Bone CT
  o Appearance of AbICA on thin-section (< 1 mm) temporal bone CT is diagnostic
  o Axial bone CT
    – AbICA appears as tubular lesion crossing middle ear from posterior to anterior
    – **Enlarged inferior tympanic canaliculus** is important observation
      □ Anteromedial to stylomastoid foramen and mastoid segment of facial nerve
    – Smaller AbICA often stenotic at point of reconnection with horizontal petrous ICA
    – Carotid foramen and vertical segment of petrous ICA are absent
  o Coronal bone CT
    – AbICA appears as round, soft tissue lesion on cochlear promontory
      □ Single slice looks disturbingly like glomus tympanicum paraganglioma
      □ **Caution**: Do not mistake AbICA for glomus tympanicum paraganglioma
      □ Tubular nature of AbICA is key observation

- Inferior tympanic canaliculus is vertical tube posterolateral to normal location of vertical segment of petrous ICA
  □ Rises at coronal level of round window niche
  o If **persistent stapedial artery** associated
    – Absent foramen spinosum
    – Enlarged anterior tympanic segment of CNVII canal
- CTA
  o Diagnostic for AbICA
  o Usually not necessary, as CT alone is diagnostic

MR Findings
- Conventional MR does not reliably identify AbICA
- MRA source images and reformatted images show aberrant nature of vessel
  o AbICA enters skull base posterior and lateral, compared to normal contralateral side
  o Frontal reformat: Petrous segment of ICA extends laterally instead of medially
    – In left ear, AbICA looks like 7
    – In right ear, AbICA looks like reverse 7

Angiographic Findings
- Frontal view: Petrous segment of ICA extends laterally instead of medially
- Lateral view: Absent extracranial course of suprabifurcation ICA (C1 segment)
  o Smaller caliber vessels arise from bifurcation posteriorly, looping back to horizontal segment of petrous ICA
    – Stenosis may be present at site of reconnection between AbICA and horizontal petrous ICA
- Conventional angiography no longer necessary to confirm imaging diagnosis
  o CTA or MRA sufficient if uncertainty arises from bone CT images

Imaging Recommendations
- Best imaging tool
  o Temporal bone CT: Tubular morphology and posterolateral position diagnostic
    – Contrast CT or CTA not necessary
- Protocol advice
  o Bone CT: < 1 mm axial and coronal images
  o If MR is used, MRA is critical component

DIFFERENTIAL DIAGNOSIS

Glomus Tympanicum Paraganglioma
- Otoscopy: Pink/red, pulsatile, retrotympanic mass
- Bone CT: Focal, ovoid mass on cochlear promontory
- T1WI C+ MR: Enhancing mass

Lateralized Internal Carotid Artery
- Otoscopy: Vague, vascular hue deep behind tympanic membrane
- Bone CT: Dehiscent lateral wall of petrous ICA genu

Petrous Internal Carotid Artery Aneurysm
- Otoscopy: Negative unless large
- Bone CT: Focal, smooth, petrous ICA canal expansion
  o ICA has normal course but focal ovoid, expansile portion
- CTA or MRA is diagnostic of nonthrombosed aneurysm

Dehiscent Jugular Bulb

- Otoscopy: Gray-blue retrotympanic mass in posteroinferior quadrant
- Bone CT: Focal absence of sigmoid plate
  - "Bud" from superolateral jugular bulb enters middle ear as "mass"

Cholesterol Granuloma in Middle Ear

- Otoscopy: Blue-black retrotympanic mass
- Bone CT: Appears identical to acquired cholesteatoma
- MR: High signal on T1 and T2 without contrast suggests diagnosis

Congenital Cholesteatoma in Middle Ear

- Otoscopy: White-tan retrotympanic mass
- Bone CT: Multilobular soft tissue middle ear mass medial to ossicles
- MR: Low T1, high T2 signal mass; DWI restricted diffusion

PATHOLOGY

General Features

- Etiology
  - Etiology of AbICA is controversial
  - Best explanation: "Alternative blood flow" theory
    - Persistence of pharyngeal artery system means C1 portion of ICA is absent
    - Mature arterial collateral system compensates for absent C1 and vertical petrous ICA segments
      - Ascending pharyngeal artery → inferior tympanic artery → caroticotympanic artery → posterolateral aspect of horizontal petrous ICA
  - Results of absent extracranial ICA C1 segment
    - Ascending pharyngeal, inferior tympanic, and caroticotympanic arteries enlarge
    - Inferior tympanic canaliculus enlarges to accommodate enlarged inferior tympanic artery
    - Bony margin of posterolateral horizontal petrous ICA canal is penetrated at site of caroticotympanic artery origin
- Associated abnormalities
  - 30% of AbICAs have **persistent stapedial artery**
    - Enlarged anterior tympanic segment of CNVII canal
    - Absent ipsilateral foramen spinosum

Gross Pathologic & Surgical Features

- Pulsatile aberrant artery is found in middle ear cavity

Microscopic Features

- Histologically normal artery

CLINICAL ISSUES

Presentation

- Most common signs/symptoms
  - Most commonly asymptomatic
    - Discovered at time of routine physical exam, during middle ear surgery, or as incidental imaging finding
  - Associated symptoms
    - Pulsatile tinnitus (PT) (pulse-synchronous sound)
      - May be subjective (only patient hears) or objective (patient and clinician hear)

- Subjective PT: Pulsatile sound may transmit directly through cochlear promontory to basal turn of cochlea
- Objective PT: When stenosis present at junction of AbICA and normal horizontal petrous ICA
  - Conductive hearing loss
  - Vertigo, otalgia rare
  - Otoscopy: Retrotympanic pink-red mass
    - Inferior aspect of tympanic membrane
    - May mimic paraganglioma

Demographics

- Age
  - Average at presentation: 40 years
- Epidemiology
  - Very rare disorder

Natural History & Prognosis

- No long-term sequelae reported with AbICA
- Poor prognosis results only if misdiagnosis → biopsy
  - Pseudoaneurysm may require endovascular repair
- If tinnitus is loud, AbICA can be debilitating

Treatment

- **No treatment** is best treatment
- Greatest risk is misdiagnosis leading to biopsy
- Most patients have minor symptoms that do not require treatment
- Persistent stapedial artery does not need to be treated

DIAGNOSTIC CHECKLIST

Image Interpretation Pearls

- Radiologist must remain firm on imaging diagnosis despite clinical impression of paraganglioma
  - Biopsy or attempted resection of misdiagnosed AbICA can be disastrous
    - Hemorrhage, stroke, or death may result from vessel injury

Reporting Tips

- Report diagnosis; offer no differential diagnosis
- Equivocal report such as "cannot exclude paraganglioma" may lead to surgical intervention

SELECTED REFERENCES

1. Becker C et al: The clinical impact of aberrant internal carotid arteries in children. Int J Pediatr Otorhinolaryngol. 78(7):1123-7, 2014
2. Honkura Y et al: Surgical treatment for the aberrant internal carotid artery in the middle ear with pulsatile tinnitus. Auris Nasus Larynx. 41(2):215-8, 2014
3. Glastonbury CM et al: Lateralized petrous internal carotid artery: imaging features and distinction from the aberrant internal carotid artery. Neuroradiology. 54(9):1007-13, 2012
4. Hatipoglu HG et al: A case of a coexisting aberrant internal carotid artery and persistent stapedial artery: the role of MR angiography in the diagnosis. Ear Nose Throat J. 90(5):E17-20, 2011
5. Sauvaget E et al: Aberrant internal carotid artery in the temporal bone: imaging findings and management. Arch Otolaryngol Head Neck Surg. 132(1):86-91, 2006
6. Roll JD et al: Bilateral aberrant internal carotid arteries with bilateral persistent stapedial arteries and bilateral duplicated internal carotid arteries. AJNR Am J Neuroradiol. 24(4):762-5, 2003
7. Lo WW et al: Aberrant carotid artery: radiologic diagnosis with emphasis on high-resolution computed tomography. Radiographics. 5(6):985-93, 1985

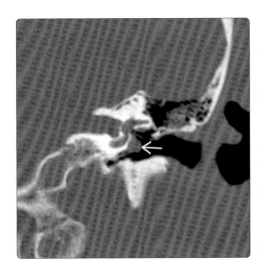
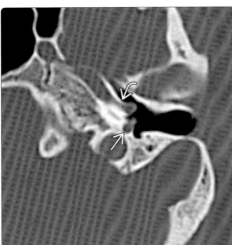

(Left) *Coronal left temporal bone CT at the level of the oval window shows the AbICA ➡ as a "mass" located on the cochlear promontory resembling a glomus tympanicum paraganglioma. Accidental biopsy of AbICA may have devastating consequences.* (Right) *Axial bone CT reveals a smaller caliber AbICA entering the middle ear cavity through an enlarged inferior tympanic canaliculus ➡, coursing across the middle ear on cochlear promontory, and reentering the horizontal petrous ICA ➡.*

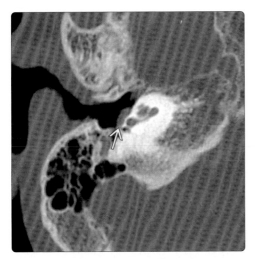
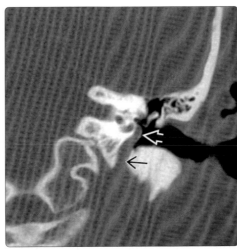

(Left) *Axial bone CT of the right ear shows the AbICA entering the posteromedial middle ear cavity ➡ and looping across the low cochlear promontory in this young adult with a vascular retrotympanic mass. Its tubular shape can help prevent a misdiagnosis.* (Right) *Coronal bone CT of the left ear shows the posterior aspect of an AbICA with its enlarged inferior tympanic canaliculus ➡ and looping course ➡ up onto the cochlear promontory. The tubular configuration of the vessel is diagnostic.*

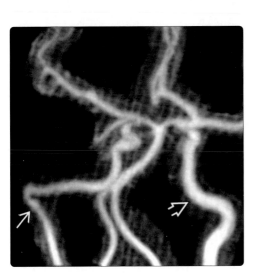
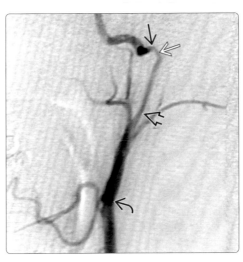

(Left) *Frontal oblique MRA shows a right ➡ AbICA with a characteristic reverse 7 shape. Note the typical configuration of the contralateral normal ICA ➡.* (Right) *Lateral internal carotid angiography of an AbICA reveals that the normal extracranial ICA is replaced by an enlarged collateral circuit, which includes the ascending pharyngeal ➡, inferior tympanic ➡, and caroticotympanic ➡ arteries. Note the caliber change from the AbICA to the horizontal petrous ICA ➡.*

TERMINOLOGY

- Persistent stapedial artery (PSA): Rare congenital vascular anomaly in which embryological stapedial artery persists

IMAGING

- Temporal bone **CT findings**
  - Enlargement of anterior tympanic segment of facial nerve canal
  - Absent foramen spinosum
    - Posterolateral from foramen ovale on axial bone CT
  - Frequently bilateral

TOP DIFFERENTIAL DIAGNOSES

- Facial nerve venous malformation ("hemangioma")
- Facial nerve schwannoma
- Perineural parotid malignancy in CNVII canal

PATHOLOGY

- Embryology-anatomy

- Primitive 2nd aortic arch gives rise to hyoid artery
- Hyoid artery gives rise to stapedial artery
- Stapedial artery divides into dorsal (**middle meningeal artery**) & ventral divisions (to maxilla & mandible)
- PSA courses from infracochlear ICA through stapedial obturator foramen
- PSA **enlarges tympanic** CNVII **canal** on its way to middle cranial fossa
- **PSA becomes middle meningeal artery**

CLINICAL ISSUES

- **Asymptomatic**; no treatment required
- Needs to be correctly identified as incidental congenital vascular anomaly on temporal bone CT

DIAGNOSTIC CHECKLIST

- If **aberrant internal carotid artery** discovered, look for associated **PSA**
- Large anterior tympanic CNVII + absent foramen spinosum = persistent stapedial artery

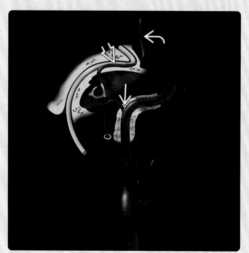
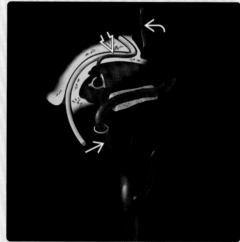

(Left) Lateral graphic shows the persistent stapedial artery (PSA) arising from the vertical segment of the petrous internal carotid artery ➡, passing through the stapes, and traveling along the tympanic segment of the facial nerve ➡ to become the middle meningeal artery ➡. (Right) Lateral graphic shows the PSA arising from the aberrant internal carotid artery ➡ and passing through the stapes to follow the anterior tympanic facial nerve segment ➡. Intracranially, the PSA becomes the middle meningeal artery ➡.

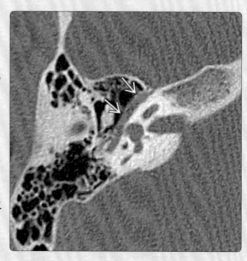
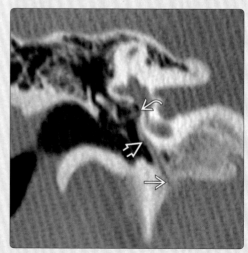

(Left) Axial right temporal bone CT reveals an enlarged tympanic segment ➡ of the intratemporal facial nerve to the PSA. (Right) Coronal bone CT of the right ear in the same patient demonstrates the PSA arising from its takeoff origin from the genu of the petrous internal carotid artery ➡, ascending on the cochlear promontory ➡, and passing through the crura of the stapes ➡ on its way to join the tympanic segment of the facial nerve canal. (Courtesy K. Funk, MD.)

Persistent Stapedial Artery

TERMINOLOGY

Abbreviations

- Persistent stapedial artery (PSA)

Definitions

- Rare congenital vascular anomaly in which embryological stapedial artery persists

IMAGING

General Features

- Best diagnostic clue
  - Enlargement of anterior tympanic segment CNVII canal + absent foramen spinosum
- Location
  - PSA passes through stapes footplate
  - Frequently bilateral
- Size
  - Doubles size of anterior CNVII tympanic segment

CT Findings

- Bone CT
  - **Absent** ipsilateral **foramen spinosum**
  - **Anterior tympanic segment** of CNVII canal enlarged
    - Separate parallel canal possible
  - Curvilinear structure crossing medial wall of middle ear cavity over cochlear promontory
  - Small canaliculus leaving carotid canal
  - PSA seen **± aberrant internal carotid artery** (AbICA)
- CTA
  - Shows absence of normal middle meningeal artery
  - PSA arising from genu of vertical & horizontal petrous internal carotid artery (ICA)

Angiographic Findings

- External carotid artery arteriogram
  - Shows absence of normal middle meningeal artery
- ICA arteriogram: PSA arising from infracochlear petrous ICA or from AbICA

Imaging Recommendations

- Best imaging tool
  - Axial & coronal temporal bone CT

DIFFERENTIAL DIAGNOSIS

Facial Nerve Venous Malformation ("Hemangioma")

- Bone CT: Intralesional ossification (50%)
- T1 C+ MR: Enhancing mass in geniculate fossa

Facial Nerve Schwannoma

- Bone CT: Tubular or focal enlargement of CNVII canal
- T1 C+ MR: Mass enhancing in CNVII canal

Perineural Parotid Malignancy, Mastoid CNVII

- Bone CT: Enlarged mastoid segment of CNVII canal
- T1 C+ MR: Enhancing tumor coming up from parotid

PATHOLOGY

General Features

- Etiology

- Stapedial artery **fails to involve** in 3rd fetal month
- Associated abnormalities
  - **AbICA**
  - Trisomy 13, 15, & 21
  - Paget disease, otosclerosis, anencephaly, neurofibromatosis
- Embryology-anatomy
  - Primitive 2nd aortic arch gives rise to hyoid artery
  - Hyoid artery gives rise to stapedial artery
  - Stapedial artery divides into dorsal (middle meningeal artery) & ventral components (to maxilla & mandible)
    - PSA courses from infracochlear ICA through stapedial obturator foramen
    - PSA **enlarges tympanic** CNVII **canal** on its way to middle cranial fossa
    - PSA becomes middle meningeal artery

Gross Pathologic & Surgical Features

- Otoendoscopy shows PSA passing through stapes

CLINICAL ISSUES

Presentation

- Most common signs/symptoms
  - **Asymptomatic** on temporal bone CT or during surgery
    - Tinnitus ± pulsatile retrotympanic red mass
- Clinical profile
  - Otoscopic exam usually normal

Demographics

- Age
  - Congenital; may be discovered at any age
- Epidemiology
  - Very rare lesion

Natural History & Prognosis

- Excellent; just needs to be left alone

Treatment

- **No treatment** is best treatment
- If presumed cause of severe pulsatile tinnitus, surgical ligation or endovascular occlusion may be considered
- PSA surgical implications
  - Can complicate stapedectomy or cholesteatoma resection
  - May prevent cochlear implantation

DIAGNOSTIC CHECKLIST

Consider

- If **AbICA** discovered, look for associated **PSA**

SELECTED REFERENCES

1. Hitier M et al: Persistent stapedial arteries in human: from phylogeny to surgical consequences. Surg Radiol Anat. 35(10):883-91, 2013
2. Koesling S et al: Vascular anomalies, sutures and small canals of the temporal bone on axial CT. Eur J Radiol. 54(3):335-43, 2005
3. Yilmaz T et al: Persistent stapedial artery: MR angiographic and CT findings. AJNR Am J Neuroradiol. 24(6):1133-5, 2003
4. Silbergleit R et al: The persistent stapedial artery. AJNR Am J Neuroradiol. 21(3):572-7, 2000
5. Moreano EH et al: Prevalence of facial canal dehiscence and of persistent stapedial artery in the human middle ear: a report of 1000 temporal bones. Laryngoscope. 104(3 Pt 1):309-20, 1994

KEY FACTS

TERMINOLOGY

- Acute coalescent otomastoiditis (ACOM): Acute middle ear-mastoid infection with progressive bony resorption and demineralization due to intramastoid empyema ± osteomyelitis

IMAGING

- Bone CT findings: Mastoid cortex ± trabecula erosions (coalescent otomastoiditis)
- CECT or enhanced MR findings of **ACOM complications**
  - **Subperiosteal abscess**: Periauricular fluid collection
  - **Bezold abscess**: Walled-off pus in and around sternocleidomastoid muscle
  - **Middle cranial fossa abscess** (epidural or temporal lobe abscess)
  - **Posterior fossa abscess** (epidural or cerebellar abscess)
  - **Thrombosed sigmoid sinus** ± **internal jugular vein**

TOP DIFFERENTIAL DIAGNOSES

- Acquired cholesteatoma
- Apical petrositis
- Temporal bone Langerhans histiocytosis
- Temporal bone rhabdomyosarcoma/metastasis

PATHOLOGY

- Common pathophysiology
  - Granulation tissue or cholesteatoma blocks aditus ad antrum and prevents mastoid air cell drainage
- Less common pathophysiology
  - Mastoid cortex remains intact with septic thrombophlebitis of **emissary veins** seeding periosteum

CLINICAL ISSUES

- Young child with days to weeks history of otalgia, postauricular swelling, fever, and otorrhea

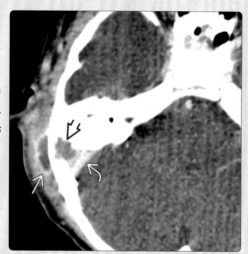
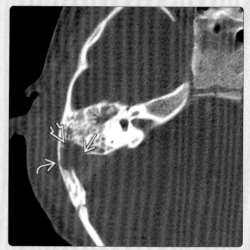

(Left) Axial CECT in a patient with postauricular tender mass, headache, and fever reveals postauricular abscess ➡ and coalescent otomastoiditis ➡, resulting in epidural extension of infection with nonthrombosed sigmoid sinus ➡. (Right) Axial bone CT of the same patient shows loss of mastoid trabecula ➡ and a dehiscent sigmoid plate ➡ diagnostic of coalescent otomastoiditis. Subtle erosion of the lateral mastoid cortex ➡ indicates continuity of mastoid infection with the postauricular abscess.

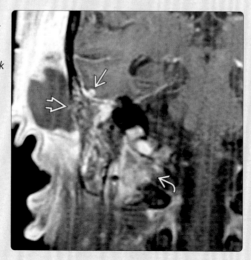
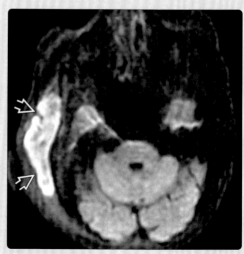

(Left) Coronal T1WI C+ FS MR reveals mastoid enhancement with a large periauricular abscess. Lateral mastoid is focally dehiscent ➡ with thick and enhancing proximal meninges ➡. Subjacent skull base enhances ➡, indicating extensive associated osteomyelitis. (Right) Axial DWI MR of the same patient reveals restricted diffusion within the extensive periauricular abscess ➡. (Courtesy N. Fischbein, MD.)

TERMINOLOGY

Abbreviations

- Acute coalescent otomastoiditis (ACOM)
- Acute otomastoiditis (AOM)

Synonyms

- Coalescent otomastoiditis with abscess

Definitions

- ACOM: Acute middle ear-mastoid (ME-M) infection with progressive bony resorption and demineralization due to intramastoid empyema ± osteomyelitis
- ACOM + abscess: Coalescent otomastoiditis with resultant **intracranial** or **extracranial** abscess
- AOM: Acute infection in ME-M without destruction of mastoid septations or cortex

IMAGING

General Features

- Best diagnostic clue
  - Rim-enhancing fluid collection adjacent to eroded mastoid cortex + mastoid air cell opacification
- Location
  - Abscess adjacent to mastoid cortical dehiscence
    - **Lateral mastoid wall**
      - □ Postauricular (thin cortical bone) abscess
      - □ Pre- or periauricular abscess
    - **Inferior mastoid wall**
      - □ Mastoid tip → Bezold abscess
      - □ Other remaining inferior mastoid cortical dehiscence → transspatial abscess
    - **Tegmen mastoideum** → temporal lobe abscess
    - **Medial mastoid wall** → posterior fossa epidural abscess, cerebellar abscess
- Size
  - Variable; usually presents with > 1-cm fluid pocket
- Morphology
  - Crescentic, lentiform, or spherical

CT Findings

- CECT
  - **Subperiosteal abscess**: Periauricular fluid collection
    - Thick, enhancing lateral wall represents inflamed periosteum
  - **Bezold abscess**: Walled-off pus in and around sternocleidomastoid muscle
  - **Middle cranial fossa abscess**
    - Epidural or temporal lobe rim-enhancing fluid
  - **Posterior fossa abscess**
    - Epidural or cerebellar rim-enhancing fluid
- Bone CT
  - ME-M opacification
  - Variable trabecular and cortical erosions (CT sign of confluent otomastoiditis)
  - Subtle to grossly **dehiscent cortex** just deep to abscess
    - Lateral mastoid cortex → subperiosteal abscess
    - Mastoid tip cortex → Bezold abscess
    - Tegmen mastoideum cortex → epidural or temporal lobe abscess
    - Medial mastoid cortex → epidural or cerebellar abscess
- CTV
  - May show thrombosed sigmoid sinus &/or internal jugular vein (IJV)

MR Findings

- T2WI FS
  - High signal fills ME-M
  - High-signal fluid in epidural or parenchymal abscess
  - Low signal intensity in sigmoid sinus or IJV if thrombus present
- DWI
  - Decreased diffusion in abscess
- T1WI C+ FS
  - Variable enhancement of ME-M
  - Rim-enhancing pus in extracranial subperiosteal, intracranial epidural, or parenchymal abscess
  - Filling defect(s) in sigmoid sinus &/or IJV if thrombus present
- MRV
  - May show dural sinus/venous thrombosis (DST/DVT)

Imaging Recommendations

- Best imaging tool
  - Temporal bone CT defines bony changes (confluence, cortical dehiscence)
    - CECT will define most infectious complications
  - Enhanced temporal bone MR more sensitive for intracranial complications (DST, meningitis, subdural empyema, parenchymal abscess)
- Protocol advice
  - Section thickness small (≤ 3 mm) for enhanced MR

DIFFERENTIAL DIAGNOSIS

Acquired Cholesteatoma

- Clinical: Retraction or rupture of tympanic membrane; may be superinfected
- Imaging: CT shows erosive mass; MR shows decreased diffusion and nonenhancing mass
- When associated with ACOM, may also cause extracranial or intracranial abscess

Apical Petrositis

- Clinical: CNVI palsy, retroauricular pain, AOM
- Imaging: CT shows coalescent changes in pneumatized petrous apex
  - T1WI C+ MR shows enhancing meninges and focal walled-off fluid in petrous apex
- In young patients, may rarely see osteomyelitis in nonpneumatized petrous apex → marrow enhancement on T1WI C+ FS MR with narrowed petrous internal carotid artery

Temporal Bone Langerhans Histiocytosis

- Clinical: Child with otorrhea and periauricular mass
- Imaging: Extensive, sometimes bilateral mastoid destruction with enhancing mass

Temporal Bone Rhabdomyosarcoma

- Clinical: Neurologic deficits common, including CNVII palsy

- Imaging: CT shows lytic bone destruction; intracranial extension
  - T1WI C+ MR shows enhancing soft tissue mass

Metastasis, Temporal Bone

- Clinical: Otorrhea, otalgia, and periauricular mass
- Imaging: Lytic bone destruction ± mass

PATHOLOGY

General Features

- Etiology
  - Inflammation, granulation tissue, or cholesteatoma blocks aditus ad antrum and prevents mastoid air cell drainage
  - Local hyperemia-acidosis creates enzymatic resorption of trabeculae (confluent otomastoiditis)
  - Subtle or gross cortical dehiscence conveys infection into adjacent tissues
  - Less common pathophysiology: Mastoid cortex remains intact with septic thrombophlebitis of **emissary veins** seeding periosteum
- Macewen triangle
  - Surgical access point to mastoid antrum at posterosuperior EAC
  - Weakest bone, loose periosteum facilitates breakout of infection in postauricular location

Gross Pathologic & Surgical Features

- Pus in mastoid, mastoid osteomyelitis, adjacent abscess cavity
- Granulation tissue or **cholesteatoma** occasionally identified in ME-M
  - More common in subacute-chronic disease
  - Requires more extensive surgery

Microscopic Features

- Polymicrobial aerobes and anaerobes
- *Streptococcus* species common

CLINICAL ISSUES

Presentation

- Most common signs/symptoms
  - Otalgia (ear pain) ± otorrhea (ear drainage)
  - Postauricular pain ± swelling
  - Fever
  - Other temporal bone signs/symptoms
    - Lateralized auricle (ear pushed outward by abscess)
    - Hearing loss: Conductive > > sensorineural
  - Intracranial complications
    - Headache, mental status changes, nausea, vomiting, and seizures
    - Nuchal rigidity and photophobia
    - Papilledema
    - CNVI palsy
- Clinical profile
  - Child with days to weeks history of otalgia, postauricular swelling, fever, and otorrhea
  - 35-70% of patients already received antibiotics for AOM
  - Postauricular edema (Griesinger sign) common in uncomplicated acute otomastoiditis (85%)

- Enhancing fluid collection needed to confirm subperiosteal abscess

Demographics

- Age
  - Infants and young children
  - If complication of acquired cholesteatoma, often older age group affected
- Epidemiology
  - 0.24% of patients with AOM develop ACOM

Natural History & Prognosis

- Isolated extracranial subperiosteal abscess
  - Excellent prognosis with prompt therapy
  - Worse if prior incomplete antibiotic therapy, virulent organism, or immunocompromised host
- Intracranial abscess (temporal lobe most common)
  - Worse prognosis
  - If concomitant complications, even worse prognosis
    - Venous sinus thrombosis
    - Epidural abscess or subdural empyema

Treatment

- Intravenous antibiotics ± tympanocentesis with myringotomy tube placement
- Surgical treatment
  - Incision and drainage of extracranial subperiosteal abscess ± canal wall up mastoidectomy
- Surgical therapy must be performed with hearing preservation in mind
  - Canal wall down mastoidectomy for cholesteatoma

DIAGNOSTIC CHECKLIST

Consider

- Seek other complications of ACOM
  - Temporal bone findings (T1WI C+ MR)
    - Facial nerve paralysis shows as enhancing CNVII
    - Labyrinthitis shows as enhancement within membranous labyrinth
    - Apical petrositis (enhancing apical air cells on MR)
  - Intracranial findings (T1WI C+ MR)
    - Subdural empyema, meningitis, brain abscess ± dural sinus, or IJV thrombosis

Image Interpretation Pearls

- MR used to distinguish between hyperintense perisinus epidural abscess and hypointense DST
- Epidural abscess is elliptical; DST is rounded/triangular

SELECTED REFERENCES

1. Funamura JL et al: Otogenic lateral sinus thrombosis: case series and controversies. Int J Pediatr Otorhinolaryngol. 78(5):866-70, 2014
2. Psarommatis IM et al: Algorithmic management of pediatric acute mastoiditis. Int J Pediatr Otorhinolaryngol. 76(6):791-6, 2012
3. Osborn AJ et al: Decisions regarding intracranial complications from acute mastoiditis in children. Curr Opin Otolaryngol Head Neck Surg. 19(6):478-85, 2011
4. Zevallos JP et al: Advanced pediatric mastoiditis with and without intracranial complications. Laryngoscope. 119(8):1610-5, 2009
5. Taylor MF et al: Indications for mastoidectomy in acute mastoiditis in children. Ann Otol Rhinol Laryngol. 113(1):69-72, 2004
6. Vazquez E et al: Imaging of complications of acute mastoiditis in children. Radiographics. 23(2):359-72, 2003

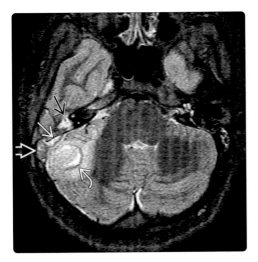

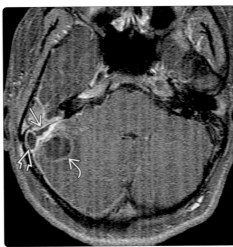

(Left) *Axial T2WI FS MR in a 15-year-old girl with mastoid tenderness and headache reveals a hyperintense epidural abscess ➡ adjacent to the mastoid cortex, hypointense sigmoid sinus thrombus ➡, and cerebellar abscess ➡ with a hypointense rim and surrounding edema. There is fluid within adjacent mastoid air cells ➡.* **(Right)** *Axial T1WI C+ MR of the same patient shows the epidural abscess ➡, sigmoid sinus thrombus ➡, and cerebellar abscess ➡ as all hypointense with peripheral enhancement.*

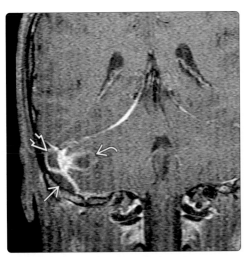

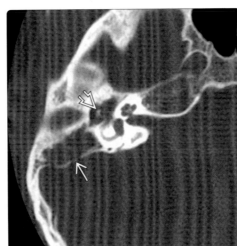

(Left) *Coronal T1WI C+ FS MR of the same patient shows the elliptical epidural abscess ➡ sitting beneath the oval thrombosed sigmoid sinus ➡. The cerebellar abscess ➡ is again seen, as well as dural and tentorial enhancement.* **(Right)** *Axial temporal bone CT of the same patient shows opacification of the middle ear space and mastoid air cells, with erosion of the posterior mastoid cortex ➡ and ossicles ➡, consistent with coalescent otomastoiditis and cholesteatoma, both confirmed at surgery.*

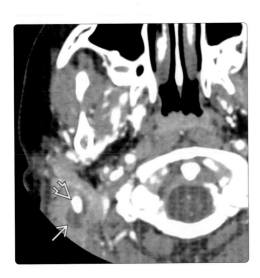

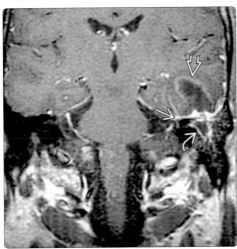

(Left) *Axial CECT in an 11-year-old girl with coalescent otomastoiditis shows there is low attenuation ➡ surrounding the mastoid process ➡ and extending along the sternocleidomastoid muscle, which is consistent with a Bezold abscess.* **(Right)** *Coronal T1WI C+ MR in a different patient reveals acute otomastoiditis with a confluent area of suppuration ➡. A direct connection between a mastoid abscess and a temporal lobe abscess ➡ is seen with associated meningitis ➡.*

Chronic Otomastoiditis With Ossicular Erosions

TERMINOLOGY

- Synonyms: Noncholesteatomatous ossicular erosion; postinflammatory ossicular erosion
- Definition: Erosive changes involving ossicles in absence of cholesteatoma in patient with history of chronic otomastoiditis (COM)

IMAGING

- Axial bone CT
  - Absence of part of posterior line of normal "2 parallel lines" of ossicles
  - Incudostapedial joint (ISJ) may be replaced by fibrous tissue
  - ISJ appears widened on axial CT
  - Erosion of cone (incus body/short process) also occurs
  - Associated findings of chronic otitis media
    - Underpneumatization of mastoid air cells
    - Inflammatory debris in middle ear and mastoid
- Coronal bone CT

  - Long process of incus most commonly absent
  - Vertical segment of **"right angle"** missing
  - Tympanic membrane retraction often present

TOP DIFFERENTIAL DIAGNOSES

- Mild congenital external ear malformation, acquired cholesteatoma + ossicular erosion, congenital middle ear cholesteatoma + ossicle erosion, postoperative ossicular loss, posttraumatic ossicular dislocation

PATHOLOGY

- COM initially causes periostitis and osteitis
- Subsequent osteoclasia and decalcification creates bone loss

CLINICAL ISSUES

- Clinical presentation: Chronic otitis media history
  - Postinflammatory conductive hearing loss
- Primary treatment: Surgical
  - Exploratory tympanotomy with ossicular reconstruction

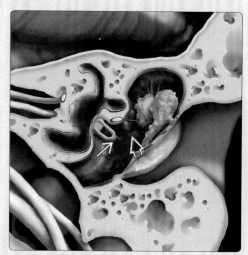

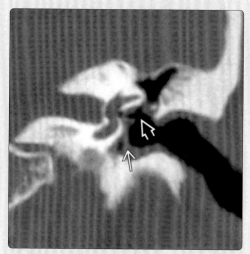

(Left) Coronal graphic of the left ear shows postinflammatory ossicular erosion of the incus long process ➡ and stapes hub ➡. Note the changes of tympanosclerosis of tympanic membrane and remaining ossicles. (Right) Coronal bone CT reveals retraction of a thickened tympanic membrane ➡ with demineralization of the long process of incus ➡. Stranding soft tissue in the middle ear is associated inflammatory debris.

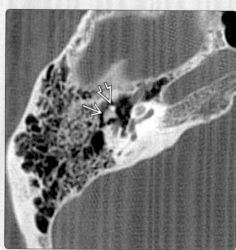

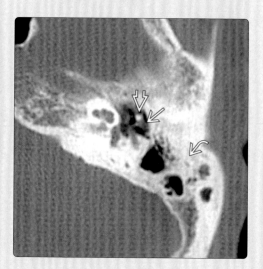

(Left) Axial bone CT shows a normal short process of the right incus ➡ and head of malleus ➡. Notice the well-pneumatized mastoid. (Right) Axial bone CT of the left ear in a patient with history of chronic otitis media demonstrates deossification of the left short process of the incus ➡. The head of the malleus ➡ is normal in density and size. The mastoid is underpneumatized ➡ from otomastoiditis during mastoid formation.

TERMINOLOGY

Abbreviations
- Chronic otomastoiditis (COM)

Synonyms
- Noncholesteatomatous ossicular erosion; postinflammatory ossicular erosion

Definitions
- Erosive changes involving ossicles in absence of cholesteatoma in patient with history of COM

IMAGING

CT Findings
- Bone CT
  - Anatomy of ossicular chain necessary to make imaging diagnosis
    - Axial CT/epitympanum: **"Ice cream cone"** (anterior "ice cream" = malleus head; posterior "cone" = incus body/short process)
    - Axial CT/mesotympanum: **"2 parallel lines"** [anterior line = tensor tympani tendon leading to malleus neck; posterior line = incus lenticular process, incudostapedial joint (ISJ), and stapes head]
    - Coronal CT through long process incus: Ossicular **"right angle"** (vertically oriented incus long process; horizontally oriented incus lenticular process)
  - Axial bone CT images
    - Absence of part of posterior line of normal "2 parallel lines"
      - ISJ may be replaced by fibrous tissue
      - ISJ appears widened on axial CT
    - Erosion of "cone" (incus body/short process) also occurs
  - Coronal bone CT images
    - Long process of incus most commonly absent
      - Vertical segment of **"right angle" missing**
    - Tympanic membrane retraction often present
  - Mastoid underpneumatization common

Imaging Recommendations
- Best imaging tool
  - Axial and coronal temporal bone CT

DIFFERENTIAL DIAGNOSIS

Mild Congenital External Ear Malformation
- Congenital hearing loss; microtia
- CT: Rotation ± fusion of ossicles

Acquired Cholesteatoma + Ossicular Erosion
- CT: Nondependent soft tissue mass is associated
  - Perforated or retracted tympanic membrane

Congenital Middle Ear Cholesteatoma + Ossicle Erosion
- CT: Soft tissue usually medial to ossicles
- Focal ossicular erosion associated

Postoperative Ossicular Loss
- Evidence for mastoidectomy/atticotomy

- CT: Stapedectomy for otosclerosis most commonly

Posttraumatic Ossicular Dislocation
- Fractured, dislocated ossicle may appear absent

PATHOLOGY

General Features
- Etiology
  - COM initiates ossicular loss
  - Initial phase: Periostitis and osteitis
  - Subsequent **osteoclasia and decalcification** creates **bone loss**
  - Incus is most vulnerable portion of ossicular chain due to tenuous blood supply

CLINICAL ISSUES

Presentation
- Most common signs/symptoms
  - Postinflammatory **conductive hearing loss**
    - Usually long history of chronic otitis media

Demographics
- Epidemiology
  - Very common clinical and CT entity

Natural History & Prognosis
- Surgical repair results variable
- Relates to severity of ossicular loss and associated tympanic membrane status
  - Involvement of malleus significant predictor of postoperative hearing outcome, independent of damage to stapes

Treatment
- Exploratory tympanotomy with ossicular reconstruction

DIAGNOSTIC CHECKLIST

Consider
- In patients with conductive hearing loss
  - Look for ossicle loss with COM
  - Then consider other diagnoses
    - **Fenestral otosclerosis**
    - Congenital ossicular malformation in **mild EAC malformation**

Image Interpretation Pearls
- Absence of segment of ossicular chain
  - Common CT finding; easily overlooked

SELECTED REFERENCES
1. Albera R et al: Ossicular chain lesions in tympanic perforations and chronic otitis media without cholesteatoma. J Int Adv Otol. 11(2):143-6, 2015
2. Blom EF et al: Influence of ossicular chain damage on hearing after chronic otitis media and cholesteatoma surgery: a systematic review and meta-analysis. JAMA Otolaryngol Head Neck Surg. 1-9, 2015
3. Swartz JD et al: Ossicular erosions in the dry ear: CT diagnosis. Radiology. 163(3):763-5, 1987

TERMINOLOGY

- Definition: Calcific, bony, or fibrous middle ear foci secondary to **suppurative** chronic otomastoiditis (COM)

IMAGING

- Bone CT: Common locations of tympanosclerotic **calcification**
  - Tympanic membrane
  - Ossicle surface
  - Stapes footplate
  - Muscle tendons
  - Ossicle ligaments
- Focal tympanosclerotic **ossifications**
  - May be seen anywhere in middle ear mastoid
- Chronic otomastoiditis findings associated

TOP DIFFERENTIAL DIAGNOSES

- Chronic otitis media
- COM with ossicular erosions
- COM with ossicular fixation
- Fenestral otosclerosis
- Ossicular prosthesis

PATHOLOGY

- Etiology: Healing response to repeated inflammatory events in middle ear mastoid
- True tympanosclerosis: Diffuse hyalinization & deposition of calcium & phosphate crystals
- New bone formation (osteoneogenesis)

CLINICAL ISSUES

- Clinical presentation
  - Severe conductive hearing loss + history of COM
  - Conductive hearing loss out of proportion to inflammatory debris
- Treatment options
  - Atticotomy with mobilization of ossicles
  - Insertion of prosthesis or homograft device

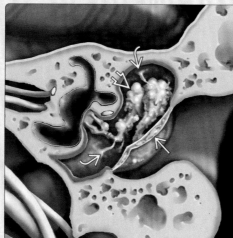
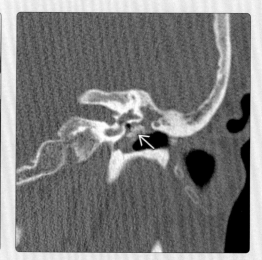

(Left) *Coronal graphic shows severe tympanosclerosis in setting of chronic otomastoiditis. Postinflammatory calcification can be seen in tympanic membrane* ➡, *ossicles* ➡, *and ossicle ligament* ➡. (Right) *Coronal bone CT reveals the ossicles as a fuzzy ball* ➡. *This appearance is due to tympanosclerotic calcific foci deposited on the surface of the middle ear ossicles.*

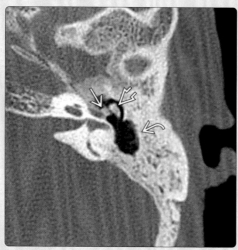
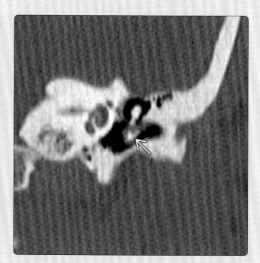

(Left) *Axial bone CT shows a focal area of ossific tympanosclerosis* ➡ *just medial to the ossicles in the medial wall of the epitympanum. Also note that the malleus-incus articulation is fused* ➡ *and the mastoid contains an antral cavity* ➡ *only.* (Right) *Coronal bone CT reveals thickening of the tympanic membrane with a linear focus of calcification* ➡ *along its surface. Tympanosclerotic calcifications can affect ligaments, tendons, ossicles, or the tympanic membrane, as in this case.*

Chronic Otomastoiditis With Tympanosclerosis

TERMINOLOGY

Abbreviations

- Chronic otomastoiditis (COM) with tympanosclerosis

Synonyms

- COM with focal calcification or ossification
- Postinflammatory ossicular fixation

Definitions

- Calcific, bony, or fibrous middle ear foci secondary to **suppurative COM**

IMAGING

General Features

- Best diagnostic clue
  - Bone CT shows high-density foci in middle ear mastoid (MEM) associated with sporadic inflammatory debris

CT Findings

- Bone CT
  - Common locations of tympanosclerotic **Ca^{++}**
    - **Tympanic membrane**
    - **Ossicle surface**
    - **Stapes footplate**
      - □ Crura and footplate thickened
      - □ Referred to as peristapedial tent
    - **Muscle tendons**
      - □ Stapedius & tensor tympani muscles
    - **Ossicle ligaments**
    - Mastoid air cells
  - Focal tympanosclerotic **ossifications**
    - Heaped up new bone (osteoneogenesis)
    - May occur anywhere in MEM
  - Chronic otomastoiditis findings
    - Heterogeneous soft tissue (inflammatory) MEM
    - Underpneumatized mastoid

DIFFERENTIAL DIAGNOSIS

Chronic Otitis Media

- Clinical: Conductive hearing loss (CHL) variable
  - COM history
- CT: Patchy, nondestructive middle ear debris
  - Debris not calcific or ossific

COM With Ossicular Erosions

- Clinical: COM + CHL
- CT: Inflammatory debris, ossicle loss

COM With Ossicular Fixation

- Clinical: COM + CHL
- CT: Focal ossicle ankylosis
  - May have component of tympanosclerosis

Fenestral Otosclerosis

- Clinical: No history of COM (well-pneumatized mastoid)
- CT: Lucency in fissula ante fenestram
  - Associated with cochlear otosclerosis

PATHOLOGY

General Features

- Etiology
  - Healing response to repeated inflammatory events
  - True calcific tympanosclerosis
    - Diffuse hyalinization & deposition of calcium & phosphate crystals
  - Ossific tympanosclerosis
    - New bone formation (osteoneogenesis)
- Associated abnormalities
  - Formed by fused collagenous fibers
    - Fibers hardened by deposition of calcium & phosphate crystals

Staging, Grading, & Classification

- 3 types of **postinflammatory ossicular fixation**
  - **Fibrous tissue fixation**
    - No calcification
    - May occur anywhere in MEM
  - **True calcific tympanosclerosis**
    - Multiple small calcifications
  - **Ossific tympanosclerosis**
    - New bone formation (osteoneogenesis)

Microscopic Features

- Calcification of previously hyalinized mucoperiosteum
- Onion skin-like lamellar arrangement

CLINICAL ISSUES

Presentation

- Most common signs/symptoms
  - Severe CHL + COM history
- Other signs/symptoms
  - Otoscopy: Thick, opaque tympanic membrane

Demographics

- Age
  - Average age at diagnosis = 35 yr
- Epidemiology
  - 10% of patients with **suppurative** COM develop tympanosclerosis

Treatment

- Atticotomy with mobilization of ossicles
  - Patients with less ossicular disease have better postsurgical hearing outcome
- Insertion of prosthesis or homograft device

DIAGNOSTIC CHECKLIST

Consider

- Fenestral otosclerosis 1st in CHL patient without COM

SELECTED REFERENCES

1. Mutlu F et al: An analysis of surgical treatment results of patients with tympanosclerosis. J Craniofac Surg. 26(8):2393-5, 2015
2. Stankovic MD: Hearing results of surgery for tympanosclerosis. Eur Arch Otorhinolaryngol. 266(5):635-40, 2009
3. Swartz JD et al: Postinflammatory ossicular fixation: CT analysis with surgical correlation. Radiology. 154(3):697-700, 1985

Pars Flaccida Cholesteatoma

TERMINOLOGY

- Pars flaccida cholesteatoma (PFC)
- "Attic" or "Prussak space" cholesteatoma

IMAGING

- Temporal bone CT: Smaller PFC
  - Soft tissue mass in Prussak space with scutum & ossicle erosions
- Temporal bone CT: Larger PFC
  - Look for lateral semicircular canal, facial nerve canal, and tegmen tympani ± mastoideum dehiscence
  - Exclude sinus tympani extension (associated with high postoperative recurrence rate)
- Temporal bone MR: Complementary; higher sensitivity & specificity than CT
  - Non-echo-planar DWI superior to conventional EPI DWI
  - May obviate need for exploratory surgery in high-risk retraction pockets or 2nd-look revision surgery

TOP DIFFERENTIAL DIAGNOSES

- Acquired pars tensa cholesteatoma
- Congenital middle ear cholesteatoma
- Middle ear cholesterol granuloma
- Glomus tympanicum paraganglioma

PATHOLOGY

- Starts at pars flaccida of tympanic membrane
- Microscopically consists of exfoliated keratin within stratified squamous epithelium

CLINICAL ISSUES

- Most common type of cholesteatoma (**80%** of all acquired cholesteatomas)
- Patient with chronic ME inflammatory disease, conductive hearing loss, & tympanic membrane (TM) abnormality
  - TM retraction: PFC **not** visible; CT must make diagnosis based on ossicle or bone loss
  - TM perforation: PFC visible; diagnosis known

(Left) Coronal graphic shows small cholesteatoma originating at pars flaccida portion of the tympanic membrane with filling of Prussak space ➡. Slight erosion ➡ with medial displacement of the head of malleus is present. (Right) Coronal bone CT reveals a small pars flaccida cholesteatoma filling the Prussak space ➡ with blunting of the scutum ➡. The head of the malleus is mildly eroded and medially displaced ➡.

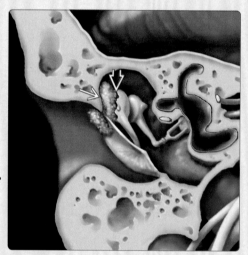
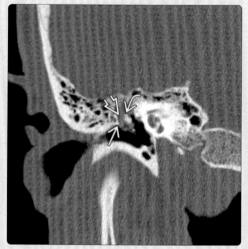

(Left) Coronal graphic shows a large pars flaccida cholesteatoma. Complications include erosion of ossicles, dehiscence of the lateral semicircular canal ➡, & scalloping of the tegmen tympani ➡. (Right) Coronal bone CT shows a large pars flaccida cholesteatoma as a soft tissue mass within the right middle ear and mastoid cavity. There is fistulation with the lateral semicircular canal ➡. Cholesteatoma is also visible protruding through the tympanic membrane perforation into the external auditory canal ➡.

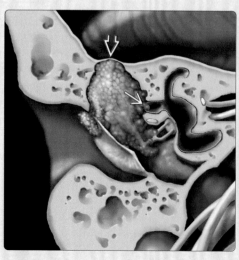
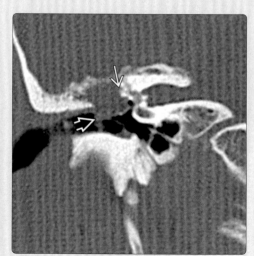

Pars Flaccida Cholesteatoma

TERMINOLOGY

Abbreviations
- Pars flaccida cholesteatoma (PFC)

Synonyms
- "Attic" or "Prussak space" cholesteatoma
- Primary acquired cholesteatoma

Definitions
- Focal accumulation of exfoliated keratin within stratified squamous epithelium, begins in Prussak space

IMAGING

General Features
- Best diagnostic clue
  - Soft tissue mass starts in Prussak space with scutum, ossicle, or lateral epitympanum wall erosion
- Location
  - From Prussak space, spreads to posterior epitympanum, posterior mesotympanum, and, less commonly, anterior epitympanum
- Size
  - From millimeters (early) to centimeters (late)
  - If neglected, may fill entire middle ear (ME) cavity & beyond
- Morphology
  - Well-circumscribed ME mass
  - Soft tissue density
  - Large lesions often associated with scar & effusion; may be less well defined

CT Findings
- CECT
  - No enhancement of cholesteatoma
    - Surrounding granulation tissue may enhance
- Bone CT
  - **Small PFC**
    - Soft tissue mass starts in **Prussak space**
    - Ossicular chain erosion in 70%
      - Long process of incus erosion more common than incus body & malleus head erosion
    - Ossicles medially displaced
    - Scutum erosion common
    - Caveat: Small cholesteatoma without bone erosion can be nonspecific on bone CT
  - **Large PFC**
    - Local extension
      - Superior extension into Prussak space & remaining epitympanum
      - Posterolateral through aditus ad antrum into mastoid antrum
      - Expansion and scalloping of ME & mastoid cavity
    - Important potential bone erosions/complications
      - Lateral semicircular canal/labyrinthine fistula
      - Tegmentum tympani & mastoideum/intracranial extension ± infection
      - CNVII canal, tympanic segment/CNVII injury
      - Focal erosions around oval or round window

MR Findings
- T1WI
  - Hypointense ME mass
- T2WI
  - Homogeneously hyperintense ME mass
- DWI
  - Hyperintense at high b values, may show true **reduced diffusivity**, as in other types of cholesteatoma or epidermoid
  - Non-echo-planar (HASTE, PROPELLER, & BLADE) DWI superior to conventional echo-planar (EP) DWI
    - May obviate need for exploratory surgery in high-risk retraction pockets or 2nd-look revision surgery
- T1WI C+
  - Nonenhancing except for peripheral rim of granulation tissue
  - If tegmen tympani erosion present, dural enhancement at bony defect

Imaging Recommendations
- Best imaging tool
  - Temporal bone CT without contrast = 1st-line test
    - Coronal CTs best show Prussak space mass, attic, and scutum
  - Temporal bone MR complementary; higher sensitivity & specificity than CT
    - Reduced diffusivity confirms PFC, delineates residual/recurrent PFC from postoperative granulation, debris
    - T1 C+ shows nonenhancing cholesteatoma vs. enhancing inflammatory tissues
      - Extratemporal infection (abscess, empyema) easily diagnosed
- Protocol advice
  - Non-echo-planar DWI more sensitive than EP DWI, less susceptibility artifact from aerated ME-mastoid
    - Reportedly detects lesion as small as 2 mm

DIFFERENTIAL DIAGNOSIS

Acquired Pars Tensa Cholesteatoma
- Otoscopy: Tympanic membrane (TM) rupture or retraction in posterosuperior pars tensa area
- Less common than pars flaccida (PF) type
- Bone CT: Sinus tympani & facial recess involvement are classic
  - Ossicles pushed laterally

Middle Ear Congenital Cholesteatoma
- Otoscopy: Tan-white mass behind **intact** TM
- Bone CT: Nondependent ME mass
  - Medial to ossicles ± ossicle erosions

Middle Ear Cholesterol Granuloma
- Otoscopy: Retrotympanic "blue" mass
- Bone CT: Ossicular & bony erosions may be similar to cholesteatoma
- MR: **Hyperintense** on T1, no reduced diffusivity

Glomus Tympanicum Paraganglioma
- Otoscopy: Retrotympanic red, pulsatile mass

- Bone CT: Focal mass on cochlear promontory; ME floor intact
- MR: T1 C+ shows avidly enhancing tumor

PATHOLOGY

General Features

- Etiology
  - Beginning at PF portion of TM
    - PF = small posterosuperior portion of TM
  - Various theories on pathogenesis
  - Retraction pocket theory (RPT), basal hyperplasia theories (BHT), & epithelial migration theory (EMT) relate best with PFC
    - RPT: Eustachian tube dysfunction → negative ME pressure → PF retraction pocket → accumulation of keratin debris → superinfection + inflammation
    - BHT: Inflammation & epidermal hyperplasia breaks basement membrane → subepithelial invasion + keratinocytic proliferation
    - EMT: Squamous epithelium of TM, particularly PF has propensity for active proliferation and medial migration when stimulated by inflammatory reaction, typically otitis media
  - Squamous epithelium + keratin accumulation forms cholesteatoma
  - Precursor retraction pocket not required for PF cholesteatoma formation, although commonly seen

Gross Pathologic & Surgical Features

- "Pearly tumor," composed of soft, waxy, white-gray or pale yellow material
- Chronic inflammatory change always present
- Erosion of ossicles, scutum, and upper part of bony tympanic annulus visible in most cases

Microscopic Features

- Stratified squamous epithelium with anucleated (dead) keratin squames
  - Content high in cholesterol crystals
- Layer of granulation tissue always present when in contact with bone
  - Seems to be cause of bone erosion

CLINICAL ISSUES

Presentation

- Most common signs/symptoms
  - Foul-smelling aural discharge
  - Conductive hearing loss (CHL)
  - Chronic ME inflammatory disease & TM retraction or perforation
- Other signs/symptoms
  - Noise- or pressure-induced vertigo (**Tullio phenomenon**) if lateral semicircular canal dehisced
- Otologic examination
  - TM retraction pocket or perforation at PF
    - If TM perforation: PFC visible
    - If TM retracted: PFC often not visible → utility of non-echo-planar DWI MR

Demographics

- Age

- May occur in children or adults
- Unusual in children < 4 years
- Cholesteatoma in children more aggressive
  - Extensive disease & recurrence common
- Epidemiology
  - Most common ME-mastoid lesion
  - Most common type of cholesteatoma (**80%** of all **acquired cholesteatomas**)

Natural History & Prognosis

- Progressive ↑ in size of cholesteatoma
  - Increasing destruction of surrounding structures, including ossicular chain, lateral semicircular canal, tegmen tympani
- CNVII involvement, venous sinus thrombosis, & intracranial extension are late complications
- Small cholesteatoma: Excellent for total eradication with normal long-term hearing
- Large cholesteatoma: Residual CHL is possible
- Recurrence rate is 5-10%

Treatment

- Early treatment of retraction pocket with tympanostomy tube may prevent cholesteatoma formation
- Surgery includes mastoidectomy & formation of common cavity between mastoid antrum & EAC
  - TM & ossicle reconstruction necessary
  - Treatment aimed at clearing cholesteatoma & infection to prevent further damage
  - Hearing improvement is secondary goal

DIAGNOSTIC CHECKLIST

Consider

- 2 clinical presentations for imaging possible cholesteatoma
  - Patient has **visible cholesteatoma**
    - Referring clinician wants to know extent & complications
  - Patient has **visible TM retraction pocket + CHL**
    - Referring clinician wants to know if cholesteatoma is present
    - Caution: If ME soft tissue seen without bone or ossicle erosion, do not suggest cholesteatoma

Image Interpretation Pearls

- When ME & mastoid completely opacified with no ossicular erosion, most likely ME effusion, not cholesteatoma

Reporting Tips

- Sinus tympani extension associated with high postoperative recurrence rate
- Lateral semicircular canal fistula & CNVII canal dehiscence warrant cautious operation

SELECTED REFERENCES

1. Li PM et al: Evaluating the utility of non-echo-planar diffusion-weighted imaging in the preoperative evaluation of cholesteatoma: a meta-analysis. Laryngoscope. 123(5):1247-50, 2013
2. Más-Estellés F et al: Contemporary non-echo-planar diffusion-weighted imaging of middle ear cholesteatomas. Radiographics. 32(4):1197-213, 2012
3. Swartz JD: Cholesteatomas of the middle ear. Diagnosis, etiology, and complications. Radiol Clin North Am. 22(1):15-35, 1984

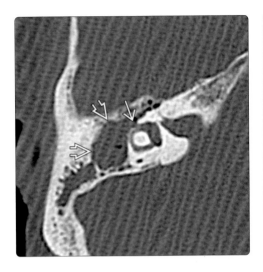

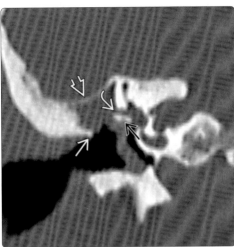

(Left) *Axial bone CT reveals a large cholesteatoma in the middle ear cavity with scalloping of the walls ➡. There is erosion of the anterior portion of the lateral semicircular canal with fistulation ➡.* (Right) *Coronal bone CT of the same patient shows that the tegmen tympani is thinned ➡ and that the lateral semicircular canal is dehiscent ➡. Saucerization of the bony tympanic CNVII canal ➡ and blunting of the scutum ➡ are also present.*

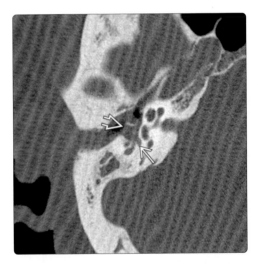

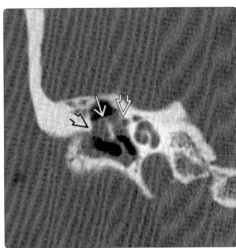

(Left) *Axial bone CT demonstrates soft tissue mass filling the tympanic cavity ➡. The soft tissue extends to the sinus tympani ➡, which is an important checkpoint as it is a surgical blind spot and often a site of recurrence. The long process of incus is eroded (not shown).* (Right) *Coronal bone CT in the same patient shows epitympanic cholesteatoma with scutum blunting ➡. The malleus is medially displaced and partially eroded ➡. The lesion abuts but does not erode into anterior tympanic CNVII ➡.*

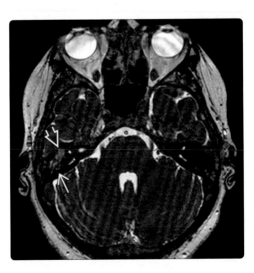

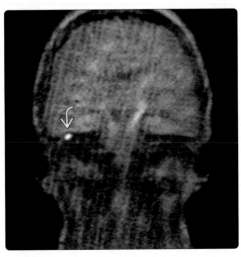

(Left) *Axial CISS in patient with pars flaccida cholesteatoma reveals slightly hyperintense fluid/soft tissue extending from Prussak space to epitympanum ➡, indistinguishable in signal intensity from mastoid effusion ➡.* (Right) *Coronal HASTE DWI demonstrates marked hyperintensity ➡, confirming cholesteatoma. Non-echo-planar diffusion pulse sequences are less degraded by susceptibility effects common to the mastoid and middle ear and are more sensitive for detection of cholesteatoma.*

Pars Tensa Cholesteatoma

TERMINOLOGY

- Abbreviation: Pars tensa cholesteatoma (PTC)
- Synonym: Secondary acquired cholesteatoma
- Definition
  - Focal accumulation of exfoliated keratin within stratified squamous epithelium at site of perforation or retraction pocket at pars tensa tympanic membrane (TM)

IMAGING

- Bone CT findings
  - Erosive mass in **posterior mesotympanum**
  - Usually found **medial** to ossicles
  - May involve sinus tympani, facial recess, and aditus ad antrum ± mastoid
  - Ossicular erosion is common along medial incus long process, stapes superstructure, and manubrium of malleus
- Axial and coronal temporal bone CT are studies of choice
- MR adjunctive; answers issues raised by bone CT

- Non-echo-planar DWI superior to conventional echo-planar DWI
  - May obviate need for 2nd-look surgery

TOP DIFFERENTIAL DIAGNOSES

- Middle ear congenital cholesteatoma
- Pars flaccida-acquired cholesteatoma
- Middle ear cholesterol granuloma
- Glomus tympanicum paraganglioma

PATHOLOGY

- Most believe is related to TM perforation at pars tensa
- Migrated/implanted epithelium through TM perforation → nidus of stratified squamous epithelium with keratin squames in middle ear → cholesteatoma

CLINICAL ISSUES

- **10-20%** of all middle ear cholesteatomas
- Significantly less common than pars flaccida cholesteatoma

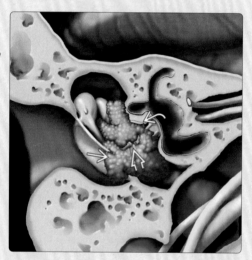
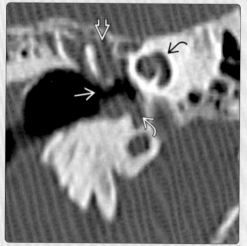

(Left) Coronal graphic of pars tensa cholesteatoma (PTC) shows the cholesteatoma extending laterally through an inferior tympanic membrane (TM) rupture ➡. The middle ear PTC erodes ossicles ➡, invades and flattens the tympanic CNVII canal ➡, and is primarily medial to the ossicles. (Right) Coronal bone CT at the level of the cochlea ▱ demonstrates a pars tensa TM perforation ➡. The most anterior aspect of the PTC is seen above ➡ and below ➡ the perforation in the middle ear cavity.

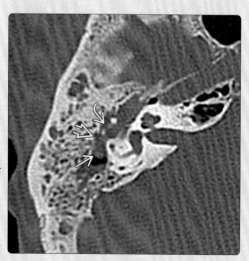
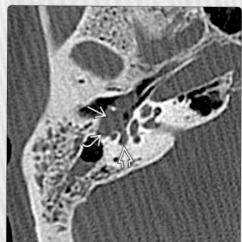

(Left) Axial bone CT in the same patient reveals the PTC eroding the short process of the incus ➡ and extending through the aditus ad antrum ➡ into the mastoid antrum ➡. (Right) Axial bone CT at the level of the oval window reveals erosion of the incus and hub of the stapes ➡, with invasion of the facial nerve recess ➡ and sinus tympani ➡. Sinus tympani involvement must be reported, as this area is blind to the surgeon and may serve as nidus for recurrence if unnoticed.

Pars Tensa Cholesteatoma

TERMINOLOGY

Abbreviations
- Pars tensa cholesteatoma (PTC)
- Middle ear (ME)

Synonyms
- Sinus cholesteatoma, due to involvement of sinus tympani
- Secondary acquired cholesteatoma

Definitions
- Focal accumulation of exfoliated keratin within stratified squamous epithelium at site of perforation or retraction pocket at pars tensa portion of tympanic membrane (TM)
  - "Tense" lower 2/3 of TM

IMAGING

General Features
- Best diagnostic clue
  - Erosive mass in posterior mesotympanum involving sinus tympani, facial nerve recess, and aditus ad antrum ± mastoid
- Location
  - Posterior mesotympanum
    - Spread posteromedially
    - In part, **medial to ossicles**
- Size
  - From several millimeters to 2-3 cm
  - Large PTC fills ME cavity
- Morphology
  - Lobular, well-circumscribed, soft tissue density mass
  - Nonenhancing, with ossicular or bone erosion
    - Bone erosion has multiple causes
      □ Inflammatory enzymatic dissolution of bone
      □ Pressure-induced bone resorption from expanding PTC

CT Findings
- CECT
  - Nonenhancing soft tissue mass
- Bone CT
  - **Small PTC**
    - Soft tissue mass begins at **posterior mesotympanum**
    - Most commonly begins at sinus tympani and facial nerve recess
    - Mass projects **medial** to ossicular chain
    - Subtle lateral displacement of ossicles
    - Early ossicular erosion from medial aspect
  - **Large PTC**
    - Fills ME cavity
    - Invades mastoid through widened aditus ad antrum
    - Ossicular erosion common
      □ Along medial incus long process, stapes superstructure, and manubrium of malleus
    - Posterior tegmen tympani and anterior tegmen mastoideum dehiscence may occur

MR Findings
- T1WI
  - Hypointense ME mass
- T2WI
  - PTC usually high signal
    - Trapped secretions of mastoid higher signal than PTC
- DWI
  - Hyperintense at high b values; may show true **reduced diffusivity**, as in other types of cholesteatoma or epidermoid)
  - Non-echo-planar (HASTE, PROPELLER, and BLADE) DWI superior to conventional echo-planar DWI;may obviate need for 2nd-look surgery
- T1WI C+
  - PTC itself **does not enhance**
  - Granulation tissue and other scar may enhance
  - Delayed (45-60 minutes) imaging may help discriminate nonenhancing PTC from surrounding inflammation, granulation, or scar
  - If tegmen erosion present, dural enhancement at bony defect
  - Shows intracranial complications

Imaging Recommendations
- Best imaging tool
  - Axial and coronal temporal bone CT is study of choice
  - T1 C+ MR to answer specific issues raised by bone CT
    - Temporal lobe extension, subperiosteal or intracranial abscess, meningitis, labyrinthitis, lateral sinus thrombosis
    - Enhancement of labyrinth suggests labyrinthitis

DIFFERENTIAL DIAGNOSIS

Middle Ear Congenital Cholesteatoma
- Otoscopy: White mass behind intact TM in children
- Bone CT: Often located posteriorly (like PTC)

Pars Flaccida-Acquired Cholesteatoma
- Otoscopy: Pars flaccida perforation or retraction pocket
- Bone CT: Prussak space mass with erosion of scutum, lateral body of incus, and head of malleus; ossicles pushed medially

Middle Ear Cholesterol Granuloma
- Otoscopy: Blue mass behind intact TM
- Bone CT: Ossicular and bony erosions may mimic cholesteatoma
- T1 MR: Hyperintense mass

Glomus Tympanicum Paraganglioma
- Otoscopy: Cherry red pulsatile mass behind intact TM
- Bone CT: Mass on cochlear promontory without ossicular erosion
- T1 C+ MR: Intense enhancement of mass

PATHOLOGY

General Features
- Etiology
  - Migration theory: TM perforation → migration of TM epidermis to ME
  - Implantation theory: Implantation of TM epidermis behind healed TM perforation, temporal bone fracture, or ME surgical site
  - Migrated/implanted stratified squamous epithelium with keratin squames is nidus of cholesteatoma

Gross Pathologic & Surgical Features

- "Pearly" tumor seen at surgery
- Well-circumscribed, soft, waxy, white material

Microscopic Features

- Stratified squamous epithelium with anucleated (dead) keratin squames
- Same histology as epidermoid and any cholesteatoma elsewhere in body

CLINICAL ISSUES

Presentation

- Most common signs/symptoms
  - Can be asymptomatic
  - History of chronic otitis media ± TM perforation
  - Progressive unilateral conductive hearing loss
  - Foul-smelling otorrhea due to infection
- Other signs/symptoms
  - Noise- or pressure-induced vertigo if labyrinthine fistula present
    - Most common at basal turn of cochlea
  - Facial nerve paresis or palsy
    - Due to pressure effect (slow onset), infection (acute onset), CNVII canal erosion
      - CNVII canal erosion more common in PTC than pars flaccida cholesteatoma
  - Otalgia, headache
    - If infected ± intracranial complication
- Otologic examination
  - Retraction pocket, perforation, or visible cholesteatoma at pars tensa
  - Edema, granulation tissue, aural polyp representing chronic inflammation
  - Sensorineural hearing loss suspicious for complication with labyrinthine fistula

Demographics

- Age
  - Occurs in children and adults
- Gender
  - M = F
- Ethnicity
  - Rare lesion in Eskimo, American Indian, and Australian children, despite ME infections
- Epidemiology
  - **10-20%** of all ME cholesteatomas
  - Significantly less common than pars flaccida cholesteatoma

Natural History & Prognosis

- Progressive enlargement with growing symptom complex due to local extension
- Small lesion
  - Excellent for total eradication and normal hearing
- Large lesion
  - Residual conductive hearing loss common
- Postoperative recurrence rate ~ 10%

Treatment

- Surgical removal of cholesteatoma requires mastoidectomy
  - Formation of common cavity between mastoid antrum and EAC
  - Canal wall up surgery: Posterior wall EAC not removed
  - Canal wall down surgery: Posterior wall EAC removed
- TM and ossicular reconstruction required for hearing restoration if ossicular chain involved

DIAGNOSTIC CHECKLIST

Consider

- PTC if CT shows that ME mass is **centered posteriorly**, extends **medial to ossicles**, and displaces ossicles laterally
- Consider PTC if bone CT shows medial ossicle erosion

Image Interpretation Pearls

- Axial and coronal CT show location and local extension best
- MR differentiates PTC from effusion, granulation, cholesterol granuloma, and glomus tympanicum
  - Enhanced T1 MR shows intracranial complication or labyrinthitis if suspected

Reporting Tips

- Sinus tympani involvement is often site of recurrence
- Presence of labyrinthine fistula, degree of posterior canal wall erosion, and mastoid aeration/sclerosis affects choice of operation
- Facial nerve canal erosion and tegmen dehiscence important for preoperative planning
- Intracranial complication requires urgent attention

SELECTED REFERENCES

1. van Egmond SL et al: A systematic review of non-echo planar diffusion-weighted magnetic resonance imaging for detection of primary and postoperative cholesteatoma. Otolaryngol Head Neck Surg. 154(2):233-40, 2016
2. Shinnabe A et al: Differences in clinical characteristics of fallopian canal dehiscence associated with pars flaccida and pars tensa cholesteatomas. Eur Arch Otorhinolaryngol. 271(8):2171-5, 2014
3. Más-Estellés F et al: Contemporary non-echo-planar diffusion-weighted imaging of middle ear cholesteatomas. Radiographics. 32(4):1197-213, 2012
4. Baráth K et al: Neuroradiology of cholesteatomas. AJNR Am J Neuroradiol. 32(2):221-9, 2011
5. Vercruysse JP et al: Magnetic resonance imaging of cholesteatoma: an update. B-ENT. 5(4):233-40, 2009
6. Jeunen G et al: The value of magnetic resonance imaging in the diagnosis of residual or recurrent acquired cholesteatoma after canal wall-up tympanoplasty. Otol Neurotol. 29(1):16-8, 2008
7. De Foer B et al: The value of single-shot turbo spin-echo diffusion-weighted MR imaging in the detection of middle ear cholesteatoma. Neuroradiology. 49(10):841-8, 2007
8. Vercruysse JP et al: The value of diffusion-weighted MR imaging in the diagnosis of primary acquired and residual cholesteatoma: a surgical verified study of 100 patients. Eur Radiol. 16(7):1461-7, 2006
9. Aikele P et al: Diffusion-weighted MR imaging of cholesteatoma in pediatric and adult patients who have undergone middle ear surgery. AJR Am J Roentgenol. 181(1):261-5, 2003
10. Gocmen H et al: Surgical treatment of cholesteatoma in children. Int J Pediatr Otorhinolaryngol. 67(8):867-72, 2003
11. Minor LB: Labyrinthine fistulae: pathobiology and management. Curr Opin Otolaryngol Head Neck Surg. 11(5):340-6, 2003
12. Williams MT et al: Detection of postoperative residual cholesteatoma with delayed contrast-enhanced MR imaging: initial findings. Eur Radiol. 13(1):169-74, 2003
13. Shohet JA et al: The management of pediatric cholesteatoma. Otolaryngol Clin North Am. 35(4):841-51, 2002
14. Yates PD et al: CT scanning of middle ear cholesteatoma: what does the surgeon want to know? Br J Radiol. 75(898):847-52, 2002

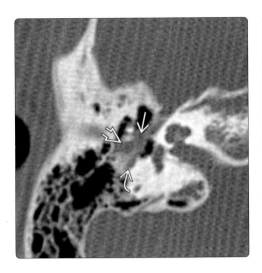
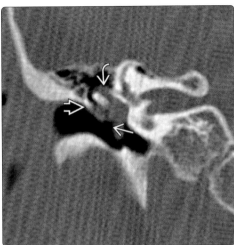

(Left) *Axial temporal bone CT reveals a smaller middle ear PTC, medial to ossicles ➡, eroding the short process of the incus ➡ and filling the sinus tympani ➡.* (Right) *Coronal temporal bone CT in the same patient shows a PTC surrounding the ossicles emanating from a tympanic membrane perforation ➡. The scutum remains intact ➡, and the bulk of the lesion is medial to the ossicles ➡, both features supporting a diagnosis of PTC.*

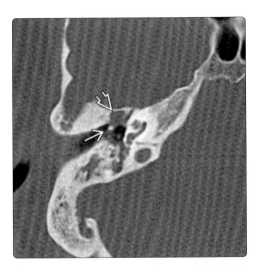
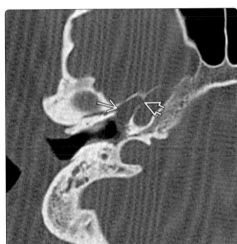

(Left) *Axial bone CT through the low mesotympanum shows thickening of the lower TM ➡ with expansile bony changes ➡ in the anterior mesotympanum. Note the underpneumatized mastoid secondary to chronic otomastoiditis.* (Right) *Axial bone CT in the same patient reveals low mesotympanum opacification with bony eustachian tube expansile remodeling ➡ along with subtle focal erosion ➡ of the lateral petrous IAC wall. PTC began in the anteroinferior TM and extended into the eustachian tube.*

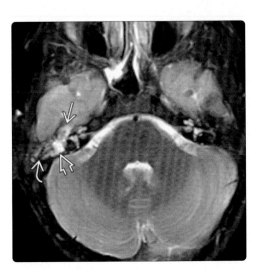
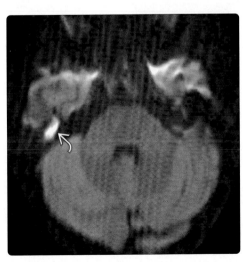

(Left) *Axial T2 FS MR in patient with chronic otitis media and PTC on otoscopic exam shows filling of the middle ear ➡ and mastoid antrum ➡ with T2 hyperintensity, as well as high signal in the mastoid air cells ➡. T2 alone cannot differentiate ear effusion from cholesteatoma.* (Right) *Axial DTI trace MR in same patient shows reduced diffusivity as marked signal hyperintensity within the middle ear and mastoid antrum ➡, differentiating cholesteatoma from background mastoid effusion.*

Mural Cholesteatoma

TERMINOLOGY

- Synonyms: Automastoidectomy; "shell" or "rind" cholesteatoma
- Rare variant of acquired cholesteatoma
- Definition: Residual cholesteatoma "rind" left behind after acquired middle ear-mastoid cholesteatoma extrudes central matrix through dehiscent **EAC bony wall**

IMAGING

- Temporal bone CT findings
  - Mastoidectomy cavity with residual soft tissue rind along cavity wall **without** history of mastoidectomy
  - Large lesion can fistulize any area of inner ear
  - Focal dehiscence of posterior or superior EAC wall

TOP DIFFERENTIAL DIAGNOSES

- Coalescent mastoiditis
- Mastoidectomy
- Keratosis obturans with automastoidectomy

PATHOLOGY

- Rind of tissue found along wall of cavity
- Only "lining" of cholesteatoma seen by pathologist
- Microscopic features: Aggressive keratinizing stratified squamous epithelium

CLINICAL ISSUES

- Long history of chronic otitis media **without** mastoidectomy
- May report material "falling out of ear"
- Older patient with chronically draining ear

DIAGNOSTIC CHECKLIST

- CT findings suggest mastoidectomy but none has occurred: Automastoidectomy
- Check for ossicle destruction, inner ear or CNVII canal dehiscence, EAC wall erosion

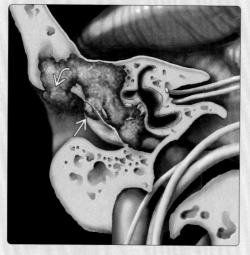
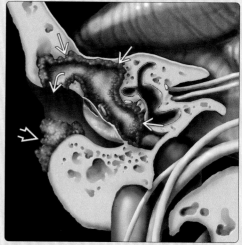

(Left) Coronal graphic shows a large cholesteatoma beginning at a pars flaccida perforation ➡. The lesion has eroded the middle ear walls, ossicles, mastoid cavity, and EAC bony walls ➡. (Right) Coronal graphic reveals that the large cholesteatoma in the previous drawing has evacuated its central material through the EAC dehiscence ➡ into the external ear canal ➡. A mural cholesteatoma is left behind as a cholesteatoma "rind" along the walls of the middle ear and mastoid ➡.

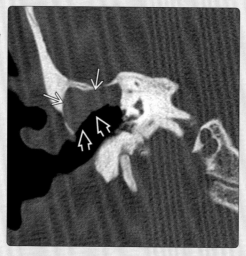
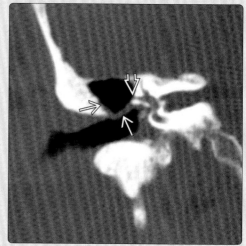

(Left) Coronal temporal bone CT demonstrates a partially extruded mural cholesteatoma ➡ in an enlarged mastoid cavity with a broad EAC posterosuperior wall dehiscence ➡. (Right) Coronal temporal bone CT shows a thin-walled mural cholesteatoma ➡ in a hollowed out mastoid cavity. Lateral semicircular canal dehiscence ➡ is present. The thickness of the mural cholesteatoma "rind" is dependent on the amount of the lesion that has been extruded.

Mural Cholesteatoma

TERMINOLOGY

Synonyms

- Automastoidectomy; "shell" or "rind" cholesteatoma

Definitions

- Residual cholesteatoma "rind" left behind after acquired middle ear-mastoid cholesteatoma extrudes central matrix through dehiscent **EAC bony wall**

IMAGING

General Features

- Best diagnostic clue
  - Mastoidectomy cavity with residual soft tissue along cavity wall **without** history of mastoidectomy
- Location
  - Middle ear & mastoid
- Size
  - Cholesteatoma "**rind**" of variable thickness

CT Findings

- Bone CT
  - "Hollowed out" middle ear-mastoid with residual **cholesteatoma** "**rind**" seen along walls of cavity
    - Variably sized mastoid cavity
  - Common cavity connects middle ear & antrum
  - Ossicles usually destroyed
  - Scutum severely truncated
  - Labyrinthine fistula often present
    - Lateral semicircular canal most common

MR Findings

- T1WI
  - Mastoid cavity appears identical to surgical defect
    - May be complicated by cephalocele
- DWI
  - Residual cholesteatoma markedly hyperintense
- T1WI C+
  - Peripheral enhancement along margin of cavity if granulation tissue present

Imaging Recommendations

- Best imaging tool
  - Temporal bone CT study of choice
- Protocol advice
  - Temporal bone CT in axial & coronal planes
  - MR with T1 C+ & DWI reserved for complicated cases

DIFFERENTIAL DIAGNOSIS

Coalescent Mastoiditis

- Middle ear cavity not enlarged
- Mastoid air cells confluent with acute otitis media
- Middle ear & mastoid completely opacified

Mastoidectomy

- Posterolateral wall of mastoid absent
- Surgical history is known

Keratosis Obturans With Automastoidectomy

- Soft tissue filling EAC ± osseous expansion
- Rare reported cases of dehiscence and automastoidectomy

PATHOLOGY

General Features

- Etiology
  - Acquired cholesteatoma begins in middle ear
  - Enlargement of cholesteatoma fills entire middle ear cavity ± mastoid antrum
  - Pressure built up with further cholesteatoma growth relieved by expulsion of content through EAC dehiscence or tympanic membrane (TM) perforation
  - Cholesteatoma matrix extrudes through perforated TM or directly into EAC
  - Outer shell/erosive membrane persists after drainage
  - Continued cavity growth from enzymatic activity

Gross Pathologic & Surgical Features

- Cholesteatoma "rind" found along wall of cavity

Microscopic Features

- Only "lining" of cholesteatoma viewable
- Aggressive keratinizing stratified squamous epithelium

CLINICAL ISSUES

Presentation

- Most common signs/symptoms
  - Long history of chronic otitis media
    - No history of mastoidectomy
    - May report material "falling out of ear"
  - Otologic exam
    - May be seen as TM perforation or draining sinus through EAC wall

Demographics

- Age
  - Usually in older patient
- Epidemiology
  - Rare variant form of acquired cholesteatoma (pars flaccida > pars tensa > mural)

Natural History & Prognosis

- Restoration of hearing difficult because of complete ossicle destruction & bone erosion

Treatment

- Surgery depends on lesion size and extent
  - Excision of tissue lining the cavity is imperative

DIAGNOSTIC CHECKLIST

Consider

- Imaging findings suggest mastoidectomy has occurred
  - **No** history of mastoidectomy; hence term **automastoidectomy**

Image Interpretation Pearls

- EAC dehiscence along with "hollowed out" mastoid + mastoid "rind" = mural cholesteatoma

SELECTED REFERENCES

1. Blake DM et al: Automastoidectomy. Ear Nose Throat J. 93(6):E53-4, 2014
2. Manasawala M et al: Imaging findings in auto-atticotomy. AJNR Am J Neuroradiol. 35(1):182-5, 2014

Middle Ear Cholesterol Granuloma

TERMINOLOGY

- Cholesterol granuloma (CG): Recurrent hemorrhage into middle ear (ME) cavity causes inflammatory mass of granulation tissue

IMAGING

- Bone CT: Smoothly **expansile mass** of ME ± mastoid air cells
- MR: **High T1** and T2 signal in ME

TOP DIFFERENTIAL DIAGNOSES

- Dehiscent jugular bulb
- Aberrant internal carotid artery
- Chronic otitis media + hemorrhage
- Pars flaccida-acquired cholesteatoma
- Paraganglioma
  - Glomus tympanicum paraganglioma
  - Glomus jugulare paraganglioma
- Encephalocele of ME

- Traumatic hemotympanum

CLINICAL ISSUES

- Clinical presentation
  - Symptoms: Conductive hearing loss
  - Otoscopy: Nonpulsating bluish discoloration of tympanic membrane = "blue" eardrum
  - Symptoms arise years after initial otitis media
- Treatment options
  - Initial surgery: Resection of wall and contents
  - Intractable disease: Mastoidectomy + ventilation tube
- Natural history
  - Most ME CGs grow over decades
- Recurrence rates for ME CG are much lower than for petrous apex CG

DIAGNOSTIC CHECKLIST

- "Blue" tympanic membrane + **expansile** bone changes (on bone CT) + **high T1** (on MR) = CG of ME

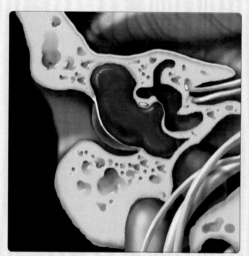
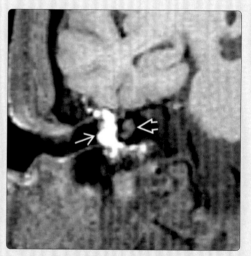

(Left) Coronal graphic depicts a large middle ear cholesterol granuloma. The entire middle ear is filled with dark brown ("chocolate") fluid with the ossicles no longer present. Otoscopy reveals a "blue-black" eardrum. (Right) Coronal T1WI MR demonstrates a retrotympanic high-signal cholesterol granuloma ➡ that causes the tympanic membrane to bulge into the external auditory canal. Notice the signal of the cochlea medially ➡. The cholesterol granuloma fills the entire middle ear cavity.

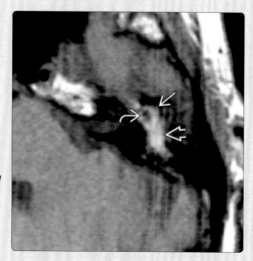
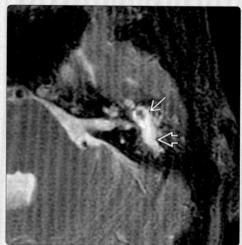

(Left) Axial T1WI MR in a patient with a "blue-black" retrotympanic lesion shows a high-signal cholesterol granuloma filling the middle ear ➡ and mastoid antrum ➡. Note the low-signal head of malleus and short process of incus ➡ visible within the lesion. (Right) Axial T2WI fat-saturated MR in the same patient reveals hyperintense cholesterol granuloma in the epitympanum ➡ and mastoid antrum ➡. Early-phase disease preserves the ossicles and shows no evidence of bony scalloping.

TERMINOLOGY

Abbreviations

- Cholesterol granuloma (CG)

Synonyms

- Cholesterol cyst, "chocolate" cyst, blue-dome cyst

Definitions

- Recurrent hemorrhage into middle ear (ME) cavity causes inflammatory mass of granulation tissue

IMAGING

General Features

- Best diagnostic clue
  - Bone CT: Smoothly **expansile mass** of ME ± mastoid cells
  - MR: **High T1** and T2 signal in ME
- Location
  - CG most commonly arises in ME
    - Also occurs in petrous apex (PA) and orbit
- Size
  - Depends on chronicity; millimeters to centimeters
- Morphology
  - Expansile nature critical to diagnosis

CT Findings

- CECT
  - May be useful to distinguish small CG from glomus tympanicum paraganglioma, which enhances briskly
- Bone CT
  - Early CG-ME bone CT findings
    - Small ME mass
    - No ossicular loss or bone remodeling
    - Difficult to make specific diagnosis
  - Late CG-ME bone CT findings
    - Opacified ME and mastoid
    - **Expansile bony changes** with scalloping
    - Ossicular displacement ± destruction

MR Findings

- T1WI
  - ↑ **signal** from paramagnetic effect of **methemoglobin**
- T2WI
  - Central ↑ signal from granulation tissue
  - Peripheral ↓ signal from hemosiderin deposition
- STIR
  - Follows T2 signal
- T1WI C+ FS
  - Inherent high T1 signal confused with enhancement
    - Compare to unenhanced T1WI
- MRA
  - May be useful to distinguish CG from vascular anomalies [e.g., aberrant internal carotid artery (ICA)]
    - CT preferred to eliminate vascular lesions

Imaging Recommendations

- Best imaging tool
  - Temporal bone CT initially
    - MR used in larger lesions
- Protocol advice
  - Remember to use axial and coronal T1 MR prior to contrast when CG ME suspected

DIFFERENTIAL DIAGNOSIS

Dehiscent Jugular Bulb

- Otoscopy: Blue-black mass in ME
- Bone CT: Absence of thin bone between jugular bulb and hypotympanum
  - Diverticulum of jugular vein extends into ME
- Thin-section CT needed for diagnosis
  - Both axial and reconstructed coronal planes useful

Aberrant Internal Carotid Artery

- Otoscopy: Pink, pulsatile mass in ME
- Bone CT: Tubular mass crosses ME cavity to rejoin horizontal petrous ICA
  - Large inferior tympanic canaliculus
- Enlarged collateral vessel traverses ME when ICA fails to develop

Chronic Otitis Media + Hemorrhage

- Otoscopy: Inflammatory tissue and blood in ME ± ruptured tympanic membrane (TM)
- Bone CT: Inflammatory tissue and blood fill ME **without** expansile bony changes
- MR: Variable T1 and T2 signal

Pars Flaccida-Acquired Cholesteatoma

- Otoscopy: TM retraction-rupture ± visible cholesteatoma
- Bone CT: Erosive ME-mastoid mass with ossicle loss
- MR: Low T1 and high T2; rim enhances on T1 C+
- Like CG-ME, associated with recurrent prior infections ± effusions
- Microscopic: Cholesteatoma lined by squamous epithelium
  - CG-ME lined with fibrous connective tissue

Paraganglioma

- Otoscopy: Red mass in middle ear
- Bone CT
  - Glomus tympanicum paraganglioma
    - On cochlear promontory
  - Glomus jugulare paraganglioma
    - Permeative bone changes, jugular foramen to ME

Encephalocele of Middle Ear

- Surgical view: Can mimic CG-ME strongly
- Bone CT: Dehiscent tegmen tympani with brain herniation into ME or mastoid cavity
- MR: Coronal T2 may define contents
- Usually posttraumatic or postsurgical

Traumatic Hemotympanum

- Otoscopy: Blood in ME from recent trauma
- Bone CT: Associated temporal bone fractures
- MR: High T1 methemoglobin does not expand ME
  - No obstruction as with CG-ME

PATHOLOGY

General Features

- Etiology
  - Still not definite

- o Obstruction-vacuum hypothesis
  - − Chronic otitis media, cholesteatoma, or previous surgery obstructs air cells of ME ± mastoid air cells
  - − Resorption of gas in obstructed air cells creates relative vacuum
  - − Decrease in pressure → mucosal engorgement → blood vessel rupture
  - − Anaerobic red blood cell degradation to cholesterol crystals incites multinucleated foreign giant cell response → inflammation with small vessel proliferation → vessel rupture
  - − Granulation tissue forms from repeated hemorrhage, expanding ME ± mastoid
- o Exposed marrow hypothesis
  - − In young adulthood, enlarging mucosa creates bony defects into hematopoietic marrow of temporal bone
  - − Recurrent microhemorrhage → accumulation of red cell degradation products
  - − Anaerobic red blood cell degradation to cholesterol crystals incites multinucleated foreign giant cell response
  - − Obstruction secondary to inflammation, rather than obstruction as primary cause
- Associated abnormalities
  - o Recurrent otitis media or effusion
  - o Cholesteatoma
  - o Benign granulation tissue
- Differences between CG-ME and CG-PA
  - o CG-ME presents with conductive hearing loss; CG-PA presents with facial pain, headache
  - o CG-ME not associated with history of cranial neuropathies; CG-PA associated with neuropathies of CNV-VII
  - o CG-ME has history of recurrent infections; CG-PA has no history of infection
  - o CG-ME has bone erosion late; large CG-PA may have extensive bone erosion
  - o CG-ME occurs in poorly pneumatized temporal bone (result of prior infections); CG-PA occurs in highly pneumatized temporal bone

Gross Pathologic & Surgical Features

- Cystic mass with fibrous capsule, filled with brownish liquid containing old blood and cholesterol crystals
- Fluid described as "crankcase oil" or "chocolate" cyst

Microscopic Features

- Lined by fibrous connective tissue
- Red blood cells
- Multinucleated giant cells surrounding cholesterol crystals embedded in connective tissue
- Hemosiderin-laden macrophages, chronic inflammatory cells, and blood vessels

CLINICAL ISSUES

Presentation

- Most common signs/symptoms
  - o Slowly progressive conductive hearing loss
  - o Other signs/symptoms
    - − Pulsatile tinnitus
    - − "Pressure on ear"

- − Otoscopy: Nonpulsating bluish discoloration of tympanic membrane = "blue" eardrum
- Clinical profile
  - o Younger to middle-aged patient with "blue" eardrum and conductive hearing loss
  - o Easily confused clinically with vascular malformation or vascular tumor
  - o History of recurrent ME infection helpful for diagnosis

Demographics

- Age
  - o Broad age range, beginning in 2nd decade
- Epidemiology
  - o CG-ME much more common than CG-PA

Natural History & Prognosis

- Great variability in growth rate of CG-ME
  - o Depends on frequency and severity of microhemorrhages within lesion
- Most CG-ME grow over decades
  - o Symptoms arise years after initial episodes of otitis media
- Recurrence rates for CG-ME much lower than for CG-PA
  - o Easier surgical exposure
- Clinical prognostic indicator
  - o Protruding TM: Poorer treatment outcome
  - o Retracted TM: Better treatment outcome

Treatment

- Initial surgery: Resection of wall and contents
- Intractable disease: Mastoidectomy + ventilation tube

DIAGNOSTIC CHECKLIST

Consider

- "Blue" TM + expansile changes (CT) + high T1 (MR) = CG-ME

Image Interpretation Pearls

- Do not mistake high T1 signal for enhancement
  - o Compare with unenhanced T1

Reporting Tips

- Note if extension into eustachian tube or mastoid
- Comment on ossicle status

SELECTED REFERENCES

1. Polo R et al: Mastoid cholesterol granuloma with posterior cranial fossa compression. Otol Neurotol. 34(7):e103-4, 2013
2. Shih TY et al: Erosive cholesterol granuloma. Otol Neurotol. 34(4):e26-7, 2013
3. Matsuda Y et al: Analysis of surgical treatment for middle-ear cholesterol granuloma. J Laryngol Otol Suppl. (31):90-6, 2009
4. Maeta M et al: Surgical intervention in middle-ear cholesterol granuloma. J Laryngol Otol. 117(5):344-8, 2003
5. Friedmann I et al: The ultrastructure of cholesterol granuloma of the middle ear: an electron microscope study. The Journal of Laryngology and Otology, 1979; Vol. 93, pp. 433-442. J Laryngol Otol. 116(11):877-81, 2002
6. Kosling S et al: CT and MR imaging after middle ear surgery. Eur J Radiol. 40(2):113-8, 2001
7. Martin N et al: Cholesterol granulomas of the middle ear cavities: MR imaging. Radiology. 172(2):521-5, 1989
8. Palva T et al: Large cholesterol granuloma cysts in the mastoid. Clinical and histopathologic findings. Arch Otolaryngol. 111(12):786-91, 1985

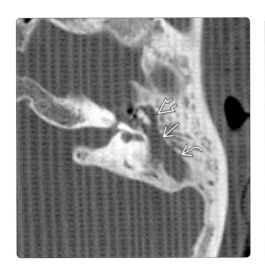

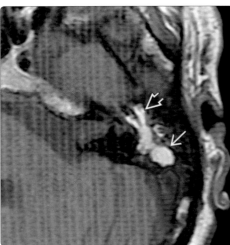

(Left) Axial bone CT shows a soft tissue mass in the epitympanum ⇒, widened aditus ad antrum ⇒, and mastoid antrum ⇒. There is no way to tell that this is a cholesterol granuloma on CT. (Right) Axial T1WI MR in the same patient reveals the high-signal cholesterol granuloma in the middle ear ⇒ and mastoid antrum ⇒. The high signal of this lesion along with the enlarged aditus ad antrum on CT is highly suggestive of the diagnosis of cholesterol granuloma.

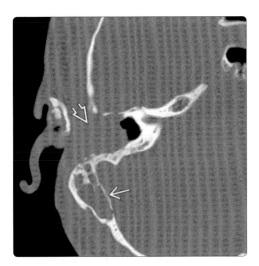

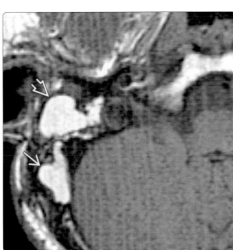

(Left) Axial bone CT reveals a postoperative temporal bone with soft tissue in the mastoid bowl and middle ear ⇒, as well as in the posterior mastoid air cells ⇒. The nature of the soft tissue cannot be determined on CT images. (Right) Axial T1 nonenhanced MR in the same patient shows a bilobed high-signal cholesterol granuloma filling the mastoid bowl ⇒ and the posterior mastoid air cells ⇒.

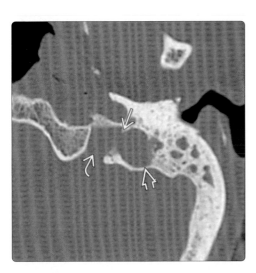

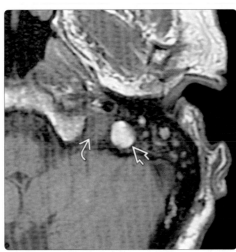

(Left) Axial bone CT in the inferior aspect of the left temporal bone reveals an expansile focus ⇒ just lateral to the jugular foramen ⇒. Notice the dehiscent lateral margin ⇒ of the jugular foramen. (Right) Axial T1WI MR in the same patient shows that the expansile lesion ⇒ just lateral to the jugular foramen ⇒ is high signal without contrast. Surgical exploration revealed a "chocolate" cyst or cholesterol granuloma.

KEY FACTS

TERMINOLOGY

- Abbreviation: Glomus tympanicum paraganglioma (GTP)
- Benign tumor arising from glomus bodies situated on **cochlear promontory**

IMAGING

- Best imaging study: Bone CT without contrast
- CT: Mass with flat base on cochlear promontory
- MR: Enhancing mass with flat base on cochlear promontory
- Floor of middle ear cavity is **intact** (if dehiscent, glomus jugulare paraganglioma)

TOP DIFFERENTIAL DIAGNOSES

- Glomus jugulare paraganglioma
- Aberrant internal carotid artery (AbICA)
- Dehiscent jugular bulb
- Congenital cholesteatoma, middle ear
- Facial nerve schwannoma, tympanic segment

PATHOLOGY

- Arise from glomus (Latin for "ball") bodies (paraganglia) found along inferior tympanic nerve (Jacobson nerve) on cochlear promontory
- GTP is most common tumor of middle ear

CLINICAL ISSUES

- Clinical presentation
  - 40- to 60-year-old woman
  - Vascular retrotympanic mass & pulsatile tinnitus
- Treatment options
  - Surgical resection
  - Approach depends on extent of GTP
- GTP may be clinically indistinguishable from glomus jugulare paraganglioma or AbICA
  - Imaging differentiates GTP from glomus jugulare paraganglioma, AbICA, and dehiscent jugular bulb

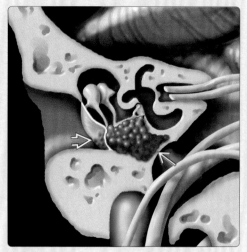
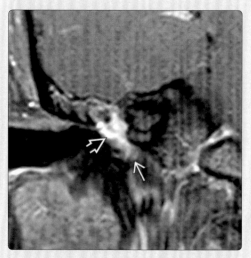

(Left) Coronal graphic shows a vascular glomus tympanicum paraganglioma (GTP) over the cochlear promontory and filling the inferior middle ear cavity. The bony floor of the middle ear cavity is intact ➡. Otoscopy reveals this tumor as a reddish, pulsatile mass behind the lower tympanic membrane ➡. (Right) Coronal T1 C+ FS MR demonstrates a large GTP filling the middle ear cavity ➡. The floor is intact ➡, separating the tumor from the jugular bulb below.

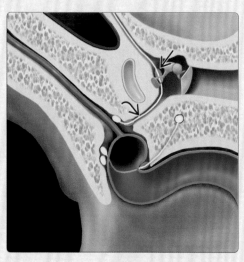
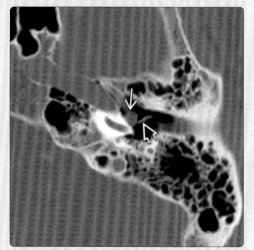

(Left) Axial graphic shows glomus bodies ➡ along course of the inferior tympanic nerve (branch of Jacobson nerve ➡) on the cochlear promontory. Glomus tympanicum tumors arise from this normal cellular collection. (Right) An axial bone CT reveals an ovoid glomus tympanicum tumor on the low cochlear promontory ➡ abutting the manubrium of the malleus ➡. The patient's history of conductive hearing loss is secondary to the restricted motion of the inferior malleus-tympanic membrane by the tumor.

TERMINOLOGY

Abbreviations

- Glomus tympanicum paraganglioma (GTP)

Synonyms

- Glomus tympanicum; chemodectoma

Definitions

- Benign tumor arising from glomus bodies situated on cochlear promontory

IMAGING

General Features

- Best diagnostic clue
  - CT: Mass with flat base on cochlear promontory
  - MR: Enhancing mass with flat base on cochlear promontory
- Location
  - Primary location: **Cochlear promontory**
  - Variant locations
    - Anterior to promontory, beneath cochleariform process
    - Inferior to promontory, in recess beneath basal turn of cochlea
- Size
  - Millimeters to ~ 2 cm
  - May be so small that nonfocused imaging causes radiologist to miss lesion altogether
- Morphology
  - Round mass with flat base most common
  - Larger lesions may fill middle ear cavity

CT Findings

- CECT
  - Difficult to identify enhancing mass in middle ear when GTP is small
- Bone CT
  - Focal mass with flat base on cochlear promontory is characteristic
  - Small GTP
    - Subtle soft tissue bump may be present on cochlear promontory
    - Projects off cochlear promontory into lower mesotympanum
    - May reach as far lateral as lower tympanic membrane (TM)
  - Large GTP
    - Fills middle ear cavity, creating attic block resulting in fluid collection in mastoid
    - Tumor margins may not be discernible on CT
    - Floor of middle ear cavity is **intact** (if dehiscent or permeative, diagnosis is glomus jugulare paraganglioma)
    - Larger lesions may show "aggressive" bone changes with permeative destruction of medial wall of middle ear cavity ± ossicles
    - Rare involvement of air cells along inferior cochlear promontory may be mistaken for invasion

MR Findings

- T1WI
  - Soft tissue intensity mass on cochlear promontory
  - Small GTP will not have high-velocity flow voids in mass
- T2WI
  - GTP has lower signal intensity compared to obstructed fluid
- T1WI C+
  - Focal enhancing mass on cochlear promontory
  - With larger obstructing GTP, contrast helps differentiate tumor from obstructed secretions
  - Utilized to determine tumor involvement of hypotympanum
- MRA
  - Does not show enlarged vessels

Angiographic Findings

- GTP arterial supply
  - **Ascending pharyngeal artery** & its inferior tympanic branch, via inferior tympanic canaliculus

Imaging Recommendations

- Best imaging tool
  - Bone CT: Bone CT without contrast best if GTP suspected clinically
  - MR: Used if GTP suspected from bone CT findings
    - Small GTP may be missed if slice thickness > 4 mm
    - May be used to confirm GTP hypotympanic involvement
  - Angiography: Unnecessary if GTP diagnosis clearly established by CT
- Protocol advice
  - Keep enhanced MR slice thickness ≤3 mm

DIFFERENTIAL DIAGNOSIS

Glomus Jugulare Paraganglioma

- Imaging: CT shows permeative change in bony floor of middle ear, involving jugular foramen
- Clinical: Red-pink mass behind TM ± pulsatile tinnitus
  - Otoscopic exam identical to GTP

Aberrant Internal Carotid Artery

- Imaging: Tubular mass crosses middle ear cavity to rejoin horizontal petrous internal carotid artery (ICA)
  - Large inferior tympanic canaliculus
- Clinical: Red-pink mass behind TM ± pulsatile tinnitus

Dehiscent Jugular Bulb

- Imaging: CT shows dehiscent sigmoid plate
  - Venous protrusion into middle ear cavity from superolateral jugular bulb
- Clinical: Asymptomatic; blue mass behind posteroinferior TM

Middle Ear Congenital Cholesteatoma

- Imaging: T1 C+ MR shows no enhancement
- Clinical: White mass behind intact TM

Facial Nerve Schwannoma, Tympanic Segment

- Imaging: Pedunculated mass from tympanic CNVII
- Clinical: Tan-white mass behind superior TM

PATHOLOGY

General Features

- Etiology
  - Arises from glomus (Latin for "ball") bodies (paraganglia) found along inferior tympanic nerve (Jacobson nerve) on cochlear promontory
    - Chemoreceptor cells derived from primitive neural crest
  - Nonchromaffin (nonsecretory) in this location
- Genetics
  - Inactivating mutation of *SDHD* gene of chromosome 11,q23 may predispose to GTP formation
- Named by location
  - GTP: Middle ear
  - Glomus jugulare paraganglioma: Jugular foramen → middle ear
  - Glomus vagale paraganglioma: Nodose ganglion of nasopharyngeal carotid space
  - Carotid body paraganglioma: In notch of carotid bifurcation

Staging, Grading, & Classification

- Glasscock-Jackson classification of GTP
  - Type I: Small mass limited to cochlear promontory
  - Type II: Tumor completely filling middle ear cavity
  - Type III: Tumor filling middle ear & extending into mastoid air cells
  - Type IV: Tumor filling middle ear & extending into mastoid ± through TM to fill EAC ± extension anterior to ICA

Gross Pathologic & Surgical Features

- Glistening, red, polypoid mass on cochlear promontory
- Fibrous pseudocapsule

Microscopic Features

- All paragangliomas have same histopathology
- Biphasic cell pattern composed of chief cells & sustentacular cells surrounded by fibromuscular stroma
- Chief cells arranged in characteristic compact cell nests or "balls" of cells, referred to as **"zellballen"**
- Immunohistochemistry: Chief cells show diffuse reaction to chromogranin
- Electron microscopy: Shows neurosecretory granules

CLINICAL ISSUES

Presentation

- Most common signs/symptoms
  - Vascular, pulsatile retrotympanic mass
    - If small: Anteroinferior quadrant of TM
    - Pneumatic otoscopy will cause blanching of mass known as Brown's sign
  - Other signs/symptoms
    - Pulsatile tinnitus (90%), conductive hearing loss (50%), facial nerve paralysis (5%)
- Clinical profile
  - 50-year-old woman with vascular retrotympanic mass & pulsatile tinnitus

Demographics

- Age
  - 66% are between 40 and 60 years of age at diagnosis
- Gender
  - M:F = 1:3
- Epidemiology
  - GTP is most common tumor of middle ear
  - GTP is rarely associated with multicentric paragangliomas

Natural History & Prognosis

- Slow-growing, noninvasive tumor
- Average time from onset of symptoms to surgical treatment is 3 years
- Complete resection yields permanent surgical cure

Treatment

- Smaller GTP lesions
  - Removed via tympanostomy through EAC
- Larger GTP lesions
  - Often require mastoidectomy
- Preoperative selective embolization not necessary
- Stereotactic radiosurgery used when conventional surgical resection is contraindicated or incomplete

DIAGNOSTIC CHECKLIST

Consider

- Be careful with initial diagnosis
  - GTP may be clinically indistinguishable from glomus jugulare paraganglioma or aberrant ICA
  - If GTP is diagnosed when glomus jugulare paraganglioma is present, incomplete surgery will result
  - If GTP is diagnosed when aberrant ICA is present, biopsy could be fatal
- Preoperative imaging must differentiate these diagnoses

Image Interpretation Pearls

- Ask referring clinician color & location of retrotympanic mass
  - Red anteroinferior mass: GTP
  - Blue posteroinferior mass: Dehiscent jugular bulb
  - Red mass crossing behind inferior TM: Aberrant ICA
  - White mass: Congenital cholesteatoma (inferior) or facial nerve schwannoma (superior)

SELECTED REFERENCES

1. Carlson ML et al: Glomus tympanicum: a review of 115 cases over 4 decades. Otolaryngol Head Neck Surg. 152(1):136-42, 2015
2. Sweeney AD et al: Glomus tympanicum tumors. Otolaryngol Clin North Am. 48(2):293-304, 2015
3. Kumar G et al: Unusual presentation of glomus tympanicum tumour: new bone formation in the middle ear. World J Clin Cases. 2(9):463-5, 2014
4. Amin MF et al: Diagnostic efficiency of multidetector computed tomography versus magnetic resonance imaging in differentiation of head and neck paragangliomas from other mimicking vascular lesions: comparison with histopathologic examination. Eur Arch Otorhinolaryngol. 270(3):1045-53, 2013
5. Karatas E et al: Promontory hemangioma mimics glomus tympanicum in the middle ear (promontory hemangioma). Eur Rev Med Pharmacol Sci. 16 Suppl 4:103-5, 2012
6. Papaspyrou K et al: Hearing results after hypotympanotomy for glomus tympanicum tumors. Otol Neurotol. 32(2):291-6, 2011

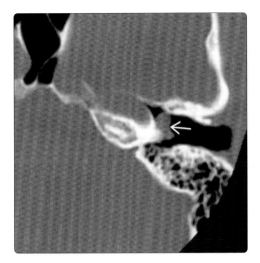
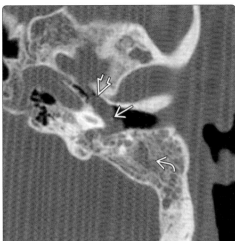

(Left) *Axial left temporal bone CT shows a multilobular soft tissue mass on the low cochlear promontory* ➡, *consistent with a diagnosis of GTP.* (Right) *CT shows this large GTP in the middle ear cavity. The lesion bulges the tympanic membrane laterally around the umbo of the manubrium* ➡. *Note extension into proximal bony eustachian tube* ➡ *and opacification of mastoid air cells* ➡ *secondary to aditus obstruction.*

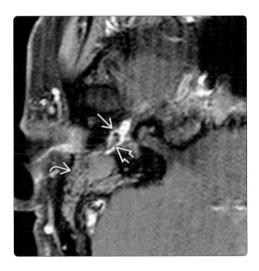
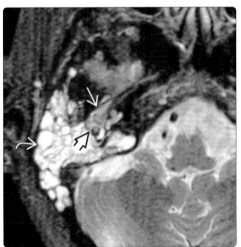

(Left) *Axial T1 C+ FS MR of the right temporal bone shows an enhancing GTP* ➡ *filling the middle ear. Note the dark ossicles embedded within the tumor* ➡. *The aditus ad antrum is obstructed, causing nonenhancing fluid* ➡ *to back up within the mastoid air cells.* (Right) *Axial T2 FS MR reveals the glomus tumor to be an intermediate signal intensity lesion in the middle ear* ➡ *compared to the very high signal obstructed mastoid secretions* ➡. *Note that the posterior margin of the mass obstructs the aditus ad antrum* ➡.

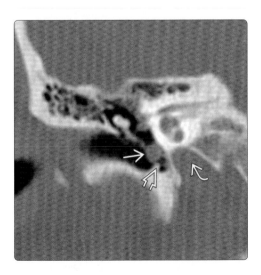
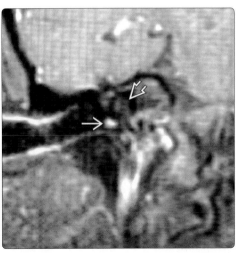

(Left) *Coronal bone CT shows a small GTP* ➡ *located on the low cochlear promontory just cephalad and medial to the tympanic annulus* ➡. *On a single coronal image, the GTP looks remarkably like an aberrant internal carotid artery (ICA), but this case shows a normal ICA* ➡ *below the cochlea.* (Right) *Coronal T1WI C+ FS MR reveals a GTP* ➡ *to be a subtle focus of enhancement inferolateral to the cochlea* ➡. *It would be easy for a radiologist to overlook such a small GTP without direction from the clinical history.*

Temporal Bone Meningioma

TERMINOLOGY

- Synonym: Intratympanic meningioma
- Definition: Meningioma involving middle ear (ME) or inner ear of temporal bone

IMAGING

- Morphology: Dural-based globular or en plaque mass
  - Extends into temporal bone via tegmen, internal carotid artery, or jugular foramen
- Bone CT findings
  - Permeative-sclerotic or **hyperostotic** changes
  - May underestimate extent of tumor
  - Intratumoral **calcification** common
  - **Ossicles intact** without destruction typically
- MR findings
  - Avidly enhancing mass involving temporal bone
  - If dural **tail** present, helps make diagnosis
- 3 principal sites of origin + specific vector of spread
  - Tegmen tympani tumor grows inferiorly into ME

- Jugular foramen tumor grows centrifugally into ME if superolateral spread present
- IAC tumor grows into inner ear
- Imaging protocol suggestion
  - Thin T1 C+ FS IAC MR best shows tumor extent
  - Especially with extensive intraosseous component

CLINICAL ISSUES

- Hearing loss patterns
  - Conductive: Tegmen tympani meningioma
  - Sensorineural: IAC meningioma
  - Mixed: Jugular foramen meningioma
- Otoscopy: Vascular retrotympanic mass if extends to ME
- Treatment: Surgical removal

DIAGNOSTIC CHECKLIST

- Identify site of origin, vector of spread, and extent
- Dural tails (MR) ± permeative sclerotic bone change (CT) may allow specific diagnosis

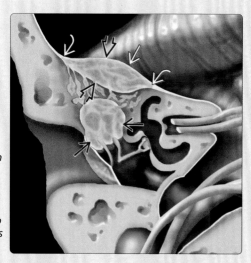
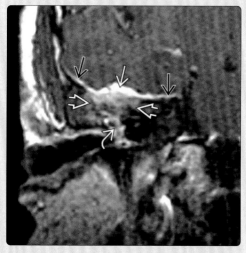

(Left) Coronal graphic of tegmen tympani meningioma reveals en plaque dural origin of the tumor ➡ with spread through the tegmen ⇨ thickened by hyperostosis into the superior middle ear cavity. The ossicles have been engulfed by the tumor ➡. Dural tails are visible along the tumor margins ➡. (Right) Coronal T1 C+ FS MR shows en plaque meningioma arising along the middle cranial fossa floor ➡. Note the enhancing dural tails ➡. Transosseous tegmen tumor ⇨ spreads into the middle ear cavity & engulfs the ossicles ➡.

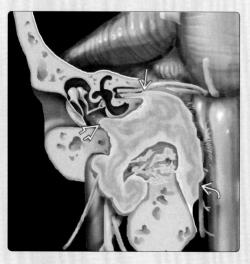
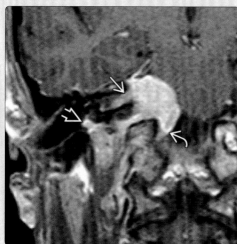

(Left) Coronal graphic of a jugular foramen meningioma depicts the centrifugal spread pattern reaching the IAC ➡, middle ear ➡, & basal cistern ➡. When a jugular foramen meningioma reaches the middle ear, it can mimic glomus jugulare paraganglioma. (Right) T1 C+ FS MR reveals extensive jugular foramen meningioma that spreads to the IAC ➡, middle ear ➡, & basal cistern ➡. Centrifugal spread pattern, dural-based morphology, & absence of flow voids suggest a diagnosis of meningioma.

TERMINOLOGY

Synonyms

- Temporal bone meningioma, intratympanic meningioma, middle ear (ME) meningioma

Definitions

- Meningioma involving temporal bone
  o May extend to ME, inner ear (IE), mastoid air cells, petrous apex air cells, internal auditory canal (IAC) &/or external auditory canal (EAC)

IMAGING

General Features

- Best diagnostic clue
  o Well-defined, **avidly enhancing** temporal bone mass
    – Best seen on T1 C+ FS MR
    – **Dural tails** highly suggestive of diagnosis
  o Bone CT shows **permeative-sclerotic** bone change
    – **Hyperostosis** is characteristic, if present
- Location
  o From 3 principal sites of origin
    – Tegmen tympani
    – Jugular foramen
    – IAC/cerebellopontine angle (CPA)
- Size
  o ME & IE component small (< 15 mm)
    – Involvement of temporal bone & beyond can be large
- Morphology
  o Dural component appears **globular** or **en plaque**
  o ME-mastoid components usually small, lobular, soft tissue masses
  o Transosseous/intraosseous component can be lobular or irregular with osseous enlargement
- **Vector of spread** characteristics from each site
  o **Tegmen tympani meningioma** spreads **inferiorly** into ME
  o **Jugular foramen meningioma** spreads **centrifugally** along dural surfaces in all directions
    – Enters ME via **superolateral** route
    – Mimics glomus jugulare paraganglioma when ME involvement occurs
  o **IAC meningioma** spreads from **CPA → IAC → intralabyrinthine structures** laterally

CT Findings

- CECT
  o 90% show strong, uniform enhancement
- Bone CT
  o General bone change findings
    – When transosseous: **Permeative-sclerotic** appearance, variable mild expansile changes
    – When adjacent to bone: Sclerotic or **hyperostotic**
  o Tegmen tympani meningioma
    – Tegmen thickens, reacts to transosseous meningioma
    – Ossicles encased with spread into ME cavity
      □ **Ossicles intact** without destruction typically
  o Jugular foramen meningoma
    – Surrounding bone shows permeative-sclerotic change

- Bone changes may **underestimate** or **overestimate tumor extent**
  o Intratumoral **calcification** common

MR Findings

- T1WI
  o Isointense to brain gray matter
- T2WI
  o Isointense or slightly higher signal than gray matter
  o If calcifications present, scattered low-intensity foci
- DWI
  o Characteristic low ADC signal intensity
- T1WI C+
  o 90% of temporal bone meningiomas strongly enhance
  o Dural component & ME/IE component enhance more strongly than intra-/transosseous components
  o If dural tail is present, may allow precise diagnosis
  o Tegmen tympani meningioma
    – En plaque dural lesion enhances avidly
    – ME-mastoid component also enhances
  o Jugular foramen meningioma
    – Enhancing mass fills jugular foramen
    – Enhancing lesion extends in all directions through bone & along dural surfaces
    – If extends to ME superolaterally, closely mimics glomus jugulare paraganglioma
      □ Usually **no flow voids**
  o IAC meningioma
    – Enhancement of vestibulocochlear (VC) apparatus ± IAC ± CPA meningioma
      □ When small, can closely mimic vestibular schwannoma
    – Intense, uniform enhancement of VC or dural tail distinguishes from schwannoma

Angiographic Findings

- Vascular tumor with immediate tumor "blush"
- **Prolonged** vascular "stain" into venous phase
- Sunburst pattern of enlarged dural feeders may occur with large tumors
- ME component may be obscured by subtraction artifact

Imaging Recommendations

- Best imaging tool
  o Combined focused imaging of temporal bone with bone algorithm CT & thin-section T1 C+ FS MR
    – Temporal bone CT
      □ Gives precise information about ossicles, CNVII
      □ In larger lesions, pattern of bone change distinguishes meningioma from other pathologies
      □ CT may underestimate tumor extent
    – Thin-section focused MR with T1 C+ fat saturated
      □ Best to show tumor within bone, dura, & ME-IE
- Protocol advice
  o Bone CT: < 1-mm axial unenhanced sections with multiplanar reformations
  o MR: ≤ 3-mm T1 FS C+ axial & coronal sequences
  o Do not ignore precontrast T1 sequences for replacement of normal fat of temporal bone
    – Do NOT use fat saturation on precontrast T1 series

DIFFERENTIAL DIAGNOSIS

Glomus Jugulare Paraganglioma

- Clinical: Red-vascular retrotympanic mass
- Temporal bone CT: Permeative-destructive bone erosion along superolateral margin of jugular bulb
- T1 MR: Jugular foramen mass with flow voids ("pepper") ± hyperintense foci ("salt") ± ME extension

Glomus Tympanicum Paraganglioma

- Clinical: Red-vascular retrotympanic mass
- Temporal bone CT: Globular mass on cochlear promontory
  - Bony floor of ME cavity intact
- T1 C+ MR: Enhancing mass on cochlear promontory

Dehiscent Jugular Bulb

- Clinical: Blue-vascular posteroinferior retrotympanic mass
- Temporal bone CT: Dehisced bony plate between jugular bulb & ME

Aberrant Internal Carotid Artery

- Clinical: Red-vascular retrotympanic mass crosses cochlear promontory
- Temporal bone CT: Tubular mass crosses ME cavity to join horizontal petrous ICA
  - Enlarged inferior tympanic canaliculus
- MRA: Asymmetric aberrant vessel

Middle Ear Cholesterol Granuloma

- Clinical: Blue-black retrotympanic mass
- Temporal bone CT: ME opacified ± ossicle destruction
- T1 MR: High signal from methemoglobin

PATHOLOGY

General Features

- Etiology
  - Arise from **arachnoid "cap" cells**
    - Embryonic migration anomaly
- Genetics
  - Long arm deletions of chromosome 22 common if associated with neurofibromatosis type 2
    - *NF2* gene inactivated in 60% of sporadic cases

Gross Pathologic & Surgical Features

- Sharply circumscribed, **unencapsulated**
- Adjacent dural thickening (collar or **tail**) is usually **reactive**, not neoplastic
- Globular (most common) or en plaque types

Microscopic Features

- Wide range of histology with little bearing on outcome
  - Meningothelial, fibrous, transitional, psammomatous, angiomatous, miscellaneous other (microcystic, chordoid, clear cell, secretory)
- Nests & whorls of "meningiomatous cells"
- Psammoma bodies: Calcifications

CLINICAL ISSUES

Presentation

- Most common signs/symptoms
  - Hearing loss

- Conductive: Tegmen tympani meningioma
- Sensorineural: IAC meningioma
- Mixed: Jugular foramen meningioma
  - Facial neuropathy rare
  - Otoscopic examination: Vascular retrotympanic mass
    - ME component may represent "tip of iceberg" for larger intracranial component
- Other signs/symptoms
  - Symptoms from larger intracranial component
    - Skull base/CPA: Complex cranial neuropathy may involve V, VII, & VIII
    - Jugular foramen: IX-XII ccranial neuropathy possible
- Clinical profile
  - Middle-aged woman with conductive hearing loss

Demographics

- Age
  - Average age at presentation = 45 years
- Gender
  - M:F = 1:3
- Epidemiology
  - 7% of intracranial meningiomas originate from anterior or posterior surface of petrous bone

Natural History & Prognosis

- Slow-growing benign tumor
- Relatively high recurrence rate due to difficulty of complete excision
- Prognosis relates to surgical outcome & complications
  - Hearing usually preserved at preoperative level
  - Facial nerve function good to acceptable
  - Chance of cranial nerve function restoration is low
  - Risk of new lower cranial nerve injury

Treatment

- Complete surgical excision
- Aggressive surgery advocated because bone invasion hard to see at surgery

DIAGNOSTIC CHECKLIST

Image Interpretation Pearls

- Identify site of origin (tegmen, jugular foramen, or IAC)
- Use imaging findings to make meningioma diagnosis
  - Morphology: Dural-based globular or en plaque mass
  - Bone CT: Permeative-sclerotic, sclerotic, or hyperostotic
  - MR: Enhancing tumor with dural tail
- Use combination of CT & MR findings to define full tumor extent

SELECTED REFERENCES

1. Thompson LD: Ear and temporal bone meningioma. Ear Nose Throat J. 95(4-5):146, 2016
2. Ricciardiello F et al: Temporal bone meningioma involving the middle ear: a case report. Oncol Lett. 10(4):2249-2252, 2015
3. Thomas AJ et al: Nonparaganglioma jugular foramen tumors. Otolaryngol Clin North Am. 48(2):343-59, 2015
4. Stevens KL et al: Middle ear meningiomas: a case series reviewing the clinical presentation, radiologic features, and contemporary management of a rare temporal bone pathology. Am J Otolaryngol. 35(3):384-9, 2014
5. Hamilton BE et al: Imaging and clinical characteristics of temporal bone meningioma. AJNR Am J Neuroradiol. 27(10):2204-9, 2006

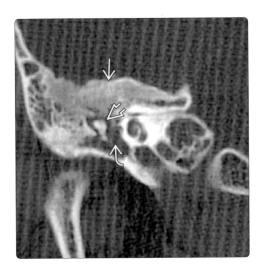

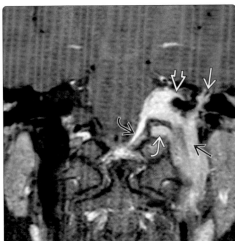

(Left) *Coronal bone CT shows thickened, sclerotic tegmen tympani ➡. Soft tissue density fills the middle ear ➡. The ossicles ➡ are encased but not eroded by this meningioma involving the middle ear.* (Right) *Coronal T1 C+ FS MR demonstrates preserved appearance of the ossicles ➡ despite surrounding invasive enhancing meningioma. Note enhancing components within the IAC ➡, hypoglossal canal ➡, jugular foramen ➡, and characteristic enhancing dural tail ➡.*

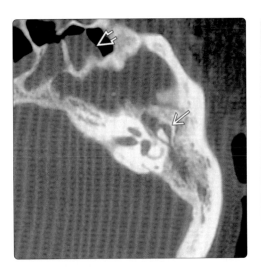

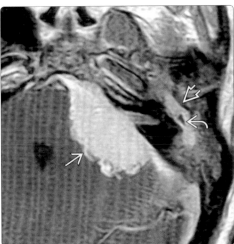

(Left) *Axial bone CT in a patient with an extensive cerebellopontine angle (CPA)-IAC meningioma (not seen) shows middle ear ➡ and sphenoid sinus ➡ opacification. Note the relative absence of bone changes that would suggest IAC &/or inner ear involvement.* (Right) *Axial T1 C+ MR reveals a large CPA and IAC meningioma ➡ extending into the middle ear ➡ to engulf the ossicles ➡. Enhanced MR is far better at determining true meningioma extent than bone CT.*

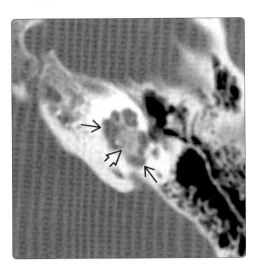

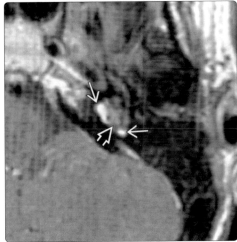

(Left) *Axial bone CT shows a rare inner ear meningioma with both lucent ➡ and sclerotic ➡ components. The lesion involves the area of the vestibule and basal turn of the cochlea. (Courtesy R. Wallace, MD.)* (Right) *Axial T1 C+ MR demonstrates a rare inner ear meningioma with enhancement ➡ of corresponding radiolucent areas on CT and relative lack of enhancement in the corresponding CT radiodense areas ➡.*

Middle Ear Schwannoma

TERMINOLOGY

- **Primary schwannoma**: Primary to middle ear (ME) cavity
  - Tympanic segment CNVII > > tympanic branch nerve (CNIX branch), chorda tympani nerve (CNVII branch)
- **Secondary schwannoma**: Arises outside ME
  - Jugular foramen schwannoma involves ME
  - Translabyrinthine CNVIII schwannoma
  - Primary inner ear schwannoma → ME

IMAGING

- Bone CT findings
  - **CNVII schwannoma**: Well-marginated mass emanating from CNVII canal
  - **Transotic intralabyrinthine schwannoma** (spread from inner ear with ME protrusion): Labyrinth erosions with mass protruding into ME via round or oval window
  - **ME schwannoma** (from chorda tympani or Jacobson nerve): Focal mass filling ME without involving CNVII canal

- T1 C+ MR findings
  - CNVII schwannoma: Enhancing mass contiguous with tympanic or mastoid CNVII
  - Transotic intralabyrinthine schwannoma: Enhancing mass contiguous with IAC & inner ear spaces
  - ME schwannoma: Mass primary to ME cavity
  - **Intramural cysts** may be visible when large

TOP DIFFERENTIAL DIAGNOSES

- Congenital ME cholesteatoma
- Glomus tympanicum paraganglioma
- Pars flaccida-acquired cholesteatoma
- ME adenoma

CLINICAL ISSUES

- Presentation: Conductive hearing loss
- Otoscopy: Fleshy-white mass behind intact TM
- Imaging depends on erosion of surrounding structures
- Treatment: Surgical removal

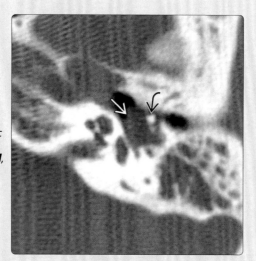
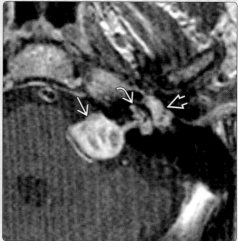

(Left) Axial temporal bone CT of the left ear reveals the middle ear component of the schwannoma ➡ pushing the ossicles laterally ➡. The mastoid air cells are opacified as a result of the aditus ad antrum block created by the schwannoma. (Right) Axial T1WI C+ MR shows a transotic schwannoma extending from the cerebellopontine angle ➡, through the inner ear ➡, and into the middle ear cavity ➡. Original clinical diagnosis in this case was congenital cholesteatoma of the middle ear.

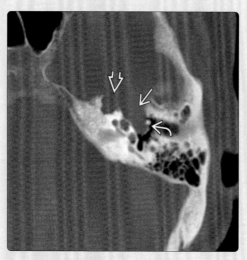
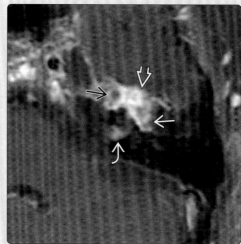

(Left) Axial bone CT reveals a facial nerve schwannoma enlarging the geniculate fossa ➡ and tympanic segment of the facial nerve canal ➡. The lesion pedunculates into the middle ear cavity, pushing the ossicles ➡ posterolaterally. (Right) Axial T1WI C+ FS MR shows the enhancing schwannoma in the geniculate ganglion ➡ with extension along the tympanic segment ➡ into the middle ear. IAC fundal tumor is also seen ➡. Note the small intramural cyst ➡.

TERMINOLOGY

Synonyms

- Facial nerve schwannoma, tympanic branch nerve schwannoma, chorda tympani schwannoma

Definitions

- **Primary schwannoma**: Tumor primary to middle ear (ME) cavity
  o Tympanic segment CNVII > > tympanic branch (CNIX branch or Jacobson nerve), chorda tympani nerve (CNVII branch)
- **Secondary schwannoma**: Arises outside ME
  o Large CNIX-XI jugular foramen schwannoma eroding into ME
  o Translabyrinthine CNVIII schwannoma
    - Cerebellopontine angle-internal auditory canal (CPA-IAC) → inner ear → ME
  o Primary inner ear schwannoma → ME

IMAGING

General Features

- Best diagnostic clue
  o T1 C+ MR shows enhancing mass in ME
- Size
  o Variable, usually < 15 mm
- Morphology
  o Well-marginated, lobular mass

CT Findings

- CECT
  o Lesion enhances with contrast
- Bone CT
  o **Facial nerve schwannoma**
    - Well-marginated mass emanating from CNVII canal
      □ Tympanic or mastoid segments
  o **Transotic intralabyrinthine schwannoma** (spread from inner ear with ME protrusion)
    - Labyrinth erosions with mass protruding into ME via round or oval window
  o **ME schwannoma** (from chorda tympani or tympanic branch nerve)
    - Well-marginated mass filling ME without involving CNVII canal

MR Findings

- T1WI C+
  o Lobulated, enhancing mass (differentiates from cholesteatoma)
    - Facial nerve schwannoma: Contiguous with tympanic or mastoid CNVII
    - Transotic intralabyrinthine schwannoma: Enhancing mass contiguous with IAC & inner ear
    - ME schwannoma: Mass primary to ME cavity
  o **Intramural cysts** may be visible when large

Imaging Recommendations

- Best imaging tool
  o T1 C+ MR thin sections through temporal bone
- Protocol advice
  o Thin-section T1 C+ MR with diffusion differentiates schwannoma from cholesteatoma
  o Thin-section bone CT in axial & coronal planes

DIFFERENTIAL DIAGNOSIS

Congenital Middle Ear Cholesteatoma

- Child or young adult with conductive hearing loss
- Otoscopy: Tan-white mass behind **intact TM**
- Bone CT: Lobulated mass, medial to ossicles
- MR: Nonenhancing ME mass
  o DWI: High signal from restricted diffusion

Glomus Tympanicum Paraganglioma

- Adult patient population
- Otoscopy: Pink-red, pulsatile mass behind intact TM
- Bone CT: Cochlear promontory mass; ME floor intact
- MR: Enhancing mass

Middle Ear Adenoma

- Rare ME tumor
- Otoscopy: Tan mass behind intact TM
- Bone CT: Remodeling or invasive-appearing ME mass
- MR: Enhancing ME mass

PATHOLOGY

General Features

- Etiology
  o Neuroectodermal origin
  o Slow-growing, encapsulated, benign lesion

Gross Pathologic & Surgical Features

- Encapsulated tan or gray neoplasm

CLINICAL ISSUES

Presentation

- Most common signs/symptoms
  o Conductive hearing loss
  o Otoscopy: Fleshy-white mass behind intact TM

Treatment

- Surgical removal

DIAGNOSTIC CHECKLIST

Consider

- If ME schwannoma diagnosis is considered
  o Is tumor from facial nerve canal?
    - Pedunculated facial nerve schwannoma
  o Is tumor primary to ME cavity?
    - ME schwannoma
    - ME adenoma
    - ME congenital cholesteatoma
    - Glomus tympanicum paraganglioma

SELECTED REFERENCES

1. Lahlou G et al: Intratemporal facial nerve schwannoma: clinical presentation and management. Eur Arch Otorhinolaryngol. ePub, 2015
2. McRackan TR et al: Primary tumors of the facial nerve. Otolaryngol Clin North Am. 48(3):491-500, 2015
3. Salzman KL et al: Intralabyrinthine schwannomas: imaging diagnosis and classification. AJNR Am J Neuroradiol. 33(1):104-9, 2012

Middle Ear Adenoma

TERMINOLOGY

- Middle ear adenoma (MEA)
  - Very rare, benign tumor of mixed exocrine & neuroendocrine origin

IMAGING

- Soft tissue mass in middle ear
- Temporal bone CT findings
  - Middle ear mass behind intact tympanic membrane (TM)
  - Indistinguishable on bone CT from glomus tympanicum & pedunculated ME schwannoma
  - Well-pneumatized mastoid (no history of chronic otitis media)
  - May show areas of **local bone invasion**
- MR findings
  - If large adenoma present, T1 C+ MR may be helpful in defining lesion extent
  - MEA **enhances** like glomus tympanicum & pedunculated CNVII schwannoma

- Enhancement excludes middle ear congenital cholesteatoma

TOP DIFFERENTIAL DIAGNOSES

- Glomus tympanicum paraganglioma
- Pedunculated facial nerve schwannoma
- Middle ear congenital cholesteatoma

CLINICAL ISSUES

- Otoscopy appearance
  - Tan-pink soft tissue mass behind intact TM
- Principal symptoms
  - Tinnitus and conductive hearing loss
  - "Ear fullness"
- Mean age at presentation: 45 years
- Natural history of tumor
  - If aggressive type, facial nerve injury possible
- Treatment options
  - Complete surgical excision = treatment of choice

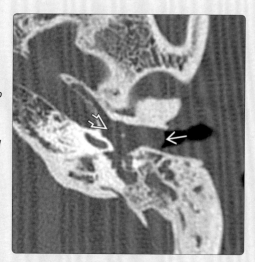
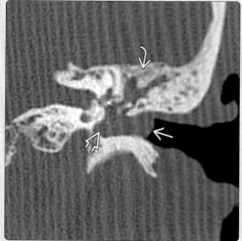

(Left) Axial bone CT through the middle ear shows a soft tissue mass filling the middle ear ⇒ with polypoid extension into the external auditory canal ➡. Mastoid opacification is present due to obstruction at the aditus ad antrum (not shown). (Right) Coronal bone CT reveals a mass filling the middle ear ⇒ and extending into the EAC ➡. Permeative changes are seen in the middle ear walls ⇒ but not to the EAC. Pathology showed the lesion to be middle ear adenoma.

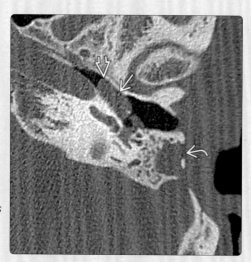
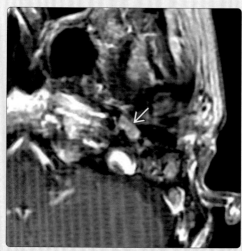

(Left) Axial bone CT through the low mesotympanum reveals a noninvasive middle ear adenoma ⇒ extending into the entrance of the bony eustachian tube ➡. Postmastoidectomy changes are also present ➡. (Right) Axial T1 C+ MR shows a well-circumscribed, enhancing lesion ➡ within the middle ear cavity. The lesion enhancement makes middle ear adenoma a possible diagnosis. Without otoscopy, one must also consider glomus tympanicum paraganglioma and middle ear schwannoma.

TERMINOLOGY

Abbreviations

- Middle ear adenoma (MEA)

Synonyms

- Adenomatous tumor of middle ear (ME)
- Middle ear carcinoid, neuroendocrine adenoma, adenomatoid tumor

Definitions

- Very rare, benign tumor arising from mucosal cells of ME having variable mixed epithelial & neuroendocrine differentiation

IMAGING

General Features

- Best diagnostic clue
  o Soft tissue mass + well-pneumatized mastoid (no chronic otitis media findings)
- Location
  o ME cavity proper (mesotympanum)
- Size
  o Early symptoms: Small (< 10 mm) at diagnosis
- Morphology
  o Often irregularly marginated

CT Findings

- CECT
  o Enhances, but difficult to see
- Bone CT
  o Mass within ME behind intact tympanic membrane (TM)
    – Indistinguishable on bone CT from glomus tympanicum & pedunculated ME schwannoma
    – May rarely show areas of local bone invasion

MR Findings

- T1WI C+
  o **Enhancing soft tissue mass** in ME

Imaging Recommendations

- Best imaging tool
  o Temporal bone CT
- Protocol advice
  o Axial & coronal bone CT images without contrast
    – If large adenoma present, T1 C+ MR may be helpful in defining lesion extent

Nuclear Medicine Findings

- Octreotide scan
  o Avid uptake similar to other neuroendocrine tumors

DIFFERENTIAL DIAGNOSIS

Glomus Tympanicum Paraganglioma

- Otoscopy: Pulsatile, red retrotympanic mass
- CT: Noninvasive cochlear promontory mass
- MR: T1 C+ MR shows enhancing mass

Pedunculated Facial Nerve Schwannoma

- Otoscopy: Avascular mass mimics congenital cholesteatoma

- T1 C+ MR: Enhancing mass connected to CNVII

Middle Ear Congenital Cholesteatoma

- Clinical: Child; no history of chronic otitis media
- CT: When large, typically erosive
- MR: T1 C+ MR shows **no** enhancement

PATHOLOGY

General Features

- Etiology
  o Benign, indolent epithelial tumors of ME that rarely invade bone
    – **Mixed exocrine & neuroendocrine** differentiation
  o MEA arises from modified respiratory mucosa

Gross Pathologic & Surgical Features

- Pink, yellow, gray, or reddish-brown firm, shimmering, soft tissue mass
- Usually poorly vascularized

CLINICAL ISSUES

Presentation

- Most common signs/symptoms
  o Otoscopy: Tan-pink soft tissue mass behind intact TM
  o Conductive hearing loss
- Other signs/symptoms
  o Ear fullness
  o Tinnitus

Demographics

- Age
  o Mean at presentation: 45 years
- Gender
  o M = F
- Epidemiology
  o Very rare ME tumor

Natural History & Prognosis

- Slow-growing benign tumor
- If aggressive type, facial nerve injury possible
- Recurrence of tumor common problem
- May progress to become malignant adenocarcinoma

Treatment

- Complete surgical excision is treatment of choice

DIAGNOSTIC CHECKLIST

Image Interpretation Pearls

- Otoscopic examination & imaging findings both nonspecific

Reporting Tips

- Describe extension outside of ME
  o Follow-up required: **20% recurrence rate**

SELECTED REFERENCES

1. Hu H et al: Neuroendocrine adenoma of middle ear with new bone formation and review of literature. Am J Otolaryngol. 37(2):108-11, 2016
2. Bierry G et al: Middle ear adenomatous tumor: a not so rare glomus tympanicum-mimicking lesion. J Neuroradiol. 37(2):116-21, 2010
3. Zan E et al: Middle ear adenoma: a challenging diagnosis. AJNR Am J Neuroradiol. 30(8):1602-3, 2009

TERMINOLOGY

- **Rhabdomyosarcoma (RMS): Rare pediatric destructive T-bone lesion**
  - Arises from embryonic skeletal muscle precursor cells or pluripotential mesenchymal cells

IMAGING

- Middle ear-mastoid or petrous apex destructive mass with variable contrast enhancement
  - Middle ear RMS often with associated external auditory canal extension (aural polyp)
  - Petrous apex RMS may be primary or spread from parameningeal RMS
  - Skull base and cranial nerve involvement common
- Both CT and MR recommended to stage skull base destruction and middle ear and intracranial extension
- T1 C+ FS MR best to detect intracranial extension via tegmen, mastoid roof, ± skull base foramina

- T2 MR helpful to differentiate obstructed mastoid secretions (more hyperintense than RMS)

TOP DIFFERENTIAL DIAGNOSES

- Acquired cholesteatoma
- Langerhans cell histiocytosis of T-bone
- Acute otomastoiditis with coalescence
- Metastatic neuroblastoma
- Cholesterol granuloma of middle ear

CLINICAL ISSUES

- Clinical presentation
  - Child (< 6 years old) with chronic otitis media
  - Other symptoms: Otorrhea, ear pain, external auditory canal polyp
- Most common soft tissue sarcoma in children
- Up to 40% of RMSs in children occurs in H&N
  - 7% of H&N RMSs occur in T-bone

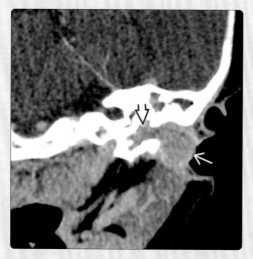
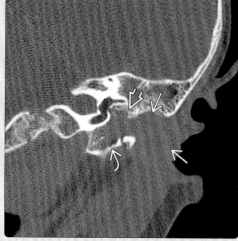

(Left) Coronal CECT in a 2-year-old child with EAC polyp and bleeding shows a lobulated mass filling and protruding from the left EAC ➡. There is also involvement of the middle ear cavity ➡. This was a rapidly growing RMS, as the clinician reported visualization of the tympanic membrane 3 weeks prior to imaging. (Right) Coronal bone CT in the same patient shows rapidly growing RMS of left EAC ➡, middle ear cavity ➡, and mastoid air cells. This tumor causes osseous erosion of the floor of the hypotympanum ➡.

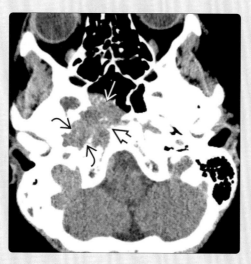
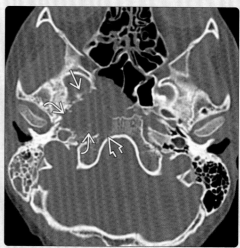

(Left) Axial NECT of the skull base of an 11-year-old boy with nasopharyngeal RMS shows superior extension of the mass into sphenoid sinus ➡, adjacent skull base/clivus ➡, and inferior aspect of petrous apex ➡. (Right) Axial bone CT in the same patient clearly defines erosion of the petrous apex ➡, clivus ➡, and middle cranial fossa floor ➡ in a patient with RMS of the nasopharynx. This is a characteristic pattern of spread in parameningeal rhabdomyosarcoma.

TERMINOLOGY

Abbreviations

- Rhabdomyosarcoma (RMS)

Definitions

- Rare **pediatric destructive T-bone lesion**
  - Arises from embryonic skeletal muscle precursor cells or pluripotential mesenchymal cells

IMAGING

General Features

- Best diagnostic clue
  - T-bone CT: Destructive middle ear-mastoid or petrous apex (PA) mass + variable contrast enhancement
  - T1 FS C+ MR: Irregular, invasive, enhancing middle ear-mastoid or PA mass in child
- Location
  - Middle ear ± mastoid or PA
    - Or direct extension from other parameningeal sites: Nasopharynx, masticator space, pterygopalatine fossa, or parapharyngeal space
  - Possible areas of extension with T-bone involvement
    - Lateral into EAC
    - Medial into IAC via CNVII canal
    - Cephalad into middle cranial fossa via mastoid or tympanic tegmen
    - Posterior into posterior cranial fossa: Direct extension or perineural spread (CNVII canal → IAC → posterior fossa)
    - Inferior into carotid space via carotid canal or jugular foramen
    - Anteroinferior into TMJ, masticator, or parotid spaces
- Size
  - Depends on tumor location; most > 3 cm
  - Fills middle ear-mastoid complex with intracranial extension
- Morphology
  - Poorly defined, locally destructive mass

CT Findings

- Middle ear-mastoid or PA destructive mass
  - Lytic, destructive bone and ossicle changes
  - Soft tissue mass with variable contrast enhancement
    - Mass may be hemorrhagic and necrotic
  - Often with associated EAC extension
  - Skull base and cranial nerve foraminal involvement common
- Nodal metastases rare at presentation unless intracranial or extracranial extension present

MR Findings

- **Iso-** to hypointense **T1**; **hyper-** to isointense **T2** mass
- Variable contrast enhancement
  - Coronal images best to detect intracranial extension via tegmen, mastoid roof ± skull base foramina
- Intracranial extension in parameningeal RMS → meningeal thickening and enhancement
  - ± enhancing intracranial mass
- T2 helpful to differentiate obstructed mastoid secretions (more hyperintense than RMS)

Nuclear Medicine Findings

- PET
  - Replacing bone scan in work-up
  - Intense FDG uptake by soft tissue tumor
  - Helpful for staging and posttreatment surveillance
    - Nodal staging
    - Distant metastases staging

Imaging Recommendations

- Best imaging tool
  - Both CT and MR recommended to stage primary mass, skull base destruction, and intracranial extension
  - Coronal T1 C+ FS MR best to identify intracranial and extracranial extension
- Protocol advice
  - Complex skull base mass with potential for intracranial extension, distant metastases, & cervical adenopathy requires careful multimodality work-up
    - Thin-section T-bone CT in axial plane, with coronal and sagittal reformations
    - Multiplanar MR pre- and postcontrast
    - Cervical adenopathy can be staged with either CECT, MR, or **PET/CT**

DIFFERENTIAL DIAGNOSIS

Pars Flaccida-Acquired Cholesteatoma

- Clinical: Pars flaccida tympanic membrane (TM) perforation or retraction ± visible cholesteatoma
- Bone CT: Scutum and ossicle erosion; soft tissue in Prussak space
  - Unless large, less extensive bone changes than RMS

Pars Tensa-Acquired Cholesteatoma

- Clinical: Pars tensa TM perforation with visible cholesteatoma
- Bone CT: Soft tissue medial to ossicles with erosions

T-Bone Langerhans Cell Histiocytosis

- Clinical: Pediatric patient with middle ear mass
  - Usually no cranial nerve palsy
- Bone CT: Destructive, enhancing T-bone mass
  - Often bilateral or with other osseous lesions

Acute Otomastoiditis With Coalescence

- Clinical: Fever, mastoid tenderness in child
- Bone CT: Opacified middle ear-mastoid
  - Mastoid trabecular breakdown mimics tumor
  - Clinical setting is key differentiator

Metastatic Neuroblastoma

- Metastatic disease to skull base frequently bilateral with enhancing masses, aggressive osseous erosion, and spiculated periosteal reaction

Middle Ear Cholesterol Granuloma

- Clinical: Retrotympanic "vascular" blue hue
  - Past history of multiple prior ear infections
- Imaging: MR shows **high T1-** and high T2-signal mass in middle ear ± mastoid

PATHOLOGY

General Features

- Etiology
  - Malignant tumor of **embryologic skeletal muscle cells** or **pluripotential mesenchymal cells**
  - Rarely radiation-induced 2nd primary neoplasm
- Genetics
  - Most cases are sporadic
  - Increased incidence in children with *p53* tumor suppressor gene mutation, Noonan syndrome, Beckwith-Wiedemann syndrome, hereditary retinoblastoma

Staging, Grading, & Classification

- **T-bone RMS** considered **parameningeal**
- International Rhabdomyosarcoma Study Group grading system used clinically
  - Group I: Completely resected localized disease
  - Group II: Completely resected regional disease or microscopic residual disease
  - Group III: Gross residual disease
  - Group IV: Distant metastases; worst prognosis

Gross Pathologic & Surgical Features

- Variable: Smooth, lobulated necrotic or hemorrhagic **or** infiltrative mass with poorly defined margins

Microscopic Features

- **Rhabdomyoblasts** in varying stages of differentiation
- Immunohistochemistry positive for desmin, vimentin, muscle-specific actin, antimyogenin and MYOD1
- 3 subtypes: Embryonal, alveolar, and pleomorphic
  - **Embryonal (ERMS)**: Most common (55%)
    - Occurs in younger children
    - Accounts for > 50% of all RMSs; 70-90% occur in H&N or genitourinary tract
  - **Alveolar (ARMS)**: 2nd most common (20%)
    - Usually occurs in older patients (15-25 years of age)
    - Most common in extremities and trunk
  - **Pleomorphic (anaplastic)**: Least common (20%)
    - Very rare; generally adults 40-60 years of age
    - Most common in extremities, rare in H&N

CLINICAL ISSUES

Presentation

- Most common signs/symptoms
  - Mimics chronic otitis media with chronic otorrhea (sometimes bloody) and ear pain
  - Other signs/symptoms
    - Aural (external auditory canal) polyp
    - Facial nerve palsy
    - Postauricular mass
- Other signs/symptoms
  - Hearing loss, headache, cervical lymph nodes
- Clinical profile
  - **Child < 6 years of age** with chronic otitis media, otorrhea, and ear pain, with EAC polyp unresponsive to medical management

Demographics

- Age

- Bimodal; children (2-5 years) and late teens (15-19 years)
  - Rarely occurs in adults
- Epidemiology
  - RMS is most common soft tissue sarcoma in children
    - Most common pediatric T-bone malignancy
  - Up to **40% of RMSs occur in H&N**
    - **Orbit**: Most common H&N site
    - **Parameningeal sites**: Middle ear, paranasal sinus, nasopharynx, masticator space, pterygopalatine fossa, parapharyngeal space
      - Intracranial extension in up to 55%
  - 7% of H&N RMSs occur in T-bone

Natural History & Prognosis

- Delay to diagnosis common
  - Child initially treated for acute or chronic otitis media
- T-bone RMS has **high probability of meningeal extension** at time of diagnosis
  - Extremely poor prognosis if intracranial spread and distant metastases present
- Embryonal type better prognosis than alveolar RMS
- Distant metastases: Lungs > > bone, liver, brain

Treatment

- T-bone RMSs are rarely resectable
  - Surgery: Biopsy or debulking
  - Multidrug chemotherapy + adjuvant radiation

DIAGNOSTIC CHECKLIST

Consider

- Clinical: Consider T-bone RMS if aural polyp or CNVII palsy found in child with chronic otitis media
- Imaging: Consider T-bone RMS if unilateral destructive T-bone mass in child
  - **Caveat**: Langerhans cell histiocytosis of T-bone can exactly mimic T-bone RMS

Image Interpretation Pearls

- Both CT & MR important for staging primary site, local disease, and nodal metastases
- Coronal plane needed to assess integrity of skull base and detect intracranial extension
  - MR is preferred modality
- PET/CT: Nodal, distant metastases & surveillance
  - Replacing bone scan in RMS work-up

Reporting Tips

- Describe location and extent of osseous destruction
  - Note intra- and extracranial extension
  - Note perivascular and perineural spread

SELECTED REFERENCES

1. Chevallier KM et al: Differentiating pediatric rhabdomyosarcoma and Langerhans cell histiocytosis of the temporal bone by imaging appearance. AJNR Am J Neuroradiol. 37(6):1185-9, 2016
2. Gluth MB: Rhabdomyosarcoma and other pediatric temporal bone malignancies. Otolaryngol Clin North Am. 48(2):375-90, 2015
3. Wolden SL et al: Local control for intermediate-risk rhabdomyosarcoma: results from D9803 according to histology, group, site, and size: a report from the Children's Oncology Group. Int J Radiat Oncol Biol Phys. 93(5):1071-6, 2015
4. Robson CD: Imaging of head and neck neoplasms in children. Pediatr Radiol. 40(4):499-509, 2010

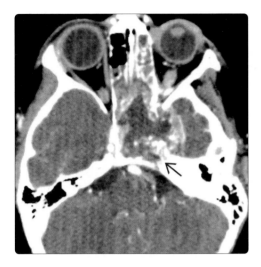

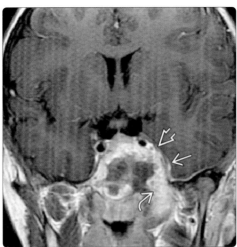

(Left) Axial CECT in a 6-year-old boy with left facial nerve palsy shows superior extension of a large, necrotic left parapharyngeal RMS invading sphenoid sinus, cavernous sinus, and middle cranial fossa, with erosion of the left petrous apex ➡. (Right) Coronal T1WI C+ MR in a patient with parapharyngeal RMS shows extension of the mass into the middle cranial fossa ➡ by direct skull base destruction ➡ as well as involvement of the left cavernous sinus ➡. Smooth interface with brain suggests no intradural extension.

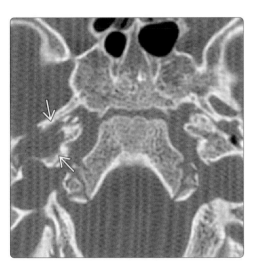

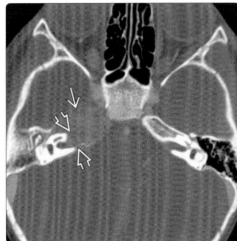

(Left) Axial bone CT in a 2 year old with chronic otitis media shows a lytic lesion in the right petrous apex ➡. Initial biopsy showed no evidence of malignancy or Langerhans cell histiocytosis. This T-bone RMS remained stable for 8 months. (Right) Axial bone CT in the same patient (with prior biopsy negative), presenting now with growing right petrous apex lesion and right facial nerve palsy, shows marked destruction of the right petrous apex ➡ with complete erosion of the walls of the right internal auditory canal ➡.

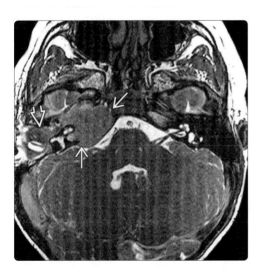

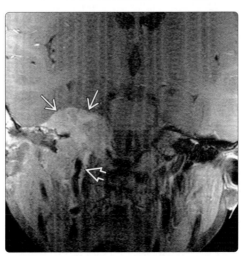

(Left) Axial T2 FSE MR shows an expansile, hypointense mass, typical of a very cellular lesion. The lesion involves the middle ear cavity ➡ and petrous apex ➡. RMS was confirmed at repeat biopsy in this 3 year old. (Right) Coronal T1WI C+ FS MR defines the intracranial extension ➡, which is common in patients with parameningeal RMS. Note also extension along the vertical segment of the petrous internal carotid artery ➡.

Temporal Bone Cephalocele

TERMINOLOGY

- Synonyms: Temporal lobe meningocele, encephalocele, or meningoencephalocele; defined by content
- Temporal bone cephalocele: Protrusion of cranial contents into middle ear (ME) or mastoid through dehiscence of tegmen

IMAGING

- CT: **Tegmen tympani** (ME roof) or **mastoideum** (mastoid roof) dehiscence
  - Tegmen defect does not necessarily result in cephalocele
- MR: Temporal lobe ± dura & CSF herniation into ME cavity or mastoid

TOP DIFFERENTIAL DIAGNOSES

- Large cholesteatoma with tegmen dehiscence
- ME cholesterol granuloma
- Temporal bone arachnoid granulation

PATHOLOGY

- Temporal bone cephalocele has multiple etiologies
  - Congenital
  - Acquired
    - Traumatic: Postsurgical or posttrauma/fracture
    - Nontraumatic: Cholesteatoma induced
    - Related to **idiopathic intracranial hypertension**
      - Obese, middle-aged women
    - Spontaneous
      - Anatomic predisposition: Thin tegmen

CLINICAL ISSUES

- Clinical presentation
  - 85% conductive or mixed hearing loss
- Treatment options
  - Immediate surgery to close defect is key
  - Threat of **meningitis** catalyzes this action
  - Treat idiopathic intracranial hypertension if present

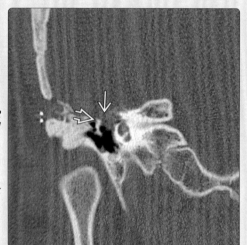
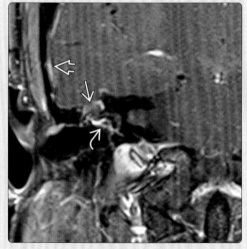

(Left) Coronal CT in a patient with history of severe temporal bone trauma and conductive hearing loss reveals a complete absence of the tegmen tympani ➡ with cephalocele surrounding the head of the malleus ➡. (Right) Coronal T1WI C+ FS MR in a patient with "fluid" behind an intact tympanic membrane shows a spontaneous tegmen tympani area cephalocele ➡. Enhancing tissue in the middle ear ➡ and dural enhancement ➡ is seen. At surgery, CSF leakage accompanied the cephalocele.

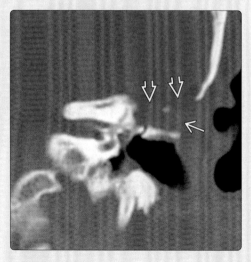
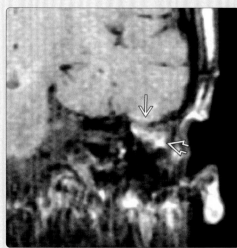

(Left) Coronal bone CT in a patient with CSF leakage following mastoidectomy demonstrates a broad tegmen dehiscence ➡ accompanied by opacification ➡ of the epitympanum and lateral mastoid air cells below the area of dehiscence. Possibility of cephalocele was raised by this coronal CT appearance. (Right) Coronal FLAIR MR in the same patient reveals a hammock-like encephalocele of the temporal lobe through tegmen rent ➡. High signal surgical fat packing is visible below the encephalocele ➡.

TERMINOLOGY

Synonyms

- Temporal lobe meningocele, encephalocele, or meningoencephalocele; defined by content

Definitions

- Protrusion of cranial contents into middle ear (ME) or mastoid through dehiscence of tegmen ± CSF leak

IMAGING

General Features

- Best diagnostic clue
  - CT: **Tegmen tympani** (ME roof) or **mastoideum** (mastoid roof) dehiscence
  - MR: CSF ± dura ± temporal lobe into ME or mastoid
- Location
  - Tegmen mastoideum > tegmen tympani
- Size
  - Few millimeter gap to centimeter or more
- Morphology
  - Hourglass or hammock shapes possible

Imaging Recommendations

- Best imaging tool
  - Temporal bone CT used initially to define bony dehiscence
  - Focused coronal T2 MR best for cephalocele contents
    - T1 C+ MR shows intracranial complication
  - Both CT & MR **coronal** views are key

CT Findings

- Bone CT
  - **Focal bone defect** in tegmen tympani or mastoideum
  - Other associated findings possible
    - Mastoidectomy or other surgical findings
    - Acute or chronic complex fractures
    - If sporadic, superior semicircular canal dehiscence may also be present
  - Opacified ME-mastoid air cells if **CSF leak**
    - CT cisternography: May be useful in localizing CSF leak

MR Findings

- T2WI
  - Small defects have dural defect → meningocele
  - Large defects may contain meningoencephalocele
    - Dura may be thin, or dural rent may be present
  - If associated dural leakage, high-signal CSF in ME-mastoid
- T1WI C+
  - Possible rim enhancement

DIFFERENTIAL DIAGNOSIS

Large Cholesteatoma With Tegmen Dehiscence

- Imaging: Nondependent soft tissue mass with ossicular erosion (on CT)
  - Restricted diffusion on DWI if large on MR

Middle Ear Cholesterol Granuloma

- Imaging: High T1 & T2 MR signal characteristic

Temporal Bone Arachnoid Granulation

- If large, may create cephalocele ± CSF leak
- Imaging: Focal cortical defect on CT
  - Enhances on T1 C+ MR

PATHOLOGY

General Features

- Etiology
  - Congenital
  - Acquired
    - Traumatic
      - □ Surgically induced: Post mastoidectomy
      - □ After severe temporal bone trauma
    - Nontraumatic
      - □ Cholesteatoma induced
    - Related to idiopathic intracranial hypertension (IIH)
    - Spontaneous
      - □ Anatomic predisposition: Thin tegmen

Gross Pathologic & Surgical Features

- Herniated brain usually nonfunctional

Microscopic Features

- Normal or necrotic CNS contents

CLINICAL ISSUES

Presentation

- Most common signs/symptoms
  - 85% conductive or mixed hearing loss
  - Complicated cephalocele
    - CSF otorrhea, meningitis, brain or epidural abscess, epilepsy
  - Obese, middle-aged women
    - Complication of IIH
- Other signs/symptoms
  - Pulsatile tinnitus, CNVII palsy, trigeminal neuralgia
  - Otoscopy: Pulsatile ME mass

Demographics

- Age
  - Usually presents > 50 years
  - Cholesteatoma & IIH groups may present earlier

Natural History & Prognosis

- Tegmen defect does not always result in cephalocele
- Delayed presentation of cephalocele develops over time with CSF pulsation, increased intracranial pressure, & low-grade inflammation

Treatment

- Immediate closure of defect is mandatory due to risk of life-threatening **meningitis**
- Treat IIH if present

SELECTED REFERENCES

1. Alonso RC et al: Spontaneous skull base meningoencephaloceles and cerebrospinal fluid fistulas. Radiographics. 33(2):553-70, 2013
2. Carlson ML et al: Temporal bone encephalocele and cerebrospinal fluid fistula repair utilizing the middle cranial fossa or combined mastoid-middle cranial fossa approach. J Neurosurg. 119(5):1314-22, 2013
3. Stucken EZ et al: The role of obesity in spontaneous temporal bone encephaloceles and CSF leak. Otol Neurotol. 33(8):1412-7, 2012

KEY FACTS

TERMINOLOGY

- Ossicular replacement prosthesis (ORP)
- **Ossiculoplasty**: Surgical reconstruction of malfunctioned ossicular chain to improve or to maintain residual conductive hearing function
- Common ORP types
  - Stapes prosthesis
  - Incus interposition graft
  - Partial ossicular replacement prosthesis
  - Total ossicular replacement prosthesis

IMAGING

- Temporal bone CT = best imaging tool
  - All or part of ossicular chain, replaced by tissue graft (autograft, homograft, autolograft) or allograft
  - CT may over- or underestimate (< 1 mm) size of metallic ORP due to metallic artifacts
  - CT may underestimate fluoroplastic portion of ORP if surrounded by soft tissue

- Allow some leeway when commenting on medial-lateral position of ORP
- **Prosthesis malfunction** findings on CT
  - Displacement, dislocation, protrusion, extrusion
  - Abnormal soft tissue-embedded ORP
  - Recurrent/progressive primary disease
    - Cholesteatoma, otosclerosis, tympanosclerosis
- Prosthetic MR safety
  - Most modern ossicular replacement prostheses are tested safe or conditional at 1.5T or 3T
  - Be sure to check specific product against known MR safety record

TOP DIFFERENTIAL DIAGNOSES

- Chronic otitis media with tympanosclerosis
- Posttraumatic incus dislocation
- Foreign body in middle ear
- Semiimplantable direct drive hearing device

(Left) Coronal graphic shows a titanium PORP ⮕ connecting the tympanic membrane (TM) to capitulum of stapes ⮕. A cartilage graft ⮕ is often placed between TM and head of prosthesis to reduce incidence of implant extrusion. Prostheses connecting any part of ossicular chain to capitulum are called PORP. (Right) Coronal graphic shows a TORP ⮕ connecting the TM to the oval window. A piston-based TORP ⮕ is used with stapedectomy. Intervening cartilage cap ⮕ is between TM and prosthesis head.

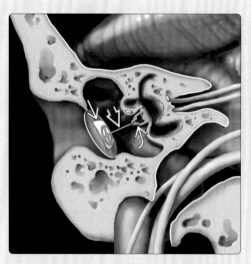
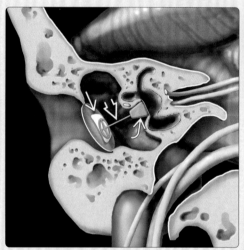

(Left) Coronal graphic shows a type of stapes piston prosthesis. The incus end ⮕ hooks to incus long process. The piston base ⮕ connects to oval window via stapedotomy. (Right) Coronal graphic reveals an example of incus interposition graft where the incus ⮕ is sculpted and rotated to connect handle of malleus to capitulum of stapes. A groove ⮕ is created in the remaining long process of incus to anchor it to the manubrium. A hole ⮕ is drilled in the incus body to accommodate the stapes capitulum.

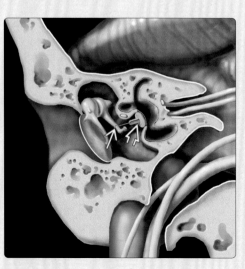
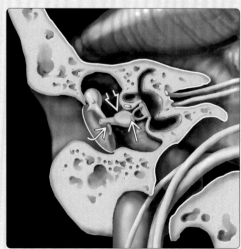

Ossicular Prosthesis

TERMINOLOGY

Synonyms

- Ossicular replacement prosthesis (ORP)

Definitions

- Ossiculoplasty: Surgical reconstruction of malfunctioned part of ossicular chain to improve or maintain conductive hearing function
- Materials: Allograft > autograft > > homograft
  - **Allograft**: Synthetic ossicular replacements (titanium)
  - **Autograft**: Patient's own ossicle used
  - **Homograft**: Radiated, frozen human ossicles
    - Homograft use ↓ ↓ in 1990s over concern of risk for disease transmission (e.g., AIDS)
  - **Autologous**: Patient's own pinna cortical bone and cartilage

4 Common ORP Types

- Stapes prosthesis
- Incus interposition graft
- Partial ossicular replacement prosthesis (PORP)
- Total ossicular replacement prosthesis (TORP)

IMAGING

General Features

- Best diagnostic clue
  - All or part of ossicular chain (OC) replaced by tissue graft (autograft, homograft, autolograft) or allograft
    - Auto-, homo-, autolograft: Ossicular bone density
    - Allograft: Metallic, soft tissue density, or combination
  - Prosthetic malfunction suggested by displacement, presence of abnormal soft tissue ± recurrence of conductive hearing loss (CHL)
  - Findings of underlying disease (e.g., otosclerosis), its complications [e.g., middle ear (ME) erosion in cholesteatoma], or related surgery (mastoidectomy) may be seen
- Location
  - Mesotympanum (ME cavity proper)

CT Findings

- Bone CT
  - **Stapes prosthesis**
    - Most commonly seen in otosclerosis setting
    - Stapes allograft connects long process of incus to stapes footplate of oval window (OW)
      - "Missing" all or part of stapes superstructure
      - OW interaction usually through hole in stapes footplate (stapedotomy)
      - OW insertion need not be central to function normally
    - Allograft materials variably visible
      - **Metallic** (titanium, stainless steel, platinum), soft tissue density (fluoroplastic), or combination
      - 4 main types: Wire loop, stapes piston > > bucket handle or homemade
      - "Anatomical" parts designated incus end (hook/clip/bucket handle), shaft and base (wire loop/piston)
  - **Incus interposition graft**
    - Most commonly seen in chronic otitis media (COM)
    - Incus **rotated and resculpted** to connect malleus with stapes capitulum
      - Normal incus is "missing"
      - Typically patient's own incus body (autograft)
      - Malleus head, cortical bone, or cartilage graft may be used if incus not available
      - Looks like "dislocated" incus if history of surgery is not known
  - **TORP or PORP**
    - More commonly seen in advanced COM or cholesteatoma
    - TORP: Replace entire OC, connect **tympanic membrane (TM) to OW**
      - "Anatomically" TORP head on TM, shaft and base on OW
      - Shaft is straight from TM to OW
    - PORP: Replace **part of OC** to **articulate with stapes superstructure**
      - Straight if connects TM to capitulum
      - Short and angled if only incudostapedial joint replaced
    - Materials: Metallic (titanium), bone density (ceramic), plastic, or combination
    - Wide variety of designs available
      - Specific name depends on manufacturer
    - TM looks thickened due to use of cartilage cap
- **Prosthetic malfunction on bone CT**
  - General CT findings
    - Dislocation/subluxation: Most commonly occurs in early postoperative period (< 6 weeks)
      - Before fibrosis secures ORP
    - Lateralization: Prosthesis drifts away, widened gap with OW
    - Protrusion: Prosthesis protrudes into vestibule (vertigo)
    - Abnormal soft tissue visible on scan
      - Embedded ORP: Represents granulation, fibrosis, or recurrent cholesteatoma
      - At oval window: Granulation-fibrosis; soft tissue develops 4-6 week after surgery (excessive stapedectomy)
    - Ankylosis with ME wall
      - Higher risk if ossicle touches ME wall and with Gelfoam (used with TORP)
    - Recurrent/progressive COM, cholesteatoma, otosclerosis
    - Surgical complications: Rare, occur early
      - Pneumolabyrinth or unexplained fluid in ME may suggest perilymph fistula
      - ME wall thickening and soft tissue may suggest postoperative otitis media
  - Specific stapes prosthesis malfunction findings
    - Necrosis of long process of incus: Related to manipulation and crimping
    - Malleoincudal joint subluxation: Abnormal torque from too long/malpositioned prosthesis
  - Specific incus interposition malfunction findings
    - Incus necrosis or recurrent cholesteatoma
  - Specific TORP/PORP malfunction findings
    - Extrusion of prosthesis through TM

□ Incidence reduced with interposing cartilage cap between TM and ORP head

Imaging Recommendations

- Best imaging tool
  - Temporal bone CT axial and coronal ~ 0.6-mm slices best for evaluating ossicle status and prosthesis complications
    - Ossicle relationships best seen on coronal CT
- TORP and PORP **MR safety**
  - Many modern prostheses are tested safe or conditional at 1.5T or 3T
  - Be sure to check specific product against known MR safety

DIFFERENTIAL DIAGNOSIS

COM With Tympanosclerosis

- If history of ossicular surgery unknown, misdiagnosis possible
- Must know normal prosthesis appearances

Posttraumatic Incus Dislocation

- Temporal bone trauma history is key
- May appear identical to incus interposition graft
- Incus may be found anywhere in middle ear or EAC

Middle Ear Foreign Body

- Clinical history is crucial

Semiimplantable Direct Drive Hearing Device

- Synonym: Active ME implantation devices
- Designed for moderate to severe sensorineural hearing loss with **intact ME ossicles**
  - May soon be used for CHL
- Implantable components consist of floating mass transducer **anchored to incus**
- Receiver in retroauricular subcutaneous layer (called vibrating ossicular replacement prosthesis or VORP)
  - Connecting wire visible

PATHOLOGY

General Features

- Etiology
  - Need for ossicular chain surgery driven by multiple clinical scenarios
    - Chronic otitis media and cholesteatoma account for **80%** of ossicular injury
    - Fenestral otosclerosis
    - COM with tympanosclerosis
    - Trauma
    - Congenital or idiopathic ossicle fusion

Gross Pathologic & Surgical Features

- Incus erosion = most commonly encountered defect
  - Incudostapedial joint erosion > absent incus > absent incus and stapes superstructure
- Stapes foot plate fixation due to otosclerosis, tympanosclerosis, or congenital stapes fixation
- Mallealincudal fixation may be congenital or due to tympanosclerosis

CLINICAL ISSUES

Presentation

- Most common signs/symptoms
  - Conductive hearing loss
- Other signs/symptoms
  - Postoperative symptoms suggesting **prosthesis malfunction**
    - Recurrent conductive hearing loss or vertigo weeks to months after surgery

Demographics

- Age
  - All ages

Natural History & Prognosis

- Early postoperative malfunction relates to surgical error or graft subluxation/dislocation
- Delayed prosthetic malfunction from mechanical failure, scarring, or recurrent/progressive disease

Treatment

- Treat recurrent otitis media ± cholesteatoma 1st
- Prosthesis malfunction requires replacement

DIAGNOSTIC CHECKLIST

Consider

- Consider prosthesis subluxation if history of recurrent CHL or vertigo

Image Interpretation Pearls

- Must have clinical and surgical history (including type of prosthesis used)
- Must have knowledge of following prior to evaluation
  - Normal ossicular anatomy
  - Normal prosthesis appearance
  - Detailed surgical history

SELECTED REFERENCES

1. Azadarmaki R et al: MRI information for commonly used otologic implants: review and update. Otolaryngol Head Neck Surg. 150(4):512-9, 2014
2. Malhotra M et al: Autologous total ossicular replacement prosthesis. J Laryngol Otol. 128(12):1050-5, 2014
3. Shellock FG et al: In vitro magnetic resonance imaging evaluation of ossicular implants at 3 T. Otol Neurotol. 33(5):871-7, 2012
4. Zeitler DM et al: Are postoperative hearing results better with titanium ossicular reconstruction prostheses? Laryngoscope. 120(1):2-3, 2010
5. Streitberger C et al: Vibrant Soundbridge for hearing restoration after chronic ear surgery. Rev Laryngol Otol Rhinol (Bord). 130(2):83-8, 2009
6. Burmeister HP et al: Three-dimensional imaging of active and passive middle ear prostheses using multislice computed tomography. J Comput Assist Tomogr. 32(2):304-12, 2008
7. Fritsch MH et al: Phylogeny of the stapes prosthesis. Otol Neurotol. 29(3):407-15, 2008
8. Rangheard AS et al: Postoperative complications in otospongiosis: usefulness of MR imaging. AJNR Am J Neuroradiol. 22(6):1171-8, 2001
9. Scheid SC et al: Pneumolabyrinth: a late complication of stapes surgery. Ear Nose Throat J. 80(10):750-3, 2001
10. Pickuth D et al: Vertigo after stapes surgery: the role of high resolution CT. Br J Radiol. 73(873):1021-3, 2000
11. Stone JA et al: CT evaluation of prosthetic ossicular reconstruction procedures: what the otologist needs to know. Radiographics. 20(3):593-605, 2000
12. Hirsch BE et al: Imaging of ossicular prostheses. Otolaryngol Head Neck Surg. 111(4):494-6, 1994

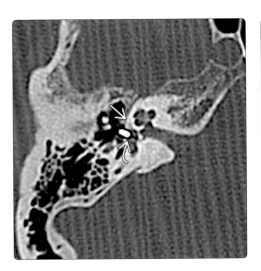

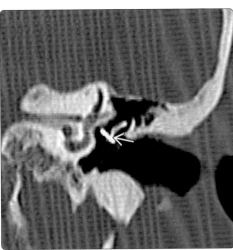

(Left) *Axial bone CT in a patient with post stapes implant vertigo and conductive hearing loss shows a stapes prosthesis protruding into the vestibule through the oval window ➡. Notice the fenestral otosclerosis plaque in the fissula ante fenestram ➡ along the anterior margin of the oval window.* (Right) *Coronal bone CT in the same patient shows that the head of stapes prosthesis ➡ articulates with the long process of incus. The oval window attachment is out of plane.*

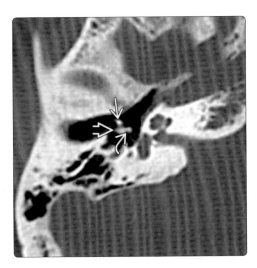

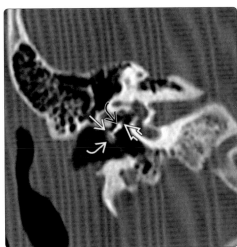

(Left) *Axial bone CT demonstrates an incus interposition graft ➡. The incus is rotated to connect the manubrium of the malleus ➡ with the capitulum of the stapes. A hole ➡ has been drilled in the incus body to receive the capitulum.* (Right) *Coronal bone CT shows a metallic PORP. The head ➡, shaft, and base ➡ project straight across to the stapes capitulum ➡. Focal soft tissue thickening at TM represents the cartilage cap ➡ commonly used with PORP and TORP to reduce risk of extrusion.*

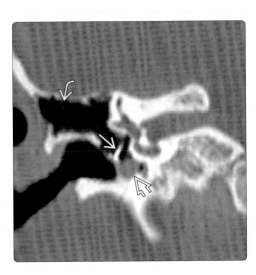

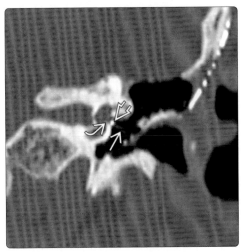

(Left) *Coronal bone CT shows a metallic PORP ➡. A soft tissue nodule ➡ with erosion of inferior tympanic annulus represents recurrent cholesteatoma. Evidence of mastoidectomy ➡ is related to previous congenital cholesteatoma excision.* (Right) *Coronal bone CT in a patient with recurrent conductive hearing loss reveals a TORP ➡ connecting TM to the oval window. Notice that the shaft has a beaded tip ➡, which is lateralized away from the oval window membrane ➡.*

Petromastoid Canal

TERMINOLOGY

- Petromastoid canal (PMC) definition: Normal temporal bone osseous canal that passes through arch of superior semicircular canal conveying subarcuate artery to otic capsule
- Synonyms: Subarcuate canal or canaliculus

IMAGING

- Osseous canal passing beneath superior semicircular canal
  - Infant: Globoid to tubular + CSF in subarachnoid space
    - Best seen on axial high resolution T2 MR
  - Adult: Linear with sclerotic margins on CT; unseen on MR

TOP DIFFERENTIAL DIAGNOSES

- Large vestibular aqueduct (IP-II)
- Prominent cochlear aqueduct
- Temporal bone fracture involving inner ear

PATHOLOGY

- Maximum size of petromastoid canal occurs at week 21 of embryonic development
  - Then ↓ in size to form subarcuate fossa & PMC
- Contains subarcuate artery & vein
- PMC in child < 2 yr of age
  - **Dural-lined subarachnoid space** connected to cerebellopontine angle cistern
- PMC in child > 2 yr of age
  - Involutes with disappearance of dura, subarachnoid space, and CSF

DIAGNOSTIC CHECKLIST

- PMC may be mistaken for pathology
  - In infant: Inner ear or petrous apex anomaly
  - In adult: Temporal bone fracture
- PMC = potential route of spread of infection

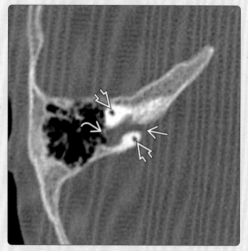
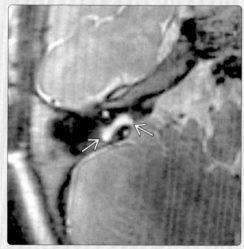

(Left) Axial bone CT in a 9 month old shows a prominent petromastoid canal extending from the medial petrous ridge ➡, beneath the superior semicircular canal ➡, to the medial mastoid antrum wall ➡. Note the thin bony wall at its medial margin. (Right) Axial T2 MR in the same infant shows the conspicuous high-signal petromastoid canal ➡. Early in life (< 2 yr of age), this developing structure is a dural-lined subarachnoid space filled with high-signal CSF that may be confused with pathology.

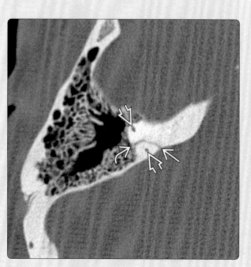
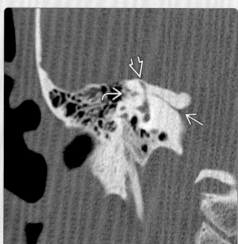

(Left) Axial temporal bone CT of adult right ear shows normal, linear, arching petromastoid canal passing from the medial petrous ridge ➡ under the superior semicircular canal ➡ to the lateral wall of the mastoid antrum ➡. (Right) Coronal CT in the same adult shows a normal curvilinear petromastoid canal passing from the subarcuate fossa of medial petrous ridge ➡ beneath the superior semicircular canal ➡ to the medial wall of the mastoid antrum ➡. PMC may be mistaken for a fracture.

Petromastoid Canal

TERMINOLOGY

Abbreviations

- Petromastoid canal (PMC)

Synonyms

- Subarcuate canal or canaliculus, subarcuate channel or tract, subarcuate artery canal

Definitions

- PMC: Normal temporal bone osseous canal that passes through arch of superior semicircular canal (SSC) conveying subarcuate artery to otic capsule

IMAGING

General Features

- Best diagnostic clue
  - Osseous canal passing through superior SSC
    - < 2 yr of age: Globoid to tubular + CSF in subarachnoid space
    - Adult: Linear (< 1 mm in width) with sclerotic margins on CT

CT Findings

- Bone CT
  - Infant under 2 yr of age
    - PMC passes under SSC
    - Measures 2-3x cross-sectional SSC dimension
  - Child > 2 yr of age
    - Adult: PMC seen as dark line passing under SSC
    - Measures ≤ cross-sectional SSC dimension

MR Findings

- T2WI
  - Infant < 2 yr of age
    - CSF intensity passage from subarcuate fossa medially to lateral wall of mastoid antrum
    - Passes under SCC
  - Child > 2 yr of age
    - PMC not visible on MR

Imaging Recommendations

- Best imaging tool
  - Temporal bone CT without contrast best shows PMC

DIFFERENTIAL DIAGNOSIS

Large Vestibular Aqueduct (IP-II)

- CT: Large bony vestibular aqueduct posterior to IAC
  - Connects to crus communis; orthogonal to PMC course
- MR: Large endolymphatic sac & duct

Prominent Cochlear Aqueduct

- May be mistaken for fracture or PMC
- CT: Parallel & inferior to IAC

Temporal Bone Fracture

- Clinical history of significant head trauma
- CT: Lacks sclerotic margins of subarcuate canaliculus
  - Air-fluid levels in middle ear cavity ± mastoid air cells
  - Pneumolabyrinth possible

PATHOLOGY

General Features

- Embryology/anatomy
  - Maximum size of subarcuate sinus occurs at week 21 of embryonic development
  - Then ↓ in size to form subarcuate fossa & PMC
    - Contains subarcuate artery & vein
    - PMC in child < 2 yr of age is **dural-lined subarachnoid space** connected to cerebellopontine angle (CPA) cistern
    - After 2 yr of age, PMC involutes with disappearance of dura, subarachnoid space, and CSF
  - Adult PMC
    - Mean length: 10.5 mm
    - ~ 50% of canals have width between 0.5-1.0 mm
    - Other 50% > 1-2 mm
  - **Subarcuate artery**
    - Subarcuate artery arises from labyrinthine artery medial to IAC
    - Labyrinthine artery arises from basilar artery or anterior inferior cerebellar artery (AICA)
    - Subarcuate artery may arise directly from AICA
    - Enters subarcuate fossa to travel in PMC
    - Supplies otic capsule, semicircular canals, & posterior wall vestibule
    - Distal branches anastomose with branches from superficial petrosal, stylomastoid, posterior meningeal, & occipital arteries

CLINICAL ISSUES

Presentation

- Most common signs/symptoms
  - Asymptomatic normal variant
- Clinical profile
  - Conspicuous structure in infant
  - May be incorrectly identified as **petrous apex or inner ear lesion**

Natural History & Prognosis

- Normal anatomic variant
- No treatment required

DIAGNOSTIC CHECKLIST

Consider

- PMC may be mistaken for pathology
  - In infant: Petrous apex or inner ear anomaly
  - In adult: Temporal bone fracture
- PMC = potential route of spread of infection

SELECTED REFERENCES

1. Mena-Domínguez EA et al: Petromastoid canal. Acta Otorrinolaringol Esp. 66(3):180, 2015
2. Koral K et al: MRI of the petromastoid canal in children. J Magn Reson Imaging. 39(4):966-71, 2014
3. Migirov L et al: Radiology of the petromastoid canal. Otol Neurotol. 27(3):410-3, 2006
4. Krombach GA et al: The petromastoid canal on computed tomography. Eur Radiol. 12(11):2770-5, 2002
5. Tekdemir I et al: The subarcuate canaliculus and its artery–a radioanatomical study. Ann Anat. 181(2):207-11, 1999

Cochlear Cleft

TERMINOLOGY

- Synonyms for cochlear cleft
  - Localized pericochlear hypoattenuating foci
  - Cochlear capsule space
- Cochlear cleft definition
  - Developmental curvilinear lucency attributed to nonosseous otic capsule space adjacent to cochlea in children

IMAGING

- Bone CT (< 1-mm thick images)
  - Bilateral > unilateral
  - C-shaped, thin, sharply defined lucency in otic capsule
  - Adjacent to middle & apical portions of first 2 cochlear turns
  - Adjacent lateral > medial aspect of cochlea
  - Anterior to oval window
  - Does not extend to oval window
- Parallel to cochlea on coronal images

- Lucency curved in shape of cochlear promontory

TOP DIFFERENTIAL DIAGNOSES

- Fenestral otosclerosis
- Cochlear otosclerosis
- Temporal bone osteogenesis imperfecta
- Postirradiated temporal bone

CLINICAL ISSUES

- Clinical presentation
  - Incidental finding in child
- Becomes less conspicuous & disappears with age
  - Medial lucency disappears 1st
- Age vs. incidence of cochlear cleft
  - **< 4 years**: Present in **~ 60%**
  - 4-7 years: Present in ~ 45%
  - 7-10 years: Present in ~ 25%
  - 10-19 years: Present in ~ 20%

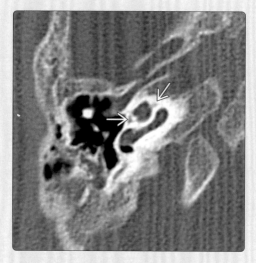
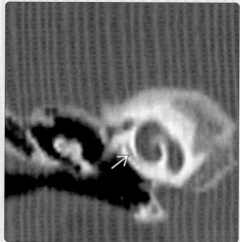

(Left) Normal temporal bone CT in 2-month-old girl with sensorineural hearing loss demonstrates well-defined curvilinear lucency ➡ within the otic capsule bone parallel to the cochlear turns. The lucency is more pronounced laterally than medially. These findings are characteristic of developmental cochlear cleft. (Right) Right ear coronal reformatted bone CT reveals the curvilinear lucency ➡ within the otic capsule bone parallel to the cochlea, just deep to the surface of the cochlear promontory.

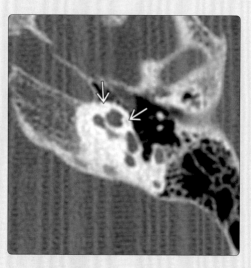
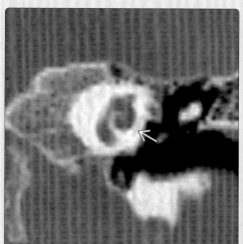

(Left) Axial bone CT in a 3-year-old boy with sensorineural hearing loss and a normal CT exam shows an evolving cochlear cleft. At this stage, a linear lucency ➡ is present medial & lateral to the apical portions of first 2 cochlear turns. (Right) Coronal CT reformation in the same patient shows a faint cochlear cleft lucent line ➡ lateral to the cochlea deep to the cochlear promontory surface.

TERMINOLOGY

Abbreviations
- Cochlear cleft (CC)

Synonyms
- Localized pericochlear hypoattenuating foci
- Cochlear capsule space

Definitions
- Developmental **curvilinear lucency** attributed to nonosseous otic capsule space adjacent to cochlea in children

IMAGING

General Features
- Best diagnostic clue
  - Sharply defined, thin, curvilinear lucency on bone CT
- Location
  - Adjacent to apical portion 1st cochlear turn

CT Findings
- Bone CT
  - Bilateral > unilateral
  - C-shaped, thin, sharply defined lucency in otic capsule
    - Adjacent to middle & apical portions of first 2 cochlear turns
      - Rarely adjacent to basal portion of 1st turn
    - Adjacent lateral > medial aspect of cochlea
    - May extend to apical turn on axial images
    - Anterior to oval window
      - Does not extend to oval window
  - Parallel to cochlea on coronal images
    - Follows shape of cochlear promontory

Imaging Recommendations
- Best imaging tool
  - Bone CT
- Protocol advice
  - < 1-mm images

DIFFERENTIAL DIAGNOSIS

Fenestral Otosclerosis
- Rare in children
- Conductive hearing loss
- CT: Focal smudgy hypodensity begins at fissula ante fenestram
  - May spread to involve round window margin, cochlear otic capsule

Cochlear Otosclerosis
- Rare in children
- Mixed hearing loss
- CT: Linear hypodensity within otic capsule

Temporal Bone Osteogenesis Imperfecta
- Generalized hypodensity, multiple skeletal fractures
- CT: Lucency of otic capsule bone
  - Cannot be differentiated from cochlear otosclerosis

Postirradiated Temporal Bone
- Radiation history; uncommon complication
- CT: Heterogeneous lucency otic capsule bone

PATHOLOGY

Staging, Grading, & Classification
- CC scoring
  - 0: Cleft not present
  - 1: No definite cleft
  - 2: Small cleft
  - 3: Moderate cleft
  - 4: Large cleft

Gross Pathologic & Surgical Features
- 2 possible explanations
  - Space in interface between inner endosteal & outer periosteal layers of otic capsule
    - **Middle layer of otic capsule bone** (endochondral + intrachondral bone) partly cartilaginous near term
    - Rapidly ossifies leaving small marrow spaces
  - Related to fissula ante fenestram
    - Fissula ante fenestram is fibrocartilaginous cleft anterior to oval window
    - Histologically aberrant bulky cartilage can form in proximity
- CC occurs in 1 of last areas of otic capsule to fully ossify
- Variation vs. delay in capsule ossification

CLINICAL ISSUES

Presentation
- Most common signs/symptoms
  - Incidental finding

Demographics
- Age
  - **< 4 years**: Present in **~ 60%**
  - 4-7 years: Present in ~ 45%
  - 7-10 years: Present in ~ 25%
  - 10-19 years: Present in ~ 20%

Natural History & Prognosis
- Becomes less conspicuous & usually disappears by 10 years of age
- Medial lucency disappears 1st

Treatment
- None; developmental variant

DIAGNOSTIC CHECKLIST

Image Interpretation Pearls
- Sharply defined lucency around cochlea in infant/young child
- Often bilateral

Reporting Tips
- Do not mistake for otosclerosis

SELECTED REFERENCES

1. Chadwell JB et al: The cochlear cleft. AJNR Am J Neuroradiol. 25(1):21-4, 2004

TERMINOLOGY

- Synonyms: Complete labyrinthine aplasia (CLA); Michel anomaly (old synonym)

IMAGING

- Bilateral or unilateral anomaly
- Temporal bone CT findings
  - Otic capsule bone: Aplasia/hypoplasia
  - Absent cochlea, vestibule, semicircular canals, & vestibular aqueduct
  - Cochlear promontory: Absent/flattened
  - Ossicles: Normal or malformed stapes
  - Tegmen tympani: Normal, low, or defective
  - Facial nerve canal: Aberrant course
  - Petrous apex: Hypoplasia
  - Internal auditory canal: Aplasia/hypoplasia
  - Carotid canal: Normal or absent
- MR: Absent vestibular & cochlear nerves

TOP DIFFERENTIAL DIAGNOSES

- Cochlear aplasia
- Common cavity
- Labyrinthine ossification, obliterative type

PATHOLOGY

- Genetic mutation (e.g., *HOXA1*), thalidomide exposure, or unknown etiology
- **Arrested otic placode development** before 3rd week of gestation

CLINICAL ISSUES

- Extremely rare anomaly
- Congenital sensorineural hearing loss
- Horizontal gaze palsy or abnormal teeth suggest underlying syndrome

DIAGNOSTIC CHECKLIST

- Often asymmetric: Contralateral common cavity, inner ear hypoplasia, or cochlear IP-I anomaly

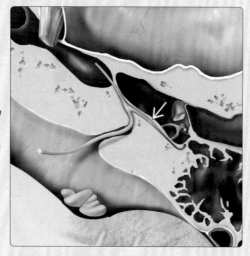
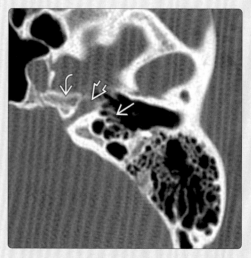

(Left) *Axial graphic depicts labyrinthine aplasia. Note the complete absence of all inner ear structures with the exception of a small IAC with only CNVII. Lateral wall of inner ear (promontory) is flattened ➡.* **(Right)** *Axial bone CT in 21-year-old woman with SNHL shows severe hypoplasia of otic capsule bone with air cells in expected location of the promontory ➡. Inner ear structures are absent. CNVII canal is present with a broadened anterior genu ➡. Note petrous apex is hypoplastic ➡, narrow in width.*

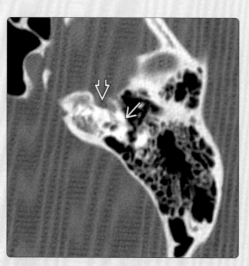
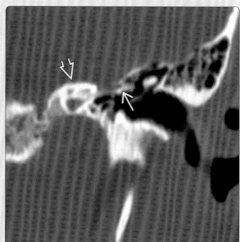

(Left) *Axial bone CT, in the same patient at a more cephalad level, shows hypoplastic otic capsule bone ➡. The anterior genu and proximal tympanic segment of the anomalous CNVII canal are visible ➡.* **(Right)** *Coronal bone CT in the same patient reveals complete absence of inner ear structures and severe hypoplasia of the otic capsule bone ➡ & petrous apex ➡. Note normal middle ear and ossicles despite complete inner ear aplasia.*

TERMINOLOGY

Synonyms
- **Complete labyrinthine aplasia** (CLA)
- Old synonym: Michel anomaly

Definitions
- **Absent cochlea, vestibule, & semicircular canals** (SCCs)

IMAGING

General Features
- Best diagnostic clue
  - Complete absence of inner ear structures
  - Absence/hypoplasia of otic capsule bone
- Morphology
  - Labyrinth fails to develop
  - Aplasia/hypoplasia of otic capsule bone

CT Findings
- Bone CT
  - Bilateral or unilateral anomaly
  - Otic capsule bone: Aplasia/hypoplasia
  - Absent cochlea, vestibule, SCC, vestibular aqueduct
  - Cochlear promontory: Absent/flattened
  - Ossicles: Normal or malformed stapes
  - Tegmen tympani: Normal, low, or defective (suggesting encephalocele)
  - Middle ear & mastoid: Normal or hypoplastic
  - Facial nerve canal: Aberrant course
  - Petrous apex: Hypoplasia
  - Internal auditory canal: Aplasia/hypoplasia
  - Jugular bulb/vein: Normal, dehiscent or stenotic + large emissary veins
  - Carotid canal: Normal or absent
  - Clivus: Normal or narrowed
  - Cervical spine: Normal or + anomalies

MR Findings
- T2WI
  - Absent membranous labyrinth
  - Absent vestibular & cochlear nerves
  - Large cerebellopontine angle cistern/arachnoid cyst
  - Pontine anomaly

Imaging Recommendations
- Best imaging tool
  - Bone CT
  - MR brain & temporal bones

DIFFERENTIAL DIAGNOSIS

Cochlear Aplasia
- **Late 3rd-week arrest**: Absent cochlea, dysmorphic vestibule, & SCC

Common Cavity
- **4th-week arrest**: Ovoid globular sac represents cochlea + vestibule

Labyrinthine Ossificans
- Postmeningitic inner ear ossification, promontory well formed

PATHOLOGY

General Features
- Etiology
  - Genetic mutation, thalidomide exposure, or unknown etiology
- Genetics
  - *FGF3* mutations: LAMM (**l**abyrinthine **a**plasia, **m**icrotia, **m**icrodontia)
  - *HOXA1* mutations: Bosley-Salih-Alorainy syndrome (BSAS) & Athabaskan brainstem dysgenesis (ABDS)
- Associated abnormalities
  - BSAS & ABDS: Congenital heart disease, horizontal gaze palsy, absent internal carotid arteries
- Embryology
  - **Arrest** of otic placode development **before 3rd gestational week**

Gross Pathologic & Surgical Features
- Failure of bony & membranous labyrinth formation

Microscopic Features
- Inner ear structures not present

CLINICAL ISSUES

Presentation
- Most common signs/symptoms
  - Congenital sensorineural hearing loss (SNHL)

Demographics
- Epidemiology
  - Extremely rare, < 1% of inner ear malformations

Treatment
- Unilateral CLA: Assess contralateral side for implantation if bilateral SNHL
- Bilateral CLA: Brainstem implantation

DIAGNOSTIC CHECKLIST

Consider
- CLA if otic capsule bone is absent/hypoplastic & cochlea, vestibule & SCC are absent

Image Interpretation Pearls
- Often asymmetric: Contralateral common cavity, inner ear hypoplasia, or cochlear IP-I anomaly

Reporting Tips
- Variable pathognomonic flattening of cochlear promontory: Subtle to marked
- Evaluate tegmen tympani integrity on coronal reformats

SELECTED REFERENCES

1. Marcus S et al: Computed tomography demonstrates abnormalities of contralateral ear in subjects with unilateral sensorineural hearing loss. Int J Pediatr Otorhinolaryngol. 78(2):268-71, 2014
2. Clemmens CS et al: Unilateral cochlear nerve deficiency in children. Otolaryngol Head Neck Surg. 149(2):318-25, 2013
3. Higley MJ et al: Bilateral complete labyrinthine aplasia with bilateral internal carotid artery aplasia, developmental delay, and gaze abnormalities: a presumptive case of a rare HOXA1 mutation syndrome. AJNR Am J Neuroradiol. 32(2):E23-5, 2011
4. Ozgen B et al: Complete labyrinthine aplasia: clinical and radiologic findings with review of the literature. AJNR Am J Neuroradiol. 30(4):774-80, 2009

Cochlear Aplasia

TERMINOLOGY

- Definition: Absent cochlea; vestibule, semicircular canals (SCC), & internal auditory canal (IAC) present in some form

IMAGING

- Cochlea: **Absent** bilaterally or unilaterally
- Cochlear nerve canal & cochlear nerve: **Absent**
- Cochlear promontory: Hypoplastic, **flattened**
- Vestibule & SCC: Often malformed, globular, & dilated or hypoplastic
- Vestibular aqueduct: **Normal**
- Facial nerve canal: **Anomalous**, obtuse angle anterior genu
- IAC: **Hypoplastic**
- Middle ear: Normal size
- Ossicles: Normal or malformed stapes
- Oval window: Normal or stenotic/atretic

TOP DIFFERENTIAL DIAGNOSES

- Labyrinthine aplasia

- ○ Cochlea, vestibule, & SCC absent
- Common cavity deformity
  - ○ Dilated cochlea & vestibule form common cavity
- Cystic cochleovestibular anomaly
  - ○ **Cochlea & vestibule are cystic with no internal architecture**
- Labyrinthine ossificans
  - ○ **Acquired sensorineural hearing loss (SNHL)**, usually postmeningitic

PATHOLOGY

- Absent cochlea, remainder of inner ear usually abnormal

CLINICAL ISSUES

- Extremely rare, congenital SNHL, usually bilateral

DIAGNOSTIC CHECKLIST

- Cochlear aplasia if no cochlea is seen on CT or T2 MR but rest of membranous labyrinth is present
- Distinguish from obliterative cochlear ossification

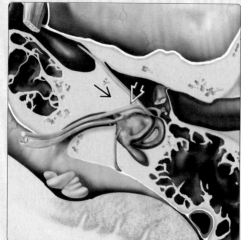
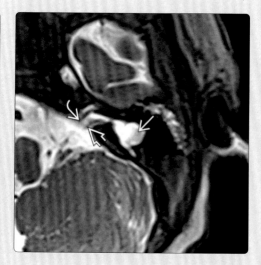

(Left) Axial graphic shows findings of cochlear aplasia, including small inner auditory canal (IAC) with absence of cochlear nerve, absent cochlea ➡, vestibular & semicircular canal malformation, & flattening of CNVII anterior genu ➡. (Right) Axial T2 SPACE in a 4-month-old girl with congenital SNHL reveals cochlear absence. There is globular vestibule-horizontal semicircular canal anomaly ➡. Short, narrow internal auditory meatus contains vestibular ➡ & facial ➡ nerves. No cochlear nerve was seen.

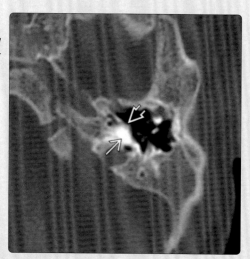
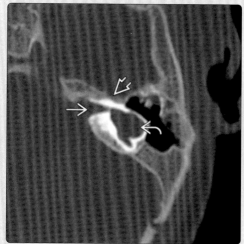

(Left) Axial bone CT in the same patient demonstrates absence of the cochlea ➡ and mild flattening of the cochlear promontory ➡. (Right) Axial bone CT in the same patient shows a globular, malformed vestibule-horizontal semicircular canal ➡. A shortened, narrowed IAC is seen ➡. An obtuse anterior genu of the facial nerve canal is partially visualized ➡ with an anomalous course of the facial nerve canal.

TERMINOLOGY

Synonyms

- Absent cochlea

Definitions

- Absent cochlea; vestibule, semicircular canals (SCC), & internal auditory canal (IAC) present in some form

IMAGING

General Features

- Best diagnostic clue
  - Absent cochlea, usually dysmorphic vestibule & SCC
- Location
  - Anterior membranous labyrinth

CT Findings

- Bone CT
  - Cochlea: **Absent**, bilaterally or unilaterally
  - Cochlear nerve canal: **Absent**
  - Cochlear promontory: Hypoplastic, flattened
  - Vestibule & SCC: Often **malformed**, globular, & dilated or hypoplastic
  - Vestibular aqueduct: **Usually normal**
  - Facial nerve canal: Anomalous, obtuse angle anterior genu
  - IAC: Usually **hypoplastic**
  - Middle ear: **Normal size**
  - Ossicles: Normal or malformed stapes
  - Oval window: Normal or stenotic/atretic
  - Round window: Atretic

MR Findings

- T2WI
  - Cochlea & cochlear nerve: Absent
  - Vestibule & SCC: Variable abnormality

Imaging Recommendations

- Best imaging tool
  - Temporal bone CT or MR

DIFFERENTIAL DIAGNOSIS

Labyrinthine Aplasia

- **Cochlea, vestibule, & SCC absent**
- Embryogenesis: Developmental arrest in 3rd gestational week

Common Cavity Deformity

- **Dilated cochlea & vestibule form common cavity**
- Embryogenesis: Developmental arrest in 4th gestational week

Cystic Cochleovestibular Anomaly

- **Cochlea & vestibule are cystic with no internal architecture**
- Embryogenesis: Developmental arrest, in 5th gestational week

Labyrinthine Ossificans

- Clinical presentation: **Acquired sensorineural hearing loss (SNHL)**, usually following meningitis

- Densely ossified membranous labyrinth, normal promontory

PATHOLOGY

General Features

- Etiology
  - Unknown
- Associated abnormalities
  - Vestibule & SSC may be dilated
- Embryology
  - Arrest of otic placode development at late 3rd gestational week

Gross Pathologic & Surgical Features

- Absent cochlea, remainder of inner ear usually present but abnormal

CLINICAL ISSUES

Presentation

- Most common signs/symptoms
  - Congenital SNHL, usually bilateral

Demographics

- Age
  - Congenital, present at birth
- Epidemiology
  - Extremely rare inner ear anomaly
  - < 1% of all inner ear congenital lesions

Treatment

- Bilateral SNHL + bilateral cochlear aplasia: Auditory brainstem implantation
- Cochlear implantation contraindicated when cochlea absent
  - Cochlear nerve absent
  - Vestibular implantation occasionally performed with some neural response, provided that audiological response is demonstrated prior to surgery

DIAGNOSTIC CHECKLIST

Consider

- Cochlear aplasia diagnosed if **no** cochlea is seen on CT or T2 MR but rest of membranous labyrinth is present
  - Important to distinguish cochlear aplasia from obliterative cochlear ossification

SELECTED REFERENCES

1. Sennaroğlu L et al: Long-term results of ABI in children with severe inner ear malformations. Otol Neurotol. ePub, 2016
2. Kontorinis G et al: Aplasia of the cochlea: radiologic assessment and options for hearing rehabilitation. Otol Neurotol. 34(7):1253-60, 2013
3. Jeong SW et al: Cochlear implantation in children with cochlear aplasia. Acta Otolaryngol. 132(9):910-5, 2012
4. Sennaroğlu L et al: A new classification for cochleovestibular malformations. Laryngoscope. 112(12):2230-41, 2002
5. Jackler RK et al: Congenital malformations of the inner ear: a classification based on embryogenesis. Laryngoscope. 97(3 Pt 2 Suppl 40):2-14, 1987

TERMINOLOGY

- Small, underdeveloped cochlea, usually < 2 turns

IMAGING

- Cochlea (variable severity)
  - Primitive single turn or bud-like
  - Small, cystic, no modiolus or interscalar septum
  - Small, + internal architecture, short modiolus
- Cochlear nerve canal: Absent, narrow, normal, wide
- Cochlear nerve: Often absent or hypoplastic
- Facial nerve canal: Aberrant course ± dehiscence
- Internal auditory canal: Normal or narrow/anomalous
- Vestibule: Normal, dilated, or hypoplastic
- Vestibular aqueduct: Normal or large

TOP DIFFERENTIAL DIAGNOSES

- Cochlear incomplete partition
  - Cochlea size is normal to large; absent interscalar septum & modiolus

- Cochlear incomplete partition
  - Deficient modiolus, absent interscalar septum between plump apical & middle turns, large vestibular aqueduct (LVA)
- Branchiootorenal syndrome
  - Hypoplastic offset middle & apical turns, ± funnel-shaped LVA
- CHARGE syndrome
  - Small/absent semicircular canal (SCC), variable cochlear hypoplasia, ± funnel-shaped LVA

CLINICAL ISSUES

- Congenital sensorineural hearing loss

DIAGNOSTIC CHECKLIST

- Consider CHARGE syndrome: Cochlear hypoplasia, cochlear nerve canal stenosis, small vestibule, & small/aplastic SCC
- Consider branchiootorenal syndrome: Tapered basal turn, hypoplastic, offset middle & apical turns

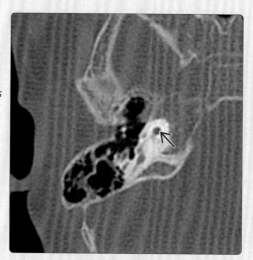
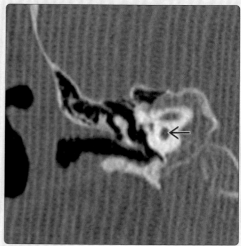

(Left) Axial bone CT in a 2.5-year-old boy with bilateral profound congenital sensorineural hearing loss shows a small bud-like structure, consistent with cochlear hypoplasia ⊸, that is isolated from the internal auditory canal (IAC). The round window is absent. (Right) Coronal CT reconstruction in the same patient shows the small bud-like hypoplastic cochlea ⊸ with no internal architecture.

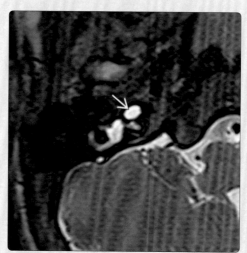
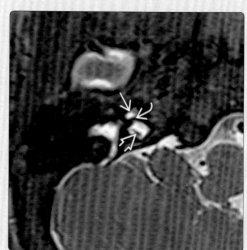

(Left) 3D T2 SPACE MR in a infant boy with bilateral profound sensorineural hearing loss shows a single, rounded cochlear turn ⊸ without a modiolus. (Right) A more cephalad image in the same infant reveals the superior aspect of the single cochlear turn ⊸. The IAC and inferior vestibular nerve ⊸ appear normal. The cochlear nerve is not identified, and the cochlear nerve canal is absent ⊸.

TERMINOLOGY

Abbreviations

- Cochlear hypoplasia (CH)

Definitions

- Cochlear underdevelopment: **Small cochlea, usually < 2 turns**

IMAGING

General Features

- Best diagnostic clue
  - Small cochlea, usually with < 2 turns
  - Cochlea often lacks internal septation

CT Findings

- Bone CT
  - Cochlear appearance
    - Spectrum of severity, sometimes asymmetric
    - **Small cochlea, usually with < 2 turns**
    - **Internal cochlear structure present or absent**
    - Primitive single turn or bud-like
    - Small, cystic, no modiolus or interscalar septum
    - Small, internal architecture present, short modiolus
  - Round window: Absent or present
  - Cochlear nerve canal: Absent, narrow, or wide
  - Internal auditory canal: Normal or narrow/anomalous
  - Vestibule: Normal, dilated, or hypoplastic
  - Semicircular canals (SCCs): Normal, dilated, hypoplastic, or absent
  - Vestibular aqueduct: Normal or large
  - Facial nerve canal: Aberrant course ± dehiscence
  - Middle ear space & contents: Usually normal

MR Findings

- Cochlea: Small, < 2 turns, internal structure present or absent
- Cochlear nerve: **Often absent or hypoplastic**

Imaging Recommendations

- Best imaging tool
  - Thin-section (≤ 1 mm) bone CT with multiplanar reformations
  - High-resolution, thin-section (≤ 1 mm) MR
- Protocol advice
  - MR 3D T2 SPACE or FIESTA for CNVIII components

DIFFERENTIAL DIAGNOSIS

Cochlear Incomplete Partition

- Cochlea normal to large in size
- Interscalar septum absent
- Modiolus absent

Cochlear Incomplete Partition

- Cochlear modiolus deficient ± plump apical and middle turns
- Deficient septation between apical & middle turns
- Enlarged bony vestibular aqueduct (on CT)
- Enlarged endolymphatic sac & duct (on MR)

Branchiootorenal Syndrome

- Tapered cochlear basal turn
- Hypoplastic, offset middle & apical cochlear turns

CHARGE Syndrome

- CH (e.g., single turn), flattened apical turn or normal-sized cochlea
- Stenotic cochlear nerve canal
- Small vestibule
- Small or absent SCCs

PATHOLOGY

General Features

- Etiology
  - Unknown etiology & syndromic forms

Staging, Grading, & Classification

- CH type I (small cochlear bud)
  - No modiolus or interscalar septum
- CH type II (small cystic cochlea)
  - No modiolus or interscalar septum
- CH type III (small cochlea, < 2 turns)
  - Shortened modiolus & interscalar septum

Gross Pathologic & Surgical Features

- Small cochlea
- Cochlea ranges from bud to usually < 2 turns
- Cochlear interscalar septum absent or present

CLINICAL ISSUES

Presentation

- Most common signs/symptoms
  - Congenital sensorineural hearing loss (SNHL)
- Other signs/symptoms
  - Varies depending on underlying etiology

Treatment

- Bilateral SNHL + mild CH: Cochlear implant if cochlear nerve present
  - High-resolution sagittal oblique 3D T2WI MR to evaluate internal auditory canal for presence of cochlear nerve

DIAGNOSTIC CHECKLIST

Consider

- CH if small cochlea with < 2 turns

Image Interpretation Pearls

- Consider CHARGE: Cochlear nerve canal stenosis, small vestibule, & SCC hypoplasia/aplasia
- Consider branchiootorenal syndrome: Tapered basal turn cochlea
  - Hypoplastic, offset middle & apical turns

SELECTED REFERENCES

1. Sennaroglu L: Cochlear implantation in inner ear malformations--a review article. Cochlear Implants Int. 11(1):4-41, 2010
2. Teissier N et al: Computed tomography measurements of the normal and the pathologic cochlea in children. Pediatr Radiol. 40(3):275-83, 2010

Common Cavity Malformation

TERMINOLOGY

- Common cavity (CC) is cystic space representing undifferentiated cochlea & vestibule

IMAGING

- **Cochlea, vestibule, & horizontal SCC**: CC, variable size
- Posterior & superior SCC: Usually absent or malformed
- IAC: Variable size, anomalous course, deficient fundus
  - Small CC: Stenotic IAC
  - Large CC: Widened IAC
- CNVIII: Small or absent components
- Facial nerve canal: Anomalous course
- Vestibular aqueduct: Not dilated, may be absent
- Ossicles: Normal or anomalous stapes & stenotic oval window

TOP DIFFERENTIAL DIAGNOSES

- Cochlear aplasia
- Cystic cochleovestibular anomaly

PATHOLOGY

- Unknown or genetic mutation
- *HOXA1* mutations: Bosley-Salih-Alorainy syndrome

CLINICAL ISSUES

- Congenital sensorineural hearing loss
- Rare: < 1% of all congenital inner ear malformations
- Bilateral profound SNHL: Successful cochlear implantation reported in common cavity anomaly
- Potential risk of recurrent meningitis for large CC & large IAC with associated perilymph fistula

DIAGNOSTIC CHECKLIST

- Common cavity if cochlea, vestibule, & horizontal SCC form single cavity without differentiation
- Consider cystic cochleovestibular anomaly if differentiated into separate but featureless cochlea & vestibule
- If IAC enters anterior CC, can be difficult to distinguish from cochlear aplasia + globular vestibule & horizontal SCC

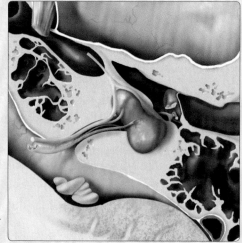
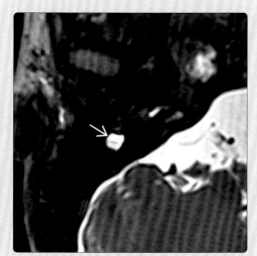

(Left) Axial graphic shows features of common cavity (CC) malformation. Note that the cochlea and vestibule are melded into 1 common cyst. Semicircular canals are not distinct from cystic vestibular component. *(Right)* Axial T2 SPACE MR in an 11-year-old boy with SNHL shows a small cyst ➡ in the expected location of the inner ear, without connection to the small IAC (not shown). It is not possible to distinguish this CC anomaly (cochlea & vestibule) from cochlear aplasia with a globular vestibule-semicircular canal anomaly.

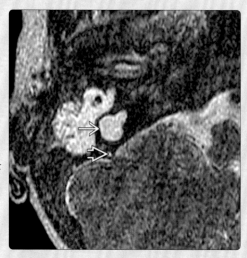
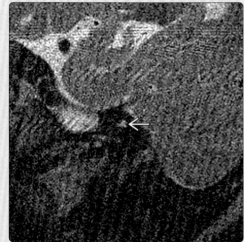

(Left) Axial 3D FIESTA image in an 18-month-old child with bilateral congenital sensorineural hearing loss demonstrates a common cavity anomaly with a cystic structure representing the vestibule, rudimentary cochlear bud, and horizontal semicircular canal ➡. There is a small posterior semicircular canal ➡. *(Right)* Oblique 2D FIESTA MR in the same patient shows a small internal auditory meatus containing only a single posteriorly located vestibular nerve ➡. No facial nerve is present.

TERMINOLOGY

Definitions

- Common cavity (CC) is cystic space representing **undifferentiated cochlea & vestibule**

IMAGING

General Features

- Best diagnostic clue
  - Featureless CC represents rudimentary cochlea, vestibule, & semicircular canals (SCCs)
- Location
  - Inner ear membranous labyrinth
- Size
  - CC: Small or large cystic structure
- Morphology
  - Ovoid cyst

CT Findings

- Bone CT
  - Unilateral or bilateral & often asymmetric
  - **Cochlea, vestibule, & horizontal SCC**: CC, variable size
  - Posterior and superior SCC: Usually absent or malformed
  - Internal auditory canal (IAC)
    - Small CC: Stenotic IAC
    - Large CC: Widened IAC
    - Defective fundus
    - Course may be anomalous
    - May enter center of CC
    - If directed to anterior aspect of CC may not be able to discriminate from cochlear aplasia
  - Facial nerve canal: Anomalous labyrinthine segment & anterior genu
  - Middle ear space & ossicles: Normal or anomalous stapes & stenotic oval window
  - Vestibular aqueduct: Not dilated, may be absent

MR Findings

- T2WI
  - High signal intensity fluid within common cavity
  - Posterior & superior SCC: Usually absent or malformed
  - IAC: Small or absent CNVIII components ± anomalous course of CNVII

Imaging Recommendations

- Best imaging tool
  - Temporal bone CT or MR
- Protocol advice
  - T2 oblique sagittal MR through IAC used to assess presence of cochlear nerve

DIFFERENTIAL DIAGNOSIS

Cochlear Aplasia

- Imaging: Absent cochlea, normal or malformed vestibule

Cystic Cochleovestibular Anomaly

- Imaging: Cochlea & vestibule are usually enlarged & cystic without internal architecture

Labyrinthine Aplasia

- Variant sometimes has tiny otocyst

PATHOLOGY

General Features

- Etiology
  - Unknown or genetic mutation
- Genetics
  - *HOXA1* mutations: Bosley-Salih-Alorainy syndrome
- Embryology
  - Developmental arrest in 4th gestational week, after differentiation of otic placode into otocyst

Microscopic Features

- May be some differentiation of organ of Corti, but neural populations are absent or low

CLINICAL ISSUES

Presentation

- Most common signs/symptoms
  - Congenital sensorineural hearing loss (SNHL)
  - Potential risk of recurrent meningitis for large CC & large IAC with associated perilymph fistula

Demographics

- Epidemiology
  - Rare: < 1% of all congenital inner ear malformations

Treatment

- Bilateral profound SNHL: Successful cochlear implantation reported in common cavity anomaly

DIAGNOSTIC CHECKLIST

Consider

- Common cavity if cochlea & vestibule form single cavity without differentiation

Image Interpretation Pearls

- Oblique sagittal T2 MR images through IAC necessary to determine presence of cochlear nerve

Reporting Tips

- Can be difficult to distinguish from cochlear aplasia + globular vestibule & horizontal SCC
- Consider cystic cochleovestibular anomaly if greater differentiation into separate but featureless cochlea & vestibule

SELECTED REFERENCES

1. Pradhananga RB et al: Long term outcome of cochlear implantation in five children with common cavity deformity. Int J Pediatr Otorhinolaryngol. 79(5):685-9, 2015
2. Beltrame MA et al: Common cavity and custom-made electrodes: speech perception and audiological performance of children with common cavity implanted with a custom-made MED-EL electrode. Int J Pediatr Otorhinolaryngol. 77(8):1237-43, 2013
3. Giesemann AM et al: From labyrinthine aplasia to otocyst deformity. Neuroradiology. 52(2):147-54, 2010
4. Bosley TM et al: The clinical spectrum of homozygous HOXA1 mutations. Am J Med Genet A. 146A(10):1235-40, 2008
5. Sennaroglu L et al: Surgical results of cochlear implantation in malformed cochlea. Otol Neurotol. 27(5):615-23, 2006
6. Sennaroglu L et al: A new classification for cochleovestibular malformations. Laryngoscope. 112(12):2230-41, 2002
7. Jackler RK et al: Congenital malformations of the inner ear: a classification based on embryogenesis. Laryngoscope. 97(3 Pt 2 Suppl 40):2-14, 1987

TERMINOLOGY

- Cochlear incomplete partition type I + dilated vestibule and horizontal semicircular canal (SCC)

IMAGING

- Cochlea: Absent internal septation & modiolus (incomplete partition type I, IP-I)
- Vestibule & SCC: Dilated vestibule & horizontal SCC form single cavity, wide communication with cochlea
- CNVII canal: Normal or mildly obtuse anterior genu angle; normal or dehiscent tympanic segment
- Internal auditory canal: Small or dilated, defective fundus
- CNVIII: Nerves hypoplastic or absent
- Vestibular aqueduct: Usually normal
- Oval window: Normal or stenotic + stapedial anomaly

TOP DIFFERENTIAL DIAGNOSES

- Cochlear aplasia
  - Absent cochlea; vestibule & SCC normal, dilated, or hypoplastic
- Common cavity
  - Cystic cochlea & vestibule form ovoid or rounded common cavity

CLINICAL ISSUES

- Presentation
  - Congenital sensorineural hearing loss
  - Isolated symptom or with syndromic features (cardiac, spine anomalies, etc.)
- Cystic cochleovestibular malformation (CCVM) accounts for < 2% of all congenital labyrinthine lesions

DIAGNOSTIC CHECKLIST

- CCVM (IP-I)
  - Figure 8 cochlea & vestibule lacking internal architecture
  - Risk of CSF leak & meningitis from translabyrinthine fistula

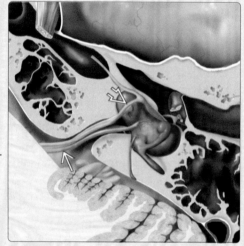
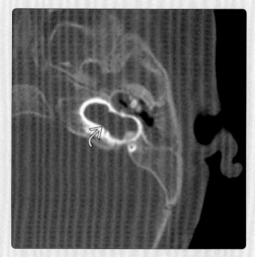

(Left) *Figure 8 morphology of featureless cochlea & vestibule is shown. Cochlear interscalar septum and modiolus are absent. CNVIII components are hypoplastic* ➡️. *Internal auditory canal is narrow & shortened. CNVII labyrinthine segment has lost its anteriorly curving shape and appears straightened* ➡️ *as it ends at the geniculate ganglion.* (Right) *Axial bone CT in a 6-month-old girl with unilateral sensorineural hearing loss (SNHL) and multiple congenital anomalies shows the typical figure 8 morphology of CCVM* ➡️.

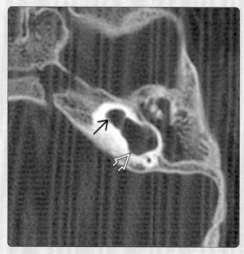
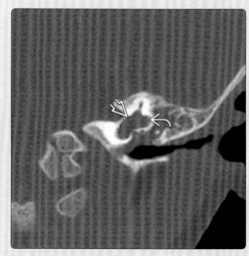

(Left) *CT in an 18-month-old boy with congenital SNHL and CCVM shows a cochlea that lacks internal architecture* ➡️, *also termed incomplete partition type I malformation. The vestibule and horizontal semicircular canal (SCC) form a single globular cavity* ➡️. *The middle ear space and mastoid air cells are opacified. This patient had a contralateral common cavity anomaly.* (Right) *Coronal bone CT in the same patient demonstrates the globular vestibule* ➡️ *and horizontal SCC* ➡️.

Cystic Cochleovestibular Malformation (IP-I)

TERMINOLOGY

Abbreviations

- Cystic cochleovestibular malformation (CCVM)

Synonyms

- Cystic cochleovestibular anomaly
- Cochlear incomplete partition type I (IP-I)

Definitions

- Arrest of inner ear development: Cochlea lacks interscalar septum & modiolus (IP-I) + dilated vestibule & horizontal semicircular canal (SCC)

IMAGING

General Features

- Best diagnostic clue
  - Cystic, featureless cochlea + dilated vestibule & horizontal SCC
- Location
  - Membranous labyrinth
- Size
  - Usually enlarged cochlea, vestibule, & horizontal SCC
- Morphology
  - Cochlea & vestibule: **Figure 8** contour, no internal features

CT Findings

- Bone CT
  - Unilateral or bilateral, often asymmetric
  - Cochlea: **Absent internal septation, absent modiolus (IP-I)**, variable size
  - Vestibule: **Dilated, enlarged communication with cochlea**
  - SCC: **Dilated horizontal SCC** forms common cavity with vestibule, anterior limb superior SCC ± dilated
  - Internal auditory canal (IAC): **Small or dilated**, defective fundus
  - CNVII canal: Normal or mildly obtuse anterior genu angle; normal or dehiscent tympanic segment
  - Vestibular aqueduct: Usually normal
  - Oval window: Normal or stenotic + stapedial anomaly

MR Findings

- T2WI
  - Cochlea + vestibule: Figure 8 contour
  - Cochlea: Lacks internal septation & modiolus
  - Vestibule & horizontal SCC: Dilated
  - CNVIII: Nerves hypoplastic or absent

Imaging Recommendations

- Best imaging tool
  - MR to identify CNVIII components
- Protocol advice
  - 3D T2 (SPACE, FIESTA): Axial & oblique sagittal

DIFFERENTIAL DIAGNOSIS

Cochlear Aplasia

- **Absent cochlea**; vestibule & SCC normal, dilated, or hypoplastic

Common Cavity

- **Cystic cochlea & vestibule** form undifferentiated or minimally differentiated common cavity

PATHOLOGY

General Features

- Etiology
  - Currently unknown
- Embryology
  - Arrest of otic placode development ~ 5th gestational week

Gross Pathologic & Surgical Features

- Cochlea & vestibule lack internal architecture

Microscopic Features

- Cochleovestibular nerves deficient
- Cochlea lacks interscalar septum & modiolus

CLINICAL ISSUES

Presentation

- Most common signs/symptoms
  - Congenital sensorineural hearing loss
  - Isolated or with syndromic features (cardiac, spine anomalies, etc.)
  - May be associated with CSF leak (from ear or nose) & meningitis from translabyrinthine fistula
  - Risk of labyrinthine ossification from meningitis

Demographics

- Epidemiology
  - Rare inner ear anomaly
  - CCVM accounts for < 2% of all congenital labyrinthine anomalies

Treatment

- If contralateral ear is normal, no treatment indicated
- Cochlear implantation
  - Some success reported if cochlear nerve present
  - Risks in CCVM: CSF leak (deficient IAC fundus), CNVII damage (dehiscent)

DIAGNOSTIC CHECKLIST

Consider

- CCVM for **figure 8** cochlea & vestibule lacking internal architecture

Image Interpretation Pearls

- MR to detect hypoplasia/aplasia of CNVIII components

Reporting Tips

- IP-I spectrum: CCVM = least differentiated manifestation; IP-I + normal vestibule = mildest manifestation

SELECTED REFERENCES

1. Wani NA et al: Recurrent meningitis in an adult secondary to an inner ear malformation: imaging demonstration. Ear Nose Throat J. 91(4):E23-6, 2012
2. Sennaroglu L et al: Surgical results of cochlear implantation in malformed cochlea. Otol Neurotol. 27(5):615-23, 2006
3. Sennaroglu L et al: Unpartitioned versus incompletely partitioned cochleae: radiologic differentiation. Otol Neurotol. 25(4):520-9; discussion 529, 2004

TERMINOLOGY

- IP-I spectrum of anomalies: Mild (cochlea lacks modiolus and interscalar septum) to severe [cystic cochleovestibular malformation (CCVM)]
- Cochlear incomplete partition type I (IP-I): Milder form of IP-I; cochlea has some external structure, variable anomaly vestibule & SCC
- CCVM: Least differentiated manifestation of IP-I involving cochlea, vestibule, & SCC

IMAGING

- IP-I has absent interscalar septum & modiolus
- Spectrum of IP-I severity
  - Amorphous sac, wide communication between cochlea & vestibule; figure 8 morphology (CCVM)
  - Some external structure, dilated vestibule, & horizontal SCC (most common)
  - External indentations suggesting cochlear turns, ± normal vestibule (rare)

- Cochlear nerve canal & IAC: Normal, wide (most common), or narrow; absent macula cribrosa
- Cochlear nerve: Usually hypoplastic or absent
- Vestibule & horizontal SCC: Usually dilated
- Vestibular aqueduct: Usually normal

TOP DIFFERENTIAL DIAGNOSES

- **Cochlear hypoplasia**: Small cochlea, < 2 turns
- **Cochlear incomplete partition type II (IP-II)**
  - Defective septation between middle & apical cochlear turns, normal basal turn
  - Large vestibular aqueduct/endolymphatic sac
- **Common cavity malformation**
  - Single cystic structure = cochlea + vestibule

CLINICAL ISSUES

- When profound bilateral SNHL: Cochlear implantation variably successful
  - Risk of CSF gusher

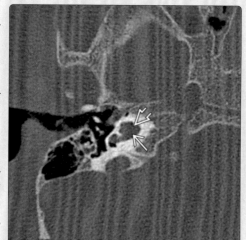
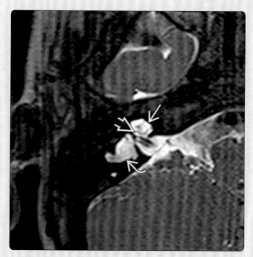

(Left) Axial bone CT in a 9-month-old girl with right SNHL shows complete absence of the cochlear modiolus ➡ & interscalar septum ➡. The anomaly affects entire cochlea. In this relatively mild & uncommon manifestation of IP-I, there is some external "shape" to the cochlea. (Right) Axial T2 MR in a 1-year-old boy with SNHL shows a large, amorphous cochlea ➡. The modiolus & osseous interscalar septum are absent. Curvilinear internal hypointensity presumably represents the spiral lamina ➡. The vestibule ➡ & lateral SCC are dilated.

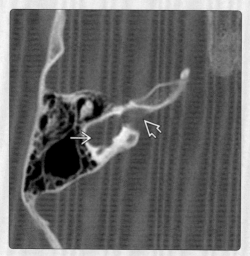
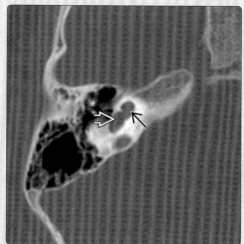

(Left) Axial bone CT in a 4-year-old boy with right SNHL shows dilatation of the vestibule & horizontal semicircular canal ➡. The vestibular aqueduct is not enlarged. The internal auditory meatus is widened ➡. (Right) Axial bone CT in the same patient shows cystic cochlea that lacks internal structure ➡. Note wide communication between the cochlea and vestibule ➡. This is the more common form of IP-I, with a cystic cochlea and dilatation of the vestibule and horizontal SCC, also referred to as CCVM.

TERMINOLOGY

Abbreviations

- Cochlear incomplete partition type I (IP-I)

Synonyms

- Cystic cochleovestibular malformation (CCVM)

Definitions

- Incomplete cochlear partition type I: Absent internal structure of entire cochlea
  - Cochlear IP-I
    - Milder form of IP-I confined to cochlea
  - CCVM
    - Least differentiated manifestation of IP-I involving cochlea, vestibule, & semicircular canals (SCCs)

IMAGING

General Features

- Best diagnostic clue
  - Cochlea lacks **interscalar septum** between basal, middle, & apical turns
    - Absent modiolus
- Size
  - Normal-sized or large cochlea
- Morphology
  - Variable morphology, unilateral or bilateral
  - Most differentiated IP-I
    - Visible external cochlear turns lacking internal interscalar septum & modiolus
    - **Normal** vestibule & SCCs
  - Least differentiated IP-I
    - Cystic featureless cochlea with cystic vestibular malformation
    - Figure 8 morphology

CT Findings

- Bone CT
  - Cochlea
    - **Malformation affects entire cochlea**
    - **Absent interscalar septum**
    - **Absent modiolus**
    - Variable external contour
      - □ Amorphous sac or external indentations suggesting cochlear turns
  - Cochlear nerve canal and internal auditory canal
    - Normal, wide, or narrow; absent macula cribrosa
  - Vestibule & horizontal SCC
    - Grossly dilated or normal
  - Vestibular aqueduct
    - Rarely enlarged
  - Middle ear and ossicles
    - Normal or oval window stenosis/atresia + abnormal stapes

MR Findings

- 3D T2 SPACE, FIESTA, or equivalent
  - Cochlea: Lacks modiolus and interscalar septum; internal curvilinear hypointensity may represent spiral lamina in mildest IP-I
  - Vestibule & horizontal SCC: Usually dilated
  - Cochlear nerve: Usually hypoplastic or aplastic

Imaging Recommendations

- Best imaging tool
  - MR: To evaluate presence & size of cochlear nerve

DIFFERENTIAL DIAGNOSIS

Cochlear Incomplete Partition Type II (IP-II)

- Normal basal turn, defective septation affects cochlear middle & apical turns
- Modiolus deficient or absent
- Large vestibular aqueduct (LVA), large endolymphatic sac

Cochlear Hypoplasia

- Small cochlea, usually with < 2 turns

CHARGE Syndrome

- Stenotic/atretic cochlear nerve canal
- Variable cochlear anomaly
- Small vestibule & small/absent SCCs
- Funnel-shaped LVA

Common Cavity Malformation

- Single cystic structure represents undifferentiated cochlea + vestibule

CLINICAL ISSUES

Presentation

- Most common signs/symptoms
  - Sensorineural hearing loss (SNHL)

Natural History & Prognosis

- Congenital SNHL
- Absent macula cribrosa & modiolus
  - Risk of CSF gusher at cochleostomy or stapedectomy
  - Risk of meningitis & postmeningitic labyrinthitis ossificans

Treatment

- Profound bilateral SNHL: Cochlear implantation with variable success
  - CSF gusher is most common surgical complication
  - Cochlear implantation more successful in IP-II group compared to IP-I group

SELECTED REFERENCES

1. Suk Y et al: Surgical outcomes after cochlear implantation in children with incomplete partition type I: comparison with deaf children with a normal inner ear structure. Otol Neurotol. 36(1):e11-7, 2015
2. Kontorinis G et al: Radiological diagnosis of incomplete partition type I versus type II: significance for cochlear implantation. Eur Radiol. 22(3):525-32, 2012
3. Sennaroglu L: Cochlear implantation in inner ear malformations--a review article. Cochlear Implants Int. 11(1):4-41, 2010
4. Chadha NK et al: Bilateral cochlear implantation in children with anomalous cochleovestibular anatomy. Arch Otolaryngol Head Neck Surg. 135(9):903-9, 2009
5. Sennaroglu L et al: Surgical results of cochlear implantation in malformed cochlea. Otol Neurotol. 27(5):615-23, 2006
6. Sennaroglu L et al: Unpartitioned versus incompletely partitioned cochleae: radiologic differentiation. Otol Neurotol. 25(4):520-9; discussion 529, 2004
7. Sennaroglu L et al: A new classification for cochleovestibular malformations. Laryngoscope. 112(12):2230-41, 2002

TERMINOLOGY

- IP-II: Incomplete partition due to deficient interscalar septum (ISS) between middle & apical cochlear turns
- Mondini anomaly (historic terminology): IP-II + large vestibular aqueduct (LVA)

IMAGING

- Cochlea
  - Absent ISS between plump middle & apical turns
  - Do not mistake osseous spiral lamina for ISS on MR
  - Smooth external contour between middle & apical turns posterolaterally (baseball cap cochlea)
  - Asymmetric scalar chambers
  - Deficient or absent modiolus
- Vestibular aqueduct/endolymphatic sac
  - Typically large (most cases) or borderline large & flared; rarely normal
- Vestibule: Normal or large
- SCC: Normal or mildly plump anterior limb lateral SCC

TOP DIFFERENTIAL DIAGNOSES

- Cochlear IP-I
- Cochlear hypoplasia
- CHARGE syndrome
- X-linked stapes gusher (DFNX2)

PATHOLOGY

- *SLC26A4* mutation (PDS gene, chromosome 7) most common
- Syndromic deafness: Pendred syndrome
- Nonsyndromic deafness: DFNB4
- ~ 20% of temporal bones with LVA have IP-II anomaly

CLINICAL ISSUES

- Bilateral or unilateral, severe or profound SNHL
- SNHL precipitated by minor trauma
- Fluctuating, progressive SNHL (or mixed hearing loss)
- Avoid contact sports & try to prevent head trauma
- Profound bilateral SNHL: **Cochlear implantation**

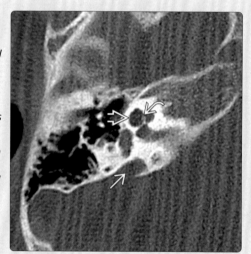
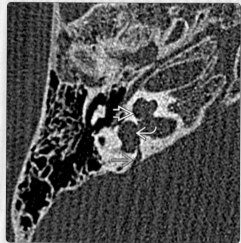

(Left) Axial bone CT in 4-year-old girl with mixed hearing loss shows large vestibular aqueduct (LVA) ➡ and an IP-II cochlear anomaly with a smooth contour laterally and deficiency of interscalar septum (ISS) between apical and middle turns ➡; modiolus is malformed ➡. (Right) Axial bone CT in a 2-year-old boy with SNHL shows mild LVA ⇨ with absence of the ISS between the plump apical and middle cochlear turns ➡ and absence of the modiolus. The cochlea resembles a baseball cap. The vestibule is mildly enlarged ➡.

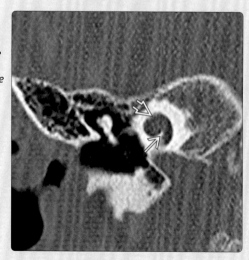
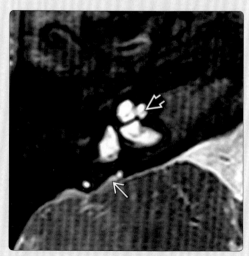

(Left) Coronal reformatted bone CT image (same patient) shows the tapered ISS between the basal and middle cochlear turns ➡. The ISS between the apical and middle turns ➡ is absent. (Right) Axial T2 SPACE MR (same patient) shows the mildly enlarged endolymphatic sac ➡. Notice again the baseball cap configuration of the cochlea, with absence of the ISS between the apical and middle cochlear turns. The osseous spiral lamina ➡ is faintly seen within the middle cochlear turn and should not be mistaken for the ISS.

TERMINOLOGY

Abbreviations

- Cochlear incomplete partition type II (IP-II)

Synonyms

- Mondini anomaly (historic terminology): IP-II + large vestibular aqueduct (LVA)

Definitions

- IP-II: Incomplete partition due to deficient interscalar septum (ISS) between middle & apical cochlear turns

IMAGING

General Features

- Best diagnostic clue
  - Temporal bone CT & T2 MR: Absent ISS between plump middle & apical cochlear turns
  - Associated LVA/large endolymphatic sac (ES)

CT Findings

- Bone CT
  - Cochlea
    - Normal basal turn
    - **Absent ISS** between **plump middle** & **apical turns**
    - Smooth external contour between middle & apical turns posterolaterally (baseball cap cochlea)
    - Asymmetric scalar chambers
    - Deficient or absent modiolus
  - Cochlear nerve canal: Normal (most) or mild stenosis
  - Vestibular aqueduct: Typically large (most) or borderline large & flared; rarely normal
  - Vestibule: Normal or large
  - Semicircular canals (SCCs): Normal or plump anterior limb lateral SCCs

MR Findings

- 3D FIESTA, T2 SPACE, or equivalent
  - Cochlea
    - Normal basal turn
    - Absent ISS between plump middle & apical turns
    - Asymmetric scalar chambers
    - Deficient or absent modiolus
  - Cochlear nerve: Usually normal
  - ES & duct: Typically large, triangular morphology
  - Vestibule & SCC: Normal or mildly enlarged vestibule; normal or plump lateral SCC

Imaging Recommendations

- Best imaging tool
  - MR: 3D T2-weighted sequence, e.g., FIESTA, SPACE, or equivalent (< 1 mm slice thickness)

DIFFERENTIAL DIAGNOSIS

Cochlear Incomplete Partition Type I

- Entire cochlea lacks internal structure

Cochlear Hypoplasia

- Small cochlea, < 2 turns, septation may be deficient

CHARGE Syndrome

- ± deficient cochlear septation; flattened/absent apical turn, cochlear nerve canal stenosis/atresia
- Funnel-shaped LVA & large ES
- Small vestibule & hypoplastic/absent SCC

X-Linked Stapes Gusher (DFNX2)

- Deficient cochlear internal septation; corkscrew cochlear morphology; absent modiolus
- Widened internal auditory canal fundus & cochlear nerve canal

PATHOLOGY

General Features

- Etiology
  - Genetic ± environmental factors produce hearing loss
  - Cochlea has microscopic infrastructural deficiencies
  - Enlarged scala media & hair cell damage
  - Susceptible to injury from mild trauma
- Genetics
  - *SLC26A4* mutation (PDS gene, chromosome 7)
    - Autosomal recessive; encodes pendrin protein
    - Syndromic deafness: Pendred syndrome (LVA + thyroid organification defect); homozygous or compound heterozygous mutations
    - Nonsyndromic deafness: DFNB4 (enlarged vestibular aqueduct syndrome) heterozygous mutations

CLINICAL ISSUES

Presentation

- Most common signs/symptoms
  - Bilateral or unilateral, severe or profound sensorineural hearing loss (SNHL)
  - SNHL precipitated by minor trauma
- Other signs/symptoms
  - Vestibular symptoms
  - Pendred syndrome: Hypothyroidism ± goiter

Natural History & Prognosis

- Fluctuating, progressive SNHL (or mixed hearing loss)

Treatment

- Avoid contact sports & try to prevent head trauma
- Profound bilateral SNHL: **Cochlear implantation**

DIAGNOSTIC CHECKLIST

Image Interpretation Pearls

- Plump apical & middle cochlear turns form single chamber; deficient or absent modiolus
- **Do not mistake osseous spiral lamina for ISS on MR**

SELECTED REFERENCES

1. Leung KJ et al: Correlation of CT, MR, and histopathology in incomplete partition-II cochlear anomaly. Otol Neurotol. 37(5):434-7, 2016
2. Griffith AJ et al: Hearing loss associated with enlargement of the vestibular aqueduct: mechanistic insights from clinical phenotypes, genotypes, and mouse models. Hear Res. 281(1-2):11-7, 2011
3. Fitoz S et al: SLC26A4 mutations are associated with a specific inner ear malformation. Int J Pediatr Otorhinolaryngol. 71(3):479-86, 2007
4. Sennaroglu L et al: Unpartitioned versus incompletely partitioned cochleae: radiologic differentiation. Otol Neurotol. 25(4):520-9; discussion 529, 2004

TERMINOLOGY

- Large vestibular aqueduct (LVA) houses enlarged endolymphatic sac and duct
- IP-II: Incomplete partition type II between middle and apical cochlear turns often seen with LVA
- IP-II + LVA: Mondini anomaly (historic terminology)

IMAGING

- Axial CT: LVA ≥ 1 mm at midpoint &/or ≥ 2 mm at operculum; short-axis CT reformat: LVA ≥ 1.2 mm at midpoint, ≥ 1.3 mm at operculum
- MR: Enlarged endolymphatic sac and duct
- Cochlea: Abnormal in ~ 75% of LVA cases
  - Absent septation between middle and apical turns
  - Deficient modiolus, asymmetric scalar chambers
- Vestibule and semicircular canal: Normal or mildly enlarged

TOP DIFFERENTIAL DIAGNOSES

- Cystic cochleovestibular malformation (IP-I)

- Cochlear hypoplasia
- CHARGE syndrome (funnel-shaped LVA)
- Branchiootorenal syndrome (funnel-shaped LVA)

PATHOLOGY

- *SLC26A4* mutations
  - Autosomal recessive, ~ 5-10% of prelingual hearing loss
  - Syndromic deafness: Pendred syndrome
  - Nonsyndromic deafness: DFNB4
  - ~ 50% of LVA patients have *SLC26A4* mutations

CLINICAL ISSUES

- Most common imaging abnormality in pediatric sensorineural hearing loss (SNHL)
- **Bilateral** anomaly (most)
- Congenital cause of acquired SNHL or mixed hearing loss
- **Progressive/fluctuating SNHL**
- Avoid contact sports and try to prevent head trauma
- Cochlear implantation for profound bilateral SNHL

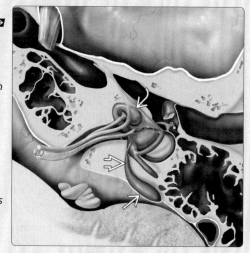
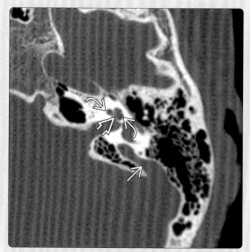

(Left) In left inner ear, large endolymphatic sac epidural ⇒ and intraosseous ⇒ components are shown. Cochlea is malformed, with absent septation between middle and apical turns, which appear bulbous ⇒. (Right) Axial temporal bone CT in a 15-year-old boy with sensorineural hearing loss (SNHL) shows a large vestibular aqueduct (LVA) ⇒. Interscalar septum is present between apical and middle cochlear turns, but modiolus is narrow ⇒ and the scalar chambers are asymmetric (posterior > anterior) ⇒.

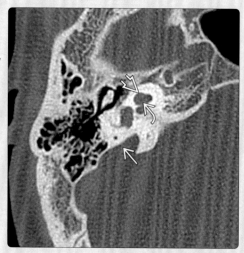
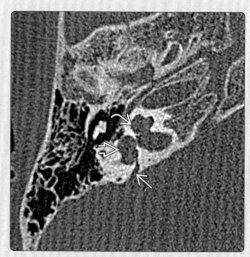

(Left) Axial temporal bone CT in a 17-year-old girl with Pendred syndrome shows an LVA ⇒ and absent septation between the middle and apical cochlear turns ⇒ with absence of the modiolus ⇒. This is typical of incomplete partition type II, which results in a baseball cap-shaped cochlea. (Right) Axial bone CT in a 3-year-old boy with SNHL and LVA ⇒ shows a typical IP-II cochlear anomaly ⇒ with plump cochlear middle and apical turns, absent modiolus, and no apical septation. The vestibule is mildly enlarged ⇒.

TERMINOLOGY

Abbreviations

- Large vestibular aqueduct (LVA)

Synonyms

- Large endolymphatic sac anomaly (LESA): T2 MR term
- Enlarged vestibular aqueduct (EVA): Temporal bone CT term
- Mondini anomaly (historic terminology): Incomplete partition type II (IP-II) + LVA

Definitions

- LVA: Enlarged bony vestibular aqueduct houses large endolymphatic sac (ES) and duct associated with variable cochlear malformation
- IP-II: Incomplete partition (deficient interscalar septum) between middle and apical cochlear turns often seen with LVA

IMAGING

General Features

- Best diagnostic clue
  - Temporal bone CT: LVA ± IP-II
  - T2 MR: Large ES ± IP-II
- Location
  - Petrous bone; bilateral or unilateral
- Size
  - Axial temporal bone CT: LVA ≥ 1 mm at midpoint, ± ≥ 2 mm at opercular margin perpendicular to long axis of vestibular aqueduct
    - Short-axis reformat: Parallel to plane of superior semicircular canal (SCC) ≥ 1.2 mm at midpoint, ≥ 1.3 mm at operculum
- Morphology
  - Axial bone CT: V-shaped, enlarged bony vestibular aqueduct (VA)
  - Axial T2 MR: Large ES along posterior wall of petrous bone, lateral to dural reflection

CT Findings

- Bone CT
  - LVA: May scallop posterior margin of petrous bone
  - Cochlea: Abnormal on CT in ~ 75% of LVA cases
    - Normal basal turn
    - Normal or **deficient septation** between **plump apical and middle turns** (IP-II)
    - **Asymmetric scalar chambers**: Anterior < posterior
    - **Deficient** (typical), absent, or normal **modiolus**
  - Vestibule: Normal or mildly enlarged; vestibular volume usually increased
  - SCC: Normal or mildly dilated
  - Middle ear space and ossicles: Normal

MR Findings

- T1WI
  - Low to intermediate signal ES visible along posterior petrous bone
- 3D SPACE, FIESTA or equivalent
  - ES and duct: Enlarged, variable signal; hypointensity attributed to hyperviscous protein

- Cochlea
  - Normal or **deficient septation** between **plump apical and middle turns** (IP-II)
  - **Asymmetric scalar chambers**: Anterior < posterior
  - **Deficient** (typical), absent, or normal **modiolus**

Imaging Recommendations

- Best imaging tool
  - High-resolution thin-section MR or temporal bone CT
- Protocol advice
  - CT: Thin-section axial temporal bone (< 1 mm), reformatted coronals, reformatted 45° transverse oblique
  - MR: 3D SPACE, FIESTA, or equivalent (< 1-mm slice thickness)

DIFFERENTIAL DIAGNOSIS

Cystic Cochleovestibular Malformation (IP-I)

- Cystic cochlea without internal structure and cystic vestibule

Cochlear Hypoplasia

- Small cochlea, usually < 2 turns

CHARGE Syndrome

- Funnel-shaped LVA, small vestibule, and small/absent SCC
- Cochlear nerve canal stenosis/atresia and thickened modiolus; occasional cochlear hypoplasia

Branchiootorenal Syndrome

- Funnel-shaped LVA, tapered basal turn, and small, offset middle and apical turns

High Jugular Bulb

- Communicates with jugular foramen, not vestibule
- Normal variation of jugular foramen anatomy

PATHOLOGY

General Features

- Etiology
  - Genetic ± environmental factors produce hearing loss
  - LVA + large ES occur during embryogenesis
  - Endolymphatic hydrops is nonspecific marker for underlying cellular/molecular lesion
    - Failed expression of *SLC26A4* → failure of fluid absorption in embryonic ES
  - Cochlea is "fragile" and susceptible to injury from mild trauma as result of microscopic infrastructural deficiencies
    - Enlargement of ELS and cochlea in affected mice → acidification and enlargement of scala media → retarded development of organ of Corti (compounded by hypothyroidism) and stria vascularis degeneration
    - Hair cell damage likely multifactorial, in part related to elevated endolymphatic Ca^{++} concentration
  - Conductive component of mixed hearing loss (MHL) due to "3rd window" effect of EVA on sound transmission in labyrinth
- Genetics
  - *SLC26A4* mutations (*PDS* gene, chromosome 7)

- ~ 50% of LVA patients have *SLC26A4* **mutations**
- Encodes pendrin protein
  - ☐ Anion transporter (chloride and iodide)
  - ☐ Expressed in thyroid, kidney, and inner ear
  - ☐ Role in endolymph homeostasis and resorption
  - ☐ Defects cause neuroepithelial damage and inner ear malformation
- **Autosomal recessive inheritance**
- *SLC26A4* mutations account for ~ 5-10% of cases of prelingual hearing loss
- Syndromic deafness: Pendred syndrome
  - ☐ Sensorineural hearing loss (SNHL) + thyroid organification defect ± goiter
  - ☐ Autosomal recessive; biallelic *SLC26A4* mutation
  - ☐ ~ 10% of hereditary deafness
- Nonsyndromic deafness: Deafness autosomal recessive 4 (DFNB4)
  - ☐ Isolated familial SNHL
  - ☐ ~ 4% of nonsyndromic deafness
  - ☐ 2nd most common cause of nonsyndromic deafness after *GJB2* mutation
  - ○ *FOXI1* mutations (less common): *SLC26A4* transcriptional activator gene
- Associated abnormalities
  - ○ **Pendred syndrome**: Goiter (2nd decade)
  - ○ Distal renal tubular acidosis (rare)
- Anatomic comments
  - ○ ES has epidural portion (larger part) and intraosseous portion
  - ○ Endolymphatic duct is short connection between crus communis and intraosseous sac
  - ○ Normal ES and duct barely visible on 3D FIESTA/SPACE MR

Gross Pathologic & Surgical Features

- Enlarged VA houses large ES found in dural sleeve in fovea in posterior wall of temporal bone

CLINICAL ISSUES

Presentation

- Most common signs/symptoms
  - ○ SNHL (or MHL)
    - Bilateral or unilateral; severe or profound
    - Fluctuating or **progressive course**
    - SNHL precipitated by minor head trauma
- Other signs/symptoms
  - ○ Tinnitus, vertigo, dizziness
  - ○ Pendred syndrome: Hypothyroidism in ~ 50%, ± goiter in adolescence

Demographics

- Age
  - ○ Prelingual or early postlingual SNHL (or MHL)
  - ○ Congenital cause of acquired SNHL
- Epidemiology
  - ○ **LVA: Most common CT/MR abnormality in pediatric SNHL**
  - ○ Bilateral (most) or unilateral anomaly

Natural History & Prognosis

- If bilateral, inevitably leads to profound SNHL

- SNHL (or MHL)
  - ○ Hearing loss may not be present until early adult life
  - ○ Fluctuating or progressive course
- ± linear relationship observed between VA width and progressive SNHL
- Prognosis best for unilateral HL or late onset HL

Treatment

- Avoid contact sports and try to prevent head trauma
- Profound bilateral SNHL: **Cochlear implantation**
  - ○ No increase in cochlear implant complications

DIAGNOSTIC CHECKLIST

Consider

- Known *SLC26A4* mutation/Pendred syndrome: Look for EVA/LESA
- EVA/LESA: Recommend *SLC26A4* testing, US thyroid, thyroid function tests, ± perchlorate discharge test
- Obtain MR if borderline VA measurements on CT

Image Interpretation Pearls

- LVA diagnosis: Look for associated cochlear anomaly

Reporting Tips

- Reformatted coronal CT or transverse oblique view differentiates LVA from high-riding jugular bulb

SELECTED REFERENCES

1. El-Badry MM et al: Evaluation of the radiological criteria to diagnose large vestibular aqueduct syndrome. Int J Pediatr Otorhinolaryngol. 81:84-91, 2016
2. Sone M et al: Endolymphatic hydrops in superior canal dehiscence and large vestibular aqueduct syndromes. Laryngoscope. 126(6):1446-50, 2015
3. Griffith AJ et al: Hearing loss associated with enlargement of the vestibular aqueduct: mechanistic insights from clinical phenotypes, genotypes, and mouse models. Hear Res. 281(1-2):11-7, 2011
4. Atkin JS et al: Cochlear abnormalities associated with enlarged vestibular aqueduct anomaly. Int J Pediatr Otorhinolaryngol. 73(12):1682-5, 2009
5. Oh SH et al: Can magnetic resonance imaging provide clues to the inner ear functional status of enlarged vestibular aqueduct subjects with PDS mutation? Otol Neurotol. 29(5):593-600, 2008
6. Ozgen B et al: Comparison of 45 degrees oblique reformats with axial reformats in CT evaluation of the vestibular aqueduct. AJNR Am J Neuroradiol. 29(1):30-4, 2008
7. Boston M et al: The large vestibular aqueduct: a new definition based on audiologic and computed tomography correlation. Otolaryngol Head Neck Surg. 136(6):972-7, 2007
8. Vijayasekaran S et al: When is the vestibular aqueduct enlarged? A statistical analysis of the normative distribution of vestibular aqueduct size. AJNR Am J Neuroradiol. 28(6):1133-8, 2007
9. Yang T et al: Transcriptional control of SLC26A4 is involved in Pendred syndrome and nonsyndromic enlargement of vestibular aqueduct (DFNB4). Am J Hum Genet. 2007 Jun;80(6):1055-63. Epub 2007 Apr 23. Erratum in: Am J Hum Genet. 81(3):634, 2007
10. Berrettini S et al: Distal renal tubular acidosis associated with isolated large vestibular aqueduct and sensorineural hearing loss. Ann Otol Rhinol Laryngol. 111(5 Pt 1):385-91, 2002
11. Miyamoto RT et al: Cochlear implantation with large vestibular aqueduct syndrome. Laryngoscope. 112(7 Pt 1):1178-82, 2002
12. Sennaroglu L et al: A new classification for cochleovestibular malformations. Laryngoscope. 112(12):2230-41, 2002
13. Pyle GM: Embryological development and large vestibular aqueduct syndrome. Laryngoscope. 110(11):1837-42, 2000
14. Davidson HC et al: MR evaluation of vestibulocochlear anomalies associated with large endolymphatic duct and sac. AJNR Am J Neuroradiol. 20(8):1435-41, 1999
15. Naganawa S et al: MR imaging of the cochlear modiolus: area measurement in healthy subjects and in patients with a large endolymphatic duct and sac. Radiology. 213(3):819-23, 1999
16. Phelps PD et al: Radiological malformations of the ear in Pendred syndrome. Clin Radiol. 53(4):268-73, 1998

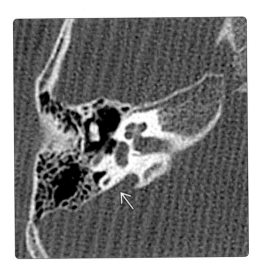

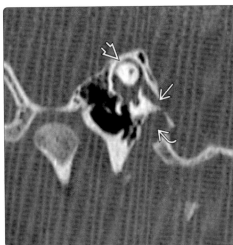

(Left) *Axial temporal bone CT in a 3-year old girl with SNHL demonstrates LVA ➡. Note the normal cochlear septation and modiolus in this patient.* (Right) *Reformatted short-axis oblique temporal bone CT in a 3-year-old girl with SNHL demonstrates the right LVA ➡ in its entirety. The reconstructed image is parallel to the plane of the superior semicircular canal ➡. The jugular bulb ➡ lies inferior to the LVA.*

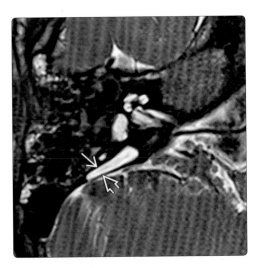

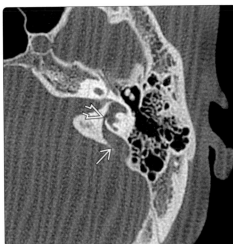

(Left) *Axial T2 SPACE MR in a 3-year-old girl with SNHL shows the hyperintense large endolymphatic sac ➡ lying lateral to the hypointense dura ➡. MR also confirms the normal internal structure of the cochlea in this patient.* (Right) *Axial temporal bone CT in 17-year-old girl with Pendred syndrome reveals the entirety of the left LVA ➡ extending from the crus communis ➡ of the vestibule to the posterior aspect of the petrous bone.*

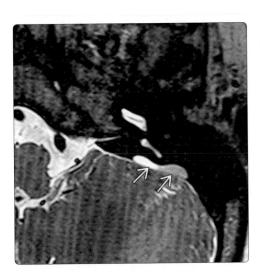

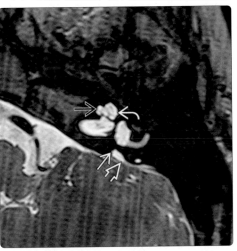

(Left) *Axial T2 SPACE in a 3-year-old boy with SNHL reveals a large ES ➡ containing variable signal intensity.* (Right) *Axial 3D FIESTA MR in a 3-year-old boy with SNHL shows a large ES ➡ lateral to the hypointense dura ➡. There is absent septation between the middle and apical cochlear turns ➡ and modiolar deficiency. The hypointense line in the center of each cochlear turn is the normal osseous spiral lamina ➡.*

TERMINOLOGY

- Stenosis or atresia of cochlear nerve canal (CNC)
- Cochlear nerve deficiency (CND): Cochlear nerve (CN) hypoplasia/aplasia

IMAGING

- CNC extends from internal auditory canal (IAC) fundus to modiolus
  - Diameter measured at narrowest point
  - **CNC stenosis**: < 1.7 mm
- Cochlea (spectrum of findings)
  - Normal
  - Normal modiolus + mildly stenotic CNC
  - Thickened modiolus + stenotic/atretic CNC
  - Cochlear anomaly + stenotic/atretic CNC
- IAC: Normal, small, absent or "duplicated" (separate CNVII canal)
- CND: CN smaller than normal CNVII (hypoplasia) or absent (aplasia)

TOP DIFFERENTIAL DIAGNOSES

- CHARGE syndrome
- Cochlear aplasia or hypoplasia

PATHOLOGY

- Unclear whether CN fails to form or forms initially then degenerates

CLINICAL ISSUES

- Presents with congenital sensorineural hearing loss (SNHL)
- ~73% incidence of CN aplasia in pediatric unilateral neural SNHL

DIAGNOSTIC CHECKLIST

- Most cases of CND have normal cochlea ± modiolar thickening ± CNC stenosis or atresia
- Assess CNs on axial & **oblique sagittal** 3D T2 SPACE/FIESTA MR sequences

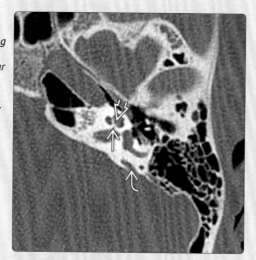
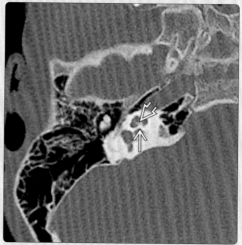

(Left) *Axial bone CT in an 11-year-old girl with profound bilateral sensorineural hearing loss (SNHL) is shown. There is severe stenosis of the cochlear nerve canal (CNC) ➡. The modiolus ➡ and scalar chambers appear asymmetric. This patient also has a mildly enlarged vestibular aqueduct ➡. (Right) Axial bone CT in a 4-year-old girl with profound right SNHL is shown. There is absence of the CNC ➡ and marked thickening of the modiolus ➡.*

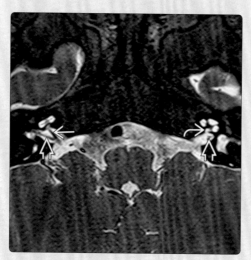
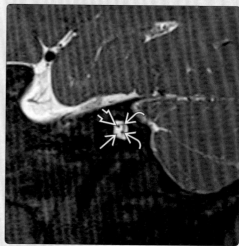

(Left) *Axial T2 SPACE MR shows a 1-year-old boy with profound left SNHL. A normal right CN ➡ and normal vestibular nerves ➡ are seen. The left CN is absent, and the left CNC is mildly stenotic ➡. (Right) Sagittal oblique T2 SPACE MR shows a 1-year-old boy with profound left SNHL. Absence of the left CN ➡ and a normal facial nerve ➡ and vestibular nerves ➡ are visible.*

TERMINOLOGY

Abbreviations

- Cochlear nerve canal (CNC)

Synonyms

- Cochlear aperture stenosis or atresia

Definitions

- CNC hypoplasia-aplasia: Narrowing or absence of CNC
- Cochlear nerve deficiency (CND): CN hypoplasia or absence (aplasia)

IMAGING

General Features

- Best diagnostic clue
  - **CND**: CN smaller than normal CNVII (hypoplasia) or absent (aplasia) on MR
  - **CNC width**: Narrowest diameter between internal auditory canal (IAC) fundus & modiolus on axial images
  - **CNC stenosis** = CNC width < 1.7 mm
  - Thickened modiolus
- Location
  - CNC extends from IAC fundus to modiolus
  - CN division of CNVIII is **anteroinferior** in IAC

Imaging Recommendations

- Best imaging tool
  - Axial & sagittal oblique 3D T2-weighted MR
- Protocol advice
  - 3D SPACE/FIESTA or analogous sequence
  - Sagittal oblique is perpendicular to plane of CNVIII

CT Findings

- Bone CT
  - **CNC**
    - Normal: In some cases of CND on MR
    - Stenosis: Severity varies
    - Atresia: Complete absence of CNC
  - **Cochlea**
    - Normal turns & normal modiolus with normal or mildly stenotic CNC
    - Normal turns & **thickened modiolus** with moderate to severe stenosis of CNC
    - Abnormal cochlea with stenotic/atretic CNC (less common) (e.g., cochlear hypoplasia)
  - Vestibule & semicircular canal (SCC): Normal (most); less commonly abnormal (e.g., syndromic etiology)
  - IAC: Normal or small, rarely separate CNVII canal ("duplicated IAC")
  - CNVII canal: Normal (most) or anomalous (rare)

MR Findings

- **CN**: Hypoplasia or aplasia
  - CNC normal: Occasional CND
  - CNC mildly stenotic: CN normal or CND
  - CNC stenotic < 1.5 mm ± thickened modiolus: CND
  - CNC stenosis + IAC narrowing: CND difficult to see on MR because of ↓ CSF around CNVIII & CNVII
- Vestibular nerves (VNs)
  - Normal IAC: VN usually normal
  - Narrow IAC: VN normal or deficient
- Cochlea, vestibule, and SCC malformation is uncommon

DIFFERENTIAL DIAGNOSIS

CHARGE Syndrome

- CNC stenosis/atresia, CNVIII deficiency, hypoplastic vestibule, absent/hypoplastic SCC

Cochlear Aplasia

- Cochlea absent

Cochlear Hypoplasia

- Small cochlea, < 2 turns

CLINICAL ISSUES

Presentation

- Most common signs/symptoms
  - Congenital sensorineural hearing loss (SNHL)
    - Unilateral > > bilateral SNHL; usually static
    - Neural-type SNHL typical of isolated CND
      - 73% incidence of CN aplasia in pediatric unilateral neural-type SNHL
  - Pediatric unilateral profound SNHL prevalence ~ 0.1-0.2%
    - ~ 50% have isolated CN hypoplasia ± CNC stenosis
  - Variable VN dysfunction

Treatment

- **Cochlear implantation contraindicated if CN absent**
  - Brainstem implantation may provide benefit

DIAGNOSTIC CHECKLIST

Consider

- CND: Most common finding in pediatric neural SNHL
- For unilateral auditory neuropathy with normal CNs, evaluate for tumor, brainstem malformation, or injury

Image Interpretation Pearls

- Most cases of CND have normal cochlea other than CNC stenosis ± modiolar thickening

Reporting Tips

- Neural SNHL: Assess CNs on MR

SELECTED REFERENCES

1. Birman CS et al: Cochlear implant outcomes in cochlea nerve aplasia and hypoplasia. Otol Neurotol. 37(5):438-45, 2016
2. Wilkins A et al: Frequent association of cochlear nerve canal stenosis with pediatric sensorineural hearing loss. Arch Otolaryngol Head Neck Surg. 138(4):383-8, 2012
3. Miyasaka M et al: CT and MR imaging for pediatric cochlear implantation: emphasis on the relationship between the cochlear nerve canal and the cochlear nerve. Pediatr Radiol. 40(9):1509-16, 2010
4. Sennaroglu L et al: Preliminary results of auditory brainstem implantation in prelingually deaf children with inner ear malformations including severe stenosis of the cochlear aperture and aplasia of the cochlear nerve. Otol Neurotol. 30(6):708-15, 2009
5. Glastonbury CM et al: Imaging findings of cochlear nerve deficiency. AJNR Am J Neuroradiol. 23(4):635-43, 2002
6. Stjernholm C et al: Dimensions of the cochlear nerve canal: a radioanatomic investigation. Acta Otolaryngol. 122(1):43-8, 2002
7. Fatterpekar GM et al: Hypoplasia of the bony canal for the cochlear nerve in patients with congenital sensorineural hearing loss: initial observations. Radiology. 215(1):243-6, 2000

TERMINOLOGY

- Definition: Hypoplasia/aplasia of 1 or multiple semicircular canals (SCCs) ± hypoplastic vestibule

IMAGING

- Hypoplastic vestibule + hypoplasia/aplasia of all SCCs in CHARGE syndrome
  - Oval window stenosis/atresia & anomalous CNVII
  - Cochlea: Variable malformation; thickened modiolus, flattened apical ± middle turns or single turn/hypoplasia
  - Cochlear nerve canal: Stenosis/atresia
  - Vestibular aqueduct: Dilated, funnel-shaped
- Hypoplasia of single SCC + normal (or large) vestibule
  - Posterior SCC (PSCC) + normal or flattened cochlear apical turn: Waardenburg & Alagille syndromes
  - PSCC + hypoplastic, offset middle & apical cochlear turns: Branchiootorenal (BOR) syndrome
  - Horizontal SCC: Oval window stenosis/atresia & anomalous ± dehiscent tympanic segment CNVII

TOP DIFFERENTIAL DIAGNOSES

- **Down syndrome**
  - Small or absent HSCC bone island; globular SCC-vestibule (anlage) anomaly
  - Cochlear nerve canal stenosis, IAC stenosis, LVA variably present
- **Labyrinthine ossificans**: Prior meningitis or surgery

DIAGNOSTIC CHECKLIST

- **CHARGE** if hypoplasia vestibule + SCC
- Axial & coronal temporal bone to assess oval window & CNVII tympanic segment
- Consider **BOR** for hypoplastic, offset middle & apical turns cochlea; look for PSCC anomaly
- Consider Waardenburg syndrome for PSCC anomaly & Hirschsprung disease
- Consider Alagille syndrome for PSCC anomaly, pulmonary stenosis, & cholestatic liver disease

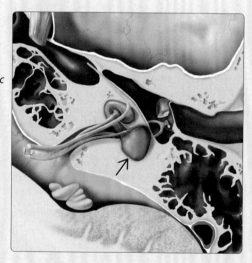
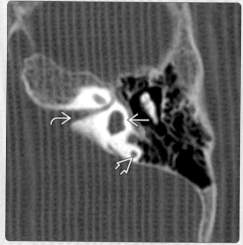

(Left) Axial graphic depicts severe, syndromic type of semicircular canal (SCC) anomaly with complete absence of all SCCs, cochlear malformation, and dysmorphic small vestibule ➡. (Right) Axial bone CT in a 12-month-old boy with profound sensorineural hearing loss shows complete absence of the horizontal SCC ➡ at the level of the vestibule. A normal posterior SCC is seen ➡. The IAC is narrow ➡.

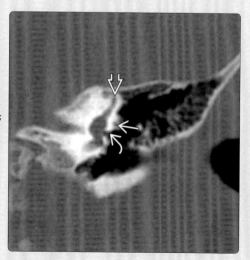
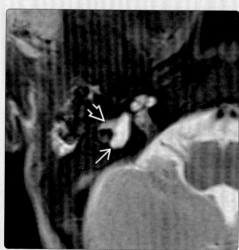

(Left) Coronal bone CT demonstrates the facial nerve canal ➡, absence of the horizontal SCC, and a normal superior SCC ➡. There is mild stenosis of the oval window ➡. (Right) Axial T2WI MR in a 1-day-old girl with Waardenburg syndrome shows a rudimentary posterior SCC bud along the posterior aspect of the vestibule ➡. A normal horizontal SCC is seen ➡.

Semicircular Canal-Vestibule Globular Anomaly

KEY FACTS

TERMINOLOGY

- Dilatation of semicircular canal (SCC) & globular vestibule
- Bone island between vestibule & affected SCC is small or absent (persistent SCC anlage anomaly)

IMAGING

- Most frequently seen SCC & vestibular anomaly
- Usually affects lateral SCC (LSCC): Last to develop
- Isolated finding or with other temporal bone anomalies
- SCC: Widened lumen of 1 limb or entire SCC; small or absent bone island
- Vestibule: Normal or large, less commonly small
- Cochlea: Normal or malformed

TOP DIFFERENTIAL DIAGNOSES

- **Large vestibular aqueduct (LVA)**
  - LVA, ± IP-II anomaly, ± globular vestibule/LSCC
- **Apert syndrome**
  - Craniosynostosis, polysyndactyly, LSCC anlage anomaly

- **Trisomy 21**
  - Vestibule normal or small; small LSCC bone island or persistent SCC anlage anomaly
- **22q11.2 deletion syndrome**
  - Vestibule normal, large or small; small LSCC bone island or persistent SCC anlage anomaly

CLINICAL ISSUES

- Mild form may be asymptomatic
- Vestibular symptoms: Normal or imbalance, vertigo
- Caloric testing: Absent or decreased caloric responses
- Hearing: Normal, sensorineural, mixed, or conductive hearing loss (ossicular or inner ear origin)

DIAGNOSTIC CHECKLIST

- LSCC + external & middle ear malformation
  - Syndromic or chromosomal/genetic anomaly
  - Craniofacial anomaly (most)
  - Toxic exposure

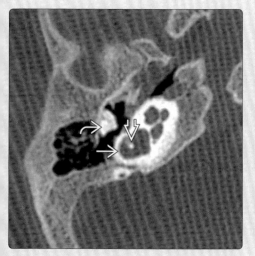
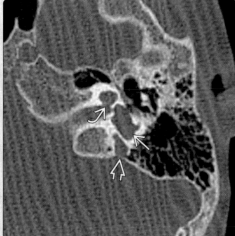

(Left) Axial bone CT in a 9-month-old boy with oculoauriculovertebral spectrum shows dilated lateral semicircular canal (LSCC) ➡ & small bone island ➡ between LSCC & globular vestibule. Malformed ossicles are fixed to lateral wall of attic ➡. (Right) Axial bone CT in 7-year-old girl with severe SNHL & in utero exposure to maternal drugs shows dilatation of posterior SCC ➡ & vestibule, & funnel-shaped large, vestibular aqueduct ➡. Cochlear modiolus ➡ & cochlear septation are deficient.

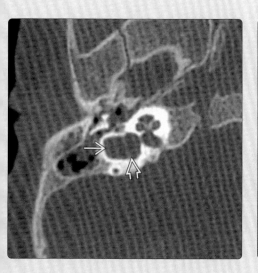
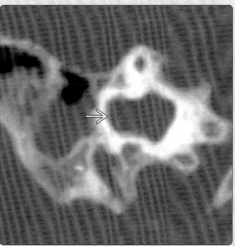

(Left) Axial bone CT in a 10-month-old girl with profound SNHL demonstrates a large, globular LSCC ➡ that communicates with a dilated vestibule ➡, forming a single cavity. (Right) Coronal CT reconstruction reveals massive dilatation of the LSCC ➡ in this patient with persistent anlage anomaly. Oval window atresia was also noted on a more anterior image (not shown).

TERMINOLOGY

- Labyrinthitis: Subacute inflammatory or infectious disease of fluid-filled spaces of inner ear

IMAGING

- **No imaging** necessary if classic presentation [unilateral sudden onset sensorineural hearing loss (SNHL)]
- MR findings
  - T1 C+ FS: Faint to moderate enhancement within inner ear fluid
  - T2: Normal high fluid signal preserved
  - T1: Normal to mildly increased signal; if hemorrhage, increased inner ear signal
- T-bone CT findings
  - Normal in acute/subacute labyrinthitis
  - Labyrinthine ossificans possible if suppurative labyrinthitis

TOP DIFFERENTIAL DIAGNOSES

- Labyrinthine ossificans
- Intralabyrinthine schwannoma
- Intralabyrinthine hemorrhage

PATHOLOGY

- Labyrinthitis classification
  - Viral labyrinthitis: Unilateral
  - Bacterial labyrinthitis: Meningogenic (bilateral) > > tympanogenic (unilateral)
  - Posttraumatic/postsurgical: Unilateral
  - Autoimmune: Related to systemic disease (bilateral)

CLINICAL ISSUES

- Viral: Sudden onset unilateral SNHL ± vertigo & tinnitus
- Bacterial: Child with bacterial meningitis → bilateral, progressive SNHL
  - Labyrinthitis ossificans possible

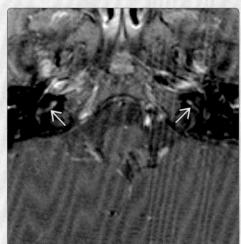
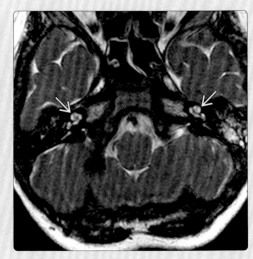

(Left) Axial T1WI C+ FS MR in a 1-year-old boy with prior history of meningitis and sensorineural hearing loss demonstrates abnormal bilateral enhancement of the basal turn of the cochlea ➡ consistent with meningogenic labyrinthitis. (Right) Axial T2WI FSE MR in a patient with bilateral labyrinthitis shows normal, hyperintense fluid within the cochlea bilaterally ➡. Normal to slightly decreased fluid signal helps distinguish labyrinthitis from labyrinthine mass(es).

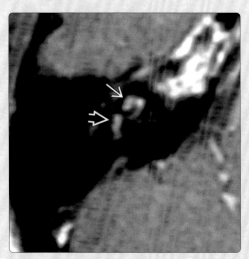
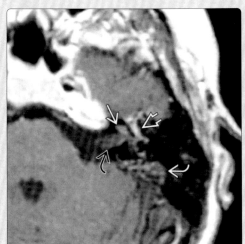

(Left) Axial T1WI C+ MR in a case of viral labyrinthitis shows pathologic enhancement of the cochlear turns ➡ and vestibule ➡ in a patient with acute onset of vertigo and hearing loss. (Right) Axial T1WI C+ MR reveals enhancement of the cochlea ➡ & internal auditory canal ➡ in a patient with bacterial otomastoiditis ➡ presenting with otalgia, CNVII palsy, and hearing loss. Tympanic CNVII is also thickened & enhancing ➡ in this example of tympanogenic labyrinthitis. (Courtesy C. Schatz, MD.)

Labyrinthitis

TERMINOLOGY

Synonyms

- Subacute labyrinthitis

Definitions

- Subacute inflammatory or infectious disease of fluid-filled spaces of inner ear (IE)
  - Labyrinthitis causes secondary changes within membranous labyrinth of IE

IMAGING

General Features

- Best diagnostic clue
  - T1 C+ MR shows **faint to moderate enhancement** within normally fluid-filled spaces of **IE**

CT Findings

- Bone CT
  - Normal in acute & subacute phases
  - If suppurative labyrinthitis (bacterial, pus producing) → **labyrinthine ossificans** (LO)
    - Initially fibrous, then ossific over weeks or years

MR Findings

- T1WI
  - Signal often normal
  - In severe, diffuse membranous labyrinthitis, may show subtle ↑ in signal
  - If intralabyrinthine hemorrhage present, ↑ in IE signal
- T2WI
  - Normal high-signal IE fluid in acute/subacute phases
    - T2 may differentiate membranous labyrinthitis from intralabyrinthine schwannoma (hypointense IE fluid)
- T1WI C+
  - Acute/subacute phases may be normal
  - Focal/diffuse faint to moderate enhancement within normally fluid-filled spaces of cochlea, vestibule, & semicircular canals
  - Enhancement may persist after symptoms resolve

Imaging Recommendations

- Best imaging tool
  - If classic clinical presentation, no imaging necessary
  - Atypical presentation: Thin-section T1 C-, T1 C+, & T2 MR are key sequences

DIFFERENTIAL DIAGNOSIS

Labyrinthine Ossificans

- Bone CT: Ossification of membranous labyrinth
- T1 C+ MR: Early phase, IE enhancement
- T2 MR: Hypointense signal replaces normal hyperintense IE fluid

Intralabyrinthine Schwannoma

- T1 C+ MR: Enhancement more intense and localized than labyrinthitis
- T2 MR: Focal decreased signal = area of enhancement

Intralabyrinthine Hemorrhage

- Underlying coagulopathy or trauma history

- T1 MR: Hyperintense precontrast T1 signal

PATHOLOGY

General Features

- Etiology
  - **Serous** or **suppurative** labyrinthitis possible
  - Etiology of IE enhancement on MR
    - Labyrinthine vasculature breakdown → neovascularization of intralabyrinthine membranes
    - Begins in subacute phase, persists for months

Microscopic Features

- Suppurative labyrinthitis → labyrinthine ossificans
- Early chronic: **Fibrous stage** shows fibroblast proliferation
- Late chronic: Ossific stage shows **LO**

CLINICAL ISSUES

Presentation

- Most common signs/symptoms
  - Sudden onset of sensorineural hearing loss (SNHL), vertigo, & tinnitus
- Labyrinthitis classification
  - **Viral labyrinthitis**
    - Sudden unilateral SNHL ± upper respiratory illness
    - Not imaged if classic presentation
    - Probably hematogenous spread
  - **Bacterial labyrinthitis**
    - Often progresses to permanent SNHL
    - **Meningogenic**: Bilateral; secondary to meningitis
      □ Primary cause of acquired childhood deafness
      □ Spreads from fundus of IAC through lamina cribrosa → vestibule **or** cochlear nerve canal → cochlea **or** cochlear aqueduct → cochlear basal turn
    - **Tympanogenic**: Unilateral; secondary to bacterial otomastoiditis
      □ Acute bacterial otomastoiditis → direct spread through round or oval window
  - **Posttraumatic/postsurgical**: Unilateral
    - Hemorrhage likely incites enhancement
    - Healing → granulation tissue ± LO
  - **Autoimmune**: Very rare, related to systemic disease

Demographics

- Any age may be affected
- Epidemiology: Viral > > bacterial labyrinthitis

Natural History & Prognosis

- Hearing loss recovery common in viral labyrinthitis
  - May be recurrent and debilitating
- Persistent SNHL common in bacterial labyrinthitis

Treatment

- Viral etiology: Steroids, vestibular suppressants, & vestibular exercises
- Bacterial: Topical & intravenous antibiotics
  - Surgical intervention when severe

SELECTED REFERENCES

1. Salzman KL et al: Intralabyrinthine schwannomas: imaging diagnosis and classification. AJNR Am J Neuroradiol. 33(1):104-9, 2012

Otosyphilis

TERMINOLOGY

- Sexually transmitted inner ear disease caused by bacterium spirochete *Treponema pallidum*

IMAGING

- Bone CT: **Moth-eaten permeative demineralization** of temporal bone (syphilitic osteitis)
  - Inner ear, middle ear-mastoid, ossicles
- T1 C+ MR: Enhancement of CNVII & CNVIII in internal auditory canal ± membranous labyrinth (syphilitic labyrinthitis-meningitis)

TOP DIFFERENTIAL DIAGNOSES

- Cochlear otosclerosis
- Temporal bone osteogenesis imperfecta
- Temporal bone Paget disease
- Temporal bone fibrous dysplasia
- Postirradiated temporal bone

PATHOLOGY

- Sexually transmitted spirochete *T. pallidum*
- **Osteitis**: Inflammatory resorptive osteitis
- **Labyrinthitis**: Obliterative endarteritis

CLINICAL ISSUES

- Diagnosis made when otologic symptoms are present with positive serology
- Hearing loss (80%) & vertigo: Often acute & fluctuating
- Simulates Ménière disease

DIAGNOSTIC CHECKLIST

- Consider: If HIV patient with hearing loss and permeative inner demineralization, test for positive syphilis serology before diagnosing otosyphilis

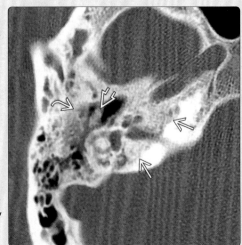

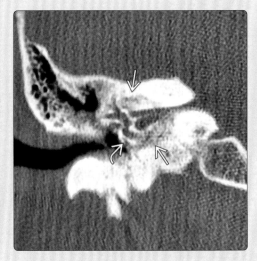

(Left) *Axial temporal bone CT shows typical findings of advanced middle and inner ear otosyphilis. There are extensive moth-eaten permeative bony changes of the inner ear ➡, middle ear mastoid ⬈, and ossicles ⬌. (Courtesy M. Sandlin, MD.)* (Right) *Coronal temporal bone CT in the same patient demonstrates permeative demineralization of the otic capsule ➡ with otosclerosis-like plaque on cochlear promontory ⬈. These findings are secondary to inflammatory resorptive osteitis.*

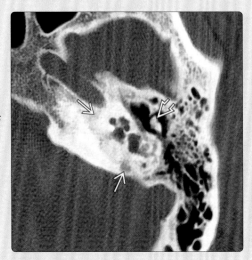

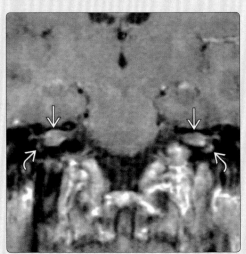

(Left) *Axial temporal bone CT shows similar but less severe changes of otosyphilis of the otic capsule ➡ and ossicles ⬌ with the remainder of the middle ear osseous structures and mastoid being normal. CT findings of the radiated temporal bone may mimic this appearance. (Courtesy M. Sandlin, MD.)* (Right) *Coronal T1 C+ MR reveals pathologic leptomeningeal enhancement in the internal auditory canals ➡ and membranous labyrinths ⬈. This is the labyrinthitis-meningitis form of otosyphilis.*

TERMINOLOGY

Synonyms

- Luetic labyrinthitis, osteitis, & meningitis

Definitions

- Sexually transmitted inner ear disease caused by bacterium spirochete *Treponema pallidum*

IMAGING

General Features

- Best diagnostic clue
  - Moth-eaten permeative demineralization of temporal bone
- Location
  - Otic capsule, internal auditory canal (IAC), & cerebellopontine angle meninges

CT Findings

- CECT
  - If contrast needed, do MR with contrast instead
- Bone CT
  - **Osteitis**: Moth-eaten permeative bone change
    - Inner ear, middle ear-mastoid, ossicles
  - **Labyrinthitis**: Not seen on temporal bone CT

MR Findings

- T1WI
  - Osteitis: Patchy areas of intermediate signal
- T2WI
  - Osteitis: If severe, patchy high signal in otic capsule
  - IAC meningeal infection: Thickened CNVII-VIII
  - Labyrinthitis: ↑ signal of inner ear fluid possible
- T1WI C+
  - Osteitis: **Patchy enhancing foci** in otic capsule
  - Labyrinthitis: Enhancement of fluid-filled spaces of inner ear
  - IAC meningitis: Enhancement of leptomeninges within IAC, including CNVII & CNVIII

Imaging Recommendations

- Best imaging tool
  - Osteitis: Axial & coronal temporal bone CT
  - Labyrinthitis & IAC meningitis: T1 C+ MR

DIFFERENTIAL DIAGNOSIS

Cochlear Otosclerosis

- Clinical: Mixed hearing loss
- Imaging: Patchy radiolucent foci throughout otic capsule
  - Ossicles not involved

Temporal Bone Osteogenesis Imperfecta

- Clinical: Children with brittle bones & blue sclera
- Imaging: Exact cochlear otosclerosis mimic except usually more severe

Temporal Bone Paget Disease

- Clinical: Affects elderly
- Imaging: Otic capsule demineralization is diffuse, involves entire skull base

Temporal Bone Fibrous Dysplasia

- Clinical: < 30-yr-old patient group
- Imaging: Ground-glass expansile bone

Postirradiated Temporal Bone

- Clinical: Post temporal bone irradiation
- Imaging: Also moth-eaten otic capsule

PATHOLOGY

General Features

- Etiology
  - Sexually transmitted spirochete *T. pallidum*

Gross Pathologic & Surgical Features

- Endolymphatic duct rarely obstructed by gumma

Microscopic Features

- Osteitis: Inflammatory resorptive osteitis
- Labyrinthitis: Obliterative endarteritis

CLINICAL ISSUES

Presentation

- Most common signs/symptoms
  - **Hearing loss** (80%) & vertigo: Often acute & fluctuating
    - Simulates Ménière disease
  - Facial palsy; meningeal signs
- Clinical profile
  - Diagnosis made when otologic symptoms are present with positive serology
  - Otosyphilis is late manifestation

Demographics

- Age
  - Older patients
- Gender
  - M > F
- Ethnicity
  - African Americans > Caucasians
- Epidemiology
  - Incidence began to ↑ in 1980s due to AIDS

Natural History & Prognosis

- After therapy, hearing loss improves in 25% of patients
- After therapy, tinnitus & vertigo improve in 75% of patients
- Best response when symptoms are fluctuating, hearing loss is < 5 yr duration, & patient is < 60 yr old

Treatment

- Antibiotics & corticosteroids

DIAGNOSTIC CHECKLIST

Consider

- If HIV patient with permeative inner demineralization, test for syphilis serology

SELECTED REFERENCES

1. Ogungbemi A et al: Computed tomography features of luetic osteitis (otosyphilis) of the temporal bone. J Laryngol Otol. 128(2):185-8, 2014
2. Phillips JS et al: Otosyphilis: a neglected diagnosis? Otol Neurotol. 35(6):1011-3, 2014

Labyrinthine Ossificans

TERMINOLOGY

- **Membranous labyrinth ossification**: Healing response to inner ear infection, inflammation, trauma, or surgery

IMAGING

- Varies with severity
  - Mild: "Enlarged" modiolus; subtle inner ear new bone
  - Severe: All inner ear fluid replaced by bone
- Temporal bone CT: **High-density** bone deposition within membranous labyrinth
- T2 MR: **Low-intensity** foci within high-signal fluid of membranous labyrinth

TOP DIFFERENTIAL DIAGNOSES

- Labyrinthine aplasia
- Cochlear aplasia
- Intravestibular lipoma
- Cochlear otosclerosis
- Labyrinthine schwannoma

PATHOLOGY

- **Fibrous stage**: Fibroblast proliferation
- **Ossific stage**: Osteoblasts forming abnormal bony trabeculae within membranous labyrinthine spaces

CLINICAL ISSUES

- Most common: Bilateral sensorineural hearing loss (SNHL) in child weeks to months after acute meningitis episode
- Less common: Unilateral SNHL with previous surgery, trauma, mastoid/middle ear infection
- Cochlear implantation used for SNHL correction if cochlear nerve is still present
- Bilateral cochlear labyrinthine ossificans (LO) is serious detriment to cochlear implantation

DIAGNOSTIC CHECKLIST

- Precochlear implant evaluation of temporal bone in children: Look for LO & inner ear congenital anomalies
- Describe LO as **cochlear** or **noncochlear**

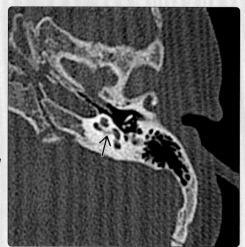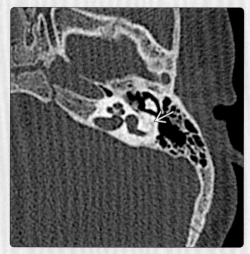

(Left) Axial bone CT in a 2-year-old boy with bilateral sensorineural hearing loss (SNHL) 7 months after an episode of bacterial meningitis shows subtle ossification at the midportion of the basal turn of the left cochlea ⊒, with sparing of the middle and apical turns. (Right) Axial bone CT in the same patient demonstrates subtotal ossification of the anterior and midportion of the lateral semicircular canal ⊒. The posterior and superior semicircular canals were also involved (not shown).

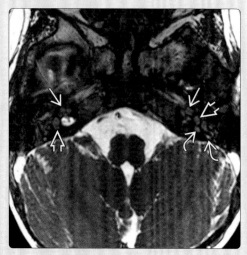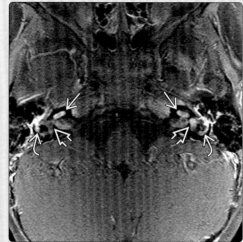

(Left) Axial thin section T2WI MR in a 2 year old with bacterial meningitis 3 weeks prior shows diffuse, bilateral decrease in normal hyperintense inner ear fluid involving the cochlea ⊒, vestibule ⊒, and visualized portions of semicircular canals ⊒. These findings are consistent with early fibroosseous replacement of normal inner ear fluid. (Right) Axial T1WI C+ FS MR in the same patient shows bilateral abnormal inner ear enhancement in the cochlea ⊒, vestibule ⊒, and lateral semicircular canal ⊒.

TERMINOLOGY

Abbreviations

- Labyrinthine ossificans (LO)

Synonyms

- Labyrinthine ossification, ossifying labyrinthitis, labyrinthitis ossificans, chronic labyrinthitis

Definitions

- Membranous labyrinth ossification as healing response to **infectious, inflammatory, traumatic, or surgical** insult to inner ear

IMAGING

General Features

- Best diagnostic clue
  - Temporal bone CT: High-density bone deposition within membranous labyrinth
  - T2 MR: Low-intensity foci within high-signal fluid of membranous labyrinth
- Location
  - **Membranous labyrinth** fluid spaces
  - **Cochlear LO**: Fluid spaces of cochlea affected
  - **Noncochlear LO**: Fluid spaces of semicircular canals (SCCs) or vestibule affected
- Morphology
  - Focal ossific plaques or diffuse ossification of membranous labyrinth

CT Findings

- CECT
  - No role in making LO diagnosis
- Bone CT
  - **Mild LO**: Fibroosseous changes result in hazy increased density within fluid spaces of membranous labyrinth & prominent-appearing modiolus
  - **Moderate LO**: Focal areas of bony encroachment on fluid spaces of membranous labyrinth
    - May be **cochlear, noncochlear**, or both
  - **Severe LO**: Membranous labyrinth completely obliterated by bone, replacing fluid spaces

MR Findings

- T2WI
  - **Mild LO**: Intermediate- & low-signal fibroosseous material partially replaces high-signal fluid spaces of membranous labyrinth
    - Associated with apparent "enlargement" of modiolus
  - **Moderate LO**: Focal areas of low-signal bone encroaching on high-signal fluid spaces of membranous labyrinth
    - May be cochlear, noncochlear, or both
  - **Severe LO**: High-signal membranous labyrinth absent, completely replaced by low-signal bone
    - Cochlear nerve often severely atrophied
- T1WI C+
  - **Membranous labyrinthitis** secondary to **infection** is usual precursor to LO
    - In this pre-LO phase, membranous labyrinth enhances, signifying active labyrinthitis

- Enhancement may be hololabyrinthine or segmental
- Enhancement may persist in ossifying stage of LO

Imaging Recommendations

- Best imaging tool
  - ≤ 1-mm thick axial & reformatted coronal temporal bone CTs are easiest imaging tools to diagnose LO
- High-resolution T2 MR imaging makes diagnosis
  - Careful inspection for absent inner ear fluid spaces
  - T2 MR imaging can show fibrous obliteration of membranous labyrinth whereas CT cannot
  - T1 C+ MR very useful in showing enhancing inner ear in pre-LO phase with labyrinthitis

DIFFERENTIAL DIAGNOSIS

Labyrinthine Aplasia

- Clinical: Sensorineural hearing loss (SNHL) present from birth
- Bone CT: **Flattening of cochlear promontory**
  - Labyrinthine aplasia: Absent cochlea, vestibule, SCCs

Cochlear Aplasia

- Clinical: SNHL present from birth
- Bone CT: Absent cochlea; flattening of cochlear promontory

Intravestibular Lipoma

- Clinical: Mild, high frequency SNHL often present
- MR imaging: **T1 high-signal** foci in vestibule
  - Cerebellopontine angle/internal auditory canal lipoma may be associated

Cochlear Otosclerosis

- Clinical: Disease of young adults
- Bone CT: Radiolucent foci in **bony labyrinth**
  - Does not encroach on membranous labyrinth, even in healing phase

Labyrinthine Schwannoma

- Clinical: Protracted history of slowly progressive unilateral SNHL
- MR imaging: T1 C+ focal intralabyrinthine enhancement
  - T2 MR shows hypointense material within enhancing portion of membranous labyrinth

PATHOLOGY

General Features

- Etiology
  - Suppurative membranous labyrinthitis → cascading inflammatory response in membranous labyrinth
    - Begins with fibrosis, progresses to ossification (as early as 4 weeks)
  - LO caused by suppurative labyrinthitis from multiple sources
    - **Meningogenic** LO: From meningitis; bilateral
    - **Tympanogenic** LO: From middle ear infection; unilateral
    - **Hematogenic** LO: From blood-borne infection such as measles or mumps (rare); bilateral
  - LO may also arise after severe trauma or temporal bone surgery

- o LO also identified as cause of SNHL in children with sickle cell anemia
  - – Hypothesis: Sequelae of arterial vasoocclusive ischemia &/or venous obstruction to inner ear
- Labyrinthitis progresses to LO when suppurative
- LO seen on temporal bone CT as early as 4 weeks after episode of meningitis

Gross Pathologic & Surgical Features

- Gross pathology of inner ear with LO shows new bone formation in membranous labyrinth
- At surgery for cochlear implantation, bony obstruction to implant entry through round window niche is observed

Microscopic Features

- **Fibrous stage**: Fibroblast proliferation
- **Ossific stage**: Osteoblasts form abnormal bony trabeculae within membranous labyrinthine spaces
  - o Scala tympani in basal turn is most frequent area of ossification in all causes of LO
  - o Meningitis → suppurative labyrinthitis associated with greatest amount of ossification

CLINICAL ISSUES

Presentation

- Most common signs/symptoms
  - o Unilateral or bilateral SNHL
  - o Other signs/symptoms
    - – Severe vertigo is infrequent but devastating
    - – Vertigo may be serious enough to require labyrinthectomy
- Clinical profile
  - o Bilateral SNHL in child weeks to months after acute meningitis episode
- Other possible patient histories
  - o Suppurative middle ear infection (tympanogenic LO)
  - o Severe bout of mumps, measles, or other viral illness (hematogenic LO)
  - o Profound head & skull base trauma (posttraumatic LO)
  - o Previous temporal bone operation (postsurgical LO)

Demographics

- Age
  - o Pediatric malady
- Epidemiology
  - o Meningogenic labyrinthitis is most common cause of acquired childhood deafness
    - – Most commonly from *Streptococcus pneumoniae* or *Haemophilus influenzae*
  - o 6-30% have some degree of hearing loss following meningitis

Natural History & Prognosis

- Gradual deterioration of hearing following ear infection (unilateral) or meningitis, blood-borne infection, head trauma, or temporal bone surgery (bilateral)
- Prognosis for SNHL is defined by response to cochlear implantation
- High-resolution axial T2WI MR shows high negative predictive value in predicting intraoperative cochlear obstruction

Treatment

- **Cochlear implantation** used for SNHL correction if cochlear nerve is still present
  - o Bilateral cochlear LO is serious detriment to cochlear implantation
    - – **Presurgical** identification of cochlear LO is key
    - – Allows planning for "drill-out" of obstructed cochlea & modifications of implant device
- "Drill-out," newer cochlear implant devices available for obstructed cochlea
  - o Scala vestibuli insertion is 1 alternative
- Labyrinthectomy used in cases of intractable vertigo

DIAGNOSTIC CHECKLIST

Consider

- In precochlear implant evaluation of temporal bone in children, look for LO & inner ear congenital anomalies
  - o Both of these diagnoses will often force surgical plan to be individualized
- LO may be contraindication to cochlear implantation or complicate surgery

Image Interpretation Pearls

- Radiologist should describe LO as **cochlear** or **noncochlear**
  - o Only describing LO of inner ear does not help cochlear implant surgeon decide what can be done
    - – Cochlear LO makes implant problematic
  - o Be specific about which noncochlear portions of membranous labyrinth are involved

SELECTED REFERENCES

1. Bloch SL et al: Labyrinthitis ossicans: on the mechanism of perilabyrinthine bone remodeling. Ann Otol Rhinol Laryngol. 124(8):649-54, 2015
2. Jiang ZY et al: Utility of MRIs in adult cochlear implant evaluations. Otol Neurotol. 35(9):1533-5, 2014
3. Lin HY et al: The incidence of tympanogenic labyrinthitis ossicans. J Laryngol Otol. 128(7):618-20, 2014
4. Young JY et al: Preoperative imaging of sensorineural hearing loss in pediatric candidates for cochlear implantation. Radiographics. 34(5):E133-49, 2014
5. Kopelovich JC et al: Early prediction of postmeningitic hearing loss in children using magnetic resonance imaging. Arch Otolaryngol Head Neck Surg. 137(5):441-7, 2011
6. Durisin M et al: Cochlear osteoneogenesis after meningitis in cochlear implant patients: a retrospective analysis. Otol Neurotol. 31(7):1072-8, 2010
7. Philippon D et al: Cochlear implantation in postmeningitic deafness. Otol Neurotol. 31(1):83-7, 2010
8. Saito N et al: Clinical and radiologic manifestations of sickle cell disease in the head and neck. Radiographics. 30(4):1021-34, 2010
9. Isaacson B et al: Labyrinthitis ossicans: how accurate is MRI in predicting cochlear obstruction? Otolaryngol Head Neck Surg. 140(5):692-6, 2009
10. Ozgen B et al: Complete labyrinthine aplasia: clinical and radiologic findings with review of the literature. AJNR Am J Neuroradiol. 30(4):774-80, 2009
11. Berrettini S et al: Scala vestibuli cochlear implantation in patients with partially ossified cochleas. J Laryngol Otol. 116(11):946-50, 2002
12. Glastonbury CM et al: Imaging findings of cochlear nerve deficiency. AJNR Am J Neuroradiol. 23(4):635-43, 2002
13. Thomas J et al: Evaluation of cochlear implantation in post-meningitic adults. J Laryngol Otol Suppl. 24:27-33, 1999
14. Johnson MH et al: CT of postmeningitic deafness: observations and predictive value of cochlear implants in children. AJNR. 16(1):103-9, 1995
15. deSouza C et al: Pathology of labyrinthine ossification. J Laryngol Otol. 105(8):621-4, 1991
16. Harnsberger HR et al: Cochlear implant candidates: assessment with CT and MR imaging. Radiology. 164(1):53-7, 1987
17. Swartz JD et al: Labyrinthine ossification: etiologies and CT findings. Radiology. 157(2):395-8, 1985

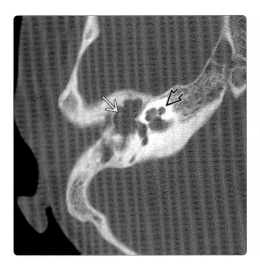
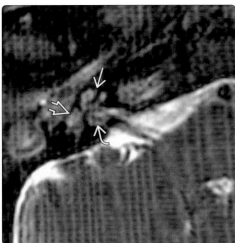

(Left) Axial bone CT in a 10-year-old boy with otomastoiditis with ossicular destruction ➡ shows a normal appearance of the cochlea ➡. (Right) Axial T2W FS MR in the same patient 5 days later demonstrates abnormal hypointense signal within the cochlea ➡, vestibule ➡, and internal auditory canal ➡ consistent with early fibroosseous replacement of normal inner ear fluid.

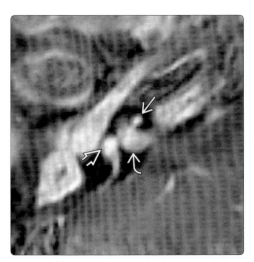
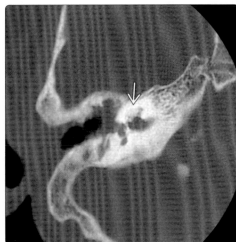

(Left) Axial T1W C+ FS MR in the same patient shows corresponding abnormal enhancement in the middle ear and mastoid as well as in the cochlea ➡, vestibule ➡, and internal auditory canal ➡. (Right) Axial bone CT in the same patient, 1 year after the infection, shows interval near-complete cochlear ossification ➡, consistent with labyrinthine ossificans (LO).

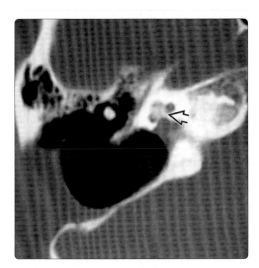
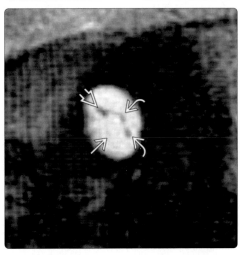

(Left) Axial right temporal bone CT in a patient with previous mastoidectomy and right SNHL shows severe osseous thickening of the cochlear modiolus ➡, which represents postoperative LO. (Right) Sagittal T2WI MR through the internal auditory canal in a patient with ipsilateral severe cochlear LO shows severe atrophy of the cochlear nerve ➡ compared with the normal facial nerve ➡ and vestibular nerves ➡, a common associated finding in severe LO.

Otosclerosis

TERMINOLOGY

- Synonym: **Otospongiosis**
- Types: Fenestral otosclerosis (FOto), cochlear otosclerosis (COto)
- Pathologic appearance of lytic spongy bone foci in bony labyrinth of unknown cause
  - Starts perifenestral (FOto), progresses to surround cochlea (FOto + COto)
- **Fissula ante fenestram**: Cleft of fibrocartilaginous tissue between inner & middle ears just anterior to oval window

IMAGING

- Best diagnostic clue: Temporal bone CT shows **lytic (otospongiotic) foci** involving bony labyrinth
- FOto: Starts at anterior margin of oval window (fissula ante fenestram)
- COto: Affects pericochlear bony labyrinth

TOP DIFFERENTIAL DIAGNOSES

- Chronic otitis media with tympanosclerosis
- Temporal bone Paget disease
- Temporal bone fibrous dysplasia
- Temporal bone osteoradionecrosis
- Temporal bone osteogenesis imperfecta

PATHOLOGY

- Enchondral layer of bony labyrinth displays spongy, vascular, decalcified, irregular bone formation

CLINICAL ISSUES

- Bilateral progressive conductive (FOto) or mixed (FOto + COto) hearing loss in young adult

DIAGNOSTIC CHECKLIST

- Typical otospongiotic plaques of "otosclerosis" are **lytic** & affect **bony** labyrinth

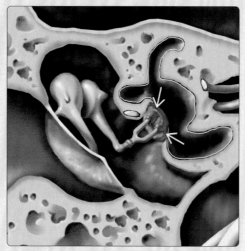
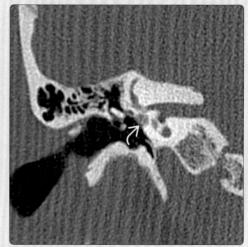

(Left) Coronal graphic illustrates findings of fenestral otosclerosis, with a "donut" otospongiotic plaque ➡ surrounding the stapes footplate in the oval window. The crisp margins of the oval window are obscured by plaque. (Right) Coronal right temporal bone CT shows a lytic focus anterior to the oval window ➡, the typical appearance and location of an otospongiotic plaque of fenestral otosclerosis.

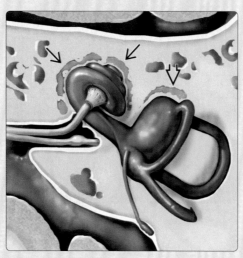
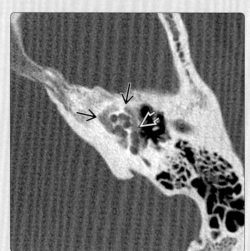

(Left) Axial graphic demonstrates a classic example of cochlear otosclerosis. Note otospongiotic plaques in halo around cochlea ➡, with concurrent fenestral otosclerosis ➡. (Right) Axial left temporal bone CT shows cochlear otosclerosis as osteolytic foci surrounding the cochlea ➡. Concurrent fenestral otosclerosis is noted as bony lucency along cochlear promontory extending from fissula ante fenestram ➡.

TERMINOLOGY

Abbreviations
- Fenestral otosclerosis (FOto)
- Cochlear otosclerosis (COto)

Synonyms
- Otospongiosis, fenestral otospongiosis, cochlear otospongiosis

Definitions
- Pathologic appearance of **lytic spongy bone foci** in bony labyrinth of unknown cause
  - Starts perifenestral (FOto), progresses to surround cochlea (FOto + COto)
- **Fissula ante fenestram**: Cleft of fibrocartilaginous tissue between inner & middle ears just anterior to oval window
  - Also called "cochlear cleft"

IMAGING

General Features
- Best diagnostic clue
  - Temporal bone CT: Lytic (otospongiotic) foci involving bony labyrinth
- Location
  - FOto: Starts at anterior margin of oval window (fissula ante fenestram)
    - May involve any bony area along medial wall of middle ear
  - COto: Affects pericochlear bony labyrinth
    - May involve any portion of bony labyrinth
- Size
  - Millimeter punctate or linear foci; may become confluent
- Morphology
  - FOto: Ovoid plaques most common
  - COto: Ovoid to linear (confluent foci)

CT Findings
- CECT
  - No role for CECT in diagnosis of otosclerosis
- Bone CT
  - **Early** temporal bone CT findings
    - Begins as radiolucent focus at oval window anterior margin (FOto)
    - Spreads to involve all margins of oval & round windows
    - May spread to inner ear otic capsule (COto)
    - Double ring sign or "halo" of radiolucency surrounds cochlea in severe COto
    - Progressive disease may involve any portion of bony labyrinth, including internal auditory canal lateral walls
  - **Late**, chronic (healing phase) temporal bone CT findings
    - FOto: "Heaped up" new bone along oval & round window margins
      - □ Healed plaque may occlude oval ± round window
    - COto: Mixed radiolucent-radiodense foci present in bony labyrinth

MR Findings
- T2WI

- Thin-section high-resolution T2 may not visualize otosclerosis, even when extensive
  - Large plaques may show subtle increased signal
- T1WI C+
  - Enhancing punctate foci in medial wall of middle ear (FOto) ± pericochlear bony labyrinth (COto)
    - Most obvious when FOto & COto combined
  - Enhancing lesions may be seen anywhere in bony labyrinth in severe cases

Imaging Recommendations
- Best imaging tool
  - Temporal bone CT
- Protocol advice
  - T1 C+ MR shows enhancing foci in active phase of otosclerosis
  - High-resolution T2 MR may miss otosclerosis

DIFFERENTIAL DIAGNOSIS

Chronic Otitis Media With Tympanosclerosis
- Clinical: Obvious chronic middle ear-mastoid inflammatory disease
- Imaging: Postinflammatory new bone deposition is not limited to oval & round windows as with most FOto
  - Seen in tympanic membrane (TM), middle ear, ossicles, & mastoids
  - New bone deposition is irregular, not smooth, in oval window area

Temporal Bone Paget Disease
- Clinical: Bone disease of old age (> 50 years)
- Imaging: Diffuse skull base involvement is rule
  - Diffuse involvement of bony labyrinth, not confined to lateral wall
  - Usually seen as diffuse temporal bone cotton wool appearance

Temporal Bone Fibrous Dysplasia
- Clinical: Bone disease of young (age < 30 years)
- Imaging: Involves all parts of temporal bone
  - Relative sparing of inner ear is rule
  - Usually sclerotic, ground-glass in appearance

Temporal Bone Osteoradionecrosis
- Clinical: History of skull base or nasopharyngeal radiation therapy
- Imaging: CT shows diffuse, permeative lucencies of otic capsule

Temporal Bone Osteogenesis Imperfecta
- Clinical: "Blue" sclera; patients with mild form develop deafness by 40 years of age
- Imaging: Looks like severe COto with more generalized demineralization of bony labyrinth

PATHOLOGY

General Features
- Etiology
  - Unknown
- Genetics
  - Sporadic or autosomal dominant gene transmission

- Bony otic capsule development: 3 layers
  - Thin inner endosteal layer
  - **Middle layer** of combined endochondral & intrachondral bone (**otosclerosis occurs here**)
  - Outer periosteal layer
- Normal otosclerosis progression
  - Begins at fissula ante fenestram (FOto)
  - Disease spreads from fissula ante fenestram posteriorly along oval window margins to round window
  - Continued active disease spreads to otic capsule (both FOto & COto present)
- Active **FOto fixes stapes footplate** in oval window niche
  - This "donut" FOto ankyloses stapes footplate
  - Pathophysiology of **conductive hearing loss**
- COto leads to sensorineural hearing loss
  - Best hypothesis: Spiral ligament becomes compromised
  - Secondary hypothesis: Toxic proteases affect cochlear nerve cells

Staging, Grading, & Classification

- Symons/Fanning CT grading system of otosclerosis (2005) has high intra- & interobserver agreement
  - Grade 1: Solely fenestral
  - Grade 2: Patchy localized cochlear disease (± fenestral involvement)
    - To basal cochlear turn (grade 2A)
    - To middle/apical turns (grade 2B)
  - Grade 3: Diffuse confluent cochlear involvement (± fenestral involvement)

Gross Pathologic & Surgical Features

- Otoscopic vascular hue behind TM = **Schwartze sign**
  - Represents active otosclerotic areas along margins of oval & round windows or just beneath cochlear promontory
- Bony ankylosis of stapes footplate is reflected as stapes immobilization when pulled on by surgeon

Microscopic Features

- Enchondral layer of bony labyrinth displays spongy, vascular, decalcified, irregular bone formation
- 3 pathologic phases of otosclerosis
  - Acute phase: Deposition of islets of osteoid tissue
  - Subacute phase: Spongiotic remodeling with osteoclasts causing focal bone resorption
  - Chronic-sclerotic phase: Osteoblasts create new bone with irregular features resembling mosaic
- **"Otospongiosis"** better describes active disease process
- Chronic, healing phase appears truly **sclerotic**
- May be histologically indistinguishable from Paget disease

CLINICAL ISSUES

Presentation

- Most common signs/symptoms
  - Bilateral progressive conductive (FOto) or mixed (FOto + COto) hearing loss
- Other signs/symptoms
  - Tinnitus (ringing in ears)
  - Otoscopy: Vascular hue behind TM = Schwartze sign
- Clinical profile

- Young adult presents with unexplained **bilateral progressive** conductive (FOto) or **mixed** (FOto + COto) **hearing loss**

Demographics

- Age
  - Appears in 2nd to 3rd decades of life
- Gender
  - M:F = 1:2
- Epidemiology
  - Occurs in 1% of population
  - Most common type of otosclerosis is **FOto alone (85%)**; COto found in 15%
  - In **adult patients** with **conductive hearing loss**, FOto responsible in ~ **90%**

Natural History & Prognosis

- FOto: Conductive hearing loss is progressive
- COto: If untreated, will gradually worsen to profound hearing loss

Treatment

- FOto: **Stapedectomy** with stapes prosthesis
  - Results negatively impacted by concurrent COto
  - If round window is obliterated, stapes prosthesis will fail
  - If narrow oval window niche height (< 1.4 mm on coronal CT reformat), stapes surgery more challenging
- Cochlear implantation
  - Used when severe FOto & COto present bilaterally resulting in profound mixed hearing loss
  - If round window obliteration present bilaterally, cochlear implantation may be more challenging
- **Fluoride** treatment if COto present
  - Early treatment can arrest progression

DIAGNOSTIC CHECKLIST

Consider

- Always check oval window anterior margin for FOto in CT evaluation of conductive hearing loss
  - Common blindspot; CT findings can be subtle
- If COto present, FOto also is present, so look for it
- Multidetector CT sometimes shows normal fissula ante fenestram on pediatric temporal bone exams as focal radiolucency

Image Interpretation Pearls

- Typical otospongiotic plaques of "otosclerosis" are lytic & affect bony labyrinth
- If bony encroachment is on membranous labyrinth, diagnosis is **labyrinthine ossificans**, not COto

Reporting Tips

- Assess oval & round window patency; narrowing or obliteration have important surgical implications

SELECTED REFERENCES

1. Ukkola-Pons E et al: Oval window niche height: quantitative evaluation with CT before stapes surgery for otosclerosis. AJNR Am J Neuroradiol. 34(5):1082-5, 2013
2. Valvassori GE: Imaging of otosclerosis. Otolaryngol Clin North Am. 26(3):359-71, 1993

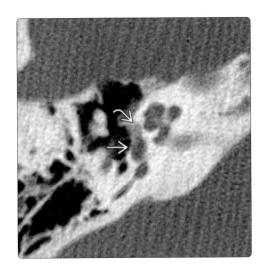

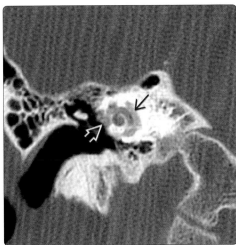

(Left) Magnified axial right temporal bone CT in a young adult with progressive conductive hearing loss demonstrates typical otospongiotic plaque of fenestral otosclerosis ➡ anterior to the oval window ➡ in the expected location of the fissula ante fenestram. (Right) Coronal right temporal bone CT in a patient with mixed hearing loss shows "halo" of radiolucency surrounding the cochlea ➡ representing cochlear otosclerosis. Also note the associated fenestral otosclerosis ➡.

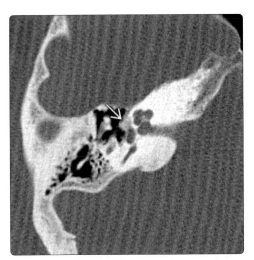

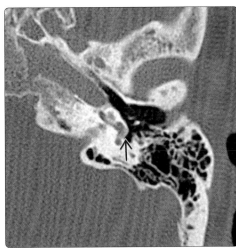

(Left) Axial right temporal bone CT reveals "heaped up" mixed sclerotic and lucent plaque ➡ anterior to the oval window and involving the fissula ante fenestram. This represents a healing (sclerotic portion) but active (lucent portion) plaque of fenestral otosclerosis. (Right) Axial left temporal bone CT demonstrates mixed lucent and sclerotic otospongiotic plaque obstructing the round window ➡. This predisposes to stapes prosthesis failure and makes cochlear implantation more challenging.

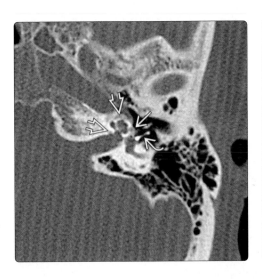

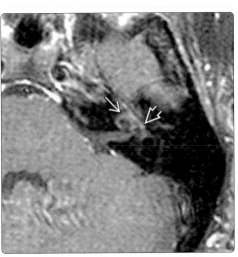

(Left) Axial left temporal bone CT shows typical lytic plaques of combined fenestral ➡ and cochlear otosclerosis ➡. The patient has undergone stapedectomy with insertion of a stapes prosthesis. Note the metallic density stapes prosthesis ➡. (Right) Axial T1WI C+ FS MR in the same patient reveals enhancement anterior to the oval window (fissula ante fenestram) ➡ and surrounding the cochlea ➡ representing active fenestral and cochlear otosclerosis, respectively.

TERMINOLOGY

- Osteogenesis imperfecta (OI): Inherited connective disorder characterized by bone fragility and fractures

IMAGING

- Skull: ± undermineralized, **wormian bones**, fractures
- Bones: Fractures ± osteopenia, ± deformity
- Mastoid and ossicles: Tendency to fracture, deformity
- Inner ear: Normal or **progressive otic capsule demineralization** (OI type I)
  - Early: Band-like pericochlear lucency
  - Late: Lucent otic capsule bone (CT), enhances on MR
- ± jugular vein stenosis and large mastoid emissary veins

TOP DIFFERENTIAL DIAGNOSES

- **Nonaccidental injury**: Unexplained fractures
- **Otosclerosis**: Demineralized otic capsule bone, may be indistinguishable
- **Paget disease**: Involves entire petrous bone, asymmetric

- **Cochlear cleft**: Faint pericochlear lucency < 4 years

PATHOLOGY

- Most OI is **autosomal dominant** (AD); *COL1A1* or *COL1A2* mutations (95%) → **defective collagen**
- **OI type I** (AD): Mild ± later onset; **fractures**, ± minimal deformity, **blue sclerae, hearing loss (HL)**
- **OI type II** (AD, AR): **Perinatal lethality**; osteopenia, severe deformity, multiple fractures
- **OI type III** (AD, AR): Progressive deformity, short stature, dentinogenesis imperfecta, ± blue sclerae
- **OI type IV** (AD): Mild/moderate deformity and fracture, mild blue sclerae, dentinogenesis imperfecta, HL

CLINICAL ISSUES

- Most common heritable connective tissue disorder
- Variable onset and severity
- **Multiple fractures from minimal trauma** ± osteopenia, deformity, short stature, blue sclerae
- HL in ~ 60%: Conductive, SNHL, or mixed ± vertigo

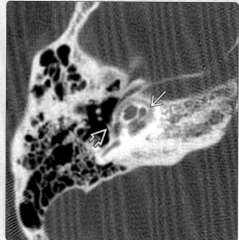
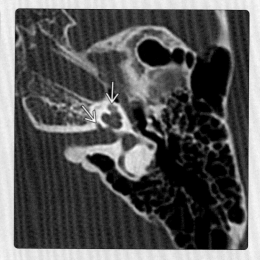

(Left) Axial right T-bone CT shows extensive otic capsule bony demineralization ⟹ of the inner ear in a patient with osteogenesis imperfecta. The posterior crus of the stapes is also thickened ⟹. *(Right)* Axial T-bone CT of another case of OI demonstrates focal otic capsule lucencies adjacent to the cochlea and internal auditory canal ⟹. OI is indistinguishable from otosclerosis on T-bone CT. Regions of demineralization may be multifocal as in this case or band-like as in previous case.

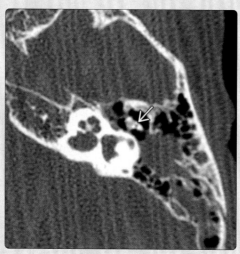
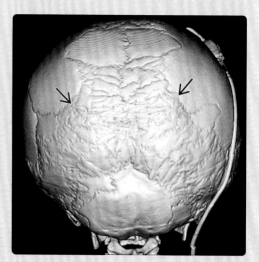

(Left) Axial bone CT in a 13-year-old boy with OI who fell and hit his head on the ground shows a fracture of the short process of the incus ⟹. In addition, there were tympanic plate and mastoid fractures. *(Right)* Posterior 3D skull reformation shows innumerable intrasutural, or wormian, bones ⟹ in a child with OI. Basilar impression and craniocervical junction stenosis result in hydrocephalus in this patient, requiring shunting. Bony demineralization and multiple old fracture deformities can often also be seen in OI.

TERMINOLOGY

Abbreviations

- Osteogenesis imperfecta (OI)

Synonyms

- OI tarda = OI type I = Van der Hoeve-de Kleyn syndrome

Definitions

- Inherited connective disorder characterized by bone fragility and fractures

IMAGING

General Features

- Best diagnostic clue
  - Multiple fractures in patient with blue sclerae
  - Demineralization of otic capsule bone indistinguishable from otosclerosis

CT Findings

- Bone CT
  - Skull: Normal or undermineralized ± deformity/fractures, wormian bones, basilar impression
  - External auditory canal (EAC): Normal or mildly stenotic
  - Ossicles
    - Tendency to fracture
    - Normal or demineralized/deformed stapedial crura
    - Normal or thinning of distal incus long process
  - Inner ear: Normal or progressive otic capsule demineralization (OI type I)
    - Early: Band-like pericochlear lucency
    - Late: Lucent otic capsule bone around cochlea, facial nerve canal, vestibule, and semicircular canal (SCC)
  - ± large mastoid emissary foramina

DIFFERENTIAL DIAGNOSIS

Nonaccidental Injury

- Unexplained fractures, ± skeletal osteopenia due to nutritional deprivation

Cochlear Otosclerosis

- Demineralization of otic capsule bone, localized without systemic bony involvement

Paget Disease, T-Bone

- ± asymmetric petrous bone demineralization in association with other skull and skeletal findings

PATHOLOGY

General Features

- Etiology
  - Genetic mutation → decreased amount of structurally normal collagen ± ↑ in structurally abnormal collagen
  - Mutations involve genes responsible for synthesis or intracellular processing of collagen
- Genetics
  - Autosomal dominant (AD), de novo genetic mutation, or autosomal recessive (AR)
  - COL1A1 (chromosome 17) or COL1A2 (chromosome 7) mutations (95%)
    - Encodes type I collagen: Most abundant protein in body, major bone protein
    - OI types I-IV (AD ± AR)
  - Mutations in encoding genes (e.g., CRTAP) that modify intracellular processing of collagen: AR, severe or lethal
    - OI types VII and VIII

Staging, Grading, & Classification

- **OI type I** (AD): **Fractures**, minimal to no deformity, **blue sclerae** ± normal stature, **hearing loss**
  - **Mild phenotype**, fractures peak in **childhood**, postmenopausal (women) and 6th decade (men)
- **OI type II** (AD, AR): Osteopenia, severe deformity, multiple fractures, platyspondyly, beaded ribs, hearing loss
  - **Severe lethal** perinatal **form**
- **OI type III** (AD, AR): Progressive deformity, very short stature, dentinogenesis imperfecta, variable scleral hue
  - **Evident at birth**
- **OI type IV** (AD): Mild/moderate deformity and fracture, variable short stature, mild blue sclerae, dentinogenesis imperfecta, hearing loss
  - **Milder phenotype**
- **OI type V** (AD): Like type IV, Ca^{++} forearm interosseous membrane, dislocated radial head, hyperplastic callus

Microscopic Features

- Deficient and abnormal ossification: Otic capsule, middle ear walls, mastoid septa, and ossicles
- Otosclerosis in OI is controversial, not seen in lethal OI III
  - Reported in OI type I adults as otospongiotic-like lesion causing stapes footplate fixation
  - Otosclerosis differs biochemically from OI

CLINICAL ISSUES

Presentation

- Most common signs/symptoms
  - **Multiple fractures from minimal trauma**
  - Osteopenia and deformity
  - Short stature, joint laxity
  - Blue sclerae
  - Hearing loss in 2/3 patients; multifactorial

Demographics

- Age
  - Symptom onset from fetus to adult depending on type
- Epidemiology
  - Most common heritable disorder of connective tissue

Treatment

- Surgical correction of ossicular fracture/stapes fixation: Results worse than non-OI patients
- Cochlear implantation: Good results but technically more difficult
- Intravenous bisphosphonate infusions

SELECTED REFERENCES

1. Swinnen FK et al: Temporal bone imaging in osteogenesis imperfecta patients with hearing loss. Laryngoscope. 123(8):1988-95, 2013
2. Pillion JP et al: Hearing loss in osteogenesis imperfecta: characteristics and treatment considerations. Genet Res Int. 2011:983942, 2011
3. Alkadhi H et al: Osteogenesis imperfecta of the temporal bone: CT and MR imaging in Van der Hoeve-de Kleyn syndrome. AJNR Am J Neuroradiol. 25(6):1106-9, 2004

Temporal Bone

TERMINOLOGY

- Intralabyrinthine schwannoma (ILS): Benign tumor arising from Schwann cells within structures of membranous labyrinth

IMAGING

- T1 C+ MR: Focal enhancing mass in membranous labyrinth
- High-resolution T2 MR: Filling defect within hyperintense perilymph
- Focal intralabyrinthine mass named by location
  - **Intracochlear**: Schwannoma within cochlea
  - **Intravestibular**: Within vestibule of inner ear
  - **Vestibulocochlear**: Involves both vestibule & cochlea
  - **Transmodiolar**: Crosses modiolus from cochlea to fundus of internal auditory canal (IAC)
  - **Transmacular**: Crosses from vestibule into fundus of IAC
  - **Transotic**: Involves inner ear, fundus of IAC to middle ear
- Use focused T1 C+ or high-resolution T2 imaging (CISS, FIESTA, 3D-TSE) of CPA-IAC to make diagnosis of ILS

TOP DIFFERENTIAL DIAGNOSES

- Labyrinthitis
- Labyrinthine ossificans
- Intralabyrinthine hemorrhage
- Facial nerve schwannoma with inner ear dehiscence

CLINICAL ISSUES

- Tumor location-specific symptoms
  - When in vestibule: Tinnitus, episodic vertigo with nausea & vomiting, mixed hearing loss
  - When in cochlea: Slowly progressive sensorineural hearing loss
- Conservative management vs. surgical resection
  - Removal if disabling symptoms (intractable vertigo)

DIAGNOSTIC CHECKLIST

- When visually interrogating MRs to "rule out acoustic schwannoma," remember to carefully evaluate inner ear fluid spaces for ILS

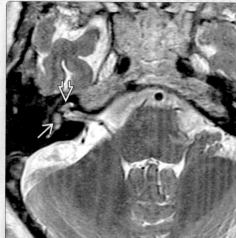
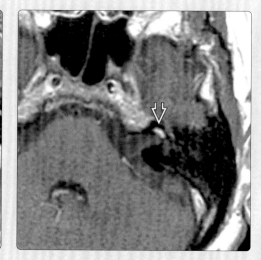

(Left) Axial T2WI MR shows a classic example of an intralabyrinthine schwannoma (ILS). This is a vestibulocochlear type as it involves both vestibule ➡ & cochlea ⇶. Note soft tissue intensity replacing the normal perilymphatic tissue of the membranous labyrinth. (Right) Axial T1WI C+ MR shows an intracochlear schwannoma as focal enhancement of the cochlea ⇶. It is important to review precontrast T1WI & T2WI to exclude intralabyrinthine hemorrhage & labyrinthitis, which may mimic this tumor.

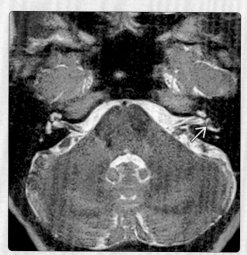
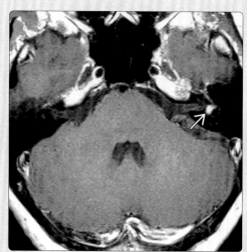

(Left) Coronal T2WI MR shows a soft tissue filling defect ➡ in the left vestibule replacing the normal high-intensity perilymphatic fluid. This intravestibular type of ILS often presents with vertigo or tinnitus. (Right) Axial T1WI C+ MR in the same patient shows intense enhancement of this intravestibular schwannoma ⇶. When these tumors are small, they may be treated conservatively unless the patient has intractable vertigo or the tumor shows signs of interval growth.

TERMINOLOGY

Abbreviations

- Intralabyrinthine schwannoma (ILS)

Synonyms

- Inner ear schwannoma

Definitions

- ILS: Benign tumor arising from Schwann cells within structures of membranous labyrinth
  - Includes schwannomas of cochlea, vestibule, or both, as well as tumors of inner ear extending to internal auditory canal (IAC) or middle ear

IMAGING

General Features

- Best diagnostic clue
  - T1 C+ MR: Focal enhancing mass in membranous labyrinth
  - High-resolution T2 MR: Filling defect within hyperintense perilymph
- Location
  - Focal intralabyrinthine mass named by location
    - **Intracochlear**: Schwannoma within cochlea
    - **Intravestibular**: Schwannoma within vestibule of inner ear
    - **Vestibulocochlear**: Schwannoma involves both vestibule & cochlea
    - **Transmodiolar**: Schwannoma crosses modiolus from cochlea to fundus of IAC
    - **Transmacular**: Schwannoma crosses from vestibule into fundus of IAC
    - **Transotic**: Schwannoma crosses entire inner ear from fundus of IAC to middle ear
- Size
  - Usually remains in millimeter range within membranous labyrinth
  - Larger lesions extend extralabyrinthine
- Morphology
  - Early, small lesions are ovoid to round
  - Older, larger lesions take on shape of portion of membranous labyrinth affected

CT Findings

- NECT
  - Typically normal, ILS not seen
- CECT
  - ILS not visible on CECT even if thin sections obtained
- Bone CT
  - Normal, unless mass projects into middle ear through round window niche
  - In very large lesions (transmodiolar, transmacular, transotic), bone erosion may be visible
  - Bone CT usually not helpful in making this diagnosis

MR Findings

- T1WI
  - Soft tissue intensity material in inner ear
  - May be mildly hyperintense to fluid of labyrinth
  - Not seen unless larger lesion is present & thinner sections are obtained
- T2WI
  - Focal low-signal mass within high-signal fluid of membranous labyrinth
- T1WI C+
  - Homogeneous enhancement of ILS
  - ILS may project multiple directions from inner ear
    - Through round window into middle ear
    - Along vestibular nerve branches into fundus of IAC = transmacular ILS
    - Through modiolus & cochlear nerve canal into IAC = transmodiolar ILS

Imaging Recommendations

- Use focused T1 C+ or high-resolution T2 imaging (i.e., CISS, FIESTA, 3D-TSE) of cerebellopontine angle (CPA)-IAC to make diagnosis of ILS
- Careful examination of all "rule out acoustic schwannoma" MR scans for presence of intralabyrinthine mass is critical
- Observe precise location of tumor
  - Consider if it involves vestibule, cochlea, or both
  - Consider if it projects into middle ear or IAC fundus
- All patients undergoing surgery for Ménière disease should undergo preoperative focused MR imaging to exclude ILS

DIFFERENTIAL DIAGNOSIS

Labyrinthitis

- Clinical: Acute onset of sensorineural hearing loss (SNHL) ± vertigo & facial neuropathy
- High-resolution T2 MR: No soft tissue intensity mass seen within high-signal inner ear fluid
- T1 C+ MR: Enhancement of most or all of membranous labyrinth

Labyrinthine Ossificans

- Clinical: History of previous meningitis or suppurative middle ear-mastoiditis
- High-resolution T2 MR: Focal low-signal areas within high-signal inner ear fluid; when fibroosseous, may mimic ILS
- T1 C+ MR: Minimal or no inner ear enhancement
- Bone CT: Encroachment on fluid of membranous labyrinth by bone

Intralabyrinthine Hemorrhage

- Clinical: Unilateral sudden onset of SNHL
- T1 MR: High-signal fluid within membranous labyrinth

Facial Nerve Schwannoma With Dehiscence Into Inner Ear

- Clinical: SNHL with associated facial neuropathy
- T1 C+ MR: Enhancing tubular mass follows course of intratemporal facial nerve canal
  - Involvement of inner ear is secondary finding
- Bone CT: Smooth enlargement of intratemporal facial nerve canal

PATHOLOGY

General Features

- Etiology

○ Tumor arises from Schwann cells wrapping distal vestibular or cochlear nerve axons within membranous labyrinth

○ Secondary endolymphatic hydrops explains Ménière symptoms

- Same pathology as other schwannomas in human body
- Intracochlear is most common type of ILS

Gross Pathologic & Surgical Features

- Tan-gray, encapsulated mass found within labyrinth

Microscopic Features

- Differentiated neoplastic Schwann cells
- Antoni A: Areas of compact, elongated cells
- Antoni B: Less densely cellular areas with tumor loosely arranged, ± clusters of lipid-laden cells
- Strong, diffuse expression of S100 protein

CLINICAL ISSUES

Presentation

- Most common signs/symptoms
  ○ Unilateral sensorineural hearing loss (SNHL)
    – Sudden onset of SNHL is extremely rare
  ○ Tumor location-specific symptoms
    – When in vestibule: Tinnitus, episodic vertigo with nausea & vomiting, mixed hearing loss (tumor impedes stapes footplate, creating element of conductive hearing loss)
    – When in cochlea: Slowly progressive SNHL
- Clinical profile
  ○ Unilateral SNHL that develops over decades

Demographics

- Age
  ○ Adults > 40
- Gender
  ○ No gender predilection
- Epidemiology
  ○ Rare lesion
  ○ Perhaps 100x less common than CPA-IAC vestibular schwannoma

Natural History & Prognosis

- Very slow-growing, benign tumor of membranous labyrinth
- History of progressive hearing loss may date back 20 years
- Often grows to fill inner ear, then stops growing
- Total deafness in ear will result eventually if untreated
- Deafness certain if tumor removed

Treatment

- Conservative management
  ○ Watchful waiting
  ○ Applied when symptoms are minor (serviceable hearing maintained) & tumor is confined to inner ear
- Surgical removal
  ○ Translabyrinthine surgery removes tumor in vestibule
  ○ Transotic surgery completed for tumors involving cochlea or middle ear
  ○ Completed if symptoms are disabling
    – Usually when there is intractable vertigo

○ If transmodiolar or transmacular extension is significant, middle cranial fossa approach may be used

○ Cochlear implantation may have role in select patients after resection

DIAGNOSTIC CHECKLIST

Consider

- ILS may be missed by excellent radiologists because they are not aware of its existence
- ILS now being diagnosed more often with high-resolution T2 imaging (CISS, FIESTA, 3D-TSE)
  ○ Increased diagnosis in part secondary to ↑ awareness of this lesion
  ○ Some ILS do not enhance robustly but can be seen on high-resolution T2 MR

Image Interpretation Pearls

- When visually interrogating MRs to "rule out acoustic schwannoma," remember to carefully evaluate inner ear fluid spaces for ILS
  ○ Unless radiologists specifically look at inner ear for focal lesions, ILS will be missed
- Once ILS is suspected, use high-resolution T2 MR to differentiate ILS from labyrinthitis
  ○ ILS will appear as soft tissue intensity lesion within high-signal inner ear fluid
  ○ Labyrinthitis will show no such focal mass within high-signal inner ear fluid

SELECTED REFERENCES

1. Frisch CD et al: Intralabyrinthine schwannomas. Otolaryngol Clin North Am. 48(3):423-41, 2015
2. Gosselin É et al: Meta-analysis on the clinical outcomes in patients with intralabyrinthine schwannomas: conservative management vs. microsurgery. Eur Arch Otorhinolaryngol. 273(6):1357-67, 2015
3. Lee JJ et al: Recovery of hearing after surgical removal of intralabyrinthine schwannoma. Laryngoscope. 125(8):1968-71, 2015
4. Slattery EL et al: Intralabyrinthine schwannomas mimic cochleovestibular disease: symptoms from tumor mass effect in the labyrinth. Otol Neurotol. 36(1):167-71, 2015
5. Dubernard X et al: Clinical presentation of intralabyrinthine schwannomas: a multicenter study of 110 cases. Otol Neurotol. 35(9):1641-9, 2014
6. Peng R et al: Intensity of gadolinium enhancement on MRI is useful in differentiation of intracochlear inflammation from tumor. Otol Neurotol. 35(5):905-10, 2014
7. Schutt CA et al: Cochlear implantation after resection of an intralabyrinthine schwannoma. Am J Otolaryngol. 35(2):257-60, 2014
8. Van Abel KM et al: Primary inner ear schwannomas: a case series and systematic review of the literature. Laryngoscope. 123(8):1957-66, 2013
9. Dubrulle F et al: Differential diagnosis and prognosis of T1-weighted post-gadolinium intralabyrinthine hyperintensities. Eur Radiol. 20(11):2628-36, 2010
10. Iseri M et al: Hearing loss owing to intralabyrinthine schwannoma responsive to intratympanic steroid treatment. J Otolaryngol Head Neck Surg. 38(3):E95-7, 2009
11. Shin YR et al: Intralabyrinthine schwannoma involving the cochlea, vestibule, and internal auditory canal: 'canalolabyrinthine schwannoma'. Eur Arch Otorhinolaryngol. 266(1):143-5, 2009
12. Jia H et al: Intralabyrinthine schwannomas: symptoms and managements. Auris Nasus Larynx. 35(1):131-6, 2008
13. Tieleman A et al: Imaging of intralabyrinthine schwannomas: a retrospective study of 52 cases with emphasis on lesion growth. AJNR Am J Neuroradiol. 29(5):898-905, 2008
14. Kennedy RJ et al: Intralabyrinthine schwannomas: diagnosis, management, and a new classification system. Otol Neurotol. 25(2):160-7, 2004
15. Mafee MF: MR imaging of intralabyrinthine schwannoma, labyrinthitis, and other labyrinthine pathology. Otolaryngol Clin North Am. 28(3):407-30, 1995

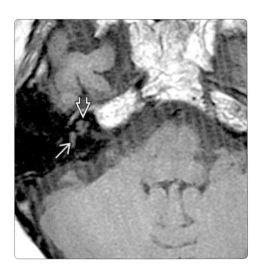

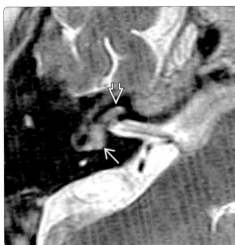

(Left) *Axial T1WI MR shows slightly hyperintense signal within the vestibule* ⮕ *and cochlea* ⮕ *of this patient with a vestibulocochlear schwannoma.* (Right) *Axial T2WI MR shows soft tissue intensity material replacing the normal fluid signal of the vestibule* ⮕ *and cochlea* ⮕ *in this patient with a vestibulocochlear type of ILS. These tumors are being recognized more frequently with the use of high-resolution T2 MR and increased awareness of the lesion.*

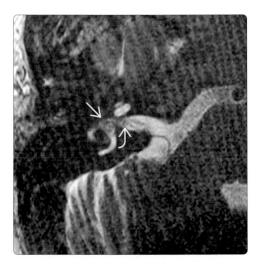

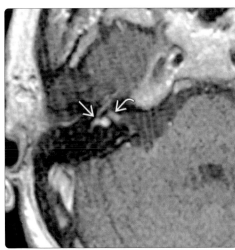

(Left) *Axial T2WI MR shows a transmacular type of ILS as soft tissue intensity material filling the vestibule* ⮕ *and coursing along the vestibular nerve branches into the distal fundus* ⮕ *of the internal auditory canal (IAC).* (Right) *Axial T1WI C+ MR in the same patient shows enhancement of both the intravestibular* ⮕ *and distal intracanalicular portion* ⮕ *of this transmacular schwannoma. The slight difference in enhancement characteristics is related to volume averaging.*

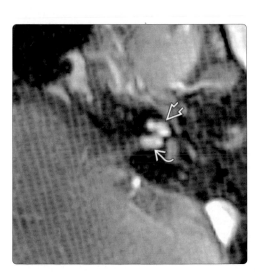

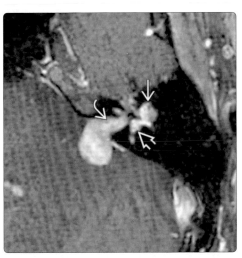

(Left) *Axial T1WI C+ MR shows enhancement of the distal IAC fundus* ⮕ *and cochlea* ⮕ *in this transmodiolar type of ILS. This tumor grew from the cochlea through the modiolus and cochlear nerve canal to reach the IAC fundus.* (Right) *Axial T1WI C+ FS MR shows the very rare transotic type of ILS. Note that the enhancing tumor extends from the CPA through the IAC* ⮕ *and also involves the inner ear* ⮕ *and middle ear* ⮕ *.*

Endolymphatic Sac Tumor

TERMINOLOGY

- Endolymphatic sac tumor (ELST)
- Papillary cystadenomatous tumor of ELS
  - Originates from epithelium of endolymphatic sac

IMAGING

- CT findings
  - **Permeative-destructive** retrolabyrinthine mass
  - Central spiculated tumor **Ca**⁺⁺ (100%)
  - Thin, **calcified rim** at posterior tumor margin
- MR findings
  - T1-hyperintense foci in 80%
  - Inhomogeneous T2 signal
  - Heterogeneous enhancement
- Angiographic findings
  - Tumors < 3 cm supplied by ECA branches
  - Tumors > 3 cm also recruit ICA branches

TOP DIFFERENTIAL DIAGNOSES

- Petrous apex cholesterol granuloma
- Glomus jugulare paraganglioma
- Petrous apex meningioma
- T-bone metastasis

PATHOLOGY

- Sporadic occurrence more common than von Hippel-Lindau disease (VHL)-associated ELST
  - **15% of VHL patients** develop **ELST**, 30% bilateral
- VHL
  - Cerebellar & spinal cord hemangioblastoma, renal cell carcinoma, pheochromocytoma
  - Kidney & pancreas cysts

CLINICAL ISSUES

- Sensorineural hearing loss = most common symptom
- Treatment: Complete surgical resection
- If sporadic ELST, check patient & family for VHL

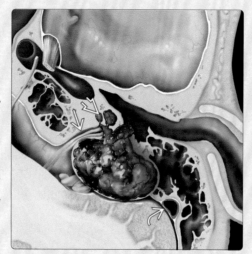
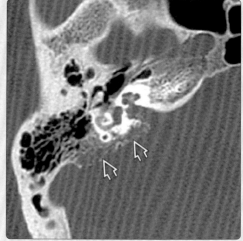

(Left) Axial graphic of T-bone illustrates typical appearance of endolymphatic sac tumor (ELST). Important features include its vascular nature, tendency to fistulize in inner ear ➡, & bone fragments within tumor matrix. Note the classic retrolabyrinthine location between the IAC ➡ and sigmoid sinus ➡. (Right) Axial bone CT shows imaging features of ELST, including tumor centered in posterior T-bone in area of fovea of the endolymphatic sac, spiculated tumor matrix Ca⁺⁺ ➡, and permeative bone changes.

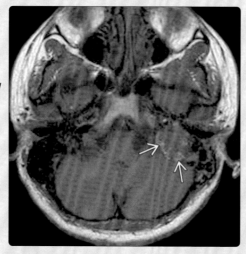
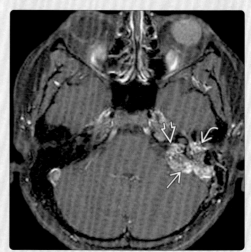

(Left) Axial T1WI MR shows an expansile, lobular mass centered in the left T-bone with areas of ↑ T1 signal, which are common in ELST and are typically peripheral in location ➡. (Right) Axial T1WI C+ FS MR in the same patient reveals the typical intense, heterogeneous contrast enhancement ➡ expected in ELST. This tumor has also grown into the left IAC ➡, middle ear ➡, & mastoid. Note diffuse abnormal signal in left globe indicating retinal angioma with detachment seen in von Hippel-Lindau disease.

TERMINOLOGY

Abbreviations

- Endolymphatic sac tumor (ELST)

Synonyms

- Adenomatous tumor of ELS, Heffner tumor

Definitions

- Papillary cystadenomatous tumor of ELS
  - Originates from epithelium of endolymphatic sac

IMAGING

General Features

- Best diagnostic clue
  - Bone CT: Central intratumoral **bone spicules** & **posterior rim Ca^{++}**
  - MR: **High-signal** foci on **unenhanced T1**
- Location
  - **Retrolabyrinthine**: Posteromedial T-bone
  - Centered in **fovea of ELS** in presigmoid, posterior surface petrous T-bone
- Size
  - Variable, but often small & detected earlier with von Hippel-Lindau disease (VHL) screening
- Morphology
  - Infiltrative, poorly circumscribed lesion

CT Findings

- Bone CT
  - **Permeative-destructive** retrolabyrinthine mass
    - Central spiculated tumor **Ca^{++} (100%)**
    - Thin, **calcified rim**, posterior margin tumor

MR Findings

- T1WI
  - **Hyperintense foci** in **80%**
    - 2° to hemorrhage, cholesterol cleft
  - Tumors > 2 cm may have **flow voids**
- T2WI
  - Inhomogeneous signal from bone fragments & cysts
- T1WI C+
  - Heterogeneous enhancement

Angiographic Findings

- Tumors < 3 cm supplied by ECA branches
- Tumors > 3 cm also recruit ICA branches

Imaging Recommendations

- Best imaging tool
  - Bone CT & T1 C+ MR (both necessary)

DIFFERENTIAL DIAGNOSIS

Petrous Apex Cholesterol Granuloma

- Bone CT: Smooth expansile margins
- MR: Entire lesion has ↑ signal on T1 & T2

Petrous Apex Meningioma

- Bone CT: Scalloped margins ± hyperostosis ± permeative sclerotic bones
- MR: T1 C+ homogeneous enhancement; dural tail; ↓ T2 SI

Glomus Jugulare Paraganglioma

- Bone CT: Permeative-destructive bone invasion without spicules
- MR: ↑ T1 foci rare; T2 flow voids very common

T-Bone Metastasis

- History of 1° tumor

PATHOLOGY

General Features

- Genetics
  - Sporadic > VHL ELST
  - *VHL* tumor suppressor gene mutated in both
- Associated abnormalities
  - VHL disease
  - 15% of VHL patients develop ELST, 30% bilateral

Staging, Grading, & Classification

- Grade I: Confined to T-bone, middle ear, ± EAC
- Grade II: Posterior cranial fossa extension
- Grade III: Posterior & middle fossa extension
- Grade IV: Clival ± sphenoid wing extension

Gross Pathologic & Surgical Features

- Heaped up tumor on posterior wall of T-bone

CLINICAL ISSUES

Presentation

- Most common signs/symptoms
  - Sensorineural hearing loss
- Other signs/symptoms
  - Tinnitus, vertigo (mimics Ménière disease)
  - Facial nerve palsy

Demographics

- Age
  - Sporadic: 40-50 years; VHL: 30 years

Natural History & Prognosis

- Prognosis excellent with complete surgical resection
  - VHL ELST found earlier (annual MR screening)
- Late recurrence possible so follow-up imaging recommended

Treatment

- Complete surgical resection
  - Preoperative embolization for larger lesions
- Radiation therapy if unresectable or nonsurgical candidate

DIAGNOSTIC CHECKLIST

Consider

- Bilateral ELST = VHL diagnosis
- If sporadic ELST, check patient & family for VHL

Image Interpretation Pearls

- Posterior wall T-bone **tumor with ↑ T1 foci = ELST**

SELECTED REFERENCES

1. Wick CC et al: Endolymphatic sac tumors. Otolaryngol Clin North Am. 48(2):317-30, 2015

Intralabyrinthine Hemorrhage

TERMINOLOGY

- Blood within normally fluid-filled spaces of labyrinth

IMAGING

- T1 MR: **High signal** within normally fluid-filled space of labyrinth
- T2 MR: Variable depending on age of hemorrhage.
- T1 C+: High signal, not to be confused with enhancement
- T1 FS: High inner ear signal remains on fat-saturated images
  - Not if intralabyrinthine lipoma present

TOP DIFFERENTIAL DIAGNOSES

- Labyrinthitis
- Vestibular schwannoma
- Intralabyrinthine schwannoma
- Congenital intralabyrinthine lipoma

PATHOLOGY

- Shortened T1 relaxation time caused by intra-/extracellular methemoglobin

CLINICAL ISSUES

- Presentation: Acute onset of unilateral sensorineural hearing loss
- History: Anticoagulant therapy, sickle cell disease, or trauma
- Prognosis: Variable return of hearing
- Treatment: Aimed at underlying condition

DIAGNOSTIC CHECKLIST

- Always perform unenhanced T1 MR & evaluate for evidence of intralabyrinthine high signal
- Differentiate from intralabyrinthine lipoma with fat-saturated images

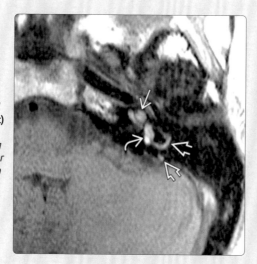
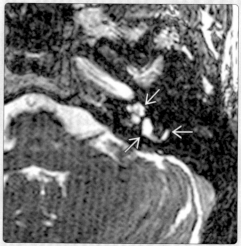

(Left) Axial T1WI MR without contrast shows the classic findings of intralabyrinthine hemorrhage (ILH), with hyperintense blood (methemoglobin) within the membranous labyrinth of the cochlea ➡, vestibule ➡, and semicircular canals ➡. (Right) Axial T2WI MR in the same patient reveals corresponding high T2 signal within the inner ear ➡. T2 signal is variable in ILH, depending on the age of the blood. When T2 signal is decreased, the diffuse involvement of the labyrinth can distinguish ILH from intralabyrinthine masses.

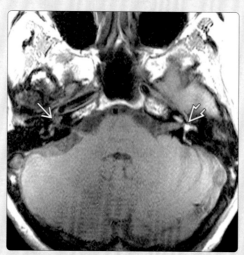
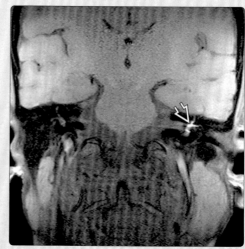

(Left) Axial T1WI MR without contrast at the level of the internal auditory canals shows hyperintense signal in the left inner ear membranous labyrinth ➡, representing ILH. Compare to normal fluid signal on the right ➡. (Right) Coronal T1WI FS MR in the same patient demonstrates that the high signal in the left inner ear ➡ is not fat, as it persists despite fat-saturation sequence. Findings exclude the possibility of intralabyrinthine lipoma and confirm the diagnosis of ILH.

TERMINOLOGY

Abbreviations

- Intralabyrinthine hemorrhage (ILH)

Synonyms

- Inner ear (IE) hemorrhage, membranous labyrinthine hemorrhage, perilymphatic labyrinthine hemorrhage

Definitions

- Blood within normally fluid-filled spaces of labyrinth

IMAGING

General Features

- Best diagnostic clue
  - **Bright signal** on **T1** nonenhanced MR of **IE**
    - IE fluid normally isointense with CSF
    - Highly proteinaceous IE contents may have identical appearance
- Location
  - Membranous labyrinth of IE
- Size
  - May be diffuse or segmental within IE spaces
- Morphology
  - Conforms to IE shape

MR Findings

- T1WI
  - High signal within normally fluid-filled space of labyrinth on nonenhanced T1
    - IE normally low signal (fluid intensity)
- T2WI
  - Variable: May be high or low depending on hemorrhage age
- T1WI C+
  - High signal already present
  - If precontrast imaging not done, may be mistaken for IE enhancement

Imaging Recommendations

- Protocol advice
  - Include at least 1 nonenhanced T1 sequence in all IE protocols

DIFFERENTIAL DIAGNOSIS

Labyrinthitis

- T1 C+ MR high signal (enhancement)
  - Focal or diffuse, usually faint
- Unenhanced T1 usually normal

Vestibular Schwannoma

- Intralabyrinthine ↑ signal on unenhanced T1 MR from high protein content
  - Often postoperative finding

Intralabyrinthine Schwannoma

- T1 C+ MR ↑ signal (focal intense enhancement)

Congenital Intralabyrinthine Lipoma

- Unenhanced T1 ↑ signal may appear identical
- T1 fat saturated: Lesion no longer seen (saturates)

PATHOLOGY

General Features

- Etiology
  - Events inciting ILH
    - Trauma
    - Anticoagulant therapy
    - Hematologic lesions: Leukemia, sickle cell anemia, & other hyperviscosity syndromes
    - Neoplasm: Endolymphatic sac tumors, sporadic or von Hippel-Lindau related
- Shortened T1 relaxation time caused by intra-/extracellular methemoglobin

CLINICAL ISSUES

Presentation

- Most common signs/symptoms
  - **Acute** onset of **unilateral sensorineural hearing loss**
    - Sudden hearing loss: Hearing loss that has evolved over hours to days
    - At least 30 decibel ↓ in threshold in 3 contiguous test frequencies over 24- to 72-hour period
- Other signs/symptoms
  - Vertigo, tinnitus
- Clinical profile
  - Patient with history of anticoagulant therapy, sickle cell disease, or trauma

Demographics

- Age
  - Possible at any age
- Ethnicity
  - Spontaneous ILH more common in African Americans due to increased incidence in sickle cell disease

Natural History & Prognosis

- Prognosis same as for underlying condition
- Return of hearing is variable

Treatment

- None unless underlying condition exists
- Treat underlying condition

DIAGNOSTIC CHECKLIST

Consider

- **Intravestibular lipoma** also has increased unenhanced T1 signal
  - Will lose its signal (saturate) on fat-saturated images

Image Interpretation Pearls

- Always perform unenhanced T1 & evaluate for evidence of intralabyrinthine high signal

SELECTED REFERENCES

1. Kaya S et al: Effects of intralabyrinthine hemorrhage on the cochlear elements: a human temporal bone study. Otol Neurotol. 37(2):132-6, 2016
2. Cervantes SS et al: Sudden sensorineural hearing loss associated with intralabyrinthine hemorrhage. Otol Neurotol. 36(8):e134-5, 2015
3. Rosado WM Jr et al: Sudden onset of sensorineural hearing loss secondary to intralabyrinthine hemorrhage: MRI findings. Ear Nose Throat J. 87(3):130-1, 2008

Semicircular Canal Dehiscence

TERMINOLOGY

- Semicircular canal dehiscence (SCCD): Defined as extreme thinning or absence of bony roof over superior (SSCC) or posterior semicircular canal

IMAGING

- Coronal T-bone CT: **≥ 2-mm** dehiscence of roof of SSCC
  - Thinning of **tegmen tympani** may be associated
- Transverse oblique T-bone CT reformats
  - In-plane view of SSCC dehiscent roof
- Axial T-bone CT
  - Provides in-plane view of dehiscence of superficial bony wall of posterior SCC

PATHOLOGY

- Unknown; developmentally thinned ± acquired component
- Results in "**unphysiological motion**" of endolymph in affected SCC
- Best hypothesis for clinical findings

- Bony opening overlying SCC creates **3rd mobile window** into inner ear
- 3rd window allows canal to respond to sound & pressure changes in membranous labyrinth

CLINICAL ISSUES

- Presenting signs and symptoms
  - Sound ± pressure-induced vestibular symptoms ± eye movements
  - Chronic disequilibrium may be debilitating
  - Oscillopsia (oscillating vision)
- **Tullio phenomenon**
  - Vertigo ± nystagmus related to sound
- Treatable form of vestibular disturbance

DIAGNOSTIC CHECKLIST

- Vestibular symptoms + positive bone CT = SCCD syndrome
- Since usually unilateral, use opposite SCC bony cover as baseline normal to compare with suspicious side

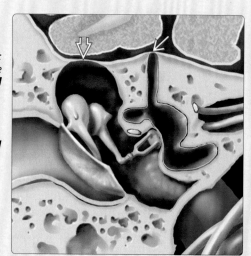
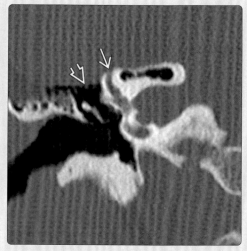

(Left) Coronal graphic illustrates the principal findings of superior semicircular canal dehiscence: Absence of bone overlying the superior semicircular canal ➡ and associated thinning of tegmen tympani ➡. (Right) Coronal T-bone CT shows no bone covering the roof of the superior semicircular canal ➡ representing superior semicircular canal dehiscence. Note thinning of the tegmen tympani ➡, a common associated finding on temporal bone CT.

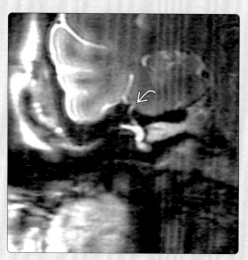
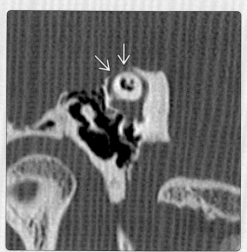

(Left) Coronal T2WI MR reveals the absence of cortical bone covering the superior semicircular canal ➡, which is diagnostic of superior semicircular canal dehiscence. (Right) T-bone CT transverse oblique reformation clearly demonstrates an in-plane view of the superior semicircular canal showing the entire extent of superior semicircular canal dehiscence ➡ in a single image.

TERMINOLOGY

Abbreviations

- Semicircular canal dehiscence (SCCD)

Definitions

- Extreme thinning or absence of bony roof over superior or posterior semicircular canal

IMAGING

General Features

- Best diagnostic clue
  - T-bone CT shows dehiscence of bone covering superior (SSCC) or posterior (PSCC) semicircular canal
- Location
  - May be bilateral
- Size
  - 2- to 4-mm dehiscent segment

CT Findings

- Bone CT
  - Coronal T-bone CT
    - **≥ 2-mm** dehiscence of roof of SSCC
    - Extreme thinning of **tegmen tympani** may be associated
  - Transverse oblique (Pöschl) T-bone CT reformats
    - Ideal for in-plane view of SSCC dehiscent roof
  - Axial T-bone CT
    - ≥ 2-mm dehiscence of superficial bony wall of PSCC

MR Findings

- T2WI
  - Thin-section, high-resolution T2 MR
    - Coronal: Absence of arcuate eminence bone covering SSCC
    - Axial: Best shows segmental absence of superficial wall of PSCC
- T1WI C+
  - Look for acoustic schwannoma as alternative explanation for vertigo

Imaging Recommendations

- Axial & coronal T-bone CTs are best test
  - Nonenhanced, bone algorithm, high-resolution (1 mm) CT
  - Oblique reconstructions in plane of SSCC or PSCC shows scope of dehiscence

DIFFERENTIAL DIAGNOSIS

Normal Thinning of SSCC or PSCC Wall

- Asymptomatic thinning of bony cover of SSCC or PSCC occurs
- Usually seen on only 1 coronal or axial CT image

PATHOLOGY

General Features

- Etiology
  - Unknown; developmental thinned ± acquired component

- Head injury or change in intracranial pressure (barotrauma) may fracture thin bone or destabilize dura over preexistent dehiscence
- Best hypothesis for clinical findings
  - Bony opening overlying SCC creates **3rd mobile window** into inner ear, allowing canal to respond to sound & pressure changes in membranous labyrinth
  - Motion at oval window (from loud noises) or ↑ intracranial pressure may then cause bowing of thin cover over SSCC or PSCC
  - Results in "**unphysiological motion**" of endolymph in affected SCC
  - Similar clinical findings described with cholesteatomas eroding horizontal SCC

Gross Pathologic & Surgical Features

- Surgical view shows absent bony cover over SSCC or PSCC

CLINICAL ISSUES

Presentation

- Most common signs/symptoms
  - Sound ± pressure-induced vestibular symptoms ± eye movements
  - Other symptoms & signs
    - Chronic disequilibrium may be debilitating
    - Oscillopsia (oscillating vision)
    - **Tullio phenomenon**: Vertigo ± nystagmus related to sound

Demographics

- Age
  - Mean: 50 years; range: 20-70 years
- Epidemiology
  - ~ 2% of population have thinning or dehiscence of bone over SSCC on autopsy; 50% bilateral
  - Recent studies suggest higher prevalence of SCCD on CT than cadaveric studies: Beware false-positives
  - SSCC dehiscence > > PSCC dehiscence

Natural History & Prognosis

- Slowly progressive symptoms

Treatment

- Treatable form of vestibular disturbance
- Earplugs & avoidance of provoking stimuli
- Surgical resurfacing of affected SCC beneficial

DIAGNOSTIC CHECKLIST

Consider

- Vestibular symptoms + positive CT = **SCCD syndrome**

Image Interpretation Pearls

- Since usually unilateral, use opposite SCC as baseline normal to compare with suspicious side

SELECTED REFERENCES

1. Klopp-Dutote N et al: A radiologic and anatomic study of the superior semicircular canal. Eur Ann Otorhinolaryngol Head Neck Dis. 133(2):91-4, 2016
2. Mong A et al: Sound- and pressure-induced vertigo associated with dehiscence of the roof of the superior semicircular canal. AJNR Am J Neuroradiol. 20(10):1973-5, 1999

TERMINOLOGY

- Cochlear implant (CI)
  - Multicomponent electronic device that provides auditory information by directly stimulating auditory fibers in cochlea

IMAGING

- Postoperative CI evaluation: T-bone CT
- Stimulation wire tip should be in basal turn or 2nd turn of cochlea
- No wire in cochlea ("empty cochlea") signifies malpositioning
- Wire fracture or kinking may be demonstrated in malfunctioning CI

CLINICAL ISSUES

- Torque experienced by CI in 1.5T MR is sufficient to cause implant movement
  - Most CI patients should **not** undergo MR

DIAGNOSTIC CHECKLIST

- Key **absolute contraindications** to CI placement
  - Cochlear or labyrinthine aplasia
  - Absent cochlear nerve
- Key **relative contraindications** to CI placement
  - Labyrinthine ossificans
  - Malformed cochlea (common cavity, cystic cochleovestibular anomaly)
  - Large endolymphatic sac anomaly
- Key findings that may complicate surgery
  - Hypoplastic mastoid process
  - Aberrant facial nerve
  - Otosclerosis
  - Otomastoiditis
  - Dehiscent jugular bulb
  - Aberrant internal carotid artery
  - Persistent stapedial artery

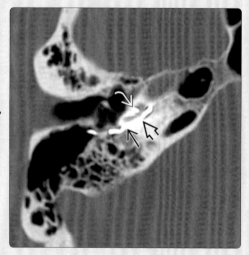 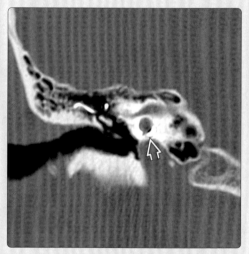

(Left) *Axial right T-bone CT shows the normal appearance and location of a cochlear implant. The wire enters the round window ⊟ and traverses the basal turn of the cochlea ⊡ to reach the cochlear 2nd turn ➡.* (Right) *Coronal T-bone CT in the same patient demonstrates normal positioning of the cochlear implant wire in the basal turn of the cochlea ➡.*

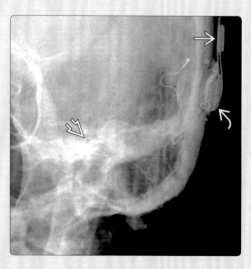 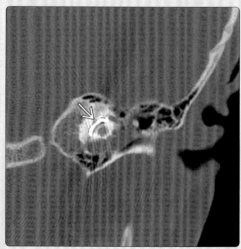

(Left) *Modified Stenvers view of the left T-bone shows the normal configuration of the distal cochlear implant wire spiraling within the cochlea ➡. The receiver ➡ and magnet ➡ are seen in profile.* (Right) *Coronal left T-bone CT shows a normally positioned cochlear implant wire in the basal turn of the cochlea ➡.*

TERMINOLOGY

Abbreviations

- Cochlear implant (CI)

Synonyms

- Cochlear electrode

Definitions

- CI: Multicomponent electronic device that provides auditory information by directly stimulating auditory fibers in cochlea
  - **Microphone**
    - External component that resides behind ear
    - Receives sound from environment
    - Transforms sound to electrical impulse
    - Transmits impulse to speech processor
  - **Speech processor**
    - External component that may be attached to microphone or worn separately in clothing
    - Custom programmed computer that emphasizes speech over other sounds
    - Digitally encodes sounds from frequency range of human speech
    - Encoding strategy depends on manufacturer
  - **Transmitter**
    - External component that resides behind ear, atop subcutaneous receiver
    - Transcutaneously sends magnetic impulses from speech processor to receiver
    - Held in place by magnet in subcutaneous receiver
  - **Receiver**
    - Thin, subcutaneous component that resides behind ear
    - Surgically implanted
    - Converts magnetic impulses from transmitter to electrical signal for stimulator wire
  - **Stimulator**
    - Wire placed inside cochlea directly stimulates spiral ganglion cells and cochlear axons
    - Stimulator wire enters cochlea via round window
    - Array of electrodes along wire appear as tiny bumps radiographically

IMAGING

General Features

- Best diagnostic clue
  - Thin, metallic wire (stimulator) with tiny beads (electrodes) extending into cochlea
  - Stimulator wire is connected to subcutaneous receiver behind ear
- Location
  - Stimulator wire should be in basal turn of cochlea, sometimes into 2nd turn
  - Enters cochlea via round window
- Size
  - Submillimeter thickness
- Morphology
  - Curvilinear with small beads on intracochlear stimulator wire

Radiographic Findings

- Modified Stenvers view of T-bone shows CI best
  - Head rotated 45° from direct AP, away from implanted ear
  - Slight head flexion

CT Findings

- Bone CT
  - Preimplant evaluation: Absolute & relative contraindications to implantation
    - Key preoperative absolute contraindication: Cochlear aplasia alone or in labyrinthine aplasia
    - Key preoperative relative contraindications: Labyrinthitis ossificans, other inner ear dysplasias
  - Preimplant CT: Findings that may complicate surgery
    - Hypoplastic mastoid process
    - Aberrant facial nerve course
    - Otomastoiditis
    - Fenestral ± cochlear otosclerosis
    - Persistent stapedial artery
    - Dehiscent jugular bulb
    - Aberrant internal carotid artery
    - Enlarged endolymphatic sac & duct
  - Postoperative search for complications
    - Key postoperative complication: **Misplaced wire** (not in cochlea)
    - Wire penetrates only partway into cochlea
    - **Broken wire**
    - Wire penetration out of inner ear

MR Findings

- T2WI
  - Must include high-resolution fluid sequence
  - Preoperative setting: Look for absolute & relative contraindications
    - Key preoperative contraindication: **Absence of cochlear nerve**
    - Absence of fluid in cochlea (e.g., labyrinthitis ossificans)
    - Ipsilateral brainstem infarct
    - Superficial siderosis
  - Postoperative setting: Traditional CI is **not** considered **safe** for 1.5T
    - Magnetic torque may dislodge CI
    - Embedded magnet causes marked field distortion

Imaging Recommendations

- Preoperative high-resolution T-bone CT and high-resolution T2 MR are complimentary
- Preoperative evaluation
  - T-bone CT
    - Adequately evaluates round window patency
    - Identifies bony phase of labyrinthitis ossificans in cochlea
    - Shows inner anomalies & anatomic variants
  - T-bone MR
    - Identifies both fibrous & ossific obstructions within cochlea
    - Can see absent or hypoplastic cochlear nerve
- Postoperative evaluation

- Modified Stenvers view of T-bone shows CI misplacement
- High-resolution T-bone CT now superior tool

DIFFERENTIAL DIAGNOSIS

Major Lesions to Identify in Preoperative CI Candidate

- Absolute contraindication diagnoses
  - Cochlear nerve & cochlear nerve canal aplasia-hypoplasia
  - Atretic cochlea
    - Labyrinthine aplasia
    - Cochlear aplasia
- Relative contraindication diagnoses
  - Malformed cochlea
    - Common cavity malformation
    - Cystic cochleovestibular malformation (IP-I)
  - Severe labyrinthine ossificans

Cochlear Nerve & Cochlear Nerve Canal Aplasia-Hypoplasia

- Imaging: Absent cochlear nerve with small IAC (congenital type)
- Embryogenesis: Cochlear nerve fails to form

Labyrinthine Aplasia

- Imaging: No cochlea or vestibule present
- Embryogenesis: Developmental arrest, 3rd gestational week

Cochlear Aplasia

- Imaging: No cochlea present
- Embryogenesis: Developmental arrest, late 3rd gestational week

Common Cavity Malformation

- Imaging: Coalesced cystic cochlea & vestibule form common cavity
- Embryogenesis: Developmental arrest in 4th gestational week

Cystic Cochleovestibular Malformation (IP-I)

- Imaging: Cochlea & vestibule cystic with no internal architecture
- Embryogenesis: Developmental arrest, 5th gestational week

PATHOLOGY

General Features

- Etiology
  - Primary causes of hearing loss = congenital, infection

Gross Pathologic & Surgical Features

- Placement of CI requires partial mastoidectomy

Microscopic Features

- Beaded appearance of stimulator wire represents individual stimulating electrodes

CLINICAL ISSUES

Presentation

- Most common signs/symptoms

- Severe to profound bilateral sensorineural hearing loss (SNHL)
- Clinical profile
  - CI candidates usually **> 2 years old** with bilateral severe SNHL
  - Must also show no benefit from conventional hearing aids

Demographics

- Epidemiology
  - Estimated 17% (36 million) of Americans reported some degree of hearing loss in 2010

Natural History & Prognosis

- Postlingually deafened patients (those who have already learned to speak, usually > 5 years old) have best CI outcome
- Postoperative complications (5%)
  - Transient CNVII paresis, imbalance, perilymph fistula, hardware failure, & skin flap problems
- 90% of CI patients report understanding basic sentences after 6 months
- Torque experienced by CI in 1.5T MR is sufficient to cause implant movement; traditional CI patients should not undergo 1.5T MR
  - MR-compatible CI is now available
  - External components should be removed in all cases

Treatment

- CI is effective rehabilitation method for profoundly hearing-impaired patients who do not benefit from hearing aids
- CI users should return to clinic at least once a year for speech processor adjustments
- Postoperative results depend on number of intracochlear electrodes
- Alternative hearing augmentation options
  - Hearing aid
  - Ossicular prosthesis
  - Auditory brainstem implant

DIAGNOSTIC CHECKLIST

Consider

- Are there any contraindications to CI placement?
- Are there any findings that might complicate surgery?
- Which side would be easier for surgeon?
- Postoperative patients: Is CI in appropriate location (basal turn of cochlea)?

SELECTED REFERENCES

1. Colby CC et al: Standardization of CT depiction of cochlear implant insertion depth. AJNR Am J Neuroradiol. 36(2):368-71, 2015
2. Fischer N et al: Radiologic and functional evaluation of electrode dislocation from the scala tympani to the scala vestibuli in patients with cochlear implants. AJNR Am J Neuroradiol. 36(2):372-7, 2015
3. Pearl MS et al: High-resolution secondary reconstructions with the use of flat panel CT in the clinical assessment of patients with cochlear implants. AJNR Am J Neuroradiol. 35(6):1202-8, 2014
4. Vlastarakos PV et al: Cochlear implantation update: contemporary preoperative imaging and future prospects - the dual modality approach as a standard of care. Expert Rev Med Devices. 7(4):555-67, 2010

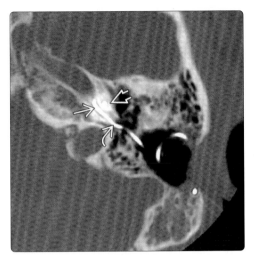

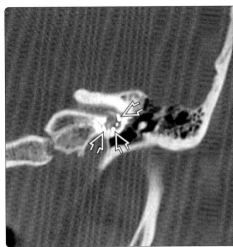

(Left) *Axial left T-bone CT demonstrates a normal cochlear implant. The wire enters the round window ➡ on its way to the basal turn of the cochlea ➡, extending well into the cochlear 2nd turn ➡. There is no evidence of wire kinking or breaking.* (Right) *Coronal T-bone CT of the same patient reveals the cochlear implant wire appropriately positioned within the cochlea. The normal beaded appearance from electrodes on the distal cochlear implant wire is well appreciated on this image ➡.*

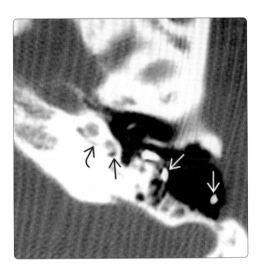

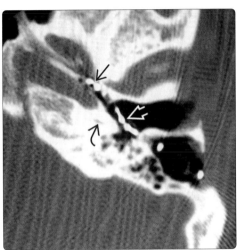

(Left) *Axial left T-bone CT reveals portions of the cochlear implant wire passing through the mastoidectomy cavity ➡ with no wire seen in the round window niche ➡ or cochlea ➡. This "empty cochlea" signifies an abnormal extracochlear location of the cochlear implant wire.* (Right) *Axial T-bone CT in the same patient demonstrates the cochlear implant wire traversing the middle ear ➡ with the tip malpositioned in the bony eustachian tube ➡. "Empty cochlea" is again partially visualized ➡.*

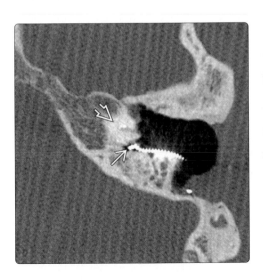

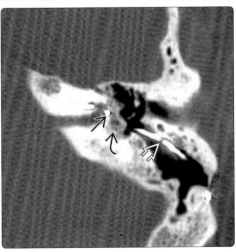

(Left) *Axial left T-bone CT of a malpositioned cochlear implant shows abnormal kinking of cochlear implant wire at round window niche ➡. Note severe obliterative labyrinthine ossificans with bone replacing the basal turn of the cochlea ➡, likely responsible for difficulty placing the cochlear implant in this case.* (Right) *Axial T-bone CT shows cochlear implant has traversed basal turn to 2nd turn ➡. Malfunction of cochlear implant is secondary to break in mastoid portion of stimulator wire ➡. Note otosclerosis ➡.*

Petrous Apex Asymmetric Marrow

TERMINOLOGY

- Synonym: Petrous apex (PA) pseudolesion
- PA asymmetric marrow: Asymmetric pneumatization of PA with nonpneumatized marrow space in opposite PA simulating mass lesion

IMAGING

- Temporal bone CT findings
  - Normal PA marrow space
  - Normal air cells visible in contralateral PA
  - **No expansile changes** present
- MR findings
  - Nonpneumatized PA contains normal fatty marrow, hyperintense on T1WI
  - Mimics cholesterol granuloma
  - Fat-saturated sequences confirm fatty nature of lesion

TOP DIFFERENTIAL DIAGNOSES

- PA cholesterol granuloma

- PA trapped fluid
- PA congenital cholesteatoma
- Apical petrositis

PATHOLOGY

- Congenital normal variant in PA pneumatization-marrow space spectrum
- Embryology-anatomy
  - **33%** have pneumatized petrous apices
  - 5% are asymmetrically pneumatized

CLINICAL ISSUES

- Clinical presentation
  - **Asymptomatic** by definition
- Patient undergoing brain MR for unrelated symptoms
  - Incidental MR finding
- Requires no treatment or follow-up
- If mentioned in radiology report, be certain to convey incidental nature

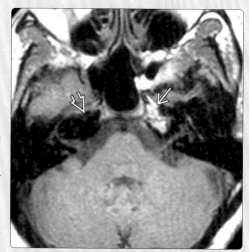
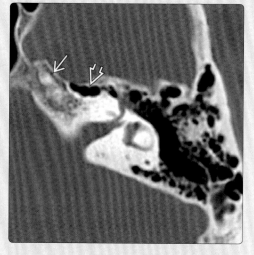

(Left) Axial T1WI MR demonstrates an irregularly shaped high-signal fatty marrow focus ➡ in the left petrous apex. The right petrous apex is low signal ➡ due to air in petrous apex air cells. Fatty marrow must not be mistaken for cholesterol granuloma. (Right) Axial bone CT in the same patient reveals only minimal petrous apex pneumatization ➡. The remainder of the petrous apex is marrow space ➡. There is no evidence for any expansile change in this area.

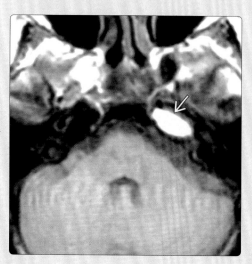
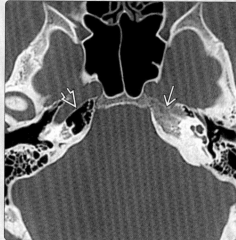

(Left) Axial T1WI MR shows a conspicuous bright lesion in the left petrous apex ➡ suspicious for cholesterol granuloma. Bone CT was ordered to further define the nature of this finding. (Right) Axial bone CT in the same patient demonstrates asymmetric marrow in the left petrous apex ➡. Notice that the opposite petrous apex is pneumatized ➡. Asymmetric fatty marrow spaces may appear quite conspicuous on T1WI MR. Review of fat-saturated MR sequences sorts this finding into the normal category.

TERMINOLOGY

Abbreviations

- Petrous apex (PA)

Synonyms

- PA pseudolesion

Definitions

- PA asymmetric marrow: Asymmetric pneumatization of PA with nonpneumatized marrow space in opposite PA simulating mass lesion

IMAGING

General Features

- Best diagnostic clue
  - Asymmetric pneumatized PA across from opposite normal PA bone marrow in absence of expansile changes

CT Findings

- CECT
  - No abnormal enhancement present
- Bone CT
  - Normal PA marrow space juxtaposed with contralateral normal PA air cells
  - **No expansile changes** present

MR Findings

- T1WI
  - Nonpneumatized PA contains normal fatty marrow, hyperintense on T1WI
    - Mimics cholesterol granuloma
  - If red marrow, may be of intermediate signal
- T2WI
  - When fatty, PA marrow will follow subcutaneous fat
- T1WI C+
  - Fat-saturated sequences remove fatty marrow high signal, confirming diagnoses of normal PA

Imaging Recommendations

- Best imaging tool
  - Most commonly **incidental finding** on brain MR
  - Temporal bone CT used to confirm marrow in PA
    - Ensures no worrisome changes to trabeculae, lack of expansile or erosive bone changes
- Protocol advice
  - Lesion is 1st suspected on MR without fat saturation
  - Use fat-saturated sequences to confirm fatty nature

DIFFERENTIAL DIAGNOSIS

Petrous Apex Cholesterol Granuloma

- Bone CT: Smooth, expansile PA mass
- MR: High signal on T1 & T2

Petrous Apex Trapped Fluid

- Bone CT: Nonexpansile, opacified PA air cells
- MR: Low or intermediate T1, high T2 signal in most cases

Petrous Apex Congenital Cholesteatoma

- Bone CT: Smooth, expansile PA lesion
- MR: Low T1, high T2 signal; nonenhancing
- DWI high signal

Apical Petrositis

- Bone CT: Destruction of PA trabecula & cortex
- MR: Thick enhancing walls with focal fluid ± dural enhancement

Petrous Apex Mucocele

- Bone CT: Smooth, expansile PA lesion
- MR: Low T1, high T2 signal; DWI low signal

PATHOLOGY

General Features

- Etiology
  - Congenital normal variant in PA pneumatization-marrow space spectrum
- Embryology-anatomy
  - **33%** have pneumatized petrous apices
  - 5% are asymmetrically pneumatized
  - PA pneumatization amount correlates with amount of mastoid aeration

CLINICAL ISSUES

Presentation

- Most common signs/symptoms
  - **Asymptomatic** by definition
- Clinical profile
  - Patient undergoing brain MR for unrelated symptoms
  - Incidental MR finding
    - PA marrow described as suspicious for cholesterol granuloma in radiology report
    - Patient is referred for surgical assessment

Natural History & Prognosis

- PA marrow remains unchanged over time
- Multiple possible morbidities from treatment of this "leave alone" lesion of PA

Treatment

- Requires no treatment or follow-up

DIAGNOSTIC CHECKLIST

Consider

- PA-asymmetric marrow is **common incidental finding** on brain MR
- May be misdiagnosed as PA cholesterol granuloma or high T1 signal trapped PA fluid
- One of "**leave alone**" lesions of PA
  - Trapped PA fluid is also "leave alone" lesion
- Misdiagnosis creates clinical confusion and potential for unnecessary treatment

SELECTED REFERENCES

1. Bag AK et al: Neuroimaging: intrinsic lesions of the central skull base region. Semin Ultrasound CT MR. 34(5):412-35, 2013
2. Connor SE et al: Imaging of the petrous apex: a pictorial review. Br J Radiol. 81(965):427-35, 2008
3. Moore KR et al: 'Leave me alone' lesions of the petrous apex. AJNR Am J Neuroradiol. 19(4):733-8, 1998
4. Virapongse C et al: Computed tomography of temporal bone pneumatization: 1. Normal pattern and morphology. AJR Am J Roentgenol. 145(3):473-81, 1985

Petrous Apex Cephalocele

TERMINOLOGY

- Synonyms: Petrous apex (PA) arachnoid cyst
- Definition: Congenital or acquired herniation of posterolateral wall of Meckel cave (MC) into PA

IMAGING

- Bone CT findings
  - Unilateral or bilateral expansile PA lesions
  - Enlarges porus trigeminus PA notch
- MR findings
  - CSF intensity ovoid PA lesion on all sequences
  - Directly communicates with MC
  - Appears to "spill out" of patulous MC

TOP DIFFERENTIAL DIAGNOSES

- PA cholesterol granuloma
- PA congenital cholesteatoma
- PA mucocele

CLINICAL ISSUES

- Common clinical presentation
  - Most commonly **incidental asymptomatic** MR finding
- Rare clinical presentation
  - Symptomatic lesion (CSF otorrhea, trigeminal neuralgia, meningitis); lesion breaks into temporal bone air cells
  - Headache from idiopathic intracranial hypertension
    - Consider if see empty sella, enlarged optic nerve CSF spaces associated with PA cephalocele (PAC)
- **No treatment** in most cases
- Surgical treatment
  - If lesion communicates with PA air cells

DIAGNOSTIC CHECKLIST

- PAC = "leave alone" lesion of PA
- PAC requires **no further work-up** or surgical intervention in most cases
- Convey incidental nature in radiologic report

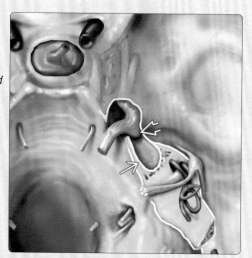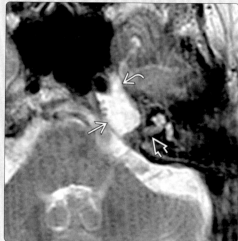

(Left) Axial graphic illustrates the herniation of a cephalocele from the Meckel cave into the petrous apex (PA) ➡. A portion of the trigeminal ganglion is depicted protruding into the cephalocele ➡. (Right) Axial T2WI MR shows a cephalocele ➡ protruding into the left PA just anteromedial to the internal auditory canal ➡. Notice the connection of the lesion to the Meckel cave ➡.

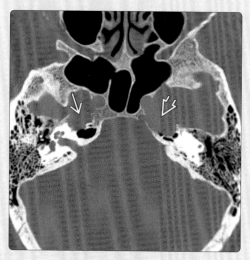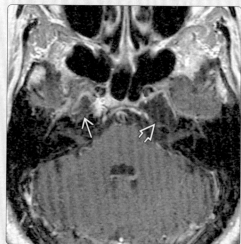

(Left) Axial bone CT demonstrates a right ➡ and left ➡ PA ovoid with scalloping lesions projecting into the PA air cells from the posterolateral Meckel cave area. Bilateral PA cephaloceles were suspected, and MR was ordered for confirmation. (Right) Axial T1WI C+ MR in the same patient reveals bilateral, left ➡ larger than right ➡, fluid intensity PA cephaloceles that arise from the inferior aspect of the Meckel cave.

TERMINOLOGY

Abbreviations

- Petrous apex (PA) cephalocele (PAC)

Synonyms

- PA arachnoid cyst, cavum trigeminale cephalocele

Definitions

- Congenital or acquired herniation of posterolateral wall of Meckel cave (MC) into PA

IMAGING

General Features

- Best diagnostic clue
  - CSF density (CT)/intensity (MR) lesion of PA that directly communicates with MC
  - Appears to "spill out" of patulous MC
- Location
  - Anteromedial PA directly adjacent to MC

CT Findings

- Bone CT
  - Unilateral or bilateral **smooth expansile** PA lesion(s)
  - **Enlarged** PA **porus trigeminus notch**
- CT cisternography
  - Contrast fills MC & PAC
  - When CSF otorrhea present, may define PAC connection to PA air cells

MR Findings

- T1WI
  - Low signal, isointense to CSF
- T2WI
  - High signal, isointense to CSF
  - Coronal best shows connection to MC
- FLAIR
  - Fluid in PAC attenuates with CSF
- T1WI C+
  - No enhancement vs. mild rim enhancement
  - If gasserian ganglion within cephalocele, will appear as enhancing component within ovoid nonenhancing lesion
    - Periganglionic venous plexus also enhances

Imaging Recommendations

- Best imaging tool
  - Focused multiplanar T2 MR makes diagnosis
  - Temporal bone CT confirms impression
  - CT cisternography if CSF otorrhea present

DIFFERENTIAL DIAGNOSIS

Petrous Apex Cholesterol Granuloma

- CT: Expansile PA lesion
- MR: T1 & T2 signal high
- Does not suppress on FLAIR

Petrous Apex Congenital Cholesteatoma

- CT: Smooth, expansile PA mass
- MR: T1 low, T2 high signal; DWI restricts

Petrous Apex Mucocele

- CT: Smooth, expansile PA lesion
- MR: T1 low, T2 high signal; DWI negative

PATHOLOGY

General Features

- Etiology
  - Congenital hypothesis
    - Developmental anomaly results in deficient dural & osseous covering of PA
    - Defect allows MC herniation into PA
  - Acquired hypothesis
    - Chronic CSF pulsations against thin anterior wall of pneumatized PA results in dehiscence
    - Eventual prolapse of meninges into PA defect
    - Idiopathic intracranial hypertension (IIH) may accelerate dehiscence
- Associated abnormalities
  - May see with IIH
    - Consider IIH diagnosis when empty sella, enlarged optic nerve CSF spaces are seen with PAC

Microscopic Features

- 1 or all 3 meningeal layers may be present

CLINICAL ISSUES

Presentation

- Most common signs/symptoms
  - **Incidental asymptomatic** MR brain finding
  - Rarely complicated by CSF otorrhea, trigeminal neuralgia, or meningitis
    - Occur when lesion breaks into temporal bone air cells
- Clinical profile
  - Common: Incidental MR finding in patient imaged for nonspecific brain indication
  - Rare: Meningitis, CSF otorrhea, or trigeminal neuralgia

Demographics

- Epidemiology
  - Uncommon incidental lesion on brain MR

Treatment

- **No treatment** in most cases
- Surgical treatment if air cell communication exists
  - Recurrent meningitis & CSF leak require surgery
  - Middle cranial fossa extradural approach
    - Repair dural defect; obliterate PA defect

SELECTED REFERENCES

1. Jamjoom DZ et al: The association between petrous apex cephalocele and empty sella. Surg Radiol Anat. 37(10):1179-82, 2015
2. Hatipoğlu HG et al: Petrous apex cephalocele and empty sella/arachnoid cyst coexistence: a clue for cerebrospinal fluid pressure imbalance? Diagn Interv Radiol. 16(1):7-9, 2010
3. Alorainy IA: Petrous apex cephalocele and empty sella: is there any relation? Eur J Radiol. 62(3):378-84, 2007
4. Moore KR et al: Petrous apex cephaloceles. AJNR Am J Neuroradiol. 22(10):1867-71, 2001
5. Vergoni G et al: Spontaneous cerebrospinal fluid rhinorrhoea in anteromedial temporal occult encephalocele. Br J Neurosurg. 15(2):156-8, 2001
6. Beaumont GD et al: Encephalocoele involving the petrous bone. Neuroradiology. 32(6):533-4, 1990

Congenital Petrous Apex Cholesteatoma

TERMINOLOGY

- Petrous apex cholesteatoma: Petrous apex (PA) focus of cholesteatoma due to **epithelial rest** of embryonal origin

IMAGING

- May simultaneously involve adjacent areas
  - Horizontal petrous internal carotid artery (ICA) canal
  - Inner ear structures (otic capsule)
  - Internal auditory canal
  - Meckel cave
  - Medial mastoid air cells
  - Facial nerve canal (labyrinthine & anterior tympanic segments)
- Bone CT: **Expansile** mass with **smooth**, **lobular bone remodeling**
  - Shows smooth, expansile, lobulated lesion of PA
- MR: Expansile PA lesion with low T1, high T2 signal but **without** enhancement

- **Restricted diffusion** (high signal on DWI) is **characteristic**

TOP DIFFERENTIAL DIAGNOSES

- PA trapped fluid
- Apical petrositis
- PA cholesterol granuloma
- PA mucocele
- Petrous ICA aneurysm

PATHOLOGY

- **Aberrant PA epithelial rest** of **exfoliated keratin** within stratified squamous epithelium
  - Growth from **progressive desquamation of epithelium**

CLINICAL ISSUES

- Clinical profile: 40-year-old adult with unilateral sensorineural hearing loss

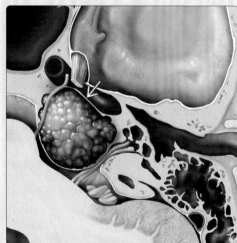
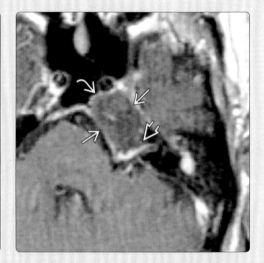

(Left) Axial graphic depicts typical petrous apex (PA) congenital cholesteatoma. Notice the benign expansile nature of the PA bone as it responds to the growing cholesteatoma. The horizontal petrous internal carotid artery (ICA) posterior wall is thinned ➡ by cholesteatoma growth. (Right) Axial T1WI C+ MR reveals a large PA cholesteatoma ➡ with minimal rim enhancement. The lesion is impinging on the internal auditory canal ➡ and sphenoid sinus ➡.

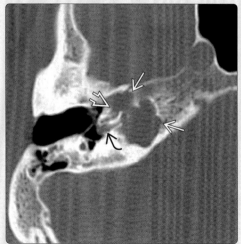
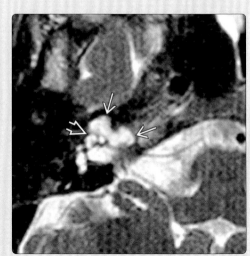

(Left) Axial bone CT in the right ear shows an expansile, smoothly marginated cholesteatoma remodeling the PA ➡ and eroding the bony labyrinth around the cochlea ➡. The cholesteatoma can also be seen emerging from the round window niche ➡. (Right) Axial T2 MR in the same patient shows the hyperintense congenital cholesteatoma eroding the PA ➡ and the bone of the cochlea ➡. PA congenital cholesteatoma often involves more than just the PA. In this case, the inner ear is affected.

TERMINOLOGY

Abbreviations
- Petrous apex cholesteatoma (PA-Chol)

Synonyms
- Congenital cholesteatoma, epidermoid cyst of petrous apex (PA)

Definitions
- PA-Chol: PA focus of cholesteatoma due to **epithelial rest** of embryonal origin

IMAGING

General Features
- Best diagnostic clue
  - Bone CT: **Expansile** mass with **smooth**, **lobular bone remodeling**
  - MR: Expansile PA lesion with low T1, high T2 signal but without enhancement
    - DWI MR sequence shows cholesteatoma as hyperintense
- Location
  - PA
  - May involve more than PA
    - Medial inner ear & internal auditory canal (IAC)
    - Medial mastoid
- Size
  - May become very large before discovered
  - 2-10 cm in maximum diameter
- Morphology
  - Ovoid to round; lobulated
  - When involves medial inner ear & mastoid with PA, may have "**dumbbell**" morphology

CT Findings
- CECT
  - PA-Chol will **not** enhance
- Bone CT
  - Shows smooth, expansile, lobulated lesion of PA
    - May simultaneously involve adjacent areas
      - Horizontal petrous internal carotid artery (ICA) canal
      - Inner ear structures (otic capsule)
      - IAC
      - Meckel cave
      - Medial mastoid air cells
      - Facial nerve canal (labyrinthine & anterior tympanic segments)

MR Findings
- T1WI
  - **Low** signal
  - May be homogeneous or heterogeneous
- T2WI
  - **High** signal
- FLAIR
  - Does not attenuate on FLAIR
  - Partial attenuation (mixed intermediate-low signal) may be seen
- DWI

- **Restricted diffusion** is **characteristic**
  - Same as congenital cholesteatoma in cerebellopontine angle (CPA) (epidermoid cyst)
- T1WI C+
  - **No** intrinsic enhancement
  - Mild rim enhancement common
- MRA
  - Large lesions may cause mass effect on horizontal petrous ICA
- MRV
  - Large lesions may compress sigmoid sinus ± jugular foramen

Angiographic Findings
- Avascular PA mass lesion

Imaging Recommendations
- Best imaging tool
  - Temporal bone CT is best initial exam
    - No contrast necessary
  - MR in axial & coronal planes used to confirm diagnosis & obtain soft tissue roadmap for surgery
    - Especially useful in large lesions
    - T1 C+ MR confirms lack of enhancement
    - Use **DWI sequence** to confirm diagnosis

DIFFERENTIAL DIAGNOSIS

Petrous Apex Trapped Fluid
- Clinical: Asymptomatic incidental finding on T2 MR
- Bone CT: Nonexpansile, opacified PA air cells
- MR: Low or intermediate T1 + high T2 signal in most cases
  - Can be high signal on T1

Apical Petrositis
- Clinical: Septic patient unless already partially treated with antibiotics
- Bone CT: Destructive PA lesion with trabecular & cortical loss
- MR: Thick enhancing walls with focal fluid
  - Dural thickening & enhancement

Petrous Apex Cholesterol Granuloma
- Clinical: Previous history of chronic otomastoiditis common
- Bone CT: Smooth, lobular expansile mass
- MR: High signal on T1 & T2
  - DWI shows no restricted diffusion

Petrous Apex Mucocele
- Bone CT: Smooth, expansile lesion
- MR: Low T1, high T2 signal
- May exactly mimic cholesteatoma of PA
  - Except **no** diffusion restriction seen on DWI MR sequence

Petrous ICA Aneurysm
- Clinical: Skull base trauma history may be present
- Bone CT: Fusiform or focal expansion centered in horizontal petrous ICA canal
- MR: Complex signal, ovoid to fusiform mass inseparable from horizontal petrous ICA

PATHOLOGY

General Features

- Etiology
  - **Aberrant PA epithelial rest** of **exfoliated keratin** within stratified squamous epithelium
    - Growth from **progressive desquamation of epithelium**
    - PA-Chol congenital, primary to PA or along labyrinthine segment of CNVII
    - PA-Chol may be part of large, multilobular lesion involving inner ear, IAC, medial mastoid
- Embryology-anatomy
  - Rests of epithelial tissue can occur in multiple locations in & around temporal bone
    - Middle ear > CPA > mastoid > PA > facial nerve canal

Gross Pathologic & Surgical Features

- Pearly white tissue within "eggshell" bone

Microscopic Features

- Sheets of stratified, keratinizing, squamous epithelium
  - No evidence of abnormal mitosis present
  - Granulation tissue & fibrosis often surround them
- Rich in cholesterol crystals

CLINICAL ISSUES

Presentation

- Most common signs/symptoms
  - Sensorineural hearing loss when large
- Other signs/symptoms
  - Peripheral facial nerve paralysis
  - Abducens nerve paralysis
  - Headache
- Clinical profile
  - 40-year-old adult with unilateral sensorineural hearing loss

Demographics

- Age
  - 20-50 years
- Epidemiology
  - Very rare PA lesion (< 1% of PA lesions)
    - Trapped fluid > > apical petrositis, cholesterol granuloma, metastases > PA congenital cholesteatoma

Natural History & Prognosis

- Very slow-growing lesion
- Complete surgical removal arrests symptom progression

Treatment

- Surgical approaches
  - Removal via transpetrous approach
  - Middle fossa approach also used

DIAGNOSTIC CHECKLIST

Consider

- Once discovery of PA **expansile lesion** occurs, sort into benign expansile & invasive expansile groups

- Invasive expansile PA group includes apical petrositis, metastases & plasmacytoma, & Langerhans cell histiocytosis
- Benign expansile PA group includes cholesteatoma, cholesterol granuloma, mucocele, petrous ICA aneurysm, PA cephalocele

Image Interpretation Pearls

- MR helpful in differentiating benign-appearing expansile PA lesions on CT
  - Congenital cholesteatoma of PA
    - T1 low, T2 high signal
    - T1 C+ MR shows no enhancement
    - FLAIR shows partial or absent attenuation
    - DWI shows **restricted diffusion**
  - Cholesterol granuloma of PA
    - T1 **high**, T2 high signal
  - Mucocele of PA
    - T1 low, T2 high signal
    - DWI shows **no** restricted diffusion
  - Petrous ICA aneurysm
    - MR sequences show **complex signal** mass centered on horizontal petrous ICA
    - Complex signal due to various ages of blood in luminal clot & turbulent flow
  - PA cephalocele
    - Look for connection to patulous Meckel cave

Reporting Tips

- Be precise about surrounding structure involvement by PA-Chol
  - Is horizontal petrous or cavernous ICA involved
  - Are CPA-IAC facial or vestibulocochlear nerves compressed
  - Is inner ear eroded
  - Is either jugular foramen or sigmoid sinus involved

SELECTED REFERENCES

1. MacKeith SA et al: Recurrent aseptic meningitis as a rare but important presentation of congenital petrous apex cholesteatoma: the value of appropriate imaging. BMJ Case Rep. 2014, 2014
2. De Foer B et al: Diffusion-weighted magnetic resonance imaging of the temporal bone. Neuroradiology. 52(9):785-807, 2010
3. Connor SE et al: Imaging of the petrous apex: a pictorial review. Br J Radiol. 81(965):427-35, 2008
4. Kojima H et al: Congenital cholesteatoma clinical features and surgical results. Am J Otolaryngol. 27(5):299-305, 2006
5. Mattox DE: Endoscopy-assisted surgery of the petrous apex. Otolaryngol Head Neck Surg. 130(2):229-41, 2004
6. Profant M et al: Petrous apex cholesteatoma. Acta Otolaryngol. 120(2):164-7, 2000
7. Chang P et al: Imaging destructive lesions of the petrous apex. Laryngoscope. 108(4 Pt 1):599-604, 1998
8. Mafee MF: MRI and CT in the evaluation of acquired and congenital cholesteatomas of the temporal bone. J Otolaryngol. 22(4):239-48, 1993
9. Atlas MD et al: Petrous apex cholesteatoma: diagnostic and treatment dilemmas. Laryngoscope. 102(12 Pt 1):1363-8, 1992
10. Ishii K et al: Middle ear cholesteatoma extending into the petrous apex: evaluation by CT and MR imaging. AJNR Am J Neuroradiol. 12(4):719-24, 1991
11. Glasscock ME 3rd et al: Petrous apex cholesteatoma. Otolaryngol Clin North Am. 22(5):981-1002, 1989
12. Rosenberg RA et al: Cholesteatoma vs. cholesterol granuloma of the petrous apex. Otolaryngol Head Neck Surg. 94(3):322-7, 1986
13. Horn KL et al: Congenital cholesteatoma of the petrous pyramid. Arch Otolaryngol. 111(9):621-2, 1985

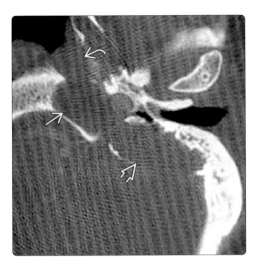

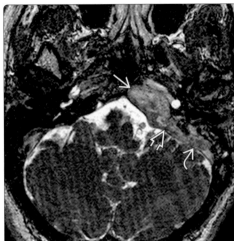

(Left) *Giant PA-medial temporal bone congenital cholesteatoma is seen on bone CT. Note the PA ➡, medial wall temporal bone ⮕, and nasopharyngeal ➶ components.* (Right) *Axial T2-CISS MR in the same patient demonstrates the intermediate-high signal large congenital cholesteatoma involving the PA ➡, medial inner ear ⮕, and mastoid ➶. The horizontal petrous ICA is bowed anteriorly by the lesion.*

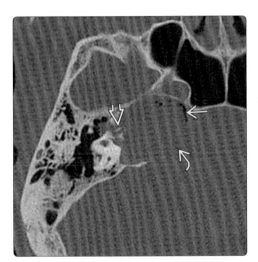

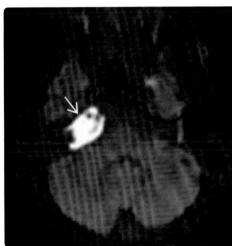

(Left) *Axial right temporal bone CT shows a smoothly enlarging petrous apex congenital cholesteatoma with intramural air ➡. The lesion is eroding the bony labyrinth of the inner ear ⮕ and dehiscing the posteromedial PA cortex ➶.* (Right) *Axial DWI MR in the same patient shows high signal (restricted diffusion) ➡ diagnostic of congenital PA cholesteatoma.*

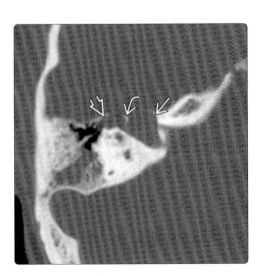

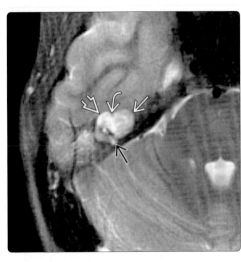

(Left) *Axial bone CT in a patient with facial nerve paresis shows an expansile lesion of the geniculate fossa ➡ and labyrinthine segment of the CN canal ➶. The congenital cholesteatoma remodels bone ➡ into the area of the medial petrous apex.* (Right) *Axial T2WI MR in the same patient reveals the congenital cholesteatoma to be high signal in the geniculate fossa ➡ and labyrinthine CN canal ➶. The PA ⮕ & superior semicircular canal ➶ are eroded by the lesion.*

Petrous Apex Trapped Fluid

TERMINOLOGY

- Definition: Sterile residual fluid collection in petrous apex (PA) air cells, sometimes resulting from remote otomastoiditis
- Also known as PA effusion

IMAGING

- Variable T1, high T2 signal in PA on MR with bone CT showing opacified PA air cells **without** trabecular loss or expansion
- Temporal bone CT findings
  - Opacified PA air cells; middle ear-mastoid clear
  - **No expansile component** to lesion
  - **No PA cortical or trabecular erosions**
- MR findings
  - T1 intermediate to high signal most common
  - High T2 signal in normal-appearing PA

TOP DIFFERENTIAL DIAGNOSES

- PA cholesterol granuloma
- PA congenital cholesteatoma
- Apical petrositis

PATHOLOGY

- Pathophysiology
  - May also follow remote otomastoiditis
  - May occur as normal developmental variant
- Sterile PA air cell fluid

CLINICAL ISSUES

- Principal presenting symptom: **None**
- Incidental finding on brain MR for unrelated symptoms
- Bone CT shows typical trapped fluid finding
- Treatment: **None**

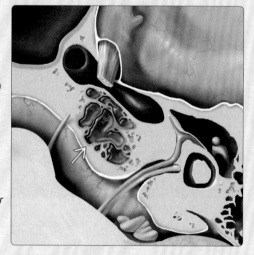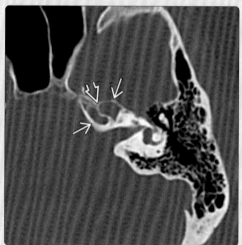

(Left) Axial graphic of the left temporal bone demonstrates fluid-filled petrous apex air cells ➡. Notice that trapped fluid in the petrous apex has no associated expansion or trabecular breakdown. (Right) Axial bone CT demonstrates a typical example of petrous apex trapped fluid as a group of nonexpansile opacified petrous apex air cells ➡ with preservation of the trabecula ➡ and cortical margins. Also notice the absence of fluid opacification of the middle ear and mastoid air cells.

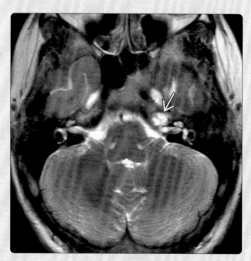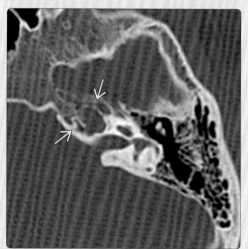

(Left) Axial T2WI MR shows a conspicuous area of high signal in the left petrous apex ➡ on brain MR performed for loss of consciousness. The radiologist queried the diagnosis of cholesterol granuloma in the radiologic report and suggested temporal bone CT for further evaluation. (Right) Axial bone CT in the same patient shows opacified air cells in the left petrous apex ➡ without evidence for expansion or trabecular loss. The diagnosis of trapped fluid was made with no follow-up recommended.

TERMINOLOGY

Abbreviations

- Trapped fluid, petrous apex (TF-PA)

Synonyms

- Petrous apex (PA) effusion

Definitions

- TF-PA: Sterile fluid in PA air cells

IMAGING

General Features

- Best diagnostic clue
  - High T2 signal in PA on MR with bone CT showing opacified PA air cells **without** trabecular loss or expansion

CT Findings

- CECT
  - No enhancement of PA or adjacent meninges
- Bone CT
  - Unilateral opacification of PA air cells
  - No PA **cortical or trabecular erosions**
  - **No expansile component** to lesion
  - Sclerotic air cell margins from presumed remote inflammation (~ 50%) or developmental variant
  - Absence of middle ear-mastoid inflammation

MR Findings

- T1WI
  - Variable PA air cell signal (protein content of fluid)
    - **Intermediate to high signal** most common
    - Heterogeneous T1 signal possible
      - □ Protein content of adjacent air cells varies
- T2WI
  - **High T2 signal**, normal-appearing PA
- T1WI C+
  - No enhancement of PA or adjacent meninges

Imaging Recommendations

- Best imaging tool
  - Bone CT after TF-PA is discovered on brain MR
- Protocol advice
  - 3-year follow-up bone CT in TF-PA with high T1 MR signal
    - Done to exclude rare possibility of transformation into cholesterol granuloma
    - Documentation of TF-PA transforming into cholesterol granuloma has not occurred

DIFFERENTIAL DIAGNOSIS

PA Cholesterol Granuloma

- Bone CT: **Expansile lesion** of PA air cells
  - Loss of PA bony trabeculae
- High T1 and high T2 MR signal

PA Congenital Cholesteatoma

- Bone CT: Smooth, **expansile lesion** of PA air cells
- MR: T1 C+ shows low-signal lesion with rim enhancement
  - No meningeal enhancement present

Apical Petrositis

- Bone CT: Trabecular and cortical erosion
- MR: Low T1 signal, high T2 signal
  - T1 C+ shows thickened, enhancing meninges with spread to adjacent structures
- Clinical setting of otomastoiditis or postmastoidectomy

PATHOLOGY

General Features

- Etiology
  - May occur as normal developmental variant
  - May also follow remote otomastoiditis
  - Sterile PA air cell fluid
- Embryology-anatomy
  - PA pneumatization required for TF-PA to occur

Microscopic Features

- Clear to xanthochromic fluid discovered at surgery

CLINICAL ISSUES

Presentation

- Most common signs/symptoms
  - Principal presenting symptom: **None**

Demographics

- Epidemiology
  - Residual fluid in PA air cells present in 1% of all head MR
  - TF-PA is most common lesion found in PA
  - TF-PA: Cholesterol granuloma of PA ratio is ~ 500:1

Natural History & Prognosis

- TF-PA remains unchanged throughout patient's life
- Rarely fluid becomes superinfected with TF-PA transforming into apical petrositis
- Theoretical possibility of rare high T1 signal lesions will transform into cholesterol granuloma

Treatment

- No therapy or follow-up is warranted for classic TF-PA

DIAGNOSTIC CHECKLIST

Image Interpretation Pearls

- Nonexpansile & nondestructive PA lesion on bone CT with uniform intermediate to high T1 & high T2 signal on MR requires **no** further work-up

SELECTED REFERENCES

1. Chapman PR et al: Petrous apex lesions: pictorial review. AJR Am J Roentgenol. 196(3 Suppl):WS26-37 Quiz S40-3, 2011
2. Lemmerling MM et al: Imaging of inflammatory and infectious diseases in the temporal bone. Neuroimaging Clin N Am. 19(3):321-37, 2009
3. Arriaga MA: Petrous apex effusion: a clinical disorder. Laryngoscope. 116(8):1349-56, 2006
4. Leonetti JP et al: Incidental petrous apex findings on magnetic resonance imaging. Ear Nose Throat J. 80(4):200-2, 205-6, 2001
5. Palacios E et al: 'Don't touch me' lesions of the petrous apex. Ear Nose Throat J. 80(3):140, 2001
6. Moore KR et al: 'Leave me alone' lesions of the petrous apex. AJNR Am J Neuroradiol. 19(4):733-8, 1998
7. Jackler RK et al: Radiographic differential diagnosis of petrous apex lesions. Am J Otol. 13(6):561-74, 1992
8. Arriaga MA et al: Differential diagnosis of primary petrous apex lesions. Am J Otol. 12(6):470-4, 1991

Petrous Apex Mucocele

TERMINOLOGY

- Mucus-containing, expanded petrous apex (PA) air cells(s) lined by secretory epithelium resulting from chronic ostial obstruction

IMAGING

- Requires pneumatized PA
- CT: Fluid-filled, **expanded PA air cell(s)**
- MR: Nonenhancing, T1 low, T2 high signal; DWI with no restricted diffusion

TOP DIFFERENTIAL DIAGNOSES

- PA trapped fluid
- PA cholesterol granuloma
- PA congenital cholesteatoma
- PA cephalocele

PATHOLOGY

- Results from **obstruction to PA air cell drainage**

- Obstruction from middle ear-mastoid infection, trauma, previous surgery
- Secretion of mucus into obstructed air cells
- Air cell expansion from pressure remodeling of wall

CLINICAL ISSUES

- Often incidental and asymptomatic
- Headache or rare cranial neuropathy from compression
- Treatment issues: Controversial if patient asymptomatic
  - Consider follow-up CT to see if mucocele increases in size
  - Surgical obliteration if enlarges

DIAGNOSTIC CHECKLIST

- When bone CT shows **expansile PA lesion**
  - Consider **mucocele** if T1 is low, T2 is high, DWI shows no restricted diffusion
  - Consider **cholesterol granuloma if T1 signal** is high
  - Consider **congenital cholesteatoma if DWI** shows **restricted diffusion**

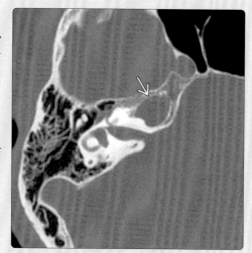

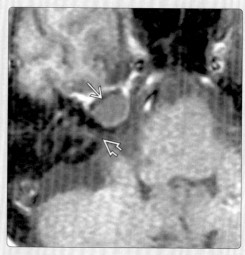

(Left) Axial bone CT shows an expansile right petrous apex (PA) lesion ➡ with loss of the normal air cell trabeculations. The differential diagnosis is congenital cholesteatoma, cholesterol granuloma, and mucocele. (Right) Axial T1WI, same patient, demonstrates an expansile PA mucocele ➡ with minimally higher signal than CSF. Note low signal CSF of internal auditory canal ➡ just posterolateral to the lesion. Low signal on T1WI excludes cholesterol granuloma.

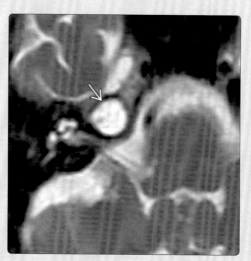

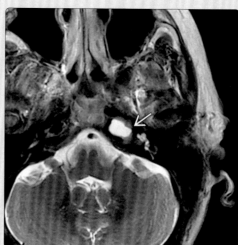

(Left) Axial T2WI MR demonstrates the PA mucocele is uniformly hyperintense ➡. DWI (not shown) had no restricted diffusion. An expansile PA lesion with low T1, high T2, and no restricted diffusion is highly suggestive of mucocele. (Right) Axial T2 MR imaging in different patient demonstrates bright T2 signal in expanded PA mucocele ➡. T1 signal was low (not a cholesterol granuloma) and there was no restricted diffusion (not a congenital cholesteatoma).

TERMINOLOGY

Definitions

- Mucus-containing, expanded petrous apex (PA) air cells(s) lined by secretory epithelium resulting from chronic ostial obstruction
  - From Latin muco = mucous + Greek kele = tumor or mucous tumor

IMAGING

General Features

- Best diagnostic clue
  - Requires pneumatized PA
  - CT: Fluid-filled, **expanded** PA air cell(s)
  - MR: T1 low, T2 high signal, DWI without increased diffusion, nonenhancing

Imaging Recommendations

- Best imaging tool
  - Temporal bone or skull base CT
  - Enhanced MR if atypical CT features
    - MR will differentiate PA mucocele from cholesterol granuloma & congenital cholesteatoma

CT Findings

- Bone CT
  - **Expanded**, opacified PA air cell(s)
  - PA cell walls are **remodeled**
    - May be thinned, focally absent, or normal thickness

MR Findings

- T1WI
  - Usually low signal
    - May be ↑ signal with increased protein content
- T2WI
  - Usually high signal
    - If inspissated mucus exists, ↓ signal
- DWI
  - No significant restricted diffusion
- T1WI C+ FS
  - May have minimal peripheral rim enhancement

DIFFERENTIAL DIAGNOSIS

Petrous Apex Cholesterol Granuloma

- Bone CT: Expansile PA air cells
- MR: ↑ signal intensity on both T1 & T2 images

Petrous Apex Trapped Fluid

- Bone CT: **Nonexpansile** air cells
- MR: T1 variable but usually ↓ signal, ↑ T2 signal

Petrous Apex Congenital Cholesteatoma

- Bone CT: Expansile PA air cells
- MR: T1 low, T2 high signal; DWI **restricted**

Petrous Apex Cephalocele

- Bone CT: Communicates with intracranial subarachnoid space or Meckel cave
  - PA wall interrupted, often at superior or posterior location
- MR: Follows CSF on all sequences

Temporal Bone Internal Carotid Artery Aneurysm

- Expansile bony petrous internal carotid artery canal, complex MR signal

PATHOLOGY

General Features

- Etiology
  - Results from **obstruction of PA air cell drainage**
    - Obstruction from middle ear-mastoid infection, trauma, previous surgery
    - Secretion of mucus into obstructed air cells
    - PA air cell expansion from pressure remodeling of wall

Microscopic Features

- Flattened, pseudostratified, ciliated columnar epithelium = mucus-secreting respiratory epithelium
- Reactive bone formation or bone remodeling of air cell wall may be present

CLINICAL ISSUES

Presentation

- Most common signs/symptoms
  - Often incidental finding on CT or MR in asymptomatic patient
  - May have headache
  - Rare cranial neuropathy from compression

Demographics

- Age
  - Most common in adults
- Epidemiology
  - Extremely rare lesion

Natural History & Prognosis

- Gradual enlargement over time

Treatment

- Controversial, especially in asymptomatic patient
- Consider follow-up CT to see if mucocele increases in size
- Surgical obliteration if enlarges

DIAGNOSTIC CHECKLIST

Consider

- When bone CT shows opacified expansile PA lesion
  - Consider **mucocele** if T1 is low, T2 is high, DWI shows no restricted diffusion
  - Consider **cholesterol granuloma if T1 signal** is **high**
  - Consider **congenital cholesteatoma if DWI** shows **restricted diffusion**

SELECTED REFERENCES

1. Razek AA et al: Lesions of the petrous apex: classification and findings at CT and MR imaging. Radiographics. 32(1):151-73, 2012
2. Chapman PR et al: Petrous apex lesions: pictorial review. AJR Am J Roentgenol. 196(3 Suppl):WS26-37 Quiz S40-3, 2011
3. Le BT et al: Petrous apex mucocele. Otol Neurotol. 29(1):102-3, 2008
4. Muckle RP et al: Petrous apex lesions. Am J Otol. 19(2):219-25, 1998

Petrous Apex Cholesterol Granuloma

TERMINOLOGY

- Petrous apex (PA) cholesterol granuloma (CG): **Expansile** PA lesion resulting from foreign body giant cell reaction to deposition of cholesterol crystals in apical air cells with fibrosis & vascular proliferation
- a.k.a. cholesterol cyst, "chocolate" cyst

IMAGING

- Temporal bone CT findings
  - **Sharply marginated**, **expansile** PA lesion
  - Trabecular breakdown with cortical thinning of PA expected
  - Larger lesions will have areas of **focal bony wall dehiscence**
- Temporal bone MR findings
  - **High T1 internal signal**
  - High T2 internal signal
  - **Peripheral low-signal hemosiderin ring** (T2)
  - No internal enhancement

TOP DIFFERENTIAL DIAGNOSES

- PA asymmetric marrow
- PA trapped fluid
- PA congenital cholesteatoma
- PA internal carotid artery aneurysm
- PA mucocele
- Apical petrositis

PATHOLOGY

- Pneumatized PA air cells **required**
- Obstruction-vacuum pathogenesis (classic hypothesis)
- Exposed bone marrow pathogenesis (recent alternative hypothesis)

CLINICAL ISSUES

- May be incidental, asymptomatic lesion
- Most common symptoms: Headache, dizziness
- If CNV-VIII affected, facial pain/weakness, diplopia, or hearing loss

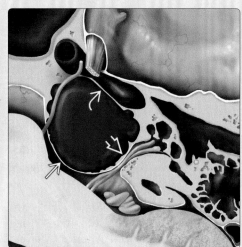
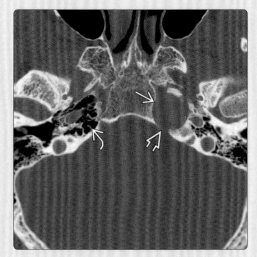

(Left) Axial graphic shows a cholesterol granuloma of the petrous apex (PA-CG). The lesion is expansile with air cell trabecular loss & "eggshell" medial cortex ➡. The lesion compresses the internal auditory canal (IAC) ➡ & thins the posterior wall of the horizontal petrous internal carotid artery (ICA) canal ➡. (Right) Axial bone CT reveals an expansile cholesterol granuloma in the left PA ➡ with marginal bone dehiscence present ➡. The right PA is well pneumatized ➡. PA-CG most commonly occurs in a pneumatized PA.

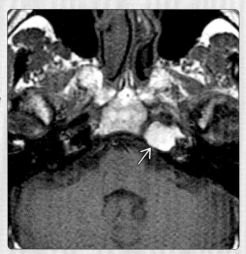
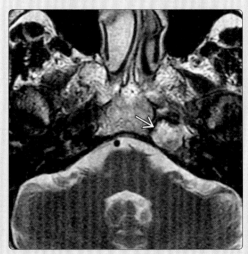

(Left) Axial T1WI unenhanced MR in the same patient shows characteristic high signal ➡ of PA-CG. If no fat saturation is applied to the enhanced sequences through this lesion, it will appear to enhance when in fact it does not. (Right) Axial T2WI MR in the same patient demonstrates the lesion has inhomogeneous high signal ➡. Cholesterol granuloma contains "old blood." The T1 signal is therefore high (methemoglobin) and T2 signal inhomogeneous (methemoglobin and hemosiderin).

Petrous Apex Cholesterol Granuloma

TERMINOLOGY

Abbreviations

- Petrous apex (PA) cholesterol granuloma (PA-CG)

Synonyms

- Cholesterol cyst, "chocolate" cyst

Definitions

- PA-CG: **Expansile** PA lesion resulting from foreign body giant cell reaction to deposition of cholesterol crystals in apical air cells with fibrosis & vascular proliferation

IMAGING

General Features

- Best diagnostic clue
  - **High T1** & T2 signal in expansile PA mass
- Location
  - PA air cells
  - When large, extends into adjacent structures
- Size
  - Ranges from small lesions confined to PA to large lobulated masses
- Morphology
  - Smooth, sharply marginated, lobulated when large

CT Findings

- Bone CT
  - **Sharply marginated**, **expansile** PA lesion
  - Trabecular breakdown with cortical thinning of PA expected
  - Larger lesions will have areas of **focal bony wall dehiscence**
  - When large, erodes regionally
    - Anteriorly to involve horizontal petrous internal carotid artery (ICA) canal
    - Medially into clivus, sphenoid sinus
    - Lateral to inner & middle ear (ME), facial nerve canal
    - Posterior to internal auditory canal & cerebellopontine angle

MR Findings

- T1WI
  - **High internal signal**
    - Secondary to presence of hemorrhage, blood breakdown products, & cholesterol crystals
    - Primary reason is most likely the presence of **paramagnetic intracellular methemoglobin**
- T2WI
  - High internal signal
  - **Peripheral low-signal hemosiderin ring**
- FLAIR
  - High signal does not attenuate (remains high)
- T1WI C+
  - No internal enhancement
  - If no T1 precontrast imaging, may be mistaken for "enhancing" lesion
- MRA
  - Useful in surgical planning, assess for involvement of petrous ICA

- Beware: Lesions with high T1 signal will appear bright on time of flight MRA; mimics aneurysm

Imaging Recommendations

- Best imaging tool
  - Combination bone CT & MR
    - Temporal bone CT evaluates bony erosion & invasion of contiguous structures
    - MR characteristic high T1 signal confirms diagnosis
- Protocol advice
  - MR imaging suggestions
    - Remember to include precontrast T1 sequences
      - □ Contrast is **not helpful** in delineating diagnosis of PA-CG
    - MRA to evaluate for involvement of petrous ICA in large lesions
  - Postoperative imaging for recurrence
    - MR more sensitive than CT for evaluation of recurrence
    - ↑ T1 signal in postoperative PA = recurrence
      - □ Beware of surgical fat packing

DIFFERENTIAL DIAGNOSIS

Petrous Apex Asymmetric Marrow

- CT: Nonexpansile fat density
- T1 MR: High signal; T2 MR: Intermediate to high signal
  - Suppresses on fat-saturated MR

Petrous Apex Trapped Fluid

- CT: Opacified air cells; **nonexpansile**; cortex & trabeculae intact
- T1 MR: Low to high signal; T2 MR: High signal
- T1 C+ MR: No contrast enhancement of lesion or meninges

Petrous Apex Congenital Cholesteatoma

- CT: Smooth, expansile margins
- T1 MR: Low to intermediate signal; T2 MR: Intermediate to high signal
- DWI: Restricted diffusion (high signal)

Petrous Apex Internal Carotid Artery Aneurysm

- CT: Smooth expansion of petrous ICA canal
- MR: Heterogeneous signal with internal flow void
- T1 C+ MR: Heterogeneous internal enhancement

Petrous Apex Mucocele

- CT: Single, expansile air cell area in PA
- MR: Low T1, high T2, nonrestricted DWI

Apical Petrositis

- CT: Permeative, destructive changes of cortex & trabeculae
- T1 MR: Low signal; T2 MR: High signal
- T1 C+ MR: Thick, enhancing rim; meninges thick & enhancing

PATHOLOGY

General Features

- Etiology
  - Obstruction-vacuum pathogenesis (classic hypothesis)
    - Otitis media creates mucosal obstruction of PA air cells causing development of vacuum

- – Vacuum phenomena leads to rupture of blood vessels & hemorrhage in PA air cells
- – Anaerobic degradation of red blood cells forms **cholesterol crystals**, which **incite foreign body giant cell infiltration**
- – Granulation tissue forms secondary to repeated hemorrhage, leading to expansile PA lesion
- o Exposed bone marrow pathogenesis (recent alternative hypothesis)
  - – Begins with mucosal penetration into PA in young adulthood
  - – Marrow exposed, which leads to sustained/repeated microhemorrhage
  - – Marrow provides lipids broken down into cholesterol crystals
- • Embryology-anatomy
  - o Pneumatized PA air cells **required**
  - o PA pneumatization occurs normally in 33% of people

Gross Pathologic & Surgical Features

- • Cystic mass **without** epithelial lining
- • Fibrous capsule filled with blue-brown liquid containing old blood & cholesterol crystals = "chocolate" cyst
- • Fluid described as "crankcase oil"

Microscopic Features

- • RBCs in various stages of degradation
- • Multinucleated giant cells surrounding cholesterol crystals embedded in fibrous connective tissue
- • Hemosiderin-laden macrophages
- • Chronic inflammatory cells & blood vessels

CLINICAL ISSUES

Presentation

- • Most common signs/symptoms
  - o May be incidental, asymptomatic lesion
  - o Headache and dizziness most common presenting symptoms
- • Other signs/symptoms
  - o Facial pain, hearing loss, or diplopia if CNV-VIII involved
- • Clinical profile
  - o Otoscopy normal unless ME involved
    - – Blue-black retrotympanic mass if in ME
  - o Audiometric exam: Sensorineural hearing loss or mixed pattern

Demographics

- • Age
  - o Young to middle-aged adults
- • Epidemiology
  - o Most common surgical lesion in PA
  - o ME-CG more common than PA-CG

Natural History & Prognosis

- • Growth rate highly variable, most stable or slow-growing
  - o Rapid growth or sudden onset new symptoms rare
- • Depends on frequency & severity of microhemorrhages
- • Most take decades to grow
  - o Symptoms show up years after initial bout of chronic otitis media
- • If adequately drained, excellent prognosis

Treatment

- • Asymptomatic patients can be safely followed with imaging
- • Traditional surgical treatment
  - o Drainage & stent placement to reestablish PA aeration via transtemporal approach
  - o Reported recurrence rate as high as 60%
- • Extended middle cranial fossa approach with extradural removal of PA-CG & obliteration of its cavity
  - o Significant decrease in recurrence rates
- • Selective transsphenoidal endoscopic drainage

DIAGNOSTIC CHECKLIST

Consider

- • Consider PA-CG in any expansile PA lesion with **high T1** & T2 signal
- • CT, MR, & MRA in preoperative planning, particularly in large lesions
- • MR best for evaluating postoperative recurrence

Image Interpretation Pearls

- • Characteristic appearance of expansile high T1 & T2 lesion differentiates from other PA lesions
- • CT most useful to evaluate bony destruction & involvement of adjacent otic capsule & carotid canal
- • Make sure to evaluate for internal flow to avoid misdiagnosing petrous ICA aneurysm

Reporting Tips

- • Specifically comment on integrity of adjacent critical structures
  - o Facial nerve canal
  - o Petrous ICA canal
  - o Internal auditory canal
  - o Inner ear otic capsule

SELECTED REFERENCES

1. Sweeney AD et al: The natural history and management of petrous apex cholesterol granulomas. Otol Neurotol. 36(10):1714-9, 2015
2. Juliano AF et al: Imaging review of the temporal bone: part I. Anatomy and inflammatory and neoplastic processes. Radiology. 269(1):17-33, 2013
3. Hoa M et al: Petrous apex cholesterol granuloma: maintenance of drainage pathway, the histopathology of surgical management and histopathologic evidence for the exposed marrow theory. Otol Neurotol. 33(6):1059-65, 2012
4. Sanna M et al: Otoneurological management of petrous apex cholesterol granuloma. Am J Otolaryngol. 30(6):407-14, 2009
5. Castillo MP et al: Petrous apex cholesterol granuloma aeration: does it matter? Otolaryngol Head Neck Surg. 138(4):518-22, 2008
6. Oyama K et al: Petrous apex cholesterol granuloma treated via the endoscopic transsphenoidal approach. Acta Neurochir (Wien). 149(3):299-302; discussion 302, 2007
7. Jackler RK et al: A new theory to explain the genesis of petrous apex cholesterol granuloma. Otol Neurotol. 24(1): 96-106; discussion 106, 2003
8. Brackmann DE et al: Surgical management of petrous apex cholesterol granulomas. Otol Neurotol. 23(4): 529-33, 2002
9. Bonneville F et al: Unusual lesions of the cerebellopontine angle: a segmental approach. Radiographics. 21(2): 419-38, 2001
10. Chaljub G et al: Magnetic resonance imaging of petrous tip lesions. Am J Otolaryngol. 20(5):304-13, 1999
11. Chang P et al: Imaging destructive lesions of the petrous apex. Laryngoscope. 108(4 Pt 1): 599-604, 1998
12. Eisenberg MB et al: Petrous apex cholesterol granulomas: evolution and management. J Neurosurg. 86(5): 822-9, 1997
13. Morrison GA et al: Cholesterol cyst and cholesterol granuloma of the petrous bone. J Laryngol Otol. 106(5): 465-7, 1992
14. Greenberg JJ et al: Cholesterol granuloma of the petrous apex: MR and CT evaluation. AJNR Am J Neuroradiol. 9(6):1205-14, 1988

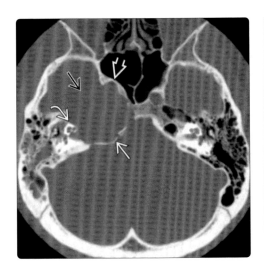

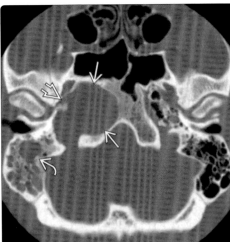

(Left) A large PA-CG is seen on bone CT as an expansile mass ➡ with a fully dehiscent anterolateral margin ➡. The lesion has broken into the IAC and is eroding the otic capsule ➡. The cavernous ICA ➡ is displaced anteriorly. (Right) A more inferior axial bone CT in the same patient again shows the PA-CG ➡ compressing the bony eustachian tube ➡. Fluid in the mastoid ➡ is secondary to eustachian tube obstruction.

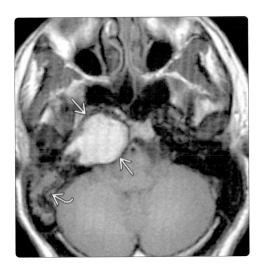

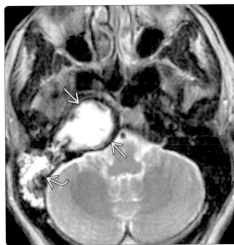

(Left) Axial T1WI MR in the same patient reveals the expansile, high-signal PA-CG ➡. The mastoid fluid ➡ is intermediate signal, most likely due to protein in the fluid. (Right) Axial T2WI MR in the same patient shows a high-signal expansile PA mass ➡. A few low-signal foci are seen within the mass secondary to hemosiderin deposits. In classic cholesterol granuloma, there is high signal on both T1 and T2. Obstructed fluid in the mastoid ➡ is also high signal.

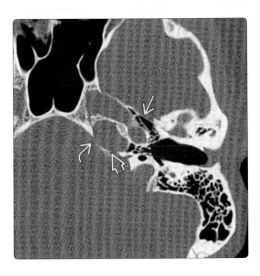

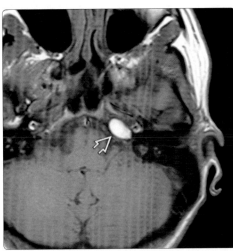

(Left) Axial bone CT in demonstrates a cholesterol granuloma as an ovoid, well-demarcated, expansile lesion ➡ in a pneumatized left PA ➡. The posterior PA wall is thinned or dehiscent ➡. (Right) Axial T1 MR in the same patient demonstrates the intrinsic T1 hyperintensity of the ovoid expansile left lesion ➡ compatible with a cholesterol granuloma.

Apical Petrositis

TERMINOLOGY

- Definition: Extension of middle ear-mastoid (ME-M) infection into pneumatized petrous apex (PA) with resulting suppurative apical petrositis

IMAGING

- Bone CT: **Trabecular breakdown ± cortical erosions** in opacified PA air cells
- Enhanced T1 findings: Early disease
  - **Rim-enhancing fluid-filled PA**
  - Adjacent **meningeal thickening**
- Enhanced T1 findings: Advanced disease
  - Thickened, C+ Meckel cave, & cavernous sinus
  - Skull base osteomyelitis (enhancing clival marrow)
  - Enhancing cranial nerves, especially CNV, CNVI
  - Petrous ± cavernous internal carotid artery spasm
  - Epidural or brain abscess

TOP DIFFERENTIAL DIAGNOSES

- PA trapped fluid
- PA metastasis
- PA cholesterol granuloma
- PA congenital cholesteatoma
- Petrooccipital fissure chondrosarcoma

PATHOLOGY

- Pathophysiology: Suppurative ME-M infection spreads via air cells or venous channels to PA

CLINICAL ISSUES

- Complete clinical syndrome = **Gradenigo syndrome**
  - Acute otomastoiditis, deep facial pain (CNV), & lateral rectus palsy (CNVI)
- Treatment: Antibiotics alone are usually sufficient
  - If severe symptoms at presentation, surgical intervention with mastoidectomy

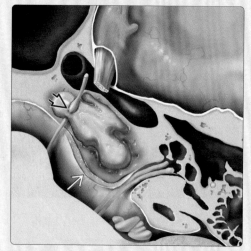
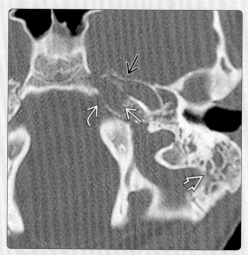

(Left) Axial graphic of the left petrous apex (PA) shows "confluent apical petrositis" with PA abscess formation. Pus surrounds the 6th cranial nerve (CN) ⇒ & associated inflammation thickens adjacent meninges ➡. (Right) Axial temporal bone CT in young patient with petrous apicitis demonstrates left PA opacification & trabecular destruction ➡, as well as cortical disruption ➡. Note accompanying mastoid opacification ⇒. Cortical irregularity of petrous carotid canal raises suspicion of spread into canal ⇒.

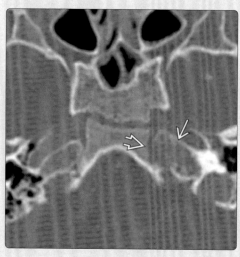
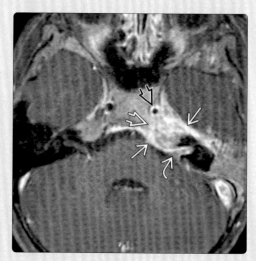

(Left) Axial bone CT in a child with full-blown Gradenigo syndrome (retroorbital pain, lateral rectus palsy, & otorrhea) reveals infection of the left PA cortical bone ➡, with infection crossing the petrooccipital fissure to involve the bone of the lateral clivus ⇒. (Right) Axial T1WI C+ FS MR in the same patient shows infection of the PA with adjacent involvement of the clivus ⇒, dura ➡, & internal auditory canal (IAC) ⇒. Note the spasm of cavernous internal carotid artery (ICA) ⇒ secondary to adjacent infectious process.

Apical Petrositis

TERMINOLOGY

Synonyms

- Confluent apical petrositis, petrous apicitis

Definitions

- Extension of middle ear-mastoid (ME-M) infection into pneumatized petrous apex (PA) with resulting suppurative apical petrositis

IMAGING

General Features

- Best diagnostic clue
  - Bone CT: **Trabecular breakdown ± cortical erosions** in opacified PA air cells
- Location
  - Both mastoid & petrous air cells usually simultaneously involved
    - Early disease confined to PA
    - Advanced disease spreads to meninges, skull base, Meckel cave, & cavernous sinus
- Morphology
  - Irregular phlegmon confined to PA until cortical breakthrough & meningeal involvement occurs

CT Findings

- CECT
  - Peripherally enhancing fluid (pus) in PA
  - Thickened & enhancing meninges
  - Advanced disease
    - Epidural or subdural abscess
    - Cavernous sinus phlegmon ± thrombosis
- Bone CT
  - Affected PA is usually pneumatized
  - Opacification of PA air cells
    - ME-M opacification usually associated
  - Destructive changes of PA = **coalescent apical petrositis**
    - **PA trabeculae lysis & focal cortical destruction**
    - Fistulization to bony labyrinth in advanced disease

MR Findings

- T1WI
  - Asymmetric low to intermediate signal in PA
- T2WI
  - High signal within marrow &/or air cells of petromastoid complex
  - **High signal** focus in **PA** where focal abscess may occur
  - Advanced disease
    - Cavernous or sigmoid sinus thrombosis
    - Epidural or brain abscess
- T1WI C+
  - **Rim-enhancing fluid-filled PA**
  - Avidly enhancing adjacent **meningeal thickening**
  - Advanced disease
    - Skull base osteomyelitis: Enhancing marrow in clivus & PA
    - Thickened, enhancing Meckel cave & cavernous sinus
    - Enhancing cranial nerves (especially CNV, CNVI)
    - Petrous ± cavernous internal carotid artery (ICA) spasm
    - Epidural, subdural, or brain abscess
- MRA
  - Severe lesions can involve adjacent skull base arteries
    - Internal carotid arteritis
    - Petrous carotid pseudoaneurysm is rare
- MRV
  - Advanced disease may cause dural venous sinus thrombophlebitis
  - Cavernous-petrosal or sigmoid sinus-jugular bulb thrombosis possible

Nuclear Medicine Findings

- Bone scan
  - Asymmetric uptake in PA on Tc-99m bone scan or gallium scan
- PET/CT
  - Avid uptake possible; do not mistake for tumor

Imaging Recommendations

- Best imaging tool
  - Initial diagnosis usually with thin-section **temporal bone CT**
  - Axial & coronal skull base T1 C+ MR with fat saturation important in evaluating intracranial complications

DIFFERENTIAL DIAGNOSIS

PA Trapped Fluid

- Clinical: Usually asymptomatic incidental finding
- CT: PA air cell trabeculae maintained; nonexpansile
- MR: Usually intermediate T1 MR signal
  - T1 signal may be high
  - High T2 signal; no meningeal enhancement

PA Metastasis

- Clinical: Lacks acute infectious symptoms
  - Systemic malignancy known
- CT: Permeative-destructive mass of PA
- MR: Infiltrative inhomogeneous enhancing PA mass

PA Cholesterol Granuloma

- CT: Trabecular breakdown & cortical expansion in PA
- MR: T1 & T2 signal high
  - T2 low signal hemosiderin rim possible

PA Congenital Cholesteatoma

- CT: Smooth, expansile PA mass
- MR: Low T1 MR signal; no meningeal enhancement
  - DWI high signal (restricted diffusion)

Petrooccipital Fissure Chondrosarcoma

- Clinical: Lacks acute infectious symptoms
- CT: Destructive mass of petrooccipital fissure often with Ca++ (50%)
- MR: Infiltrative inhomogeneous enhancing petrooccipital fissure mass

PATHOLOGY

General Features

- Etiology
  - Acute or chronic suppurative ME-M infection spreads via air cells or venous channels to PA

- o Infection of PA air cells causes coalescence with breakdown of trabeculae ± cortical loss
- o Thrombophlebitis or direct extension to adjacent structures, including meninges, Meckel cave, & cavernous sinus
- Embryology-anatomy
  - o **Pneumatized PA** present in ~ **33%** of patients
  - o PA pneumatization required for apical petrositis to occur in most cases
  - o In rare nonpneumatized PA, spread via fascial planes, vascular channels, or directly through osteomyelitic bone

Gross Pathologic & Surgical Features

- Soft osteomyelitic bone with pockets of purulent material within confluent PA air cells
- Air cell tracks from mastoid to PA filled with pus & granulation tissue
- Phlegmon thickens & inflames adjacent meninges

Microscopic Features

- Offending organism often not cultured secondary to preoperative broad spectrum antibiotics
  - o Flora of acute infection similar to otomastoiditis
    - Acute pathogens: *Haemophilus influenzae*
  - o Chronic apical petrositis associated with chronic suppurative otomastoiditis
    - Chronic pathogens: *Pseudomonas aeruginosa*, *Proteus* spp.

CLINICAL ISSUES

Presentation

- Most common signs/symptoms
  - o Otorrhea associated with deep facial, ear, or retroorbital pain
- Other signs/symptoms
  - o Symptoms variable; may be subtle, appearing gradually or acutely
    - Acute onset of deep facial pain & otorrhea following acute otomastoiditis
    - Insidious onset of cranial neuropathy (especially CNV) & otorrhea with chronic suppurative ear
    - Other cranial neuropathies (CNVI, VII, & VIII)
    - Fever, hearing loss, & diplopia
- Clinical profile
  - o Complete clinical syndrome = **Gradenigo syndrome**
    - Classic clinical triad associated with apical petrositis
    - Rare presentation
    - Acute otomastoiditis, deep facial pain (CNV), & lateral rectus palsy (CNVI)

Demographics

- Age
  - o Child or adolescent with acute otomastoiditis
  - o Adult with chronic suppurative ear or following mastoidectomy
- Epidemiology
  - o Rare in postantibiotic era

Natural History & Prognosis

- Prognosis excellent given adequate surgical drainage & aggressive antibiotics

- Progresses to obtundation & death if untreated (common in preantibiotic era)

Treatment

- Antibiotics alone usually sufficient
  - o Used when severe symptoms not yet present
  - o Addition of tympanostomy tube may improve symptoms
- If severe symptoms at presentation, surgical intervention with mastoidectomy
  - o Surgery follows air cell tracks to PA
- Multiple surgical options have been described
  - o Simple vs. radical mastoidectomy & middle cranial fossa approach

DIAGNOSTIC CHECKLIST

Consider

- Initial imaging with thin-section nonenhanced temporal bone CT
- MR with multiplanar, fat-saturated, enhanced images are most effective way to evaluate for intracranial complications

Image Interpretation Pearls

- Temporal bone CT to evaluate for subtle trabecular ± cortical erosion & involvement of middle & inner ear
- To differentiate from other PA lesions, look for peripheral PA/meningeal enhancement & correlate with clinical history
- Evaluate vascular structures adjacent to PA for involvement: ICA, dural venous sinuses, cavernous sinus

SELECTED REFERENCES

1. Choi KY et al: Petrositis with bilateral abducens nerve palsies complicated by acute otitis media. Clin Exp Otorhinolaryngol. 7(1):59-62, 2014
2. Kong SK et al: Acute otitis media-induced petrous apicitis presenting as the Gradenigo syndrome: successfully treated by ventilation tube insertion. Am J Otolaryngol. 32(5):445-7, 2011
3. Ibrahim M et al: Diffusion-weighted MRI identifies petrous apex abscess in Gradenigo syndrome. J Neuroophthalmol. 30(1):34-6, 2010
4. Lemmerling MM et al: Imaging of inflammatory and infectious diseases in the temporal bone. Neuroimaging Clin N Am. 19(3):321-37, 2009
5. Connor SE et al: Imaging of the petrous apex: a pictorial review. Br J Radiol. 81(965):427-35, 2008
6. Fournier HD et al: Surgical anatomy of the petrous apex and petroclival region. Adv Tech Stand Neurosurg. 32:91-146, 2007
7. Koral K et al: Petrous apicitis in a child: computed tomography and magnetic resonance imaging findings. Clin Imaging. 30(2):137-9, 2006
8. Lee YH et al: CT, MRI and gallium SPECT in the diagnosis and treatment of petrous apicitis presenting as multiple cranial neuropathies. Br J Radiol. 78(934):948-51, 2005
9. Park SN et al: Cavernous sinus thrombophlebitis secondary to petrous apicitis: a case report. Otolaryngol Head Neck Surg. 128(2): 284-6, 2003
10. Mathew L et al: Gradenigo's syndrome: findings on computed tomography and magnetic resonance imaging. J Postgrad Med. 48(4): 314-6, 2002
11. Price T et al: Abducens nerve palsy as the sole presenting symptom of petrous apicitis. J Laryngol Otol. 116(9): 726-9, 2002
12. Somers TJ et al: Chronic petrous apicitis with pericarotid extension into the neck in a child. Ann Otol Rhinol Laryngol. 110(10): 988-91, 2001
13. Dave AV et al: Clinical and magnetic resonance imaging features of Gradenigo syndrome. Am J Ophthalmol. 124(4): 568-70, 1997
14. Murakami T et al: Gradenigo's syndrome: CT and MRI findings. Pediatr Radiol. 26(9): 684-5, 1996
15. Hardjasudarma M et al: Magnetic resonance imaging features of Gradenigo's syndrome. Am J Otolaryngol. 16(4): 247-50, 1995
16. Frates MC et al: Petrous apicitis: evaluation by bone SPECT and magnetic resonance imaging. Clin Nucl Med. 15(5): 293-4, 1990
17. Chole RA: Petrous apicitis: surgical anatomy. Ann Otol Rhinol Laryngol. 94(3): 251-7, 1985
18. Contrucci RB et al: Petrous apicitis. Ear Nose Throat J. 64(9): 427-31, 1985

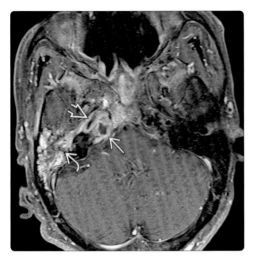

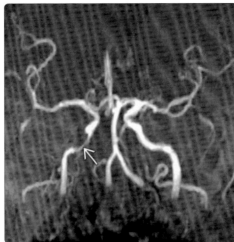

(Left) *Axial T1WI C+ FS MR in a patient with severe headache associated with suppurative otomastoiditis* ⬈ *shows rim-enhancing pus in confluent PA air cells* ⮕*. The horizontal petrous ICA has thick enhancing phlegmon along its margins* ⮕. (Right) *Coronal MRA in the same patient reveals a long segment of horizontal-cavernous ICA narrowing* ⮕ *secondary to carotid canal phlegmon associated with the confluent apical petrositis & suppurative otomastoiditis.*

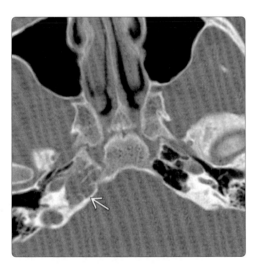

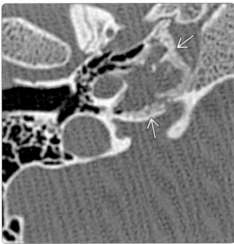

(Left) *Axial bone CT in a patient with trapped fluid in PA on head MR shows opacification of PA air cells* ⮕ *with no trabecular loss. The imaging diagnosis was uncomplicated trapped fluid.* (Right) *Axial bone CT in same patient, now with new severe headache 2 years after initial diagnosis of trapped fluid, shows loss of PA trabeculae & cortical thickening* ⮕. *The presumptive imaging diagnosis of superinfection of trapped fluid was made, & symptoms responded to antibiotics.*

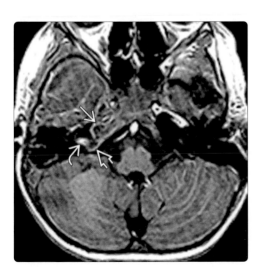

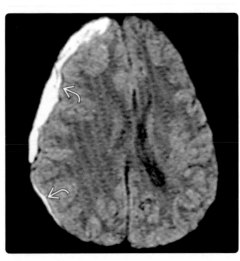

(Left) *Axial T1WI C+ MR in a child presenting with headache & fever demonstrates rim-enhancing pus* ⮕ *in the right PA & area of the porus acusticus* ⮕. *Focal enhancement in the right IAC* ⮕ *indicates that the infection has caused focal meningitis.* (Right) *Axial DWI MR in the same patient at the level of the lateral ventricles shows restricted diffusion caused by frontoparietal subdural empyema* ⮕.

TERMINOLOGY

- Rare congenital or acquired aneurysm of petrous internal carotid artery (ICA)

IMAGING

- Rarity makes errors in imaging diagnosis common
- Complex expansile mass of petrous ICA canal with internal flow on CTA, MRA, or angio
  - Size: Variable; 1-5 cm
  - Shape: Focal ovoid to fusiform
- Bone CT findings
  - **Ovoid** or **fusiform** enlargement of petrous ICA canal
  - **Curvilinear calcifications** in aneurysm wall
- CTA: **Aneurysmal dilation** of petrous ICA is **diagnostic**
- MR findings
  - T1: **Complex signal mass**
  - High signal: Intraluminal clot, slow flow
  - Low signal: Wall calcification, high flow

TOP DIFFERENTIAL DIAGNOSES

- Petrous apex cholesterol granuloma
- Aberrant ICA
- Dehiscent jugular bulb

PATHOLOGY

- **Congenital aneurysm** (true aneurysm)
  - Forms at congenital weakness at origin of obliterated embryologic vessel (caroticotympanic)
- **Acquired aneurysm** (false or pseudoaneurysm)
  - Posttraumatic, postinfectious, postradiation

CLINICAL ISSUES

- Sensorineural hearing loss, Horner syndrome, pulsatile tinnitus, stroke
- Gradual enlargement; progressive risk of rupture
- **Endovascular therapy**: Obliteration or stent placement

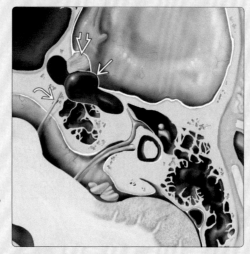
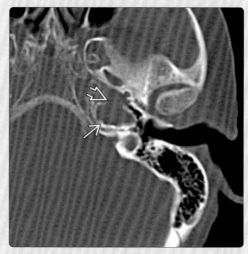

(Left) Axial graphic through the left temporal bone shows focal aneurysmal dilation ⇨ of the horizontal petrous internal carotid artery (ICA). Note the proximity to the trigeminal nerve ⇨ and the abducens nerve ⇨ to the petrous ICA aneurysm. (Right) Axial bone CT in a patient presenting with recurrent transient ischemic attacks shows an expansile ovoid lesion ⇨ in the left petrous apex (PA). Note the anterior wall dehiscence ⇨ where the aneurysm connects to the horizontal petrous ICA.

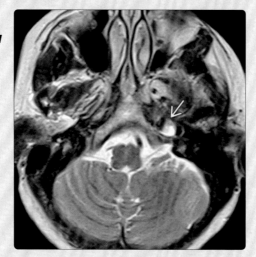
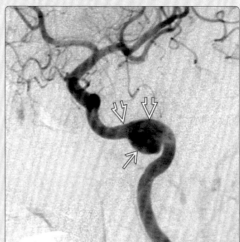

(Left) Axial T2WI MR in the same patient demonstrates a complex signal ovoid mass ⇨ in the PA. Without CTA or MRA, it might be possible to mistake this petrous ICA aneurysm for a cholesterol granuloma. (Right) Oblique left ICA angiogram in the same patient reveals the PA aneurysm ⇨ projecting off the undersurface of the horizontal petrous ICA ⇨.

TERMINOLOGY

Definitions

- Rare congenital or acquired aneurysm of petrous internal carotid artery (ICA)

IMAGING

General Features

- Best diagnostic clue
  - Complex expansile mass of petrous ICA canal with internal flow on CTA, MRA, or angio
- Location
  - **Horizontal petrous ICA** most common location
- Size
  - Variable: 1-5 cm

CT Findings

- Bone CT
  - **Ovoid** or **fusiform** enlargement of petrous ICA canal
  - **Curvilinear calcifications** in aneurysm wall
  - May appear destructive
    - Extensive bone loss/remodeling possible
- CTA
  - **Aneurysmal dilation** of petrous ICA is **diagnostic**

MR Findings

- T1WI
  - **Complex signal mass**
    - High signal: Intraluminal clot, slow flow
    - Low signal: Wall calcification, high flow
- T2WI
  - Complex signal mass with peripheral hemosiderin
  - Internal flow voids produce swirl pattern
- T1WI C+
  - Diffusely enhancing complex mass within petrous apex (PA)
- MRA
  - Enlarged, irregular area along petrous ICA
  - Often smaller than actual aneurysm since only lumen with flowing blood is seen

Angiographic Findings

- Lumen of petrous ICA aneurysm is visible
- May underestimate aneurysm size

Imaging Recommendations

- Best imaging tool
  - CTA is best exam
    - Diagnostic of aneurysm with precise localization along petrous ICA
    - Bone CT from CTA shows skull base anatomy
  - Angiography for treatment not diagnosis

DIFFERENTIAL DIAGNOSIS

Petrous Apex Cholesterol Granuloma

- Bone CT: Expansile PA mass
- MR: Hyperintense T1 & T2 signal in PA

Aberrant Internal Carotid Artery

- Bone CT: Tubular mass crosses middle ear cavity to rejoin horizontal petrous ICA

- CTA or MRA: Artery enters middle ear posterolateral to normal entry point however

Dehiscent Jugular Bulb

- Bone CT: Focal absence of sigmoid plate connects jugular bulb to middle ear "mass"
- CTA or MRV: Coronal reprojection shows "bud" off superolateral jugular bulb

PATHOLOGY

General Features

- Etiology
  - **Congenital aneurysm** (true aneurysm)
    - Forms at congenital weakness at origin of obliterated embryologic vessel (caroticotympanic)
  - **Acquired aneurysm** (false or pseudoaneurysm)
    - Posttraumatic, postinfectious, postradiation
    - Rarely atherosclerotic in this location
- Associated abnormalities
  - Congenital aneurysm associated with multiple additional intracranial aneurysms

CLINICAL ISSUES

Presentation

- Most common signs/symptoms
  - Sensorineural hearing loss
- Other signs/symptoms
  - Horner syndrome
  - Pulsatile tinnitus
  - Transient ischemic attacks; stroke

Demographics

- Age
  - Congenital aneurysm: Childhood or adolescence
  - Acquired pseudoaneurysm: Any age
- Epidemiology
  - Very rare lesion: **Errors in diagnosis common**

Natural History & Prognosis

- Gradual enlargement; progressive risk of rupture

Treatment

- **Endovascular therapy**
  - Allows for pretreatment ICA occlusion trial
  - Balloon trapping or aneurysmal obliteration with ICA preservation
  - **Endovascular stent placement** across aneurysm is viable option
- Surgical therapy no longer preferred 1st approach
  - When necessary, includes ICA sacrifice ± ECA-ICA bypass

SELECTED REFERENCES

1. Shapiro M et al: Toward an endovascular internal carotid artery classification system. AJNR Am J Neuroradiol. 35(2):230-6, 2014
2. Liu JK et al: Aneurysms of the petrous internal carotid artery: anatomy, origins, and treatment. Neurosurg Focus. 17(5):E13, 2004
3. Love MH et al: Case report: giant aneurysm of the intrapetrous carotid artery presenting as a cerebellopontine angle mass. Clin Radiol. 51(8): 587-8, 1996
4. Halbach VV et al: Aneurysms of the petrous portion of the internal carotid artery: results of treatment with endovascular or surgical occlusion. AJNR Am J Neuroradiol. 11(2):253-7, 1990

TERMINOLOGY

- Definition: Normal contrast enhancement (CE) on T1 C+ MR along course of intratemporal facial nerve (CNVII) without abnormal bony changes on bone CT

IMAGING

- T1 C+ MR enhancement along CNVII
  - Mastoid > geniculate ganglion > tympanic segments
- Bone CT: Normal CNVII canal

TOP DIFFERENTIAL DIAGNOSES

- Bell palsy
- Perineural parotid tumor of intratemporal CNVII
- Facial nerve schwannoma within temporal bone

PATHOLOGY

- Lush **circumneutral arteriovenous plexus** surrounds CNVII within temporal bone
  - Labyrinthine segment is **least** well vascularized

CLINICAL ISSUES

- Clinical presentation: **Asymptomatic** by definition
- Treatment options
  - None; do not mistake for Bell palsy
- Imaging recommendations
  - Bone CT used when asymmetric CE is marked to rule out underlying bony changes
  - If CNVII bony canal is enlarged, consider CNVII schwannoma or perineural tumor

DIAGNOSTIC CHECKLIST

- Asymmetric CE along canalicular (internal auditory canal), labyrinthine segment, or extracranial (parotid) CNVII segments **not** normal
- Higher field strength (3T) ± IR-FSPGR MR sequences makes normal CNVII CE more conspicuous
- If fundal vestibular schwannoma present, labyrinthine segment of CNVII may enhance normally
  - Arteriovenous plexus congestion is likely cause

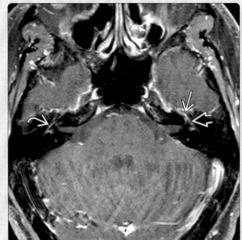
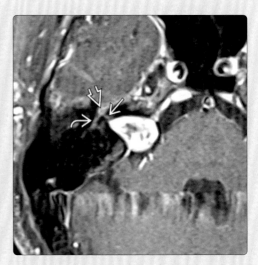

(Left) Axial T1WI C+ FS MR through the internal auditory canals reveals a normal geniculate ganglion ➡ and anterior tympanic segment CNVII ➡ enhancement on the left. On the right, normal anterior tympanic segment enhancement ➡ is visible. (Right) Axial T1WI C+ FS MR in a patient with right vestibular schwannoma demonstrates increased enhancement of the labyrinthine ➡ CNVII, geniculate ganglion ➡, and anterior tympanic segment ➡ CNVII.

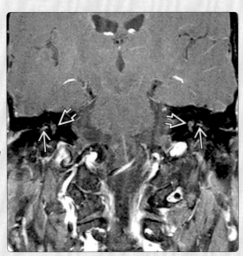
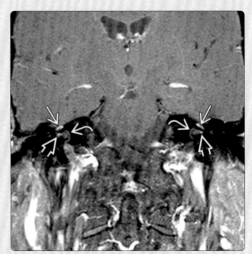

(Left) Coronal T1WI C+ FS MR at the level of the vestibules ➡ reveals normal enhancement of the midtympanic segment of the facial nerves ➡. (Right) Coronal T1WI C+ FS MR in the same patient shows the normal geniculate ganglion enhancement ➡ just superior to the cochleas ➡. Note that the tensor tympani muscles ➡ both also enhance. With 3T imaging, more normal enhancement of structures within the temporal bone is seen.

Intratemporal Facial Nerve Enhancement

TERMINOLOGY

Definitions

- Normal contrast enhancement (CE) on T1 C+ MR along course of intratemporal facial nerve (CNVII) without abnormal bony changes

IMAGING

General Features

- Best diagnostic clue
  - T1 C+ MR CE along CNVII geniculate ganglion, tympanic, & mastoid segments without bony CNVII canal changes
- Location
  - Geniculate ganglion, tympanic, & mastoid segments

CT Findings

- Bone CT
  - Normal bony intratemporal CNVII canal

MR Findings

- T1WI
  - Normal CNVII will produce increased signal on T1 C- compared with surrounding osseous structures
- T1WI C+
  - Normal CE along portions of CNVII (1.5T spin-echo CE T1)
    - Mastoid > geniculate ganglion > tympanic segments
    - Usually symmetrical side-to-side
- MR field strength & sequence summary
  - 1.5T MR: CE of CNVII canalicular & labyrinthine segments not seen
  - 3.0T MR: CE of CNVII may be normally seen in any segment **including** canalicular (15%) & labyrinthine (5%)
    - Mastoid (100%), geniculate (75%), tympanic (40%)
  - Comparing CE spin-echo to CE inversion recovery-prepared fast spoiled gradient-echo (IR-FSPGR)
    - IR-FSPGR: Greater CNVII signal intensity, all segments
    - In absence of facial neuropathy & side-to-side symmetry, this finding should be considered normal

Imaging Recommendations

- Best imaging tool
  - Normal CE seen best on 3-mm axial & coronal spin-echo T1 C+ MR at 3.0T

DIFFERENTIAL DIAGNOSIS

Bell Palsy

- Clinical: Acute onset of unilateral peripheral CNVII paralysis
- T1 C+ MR: Intense enhancement of intratemporal CNVII
  - "Tuft" of internal auditory canal fundal enhancement highly suggestive
- Bone CT: CNVII bony canal normal

Perineural Parotid Tumor of Intratemporal CNVII

- Clinical: Parotid mass + CNVII paralysis
- T1 C+ MR: Focal enhancement spreading from invasive parotid mass into mastoid CNVII segment
- CT: Enlarged bony mastoid segment of CNVII canal
  - Fat in stylomastoid foramen replaced by tissue

Facial Nerve Schwannoma of Intratemporal CNVII

- Clinical: Hearing loss ± peripheral CNVII paresis late
- Most frequently found in geniculate fossa
- T1 C+ MR: Focal enhancing mass along CNVII course
- Bone CT: Enlargement of intratemporal CNVII canal

PATHOLOGY

General Features

- Embryology/anatomy
  - Lush **arteriovenous plexus** surrounds CNVII within temporal bone
    - Labyrinthine segment is least well vascularized

Gross Pathologic & Surgical Features

- Arteriovenous plexus consists of combination of relatively large arteries & veins in capillary plexus

Microscopic Features

- Dense CNVII circumneutral arteriovenous plexus predominantly located in geniculate ganglion, tympanic, & mastoid segments ± greater superficial petrosal nerve

CLINICAL ISSUES

Presentation

- Most common signs/symptoms
  - **Asymptomatic** by definition
- Clinical profile
  - CNVII normal enhancement seen incidentally during T1 C+ MR imaging work-up for unrelated clinical findings

Demographics

- Epidemiology
  - Majority of patients have normal CE along ≥ 1 segment of intratemporal CNVII

Natural History & Prognosis

- Normal CNVII enhancement will not change over time

Treatment

- None; do not mistake for Bell palsy
- Bone CT used when asymmetric CNVII enhancement is marked to rule out underlying bony changes

DIAGNOSTIC CHECKLIST

Consider

- Significant CE along cisternal, labyrinthine segment or extracranial mastoid CNVII segments **not** normal
- Higher field strength (3T) and IR-FSPGR MR sequences make normal CNVII CE more conspicuous
- If fundal vestibular schwannoma present, labyrinthine segment of CNVII may enhance normally
  - Arteriovenous plexus congestion is likely cause

SELECTED REFERENCES

1. Dehkharghani S et al: Redefining normal facial nerve enhancement: healthy subject comparison of typical enhancement patterns–unenhanced and contrast-enhanced spin-echo versus 3D inversion recovery-prepared fast spoiled gradient-echo imaging. AJR Am J Roentgenol. 202(5):1108-13, 2014
2. Hong HS et al: Enhancement pattern of the normal facial nerve at 3.0 T temporal MRI. Br J Radiol. 83(986):118-21, 2010
3. Tabuchi T et al: Vascular permeability to fluorescent substance in human cranial nerves. Ann Otol Rhinol Laryngol. 111(8):736-7, 2002
4. Martin-Duverneuil N et al: Contrast enhancement of the facial nerve on MRI: normal or pathological? Neuroradiology. 39(3):207-12, 1997

Middle Ear Prolapsing Facial Nerve

TERMINOLOGY

- Definition: Midtympanic facial nerve (CNVII) segment protrudes through bony dehiscence
  - **CNVII dehiscence** refers only to segmental absence of bony covering of CNVII
  - **Prolapsing CNVII**: CNVII protrudes through dehiscence in tympanic CNVII canal

IMAGING

- **Incidental finding** on temporal bone CT
  - Tubular soft tissue extends from midtympanic CNVII into oval window niche
- Coronal bone CT
  - Soft tissue mass in oval widow niche
  - Along undersurface of lateral semicircular canal
  - Contiguous with midtympanic segment of CNVII
- Axial bone CT
  - Hammock-like CNVII spanning middle ear cavity under lateral semicircular canal

TOP DIFFERENTIAL DIAGNOSES

- Intratemporal facial nerve schwannoma
- Oval window atresia
- Congenital cholesteatoma in facial nerve canal
- Persistent stapedial artery

CLINICAL ISSUES

- Clinical presentation
  - Most commonly **asymptomatic**
  - Rarely conductive hearing loss present from impingement on stapes
- Treatment option
  - None; do not mistake for small CNVII schwannoma

DIAGNOSTIC CHECKLIST

- Warning to radiologist
  - Prolapsed CNVII in peril during stapedectomy
  - Report and call this finding to ear surgeon

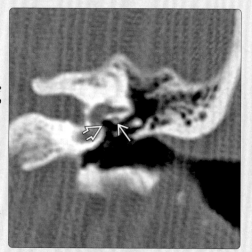
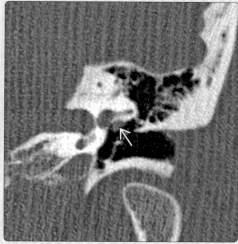

(Left) Coronal left ear temporal bone CT shows the normal tympanic segment of the facial nerve in cross section ⇒ along the undersurface of the lateral semicircular canal. Note subtle bone covering and relationship to the oval window niche ⇒. (Right) Coronal left ear temporal bone CT reveals a focal mass projecting from the midtympanic facial nerve ⇒. Lesion is prolapsed facial nerve, not a facial nerve schwannoma. Facial nerve prolapse can create significant surgical difficulties during stapedectomy.

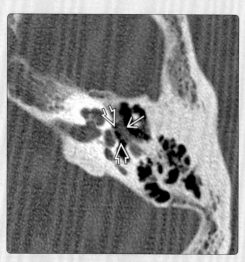
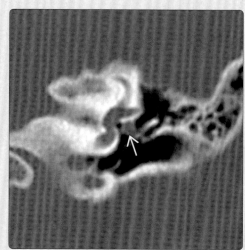

(Left) Axial bone CT in the same patient demonstrates the hammock-like protruding tympanic segment of CNVII ⇒ strung across middle ear cavity. Notice that CNVII touches the crura ⇒ of the stapes, explaining the conductive hearing loss presentation. (Right) Coronal left ear temporal bone CT shows a round soft tissue mass ⇒ projecting off the midtympanic segment of CNVII. Enhanced MR can differentiate protrusion of CNVII (no enhancement) vs. facial nerve schwannoma (enhancement).

TERMINOLOGY

Definitions

- Midtympanic facial nerve (CNVII) segment protrudes through bony dehiscence
- **CNVII dehiscence** refers only to segmental absence of bony covering of CNVII
- **Prolapsing CNVII**: CNVII protrudes through dehiscence

IMAGING

General Features

- Best diagnostic clue
  - Tubular soft tissue extends from midtympanic CNVII into oval window niche (CT)
- Location
  - Undersurface of lateral semicircular canal (LSC) → oval window niche
- Size
  - Variable; may be subtle or appear mass-like (2-3 mm) within oval window niche
- Morphology
  - Smooth, tubular appearance

CT Findings

- Bone CT
  - Coronal: Soft tissue mass in oval widow niche
    - Along undersurface of LSC
    - Contiguous with midtympanic segment of CNVII
  - Axial: Hammock-like CNVII spanning middle ear cavity under LSC
  - Simple dehiscence (uncovered CNVII) poorly seen unless CNVII prolapsed through dehiscence

MR Findings

- No abnormality identified
- T1 C+ is normal excluding facial nerve schwannoma

Imaging Recommendations

- Best imaging tool
  - Axial & coronal thin-section temporal bone CT
    - Best seen on **coronal** at level of oval window
- Protocol advice
  - When protruding CNVII is mass-like, use contrast-enhanced MR to exclude CNVII schwannoma
    - Facial nerve schwannoma enhances

DIFFERENTIAL DIAGNOSIS

Intratemporal Facial Nerve Schwannoma

- Clinical: Hearing loss > > facial nerve palsy
- CT: Tubular enlargement of CNVII canal
  - Geniculate fossa > tympanic > mastoid segments
- MR: Enhancing tubular mass enlarges CNVII canal

Oval Window Atresia

- Clinical: Conductive hearing loss
- ± EAC atresia
- CT: Facial nerve tympanic segment ectopic
  - Tympanic CNVII in oval window niche

Congenital Cholesteatoma in Facial Nerve Canal

- Rare congenital cholesteatoma type

- CT: Enlargement of CNVII bony canal
  - Most commonly geniculate ganglion area

Persistent Stapedial Artery

- Asymptomatic vascular variant
- CT: Absent foramen spinosum
  - Tubular lesion on cochlear promontory
  - Large anterior tympanic segment CNVII

PATHOLOGY

General Features

- Etiology
  - Congenital/developmental
  - Can be acquired from cholesteatoma

CLINICAL ISSUES

Presentation

- Most common signs/symptoms
  - **Asymptomatic** most commonly
  - Rarely conductive hearing loss: Impingement on stapes
- Clinical profile
  - **Incidental finding** on temporal bone CT
    - Critical to communicate its presence to surgeon prior to middle ear exploration
    - Easy to injure facial nerve during stapedectomy if CNVII prolapse is present

Demographics

- Age
  - All ages; congenital lesion
- Epidemiology
  - Simple dehiscence without protrusion ~ 50% of cases
  - Prolapsing facial nerve is rare (~ 1% of cases)

Natural History & Prognosis

- Excellent if left alone

Treatment

- Careful avoidance at time of middle ear surgery

DIAGNOSTIC CHECKLIST

Image Interpretation Pearls

- Prolapse often associated with absence of notch defect along undersurface of LSC
- If notch is seen, consider alternative explanation

Reporting Tips

- Caveat: Prolapsed CNVII in peril during stapedectomy
- Report and call this finding to ear surgeon

SELECTED REFERENCES

1. Yetiser S: The dehiscent facial nerve canal. Int J Otolaryngol. 679708, 2012
2. Yu Z et al: The value of preoperative CT scan of tympanic facial nerve canal in tympanomastoid surgery. Acta Otolaryngol. 131(7):774-8, 2011
3. Di Martino E et al: Fallopian canal dehiscences: a survey of clinical and anatomical findings. Eur Arch Otorhinolaryngol. 262(2):120-6, 2005
4. Park GC et al: Dehiscence of the tympanic segment of the facial nerve. Otolaryngol Head Neck Surg. 123(4):522, 2000
5. Tange RA et al: Dehiscences of the horizontal segment of the facial canal in otosclerosis. ORL J Otorhinolaryngol Relat Spec. 59(5):277-9, 1997
6. Swartz JD: The facial nerve canal: CT analysis of the protruding tympanic segment. Radiology. 153(2):443-7, 1984

Bell Palsy

TERMINOLOGY

- Bell palsy (BP): Herpetic peripheral facial nerve paralysis secondary to herpes simplex virus

IMAGING

- T1WI C+ fat-saturated MR: Fundal tuft and labyrinthine segment CNVII show intense asymmetric enhancement
  - Entire intratemporal CNVII may enhance
- Imaging note: Classic rapid-onset BP requires **no imaging** in initial stages
- If **atypical BP**, search with imaging for underlying lesion

TOP DIFFERENTIAL DIAGNOSES

- Normal enhancement of intratemporal CNVII
- Ramsay Hunt syndrome
- Facial nerve schwannoma
- Facial nerve venous malformation (hemangioma)
- Perineural tumor from parotid

PATHOLOGY

- Etiology-pathogenesis (current hypothesis)
  - Latent **herpes simplex** infection of geniculate ganglion with reactivation and spread of inflammatory process along proximal and distal intratemporal facial nerve fibers

CLINICAL ISSUES

- Classic clinical presentation
  - Acute-onset peripheral CNVII paralysis (36-hr onset)
- Medical therapy for BP
  - Tapering course of prednisone; begin within 3 days of symptoms for best result
  - Antiviral agents no longer used
- Surgical therapy for BP is controversial
  - Profound denervation (> 95%) treated with facial nerve decompression from internal auditory canal fundus to stylomastoid foramen

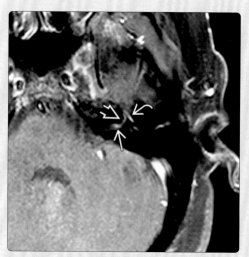
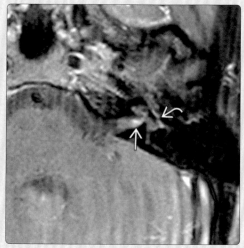

(Left) *Axial T1WI C+ FS MR shows classic findings of Bell palsy with the internal auditory canal (IAC) fundal tuft sign ➡, labyrinthine ➡, and tympanic ➡ facial nerve segment enhancement.* (Right) *Axial T1WI C+ FS MR in the same patient again shows the IAC fundal tuft sign ➡ and tympanic segment of the facial nerve enhancement ➡. Remember that the geniculate ganglion and posterior genu/upper mastoid segment of the facial nerve may normally enhance.*

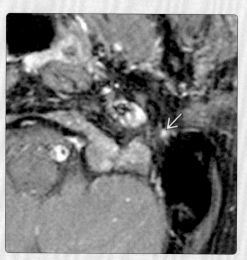
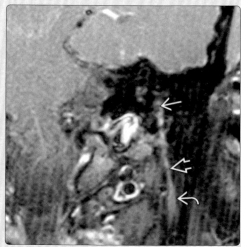

(Left) *Axial T1WI C+ FS MR in the same patient through the stylomastoid foramen demonstrates an enhancing, slightly enlarged facial nerve ➡. Swelling of the facial nerve is possible outside the bony facial nerve canal within the temporal bone.* (Right) *Coronal T1WI C+ FS MR in the same patient reveals avid enhancement in the mastoid ➡, stylomastoid ➡, and extracranial facial nerve ➡ in this patient with typical Bell palsy.*

TERMINOLOGY

Abbreviations
- Bell palsy (BP)

Synonyms
- Herpetic facial paralysis

Definitions
- BP (original definition): Idiopathic acute onset of lower motor neuron facial paralysis
- BP (modern definition): Herpetic facial paralysis secondary to herpes simplex virus

Other Facts
- Named after Sir Charles Bell (1774-1842), who 1st described BP syndrome

IMAGING

General Features
- Best diagnostic clue
  - Fundal **tuft** and labyrinthine segment CNVII intense asymmetric enhancement on T1WI C+ MR
- Location
  - Fundal and labyrinthine segment CNVII most affected
  - Often involves entire intratemporal CNVII
    - Intraparotid segment less commonly affected
- Size
  - CNVII swells within facial nerve canal

CT Findings
- Bone CT
  - Normal facial nerve canal
    - If enlargement present, **not** BP

MR Findings
- T2WI
  - Brain normal; no high-signal lesions
  - High-resolution thin-section T2 or T2*GRE may show internal auditory canal (IAC) CNVII enlargement
- T1WI C+
  - Uniform, contiguous CNVII enhancement
    - CNVII: Normal in size within bony canal
    - CNVII: Conspicuous high signal appears slightly enlarged
    - Enhancement pattern is linear, not nodular
  - Enhancement usually present from distal IAC through labyrinthine segment, geniculate ganglion, and anterior tympanic segment
    - **Tuft** of enhancement in IAC fundus (premeatal segment) along with C+ of labyrinthine segment of CNVII are distinctive MR findings
    - Mastoid CNVII enhances less frequently
    - Enhancement of intraparotid CNVII infrequent

Imaging Recommendations
- Best imaging tool
  - Thin-section fat-saturated T1WI C+ MR focused to IAC and temporal bone
  - Temporal bone CT: Only used if MR creates suspicion of enlarged CNVII canal or focal lesion
- Classic rapid-onset BP requires **no imaging** in initial stages

- 90% of BP patients recover spontaneously in < 2 months
- If decompressive surgery is anticipated, MR imaging is warranted to ensure that no other lesion is causing CNVII paralysis
- If **atypical BP**, search for underlying lesion
  - Atypical BP
    - Slowly progressive CNVII palsy
    - Facial hyperfunction (spasm) preceding BP
    - Recurrent CNVII palsies
    - BP with any other associated cranial neuropathies
    - CNVII paralysis persisting or deepening > 2 months

DIFFERENTIAL DIAGNOSIS

Normal Enhancement of Intratemporal CNVII
- Clinical: No facial nerve symptoms
- T1WI C+ MR: Mild, linear, discontinuous enhancement of anterior and posterior genus of intratemporal CNVII
  - IAC and labyrinthine CNVII segments normal

Ramsay Hunt Syndrome
- Clinical: Peripheral CNVII paralysis with CNVIII associated symptoms
  - External auditory canal (EAC) hemorrhagic vesicular rash
  - Varicella-zoster virus infection = cause
- T1WI C+ MR: Linear, continuous enhancement of fundal IAC and intratemporal CNVII
  - Enhancement of inner ear structures and vestibulocochlear nerve variable

Facial Nerve Schwannoma
- Clinical: Hearing loss more common than CNVII palsy
- T1WI C+ MR: Well-circumscribed, tubular, C+ mass within enlarged CNVII canal most commonly centered on geniculate ganglion

Facial Nerve Venous Malformation ("Hemangioma")
- Clinical: CNVII paralysis occurs when lesion is small
- Bone CT: May show intratumoral bone spicules
- T1WI C+ MR: Poorly circumscribed, enhancing mass commonly found in geniculate fossa

Perineural Tumor From Parotid
- Clinical: Parotid malignancy usually palpable
- Imaging: Invasive parotid mass is present
  - Tissue-filled stylomastoid foramen
  - CNVII is enlarged from distal to proximal with associated mastoid air cell invasion

PATHOLOGY

General Features
- Etiology
  - Etiology-pathogenesis (current hypothesis)
    - Latent herpes simplex infection of geniculate ganglion with reactivation and spread of inflammatory process along proximal and distal CNVII fibers
    - Pathophysiology: Formation of intraneural edema in neuronal sheaths caused by breakdown of blood-nerve barrier and by venous congestion in epineural and perineural venous plexus
- Intratemporal CNVII normal anatomy
  - CNVII normal C+ at its anterior and posterior genus

Brackman Facial Nerve Grading System

Grade	Description of Facial Paralysis	Measurement**	Function %	Estimated Function %
I	Normal	8/8	100	100
II	Slight	7/8	76-99	80
III	Moderate	5/8-6/8	51-75	60
IV	Moderately severe	3/8-4/8	26-50	40
V	Severe	1/8-2/8	1-25	20
VI	Total	0/8	0	0

*** Facial nerve injury is measured by the superior movement of the midportion of the upper eyebrow and the lateral movement of the oral commissure. For each 0.25 cm of upward motion for both eyebrow and oral commissure, a scale of 1 is assigned up to 1 cm. The points are then added together. A total of 8 points can be obtained if both the eyebrow and the oral commissure both move 1 cm. Adapted from House JW et al: Facial nerve grading system. Otolaryngol Head Neck Surg. 93(2):146-7, 1985.*

- o C+ from robust circumneural arteriovenous plexus
- o Familiarity with normal patterns of intratemporal CNVII C+ allows radiologist to identify abnormal C+ seen with BP

Gross Pathologic & Surgical Features

- CNVII edema peaks at 3 weeks after symptom onset

Microscopic Features

- Herpes simplex DNA recovered from CNVII

CLINICAL ISSUES

Presentation

- Most common signs/symptoms
  - o Acute-onset peripheral CNVII paralysis (36-hour onset)
- Clinical profile
  - o Healthy adult with acute unilateral CNVII paralysis
    - — More common in diabetic patients
- Other signs/symptoms
  - o Viral prodrome often reported before BP onset
  - o 70%: Taste alterations days before CNVII paralysis
  - o 50%: Pain around ipsilateral ear (not severe)

Demographics

- Age
  - o All ages affected; incidence peaks in 5th decade
- Epidemiology
  - o Herpetic facial paralysis thought to be responsible for ~ 75% of peripheral CNVII paralysis cases
  - o Annual BP incidence: 10-50/100,000 persons

Natural History & Prognosis

- 80% of BP patients spontaneously recover all of CNVII function without therapy in 1st 2 months
  - o 15% partially recover; 5% show no recovery

Treatment

- Test for diabetes and Lyme disease
- Medical therapy for BP
  - o Tapering course of prednisone; begin within 3 days of symptoms for best result
  - o Acyclovir or valacyclovir (antivirals) no longer used
- Surgical therapy for BP is controversial

- o Profound denervation (> 95%) treated with CNVII decompression, fundus to stylomastoid foramen
- o Decompression performed within 2 weeks of onset of total paralysis for maximal effect
- Intensity, pattern ± location of enhancement on T1WI C+ MR **not** helpful in predicting individual patient outcome
- Older patients: Lower rate of complete CNVII recovery

DIAGNOSTIC CHECKLIST

Consider

- **No** imaging necessary for typical BP
  - o MR imaging reserved for **atypical** BP
- Abnormal CNVII C+ on MR may persist well beyond clinical improvement or full recovery
- Not all intratemporal facial nerves enhance in BP
  - o < 10 days following onset of BP, CNVII often normal

Image Interpretation Pearls

- Tuft of IAC fundal C+ associated with labyrinthine segment CNVII C+ without associated focal lesion is highly suggestive of BP

Reporting Tips

- Remember to comment on parotid as normal
- Also note absence of focal CNVII lesions

SELECTED REFERENCES

1. Hohman MH et al: Etiology, diagnosis, and management of facial palsy: 2000 patients at a facial nerve center. Laryngoscope. 124(7):E283-93, 2014
2. Baugh RF et al: Clinical practice guideline: Bell's palsy. Otolaryngol Head Neck Surg. 149(3 Suppl):S1-27, 2013
3. Kim IS et al: Correlation between MRI and operative findings in Bell's palsy and Ramsay Hunt syndrome. Yonsei Med J. 48(6):963-8, 2007
4. Kress B et al: Bell palsy: quantitative analysis of MR imaging data as a method of predicting outcome. Radiology. 230(2):504-9, 2004
5. Unlu Z et al: Serologic examinations of hepatitis, cytomegalovirus, and rubella in patients with Bell's palsy. Am J Phys Med Rehabil. 82(1):28-32, 2003
6. Adour KK: Medical management of idiopathic (Bell's) palsy. Otolaryngol Clin North Am. 24(3):663-73, 1991
7. Schwaber MK et al: Gadolinium-enhanced magnetic resonance imaging in Bell's palsy. Laryngoscope. 100(12):1264-9, 1990
8. Tien R et al: Contrast-enhanced MR imaging of the facial nerve in 11 patients with Bell's palsy. AJNR Am J Neuroradiol. 11(4):735-41, 1990
9. Daniels DL et al: MR imaging of facial nerve enhancement in Bell palsy or after temporal bone surgery. Radiology. 171(3):807-9, 1989
10. Matsumoto Y et al: Facial nerve biopsy for etiologic clarification of Bell's palsy. Ann Otol Rhinol Laryngol Suppl. 137:22-7, 1988

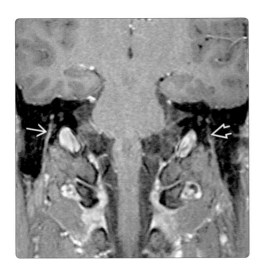

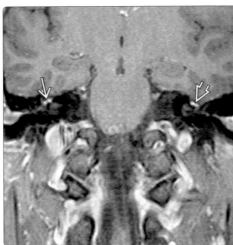

(Left) *Coronal T1WI C+ FS MR in a patient with right Bell palsy shows asymmetric right mastoid CN avid enhancement ➡ compared to minimal enhancement on the left ➡.* (Right) *Coronal T1WI C+ FS MR in the same patient shows similar enhancement of the right ➡ compared to the left ➡ geniculate ganglion. This can be explained by the fact that the geniculate ganglion, along with the posterior genu/upper mastoid facial nerve, may normally enhance.*

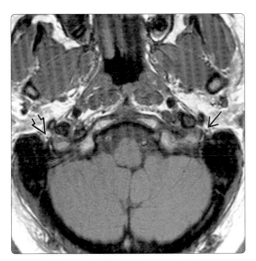

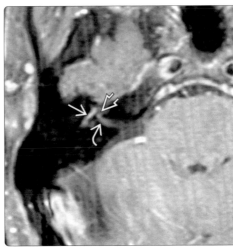

(Left) *Axial T1WI MR in a patient with left Bell palsy reveals that the left facial nerve in the stylomastoid foramen ➡ is larger than the right ➡. The injured left facial nerve swells when it is not confined by the intratemporal bony facial nerve canal.* (Right) *Axial T1WI C+ FS MR in a patient with right-sided Bell palsy demonstrates typical findings of enhancing tympanic ➡ and labyrinthine ➡ segments of the facial nerve. Notice the more subtle IAC fundus tuft sign ➡.*

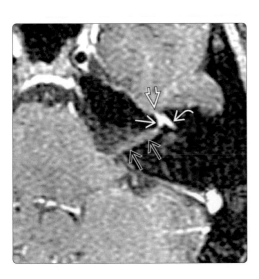

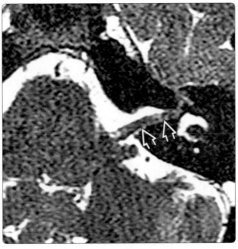

(Left) *Axial T1WI C+ FS MR in a patient with profound, unremitting Bell palsy shows intense enhancement of the labyrinthine ➡, geniculate ganglion ➡, and anterior tympanic portions ➡ of the facial nerve. The IAC tuft spreads along the IAC facial nerve as more subtle enhancement ➡, reaching the porus acusticus.* (Right) *Axial thin-section (1 mm) T2WI FS MR in the same patient reveals a swollen intracanalicular facial nerve ➡ through the IAC.*

Temporal Bone Facial Nerve Venous Malformation (Hemangioma)

TERMINOLOGY

- Facial nerve venous malformation (FNVM)
- Older terms: Facial nerve hemangioma/ossifying hemangioma
- Definition: Benign developmental lesion near intratemporal CNVII in geniculate fossa area

IMAGING

- Bone CT
  - **Honeycomb high-density matrix** lesion (50%)
  - Most commonly located in geniculate fossa
- T1 C+ FS MR
  - Enhancing geniculate ganglion area lesion
  - Usually with irregular margins

TOP DIFFERENTIAL DIAGNOSES

- Normal intratemporal facial nerve enhancement
- Intratemporal facial nerve schwannoma
- Bell palsy

- Perineural parotid malignancy on intratemporal CNVII
- Congenital cholesteatoma within intratemporal CNVII canal

PATHOLOGY

- **Immunohistochemical markers** critical to correct venous malformation (hemangioma) diagnosis
  - Endothelial lining of vascular channels stain negatively for hemangioma-associated markers (**GLUT1 and LeY**)
  - **Podoplanin** staining utilizing D2-40 antibody **negativity** excludes lymphatic malformation

CLINICAL ISSUES

- Intratemporal FNVM produces **peripheral CNVII paralysis** early in its natural history
  - Caveat: May be described as "**atypical Bell palsy**"
- Treatment: Perform surgery as soon as possible
  - Final CNVII function depends on duration of preoperative CNVII deficit
  - Smaller lesion are extraneural, larger lesion invade CNVII

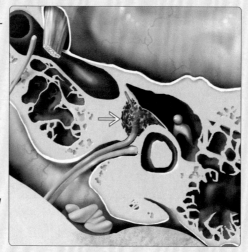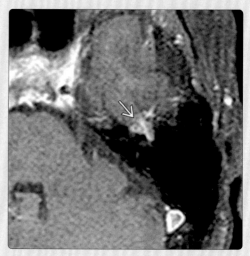

(Left) *Axial graphic illustrates a classic example of a medium-sized facial nerve venous malformation (FNVM) centered in the geniculate fossa ⇥ of the temporal bone. Notice the honeycomb bone within the lesion matrix.* (Right) *Axial T1 C+ MR with fat saturation in a patient with a left atypical Bell palsy reveals a classic left geniculate fossa enhancing FNVM ⇥. Punctate areas of high density on bone CT (not shown) confirmed this imaging impression.*

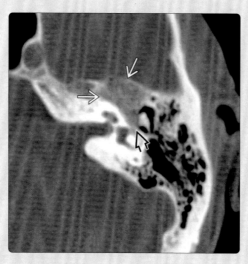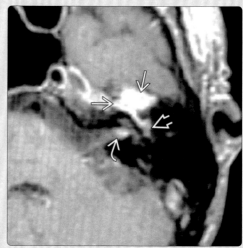

(Left) *Axial bone CT demonstrates the honeycombing appearance of FNVM centered in the geniculate fossa ⇥. Note extension of the lesion along the proximal tympanic CNVII segment ⇥.* (Right) *Axial T1 C+ MR in the same patient shows a poorly marginated, avidly enhancing lesion in the geniculate fossa ⇥. Note extension along the tympanic segment of CNVII ⇥ and into the fundus of the internal auditory canal (IAC) ⇥. IAC extension occurred via the labyrinthine segment of CNVII (not shown).*

TERMINOLOGY

Abbreviations

- Facial nerve venous malformation (FNVM)

Synonyms

- Facial nerve hemangioma/ossifying hemangioma
  - Historic terms for FNVM

Definitions

- FNVM: Benign developmental lesion near intratemporal facial nerve in geniculate fossa area

IMAGING

General Features

- Best diagnostic clue
  - **Honeycomb high-density matrix** lesion in geniculate fossa area (bone CT)
  - Enhancing geniculate ganglion area lesion with irregular margins on T1 C+ MR
- Location
  - **Geniculate fossa area** > > internal auditory canal (IAC)
- Size
  - Range: 2 mm to 2 cm
  - Small at presentation, **often < 1 cm**
- Morphology
  - Irregular, invasive-appearing margins typical

CT Findings

- Bone CT
  - Poorly marginated lesion of geniculate fossa
  - Larger lesions affect adjacent temporal bone
    - Anteromedial to geniculate fossa
    - Labyrinthine segment CNVII → IAC
      - □ Dumbbell lesion appearance
  - Amorphous **honeycomb bone changes** are distinctive
    - Present in 50% of all lesions
    - Seen in 100% of larger lesions
  - Punctate high-density foci also possible

MR Findings

- T1WI
  - Mixed signal lesion with foci of low signal within lesion matrix (ossific matrix)
- T2WI
  - High-signal lesion with foci of low signal within lesion matrix
- FLAIR
  - Mixed intermediate & high-signal lesion
- T1WI C+
  - **Avid lesion enhancement** is rule
  - Perineural spread from geniculate ganglion
    - Posterolateral along tympanic segment CNVII
    - Posteromedial along labyrinthine segment CNVII → IAC
      - □ **Dumbbell** appearance possible
  - Fundal IAC FNVM, exactly mimics vestibular schwannoma
    - Ovoid, well-demarcated, enhancing IAC mass
    - Low-signal foci may distinguish FNVM from vestibular schwannoma

Imaging Recommendations

- Best imaging tool
  - Imaging indicates CNVII (**facial nerve paresis**) or CNVIII (hearing loss) dysfunction
  - 1st exam: Thin-section **T1 C+ MR** focused to CPA-IAC-inner ear
  - If MR negative or shows equivocal small area of enhancement along intratemporal CNVII, recommend **temporal bone CT**
    - Bone CT may show small FNVM in geniculate fossa
    - Inspect intratemporal CNVII canal carefully for 1-2 mm FNVM

DIFFERENTIAL DIAGNOSIS

Normal Intratemporal Facial Nerve Enhancement

- Clinical: Asymptomatic
- Imaging: T1 C+ MR shows normal enhancement of geniculate ganglion, anterior tympanic CNVII, &/or mastoid segment CNVII
- Comment: Sometimes mistaken for facial nerve pathology

Intratemporal Facial Nerve Schwannoma

- Clinical: Hearing loss ± gradual onset of CNVII paralysis
- Imaging: T1 C+ MR reveals tubular enhancing mass, smoothly enlarging CNVII canal (bone CT)
- Comment: Most commonly centered in geniculate ganglion like FNVM

Bell Palsy

- Clinical: Acute onset of peripheral CNVII paralysis
- Imaging: T1 C+ MR shows prominent enhancement of all or most of intratemporal CNVII
  - IAC enhancing tuft often present
- Comment: No focal mass; bone CT normal

Perineural Parotid Malignancy on Intratemporal CNVII

- Clinical: Parotid malignancy in history, palpable or subclinical
- Imaging: T1 C+ MR shows invasive parotid mass
  - Stylomastoid foramen is tissue filled
  - CNVII enlarged & enhancing from distal to proximal
  - CNVII may be involved to CPA-IAC
  - Mastoid air cell invasion also possible
- Comment: Continuous linear nature different from focal FNVM

Congenital Cholesteatoma Within Intratemporal CNVII Canal

- Clinical: Avascular mass behind intact tympanic membrane
- Imaging: T1 C+ MR shows nonenhancing middle ear mass tracking along CNVII canal
- Comment: Involvement of facial nerve canal rare with this lesion

PATHOLOGY

General Features

- Etiology
  - Benign congenital venous malformation arising out of sites of anastomoses between feeding arteries in temporal bone

Staging, Grading, & Classification

- Classification for vascular lesions based on clinical, histopathological, and cytological features was introduced by Mulliken & Glowacki in 1982
  - **Malformation** term used for errors of vascular morphogenesis that develop in utero and persist postnatally
  - **Hemangioma** term reserved for benign vascular tumors that arise by cellular hyperplasia

Gross Pathologic & Surgical Features

- Richly vascular lesion without large feeding vessels

Microscopic Features

- H&E: Nonencapsulated venous malformation composed of dilated vascular channels of varying sizes
  - Widely ectatic vascular channels rimmed by thin smooth muscle coats without evident elastic laminae
  - Flattened & mitotically quiescent endothelial cells
- Venous malformations = low-flow lesions
- Ossifying type: Lesion has spicules of lamellar bone
  - When seen, called **ossifying venous malformation**
- **Immunohistochemical markers** critical to correct venous malformation diagnosis
  - Endothelial lining of vascular channels stain negatively for hemangioma-associated markers (**GLUT1 and LeY antigen**)
  - Venous vs. lymphatic malformation endothelial differentiation
    - **Podoplanin** staining utilizing D2-40 antibody **negative** for endothelial cells confirms lack of lymphatic differentiation

CLINICAL ISSUES

Presentation

- Most common signs/symptoms
  - Intratemporal FNVM produces **peripheral CNVII paralysis** early in its natural history
    - Occurs early because of intimate relationship between CNVII & FNVM
    - Onset of CNVII paralysis usually acute: May be slowly progressive or intermittent
    - Caveat: May be described as "**atypical Bell palsy**"
  - IAC facial nerve venous malformation
    - Sensorineural hearing loss may be more prominent symptom
    - IAC lesion with CNVII symptoms, consider FNVM
- Other signs/symptoms
  - Hemifacial spasm may progress to CNVII paralysis

Demographics

- Age
  - Wide range but usually adults
- Epidemiology
  - Rare lesion
    - 0.7% of all temporal bone lesions
  - Slightly less common than CNVII schwannoma

Natural History & Prognosis

- FNVM = slowly growing lesion
  - Proportional growth is norm
  - Disproportionate growth can occur secondary to infection, trauma, hormonal influences, or progressive hemodynamic forces
- Prognosis related to size at diagnosis, severity and duration of preoperative CNVII paralysis
- After surgery, full CNVII function rarely regained

Treatment

- Surgery done as soon as possible
  - Final facial nerve function depends on duration of preoperative CNVII deficit
- Surgical alternatives
  - Middle cranial fossa (MCF) approach for lesions confined to geniculate fossa
  - MCF-transmastoid approach for lesion of geniculate fossa and tympanic segment CNVII
- Small FNVM are extraneural
  - Resection with preservation of CNVII function = goal
    - Even with small lesions, rarely achieved
- Larger FNVM invades facial nerve
  - Segmental facial nerve resection completed
  - Followed by primary or cable graft repair of CNVII
  - When necessary, yields poorer outcome

DIAGNOSTIC CHECKLIST

Consider

- FNVM presents with CNVII dysfunction when small
  - Since early removal is best chance at CNVII preservation, radiologist must make diagnosis of subtle lesions
  - Caveat: **Small FNVM** may be **subtle** on T1 C+ **MR**
    - Use CT liberally in negative or equivocal MR

Image Interpretation Pearls

- Poorly circumscribed, C+ lesion in geniculate fossa in setting of CNVII paralysis is most likely FNVM

SELECTED REFERENCES

1. Yue Y et al: Retrospective case series of the imaging findings of facial nerve hemangioma. Eur Arch Otorhinolaryngol. 272(9):2497-503, 2015
2. Ma X et al: Facial nerve preservation in geniculate ganglion hemangiomas. Acta Otolaryngol. 134(9):974-6, 2014
3. Benoit MM et al: Facial nerve hemangiomas: vascular tumors or malformations? Otolaryngol Head Neck Surg. 142(1):108-14, 2010
4. Greene AK et al: Intraosseous "hemangiomas" are malformations and not tumors. Plast Reconstr Surg. 119(6):1949-50; author reply 1950, 2007
5. Isaacson B et al: Hemangiomas of the geniculate ganglion. Otol Neurotol. 26(4):796-802, 2005
6. Bernardeschi D et al: Vascular malformation (so-called hemangioma) of Scarpa's ganglion. Acta Otolaryngol. 124(9):1099-102, 2004
7. Achilli V et al: Facial nerve hemangioma. Otol Neurotol. 23(6):1003-4, 2002
8. Friedman O et al: Temporal bone hemangiomas involving the facial nerve. Otol Neurotol. 23(5):760-6, 2002
9. Salib RJ et al: The crucial role of imaging in detection of facial nerve haemangiomas. J Laryngol Otol. 115(6):510-3, 2001
10. Dufour JJ et al: Intratemporal vascular malformations (angiomas): particular clinical features. J Otolaryngol. 23(4):250-3, 1994
11. Martin N et al: Haemangioma of the petrous bone: MRI. Neuroradiology. 34(5):420-2, 1992
12. Shelton C et al: Intratemporal facial nerve hemangiomas. Otolaryngol Head Neck Surg. 104(1):116-21, 1991
13. Lo WW et al: Intratemporal vascular tumors: detection with CT and MR imaging. Radiology. 171(2):445-8, 1989
14. Curtin HD et al: "Ossifying" hemangiomas of the temporal bone: evaluation with CT. Radiology. 164(3):831-5, 1987
15. Mulliken JB et al: Hemangiomas and vascular malformations in infants and children: a classification based on endothelial characteristics. Plast Reconstr Surg. 69(3):412-22, 1982

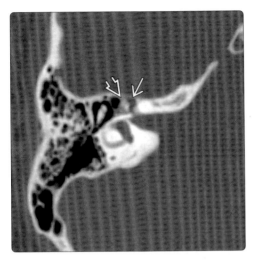

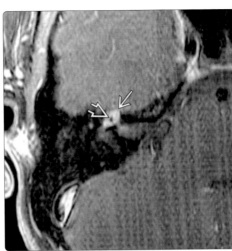

(Left) Axial bone CT in a patient with right facial nerve palsy shows a small FNVM in the geniculate fossa ➡. Notice the punctate ossific foci ➡ within the lesion. This finding allows differentiation of FNVM from facial nerve schwannoma, which also occurs most frequently in the geniculate fossa. (Right) Axial T1 C+ MR with fat saturation in the same patient reveals FNVM ➡ enhancing in the geniculate ganglion. The punctate ossific area is seen as an intralesional low-signal focus ➡.

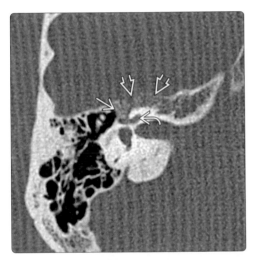

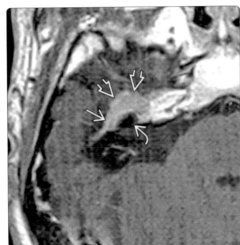

(Left) Axial bone CT through the right temporal bone demonstrates a medium-sized FNVM in the geniculate fossa ➡ with extension along the anteromedial surface of the temporal bone ➡. The crescentic shape of this lesion arching around the cochlea ➡ medially on the anterior temporal bone surface is typical of FNVM. (Right) Axial T1 C+ MR in the same patient shows diffuse FNVM enhancement in the geniculate fossa ➡, arching around the cochlea ➡ along the anteromedial temporal bone surface ➡.

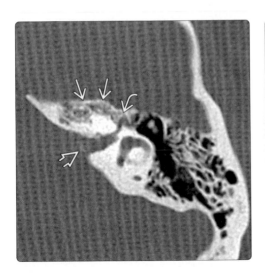

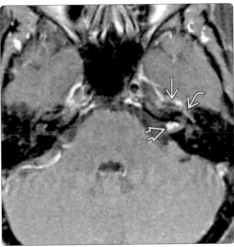

(Left) Axial bone CT shows an FNVM within the anteromedial temporal bone ➡ and in the bone surrounding the geniculate fossa ➡. Subtle foci of increased density ➡ are also seen in the IAC. (Right) Axial T1 C+ FS MR in the same patient shows the venous malformation enhancing in anteromedial temporal bone ➡, around geniculate ganglion ➡, and in IAC ➡. IAC lobe of FNVM occurs due to extension along the labyrinthine segment of CNVII (not shown).

KEY FACTS

TERMINOLOGY

- Facial nerve schwannoma (FNS): Rare benign tumor of Schwann cells that invests intratemporal facial nerve (CNVII)

IMAGING

- Temporal bone CT: Tubular mass spanning multiple intratemporal CNVII segments with smooth enlargement of bony CNVII canal
  - > 90% of FNS span ≥ 3 intratemporal CNVII segments
- T1 C+ MR: Homogeneously enhancing tubular mass ± intramural cysts
- Temporal bone CT appearance dictated by specific location
  - **Geniculate fossa FNS**: Ovoid smooth enlargement of geniculate fossa with projections into labyrinthine ± anterior tympanic segments of CNVII
  - **Tympanic segment FNS**: Pedunculated FNS emanates from tympanic CNVII into middle ear

  - **Mastoid segment FNS**: Either tubular with sharp margins or globular with irregular margins (breaks into mastoid air cells)
  - **Greater superficial petrosal nerve (GSPN) schwannoma**: Enlargement of GSPN canal; middle cranial fossa mass

TOP DIFFERENTIAL DIAGNOSES

- Normal intratemporal facial nerve enhancement
- Bell palsy (herpetic facial paralysis)
- Intratemporal facial nerve venous malformation
- Intratemporal CNVII perineural malignancy

CLINICAL ISSUES

- Symptoms: Hearing loss (70%), CNVII paresis (50%)
- Treatment options
  - Conservative: Observation
  - Surgical treatment: Complete removal is goal
  - Radiotherapy: May be viable treatment option

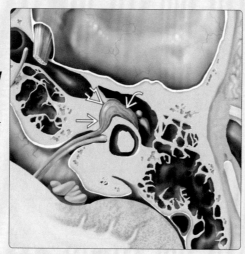
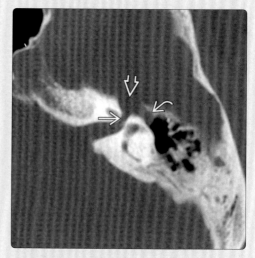

(Left) Axial graphic shows a tubular facial nerve schwannoma (FNS) involving the labyrinthine ➡ segment, geniculate ganglion ⤴, and anterior tympanic segment ➡ of the intratemporal facial nerve. (Right) Axial bone CT in a patient with CNVII paresis shows tubular enlargement of the distal labyrinthine segment ➡, geniculate fossa ⤴, and anterior tympanic segment ➡ of the CNVII canal. Involvement of multiple segments of the facial nerve, as in this case, is highly suggestive of FNS.

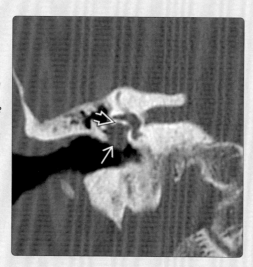
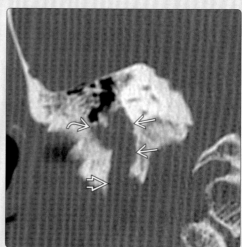

(Left) Coronal bone CT in the same patient reveals the FNS involving the midtympanic segment ⤵ of the facial nerve. Notice that the facial nerve bony canal "opens" into the middle ear mass ➡. (Right) Coronal bone CT in the same patient demonstrates that the FNS also involves the mastoid CNVII ➡, exiting the enlarged stylomastoid foramen ➡ inferiorly. The tumor has broken into adjacent air cells ➡ on its lateral margin.

TERMINOLOGY

Abbreviations

- Facial nerve schwannoma (FNS)

Synonyms

- Facial neuroma, facial neurilemmoma

Definitions

- FNS: Rare benign tumor of Schwann cells that invests intratemporal facial nerve (CNVII)

IMAGING

General Features

- Best diagnostic clue
  - Temporal bone CT: Tubular mass spanning multiple intratemporal CNVII segments with smooth enlargement of bony CNVII canal
  - T1 C+ MR: Homogeneously enhancing tubular mass ± intramural cysts
- Location
  - Most common location: Geniculate ganglion
  - > 90% of FNS span ≥ 3 intratemporal CNVII segments
- Size
  - Often long (multiple centimeters)
  - Cross-sectional measurement usually < 1 cm
- Morphology
  - Location dependent
    - Geniculate fossa: Ovoid or triangular
    - Greater superficial petrosal nerve (GSPN): Ovoid, projects into middle cranial fossa
    - Tympanic CNVII: Lobulates into middle ear
    - Mastoid CNVII: Irregular margin if breaks into surrounding air cells
    - Parotid CNVII: Tubular or ovoid mass along CNVII intraparotid course
  - Tubular shape along multiple CNVII segments

CT Findings

- CECT
  - No role for CECT in this diagnosis
  - Use enhanced MR instead
- Bone CT
  - General temporal bone CT appearances
    - Tubular enlargement of CNVII canal
    - Bony margins are smooth, benign-appearing
  - Temporal bone CT appearance is dictated by specific location of FNS along CNVII
    - **Geniculate fossa FNS**: Ovoid smooth enlargement of geniculate fossa
      - □ Tumor projects into labyrinthine ± anterior tympanic segments of CNVII
    - **Tympanic segment FNS**: Pedunculated FNS emanates from tympanic segment of CNVII into middle ear cavity
    - **Mastoid segment FNS**: Either tubular with sharp margins or globular with irregular margins
      - □ Shape depends on whether FNS breaks into surrounding mastoid air cells
    - **GSPN schwannoma**: Ovoid enlargement of GSPN canal anteromedial to geniculate fossa

MR Findings

- T1WI
  - Intermediate to low-signal lesion
- T2WI
  - High-signal lesion
- T1WI C+
  - **Geniculate ganglion FNS**: Ovoid, enhancing mass in enlarged geniculate fossa
    - Tumor tails project into labyrinthine ± anterior tympanic segments of CNVII
  - **Tympanic segment FNS**: Pedunculates into middle ear cavity
  - **Mastoid segment FNS**
    - Either tubular with sharp margins or globular with irregular margins
    - Depends on whether it breaks into surrounding mastoid air cells
  - **GSPN schwannoma**
    - Diagnosed when enhancing mass is seen in location of GSPN
    - Just anteromedial to geniculate fossa
    - Middle cranial fossa enhancing mass with connection to geniculate fossa
    - May be difficult to establish extraaxial nature of this schwannoma

Imaging Recommendations

- Best imaging tool
  - Patient presents with hearing loss ± CNVII paresis
    - Start with thin-section T1 C+ fat-saturated MR in axial & coronal plane through internal auditory canal (IAC) & temporal bone
    - If intratemporal, tubular enhancing mass is diagnosed on MR, then temporal bone CT helps delineate nature of lesion based on bone changes

DIFFERENTIAL DIAGNOSIS

Normal Intratemporal Facial Nerve Enhancement

- Clinical: Asymptomatic
- Temporal bone CT: Intratemporal CNVII canal is normal
- T1 C+ MR: Geniculate ganglion, anterior tympanic ± mastoid segments enhance normally
  - Labyrinthine CNVII does not enhance normally

Bell Palsy (Herpetic Facial Paralysis)

- Clinical: Sudden onset of peripheral CNVII paralysis
- Temporal bone CT: Normal intratemporal CNVII canal
- T1 C+ MR: Intratemporal + IAC fundal CNVII enhancement

Intratemporal Facial Nerve Venous Malformation

- Clinical: Sudden unilateral peripheral CNVII paralysis
- Temporal bone CT: Intratumoral honeycomb or bone spicules
- T1 C+ MR: Poorly circumscribed, geniculate fossa enhancing mass

Intratemporal CNVII Perineural Malignancy

- Clinical: Known or recurrent parotid malignancy
- Temporal bone CT: Mastoid CNVII canal is enlarged but less than in FNS
- T1 C+ MR: Infiltrating parotid mass is present

PATHOLOGY

General Features

- Etiology
  - Slowly growing, benign tumor from Schwann cells investing intratemporal CNVII
- Genetics
  - If multiple schwannomas ± meningiomas, think neurofibromatosis 2 (NF2)
- Associated abnormalities
  - NF2: Bilateral vestibular schwannomas; other schwannoma & meningioma possible

Gross Pathologic & Surgical Features

- Tan, ovoid-tubular, encapsulated mass
- Arises from outer nerve sheath layer of CNVII, expanding eccentrically away from nerve

Microscopic Features

- Benign encapsulated tumor made up of bundles of spindle-shaped Schwann cells forming whorled pattern
- Cellular architecture consists of densely cellular (Antoni A) areas ± loose, myxomatous (Antoni B) areas
- S100 protein stain: Strongly & diffusely positive in both nucleus & cytoplasm
- May display **intramural cystic changes**

CLINICAL ISSUES

Presentation

- Most common signs/symptoms
  - Hearing loss present in ~ 70%
  - Facial nerve symptoms present in ~ 50%
    - CNVII weakness or paralysis > involuntary facial movements
    - Bell palsy-like CNVII paralysis is rare
  - Ear ± facial pain
- Other signs/symptoms
  - Cerebellopontine angle (CPA)-IAC FNS: Sensorineural hearing loss, vertigo, & tinnitus
  - Larger tympanic & mastoid segments FNS
    - Avascular retrotympanic mass
    - Conductive hearing loss

Demographics

- Age
  - Mean age at presentation: 50 years
- Epidemiology
  - FNS is rare tumor (< 1% of intrapetrous tumors)
    - Within temporal bone > > intraparotid > CPA-IAC

Natural History & Prognosis

- Slow-growing benign tumor
- Eventually enlarges sufficiently to cause hearing loss & other cranial neuropathy
- Some tumors (< 10%) do not grow or become symptomatic

Treatment

- **Conservative management**
  - If CNVII paralysis is absent or mild when diagnosed, surgical cure can be worse than disease

- Incomplete recovery of full CNVII function may occur despite surgical restoration of CNVII continuity
  - Follow until CNVII symptoms begin to develop
  - Treatment used in elderly patients
- **Surgical treatment**
  - Goal = complete FNS removal with preservation of hearing & CNVII function restoration
  - Size-specific surgical techniques
    - Large FNS: Remove tumor + CNVII cable graft
    - Small FNS (< 1 cm): CNVII transposition with primary anastomosis
  - Location-specific surgery
    - Labyrinthine or geniculate FNS: Middle cranial fossa & transmastoid approaches combined
    - Tympanic-mastoid FNS: Transmastoid alone
- **Radiotherapy**
  - Early evidence suggests stereotactic radiotherapy may be alternative to surgery
  - Surgery then reserved for radiotherapy failures
  - Large series needed to confirm this therapy option

DIAGNOSTIC CHECKLIST

Consider

- Older patients with FNS often followed, not operated
- Younger patients without CNVII paresis often followed

Image Interpretation Pearls

- Intratemporal FNS: Segmental, tubular enlargement of CNVII canal
  - Distinctive imaging findings depending on segment of CNVII involved
- CPA-IAC FNS: Exactly mimics vestibular schwannoma if no extension into labyrinthine segment CNVII occurs
  - If present, labyrinthine segment tail makes imaging diagnosis
- Intraparotid FNS: Tubular mass in parotid coursing lateral to retromandibular vein
  - If present, mastoid segment tail suggests diagnosis
  - Differentiate from perineural parotid malignancy

SELECTED REFERENCES

1. Bäck L et al: Management of facial nerve schwannoma: a single institution experience. Acta Otolaryngol. 130(10):1193-8, 2010
2. Chao WC et al: Facial nerve schwannoma. Otolaryngol Head Neck Surg. 141(1):146-7, 2009
3. Madhok R et al: Gamma knife radiosurgery for facial schwannomas. Neurosurgery. 64(6):1102-5; discussion 1105, 2009
4. Thompson AL et al: Magnetic resonance imaging of facial nerve schwannoma. Laryngoscope. 119(12):2428-36, 2009
5. Stasolla A et al: Dural tail: another face of facial nerve schwannoma? AJNR Am J Neuroradiol. 27(9):1804; author reply 1805, 2006
6. Wiggins RH 3rd et al: The many faces of facial nerve schwannoma. AJNR Am J Neuroradiol. 27(3):694-9, 2006
7. Liu R et al: Facial nerve schwannoma: surgical excision versus conservative management. Ann Otol Rhinol Laryngol. 110(11):1025-9, 2001
8. Salzman KL et al: Dumbbell schwannomas of the internal auditory canal. AJNR Am J Neuroradiol. 22(7):1368-76, 2001
9. McMenomey SO et al: Facial nerve neuromas presenting as acoustic tumors. Am J Otol. 15(3):307-12, 1994
10. Parnes LS et al: Magnetic resonance imaging of facial nerve neuromas. Laryngoscope. 101(1 Pt 1):31-5, 1991
11. Inoue Y et al: Facial nerve neuromas: CT findings. J Comput Assist Tomogr. 11(6):942-7, 1987

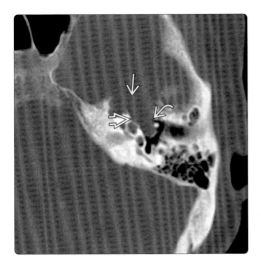

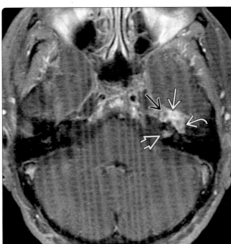

(Left) *Axial bone CT reveals an enlarged geniculate fossa mass* ➡️ *with the tumor extending along the anterior tympanic CNVII* ➡️, *displacing the ossicles laterally. The lateral surface of the otic capsule is thinned* ➡️ *by the FNS.* (Right) *Axial T1 C+ fat-saturated MR in the same patient shows the enhancing FNS centered in the geniculate ganglion* ➡️. *The tumor extends along the CNVII tympanic segment* ➡️ *as well as into the internal auditory canal* ➡️ *via the labyrinthine segment of CNVII. Note medial intramural cyst* ➡️.

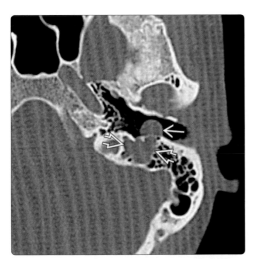

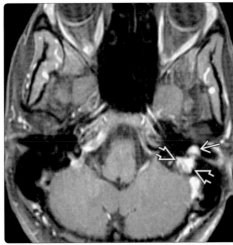

(Left) *Axial bone CT in a patient with an external auditory canal (EAC) polyp* ➡️ *shows an irregular mass* ➡️ *centered in the area of the mastoid segment of CN that appears contiguous.* (Right) *Axial T1WI C+ FS MR in the same patient reveals the enhancing FNS in the CNVII mastoid segment* ➡️, *projecting through a bony dehiscence into the EAC* ➡️.

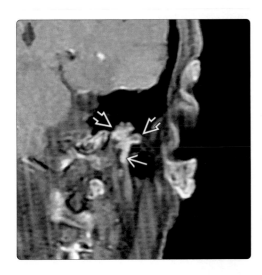

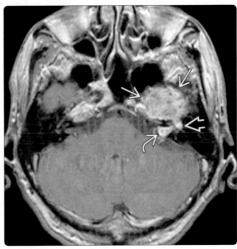

(Left) *Coronal T1WI C+ FS MR in a patient with conductive hearing loss & facial twitching shows a multilobular enhancing FNS* ➡️ *that has broken into mastoid air cells & projects inferiorly along the mastoid CN segment* ➡️. (Right) *Axial T1 C+ MR shows an enhancing mass* ➡️ *projecting into the medial middle cranial fossa from the greater superficial petrosal nerve. FNS diagnosis is suggested if the projections along the tympanic CNVII* ➡️ *& along the labyrinthine CNVII into the internal auditory canal* ➡️ *are seen.*

TERMINOLOGY

- Perineural tumor (PNT) on CNVII in T-bone: Local extension of malignant tumor along intratemporal CNVII

IMAGING

- Best clue: Poorly circumscribed, enhancing, tubular lesion extending from intraparotid tumor through stylomastoid foramen (SMF) to involve at least mastoid CNVII segment
  - **Contiguous spread** or **skip lesions** along CNVII
  - Image entire CNVII from end organ to brain stem
- T-bone CT findings
  - Intratemporal CNVII PNT may be difficult to detect
  - Mastoid CNVII canal may be slightly enlarged
  - Adjacent air cell opacification
- MR findings
  - Loss of SMF fat best seen on axial T1 MR
  - Axial images best delineate tympanic, geniculate ganglion, & labyrinthine CNVII PNT

- Coronal & sagittal images through T-bone best show PNT extending through SMF into mastoid CNVII segment

TOP DIFFERENTIAL DIAGNOSES

- Bell palsy
- T-bone CNVII venous malformation ("hemangioma")
- T-bone CNVII schwannoma
- Transmodiolar cochlear nerve schwannoma
- Ramsay Hunt syndrome

CLINICAL ISSUES

- Clinical presentation
  - Asymptomatic (60%) but with imaging findings
  - Progressive peripheral CNVII paresis or paralysis in adult
- Treatment options
  - Surgery combined with postoperative radiation therapy
  - 1° radiation therapy with neutron or proton beams may be indicated for surgically unresectable tumors

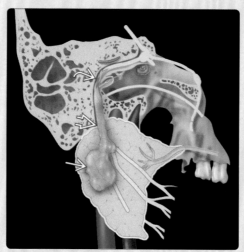
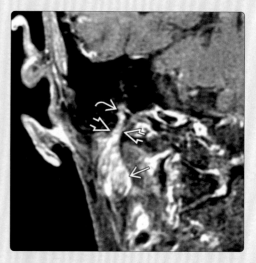

(Left) Sagittal graphic depicts an intraparotid neoplasm ➡ spreading along CNVII through the stylomastoid foramen ➡. Note that it travels superiorly on the mastoid segment of CNVII to the posterior genu ➡. (Right) Coronal T1 C+ MR shows parotid adenoid cystic carcinoma ➡ spreading along proximal extracranial CNVII through the stylomastoid foramen ➡ then up the mastoid segment of CNVII ➡.

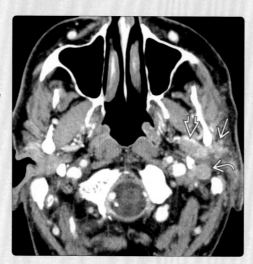
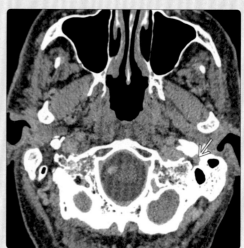

(Left) Axial CECT shows infiltrating parotid adenoid cystic carcinoma ➡ with perineural spread along the auriculotemporal nerve ➡. Perineural spread along intraparotid CNVII is seen as a round lesion ➡ in the fat just below the stylomastoid foramen. (Right) Axial CECT demonstrates an enlarged facial nerve from a perineural tumor ➡ in the left stylomastoid foramen in this patient with primary parotid adenoid cystic carcinoma.

TERMINOLOGY

Abbreviations
- Perineural tumor spread (PNT) on intratemporal facial nerve (CNVII)

Synonyms
- Neurotropic spread on intratemporal facial nerve

Definitions
- Local tumor extension along intratemporal CNVII

IMAGING

General Features
- Best diagnostic clue
  - Poorly circumscribed, enhancing, invasive mass arising within parotid gland extending through stylomastoid foramen (SMF) to involve mastoid CNVII segment
- Location
  - Extracranial & intracranial
  - Malignant primary parotid tumor or parotid metastasis can cause CNVII PNT
  - PNT can extend along entire course CNVII from end organ to nucleus in brainstem
- Size
  - Cross section size: Variable but larger than normal nerve
  - Length: May be many centimeters in length
- Morphology
  - Tubular enlargement of intratemporal CNVII
    - Contiguous spread along CNVII with radiographic **skip lesions** possible

CT Findings
- CECT
  - Delineates intraparotid malignancy
  - Tumor replacing SMF fat pad
  - Intratemporal CNVII PNT may be difficult to detect
  - Chronic denervation atrophy of mm facial expression
    - Early & subacute denervation not seen on CT
- Bone CT
  - Asymmetric widening of SMF & mastoid CNVII canal
  - Adjacent mastoid air cells may show tumor invasion

MR Findings
- T1WI
  - Infiltrating parotid malignancy
  - Loss of fat in "bell" of SMF
    - Best seen on axial T1 MR images
  - ↑ signal in chronic denervated mm facial expression
- T2WI
  - High-resolution (≤ 3 mm) T2 defines internal auditory canal (IAC) PNT if present
    - Fundal CNVII appears thickened
      - May connect to enlarged labyrinthine segment CNVII
    - ↑ T2 signal in intratemporal segment
- T2WI FS
  - ↑ T2 signal in subacute muscle denervation
    - Acute denervation not recognized because mm too small
- T1WI C+

- Abnormally enlarged & enhancing intratemporal CNVII
- PNT may involve mastoid & tympanic segments of CNVII, geniculate ganglion, & labyrinthine segment CNVII
- PNT may extend into IAC fundus as enhancing nodule
- PNT can travel along CNVII → CNV3 via **auriculotemporal nerve**

Nuclear Medicine Findings
- PET/CT rarely detects PNT
  - Because small volume of tumor along nerve or tumor not classically FDG avid [e.g., adenoid cystic carcinoma (ACCa)]

Imaging Recommendations
- Best imaging tool
  - Enhanced, multiplanar MR ± fat saturation
    - Defines scope of intraparotid malignancy
    - Best depicts intratemporal CNVII PNT
    - Shows denervation atrophy mm facial expression
  - Temporal bone CT is best to evaluate osseous SMF & intratemporal CNVII canal
    - Also helpful in evaluating subtle involvement of adjacent structures
      - Adjacent middle ear & mastoid air cells
      - Medial external auditory canal
- Protocol advice
  - Some 3T sequences exaggerate artifact with fat-saturation images and may render images of intratemporal CNVII uninterpretable
  - Scan must include entire course CNVII from nucleus → end organ

DIFFERENTIAL DIAGNOSIS

Bell Palsy
- Abrupt onset of peripheral CNVII paralysis
  - Self-limiting process: Generally resolves in 6 weeks
- Imaging: Intratemporal facial nerve asymmetric enhancement ± IAC fundal tuft on T1 C+ MR

T-Bone CNVII Venous Malformation ("Hemangioma")
- CNVII paralysis early in disease process
- Imaging: Infiltrating focal enhancing CNVII lesion in geniculate fossa on T1 C+ MR
  - T-bone CT: 50% with honeycomb bone pattern

T-Bone CNVII Schwannoma
- Hearing loss >> CNVII paralysis
- Imaging: Tubular enhancing mass along course of intratemporal CNVII on T1 C+ MR
  - T-bone CT: Fusiform enlargement of intratemporal CNVII canal; most commonly at geniculate ganglion

Transmodiolar Cochlear Nerve Schwannoma
- Slowly progressive sensorineural hearing loss; no CNVII paralysis
- Imaging: Dumbbell-shaped enhancing mass extending from cochlea through cochlear aperture into IAC fundus on T1 C+ MR

Ramsay Hunt Syndrome
- CNVII palsy + painful vesicles about ear

- Imaging: Enhancement of intratemporal CNVII

PATHOLOGY

General Features

- Etiology
  - Any parotid malignancy → PNT via direct invasion CNVII
  - Skin cancer [squamous cell carcinoma (SCCa), melanoma] → PNT
    - Direct extension along CNVII
    - More commonly CNV → CNVII via **auriculotemporal nerve**
  - Neurotropic tumors
    - ACCa: Salivary
    - SCCa: Skin
      - □ Less neurotropic but most common H&N cancer
    - Desmoplastic melanoma: Skin
    - Lymphoma
- Associated abnormalities
  - **Retrograde** PNT (toward CNS) **> antegrade** (away CNS)
  - PNT CNVII: **Contiguous** or radiographic **skip areas**

Staging, Grading, & Classification

- Staging criteria: Salivary gland tumor with perineural tumor on facial nerve
  - **T4**: Tumor **invades CNVII**
  - Stage IV: T4, any nodes, any metastases

Gross Pathologic & Surgical Features

- PNT can occur early in H&N cancers
- PNT can be extensive without local invasion of adjacent structures or significant lymphadenopathy

Microscopic Features

- Tumor 1st grows along CNVII sheath; eventually invades nerve

CLINICAL ISSUES

Presentation

- Most common signs/symptoms
  - Asymptomatic (60%) but with imaging findings
  - **Progressive peripheral CNVII paresis or paralysis**
    - Often preceded by facial twitching
  - Palpable parotid mass (not always)
- Other signs/symptoms
  - Burning or stinging facial or ear pain
  - Formication (sensation of ants crawling)
- Clinical profile
  - Adult + parotid mass + ipsilateral CNVII paralysis
  - May confuse with Bell palsy
    - High index of suspicion if parotid or skin cancer history

Demographics

- Age
  - 40-60 year olds
- Epidemiology
  - ACCa is most common parotid malignancy to show PNT along CNVII
  - SCCa is most common H&N cancer showing PNT spread
  - Other malignancies with CNVII PNT
    - Primary or secondary (from skin) SCCa or melanoma

- Non-Hodgkin lymphoma
- Mucoepidermoid carcinoma

Natural History & Prognosis

- PNT presence = ↑ risk local recurrence of primary tumor
- Carcinomas with PNT usually have relentless progression
- CNVII PNT can lead to serious physical deformity
- H&N neoplasms can exist within nerves for years without symptoms
  - Especially true in low-grade ACCa
- Diagnosis is frequently delayed, & outcome is poor once clinical manifestations arise
- 5-year overall survival: Poor
- Parotid ACCa has distinct clinical behavior
  - 65% overall 10-year survival rate
  - Recurrence depends on stage > histologic grade
  - Often indolent & slow growing
  - Long-term (> 10 year) imaging follow-up is recommended given tendency of ACCa to recur late

Treatment

- Treatment & prognosis altered by PNT
- Surgery combined with postoperative radiation therapy
- 1° radiation therapy with neutron or proton beams may be indicated for surgically unresectable tumors

DIAGNOSTIC CHECKLIST

Consider

- Imaging findings of PNT may be subtle
  - **Caveat**: If radiologist does not think to search for PNT when suspected parotid malignancy is seen, diagnosis of PNT is usually missed
    - Identification of PNT & its extent on imaging is critical to patient's chances of cure
  - Beware Bell palsy diagnosis

Image Interpretation Pearls

- If invasive parotid space lesion seen on imaging, radiologist must search for intratemporal PNT on CNVII
- MR more sensitive than CECT in detecting PNT along intratemporal CNVII
- If SMF fat is invaded, dedicated T-bone CT & enhanced MR to assess extent of CNVII PNT
- There may be radiologic **skip areas** along CNVII
  - Visually interrogate entire CNVII from nucleus/brainstem → end organ

SELECTED REFERENCES

1. Carlson ML et al: Occult temporal bone facial nerve involvement by parotid malignancies with perineural spread. Otolaryngol Head Neck Surg. 153(3):385-91, 2015
2. Mantravadi AV et al: Lateral temporal bone and parotid malignancy with facial nerve involvement. Otolaryngol Head Neck Surg. 144(3):395-401, 2011
3. Raghavan P et al: Imaging of the facial nerve. Neuroimaging Clin N Am. 19(3):407-25, 2009
4. Selcuk A et al: Adenoid cystic carcinoma of the parotid gland presenting as temporal bone neoplasm: a case report. B-ENT. 3(3):153-6, 2007
5. Terhaard C et al: Facial nerve function in carcinoma of the parotid gland. Eur J Cancer. 42(16):2744-50, 2006
6. Chang PC et al: Perineural spread of malignant melanoma of the head and neck: clinical and imaging features. AJNR Am J Neuroradiol. 25(1):5-11, 2004
7. Fischbein NJ et al: MR imaging in two cases of subacute denervation change in the muscles of facial expression. AJNR Am J Neuroradiol. 22(5):880-4, 2001

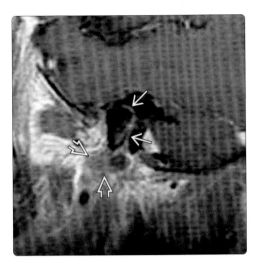

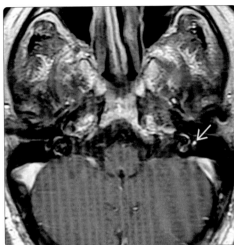

(Left) *Sagittal T1WI MR shows subtle diffuse enlargement and enhancement of the left intratemporal facial nerve* ➔ *from primary parotid acinic cell carcinoma* ➔ *noted adjacent to the stylomastoid foramen.* (Right) *Axial T1WI C+ MR shows subtle asymmetric enlargement and enhancement of the mastoid segment of CNVII* ➔ *from left parotid acinic cell carcinoma.*

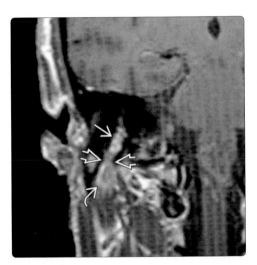

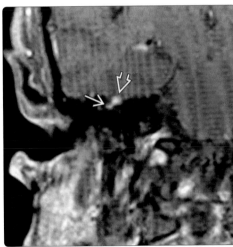

(Left) *Coronal T1WI C+ MR demonstrates primary parotid malignancy* ➔ *entering the right stylomastoid foramen* ➔ *and extending along the mastoid segment of CNVII* ➔*.* (Right) *Coronal T1WI C+ MR reveals a skip lesion of perineural tumor involving the right anterior tympanic* ➔ *and labyrinthine* ➔ *segments of CNVII in a patient with primary parotid malignancy. The intervening tympanic segment (not shown) appeared normal, hence the term skip lesion.*

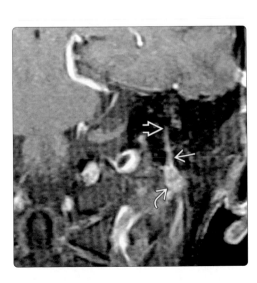

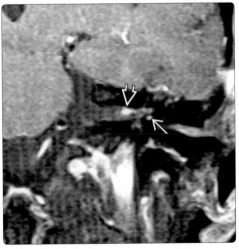

(Left) *Coronal T1WI C+ MR shows a small primary parotid acinic cell carcinoma* ➔ *at the level of the stylomastoid foramen. Notice the perineural tumor extending along the mastoid segment of CNVII* ➔ *to the posterior genu* ➔*.* (Right) *Coronal T1WI C+ MR shows perineural spread in the midtympanic CNVII* ➔ *and anterosuperior fundus of the internal auditory canal* ➔ *in a patient with a small primary parotid acinic cell carcinoma. It is unusual for such a small parotid malignancy to have this amount of perineural tumor spread along CNVII.*

Temporal Bone CSF Leak

TERMINOLOGY

- CSF leak into middle ear (ME) cavity
- Leak of CSF either from congenital or acquired tegmen or inner ear (IE) defect

IMAGING

- Axial bone CT (≤ 1 mm) + coronal reformats
  - Coronal best shows tegmen defect
- Bone CT findings
  - Opacified ME-mastoid air cells
  - Tegmen defect: Isolated or with **cephalocele**
  - Possible associated findings: Fracture, arachnoid granulation or osseous dural defect, postsurgical findings, IE anomaly
- MR findings if suspect cephalocele
  - T2 coronal: Meningocele (fluid-filled sac) or encephalocele (brain)
  - Extends through tegmen defect into ME
- Imaging recommendations

- CT: Include all paranasal sinuses & both temporal bones

TOP DIFFERENTIAL DIAGNOSES

- Rhinorrhea without CSF leak
  - Cribriform plate, ethmoid roof, sphenoid sinus walls intact on HRCT
  - β2-transferrin negative
- Otorrhea without CSF leak

CLINICAL ISSUES

- Watery fluid leaking from nose or external auditory canal
- Fluid positive for β2-transferrin = CSF protein
- Obesity with increased intracranial hypertension (IIH) increasing in frequency

DIAGNOSTIC CHECKLIST

- Consider temporal bone as source of leak even if CSF dripping from nose
- Multiple and bilateral defects common in posttraumatic or IIH patients

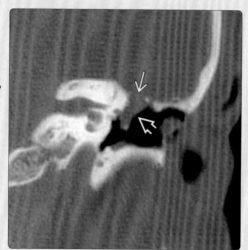
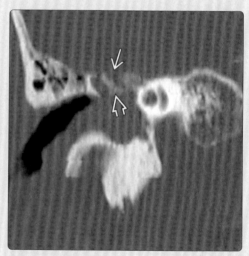

(Left) Coronal bone CT of left ear in patient with CSF leak shows tegmen tympani dehiscence ➡ & cephalocele projecting into middle ear behind tympanic membrane ⇒. High-resolution coronal T2 MR would determine type of cephalocele. (Right) Coronal bone CT, right ear, reveals comminuted posttraumatic tegmen fracture ➡ with bone fragments ⇒ in epitympanum. Some CSF leaks resolve spontaneously, but a defect this large will likely need surgery. MR can best characterize soft tissue/fluid filling middle ear.

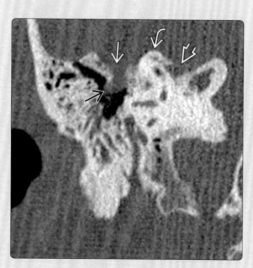
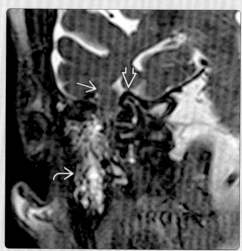

(Left) Coronal bone CT, right ear, in an 80 year old with spontaneous CSF leak ➡ shows 2 areas of dehiscence on either side of arcuate eminence ➡: Lateral tegmen roof dehiscence ⇒ & medial petrous apex roof dehiscence ⇒. (Right) Coronal T2WI FS MR in same patient reveals that tegmen dehiscence lateral to arcuate eminence ⇒ is accompanied by an encephalocele involving a inferior temporal gyrus ➡. Note CSF ➡ high signal in mastoid air cells.

TERMINOLOGY

Synonyms

- CSF otorhinorrhea, CSF fistula

Definitions

- Leak of cerebrospinal fluid (CSF) either from acquired tegmen defect or congenital inner ear (IE) defect
  - Acquired **tegmen tympani** or **mastoideum** defect, resulting in leak of CSF into middle ear (ME)
    - 2 main patient populations: Posttraumatic or idiopathic intracranial hypertension (IIH)
  - Congenital IE anomaly with **perilymph fistula with CSF leak** into ME cavity

IMAGING

General Features

- Best diagnostic clue
  - Opacified ME cavity with bony defect in tegmen
- Location
  - Tegmen tympani or mastoideum

CT Findings

- Bone CT
  - Opacified ME-mastoid from CSF
  - Possible causal findings
    - Previous temporal bone surgery or fracture
    - Osseous dural defect (pit, arachnoid granulation) of tegmen or posterior wall common in IIH
    - Congenital IE malformation with absent modiolus, perilymph fistula

MR Findings

- T2WI
  - Fluid-filled ME-mastoid complex with dehiscent tegmen ± **cephalocele**
    - Meningocele (CSF) or encephalocele (brain)
  - Traction encephalomalacia of adjacent brain from sag into bone defect common secondary finding
- T1WI C+
  - Thin dural enhancement at site of bone defect common even without infection/meningitis

Imaging Recommendations

- Best imaging tool
  - High-resolution, noncontrast temporal bone CT
- Protocol advice
  - Axial MDCT (≤ 1 mm); reformat coronals
  - Include all paranasal sinuses & both temporal bones as multiple defects can occur
    - Multiple defects common in posttrauma patient and IIH
  - Heavily T2-weighted multiplanar, especially coronal, sequences best show associated cephalocele
  - Rarely, CT cisternography if CT normal or multiple bone defects that could be source of leak

DIFFERENTIAL DIAGNOSIS

Rhinorrhea

- Vasomotor rhinitis, posttraumatic autonomic dysfunction may mimic CSF leak

Otorrhea

- Otitis media with TM perforation, otitis externa, or external auditory canal (EAC) foreign body may all mimic CSF leak

PATHOLOGY

General Features

- Etiology
  - Traumatic: Most temporal bone CSF leaks are traumatic (motor vehicle accident, GSW)
  - Tegmen defects increasing because of increasing obesity and IIH
  - Congenital: IE malformation + perilymph fistula

CLINICAL ISSUES

Presentation

- Most common signs/symptoms
  - Watery fluid leaking from nose or EAC
- Other signs/symptoms
  - Laboratory tests for CSF: β2-transferrin = protein found in CSF, newer β trace protein test
    - Reliable test; only few drops of fluid needed
  - Ascending meningitis less common now due to early recognition & imaging after trauma
  - Posttraumatic
    - Conductive or sensorineural hearing loss, vertigo, CNVII paresis (temporal bone injuries)

Demographics

- Epidemiology
  - 2-9% of patients with head injury have CSF leak
  - Obese, middle-aged women with IIH

Natural History & Prognosis

- Posttraumatic: Up to 85% resolve spontaneously within 7 days; almost all within 6 months
- IIH: May require skull base repair, followed by treatment for increased intracranial pressure and weight reduction

Treatment

- Posttraumatic: Bed rest, lumbar drain
- IIH: Middle fossa or mastoid approach for temporal bone leaks

DIAGNOSTIC CHECKLIST

Consider

- Temporal bone as leak source even if CSF from nose
  - ME CSF →eustachian tube → nasopharynx
  - If β2-transferrin positive, find leak!

Reporting Tips

- Size of bone defect and presence of cephalocele critical to report
- If patient infected from ascending meningitis, check for empyema or abscess

SELECTED REFERENCES

1. Brainard L et al: Association of benign intracranial hypertension and spontaneous encephalocele with cerebrospinal fluid leak. Otol Neurotol. 33(9):1621-4, 2012
2. Patel A et al: Management of temporal bone trauma. Craniomaxillofac Trauma Reconstr. 3(2):105-13, 2010

TERMINOLOGY

- Temporal bone arachnoid granulation (AG): **Nonvenous sinus-related** (aberrant) pseudopodial **pia-arachnoid projection** into tegmen tympani or posterior wall of temporal bone

IMAGING

- Bone CT findings
  - Ovoid/tubular scalloping erosion in temporal bone wall
- MR findings
  - Nonenhancing low signal (T1 C+)
  - High T2 signal lesion
- Locations
  - Lateral 1/3 of posterior temporal bone wall
    - Between posterior semicircular canal & anterior margin of sigmoid sinus
  - Tegmen tympani & mastoideum: Hard to see on CT MR
- Size variation of posterior wall AG
  - Few millimeters to 2-3 centimeters (**giant AG**)

TOP DIFFERENTIAL DIAGNOSES

- Endolymphatic sac tumor
- Large vestibular aqueduct (incomplete partition type II)
- Skull base dural AV fistula

PATHOLOGY

- **Temporal bone AG** = form of **aberrant AG**
  - Aberrant AG = AG that penetrates dura but **fails to reach venous sinus**
  - CSF pulsations suspected to enlarge AG causing arachnoid pouch to bulge into temporal bone
    - Idiopathic intracranial hypertension may accelerate

CLINICAL ISSUES

- **Incidental asymptomatic** finding
  - Rarely CSF leak associated ± meningitis
- Posterior wall AG **prevalence ↑ with age**
- On bone CT, posterior wall AG seen in **2.5%** of patients
- Treatment: None unless CSF leak associated

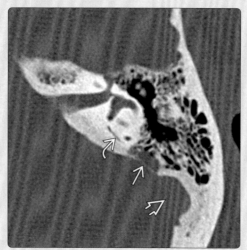
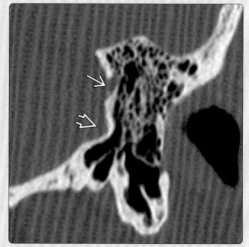

(Left) *Axial bone CT of the left ear in patient with right ear symptoms shows a medium-sized incidental arachnoid granulation in the medial mastoid wall ➡ projecting into the mastoid air cells. Note the proximity of the sigmoid sinus ➡ and bony vestibular aqueduct ➡. (Right) Short-axis oblique bone CT of the left temporal bone reveals a small arachnoid granulation ➡ in the medial mastoid wall. Note that the lesion is on the superior margin of the sigmoid sinus ➡.*

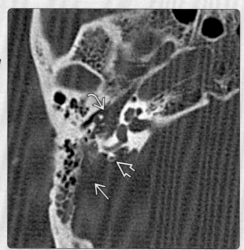
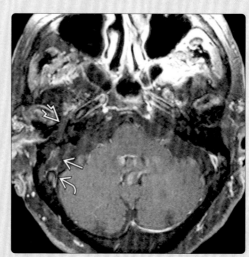

(Left) *Axial bone CT of the right temporal bone in a patient with clinically obvious CSF leak demonstrates a giant AG eroding the medial mastoid wall ➡. The posterior semicircular ➡ canal appears to float in the AG. The middle ear is full of fluid (CSF) ➡. (Right) Axial T1WI C+ fat-saturated MR in the same patient reveals the giant arachnoid granulation ➡ as a lobular fluid signal structure with subtle rim enhancement. The middle ear fluid is low signal ➡. Note the proximity of the sigmoid sinus ➡ to the giant AG.*

TERMINOLOGY

Abbreviations

- Arachnoid granulation (AG)

Synonyms

- Aberrant AG, osteodural defects
- When large → giant AG

Definitions

- Temporal bone AG: **Nonvenous sinus-related** (aberrant) pseudopodial **pia-arachnoid projection** into tegmen tympani or posterior wall of temporal bone

IMAGING

General Features

- Best diagnostic clue
  - Bone CT: Scalloped lucency in temporal bone wall; ovoid or tubular; multilobular when large
  - MR: Nonenhancing low signal (T1 C+), high T2 signal lesion
- Location
  - Tegmen tympani
  - Lateral 1/3 of posterior temporal bone wall
    - Between posterior semicircular canal & anterior margin of sigmoid sinus
    - At axial level of crus communis
- Size
  - Tegmen tympani AG: Millimeters
  - Posterior wall AG: Few millimeters to 2-3 centimeters (**giant AG**)

CT Findings

- Bone CT
  - Tegmen tympani AG
    - Small size & variable ossification of tegmen makes it **difficult to see** with CT
  - Posterior wall AG
    - Ovoid or tubular lucency in medial mastoid wall
      □ Multilobular when large
    - Mastoid cortex with focal erosion
    - AG may project into medial mastoid air cells

MR Findings

- T1WI C+ FS
  - Ovoid or tubular (fluid) signal lesion of posterior mastoid wall
  - No or subtle rim enhancement
    - No nodular enhancement
- CISS or FIESTA
  - High (fluid) signal lesion

Imaging Recommendations

- Best imaging tool
  - Bone CT best characterizes AG

DIFFERENTIAL DIAGNOSIS

Endolymphatic Sac Tumor

- Centered in fovea of endolymphatic sac, posterior wall
- CT: Spiculated or coarse calcifications within tumor matrix
  - Thin Ca^{++} along posterior margin

- MR: T1 high-signal foci from trapped blood products

Large Vestibular Aqueduct (Incomplete Partition Type II)

- CT: Enlarged bony vestibular aqueduct
- MR: Enlarged endolymphatic sac

Dural AV Fistula, Skull Base

- CT: Transosseous collaterals traverse posterior mastoid
- MR: Recanalized, irregular transverse-sigmoid sinus

PATHOLOGY

General Features

- Etiology
  - Unknown why AG can occur without venous sinus communication
    - May represent aborted attempt by AG to enter sigmoid sinus to resorb CSF
  - **Temporal bone AG** = form of **aberrant AG**
    - Defined as AG that penetrates dura but **fails to reach venous sinus**
    - CSF pulsations suspected to enlarge AG causing arachnoid pouch to bulge into temporal bone
      □ Idiopathic intracranial hypertension may facilitate AG growth
    - Rarely with arachnoid pouch enlargement, rupture results in CSF leak into mastoid temporal bone

Gross Pathologic & Surgical Features

- **Osteodural defect** with arachnoid pouch

Microscopic Features

- Arachnoid villi with central core of loose connective tissue, peripheral zone of dense connective tissue

CLINICAL ISSUES

Presentation

- Most common signs/symptoms
  - **Incidental asymptomatic** finding
- Other signs/symptoms
  - Rarely CSF leak associated ± meningitis

Demographics

- Epidemiology
  - Tegmen tympani AG > > posterior wall AG
  - Posterior wall AG **prevalence ↑ with age**
  - Can see posterior wall AG on CT in **~ 2.5%** of patients

Treatment

- None unless CSF leak associated
- CSF leak treatment
  - Canal wall up mastoidectomy with repair of dural defect with tissue graft

SELECTED REFERENCES

1. Junet P et al: Spontaneous osteo-dural fistulae of petrous bone posterior wall. Eur Ann Otorhinolaryngol Head Neck Dis. 130(6):341-3, 2013
2. Lee MH et al: Prevalence and appearance of the posterior wall defects of the temporal bone caused by presumed arachnoid granulations and their clinical significance: CT findings. AJNR Am J Neuroradiol. 29(9):1704-7, 2008
3. VandeVyver V et al: Arachnoid granulations of the posterior temporal bone wall: imaging appearance and differential diagnosis. AJNR Am J Neuroradiol. 28(4):610-2, 2007

Temporal Bone Fibrous Dysplasia

TERMINOLOGY

- FD definition: Congenital disorder with **defect in osteoblastic differentiation & maturation** resulting in progressive replacement of normal cancellous bone by mixture of **fibrous tissue** & **immature woven bone**

IMAGING

- Bone CT shows **expansile ground-glass** bony matrix
  - Expansile lesion centered in medullary space with variable attenuation
  - **Pagetoid (mixed) pattern (50%)**: Mixed radiopacity & radiolucency
  - **Sclerotic FD (25%)**: Ground-glass density
  - **Cystic FD (25%)**: Centrally lucent lesions with thinned but sclerotic borders
- T1 MR: Expansile lesion with ↓ signal
- T2 MR: ↓ signal in ossified ± fibrous areas
- T1 C+ FS MR: Diffuse, rim, or no enhancement possible

TOP DIFFERENTIAL DIAGNOSES

- Temporal bone Paget disease
- Skull base giant cell tumor
- Temporal bone meningioma
- Temporal bone metastasis

PATHOLOGY

- Benign **tumor-like lesion** of bone with local arrest of normal structural/architectural development
  - Contains fibrous tissue (spindle cell stroma) with intramural woven bone trabeculae

CLINICAL ISSUES

- Clinical setting
  - Young affected (< 30 yr old)
  - Often asymptomatic lesion when small
- Natural history
  - Most spontaneously cease to grow by age 25-30 yr

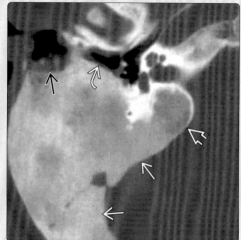
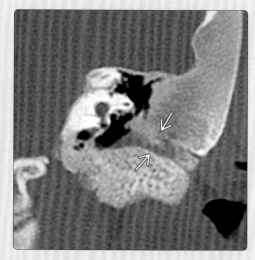

(Left) Axial bone CT reveals the common sclerotic variety of fibrous dysplasia (FD) involving the mastoid ➡ and inner ear ➡ and encroaching on the posterior middle ear. FD expansion causes external auditory canal (EAC) stenosis ➡. Anterolaterally, note previous biopsy site ➡. (Right) Coronal bone CT shows sclerotic FD that has expanded to occlude the EAC ➡. Clinically significant conductive hearing loss can be expected. Otoscopy reveals finding similar to congenital EAC malformation.

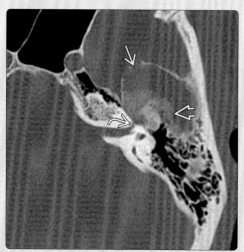
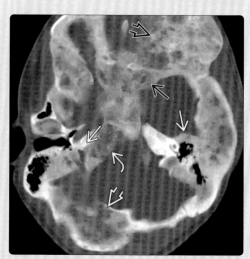

(Left) Axial left temporal bone CT reveals aggressive-appearing anterior left temporal bone foci of cystic FD ➡. Subtle ground-glass component ➡ is visible within the lesion. Note the labyrinthine segment of the facial nerve canal is visible ➡, but the lesion involves the geniculate fossa. (Right) Axial bone CT shows polyostotic fibrous dysplasia affecting both temporal bones ➡. Multiple other foci are apparent, including the right occipital bone ➡, clivus ➡, sphenoid bone ➡, and frontal bone ➡.

TERMINOLOGY

Abbreviations

- Fibrous dysplasia (FD)

Definitions

- Congenital disorder with **defect in osteoblastic differentiation & maturation** resulting in progressive replacement of normal cancellous bone by mixture of **fibrous tissue** & **immature woven bone**

IMAGING

General Features

- Best diagnostic clue
  - Bone CT shows **expansile ground-glass** bony matrix
- Location
  - May affect any bone in body
- Size
  - Localized or diffuse
  - Lesions may reach many cm in size
- Morphology
  - FD conforms to general shape of affected bone

CT Findings

- Bone CT
  - **Expansile lesion** centered in medullary space with variable attenuation
    - **Pagetoid (mixed) pattern (50%)**: Mixed radiopacity & radiolucency
    - **Sclerotic FD (25%)**: Ground-glass density
    - **Cystic FD (25%)**: Centrally lucent lesions with thinned but sclerotic borders

MR Findings

- T1WI
  - Expansile lesion with ↓ signal
- T2WI
  - ↓ signal in ossified ± fibrous areas
- T1WI C+
  - Diffuse, rim or limited enhancement possible
  - Active phase: Heterogeneous enhancement typical
    - May appear aggressive when present

Nuclear Medicine Findings

- Bone scan
  - ↑ radionuclide accumulation, perfusion, & delayed phase
  - Nonspecific; sensitive to locations in polyostotic FD
- PET
  - Can be variably hot on FDG PET
    - Should not be mistaken for metastasis

Imaging Recommendations

- Best imaging tool
  - Bone CT is key to making correct diagnosis

DIFFERENTIAL DIAGNOSIS

Temporal Bone Paget Disease

- Presents in elderly
- Cotton-wool CT appearance
- Pagetoid ground-glass FD mimics Paget disease
- Involves temporal bone & calvarium, not craniofacial area

Skull Base Giant Cell Tumor

- May mimic sclerotic FD on bone CT
- Hypointense on T2 MR (hemosiderin deposition)

Temporal Bone Meningioma

- Intraosseous meningioma mimics FD on bone CT
- En plaque soft tissue mass seen on MR

Temporal Bone Metastasis

- Mixed sclerotic-destructive metastasis mimics FD
- Prostate & breast carcinoma most common

PATHOLOGY

General Features

- Etiology
  - Benign **tumor-like lesion** of bone with local arrest of normal structural/architectural development
- Genetics
  - Sporadic gene mutation of *GNAS1* gene

Microscopic Features

- FD lesion contains fibrous tissue (spindle cell stroma) with intramural woven bone trabeculae

CLINICAL ISSUES

Presentation

- Most common signs/symptoms
  - Bulging of temporal area
  - Stenosis of EAC with recurrent otitis
  - Hearing loss: Conductive, sensorineural, or mixed

Demographics

- Age
  - Active in young, typically quiescent after puberty
  - Young affected (< 30 yr old)
- Gender
  - M:F = 1:3
- Epidemiology
  - Monostotic FD is 6x more common than polyostotic

Natural History & Prognosis

- Monostotic craniofacial FD has excellent prognosis
- Most spontaneously cease to grow by age 25-30 yr
- Polyostotic FD rarely life threatening but has poorer prognosis

Treatment

- Aggressive surgical management not recommended in most cases

SELECTED REFERENCES

1. Yang H et al: Surgical treatment of monostotic fibrous dysplasia of the temporal bone: a retrospective analysis. Am J Otolaryngol. 33(6):697-701, 2012
2. Kim YH et al: Role of surgical management in temporal bone fibrous dysplasia. Acta Otolaryngol. 129(12):1374-9, 2009
3. Jee WH et al: Fibrous dysplasia: MR imaging characteristics with radiopathologic correlation. AJR Am J Roentgenol. 167(6):1523-7, 1996
4. Brown EW et al: Fibrous dysplasia of the temporal bone: imaging findings. AJR Am J Roentgenol. 164(3):679-82, 1995
5. Megerian CA et al: Fibrous dysplasia of the temporal bone: ten new cases demonstrating the spectrum of otologic sequelae. Am J Otol. 16(4):408-19, 1995

TERMINOLOGY

- Paget disease (PD) definition: Bone dysplasia characterized by **excessive remodeling** of bone resulting from alternating waves of osteoclastic & osteoblastic activity

IMAGING

- Location of involvement of PD
  - Calvarium > cranial base > temporal bone
- Bone CT
  - Calvarium & cranial base: Diffuse thickening with mixed-density bone
  - Temporal bone: Sclerotic & erosive bone change affecting all areas
    - Includes otic capsule when advanced
  - External auditory canal: Tortuosity & stenosis
  - Middle ear: Middle ear cavity constriction; ossicles & ligaments with pagetoid changes
  - Inner ear/otic capsule: Otic capsule demineralization (peripheral to central) involves all 3 layers

- Internal auditory canal (IAC): Enlarging bone narrows IAC and compresses CNVII & CNVIII
- MR: Diminished T1 signal of enlarged bones
  - T1 C+ FS: Avid enhancement

TOP DIFFERENTIAL DIAGNOSES

- Temporal bone fibrous dysplasia
- Temporal bone osteoradionecrosis
- Otosclerosis

CLINICAL ISSUES

- Clinical presentation
  - Progressive bilateral mixed hearing loss → deafness
  - Conductive hearing loss: Ossicles & ligaments affected
  - Sensorineural hearing loss: Otic capsule erosions; IAC compression
- Age at presentation
  - > 40 years of age
  - Compare to < 30 years for fibrous dysplasia

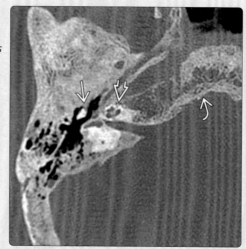
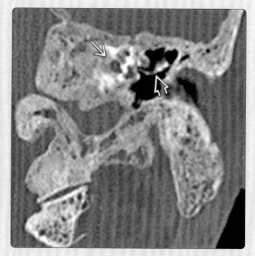

(Left) Axial right ear temporal bone CT shows Paget disease causing diffusely thickened bones of the clivus ➡, petrous apex, and bones around the middle and inner ear. Notice the thickened ligament ➡ connected to the malleus and the erosion of the otic capsule ➡. (Right) Coronal bone CT in the opposite ear in the same patient reveals diffuse bony enlargement of all bones of the skull base and temporal bone. Erosive changes ➡ of the otic capsule and thickening of the ossicles ➡ are evident.

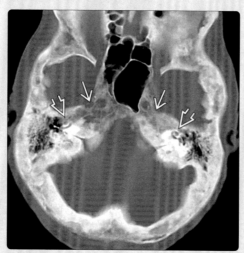
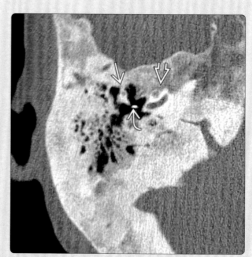

(Left) Axial bone CT shows diffuse enlarged bones of the skull base with a cotton wool pattern appearance. The petrous apices ➡ are enlarged but demineralized, which indicates that earlier, more active disease is present. The anteromedial otic capsules are eroded ➡. (Right) Axial bone CT of the right ear in a patient with hearing loss shows malleal ligament ossification ➡ as well as subacute erosive phase of Paget disease affecting the otic capsule ➡. Stapedectomy with stapes prosthesis ➡ had been performed.

TERMINOLOGY

Abbreviations
- Paget disease (PD)

Synonyms
- Osteitis deformans

Definitions
- Bone dysplasia characterized by **excessive remodeling** of bone resulting from alternating waves of osteoclastic & osteoblastic activity

IMAGING

General Features
- Best diagnostic clue
  - Bone CT
    - Calvarium & skull base: Diffuse thickening with mixed density bone
    - Temporal bone: Sclerotic & erosive bone change in all areas
- Location
  - Calvarium > cranial base > temporal bone

CT Findings
- Bone CT
  - **External auditory canal** (EAC) & **middle ear**
    - EAC tortuosity & stenosis
    - Middle ear cavity constriction
    - Ossicles & ligaments with pagetoid changes
  - **Inner ear/otic capsule**
    - Otic capsule demineralization (peripheral to central) **involves all 3 layers**
      - □ Periosteum → endochondral → endosteum
  - **Internal auditory canal** (IAC)
    - Enlarging bone narrows IAC
  - **Skull base & calvarium**
    - Diffuse inhomogeneous **thickening** of cranial base & calvarium

MR Findings
- T1WI
  - Diminished T1 signal
    - Marrow replacement by fibrous tissue
  - Heterogeneous patchy T1 hyperintense signal
    - Areas of hemorrhage & slow flow in vascular channels
- T1WI C+
  - Heterogeneous enhancement within thickened calvarium, skull base ± temporal bone possible
    - Secondary to hypervascular nature
  - Meningeal enhancement has also been reported
    - May reflect ↑ metabolism & blood flow

Imaging Recommendations
- Best imaging tool
  - Temporal bone CT only study needed to make diagnosis

DIFFERENTIAL DIAGNOSIS

Temporal Bone Fibrous Dysplasia
- Clinical: Younger patient
- CT: Increased bone volume

- Commonly involves facial bones

Temporal Bone Osteoradionecrosis
- CT: Unilateral demineralization similar to acute PD
  - Not thickened or diffuse like PD

Otosclerosis
- Clinical: Much younger patient compared with PD
- CT: Multifocal otic capsule demineralization
  - Usually bilateral, symmetric
  - Adjacent skull base & calvarium normal

PATHOLOGY

General Features
- Etiology
  - Unknown; nuclear viral inclusions suggest viral etiology
  - Progressive osteodystrophy with **monostotic** & **polyostotic** varieties
- Genetics
  - Mostly sporadic
  - 15% autosomal dominant inheritance pattern
    - Defects in chromosome 6 & 18q implicated
- Associated abnormalities
  - Characteristic involvement of vertebrae, pelvis, & long bones
  - In temporal bone, marrow-containing structures are involved 1st
    - Petrous apex undergoes initial changes
  - Demineralization of otic capsule & encroachment upon middle ear structures occur late

CLINICAL ISSUES

Presentation
- Most common signs/symptoms
  - Mixed hearing loss
- Other signs/symptoms
  - Tinnitus (intraosseous arteriovenous shunts)
  - Vertigo, hemifacial spasm, trigeminal neuralgia
- Laboratory abnormalities
  - ↑ serum alkaline phosphatase
  - ↑ urinary hydroxyproline

Demographics
- Age
  - > 40 years of age
- Gender
  - M:F = 4:1

Natural History & Prognosis
- Disorder usually progressive despite therapy
- Progressive bilateral mixed hearing loss → deafness

Treatment
- Calcitonin, diphosphonates, mithramycin

SELECTED REFERENCES

1. Bahmad F Jr et al: Paget disease of the temporal bone. Otol Neurotol. 28(8):1157-8, 2007
2. Van der Stappen A et al: Paget disease of the skull and temporal bone. JBR-BTR. 88(3):156-7, 2005
3. Tehranzadeh J et al: Computed tomography of Paget disease of the skull versus fibrous dysplasia. Skeletal Radiol. 27(12):664-72, 1998

Temporal Bone Langerhans Cell Histiocytosis

TERMINOLOGY

- Synonyms: Dendritic cell histiocytosis, histiocytosis X, eosinophilic granuloma (EG), Hand-Schüller-Christian disease (HSCD), Abt-Letterer-Siwe disease (ALSD)
- Proliferative disorder of Langerhans-type histiocytes, which form granulomas in T-bone & surrounding soft tissues

IMAGING

- Well-defined lytic lesions of T-bone with associated enhancing soft tissue masses
  - **Squamous & mastoid bones** > petrous apex
- Both enhanced CT & MR often performed in complex cases
  - Bone CT best for evaluating osseous structures
  - MR best for soft tissue evaluation

TOP DIFFERENTIAL DIAGNOSES

- Coalescent otomastoiditis
- T-Bone rhabdomyosarcoma
- T-Bone metastasis

PATHOLOGY

- Poorly understood pathology with histiocyte proliferation and infiltration
- Old classification system: 3 groups
  - EG
  - HSCD
  - ALSD
- New classification system based on risk factors
  - Multifocal involvement, young age, multiorgan dysfunction, disease relapse

CLINICAL ISSUES

- Otologic symptoms in **25%** of T-bone cases
  - **Conductive hearing loss ± otorrhea**
- T-bone presents in **1st decade** of life
- Other symptoms: Otalgia, vertigo, otitis media ± externa, periauricular soft tissue swelling, CNVII palsy, sensorineural hearing loss, aural polyp

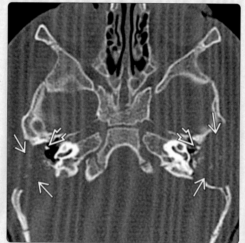
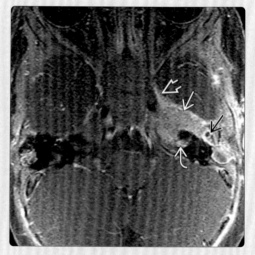

(Left) Axial bone CT in a 2-year-old girl with bilateral otorrhea shows well-defined destructive lesions of LCH involving bilateral mastoid and left squamous temporal bones ➡, opacified middle ear cavities, and near-complete ossicular destruction ➡. The lesions lack the typical aggressive periosteal reaction of metastatic neuroblastoma. (Right) Axial T1 C+ FS MR shows enhancing LCH extending into the left middle cranial fossa ➡, cavernous sinus ➡, and internal auditory canal ➡. The ossicles are encased ➡ by tumor.

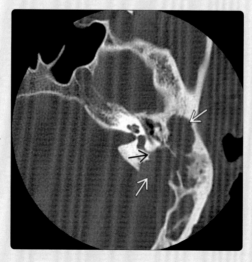
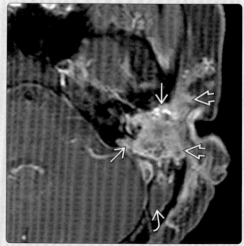

(Left) Axial bone CT demonstrates sharply punched-out lytic destruction of the left T-bone due to LCH ➡, including involvement of the otic capsule ➡ (which is uncommonly eroded by most processes). (Right) Axial T1 C+ FS MR shows extensive enhancement within the left T-bone ➡ due to involvement by LCH, with extension into the adjacent extracranial soft tissues ➡. Trapped mastoid fluid is noted posteriorly ➡.

TERMINOLOGY

Abbreviations

- Langerhans cell histiocytosis (LCH)

Synonyms

- T-bone dendritic cell histiocytosis (DCH), histiocytosis X, eosinophilic granuloma, Hand-Schüller-Christian disease, Letterer-Siwe disease, Abt-Letterer-Siwe disease, Hashimoto-Pritzker

Definitions

- Proliferation of dendritic cell histiocytes, which form granulomas within any organ system, including T-bone

IMAGING

General Features

- Best diagnostic clue
  - Well-defined **lytic bone** lesion, usually with **enhancing soft tissue** mass
- Location
  - Squamous & mastoid T-bone > petrous apex

CT Findings

- Bone CT
  - Variable lytic **punched-out** lesions
    - Usually geographic osseous destruction of mastoid &/or squamous portions of T-bone
    - May involve petrous apex, otic capsule, ± ossicles
  - Beveled margins of lytic lesions
    - More common in calvarium
    - May also have sclerosis (more common appearance of skull base lesions)
  - May have diffuse T-bone osseous destruction

MR Findings

- T1WI
  - Marrow replacement process of T-bone
  - Hypointense or isointense to muscle T-bone lesion ± soft tissue component
    - ± ↑ **T1** signal (lipid-laden macrophages)
    - ± **blood products** within soft tissue mass
- T2WI
  - Iso- to hyperintense soft tissue mass
  - **Fluid-fluid levels** may be present
- T1WI C+ FS
  - Avid, heterogeneous soft tissue enhancement
    - Well-defined or poorly defined margins
  - ± intracranial spread with dural enhancement

Imaging Recommendations

- Best imaging tool
  - Bone CT ± enhanced MR

DIFFERENTIAL DIAGNOSIS

Coalescent Otomastoiditis

- Acute infection of middle ear & mastoid air cells
- Progressive resorption of mastoid osseous septa

T-Bone Rhabdomyosarcoma

- Soft tissue sarcoma arising from rhabdomyoblasts

- Invasive heterogeneous soft tissue mass in child, usually with osseous destruction

T-Bone Metastasis

- Destructive T-bone lesion (e.g., neuroblastoma)

PATHOLOGY

General Features

- Etiology
  - Poorly understood pathology with histiocyte proliferation and infiltration
    - **Neoplastic or inflammatory**
- Associated abnormalities
  - Hypothalamic-pituitary disease
    - Presents with symptoms of **diabetes insipidus**
      - Absent posterior pituitary hyperintensity on T1 MR
      - Thick, enhancing infundibulum
  - Cerebral abnormalities
    - Cerebral, cerebellar, and brainstem

Staging, Grading, & Classification

- **Old classification**: 3 groups
  - Eosinophilic granuloma
  - Hand-Schüller-Christian disease
  - Abt-Letterer-Siwe disease
- **New classification system** based on risk factors
  - Multifocal involvement, young age, multiorgan dysfunction, disease relapse

Microscopic Features

- Electron microscopy shows **Birbeck granules** & elongated tennis racket-shaped cytoplasmic inclusion

CLINICAL ISSUES

Presentation

- Most common signs/symptoms
  - **Conductive hearing loss ± otorrhea**

Demographics

- Age
  - T-bone LCH typically presents in 1st decade
    - Inverse relationship between age of presentation & severity of disease

Natural History & Prognosis

- **90% cure** rate for **unifocal** disease of T-bone
- Multifocal & systemic LCH: Mortality up to 18%

Treatment

- Depends on symptoms, location, & extent of disease

SELECTED REFERENCES

1. Chevallier KM et al: Differentiating pediatric rhabdomyosarcoma and Langerhans cell histiocytosis of the temporal bone by imaging appearance. AJNR Am J Neuroradiol. 37(6):1185-9, 2016
2. Modest MC et al: Langerhans cell histiocytosis of the temporal bone: A review of 29 cases at a single center. Laryngoscope. 126(8):1899-904, 2015
3. Nabavizadeh SA et al: CT and MRI of pediatric skull lesions with Fluid-Fluid Levels. AJNR Am J Neuroradiol. 35(3):604-8, 2014
4. Radhakrishnan R et al: Petrous apex lesions in the pediatric population. Pediatr Radiol. 44(3):325-39; quiz 323-4, 2014
5. Coleman MA et al: Bilateral temporal bone langerhans cell histiocytosis: radiologic pearls. Open Neuroimag J. 7:53-7, 2013

Temporal Bone Metastasis

TERMINOLOGY

- Hematogenous spread from distant primary neoplasm
- Bony metastatic disease to petrous apex (PA) or mastoid/middle ear

IMAGING

- PA most common site
- Bone CT
  - Focal **lytic** or **permeative**, rarely **blastic** lesion
  - Commonly other bone metastases
  - Subtle appearance in pneumatized portions of T-bone
  - Enhances significantly in most cases
  - CT differentiates benign lesions (fibrous dysplasia, osteoma)
- MR
  - T1: Lesion hypointense to normal fatty marrow
  - T1 C+ FS: Delineates tumor vs. normal fatty marrow

TOP DIFFERENTIAL DIAGNOSES

- Apical petrositis
- Cholesterol granuloma of PA
- Langerhans cell histiocytosis of T-bone
- Plasmacytoma of T-bone

CLINICAL ISSUES

- Often asymptomatic
  - Hearing loss if any symptoms
  - CN palsy (CNVIII > CNVII > CNV or CNVI)
- Breast > lung > renal > prostate cancer origin
- Neuroblastoma and leukemia most common in children

DIAGNOSTIC CHECKLIST

- Remember background PA marrow/pneumatization is commonly asymmetric
- Isolated T-bone lesion is less likely to be metastasis
- Look for dura, dural venous sinus, and brain invasion

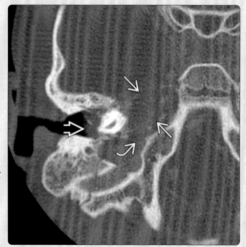
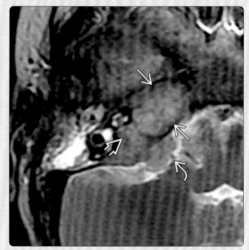

(Left) T-bone CT in an infant with right CNVII palsy shows permeative, lytic petrous apex destruction ➡ with sparing of the dense otic capsule bone. The tumor extends into the middle ear cavity ➡ & erodes the anterior wall of the jugular foramen ➡. (Right) Axial T2WI FS MR in the same patient shows a hypointense petrous apex mass ➡, consistent with a cellular tumor. It extends into the right IAC ➡ and cerebellopontine angle ➡. Biopsy revealed neuroblastoma. Subsequent imaging revealed an adrenal primary.

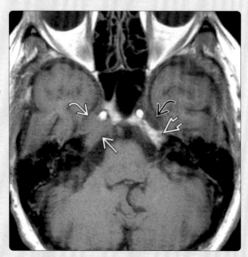
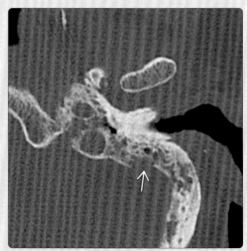

(Left) Axial T1WI MR shows typical appearance of right petrous apex metastasis replacing fatty marrow ➡ with expansion into right Meckel cave ➡ in this patient with right facial numbness. On left, note normal marrow signal in petrous apex ➡ & CSF Meckel cave ➡. (Right) Osseous mastoid bone metastasis, with cortical destruction of the inner cortex/sigmoid plate ➡, puts the sigmoid sinus at risk for invasion/thrombosis. Smaller metastases are easily missed, secondary to aerated/varied appearance of the T-bone.

TERMINOLOGY

Definitions

- Hematogenous spread to T-bone from distant primary neoplasm
- Bony metastatic disease to petrous apex (PA) or mastoid/middle ear

IMAGING

General Features

- Best diagnostic clue
  - Bone CT shows focal destructive lesion of T-bone
- Location
  - PA most common
- Size
  - Variable, 2-8 cm
- Morphology
  - Lytic, permeative destruction, ± poorly defined margins

CT Findings

- CECT
  - Soft tissue component enhances significantly in most cases
- Bone CT
  - **Lytic or permeative**, rarely **blastic** lesion
    - Commonly has other bone metastases
  - T-bone cortex is destroyed
  - Subtle appearance in pneumatized portions of T-bone

MR Findings

- T1WI
  - Nonspecific, low to intermediate signal
    - Lower signal metastasis easily distinguished from adjacent normal adult fatty marrow
- T2WI
  - Variable, may be hyper- or hypointense
    - Depends upon cellularity of primary lesion
- T1WI C+
  - Variable enhancement; may blend with normal fatty marrow
  - Fat saturation to exclude normal fatty marrow
  - Thin dural enhancement likely reactive
  - Thick nodular or irregular dural enhancement likely transdural tumor

Nuclear Medicine Findings

- Bone scan
  - Abnormal nonspecific ↑ radiotracer
- PET
  - Positive in T-bone, other bones, and primary

Imaging Recommendations

- Best imaging tool
  - Both CT & MR necessary if surgical resection considered
- Protocol advice
  - T1 MR: Lesion hypointense to normal fatty marrow
  - T1 C+ FS MR: Differentiates tumor from normal fatty marrow & shows intracranial extension

DIFFERENTIAL DIAGNOSIS

Confluent Apical Petrositis

- Clinical: Infectious symptoms
- Imaging: Destructive lesion of PA + dural thickening

PA Cholesterol Granuloma

- Clinical: History of chronic otitis media
- Imaging: Expansile PA lesion; high signal on T1

T-Bone Langerhans Cell Histiocytosis

- Clinical: Pediatric patient
- Imaging: Destructive mastoid/middle ear mass

T-Bone Plasmacytoma

- Clinical: Often with multiple myeloma
- Imaging: Destructive PA lesion

PATHOLOGY

General Features

- Etiology
  - Marrow-filled PA may predispose to metastases
- Must exclude direct extension from local primary (nasopharynx, parotid, maxillary sinus, external ear)

CLINICAL ISSUES

Presentation

- Most common signs/symptoms
  - Hearing loss most common symptom
  - Asymptomatic or skull base/ear pain
- Other signs/symptoms
  - CN palsy (CNVIII > CNVII > CNV or CNVI)

Demographics

- Epidemiology
  - Breast > lung > renal > prostate cancer origin in adults
  - Neuroblastoma and leukemia most common in children

Natural History & Prognosis

- Poor, depends on primary tumor type

Treatment

- Surgery if tumor isolated to mastoid/middle ear
- Palliative depending on primary tumor type and other metastases

DIAGNOSTIC CHECKLIST

Image Interpretation Pearls

- Remember: PA marrow/pneumatization commonly asymmetric
- Isolated T-bone lesion is less likely to be metastasis

Reporting Tips

- Look for dura, dural venous sinus, and brain invasion

SELECTED REFERENCES

1. Wierzbicka M et al: Efficacy of petrosectomy in malignant invasion of the temporal bone. Br J Oral Maxillofac Surg. ePub, 2016
2. Morris LG et al: Predictors of survival and recurrence after temporal bone resection for cancer. Head Neck. 34(9):1231-9, 2012
3. Connor SE et al: Imaging of the petrous apex: a pictorial review. Br J Radiol. 81(965):427-35, 2008

Temporal Bone Osteoradionecrosis

TERMINOLOGY

- Radiation-induced injury to temporal bone

IMAGING

- Bone CT findings
  - **Moth-eaten destruction** of temporal bone and adjacent skull base ± **sequestrum**
- T2 MR findings
  - High-signal mucosal injury of external auditory canal (EAC), middle ear cavity, mastoid
  - High signal of adjacent brain → radiation necrosis
  - Meningitis, abscess, dural sinus thrombosis

TOP DIFFERENTIAL DIAGNOSES

- Malignant external otitis
- Coalescent mastoiditis
- Aggressive cholesteatoma
- EAC carcinoma
- Paget disease

PATHOLOGY

- **Avascular bone necrosis** from **obliterative endarteritis**
- Susceptible to infection, which accelerates ORN

CLINICAL ISSUES

- Presentation: Otalgia, otorrhea, hearing loss after regional radiation therapy (RT)
- Occurs few months to many years post RT (> 60 Gy)
  - Most common in setting of RT for parotid, EAC, or nasopharynx carcinoma
- Treatment options
  - Conservative management: 1st-line option
  - Surgical management and adjuvant therapy as indicated
  - Pentoxifylline, vitamin E, and clodronate (PENTOCLO) for prevention and treatment

DIAGNOSTIC CHECKLIST

- CT for bone changes, extent of involvement; MR for complications

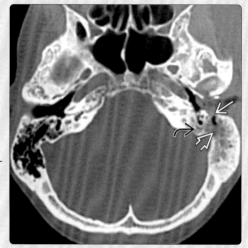
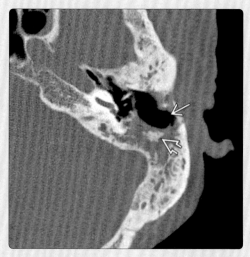

(Left) Axial bone CT reveals abnormal soft tissue ➡ filling the left external auditory canal (EAC) and mastoid air cells with obvious destruction of the posterior EAC wall and mastoid septations ➡. Note mixed sclerotic and lytic ▱ bone. Findings represent classic appearance of temporal bone osteoradionecrosis. (Right) Axial bone CT shows radiation-induced necrosis of the bony EAC ➡ and confluent destruction of mastoid air cells. Note "floating" bony sequestrum ➡, all indicating severe osteoradionecrosis.

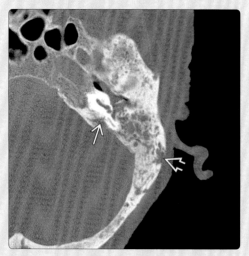
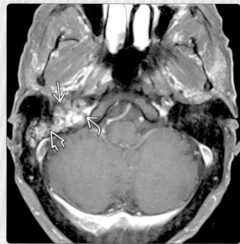

(Left) Axial bone CT shows diffuse opacification of the middle ear and mastoid in association with permeative-destructive bony changes in this previously radiated patient. Focal bone necrosis is seen in petrous bone ➡ and lateral mastoid cortex ➡. (Right) Axial T1 C+ FS MR in a previously radiated patient reveals nonspecific enhancing tissue in the middle ear ➡, mastoid ➡, and petrous apex ➡. Although radiation changes can be suggested by MR, ORN of bone is a diagnosis best made by temporal bone CT.

TERMINOLOGY

Abbreviations

- Osteoradionecrosis (ORN)

Synonyms

- Radiation osteitis, radiation necrosis, irradiation osteomyelitis, avascular bone necrosis

Definitions

- Radiation-induced injury to temporal bone
  - Localized (more common): Limited to external auditory canal (EAC)
  - Diffuse: Involves mastoid septations and middle ear cavity (MEC), possibly skull base

IMAGING

General Features

- Best diagnostic clue
  - Bone CT shows moth-eaten demineralization and destruction of temporal bone ± sequestrum

CT Findings

- CECT
  - Mucosal involvement may enhance
  - Contrast not needed to make diagnosis
- Bone CT
  - Diffuse mucosal thickening in EAC, MEC, and mastoid
  - **Permeative bone destruction ± sequestrum**

MR Findings

- T2WI
  - Nonspecific high signal in EAC, MEC, and mastoid
  - High-signal adjacent brain indicates **cerebral radiation necrosis**
- T1WI C+
  - Variable enhancement in osteitic bone
  - Mucosal injury will enhance

Imaging Recommendations

- Best imaging tool
  - Temporal bone CT
- Protocol advice
  - Thin-section axial and coronal bone CT
  - MR for complications
    - Cerebral radiation injury
    - Meningitis or abscess
    - Dural sinus thrombosis

DIFFERENTIAL DIAGNOSIS

Necrotizing External Otitis

- Immunocompromised, often diabetic patient; no radiation history
- EAC soft tissue and bone infection

Coalescent Mastoiditis

- Disruption of mastoid septa in acute/chronic otomastoiditis

Aggressive Cholesteatoma

- Cholesteatoma seen at otoscopy; no radiation history
- CT: Otic capsule invasion late finding

Paget Disease

- Bilateral sensorineural hearing loss
- Entire cranial base usually involved

EAC Carcinoma

- Skin lesion of EAC
- No prior radiation therapy (RT)

PATHOLOGY

General Features

- Etiology
  - Radiation dose > 60 Gy
  - **Avascular bone necrosis** from obliterative endarteritis
  - Susceptible to infection, which accelerates ORN
- Temporal bone at higher risk for ORN
  - Poorly vascularized bone
  - Thin protective overlying soft tissue
  - Exposure to respiratory pathogens via eustachian tube

Gross Pathologic & Surgical Features

- **Dead bone** and **soft tissue fibrosis**

CLINICAL ISSUES

Presentation

- Most common signs/symptoms
  - Purulent, foul-smelling otorrhea with spicules of exposed bone
  - Hearing loss
- Intracranial complications
  - Meningitis, abscess, sinus thrombosis, CSF leak

Natural History & Prognosis

- Occurs few months to many years post RT
  - More commonly in setting of parotid, EAC, or nasopharynx cancer
- Mastoid air cell destruction: Poor prognostic indicator

Treatment

- Conservative: Initial management for most patients
  - Local debridement of EAC
  - Antibiotics; otic prep (may need systemic treatment)
  - Pentoxifylline, vitamin E, and clodronate (PENTOCLO)
- Surgical: If conservative management fails
  - **Resect all necrotic tissue** ± repair with vascularized flap
  - Adjuvant PENTOCLO ± hyperbaric oxygen

DIAGNOSTIC CHECKLIST

Image Interpretation Pearls

- CT for bone changes; MR for soft tissue complications

SELECTED REFERENCES

1. Glicksman JT et al: Pentoxifylline-tocopherol-clodronate combination: a novel treatment for osteoradionecrosis of the temporal bone. Head Neck. 37(12):E191-3, 2015
2. Kammeijer Q et al: Treatment outcomes of temporal bone osteoradionecrosis. Otolaryngol Head Neck Surg. 152(4):718-23, 2015
3. Ahmed S et al: CT findings in temporal bone osteoradionecrosis. J Comput Assist Tomogr. 38(5):662-6, 2014

SECTION 26
CPA-IAC

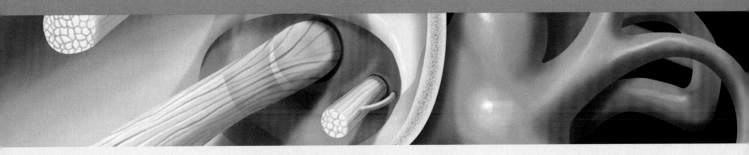

Terminology

The contents of the cerebellopontine angle (CPA) and internal auditory canal (IAC) cisterns include the facial nerve (CNVII), the vestibulocochlear nerve (CNVIII), and the anterior inferior cerebellar artery (AICA) loop. The bony IAC, its fundal crests (vertical and horizontal), and its opening in the porus acusticus are also included as part of this discussion.

Embryology

The temporal bone forms as 3 distinct embryological events: (1) The external and middle ear, (2) the inner ear, and (3) the IAC. The practical implications of these 3 related but separate embryological events are that the presence or absence of the IAC is independent of the development of the inner, middle, or external ear.

The IAC develops in response to formation and migration of the facial and vestibulocochlear nerves through this area. IAC size depends on the number of migrating nerve bundles. The fewer the nerve bundles, the smaller the IAC. If the IAC is very small and only 1 nerve is seen, it is usually the facial nerve.

Imaging Anatomy of Cochlea-IAC-CPA

The cochlear nerve portion of the vestibulocochlear nerve begins in the modiolus of the cochlea where the bipolar **spiral ganglia** are found. Distally projecting axons reach the organ of Corti within the scala media. Proximally projecting axons coalesce to form the cochlear nerve itself within the fundus of the IAC.

CNVIII in the IAC and CPA cisterns is made up of vestibular (balance) and cochlear (hearing) components. The cochlear nerve is located in the anteroinferior quadrant of the IAC. In the region of the porus acusticus, the cochlear nerve joins the superior and inferior vestibular nerve bundles to become the vestibulocochlear nerve in the CPA cistern.

The vestibulocochlear nerve crosses the CPA cistern as the posterior nerve bundle (CNVII is the anterior nerve bundle) to enter the brainstem at the junction of the medulla and pons. The entering cochlear nerve fibers pierce the brainstem and bifurcate to form synapses with both the **dorsal** and the **ventral cochlear nuclei**. These 2 nuclei are found on the lateral surface of the inferior cerebellar peduncle. Their location can be accurately determined by looking at high-resolution T2 axial images and identifying the contour of the inferior cerebellar peduncle. The entering vestibular nerve fibers divide into 4 branches to form synapses with the superior, inferior, medial, and lateral nuclei. The vestibular nuclei are clustered in the inferior cerebellar peduncle just anteromedial to the cochlear nuclei.

Remembering the normal orientation of nerves within the IAC cistern is assisted by the mnemonic "7-Up, Coke down." CNVII is found in the anterosuperior quadrant, whereas the cochlear nerve is confined to the anteroinferior quadrant. Given this information, it is simple to remember that the superior vestibular nerve (SVN) is posterosuperior, while the inferior vestibular nerve (IVN) is posteroinferior.

Other normal structures to be aware of in the IAC include the **horizontal crest** (crista falciformis) and the **vertical crest** ("Bill's bar"). The horizontal crest is a medially projecting horizontal bony shelf in the IAC fundus that separates the CNVII and SVN above from the cochlear nerve and IVN below. The vertical crest is found between CNVII and the SVN along the superior fundal bony wall. The horizontal crest is easily

seen on both bone CT and high-resolution MR. The vertical crest is more readily seen on bone CT.

Openings from the IAC fundus into the inner ear are numerous. The largest is the anteroinferior **cochlear nerve canal**, which conveys the cochlear nerve from the modiolus to the IAC fundus. Anterosuperiorly, the **meatal foramen** opens into the labyrinthine segment of CNVII. The **macula cribrosa** is the multiply perforated bone that separates the vestibule of the inner ear from the IAC fundus.

Other nonneural normal anatomy of interest in the CPA cistern includes the AICA loop, flocculus, and choroid plexus. The **AICA** arises from the basilar artery, courses superolaterally into the CPA cistern, and then travels into the IAC cistern. Within the IAC, the AICA feeds the internal auditory artery of the cochlea. The AICA loop in the IAC or CPA cisterns may mimic a cranial nerve bundle on high-resolution T2WI MR. AICA vascular territory includes the cochlea, flocculus of the cerebellum, and anterolateral pons in the area of cranial nerve nuclei for CNV, CNVII, and CNVIII. The **flocculus** is a lobule of the cerebellum that projects into the posterolateral CPA cistern. The 4th ventricle **choroid plexus** typically passes through the foramen of Luschka in the CPA cistern.

Imaging Techniques & Indications

The principal clinical indication requiring radiologists to examine the CPA-IAC is **sensorineural hearing loss (SNHL)**. Three principal parameters must be satisfied when completing the MR study in SNHL: (1) Use contrast-enhanced T1 fat-saturated thin-section sequences through the CPA-IAC to identify enhancing lesions in this location, (2) utilize high-resolution T2-weighted sequences to answer presurgical questions when a mass lesion is found, and (3) screen the brain for intraaxial causes, such as multiple sclerosis.

The gold standard for imaging patients with acquired SNHL is enhanced thin-section (≤ 3 mm) axial and coronal fat-saturated MR through the CPA-IAC. With these enhanced sequences, it is highly unlikely that a lesion causing SNHL will be missed. Be sure to obtain an axial or coronal precontrast T1 sequence and use fat saturation when contrast is applied to avoid the rare but troublesome mistake of calling a CPA-IAC lipoma a vestibular schwannoma. In the absence of fat saturation, the inherent high signal of lipoma will appear to enhance, leading to the misdiagnosis of vestibular schwannoma.

High-resolution T2-weighted thin-section (≤ 1 mm) MR sequences (CISS, FIESTA, T2 space) in the axial and coronal planes can be used as a screening exam without contrast to identify patients with mass lesions in the CPA-IAC area. However, these sequences are currently more commonly used as supplements when vestibular schwannoma is found on the enhanced T1 sequences to answer specific surgically relevant questions: What size is the fundal cap? What is the nerve of origin? Does the lesion enter the cochlear foramen?

Whenever MR is ordered for SNHL, remember to include whole-brain FLAIR, GRE, and DWI sequences. FLAIR will identify the rare multiple sclerosis patient presenting with SNHL as well as other intraaxial causes. GRE will demonstrate micro- or macrohemorrhage within a vestibular schwannoma and may help with aneurysm diagnosis when blooming of blood products or calcium in an aneurysm wall is seen. When

CPA Mass Differential Diagnosis

Pseudolesions	Vascular
Asymmetric cerebellar flocculus	Aneurysm (vertebrobasilar, posterior and anterior inferior cerebellar artery)
Asymmetric choroid plexus	Arteriovenous malformation
High jugular bulb	**Benign tumor**
Jugular bulb diverticulum	Choroid plexus papilloma
Marrow foci around internal auditory canal	Facial nerve schwannoma
Congenital	Hemangioblastoma, cerebellum
Arachnoid cyst	IAC hemangioma (venous malformation)
Epidermoid cyst	Meningioma
Lipoma	Vestibular schwannoma
Neurofibromatosis type 2	**Malignant tumor**
Infectious	Brainstem glioma, pedunculated
Cysticercosis	Ependymoma, pedunculated
Meningitis	Melanotic schwannoma
Inflammatory	Metastases, systemic or subarachnoid spread ("drop")
Idiopathic intracranial pseudotumor	
Sarcoidosis	

DWI shows restricted diffusion in a CPA mass, the diagnosis of **epidermoid** is easily made.

Approaches to Imaging Issues of CPA-IAC

Approach to Sensorineural Hearing Loss in Adult

Unilateral SNHL in an otherwise healthy adult is evaluated with an enhanced thin-section fat-saturated T1WI MR of the CPA-IAC area, with high-resolution T2WI sequences providing help in surgical planning if a lesion is identified. Despite audiometric and brainstem-evoked response testing in the otolaryngology clinic, positive MR studies for lesions causing the SNHL are infrequent (< 5% even in highly screened patient groups). **Vestibular schwannoma** is by far the most common cause of unilateral SNHL (about 90% of lesions found with MR). It is important for the radiologist to become familiar with the wide range of appearances of vestibular schwannoma, including intramural cystic change, micro- and macroscopic hemorrhage, and associated arachnoid cyst.

Meningioma, epidermoid cyst, and CPA aneurysm are responsible for about 8% of lesions found in adult patients with SNHL. A long list of rare lesions, including otosclerosis, facial nerve, labyrinthine and jugular foramen schwannomas, IAC hemangioma, CPA metastases, labyrinthitis, sarcoidosis, lipoma, and superficial siderosis, make up < 2% of lesions causing unilateral SNHL in an adult that are found by MR.

Approach to Sensorineural Hearing Loss in Child

When a child presents with unilateral or bilateral SNHL, the emphasis in the imaging work-up veers away from the typical adult tumor causes. Instead, congenital inner ear or CPA-IAC lesions are sought as the cause of the hearing loss. Complications of suppurative labyrinthitis (labyrinthine ossificans) are also included in the differential diagnosis.

When the child's presentation is bilateral profound SNHL, imaging is usually obtained as part of the work-up for possible **cochlear implantation**. High-resolution T2 MR imaging is obtained in the axial and **oblique sagittal** planes to look for

inner ear anomalies and labyrinthine ossificans as well as the presence or absence of a cochlear nerve in the IAC. If complex congenital inner ear disease is found, bone CT is often obtained to further define the inner ear fluid spaces and look for an absent cochlear nerve canal.

In reviewing the MR and CT in a child with SNHL, it is important to accurately describe any inner ear congenital anomaly, if present. If there is a history of meningitis, labyrinthine ossificans may be present. Look for bony encroachment on the fluid spaces of the inner ear. In particular, make sure the basal turn of the cochlea is open because occlusion by bony plaque may thwart successful cochlear implantation. Check the T2 oblique sagittal MR images for the presence of a normal cochlear nerve. If absent, cochlear implantation results may be negatively affected. Finally, look carefully at the IAC and CPA for signs of epidermoid cyst (restricted diffusion on DWI), lipoma (high signal on T1 precontrast sequences), and neurofibromatosis type 2 (bilateral CPA-IAC vestibular or facial schwannoma).

Selected References

1. Giesemann AM et al: The vestibulocochlear nerve: aplasia and hypoplasia in combination with inner ear malformations. Eur Radiol. 22(3):519-24, 2012
2. Burmeister HP et al: Identification of the nervus intermedius using 3T MR imaging. AJNR Am J Neuroradiol. 32(3):460-4, 2011
3. Sheth S et al: Appearance of normal cranial nerves on steady-state free precession MR images. Radiographics. 29(4):1045-55, 2009
4. Trimble K et al: Computed tomography and/or magnetic resonance imaging before pediatric cochlear implantation? Developing an investigative strategy. Otol Neurotol. 28(3):317-24, 2007
5. Rabinov JD et al: Virtual cisternoscopy: 3D MRI models of the cerebellopontine angle for lesions related to the cranial nerves. Skull Base. 14(2):93-9; discussion 99, 2004
6. Daniels RL et al: Causes of unilateral sensorineural hearing loss screened by high-resolution fast spin echo magnetic resonance imaging: review of 1,070 consecutive cases. Am J Otol. 21(2):173-80, 2000
7. Schmalbrock P et al: Assessment of internal auditory canal tumors: a comparison of contrast-enhanced T1-weighted and steady-state T2-weighted gradient-echo MR imaging. AJNR Am J Neuroradiol. 20(7):1207-13, 1999

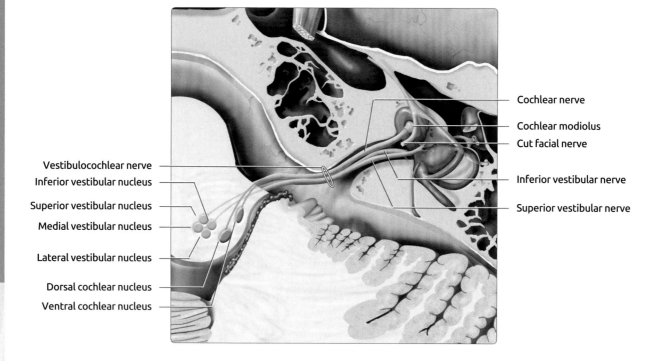

Cochlear nerve

Cochlear modiolus

Cut facial nerve

Inferior vestibular nerve

Superior vestibular nerve

Vestibulocochlear nerve

Inferior vestibular nucleus

Superior vestibular nucleus

Medial vestibular nucleus

Lateral vestibular nucleus

Dorsal cochlear nucleus

Ventral cochlear nucleus

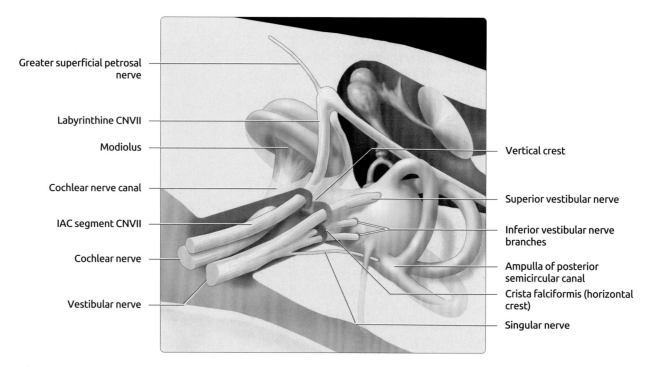

Greater superficial petrosal nerve

Labyrinthine CNVII

Modiolus

Cochlear nerve canal

IAC segment CNVII

Cochlear nerve

Vestibular nerve

Vertical crest

Superior vestibular nerve

Inferior vestibular nerve branches

Ampulla of posterior semicircular canal

Crista falciformis (horizontal crest)

Singular nerve

(Top) *Axial graphic depicts the vestibulocochlear nerve (CNVIII). The cochlear component of CNVIII begins in bipolar cell bodies within the spiral ganglion in the modiolus. Central fibers run in the cochlear nerve to the dorsal and ventral cochlear nuclei on the lateral margin of the inferior cerebellar peduncle. Inferior and superior vestibular nerves begin in cell bodies in the vestibular ganglion; from there, they course centrally to 4 vestibular nuclei.* (Bottom) *Graphic shows the normal facial nerve and vestibulocochlear nerve in the internal auditory canal (IAC) and temporal bone. Notice that by the mid IAC, there are 4 main nerves present, including the facial, cochlear, superior vestibular, and inferior vestibular nerves. The singular nerve branches off the inferior vestibular nerve midway through the IAC on its way to the ampulla of the posterior semicircular canal. Multiple inferior vestibular nerve branches pierce the macular cribrosa, as does the superior vestibular nerve, on their way to the vestibule.*

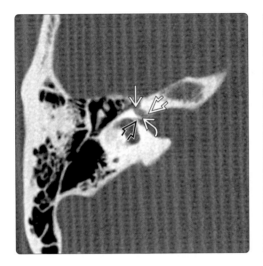

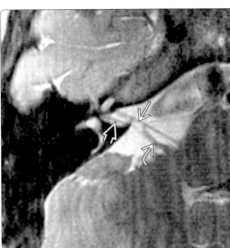

(Left) *Axial bone CT through the superior IAC reveals the labyrinthine segment of CNVII* ➡, *the meatal foramen* ⮞, *the vertical crest* ➡, *and the superior vestibular nerve* ⇨ *connecting the IAC to the vestibule through the macula cribrosa.* **(Right)** *Axial T2WI MR through the superior IAC shows the anterosuperior CNVII* ➡, *the superior vestibular nerve* ⮞, *and the vestibulocochlear nerve* ⮞.

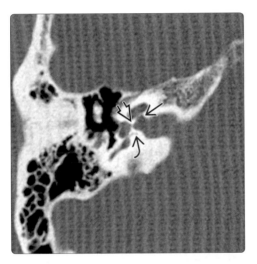

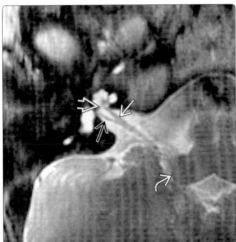

(Left) *Axial bone CT through the mid IAC shows the cochlear nerve canal* ⮕, *inferior vestibular nerve leaving the fundus* ⮞, *and singular nerve canal containing the posterior branch of the inferior vestibular nerve* ⮕. **(Right)** *Axial T2WI MR through the inferior IAC reveals the cochlear nerve* ➡ *projecting into the cochlear nerve canal* ⮞. *Dorsal and ventral cochlear nuclei are not seen but are known to reside in the lateral inferior cerebellar peduncle margin* ⮞. *Note the inferior vestibular nerve* ⮕.

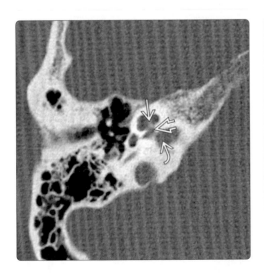

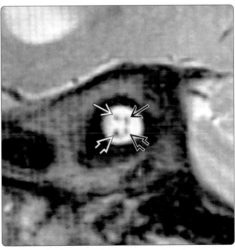

(Left) *Axial bone CT through the inferior IAC demonstrates the cochlear modiolus as a high-density structure at the cochlear base* ⮞. *The cochlear nerve canal* ⮞ *and the fundus of the IAC* ⮞ *are also labeled.* **(Right)** *Oblique sagittal T2WI MR shows the 4 nerve bundles of the mid IAC cistern. CNVII is anterosuperior* ⮞, *the cochlear nerve is anteroinferior* ⮞, *and the superior* ⮕ *and inferior* ⮞ *vestibular nerves are posterosuperior and posteroinferior, respectively.*

TERMINOLOGY

- Definition: Congenital inclusion of ectodermal epithelial elements during neural tube closure

IMAGING

- CPA cisternal **insinuating** mass with high signal on DWI MR
  - 90% intradural, 10% extradural
  - Margins usually scalloped or irregular
  - Cauliflower-like margins with "fronds" possible
- TI and T2: Isointense or slightly hyperintense to CSF
- DWI: **Restricted diffusion** makes diagnosis

TOP DIFFERENTIAL DIAGNOSES

- Arachnoid cyst in CPA
- Cystic neoplasm in CPA
  - Cystic vestibular schwannoma
  - Cystic meningioma
  - Infratentorial ependymoma
  - Pilocytic astrocytoma

- Neurenteric cyst
- Neurocysticercosis, CPA

PATHOLOGY

- Surgical appearance: Pearly white CPA cistern mass
- Cyst wall: Internal layer of stratified squamous epithelium covered by fibrous capsule

CLINICAL ISSUES

- Clinical presentation
  - Principal presenting symptom: Dizziness and headache
    - Sensorineural hearing loss also common
  - If extends to lateral pons: Trigeminal neuralgia
  - Rarer symptoms: Facial palsy, seizure
- Treatment: Complete surgical removal is goal
  - If adherent to neural structures, complete removal may not be possible
  - If recurs, takes many years to grow
  - DWI MR key to diagnosing recurrence

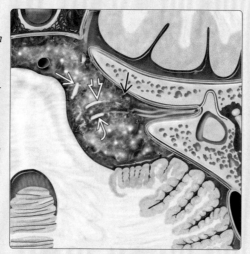
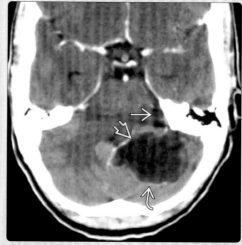

(Left) Axial graphic shows a large cerebellopontine angle (CPA) epidermoid cyst within a typical bed of pearls appearance. Note that the V, ➡, VII ➡, and VIII ➡ cranial nerves along with the anterior inferior cerebellar artery loop ➡ are characteristically engulfed by this insinuating mass. (Right) Axial CECT shows a large CPA epidermoid cyst ➡. Note that this nonenhancing low-density lesion appears to invade the left cerebellar hemisphere ➡. Minimal rim enhancement is visible along the posterior margin of the cyst ➡.

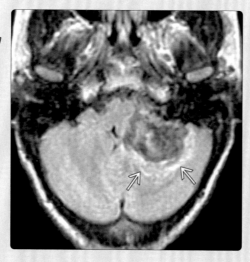
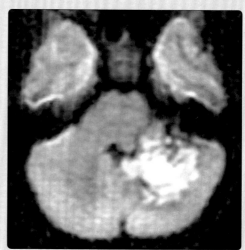

(Left) Axial FLAIR MR of the same patient shows "incomplete" or partial nulling of the signal of this large epidermoid cyst. Associated high signal ➡ along the deep margins of the lesion is most likely due to gliosis of the cerebellar hemisphere. (Right) Axial DWI MR in the same patient reveals the expected high signal from epidermoid cyst diffusion restriction. DWI sequence allows straightforward differentiation of this epidermoid cyst from an arachnoid cyst.

TERMINOLOGY

Synonyms

- Epidermoid tumor, primary cholesteatoma, or epithelial inclusion cyst

Definitions

- Congenital **inclusion** of ectodermal epithelial elements during neural tube closure

IMAGING

General Features

- Best diagnostic clue
  - Cerebellopontine angle (CPA) cistern **insinuating** mass with high signal on DWI MR
    - Engulfs cranial nerves (7th and 8th) and anterior inferior cerebellar artery (AICA) loop
- Location
  - 90% intradural, 10% extradural
    - Posterior fossa location most common
      - CPA ~ 40%; 4th ventricle ~ 20%
- Size
  - Wide range: 1- to 8-cm diameter or more
- Morphology
  - Insinuating mass in cisterns
  - Margins usually scalloped or irregular
    - Cauliflower-like margins with "fronds" possible
  - When large, compresses or invades brainstem ± cerebellum

CT Findings

- NECT
  - Similar density to CSF
  - Calcification in 20%, usually margins
  - Pressure erosion of temporal bone and skull base may occur
  - Rare variant: "Dense epidermoid"
    - 3% of intracranial epidermoids
    - From protein, cyst debris saponification to calcium soaps or iron-containing pigment
- CECT
  - No enhancement is rule
    - Sometimes margin of cyst minimally enhances

MR Findings

- T1WI
  - Isointense or slightly hyperintense to CSF
  - If hyperintense, term "dirty CSF" has been applied
  - Rare variant: "White epidermoid" with high T1 compared to brain
    - Secondary to high triglycerides and unsaturated fatty acids
    - Caveat: If lesion in prepontine cistern, consider neuroepithelial cyst diagnosis
  - Epidermoid with hemorrhage
    - Mixed low- and high-signal areas
    - High signal secondary to methemoglobin
- T2WI
  - Isointense to hyperintense to CSF
  - "White epidermoid": Low T2 signal

- FLAIR
  - Does not null (attenuate) like CSF or arachnoid cyst
- DWI
  - **Restricted diffusion** on DWI or DTI **makes diagnosis**
    - Secondary to high fractional anisotropy from diffusion along 2D geometric plane
      - Due to microstructure of parallel-layered keratin filaments and flakes
  - Apparent diffusion coefficient (ADC) = low signal
  - High-signal foci on DWI trace images in surgical bed indicates recurrence
- T1WI C+
  - No enhancement is rule
  - Subtle marginal enhancement may occur (25%)
- MRA
  - Vessels of CPA may be displaced or engulfed
  - Artery wall dimension not affected
- MRS
  - Resonances from lactate
  - No NAA, choline, or lipid

Imaging Recommendations

- Best imaging tool
  - Brain MR with FLAIR, DWI, and T1WI C+ sequences
- Protocol advice
  - DWI sequences make diagnosis
  - If looking for recurrence, DWI (DTI) is best sequence

DIFFERENTIAL DIAGNOSIS

Arachnoid Cyst in Cerebellopontine Angle

- Displaces, does not engulf, adjacent structures
- Isointense to CSF on all standard MR sequences
  - T2 higher signal possible; if no CSF pulsations
- Completely nulls on FLAIR (low signal)
- Hypointense (no restricted diffusion) on DWI trace MR
  - Contains highly mobile CSF
  - ADC = stationary water

Cystic Neoplasm in Cerebellopontine Angle

- Cystic vestibular schwannoma
- Cystic meningioma in CPA
- Infratentorial ependymoma
  - Pedunculates from 4th ventricle
- Pilocytic astrocytoma
  - Pedunculates from cerebellum
- All show some areas of enhancement on T1WI C+ MR

Neurenteric Cyst

- Most common prepontine cistern in location
- T1 high signal (might mimic "white epidermoid")
- T2 signal often low

Neurocysticercosis in Cerebellopontine Angle

- Partially enhances
- Density/signal intensity does not precisely follow CSF
- Adjacent brain edema or gliosis common

PATHOLOGY

General Features

- Etiology

- Congenital **inclusion of ectodermal elements** during neural tube closure
  - 3rd to 5th week of embryogenesis
- CPA lesion derived from 1st branchial groove cells

Gross Pathologic & Surgical Features

- **Pearly white mass** in CPA
- Surgeons refer to it as "beautiful tumor"
- Lobulated, cauliflower-shaped surface features
- Insinuating growth pattern in cisterns
  - Engulfs cisternal vessels and nerves
    - May become adherent
- Lesion filled with soft, waxy, creamy, or flaky material

Microscopic Features

- Cyst wall: Internal layer of stratified squamous epithelium covered by fibrous capsule
- Cyst contents: Solid crystalline cholesterol, keratinaceous debris
  - **No** dermal appendages (hair follicles, sebaceous glands, or fat)
  - If any of these present, consider dermoid
- Grows in successive layers by desquamation of squamous epithelium from cyst wall
  - Conversion to keratin/cholesterol crystals forms concentric lamellae

CLINICAL ISSUES

Presentation

- Most common signs/symptoms
  - Principal presenting symptoms: Dizziness
  - Other symptoms depend on location, growth pattern
    - Sensorineural hearing loss: Common symptom
    - Trigeminal neuralgia (tic douloureux): If extends to lateral pontine CNV root entry zone
    - Seizures: If extends superiorly through incisura to temporomesial location
  - Symptoms usually present for > 4 years before diagnosis
- Clinical profile
  - 40-year-old patient with minor symptoms and large lesion discovered in CPA on MR
  - Asymptomatic patient shows incidental hyperintense lesion in CPA on DWI MR sequence

Demographics

- Age
  - Although congenital, presents in adult life
  - Broad presentation: 20-60 years
    - Peak age: 40 years
- Epidemiology
  - 3rd most common CPA mass
  - 1% of all intracranial tumors

Natural History & Prognosis

- Slow-growing congenital lesions that remain clinically silent for many years
- Smaller cisternal lesions are readily cured with surgery
- Larger lesions with upward supratentorial herniation are more difficult to completely remove
  - Larger lesions have more significant surgical complications

Treatment

- Complete surgical removal is goal
  - If large, near-total removal is prudent surgical choice
    - Aggressive total removal may cause significant cranial neuropathy
    - Used when capsule is adherent to brainstem and cranial nerves
- If recurs, takes many years to grow
  - DWI MR key to diagnosing recurrence

DIAGNOSTIC CHECKLIST

Consider

- MR diagnosis based on
  - Insinuating CPA lesion
  - Low signal on T1, high on T2 (similar but not identical to CSF)
  - No or partial nulling on FLAIR
  - Hyperintense on DWI trace images

Image Interpretation Pearls

- **Diffusion MR** imaging sequence is **key to correct diagnosis**

Reporting Tips

- Be sure to report prepontine or medial middle cranial fossa extension if present

SELECTED REFERENCES

1. Gopalakrishnan CV et al: Long term outcome in surgically treated posterior fossa epidermoids. Clin Neurol Neurosurg. 117:93-9, 2014
2. Schiefer TK et al: Epidermoids of the cerebellopontine angle: a 20-year experience. Surg Neurol. 70(6):584-90; discussion 590, 2008
3. Bonneville F et al: Imaging of cerebellopontine angle lesions: an update. Part 2: intra-axial lesions, skull base lesions that may invade the CPA region, and non-enhancing extra-axial lesions. Eur Radiol. 17(11):2908-20, 2007
4. Dutt SN et al: Radiologic differentiation of intracranial epidermoids from arachnoid cysts. Otol Neurotol. 23(1):84-92, 2002
5. Kobata H et al: Cerebellopontine angle epidermoids presenting with cranial nerve hyperactive dysfunction: pathogenesis and long-term surgical results in 30 patients. Neurosurgery. 50(2):276-85; discussion 285-6, 2002
6. Dechambre S et al: Diffusion-weighted MRI postoperative assessment of an epidermoid tumour in the cerebellopontine angle. Neuroradiology. 41(11):829-31, 1999
7. Ochi M et al: Unusual CT and MR appearance of an epidermoid tumor of the cerebellopontine angle. AJNR Am J Neuroradiol. 19(6):1113-5, 1998
8. Talacchi A et al: Assessment and surgical management of posterior fossa epidermoid tumors: report of 28 cases. Neurosurgery. 42(2):242-51; discussion 251-2, 1998
9. Timmer FA et al: Chemical analysis of an epidermoid cyst with unusual CT and MR characteristics. AJNR Am J Neuroradiol. 19(6):1111-2, 1998
10. Ikushima I et al: MR of epidermoids with a variety of pulse sequences. AJNR Am J Neuroradiol. 18(7):1359-63, 1997
11. Kallmes DF et al: Typical and atypical MR imaging features of intracranial epidermoid tumors. AJR Am J Roentgenol. 169(3):883-7, 1997
12. Tien RD et al: Variable bandwidth steady-state free-precession MR imaging: a technique for improving characterization of epidermoid tumor and arachnoid cyst. AJR Am J Roentgenol. 164(3):689-92, 1995
13. Gao PY et al: Radiologic-pathologic correlation. Epidermoid tumor of the cerebellopontine angle. AJNR Am J Neuroradiol. 13(3):863-72, 1992
14. Tsuruda JS et al: Diffusion-weighted MR imaging of the brain: value of differentiating between extraaxial cysts and epidermoid tumors. AJNR Am J Neuroradiol. 11(5):925-31; discussion 932-4, 1990
15. Tampieri D et al: MR imaging of epidermoid cysts. AJNR Am J Neuroradiol. 10(2):351-6, 1989

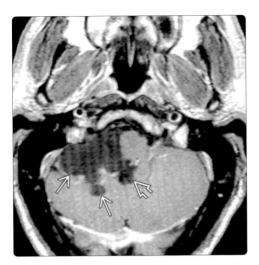

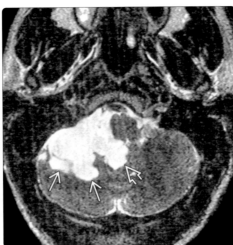

(Left) *Axial T1WI C+ MR demonstrates a large, insinuating, right CPA cistern epidermoid cyst ➡. Note the low signal with lack of enhancement of the lesion. The cyst insinuates into the cerebellar hemisphere and foramen of Luschka ⇉.* (Right) *Axial T2WI MR in the same patient reveals a large, insinuating epidermoid cyst with typical high T2 signal and invagination into the cerebellar hemisphere ➡ and foramen of Luschka ⇉.*

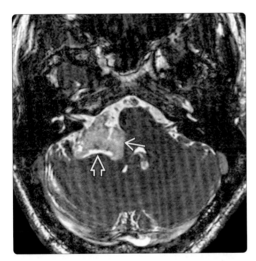

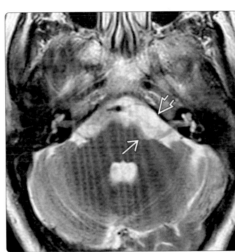

(Left) *Axial T2 FS thin-section high-resolution MR shows a right CPA epidermoid cyst. Note the cauliflower-like surface architecture. This lesion is compressing the brachium pontis ➡ and adjacent cerebellar hemisphere ⇉.* (Right) *Axial T2WI MR shows slight widening of the left CPA cistern ⇉ with minimal mass effect on the brachium pontis ➡, but no definite lesion is visible. In a patient with left sensorineural hearing loss, arachnoid cyst or epidermoid cyst should be considered.*

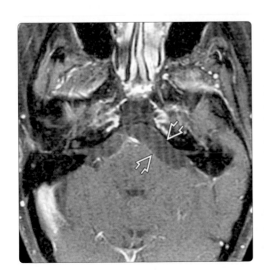

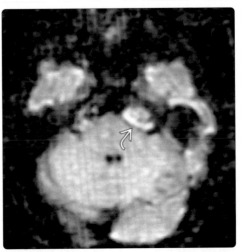

(Left) *Axial T1WI C+ FS MR in the same patient again reveals a widened CPA cistern ⇉ but no evidence of enhancing tumor. If an epidermoid cyst is present in the enlarged cistern, DWI sequences will be positive with restricted diffusion making the diagnosis.* (Right) *Axial DWI MR in the same patient demonstrates the characteristic restricted diffusion of the epidermoid cyst ➡ in the left CPA cistern. Without DWI information, the lesion could have been missed altogether.*

TERMINOLOGY

- Arachnoid cyst (AC) definition: Developmental arachnoid duplication anomaly creating CSF-filled sac

IMAGING

- Sharply demarcated ovoid extraaxial cisternal cyst with imperceptible walls with CSF density (CT) or intensity (MR)
- AC signal parallels (is isointense) CSF on **all** MR sequences
- Complete fluid attenuation on FLAIR MR
- **No** diffusion restriction on DWI MR imaging

TOP DIFFERENTIAL DIAGNOSES

- Epidermoid cyst in cerebellopontine angle (CPA)
- Cystic vestibular schwannoma
- Neurenteric cyst
- Cystic meningioma in CPA
- Cystic infratentorial ependymoma
- Cerebellar pilocytic astrocytoma

CLINICAL ISSUES

- Clinical presentation
  - Small AC: Asymptomatic, incidental finding (MR)
  - Large AC: Mostly asymptomatic
    - Symptoms may arise from direct compression ± ↑ intracranial pressure
- Natural history
  - Vast majority of ACs **do not** enlarge over time
- Treatment options
  - Most cases require **no** treatment
  - Treatment is highly selective process

DIAGNOSTIC CHECKLIST

- Differentiate AC from epidermoid cyst
- AC: No restriction on DWI = best clue
- Reporting tip: Since AC is usually not treated surgically, avoid offering any differential diagnosis when imaging findings diagnose AC

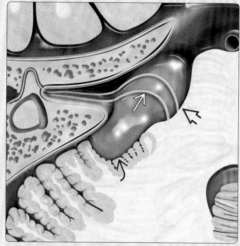
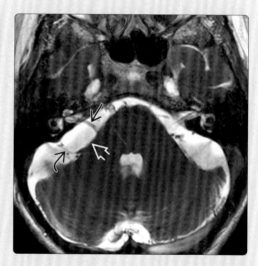

(Left) *Axial graphic of an arachnoid cyst in the cerebellopontine angle (CPA) shows a thin, translucent wall. Notice the cyst bowing the VII and VIII cranial nerves anteriorly ➡ and effacing of the brainstem ➡ and cerebellum ➡. (Right) Axial T2WI MR reveals a right CPA arachnoid cyst causing bowing of the facial and vestibulocochlear nerves anteriorly ➡, small bridging veins posteriorly ➡, and flattening of the lateral margin of the brachium pontis ➡.*

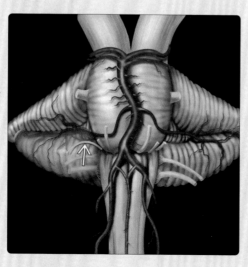
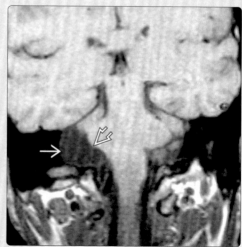

(Left) *Coronal graphic of a CPA arachnoid cyst depicts a typical translucent cyst wall. CNVII and CNVIII are pushed by the cyst ➡ without being engulfed by it. In an epidermoid cyst, cranial nerves are usually engulfed. (Right) Coronal T1WI MR demonstrates a small CSF intensity CPA arachnoid cyst ➡ with subtle mass effect on the adjacent brainstem ➡. Complete fluid attenuation on FLAIR MR helps differentiate this lesion from an epidermoid cyst, which is the primary imaging differential diagnosis.*

TERMINOLOGY

Abbreviations

- Arachnoid cyst (AC)

Synonyms

- Primary or congenital AC, subarachnoid cyst

Definitions

- Developmental arachnoid duplication anomaly creating **intraarachnoid** CSF-filled sac

IMAGING

General Features

- Best diagnostic clue
  - Sharply demarcated ovoid or lentiform extraaxial cisternal cyst with imperceptible walls with CSF density (CT) or signal intensity (MR)
  - AC signal parallels CSF (is isointense to CSF) on all MR sequences
    - **Complete fluid attenuation** on FLAIR MR
    - **No diffusion restriction** on DWI MR imaging
- Location
  - 10-20% of all ACs occur in posterior fossa
    - Cerebellopontine angle (CPA) = most common infratentorial site
    - **10%** found in CPA
  - Spread patterns
    - Most remain confined to CPA (60%)
    - May spread dorsally along brainstem (25%)
    - Rarely spread into internal auditory canal (IAC)
- Size
  - Broad range: 1 cm to giant (> 8 cm)
  - In posterior fossa, when very large may be symptomatic
  - When large, will exert mass effect on vestibulocochlear and facial nerves, adjacent brainstem, and cerebellum
- Morphology
  - Sharply demarcated with broad-arching margins
  - Displaces, does not engulf, surrounding structures
  - Pushes cisternal structures but does not insinuate
    - Epidermoid cyst insinuates adjacent structures

CT Findings

- NECT
  - Density same as CSF
  - Rare high density from hemorrhage or proteinaceous fluid
- CECT
  - No enhancement of cavity or wall
- Bone CT
  - Rarely causes expansile remodeling of bone
    - Seen mostly in children
- CT cisternography
  - May show connection to subarachnoid space

MR Findings

- T1WI
  - Low-signal AC is isointense to CSF
- T2WI
  - High-signal lesion isointense to CSF
    - May have brighter signal than CSF

- Cyst fluid lacks CSF pulsations
  - Well-circumscribed lesion
    - Compresses adjacent CNVII-VIII bundle, brainstem, and cerebellum when large
- FLAIR
  - Suppresses AC fluid completely
- DWI
  - No diffusion restriction
- T1WI C+
  - No enhancement seen
- High-resolution, thin-section MR (CISS, FIESTA, T2 space)
  - Help define cyst wall, relationship to adjacent structures (CNVII, CNVIII, anterior inferior cerebellar artery, etc.)
- Phase-contrast cine MR
  - Flow quantification can sometimes distinguish AC from subarachnoid space
  - May rarely show connection between AC and cistern

Ultrasonographic Findings

- Grayscale ultrasound
  - Shows hypoechoic AC in infants < 1 year of age
  - Larger AC diagnosed in utero

Imaging Recommendations

- Best imaging tool
  - MR ± contrast
- Protocol advice
  - Add FLAIR (suppresses)
  - Add DWI (no restricted diffusion)

DIFFERENTIAL DIAGNOSIS

Epidermoid Cyst in CPA

- Major lesion of differential concern in setting of AC
- FLAIR: Incomplete fluid attenuation
- DWI: Restricted diffusion (high signal)
- Morphology: Insinuates into adjacent CSF spaces

Cystic Vestibular Schwannoma in CPA-IAC

- Intramural or marginal cysts seen in larger lesions
- Foci of enhancing tumor always present on T1WI C+ MR
- Rarely, larger lesions have associated AC

Cystic Meningioma in CPA-IAC

- Rare meningioma variant
- Dural tails, asymmetry to IAC still present with mixed enhancement on T1WI C+ MR

Neurenteric Cyst

- Rare prepontine cistern near midline
- Often contains proteinaceous fluid (↑ on T1WI MR)

Cystic Infratentorial Ependymoma

- Ependymoma pedunculates from 4th ventricle via foramen of Luschka
- 50% calcified
- Cystic and solid enhancing components

Cerebellar Pilocytic Astrocytoma

- Cystic tumor in cerebellar hemisphere
- Enhancing mural nodule

PATHOLOGY

General Features

- Etiology
  - Embryonic meninges fail to merge
    - Remain separate as **duplicated** arachnoid
    - Split arachnoid contains CSF
  - 2 types
    - Noncommunicating; most common type
    - Communicating with subarachnoid space/cistern
- Genetics
  - Usually sporadic; rarely familial
  - Inherited disorders of metabolism
    - "Sticky" leptomeninges: Mucopolysaccharidoses
- Associated abnormalities
  - Vestibular schwannoma has AC associated in 0.5%

Gross Pathologic & Surgical Features

- Fluid-containing cyst with translucent membrane
- Displaces adjacent vessels or cranial nerves

Microscopic Features

- Thin wall of flattened but normal arachnoid cells

CLINICAL ISSUES

Presentation

- Most common signs/symptoms
  - Small AC: **Asymptomatic, incidental** finding (MR)
  - Large AC: Symptoms from direct compression ± ↑ intracranial pressure
  - Pediatric AC associated with higher symptom rate
- Other signs/symptoms
  - Defined by location and size
    - Headache
    - Dizziness, tinnitus ± sensorineural hearing loss
      - □ Rarely facial nerve symptoms
    - Hemifacial spasm or trigeminal neuralgia
- Clinical profile
  - Adult undergoing brain MR for unrelated symptoms

Demographics

- Age
  - May be initially seen at any age
    - 75% of AC identified in childhood
- Gender
  - M:F = 3:1
- Epidemiology
  - Most common congenital intracranial cystic lesion
  - Accounts for 1% of intracranial masses

Natural History & Prognosis

- Most ACs **do not enlarge** over time
  - Infrequently enlarge via CSF pulsation through ball-valve opening into AC
  - Hemorrhage with subsequent ↓ in size reported
- If surgery is limited to AC where symptoms are clearly related, prognosis is excellent
- Radical cyst removal may result in cranial neuropathy ± vascular compromise

Treatment

- Most cases require **no treatment**
  - Pediatric AC more commonly treated than adult AC
- Surgical intervention is highly selective process
  - Reserved for cases where clear symptoms can be directly linked to AC anatomic location
  - Endoscopic cyst decompression via fenestration
    - Least invasive initial approach

DIAGNOSTIC CHECKLIST

Consider

- Differentiate AC from epidermoid cyst
  - AC: No restriction on DWI = best clue
- Determine if symptoms match location of AC before considering surgical treatment

Image Interpretation Pearls

- AC signal follows CSF on all MR sequences
  - Remember T2 signal may be higher than CSF from lack of CSF pulsation
- **DWI** sequence shows AC as **low signal**
- **FLAIR** sequence shows AC as **low signal**
- **No** enhancement of AC, including wall, is expected
  - Nodular enhancement suggests alternative diagnosis

Reporting Tips

- Since AC is usually not treated surgically, avoid offering any differential diagnosis when imaging findings diagnose AC

SELECTED REFERENCES

1. Gangemi M et al: Endoscopy versus microsurgical cyst excision and shunting for treating intracranial arachnoid cysts. J Neurosurg Pediatr. 8(2):158-64, 2011
2. Jayarao M et al: Recovery of sensorineural hearing loss following operative management of a posterior fossa arachnoid cyst. Case report. J Neurosurg Pediatr. 4(2):121-4, 2009
3. Boutarbouch M et al: Management of intracranial arachnoid cysts: institutional experience with initial 32 cases and review of the literature. Clin Neurol Neurosurg. 110(1):1-7, 2008
4. Helland CA et al: A population-based study of intracranial arachnoid cysts: clinical and neuroimaging outcomes following surgical cyst decompression in children. J Neurosurg. 105(5 Suppl):385-90, 2006
5. Osborn AG et al: Intracranial cysts: radiologic-pathologic correlation and imaging approach. Radiology. 239(3):650-64, 2006
6. Tang L et al: Diffusion-weighted imaging distinguishes recurrent epidermoid neoplasm from postoperative arachnoid cyst in the lumbosacral spine. J Comput Assist Tomogr. 30(3):507-9, 2006
7. Alaani A et al: Cerebellopontine angle arachnoid cysts in adult patients: what is the appropriate management? J Laryngol Otol. 119(5):337-41, 2005
8. Yildiz H et al: evaluation of communication between intracranial arachnoid cysts and cisterns with phase-contrast cine MR imaging. AJNR Am J Neuroradiol. 26(1):145-51, 2005
9. Boltshauser E et al: Outcome in children with space-occupying posterior fossa arachnoid cysts. Neuropediatrics. 33(3):118-21, 2002
10. Dutt SN et al: Radiologic differentiation of intracranial epidermoids from arachnoid cysts. Otol Neurotol. 23(1):84-92, 2002
11. Gangemi M et al: Endoscopic surgery for large posterior fossa arachnoid cysts. Minim Invasive Neurosurg. 44(1):21-4, 2001
12. Samii M et al: Arachnoid cysts of the posterior fossa. Surg Neurol. 51(4):376-82, 1999
13. Jallo GI et al: Arachnoid cysts of the cerebellopontine angle: diagnosis and surgery. Neurosurgery. 40(1):31-7; discussion 37-8, 1997
14. Higashi S et al: Hemifacial spasm associated with a cerebellopontine angle arachnoid cyst in a young adult. Surg Neurol. 37(4):289-92, 1992
15. Babu R et al: Arachnoid cyst of the cerebellopontine angle manifesting as contralateral trigeminal neuralgia: case report. Neurosurgery. 28(6):886-7, 1991

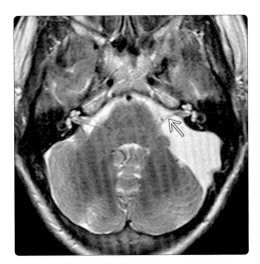
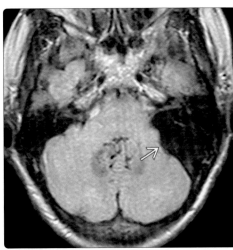

(Left) Axial T2WI MR shows a high-signal, large arachnoid cyst enlarging the left CPA cistern. The facial and vestibulocochlear nerves are visible bowing over the anteromedial surface of the arachnoid cyst ➡. (Right) Axial FLAIR MR in the same patient shows the low-signal arachnoid cyst ➡ and complete fluid attenuation. FLAIR suppression is expected as the arachnoid cyst is essentially CSF collecting between arachnoid layers.

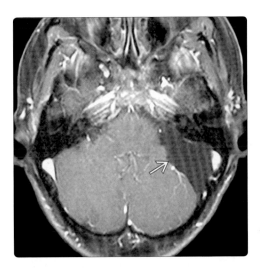
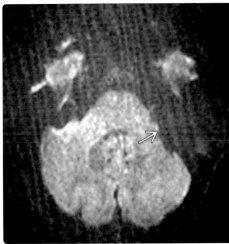

(Left) Axial T1WI C+ FS MR in the same patient demonstrates that the CPA arachnoid cyst ➡ does not enhance. (Right) Axial DWI MR in the same patient shows that the arachnoid cyst ➡ has no associated signal (no restricted diffusion). If this were an epidermoid cyst, high signal on DWI (restricted diffusion) would be present. DWI is the best way to differentiate an arachnoid cyst from an epidermoid cyst.

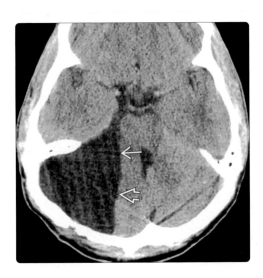
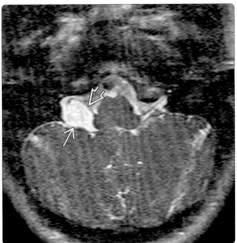

(Left) Axial NECT through the upper CPA cistern shows a large low-density arachnoid cyst causing flattening of the lateral brachium pontis ➡ and cerebellar hemisphere ➡. (Right) Axial T2WI FS MR demonstrates an incidental hyperintense CPA arachnoid cyst ➡ found at the time of imaging for headache. This lenticular-shaped lesion displaces the glossopharyngeal nerve (CNIX) anteriorly ➡. These small lesions require no additional imaging or treatment.

Lipoma in CPA-IAC

TERMINOLOGY

- Lipoma in CPA-IAC: Nonneoplastic mass of adipose tissue in CPA-IAC area

IMAGING

- Focal benign-appearing CPA-IAC mass, which follows fat density (CT) and intensity (MR)
- Concurrent intralabyrinthine deposit may be seen in association with CPA-IAC lipoma
- MR: Hyperintense CPA mass (parallels subcutaneous and marrow fat intensity)
  - Becomes **hypointense** with **fat saturation**
  - Caveat: Fat-saturated MR sequences avoid mistaking lipoma for "enhancing CPA mass"

TOP DIFFERENTIAL DIAGNOSES

- Hemorrhagic vestibular schwannoma
- Aneurysm in CPA-IAC
- Neurenteric cyst
- Ruptured dermoid cyst

PATHOLOGY

- Aberrant differentiation of embryonic meninx primitiva (meningeal precursor tissue)
- Lipoma composed of mature lipocytes (fat cells)

CLINICAL ISSUES

- Most common presentation: Adult presenting with unilateral sensorineural hearing loss
  - CNVIII compression: Tinnitus (40%), vertigo (45%)
  - Compression of CNV root entry zone: Trigeminal neuralgia (15%)
  - Compression of CNVII root exit zone: Hemifacial spasm, facial nerve weakness (10%)
  - Incidentally seen on brain CT or MR completed for unrelated reasons (33%)
- Treatment: **No treatment** is best treatment
  - If surgery required (cranial neuropathy), subtotal resection (debulking) only recommended

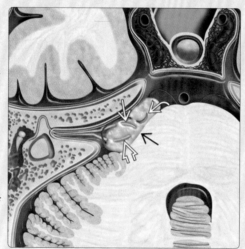
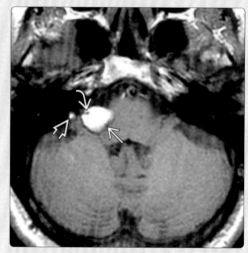

(Left) Axial graphic shows a cerebellopontine angle (CPA) lipoma ⮕ abutting the lateral pons. Notice that the facial nerve ⮕, vestibulocochlear nerve ⮕, and anterior inferior cerebellar artery (AICA) loop ⮕ all pass through the lipoma on their way to the internal auditory canal (IAC). (Right) Axial T1WI MR shows a right CPA lipoma ⮕ adherent to the lateral pontine pial surface. Note the 2nd smaller lipoma ⮕ along the lateral margin of the IAC. A portion of the AICA loop ⮕ passes through the anterolateral lipoma.

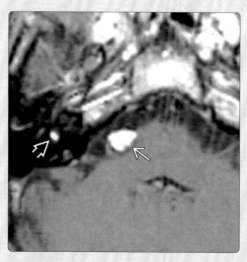
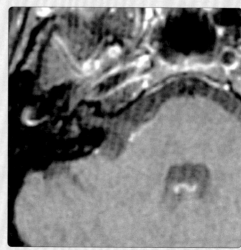

(Left) Axial T1WI MR reveals a hyperintense CPA lipoma ⮕ abutting the lateral pons. Note the 2nd ⮕ focus of hyperintensity representing a small intravestibular lipoma. Such intralabyrinthine lipomas are very rare and may exist with or without CPA lipoma. (Right) Axial T1WI C+ FS MR in the same patient shows both lesions have disappeared. Fat-saturation MR sequences are key to confirming the diagnosis of lipoma and to avoid mistaking a lipoma for an enhancing CPA mass.

TERMINOLOGY

Synonyms

- Congenital lipoma, lipomatous hamartoma

Definitions

- Lipoma in cerebellopontine angle (CPA)-internal auditory canal (IAC): **Nonneoplastic** mass of adipose tissue in CPA-IAC area
  - Congenital malformation; not true neoplasm

IMAGING

General Features

- Best diagnostic clue
  - Focal benign-appearing CPA-IAC mass, which follows fat density (CT) and intensity (MR)
- Location
  - 20% of intracranial lipomas are infratentorial
  - Primary location = CPA cistern
    - May be in IAC only
    - Concurrent **intralabyrinthine lipoma** may be present
      - □ Isolated intralabyrinthine lipoma also possible
- Size
  - Range: 0.5-5.0 cm in maximum diameter
    - May be as small as few millimeters
- Morphology
  - Lobulated pial-based fatty mass
    - Characteristically encases facial nerve (CNVII), vestibulocochlear nerve (CNVIII), anterior inferior cerebellar artery (AICA) loop
  - Small lesions
    - Linear along course of CNVII and CNVIII in CPA
    - Ovoid within CPA cistern; tubular within IAC
  - Large lesions
    - Broad-based hemispherical shape adherent to lateral pontine pial surface

CT Findings

- NECT
  - **Low-density** CPA-IAC mass
  - Measure mass using Hounsfield units (HU) if uncertain
    - HU range: **-50 to -100 HU**
  - IAC lipoma may create bulbous bone CT appearance
- CECT
  - Lesion does **not** enhance

MR Findings

- T1WI
  - **Hyperintense** CPA-IAC mass (parallels subcutaneous and marrow fat intensity)
    - Noncontiguous 2nd fatty lesion in inner ear may be present
  - Becomes **hypointense** with fat-saturation MR sequences
- T2WI
  - Intermediate "fat intensity" lesion
  - Conspicuous **chemical shift artifact** (frequency-encoding direction)
  - Signal parallels subcutaneous and marrow fat
- STIR
  - Hypointense due to STIR inherent fat suppression

- FLAIR
  - Hyperintense compared to cisternal CSF
- T1WI C+
  - Lesion already hyperintense on precontrast images
  - Use fat-saturated T1WI C+ sequence
    - Lesion **"disappears"** secondary to **fat saturation** aspect of this MR sequence
    - No enhancement in region of lesion is present

Imaging Recommendations

- Best imaging tool
  - **MR** is 1st study ordered when symptoms suggest possibility of CPA-IAC mass
  - CT can easily confirm diagnoses by measuring HU if some confusion on MR images persists
- Protocol advice
  - When T1WI C+ MR focused to CPA area is anticipated, need at least 1 **precontrast T1 sequence**
    - Precontrast T1 sequence helps distinguish fatty and hemorrhagic lesions from enhancing lesions
    - Fatty lesions include lipoma and dermoid
    - Hemorrhagic lesions with methemoglobin high signal include aneurysm and venous varix
  - Once high signal is seen on precontrast T1 sequence, **fat-saturated sequences** distinguish fat from hemorrhage
    - **Caveat**: Fat saturation avoids mistaking lipoma for "enhancing CPA mass" (vestibular schwannoma)

DIFFERENTIAL DIAGNOSIS

Hemorrhagic Vestibular Schwannoma

- Rare manifestation of common lesion
- Patchy intraparenchymal hyperintensity on T1WI MR
- Hyperintensities persist with fat-saturated sequences
- T2* GRE shows blooming of intralesional hemorrhage

Aneurysm in CPA-IAC

- CPA aneurysm may have complex signal
  - Posterior inferior cerebellar artery aneurysm most common > vertebral artery > AICA
- Rarely enters IAC (AICA)
- Ovoid CPA mass with calcified rim (CT) and complex layered signal (MR)
- MR signal complex with high-signal areas from methemoglobin in aneurysm lumen or wall
  - Does not fat saturate

Neurenteric Cyst

- Most common in prepontine cistern
- Contains proteinaceous fluid (hyperintense on T1WI MR)
- Does not fat saturate

Ruptured Dermoid Cyst

- Ectodermal inclusion cyst
- Original location usually midline
- Rupture spreads fat droplets into subarachnoid space
- Rupture may lead to chemical meningitis

PATHOLOGY

General Features

- Etiology
  - Best hypotheses for congenital lipoma

- – Aberrant differentiation of meninx primitiva (neural crest derived mesenchymal anlage)
    - ▫ Responsible for development of pia, arachnoid, dura, and subarachnoid cisterns
    - ▫ Maldifferentiates into fat instead
  - – Hyperplasia of fat cells normally **within pia**
- Genetics
  - ○ No known defects in sporadic CPA lipoma
  - ○ Epidermal nevus syndrome has CPA lipomas as part of complex congenital anomalies
- Associated abnormalities
  - ○ 2nd fatty lesion may occur in inner ear

Gross Pathologic & Surgical Features

- Soft, yellowish mass attached to leptomeninges
  - ○ Sometimes adherent to lateral pontine pia
- May incorporate CNVII and CNVIII with dense adhesions
  - ○ AICA loop may also be engulfed

Microscopic Features

- Histologically normal lipocytes in atypical location
- Highly vascularized adipose tissue
- Mature lipocytes; mitoses rare

CLINICAL ISSUES

Presentation

- Most common signs/symptoms
  - ○ Unilateral sensorineural hearing loss (60%)
- Clinical profile
  - ○ Adult presenting with slowly progressive unilateral sensorineural hearing loss
- Other signs/symptoms
  - ○ Incidentally on brain CT or MR (33%)
  - ○ CPA lipoma symptoms
    - – CNVIII compression: Sensorineural hearing loss (60%), tinnitus (40%), vertigo (40%)
    - – Compression of CNV root entry zone: **Trigeminal neuralgia** (15%)
    - – Compression of CNVII root exit zone: **Hemifacial spasm**, facial nerve weakness (10%)
  - ○ Internal auditory canal lipoma symptoms
    - – Sensorineural hearing loss, tinnitus, and vertigo only

Demographics

- Age
  - ○ Range at presentation: 8-60 years
  - ○ Mean age at presentation: 45 years
- Epidemiology
  - ○ Lipomas occur less frequently in CPA than epidermoid and arachnoid cysts
    - – Epidermoid cyst > arachnoid cyst > > lipoma
  - ○ CPA lipoma represents 10% of all intracranial lipomas
    - – Interhemispheric (45%), quadrigeminal/superior cerebellar (25%), suprasellar/interpeduncular (15%), sylvian cisterns (5%)

Natural History & Prognosis

- Usually does not grow over time
  - ○ Lesion consists of mature lipocytes
  - ○ Growth has been seen in pediatric lesions
  - ○ Growth reported in obese or steroid treated patients

- Stability confirmed with follow-up examinations

Treatment

- Primum non nocere ("1st, do no harm") is guiding principle
  - ○ **No treatment** is best treatment
- Conservative therapy recommendations
  - ○ Medical therapy: Trigeminal neuralgia, hemifacial spasm
  - ○ Discontinue steroid treatment if present; weight loss
- **Surgical removal** is **no longer recommended**
  - ○ Injury to CNVII, CNVIII, or AICA common
  - ○ Historically, 70% of postoperative patients had new postoperative deficits
- Surgical intervention if CNV or CNVII decompression needed
  - ○ Subtotal removal (debulking) only recommended

DIAGNOSTIC CHECKLIST

Consider

- When high-signal lesion is seen in CPA-IAC on T1WI unenhanced MR, 3 explanations to consider
  - ○ Fatty lesion
    - – Lipoma most common (will fat saturate)
  - ○ Hemorrhagic lesion
    - – Aneurysm wall clot or clotted venous varix (dural AVF)
    - – Rare hemorrhagic acoustic schwannoma
    - – Hemorrhage will not fat saturate
  - ○ Highly proteinaceous fluid
    - – Neurenteric cyst (usually in prepontine cistern)
    - – High protein hyperintensity will not fat saturate

Image Interpretation Pearls

- Once high signal lesion is seen in CPA on precontrast T1WI MR, use **fat-saturation** sequences to confirm diagnosis

Reporting Tips

- Report size and extent of lipoma
  - ○ Check inner ear for 2nd lesion
- Report CNVII, CNVIII, and AICA loop engulfed by lipoma

SELECTED REFERENCES

1. Bacciu A et al: Lipomas of the internal auditory canal and cerebellopontine angle. Ann Otol Rhinol Laryngol. 123(1):58-64, 2014
2. White JR et al: Lipomas of the cerebellopontine angle and internal auditory canal: Primum Non Nocere. Laryngoscope. 123(6):1531-6, 2013
3. Mukherjee P et al: Intracranial lipomas affecting the cerebellopontine angle and internal auditory canal: a case series. Otol Neurotol. 32(4):670-5, 2011
4. Sade B et al: Cerebellopontine angle lipoma presenting with hemifacial spasm: case report and review of the literature. J Otolaryngol. 34(4):270-3, 2005
5. Dahlen RT et al: CT and MR imaging characteristics of intravestibular lipoma. AJNR Am J Neuroradiol. 23(8):1413-7, 2002
6. Kato T et al: Trigeminal neuralgia caused by a cerebellopontine-angle lipoma: case report. Surg Neurol. 44(1):33-5, 1995

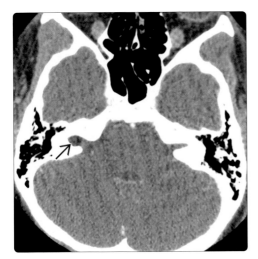
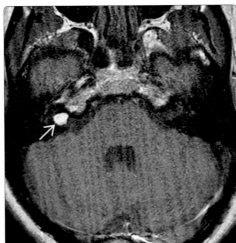

(Left) Axial CECT reveals a fat-density lesion ➡ in the fundus of the right IAC. The bone shape in this area is bulbous in comparison to the opposite normal IAC, suggesting a congenital origin of the lesion. (Right) Axial T1WI MR in the same patient shows the expected hyperintense fundal intracanalicular congenital lipoma ➡. Lipoma of the CPA-IAC area may be found in the CPA, IAC, and, rarely, in the inner ear.

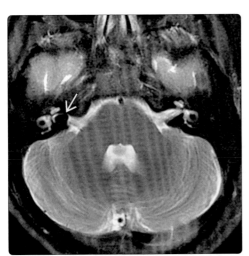
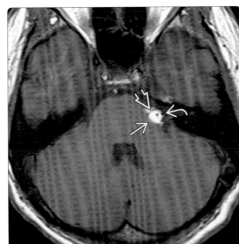

(Left) Axial T2WI fat-saturated MR in the same patient shows the lipoma in the IAC fundus as a low-signal filling defect ➡ in the high signal surrounding CSF. (Right) Axial T1 MR in a 30-year-old patient with sensorineural hearing loss and trigeminal neuralgia shows a hyperintense CPA lipoma abutting the lateral pons ➡. The linear hypointense line ➡ is the proximal facial nerve (CNVII), while the hypointense dots within the lateral aspect of the lipoma ➡ are AICA loops.

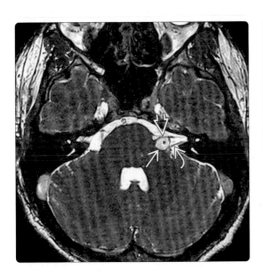
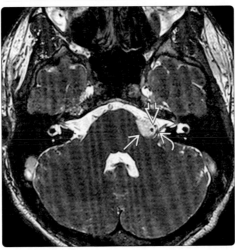

(Left) Axial CISS MR in same patient better demonstrates the lipoma adherent to the lateral pons ➡. Note the lesion engulfs the proximal CNVII ➡ and superior vestibular CNVIII ➡. AICA loop is the hypointense dot in the center of the lipoma. (Right) Axial CISS MR in the same patient slightly inferior to the previous image shows the lipoma ➡ surrounding the AICA loops ➡ and superior vestibular branch of the CNVIII ➡. The possibility of CNVII and CNVIII injury and AICA stroke preclude surgery in this patient.

IAC Venous Malformation

TERMINOLOGY

- IAC-VM: Benign developmental lesion associated with CNVII in IAC
  - May extend to geniculate ganglion
- IAC "hemangioma" is misnomer for IAC-VM

IMAGING

- Temporal bone CT findings
  - **Stippled ossifications** in lesion matrix
- Enhanced T1 MR findings
  - Enhancing IAC mass (< 10 mm) in fundus
  - Focal intralesional low-signal foci possible
  - If extends along labyrinthine CNVII to geniculate ganglion, creates **dumbbell** appearance

TOP DIFFERENTIAL DIAGNOSES

- CPA-IAC meningioma
- Vestibular schwannoma
- CPA-IAC facial nerve schwannoma

- CPA-IAC metastases

PATHOLOGY

- Etiology
  - Benign congenital VM arising in close approximation to CNVII in IAC
  - "Malformation" is term used for **errors of vascular morphogenesis** that develop in utero and persist postnatally
- Microscopic features
  - Immunohistochemical markers critical to VM diagnosis
  - Endothelial lining of vascular channels **stain negatively** for hemangioma-associated markers (**GLUT1 & LeY** antigen)

DIAGNOSTIC CHECKLIST

- IAC enhancing mass + CNVII paralysis ± punctate ossifications = IAC VM

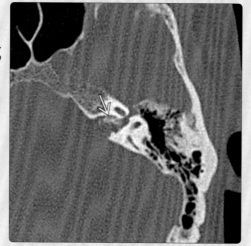
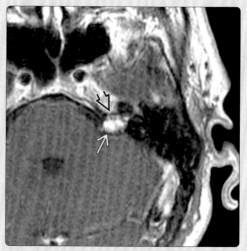

(Left) Axial bone CT shows typical CT stippled ossifications ➡ in the matrix of an IAC-VM ("hemangioma"). When found, ossifications help differentiate IAC-VM from IAC acoustic schwannoma. (Right) Axial T1WI C+ MR in the same patient demonstrates an enhancing IAC-VM ➡. The low-signal foci ⇴ along the anterior margin of the lesion are secondary to intratumoral ossifications.

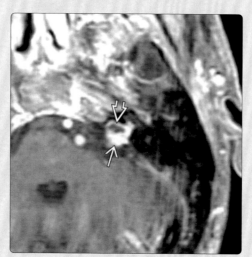
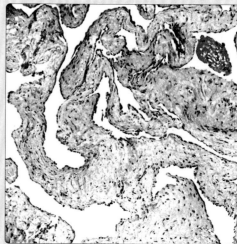

(Left) Axial T1WI C+ FS MR reveals an enhancing IAC-VM ➡ with an area of low signal along the anterior margin of the lesion ⇴ secondary to intratumoral ossification. (Right) Micropathology shows dilated vascular spaces with collagenous walls lined by a single layer of endothelium. The endothelial lining stains negative for GLUT1 and LeY antigens. These antigens are considered hemangioma-associated markers.

TERMINOLOGY

Abbreviations

- Internal auditory canal venous malformation (IAC-VM)

Synonyms

- "Hemangioma" and "cavernous hemangioma" are misnomers; cavernous malformation

Definitions

- IAC-VM: Benign developmental lesion associated with CNVII in IAC; may extend to geniculate ganglion

IMAGING

General Features

- Best diagnostic clue
  - **Stippled ossifications** in lesion matrix
- Location
  - IAC ± labyrinthine CNVII ± geniculate ganglion
- Size
  - Small at presentation; **< 10 mm**
- Morphology
  - Ovoid to fusiform; may have irregular margins

CT Findings

- Bone CT
  - Fundal IAC mass < 10 mm
  - **Stippled ossifications** often present
    - No hyperostosis of IAC bony walls
  - IAC flaring when lesion is larger

MR Findings

- T2WI
  - IAC mass < 10 mm
  - Intermediate signal with focal low-signal foci
- T2* GRE
  - Blooming of intralesional ossifications possible
- T1WI C+ FS
  - Enhancing IAC mass (< 10 mm) in fundus
  - Focal intralesional low-signal foci possible

Imaging Recommendations

- Best imaging tool
  - High-resolution CISS or FIESTA MR
    - Enhanced T1 fat saturated also
  - Temporal bone CT to verify ossifications

DIFFERENTIAL DIAGNOSIS

CPA-IAC Meningioma

- Most important lesion to differentiate from IAC-VM because it may also have low-signal foci
- Enhancing IAC lesion ± **hyperostotic bony walls** ± calcification

Vestibular Schwannoma

- Enhancing IAC lesion **without** ossifications
- If larger, symmetric projection from porus acusticus to CPA cistern

CPA-IAC Facial Nerve Schwannoma

- Enhancing CPA-IAC mass

- Facial nerve labyrinthine segment tail is key

CPA-IAC Metastases

- Pial type: Thickens CNVII & CNVII in IAC; enhances
- Dural type: Diffuse smooth or nodular thickening of IAC-CPA dura; enhances

PATHOLOGY

General Features

- Etiology
  - Benign congenital VM arising in close approximation to IAC CNVII
    - "Malformation" used for in utero **errors of vascular morphogenesis** that persist postnatally

Microscopic Features

- H&E: Nonencapsulated VM composed of dilated vascular channels of varying sizes
  - Widely ectatic vascular channels rimmed by smooth muscle coats without elastic laminae
  - Flattened & mitotically quiescent endothelial cells
  - Intralesional ossification often seen
- Immunohistochemical markers critical to VM diagnosis
  - Endothelial lining of vascular channels **stain negatively** for hemangioma-associated markers (**GLUT1 & LeY antigen**)

CLINICAL ISSUES

Presentation

- Most common signs/symptoms
  - Hearing loss associated with **CNVII paralysis**
  - Hearing loss may come on rapidly

Demographics

- Epidemiology
  - Rare (< 1% of IAC masses)

Natural History & Prognosis

- Adult-onset progressive hearing loss ± CNVII paralysis

Treatment

- Nerve-sparing surgical resection
- Rarely, CNVII graft necessary when CNVII invaded

DIAGNOSTIC CHECKLIST

Consider

- IAC enhancing mass + CNVII paralysis ± punctate ossifications = IAC-VM

SELECTED REFERENCES

1. Oldenburg MS et al: Cavernous hemangiomas of the internal auditory canal and cerebellopontine angle. Otol Neurotol. 36(1):e30-4, 2015
2. Benoit MM et al: Facial nerve hemangiomas: vascular tumors or malformations? Otolaryngol Head Neck Surg. 142(1):108-14, 2010
3. Greene AK et al: Intraosseous "hemangiomas" are malformations and not tumors. Plast Reconstr Surg. 119(6):1949-50; author reply 1950, 2007
4. Di Rocco F et al: Cavernous malformation of the internal auditory canal. Acta Neurochir (Wien). 148(6):695-7, 2006
5. Bernardeschi D et al: Vascular malformation (so-called hemangioma) of Scarpa's ganglion. Acta Otolaryngol. 124(9):1099-102, 2004
6. Omojola MF et al: CT and MRI features of cavernous haemangioma of internal auditory canal. Br J Radiol. 70(839):1184-7, 1997

TERMINOLOGY

- Definition: Acute or chronic infectious infiltrate of pia, arachnoid, & CSF in vicinity of T-bone, internal auditory canal (IAC), and cerebellopontine angle (CPA)

IMAGING

- CT shows underlying lesion causing meningitis ± CSF leak
  - Congenital: Inner ear lesions, cephalocele, patent petromastoid canal
  - Acquired: Coalescent mastoiditis or apical petrositis
  - Acquired: Tegmen or posterior wall arachnoid granulations
  - Acquired: T-bone fractures of tegmen or IE
- MR may show meningitis
  - Meningeal exudate + brain surface C+
    - Thickened meninges: Local or diffuse
  - Hyperintensity in posterior fossa sulci ± cisterns

TOP DIFFERENTIAL DIAGNOSES

- Meningeal metastases
- Neurosarcoidosis, CPA-IAC
- Increased FLAIR signal in CSF from acute stroke, subarachnoid hemorrhage, or artifact

PATHOLOGY

- Meningitis focused along deep surfaces of T-bone or in floor of middle cranial fossa is secondary to T-bone disease until proven otherwise
- Complications: Cerebritis, abscess, empyema, ventriculitis
- Cerebrovascular complications: Venous sinus or arterial thrombosis

CLINICAL ISSUES

- Meningitis = clinical/laboratory diagnosis
- Meningitis **not** imaging diagnosis
- Imaging used to identify underlying lesions

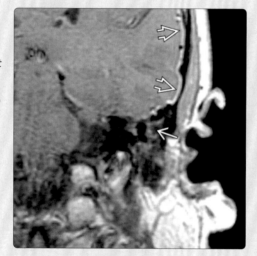
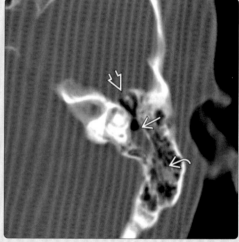

(Left) Coronal T1WI C+ MR shows enhancing mastoid tissue ➡ along with meningeal enhancement (meningitis) ➡ in this patient with severe headache and recurrent otomastoiditis. (Right) Axial bone CT through the left T-bone in the same patient demonstrates an air-fluid level in mastoid ➡ with thinning of the anterior epitympanic recess wall ➡. Notice the partial opacification of the mastoid air cells ➡. In this case, bacterial otomastoiditis spread locally to cause the meningitis.

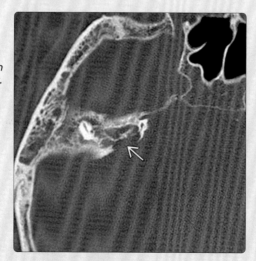
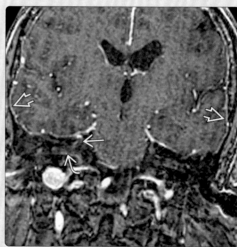

(Left) Axial bone CT of the right T-bone in this patient with CSF-proven meningitis reveals an arachnoid granulation ➡ in the location of the subarcuate canaliculus. CSF otorrhea was present. (Right) Coronal T1 C+ fat-saturated MR in the same patient after antibiotic treatment shows the arachnoid granulation as a focal fluid collection ➡ just above the right internal auditory canal ➡. Notice the diffuse leptomeningeal enhancement ➡ sometimes seen in the setting of meningitis.

TERMINOLOGY

Synonyms

- Leptomeningitis, infectious meningitis

Definitions

- Acute or chronic infectious infiltrate of pia, arachnoid, & CSF in vicinity of T-bone, internal auditory canal (IAC), & cerebellopontine angle (CPA)
- Classified as acute pyogenic (bacterial), lymphocytic (viral), or chronic (tuberculous or granulomatous)

IMAGING

General Features

- Best diagnostic clue
  - Positive CSF by lumbar puncture

Imaging Recommendations

- Protocol advice
  - MR with FLAIR, DWI, T1WI C+
  - CISS or FIESTA sequence aimed at T-bone
    - May show predisposing arachnoid granulations, cephalocele, or inner ear (IE) malformation

CT Findings

- Bone CT
  - Underlying lesion causing CSF leak & meningitis
  - Congenital predisposing lesions
    - Congenital IE lesions, cephalocele, patent petromastoid canal
  - Acquired predisposing lesions
    - Tegmen tympani/mastoideum or posterior wall arachnoid granulations
    - T-bone fractures of tegmen or IE
    - Confluent otomastoiditis or apical petrositis

MR Findings

- T2WI
  - Meningitis: Hyperintense exudate lines CPA-IAC ± deep t-bone meningeal surfaces
  - T-bone: High signal in middle ear if CSF leak
- FLAIR
  - Meningitis: **Hyperintense signal in sulci & cisterns** of posterior fossa and middle cranial fossa
  - Delayed C+ FLAIR most sensitive
- DWI
  - **Detects complications**: Vascular complications, empyema, abscess
- T1WI C+
  - Meningitis: Meningeal exudate + brain surface C+
    - Thickened meninges: Local or diffuse
  - T-bone: Focal meningeal thickening + enhancement within T-bone may localize primary infection site
- CISS, FIESTA, or T2 Space
  - Thin-section imaging may show predisposing arachnoid granulations, IE malformation, cephalocele

DIFFERENTIAL DIAGNOSIS

Meningeal Metastases

- Primary tumor usually known (exception: NHL)

Neurosarcoidosis

- Leptomeningeal nodular or lacy enhancement
- T-bone is uninvolved

Increased FLAIR Signal in Cerebrospinal Fluid

- Nonspecific MR finding: Subarachnoid hemorrhage, artifact, acute stroke venous congestion, high inspired oxygen, or retained MR contrast in CSF

PATHOLOGY

General Features

- Etiology
  - Meningitis focused along deep surfaces of T-bone or in floor of middle cranial fossa is secondary to T-bone disease until proven otherwise

Gross Pathologic & Surgical Features

- Looks similar to whatever infectious agent there is
- Cisterns, sulci filled with cloudy CSF, then purulent exudate
- Pia-arachnoid thickened

Microscopic Features

- Meningeal exudate: White cells, fibrin, bacteria

CLINICAL ISSUES

Presentation

- Most common signs/symptoms
  - Meningitis = clinical/laboratory diagnosis
  - CSF leak into middle ear + meningitis
    - Otalgia, ↓ hearing, bulging tympanic membrane with retrotympanic fluid
    - Headache, fever, nuchal rigidity, ± ↓ mental status ± seizures (30%)
- Clinical profile
  - CSF shows ↑ white blood cells
    - ↑ CSF protein, ↓ glucose (infectious meningitis)

Natural History & Prognosis

- Effective antimicrobial agents have ↓ but not eliminated morbidity & mortality (~ 20%)

Treatment

- Intravenous antibiotics
- Surgical treatment varies with cause
  - Acute T-bone infections
  - T-bone fractures with meningitis ± CSF leak
  - Underlying lesions causing meningitis ± CSF leak (arachnoid granulations, congenital IE lesions, cephalocele)

SELECTED REFERENCES

1. Oliveira CR et al: Brain magnetic resonance imaging of infants with bacterial meningitis. J Pediatr. 165(1):134-9, 2014
2. Mohan S et al: Imaging of meningitis and ventriculitis. Neuroimaging Clin N Am. 22(4):557-83, 2012
3. Tebruegge M et al: Epidemiology, etiology, pathogenesis, and diagnosis of recurrent bacterial meningitis. Clin Microbiol Rev. 21(3):519-37, 2008
4. Migirov L: Computed tomographic versus surgical findings in complicated acute otomastoiditis. Ann Otol Rhinol Laryngol. 112(8):675-7, 2003
5. Quiney RE et al: Recurrent meningitis in children due to inner ear abnormalities. J Laryngol Otol. 103(5):473-80, 1989
6. Vermeersch H et al: The temporal bone as route of infection in recurrent meningitis. J Otolaryngol. 9(3):199-201, 1980

Ramsay Hunt Syndrome

TERMINOLOGY

- Ramsay Hunt syndrome (RHS): Varicella-zoster virus infection involving sensory fibers of CNVII & CNVIII & portion of **external ear** supplied by auriculotemporal nerve

IMAGING

- Imaging diagnosis: Pathologic enhancement on T1 C+ MR of CNVII ± CNVIII in IAC fundus along with all or part of membranous labyrinth
- Enhanced MR findings by location
  - External ear: Enhancing external ear vesicles & associated inflammation
  - Intratemporal CNVII: Entire intratemporal CNVII enhancement typical
  - Membranous labyrinth: Fluid spaces of cochlea, vestibule, & semicircular canals may all be variably affected
  - IAC: Linear to fusiform enhancement in internal auditory canal (IAC) fundus (CNVII & CNVIII)
  - Brainstem: Facial nucleus in brainstem enhances infrequently in RHS

TOP DIFFERENTIAL DIAGNOSES

- Bell palsy
- Meningitis
- Neurosarcoidosis in cerebellopontine angle-IAC

CLINICAL ISSUES

- Clinical presentation
  - CNVII palsy & sensorineural hearing loss associated with external ear vesicular rash
  - Fever, vertigo, nausea, & vomiting
  - Deep, burning pain in ear
- Treatment options
  - Conservative management 1st
  - Pharmacologic treatment as indicated
    - Corticosteroids ± acyclovir (↓ pain; improves CNVII function)

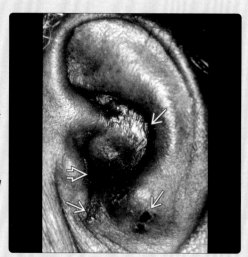
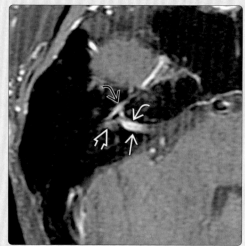

(Left) Clinical photograph of the external ear demonstrates a hemorrhagic vesicular rash affecting the auricle ➡ and external auditory canal ➡. This often painful rash, along with facial and vestibulocochlear neuropathy, makes the clinical diagnosis of Ramsay Hunt syndrome (RHS) obvious. (Right) Axial T1WI C+ FS MR in a RHS patient shows linear enhancement of CNVII in the IAC fundus ➡ extending into the labyrinthine and tympanic segments ➡. The superior vestibular nerve also enhances in the IAC fundus ➡ and on into the vestibule ➡.

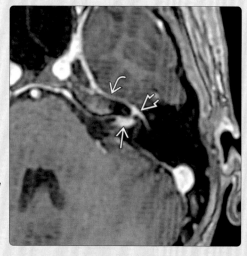
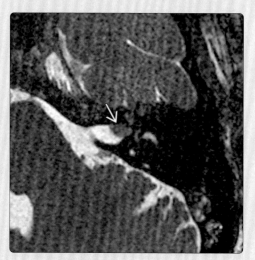

(Left) Axial SPGR C+ reveals enhancement of the left IAC fundus ➡ as well as enhancement of the labyrinthine segment, geniculate ganglion, and anterior tympanic segment of CNVII ➡. In addition, the greater superficial petrosal nerve branch of CNVII ➡ enhances along the anterior margin of the petrous apex. (Right) Magnified axial T2WI FS MR in the same patient shows the thickened, inflamed CNVII and CNVIII as brain intensity material ➡ in the fundus of the IAC.

TERMINOLOGY

Abbreviations

- Ramsay Hunt syndrome (RHS)

Synonyms

- Herpes zoster oticus

Definitions

- RHS: Varicella-zoster virus infection involving sensory fibers of CNVII & CNVIII & portion of **external ear** supplied by auriculotemporal nerve

IMAGING

General Features

- Best diagnostic clue
  - Pathologic enhancement on T1 C+ MR of CNVII ± CNVII in internal auditory canal (IAC) fundus along with all or part of membranous labyrinth
- Morphology
  - Linear or fusiform IAC enhancement is rule

MR Findings

- T2WI
  - High-resolution (≤ 2 mm) T2
    - Fundal cranial nerves VII & VIII thickened
    - When severe, may mimic fundal vestibular schwannoma
- FLAIR
  - Parenchymal brain normal
- T1WI C+
  - External ear
    - Enhancing external ear vesicles & associated inflammation
  - Intratemporal facial nerve
    - Entire intratemporal CNVII enhancement typical
      - □ **Labyrinthine segment** CNVII & geniculate ganglion reliably enhance
  - Membranous labyrinth
    - Fluid spaces of cochlea, vestibule, & semicircular canals may all be variably affected
      - □ Cochlear portion enhances most commonly
    - Membranous labyrinth enhancement may **not** be present even when hearing loss & vertigo present
  - IAC
    - Linear to globoid C+ in IAC fundus (CNVII & CNVIII)
    - IAC enhancement **not** always present even with sensorineural hearing loss ± vertigo
  - Brainstem
    - Facial nucleus in brainstem enhances rarely in RHS

Imaging Recommendations

- Best imaging tool
  - Whole-brain MR with enhanced sequences focused on cerebellopontine angle-IAC & temporal bone
  - Findings best seen on **fat-saturated** T1 C+ MR images
- Protocol advice
  - If external ear vesicular rash is clinically apparent, **no imaging is necessary** to investigate associated CNVII & CNVIII palsies

DIFFERENTIAL DIAGNOSIS

Bell Palsy

- Enhancement of CNVII; not membranous labyrinth or CNVIII
- Fundal CNVII enhancing "tuft"
- IAC enhancement usually less intense than RHS

Meningitis

- Headache, stiff neck, fever
- Thickened, diffusely enhancing meninges
- Cerebrospinal fluid analysis may be revealing

PATHOLOGY

General Features

- Etiology
  - Classic hypothesis: Virus remains dormant within geniculate ganglion with periodic **reactivation**
    - Varicella-zoster virus can be cultured from vesicles or from saliva

CLINICAL ISSUES

Presentation

- Most common signs/symptoms
  - Facial palsy & sensorineural hearing loss associated with external ear vesicular rash
- Other signs/symptoms
  - Fever, vertigo, nausea, & vomiting
  - Deep, burning pain in ear

Natural History & Prognosis

- Ear pain followed in ~ 7 days by erythematous vesicular rash of external ear
- Cranial neuropathies appear after onset of ear pain
  - Appear before or after vesicular eruption
  - When before, imaging may be done to look for etiology of cranial nerve VII palsy

Treatment

- Conservative management 1st
  - Warm compresses & analgesics
  - Cornea care for facial paralysis
- Pharmacologic treatment
  - Corticosteroids ± acyclovir (↓ pain, improves CNVII function)

DIAGNOSTIC CHECKLIST

Consider

- MR imaging should be done only when clinical presentation is atypical

SELECTED REFERENCES

1. Chung MS et al: The clinical significance of findings obtained on 3D-FLAIR MR imaging in patients with Ramsay-Hunt syndrome. Laryngoscope. 125(4):950-5, 2015
2. Iwasaki H et al: Vestibular and cochlear neuritis in patients with Ramsay Hunt syndrome: a Gd-enhanced MRI study. Acta Otolaryngol. 133(4):373-7, 2013
3. Sartoretti-Schefer S et al: Ramsay Hunt syndrome associated with brain stem enhancement. AJNR Am J Neuroradiol. 20(2):278-80, 1999
4. Sartoretti-Schefer S et al: Idiopathic, herpetic, and HIV-associated facial nerve palsies: abnormal MR enhancement patterns. AJNR Am J Neuroradiol. 15(3):479-85, 1994

TERMINOLOGY

- Neurosarcoidosis: Systemic disorder with **noncaseating epithelioid cell granulomas** of multiple organ systems

IMAGING

- MR findings
  - Multifocal enhancing meningeal masses
  - Other intracranial locations
    - Optic chiasm, hypothalamus, infundibulum
    - Cranial nerves (CNII > CNV > CNVII and VIII)
- **T2**: **Hypointense** or **hyperintense** meningeal foci
  - Hypointense: Fibrocollagenous tissue
  - Hyperintense: Inflammatory tissue
- T1 C+: Nodular or linear dural enhancing lesions

TOP DIFFERENTIAL DIAGNOSES

- Multiple meningiomas
- CPA-IAC metastases
- Idiopathic extraorbital inflammation (pseudotumor)

- Meningitis

PATHOLOGY

- **Noncaseating granulomas** are characteristic

CLINICAL ISSUES

- African Americans affected more frequently
- Systemic sarcoidosis: Pulmonary symptoms
- CNS sarcoidosis symptoms
  - Visual loss and pituitary dysfunction
  - Cranial neuropathy: CNII > > CNV > **CNVII and VIII**
- Laboratory findings are confirmatory
  - Kveim-Siltzbach skin test positive in 85%
  - Serum ACE levels elevated in < 50%
  - Use modified Zajicek criteria for diagnosis
    - Divides into confirmed, probable, and possible
- Treatment options
  - Steroids ± immunomodulators
  - 50% of neurosarcoidosis progresses despite treatment

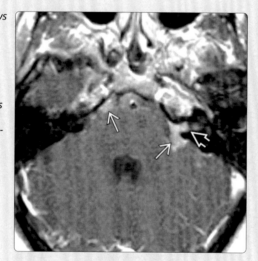
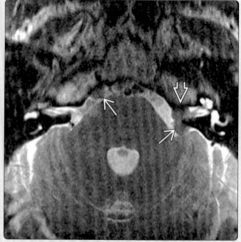

(Left) Axial T1WI C+ MR shows multifocal enhancing meningeal nodules ➡. The lesion in the left CPA enters the IAC ➡. Inflammatory diseases (Wegener granulomatosis, intracranial pseudotumor, granulomatous infection) and diffuse meningeal malignancies (non-Hodgkin lymphoma, metastases) are part of the differential diagnosis. (Right) Axial thin-section T2WI MR in the same patient reveals multifocal hypointense meningeal nodules ➡ with left IAC involvement ➡.

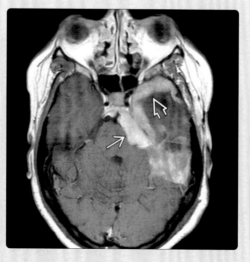
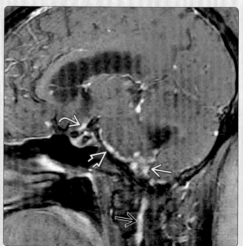

(Left) Axial T1WI C+ MR demonstrates an extensive, contiguous sarcoid meningeal lesion with a conspicuous CPA component ➡ mimicking en plaque meningioma. The meninges that line the middle cranial fossa are diffusely affected ➡. (Right) Sagittal T1WI C+ FS MR demonstrates leptomeningeal (primarily pial) enhancing sarcoid nodules in the CPA ➡ along brainstem surface ➡ and in the hypothalamus ➡. Also notice the meningeal lesion ➡ along anterior surface of cervical spinal canal.

TERMINOLOGY

Definitions

- Systemic disorder with **noncaseating epithelioid cell granulomas** of multiple organ systems

IMAGING

General Features

- Best diagnostic clue
  - Solitary or multifocal enhancing meningeal mass(es) + abnormal CXR
- Location
  - **Dural** (~ 35%), **leptomeningeal** (~ 35%) > subarachnoid/perivascular spaces

MR Findings

- FLAIR
  - 50% have periventricular hyperintense lesions
    - Can infiltrate perivascular (Virchow-Robin) spaces
    - May cause vasculitis/angiitis of white matter
  - Hydrocephalus, lacunar infarcts
- T1WI C+
  - Nodular or linear dural enhancing lesions
  - Leptomeningeal disease spreads via perivascular spaces into brain
  - Cranial nerve enhancement

Imaging Recommendations

- Best imaging tool
  - MR with FLAIR & T1 C+ sequences
- Protocol advice
  - Include T1 C+ MR thin-sections through CPA

DIFFERENTIAL DIAGNOSIS

Multiple Meningiomas

- Clinical: Absent systemic manifestations of sarcoidosis
- Multifocal enhancing dural masses
- No parenchymal or subarachnoid space findings

CPA-IAC Metastases

- Clinical: Primary neoplasm known
- Nodular meningeal metastases < diffuse
- When nodular, T1 C+ MR appearance is similar to sarcoidosis

Idiopathic Extraorbital Inflammation (Pseudotumor)

- Usually unifocal enhancing meningeal mass

PATHOLOGY

General Features

- Etiology
  - Pathophysiology unknown
- Genetics
  - Sarcoidosis occurs in families
  - Genetic polymorphisms of MHC are associated with ↑ risk of disease
- General pathology issues
  - Diagnosis often made after biopsy of skin lesions

Gross Pathologic & Surgical Features

- Granulomatous leptomeningitis (most common) or dural-based solitary mass (diffuse > nodular)
- May infiltrate along perivascular spaces

Microscopic Features

- **Noncaseating granulomas** are characteristic
  - Compact, radially arranged epithelioid cells with pale-staining nuclei

CLINICAL ISSUES

Presentation

- Most common signs/symptoms
  - CNS sarcoidosis
    - Visual loss
    - Pituitary/hypothalamic dysfunction
    - Cranial neuropathy: CNII > > CNV > CNVII and CNVIII
    - Headache, seizures, encephalopathy, dementia
  - CPA-IAC: Unilateral sensorineural hearing loss (SNHL) ± facial neuropathy
- Clinical profile
  - Adult with visual loss, central diabetes insipidus, and unilateral SNHL
- Laboratory findings are confirmatory
  - Kveim-Siltzbach skin test positive in 85%
  - Serum ACE levels elevated in < 50%
  - Use modified Zajicek criteria for diagnosis
    - Divides into confirmed, probable, and possible

Demographics

- Age
  - Bimodal: Initial peak 20-29 years; later peak > 50 years
- Ethnicity
  - USA: Risk in **African Americans** 3x that of Caucasians
- Epidemiology
  - CNS sarcoid: ~ **25%** of systemic sarcoidosis patients

Natural History & Prognosis

- 2/3 have self-limited monophasic illness
  - Remainder have relapsing or chronic course
- > 50% recover without significant morbidity

Treatment

- No known cure; goal is alleviation of symptoms
- Prompt administration of steroids ± immunomodulators
  - Immunosuppressive therapy when disabling disease
- 50% of neurosarcoidosis progress despite therapy

DIAGNOSTIC CHECKLIST

Image Interpretation Pearls

- When multiple "meningiomas" identified in patient with systemic disease, think sarcoidosis
- When bilateral IAC lesions identified in adult (not neurofibromatosis type 2), consider neurosarcoidosis or metastases

SELECTED REFERENCES

1. Carlson ML et al: Cranial base manifestations of neurosarcoidosis: a review of 305 patients. Otol Neurotol. 36(1):156-66, 2015
2. Hebel R et al: Overview of neurosarcoidosis: recent advances. J Neurol. 262(2):258-67, 2015

Vestibular Schwannoma

TERMINOLOGY

- Vestibular schwannoma (VS): Benign tumor from Schwann cells that wrap vestibular CNVIII branches in CPA-IAC

IMAGING

- T1WI fat-saturated enhanced MR = gold standard
  - Focal, enhancing mass of CPA-IAC cistern centered on porus acusticus
  - Small VS: Ovoid enhancing intracanalicular mass
  - Large VS: Ice cream on cone shape in CPA and IAC
  - 15% with intramural cysts (low-signal foci)
  - 0.5% with associated arachnoid cyst/trapped CSF
- High-resolution T2 space, CISS, or FIESTA: Filling defect in hyperintense cerebrospinal fluid of CPA-IAC cistern
- FLAIR: ↑ cochlear signal from ↑ protein
- T2* GRE: Microhemorrhages ↓ signal foci (common)
  - Characteristic VS finding when present
  - Not seen in meningioma

TOP DIFFERENTIAL DIAGNOSES

- Meningioma in CPA-IAC
- Epidermoid cyst in CPA
- Aneurysm in CPA
- Facial nerve schwannoma in CPA-IAC
- Metastases in CPA-IAC

PATHOLOGY

- Benign tumor arising from vestibular portion of CNVIII at glial-Schwann cell junction

CLINICAL ISSUES

- Demographics and symptoms
  - Adults with unilateral sensorineural hearing loss
- Surgical approaches
  - Translabyrinthine resection if no hearing
  - Middle cranial fossa approach for IAC VS
  - Retrosigmoid approach when CPA involved
- Fractionated or stereotactic radiosurgery

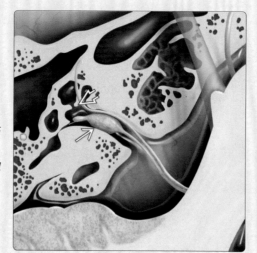
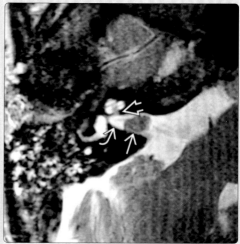

(Left) Axial graphic shows small intracanalicular vestibular schwannoma ➡ arising from the superior vestibular nerve. Notice that the cochlear nerve canal is uninvolved ⇒. (Right) Axial T2WI MR reveals a small intracanalicular vestibular schwannoma ➡ visualized as a soft tissue intensity mass surrounded by high-intensity CSF. The cochlear nerve canal ⇒ is not involved, and an 8-mm fundal cap ➡ is present.

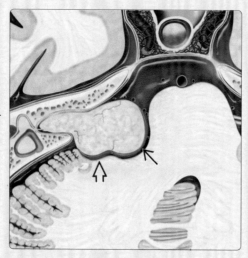
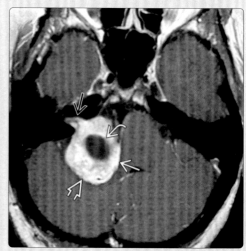

(Left) Axial graphic of a large vestibular schwannoma reveals the typical ice cream on cone CPA-IAC morphology. Mass effect on the middle cerebellar peduncle ➡ and cerebellar hemisphere ⇒ is evident. (Right) Axial T1WI C+ MR demonstrates a large CPA-IAC vestibular schwannoma compressing the middle cerebellar peduncle ➡ and cerebellar hemisphere ⇒. Enhancement within the IAC ➡ and the large intramural cyst ➡ makes the imaging diagnosis certain.

TERMINOLOGY

Abbreviations

- Vestibular schwannoma (VS)

Synonyms

- Acoustic schwannoma, acoustic neuroma, acoustic tumor
  - Uncommon names: Neurinoma, neurilemmoma

Definitions

- Benign tumor arising from Schwann cells that wrap vestibular branches of CNVIII in CPA-IAC

IMAGING

General Features

- Best diagnostic clue
  - Avidly enhancing cylindrical (IAC) or **ice cream on cone** (CPA-IAC) mass
- Location
  - Small lesions: Intracanalicular
  - Large lesions: Intracanalicular with CPA cistern extension
- Size
  - Small lesions: 2-10 mm
  - Larger lesions: Up to 5 cm in maximum diameter
- Morphology
  - Small and intracanalicular VS: Ovoid mass
  - Large VS: Ice cream (CPA) on cone (IAC)

CT Findings

- CECT
  - Well-delineated, enhancing mass of CPA-IAC cistern
  - Calcification not present (compared to CPA meningioma)
  - May flare IAC when large
  - Smaller intracanalicular lesions (< 5 mm) may be missed with CECT

MR Findings

- T1WI
  - Usually isointense with brain
  - ↑ signal foci if rare hemorrhage present
    - Microhemorrhages more common but not seen on T1
- T2WI FS
  - High-resolution T2 space, CISS, or FIESTA: Filling defect in ↑ signal cerebrospinal fluid (CSF) of CPA-IAC cistern
    - Small lesion: Ovoid filling defect in ↑ signal CSF of IAC
    - Large lesion: Ice cream on cone filling defect in CPA-IAC
- FLAIR
  - ↑ cochlear signal from ↑ perilymph protein
- T2* GRE
  - **Microhemorrhage** low-signal foci common
    - Not seen in meningioma unless sufficient intramural calcifications present to cause blooming
- T1WI C+ FS
  - Focal, enhancing mass of CPA-IAC cistern centered on porus acusticus
  - 100% enhance strongly
  - **15%** with **intramural cysts** (low-signal foci)
  - Dural tails rare (compared to meningioma)
- Other MR findings
  - < 1%: Macroscopic intratumoral hemorrhage
  - 0.5% with associated arachnoid cyst/trapped CSF

Imaging Recommendations

- Best imaging tool
  - Gold standard is full-brain FLAIR MR with axial and coronal thin-section T1WI C+ FS MR of CPA-IAC
- Protocol advice
  - High-resolution T2 space, CISS, or FIESTA MR of CPA-IAC is only screening exam for VS
    - Used for uncomplicated unilateral sensorineural hearing loss (SNHL) in adult
    - Not useful for postoperative follow-up imaging

DIFFERENTIAL DIAGNOSIS

Meningioma in CPA-IAC

- Intracanalicular meningioma may mimic VS (rare)
- CECT: Calcified dural-based mass eccentric to porus acusticus
- T1WI C+ MR: Broad dural base with associated dural tails
- T2* GRE: Typically **no** microhemorrhages seen

Epidermoid Cyst in CPA

- May mimic rare cystic VS
- Insinuating morphology
- T1WI C+ MR: Nonenhancing CPA mass
- DWI: **Diffusion restriction** (high signal) diagnostic

Arachnoid Cyst in CPA

- Well-marginated CPA lesion: Does not enter IAC
- Follows CSF signal on all MR sequences
- DWI: No restricted diffusion

Aneurysm in CPA

- Ovoid to fusiform **complex signal** CPA mass

Facial Nerve Schwannoma in CPA-IAC

- When confined to CPA-IAC, may exactly mimic VS
- Look for labyrinthine segment **tail** to differentiate

Metastases in CPA-IAC

- May have bilateral meningeal involvement
  - Beware of misdiagnosing as neurofibromatosis type 2 (NF2)

PATHOLOGY

General Features

- Etiology
  - Benign tumor arising from vestibular portion of CNVIII at glial-Schwann cell junction
    - Rare in cochlear portion CNVIII
- Genetics
  - Inactivating mutations of *NF2* tumor suppressor gene in 60% of sporadic VS
  - Loss of chromosome 22q also seen
  - Multiple or bilateral schwannomas = NF2
- Associated abnormalities
  - Arachnoid cyst (0.5%)
  - At surgery may be arachnoid cyst or trapped CSF

Staging, Grading, & Classification

- WHO grade I lesion

Gross Pathologic & Surgical Features

- Tan, round-ovoid, encapsulated mass
- Arises eccentrically from CNVIII at glial-Schwann cell junction
  - Glial-Schwann cell junction usually at porus acusticus

Microscopic Features

- Differentiated Schwann cells in collagenous matrix
- Areas of compact, elongated cells = Antoni A
  - Most VS composed mostly of Antoni A cells
- Areas less densely cellular with tumor loosely arranged, ± clusters of lipid-laden cells = Antoni B
- Strong, diffuse expression of S100 protein
- No necrosis; instead intramural cysts
- < 1% hemorrhagic

CLINICAL ISSUES

Presentation

- Most common signs/symptoms
  - Adults with unilateral SNHL
- Clinical profile
  - Slowly progressive SNHL
  - Laboratory
    - Brainstem electric response audiometry (BERA) most sensitive preimaging test for VS
    - Screening MR could replace BERA
- Other symptoms
  - Small VS: Tinnitus (ringing in ear); disequilibrium
  - Large VS: Trigeminal ± facial neuropathy possible

Demographics

- Age
  - Adults (rare in children unless NF2)
  - Peak age = 40-60 yr
  - Age range = 30-70 yr
- Epidemiology
  - Most common lesion in unilateral SNHL **(> 90%)**
  - Most common CPA-IAC mass (85-90%)
  - 2nd most common extraaxial neoplasm in adults

Natural History & Prognosis

- 60% of VS are slow growing (< 1 mm/yr)
- 10% of VS grow rapidly (> 3 mm/yr)
- 60% of VS grow slowly; can be followed with imaging
  - Used in > 60 yr olds, poor health, small tumor size, patient preference
- Successful surgical removal of VS will not restore any hearing already lost
- Negative prognostic imaging findings for hearing preservation
  - Size > 2 cm
  - VS involves IAC fundus ± cochlear aperture

Treatment

- **Translabyrinthine** resection if no hearing preservation possible
- **Middle cranial fossa** approach for intracanalicular VS
  - Especially lateral IAC location
- **Retrosigmoid approach** when CPA or medial IAC component present

- Fractionated or stereotactic radiosurgery
  - Gamma knife: Low-dose, sharply collimated, focused cobalt-60 treatment
  - Used when medical contraindications to surgery and residual postoperative VS
  - Can be used as 1st treatment

DIAGNOSTIC CHECKLIST

Consider

- Consider using high-resolution T2 space, CISS, or FIESTA MR as screening for VS
- Thin-section, T1WI enhanced, fat-saturated axial and coronal MR = gold standard imaging approach

Image Interpretation Pearls

- Unilateral well-circumscribed IAC or CPA-IAC mass should be considered VS until proven otherwise
- Always make sure there is no labyrinthine tail on all VS to avoid misdiagnosing facial nerve schwannoma

Reporting Tips

- Comment on tumor size ± CPA involvement
- Does VS involve cochlear nerve canal or IAC fundus
- How large in millimeters is fundal cap
- Is hemorrhage, intramural cyst, or arachnoid cyst/trapped CSF present within or associated with VS
- When small, comment on nerve of origin if possible

SELECTED REFERENCES

1. Oh JH et al: Clinical application of 3D-FIESTA image in patients with unilateral inner ear symptom. Korean J Audiol. 17(3):111-7, 2013
2. Tomogane Y et al: Usefulness of PRESTO magnetic resonance imaging for the differentiation of schwannoma and meningioma in the cerebellopontine angle. Neurol Med Chir (Tokyo). 53(7):482-9, 2013
3. Bakkouri WE et al: Conservative management of 386 cases of unilateral vestibular schwannoma: tumor growth and consequences for treatment. J Neurosurg. 110(4):662-9, 2009
4. Fukuoka S et al: Gamma knife radiosurgery for vestibular schwannomas. Prog Neurol Surg. 22:45-62, 2009
5. Bhadelia RA et al: Increased cochlear fluid-attenuated inversion recovery signal in patients with vestibular schwannoma. AJNR Am J Neuroradiol. 29(4):720-3, 2008
6. Ferri GG et al: Conservative management of vestibular schwannomas: an effective strategy. Laryngoscope. 118(6):951-7, 2008
7. House JW et al: False-positive magnetic resonance imaging in the diagnosis of vestibular schwannoma. Otol Neurotol. 29(8):1176-8, 2008
8. Meijer OW et al: Tumor-volume changes after radiosurgery for vestibular schwannoma: implications for follow-up MR imaging protocol. AJNR Am J Neuroradiol. 29(5):906-10, 2008
9. Thamburaj K et al: Intratumoral microhemorrhages on T2*-weighted gradient-echo imaging helps differentiate vestibular schwannoma from meningioma. AJNR Am J Neuroradiol. 29(3):552-7, 2008
10. Maire JP et al: Twenty years' experience in the treatment of acoustic neuromas with fractionated radiotherapy: a review of 45 cases. Int J Radiat Oncol Biol Phys. 66(1):170-8, 2006
11. Furuta S et al: Prediction of the origin of intracanalicular neoplasms with high-resolution MR imaging. Neuroradiology. 47(9):657-63, 2005
12. Dubrulle F et al: Cochlear fossa enhancement at MR evaluation of vestibular Schwannoma: correlation with success at hearing-preservation surgery. Radiology. 215(2):458-62, 2000
13. Nakamura H et al: Serial follow-up MR imaging after gamma knife radiosurgery for vestibular schwannoma. AJNR Am J Neuroradiol. 21(8):1540-6, 2000
14. Allen RW et al: Low-cost high-resolution fast spin-echo MR of acoustic schwannoma: an alternative to enhanced conventional spin-echo MR? AJNR Am J Neuroradiol. 17(7):1205-10, 1996

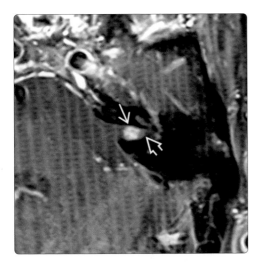
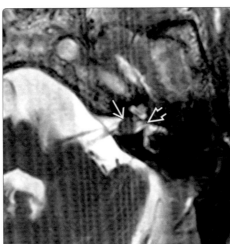

(Left) Axial T1WI C+ FS MR in a patient with left sensorineural hearing loss shows a small enhancing vestibular schwannoma ⇒ within the IAC with a 3-mm fundal CSF cap ⇨ lateral to the tumor. (Right) Axial CISS MR in the same patient reveals a filling defect ⇒ within the high-signal CSF in the IAC. The vestibular schwannoma is easily diagnosed with CISS imaging. The fundal CSF cap ⇨ is more readily seen with T2 or CISS MR.

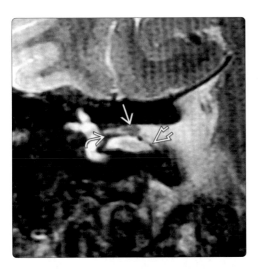
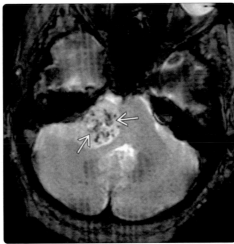

(Left) Coronal high-resolution thin-section T2WI MR demonstrates a 2-mm superior vestibular schwannoma ⇒. The lesion is seen superior to the crista falciformis ⇨ with the anterior inferior cerebellar artery loop ⇨ visible in the lateral IAC. (Right) Axial T2* GRE MR reveals punctate microhemorrhages ⇒ in the CPA component of a larger vestibular schwannoma. When present this finding is highly suggestive of vestibular schwannoma.

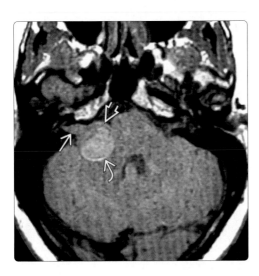
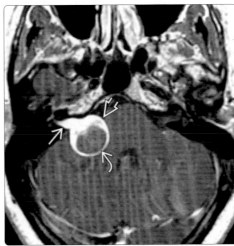

(Left) Axial T1WI MR reveals the IAC ⇒ and CPA ⇨ components of a larger vestibular schwannoma. Increased signal in the medial CPA portion of this tumor ⇒ is due to methemoglobin from a subacute intratumoral hemorrhage. (Right) Axial T1WI C+ MR in the same patient shows an enhancing vestibular schwannoma with IAC ⇒ and CPA ⇨ components. The medial CPA intramural cystic change ⇒ is due to hemorrhage.

Infantile Hemangioma and PHACES Association

TERMINOLOGY

- **PHACES**: Association of craniofacial hemangioma and 1 or more features listed in PHACES acronym
  - **P**osterior fossa malformations
  - **H**emangioma
  - **A**rterial lesions
  - **C**ardiac abnormalities/aortic coarctation
  - **E**ye abnormalities
  - **S**ternal defects or supraumbilical raphe

IMAGING

- **Proliferating regional or midline cervicofacial hemangioma**: Lobulated or plaque-like, prominent vascularity
- Unilateral cerebellar hypoplasia and prominent retrocerebellar CSF space
- Widened IAC ± hemangioma ± persistent stapedial artery
- Hypoplasia, aplasia, aberrancy, ectasia, tortuosity, & stenoocclusive changes of major cerebral arteries

TOP DIFFERENTIAL DIAGNOSES

- Sturge-Weber syndrome
- Schwannoma

PATHOLOGY

- Suspected genetic defect with possible environmental factors

CLINICAL ISSUES

- Hemangioma appears at birth or in neonate
- Gender: 80-90% female
- Cutaneous: Large regional or midline craniofacial hemangioma (20% of patients have PHACES)

DIAGNOSTIC CHECKLIST

- Consider PHACES association with large regional or midline cervicofacial hemangioma
- Look for ipsilateral cerebellar hemisphere anomaly of PHACES clinically mistaken for Sturge-Weber syndrome with port-wine stain

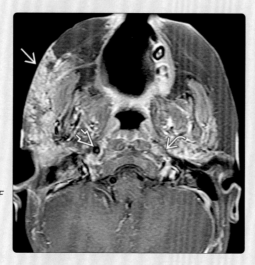
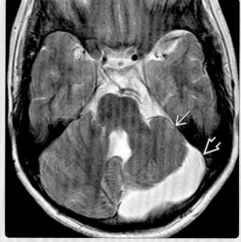

(Left) Axial T1WI C+ FS MR shows an enhancing right facial hemangioma ➡ with cutaneous and subcutaneous involvement. A normal right internal auditory canal (ICA) flow void is seen ➡. There is no left ICA flow void as a result of ICA atresia ➡. *(Right)* Axial T2WI MR in the same patient reveals cerebellar hypoplasia and cerebellar cortical malformation ➡ with a prominent retrocerebellar CSF space ➡. The ventral aspect of the pons is flattened and small.

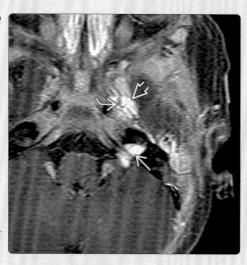
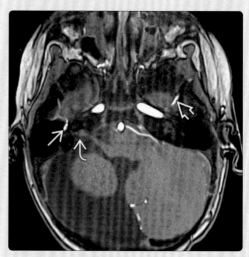

(Left) Three-week-old boy with left facial palsy shows avidly enhancing masses within the left IAC ➡ and cavernous sinus ➡, with a prominent flow void within the left cavernous sinus mass ➡. The IAC mass mimics a schwannoma. These hemangiomas involuted after the 1st year of life. *(Right)* Axial MRA of an infant girl with PHACES and right cerebellar hypoplasia is shown. There is a right persistent stapedial artery ➡. Note the normal left middle meningeal artery ➡. The right OIAC ➡ is widened.

TERMINOLOGY

Definitions

- Infantile hemangioma: Most common benign vascular tumor of infancy; proliferating and involuting phases
- **PHACES** acronym
  - **P**osterior fossa malformations
  - **H**emangioma
  - **A**rterial lesions
  - **C**ardiac abnormalities/aortic coarctation
  - **E**ye abnormalities
  - **S**ternal defects or supraumbilical raphe

IMAGING

General Features

- Best diagnostic clue
  - **Cervicofacial hemangioma**: Single or multiple; regional or midline
  - Posterior fossa anomaly
    - Unilateral (or bilateral) cerebellar hypoplasia ± malformation, prominent retrocerebellar CSF space
  - Cerebrovascular arterial findings
  - Cardiovascular findings
  - Sternal anomaly and supraumbilical raphe

Imaging Recommendations

- Best imaging tool
  - MR/MRA for hemangioma extent and CNS findings
- Protocol advice
  - Fat-suppressed T2, T1, fat-suppressed T1 C+
  - MRA: 3D TOF MRA brain and neck

CT Findings

- Hemangioma: Enhances intensely
- Small petrous internal carotid artery (ICA) canal
- Widened internal auditory canal (IAC) ipsilateral to cerebellar hypoplasia
- Persistent stapedial artery, absent foramen spinosum

MR Findings

- **Proliferating hemangioma**: Lobulated, intermediate signal on T2WI MR, **prominent flow voids**, **intense enhancement**
- **Involuting hemangioma**: Smaller, **less prominent flow voids**, increased fibrofatty tissue, **less enhancement**
- Multiple hemangiomas: Can involve CNS
  - Temporal bone locations: Pinna, external auditory canal, middle ear, & IAC
    - **IAC hemangioma simulates schwannoma**
- Brain MR
  - **Cerebellar hypoplasia** ± malformation (unilateral > bilateral) and prominent retrocerebellar CSF space
  - Agenesis/hypogenesis of corpus callosum ± lipoma
  - Polymicrogyria
  - **Arterial ischemic infarctions**
- MRA
  - Hypoplasia/aplasia, aberrant origin or course, kinking, tortuosity, loops, ectasia, or aneurysm of ICAs or vertebral arteries
  - **Persistent fetal connections** (e.g., persistent stapedial artery)
  - Stenoocclusive change with moyamoya collaterals

DIFFERENTIAL DIAGNOSIS

Sturge-Weber Syndrome

- Facial capillary-venular port-wine stain

Vestibular Schwannoma

- Older child; enhancing tumor lacks marked vascularity

PATHOLOGY

General Features

- Etiology
  - Neurocutaneous syndrome, currently of uncertain etiology and pathogenesis

Staging, Grading, & Classification

- Hemangioma: Classified as proliferating, involuting, or completely/incompletely regressed

Gross Pathologic & Surgical Features

- Birth: Cutaneous stain; congenital hemangioma uncommon
- 0-1 yr old: Proliferating hemangioma
  - Cutaneous: Crimson, raised, bosselated, or plaque-like
  - Subcutaneous: Bluish, raised, warm skin over mass

CLINICAL ISSUES

Presentation

- Most common signs/symptoms
  - Plaque-like cutaneous craniofacial hemangioma: Typically supraorbital, cheek, beard-like, or midline; L > R
  - Cardiac & aortic: Cardiac failure, cardiac tamponade
  - Neurologic: Developmental delay, seizures, headaches, stroke
- Other signs/symptoms
  - Sternal pit, sternal cleft, supraumbilical raphe

Demographics

- Hemangioma appears at birth or in neonate
- Incidence ~ 5%; ~ 80-90% female
- PHACES: Uncommon but not rare

Natural History & Prognosis

- Variable prognosis, depends on type & severity of anomalies

Treatment

- Propranolol: Accelerates involution
- Neurosurgical revascularization

SELECTED REFERENCES

1. Meltzer DE et al: Enlargement of the internal auditory canal and associated posterior fossa anomalies in PHACES association. AJNR Am J Neuroradiol. 36(11):2159-62, 2015
2. Hess CP et al: Cervical and intracranial arterial anomalies in 70 patients with PHACE syndrome. AJNR Am J Neuroradiol. 31(10):1980-6, 2010
3. Metry D et al: Consensus statement on diagnostic criteria for PHACE syndrome. Pediatrics. 124(5):1447-56, 2009
4. Oza VS et al: PHACES association: a neuroradiologic review of 17 patients. AJNR Am J Neuroradiol. 29(4):807-13, 2008
5. Frieden IJ et al: PHACE syndrome. The association of posterior fossa brain malformations, hemangiomas, arterial anomalies, coarctation of the aorta and cardiac defects, and eye abnormalities. Arch Dermatol. 132(3):307-11, 1996
6. Pascual-Castroviejo I et al: Hemangiomas of the head, neck, and chest with associated vascular and brain anomalies: a complex neurocutaneous syndrome. AJNR Am J Neuroradiol. 17(3):461-71, 1996

TERMINOLOGY

- Definition: Benign, unencapsulated neoplasm arising from meningothelial arachnoid cells of CPA-IAC dura

IMAGING

- 10% occur in posterior fossa
- When in CPA, asymmetric to IAC porus acusticus
- NECT: 25% calcified; 2 types seen
  ○ Homogeneous, sand-like (psammomatous)
  ○ Focal sunburst, globular, or rim pattern
- Bone CT: Hyperostotic or permeative-sclerotic bone changes possible (en plaque type)
- T2WI MR: Pial blood vessels seen as surface flow voids between tumor and brain
  ○ High signal crescent from CSF ("CSF cleft")
- T1WI C+ MR: Enhancing dural-based mass with dural tails centered along posterior petrous wall
  ○ When IAC tail present, usually dural reaction, not tumor

TOP DIFFERENTIAL DIAGNOSES

- Vestibular schwannoma
- Epidermoid cyst, CPA-IAC
- Dural metastases, CPA-IAC
- Sarcoidosis, CPA-IAC
- Idiopathic inflammatory pseudotumor

CLINICAL ISSUES

- 2nd most common CPA tumor
- Slow-growing tumor, displacing adjacent structures
- Often found as incidental brain MR finding
- < 10% symptomatic
  ○ Usually do not cause sensorineural hearing loss
- Treatment
  ○ Follow with imaging if smaller size and older patient
  ○ Surgical removal if medically safe
  ○ Adjunctive radiation therapy with incomplete surgery

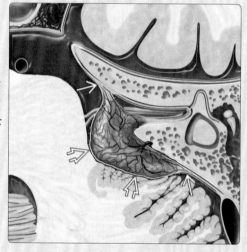
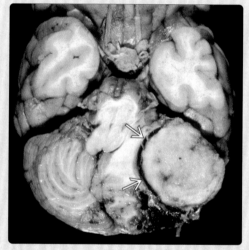

(Left) Axial graphic at level of the IAC shows a large CPA meningioma causing mass effect on the brainstem and cerebellum. Notice the broad dural base creating the shape of a mushroom cap. Dural tails ➡ are present in ~ 60% of cases, typically representing reactive rather than neoplastic change. CSF-vascular cleft is also visible ➡. (Right) Gross pathologic section viewed from below shows a large CPA meningioma with a broad dural base compressing the cerebellum. The specimen demonstrates a CSF-vascular cleft ➡.

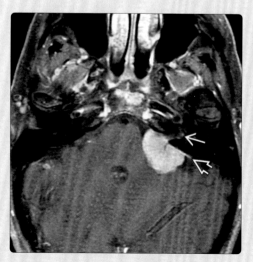
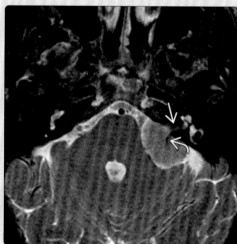

(Left) Axial T1WI C+ FS MR through the IAC shows a meningioma overlying the porus acusticus. Note the dural tail ➡ extending along the temporal bone posterior wall. A dot of enhancement in the IAC fundus ➡ suggests that the low signal area in the IAC is a nonenhancing meningioma. (Right) Axial T2WI FS MR in the same patient reveals a high-velocity flow void ➡ representing a dural artery feeder penetrating the meningioma core. Low signal in the IAC ➡ is a intracanalicular meningioma.

TERMINOLOGY

Definitions

- Benign, unencapsulated neoplasm arising from meningothelial arachnoid cells of CPA-IAC dura

IMAGING

General Features

- Best diagnostic clue
  - CPA dural-based enhancing mass with **dural tails**
- Location
  - 10% occur in posterior fossa
  - When in CPA, **asymmetric** to IAC porus acusticus
- Size
  - Broad range; usually 1-8 cm but may be larger
  - Generally significantly larger than vestibular schwannoma at presentation
- Morphology
  - 3 distinct morphologies
    - "Mushroom cap" (hemispherical) with broad base towards posterior petrous wall (75%)
    - Plaque-like (en plaque), ± bone invasion with hyperostosis (20%)
    - Ovoid mass mimics vestibular schwannoma (5%)
  - Larger lesions often herniate superiorly through incisura into medial middle cranial fossa

CT Findings

- NECT
  - 25% isodense, 75% hyperdense
  - 25% calcified; 2 types seen
    - Homogeneous, sand-like (psammomatous)
    - Focal sunburst, globular, or rim pattern
- CECT
  - > 90% strong, uniform enhancement
- Bone CT
  - Hyperostotic or permeative-sclerotic bone changes possible (en plaque type)
  - IAC flaring is rare (cf. vestibular schwannoma)

MR Findings

- T1WI
  - Isointense or minimally hyperintense to gray matter
  - When tumor has calcifications or is highly fibrous, hypointense areas are visible
- T2WI
  - Wide range of possible signals on T2 sequence
    - Isointense or hypointense CPA mass (compared to gray matter) is most likely meningioma
    - Focal or diffuse parenchymal low signal seen if calcified or highly fibrous
  - **CSF-vascular cleft**
    - Pial blood vessels seen as surface flow voids between tumor and brain
    - High-signal crescent from CSF
  - Tumor arterial feeders seen as arborizing flow voids
  - High signal in adjacent brainstem or cerebellum
    - Represents peritumoral brain edema
    - Correlates with pial blood supply
    - Signals problems with safe removal

- T2* GRE
  - Calcifications may bloom
- T1WI C+
  - Enhancing **dural-based mass** with **dural tails** centered along posterior petrous wall
    - > 95% enhance strongly
    - Heterogeneous enhancement when large
  - Dural tail in ~ 60%
    - Represents **reactive** rather than neoplastic change in most cases
    - When extending into IAC, may mimic IAC component of vestibular schwannoma
  - En plaque: Sessile, thickened enhancing dura

Angiographic Findings

- Digital subtraction angiography
  - Dural vessels supply tumor center, **pial vessels** supply **tumor rim**
  - Sunburst pattern: Enlarged dural feeders
  - Prolonged vascular "stain" into venous phase
- Interventional: Preoperative embolization
  - ↓ operative time and blood loss
  - Particulate agents favored (e.g., polyvinyl alcohol)
  - Optimal interval between embolization and surgery is 7-9 days
    - Allows for greatest tumor softening

Imaging Recommendations

- Best imaging tool
  - Enhanced MR focused to posterior fossa
  - Bone CT if bone invasion suspected on MR
- Protocol advice
  - Full brain T2 ± FLAIR shows brain edema best

DIFFERENTIAL DIAGNOSIS

Vestibular Schwannoma

- Intracanalicular 1st, then CPA extension
- Intracanalicular meningioma may mimic

Epidermoid Cyst, CPA-IAC

- Near CSF signal insinuating mass on MR
- DWI high signal characteristic

Dural Metastases, CPA-IAC

- May be bilateral in CPA area
- Multifocal meningeal involvement

Sarcoidosis, CPA-IAC

- Often multifocal, dural-based foci
- Look for infundibular stalk involvement

Idiopathic Inflammatory Pseudotumor

- Diffuse or focal meningeal thickening
- CPA involvement is rare

PATHOLOGY

General Features

- Etiology
  - Arises from arachnoid ("cap") meningothelial cells
  - Radiation therapy (XRT) predisposes

    – Most common radiation-induced tumor; latency 20-35 years
- Genetics
  - Long arm deletions of chromosome 22 are common
  - *NF2* gene inactivated in 90% of sporadic cases
  - May have progesterone, prolactin receptors; may express growth hormone
- Associated abnormalities
  - Neurofibromatosis type 2 (NF2)
    - 10% of multiple meningiomas have NF2
    - Meningioma + schwannoma = NF2
    - Multiple inherited schwannomas, meningiomas, and ependymomas (MISME)

Staging, Grading, & Classification
- WHO grading classification (grades I-III)
  - Typical meningioma (grade I, benign) = 90%
  - Atypical meningioma (grade II) = 9%
  - Malignant (anaplastic) meningioma (grade III) = 1%

Gross Pathologic & Surgical Features
- "Mushroom cap" (globose, hemispherical) morphology most common (75%)
- En plaque morphology (20%) also seen in CPA
- Sharply circumscribed, unencapsulated
- Adjacent dural thickening (collar or tail) is usually reactive, not neoplastic

Microscopic Features
- Subtypes (wide range of histology with little bearing on imaging appearance or clinical outcome)
  - Meningothelial (lobules of meningothelial cells)
  - Fibrous (parallel, interlacing fascicles of spindle-shaped cells)
  - Transitional (mixed; "onion-bulb" whorls and lobules)
  - Angiomatous (↑ vascular channels), not equated with obsolete term "angioblastic meningioma"
  - Lipoblastic: Metaplasia into adipocytes; large triglyceride fat droplets
  - Miscellaneous forms (microcystic, chordoid, clear cell, secretory, lymphoplasmacyte-rich, etc.)

CLINICAL ISSUES

Presentation
- Most common signs/symptoms
  - Incidental brain MR finding
  - < 10% symptomatic
- Clinical profile
  - Adult undergoing brain MR for unrelated indication

Demographics
- Age
  - Middle-aged, elderly; peak = 60 years old
  - If found in children, consider possibility of NF2
- Gender
  - M:F = 1:1.5-3
- Ethnicity
  - More common in African Americans
- Epidemiology
  - Accounts for ~ 20% of primary intracranial tumors
    - Most common primary nonglial tumor

- 1-1.5% prevalence at autopsy or imaging
- 10% multiple (NF2; multiple meningiomatosis)
- 2nd most common CPA-IAC mass

Natural History & Prognosis
- Slow-growing tumor
- Compresses rather than invades structures
- Negative prognostic findings on MR
  - Peritumoral edema in adjacent brainstem
  - Significant subjacent bone invasion

Treatment
- Asymptomatic: Follow with serial imaging if smaller tumor or older patient
- Surgical removal if medically safe
  - Complete surgical removal possible in 95% when tumor does not invade skull base
- Radiation therapy
  - Adjunctive therapy with incomplete surgery
  - Primary therapy if extensive skull base invasion

DIAGNOSTIC CHECKLIST

Consider
- Meningioma when MR shows hemispherical, dural-based enhancing CPA mass with dural tails
- Meningioma when CPA mass is large but asymptomatic

Image Interpretation Pearls
- Focal or diffuse hypointensity on T2 in CPA mass suggests meningioma
- Dural tail in IAC suggests meningioma

Reporting Tips
- Report extent of meningioma, including intraosseous component
  - Mention cranial nerves in area of involvement
  - Note any brainstem or brain edema indicating pia-arachnoid involvement

SELECTED REFERENCES

1. Park SH et al: Stereotactic radiosurgery for cerebellopontine angle meningiomas. J Neurosurg. 120(3):708-15, 2014
2. Agarwal V et al: Cerebellopontine angle meningiomas: postoperative outcomes in a modern cohort. Neurosurg Focus. 35(6):E10, 2013
3. Zeidman LA et al: Growth rate of non-operated meningiomas. J Neurol. 255(6):891-5, 2008
4. Nakamura M et al: Facial and cochlear nerve function after surgery of cerebellopontine angle meningiomas. Neurosurgery. 57(1):77-90; discussion 77-90, 2005
5. Roser F et al: Meningiomas of the cerebellopontine angle with extension into the internal auditory canal. J Neurosurg. 102(1):17-23, 2005
6. Asaoka K et al: Intracanalicular meningioma mimicking vestibular schwannoma. AJNR Am J Neuroradiol. 23(9):1493-6, 2002
7. Filippi CG et al: Appearance of meningiomas on diffusion-weighted images: correlating diffusion constants with histopathologic findings. AJNR Am J Neuroradiol. 22(1):65-72, 2001
8. Kuratsu J et al: Incidence and clinical features of asymptomatic meningiomas. J Neurosurg. 92(5):766-70, 2000
9. Yoshioka H et al: Peritumoral brain edema associated with meningioma: influence of vascular endothelial growth factor expression and vascular blood supply. Cancer. 85(4):936-44, 1999
10. Haught K et al: Entirely intracanalicular meningioma: contrast-enhanced MR findings in a rare entity. AJNR Am J Neuroradiol. 19(10):1831-3, 1998

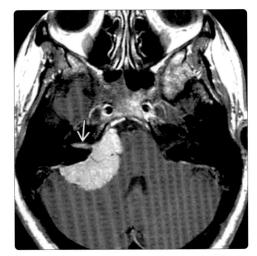

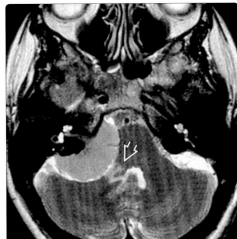

(Left) *Axial T1WI C+ MR demonstrates a large CPA meningioma with an IAC component* ➡. *This degree and depth of IAC enhancement usually signifies tumor rather than dural reaction.* (Right) *Axial T2WI MR in the same patient reveals high signal in the adjacent brachium pontis* ➡. *Pial invasion by the meningioma is likely. This MR finding is predictive of an increased risk of complications when surgical removal occurs.*

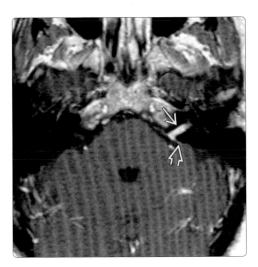

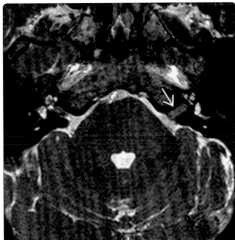

(Left) *Axial T1WI C+ MR shows an enhancing intracanalicular mass* ➡. *Subtle dural tails* ➡ *along the posterior margin of the porus acusticus suggest but do not definitively diagnose meningioma.* (Right) *Axial T2WI MR in the same patient reveals the intracanalicular meningioma* ➡ *as low signal tissue filling the IAC. Often IAC meningioma cannot be reliably distinguished from IAC vestibular schwannoma, the most common lesion in this location.*

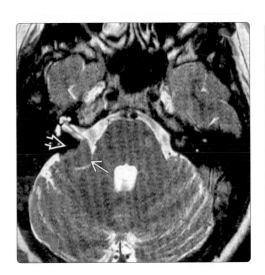

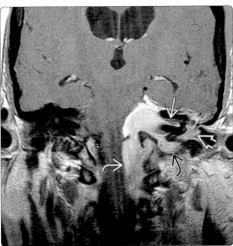

(Left) *Axial T2WI MR shows a gray matter signal intensity meningioma* ➡ *abutting the posterior wall of the temporal bone. Note the underlying dark signal of bony hyperostosis* ➡. *Despite the tumor abutting CNVII-III along the posterior margin of the porus acusticus, the patient did not have hearing loss.* (Right) *Coronal T1WI C+ MR shows a large enhancing CPA meningioma. Note that the IAC* ➡, *middle ear* ➡, *and jugular foramen* ➡ *are filled with tumor. Tumor extends through the foramen magnum* ➡.

KEY FACTS

TERMINOLOGY

- Abbreviation: Facial nerve schwannoma (FNS)
- FNS definition: Rare benign tumor of Schwann cells that surround CNVII in CPA-IAC ± labyrinthine CNVII

IMAGING

- Temporal bone CT findings
  - ↑ size of labyrinthine CNVII canal ± geniculate fossa
- MR findings
  - T1 C+ MR: CPA-IAC-labyrinthine CNVII canal C+ mass

TOP DIFFERENTIAL DIAGNOSES

- Bell palsy (herpetic facial paralysis)
- Vestibular schwannoma
- CPA-IAC meningioma
- Neurofibromatosis type 2

PATHOLOGY

- Tumor of Schwann cells lining CNVII

- Neurofibromatosis type 2
  - **Bilateral** CPA-IAC schwannomas
  - May be of **vestibular** or **facial** nerve origin

CLINICAL ISSUES

- Clinical presentation
  - Sensorineural hearing loss (SNHL)
  - Facial nerve paralysis
  - SNHL & facial nerve paralysis similar in frequency
- Treatment options
  - Conservative management: Do nothing until CNVII paralysis present
  - Surgical management: Used when CNVII paralysis + other symptoms evolving
    - Debulking also effective
  - Stereotactic radiosurgery
    - Used for poor surgical candidates
    - Recent use in small- to medium-sized FNS with CNVII function and hearing relatively preserved

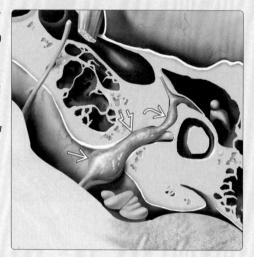
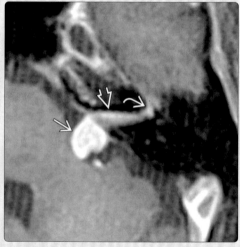

(Left) Axial graphic of a larger facial nerve schwannoma (FNS) shows CPA ("ice cream") ➡ & IAC ("cone") ➡ components that mimic vestibular schwannoma. The labyrinthine segment of facial nerve involvement ➡ makes the diagnosis. (Right) Axial T1WI C+ fat-saturated MR in a patient with unilateral sensorineural hearing loss shows FNS with CPA ➡ & IAC ➡ components. Note the labyrinthine segment facial nerve tail ➡, which differentiates FNS from vestibular schwannoma.

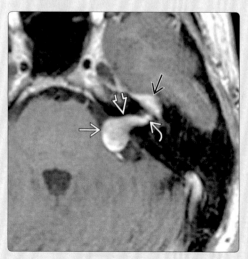
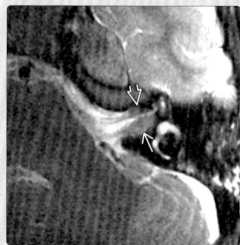

(Left) Axial T1WI C+ MR in a patient with facial paresis reveals a C+ FNS that involves the CPA ➡, IAC ➡, labyrinthine segment ➡, & geniculate ganglion ➡ of CNVII. When the FNS is confined to IAC only, it exactly mimics vestibular schwannoma. (Right) Axial thin-section magnified T2 MR of left IAC fundus in a patient with neurofibromatosis type 2 (NF2) shows the superior vestibular nerve ➡ & facial nerve schwannomas ➡. Caveat: In NF2, not all IAC lesions are vestibular schwannoma.

TERMINOLOGY

Abbreviations

- Facial nerve schwannoma (FNS)

Synonyms

- Facial neuroma, facial neurilemmoma

Definitions

- FNS: Rare benign tumor of Schwann cells that surround facial nerve in cerebellopontine angle (CPA)-internal auditory canal (IAC)

IMAGING

General Features

- Best diagnostic clue
  - CPA-IAC mass + **tail in labyrinthine CNVII canal**
- Location
  - CPA-IAC & labyrinthine segment of CNVII canal
- Morphology
  - Large: CPA-IAC ice cream on cone shape with comma-shaped tail in labyrinthine segment CNVII
  - Small: IAC mass curves into labyrinthine tail (may be in IAC CNVII only mimicking vestibular schwannoma)

CT Findings

- Bone CT
  - ↑ size labyrinthine CNVII canal ± geniculate fossa

MR Findings

- T1WI C+
  - CPA-IAC-labyrinthine canal enhancing mass
    - ± **intramural cystic change**
- CISS, FIESTA, T2 Space
  - FNS CPA-IAC = mass displacing high-signal CSF

Imaging Recommendations

- Best imaging tool
  - CNVII or CNVIII symptoms 1st studied with contrast-enhanced T1 MR
    - Axial ≤ 3-mm T1 C+ MR; axial & coronal of CPA-IAC
  - Bone CT: Verify MR suspicion of ↑ size labyrinthine CNVII

DIFFERENTIAL DIAGNOSIS

Bell Palsy (Herpetic Facial Paralysis)

- T1 C+ MR: Prominent enhancement of intratemporal CNVII with IAC fundal tuft

Vestibular Schwannoma

- T1 C+ MR: CPA-IAC enhancing mass without labyrinthine canal tail

CPA-IAC Meningioma

- T1 C+ MR: Dural-based, eccentric CPA enhancing mass with dural tail projecting into IAC

PATHOLOGY

General Features

- Etiology
  - Tumor of Schwann cells investing CNVII
- Genetics

- Multiple schwannomas = neurofibromatosis 2 (NF2)
- Associated abnormalities
  - **NF2**: Bilateral vestibular schwannoma; other CN schwannoma, meningiomas also seen

Gross Pathologic & Surgical Features

- From outer nerve sheath layer

Microscopic Features

- Encapsulated; bundles of spindle-shaped Schwann cells forming whorled pattern
- Cellular architecture: Densely cellular (**Antoni A**) areas ± loose, myxomatous (**Antoni B**) areas

CLINICAL ISSUES

Presentation

- Most common signs/symptoms
  - Sensorineural hearing loss ~ facial nerve paralysis
  - Other symptoms: Vertigo, hemifacial spasm

Demographics

- Age
  - Average age at presentation: ~ **50 yr**
- Epidemiology
  - Rare tumor (temporal bone > CPA-IAC > parotid)

Natural History & Prognosis

- CNVII paralysis takes years to develop
- Surgical cure can be worse than disease

Treatment

- Conservative: Do nothing until CNVII paralysis present
  - Some do not grow; some never become symptomatic
- Surgery when CNVII paralysis + other symptoms evolving
  - Goal: Complete tumor removal + preservation of hearing & restoration of CNVII function
- Stereotactic radiosurgery
  - Used as primary treatment for small- to medium-sized FNS when CNVII function and hearing relatively preserved

DIAGNOSTIC CHECKLIST

Consider

- Thin-section imaging shows labyrinthine tail

Image Interpretation Pearls

- CPA-IAC FNS exactly mimics vestibular schwannoma if no labyrinthine tail present

SELECTED REFERENCES

1. Moon JH et al: Gamma Knife surgery for facial nerve schwannomas. J Neurosurg. 121 Suppl:116-22, 2014
2. Mowry S et al: Surgical management of internal auditory canal and cerebellopontine angle facial nerve schwannoma. Otol Neurotol. 33(6):1071-6, 2012
3. Wiggins RH 3rd et al: The many faces of facial nerve schwannoma. AJNR Am J Neuroradiol. 27(3):694-9, 2006
4. Liu R et al: Facial nerve schwannoma: surgical excision versus conservative management. Ann Otol Rhinol Laryngol. 110(11):1025-9, 2001
5. Yokota N et al: Facial nerve schwannoma in the cerebellopontine cistern. Findings on high resolution CT and MR cisternography. Br J Neurosurg. 13(5):512-5, 1999
6. McMenomey SO et al: Facial nerve neuromas presenting as acoustic tumors. Am J Otol. 15(3):307-12, 1994

TERMINOLOGY

- Definition: CPA-IAC metastases refers to systemic or CNS neoplasia affecting area of CPA-IAC

IMAGING

- 4 major sites: Leptomeningeal (pia-arachnoid), dura, flocculus, and choroid plexus
- T1WI C+ MR
  - **Leptomeningeal metastases**: Diffuse thickening and enhancement of cranial nerves in IAC
  - **Dural metastases**: Thickened enhancing dura; may be diffuse or focal
  - **Floccular metastases**: Enhancing floccular mass extends into CPA cistern
  - **Choroid plexus metastases**: Enhancing nodular lesion along normal course of choroid plexus
  - Focal, enhancing brain metastases may be present
- FLAIR MR
  - Parenchymal brain metastases usually high signal

TOP DIFFERENTIAL DIAGNOSES

- Bilateral vestibular schwannoma (NF2)
- Sarcoidosis
- Meningitis
- Ramsay Hunt syndrome

CLINICAL ISSUES

- Rapidly progressive unilateral or bilateral facial nerve paralysis and sensorineural hearing loss
- Patient with past history of treated malignancy

DIAGNOSTIC CHECKLIST

- If trying to diagnose bilateral "vestibular schwannoma" in adult as NF2, probably CPA metastases instead
- Rapidly progressive CNVII and CNVIII palsies + CPA mass suggests metastatic focus
  - Vestibular schwannoma rarely causes CNVII palsy

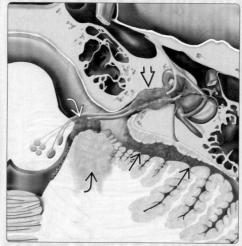
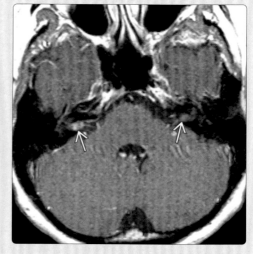

(Left) Axial graphic depicts the 4 major types of CPA-IAC area metastases. Along the posterolateral margin of the IAC, thickened dural metastases ⇨ are visible. Within the IAC metastatic leptomeningeal (pia-arachnoid) ⇨ involvement is present. Choroid plexus ⇨ and floccular ⇨ metastases are also depicted. (Right) Axial T1WI C+ MR shows bilateral leptomeningeal breast carcinoma metastases ⇨ within the internal auditory canals. The left-sided disease is more subtle than the right.

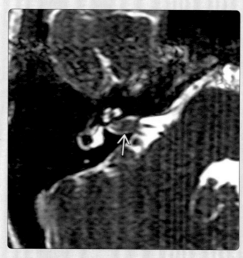
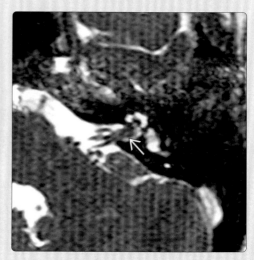

(Left) Axial T2WI MR demonstrates right IAC leptomeningeal metastatic foci as thickening of the branches of CNVII and CNVIII ⇨ within the internal auditory canal. (Right) Axial T2WI MR reveals left IAC metastatic disease as subtle thickening of the branches of CNVII and CNVIII ⇨ within the internal auditory canal. In an adult patient with suspected "bilateral vestibular schwannoma," consider metastatic disease rather than NF2.

TERMINOLOGY

Abbreviations

- Metastases (mets)

Synonyms

- Leptomeningeal carcinomatosis, meningeal carcinomatosis, carcinomatous meningitis
  - All of above terms are misnomers for following reasons
    - Neoplasms are not always carcinomas
    - Pachymeninges (dura) and leptomeninges (pia + arachnoid) are often both involved
    - Usually does not contain inflammatory component
      - -itis suffix makes no sense

Definitions

- CPA-IAC metastases: Systemic or central nervous system (CNS) neoplasia affecting area of CPA-IAC

IMAGING

General Features

- Best diagnostic clue
  - Multiple enhancing masses on T1WI C+ MR
- Location
  - 4 major sites: **Leptomeningeal (pia-arachnoid), dura, flocculus, and choroid plexus**
  - Primary site locations
    - Primary tumors: Breast, lung, and melanoma
    - Meningeal lymphoproliferative malignancy
      - Lymphoma and leukemia
    - Primary CNS tumor seeds basal cisterns via cerebrospinal fluid (CSF) pathways: "Drop" metastases
- Size
  - Often small (< 1 cm)
    - Metastases cause symptoms early
- Morphology
  - Leptomeningeal: Thickened CNVII and CNIII in IAC
  - Dura: Diffuse dural thickening (pachymeninges)
  - Flocculus: Enlarged flocculus with associated brain edema; mass extends into CPA cistern
  - Choroid plexus: Nodular thickening

CT Findings

- CECT
  - Unilateral or bilateral dural enhancement along CPA
  - CT shows metastases only when larger ± multiple

MR Findings

- T1WI
  - Focal dural thickening isointense to gray matter
- T2WI
  - High-resolution T2 MR
    - Leptomeningeal metastases: CNVII and CNVIII thickening
    - Floccular metastases: ↑ signal edema associated
- FLAIR
  - Larger CPA-IAC metastases may cause ↑ signal in adjacent brainstem ± cerebellum
  - Floccular metastases seen as ↑ signal
- T1WI C+

- o **Leptomeningeal metastases**: Diffuse thickening and enhancement of cranial nerves in IAC
    - Late finding shows plug of enhancing tissue in IAC
    - Unilateral or bilateral
  - o **Dural metastases**: Thickened enhancing dura; may be focal or diffuse
    - Associated with other dural or skull lesions
  - o **Floccular metastases**: Enhancing floccular mass
  - o **Choroid plexus metastases**: Enhancing nodular lesion along normal course of choroid plexus
    - Lateral recess 4th ventricle → foramen of Luschka → inferior CPA cistern
  - o Focal, enhancing brain metastases may be present

Imaging Recommendations

- Best imaging tool
  - T1WI C+ MR of posterior fossa is best imaging tool and sequence
  - Whole-brain FLAIR and T1WI C+ for associated brain metastases
- Protocol advice
  - Axial and coronal planes recommended

DIFFERENTIAL DIAGNOSIS

Bilateral Vestibular Schwannoma (NF2)

- Younger patients; no history of malignancy
- T1WI C+ MR shows bilateral CPA-IAC enhancing masses
  - Mimics bilateral leptomeningeal metastases
- Other cranial nerve schwannoma ± meningiomas possible

Sarcoidosis, CPA-IAC

- ↑ erythrocyte sedimentation rate (ESR) and serum angiotensin converting enzyme (ACE)
- T1WI C+ MR may be identical to metastases when multifocal meningeal type
  - May be bilateral CPA lesions mimicking neurofibromatosis 2 (NF2) or metastases
  - May be single, en plaque focus mimicking meningioma
- Look for infundibular stalk involvement

Meningitis, CPA-IAC

- Bacterial meningitis
- Fungal meningitis
- Tuberculous meningitis
- T1WI C+ MR may be identical to CPA-IAC metastases
- Clinical information and CSF evaluation are key

Ramsay Hunt Syndrome

- External ear vesicular rash
- T1WI C+ MR shows enhancement in IAC fundus and inner ear ± CNVII
  - Mimics unilateral leptomeningeal metastasis

PATHOLOGY

General Features

- Etiology
  - Metastatic tumor involves leptomeningeal or dural surfaces of CPA-IAC
    - Leptomeningeal metastases follow CNVII and CNVIII into IAC
  - Metastatic tumor deposits in flocculus or choroid plexus

- Routes of spread
  - Extracranial neoplasm spreads hematogenously to meninges
  - CSF spread from intracranial or intraspinal neoplasm is less common
- Associated abnormalities
  - Multiple other pial or dural metastatic foci
  - Parenchymal brain metastases also possible
    - Pia + arachnoid = **leptomeninges**
- Key anatomy: Meninges has 3 discrete layers
  - **Dura** (pachymeninges): Dense connective tissue attached to calvarium
  - **Arachnoid**: Interposed between pia and dura
  - **Pia**: Clear membrane firmly attached to surface of brain; extends deeply into sulci

Gross Pathologic & Surgical Features

- Diffuse, nodular ± discrete

Microscopic Features

- Common tissue types found
  - Solid tumors = breast, lung, and melanoma
    - All involve both leptomeninges and pachymeninges
  - Lymphoproliferative malignancy = lymphoma and leukemia
    - Involve both leptomeninges and pachymeninges
  - "Drop" metastases from CNS tumors
    - Medulloblastoma, ependymoma, glioblastoma multiforme

CLINICAL ISSUES

Presentation

- Most common signs/symptoms
  - **Rapidly progressive** unilateral or bilateral facial nerve (CNVII) paralysis and sensorineural hearing loss (CNVIII)
- Other signs/symptoms
  - Vertigo and polycranial neuropathy
- Clinical profile
  - Patient with past history of treated malignancy

Demographics

- Age
  - Older adults
- Epidemiology
  - Increasingly more common neurologic complication of systemic cancer
    - Due to increase in survival rate of cancer patients

Natural History & Prognosis

- Meningeal metastases usually late-stage finding
- Poor prognosis as patients have advanced, incurable disease by definition

Treatment

- No curative treatments available
- Therapies aimed at preserving neurologic function and improving quality of life
- Treatments are same as for underlying neoplasm
  - Radiotherapy ± chemotherapy depending on tissue type
- Surgery will rarely play role at this stage
  - Solitary melanoma metastases may be exception

- If any question of diagnosis, excisional biopsy necessary

DIAGNOSTIC CHECKLIST

Consider

- If trying to diagnose bilateral "vestibular schwannoma" in adult as NF2, probably CPA metastases instead
- Rapidly progressive CNVII palsy + sensorineural hearing loss with CPA mass suggests metastatic focus
  - Vestibular schwannoma rarely causes CNVII palsy

Image Interpretation Pearls

- If suspect CPA-IAC metastasis from T1WI C+ MR appearance or history of known malignancy, make sure to review
  - Extracranial and calvarial structures for other lesions to confirm diagnosis
  - Look for involvement of other meningeal sites, such as parasellar, other basal meninges
  - Parenchymal brain for abnormal FLAIR high signal ± enhancing lesions on T1WI C+ sequences

SELECTED REFERENCES

1. Lee EK et al: Intracranial metastases: spectrum of MR imaging findings. Acta Radiol. 53(10):1173-85, 2012
2. Warren FM et al: Imaging characteristics of metastatic lesions to the cerebellopontine angle. Otol Neurotol. 29(6):835-8, 2008
3. Siomin VE et al: Posterior fossa metastasis: risk of leptomeningeal disease when treated with stereotactic radiosurgery compared to surgery. J Neurooncol. 67(1-2):115-21, 2004
4. Soyuer S et al: Intracranial meningeal hemangiopericytoma: the role of radiotherapy: report of 29 cases and review of the literature. Cancer. 100(7):1491-7, 2004
5. Kesari S et al: Leptomeningeal metastases. Neurol Clin. 21(1):25-66, 2003
6. Krainik A et al: MRI of unusual lesions in the internal auditory canal. Neuroradiology. 43(1):52-7, 2001
7. Schick B et al: Magnetic resonance imaging in patients with sudden hearing loss, tinnitus and vertigo. Otol Neurotol. 22(6):808-12, 2001
8. Whinney D et al: Primary malignant melanoma of the cerebellopontine angle. Otol Neurotol. 22(2):218-22, 2001
9. Cha ST et al: Cerebellopontine angle metastasis from papillary carcinoma of the thyroid: case report and literature review. Surg Neurol. 54(4):320-6, 2000
10. Shen TY et al: Meningeal carcinomatosis manifested as bilateral progressive sensorineural hearing loss. Am J Otol. 21(4):510-2, 2000
11. Zamani AA: Cerebellopontine angle tumors: role of magnetic resonance imaging. Top Magn Reson Imaging. 11(2):98-107, 2000
12. Lewanski CR et al: Bilateral cerebellopontine metastases in a patient with an unknown primary. Clin Oncol (R Coll Radiol). 11(4):272-3, 1999
13. Swartz JD: Meningeal metastases. Am J Otol. 20(5):683-5, 1999
14. Arriaga MA et al: Metastatic melanoma to the cerebellopontine angle. Clinical and imaging characteristics. Arch Otolaryngol Head Neck Surg. 121(9):1052-6, 1995
15. Kingdom TT et al: Isolated metastatic melanoma of the cerebellopontine angle: case report. Neurosurgery. 33(1):142-4, 1993
16. Mark AS et al: Sensorineural hearing loss: more than meets the eye? AJNR Am J Neuroradiol. 14(1):37-45, 1993
17. Yuh WT et al: Metastatic lesions involving the cerebellopontine angle. AJNR Am J Neuroradiol. 14(1):99-106, 1993
18. Lee YY et al: Loculated intracranial leptomeningeal metastases: CT and MR characteristics. AJR Am J Roentgenol. 154(2):351-9, 1990
19. Maiuri F et al: Cerebellar metastasis from prostatic carcinoma simulating, on CT-scan, a cerebellopontine angle tumor. Case report. Acta Neurol (Napoli). 11(1):21-4, 1989
20. Gentry LR et al: Cerebellopontine angle-petromastoid mass lesions: comparative study of diagnosis with MR imaging and CT. Radiology. 162(2):513-20, 1987

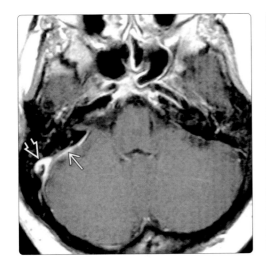

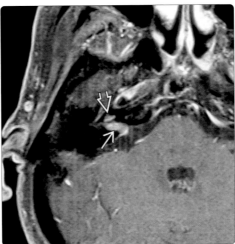

(Left) *Axial T1WI C+ MR reveals dural lung carcinoma metastases ⇒ in the CPA region. The enhancing, thickened dura should be distinguished from the enhancement in the normal sigmoid sinus ⇒. CSF examination was positive for malignant cells.* (Right) *Axial T1WI C+ FS MR shows an enhancing metastasis in the right IAC ⇒ with extension of enhancing tissue through the cochlear nerve canal, across the modiolus into the membranous labyrinth of the cochlea ⇒.*

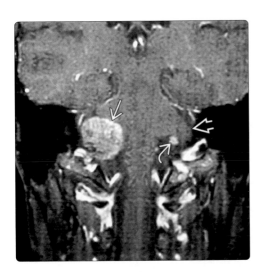

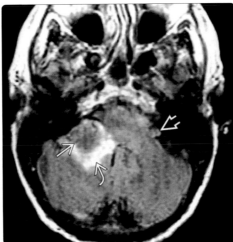

(Left) *Coronal T1WI C+ MR depicts an enhancing breast carcinoma metastasis ⇒ centered within the right flocculus. Note the normal flocculus ⇒ and cisternal choroid plexus ⇒.* (Right) *Axial FLAIR MR in the same patient shows the mass ⇒ to be slightly lower in signal than the adjacent gray matter. Vasogenic edema within the brachium pontis and cerebellum ⇒ is seen as high signal. The left flocculus ⇒ is normal.*

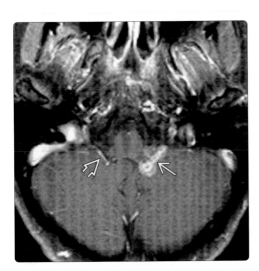

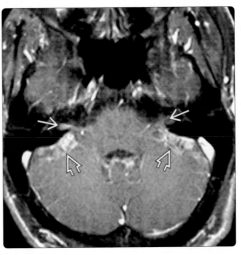

(Left) *Axial T1WI C+ FS MR in a patient with known metastatic rectal carcinoma shows an enhancing metastasis ⇒ of the choroid plexus projecting into the low CPA cistern through the foramen of Luschka. The normal right choroid plexus ⇒ is seen.* (Right) *Axial T1WI C+ FS reveals bilateral CPA-IAC "drop" metastases from a supratentorial glioblastoma multiforme. Bilateral IAC enhancing metastases ⇒ are seen along with multiple leptomeningeal metastases on the cerebellar surface ⇒.*

TERMINOLOGY

- Definition: Vascular loop compressing trigeminal nerve (CNV) at its root entry zone (REZ) or preganglionic segment (PGS)

IMAGING

- High-resolution MR: Serpiginous asymmetric signal void (vessel) in CPA CNV REZ or PGS
  - CNV PGS atrophy: Severe, prolonged compression; compressing vessel will bow PGS
- Offending vessels: **Superior cerebellar artery** (55%) > AICA (10%) > basal artery (5%) > variant vein (5%) > other

TOP DIFFERENTIAL DIAGNOSES

- Aneurysm in CPA-IAC
- Arteriovenous malformation in CPA
- Sevelopmental venous anomaly in posterior fossa

PATHOLOGY

- CNV REZ or PGS experiences "irritation" from vessel

CLINICAL ISSUES

- Trigeminal neuralgia symptoms
  - Lancinating pain following V2 ± V3 distributions
  - May occur spontaneously or in response to "trigger" from tactile stimulation
- Treatment: Begin with conservative drug therapy; microvascular decompression or focused radiotherapy (~ 70% long-term success rate)

DIAGNOSTIC CHECKLIST

- 1st look for multiple sclerosis or DVA with draining vein along PGS
  - Also check for cisternal mass: Schwannoma, meningioma, epidermoid
- Next, follow CNV distally into cavernous sinus & face
  - Exclude perineural tumor, malignancies of face
- Lastly, view high-resolution thin-section MR for causal vessel
  - Causal vessel will bow PGS or deform REZ

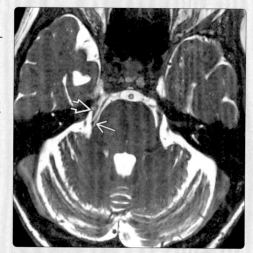
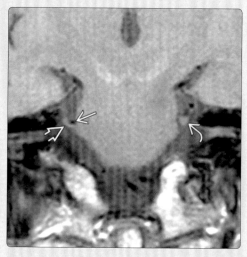

(Left) Axial T2WI MR in this patient with right trigeminal neuralgia (TN) shows the low-signal superior cerebellar artery ➡ impinging on the root entry zone of the preganglionic segment ➡ of the trigeminal nerve. (Right) Coronal T1WI MR in the same patient reveals the superior cerebellar artery ➡ compressing & deforming the right proximal preganglionic segment of CNV ➡. Notice the larger, normal left preganglionic CNV ➡. indicating that atrophy is a feature of the affected right side.

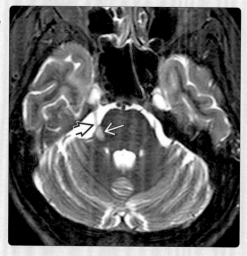
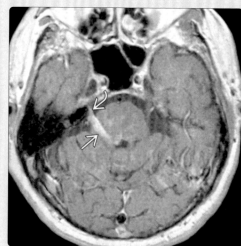

(Left) Axial T2WI FS MR in a patient with right TN reveals a multiple sclerosis lesion ➡ involving the lateral pons at the root entry zone of the trigeminal nerve ➡. Rarely, cisternal masses or MS may present with TN. (Right) Axial T1WI C+ MR in a patient with right TN shows a developmental venous anomaly of the cerebellum draining through the lateral pons ➡ & root entry zone ➡ of CNV. Less than 5% of patients with TN have a venous explanation for their symptoms.

TERMINOLOGY

Abbreviations

- Trigeminal neuralgia (TN)

Synonyms

- Tic douloureux, trigeminal nerve vascular loop syndrome, trigeminal nerve hyperactive dysfunction syndrome

Definitions

- Vascular loop compressing trigeminal nerve at its root entry zone (REZ) or preganglionic segment (PGS)

IMAGING

General Features

- Best diagnostic clue
  - High-resolution MR shows serpentine asymmetric signal void (vessel) in cerebellopontine angle (CPA) CNV REZ or PGS
- TN offending vessels: Superior cerebellar artery (SCA) > anterior inferior cerebellar artery (AICA) > basal artery > petrosal vein

MR Findings

- FLAIR
  - Multiple sclerosis (MS) may present with TN
- DWI
  - Hyperintense cisternal mass diagnoses epidermoid
- T1WI C+
  - In vascular loop-caused TN, CNV PGS does **not** enhance
  - May show rare venous cause of TN or perineural tumor
  - Rare cisternal mass possible
- High-resolution MR (CISS, FIESTA, T2 space, other)
  - Causal vessel compressing CNV REZ or PGS (vessel bows PGS or deforms REZ if cause of neurovascular conflict)
  - CNV PGS atrophy: When compression severe, prolonged
- MRA: Source images most helpful

Imaging Recommendations

- Best imaging tool
  - High-resolution MR for imaging of causal vascular loop

DIFFERENTIAL DIAGNOSIS

Aneurysm in CPA-IAC

- AICA or vertebral artery aneurysm
- Oval complex signal mass
- Rarely causes TN

Arteriovenous Malformation in Cerebellopontine Angle

- Much larger vessels (arteries & veins) with nidus
- Rare in posterior fossa

Developmental Venous Anomaly in Posterior Fossa

- Larger vessels (veins)
- CPA rare as venous drainage route
- Rarely causes venous compression-induced TN

PATHOLOGY

General Features

- Etiology

- CNV REZ or PGS vascular compression → **atrophy**
- Atrophy secondary to axonal loss & demyelination
- Atrophy → abnormal contacts among nerve fibers
  - Abnormal contacts cause paroxysmal pain of TN

Microscopic Features

- Myelin cover of proximal CNV is breached

CLINICAL ISSUES

Presentation

- Most common signs/symptoms
  - Lancinating pain following V2 ± V3 distributions; spontaneous or in response to tactile stimulation

Demographics

- Age
  - Older patients (usually > 65 years)
- Epidemiology
  - 5:100,000

Natural History & Prognosis

- Prognosis: ~ 70% pain-free 10 years after surgery or radiotherapy

Treatment

- Begin with conservative drug therapy
- Other treatments if conservative therapy fails: Focused radiotherapy (Gamma knife), microvascular decompression

DIAGNOSTIC CHECKLIST

Consider

- Many normal vessels in CPA cistern; look for asymmetric vessel with visible compression

Image Interpretation Pearls

- 1st look for MS, pontine developmental venous anomaly, cisternal masses
- Follow CNV distally into cavernous sinus & face
  - Exclude perineural tumor, malignancies of face
- View high-resolution MR for neurovascular conflict

SELECTED REFERENCES

1. Lee JK et al: Long-term outcome of gamma knife surgery using a retrogasserian petrous bone target for classic trigeminal neuralgia. Acta Neurochir Suppl. 116:127-35, 2013
2. Lutz J et al: Trigeminal neuralgia due to neurovascular compression: high-spatial-resolution diffusion-tensor imaging reveals microstructural neural changes. Radiology. 258(2):524-30, 2011
3. Kabatas S et al: Microvascular decompression as a surgical management for trigeminal neuralgia: long-term follow-up and review of the literature. Neurosurg Rev. 32(1):87-93; discussion 93-4, 2009
4. Satoh T et al: Severity analysis of neurovascular contact in patients with trigeminal neuralgia: assessment with the inner view of the 3D MR cisternogram and angiogram fusion imaging. AJNR Am J Neuroradiol. 30(3):603-7, 2009
5. Sindou M et al: Microvascular decompression for primary trigeminal neuralgia: long-term effectiveness and prognostic factors in a series of 362 consecutive patients with clear-cut neurovascular conflicts who underwent pure decompression. J Neurosurg. 107(6):1144-53, 2007
6. Yoshino N et al: Trigeminal neuralgia: evaluation of neuralgic manifestation and site of neurovascular compression with 3D CISS MR imaging and MR angiography. Radiology. 228(2):539-45, 2003
7. Hutchins LG et al: Trigeminal neuralgia (tic douloureux): MR imaging assessment. Radiology. 175(3):837-41, 1990

TERMINOLOGY

- Definition: Vascular loop compressing facial nerve at its root exit zone within cerebellopontine angle (CPA) cistern causing hemifacial spasm

IMAGING

- High-resolution T2WI MR or source MRA images show serpentine asymmetric signal void (vessel) in medial CPA
  - AICA (50%) > PICA (30%) > VA (15%) > vein (5%)

TOP DIFFERENTIAL DIAGNOSES

- Aneurysm, CPA-internal auditory canal
- Arteriovenous malformation, CPA
- Developmental venous anomaly, posterior fossa

PATHOLOGY

- CNVII bundle experiences "irritation" from vessel
- Rare, nonvascular causes of hemifacial spasms (HFS)
  - Multiple sclerosis

- Cisternal masses
  - Epidermoid, meningioma, schwannoma
- Temporal bone and parotid lesions
  - Perineural CNVII malignancy

CLINICAL ISSUES

- Clinical presentation
  - Unilateral involuntary facial spasms (HFS)
  - HFS begins with orbicularis oculi spasms
  - Tonic-clonic bursts become constant over time

DIAGNOSTIC CHECKLIST

- Positive MR findings present in ~ 50% HFS patients
- First look for cisternal mass lesions, multiple sclerosis
- Then follow CNVII distally into temporal bone and parotid
  - Exclude CNVII venous malformation, parotid malignancy
- Determine if MRA source images or high-resolution T2WI images identify causal vessel
  - Negative MR does not preclude surgical therapy

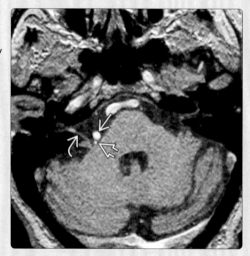

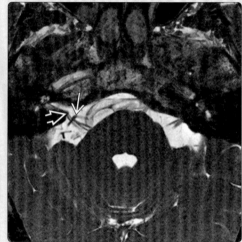

(Left) Axial MRA source image in a patient with right hemifacial spasm shows a tortuous right vertebral artery ➡ and associated PICA ➡ pushing on the root exit zone of the facial nerve. The facial nerve is visible in the cerebellopontine angle (CPA) cistern ➡. (Right) Axial CISS MR through the CPA cisterns in a patient with right hemifacial spasm demonstrates a PICA loop ➡ pushing the cisternal CNVII and CNVII posteriorly, causing them to drape over the posterior margin of the porus acusticus ➡.

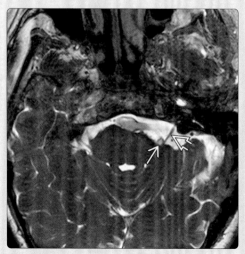

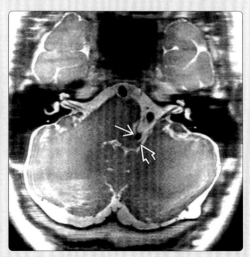

(Left) Axial CISS MR in a patient with left hemifacial spasm reveals the left vertebral artery ➡ looping into the CPA cistern where it impinges on the proximal facial nerve ➡ at the root exit zone. (Right) Axial T2WI MR reveals a dolichoectatic vertebral artery ➡ impinging on the root exit zone ➡ of the facial nerve in the medial CPA cistern in this patient with hemifacial spasm. Approximately 50% of patients with hemifacial spasm have positive MR findings, typically on thin-section T2 or MRA sequences.

TERMINOLOGY

Abbreviations

- Hemifacial spasm (HFS)

Synonyms

- Facial nerve vascular loop syndrome, facial nerve hyperactive dysfunction syndrome

Definitions

- Vascular loop compressing facial nerve at its root exit zone within cerebellopontine angle (CPA) cistern causing hemifacial spasm

IMAGING

General Features

- Best diagnostic clue
  o High-resolution T2WI MR shows serpentine asymmetric signal void (vessel) in medial CPA
- Location
  o Loop in medial CPA cistern at CNVII root exit zone
- HFS offending vessels: AICA (50%), PICA (30%), VA (15%), vein (5%)

MR Findings

- T2WI
  o High-resolution T2WI: Vessel best seen as low-signal tube coursing through high-signal CSF
- FLAIR
  o Adjacent brain most commonly normal
  o Multiple sclerosis may present with HFS
- MRA
  o Source images most helpful

Imaging Recommendations

- Best imaging tool
  o Thin-section high-resolution T2WI MR of CPA allows best vascular loop visualization
- Protocol advice
  o Begin with whole-brain T2 or FLAIR sequence to exclude multiple sclerosis
  o Follow with axial and coronal T1WI C+ FS of brainstem and CPA cistern, including deep face
    – Look for asymmetric venous cause
    – Look for cisternal or perineural tumor, cranial neuritis
  o High-resolution T2WI of brainstem and CPA cistern next
    – Best sequence to look for causal artery

DIFFERENTIAL DIAGNOSIS

CPA-IAC Aneurysm

- PICA or vertebral artery aneurysm
- Oval complex signal mass

CPA Arteriovenous Malformation

- Larger vessels (arteries and veins) with nidus
- Rare in posterior fossa

Posterior Fossa Developmental Venous Anomaly

- Larger vessels (veins)
- CPA rare as venous drainage route
- Rarely causes venous compression with HFS

PATHOLOGY

General Features

- Etiology
  o CNVII bundle experiences "irritation" from vessel
    – Brainstem nuclei secondarily affected
    – Abnormal brainstem response (ABR)

Microscopic Features

- Myelin cover on proximal CNVII breached

CLINICAL ISSUES

Presentation

- Most common signs/symptoms
  o HFS: Unilateral involuntary facial spasms
    – Begins with orbicularis oculi spasms
    – **Tonic-clonic bursts** become constant

Demographics

- Age
  o Older patients (usually > 65 years)
- Epidemiology
  o < 1:100,000

Natural History & Prognosis

- 90% symptom-free ≥ 5 years after surgery

Treatment

- Local injections of botulinum toxin
  o 85% of patients obtain significant relief from local injections
  o Repeat treatment every 4 months
- **Microvascular decompression** as needed
  o Provides permanent relief in 90% of patients

DIAGNOSTIC CHECKLIST

Consider

- Positive MR findings present in ~ 50% of HFS patients

Image Interpretation Pearls

- First look for cisternal mass lesions, multiple sclerosis
- Follow CNVII distally into temporal bone and parotid
  o Exclude CNV11 hemangioma, parotid malignancy
- Review MRA and high-resolution T2WI for causal vessel
  o Negative MR does **not** preclude surgical therapy

SELECTED REFERENCES

1. Garcia M et al: High-resolution 3D-constructive interference in steady-state MR imaging and 3D time-of-flight MR angiography in neurovascular compression: a comparison between 3T and 1.5T. AJNR Am J Neuroradiol. 33(7):1251-6, 2012
2. Huh R et al: Microvascular decompression for hemifacial spasm: analyses of operative complications in 1582 consecutive patients. Surg Neurol. 69(2):153-7; discussion 157, 2008
3. Lee MS et al: Clinical usefulness of magnetic resonance cisternography in patients having hemifacial spasm. Yonsei Med J. 42(4):390-4, 2001
4. Yamakami I et al: Preoperative assessment of trigeminal neuralgia and hemifacial spasm using constructive interference in steady state-three-dimensional Fourier transformation magnetic resonance imaging. Neurol Med Chir (Tokyo). 40(11):545-55; discussion 555-6, 2000
5. Mitsuoka H et al: Delineation of small nerves and blood vessels with three-dimensional fast spin-echo MR imaging: comparison of presurgical and surgical findings in patients with hemifacial spasm. AJNR Am J Neuroradiol. 19(10):1823-9, 1998

TERMINOLOGY

- Focal ballooning or fusiform dilatation of posterior inferior cerebellar artery (PICA), vertebral artery (VA), or anterior inferior cerebellar artery (AICA) in CPA-IAC cistern

IMAGING

- CPA aneurysm incidence: PICA > VA > AICA
  - 10% all intracranial aneurysms are vertebrobasilar
- CPA-IAC aneurysm: Mass with **calcified rim** (CT) or layered **complex signal** in wall (MR)
- CECT of partially thrombosed aneurysm
  - Complex mass with central or eccentric enhancing lumen, nonenhancing mural thrombus
  - Often has **calcified rim**
- CTA: Shows neck & originating artery (PICA, VA, AICA)
- MR findings
  - MR complex signal from Ca^{++}, clot, flow
  - T1: **Subacute luminal clot** is **hyperintense** secondary to methemoglobin T1 shortening

- T2: Signal varies from hypointense flow void to **complex mixed signal** appearance
- Angiogram: Visible lumen may be smaller than overall aneurysm if clot is present
  - May **underestimate** aneurysm size

TOP DIFFERENTIAL DIAGNOSES

- Vertebrobasilar dolichoectasia
- Dural AV fistula + venous varix
- Arteriovenous malformation

CLINICAL ISSUES

- Clinical presentation
  - Sensorineural hearing loss (70%)
  - Headache from subarachnoid hemorrhage (50%)
  - Hemifacial spasm or facial nerve palsy
- Treatment options
  - Surgical clipping
  - Endovascular coiling depending on configuration

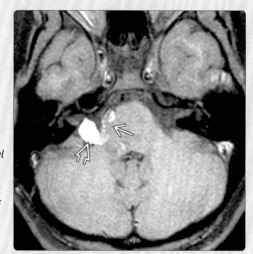
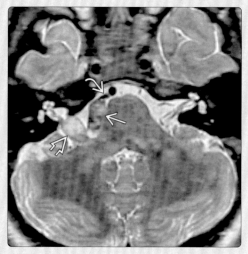

(Left) *Axial T1WI shows a tubular hyperintense mass extending laterally from the basilar artery into the CPA cistern. The more medial portion of the mass shows complex signal from flow & subacute clot ⇨, while the more lateral component is completely thrombosed & filled with high-signal subacute clot ⇨. (Right) Axial T2WI MR in the same patient reveals the patent PICA-AICA complex takeoff from the basilar artery ⇨ with area of partial ⇨ & complete thrombosis ⇨ of the aneurysm.*

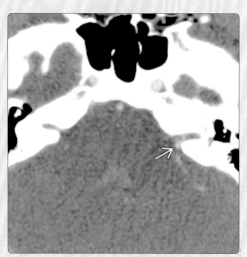
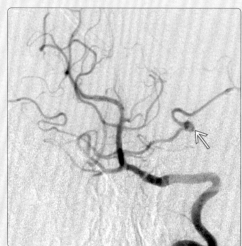

(Left) *Axial CTA image through the IAC demonstrates a focal area of enhancement on the posterior margin of the porus acusticus ⇨. (Right) Anteroposterior left vertebral angiogram in the same patient demonstrates the AICA aneurysm ⇨ looping into the vicinity of the internal auditory canal. AICA aneurysm in the CPA-IAC is the rarest of the aneurysms affecting the CPA-IAC area.*

TERMINOLOGY

Definitions

- Focal ballooning or fusiform dilatation of posterior inferior cerebellar artery (PICA), vertebral artery (VA), or anterior inferior cerebellar artery (AICA) in CPA-IAC cistern

IMAGING

General Features

- Best diagnostic clue
  - CPA mass with **calcified rim** (CT) or layered **complex signal** in wall (MR)
- Location
  - CPA aneurysms from PICA > VA > AICA
- Size
  - Millimeters to centimeters
- Morphology
  - **Round, ovoid,** or **fusiform**-shaped

CT Findings

- CECT
  - Patent aneurysm
    - Well-delineated iso- to hyperdense extraaxial mass with strong, uniform enhancement
  - Partially thrombosed aneurysm
    - Complex mass with central or eccentric enhancing lumen, nonenhancing mural thrombus; often has **calcified rim**
  - Completely thrombosed aneurysm
    - No enhancing lumen
- CTA
  - Shows neck & originating artery (PICA, VA, AICA)

MR Findings

- T1WI
  - **Subacute luminal clot** is **hyperintense** secondary to **methemoglobinT1 shortening**
- T2WI
  - Phase artifact across from patent aneurysm common
  - Signal varies from hypointense flow void to **complex mixed signal** appearance
    - Varies with flow rate & age of luminal thrombus; complex signal from Ca++, clot, flow
- T2* GRE
  - Calcified wall & luminal clot may bloom
- T1WI C+
  - Aneurysm lumen enhances if slow flow present
- MRA
  - May delineate relationship with parent vessel

Angiographic Findings

- Visible lumen may be smaller than overall aneurysm if clot is present (angiogram may **underestimate** aneurysm size)
- Angiography delineates precise vascular relationships

Imaging Recommendations

- Best imaging tool
  - Once CT or MR suggests aneurysm, confirm with CTA or angiography

DIFFERENTIAL DIAGNOSIS

Vertebrobasilar Dolichoectasia

- MRA reprojections or source images show no aneurysm

Dural Atrioventricular Fistula + Venous Varix

- Angiogram delineates best
- MR venography may help delineate

Arteriovenous Malformation

- Large feeding arteries + nidus

PATHOLOGY

General Features

- Etiology
  - Inherited factors + hemodynamic-induced degenerative changes in vessel wall often combine to form aneurysm
- Genetics
  - Aneurysm propensity has hereditary driver

Gross Pathologic & Surgical Features

- Saccular: Berry-like outpouching of artery wall
- Fusiform: Enlarged, ectatic atherosclerotic artery

Microscopic Features

- Lacks internal elastic lamina & smooth muscle layers
- Degenerative changes in parent vessel common
- Thrombus, atherosclerosis are common

CLINICAL ISSUES

Presentation

- Most common signs/symptoms
  - Unilateral sensorineural hearing loss (SNHL) (70%)
- Other signs/symptoms
  - Headache from subarachnoid hemorrhage (50%); hemifacial spasm or facial nerve palsy; tinnitus, vertigo
- Clinical profile
  - Middle-aged patient, unilateral SNHL

Demographics

- Age
  - 40-60 yr
- Epidemiology
  - CPA aneurysms account for ≤ 1% of CPA masses
  - 10% of all intracranial aneurysms are vertebrobasilar

Natural History & Prognosis

- Larger aneurysms rupture more frequently
- Left unclipped, aneurysm rupture growing possibility

Treatment

- Endovascular coiling vs. surgical clipping

DIAGNOSTIC CHECKLIST

Image Interpretation Pearls

- CT: Rim calcification in CPA mass suggests aneurysm
- MR: Complex signal in CPA mass suggests aneurysm

SELECTED REFERENCES

1. Cianfoni A et al: Clinical presentation of cerebral aneurysms. Eur J Radiol. Epub ahead of print, 2012

TERMINOLOGY

- Superficial siderosis (SS) definition: Recurrent subarachnoid hemorrhage (SAH) causes hemosiderin deposition on surface of brain, brainstem, and cranial nerve leptomeninges

IMAGING

- Nonenhanced CT findings
  - Slightly hyperdense rim over brain surface
  - Brainstem high-density line most evident
  - **Caveat**: Do not mistake high-density rim on brain surfaces as SAH
- MR findings
  - In diffuse disease, ventricle surfaces, brain, brainstem, cerebellum, and cervical spine all have hypointense hemosiderin rim
  - Contours of brain and cranial nerves outlined by **hypointense rim** on T2 or T2* GRE MR images
  - CNVIII appears darker and thicker than normal

- GRE: Most sensitive to hemosiderin deposition on CNS surfaces (blooming dark signal)
- Once diagnosis of SS is made, search for cause of recurrent SAH must commence
  - Whole-brain MR with contrast and MRA
  - Total spine MR if brain negative for underlying lesion

PATHOLOGY

- SAH deposits hemosiderin on meningeal lining of CNS
- Affects brain, brainstem, cranial nerves, and spinal cord
- Causes of recurrent SAH
  - Trauma: Nerve root avulsion, head injury, SDH
  - Bleeding neoplasm: Brain or spine
  - Arteriovenous or cavernous malformation
  - Aneurysm
  - Surgical sites (brain or spine)
  - Amyloid angiopathy
  - Vasculitis
  - Meningocele

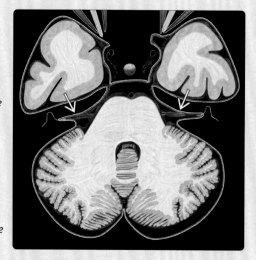
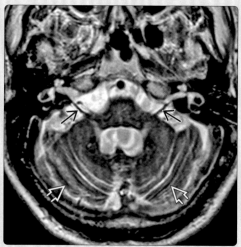

(Left) *Axial graphic shows darker brown hemosiderin staining on all surfaces of the brain, meninges, and cranial nerves. Notice that cranial nerves VII and VIII in the cerebellopontine angle-internal auditory canal ➡ are particularly affected.* (Right) *Axial T2WI MR reveals superficial siderosis in the posterior fossa. Both vestibulocochlear nerves (CNVIII) are seen as very low-signal lines in the cerebellopontine angle cisterns ➡. Also observe low signal along the surface of the cerebellar folia ➡.*

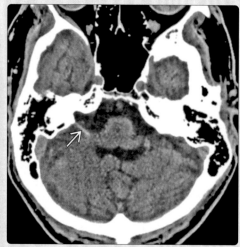
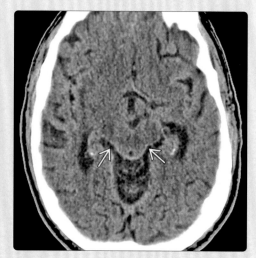

(Left) *Axial NECT demonstrates findings of superficial siderosis as a high-density right vestibulocochlear nerve ➡. CT is often normal in patients with this disease as the fine siderosis coating on the cranial nerves, brain, and brainstem may not be dense enough to see.* (Right) *Axial NECT in this patient with superficial siderosis shows linear high density along the surface of the midbrain ➡. This is not an artifact or subarachnoid hemorrhage but hemosiderin deposition on the surface of the midbrain.*

TERMINOLOGY

Abbreviations

- Superficial siderosis (SS)

Synonyms

- Siderosis, central nervous system siderosis

Definitions

- Recurrent subarachnoid hemorrhage (SAH) causes **hemosiderin deposition** on surface of brain, **brainstem**, and **cranial nerve leptomeninges**

IMAGING

General Features

- Best diagnostic clue
  - Contours of brain and cranial nerves outlined by **hypointense rim** on T2 or T2* GRE MR images
- Location
  - Cerebral hemispheres, cerebellum, brainstem, cranial nerves, and spinal cord may all be affected
- Size
  - Linear low signal along CNS surfaces varies in thickness but is usually ≤ 2 mm
- Morphology
  - Curvilinear dark lines on CNS surfaces

CT Findings

- NECT
  - Cerebral and **cerebellar atrophy**
    - Especially marked in posterior fossa
      □ Cerebellar sulci often disproportionately large
  - **CNVIII** may be **hyperdense**
  - Slightly hyperdense rim over brain surface
    - Brainstem changes most evident
    - CT relatively insensitive to SS compared to MR
    - **Caveat**: Do not mistake high-density rim on brain surfaces as subarachnoid hemorrhage
- CECT
  - No enhancement typical

MR Findings

- T1WI
  - Hyperintense signal may be seen on CNS surfaces
- T2WI
  - High-resolution, thin-section T2 MR of CPA-IAC
    - **CNVIII** appears **hypointense**, thicker than normal
    - Adjacent cerebellar structures and brainstem show low-signal surfaces
    - Less easily seen than on T2* GRE images
  - In diffuse disease, ventricle, brain, brainstem, cerebellum, and cervical spine surfaces all have hypointense hemosiderin rim
  - Vermian and cerebellar atrophy most prominent
- FLAIR
  - Dark border on local surface of brain, brainstem, cerebellum, and cranial nerves
- T2* GRE
  - More sensitive to hemosiderin deposition on CNS surfaces than T2 sequence
  - **Blooming** dark signal

- Makes SS appear more conspicuous, thicker
- T1WI C+
  - Surface of CNS does not enhance
- MR findings do not correlate with severity of disease

Imaging Recommendations

- Best imaging tool
  - Brain MR with posterior fossa focus
    - Once diagnosis of SS is made, **search for cause** of recurrent SAH must commence
    - Whole-brain MR with contrast and MRA
    - Then total spine MR if brain negative for underlying lesion
- Protocol advice
  - Brain MR
    - Unenhanced MR with FLAIR initially
    - If SS suspected, add T2* GRE sequences to confirm

DIFFERENTIAL DIAGNOSIS

"Bounce Point" Artifact

- Mismatch between repetition time and inversion time on inversion recovery T1 and FLAIR sequences
- Imaging clue: Not present on all sequences

Brain Surface Vessels

- Normal or abnormal surface veins
- Linear, focal area of low signal on brain surface

Neurocutaneous Melanosis

- Congenital syndrome
- Large or multiple congenital melanocytic nevi
- Benign or malignant pigment cell tumors of leptomeninges may be low signal on surface of brain
- T1 high signal diffusely in pia-arachnoid
- T2 low signal diffusely in pia-arachnoid

Meningioangiomatosis

- Hamartomatous proliferation of meningeal cells via intraparenchymal blood vessels into cerebral cortex
- Leptomeninges are thick and infiltrated with fibrous tissue
- May be calcified

PATHOLOGY

General Features

- Etiology
  - Repeated SAH deposits hemosiderin on meningeal lining of CNS
    - Affects brain, brainstem, cerebellum, cranial nerves, and spinal cord
  - Hemosiderin is cytotoxic to neurons
    - "Free" iron with excess production of hydroxyl radicals is best current hypothesis explaining cytotoxicity
  - CNVIII is extensively lined with CNS myelin, which is supported by hemosiderin-sensitive microglia
    - Increased exposure in CPA cistern
- Associated abnormalities
  - **Causes of recurrent SAH**
    - Intradural surgical sites (brain or spine)
    - Traumatic
      □ Cervical nerve root avulsion

□ Multiple episodes of head injury
□ Subdural hematoma
– Bleeding neoplasm (brain or spine)
– Arteriovenous malformation (AVM)
– Cavernous malformation
– Aneurysm
– Amyloid angiopathy
– Vasculitis
– Meningocele

Gross Pathologic & Surgical Features

- Dark brown discoloration of leptomeninges, ependyma, and subpial tissue
- Causes of recurrent SAH found in ~ 70%
  ○ Dural pathology (70%)
    – Traumatic cervical nerve root avulsion
    – CSF cavity lesion (surgical cavity) with "fragile" neovascularity most common
  ○ Bleeding neoplasms (15%)
    – Ependymoma, oligodendroglioma, astrocytoma, etc.
  ○ Vascular abnormalities (10%)
    – AVM or aneurysm
    – Multiple cavernous malformations near brain surface
  ○ Amyloid angiopathy in elderly patients (< 5%)

Microscopic Features

- **Hemosiderin staining** of meninges & subpial tissues to 3-mm depth
- Thickened leptomeninges
- Cerebellar folia: Loss of Purkinje cells and Bergmann gliosis

CLINICAL ISSUES

Presentation

- Most common signs/symptoms
  ○ **Bilateral sensorineural hearing loss** (SNHL) in 95%
- Clinical profile
  ○ Past history of trauma or intradural surgery common
    – Past history of SAH rare
  ○ Classic presentation is adult patient with bilateral SNHL and ataxia
  ○ Seen less commonly as late complication of treated childhood cerebellar tumor
- Laboratory
  ○ CSF from lumbar puncture
    – High protein (100%)
    – Xanthochromic (75%)
- Other symptoms
  ○ **Ataxia** (88%)
  ○ **Bilateral hemiparesis**
  ○ Hyperreflexia, bladder disturbance, anosmia, **dementia**, & headache
    – Anosmia: CNI very sensitive to hemosiderin deposition
  ○ Presymptomatic phase averages 15 years

Demographics

- Age
  ○ Broad range: Neonate to elderly
- Gender
  ○ M:F = 3:1
- Epidemiology

○ Rare chronic progressive disorder
○ 0.15% of patients undergoing MR

Natural History & Prognosis

- Bilateral worsening SNHL and ataxia within 15 years of onset
- Deafness almost certain if unrecognized
- 25% bedridden within years after 1st symptom (adults)
  ○ Result of cerebellar ataxia, myelopathic syndrome, or both

Treatment

- Treat source of bleeding
  ○ Surgically remove source of bleeding (surgical cavity, tumor)
  ○ Endovascular therapy for AVM and aneurysm
- Cochlear implantation for SNHL
  ○ Cochlear implants may not work if CNVIII damage is severe

DIAGNOSTIC CHECKLIST

Consider

- Remember that SS is effect, not cause
- Look for source of recurrent SAH in spine or brain
- MR findings do not correlate with severity of patient's symptoms
  ○ MR diagnosis may be made in absence of symptoms

Image Interpretation Pearls

- CNS surfaces including cranial nerves that appear "outlined in black" on T2 MR

Reporting Tips

- Describe individual findings of SS
- Describe any possible sites of chronic SAH
- If no site of SAH visible, recommend full spine MR in search of SAH site
  ○ Treatment of SAH site may arrest progression of associated symptoms

SELECTED REFERENCES

1. Charidimou A et al: Cortical superficial siderosis: detection and clinical significance in cerebral amyloid angiopathy and related conditions. Brain. 138(Pt 8):2126-39, 2015
2. Kishimoto I et al: Clinical features of rapidly progressive bilateral sensorineural hearing loss. Acta Otolaryngol. 134(1):58-65, 2014
3. Tyler GK et al: Systematic review of outcome of cochlear implantation in superficial siderosis. Otol Neurotol. 33(6):976-82, 2012
4. Nadol JB Jr et al: Temporal bone histopathology in a case of sensorineural hearing loss caused by superficial siderosis of the central nervous system and treated by cochlear implantation. Otol Neurotol. 32(5):748-55, 2011
5. Linn J et al: Prevalence of superficial siderosis in patients with cerebral amyloid angiopathy. Neurology. 74(17):1346-50, 2010
6. Koeppen AH et al: The pathology of superficial siderosis of the central nervous system. Acta Neuropathol. 116(4):371-82, 2008
7. Kumar N: Superficial siderosis: associations and therapeutic implications. Arch Neurol. 64(4):491-6, 2007
8. Dhooge IJ et al: Cochlear implantation in a patient with superficial siderosis of the central nervous system. Otol Neurotol. 23(4):468-72, 2002
9. Hsu WC et al: Superficial siderosis of the CNS associated with multiple cavernous malformations. AJNR Am J Neuroradiol. 20(7):1245-8, 1999
10. Weller M et al: Elevated CSF lactoferrin in superficial siderosis of the central nervous system. J Neurol. 246(10):943-5, 1999
11. Castelli ML et al: Superficial siderosis of the central nervous system: an underestimated cause of hearing loss. J Laryngol Otol. 111(1):60-2, 1997
12. Bracchi M et al: Superficial siderosis of the CNS: MR diagnosis and clinical findings. AJNR Am J Neuroradiol. 14(1):227-36, 1993

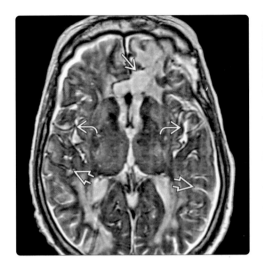

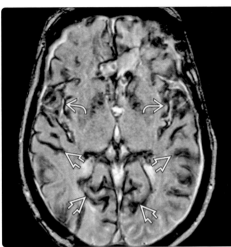

(Left) *Months after the surgical removal of a frontal lobe melanoma metastasis in this patient, axial T2WI MR shows the surgical cavity ➡ and subtle low signal lining the sulci ➡ and sylvian fissures ➡, secondary to superficial siderosis.* (Right) *Axial T2* GRE MR in the same patient demonstrates much more obvious siderosis involving the sylvian fissures ➡ and sulci ➡. GRE T2* sequences cause hemosiderin deposits to bloom, increasing the conspicuity of this disease.*

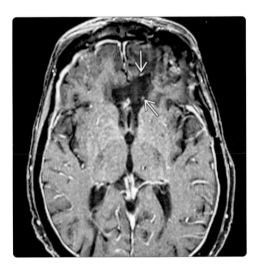

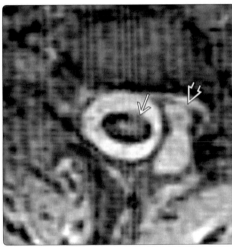

(Left) *Axial T1WI C+ FS MR in the same patient reveals focal areas of enhancement in the surgical cavity ➡. These are granulation tissue foci along the margin of the surgical site that likely continue to chronically ooze blood, causing superficial siderosis.* (Right) *Axial T2WI MR in a patient with cervical trauma shows interruption of hemosiderin hypointense rim ➡ due to the absence of spinal cord pia mater at the root avulsion site. Note the pseudomeningocele ➡. (Courtesy N. Kumar, MD.)*

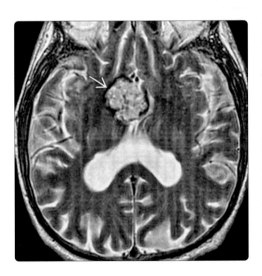

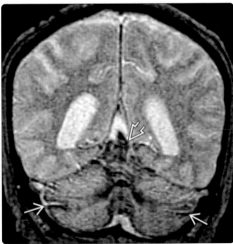

(Left) *Axial T2WI MR reveals the popcorn ball appearance of a classic Zabramski type 2 cavernous malformation ➡. A complete hemosiderin rim surrounds the lesion as a hypointense line.* (Right) *Coronal T2* GRE in the same patient demonstrates extensive superficial siderosis in the posterior fossa. Blooming of the hemosiderin on the surfaces is seen as a hypointense outline. The superior vermis ➡ as well as the cerebellar folia ➡ are involved.*

INDEX

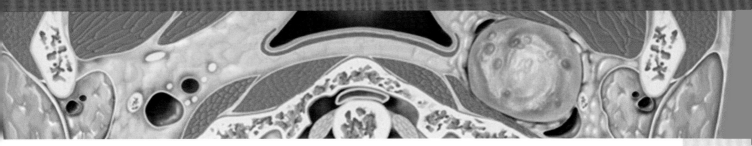

INDEX

INDEX

INDEX

INDEX

N

INDEX

INDEX

INDEX

INDEX

W

X